EDITED BY
ROBERT W. KIRK, D.V.M.

Professor of Medicine
New York State College of Veterinary Medicine
Cornell University
Ithaca, New York
Special Therapy

Consulting Editors

FREDERICK W. OEHME
Chemical and Physical Disorders

N. EDWARD ROBINSON
Respiratory Diseases

STEPHEN J. ETTINGER
Cardiovascular Diseases

VICTOR PERMAN
Hemolymphatic Disorders and Oncology

RICHARD E.W. HALLIWELL
Dermatologic Diseases

CHARLES L. MARTIN
Ophthalmologic Diseases

MURRAY E. FOWLER
Diseases of Caged Birds and Exotic Pets

ALEXANDER DE LAHUNTA
Neurologic and Musculoskeletal Disorders

DONALD R. STROMBECK
Gastrointestinal Disorders

JOHN A. MULNIX
Endocrine and Metabolic Disorders

CARL A. OSBORNE
Genitourinary Disorders

FREDRIC W. SCOTT
Infectious Diseases

CURRENT VETERINARY THERAPY VII

SMALL ANIMAL PRACTICE

1980

W. B. SAUNDERS COMPANY · PHILADELPHIA · LONDON · TORONTO

W. B. Saunders Company: West Washington Square
Philadelphia, PA 19105

1 St. Anne's Road
Eastbourne, East Sussex BN21, 3UN, England

1 Goldthorne Avenue
Toronto, Ontario M8Z 5T9, Canada

Listed here is the latest translated edition of this book
with the language of the translation and the publisher.

Spanish (3rd edition) — Editorial Continental, Mexico

Japanese (4th edition) — Ishiyaku Publishers, Inc., Tokyo, Japan

Current Veterinary Therapy, VII   ISBN   0-7216-5471-1

Last digit is the print number: 9   8   7   6   5   4   3   2   1

CONTRIBUTORS

MELVIN K. ABELSETH, D.V.M., Ph.D., Director, Laboratories for Veterinary Science, Division of Laboratories and Research, New York State Department of Health, Albany, New York.

GRAEME S. ALLAN, M.V.Sc.; Diplomate, American College of Veterinary Radiology; Assistant Professor of Radiology, New York State College of Veterinary Medicine, Cornell University, Ithaca, New York.

GARY L. ANDERSEN, D.V.M., M.S., Clinician, Military Working Dog Veterinary Service, Wilford Hall Medical Center, Lackland Air Force Base, San Antonio, Texas.

AMY H. ANSFIELD, R.R.T., Instructor in Respiratory Therapy, Pruett College, Concord, California; Supervisor, Respiratory Therapy Department, Herrick Memorial Hospital, Berkeley, California.

MAX J. G. APPEL, D.Vet.Med., Ph.D., Professor of Virology, New York State College of Veterinary Medicine, Cornell University, Ithaca, New York.

ARTHUR L. ARONSON, D.V.M., Ph.D., Professor of Pharmacology, New York State College of Veterinary Medicine, Cornell University, Ithaca, New York.

CLARKE E. ATKINS, D.V.M.; Diplomate, American College of Veterinary Internal Medicine; Assistant Professor of Small Animal Medicine, School of Veterinary Medicine, Oklahoma State University, Stillwater, Oklahoma.

MARIE H. ATTLEBERGER, D.V.M., Ph.D., Associate Professor of Microbiology, School of Veterinary Medicine, Auburn University, Auburn, Alabama.

E. MURL BAILEY, Jr., D.V.M., Ph.D.; Diplomate, American Board of Veterinary Toxicology; Associate Professor of Veterinary Toxicology, Department of Veterinary Physiology and Pharmacology, College of Veterinary Medicine, Texas A and M University, College Station, Texas.

RALPH E. BARRETT, D.V.M.; Diplomate, American College of Veterinary Internal Medicine; Veterinary Internist, Sacramento Animal Medical Group, Carmichael, California.

JEANNE A. BARSANTI, D.V.M., M.S.; Diplomate, American College of Veterinary Internal Medicine; Assistant Professor, Department of Small Animal Medicine, College of Veterinary Medicine, University of Georgia; Small Animal Clinician, University of Georgia Teaching Hospital, Athens, Georgia.

BRUCE E. BELSHAW, D.V.M.; Diplomate, American College of Veterinary Pathologists; Small Animal Clinic, State University of Utrecht, Utrecht, The Netherlands.

JOHN BENTINCK-SMITH, D.V.M.; Diplomate, American College of Veterinary Pathologists; Professor of Clinical Pathology, New York State College of Veterinary Medicine, Cornell University, Ithaca, New York.

STEPHEN BISTNER, D.V.M.; Diplomate, American College of Veterinary Ophthalmologists; Associate Professor, Department of Clinical Medicine, School of Veterinary Medicine, University of Minnesota, St. Paul, Minnesota.

GARY R. BOLTON, D.V.M.; Diplomate, American College of Veterinary Internal Medicine (Cardiology); Associate Professor of Medicine and Cardiology, New York State College of Veterinary Medicine, Cornell University, Ithaca, New York.

JOHN D. BONAGURA, D.V.M., M.Sc.; Diplomate, American College of Veterinary Internal Medicine (Cardiology, Internal Medicine); Assistant Professor, Department of Veterinary Clinical Sciences, The Ohio State University, College of Veterinary Medicine; Internist, The Ohio State University Veterinary Teaching Hospital, Columbus, Ohio.

BETSY R. BOND, D.V.M., Assistant Professor of Small Animal Medicine, Washington State University, College of Veterinary Medicine, Pullman, Washington.

KENNETH C. BOVÉE, D.V.M., M.Med.Sci.; Diplomate, American College of Veterinary Internal Medicine; Professor of Medicine, University of Pennsylvania School of Veterinary Medicine, Philadelphia, Pennsylvania.

JAMES J. BRACE, D.V.M.; Diplomate, American College of Veterinary Internal Medicine; Associate Professor of Medicine, University of Tennessee, College of Veterinary Medicine, Department of Urban Practice, Knoxville, Tennessee.

DAVID B. BRUNSON, D.V.M., M.S.; Diplomate, American College of Veterinary Anesthesiologists; Assistant Professor of Anesthesiology, Michigan State University, College of Veterinary Medicine, East Lansing, Michigan.

WILLIAM B. BUCK, D.V.M., M.S.; Diplomate, American Board of Veterinary Toxicology; Professor of Toxicology, University of Illinois, College of Veterinary Medicine, Department of Veterinary Biosciences, Urbana, Illinois.

THOMAS J. BURKE, D.V.M., M.S., Associate Professor, University of Illinois, Urbana, Illinois; Consultant, Capitol Illini Veterinary Hospitals, Springfield, Illinois.

COLIN F. BURROWS, B.Vet.Med., M.R.C.V.S.; Diplomate, American College of Veterinary Internal Medicine; Assistant Professor of Medicine, University of Pennsylvania, School of Veterinary Medicine, Philadelphia, Pennsylvania.

MITCHELL BUSH, D.V.M., Head, Office of Animal Health, National Zoological Park, Smithsonian Institution, Washington, D.C.

NED BUYUKMIHCI, V.M.D.; Diplomate, American College of Veterinary Ophthalmologists; Assistant Professor of Ophthalmology, University of California, School of Veterinary Medicine, Department of Surgery, Davis, California.

LEWIS H. CAMPBELL, D.V.M.; Diplomate, American College of Veterinary Ophthalmologists; Animal Eye Clinic, Los Altos, California.

CHARLES C. CAPEN, D.V.M., Ph.D.; Diplomate, American College of Veterinary Pathologists; Professor of Veterinary Pathobiology, The Ohio State University, College of Veterinary Medicine; Consulting Clinician, The Ohio State University Veterinary Hospital, Columbus, Ohio.

LELAND E. CARMICHAEL, D.V.M., Ph.D.; Diplomate, American College of Veterinary Microbiologists; Professor of Virology, New York State College of Veterinary Medicine, Cornell University, Ithaca, New York.

THOMAS L. CARSON, D.V.M., Ph.D.; Diplomate, American Board of Veterinary Toxicology; Associate Professor of Veterinary Pathology, Iowa State University, College of Veterinary Medicine, Veterinary Diagnostic Laboratory, Ames, Iowa.

DENNIS D. CAYWOOD, D.V.M., M.S., Assistant Professor of General and Orthopedic Surgery, Department of Small Animal Clinical Sciences, College of Veterinary Medicine, University of Minnesota, St. Paul, Minnesota.

DENNIS J. CHEW, D.V.M.; Diplomate, American College of Veterinary Internal Medicine; Assistant Professor, Department of Veterinary Clinical Sciences, College of Veterinary Medicine, The Ohio State University, Columbus, Ohio.

ANNE M. CHIAPELLA, D.V.M.; Diplomate, American College of Veterinary Internal Medicine; Associate in Small Animal Medicine, School of Veterinary Medicine, University of Pennsylvania; Small Animal Clinic, University of Pennsylvania, Philadelphia, Pennsylvania.

DAVID B. CHURCH, B.V.Sc., Department of Veterinary Clinical Studies, University of Sydney; Attending Clinician, University of Sydney Veterinary Hospital and Clinic, Sydney, N.S.W., Australia.

MICHAEL T. COLLINS, D.V.M., Ph.D., Assistant Professor, Department of Microbiology, College of Veterinary Medicine and Biomedical Sciences, Colorado State University, Fort Collins, Colorado.

RALPH S. COOPER, D.V.M., Veterinary Medical Officer IV (Pathology), State of California Department of Food and Agriculture, Division of Animal Industry, Veterinary Laboratory Services, San Gabriel, California.

LARRY M. CORNELIUS, D.V.M., Ph.D.; Diplomate, American College of Veterinary Internal Medicine; Associate Professor of Internal Medicine, University of Georgia, College of Veterinary Medicine, Department of Small Animal Medicine and Surgery; Internist, Veterinary Medical Teaching Hospital, Athens, Georgia.

GERALD E. COSGROVE, M.D., Pathologist, Zoological Society of San Diego, San Diego, California.

SUSAN M. COTTER, D.V.M.; Diplomate, American College of Veterinary Internal Medicine; Staff Member in Internal Medicine, Angell Memorial Animal Hospital; Research Associate in Oncology, Harvard School of Public Health, Boston, Massachusetts.

DAVID COVITZ, D.V.M.; Diplomate, American College of Veterinary Ophthalmologists; Clinical Assistant Professor, Yale University School of Medicine, Section of Comparative Medicine, New Haven, Connecticut; Private Practice in Ophthalmology, Meadow Veterinary Hospital, White Plains, New York.

LARRY D. COWGILL, D.V.M., Ph.D.; Diplomate, American College of Veterinary Internal Medicine; Assistant Professor of Medicine, School of Veterinary Medicine, University of California; Small Animal Medicine Service, Veterinary Medical Teaching Hospital, University of California, Davis, California.

VICTOR S. COX, D.V.M., Ph.D., Associate Professor of Anatomy, Department of Veterinary Biology, College of Veterinary Medicine, University of Minnesota, St. Paul, Minnesota.

STANLEY R. CREIGHTON, D.V.M.; Diplomate, American College of Veterinary Internal Medicine; Brentwood Pet Clinic, Los Angeles, California.

STEVEN E. CROW, D.V.M.; Diplomate, American College of Veterinary Internal Medicine; Assistant Professor, Michigan State University, College of Veterinary Medicine; Staff Internist and Clinical Oncologist, Veterinary Clinical Center, Michigan State University, East Lansing, Michigan.

WAYNE CROWELL, D.V.M., Ph.D.; Diplomate, American College of Veterinary Pathologists; Associate Professor, Department of Veterinary Pathology, College of Veterinary Medicine, University of Georgia, Athens, Georgia.

MARK V. DAHL, M.D., Associate Professor of Dermatology, University of Minnesota Medical School, Minneapolis, Minnesota.

LLOYD E. DAVIS, D.V.M., Ph.D., Professor of Clinical Pharmacology, University of Illinois College of Veterinary Medicine; Staff, Veterinary Medical Teaching Hospital, University of Illinois, Urbana, Illinois.

ALEXANDER DE LAHUNTA, D.V.M., Ph.D.; Diplomate, American College of Veterinary Internal Medicine (Neurology); Chairman, Department of Clinical Sciences; Professor of Anatomy; Director, Teaching Hospital, New York State College of Veterinary Medicine, Cornell University, Ithaca, New York.

PAUL F. DICE, II, V.M.D., M.S.; Diplomate, American College of Veterinary Ophthalmologists; Animal Eye Clinic, Seattle, Washington.

ROBERT A. DIETERICH, D.V.M., Professor of Veterinary Science, Institute of Arctic Biology, University of Alaska; Chairman, Program in Veterinary Sciences and Wildlife Diseases, Fairbanks, Alaska.

RAY DILLON, D.V.M., M.S.; Diplomate, American College of Veterinary Internal Medicine; Assistant Professor, Department of Small Animal Surgery and Medicine, Auburn University, Auburn, Alabama.

MARTIN R. DINNES, D.V.M., Chief of Service, Zoo and Aquatic Animal Medicine, West Los Angeles Veterinary Medical Group, Los Angeles, California; Dinnes Memorial Veterinary Hospital, International Zoo Veterinary Group, Encino, California.

EDWARD F. DONOVAN, D.V.M.; Diplomate, American College of Veterinary Internal Medicine; Professor of Veterinary Medicine, College of Veterinary Medicine, The Ohio State University, Columbus, Ohio.

IAN DAVID DUNCAN, B.V.M.S., Ph.D., M.R.C.V.S., Department of Neurology, The Montreal General Hospital, McGill University, Montreal, Quebec, Canada.

L. REED ENOS, Pharm.D., Lecturer, Department of Medicine, School of Veterinary Medicine, University of California, Davis; Clinical Instructor, Division of Clinical Pharmacy, School of Pharmacy, University of California, San Francisco; Chief Pharmacist, Veterinary Medical Teaching Hospital, University of California, Davis, California.

STEPHEN J. ETTINGER, D.V.M.; Diplomate, American College of Veterinary Internal Medicine (Cardiology and Internal Medicine); California Animal Hospital, Inc., Los Angeles, California.

PETER EYRE, B.V.M.S., Ph.D., M.R.C.V.S., F.A.C.V.P.T., Professor of Pharmacology, Department of Biomedical Sciences, Ontario Veterinary College, University of Guelph, Guelph, Ontario, Canada.

BRIAN R. H. FARROW, B.V.Sc., Ph.D., M.A.C.V.Sc., M.R.C.V.S., Associate Professor of Veterinary Medicine, Department of Veterinary Clinical Studies, University of Sydney, Sydney, N.S.W., Australia.

CHARLES S. FARROW, D.V.M., Associate Professor of Radiology, Western College of Veterinary Medicine, University of Saskatchewan; Staff Radiologist and Medical Consultant in Respiratory Disease, Saskatoon, Saskatchewan, Canada.

BERNARD F. FELDMAN, D.V.M., Ph.D., Assistant Professor of Clinical Pathology, School of Veterinary Medicine, University of California, Davis, California.

EDWARD CHARLES FELDMAN, D.V.M.; Diplomate, American College of Veterinary Internal Medicine; Assistant Professor of Veterinary Medicine, School of Veterinary Medicine, University of California, Davis;

Veterinary Medical Teaching Hospital, Davis, California.

DELMAR R. FINCO, D.V.M., Ph.D.; Diplomate, American College of Veterinary Internal Medicine; Professor, College of Veterinary Medicine, University of Georgia; Veterinary Medical Teaching Hospital, University of Georgia, Athens, Georgia.

RICARDO FLORES-CASTRO, M.V.Z., D.V.M., Ph.D., Professor of Bacteriology, U.N.A. (Cuotitlan), Mexico City, Mexico; Instituto Nacional Investigaciones Pecuarias, Palo Alto (D.F.), Mexico.

RICHARD B. FORD, D.V.M., M.S., Assistant Professor of Internal Medicine, Purdue University, West Lafayette, Indiana.

ARTHUR S. FOUTZ, Ph.D., Research Associate, Department of Psychiatry, Stanford University School of Medicine, Stanford, California.

MURRAY E. FOWLER, D.V.M.; Diplomate, American Board of Veterinary Toxicology and American College of Veterinary Internal Medicine; Professor of Veterinary Medicine, School of Veterinary Medicine, University of California, Davis; Chief of Service, Zoological Medicine, Veterinary Medical Teaching Hospital, University of California, Davis, California.

JAMES G. FOX, D.V.M., M.S., Associate Professor of Comparative Medicine, Division of Laboratory Animal Medicine, Massachusetts Institute of Technology, Cambridge; Staff Affiliate, Angell Memorial Animal Hospital, Boston, Massachusetts.

FREDRIC L. FRYE, D.V.M., M.S., Consultant, U.S. Public Health Service Hospital, San Francisco, California; Valley Veterinary Hospital, Walnut Creek, California.

CHARLES E. GALVIN, D.V.M., Veterinary Hospital of Ignacio, Ignacio, California.

JAMES R. GANNON, B.V.Sc., F.A.C.V.Sc., Victoria, Australia.

KIRK N. GELATT, V.M.D.; Diplomate, American College of Veterinary Ophthalmology; Professor of Comparative Ophthalmology, College of Veterinary Medicine, University of Florida; Veterinary Medical Teaching

Hospital, Ophthalmology Service, Gainesville, Florida.

LAWRENCE T. GLICKMAN, V.M.D., Dr.P.H., Assistant Professor of Epidemiology and Preventive Medicine, New York State College of Veterinary Medicine, Cornell University, Ithaca, New York.

REBECCA ELAINE GOMPF, D.V.M., M.S., Assistant Professor of Medicine and Cardiology, College of Veterinary Medicine, University of Tennessee; Veterinary Teaching Hospital, University of Tennessee, Knoxville, Tennessee.

T. GOPAL, B.V.Sc., Ph.D., Scientist, CSIR Pool. Department of Pathology, Veterinary College, University of Agricultural Sciences, Hebbal, Bangalore, India.

DAVID L. GRAHAM, D.V.M., Ph.D.; Diplomate, American College of Veterinary Pathologists; Professor of Veterinary Pathology, College of Veterinary Medicine, Iowa State University, Ames, Iowa.

ROBERT A. GREEN, D.V.M., Ph.D.; Diplomate, American College of Veterinary Pathologists; Associate Professor, Department of Veterinary Pathology, Texas A and M University; Clinical Pathologist, Texas A and M Veterinary Teaching Hospital, College Station, Texas.

RICHARD W. GREENE, D.V.M.; Diplomate, American College of Veterinary Surgeons; New Rochelle Animal Hospital, New Rochelle, New York

IAN RONALD GRIFFITHS, B.V.M.S., Ph.D., F.R.C.V.S., Senior Lecturer, Surgery Department, Glasgow University Veterinary School, Bearsden, Glasgow, Scotland.

LESLIE RAYMOND GRONO, B.V.Sc., Ph.D., M.A.C.V.Sc., Reader in Veterinary Surgery, Department of Veterinary Surgery, University of Queensland, St. Lucia, Brisbane, Australia.

DONALD P. GUSTAFSON, D.V.M., Ph.D.; Diplomate, American College of Veterinary Microbiologists; Professor of Virology, Purdue University, School of Veterinary Medicine, West Lafayette, Indiana.

ROBERT MILTON GWIN, D.V.M., M.S.; Diplomate, American College of Veterinary Ophthalmologists; Assistant Professor of Comparative Ophthalmology, College of Veterinary Medicine, University of Florida, Gainesville, Florida.

RICHARD E. W. HALLIWELL, Vet.M.B., Ph.D.; Diplomate, American College of Veterinary Internal Medicine (Dermatology); Associate Professor and Chairman, Department of Medical Sciences, College of Veterinary Medicine, University of Florida, Gainesville, Florida

ROBERT F. HAMMER, D.V.M., Ph.D., Associate Professor, Department of Veterinary Biology, College of Veterinary Medicine, University of Minnesota, St. Paul, Minnesota.

ROBERT M. HARDY, D.V.M., M.S.; Diplomate, American College of Veterinary Internal Medicine; Associate Professor, Department of Small Animal Clinical Sciences, College of Veterinary Medicine, University of Minnesota, St. Paul, Minnesota.

JAMES M. HARRIS, D.V.M., Montclair Veterinary Clinic and Hospital, Oakland, California.

JOHN W. HARVEY, D.V.M., Ph.D.; Diplomate, American College of Veterinary Pathologists (Veterinary Clinical Pathologist); Associate Professor, College of Veterinary Medicine, University of Florida; Chief, Clinical Pathology Service, Veterinary Medical Teaching Hospital, Gainesville, Florida.

DAVID W. HAYDEN, D.V.M., Ph.D.; Diplomate, American College of Veterinary Pathologists; Associate Professor of Veterinary Pathology, Department of Veterinary Pathobiology, College of Veterinary Medicine, University of Minnesota, St. Paul, Minnesota.

MARY A. HERRON, D.V.M., Ph.D., Associate Professor, College of Veterinary Medicine, Texas A and M University, College Station, Texas.

HENRY L. HIRSCHHORN, B.V.Sc., Director, Pittwater Animal Hospital, Warriewood, N.S.W., Australia.

DWIGHT C. HIRSH, D.V.M., Ph.D., Associate Professor of Microbiology, Department of Veterinary Microbiology, School of Veterinary Medicine, University of California, Davis; Chief, Microbiology Service, Veterinary Medical Teaching Hospital, University of California, Davis, California.

STEPHEN B. HITCHNER, V.M.D.; Diplomate, American College of Veterinary Microbiologists; Professor of Avian Diseases, New York State College of Veterinary Medicine, Cornell University; Staff, Small Animal Hospital, New York State College of Veterinary Medicine, Cornell University, Ithaca, New York.

RICHARD E. HOFFER, D.V.M., M.S.; Diplomate, American College of Veterinary Surgeons; Research Associate Professor of Surgery, Division of Artificial Internal Organs, School of Medicine, University of Utah; Surgical Consultant, Salt Lake City, Utah.

DOROTHY F. HOLMES, D.V.M., Ph.D., Senior Research Associate, Department of Microbiology, New York State College of Veterinary Medicine, Cornell University, Ithaca, New York.

JEAN HOLZWORTH, D.V.M.; Diplomate, American College of Veterinary Internal Medicine; Clinical Staff, Angell Memorial Animal Hospital, Boston, Massachusetts.

EDWARD A. HOOVER, D.V.M., Ph.D., Professor, Department of Veterinary Pathobiology, College of Veterinary Medicine, The Ohio State University, Columbus, Ohio.

BARRY R. HORN, M.D., Assistant Clinical Professor of Medicine, University of California, San Francisco; Associate Medical Director, Pulmonary Medicine Department, Herrick Memorial Hospital, Berkeley, California.

WILLIAM E. HORNBUCKLE, D.V.M., Assistant Professor of Small Animal Medicine, New York State College of Veterinary Medicine, Cornell University, Ithaca, New York.

KATHERINE ALBRO HOUPT, V.M.D., Ph.D., Assistant Professor of Physiology, New York State College of Veterinary Medicine, Cornell University; Behavioral Consultant, Veterinary Hospital, New York State College of Veterinary Medicine, Cornell University, Ithaca, New York.

PETER J. IHRKE, V.M.D., Assistant Professor of Dermatology and Allergy, Department of Medicine, School of Veterinary Medicine, University of California, Davis; Veterinary

Medical Teaching Hospital, University of California, Davis, California.

JAN E. ILKIW, B.V.Sc., Ph.D., Dip. Vet. An., M.A.C.V.Sc., Lecturer, Department of Veterinary Clinical Studies, University of Sydney, Sydney, N.S.W., Australia.

KATHRYN ANNE INGRAM, D.V.M., Shea Animal Hospital, Phoenix, Arizona.

DENNIS A. JACKSON, D.V.M., M.S., Assistant Professor of Surgery, College of Veterinary Medicine, University of Illinois, Urbana, Illinois.

WILLIAM F. JACKSON, D.V.M., M.S.; Diplomate, American College of Veterinary Ophthalmologists and American College of Veterinary Surgeons; Adjunct Clinical Professor, University of Florida, Gainesville; Practitioner, Lakeland, Florida.

ELLIOTT R. JACOBSON, D.V.M., Ph.D., Assistant Professor of Laboratory Animal and Wildlife Medicine, College of Veterinary Medicine, University of Florida; Wildlife Clinician, Veterinary Medical Teaching Hospital, University of Florida, Gainesville, Florida.

RICHARD H. JACOBSON, Ph.D., Assistant Professor of Immunoparasitology, New York State College of Veterinary Medicine, Cornell University, Ithaca, New York.

KARIM JERAJ, B.V.Sc., Research Associate in Pediatric Nephrology, Department of Pediatrics, College of Medicine, University of Minnesota, Minneapolis; Research Associate, Department of Small Animal Clinical Sciences, College of Veterinary Medicine, University of Minnesota, St. Paul, Minnesota.

ROGER K. JOHNSON, D.V.M.; Diplomate, American College of Veterinary Internal Medicine; Encino Veterinary Clinic, Walnut Creek, California.

GARY R. JOHNSTON, D.V.M., M.S., Assistant Professor of Radiology, Department of Small Animal Clinical Sciences, College of Veterinary Medicine, University of Minnesota, St. Paul, Minnesota.

SHIRLEY D. JOHNSTON, D.V.M., M.S., Resident in Theriogenology, Department of Large Animal Clinical Sciences, College of Veterinary Medicine, University of Minnesota, St. Paul Minnesota.

JANINE B. KASPER, D.V.M., Instructor in Small Animal Medicine, School of Veterinary Medicine, University of California, Davis, California.

JOHN D. KELLY, B.V.Sc., Ph.D., M.R.C.V.S., Officer in Charge, Regional Veterinary Laboratory, Victorian Department of Agriculture, Bendigo, Australia.

SUZANNE KENNEDY, D.V.M., Assistant Professor, Department of Environmental Medicine, College of Veterinary Medicine, University of Tennessee, Knoxville; Veterinarian, Knoxville Zoological Park, Knoxville, Tennessee.

KERRY L. KETRING, D.V.M.; Diplomate, American College of Veterinary Ophthalmologists; Private Practitioner in Ophthalmology, Cincinnati, Ohio.

ROBERT W. KIRK, D.V.M.; Diplomate, American College of Veterinary Internal Medicine (Dermatology); Professor of Medicine, New York State College of Veterinary Medicine, Cornell University, Ithaca, New York.

JEFFREY S. KLAUSNER, D.V.M., M.S.; Diplomate, American College of Veterinary Internal Medicine; Assistant Professor, Department of Small Animal Clinical Sciences, College of Veterinary Medicine, University of Minnesota, St. Paul, Minnesota.

LAWRENCE J. KLEINE, D.V.M., M.S.; Diplomate, American College of Veterinary Radiology; Director of Radiology, Angell Memorial Animal Hospital, Boston, Massachusetts.

KENNETH W. KNAUER, D.V.M., M.S.; Diplomate, American College of Veterinary Internal Medicine; Associate Professor of Small Animal Medicine and Surgery, College of Veterinary Medicine, Texas A and M University; Chief of Medicine and Cardiologist, Department of Small Animal Medicine and Surgery, Veterinary Medical Teaching Hospital, Texas A and M University, College Station, Texas.

SETH A. KOCH, V.M.D., M.M.Sc.; Diplomate, American College of Veterinary Ophthalmologists; Alexandria, Virginia.

RONALD J. KOLATA, D.V.M., M.S.; Diplomate, American College of Veterinary Surgeons; Assistant Professor, Department of Small Animal Medicine, College of Veterinary Medicine, University of Georgia, Athens, Georgia.

DAVID F. KOWALCZYK, V.M.D., Ph.D., Assistant Professor of Pharmacology and Toxicology, University of Pennsylvania School of Veterinary Medicine, Philadelphia, Pennsylvania.

D. J. KRAHWINKEL, Jr , D.V.M., M.S.; Diplomate, American College of Veterinary Anesthesiologists and American College of Veterinary Surgeons; Associate Professor of Surgery, College of Veterinary Medicine, University of Tennessee; Director of Surgical Services, Veterinary Teaching Hospital, University of Tennessee, Knoxville, Tennessee.

RAYMOND A. KRAY, D.V.M., Kray Veterinary Clinic for Birds, Burbank, California.

GAIL A. KUNKLE, D.V.M., Associate in Dermatology, University of Pennsylvania, School of Veterinary Medicine; Clinical Dermatologist, Small Animal Clinic, Philadelphia, Pennsylvania.

ARTHUR L. LAGE, D.V.M.; Diplomate, American College of Veterinary Internal Medicine; Assistant Professor of Veterinary Medicine, Harvard Medical School, Boston, Massachusetts; Director of Medicine, South Shore Veterinary Associates, South Weymouth, Massachusetts.

ROLF E. LARSEN, D.V.M., Ph.D., Assistant Professor, University of Florida, College of Veterinary Medicine, Gainesville, Florida.

DANIEL C. LAUGHLIN, M.Ed., D.V.M., Director, Exotic Animal Veterinary Services Ltd., Riverside, Illinois; Research Associate, The Arthritis Institute of the National Orthopaedic and Rehabilitation Hospital, Arlington, Virginia.

J. DANIEL LAVACH, D.V.M., M.S.; Diplomate, American College of Veterinary Ophthalmologists; Assistant Professor of Comparative Ophthalmology, College of Veterinary Medicine, University of Florida; Ophthalmology Service, Veterinary Medical Teaching Hospital, Gainesville, Florida.

GEORGE E. LEES, D.V.M., M.S.; Diplomate, American College of Veterinary Internal Medicine; Assistant Professor, Department of Small Animal Clinical Sciences, College of Veterinary Medicine, University of Minnesota, St. Paul, Minnesota.

ALFRED M. LEGENDRE, D.V.M., M.S.; Diplomate, American College of Veterinary Internal Medicine; Associate Professor, University of Tennessee, College of Veterinary Medicine, Knoxville, Tennessee.

LON D. LEWIS, D.V.M., Ph.D., Associate Professor, Mark L. Morris Chair in Clinical Nutrition, Department of Clinical Sciences, College of Veterinary Medicine and Biomedical Sciences, Colorado State University, Fort Collins, Colorado.

GERALD V. LING, D.V.M., Associate Professor, School of Veterinary Medicine, University of California, Davis; Section of Small Animal Internal Medicine, Veterinary Medical Teaching Hospital, University of California, Davis, California.

ALAN J. LIPOWITZ, D.V.M., M.S.; Diplomate, American College of Veterinary Surgeons; Associate Professor of Surgery and Head, Division of Small Animal Surgery, Department of Small Animal Clinical Sciences, College of Veterinary Medicine, University of Minnesota, St. Paul, Minnesota.

MICHAEL D. LORENZ, D.V.M.; Diplomate, American College of Veterinary Internal Medicine; Associate Professor, University of Georgia, College of Veterinary Medicine; Chief, Small Animal Medicine, University of Georgia Veterinary Medical Teaching Hospital, Athens, Georgia.

DONALD G. LOW, D.V.M., Ph.D.; Diplomate, American College of Veterinary Internal Medicine; Professor of Veterinary Medicine, University of California, School of Veterinary Medicine, Davis; Director, Veterinary Medical Teaching Hospital, University of California, Davis, California.

LINDA J. LOWENSTINE, D.V.M.; Diplomate, American College of Veterinary Pathologists; Postgraduate Research Pathologist, Experimental Pathology, California Primate Research Center, University of California, Davis, California.

ALEID A. M. E. LUBBERINK, D.V.M., Ph.D., Lecturer, Small Animal Clinic; Veterinary Faculty, University of Utrecht, Utrecht, The Netherlands.

SCOTT E. McDONALD, D.V.M., Resident in Exotic Animal Medicine, School of Veterinary Medicine, University of California, Davis, California.

E. GREGORY MacEWEN, V.M.D.; Diplomate, American College of Veterinary Internal Medicine; Head, Donaldson-Atwood Cancer Clinic; Staff, Department of Medicine, The Animal Medical Center; Research Associate, Memorial Sloan-Kettering Cancer Center, New York, New York.

PATRICK J. McKEEVER, D.V.M., M.S., Associate Professor of Comparative Dermatology, Department of Small Animal Clinical Sciences, College of Veterinary Medicine, University of Minnesota; University of Minnesota Veterinary Teaching Hospital, St. Paul, Minnesota.

BRENDAN C. McKIERNAN, D.V.M., Assistant Professor, College of Veterinary Medicine, University of Illinois; Small Animal Medical Clinician, Veterinary Medical Teaching Hospital, Urbana, Illinois.

BRIAN J. McLEAVEY, B.V.Sc., Small Animal Practitioner, Christchurch, New Zealand.

BRUCE R. MADEWELL, V.M.D., M.S.; Diplomate, American College of Veterinary Internal Medicine; Assistant Professor, School of Veterinary Medicine, University of California, Davis; Small Animal Clinics, Davis, California.

CHARLES L. MARTIN, D.V.M., M.S.; Diplomate, American College of Veterinary Ophthalmologists; Professor, Department of Small Animal Medicine, College of Veterinary Medicine, University of Georgia, Athens, Georgia.

SHARRON L. MARTIN, D.V.M., M.S., Professor of Veterinary Clinical Sciences, College of Veterinary Medicine, The Ohio State University; Attending Clinician, The Veterinary Hospital of the Ohio State University, Columbus, Ohio.

GAVIN L. MEERDINK, D.V.M., Associate Professor, Animal Health Diagnostic Laboratory and Department of Large Animal Surgery and Medicine, Michigan State University, East Lansing, Michigan.

JAN C. MEIJER, D.V.M., Veterinary Faculty, Small Animal Clinic, University of Utrecht, Utrecht, The Netherlands.

DENNIS J. MEYER, D.V.M.; Diplomate, American College of Veterinary Internal Medicine; Assistant Professor of Small Animal Medicine and Clinical Pathology, College of Veterinary Medicine, University of Florida, Gainesville, Florida.

WILLIAM H. MILLER, Jr., V.M.D., Instructor in Dermatology, School of Veterinary Medicine, University of Pennsylvania; Small Animal Hospital, Philadelphia, Pennsylvania.

MERRILL M. MITLER, Ph.D., Research Associate Professor, Department of Psychiatry, State University of New York at Stony Brook, Long Island, New York.

RONALD L. MULL, D.V.M., Ph.D.; Diplomate, American Board of Veterinary Toxicology; Associate Study Director, Toxicology Research, Medical Research Division, American Cyanamid Company, Lederle Laboratories, Pearl River, New York.

GEORGE H. MULLER, D.V.M.; Diplomate, American College of Veterinary Internal Medicine (Dermatology); Clinical Professor of Dermatology, Department of Dermatology, Stanford University Medical School, Stanford, California.

JOHN A. MULNIX, D.V.M., M.S., Private Practitioner, Anderson Animal Hospital, Denver, Colorado, and Moore Animal Hospital, Fort Collins, Colorado.

JOAN A. O'BRIEN, V.M.D.; Diplomate, American College of Veterinary Internal Medicine; Professor of Medicine and Chief of Small Animal Medicine, School of Veterinary Medicine, University of Pennsylvania; Associate Professor of Otorhinolaryngology, Hahnemann Hospital and University of Pennsylvania Hospital, Philadelphia, Pennsylvania.

FREDERICK W. OEHME, D.V.M., D.Med. Vet., Ph.D.; Diplomate, American Board of Veterinary Toxicology; Professor of Toxicology, Medicine, and Physiology and Director,

Comparative Toxicology Laboratory, Kansas State University, College of Veterinary Medicine; Clinical Toxicologist, Veterinary Medical Center, Kansas State University, Manhattan, Kansas.

JOHN E. OLIVER, Jr., D.V.M., Ph.D.; Diplomate, American College of Veterinary Internal Medicine (Neurology); Professor, Department of Small Animal Medicine and Department of Veterinary Physiology and Pharmacology, College of Veterinary Medicine, University of Georgia; Neurologist, University of Georgia Veterinary Medical Teaching Hospital, Athens, Georgia.

PATRICIA N. S. OLSON, D.V.M., M.S., Clinical Director, Rothgerber Endocrinology Laboratory, Department of Physiology and Biophysics, Colorado State University; Veterinary Teaching Hospital, Fort Collins, Colorado.

STEN-ERIK OLSSON, V.M.D., M.D., Ph.D., Dr.Sc.h.c., Head, Division of Radiation Protection Medicine, The Swedish Radiation Protection Institute; Docent in Experimental Surgery, Medical College of the Caroline Institute, Stockholm, Sweden; Consultant in Radiology and Comparative Orthopedics, College of Veterinary Medicine, University of Florida, Gainesville, Florida; Formerly, Professor of Clinical Radiology, The Royal Veterinary College, Stockholm, Sweden.

CARL A. OSBORNE, D.V.M., Ph.D.; Diplomate, American College of Veterinary Internal Medicine; Professor and Chairman, Department of Small Animal Clinical Sciences, College of Veterinary Medicine, University of Minnesota, St. Paul, Minnesota; Professor, Department of Pediatrics, College of Medicine, University of Minnesota, Minneapolis, Minnesota.

GARY D. OSWEILER, D.V.M., Ph.D.; Diplomate, American Board of Veterinary Toxicology; Professor, College of Veterinary Medicine, University of Missouri; Veterinary Medical Diagnostic Laboratory, Columbia, Missouri.

JANIS EILEEN OTT, D.V.M., Staff Veterinarian, Brookfield Zoo, Chicago Zoological Park, Brookfield, Illinois.

ALAN J. PARKER, Ph.D., M.R.C.V.S.; Diplomate, American College of Veterinary Internal Medicine (Neurology); Associate Professor of Medicine, College of Veterinary Medicine, University of Illinois; Neurologist, Department of Veterinary Clinical Medicine, University of Illinois, Urbana, Illinois.

HAROLD R. PARKER, D.V.M., Ph.D., Professor of Surgery, School of Veterinary Medicine, University of California, Davis; Supervisor, Intensive Care Unit, Veterinary Medical Teaching Hospital, Davis, California.

DONALD F. PATTERSON, D.V.M., D.Sc.; Diplomate, American College of Veterinary Internal Medicine (Cardiology); Professor of Medicine, School of Veterinary Medicine, University of Pennsylvania; Chief, Section of Medical Genetics, Small Animal Hospital, University of Pennsylvania, Philadelphia, Pennsylvania.

JAMES M. PATTERSON, D.V.M.; Diplomate, American College of Veterinary Internal Medicine; Associate Professor of Veterinary Medicine, Ontario Veterinary College, Guelph, Ontario, Canada.

NIELS C. PEDERSEN, D.V.M., Ph.D., Associate Professor, School of Veterinary Medicine, University of California, Davis; Small Animal Clinics, Davis, California.

ROBERT LOUIS PEIFFER, Jr., D.V.M.; Diplomate, American College of Veterinary Ophthalmologists; Assistant Professor and Director of Laboratories, Departments of Ophthalmology and Pathology, School of Medicine, University of North Carolina, Chapel Hill, North Carolina.

PAUL LEONARD PEMBERTON, B.V.Sc., Lecturer, University of Sydney, Department of Animal Husbandry, Faculty of Veterinary Science; Private Practitioner, Sydney, N.S.W., Australia.

VICTOR PERMAN, D.V.M., Ph.D.; Diplomate, American College of Veterinary Pathologists; Professor, Department of Pathobiology, College of Veterinary Medicine, University of Minnesota; Staff, University of Minnesota Teaching Hospital, St. Paul, Minnesota.

GUY L. PIDGEON, D.V.M., Assistant Professor, Auburn University, Auburn, Alabama.

DAVID JAMES POLZIN, D.V.M., Resident in Internal Medicine and Urology, Department of Small Animal Clinical Sciences, College

of Veterinary Medicine, University of Minnesota, St. Paul, Minnesota.

R. LEE PYLE, V.M.D., M.S.; Diplomate, American College of Veterinary Internal Medicine (Cardiology); Associate Professor, College of Veterinary Medicine, Mississippi State University, Mississippi State, Mississippi.

A. H. REBAR, D.V.M., Ph.D.; Diplomate, American College of Veterinary Pathologists (Veterinary Clinical Pathologist); Associate Professor of Veterinary Clinical Pathology; School of Veterinary Medicine, Purdue University, West Lafayette, Indiana.

LLOYD M. REEDY, D.V.M.; Diplomate, American College of Veterinary Internal Medicine (Dermatology); Clinical Assistant Professor of Comparative Medicine, University of Texas, Southwestern Medical School; Animal Dermatology Clinic, Dallas, Texas.

RON C. RIIS, D.V.M., M.S.; Diplomate, American College of Veterinary Ophthalmologists; Assistant Professor of Veterinary Medicine, New York State College of Veterinary Medicine, Cornell University, Ithaca, New York.

AD RIJNBERK, D.V.M., Ph.D., Professor, Small Animal Clinic, State University of Utrecht, Utrecht, The Netherlands.

EDWARD LEE ROBERSON, M.A.T., D.V.M., Ph.D., Associate Professor of Parasitology, College of Veterinary Medicine, University of Georgia, Athens, Georgia.

NORMAN EDWARD ROBINSON, B.Vet.Med., Ph.D., M.R.C.V.S., Professor, Department of Physiology, Michigan State University, East Lansing, Michigan.

WALTER J. ROSSKOPF, Jr., D.V.M., Animal Medical Centre of Lawndale, Hawthorne, California.

JAMES CHARLES ROUSH, II, D.V.M., Research Associate in Biology, University of California, Santa Cruz; Director of Surgical Service, Santa Cruz Veterinary Hospital, Santa Cruz, California.

ROBERT ALLEN RUSHMER, V.M.D., Assistant Professor, University of Pennsylvania, School of Veterinary Medicine, Kennett Square, Pennsylvania.

WILLIAM C. SATTERFIELD, D.V.M., Faculty, Tufts University, School of Veterinary Medicine; Director of Biomedical Activities,

Boston Zoological Society, Boston, Massachusetts.

RANDALL H. SCAGLIOTTI, D.V.M., M.S.; Diplomate, American College of Veterinary Ophthalmologists; Assistant Clinical Professor, School of Veterinary Medicine, University of California, Davis; Staff Ophthalmologist, Sacramento Animal Medical Group, Carmichael, California.

MICHAEL SCHAER, D.V.M.; Diplomate, American College of Veterinary Internal Medicine; Associate Professor and Chief, Small Animal Medical Services, College of Veterinary Medicine, University of Florida, Gainesville, Florida.

WILLIAM D. SCHALL, D.V.M.; Diplomate, American College of Veterinary Internal Medicine; Associate Professor of Internal Medicine, College of Veterinary Medicine, Michigan State University; Internist, Veterinary Clinical Center, East Lansing, Michigan.

GRETCHEN M. SCHMIDT, D.V.M.; Diplomate, American College of Veterinary Ophthalmologists; Assistant Professor, Michigan State University, Veterinary Teaching Hospital, East Lansing, Michigan.

NORMAN R. SCHNEIDER, D.V.M., M.S.; Diplomate, American Board of Veterinary Toxicology; Associate Professor, Department of Veterinary Science, Institute of Agriculture and Natural Resources, University of Nebraska, Lincoln, Nebraska.

STEPHEN M. SCHUCHMAN, D.V.M., Boulevard Pet Hospital, Castro Valley, California.

RONALD DAVID SCHULTZ, Ph.D., Professor of Immunology, School of Veterinary Medicine, Auburn University, Auburn, Alabama.

WAYNE S. SCHWARK, D.V.M., Ph.D., Associate Professor of Pharmacology, New York State College of Veterinary Medicine, Cornell University, Ithaca, New York.

DOROTHEA SCHWARTZ-PORSCHE, Prof. Dr.Med.Vet., Professor of Veterinary Medicine, Small Animal Clinic, Free University of Berlin, Berlin, Germany.

DANNY W. SCOTT, D.V.M.; Diplomate, American College of Veterinary Internal Medicine (Dermatology); Associate Professor of Medi-

cine, New York State College of Veterinary Medicine, Cornell University, Ithaca, New York.

FREDRIC W. SCOTT, D.V.M., Ph.D.; Diplomate, American College of Veterinary Microbiologists; Professor of Virology, New York State College of Veterinary Medicine, Cornell University; Director, Cornell Feline Research Laboratory, Cornell University, Ithaca, New York.

RICHARD C. SCOTT, D.V.M.; Diplomate, American College of Veterinary Internal Medicine; Staff, Department of Medicine, Animal Medical Center, New York, New York.

GENE P. SEARCY, D.V.M., Ph.D.; Diplomate, American College of Veterinary Pathologists (Veterinary Clinical Pathologist); Professor of Pathology, Western College of Veterinary Medicine, Saskatoon, Saskatchewan, Canada.

CHARLES JEROME SEDGWICK, D.V.M., Assistant Professor, School of Veterinary Medicine, University of California, Davis, California.

DAVID FRANK SENIOR, B.V.Sc.; Diplomate, American College of Veterinary Internal Medicine; Assistant Professor of Medicine, College of Veterinary Medicine, University of Florida, Gainesville, Florida.

CHARLES E. SHORT, D.V.M., M.S.; Diplomate, American College of Veterinary Anesthesiologists; Professor and Chief, Anesthesiology, Department of Clinical Sciences, New York State College of Veterinary Medicine, Cornell University, Ithaca, New York.

SAM SILVERMAN, D.V.M.; Diplomate, American College of Veterinary Radiology; Associate Clinical Professor of Radiology, University of California, Davis; Staff Radiologist, Ocean Avenue Veterinary Hospital, San Francisco, California.

ERWIN SMALL, D.V.M., M.S.; Diplomate, American College of Veterinary Internal Medicine (Dermatology); Professor of Veterinary Medicine, College of Veterinary Medicine, University of Illinois; Chief of Medicine, Small Animal Section, University of Illinois, Urbana, Illinois.

LAWRENCE R. SOMA, V.M.D.; Diplomate, American College of Veterinary Anesthesiologists; Professor of Anesthesiology, Department of Clinical Studies, School of Veterinary Medicine, University of Pennsylvania, Philadelphia, Pennsylvania.

GLEN L. SPAULDING, D.V.M.; Diplomate, American College of Veterinary Internal Medicine; Assistant Professor of Medicine, New York State College of Veterinary Medicine, Cornell University, Ithaca, New York.

ROSS STAADEN, B.V.Sc., Practitioner; Graduate Student in Veterinary Studies, Murdoch University, Perth, Western Australia.

BARBARA SYDNEY STEIN, D.V.M., Director, Chicago Cat Clinic, Chicago, Illinois.

JERRY B. STEVENS, D.V.M., Ph.D., Professor, Department of Veterinary Pathobiology, College of Veterinary Medicine, University of Minnesota, St. Paul, Minnesota.

DONALD R. STROMBECK, D.V.M., Ph.D., Professor of Veterinary Medicine, School of Veterinary Medicine, University of California, Davis; Chief, Small Animal Medicine Service, Veterinary Medical Teaching Hospital, University of California, Davis, California.

PETER F. SUTER, D.Med.Vet.; Diplomate, American College of Veterinary Radiology; Professor of Radiology, School of Veterinary Medicine, University of California, Davis; Radiology Service, Small Animal Clinic, Veterinary Medical Teaching Hospital, University of California, Davis, California.

CAROL M. SZYMANSKI, D.V.M.; Diplomate, American College of Veterinary Ophthalmologists; Assistant Professor, College of Veterinary Medicine, Ohio State University, Columbus, Ohio.

DAVID H. TAYLOR, D.V.M., Private Practitioner, Syracuse, New York.

PETER THERAN, V.M.D.; Diplomate, American College of Veterinary Internal Medicine; Assistant Chief of Staff, Angell Memorial Animal Hospital, Boston, Massachusetts.

WILLIAM P. THOMAS, D.V.M.; Diplomate, American College of Veterinary Internal Medicine (Cardiology); Assistant Professor of Medicine, School of Veterinary Medicine, University of California, Davis; Chief, Cardiology Service, Veterinary Medical Teaching

Hospital, University of California, Davis, California.

JERRY A. THORNHILL, D.V.M.; Diplomate, American College of Veterinary Internal Medicine; Assistant Professor of Medicine, Purdue University, School of Veterinary Medicine, West Lafayette, Indiana.

LAWRENCE P. TILLEY, D.V.M.; Diplomate, American College of Veterinary Internal Medicine (Cardiology); Adjunct Assistant Professor, Department of Pharmacology, College of Physicians and Surgeons, Columbia University; Staff Cardiologist, The Animal Medical Center, New York, New York.

TERESA L. TOMCHICK, D.V.M., Staff Surgeon, South Hill Veterinary Clinic, Puyallup, Washington.

A. J. VENKER–VAN HAAGEN, Small Animal Clinic, State University of Utrecht, Utrecht, The Netherlands.

LARRY J. WALLACE, D.V.M., M.S.; Diplomate, American College of Veterinary Surgeons; Professor of Surgery, Department of Small Animal Clinical Sciences, College of Veterinary Medicine, University of Minnesota, St. Paul, Minnesota.

RICHARD WALSHAW, B.V.M.S., M.R.C.V.S., Assistant Professor, College of Veterinary Medicine, Michigan State University; Staff Surgeon, General Surgery, Veterinary Clinical Center, Michigan State University, East Lansing, Michigan.

RICHARD C. WEISS, V.M.D., Postdoctoral Fellow, Department of Microbiology, New York State College of Veterinary Medicine, Cornell University, Ithaca, New York.

R. DAVID WHITLEY, D.V.M., NIH Fellow in Comparative Ophthalmology, College of Veterinary Medicine, University of Florida; Ophthalmology Service, Veterinary Medical Teaching Hospital, Gainesville, Florida.

STEPHEN R. WIGHTMAN, D.V.M., M.S., Senior Veterinarian, Toxicology Division, Lilly Research Laboratories, Greenfield, Indiana.

ROBERT J. WILKINS, B.V.Sc.; Diplomate, American College of Veterinary Pathologists (Veterinary Clinical Pathologist); Staff Clinical Pathologist, Animal Medical Center, New York, New York.

TON (A.) WILLEMSE, D.V.M., Dermatologist, University Clinic of Small Animal Medicine, University of Utrecht, Utrecht, The Netherlands.

JEFFREY F. WILLIAMS, B.V.Sc., Ph.D., Professor, Department of Microbiology and Public Health, Michigan State University, East Lansing, Michigan.

JAMES W. WILSON, D.V.M., M.S.; Diplomate, American College of Veterinary Surgeons; Roseville, Minnesota.

MILTON WYMAN, D.V.M., M.S.; Diplomate, American College of Veterinary Ophthalmologists; Professor and Chief, Comparative Ophthalmology, College of Veterinary Medicine, The Ohio State University, Columbus, Ohio.

ROBERT D. ZENOBLE, D.V.M., M.S.; Diplomate, American College of Veterinary Internal Medicine; Assistant Professor, Department of Veterinary Clinical Sciences, College of Veterinary Medicine, Iowa State University, Ames, Iowa.

JAMES F. ZIMMER, D.V.M., Ph.D., Assistant Professor of Medicine, New York State College of Veterinary Medicine, Cornell University, Ithaca, New York.

PREFACE

Current Veterinary Therapy continues to be a text written for clinicians by clinicians. It remains a useful tool only as long as it fills the needs of people who are practicing veterinary medicine. We ask for your suggestions of ways we can improve the presentation of information.

This volume has placed more emphasis on illustrations, radiographs, drugs, and diagnostic algorithms. The contrast between the depth and the volume of information presented here and in the first edition is graphic. Our growth as a profession, with new knowledge and techniques, has been impressive. We hope this text continues to be useful to you.

As always, the editor is grateful to each contributor and hopes there is a special place in heaven for each dedicated consulting editor. We have a very special thank-you for the staff of W. B. Saunders — particularly Carroll Cann, good friend and colleague.

ROBERT W. KIRK, D.V.M.
Ithaca, New York

CONTENTS

SECTION 1
SPECIAL THERAPY
Robert W. Kirk
Consulting Editor

ANTIMICROBIAL THERAPY...................... 2
Lloyd E. Davis

DIAGNOSTIC CYTOLOGY IN VETERINARY
PRACTICE: CURRENT STATUS AND
INTERPRETIVE PRINCIPLES 16
A. H. Rebar

FEVERS OF UNKNOWN ORIGIN IN
DOGS AND CATS 28
Anne M. Chiapella

SHOCK: PATHOPHYSIOLOGY AND
MANAGEMENT 32
Ronald J. Kolata, Colin F. Burrows,
and Lawrence R. Soma

FLUID AND ELECTROLYTE THERAPY....... 49
Charles E. Short

PHYSICAL FITNESS AND TRAINING FOR
DOGS 53
Ross Staaden

CRYOTHERAPY................................. 65
R. E. Hoffer

PREVENTIVE MEDICINE IN KENNEL
MANAGEMENT 67
Lawrence T. Glickman

PEDIATRICS.................................... 77
Erwin Small

A CATALOG OF GENETIC DISORDERS
OF THE DOG 82
Donald F. Patterson

SECTION 2
CHEMICAL AND PHYSICAL DISORDERS
Frederick W. Oehme
Consulting Editor

EMERGENCY AND GENERAL TREAT-
MENT OF POISONINGS........................... 105
E. Murl Bailey

USE OF LABORATORIES FOR THE
CHEMICAL ANALYSIS OF TISSUES 115
William B. Buck

COMMON POISONINGS IN SMALL
ANIMAL PRACTICE 122
Gary D. Osweiler

STRYCHNINE POISONING........................ 129
Gary D. Osweiler

WARFARIN AND OTHER ANTI-
COAGULANT POISONINGS 131
Robert A. Green and William B. Buck

METALDEHYDE POISONING 135
Ronald L. Mull

LEAD POISONING 136
David F. Kowalczyk

LEAD POISONING IN NEW ZEALAND........ 141
Brian J. McLeavey

ANTIFREEZE (ETHYLENE GLYCOL)
POISONING 144
Frederick W. Oehme

ORGANOPHOSPHATE AND CARBAMATE
INSECTICIDE POISONING 147
Thomas L. Carson

COMMON POTENTIAL SOURCES OF
SMALL ANIMAL POISONINGS 149
  Gary D. Osweiler

ADVERSE DRUG REACTIONS 155
  Arthur L. Aronson and
  Wayne S. Schwark

TERATOGENESIS AND MUTAGENESIS 161
  Norman R. Schneider

CARCINOGENESIS 172
  T. Gopal

BITES AND STINGS OF VENOMOUS
ANIMALS 174
  G. L. Meerdink

SNAKEBITE IN AUSTRALIA AND
NEW GUINEA 179
  Henry L. Hirschhorn

NEAR-DROWNING (WATER
INHALATION) 182
  Charles S. Farrow

INHALATION INJURY 186
  Charles S. Farrow

THERMAL INJURY 191
  Patrick J. McKeever

HEAT STROKE (HEAT STRESS,
HYPERPYREXIA) 195
  William D. Schall

ACCIDENTAL HYPOTHERMIA 197
  R. D. Zenoble

COLD INJURY (HYPOTHERMIA,
FROSTBITE, FREEZING) 199
  Robert A. Dieterich

EMERGENCY KIT FOR TREATMENT OF
SMALL ANIMAL POISONING (ANTIDOTES,
DRUGS, EQUIPMENT) 201
  Frederick W. Oehme

CLINICAL PHARMACOLOGY OF THE
RESPIRATORY SYSTEM 208
  Lloyd E. Davis

CANINE UPPER RESPIRATORY
DISEASE 214
  Richard Walshaw and
  Richard B. Ford

FELINE UPPER RESPIRATORY
DISEASE 224
  Richard B. Ford and
  Richard Walshaw

DISEASES OF THE CANINE AND FELINE
TRACHEOBRONCHIAL TREE 229
  Brendan McKiernan

CANINE AND FELINE PNEUMONIA 235
  Brendan McKiernan

PULMONARY EDEMA 243
  John D. Bonagura

NEOPLASMS OF THE RESPIRATORY
TRACT 249
  Steven E. Crow

PLEURAL EFFUSIONS 253
  Stanley R. Creighton and
  Robert J. Wilkins

PARASITIC DISEASES OF THE
RESPIRATORY TRACT 262
  J. F. Williams

THORACIC TRAUMA 268
  D. J. Krahwinkel, Jr.

THERAPY FOR RESPIRATORY
EMERGENCIES 277
  Charles E. Short

INTERPRETATION OF PULMONARY
RADIOGRAPHS 279
  Peter F. Suter

LARYNGEAL PARALYSIS IN YOUNG
BOUVIERS 290
  A. J. Venker-van Haagen

SECTION
3

RESPIRATORY DISEASES
N. Edward Robinson
Consulting Editor

A DIAGNOSTIC APPROACH TO
RESPIRATORY DISEASE 203
  Joan A. O'Brien

SECTION
4

CARDIOVASCULAR DISEASES
Stephen J. Ettinger
Consulting Editor

CARDIOPULMONARY RESUSCITATION
FOR PEOPLE 293
  Barry R. Horn and Amy H. Ansfield

CARDIAC ARREST 297
   Stephen J. Ettinger

VALVULAR HEART DISEASE 297
   Kenneth W. Knauer

CARDIOMYOPATHY IN THE DOG AND
CAT.. 307
   Betsy Bond and Lawrence P. Tilley

MYOCARDIAL DISEASE 316
   David B. Church

PERICARDIAL DISEASE........................ 321
   Rebecca E. Gompf

CANINE HEARTWORM DISEASE............... 326
   John D. Kelly

COR PULMONALE............................. 335
   Glen L. Spaulding

DISEASES OF PERIPHERAL
LYMPHATICS: LYMPHEDEMA 337
   P. F. Suter

INFLUENCE OF NON-CARDIAC DISEASE
ON THE HEART.............................. 340
   Edward C. Feldman

CARDIOVASCULAR SYSTEM OF THE
RACING DOG 347
   Ross Staaden

PHARMACODYNAMICS OF DIGITALIS,
DIURETICS, AND ANTIARRHYTHMIC
DRUGS..................................... 352
   Lloyd E. Davis

ACUTE HEART FAILURE 359
   John Bonagura

LONG-TERM THERAPY OF CHRONIC
CONGESTIVE HEART FAILURE IN
THE DOG AND CAT 368
   William P. Thomas

BRADYCARDIA............................... 376
   G. R. Bolton

TACHYARRHYTHMIA 381
   R. Lee Pyle

SECTION
5
HEMOLYMPHATIC DISORDERS AND ONCOLOGY
Victor Perman
Consulting Editor

LABORATORY DIAGNOSIS OF
IMMUNOLOGIC DISORDERS.................... 390
   Ronald D. Schultz

FELINE LEUKEMIA VIRUS DISEASE
COMPLEX.................................. 404
   Niels C. Pedersen and
   Bruce R. Madewell

FELINE HEMOBARTONELLOSIS 410
   John W. Harvey

BONE MARROW FAILURE IN THE DOG
AND CAT.................................. 413
   Gene P. Searcy

HEINZ BODY HEMOLYTIC ANEMIAS
AND METHEMOGLOBINEMIAS................. 417
   George E. Lees

CANINE LYMPHOSARCOMA 419
   E. Gregory MacEwen

CANCER CHEMOTHERAPY 423
   E. Gregory MacEwen

IMMUNOTHERAPY OF MALIGNANT
DISEASE 426
   E. Gregory MacEwen

SECTION
6
DERMATOLOGIC DISEASES
R. E. W. Halliwell
Consulting Editor

AUTOIMMUNE SKIN DISEASES................. 432
   R. E. W. Halliwell

THE DIFFERENTIAL DIAGNOSIS OF
FACIAL DERMATITIS 436
   Danny W. Scott

CANINE NASAL SOLAR DERMATITIS 440
   Peter J. Ihrke

SUBCORNEAL PUSTULAR DERMATOSIS
AND DERMATITIS HERPETIFORMIS.......... 443
   Patrick J. McKeever and
   Mark V. Dahl

THE MANAGEMENT OF FLEA ALLERGY
DERMATITIS 446
    Michael D. Lorenz

THE DIAGNOSIS OF CANINE ATOPIC
DISEASE 450
    Lloyd M. Reedy

THE TREATMENT OF CANINE ATOPIC
DISEASE 453
    Gail A. Kunkle

DRUG ERUPTION 458
    Danny W. Scott

OTITIS EXTERNA 461
    L. R. Grono

CANINE PODODERMATITIS.................... 467
    Danny W. Scott

CRUSTING DERMATOSES IN CATS 469
    Ton (A.) Willemse

ZINC-RESPONSIVE DERMATOSES
IN DOGS 472
    Gail A. Kunkle

SUBCUTANEOUS AND OPPORTUNISTIC
MYCOSES, THE DEEP MYCOSES, AND
THE ACTINOMYCETES 477
    Marie H. Attleberger

HEREDITARY HAIR AND PIGMENT
ABNORMALITIES.................................. 487
    George H. Muller

FELINE ALOPECIAS 490
    Robert W. Kirk

CANINE CUTANEOUS LYMPHOMAS 493
    William H. Miller, Jr.

CRYOTHERAPY IN SMALL ANIMAL
DERMATOLOGY................................... 495
    Ton (A.) Willemse

PHARMACOLOGY OF ANTIPRURITIC
DRUGS.. 497
    Peter Eyre

SECTION
7
OPHTHALMOLOGIC DISEASES
Charles L. Martin
Consulting Editor

THE OPHTHALMIC EXAMINATION AND
ANAMNESIS 505
    Charles L. Martin

NEURO-OPHTHALMOLOGY 510
    Randall H. Scagliotti

OCULAR THERAPEUTICS 517
    Stephen Bistner

ALGORITHMS FOR OPHTHALMOLOGIC
PROBLEMS 528
    Gretchen Schmidt

OCULAR EMERGENCIES 542
    Milton Wyman

DISEASES OF THE EYELIDS..................... 546
    Kerry L. Ketring

DISEASES OF THE CONJUNCTIVA............. 550
    Lewis H. Campbell

DISEASES OF THE LACRIMAL
APPARATUS 553
    David Covitz

DISEASES OF THE CORNEA 558
    Robert M. Gwin

DISEASES OF THE LENS......................... 565
    R. C. Riis

DISEASES OF THE ANTERIOR UVEA......... 570
    Kirk N. Gelatt, J. Daniel Lavach,
    and R. David Whitley

CANINE AND FELINE GLAUCOMA............ 576
    Paul F. Dice, II

DISEASES OF THE VITREOUS, RETINA,
AND CHOROID 579
    Ned Buyukmihci

DISEASES OF THE ORBIT 583
    Seth Koch

INTRAOCULAR AND ORBITAL
NEOPLASIA... 585
    Carol Szymanski

OPHTHALMIC DISORDERS OF PROVEN
OR SUSPECTED GENETIC ETIOLOGY
IN THE DOG AND CAT 587
    Robert L. Peiffer, Jr.

THE EYE AND SYSTEMIC DISEASE 593
    Charles L. Martin

SECTION
8
DISEASES OF CAGED BIRDS AND EXOTIC PETS
Murray E. Fowler
Consulting Editor

INTRODUCTION 601
    Murray E. Fowler

VETERINARY INVOLVEMENT IN
REHABILITATION CENTERS 601
    Raymond A. Kray

MYCOBACTERIAL INFECTIONS IN
NON-DOMESTIC ANIMALS 604
    Suzanne Kennedy

MEDICAL CARE OF TROPICAL FISH........ 606
    Michael Thomas Collins

AMPHIBIAN CARE AND DISEASES 616
    Gerald E. Cosgrove

ANESTHESIA OF REPTILES 618
    Charles J. Sedgwick

SURGERY IN CAPTIVE REPTILES 620
    Fredric L. Frye

INFECTIOUS DISEASES OF REPTILES 625
    Elliot R. Jacobson

RESPIRATORY DISEASE IN REPTILES 633
    Murray E. Fowler

MEDICAL CARE OF AQUATIC
TURTLES............................... 637
    W. J. Rosskopf, Jr.

ANTIBIOTIC THERAPY IN REPTILES 647
    Mitchell Bush

AVIAN RADIOGRAPHIC TECHNIQUE
AND INTERPRETATION 649
    Sam Silverman

ANESTHESIA OF CAGED BIRDS................ 653
    Charles J. Sedgwick

OTOSCOPE TECHNIQUE FOR SEXING
BIRDS 656
    Kathryn A. Ingram

DIAGNOSTIC LAPAROSCOPY IN BIRDS 659
    William C. Satterfield

AVIAN ORTHOPEDICS.......................... 662
    James C. Roush, II

FOREIGN DISEASES AND IMPORTED
BIRDS 674
    Linda J. Lowenstine

PSITTACOSIS—AN EVER-PRESENT
PROBLEM IN CAGED BIRDS 677
    Ralph Cooper

MANAGEMENT OF OIL-SOAKED BIRDS 687
    James M. Harris

CARE AND TREATMENT OF CAPTIVE
WILD BIRDS 692
    Charles Galvin

RESPIRATORY DISEASE IN
PSITTACINE BIRDS 697
    Scott E. McDonald

ACUTE AVIAN HERPESVIRUS
INFECTIONS 704
    David L. Graham

ANESTHESIA FOR RABBITS AND
RODENTS 706
    Charles J. Sedgwick

MEDICAL CARE OF NON-DOMESTIC
CARNIVORES................................. 710
    Martin R. Dinnes

VIRUS DISEASES OF PRIMATES—THEIR
HAZARDS TO HUMAN HEALTH 733
    Janis E. Ott

INDIVIDUAL CARE AND TREATMENT
OF RABBITS, MICE, RATS, GUINEA
PIGS, HAMSTERS, AND GERBILS............. 741
    Stephen M. Schuchman

SECTION
9

NEUROLOGIC AND MUSCULO-SKELETAL DISORDERS

Alexander de Lahunta
Consulting Editor

CEREBROSPINAL FLUID ANALYSIS........... 769
James W. Wilson

BOTULISM, TICK PARALYSIS, AND
ACUTE POLYRADICULONEURITIS
(COONHOUND PARALYSIS)...................... 773
Jeanne A. Barsanti

TICK PARALYSIS IN AUSTRALIA.............. 777
Jan E. Ilkiw

INFLAMMATORY MUSCLE DISEASE
IN THE DOG 779
I. D. Duncan and I. R. Griffiths

EXERTIONAL RHABDOMYOLYSIS
(MYOGLOBINURIA) IN THE RACING
GREYHOUND 783
James R. Gannon

MYOTONIA IN THE DOG........................ 787
I. D. Duncan

EPISODIC WEAKNESS 791
Brian R. H. Farrow

CANINE POLYARTHRITIS 795
Ralph E. Barrett

CANINE HIP DYSPLASIA........................ 802
Sten-Erik Olsson

OSTEOCHONDROSIS IN THE DOG............ 807
Sten-Erik Olsson

INTRACRANIAL INJURY.......................... 815
J. E. Oliver, Jr.

STORAGE DISEASES.............................. 821
Brian R. H. Farrow

CANINE HEPATIC ENCEPHALOPATHY 822
Ralph E. Barrett

TREATMENT OF FELINE AND CANINE
SEIZURE DISORDERS 830
Alan J. Parker

DIAGNOSIS AND TREATMENT OF
NARCOLEPSY IN ANIMALS 837
Merrill M. Mitler and
Arthur S. Foutz

CLINICAL BEHAVIORAL PROBLEMS:
AGGRESSION... 841
Katherine A. Houpt

FELINE AND CANINE BEHAVIOR
CONTROL: PROGESTIN THERAPY 845
Paul L. Pemberton

SECTION
10

GASTROINTESTINAL DISORDERS

Donald R. Strombeck
Consulting Editor

THE ORAL CAVITY................................ 855
Ray Dillon

CLINICAL PATHOLOGY OF THE LIVER 875
Bernard F. Feldman

MANAGEMENT OF CANINE CHRONIC
ACTIVE HEPATITIS................................ 885
Donald R. Strombeck

FELINE LIVER DISEASE 891
William E. Hornbuckle and
Graeme S. Allan

ACUTE GASTRIC DILATION—
VOLVULUS 896
Donald R. Strombeck

MICROBIOLOGY OF THE GASTRO-
INTESTINAL TRACT: MICROFLORA AND
IMMUNOLOGY...................................... 901
Dwight C. Hirsh

THE USE OF ANTIMICROBIAL DRUGS
IN THE TREATMENT OF GASTRO-
INTESTINAL DISORDERS........................ 913
Dwight C. Hirsh and L. Reed Enos

MANAGEMENT OF DIARRHEA:
MOTILITY MODIFIERS AND ADJUNCT
THERAPY 914
Donald R. Strombeck

DIET AND NUTRITION IN THE MANAGE-
MENT OF GASTROINTESTINAL
PROBLEMS 919
Donald R. Strombeck

MALASSIMILATION SYNDROME:
MALDIGESTION/MALABSORPTION............ 930
Guy Pidgeon

GASTROINTESTINAL PARASITISM............. 935
Edward L. Roberson and
Larry M. Cornelius

THE MANAGEMENT OF COLITIS............. 948
Michael D. Lorenz

PERIANAL FISTULAS............................ 952
Richard E. Hoffer

GASTROINTESTINAL FIBEROPTIC
ENDOSCOPY 954
James F. Zimmer

GASTROINTESTINAL BIOPSY
TECHNIQUES 962
Janine B. Kasper and
Ann M. Chiapella

LAPAROSCOPY IN SMALL ANIMAL
MEDICINE 969
J. M. Patterson

SECTION
11
ENDOCRINE AND METABOLIC DISORDERS
John A. Mulnix
Consulting Editor

CANINE HYPERADRENOCORTICISM 975
Jan C. Meijer

THERAPY FOR SPONTANEOUS
HYPERADRENOCORTICISM 979
Aleid A. M. E. Lubberink

HYPOADRENOCORTICISM........................ 983
Michael Schaer

SYSTEMIC GLUCOCORTICOID
THERAPY 988
Danny W. Scott

HYPOTHYROIDISM 994
Bruce E. Belshaw and Ad Rijnberk

FELINE HYPERTHYROIDISM.................... 998
Peter Theran and Jean Holzworth

PRIMARY HYPOPARATHYROIDISM 1000
Dennis J. Meyer

PRIMARY HYPERPARATHYROIDISM 1003
Alfred M. Legendre

DIABETES INSIPIDUS 1005
Dorothea Schwartz-Porsche

DIABETES MELLITUS 1011
Edward Charles Feldman

DIABETIC KETOACIDOSIS 1016
William D. Schall and
Larry M. Cornelius

FUNCTIONAL PANCREATIC ISLET CELL
ADENOCARCINOMA IN THE DOG............. 1020
Dennis D. Caywood and
James W. Wilson

NON-NEOPLASTIC CAUSES OF
CANINE HYPOGLYCEMIA........................ 1023
Roger K. Johnson and
Clarke E. Atkins

PUERPERAL TETANY 1027
S. L. Martin and C. C. Capen

THE OVARY, OVARIAN HORMONES,
AND CONTRACEPTIVES........................... 1030
P. N. S. Olson

OBESITY 1034
Gary L. Andersen and Lon D. Lewis

SECTION
12
GENITOURINARY DISORDERS
Carl A. Osborne
Consulting Editor

THE KIDNEYS

URINARY SYSTEM EMERGENCIES 1042
James J. Brace and
Dennis J. Chew

TOXIC NEPHROPATHY 1047
Jerry A. Thornhill

GLOMERULONEPHROPATHY AND THE
NEPHROTIC SYNDROME 1053
Carl A. Osborne and Karim Jeraj

RENAL AMYLOIDOSIS............................ 1063
J. A. Barsanti and Wayne Crowell

HYPERCALCEMIC NEPHROPATHY AND
ASSOCIATED DISORDERS........................ 1067
Dennis J. Chew and
Charles C. Capen

HYDRONEPHROSIS................................. 1073
James J. Brace

FANCONI SYNDROME IN THE DOG........... 1075
    K. C. Bovée

CHRONIC TUBULAR-INTERSTITIAL
DISEASE OF THE KIDNEY...................... 1076
    Richard C. Scott

OVERVIEW OF THE UREMIC SYNDROME... 1079
    K. C. Bovée

WATER DEPRIVATION AND VASO-
PRESSIN CONCENTRATION TESTS IN THE
DIFFERENTIATION OF POLYURIC
SYNDROMES 1080
    Robert M. Hardy and
    Carl A. Osborne

NEONATAL CLINICAL NEPHROLOGY........ 1085
    Arthur L. Lage

MANAGEMENT OF OLIGURIC AND
ANURIC RENAL FAILURE........................ 1087
    Larry D. Cowgill

INTENSIVE DIURESIS IN POLYURIC
RENAL FAILURE 1091
    Delmar R. Finco and Donald G. Low

MEDICAL MANAGEMENT OF POLYURIC
RENAL FAILURE: SALT AND SODIUM
BICARBONATE....................................... 1094
    Larry D. Cowgill and
    Donald G. Low

CONSERVATIVE MANAGEMENT OF
POLYURIC PRIMARY RENAL FAILURE:
DIET THERAPY..................................... 1097
    David J. Polzin and Carl A. Osborne

MEDICAL MANAGEMENT OF POLYURIC
RENAL FAILURE: ANABOLIC AGENTS....... 1102
    Donald G. Low

MEDICAL MANAGEMENT OF CHRONIC
RENAL FAILURE: CONTROL OF
HYPERPHOSPHATEMIA........................... 1103
    K. C. Bovée

NUTRITION DURING THE UREMIC
CRISIS 1104
    Delmar R. Finco

CURRENT STATUS OF PERITONEAL
DIALYSIS 1106
    Harold R. Parker

CURRENT STATUS OF VETERINARY
HEMODIALYSIS 1111
    Larry D. Cowgill

DRUG THERAPY IN RENAL
DISORDERS 1114
    Lloyd E. Davis

ANESTHESIA IN RENAL FAILURE............. 1117
    David B. Brunson

THE URINARY TRACT

NEUROGENIC URINARY INCONTINENCE ... 1122
    John E. Oliver, Jr., and
    Carl A. Osborne

NON-NEUROGENIC URINARY
INCONTINENCE 1128
    Carl A. Osborne, John E. Oliver, Jr.,
    and David E. Polzin

CANINE POLYPOID CYSTITIS 1137
    Shirley D. Johnston, Carl A. Osborne,
    and Jerry B. Stevens

RUPTURE OF THE CANINE URINARY
BLADDER 1139
    Colin F. Burrows and
    Ronald J. Kolata

PARASITES OF THE CANINE URINARY
TRACT 1141
    David F. Senior

CONGENITAL DISEASES OF THE
URACHUS... 1143
    Jeffrey S. Klausner, Carl A. Osborne,
    Jerry B. Stevens, and James W. Wilson

MEDICAL MANAGEMENT OF
PROSTATIC DISEASE.............................. 1146
    William E. Hornbuckle and
    Lawrence J. Kleine

CYSTOCENTESIS.................................... 1150
    Carl A. Osborne, George E. Lees,
    and Gary R. Johnston

SCREENING TESTS FOR THE DETECTION
OF SIGNIFICANT BACTERIURIA................ 1154
    Jeffrey S. Klausner, Carl A. Osborne,
    and Jerry B. Stevens

URINARY TRACT INFECTIONS 1158
    Delmar R. Finco

CHOICE OF ANTIMICROBIAL AGENTS
IN THE TREATMENT OF URINARY
TRACT INFECTIONS 1162
    Gerald V. Ling

ANCILLARY TREATMENT OF URINARY
TRACT INFECTIONS 1164
  Carl A. Osborne, Jeffrey S. Klausner,
  Robert M. Hardy, and George E. Lees

STRUVITE UROLITHIASIS 1168
  Jeffrey S. Klausner and
  Carl A. Osborne

URATE UROLITHIASIS 1172
  Jerry A. Thornhill

CYSTINURIA AND CYSTINE
UROLITHIASIS 1175
  Arthur L. Lage

CALCIUM OXALATE UROLITHIASIS 1177
  Carl A. Osborne and
  Jeffrey S. Klausner

CANINE SILICA UROLITHIASIS 1184
  Carl A. Osborne, Robert F. Hammer,
  and Jeffrey S. Klausner

FELINE CYSTIC CALCULI 1187
  Richard W. Greene

FELINE UROLOGIC SYNDROME:
MANAGEMENT OF THE CRITICALLY ILL
PATIENT 1188
  Delmar R. Finco

FELINE UROLOGIC SYNDROME:
REMOVAL OF URETHRAL OBSTRUCTIONS
AND USE OF INDWELLING URETHRAL
CATHETERS 1191
  George E. Lees and Carl A. Osborne

FELINE UROLOGIC SYNDROME: MEDICAL
ASPECTS OF PROPHYLAXIS 1196
  Carl A. Osborne and George E. Lees

FELINE UROLOGIC SYNDROME:
SURGICAL ASPECTS OF PROPHYLAXIS 1201
  Teresa L. Tomchick and
  Richard W. Greene

NEOPLASMS OF THE CANINE AND
FELINE URINARY TRACTS 1203
  Dennis D. Caywood, Carl A. Osborne,
  and Gary R. Johnston

THE GENITAL SYSTEM

DYSTOCIA 1212
  Edward F. Donovan

ACUTE METRITIS 1214
  Alan J. Lipowitz and Rolf E. Larsen

CANINE PYOMETRA 1216
  Robert M. Hardy and David F. Senior

CANINE VAGINITIS 1219
  Patricia N. S. Olson

VAGINAL HYPERPLASIA AND UTERINE
PROLAPSE 1222
  R. Allen Rushmer

NON-NEOPLASTIC DISORDERS OF THE
MAMMARY GLANDS 1224
  Shirley D. Johnston and
  David W. Hayden

MANAGEMENT OF CANINE
INFERTILITY 1226
  Rolf E. Larsen and
  Shirley D. Johnston

PROGNOSIS AND MANAGEMENT OF
FELINE INFERTILITY 1231
  Mary A. Herron and
  Barbara Stein

PREVENTION OF ESTRUS 1237
  Thomas J. Burke

PREGNANCY PREVENTION AND
TERMINATION 1239
  William F. Jackson and
  Shirley D. Johnston

PSEUDOHERMAPHRODITISM 1241
  Dennis A. Jackson

CANINE CRYPTORCHIDISM 1244
  Larry J. Wallace and Victor S. Cox

SECTION
13
INFECTIOUS DISEASES
Fredric W. Scott
Consulting Editor

THEORY AND PRACTICE OF
IMMUNIZATION 1248
  Ronald D. Schultz

UPDATE ON CANINE IMMUNIZATION 1252
  Ronald D. Schultz, Max Appel,
  Leland E. Carmichael, and
  Brian Farrow

UPDATE ON FELINE IMMUNIZATION 1256
  Fredric W. Scott

IMMUNIZATION OF EXOTIC CATS 1258
  Daniel C. Laughlin

RABIES: IMMUNIZATION AND PUBLIC
HEALTH ASPECTS 1261
  Melvin K. Abelseth

PET-ASSOCIATED ZOONOSES 1265
  Dorothy N. Holmes

CONTROL OF CANINE INFECTIOUS
DISEASES IN ADOPTION SHELTERS 1268
  David H. Taylor

CONTROL OF FELINE INFECTIOUS
DISEASES IN CATTERIES AND
ADOPTION SHELTERS 1270
  Jean Holzworth

CONTROL OF INFECTIOUS DISEASES
IN AVIARIES AND PET SHOPS 1273
  Stephen B. Hitchner

CANINE RESPIRATORY DISEASE
COMPLEX 1276
  Glen L. Spaulding

FELINE RESPIRATORY DISEASE
COMPLEX 1279
  Barbara S. Stein

CANINE DISTEMPER 1284
  Brian R. H. Farrow

FELINE PANLEUKOPENIA 1286
  Susan M. Cotter

FELINE INFECTIOUS PERITONITIS 1288
  Richard C. Weiss and Fredric W. Scott

CANINE VIRAL ENTERITIS..................... 1292
  Leland E. Carmichael and
  Max J. Appel

PSEUDORABIES IN DOGS AND CATS 1296
  D. P. Gustafson

FELINE PNEUMONITIS 1299
  Edward A. Hoover

CANINE BRUCELLOSIS 1303
  Ricardo Flores-Castro and
  Leland E. Carmichael

FELINE SALMONELLOSIS........................ 1305
  James G. Fox

TOXOPLASMOSIS — FELINE INFECTIONS
AND THEIR ZOONOTIC POTENTIAL.......... 1307
  Richard H. Jacobson

FELINE CYTAUXZOONOSIS 1312
  Stephen R. Wightman

KITTEN MORTALITY COMPLEX 1313
  Fredric W. Scott

SHIPPING REGULATIONS FOR SMALL
ANIMALS.. 1316
  Robert W. Kirk

APPENDICES
Robert W. Kirk
Consulting Editor

TABLES OF NORMAL PHYSIOLOGICAL
DATA: ELECTROCARDIOGRAPHY 1319

TABLES FOR CONVERSION OF WEIGHT
TO BODY-SURFACE AREA IN SQUARE
METERS FOR DOGS 1320

A ROSTER OF NORMAL VALUES FOR
DOGS AND CATS 1321
  John Bentinck-Smith

TABLE OF COMMON DRUGS:
APPROXIMATE DOSES 1331

INDEX.. 1341

NORMAL CLINICAL PATHOLOGY
DATA .... Back End Sheet

NOTICE

Extraordinary efforts have been made by the authors, the editors, and the publisher of this book to insure that dosage recommendations are precise and in agreement with standards officially accepted at the time of publication.

It does happen, however, that dosage schedules are changed from time to time in the light of accumulating clinical experience and continuing laboratory studies. This is most likely to occur in the case of recently introduced products.

It is urged, therefore, that you check the manufacturer's recommendations for dosage, especially if the drug to be administered or prescribed is one that you use only infrequently or have not used for some time.

In addition, some drugs mentioned have been used by the authors as experimental drugs. Others have been used after official clearance for use in one species but not in others described here. This is particularly true for rare and exotic species. In these cases the authors have reported on their own considerable experience, but readers are urged to view the recommendations with discretion and precaution.

THE EDITORS

Section
1

SPECIAL
THERAPY

ROBERT W. KIRK, D.V.M.
Consulting Editor

Antimicrobial Therapy... 2
Diagnostic Cytology in Veterinary Practice: Current Status and
    Interpretive Principles.. 16
Fevers of Unknown Origin in Dogs and Cats 28
Shock: Pathophysiology and Management 32
Fluid and Electrolyte Therapy 49
Physical Fitness and Training for Dogs.................................. 53
Cryotherapy 65
Preventive Medicine in Kennel Management............................... 67
Pediatrics 77
A Catalog of Genetic Disorders of the Dog 82

Additional Pertinent Information found in **Current
Veterinary Therapy VI:**

Bolton, Gary R., D.V.M.: Aerosol Therapy, p. 12.
Finco, Delmar R., D.V.M.: Fluid Therapy, p. 3.
Morris, M. L., Jr. D.V.M.: Index of Dietetic Management,
    p. 59.
Mosier, J. E., D.V.M.: Causes and Treatment of Neonatal
    Death, p. 44.

ANTIMICROBIAL THERAPY

LLOYD E. DAVIS, D.V.M.
Urbana, Illinois

Antimicrobial agents are among the most frequently used and misused drugs in veterinary medical practice. Overuse of antibiotics, as with other drugs, is encouraged by forces such as operant conditioning, conditioning by advertising, client pressure, and fear of litigation. In response to this demand, the annual production of antimicrobial drugs in the U.S. is in excess of 26,000 tons (1971 data). This greatly exceeds any rational medical need.

Drugs are inherently neither good nor bad. Whether they are boon or bane to the patient depends on how the veterinarian employs them in his or her practice. Data on the prescribing and dispensing practice of veterinarians are not available, but the performance of physicians may be instructive. A study conducted by Roberts and Visconti (1972) analyzed the records of 340 human patients who had received antibacterial therapy during their hospitalization. A team of experts judged that the prescriptions had been rational in 12.9 percent of the cases, questionable in 21.5 percent, and completely irrational in 65.6 percent of the cases. Of the 340 patients, 48 developed an adverse drug reaction during the course of therapy. In 92 percent of patients suffering a drug reaction, the prescribed treatment was rated as questionable or clearly irrational. I suspect that studies of performance in veterinary medicine would yield results not any more favorable to the patient.

Melmon and Morrelli (1978) pointed out that inappropriate use of drugs may result in:

1. Delay in diagnosis
2. Lack of effective therapy for a life-threatening but curable disease
3. The production of severe toxicity
4. Prolongation of a disease state
5. The development of a disorder to which a patient would otherwise not be subject.

All these results have been observed in veterinary clinical practice. Inappropriate selection of an antimicrobial drug will lead to a delay in diagnosis by interference with subsequent laboratory procedures for the identification of the etiologic agent. The fact that one has committed oneself to inappropriate therapy tends to remove the motivation to delve deeper into other possible causes for a patient's illness. In addition, the veterinarian may induce severe toxic reactions through drug interactions or direct adverse effects of the drug therapy. Antibacterial drugs can prolong the course of diarrhea by inducing suprainfections within the intestinal tract. A recent example of the fifth aforementioned result was a canine patient that was treated with isoniazid for an undiagnosed respiratory disease. The dog developed thrombocytopenic purpura in response to the drug and died.

A rational approach to antimicrobial therapy entails choosing the proper drug to be administered by a dosage regimen appropriate to the species after due consideration of potential benefits and risks. Prerequisites to rational therapy include a diagnosis, understanding of the pathophysiology of the disease and pharmacology of the drug, and the establishment of therapeutic objectives. These factors should be considered within an ethical framework, and the practitioner should base his or her decisions on the welfare of the patient rather than on conditioned behavior.

CONSIDERATIONS IN THE SELECTION OF AN ANTIMICROBIAL DRUG FOR THERAPY

DOCUMENTATION OF INFECTION

Establishment of an etiologic diagnosis is essential to the selection of the most effective chemotherapeutic agent for the infection. Samples for submission to the laboratory should be collected prior to instituting any therapy. The nature of these samples will vary, depending on the anatomic locus of infection and the nature of the infectious process. Multiple blood samples (5 to 10 ml) should be collected at one- to two-hour intervals from patients with serious systemic infections. Frequently, several days may be required to grow out the pathogen from blood. Samples of exudates, urine, cerebrospinal fluid, transtracheal aspirates, or synovial fluid should be submitted to the laboratory for culture and sensitivity tests. At the time of collection, it is wise to stain a smear of exudate

2

or sediment (following centrifugation) with Gram's stain and examine it microscopically. This can provide immediate information concerning the presence of bacteria and the general nature of the pathogen (gram-positive or negative, bacilli or cocci). Such information will greatly improve one's ability to select a drug that is likely to be effective for the initial treatment of an infection. A convenient control of the staining procedure is to scrape one's own teeth and place this specimen on the edge of the slide prior to staining (the human mouth contains an abundance of both gram-positive and negative bacteria).

The importance of documentation that a bacterial infection exists cannot be overemphasized. The most common error observed in a referral practice setting is that veterinarians treat patients that have viral, mycotic, neoplastic, or parasitic diseases with several antimi-

Table 1. *Possible Etiologic Agents in Typical Clinical Infections*

DIAGNOSIS	COMMONLY ISOLATED ORGANISMS
Stomatitis	*Streptococcus*, Staphylococcus*, Proteus, Pseudomonas, Escherichia coli, Fusobacterium fusiforme, Candida albicans*
Tonsillitis, pharyngitis	*Streptococcus*, Staphylococcus*
Bronchitis, pneumonia	*Bordetella bronchiseptica*, Pseudomonas aeruginosa, Klebsiella, Staphylococcus aureus, Streptococcus pyogenes,* viruses
Pyothorax	*Pasteurella multocida*, Escherichia coli*, Streptococcus, Staphylococcus, Nocardia,* viruses
Pyodermas	*Staphylococcus aureus, Streptococcus*, Proteus*, Pseudomonas, Corynebacterium, Escherichia coli*, Enterobacter aerogenes*
Vulvitis, vaginitis	*Proteus mirabilis*, Escherichia coli*, Streptococcus*
Metritis—chronic	*Streptococcus*, Brucella canis, Escherichia coli, Haemophilus*
″ —acute	*Streptococcus*, Proteus mirabilis, Escherichia coli*
Pyometra	*Escherichia coli*, Streptococcus*
Balanoposthitis	*Escherichia coli*, Klebsiella, Enterobacter, Proteus, Pseudomonas, Staphylococcus*
Cystitis	*Escherichia coli*, Proteus mirabilis*, Pseudomonas*, Streptococcus, Staphylococcus*
Prostatitis	*Escherichia coli*, Proteus, Pseudomonas, Streptococcus, Staphylococcus*
Infectious enteritis	*Salmonella*, Escherichia coli*, Pseudomonas (?Streptococcus, Proteus), Giardia,* coccidia, distemper virus
Superficial ocular infections	*Staphylococcus, Streptococcus*
Osteomyelitis	*Staphylococcus aureus*, Escherichia coli*, Streptococcus, Proteus*
Wound infections	*Staphylococcus*,* coliforms**, Clostridium*
Bacterial endocarditis	*Streptococcus*, Escherichia coli, Pseudomonas, Staphylococcus*
Puppy septicemias	*Streptococcus*, Escherichia coli*, Proteus mirabilis, Pseudomonas aeruginosa, Staphylococcus,* viruses
Otitis media	*Staphylococcus*, Streptococcus*, Pityrosporum, Pseudomonas, Escherichia coli, Proteus mirabilis*
Otitis externa	*Staphylococcus aureus*, Streptococcus*, Pityrosporum*;* secondary: *Proteus mirabilis, Pseudomonas*, Corynebacterium, Bacillus subtilis, Candida albicans*
Burns	*Pseudomonas*, Proteus, Escherichia coli, Staphylococcus*

Modified from Aronson and Kirk, 1975.
*Most commonly isolated.

Table 2. *Use of Antimicrobial Agents for Treatment of Infections*

ORGANISM	DISEASE	DRUGS OF CHOICE	ALTERNATIVE DRUGS
Actinomyces	Actinomycosis	Penicillin G*	Tetracyclines
Bacillus anthracis	Anthrax	Penicillin G	Erythromycin, tetracyclines
Blastomyces, Candida, Coccidioides, Histoplasma, Cryptococcus, Mucor, Aspergillus	Pneumonia, skin and soft tissue lesions, bone lesions, disseminated disease	Amphotericin B	2 hydroxystilbamide† (*Blastomyces*), flucytosine† (*Candida, Cryptococcus*)
Bordetella bronchiseptica	Respiratory infections	Tetracyclines	Chloramphenicol
Brucella canis	Abortions	Tetracyclines with streptomycin	——
Chlamydia psittaci	Respiratory infections, conjunctivitis	Tetracyclines	Chloramphenicol
Clostridium tetani	Tetanus	Penicillin G*	Erythromycin
Clostridia, other	Gas gangrene	Penicillin G*	Tetracyclines
Coccidia	Coccidiosis	Sulfonamides	Nitrofurazone
Escherichia coli	Urinary tract infections	Nitrofurantoin, sulfonamides, ampicillin	Cephalosporins, chloramphenicol, tetracyclines
	Other infections	Ampicillin, chloramphenicol tetracyclines	Aminoglycosides, polymyxins
Fusobacterium	Ulcerative stomatitis	Penicillin G	Tetracyclines, metronidazole
Giardia	Enteritis	Metronidazole	Quinacrine, glycobiarsol
Haemobartonella	Infectious anemia	Tetracyclines‡	Chloramphenicol‡
Klebsiella, Enterobacter	Respiratory, urinary tract infections	Kanamycin, gentamicin	Cephalosporins, chloramphenicol
Leptospira	Leptospirosis	Penicillin G with streptomycin	Tetracyclines
Microsporum, Trichophyton, Epidermophyton	Skin, hair and nail bed infections	Griseofulvin	——
Mycobacterium	Tuberculosis	Isoniazid with streptomycin or p-aminosalicylic acid	——
Mycoplasma	Respiratory infection(?), conjunctivitis	Tetracyclines	Chloramphenicol, macrolides
Neorickettsia	Salmon disease	Tetracyclines	Chloramphenicol
Nocardia	Nocardiosis	Sulfonamide–trimethoprim*	Chloramphenicol, tetracyclines
Pasteurella multocida	Abscesses, respiratory infections	Penicillin G*	Tetracyclines, ampicillin
Pentatrichomonas	Trichomonal enteritis	Metronidazole	Glycobiarsol

Modified from Aronson and Kirk 1975.

*Large dosage.

†Used to treat these infections in man; efficacy in dogs and cats uncertain.

‡Efficacy questionable.

§Urinary tract infections only.

Continued on next page

Table 2. *Use of Antimicrobial Agents for Treatment of Infections (Continued)*

ORGANISM	DISEASE	DRUGS OF CHOICE	ALTERNATIVE DRUGS
Pityrosporum	Skin and ear infections	2% "tame" iodine or 25% glyceryl triacetate topically	—
Proteus mirabilis	Urinary tract and soft tissue infections	Ampicillin, chloramphenicol, nitrofurantoin§	Cephalosporins, aminoglycosides
Pseudomonas aeruginosa	Urinary tract and soft tissue infections, burns	Polymyxins, gentamicin	Carbenicillin, plus gentamicin chloramphenicol
Salmonella	Gastroenteritis	Chloramphenicol	Ampicillin, nitrofurans
Staphylococcus aureus	Pyoderma, endocarditis, osteomyelitis, soft tissue infections	Penicillin G sensitive: penicillin G Penicillin G resistant: cloxacillin, macrolides	Ampicillin, macrolides, lincomycin Cephalosporins, chloramphenicol, lincomycin
Streptococcus	Urinary tract infections, otitis, soft tissue infections, upper respiratory infections	Penicillin G	Ampicillin, cephalosporins, erythromycin
Toxoplasma	Toxoplasmosis	Pyrimethamine with sulfonamide	—

§Urinary tract infections only.

crobial drugs prior to referral. These animals frequently have adverse reactions to the drugs and a multiply-resistant microbial flora. The only pathogens susceptible to antimicrobial therapy are bacteria, yeasts, chlamydia, rickettsia, and certain protozoa.

The presence of fever or changes in the differential blood cell count are not, in themselves, adequate evidence that a patient has a bacterial infection requiring chemotherapy. Fever can be caused by immune-mediated diseases, neoplasms, drug reactions, exercise, excitement, increased environmental temperature, and dehydration. Neutrophilia can be produced by causes other than a suppurative process.

Certain considerations are helpful as clues to possible etiology that might permit more rational therapy. The site of origin of the infection may lead one to suspect involvement of certain types of organisms; e.g., infections of surgical wounds might be expected to be caused by gram-positive bacteria from the surrounding skin, whereas infections of the urogenital system or perineum might be expected to be associated with gram-negative organisms. The character of onset of fever may provide information relative to etiology. A gradual, stepwise climb to a peak is most often associated with gram-positive pathogens,

whereas an abrupt, rapid rise to a peak is most often indicative of sepsis caused by gramnegative organisms. The most commonly encountered pathogens in a small animal practice are listed in Tables 1 and 2.

DRUG SELECTION

Once the clinician has documented the presence of an infection by a susceptible pathogen, he is in a position to select the most appropriate drug for therapy. Suggestions are provided in Tables 3 and 4 relative to some possible choices for treating infections caused by specific pathogens. In addition to susceptibility of the organism to the drug, one must consider various pharmacologic factors, comparative toxicity, and cost of drugs likely to be effective.

To be effective, the drug must reach the site of infection at concentrations high enough to destroy or inhibit the infecting organism. Consideration should be given to drug absorption from the route of administration. Many drugs are poorly absorbed from the gut (aminoglycosides, acid-labile penicillins, some nitrofurans and cephalosporins, polymyxins, and tetracyclines, under certain circumstances). This would obviate this route for the treatment of

Table 3.   *Properties of Some Antimicrobial Drugs**

I. PENICILLINS	Bactericidal drugs, toxic effects rare. Excretion mainly renal, hindered by probenecid orally (occasionally useful when treating systemic infections with expensive penicillins).
Penicillin G (benzylpenicillin)	Active mainly against gram-positive organisms, also against some gram-negative species at higher concentrations (e.g., in urine). Drug of choice against most gram-positive pathogens, except strains of *Staphylococcus aureus* producing penicillinase. Available in 3 parenteral forms—Na or K salt (short-acting), procaine salt (duration about 24 hours at usual doses) and benzathine or benethamine salt (low blood levels for at least 5 days after single injection, which is inadequate for less susceptible microbes). Should not be given to guinea pigs.
A. Acid-resistant Penicillin V (phenoxymethylpenicillin), phenethicillin	Similar activity to penicillin G against gram-positive organisms, but preferred for oral dosage because of greater resistance to gastric acid.
B. Staphylococcal penicillinase–resistant Cloxacillin, oxacillin, nafcillin, methicillin	Generally less active than penicillin G, indicated only for infections caused by penicillinase-producing strains of *S. aureus*. Methicillin must be given parenterally, the others orally or parenterally.
C. Wide-spectrum Ampicillin	Compared with penicillin G, ampicillin is slightly less active against gram-positive bacteria but more active against gram-negative bacilli. Given orally or parenterally.
Hetacillin	Similar properties, hydrolyzed to ampicillin *in vivo*, given orally.
Amoxicillin	Similar spectrum to ampicillin but has better bioavailability, orally.
Carbenicillin	Expensive, parenteral use only, may be useful for systemic or urinary tract infections caused by gentamicin-resistant *Pseudomonas aeruginosa, Proteus* spp.
II. CEPHALOSPORINS	Bactericidal, active against many gram-positive and gram-negative bacteria. Useful against penicillin-resistant staphylococci, gram-negative bacteria (mainly in urinary tract), and as substitutes for penicillin in penicillin-sensitive patients.
Cephaloridine	Administered intramuscularly. High doses nephrotoxic.
Cephalothin	Administered IM
Cephalexin	Administered orally, well absorbed.
III. AMINOGLYCOSIDES	Bactericidal, active against gram-negative bacteria, mycobacteria, some staphylococci. Absorption from gut minimal—administered parenterally for systemic or urinary tract infections (antibacterial activity enhanced in alkaline urine), orally for gut antisepsis. Excretion mainly renal. Toxic effects: damage to eighth cranial nerve (deafness, vestibular disturbance); renal damage; neuromuscular blockade.
Streptomycin, dihydrostreptomycin	Identical activity; dihydrostreptomycin used in most veterinary preparations, but no longer recommended for people because it causes deafness more frequently than streptomycin. Bacterial strains resistant to these two emerge rapidly during treatment.
Neomycin	Similar activity but more toxic than streptomycin. Prolonged high oral dosage of neomycin (or kanamycin) may cause diarrhea, malabsorption (reversible), suprainfections.
Kanamycin	Safer systemically than neomycin, but more expensive.
Gentamicin	More active than other aminoglycosides against many microbes, expensive—practicable only for gram-negative pathogens resistant to other aminoglycosides, polymyxins.
IV. TETRACYCLINES	Bacteriostatic, active against many gram-positive and gram-negative bacteria, also mycoplasmas, rickettsias and chlamydia. Administration: oral route usually preferred, but absorption is incomplete and hindered by food or divalent cations. Intramuscular injection often painful, some intravenous formulations available. Widely distributed in body, deposited in growing bone and teeth (but not necessarily active there). Excretion: mainly urine, also bile. Toxicity: gastrointestinal disturbances, necrosis at injection sites, hyperthermia, discolored teeth (if given to neonates or during gestation). Use in renal failure contraindicated because of their antianabolic effect and delayed excretion (except doxycycline). Fanconi syndrome with outdated products.

Continued on next page

Table 3. *Properties of Some Antimicrobial Drugs (Continued)*

Tetracycline, oxytetracycline, chlortetracycline, demethylchlortetracycline (*Also* rolitetracycline, methacycline, minocycline)	Most commonly used tetracyclines in veterinary practice— cheaper than many of the newer derivatives (rolitetracycline, methacycline, minocycline) which offer few advantages.
Doxycycline	Low dosage form, once daily administration, may be safe in patients with renal failure.
Demeclocycline	May induce nephrogenic diabetes insipidus.
V. MACROLIDES	Bacteriostatic, active mainly against gram-positive cocci and clostridia, some effect against mycoplasmas, rickettsias and chlamydia.
Erythromycin	Usually second choice to penicillin G or V, which are cheaper. Generally administered orally, occasionally intramuscularly (causes pain) or intravenously. Excreted in urine and bile. Side-effects uncommon in animals, in people sometimes gastrointestinal upsets or hepatopathy with the estolate ester.
Tylosin (*Rarely used:* oleandomycin, triacetyloleandomycin, spiramycin)	Similar indications to erythromycin. Other macrolides rarely used.
VI. POLYMYXINS	Bactericidal, active against gram-negative bacilli, including *Pseudomonas aeruginosa* but not *Proteus* spp. Not absorbed from gut. Administered parenterally for systemic or urinary tract infections as *polymyxin B* sulfate, or methanesulfonate derivative of *colistin (polymyxin E)*. Excreted mainly in urine. Toxicity: renal damage, neurotoxicity (drowsiness, ataxia, neuromuscular blockade). Gentamicin is less toxic and has tended to supplant polymyxins but polymyxins may be preferred on the basis of cost.
Polymyxin B Colistin	
VII. MISCELLANEOUS ANTIBIOTICS	
Chloramphenicol	Bacteriostatic, active against many gram-positive and gram-negative bacteria, as well as mycoplasmas, rickettsias, *Bacteroides* spp. and *Chlamydia*. Oral administration: satisfactory for routine therapy, well absorbed. Given as tablets, capsules (absorption unimpeded by food) or suspensions of palmitate ester (provides similar blood levels to capsules at equivalent dosage). Parenteral administration: solutions in nonaqueous solvents, or solutions of succinate ester. Excretion: 5–10% eliminated in urine as active antibiotic, the rest metabolized by liver. Toxicity: depression, decreased food intake and reversible bone marrow suppression may occur at therapeutic dose rates in cats and at higher dosages in dogs. Inhibition of metabolism of many drugs. Inhibits immune response. Animals should not be immunized while receiving chloramphenicol.
Lincomycin	Bacteriostatic, active mainly against gram-positive bacteria and some mycoplasmas. Indications and usefulness similar to erythromycin, which is cheaper. For staphylococcal infections, combined use with another antistaphylococcal agent advised because lincomycin resistance emerges readily. Excreted mainly in urine. Toxicity: hemorrhagic diarrhea may occur in dogs. The drug may be fatal to horses and rabbits.
Clindamycin (clinimycin)	A derivative of lincomycin, more active, some pharmacologic advantages, may eventually replace lincomycin. May be especially useful in infections due to *Actinomyces* spp. or *Bacteroides* spp.
Amphotericin B	Fungicidal, active against many fungi causing deep mycotic infections. Administration: intravenous or intraperitoneal route, prolonged course. Very toxic, low margin of safety, causes renal damage, vomiting, abdominal pain. Indications: blastomycosis, coccidioidomycosis, histoplasmosis, disseminated candidiasis, cryptococcosis, sporotrichosis, mucormycosis, aspergillosis.
Nystatin	Fungicidal, similar spectrum of activity to amphotericin B. Too toxic for parenteral use, not absorbed from the gut. Indications: topically or by mouth for superficial or intestinal candidiasis. Routine prophylactic use during tetracycline therapy (intended to prevent *Candida albicans* overgrowth) probably unwarranted.
Griseofulvin	Fungistatic. Indicated for dermatophyte infections of hair, skin, nails. Administered orally, absorption promoted by high fat diet. Teratogenic, avoid in pregnancy. Not effective topically.

Continued on next page

Table 3. *Properties of Some Antimicrobial Drugs (Continued)*

VIII. SULFONAMIDES	Bacteriostatic, active against many gram-positive and gram-negative bacteria, some chlamydia and some protozoa. Generally less active than antibiotics but relatively inexpensive. Administration: usually oral, some parenteral forms available. Excretion: mainly renal. Toxicity: a variety of effects recognized, generally uncommon with correct dosage; crystalluria and renal damage avoided with highly soluble sulfonamides, alkaline urine (increases solubility), high urine flow rate. Several types available:
Sulfamethizole, sulfisoxazole (sulfafurazole)	*Short-acting*: rapidly absorbed and excreted, highly soluble, commonly used for urinary tract infections.
Sulfadiazine, sulfamethazine, sulfa-merazine, triple sulfonamide mixtures	*Intermediate*: rapidly absorbed but more slowly excreted, used for systemic or urinary tract infections.
Sulfadimethoxine, sulfamethoxypyridazine	*Long-acting*: very slow excretion, used for systemic infections if once daily dosage advantageous.
Phthalylsulfathiazole	*Poorly Absorbed*: used for topical effect in bowel.
IX. SULFONAMIDE POTENTIATORS	The action of sulfonamides against many microbes is potentiated by combined therapy with other drugs acting on the same metabolic sequence as sulfonamides. Combinations of *trimethoprim* and sulfonamide regularly show synergistic action against many bacteria *in vitro*—often producing a bactericidal effect where each drug alone was bacteriostatic. Clinical trials have generally confirmed the potentiation, but synergy should not be expected universally during therapy because the conditions required for it to occur may not always be present *in vivo*. Veterinary preparations currently available contain trimethoprim and sulfonamide (usually sulfadiazine) in 1:5 ratio. Indications: as for broad-spectrum antibiotics. Toxicity: possibility of folate deficiency.
Trimethoprim	
Pyrimethamine	Potentiates the action of sulfonamides against protozoa, may be used with sulfonamides for toxoplasmosis, coccidiosis. Toxicity: folate deficiency.

*Adapted from Watson, A. D. J., *Current Veterinary Therapy VI*.

systemic diseases. Absorption from muscle or subcutaneous sites may be poor in animals that are in shock or severely debilitated. In general, severe infections should be treated with parenterally administered drugs followed by oral administration during the convalescent phase. As an example, for a severe staphylococcal infection, one might select cephalothin for parenteral administration followed by cephalexin tablets after the infection is controlled. In acute sepsis, continuous intravenous infusion of an appropriate drug might be considered. Rates of infusion necessary to maintain constant blood concentrations can be calculated easily using data presented in Table 5. When the rate of input of a drug into the circulation is equal to the rate of elimination, there will be no net change in concentration. To determine this rate, simply multiply the usual dose of the drug times the value of k_e for the drug. For example, from Table 4 we find the recommended dose of sodium penicillin G to be 20,000 units per kg, and the value for the rate constant (sixth column of Table 5) is 1.386 hr.$^{-1}$ Thus, 20,000 × 1.386 = 27,720 units/kg/hr, which for a 20-kg dog would be an infusion rate of about 550,000 units/hr. If one simply infused this solution, it would require two hours (four half-lives) to reach 92 percent of a plateau concentration. Since our patient is in urgent need of therapy, we would administer an intravenous bolus of sodium penicillin G at a dosage of 20,000 u/kg (400,000 units) followed immediately with the infusion at a rate of 550,000 u/hr. This would immediately establish therapeutic concentrations of penicillin in the blood and would maintain them at that level for as long as we infused the drug. When the infusion is stopped, the plasma concentrations of penicillin will decline with a half-life of 30 minutes.

Another factor to be considered in selecting a drug is its distribution in the body. The tissue distribution of several antimicrobial drugs is shown in Table 6. For most body tissues, the permeation of various drugs is not a limiting factor in selecting a drug for therapy. Several of the commonly used antibacterial drugs will not enter freely into the brain, aqueous humor, prostate gland, bone, synovial fluid, or serosal fluids. In such circumstances, it would be appropriate to consider an alternative drug, shown to be active against the pathogen, or to increase the dosage of the drug initially selected.

Knowledge of routes of elimination of antimicrobial drugs is essential to selection of drugs for therapy. Drugs that are excreted un-

Table 4. *Conventional Regimens for Some Antimicrobial Drugs in Dogs and Cats*

DRUG	DOSAGE	ROUTE	REPEAT DOSE
Amphotericin B	0.5 to 1.0 mg./kg.	IV	see below*
Ampicillin	10 to 20 mg./kg.	PO	6 hours
	5 to 10 mg./kg.	IV,IM,SC	6 hours
Amoxicillin	11 mg./kg.	PO, IM	12 hrs
Carbenicillin	15 mg./kg.	IV	8 hours
Cephalexin	30 mg./kg.	PO	12 hours
Cephaloridine	10 mg./kg.	IM,SC	8 to 12 hours
Cephalothin	35 mg./kg.	IM,SC	8 hours
Chloramphenicol	50 mg./kg.	PO, IV,IM,SC	8 hours (Dog), 12 hours (Cat)
Chlortetracycline	20 mg./kg.	PO	8 hours
Cloxacillin	10 mg./kg.	PO,IV,IM	6 hours
Colistin	1 mg./kg.	IM	6 hours
Dihydrostreptomycin	20 mg./kg.	PO	6 hours (not absorbed)
	10 mg./kg.	IM,SC	8 hours
Erythromycin	10 mg./kg.	PO	8 hours
Framycetin	20 mg./kg.	PO	6 hours (not absorbed)
Gentamicin	4 mg./kg.	IM,SC	12 hours first day, then 24 hours
Griseofulvin	20 mg./kg.	PO	24 hours, with fat
	140 mg./kg.	PO	1 week, with fat
Hetacillin	10 to 20 mg./kg.	PO	8 hours
Kanamycin	10 mg./kg.	PO	6 hours (not absorbed)
	7 mg./kg.	IM,SC	6 hours
Lincomycin	15 mg./kg.	PO	8 hours
	10 mg./kg.	IV,IM	12 hours
Methicillin	20 mg./kg.	IV,IM	6 hours
Metronidazole	60 mg./kg.	PO	24 hours
Nafcillin	10 mg./kg.	PO,IM	6 hours
Neomycin	20 mg./kg.	PO	6 hours (not absorbed)
	10 mg./kg.	IM,SC	12 hours
Nitrofurantoin	4 mg./kg.	PO	8 hours
	3 mg./kg.	IM	12 hours
Nystatin	100,000 U	PO	6 hours (not absorbed)
Oxacillin	10 mg./kg.	PO,IV,IM	6 hours
Oxytetracycline	20 mg./kg.	PO	8 hours
	7 mg./kg.	IV,IM	12 hours
Penicillin G,Na or K	40,000 U/kg.	PO	6 hours (not with food)
	20,000 U/kg.	IV,IM,SC	4 hours
Penicillin G, benethamine	40,000 U/kg.	IM	5 days
Penicillin G, procaine	20,000 U/kg.	IM,SC	12 to 24 hours
Penicillin V	10 mg./kg.	PO	8 hours
Phenethicillin	10 mg./kg.	PO	8 hours
Phthalylsulfathiazole	50 mg./kg.	PO	6 hours (not absorbed)
Polymyxin B	2 mg (20,000 U)/kg.	IM	12 hours
Pyrimethamine	1 mg./kg.	PO	24 hours for 3 days, then
	0.5 mg./kg.	PO	24 hours
Streptomycin	20 mg./kg.	PO	6 hours (not absorbed)
	10 mg./kg.	IM,SC	8 hours
Sulfadiazine, sulfamerazine, sulfamethazine	50 mg./kg.	PO,IV	12 hours
Sulfadimethoxine	25 mg./kg.	PO,IV,IM	24 hours
Sulfamethizole, sulfisoxazole	50 mg./kg.	PO	8 hours
Sulfasalazine	15 mg./kg.	PO	6 hours (Dog only)
Tetracycline	20 mg./kg.	PO	8 hours
	7 mg./kg.	IV,IM	12 hours
Trimethoprim plus sulfadiazine	30 mg./kg.	PO	12 hours
Trimethoprim plus sulfadoxine	15 mg.(combined)/kg.	IV,IM	24 hours
Tylosin	10 mg./kg.	PO	8 hours
	5 mg./kg.	IV,IM	12 hours

*Amphotericin B must be diluted with 5% dextrose and water. It can be given IV 2 to 3 times weekly. It is very toxic; stop treatment if vomiting, proteinuria or an increase in BUN develops. Toxicity may preclude its use in cats.

Table 5. Pharmacokinetic Data for Selected Antimicrobial Drugs in Dogs*

DRUGS	% ABSORBED	ABSORPTION HALF-LIFE (Hr)	V_D (% of Body Wt.)	ELIMINATION HALF-LIFE (Hr)	K_E (Hr^{-1})
Amoxicillin, PO	80	0.5	20	1.5	0.462
Ampicillin, IM	100	0.3	40	1.5	0.462
Ampicillin, PO	50	0.5	40	1.5	0.462
Carbenicillin, IM	—	—	20	1.5	0.462
Cephalothin, IM	100	0.3	30	0.5	1.386
Chloramphenicol succinate, IM	70	0.3	177	4.2	0.165
Chloramphenicol, PO	100	1.0	177	4.2	0.165
Cloxacillin, IM	—	—	20	0.5	1.386
Erythromycin, PO	60	1.5	70	1.5	0.462
Gentamicin, IM	100	0.2	20	1.5	0.462
Kanamycin, IM	100	0.2	20	2.0	0.347
Methicillin, IV	—	—	20	0.5	1.386
Metronidazole, PO	100	0.5	90	4.4	0.158
Oxacillin, IM	100	0.3	30	0.5	1.386
Oxacillin, PO	50	0.5	30	0.5	1.386
Oxytetracycline, PO	—	—	90	5.0	0.139
Potassium Pen. G, IM	100	0.2	30	0.5	1.386
Potassium Pen. G, PO	25	0.5	30	0.5	1.386
Procaine Pen. G, IM	100	4.0	30	0.5	1.386
Streptomycin, IM	100	0.3	20	2.5	0.277
Sulfadimethoxine	30	1.5	40	13.2	0.053
Sulfamethazine, PO	100	0.5	70	6.0	0.116
Sulfisoxazole, PO	—	—	30	4.5	0.154
Tetracycline, PO	70	0.5	120	7.0	0.099
Trimethoprim	—	—	400	3.9	0.178
Tylosin, IM	100	0.25	170	0.9	0.770

*From: Dr. G. C. Conzelman, Jr., School of Veterinary Medicine, University of California, Davis, CA. Personal communication. V_d = volume of distribution; k_e = rate constant of elimination.

changed by the kidneys — such as penicillins, aminoglycosides, and certain tetracyclines or sulfonamides — must be used with caution and with dosage modification in patients with impaired renal function. Conversely, those compounds metabolized or eliminated by the liver (chlortetracycline and chloramphenicol) should be avoided in patients with hepatic dysfunction. In treating urinary tract or biliary infections, it is desirable to use an effective drug that is eliminated unchanged by these routes.

If everything else is equal, the least toxic and lowest priced drug should be used to accomplish therapeutic objectives. Very seldom are combinations of antibacterial drugs needed in practice. The fewer drugs employed in a given patient, the less likelihood there will be of producing adverse reactions in the animal as a result of drug interactions or other untoward effects. In some circumstances, the simultaneous use of two antimicrobial drugs can be advantageous due to synergy. Some examples are (1) penicillin and streptomycin in endocarditis caused by *E. coli,* (2) polymyxin and sulfonamides in urinary tract infections caused by certain strains of *Proteus,* (3) carbenicillin and gentamicin for gentamicin-resistant *Pseudomonas* infections, (4) cephalo-

thin and gentamicin for infections by resistant *E. coli, Klebsiella,* or *Proteus* spp., and (5) a sulfonamide with trimethoprim for nocardiosis. These drugs should be employed separately and administered according to the usual dosage regimens for each drug. The only fixed dosage combination product that the author advocates is the combination of a sulfonamide with trimethoprim.

PITFALLS IN ANTIMICROBIAL THERAPY

The other half of the benefit-risk equation for antimicrobial chemotherapy involves hazards associated with the use of the various members of this class of drugs in patients. Risks can be divided for discussion into therapeutic failures and direct pharmacologic hazards presented by the presence of the drug in the patient.

FREQUENTLY ENCOUNTERED CAUSES OF THERAPEUTIC FAILURE

Failure of a patient to respond to drug therapy can be of considerable importance to a patient and its owner when therapy is urgently needed. Some common causes of failure are

Table 6. *Tissue Distribution of Several Antimicrobial Drugs**

TISSUE	PENICILLINS	STREPTOMYCIN	TETRACYCLINES	SULFONAMIDES	ERYTHROMYCIN	CHLORAMPHENICOL	NOVOBIOCIN	LINCOMYCIN
Prostate	Low	Negligible	++++	++	++++	++	-	+++
Synovial Fluid	Low	++	Low	++	++	+++	++	+++
Peritoneal Fluid	Low	+++	Low	+++	++	+++	++	++++
Pleural Fluid	Low	+++	Low	+++	+++	+++	++	++++
Bile	++	+++	++	++++	++	Low	++	+++
Urine	+++	+++	++		Low	++	Negligible	+
Brain	Negligible	Negligible	Negligible	Some Compounds	+	+++	Negligible	Negligible
Eye (aqueous)	Negligible	+++	Low	Some Compounds	Negligible	++	Negligible	Negligible
Lung	++	++	+++	+++	+++	+++	Low	+++
Kidneys	+++	+	+++	+++	+++	+++	++	+++
Liver	+++	++	+++	++	+++	+++	+++	+++
Skin	+++	++	+++	+++	++	+++	++	+++
Intestine	Low	++	+++	+++	Low	++	-	+
Milk	Low	+++	+++	Low	Low	+	-	++
Bone	Low	-	+++		-	-	++	+++
Muscle	++	++	++	+++	+++	++	-	++
Fetus	Low	++	+++	+++	+	+	-	
Intracellular	No	No	Yes	Yes	No	Yes	-	Yes
Elimination								
Renal	+++	+++	+++	+++	Low	Low	Low	+++
Biliary	Low	Low	++	++	++++	++	++	++
Biotransformation	+	No	+	+	-	+++	-	-

*Concentrations of antimicrobial drugs found in various tissues and the principal route of elimination are indicated in relative terms. Negligible = nil; ++++ = concentrations higher than those found in other tissues or principal route of elimination. From Davis, L. E.: Syllabus on Clinical Pharmacology and Therapeutics. Colorado State University, Fort Collins, 1976.

Table 7. *Frequent Causes of Failure of Antimicrobial Therapy**

1. Pharmacologic factors
    Drug interactions
    Inactivation due to incompatibilities
2. Presence of nondraining, deep-seated abscess
3. Obstruction to natural drainage of an infected area
4. Presence of a foreign body
    Soft tissues
    Bronchus
    Cystic calculi
5. Emergence of drug resistance
6. Antagonism from simultaneously administered antibiotics
7. Protection of a penicillin-susceptible pathogen on mucosal surfaces by a penicillinase-producing member of the normal host flora
8. Elimination of competing normal bacterial flora
9. Diseases impairing normal host defenses
10. Incorrect diagnoses
    Underlying noninfectious disease
    Drug reactions may mimic signs of infectious disease
11. Presence of nontreatable diseases
    Viral, neoplastic, immune-mediated
12. Incorrect dosage or route of administration

---

*Adapted from Davis, L.E.: Rational Therapy with Newer Antibacterial Drugs. Proc. 45th Ann. Meet. Amer. Animal Hospital Assoc., 1978, p. 72.

listed in Table 7. These various possibilities should be considered and investigated in patients with documented infections that are not responding to properly chosen drug therapy.

PHARMACOLOGIC HAZARDS OF ANTIMICROBIAL THERAPY

Three principal mechanisms of toxicity produced by antimicrobial drugs are (1) dose-related toxicity, which can generally be predicted and which is related to overdosage or impaired pathways of drug elimination, (2) idiosyncratic or allergic reactions, which are not dose-related and cannot often be predicted, and (3) drug interactions, which can be anticipated and prevented.

Dose-related toxicity will vary depending on the chemical class of drug involved, and it will be manifested by organ toxicity. Neurotoxic antibiotics include the aminoglycosides, which will selectively damage either the vestibular or auditory nucleus of the eighth cranial nerve; the penicillins, which will cause convulsions if directly applied to nervous tissue; and drugs such as nitrofurantoin, which will elicit vomition by stimulating the chemoreceptor trigger zone in the medulla. Nephrotoxic drugs can (1) decrease the glomerular filtration rate (GFR) and damage renal tubules (aminoglycosides, polymyxins, ampho-

tericin B, cephaloridine), (2) cause lower nephron nephrosis secondary to crystalluria (sulfonamides), or (3) produce renal tubular acidosis (amphotericin B or outdated tetracycline preparations). Hepatotoxic drugs include isoniazid, oxacillin, and erythromycin estolate. Tetracyclines can produce fulminant fatty metamorphosis of the liver in bitches late in pregnancy. This is a rapidly fatal condition that is not observed in dogs or non-pregnant bitches. Hematologic disorders include dose-related neutropenia with chloramphenicol, thrombocytopenia produced by isoniazid or chloramphenicol, and hemolytic anemia associated with nitrofurantoin and sulfonamides.

Chloramphenicol can suppress antibody production and may interfere with the development of active immunity. Until this situation is clarified, it would be wise not to immunize dogs or cats during a period of treatment with chloramphenicol.

Some antibiotics can be enterocolotoxic, and these include the broad spectrum antibiotics lincomycin, clindamycin, and ampicillin. These effects are mediated, in part, by their alteration of the flora of the gut. The pathogenesis of hemorrhagic diarrhea associated with ampicillin has not been clarified. It has been demonstrated in experiments with hamsters that lincomycin produces pseudomembranous colitis by suppression of normal competing flora, which permits overgrowth by a fastidious, exotoxin-producing *Clostridium*. It is this exotoxin that induces the characteristic lesions. Lincomycin should not be used in rabbits, horses, or, perhaps, hamsters. Pulmonary infiltrates may occur in animals treated with nitrofurantoin.

Tetracyclines administered during pregnancy or the neonatal period may cause enamel hypoplasia of the developing teeth and interfere with long bone growth. This group of antibiotics exerts an antianabolic effect by inhibiting protein synthesis. By virtue of this action, they can exacerbate uremia in patients with impaired renal function, and when employed in combination with high doses of corticosteroids, they can produce rapid development of severe cachexia.

Allergic reactions to antimicrobial drugs can manifest themselves in a variety of ways including anaphylaxis, urticaria, angioneurotic edema, serum sickness, purpura, eosinophilia, drug fever, and positive Coomb's tests. This type of drug reaction sometimes can be very misleading to the clinician. Production of fever by the drug might be interpreted as a worsening of the infectious process being treated. Observation of eosinophilia or a positive Coomb's test might cause the physician to question his original diagnosis of a bacterial infection, which was correct, and lead him to suspect a parasitic or primary immune-mediated disease. The key diagnostic features of an allergic drug reaction are (1) it is not dose-related, (2) the clinical signs abate upon withdrawal of the drug, and (3) some allergic manifestation will occur upon challenge with the same or similar drug. In a patient with no prior history of allergy, allergic reactions will be entirely unpredictable. The author is aware of healthy animals that were given antibiotics prophylactically and that died of anaphylactic reactions. In case of an acute allergic reaction such as anaphylaxis, urticaria, laryngeal edema, or angioneurotic edema, one should *immediately administer epinephrine* intravenously or intramuscularly. Corticosteroids or antihistaminics are not effective in this situation. Administration of an antihistaminic is of value after the reaction has been controlled with epinephrine, in order to prevent a relapse.

A variety of drug-drug interactions can occur between various antibiotics and other drugs. A complete discussion of drug interactions is beyond the scope of this chapter. (For detailed information and reference, the reader is referred to Martin's book listed in the references.) Some of the more common interactions with which the veterinarian should be familiar will be discussed here.

Chloramphenicol and the tetracyclines inhibit microsomal enzymes in the liver that metabolize a variety of drugs. If a second, pharmacologically active drug were administered to a patient receiving one of these drugs, the pharmacokinetics of the second drug would be modified, thus leading to accumulation or prolongation of its effect. Sleeping time with barbiturates is increased with the result that recovery from anesthesia will be prolonged. I have seen four cases of acute digitalis toxicity in dogs being digitalized while receiving chloramphenicol.

Interactions can occur that will influence renal excretion of antimicrobial drugs. Probenicid and thiazide diuretics can compete with the penicillins for active transport by the proximal tubules and prolong the elimination rate of the penicillins. Drugs with a high affinity for binding with albumin (e.g., phenylbutazone) can displace highly protein-bound antimicrobial drugs, such as sulfadimethoxine, which are excreted by glomerular filtration. This will cause more rapid excretion of the antimicrobial drug with resultant lower plasma concentrations. Displacement of drugs from protein will increase the concentration of unbound drug in the plasma, which is free to diffuse into tissues. Furosemide is normally about 98 percent bound to serum albumin and is potentially ototoxic. If this drug were displaced by an aminoglycoside, the two drugs may have additive effects and cause hearing loss.

A serious and not uncommon interaction occurs between anesthetic agents and some other drugs with the aminoglycoside antibiotics to block the myoneural junction and inhibit the release of acetylcholine from motor nerve endings. This curariform effect results in paralysis of skeletal muscle with apnea. It is most commonly observed with administration of neomycin or polymyxin in animals during surgery. The use of aminoglycosides in patients receiving anesthetic agents, muscle relaxants, quinidine, promethazine, or sodium citrate (blood transfusions) should be avoided. Should paralysis occur under these circumstances, the cause should be recognized as a drug interaction because it is reversible, and prompt action can be lifesaving. Paralysis may be corrected by administration of calcium gluconate solution or neostigmine.

Another common interaction can occur in the gastrointestinal tract to impair the absorption of certain antibiotics. The administration of anticholinergic drugs (such as atropine) will delay gastric emptying and increase the destruction of orally administered penicillins. Antacids, dairy products, and iron salts will impair absorption of tetracyclines. Antidiarrheal preparations containing kaolin, pectin, or bismuth will decrease the absorption of lincomycin and erythromycin from the gut. Slow absorption due to interactions of antimicrobial drugs with other drugs or foods will result in inadequate blood concentrations, slow onset of action, and sustained release with possible prolonged undesirable effects. Some suggestions for minimizing the chance of an interaction are:

1. Whenever possible, avoid multiple drug therapy
2. Avoid combination products
3. With oral dosage forms, adjust the regimen relative to feeding times; e.g., tetracyclines are better given between meals
4. Avoid simultaneous use of drugs that might be antagonistic; e.g., tetracyclines and penicillins
5. Try to minimize the personal formulary to a point at which you are thoroughly familiar with each drug
6. When in doubt, consult a pharmacist.

SOME NEWER ANTIMICROBIAL DRUGS

There have been few really new entities since the last edition of this book. The newest major concept to appear in recent years is that of potentiated sulfonamides such as sulfadiazine-trimethoprim, sulfadimethoxine-ormetoprim, and sulfonamide-pyrimethamine combinations. Newer penicillins — cephalosporins, aminoglycosides, sulfonamides, and tetracyclines — should be mentioned, although experience with them in small animal practice has been limited.

PENICILLINS

The penicillins can be classified conveniently into (1) the various salts and esters of penicillin G that are susceptible to degradation by penicillinase and are acid-labile; (2) the penicillinase-resistant semi-synthetic penicillins; (3) the acid-stable oral penicillins, and (4) the extended spectrum semi-synthetic penicillins. For treatment of infections caused by susceptible organisms, penicillin G remains the drug of choice because it has the greatest antimicrobial activity of all. One should have a definite objective in mind when using other members of the group such as in treatment of penicillin-resistant staphylococcal infections, in oral therapy, or in treatment of susceptible gram-negative infections. If an animal has a history of being allergic to penicillin G, all penicillins should be avoided, and alternative drugs such as erythromycin or cephalosporins should be considered. A common error is the selection of an extended spectrum. penicillin such as ampicillin for the treatment of staphylococcal infections. These drugs (ampicillin, amoxicillin, carbenicillin) are susceptible to destruction by penicillinase.

The only indication for the penicillinase-resistant penicillins is treatment of resistant staphylococcal infections such as pyoderma. Drugs available include methicillin, oxacillin, cloxacillin, dicloxacillin, flucloxacillin, and nafcillin. The cloxacillins are available in oral dosage forms only, methicillin must be given parenterally, and oxacillin and nafcillin are available for injection or oral use.

Amoxicillin is similar to ampicillin in its spectrum of activity and pharmacokinetic characteristics. It has a major advantage in that the bioavailability following oral administration is twice that of ampicillin. Like other penicillins, amoxicillin has a low order of toxicity in animals that are not allergic. Amoxicillin is available as an oral tablet, an oral suspension, and a suspension for injection.

Carbenicillin is available as the disodium salt for parenteral use and as carbenicillin indanyl for oral administration. The only indication for its use is treatment of infections caused by gentamicin-resistant *Proteus* or *Pseudomonas*. There is rapid development of resistance when carbenicillin is used alone, and the drugs are quite expensive. Carbenicillin is destroyed by penicillinase and the drug is acid-labile.

CEPHALOSPORINS

The cephalosporins are classified according to their relative susceptibility to beta lactamases. Those resistant to gram-negative beta lactamases include cefoxitin, cefamandole, cefatrizine, and cephanone. Drugs resistant to staphylococcal beta lactamase are cephalothin, cephalexin, cefazolin, cephapirin, cephaloridine, and cephadrine. As a group, the cephalosporins are active against streptococcus spp., staphylococci, *Clostridia, Salmonella, Proteus mirabilis, Shigella,* 75 percent of strains of *E. coli,* 60 percent of *Paracolon,* 50 percent of *Hemophilus,* and most strains of *Klebsiella.* They are not active against other species of *Proteus, Pseudomonas, Aerobacter, Pasteurella,* or *Bacteroides,* or enterococci.

Allergic reactions have been the principle adverse reaction to drugs of this group. Cephaloridine is nephrotoxic and should be replaced in our armamentarium by cephalothin or cefazolin for parenteral use. Cefazolin has the advantage over cephalothin of a longer half-life (1.8 hours compared with 0.5 hours) and is less painful when injected intramuscularly. Both are cleared by the kidney and are useful for urinary tract infections. Outpatient therapy can be continued by prescribing cephalexin or cephadrine capsules or oral suspension.

AMINOGLYCOSIDES

The individual aminoglycosides share the common pharmacologic characteristics of the group (Table 3). Two new members of this group have become available in recent years, tobramycin and amikacin. The pharmacology of tobramycin is similar to that of gentamicin, but it is more active against *Pseudomonas aeruginosa.* Amikacin is a new semi-synthetic derivative of kanamycin. It is active against a number of gram-negative organisms that have become resistant to other aminoglycoside antibiotics. For this reason, the value of amikacin must be preserved by not subjecting it to indiscriminate use. Both tobramycin and amikacin are very expensive drugs.

TETRACYCLINES

The newer tetracyclines such as demeclocycline, doxycycline, and minocycline differ from the older drugs of the group by being more extensively protein bound in the plasma. This results in longer half-lives and a longer interval between doses. They are no more effective than the older tetracyclines but are considerably more expensive. Doxycycline is not excreted into the urine to any extent and may offer an advantage in the management of susceptible infections in patients with impaired renal function. Demeclocycline may cause photosensitive reactions in the skin and has the unusual property of inducing nephrogenic diabetes insipidus. Apparently, this latter effect is the result of interference with the action of antidiuretic hormone on the collecting ducts of the kidney.

SULFONAMIDES

The sulfonamides are probably the most underrated drugs in our armamentarium. They are capable of a wide spectrum of activity, are relatively inexpensive, and have comparatively low toxicity. The mechanism of action is the inhibition of the conversion of para-aminobenzoic acid to dihydrofolate in the synthesis of folate coenzymes by susceptible bacteria. Because of this common mechanism of action, there is almost perfect cross-resistance observed in members of this group because once a strain of organism develops alternative metabolic pathways for the synthesis of dihydrofolate, none of the sulfonamides will be effective.

Newer drugs that are available include silver sulfadiazine (Silvadene®), sulfasalazine (Azulfidine®), mafenide (Sulfamylon®), and the potentiated sulfonamide combinations. Silver sulfadiazine is a topical preparation in a water-miscible cream base that is bactericidal against many gram-negative and gram-positive bacteria and some yeasts. It has been employed primarily for the treatment of infections associated with thermal burns. Mafenide is a topical sulfonamide available in a cream base. It inhibits growth of a wide spectrum of gram-positive and gram-negative organisms. It may be irritating and can cause pain when applied to inflamed cutaneous surfaces. Sulfasalazine is sulfapyridine connected through an azo linkage to salicylic acid. After oral administration, about one-third is absorbed from the small intestine and the remainder passes to the colon, where the azo bond is reduced by bacterial enzymes. Sulfapyridine and 5-amino salicylic acid are released within the colon. This drug may be of value in the treatment of colitis in dogs. It is not clear whether the beneficial effect in human patients is due to the antimicrobial action of the sulfonamide or the anti-inflammatory action of the salicylate. Adverse reactions that have occurred in people include allergic reactions, agranulocytosis, thrombocytopenia, Heinz body anemia, nephrosis, hepatitis, pancreatitis, and CNS reactions. The most common disturbances were anorexia, nausea, and vomiting. Sulfasalazine is available as 500 mg scored tablets and 500 mg enteric coated tablets. Its use has not been established in veterinary medical practice.

Potentiated sulfonamides include sulfadiazine-trimethoprim (Tribrissen®), sulfadimethoxine-ormetoprim (RO-0037), and sulfonamide-pyrimethamine combinations. These drugs were originally developed as antimalarials. As discussed, sulfonamides inhibit the conversion of PABA to dihydrofolate, whereas the pyrimidines inhibit dihydrofolate reductase, which is the next step in the synthesis of folinic acid. By inhibiting two sequential steps in the synthesis of tetrahydrofolate, the combination drug has a greatly decreased frequency of inducing development of resistant strains of organism and the action becomes bactericidal. The basis for the selective toxicity of the trimethoprim or pyrimethamine for bacterial or protozoal cells resides in differences in binding among the dihydrofolate reductases from mammalian, protozoal, and bacterial organisms. It requires 60,000 times the concentration of trimethoprim to inhibit the mammalian enzyme as compared with bacterial reductase, and 4500 times as much as compared to protozoal enzyme. The case with pyrimethamine is different, as the protozoal enzyme is 3600 times as sensitive as the bacterial enzyme. Consequently, pyrimethamine cannot be used as an antibacterial agent.

The diaminopyrimidines should always be used in combination with sulfonamides because of the unique potentiating effect. Resistance can develop rapidly in organisms exposed to the pyrimidines alone. It has been established that the optimal ratio of sulfonamide to trimethoprim is 20:1 for maximal potentiation. The dosage forms of the combination product contain the active drugs in appropriate ratio to achieve this optimum ratio in the patient.

The spectrum of activity includes *Proteus*, *Pasteurella*, *E. coli*, *Salmonella*, *Klebsiella*, *Actinobacillus*, enterococci, *Bordatella* (50 percent of strains), Streptococci, Staphylococci, and *Nocardia*. The drug is widely distributed in the body, and trimethoprim actually will concentrate in the prostate gland. Currently, these drugs are available in oral dosage forms only. An injectable dosage form is available for investigational use.

The drug is dosed on the basis of the sulfonamide at 30 mg/kg every 12 hours for most infections. We have successfully treated two cases of nocardiosis with the potentiated sulfonamides: one a case of disseminated pleural and mediastinal nocardiosis in a dog and the other nocardial pneumonitis in a horse. The drug was employed at three times the usual dose for periods of 30 days. Folinic acid supplementation was required in the dog to prevent suppression of erythropoiesis. In cases of prolonged therapy, it is advisable to perform periodic hematologic studies. Pyrimethamine in combination with a sulfonamide is probably the treatment of choice for toxoplasmosis.

The potentiated sulfonamides have a high therapeutic index and adverse reactions have not been reported aside from dose-related anemia. Any of the adverse reactions associated with sulfonamides might be expected to occur as the drug receives wider usage.

SUPPLEMENTAL READING

Baggot, J. D.: *Principles of Drug Disposition in Domestic Animals*. Philadelphia, W. B. Saunders Co., 1977.

Braude, A. I.: *Antimicrobial Drug Therapy*. Vol. III in Smith, L. H., (ed.): Major Problems in Internal Medicine. Philadelphia, W. B. Saunders Co., 1976.

Garrod, L. P., and O'Grady, F.: *Antibiotic and Chemotherapy*. Edinburgh, E. & S. Livingstone, 1971.

Kagan, B. M.: *Antimicrobial Therapy*. Philadelphia, W. B. Saunders Co., 1970.

Martin, E. W.: *Hazards of Medication*. Philadelphia, J. B. Lippincott Co., 1971.

Melmon, K. L., and Morrelli, H. F.: *Clinical Pharmacology: Basic Principles in Therapeutics*, 2nd ed. New York, Macmillan, 1978.

Pratt, W. B.: *Chemotherapy of Infection*. New York, Oxford University Press, 1977.

Proceedings of the International Veterinary Symposium on Amoxicillin. Spec. Suppl., Vet. Med. Small Anim. Clin. 72:677–804, 1977.

Proceedings of a Symposium on Trimethoprim / Sulfadiazine. Research Triangle Park, N. C., Burroughs Wellcome Co., 1978. (Available upon request to the Company.)

Roberts, A. W., and Visconti, J. A.: The rational and irrational use of systemic antimicrobial drugs. Am. J. Hosp. Pharm. 29:1054, 1972.

Spinelli, J. S., and Enos, L. R.: *Drugs in Veterinary Practice*. St. Louis, C. V. Mosby Co., 1978. (Particularly recommended for veterinary technicians.)

Youmans, C. P., Paterson, P. Y., and Sommers, H. M.: The Biologic and Clinical Basis of Infectious Diseases. Philadelphia, W. B. Saunders Co., 1975.

DIAGNOSTIC CYTOLOGY IN VETERINARY PRACTICE: CURRENT STATUS AND INTERPRETIVE PRINCIPLES

A.H. REBAR, D.V.M.
Lafayette, Indiana

Proper therapy depends upon proper diagnosis; any diagnostic technique or group of techniques that aids the clinician in reaching a proper diagnosis is therefore appropriately discussed in a book such as *Current Veterinary Therapy*. Over the years, a number of new diagnostic aids have emerged and have been reviewed in previous editions of this text. One group of diagnostic procedures that has not yet been collectively reviewed is diagnostic cytology.

Diagnostic cytology may be defined as the study or evaluation of cells that are sloughed into body cavities, lost from body surfaces, or obtained from solid tissues or organs by fine needle aspiration or impression smear techniques. Diagnostic veterinary cytology is a relatively new discipline; nevertheless, tremendous strides have been made in the area. It is the purpose of this article to summarize these advancements by outlining the principles of cytologic evaluation and discussing the use of cytology in veterinary practice.

GENERAL PRINCIPLES OF CYTOLOGIC EVALUATION

The primary goal of the cytologist is to define a cytologic response as a normal cell population, a hyperplastic or benign neoplastic population, a malignant neoplastic population, or an inflammatory cell population (Fig. 1). If the reaction is inflammatory, an attempt is made to classify the reaction as to type (for example, acute versus chronic) and to identify etiologic agents. In order for such evaluations to be made, cytologic specimens must be of high quality. The following paragraphs detail collection and staining techniques that generally provide cytologic specimens of the quality required. The criteria used to differentiate the various cytologic responses are also described.

SPECIMEN COLLECTION AND PREPARATION

Probably the most useful collection technique for the practicing veterinarian is fine nee-

dle aspiration. Fine needle aspiration can be done on an awake animal in the examining room, and it involves minimal time and expense. The technique is of value in obtaining high quality cytologic specimens from oral and cutaneous lesions and masses, enlarged lymph nodes, and palpable internal masses.

Fine needle aspiration is best performed with a 20- or 23-gauge needle and a 12-cc syringe. The lesion to be aspirated is cleansed and prepared as for surgery. The needle is then introduced into the lesion and negative pressure is applied via the syringe. To assure that a representative sample is obtained from the lesion, the needle should be redirected into the lesion several times as negative pressure is continuously applied. It should be emphasized that in many instances, *no* material will be aspirated into the syringe. Nevertheless, adequate tissue fluid and cells will have been aspirated into the needle to allow cytologic interpretation.

After aspiration is complete, negative pressure is released from the syringe and the needle is withdrawn from the mass. If negative pressure is not released before withdrawal, material will be aspirated from the needle into the syringe and it will be difficult to force the aspirated material onto slides.

The needle is then separated from the syringe and the syringe is filled with air. The needle is

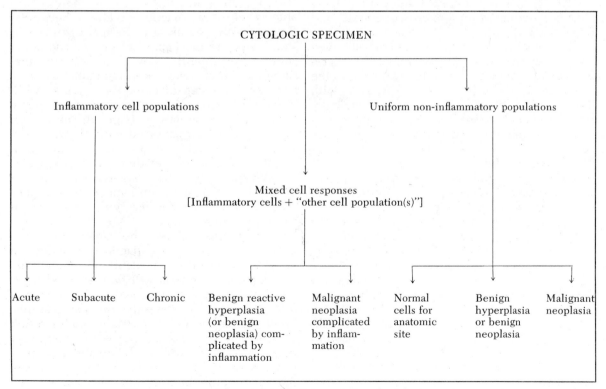

Figure 1. General approach to the interpretation of cytologic specimens.

reattached and its contents are forcefully expressed onto one or more microscope slides. Several "squash preps" are prepared by placing a second slide at right angles across the aspirated material. When the aspirated fluid has spread between the two slides, they are gently drawn apart, creating two useable slides. Fine needle aspiration technique and preparation of squash prep slides are well illustrated elsewhere (Rebar, 1978).

Cytologic specimens from animals presenting with hydrothorax and ascites may be collected by thoracentesis and abdominal paracentesis respectively. Thoracentesis and abdominal paracentesis are really nothing more than fine needle aspiration biopsy of the pleural and peritoneal cavities. In the dog, an 18-gauge 1 to 1½-inch needle and a 12 to 50-cc syringe are employed. A three-way valve is often helpful.

Thoracentesis is most commonly done in the sixth or seventh intercostal space on the right side with the animal in a standing position. The site should be prepared as for surgery. While general anesthesia is not necessary, local anesthesia is recommended in order to reduce the likelihood of sudden movement when the needle penetrates the thoracic wall. Fluid should be collected aseptically. A portion is saved for culture and a portion is transferred to an EDTA tube for physical and cytologic evaluation. Cytologic specimens are prepared by centrifuging the EDTA sample to obtain a sediment, placing a drop of sediment on a microscope slide, and preparing a smear.

Abdominal paracentesis is also best achieved with the animal in a standing position. The preferred site is approximately 1 cm anterior to the umbilicus to the right of the midline. As with thoracentesis, the aspiration site is surgically prepped. Local anesthesia is generally not necessary for abdominal paracentesis. Fluids are collected and processed in the same manner as is thoracentesis fluid.

In both abdominal paracentesis and thoracentesis, positioning of the needle is important in obtaining satisfactory fluid samples. The beveled edge of the needle should always be directed outward (away from the body cavity). If the beveled (luminal) side of the needle is directed into the body cavity, it may be easily occluded by mesenteric fat in the abdominal cavity or pulmonary tissue in the thoracic cavity. Such occlusions can prevent fluid from being aspirated. As with fine needle aspiration technique, thoracentesis and abdominal paracentesis have been illustrated elsewhere (Osborne et. al, 1973; Rebar, 1978; Schall, 1974; Scott et. al, 1974).

Fine needle aspiration, thoracentesis, and ab-dominal paracentesis are by far the most commonly used cytologic sampling techniques. Procedures for cerebrospinal fluid collection, synovial fluid collection, transtracheal aspiration, impression smear preparation, and prostatic massage have all been detailed elsewhere and will not be dealt with here (Coles, 1971; Coles, 1974; Rebar, 1978).

After cytologic slides have been prepared, they must be stained before they are examined. Considerable controversy has developed concerning the proper staining techniques to be employed. A number of individuals have suggested that New Methylene Blue or Romanowsky stains (Wright's stain, quick stains such as Harleco's Diff Quik, etc.) are quite satisfactory for diagnostic veterinary cytology (Duncan and Prasse, 1977; Perman, 1966; Perman, 1971; Perman and Cornelius, 1971; Prasse and Duncan, 1976; Rebar, 1978; Stevens et al, 1974), whereas others have advocated the use of Papanicolaou-type stains (Sano's trichrome or the Rapid Trichrome) in all instances (Roszel, 1967; Roszel, 1970; Roszel, 1975).

In the author's experience, both stains have a definite role in veterinary cytology. In general, however, the author prefers the Romanowsky stains for most purposes for a number of reasons. Since air-dried specimens may be adequately stained by Romanowsky techniques, and since many reliable quick stains are available, the Romanowsky stains are more adaptable to veterinary practice situations. Secondly, Romanowsky stains are better cytoplasmic stains than are the Papanicolaou and trichrome stains. Consequently, they afford better evaluation of cytologic changes in inflammatory reactions than do Papanicolaou-type stains. Additionally, microorganisms and metachromatic cytoplasmic granulation (e.g., in mast cell tumors) are both visualized with Romanowsky stains. Finally, Romanowsky stains are traditionally used for the evaluation of peripheral blood smears; therefore, most veterinary practitioners have the stains on hand in their clinics and are somewhat familiar with cytomorphology under these stains.

The principal value of the Papanicolaou and trichrome stains is in the diagnosis of malignant neoplasia. Papanicolaou stains are principally nuclear stains, and (as will be discussed later) the criteria that define malignant neoplasia refer primarily to abnormal nuclear features. Since Romanowsky stains stain nuclei rather coarsely, these abnormal nuclear features may be more readily visible with Papanicolaou-type stains. Nevertheless, in most instances, the author has found the Romanowsky stains to be perfectly adequate for the diagnosis of malignant neoplasia and has therefore relied upon Papanicolaou stains primarily as a backup (and very useful) special stain.

Several features of the Papanicolaou stains make them difficult to use in veterinary practive. Firstly, all specimens must be immediately wet-fixed either in alcohol or with a spray fixative as soon as they are collected. Secondly, the staining procedures are considerably more complex than are those for the Romanowsky stains. Roszel (1975) published a modified rapid trichrome method that can be adapted to practice situations. Individuals interested in pursuing the use of Papanicolaou-type stains in diagnostic veterinary cytology should consult the several excellent review articles available (Roszel, 1967; Roszel, 1975). The interpretive discussions that follow here refer exclusively to specimens stained with Wright's stain or other Romanowsky stains.

SPECIMEN INTERPRETATION

As mentioned previously, the principal use of cytology is in the differentiation of inflammatory, neoplastic, and hyperplastic cellular reactions (see Fig. 1). Such differentiation can usually be accomplished by applying the basic interpretive principles outlined in the following paragraphs.

CYTOLOGY OF INFLAMMATION

Inflammatory reactions are cytologic responses in which inflammatory cells — neutrophils, eosinophils, lymphocytes, monocytes, or macrophages — are the predominant cells seen. Inflammatory reactions may be further classified as acute, subacute (chronic active), chronic, or granulomatous (Table 1).

In acute inflammation, neutrophils account for 70 percent or more of all inflammatory cells. The remaining cells usually include varying numbers of lymphocytes, eosinophils, and macrophages. Acute inflammation may be either non-degenerative or degenerative. In non-degenerative reactions, the neutrophils are unaltered (resembling those in the peripheral blood) or exhibit only the aging change of nuclear hypersegmentation (Fig. 2). In contrast, in degenerative reactions, both neutrophil nuclei and cytoplasm are abnormal. Nuclear changes are those of cellular death — pyknosis, karyorrhexis, and karyolysis (Fig. 3). Cytoplasmic changes include basophilia and vacuolation.

Acute degenerative inflammation reflects the action of toxins on infiltrating neutrophils; it is almost invariably associated with bacterial infections. Consequently, whenever degenerate neutrophils are seen in a cytologic specimen, a bacterial etiologic agent should also be sought. In contrast, acute non-degenerative inflamma-

Table 1. *Cytologic Classification of Inflammation*

INFLAMMATORY CLASSES	CELL POPULATIONS	MORPHOLOGIC SUBTYPES	POSSIBLE ETIOLOGIES
Acute	>70% neutrophils	Non-degenerate — neutrophils resemble those of peripheral blood or feature hyper-segmented nuclei	Severe irritant
		Degenerate — neutrophils exhibit karyolysis, pyknosis, and karyorrhexis; cytoplasmic basophilia and vacuolation	Pyogenic bacteria
		Eosinophilic — large numbers of eosinophils	Parasites
Subacute (Chronic active)	50–70% neutrophils, 30–50% monocytes and macrophages		Resolving acute response
			Irritant of intermediate severity
Chronic	>50% macrophages	Granulomatous — epithelioid cells and/or giant cells	Resolving acute response
			Low grade irritant: foreign body systemic mycosis

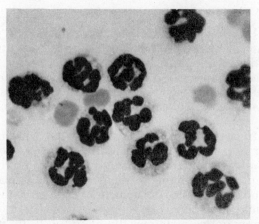

Figure 2. Acute non-degenerative inflammation. Hypersegmented neutrophils are the predominant cells seen.

tion is usually associated with severe irritation of a non-infectious nature. It should be emphasized that this separation of acute degenerative from acute non-degenerative inflammation is a generalization and therefore somewhat artificial; for example, nocardiosis is characterized by acute degenerative inflammation in areas immediately adjacent to bacterial colonies and an acute non-degenerative response in areas in which no bacteria are seen.

Separating inflammatory responses into degenerative and non-degenerative classifications may also be of prognostic value. This can be best illustrated by considering the cytologic responses encountered in peritoneal fluids associated with intestinal vascular accidents such as volvulus or intussusception. In these conditions, the principal lesion is infarction of the intestinal wall. Early in the course of the dis-

ease process, there is severe irritation of the intestinal wall and an acute irritative peritonitis results. Cytologically, this is reflected as acute non-degenerative inflammation. As the process continues, however, the lesion becomes more severe and life-threatening. Stasis of gut contents generally occurs in the infarcted segment. This is often accompanied by bacterial proliferation and toxin production. Additionally, if infarction of the intestinal wall is complete, necrosis of the wall occurs and bacterial toxins and bacteria are leaked into the peritoneal cavity, causing acute septic peritonitis. Cytologically, the response is one of acute degenerative inflammation. In the author's experience, the prognosis for surgical correction at this point is considerably more guarded than for the same disease process when only non-degenerative neutrophils are observed.

Chronic active inflammatory responses are defined as those responses in which 50 to 70 percent of the inflammatory cells are neutrophils and the bulk of the remaining inflammatory cells are monocytes and macrophages (Fig. 4). Such reactions reflect less severe irritation than do acute inflammatory responses. They may represent a stage in the resolution of a more acute lesion or simply a tissue response to a less irritating etiologic agent than pyogenic bacteria. Systemic mycotic agents such as *Histoplasma capsulatum* or *Blastomyces dermatitidis* commonly elicit chronic active inflammatory responses. Since chronic active inflammatory responses virtually always reflect less severe irritation than do acute responses, they are only rarely degenerative. (It is important to recognize that the degenerative nature of an inflammatory reaction is evaluated strictly on the basis of *neutrophil* morphology; monocyte and macrophage morphology are *not* considered.)

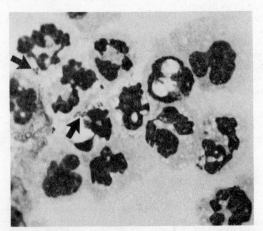

Figure 3. Acute degenerative inflammation. Nuclei are swollen and more palely stained than in Figure 2 and are undergoing acute degeneration. The cytoplasm of many neutrophils is vacuolated. Bacterial rods (*arrows*) are seen in a number of vacuolated neutrophils.

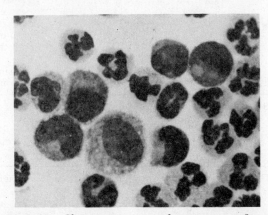

Figure 4. Chronic active non-degenerative inflammation. Monocytes are present in equal numbers with nondegenerate neutrophils.

Chronic inflammatory responses are those in which over 50 percent of the inflammatory cells are monocytes and macrophages. These responses imply low-grade irritation and again are commonly seen with systemic mycotic agents or non-infectious foreign bodies. They may also represent the resolution phase of a previously more active reaction.

Granulomatous inflammation represents a specific category of chronic inflammation that is occasionally recognized cytologically. Inflammatory giant cells and epithelioid cells (see Fig. 11) are the hallmark of granulomatous inflammation. When granulomatous inflammation is observed, an etiologic agent such as the systemic mycotic agents or a foreign body almost certainly can be identified.

Eosinophilic exudates (inflammatory responses containing large numbers of eosinophils) merit specific consideration. Eosinophils are occasionally seen in large numbers in fine needle aspirates from focal inflammatory skin lesions in cats, including feline rodent ulcers (eosinophilic granulomas). Aspirates of lick granulomas in dogs may also contain significant numbers of eosinophils. Since mast cell neoplasms may also contain large numbers of eosinophils, care must be taken to distinguish these two conditions in the dog. In horses, fine needle aspirates of cutaneous parasitic lesions (cutaneous habronemiasis or onchocercosis) often contain significant numbers of eosinophils. Microfilariae are occasionally seen in aspirates of onchocercosis.

The author has also seen several eosinophilic exudates involving the pleural or peritoneal cavities in horses and dogs. In dogs, these exudates have been associated with heartworm disease or disseminated mast cell neoplasia. In horses exhibiting acute colic secondary to verminous arteritis, eosinophilic peritoneal exudates are commonly encountered. In general, eosinophilic exudates are most prevalent in parasitic infestations or allergic phenomena.

CYTOLOGY OF MALIGNANT NEOPLASIA

Neoplastic processes may be either benign or malignant. It is virtually impossible to differentiate between benign neoplasia and hyperplasia cytologically, and these benign processes will therefore be discussed together in a later section. Malignant neoplastic processes are identified through the recognition of specific malignant criteria exhibited by the cell population under consideration, which may be loosely classified into four categories: (1) general criteria, (2) nuclear criteria, (3) cytoplasmic criteria, and (4) structural criteria (Papanicolaou, 1954; Roszel, 1967; Roszel, 1975; Duncan and Prasse, 1977) (Table 2).

General criteria of malignancy refer to the appearance of the cell population as a whole. Malignant neoplastic processes are generally characterized as a *uniform* population of *pleomorphic* cells; that is, cells usually appear to be of a single cell type (for example, all mast cells or all spindle-shaped connective tissue cells) that exhibits variable cell size and variable nuclear size. These features can generally be recognized at low magnification and represent the first suggestion that the cytologic diagnosis is

Table 2. *Cytologic Criteria of Malignancy*

MALIGNANT CRITERIA	CYTOLOGIC FEATURES
General	Uniform population of pleomorphic cells — can be assessed at low magnification
Nuclear	Abnormal mitoses Variable nuclear size Variable nuclear/cytoplasmic ratios Multiple nucleoli Large irregularly shaped nucleoli Coarse chromatin patterns Irregular prominence of nuclear margin
Cytoplasmic	Basophilia Vacuolation
Structural	Carcinoma — round to oval cells arranged in sheets of acinar patterns Sarcoma — spindle shaped cells Discrete cell tumor — individual round or oval cells

one of malignant neoplasia. Although such pleomorphism in a uniform population of cells is easy to recognize in uncomplicated cases, the presence of large numbers of inflammatory cells may mask neoplasia. Therefore, whenever an inflammatory response is associated with a population of non-inflammatory cells, the non-inflammatory cells should be carefully scrutinized for evidence of malignancy. Inflammatory cells are commonly encountered in large numbers in cytologic preparations from oral or skin neoplasms with ulcerated surfaces.

Nuclear criteria of malignancy are the most important criteria employed in identifying a malignant neoplasm cytologically. Evaluation of nuclei for malignancy is best performed under oil immersion. Features suggesting malignancy (in Romanowsky stained preparations) include multiple nucleoli, large irregularly shaped nucleoli, coarse chromatin patterns (areas within the nucleus that stain intensely, as well as other areas that are virtually unstained or only poorly stained), irregularities and indentations in the nuclear membrane, and variable nuclear/cytoplasmic ratios among the cells seen. Mitotic figures per se are not a criterion of malignancy, as they may be seen in hyperplastic cell populations (e.g., lymph node hyperplasia); however, abnormal mitoses (e.g., three or more planes of division) are a feature of malignancy. Multinucleated tumor cells are occasionally seen, but giant cells may also occur in inflammatory reactions (granulomatous inflammation). The author suggests that three or four such nuclear alterations be identified before the diagnosis of malignancy is suggested.

Cytoplasmic criteria of malignancy are considerably less important in establishing a diagnosis of malignant neoplasia, but they do provide supportive evidence. These include cytoplasmic basophilia, cytoplasmic vacuolation, and variation in amounts of cytoplasm. Cytoplasmic features of malignancy suggest the primitive nature of the neoplastic population; for example, cytoplasmic basophilia results from a high cytoplasmic content of RNA, a constant feature of young proliferating cells.

After the nuclear and cytoplasmic criteria of malignancy have been used to establish the cytologic diagnosis of malignant neoplasia, the structural features of the neoplastic cells may be evaluated in an attempt to classify the tumor as a carcinoma, sarcoma, or discrete cell neoplasm. Carcinomas are neoplasms of epithelial cell origin. Normal epithelial cells are generally adherent to one another, and this property is generally reflected in cytologic preparations from epithelial cell neoplasms. Carcinoma cells are generally round to oval, and they are arranged

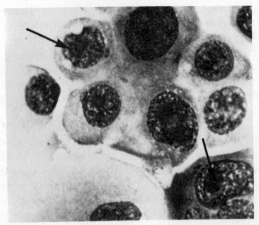

Figure 5. Cytology of carcinoma. A cluster of carcinoma cells is seen. Malignant features include variable cell size, variable nuclear-cytoplasmic ratios, coarse nuclear chromatin, and prominent large nucleoli (*arrows*).

in sheets and clusters (Fig. 5). Cells from neoplasms of glandular epithelium (adenocarcinomas) are often arranged in acinar patterns around a central lumen. Adenocarcinoma cells also often contain large vacuoles containing secretory products.

Sarcomas are neoplasms of cells of connective tissue origin. Connective tissue cells generally are embedded in a matrix that they themselves secrete. Consequently, aspirates or imprints from sarcomatous masses are generally less cellular than cytologic preparations made from epithelial or discrete cell neoplasms. Structurally, connective tissue cells are usually spindle shaped or flame shaped (cells with tails), and this morphology is also typical of sarcomatous cells (Fig. 6).

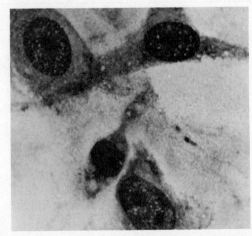

Figure 6. Cytology of sarcoma. Several malignant spindle-shaped cells (cells with cytoplasmic tails) are seen. Malignant features include variable cell size, variable nuclear-cytoplasmic ratios, coarse nuclear chromatin patterns, and prominent nucleoli.

The sarcomas of veterinary significance include osteosarcoma, fibrosarcoma, liposarcoma, hemangiosarcoma, melanosarcoma, and chondrosarcoma. Osteosarcoma and chondrosarcoma cells are more commonly flame shaped than spindle shaped. In addition, aspirates from these two neoplasms may contain considerable matrix material — eosinophilic osteoid in the case of osteosarcoma and metachromatic (purple) chondroid in the case of chondrosarcoma. The cytoplasmic margin of osteosarcoma cells is often irregular and vacuolated. Melanosarcoma has several distinguishing cytologic features. Of principal importance is the presence of brown to black cytoplasmic granules (melanin) of variable size and shape. In addition, melanosarcomas are often composed of cells of two shapes: spindle and round to oval (epithelioid). Fibrosarcoma, hemangiosarcoma, and liposarcoma may be indistinguishable cytologically. All are composed of basically spindle-shaped cells. Aspirates from hemangiosarcoma usually contain considerably more blood than the other sarcomatous masses. Liposarcoma cells may contain large lipid-filled vacuoles that may be demonstrated with lipid stains such as oil red O or the Sudan stains. Illustrations of the various sarcoma cells can be found elsewhere (Duncan and Prasse, 1977; Rebar, 1978).

The discrete cell neoplasms constitute a rather large group of tumors of veterinary importance. Included among these are malignant lymphomas, mast cell tumors, histiocytomas, and transmissible venereal tumors. Structurally, discrete cell neoplasms are seen cytologically as neoplasms made of individual round or oval cells with no adherence between cells and no ordered arrangement of cells (such as cluster formation) (Fig. 7). Distinguishing features of the individual discrete cell neoplasms have been illustrated and described elsewhere (Rebar, 1978).

CYTOLOGY OF REACTIVE HYPERPLASIA AND BENIGN NEOPLASIA

Inflammatory cytologic responses may be easily differentiated from neoplastic cytologic responses *as long as the reactions are uncomplicated*. Unfortunately, however, this is not always the case, and the cytologist is often faced with the problem of distinguishing reactive hyperplasia secondary to inflammation from malignant neoplasia. While there are no foolproof rules that may be applied to accomplish this separation, the practitioner is aided by understanding clearly those situations in which reactive hyperplasia is likely to occur and by recognizing morphologic similarities and differences between hyperplastic and malignant cells.

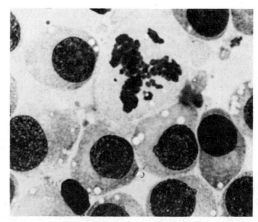

Figure 7. Cytology of discrete cell neoplasia (canine transmissible venereal tumor). The aspirate consists of individual round or oval cells without intercellular adhesions. An abnormal mitotic figure (three planes of division) is seen.

Reactive hyperplasia can occur whenever there is irritation or injury of normal tissue. For example, irregular cutaneous wounds heal by the process of scab formation, epithelial cell hyperplasia, and granulation tissue and scar formation in the dermis. Granulation tissue formation is actually hyperplasia of fibroblasts and vascular tissue. Similarly, oral or cutaneous ulceration secondary to localized bacterial infection and acute inflammation is accompanied by reactive hyperplasia of both superficial epithelial cells and underlying dermal connective tissue. Cytologic specimens collected from such lesions may therefore be expected to contain a population of hyperplastic epithelial cells or hyperplastic fibroblasts or both.

Fluid specimens collected from body cavities, synovial joints, or the respiratory tract may also be expected to contain hyperplastic cells whenever there is continuous irritation or injury to the cells lining the spaces from which the fluid is being collected. For example, in congestive heart failure, the simple presence of ascitic fluid in the peritoneal cavity causes continuous irritation to the mesothelial cells lining the peritoneal space. As a result, these mesothelial cells proliferate, and clusters of them are sloughed into the peritoneal fluid. Reactive (hyperplastic) mesothelial cells therefore constitute the principal nucleated cellular constituent seen in ascites of congestive heart failure. As might be expected, any inflammatory condition involving the body cavities also causes irritation to the mesothelial lining cells, and a distinct population of reactive mesothelial cells is expected in cytologic specimens.

Synovial lining cells react in a similar fashion to continued irritation. Smears of synovial fluid from joints involved with chronic suppurative arthritis often contain a significant population of large irregular mononuclear cells with abundant basophilic cytoplasm. While it is likely that a portion of these cells are derived from blood monocytes, it is equally probable that many represent reactive (hyperplastic) synovial lining cells that have sloughed into the joint space. In chronic degenerative joint disease, hydroarthrosis, and chronic rheumatoid arthritis, proliferation of synovial lining cells is expected. This proliferation is of course reflected by increased numbers of lining cells in synovial fluid specimens.

Transtracheal washes from animals suffering from chronic respiratory disease often contain numerous features of reactivity and hyperplasia. Irritated ciliated columnar respiratory epithelial cells that readily lose their cilia and nonciliated columnar cells may be seen. Additionally, irritated respiratory lining cells undergo both squamous metaplasia (transformation) and reactive hyperplasia; sheets of round to oval epithelial cells with central nuclei and abundant cytoplasm are consequently seen.

Having defined the general conditions under which reactive hyperplasia is likely to occur, it is now essential to consider the morphologic features that characterize hyperplastic cells. It should be apparent from the preceding paragraphs that reactive hyperplastic cells are a young, active, and proliferative cell population; their cytologic appearance reflects both their youth and their functional activity. Consequently, hyperplastic cells generally feature large vesicular (palely or delicately stained) nuclei usually with plainly visible single or multiple nucleoli. Multiple nucleoli indicate active RNA synthesis. Cytoplasm is generally more basophilic than in mature cells, reflecting a high cytoplasmic RNA content. Nuclear/cytoplasmic ratio is usually high in hyperplastic cells and normal mitotic figures may be seen.

A glance at Table 3 will remind the reader that all the features just ascribed to hyperplastic reactive cells may also be seen in malignant cell populations. The cytologic differentiation between benign hyperplasia (or neoplasia) and malignant neoplasia is therefore a matter of degree. In hyperplastic reactions, four clear criteria of malignancy cannot be identified. For example, although multiple nucleoli are seen in nuclei of hyperplastic cells, they are regularly (round) rather than irregularly (triangular or trapezoidal) shaped, as in malignant cells. Similarly, although mitoses are seen in hyperplasia, they are always normal. Hyperplastic cells feature a high nuclear/cytoplasmic ratio, but they generally exhibit a relatively uniform nuclear/cytoplasmic ratio among all the cells of the hyperplastic population. This is in direct contrast to the high degree of variability in nuclear/cytoplasmic ratio seen among the cells of a blatantly malignant population.

Obviously, differentiating hyperplasia from neoplasia is a difficult procedure, and great caution should be exercised in questionable cases. Wherever possible, cytologic diagnoses should be confirmed by histopathology.

APPLICATION OF INTERPRETIVE PRINCIPLES: EVALUATION OF LYMPH NODE ASPIRATES

As mentioned previously, the interpretive principles can be applied to the cytologic evaluation of cutaneous and oral lesions, pleural and peritoneal effusions, cerebrospinal fluid, synovial fluid, transtracheal wash fluid, and even various internal organ systems. It is beyond the scope of this discussion to consider specific features of cytologic interpretation in each of these cases. For this purpose, the reader is referred to a number of other more specific references

---

Table 3.   *A Cytologic Comparison of Hyperplasia and Neoplasia*

FEATURES OF BOTH HYPERPLASTIC AND NEOPLASTIC CELLS
1. Multiple nucleoli
2. Increased mitoses
3. Cytoplasmic basophilia

DIFFERENTIAL FEATURES OF HYPERPLASIA AND NEOPLASIA

Hyperplasia	*Neoplasia*
1. All mitoses normal	1. Abnormal mitoses may be seen
2. Constant nuclear/cytoplasmic ratios for cells of same age	2. Variable nuclear/cytoplasmic ratios
3. Multiple nucleoli generally regular in shape	3. Nucleoli often bizarre and irregular in shape

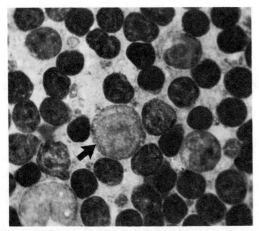

Figure 8. Normal lymph node cytology. Small lymphocytes predominate. A large pale-staining lymphoblast (*arrow*) is also seen.

(Duncan and Prasse, 1977; Perman, 1966; Perman, 1971; Perman and Cornelius, 1971; Prasse and Duncan, 1976; Rebar, 1978; Roszel, 1967; Roszel, 1970; Roszel, 1975). Nevertheless, it is appropriate to underscore and exemplify the general principles of interpretive cytology by considering in detail the diagnostic cytology of at least one specific system. For this reason, the remainder of this paper will consider the cytologic evaluation of fine needle aspiration lymph node biopsy.

Before considering pathologic cytology of lymph nodes, it is necessary to define normal lymph node cytology (Fig. 8). Aspirates from normal lymph nodes contain mixed cell populations in which small lymphocytes are the predominant cell (> 80 per cent of all cells). Small lymphocytes are round cells approximately 8 to 10 μ in diameter that contain round, densely stained nuclei with a scant rim of pale basophilic cytoplasm. Nucleoli are rarely visible. Prolymphocytes constitute the second most prevalent cell type in normal nodes. Prolymphocytes (10 to 15 μ in diameter) are larger than small lymphocytes and contain larger, more vesicular nuclei and more abundant basophilic cytoplasm. As with small lymphocytes, nucleoli are not seen. Lymphoblasts are even less prevalent than prolymphocytes, constituting 1 per cent or less of all cells seen. Lymphoblasts are large cells (up to 30 μ in diameter) with large pale vesicular nuclei in which single to multiple nucleoli are visualized. Cytoplasm is relatively scant and basophilic.

It should be emphasized that not all aspirated lymphoid cells can be classified. The aspiration technique is somewhat traumatic and a number of cells are ruptured. These ruptured cells are seen as naked nuclei, the origin of which cannot be determined. Consequently, only intact cells with clearly recognized cytoplasmic boundaries should be evaluated.

In addition to lymphocytic cells, other cell types may be seen in lymph node aspirates in small numbers. Plasma cells, mast cells, and macrophages may all be seen in low numbers. Macrophages are often very active, containing cytoplasmic vacuoles filled with cellular debris or brown-black hemosiderin (iron) granules. Rare neutrophils may also be seen.

Hyperplastic lymph node aspirates are similar morphologically to aspirates from normal nodes in that all the aforementioned populations are seen. However, there is a shift in the relative numbers of the different cell types. Small lymphocytes continue to predominate, but in general, the cell populations are "left-shifted"; increased numbers of prolymphocytes and lymphoblasts are present. In addition, mitotic figures, which are rarely encountered in normal lymph node aspirates, are observed with some frequency.

Simple lymph node hyperplasia is rarely seen. A much more commonly observed phenomenon is reactive lymph node hyperplasia. Reactive hyperplasia implies antigenic stimulation of the involved node. Cytologically reactive hyperplasia exhibits all the features of simple hyperplasia. However, the striking feature is the presence of large numbers of plasma cells and plasmacytoid prolymphocytes and lymphoblasts; that is, precursors that are obviously differentiating into plasma cells (Fig. 9). In some instances, plasma cells containing numerous vacuoles (presumably filled with immunoglobulin) are observed. These cells are known as Mott cells; cells containing immunoglobulin

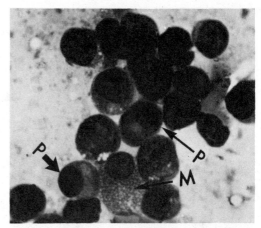

Figure 9. Reactive lymph node hyperplasia. Several mature plasma cells (*P*) as well as plasmacytoid lymphocytes are seen. A Mott cell (*M*) distended with Russell bodies is seen at bottom.

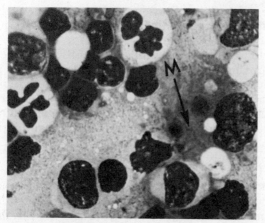

Figure 10. Subacute lymphadenitis. Neutrophils and macrophages (*M*) are admixed with small lymphocytes. The cytoplasm of the macrophage contains much-phagocytized cytoplasmic debris.

crystals may also be observed. In the author's experience, reactive hyperplasia has been most commonly seen in superficial lymph nodes that drain chronic inflammatory dermal lesions. For example, reactive hyperplasia of superficial lymph nodes is a common accompaniment of canine demodicosis and flea bite dermatitis.

Inflammatory lesions of lymph nodes (lymphadenitis) may be classified as acute, subacute, chronic, or granulomatous on the basis of the predominant inflammatory cell type infiltrating the node. Acute lymphadenitis aspirates contain large numbers of neutrophils and suggest severe irritation. Bacterial agents should always be suspected and in some cases may even be seen. Subacute lymphadenitis exhibits increased numbers of both neutrophils and macrophages and is usually associated with less

severe irritation than is acute inflammation (or a more prolonged time course). Subacute lymphadenitis is usually accompanied by reactive hyperplasia of lymphoid elements (Fig. 10). Chronic lymphadenitis is characterized by a marked increase in nodal macrophage numbers. Granulomatous lymphadenitis is a special form of chronic inflammatory response characterized by the presence of either inflammatory giant cells or epithelioid cells or both (Fig. 11). In both chronic and granulomatous lymphadenitis, the inciting irritation is low grade and etiologic agents such as systemic mycotic agents or foreign bodies should be sought (see Fig. 11).

Neoplastic processes in lymph nodes may be either primary or metastatic. In primary neoplastic disease (malignant lymphoma), the striking cytologic feature is the presence of a remarkably uniform population of round cells, which may be classified as either bizarre lymphoblasts or prolymphocytes (Fig. 12). This uniformity of cell type contrasts sharply with the heterogeneous cell populations seen in normal nodes and non-neoplastic reactions. Examination of lymphomatous aspirates at high magnification reveals many of the nuclear and cytoplasmic criteria of malignancy described previously; those seen most frequently include variable cell size, variable nuclear size, variable nuclear/cytoplasmic ratio, large prominent nucleoli, and prominent cytoplasmic basophilia and vacuolation (see Fig. 12).

Metastatic neoplastic disease is characterized cytologically by the presence of an aberrant cell population in lymph node aspirates; metastatic foci may consist of spindle-shaped cells (sarcoma), clusters or sheets of round or oval cells (carcinoma), or individual round or oval cells (discrete cell tumors such as mastocytoma) (Fig.

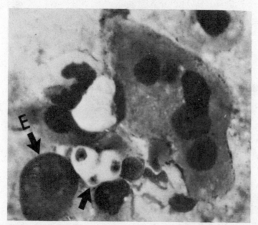

Figure 11. Granulomatous lymphadenitis. This reaction was seen in response to the systemic mycotic agent *Cryptococcus neoformans* (*arrow*). A giant cell is seen at right. A large epithelioid cell (*E*) is also present.

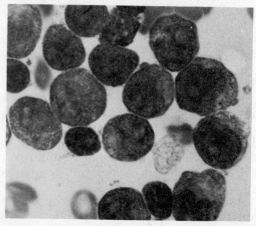

Figure 12. Malignant lymphoma. Aspiration from involved nodes revealed a uniform population of variably sized lymphoblastic cells with irregular nuclear boundaries and very prominent nucleoli.

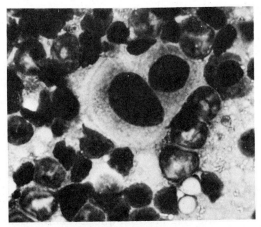

Figure 13. Metastatic lymph node neoplasia. This aspirate was taken from a node of the dog suffering from the carcinoma illustrated in Figure 5. Two malignant epithelial cells are surrounded by normal lymphoid elements.

13). As in primary neoplastic disease, several criteria of malignancy should be identified in the aberrant cell population. Reactive and hyperplastic changes may also be identified in the lymphoid elements aspirated from the more normal portions of the node.

SUMMARY

The preceding paragraphs have outlined the basic interpretive principles that are used to evaluate cytologic specimens and the application of these principles to the interpretation of cytologic specimens in a specific organ system. It is hoped that this discussion has pointed out the value of diagnostic cytology to the veterinary practitioner and the relative ease with which cytology can be used in clinical veterinary medicine. In many cases, cytologic evaluation provides definitive diagnostic information; in other cases, cytologic findings may be merely suggestive. Whenever cytologic findings are equivocal, excision biopsy and histopathology should be relied upon for confirmation.

SUPPLEMENTAL READING

Coles, E.H.: Cerebrospinal fluid. In Kaneko, J.J., and Cornelius, C.E. (eds.): *Clinical Biochemistry of Domestic Animals*, Vol. II. New York, Academic Press, 1971.

Coles, C.H.: *Veterinary Clinical Pathology*, 2nd ed. Philadelphia, W.B. Saunders Co., 1974.

Duncan, J.R., and Prasse, K.W.: *Veterinary Laboratory Medicine*. Ames, Iowa State University Press, 1977.

Osborne, C.A., Perman, V., and Low, D.G.: Clinical and laboratory evaluation of abnormal body fluid accumulations. I, Techniques of paracentesis. Proc. Amer. Animal Hosp. Assoc. 1973.

Papanicolaou, G.N.: *Atlas of Exfoliative Cytology*. Cambridge, Harvard University Press, 1954.

Perman, V.: Diagnostic cytology in canine medicine. 16th Gaines Symposium, 6–14, 1966.

Perman, V.: Transudates and exudates. In Kaneko, J.J., and Cornelius, C.E. (eds.): *Clinical Biochemistry of Domestic Animals*, Vol. II. New York, Academic Press, 1971.

Perman, V., and Cornelius, C.E.: Synovial fluid. In Kaneko, J.J., and Cornelius, E.C. (eds.): *Clinical Biochemistry of Domestic Animals*, Vol. II. New York, Academic Press, 1971.

Prasse, K.W., and Duncan, J.R.: Laboratory diagnosis of pleural and peritoneal effusions. Vet. Clin. North Am. 6:625–636, 1976.

Prasse, K.W., and Duncan, J.R.: Cytologic examination of the skin and subcutis. Vet. Clin. North Am. 6:637–646, 1976.

Rebar, A.H.: *Handbook of Veterinary Cytology*. St. Louis, Ralston Purina Co., 1978.

Roszel, J.F.: Exfoliative cytology in diagnosis of malignant canine neoplasms. Vet. Scope 12:14–20, 1967.

Roszel, J.F.: Genital cytology of the bitch. Vet. Scope 19:3–13, 1975.

Roszel, J.F.: Membrane filtration of canine and feline cerebrospinal fluid for cytologic evaluation. JAVMA 160:720–724, 1970.

Schall, W.D.: Thoracentesis. Vet. Clin. North Am. 4:2 395–401, 1974.

Scott, R.C., Wilkins, R.J., and Greene, R.W.: Abdominal paracentesis and cystocentesis. Vet. Clin. North Am. 4:2 413–417, 1974.

Stevens, J.B., Perman, V., and Osborne, C.A.: Biopsy sample management, staining, and examination. Vet. Clin. North Am. 4:2 233–253, 1974.

FEVERS OF UNKNOWN ORIGIN IN DOGS AND CATS

ANNE M. CHIAPELLA, D.V.M.
Philadelphia, Pennsylvania

Fever of unknown origin (FUO) implies a continuous or intermittent elevated temperature of 39.7° C (103° F) or greater that is associated with an illness of two to three weeks duration or longer. Fever is a common presenting sign of disease in animals and is usually due to transient bacterial or viral infection. Most fevers resolve spontaneously or with minimal therapy, but when FUO occurs, it may be one of the most challenging diagnostic problems in veterinary medicine.

TEMPERATURE REGULATING MECHANISMS

Normal temperature regulation involves a dynamic balance between heat loss from skin and lungs and heat production by skeletal muscle and the liver. Control of body temperature is centered in the thermoregulatory center of the rostral hypothalamus (pre-optic area). This area acts like a thermostat with a "set point" temperature. Changes in body temperature are compared with the set point, and the autonomic nervous system or motor outflow tracts to muscle are then activated to preserve, generate, or dissipate heat.

Fever is due to a rise in the set point temperature with subsequent activation of systems to create heat; the body's temperature then increases to the new set point.

Endogenous pyrogen (EP) is the mediator of fever. EP is a protein produced and released from phagocytic cells such as polymorphonuclear leukocytes, monocytes, and tissue macrophages. The known stimuli of EP release from these cells include viruses, gram-positive bacteria, endotoxins, fungi, yeast, and antigen-antibody complexes. Lymphocytes involved in hypersensitivity reaction secrete lymphokines that provoke the production of EP by monocytes.

CLASSIFICATIONS OF FUO IN THE DOG

The causes of FUO differ between dogs and cats (Tables 1 and 2). The reader is referred to other chapters concerning specific diseases for more complete discussions on presentation, diagnosis, and treatment. The major causes of FUO in the dog are immune-mediated disease (collagen vascular disease), systemic and localized infections, and neoplastic disease.

Immune-mediated diseases frequently present with muscle wasting, shifting leg lameness, joint effusions, limb edema, and FUO. Systemic lupus erythematosus (SLE) is a multisystemic disease, commonly presenting as polyarthritis

Table 1. Causes of FUO in the Dog

IMMUNE MEDIATED DISEASE
(COLLAGEN VASCULAR DISEASE)
Systemic lupus erythematosus, especially polyarthritis
Rheumatoid arthritis

INFECTION
Systemic
Subacute bacterial endocarditis
Systemic fungal infections and *Actinomyces* spp.
Rickettsial disease: *Ehrlichia*, salmon poisoning agents, *Rickettsia rickettsi*
Others: Toxoplasmosis, brucellosis, protozoa (*Babesia*), mycobacterium, leptospirosis
Localized
Urogenital: pyelonephritis, prostatic abscess
Pulmonary: lung abscess, pyothorax, pneumonia
Hepatic: abscess or cholangitis
Other visceral abscess: pancreatic or localized peritonitis

NEOPLASIA
Lymphosarcoma, especially with hepatic involvement
Leukemia, myeloma, and other myeloproliferative diseases
Intracranial tumors (hypothalamic)
Others, especially hepatic neoplasia

OTHERS
Granulomatous bowel disease
Skeletal disease: idiopathic polyarthritis, hypertrophic osteodystrophy, osteomyelitis
Hepatic disease with necrosis or endotoxemia
Drug fever: tetracycline
Nodular panniculitis
Pulmonary emboli
Hyperthyroidism
Pyogranuloma (organs or masses)

UNDIAGNOSED

Table 2. *Causes of FUO in Cats*

INFECTIONS
Systemic
    FeLV-related disease
    Feline infectious peritonitis
    Toxoplasmosis
    Systemic fungal disease
Localized
    Similar to the dog
    Cat bite abscesses

IMMUNE MEDIATED DISEASE (COLLAGEN VASCULAR
    DISEASE)
    Systemic lupus erythematosus (rare)
    Polyarthritis

NEOPLASIA (USUALLY FeLV-RELATED)
    Lymphosarcoma
    Myeloproliferative disease

OTHERS
    Pansteatitis
    Drug fever: tetracyclines
    Hyperthyroidism

UNDIAGNOSED

with fever. Less frequently, autoimmune hemolytic anemia and idiopathic thrombocytopenic purpura are seen. Other manifestations of this disease are erosive skin lesions (discoid lupus), neurologic abnormalities, and polymyositis.

Systemic and localized infection may be the cause of FUO. Because of related therapeutic implications — e.g., the need for antibiotics — infections must be a primary consideration. The major systemic infections causing FUO in the dog are bacterial endocarditis and fungal diseases (including actinomyces spp.). Animals with endocarditis may present with a shifting leg lameness and joint effusion, a clinical picture very similar to that of an immune-mediated polyarthritis. Particular attention must be given to recent surgical or medical diseases, as the source of the infection is frequently an organ involved in a recent disease process.

Systemic fungal diseases often have a persistent or intermittent fever associated with chronic wasting disease. Osteomyelitis and chronic coughing or other respiratory signs are commonly seen; however, any organ may be involved. Rickettsial diseases, especially ehrlichiosis, are associated with fever and hematologic abnormalities. Neutropenia, thrombocytopenia, and, later, anemia are seen with ehrlichiosis infections.

Localized infections associated with FUO are common in the pulmonary and urogenital systems. Persistent fevers may be seen in pneumonia and pyothorax. Pneumonias associated with fever include those resistant to antibiotics, such as toxoplasma and fungal pneumonia. Dogs with distemper are frequently immunosuppressed and develop bacterial pneumonias with persistent fevers.

Fever may be a cardinal sign of neoplastic disease, especially lymphosarcoma. Primary hepatic lymphosarcoma has been the cause of FUO in the author's experience, but it can be difficult to diagnose because of marginal hepatomegaly and minor changes in liver enzyme values. A liver biopsy is needed to make the diagnosis. An atypical lymphosarcoma has presented as a severe diffuse interstitial lung · disease associated with dyspnea and fever. Hemopoietic neoplasia that affects the bone marrow may cause pancytopenia or neutropenia, which facilitates secondary infection. Fever associated with neoplastic diseases often results from secondary infections or extensive necrosis in the tumor itself.

Many miscellaneous diseases can cause FUO. Inflammatory bowel disease with abdominal pain but few gastrointestinal signs has presented with persistent fever. Skeletal diseases such as hypertrophic osteodystrophy and polyarthritis are commonly associated with fever and lameness. Drug fevers have been reported in dogs receiving tetracyclines. Antibiotics, anticonvulsants, and antiarrhythmic drugs have caused fevers and lupuslike syndromes in humans. As yet, these syndromes have not been reported in the dog and cat. Many hepatic diseases may be associated with fever. Active hepatic necrosis and intermittent endotoxemia are thought to cause fever in liver diseases. Some dogs with FUO will remain undiagnosed, and the fever may resolve spontaneously.

DIAGNOSIS OF FUO IN THE DOG

Diagnosis of FUO in the dog depends upon the presenting signs, case history, and physical examination. The clinician must recognize that many diagnoses are made because new signs of disease develop; therefore, serial examinations of the patient are imperative. Careful histories and physical examinations should be performed with consideration of prior trauma, surgery, or medical disorders. Detailed examinations of the cardiovascular system, pulmonary system, musculoskeletal system, and abdomen are particularly important. Daily examinations are performed with emphasis on cardiac auscultation (murmurs changing in intensity or timing in endocarditis). Later developments in endocarditis include signs of bacterial embolization: petechiation, splenomegaly, microscopic hematuria, and retinal hemorrhages. The clinician must determine from this information if a potentially life-threatening disease is present. This will dictate the urgency and nature of subsequent procedures.

Diagnostic tests such as hemograms, urinalyses, and pertinent biochemical assays are performed frequently. The diagnosis may become obvious when a previously negative laboratory test becomes positive. An electrocardiogram should be performed frequently, as arrhythmias due to secondary myocarditis may develop. Joint aspiration and cultures of the aspirate are performed routinely in cases of FUO; many diseases, particularly the immune-mediated diseases and bacterial endocarditis, are associated with polyarthritis and fever. Bone marrow aspiration is indicated if pancytopenia or neutropenia is evident in the hemogram. Neutrophils and monocytes should be carefully examined for *Ehrlichia canis*; titers for *E. canis* are indicated if pancytopenia, hyperglobulinemia, or epistaxis are seen. Tests for antinuclear antibody (ANA) and LE cell preparations are performed routinely and repeated periodically at intervals of two to four weeks, since they may become positive with time. Occasionally, a positive ANA has been seen in bacterial endocarditis; therefore, the presence of immune-mediated disease should be documented by biopsy and immunofluorescence of affected tissue (skin, kidney, muscle). Bacterial cultures should also be negative.

Thoracic radiographs are indicated in animals with respiratory signs or suspected fungal diseases. Transtracheal and transthoracic aspirations with culture should be performed if indicated. If pneumonia is seen, red cells should be examined for distemper inclusions. Abdominal radiographs help identify organs (liver, prostate, and kidneys) commonly involved in FUO cases. Animals with abdominal pain, persistent pyuria, or biochemical values indicative of liver disease warrant radiographic examination of the abdomen.

Bacterial and fungal cultures are important because infection is a common cause of pyrexia. Bacterial cultures should be made of urine and joint fluid. Fungal and bacterial cultures should be performed on bronchial secretions, pleural effusion, and skin lesions or exudates when applicable. Skin lesions associated with FUO should be biopsied and cultured to differentiate nodular panniculitis from cutaneous fungal involvement (*Nocardia asteroides*, *Sporothrix schenckii*). Biopsies will reveal areas of fat necrosis without granuloma formation in panniculitis. Since cultures of joint aspirates are frequently negative in suspected cases of bacterial endocarditis, cultures of the synovium may be indicated.

Blood cultures are indicated in FUO cases, especially if the fever is somewhat responsive to antibiotics. Many animals with fever receive antibiotics that are inhibitory to bacterial growth in culture; hence, these drugs should be discontinued for two to seven days before blood cultures are made. If the disease is life threatening, cultures may be made immediately. Bacteremia in intravascular infections is continuous but often of a low magnitude. Consequently, multiple cultures are necessary. Intermittent bacteremias precede fevers by several hours; cultures must be taken as the temperature is rising. A dilution of 1:10 to 1:20 blood to culture medium is desirable to decrease antibiotic residue and the normal bacteriostatic effects of plasma. Casein soy broth with a CO_2 vacuum and .025 percent sodium polyanetholesulfonate (50 ml)* is recommended for larger dogs. Supplemented peptone broth (20 ml)† is used for blood cultures in smaller animals. *Streptococcus, Proteus, E. coli, Pseudomonas, Bacteroides,* and *Staphylococcus aureus* are recognized pathogens when cultured from the blood. However, many organisms may become pathogenic in immunosuppressed hosts or when introduced by intravenous line contamination. Negative blood cultures are quite common in endocarditis because of prior antibiotic therapy, improper culture techniques, or improper culture media.

Biopsies with histologic examination and culture of involved tissues have been particularly helpful in the diagnosis of FUO. Special histologic stains may be necessary to document some organisms. Percutaneous liver biopsies are indicated when biochemical evaluations suggest hepatic disease. Exploratory laparotomy is indicated when the physical examination, biochemical evaluation, and radiographic studies suggest abdominal organ involvement. Multiple organ biopsies with culture of involved tissue is recommended when exploratory laparotomy is performed.

Careful observation of the animal for new signs is recommended if the animal is stable or improving, but more drastic, aggressive diagnostic procedures should be performed when the animal's condition is deteriorating. Therapeutic trials of antibiotics and steroids are often misleading and should be avoided without strong clinical justification.

---

*Casein soy broth (TSB): available from Gib Co., 3175 Staley Rd., Grand Island, Ill. 64072

†Peptone broth: available from Becton-Dickenson Co., Ralston, N.J. 07070

CLASSIFICATION OF FUO IN THE CAT

The most common causes of FUO in the cat are systemic viral infections. Fevers due to feline infectious peritonitis (FIP) and feline leukemia (FeLV)-related diseases are frequently unresponsive to antibiotics; they occur primarily in young cats, although all ages may be affected. Fungal diseases and toxoplasmosis may also cause fever in cats. The aforementioned diseases are all multi-systemic; therefore, clinical signs will vary depending on the organ involved. Other causes of FUO in cats include drug fever, polyarthritis, pansteatitis and non-resolving cat bite abscesses. Drug fevers in cats have been reported to occur with the tetracyclines. A polyarthritis syndrome, similar to rheumatoid arthritis in dogs, has been documented in cats, but its etiology remains unknown. Pansteatitis is a disease associated with low-grade persistent fever, pain on palpation of fat, lumpy fat, and regenerative leukocytosis. Cat bite abscesses that fail to resolve may cause fevers and are sometimes associated with positive FeLV tests or uncommon organisms.

DIAGNOSIS OF FUO IN THE CAT

Methods for diagnosis of FUO in cats are similar to those used in dogs. Emphasis is placed on history, physical examination, and total body radiography. Ocular examination is routinely performed, since many systemic diseases involve the eye. Prior exposure of a cat that develops FUO to cats with known FeLV-related disease or FIP may be historically important. The initial laboratory evaluation should include a hemogram, urinalysis, FeLV test, FIP titer, and serum protein electrophoresis. Results of the FeLV test and FIP antibody titer must be interpreted in light of the clinical findings. These viruses are ubiquitous in nature, and a positive test result does not necessarily indicate a viral etiology for the fever. Serial toxoplasma and FIP titers should be performed; rising titers may indicate an active infection. Pansteatitis is diagnosed by biopsy of affected fat; histology shows fat necrosis and ceroid deposition. A definitive diagnosis of fungal disease is usually made by identification of the organism in purulent material, by culture and isolation, or by biopsy of infected tissue with microscopic identification of organisms.

SUMMARY

The causes of fevers of unknown origin vary considerably between dogs and cats. Immune-mediated diseases, infections, and neoplasms are common in the dog. Viral-related diseases are common in the cat. Clues to the cause of FUO originate from the history and physical examination. The clinician must keep the owner aware of the difficulties in and the expense of the diagnosis of FUO. This, unfortunately, may be a limiting factor in many instances.

Non-invasive procedures (laboratory evaluations, cultures, radiography) and minor procedures (bone marrow and joint aspiration) are performed initially. A definitive diagnosis may be made because of the development of new signs or changes in laboratory and radiographic findings. More invasive procedures (percutaneous biopsy and exploratory laparotomy) are delayed unless the animal's condition is deteriorating.

SUPPLEMENTAL READING

Dinarello, C. A., and Wolff, S. M.: Pathogenesis of fever in man. N. Engl. J. Med. 298 (11):607–612, 1978.
Jacoby, G. E.: Fevers of undetermined origin. N. Engl. J. Med. 289:1407–1410, 1973.
Pederson, W. H., Weisner, K., and Castles, J. J.: Non-infectious canine arthritis: the inflammatory non-erosive arthritides. J. Am. Vet. Med. Assoc. 169:304–310, 1976.
Scott, D. W.: The systemic mycoses; Nocardiosis and actinomycosis. In Kirk, Robert W. (ed.): *Current Veterinary Therapy.* VI. Philadelphia, W. B. Saunders Co., 1977.
Vickery, D. M., and Quinnell, R. K.: Fever of unknown origin. JAMA 238:2188, 1977.
Washington, J. A.: Blood cultures. Mayo Clin. Proc. 50:91–97, 1975.

SHOCK: PATHOPHYSIOLOGY AND MANAGEMENT

RONALD J. KOLATA, D.V.M.,
Athens, Georgia

COLIN F. BURROWS, B. Vet. Med.,
and LAWRENCE R. SOMA, V.M.D.
Philadelphia, Pennsylvania

INTRODUCTION

Shock is a clinical state, the central feature of which is ineffective tissue blood flow and cellular hypoxia. The course and outcome of shock depend on a number of factors, including its etiology, the time from onset to recognition and treatment, and any underlying disease process. An animal in shock demonstrates progressive dysfunction of many organs at the macro-, micro-, and biochemical levels.

Many individual organs and metabolites have been studied in the hope that a specific organ or substance could be incriminated as the major contributor to the progressive nature of shock. In many instances, a "target organ" has been identified that, in a particular shock model, supposedly contributes more than any other to the eventual demise of the patient. While this may be true in the experimental model, it is seldom true in the clinical situation.

The use of a variety of experimental animals in attempts to define general concepts can be misleading. It might be concluded, for example, that a standardized form of hemorrhagic shock would have similar physiologic and pathologic manifestations in a diverse number of species. However, the effects of hemorrhagic hypotension can be very different in different species, and extrapolation of information from controlled experiments to clinical situations can lead to false assumptions.

One of the more difficult aspects of the clinical management of shock is the evaluation of therapy, especially when assessment is limited to clinically applicable methods. It is difficult to establish what phase of shock a patient is in when presented. This is different from the experimental model, in which the insult can be graded and procedures can be standardized. In most models, the refractory or irreversible phase of shock is defined by rather clear-cut physiologic or biochemical changes. In clinical situations in which insults may be multiple and the time from onset to presentation is variable, it takes a period of evaluation and therapy to establish the phase of shock.

As a prelude to discussion of therapy, some basic concepts of shock pathophysiology will be presented. These will enable the reader to approach shock therapy with an understanding of the underlying physiologic changes.

DEFINITION OF THE SYNDROME

The word *shock* has been used for at least a century to describe a condition that can be initiated by a number of insults (Table 1). Despite its many causes, the syndrome called shock can be described by a small number of commonly recognizable signs. This does not imply that all causes produce identical physiologic changes, but it does imply that when the changes are severe enough, homeostasis is disrupted to a degree that produces the cluster of signs recognized as shock. Shock is produced when (1) the circulating volume is reduced, as in hemorrhage or dehydration, (2) left ventricular work is decreasing, as in heart failure, and (3) blood flow is maldistributed, as in sepsis. Irrespective of the initiating insult, shock is a condition in which the overriding defect is inadequate tissue perfusion. Poor perfusion results in tissue ischemia with dis-

Table 1. Causes of Shock

Hemorrhage
Fluid loss
Trauma
Sepsis
Toxins
Adrenal insufficiency
Cardiac failure
Anaphylaxis

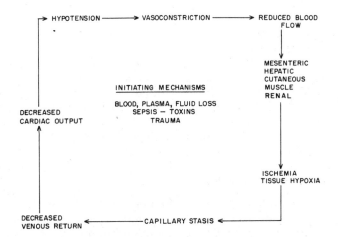

Figure 1. Schematic representation of overall cardiovascular changes associated with the shock state.

ruption of cellular functions. If a sufficient volume of tissue is underperfused for a sufficient period, generalized and in some instances irreversible changes take place in the animal. Shock can be defined then as a physical state arising from inadequate tissue perfusion.

DYNAMICS OF SHOCK

In shock produced by acute blood loss, by a slow fluid loss as in severe vomiting or diarrhea, or by a combination of vasomotor and fluid alterations as in sepsis, a common pathway of circulatory failure evolves (Fig. 1).

Reflex adjustment attempts to compensate for the descrepancy between the available circulating fluid volume and the available vascular space. There is an attempt to maintain cardiac output by a sympathetically mediated increase in heart rate and contractility and an increased arteriolar constriction within specific organs. In addition, blood reserves in the capacitance vessels, spleen, and liver are mobilized. These adjustments result in redistribution of blood volume and flow to those organs immediately essential to life — i.e., heart, brain, and adrenal glands. The arterial flow to the liver, a vital organ, is preserved, but its portal venous flow is drastically reduced. This redistribution is achieved by reduction in perfusion of organs not immediately essential to life — i.e., kidney, spleen, GI tract, muscles, and skin.

Initially, this generalized vasomotor response is beneficial, but it becomes deleterious if it is prolonged, as adverse changes take place at the microcirculatory and cellular levels in the underperfused organs. Adverse changes include loss of circulatory autoregulation, cessation of spontaneous vasomotion, and a progressive decline in cellular energy production (Fig. 2). These result in loss of plasma volume and in further decline in perfusion of the already underperfused tissues. Flow to vital organs is consequently decreased to a

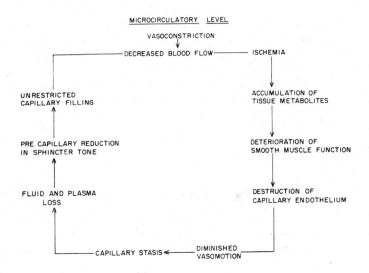

Figure 2. Schematic representation of alterations occurring at the microcirculatory level.

level at which their functions begin to deteriorate. At this level of generalized circulatory failure, the animal begins to enter a phase of shock defined in the experimental model as irreversible. This phase is progressive and ends with the death of the animal, as no known treatment can sustain its life. Although not seen as such, this phase surely exists in clinical shock but cannot be defined as it is in the experimental model.

METABOLISM IN SHOCK

Inadequate tissue perfusion results in decreased delivery of oxygen and energy substrates to the cell and decreased removal of the products of metabolism. Forced to function anaerobically, the glycolytic cycle produces less than optimal amounts of ATP and an excess of lactic acid. Deficiency of ATP impairs all energy-dependent cell functions. Probably the most important effect is on the transport of sodium and potassium, since movement of these ions is linked to maintenance of cell hydration, the electrochemical gradient, and the transport of energy substrates. Impaired sodium and potassium transport results in edema of the cell with disruption of organelles and decreased substrate transport. These lead to a further decline in energy production, and a self-energizing cycle of decreasing cell function is begun. The excess production of lactic acid causes intracellular acidosis and extracellular acidemia, which are compounded by the reduction in lactate removal caused by the poor tissue perfusion.

Intracellular acidosis is implicated in the disruption of lysosomes. The release of lysosomal proteases in turn generates vasoactive peptides such as bradykinin and toxic factors such as myocardial depressant factor (MDF). The vasoactive peptides cause local vascular changes that degrade the already inadequate tissue perfusion. MDF directly decreases cardiac contractility and further reduces cardiac output and thereby tissue perfusion.

In addition, cellular injury (especially of the GI epithelium) allows the escape of bacteria and the absorption of their toxins into the blood stream. All these adverse events interact in complementary ways and ultimately result in irreversible changes.

REGIONAL BLOOD FLOW

Changes in regional blood flow are an important consideration in the pathophysiology of shock, and much work has been done to determine the changes occurring in the various vascular beds. Among the most important are the cerebral, coronary, and splanchnic circulations.

CEREBRAL CIRCULATION

Measurements of cerebral blood flow in shock show a selective preservation of the cerebral circulation as compared with other organs until arterial pressure declines below 50 mm Hg. Despite compensating mechanisms to sustain cerebral flow, it is reduced at these pressures. In the experimental dog, a reduction of arterial pressure to a mean of between 45 and 50 mm Hg produces a transitory excitement followed by unconsciousness. Despite the reduced perfusion pressure, permanent ischemic brain damage occurs only when arterial pressure remains below this level for an extended period. After resuscitation, the dogs regain consciousness and show a normal degree of alertness.

Ischemic brain damage is produced if the arterial pressure is maintained at 30 to 35 mm Hg for more than two hours. Dogs exposed to this degree of hypotension will survive for at least 24 hours after resuscitation, but irreversible neuronal and microvascular injury has occurred. The importance of the direct effect of shock on the brain relative to survival is not clear. This is because of the difficulty in differentiating the effects of impaired CNS function from the effects of local ischemia on other organs.

CORONARY CIRCULATION AND MYOCARDIAL FUNCTION

Coronary circulation (like cerebral) is preferentially preserved in shock. Coronary flow is well maintained when the mean arterial pressure is above 70 mm Hg. But as pressure falls, so does coronary flow. Compensation for hypotension comes about by a dilation of the coronary bed and an elevation of coronary flow relative to cardiac output. In experimental hemorrhagic shock, there is little change in coronary flow following a 34 percent reduction in cardiac output. A 50 percent reduction in cardiac output results in a 40 percent decrease in coronary flow; a 70 percent reduction in cardiac output results in only a 50 percent decrease in coronary flow. However, despite the relative maintenance of coronary flow at this level of cardiac output, the ability to compensate for additional stress is minimal. Therefore, rapid movement of the animal, administration of depressant drugs, and induction of anesthesia can profoundly decrease coronary flow and result in acute myocardial hypoxia.

Many factors have been implicated in the progressive decline of cardiac function seen in shock. These include reduced coronary perfusion, reduced venous return, insufficient coronary perfusion pressure, reduced coronary oxygen tension, acidemia, blood-borne toxins, and combinations of these. One toxin, designated myocardial depressant factor (MDF), coming from the ischemic pancreas, has been shown to reduce cardiac contractility. It has been proved to be present in the later stages in all forms of shock and may play an important role in the irreversibility of shock.

Although depression of cardiac function is observed in shock, studies of ventricular function following volume replacement show that the heart is capable of responding to a volume load. Cardiac output and stroke work can be increased by massive infusion of fluid or blood over a short period, even in the irreversible stage of shock. Myocardial stores of ATP, creatine phosphate, and glucose are not depleted, indicating that energy synthesis and storage are not significantly altered during shock. Myocardial function is sustained for as long as venous return is adequate. Diminished venous return due to peripheral vascular fluid leakage seems to be the crucial factor in the final deterioration of cardiac function and tissue perfusion.

SPLANCHNIC CIRCULATION

Splanchnic blood volume represents about 20 percent of the dog's total blood volume and is a potential source of blood for redistribution. Splanchnic circulation is made up of the mesenteric or gastrointestinal, splenic, and hepatic circulations. Flow to all these organs is reduced during shock.

The hepatic arterial flow is maintained but the portal flow is drastically reduced. In mild hemorrhage, few changes in hepatic function are seen, but in severe hemorrhage, hepatic hypoxia and decreased function occur.

Mesenteric blood flow is greatly decreased during shock, to a greater degree than is cardiac output. When mesenteric blood flow reduction is severe and sustained, intestinal and pancreatic ischemia ensue. Pancreatic ischemia results in release of lysosomal proteases and MDF into the circulation. Intestinal ischemia results in damage to the intestinal epithelium and villi and in release of lysosomal proteases. If the experimental animal is sacrificed during the early phases of shock, prior to reinfusion of blood, the GI tract is found to be pale and reduced in volume. Microscopically, the submucosal structures are intact, but changes are noted in the mucosal architecture with sloughing of the tips of villi. The microvasculature is devoid of red blood cells (RBCs). However, after blood volume replacement, the GI tract becomes congested and blood and fluid are lost into the gut lumen. Microscopic changes include venous congestion, submucosal hemorrhage and edema and microthrombi in villous capillaries. This is the so called shock gut seen in irreversible canine shock (Fig. 3). It has been shown that this hemorrhagic enteritis can be eliminated if, prior to shock, the pancreas is removed, its duct is ligated, or a trypsin inhibitor (Trasylol®) is given into the lumen of the bowel. The clinical significance of these maneuvers is uncertain.

PULMONARY FUNCTION

Three overlapping categories of pulmonary involvement related to trauma and shock can be distinguished in the dog. Obviously in many clinical cases, the categorization may not be absolute, and there is inherent danger in attempting such distinction. However, categorization permits discussion of the disparate pathophysiologic mechanisms involved. The three categories of pulmonary involvement are (1) progressive pulmonary insufficiency, (2) non-penetrating blunt pulmonary trauma, and (3) pulmonary damage related to refractory or irreversible shock.

PROGRESSIVE PULMONARY INSUFFICIENCY (PPI)

The effect of cardiovascular shock on pulmonary function has been the subject of extensive clinical and experimental investigations in various species. A major area of consideration has been post-traumatic pulmonary failure or progressive pulmonary insufficiency, a condition first described during the late 1960's. Since then it has become a prominent syndrome, owing primarily to more effective initial shock therapy. Following severe trauma, hemorrhage, sepsis, burns, or major operations, more patients are surviving the initial insult, but a certain percentage progress to pulmonary insufficiency and may die of hypoxia. Cases have also been seen in veterinary medicine, owing to the marked improvement in shock therapy and intensive patient care.

Progressive pulmonary insufficiency is a consequence of severe shock and follows successful resuscitation. The time period may be

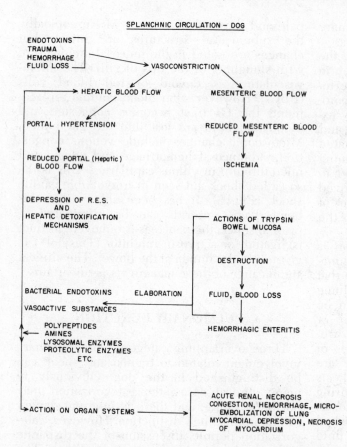

Figure 3. Schematic representation of the cycle of changes in the splanchnic circulation of the dog in the refractory or irreversible stage of shock, and their effect on other organ systems.

from a few hours to five days after injury. The cases observed in this clinic showed evidence of pulmonary failure within 48 hours. There is considerably more clinical experience in man, and the syndrome is characterized as having four somewhat separable phases.

Phase one is the injury and resuscitation period, which includes the low flow aspects of the shock state; transfusion of large volumes of fluid, blood, or plasma; and the reestablishment of circulatory homeostasis. It may also include surgery, anesthetic agents, depressants, and various other drugs (Table 2). Recovery from the initial insult may proceed uneventfully. A favorable response is maintenance of circulating homeostasis without fluid and drug support, reestablishment of near normal acidbase balance, and urinary output and maintenance of adequate arterial oxygen tension without oxygen therapy or support of ventilation.

Phase two is associated with continued cardiovascular stability, but with deterioration in the respiratory status. The initial indication of a respiratory problem is continuous hyperventilation and borderline arterial oxygen tensions. When 100 percent oxygen is administered, an increase in oxygen tension occurs but not to levels appropriate to the inspired

gas mixture. A respiratory alkalemia exists because of the continuous hyperventilation. This phase is difficult to detect if blood gas data are not obtained and the response to administration of increased concentrations of oxygen is not evaluated.

Phase three is a progression of respiratory difficulty and includes an increase in tidal volume, hypocarbia, and hypoxemia. Pulmonary crackles become detectable, and radiographic signs of diffuse interstitial alveolar involvement are seen. There is a continuous fall in arterial

Table 2.   *Causative Factors Progressive in Pulmonary Insufficiency*

1. Ischemic pulmonary injury
2. Pulmonary infection
3. Sepsis
4. Aspiration
5. Fluid overload
6. Microemboli
   a. Fat emboli
   b. Multiple transfusions
   c. Intravascular coagulation
   d. Tissue trauma
7. Oxygen toxicity
8. Microatelectasis
9. Cerebral trauma

oxygen tension despite 100 percent oxygen therapy and controlled ventilation.

Phase four is terminal hypoxia and hypercarbia with complete pulmonary failure and cardiac arrest. The cause of progressive pulmonary insufficiency is not clearly defined, and many factors have been implicated (Table 2). The most consistent factors appear to be overhydration, microemboli, and sepsis. Careful control of the factors favoring the development of PPI is important, since it is extremely difficult to treat when established. Fluid therapy should be monitored to avoid overhydration, and diuretics should be given if pulmonary crackles develop. Filtration of stored blood through a micropore filter during transfusion eliminates exogenous microemboli. Respiratory care in the form of frequent positional changes, coupage, and periodic induction of coughing is helpful in preventing retention of secretions, hypostatic congestion, and atelectasis.

NON-PENETRATING BLUNT PULMONARY TRAUMA

Injuries of the thorax and upper abdomen caused by automobile accidents or other impact or crushing trauma are commonly seen in small animals. In injuries causing pneumothorax, hemothorax, or diaphragmatic rupture, the degree of respiratory distress is related to the extent of lung collapse. The animal may have incurred other injuries that will influence the prognosis, but it is generally favorable subsequent to removal of air or blood and reexpansion of the lung; these injuries seldom involve the lung directly.

Pulmonary contusion results from direct blunt trauma transmitted to the underlying lung, producing rapid compression and reexpansion. Disruption of the pulmonary parenchyma causes tearing of alveoli and small pulmonary capillaries, with interstitial and intra-alveolar hemorrhage. A major vessel tear causes a hematoma. Signs of pulmonary contusion are tachypnea, crackles, and hemoptysis. The radiographic appearance is one of parenchymal consolidation in a pattern inconsistent with pulmonary edema, pneumonia, or aspiration. The prognosis can be good, depending upon the extent of lung involvement. The injury may be so mild that the diagnosis is based solely on radiographic examination. Hemorrhage into an airway with crackles and hemoptysis has a very poor prognosis.

Trauma in both the chest and upper abdomen may cause hepatic damage and hemorrhage. Often, the abdominal hemorrhage becomes the prime concern, and the pulmonary involvement becomes obvious only during the resuscitative or operative period. The sequence of events is (1) severe trauma to chest and upper abdomen, (2) hepatic damage, (3) general anesthesia and surgical manipulation of the liver, and (4) respiratory failure and death. At necropsy, the lungs do not collapse; they are heavy and congested and show interstitial and intraalveolar hemorrhage.

Surgical manipulation of the liver seems to be instrumental in pulmonary involvement and has been observed in man — in this hospital — and in the experimental dog. During surgical repair, emboli of liver tissue, bile salts, and toxic or vasoactive substances are released into the vena cava and pass to the lung, resulting in pulmonary insufficiency.

PULMONARY DAMAGE RELATED TO IRREVERSIBLE SHOCK

Abundant literature exists in reference to pulmonary damage secondary to hemorrhagic, septic, and traumatic shock and shock produced by regional ischemia. The pulmonary pathology includes atelectasis, congestion, alveolar and parenchymal edema, and hemorrhage. Pathologic changes are related to the severity and length of the shock state. Contrary to progressive pulmonary insufficiency, the pulmonary lesions are contributory to but are not the primary cause of death. The pathologic changes are part of the overall generalized effect of the shock state on body systems. The two mechanisms that may be involved in the pulmonary pathologic changes in dogs in shock are (1) release and absorption of toxins, vasoactive substances, and metabolites from ischemic and damaged tissue (see Fig. 3) and (2) infusion of stored blood that contains particulate debris and platelet microaggregations.

In the dog, experimental pulmonary lesions can be prevented by blockage of the actions of trypsin on the gastrointestinal tract. In the clinical situation, pulmonary lesions can be minimized by quickly reestablishing normal blood flow to damaged and ischemic tissues.

The filtration of blood through fiberglass filters (Pall) prevents pulmonary damage during shock. This is through the removal of the microaggregates that would otherwise be filtered by the lung.

RENAL FUNCTION

Acute failure of renal function in shock is fortunately an uncommon occurrence. It is seen mainly (1) in the older animal with a reduced nephron population, (2) when severe tissue damage has occurred, resulting in the presence of circulating myoglobin and hemoglobin, and (3) in dogs with a combination of hypovolemia and endotoxemia such as can occur in pyometra. The exact pathogenesis of shock-induced renal failure is unclear, but it is generally agreed that prolonged hypotension and poor renal perfusion are the principal factors. Associated with this is the activity of vasoactive hormones such as renin-angiotensin and the catecholamines. Renal vasoconstriction is typically patchy and confined to the cortex, and it may persist even after the return of systemic blood pressure to normal. If vasoconstriction persists for more than 12 to 24 hours, renal tubular damage occurs.

The changes brought about by prolonged vasoconstriction are manifested clinically by oliguria, isosthenuria, glycosuria, and the presence of renal tubular cells in the urinary sediment. Confirmation can be made from the clinical signs of increasing depression, the onset of vomition, and signs compatible with metabolic acidosis. Laboratory confirmation is made by increases in serum creatinine, serum potassium, and blood urea nitrogen.

In most cases, the changes produced by prolonged hypotension are reversible, and it is uncommon for oliguric renal failure to occur in the shocked animal if adequate volume replenishment is initiated early.

CLINICAL SIGNS AND INITIAL EVALUATION

The initial evaluation of the animal in shock requires only a few moments and yet is of vital importance in estimating the severity of the shock state and in formulating immediate resuscitative procedures. A rapid physical examination is made almost subconsciously by the experienced clinician, who will examine such factors as the color and refill time of the mucous membranes, state of hydration, character and rate of the pulse, rate and rhythm of the heart, and respiration and mental state of the patient. The more abnormal these are, the more severe the state of shock.

The classic signs of shock are related primarily to the integrity and function of the cardiovascular system (Table 3). Tachycardia is often present, reflecting the response of the system to a decreased blood volume. Hypotension is evidenced by a narrowing of the pulse pressure and absence of a pulse in small peripheral arteries such as the labial or dorsal pedal. The mucous membranes may be pale or muddy and usually have a slow refill time.

Table 3. *Signs of Shock*

1. Tachycardia
2. Hypotension
   a. Reduced pulse pressure
   b. Poor capillary refill
   c. Muscle weakness
   d. Cold extremities
3. Depressed sensorium
4. Hyperventilation
5. Decreased urinary output

If refill time is longer than two seconds, peripheral perfusion is inadequate. Mucous membrane color is of limited use in evaluating the state of shock. Evidence of peripheral and cutaneous vasoconstriction can be detected by palpation of cold extremities. Body temperature varies widely and is consequently of limited use in evaluation. Hyperventilation, which is present in even the mildest shock case, results from acidemia, pain, fear, excitement, hypotension, and hypoxia. The character, rate, rhythm, and sounds of respiration are important in estimating the extent of pulmonary involvement. Cerebral hypoxia is manifested by a depressed sensorium and in severe shock by dilated pupils. Inadequate muscle perfusion is reflected by generalized weakness.

The severity of the shock state can only be estimated by considering and evaluating all the above parameters. After initial evaluation and resuscitation, a more detailed examination must be made. This includes an accurate history and a thorough examination to facilitate decisions regarding specific therapy or further diagnostic procedures.

TREATMENT OF SHOCK

Many factors determine the treatment of shock, and each patient requires management on an individual basis. Because of the rapid changes in body functions, management necessitates continuous monitoring and intensive patient care. Therapy may have to be altered repeatedly, since shock is never a self-limiting disease in which therapy can be prescribed and administered on a timed basis until a cure is achieved. Etiology will obviously determine definitive therapy, but there are a number of specific treatments that are carried out as part of the initial therapy of any type of shock.

PRIORITIES OF SHOCK MANAGEMENT

The essential steps in the initial management of the shocked patient are:

1. Insure adequate ventilation and oxygenation.

2. Arrest hemorrhage if present.
3. Initiate volume replacement.

After these initial procedures have been carried out, reevaluation will be necessary to identify the requirements for further therapy. This may include one or more of the following:

1. Regulation of acid-base disturbances.
2. Glucocorticosteroids.
3. Antibiotics.
4. Mannitol.
5. Vasoactive drugs.
6. Oxygen.

SPECIFIC THERAPY

AIRWAY

Deficient ventilation is a serious factor contributing to the unfavorable course of shock and may be caused by many factors — e.g., airway obstruction, pulmonary trauma, splinting of respiratory muscles, and central nervous system depression. Animals with thoracic trauma may have pulmonary parenchymal hemorrhage, pneumothorax, hemothorax, or ruptured diaphragm. All can contribute to hypoxia and respiratory acidosis, exacerbating the concomitant metabolic acidosis.

If, on presentation, the patient shows signs of respiratory distress, the first and most important step is to insure an adequate airway. Endotracheal intubation is the most rapid method; a cuffed tube is essential to prevent aspiration and enables the use of assisted or controlled ventilation if required. Suction should be employed to clear the tracheobronchial tree of excessive mucus, blood, or foreign material. If the patient has been successfully intubated, resistance to the tube can be overcome by taping the mouth shut and using a tape roll as a bite block. If ventilation is inadequate, it should be assisted with the use of a self-inflating bag or mechanical ventilator. In many cases, the addition of oxygen to the spontaneously breathing animal may be sufficient to abolish hypoxia. If the animal is conscious and ventilating, oxygen can be administered by intratracheal catheter or mask. Respiratory distress may also be due to pleural rupture or pulmonary contusion, but in these cases, oxygen administration alone will not completely reverse the dyspnea. Since auscultation, percussion, and thoracocentesis are sufficient to diagnose pneumothorax, corrective measures should be initiated immediately without confirmatory radiographic examination.

Treatment of pneumohemothorax is straightforward. The chest is clipped and prepared with alcohol and iodine. A 16-gauge plastic catheter is inserted bilaterally at midlevel through the seventh or eighth interspace into the thoracic cavity, and air or blood is aspirated. This therapy usually suffices, but chest tube drainage can be established later if air or blood loss is excessive.

CONTROL OF HEMORRHAGE

Any obvious hemorrhage should be controlled by direct pressure, bandaging, or ligation. Internal hemorrhage may warrant immediate surgical intervention during a period of intensive fluid replacement.

VOLUME REPLACEMENT

Reestablishment of adequate tissue perfusion is the key to the successful treatment of any form of shock. In most types, this is achieved by the administration of crystalloids, blood, or plasma. In cardiogenic and some cases of septic shock, however, rapid fluid replenishment, although important, is not always a major initial consideration.

CRYSTALLOIDS

Lactated Ringer's solution has been commonly used for resuscitation, but several better balanced multielectrolyte solutions are now available. Besides some changes in ionic concentration and a higher osmolarity, the most important change in these fluids is the substitution of gluconate or acetate for lactate. These solutions are recommended in large volumes for initial resuscitation.

Adequate tissue oxygenation results from a combination of perfusion and hemoglobin oxygen saturation. There is, therefore, a limit to the amount of crystalloid that can be infused without hemodilution and a reduction in oxygen delivery, which occurs at hematocrits below 20 percent. At hematocrits above 50 percent, blood viscosity is increased, with a subsequent decrease in tissue perfusion; oxygen delivery is reduced despite high hemoglobin levels. While a balanced salt solution is adequate for replacement in most shocked animals, some diseases require definitive ion replacement. A guide to these is given in Table 4.

REPLACEMENT THERAPY

Assessment of Volume Requirement. Clinical estimations of fluid and blood loss are inaccurate and generally low. Many techniques

Table 4. Guide to Fluid and Electrolyte Therapy in Common Shock States

1. *Hypovolemic and Hemorrhagic Shock:*
   Give balanced electrolyte solution in mild shock and whole blood or packed cells if the hematocrit falls below 25%. Give plasma if total solids fall below 4 gm/100 ml. If the patient is azotemic, give a potassium-free solution until diuresis occurs or the serum potassium concentration is ascertained.
2. *Severe Diarrhea:*
   Give a balanced electrolyte solution. Sodium bicarbonate if acidotic, and potassium chloride supplementation after diuresis occurs.
3. *Severe Vomiting:*
   Give normal saline. Add KCl after diuresis up to a maximum of 40 mEq/l for maintenance.
4. *Renal Failure:*
   Avoid potassium-containing solutions. Give NaCl or ½ strength dextrose and saline until serum potassium concentration is ascertained or diuresis occurs. Animals with chronic renal failure are potassium-depleted. Avoid potassium-containing fluids until shock is controlled and the serum potassium concentration is ascertained. Potassium supplementation may be required.
5. *Ketoacidotic Diabetics:*
   Give normal saline. Add KCl when diuresis occurs. Large quantities of supplemental potassium will be required, because diabetics are potassium-depleted and insulin lowers serum potassium concentrations.
6. *Pancreatitis and Peritonitis:*
   Balanced electrolyte solution. Supplemental potassium will be required. Give plasma if total solids fall below 4 gm/100 ml.

and sample calculations for estimating fluid deficit have been quoted in the veterinary literature. However, at best, these give a very rough assessment and invariably underestimate fluid requirements. This is because they use the normal animal as the basis for their assumptions. It is advisable to ignore such calculations and adopt an open-minded approach to the question of replacement volume in shock. Obviously, a rough volume will have been assessed from such factors as the size of the patient, the nature and severity of the shock state, and such criteria as skin turgor and initial hematocrit (Hct), but the exact volume can only be assessed according to the response of the patient as fluids are infused. The technique is in effect a titration of fluid volume against the various monitoring techniques to be described later. Thus, in traumatic shock, a return of heart rate, capillary refill, and urine output toward normal might be considered the endpoint, whereas in the severely dehydrated patient, a return of Hct, total solids (TS), vital signs, and urine output toward normal would indicate adequate volume replacement.

Route of Administration. In the severely depleted patient, fluids should be given as rapidly as possible. This is best achieved with a short (over-the-needle) 16- or 18-gauge catheter in a peripheral vein. In large dogs, two such catheters should be inserted. If central venous pressure is to be measured, a central venous catheter should be inserted when convenient. In most animals, a 17-gauge through-the-needle catheter (e.g., Intracath®) can be used, but in obese dogs and in some cats, direct visual insertion of the catheter into the jugular vein by cutdown catheterization is indicated.

As the monitored parameters begin to return to normal, the rate of administration can be slowed accordingly.

Maintenance Therapy and Replacement of Ongoing Losses. Following the return of blood volume to normal, the patient should continue to receive fluids but at a slower rate. Most shock patients continue to lose body fluids at a faster than normal rate because of increased capillary permeability together with increased renal and respiratory losses. Although ADH secretion is increased as a result of hypotension, the kidneys are unable to produce maximally concentrated urine because of changes in renal blood flow that result in reduced medullary osmolarity. The increased respiratory rate of shocked animals results in additional respiratory water loss.

Maintenance volumes of up to 80 ml/kg/24 hours (double the normal value) are usually indicated to replace these losses. Fluids should be given at this rate for one to three days and reduced as the patient returns to homeostasis. In animals with diseases associated with an excessive ongoing fluid loss such as peritonitis or diarrhea,, additional volume replacement is indicated.

Hypokalemia is a common finding in the post-shock state, particularly if adequate volume replacement has been given. While not too important in mild shock, hypokalemia can markedly increase morbidity and recovery time in severely shocked animals. Commercially available fluids contain insufficient potassium to correct this deficit, and for this reason, if the animal is not eating, extra potassium chloride should be added to the maintenance fluids. Provided that the animal is producing urine, 20 mEq of KCl should be added to every 500 ml of fluid. This is a safe amount and prevents hypokalemia in all but the most severely affected animal.

Blood. Whole blood or packed cells are indicated in severe hemorrhagic and traumatic shock. The need for blood cannot be determined from the initial hematocrit, and the decision to transfuse is usually a matter of clinical judgment. Animals with hemorrhage of up to 30 percent of blood volume (a category in which most hemorrhagic shock patients fall) do not generally require transfusion, as crystalloid replacement alone is adequate. Blood transfusion after initial replacement therapy should be considered if hemorrhage is severe, and when the Hct decreases below 20 percent during resuscitation. Blood should be stored in citrate-phosphate-dextrose (CPD), be from an A-negative donor, or be cross-matched before administration.

Platelet aggregations, fibrin particles, and other microparticles that accumulate in stored blood have a deleterious effect upon the pulmonary circulation, especially in animals with preexisting pulmonary damage. To obviate this potentially dangerous phenomenon, blood should be fresh, transfused into an artery, or filtered through commercially available microfilters, which are much finer than the filters on blood administration sets.

Plasma. Plasma is essential to maintain oncotic pressure in shock involving severe protein loss such as that which occurs in peritonitis and large volume hemorrhage. It should be given in sufficient quantity to return plasma protein levels toward normal.

Colloids. Therapy with high molecular weight solutions (dextran) has been advocated but is now out of favor in the therapy of most types of shock. Dextrans exert an osmotic effect and rapidly expand the circulating blood volume at the expense of the extracellular fluid; they should therefore be administered together with a balanced salt solution. They are indicated to maintain serum oncotic pressure when plasma is unavailable.

FURTHER THERAPY

REGULATION OF ACID-BASE DISTURBANCES

Most shock states are associated with a metabolic acidosis, the degree of acidemia being related to the extent and duration of tissue hypoperfusion. If capable, the shocked animal hyperventilates, often to the extent of being alkalotic on presentation, especially those in traumatic or hemorrhagic shock. The increased ventilation is a response to hypotension, excitement, and the developing metabolic acidosis. The ventilatory response, however, is never sufficient to counter fully the metabolic acidosis that develops during severe hypoperfusion states.

Acidosis will be exacerbated in the comatose, anesthetized (spontaneously breathing) patient or in those with severe thoracic trauma. Massive blood transfusions also contribute to the metabolic acidosis.

Recovery from this acid-base disturbance can proceed rapidly following the restoration of tissue perfusion and cardiovascular function. Carbon dioxide will be eliminated by the respiratory system, and the liver rapidly metabolizes lactate and any transfused citrate.

Adjustment of acid-base status is best done after the measurement of arterial pH and PCO_2 and the circulation of bicarbonate concentrations and base deficit. The amount necessary to adjust pH to near normal levels is estimated from measured values, and a calculated amount of sodium bicarbonate is given intravenously.* Since blood gas and pH analyses are not often available to the practitioner, sodium bicarbonate solution should be administered at a dosage of 1 to 4 mEq/kg according to the apparent severity of the animal's condition. Half the amount should be given slowly intravenously and the remainder should be added to the intravenous fluid and given over the next four to six hours. A mild degree of acidosis is not deleterious or in need of correction. The majority of shocked animals seen in clinical practice do not require bicarbonate therapy.

GLUCOCORTICOSTEROIDS

Examination of data relating to the use of glucocorticosteroids in shock shows that these drugs have many desirable effects. They help preserve the integrity of cell and cell organelle membranes, favorably alter cellular metabolism, improve oxygen transport, alter microvascular hemodynamics, and decrease anaphylotoxin production in septic shock.

Despite recognition of these effects, controversy still exists over the efficacy of glucocorticosteroids in every shock state. This controversy results from the large number of different shock models and experimental protocols and the paucity of objective clinical data confirming their value. Although definitive information describing the role of glucocorticosteroids in the treatment of all shock states is still unavailable, these drugs have been shown to be of some value in the treatment of septic and cardiogenic shock. Their use in other shock states, however, is not contraindicated.

---

*The bicarbonate requirement is calculated from the following equation: bicarbonate deficit (mEq/liter) = base deficit (mEq/liter) $\times$ 0.3 $\times$ body weight in kg.

Massive (pharmacologic) doses of the aqueous soluble salts of these drugs must be given very early in the course of treatment to be of maximal benefit.

It has been shown experimentally that if non-pharmacologic doses are used, few of the biochemical defects caused by shock will be reversed or eliminated, and survival of the test animals will be similar to that of the untreated animals. Pharmacologic doses are hydrocortisone, 150 to 300 mg/kg; prednisolone, 15 to 30 mg/kg; and dexamethasone, 4 to 8 mg/kg. These doses are not harmful if given for short periods (24 to 48 hours) and can be withdrawn without tapering. These drugs are available for intravenous administration as the water-soluble sodium succinate and phosphate salts. Dexamethasone is also available in a polyethylene glycol suspension (Azium®). Aqueous solutions are expensive but are necessary to achieve rapidly the necessary high tissue concentrations. Because of the economic constraints of veterinary practice, the slower acting and less expensive dexamethsaone suspension (Azium), though less than ideal, can be given concurrently with a loading dose of the aqueous salt. The suspension should be given every four hours for as long as is necessary.

While use of glucocorticosteroids may be a valuable adjunct in the treatment of shock, it is important to recognize that they are no substitute for specific shock therapy.

Glucose. Hypoglycemia and hypoinsulinemia are seen in severe septic shock. Clinical and experimental studies report that administration of glucose-insulin-potassium will cause improvement of hemodynamic parameters during sepsis and endotoxemia. Experience with several animals with clinical sepsis has shown that the mixture of 3 gm of glucose, 1 unit of regular insulin, and 0.5 mEq of potassium per Kg of body weight in 250 to 500 cc of normal saline infused at a rate that will deliver 0.5 to 1 gm of glucose/Kg/hr is a useful adjunct in treatment of these animals. Animals receiving this mixture in addition to volume replacement, antibiotics, and surgical drainage showed subjective and objective improvement in some hemodynamic parameters. Their heart rates decreased to the normal range and peripheral perfusion improved as evidenced by creased toe web temperature. This infusion should be continued until the animal is stabilized.

ANTIBIOTICS

The precise role of bacteria and their products in the genesis of clinical shock from causes other than sepsis remains to be elucidated. Broad-spectrum antibiotic therapy is recommended for purely prophylactic reasons, however, following extensive tissue damage and operative procedures. Septic shock cannot be effectively treated until infection is controlled, and in such cases, broad-spectrum bactericidal antibiotics such as gentamicin, kanamycin, cephalosporin, or ampicillin should be given intravenously in high doses. Specific antibiotic therapy is indicated after the offending organism has been identified and its sensitivity has been determined.

MANNITOL

Renal blood flow ceases when blood pressure falls below 50 to 60 mm Hg. The functional result of this is oliguria or anuria. The canine and feline kidney is able to survive several hours of markedly reduced blood flow, and in most animals, the defect is only temporary, urine output being restored with the re-establishment of normal blood pressure and renal perfusion. To establish urine output, mannitol should be given only after circulatory stability is achieved and when there is no evidence of lower urinary tract injury. The effect of mannitol is fourfold: (1) it increases circulating blood volume by an osmotic effect, (2) it retains water within the proximal nephrons, (3) it has a direct effect in increasing renal blood flow and, (4) it reduces renal cellular edema. Mannitol, which is available as a 25 percent solution, should be diluted with an equal volume of normal saline and given intravenously (0.5 to 2.0 gm/kg). Dosage should not exceed 2 gm/kg in a 24-hour period. If diuresis is not evident within an hour, furosemide should be given intravenously at a dose of 2 mg/kg; if not effective, the dose should be doubled.

VASOACTIVE DRUGS

The use of vasopressors has declined as a more rational approach to shock therapy has developed. These drugs should never be used in the initial therapy of hypovolemic or septic shock and should be reserved for extreme situations in which cardiovascular collapse is imminent.

The use of vasodilators such as chlorpromazine or isoproterenol has been suggested for some types of shock; their use is based on the assumption that restoration of blood flow through the tissues rather than the artificial maintenance of arterial pressure is the therapeutic aim. Use of these agents is indicated only after adequate fluid replacement, since they exacerbate hypotension and cardiovascular collapse in the hypovolemic patient. They are indicated in septic shock, especially in the later phases, but have no role in initial shock therapy.

Isoproterenol is a beta stimulator that can be diluted in saline and used as a continuous IV drip (Table 5) in septic, traumatic, and hypovolemic shock. It increases myocardial contractility and is a vasodilator. Since both these actions result in increased tissue perfusion, isoproterenol is a useful drug in refractory shock. It can induce arrhythmias, and thus the heart rate and rhythm must be monitored closely. The rate of administration should be adjusted so that, depending on the size of the patient, the heart rate does not rise above 160 to 200 beats/minute.

Dopamine, a precursor of norepinephrine, has been recommended for the treatment of shock, particularly in patients not responding to volume expansion. Its effects are similar to but somewhat more selective than those of isoproterenol. Dopamine increases cardiac output and, at low concentrations, causes vasodilation of the renal and mesenteric vascular beds. Like isoproterenol, it is diluted and given in a continuous IV drip.

OXYGEN THERAPY

Oxygen is indicated whenever a reduced arterial oxygen tension has been measured or is suspected. Hypoxemia is manifested by tachypnea, the presence of ventricular arrhythmias, restlessness, and occasionally cyanosis — even when blood volume is adequate. These clinical signs must be used in lieu of blood gas measurements, since the necessary equipment is not available in most veterinary practices. However, a blood oxygen analyzer that

Table 5.   *Vasoactive Drugs*

Vasopressors	*Dose*
1. Methoxamine HCl	0.2 mg/kg IV or IM
2. Ephedrine HCl	10-20 mg IV or IM
3. Levarterenol bitartrate	(0.2% solution) 1-2 ml diluted in 100 ml IV slowly
Vasodilators	
1. Isoproterenol HCl°	(0.02% solution) 0.05-0.10 ml diluted in 100 ml IV slowly
2. Dopamine	10 mg diluted in 100 ml saline given at the rate of 5µgm/kg/min IV
3. Chlorpromazine HCl	0.5-1 mg/kg IV slowly

°Isoproterenol lowers peripheral vascular resistance and diastolic pressure falls, but the positive inotropic and chronotropic actions of the drug maintain or raise the systolic pressure, although mean pressure is reduced.

is simple to operate is available commercially. This machine can be used to diagnose hypoxia and to monitor subsequent therapy. An increase in the inspired oxygen concentration from 20 to 30 or 40 percent provides adequate tissue oxygenation in most cases of hypoxia. However, in some animals, 100 percent oxygen with controlled ventilation may be necessary. Oxygen therapy in the conscious animal must be a compromise between the patient's requirements and the amount of restraint it will tolerate. Several techniques of oxygen administration are available.

Intratracheal Catheters. This technique is extremely well tolerated by most animals and is one of the most efficacious and economic methods for long-term administration. After appropriate skin preparation and infiltration of a local anesthetic, a 14- or 16-gauge, 6- to 8-inch plastic catheter is inserted percutaneously into the trachea in the ventral midline of the neck in the midcervical region. The catheter is attached to an oxygen delivery tube and taped to the neck. For long-term administration (> 4 hours), oxygen must be humidified in order to prevent ciliary damage and dehydration through drying of the respiratory mucous membranes. This is best achieved by passing the oxygen through a commercially available humidification unit. Depending on size and respiratory rate, flow rates of 0.5 to 3.0 liters/minute are adequate.

Nasal Catheters. This technique is effective for short-term administration in the depressed patient. A soft 5 to 8 French rubber catheter is coated with local anesthetic cream and passed up the nose so that the tip comes to lie in the nasopharynx. The catheter is then taped in place. Before insertion, the catheter should be measured against the patient and marked to insure accurate placement in the nasopharynx. Flow rates of 2 to 4 liters/minute are generally adequate. This technique should not be used for more than four hours without humidified oxygen.

Masks. Masks are useful in emergency situations when intubation is difficult or impractical. They require high flow rates to prevent carbon dioxide accumulation and have the disadvantage that many patients resent them, struggle, and negate the benefits of additional oxygen.

Oxygen Compartments. Mobile oxygen compartments consisting of a sealed cage, air conditioner, CO_2 absorber, humidifier, thermostat, and oxygen analyzer are now commercially available. These units enable the temperature, humidity, and oxygen concentration within the sealed cage to be accurately regulated.

Sealed oxygen cages have no humidity or

temperature control but are much cheaper. Oxygen concentrations are related to flow, size of cage, and frequency of opening. Overheating of the patient is common in these units.

A pediatric incubator is useful for oxygen supplementation in the small dog, cat, or exotic animal. These units have a more effective temperature and humidity control but suffer many of the same disadvantages as oxygen cages.

Oxygen concentrations above 40 percent are rarely achieved in any of these units; although this concentration is adequate for most patients, oxygenation ultimately depends upon the ventilatory capacity of the patient. If oxygenation is inadequate, controlled ventilation should be considered.

GENERAL PRECAUTIONS IN SHOCK THERAPY

1. *Never permit unnecessary movement of the patient.* Rapid changes in position, such as lifting, rotation, or rapid movement on a cart, are contraindicated. Shocked animals' compensatory reflex mechanisms for both cardiovascular and respiratory adjustment are minimal; positional changes that are of no consequence in the normal animal can be disastrous in the shock state.

2. *Never delay therapy.* Always insure an adequate airway and administer intravenous fluids. If surgery is needed, it should be limited to procedures essential for correction of the initiating factors. Additional diagnostic procedures such as radiographic axamination should only follow initial resuscitative procedures.

3. *Delay analgesic administrations.* Analgesics and sedatives should not be given until the condition of the animal has been carefully assessed and volume replacement has been initiated. All narcotics, tranquilizers, and barbiturates depress cardiovascular and respiratory function. Restlessness and delirium may be due to hypoxia, not discomfort or pain, indicating the need for oxygen, not depressants.

4. *Never subject the animal to deep planes of anesthesia.* All the currently used inhalation anesthetics depress the sympathetic nervous and cardiovascular systems. As with the administration of other depressants, anesthesia must be administered carefully and only in concentrations that will produce the minimal necessary plane. *No* situation requires immediate surgical treatment before an airway is established, external hemorrhage is controlled, and volume replacement is commenced.

EPILOG TO THERAPY

It is not enough to give the shocked patient intravenous fluids, place it in a cage, and leave observation and care to a less skilled person. Proper care demands intensive therapeutic and nursing support. After initial resuscitation and therapy, continuous attention to the patient's comfort, warmth, nutrition, oxygenation, and hydration often make the difference between life and death. The therapy of shock may last from a few hours to several days. Close observation and therapy must not cease until the patient is stable. Stability is evidenced by the maintenance of cardiovascular function without fluid or drug support, a return of normal urine output, maintenance of adequate oxygenation at normal ventilatory rates, and improvement of acid-base balance.

SUMMARY OF SHOCK THERAPY

1. Insure adequate airway and ventilation.
2. Control serious external hemorrhage.
3. Place large-bore catheter in a peripheral vein. Obtain a blood sample for basic biochemical data, Hct, TS, and crossmatching.
4. Begin volume replacement at a rate commensurate with degree of hypotension.
5. Conduct rapid physical examination. Decide on further diagnostic and therapeutic procedures.
6. Insert catheters to monitor CVP and urine output.
7. Determine response to initial therapy; record all parameters monitored and treatment given.
8. Begin appropriate adjunctive therapy:
   a. Acid-base correction
   b. Antibiotics
   c. Steroids.
9. Give blood or plasma, if indicated.
10. Reassess animal's condition after therapy and reevaluate diagnosis as necessary.

MONITORING TECHNIQUES

Monitoring, derived from the Latin *monere*— to warn — is the observation, measurement, and recording of clinical and physiologic variables. Shocked patients present a complex of constantly changing physiologic functions, and it is essential for the clinician to be continually aware of these so that therapy can be changed in response to the patient's changing needs. For these reasons, monitoring must be considered an integral part of shock therapy.

Monitoring can conveniently be divided into two types: clinical, which requires skilled staff but very little equipment, and physiologic, which requires more equipment but which reveals correspondingly more information on specific organ function.

CLINICAL MONITORING

Temperature. The temperature of the shocked patient can vary widely. Temperature is best monitored with a continuously recording electronic thermometer and thermistor probe, since this avoids repeatedly disturbing the patient. If the temperature falls below 100°F, the patient should be warmed, using a heating pad, blanket, or lamp. Replacement fluids are best prewarmed to 37°C, since cold fluids further reduce body temperature, especially when given in large volumes.

Subjective evaluation of the temperature of the extremities of patients in shock is a time-honored means of assessing peripheral circulation. Skin temperature correlates well with cardiac output and peripheral blood flow and can be used as a means of prognosis during treatment. This technique is valuable in veterinary practice because it is rapidly performed, is non-invasive, and does not require highly skilled personnel or expensive equipment.

The maximal value of this technique is achieved if frequent measurements are made and recorded during resuscitation. Temperature can be taken either with an electronic thermometer and thermistor probe or with a mercury thermometer having a range of 15 to 45°C (70 to 110°F).

Measurements are most conveniently made in the toe web of a rear paw. The temperature recorded at this site is usually between 1 and 5°C (2 and 9°F) less than that of the rectum and approximately 13 to 20°C (24 to 30°F) greater than room temperature (20 to 23°C) (68 to 72°F). During shock, the toe web/rectal temperature difference is greater than 5°C (9°F). The greater the difference, the greater the reduction in cardiac output and consequently in peripheral blood flow. As the animal responds favorably to treatment, cardiac output increases, peripheral circulation is improved, and the temperature differential returns toward normal. These measurements provide accurate prognostic information regarding the effectiveness of therapy.

Pulse. The return of pulse rate, rhythm and character toward normal as therapy progresses in the shocked patient is a good prognostic sign. After homeostasis is achieved, changes in the pulse can be the first sign of infection, hypoxia, or ongoing fluid loss. For these reasons, it is important that the pulse be checked and findings be recorded frequently throughout therapy. Because of the redistribution of blood flow in shock, it is advisable to check the pulse in more than one site. For example, while a pulse may still be detected in the femoral artery, its absence in a peripheral artery is indicative of serious hypovolemia or intense vasoconstriction.

Respiration. Changes in rate, rhythm, and character should be noted carefully. A gradual increase in rate may be the first sign of hypoxia or of the development of pulmonary diseases such as shock lung, pulmonary edema, aspiration pneumonia, or secondary pneumonia. Regular auscultation of all lung fields is important. Fluid rates or an increased harshness in the respiratory sounds can be the first sign of overhydration, incipient pulmonary disease, or a failing myocardium. Most shocked patients will show an initial increase in the rate and depth of ventilation unless they are depressed or injured to such an extent that they cannot respond. A return of rate and tidal volume toward normal is a favorable prognostic sign.

Palpation. Palpation tends to be neglected as a monitoring technique in the critical patient. Palpation can be used as a rough assessment of the temperature of the extremities. In the hypovolemic animal, the extremities are cool, indicating lowered peripheral perfusion; rewarming is an indication of an improved circulation, a favorable response to therapy, and an increased heat loss to the environment. Careful palpation of the extremities is also useful in detecting edema. Asymmetrical temperature differences may indicate inflammation or locally impaired circulation.

Capillary Refill. Capillary refill is an indication of peripheral perfusion. A refill time of more than two seconds is abnormal, indicating hypotension, hypovolemia, or peripheral vasoconstriction. Injected membranes indicate sepsis or polycythemia, whereas pale membranes indicate anemia or poor tissue perfusion. Membrane color is a poor indicator of tissue perfusion and oxygenation. Cyanosis is usually a very late indicator of hypoxemia.

PHYSIOLOGIC MONITORING

Hematocrit and Total Solids. The serial measurement of these parameters is one of the simplest and most effective shock monitoring techniques. Although individually these parameters provide little definitive information about the circulating blood volume, when used conjointly, they provide some of the information necessary to manipulate volume replacement efficiently. The hematocrit (normal 35 to 48 percent) is important in determining changing red cell plasma ratios, and the total solids (normal 5.5 to 8.0 gm/100 ml) are rough indicators of plasma protein concentration.

Serial measurements are indicated in all shock patients. If the animal has suffered water loss, both the hematocrit Hct) and the total solids (TS) will be increased. In cases of plasma loss through exudation such as in peritonitis or thermal burns, the Hct is increased whereas the TS may be normal or low. In hypovolemia with anemia, the Hct may be misleadingly normal and the TS is usually increased. The Hct and TS are not markedly changed in early hemorrhagic shock; these values fall only as fluid compartment shifts compensate for loss of blood volume or as crystalloid replacement therapy progresses. The initial Hcts cannot therefore be used to assess the extent of hemorrhage. Following therapy, the TS returns to normal more rapidly than does the Hct, and a steady or increasing TS therefore provides an early indication that transcapillary loss may have ceased.

The difference in Hct between a peripherally and a centrally drawn blood sample can be of prognostic value in assessing the response to therapy. Normally, the central Hct is about 3 percent less than the peripheral Hct. Differences in excess of this indicate peripheral hypoperfusion. If the differential continuously increases, the prognosis is grave. Most often, this can be deduced from other signs, but, on the other hand, a narrowing may be among the first indications of an improved peripheral circulation.

During volume replacement, serial Hct and TS determinations will indicate whether the most appropriate replacement fluid is blood, plasma, or a balanced salt solution. The Hct and TS should be maintained within the normal range, if possible, but a decrease in Hct to 20 percent can be tolerated without a significant decrease in tissue oxygen delivery in animals with normal pulmonary function. Pulmonary edema is not usually a threat until the TS falls below 3.5 gm/100 ml. Conversely, the Hct should not be permitted to rise above 50 percent, since tissue perfusion is decreased and cardiac work is increased because of the increased blood viscosity.

Electrocardiogram. Ideally, an electrocardiogram should be taken for all shocked animals at or soon after admission to act as a baseline with which to compare later changes. This is especially true of those with thoracic trauma. Depending on the cause of shock, animals can demonstrate a wide range of electrocardiographic abnormalities. Most result from electrolyte imbalances, hypoxia, or cardiac contusion. Tachycardia can result from pain, fever, anoxia, or hypovolemia. Premature ventricular contractions (PVCs) and changes in the S-T Segment and in the T-wave are seen in hypoxia and cardiac contusion. Oxygen therapy may eliminate arrhythmias caused by hypoxia. If abnormalities are detected, a complete diagnostic electrocardiogram should be taken, but for monitoring, lead II is sufficient.

Central Venous Pressure. The measurement of central venous pressure (CVP) has become an invaluable aid in estimating the fluid requirements of the shocked patient. It is measured from the anterior vena cava and depends on the volume of blood returning to the heart (the effective blood volume) and the efficiency of the cardiac pump. An alteration in either of these factors will tend to change the CVP. A low CVP implies a deficit in the circulating blood volume (note that it only *implies* a deficit, it does not indicate one), and a high CVP implies a failing myocardium or fluid overload. CVP measurement should always be used in the severely shocked patient or when a patient fails to respond to what is believed to be adequate volume replacement. The CVP is particularly helpful in the older animal or when cardiac failure complicates the clinical picture.

The CVP is measured using a catheter inserted via the external jugular vein into the anterior vena cava. The strictest aseptic precautions should be used whenever a catheter is introduced. Failure to do so has resulted in a large number of cases of fatal bacteremia from infected catheters. Several varieties of plastic catheters and cannulae for recording CVP are produced commercially. The shortest catheter that will reach the anterior vena cava should be used, because the sensitivity of CVP recording and the rate at which intravenous fluids can be given through the catheter are a function of its length and diameter. In addition, myocardial injury due to the introduction of too long a catheter has been reported. A saline manometer is the simplest and cheapest method of recording central venous pressure. Its two main disadvantages are that it does not permit a permanent continuous record to be made and that a rise in pressure fills the catheter with blood, which is liable to clot. After insertion, the intravenous catheter is connected via a three-way stopcock to the manometer, and the third limb of the stopcock is connected to an infusion set from which the system can be primed and infusions can be given when a recording is not being taken. A fluctuation of 2 to 5 mm in the saline level with each respiration indicates that the catheter tip is correctly sited and that an accurate reading is being taken.

The actual level of CVP recorded varies widely from individual to individual and also depends on the level at which the zero of the manometer is set. The most satisfactory zero level is the center of the sternum with the dog or cat lying on its side. With this as zero, the CVP of the dog or cat normally varies between 0 and 5 cm of water. Values consistently above 8 to 10 cm usually indicate an expanded blood volume, and if this value is obtained, fluid administration should be slowed or stopped. Values above 15 cm water indicate right heart failure. A rising CVP in the face of falling blood pressure, reduced palpable pulse pressure, increased capillary refill time, and rales indicates myocardial failure, overhydration, or cardiac tamponade.

Several factors should be borne in mind when evaluating CVP:

1. Use trends rather than single values.
2. Measure at the same level with the patient in the same position.
3. Changes of less than 3 cm water between readings, unless consistent, are not significant and can be due to positional changes.
4. The CVP fluctuates markedly in sequence with respiration when controlled ventilation is used.
5. Vasoactive drugs can cause a venoconstriction that can result in a large incremental rise in CVP.
6. Mechanical occlusion of the catheter by clots or kinks can cause a false elevation of CVP. If the column of fluid does not fluctuate freely with respiration during measurement, mechanical flaws should be suspected.
7. When not in use, the catheter should be flushed with heparinized saline (2000 IU/liter every 6 hours) to prevent clot formation.

Urine Output. The rate of urine production is proportional to the GFR and is therefore a measure of renal perfusion and, indirectly, of arterial blood pressure. GFR is maintained at a constant level over a wide range of blood pressures but ceases when arterial pressure falls below 60 mm Hg. Reduced urine output is therefore an indicator of reduced organ perfusion and hypotension; likewise, a return of urine output in a previously anuric animal is a good prognostic sign.

Urine output is best monitored with an indwelling urinary catheter. It is far better to possess accurate knowledge of the rate of urine formation than to adopt a wait-and-see attitude or attempt to ascertain whether the animal is forming urine by palpating the bladder or compressing the abdomen. By the time oliguria has been confirmed using these latter techniques, it may well be too late to reestablish renal function pharmacologically.

In the male dog, catheter placement is simple. A soft rubber urinary catheter is inserted and secured by means of a piece of tape attached to the end of the catheter. The tape is then sutured to the prepuce. A pediatric 8 French Foley catheter is suitable for most female dogs. A length of stainless steel wire placed in the catheter lumen adds stability to facilitate insertion. After catheter placement, the bladder should be emptied of all urine and monitoring should be started. For continuous measurement, the catheter is attached to a fluid delivery tube and an empty intravenous fluid bottle, which acts as a graduated collection reservoir. For intermittent measurement (in the more active patient), the catheter can be occluded with a plastic plug (needle cover or venoset cover) and emptied hourly with a syringe and three-way stopcock.

The normal cat or dog should produce 0.5 to 1.0 ml of urine/kg body weight/hour. If this volume is not produced after fluid volume expansion has been achieved and blood pressure has returned to normal, a test does of a diuretic such as mannitol or furosemide should be considered, provided that the bladder is not ruptured.

Sterile technique is vital in urinary catheter placement. In order to minimize the chance of infection, the catheter should be removed as soon as the patient is stable; i.e., when urine production has been normal for several hours or when the patient is able to urinate without soiling itself.

Blood Pressure. Blood pressure monitoring by either direct or indirect means is a feasible and clinically useful technique. Direct monitoring requires arterial catheterization, but the measurements are accurate and the catheter can also be used to obtain arterial blood samples. An 8-inch 16- to 19-gauge catheter is placed either percutaneously or by cutdown into the femoral artery. An injection cap is applied to the catheter and both are then taped to the animal's leg. An 18-gauge needle attached by a short length of tubing to a sphygmomanometer is inserted through the injection cap, permitting measurements to be made as necessary. When not is use, the catheter should be flushed with heparinized saline solution every four hours to prevent occlusion.

Indirect measurements of blood pressure can be made from the dorsal pedal artery using an Arteriosonde® sphygmomanometer or an ultrasonic flow detector and an aeronoid sphygmomanometer. This device is not highly accurate but provides clinically useful information. The pressure obtained depends to some extent on the method of measurement, but the range 90 to 140 mm Hg is considered normal in the dog and cat. As with CVP measurement, however, it is not the specific value that is important but the return to the normal range as therapy progresses.

Blood pressure can also be estimated by palpation. Although the values obtained are only approximations, the technique is clinically useful. If the femoral pulse is absent or very difficult to detect, blood pressure is 50 mm Hg or less. If the femoral pulse is detectable but weak and the dorsal pedal pulse is absent or barely detectable, the blood pressure is between 50 and 70 mm Hg.

Blood Chemistries. Except in simple hemorrhagic shock, blood chemical changes should be monitored. A knowledge of the specific disturbance associated with individual diseases is obviously essential, but some disturbances are common to many diseases and should be monitored routinely. Included in the parameters that might be monitored at least once daily are electrolytes (Na^+, K^+, Cl^-), enzymes (SGPT, SAP), and creatinine and/or BUN. Commercial "profiles," which are often cheaper than the cost of individual tests, provide a good method of monitoring these biochemical changes.

CONCLUSIONS

Although physiologic monitoring is a valuable adjunct to patient care, it cannot replace close patient observation by trained personnel. Every shocked patient needs continuous monitoring until it is stable, but the extent and type must be adapted to the patient's requirements. No matter what parameters are monitored, it is mandatory that they be recorded and form a part of the patient's hospital records. It is of vital importance to keep a record of all signs, monitored parameters, laboratory studies, and therapy. One person cannot remember all the facts pertinent to a case. If an adequate record is kept, trends can be noted and appropriate therapeutic measures can be taken. Many expensive and complex monitoring devices are available, but, as with all sophisticated equipment, they are no substitute for clinical acumen and careful patient observation.

List of Equipment Described in Text:

Ambubag: Airshields Inc., Hatboro, PA.

Arteriosonde Sphygmomanometer: Hoffmann LaRoche, Inc., Cranbury, NJ.

Azium (dexamethasone): Schering Pharmaceuticals, Bloomfield, NJ.

Chest Trocar and Cannula: Sherwood Medical Industries, Ltd., St. Louis, MO.

Continuous Recording Thermometer: Yellow Springs Corp., A.H. Thomas, Philadelphia, PA.

Cutdown Catheter: Becton-Dickinson, Rutherford, NJ.

CVP Manometer Set: Bard-Parker (division of Becton-Dickinson), Rutherford, NJ.

Foley Catheter: (8 Fr. Pediatric) Bard-Parker (division of Becton-Dickinson), Rutherford, NJ.

Goldberg Refractometer: American Optical Company, Buffalo, NY.

Injection Cap: Becton-Dickinson, Rutherford, NJ.

Intensive Care Oxygen Therapy Unit: Kirschner Scientific, Seattle, WA.

Intracath (through-the-needle catheter): Deseret Pharmaceutical Company, Sandy, UT.

Jet Humidifier: #217-6003-800 (oxygen humidification unit), Ohio Medical Products, Madison WI.

Longdwell Catheter (over-the-needle catheter): Becton-Dickinson, Rutherford, NJ.

Oxygen Analyzer: Biomarine Industries, Malvern, PA.

Pall Filter: Pall Corporation, Glen Cove, Long Island, NY.

Rubber Urinary Catheter: Sherwood Medical Industries, Ltd., St. Louis, MO.

Sphygomomanometer: 9068D Medisco Inc., Broadway, New York, NY.

Squeeze Bag and Non-rebreathing Valve: North American Drager, Telford, PA.

Temperature Pads: Gaymar Ind., Buffalo, NY.

Ultrasonic Doppler Flow Detector: Parks Electronics Laboratory, Beaverton, Oregon.

FLUID AND ELECTROLYTE THERAPY

CHARLES E. SHORT, D.V.M.
Ithaca, N.Y.

In using appropriate fluid therapy in small animals, it is important not only to apply scientific rationale to the utilization of various fluids to achieve the well being of the patient, but also to utilize appropriate methods of preparing the subject for receiving fluids and to monitor the patient properly in order to achieve the best results. In veterinary medicine, a wide range of approaches and rationale have been used. Some practitioners have even used alpha blocking agents to allow hyperhydration of individual subjects. In some instances, the overambitious utilization of fluids has continued past the time when the animal could adequately consume fluids orally. In other instances, appropriate analyses of electrolytes have been made and correct electrolyte and fluid therapy have been administered but without regard for the need to supply adequate calories.

Fluid therapy in small animal subjects is indeed a challenge. One of the initial problems that is encountered is the proper placement of catheters. Another is the maintenance of the animal in a position and in an environment in which fluids may be administered at appropriate rates over sufficient periods with adequate monitoring. One often finds that the predominant fluids that are administered to small animals are those that are given during anesthesia and surgery. This does not take into account the need for fluid therapy preoperatively, postoperatively, or in disease problems for which surgical intervention is not appropriate.

PLACEMENT OF CATHETERS

Prior to the placement of an intravenous catheter, the skin in the area in which the catheter is to be placed should be carefully prepared. The venapuncture site can be either in the neck region over the jugular vein or in the extremities in the area of the cephalic or saphenous vein. The principal problems of using the jugular vessel in the dog and cat are (1) difficulty in placement of the catheter and (2) maintenance of a patent catheter owing to the looseness of skin and the excessive amount of subcutaneous tissue that allows the catheter to move. This can frequently cause contamination of the catheter site, interference with fluid flow, or displacement of the catheter from excessive bending of the head, neck, or legs. After the catheter site has been chosen, a sufficient area of hair should be clipped so a sterile prep can be made and the catheter can be placed without contamination of the site or the catheter. The site is treated with iodine-type surgical prep materials in a fashion similar to that for a surgical procedure.

SECTION OF INTRAVENOUS CATHETERS

Two types of catheters are commercially available: the catheter over the needle and the catheter through the needle. The catheter over the needle enables the clinician to place a larger bore catheter in a given vessel, since the catheter is the largest object that will be inserted. The catheter through the needle results in a small catheter being placed in the vessel. In this case, when the needle is removed, some hemorrhage will occur and a hematoma will usually form. Commercially prepared catheters from companies such as Abbott, Johnson & Johnson, and Sherwood come in a wide range of sizes in both diameter and length. The normal size utilized for cats is listed as feline, or 22- to 18-gauge catheters. In the dog, small catheters may be utilized for small breeds, with up to 14 gauge possible in large subjects. The catheter is placed in a manner similar to that for an intravenous injection. The catheter is advanced with a needle in place one-half to one inch into the vessel. The needle is then held in place while the catheter is advanced over the needle into the vessel. It is maintained in position by the use of adhesive tape. We recommend that antibiotic or antiseptic ointment be applied at the junction of the catheter and the skin. The catheter may then be attached to the administration set for the intravenous fluid or may be capped after it has been filled with heparinized saline. If catheters are to be left in place for extended periods without fluids running, heparinized saline must be added to avoid clotting.

The catheter through the needle is enclosed

in a sterile plastic sleeve. The catheter is maintained inside the needle and the needle is placed through the skin, penetrating into the jugular vein while the head is extended. Then the catheter is pushed through the needle and advanced into the jugular vessel. Frequently, the catheter will enter the right heart before its full length can be advanced inside the vessel. When this occurs, it is advantageous to remove the metal stylus in order to allow flexibility of the catheter. The catheter should not be further advanced, as it will traumatize the cardiovascular system. In smaller animals, especially those with shorter necks, the shorter catheter over the needle may be utilized for jugular catheters as well. Once the jugular catheter is placed, antibiotic or antiseptic ointment should again be utilized at the junction of catheter and skin. The catheter should be taped in place and then bandaged. Efforts should be made to incorporate the hair on the opposite side of the neck into the bandage to assist in anchoring the bandage and to help prevent dislodging the catheter from the neck. The commercially available catheters that are used for jugular catheterization are usually easily placed. However, some of the brands (Bard) are relatively stiff and can be traumatizing. Other brands have a tendency to be soft and are prone to bend. With either type catheter, utilization for more than 48 hours is not recommended due to likelihood of contamination and phlebitis.

FACTORS TO BE CONSIDERED IN DETERMINING FLUID THERAPY

After the catheter has been placed, fluids are administered. A number of decisions have to be made about fluid therapy, including the type of fluid and electrolyte mixture to be used and the volume and rate of administration. One should also consider the tonicity of the fluid, the calories needed, the acid-base status of the patient, the extent of dehydration, and the status of cardiovascular and renal function. The route of administration is usually intravenous, since in most instances when the animal is capable of utilizing oral fluids, fluid therapy is not a major concern. With severe needs, parenteral fluids may be administered by injection and usually by the intravenous route. Subcutaneous or intraperitoneal routes are seldom satisfactory ways to maintain fluid and electrolyte balance.

Table 1 illustrates the composition of commonly used fluids. First, the patient's status of hydration is determined. Clinical dehydration can be observed after 5 percent or more of the body fluid has been lost. Below this level, it is clinically difficult to detect dehydration. At 5 to 6 percent dehydration, one will probably observe slight changes in skin condition and dry mucous membranes. From 7 to 9 percent, there is a definite change in the elasticity of the skin with a slow capillary refill time. At 10 to 12 percent dehydration, there will be pronounced changes in the elasticity of the skin with an incomplete return to normal position after it has been moved. At 12 to 15 percent dehydration, one may observe vascular collapse.

In addition to the outward signs of dehydration, laboratory determinations are of great benefit. The determination of plasma osmolarity or tonicity is of special value. The normal value is 288 to 305 mOsm/kg, and this increases as the animal dehydrates. The urine osmolarity in a normal subject will range from 500 to 1200 mOsm/kg. With extreme diuresis, one could expect 50 mOsm/kg, and with oliguria, the levels may rise to 2000 to 2400 mOsm/kg. If the level is more than 2400 mOsm/kg, there is a severe water deficit. The packed cell volume will usually increase during dehydration; however, one should not ignore the fact that changes may be the result of anemia. Total serum protein usually increases with dehydration also, but again, the animal may have sufficient fluids but be hypoproteinemic. One should also remember that obese patients maintain elasticity of the skin despite dehydration. It is also more difficult to determine the state of dehydration in long haired dogs and cats versus the short haired breeds because it is not as apparent. The patient should be weighed accurately before determining the amount of fluid to give.

DETERMINATION OF FLUID VOLUME NEEDED

After it is decided that the animal is dehydrated and should receive fluid therapy, three factors are important in determining the volume of fluid to administer: the maintenance needs, the existing deficit, and the continuing losses. In the patient with a normal temperature, an average volume of 44 ml/kg/day is satisfactory for fluid maintenance. If there is an elevated body temperature, fluid volumes should be increased by 50 percent so that the febrile animal receives 66 ml/kg/day for maintenance.

The continuing losses of fluid from tissue damage or fluid loss during surgery should be estimated. Urine output, usually from 1.0 to 2.2 ml/kg/day, should be considered part of continuing fluid loss.

After the volume of fluid needed has been estimated, the type of fluid needed is determined. Without knowing serum levels, one can-

Table 1. *Typical Intravenous Fluids and Their Contents*

FLUID	TOXICITY	CALORIES PER LITER	Na	IONS (MEQ) K	IONS (MEQ) Ca	Mg	Cl	BICARBONATE mEq
Lactated Ringer's	Isotonic	9	131	4	3	0	110	28
Dextrose 5% in half-strength saline	Hypertonic	170	77	0	0	0	77	0
Dextrose 2.5% in half-strength saline	Isotonic	85	77	0	0	0	77	0
Dextrose 2.5% in half-strength Lactated Ringer's	Isotonic	89	65	2	1	0	54	0
Normal Saline	Isotonic	0	155	0	0	0	155	0
Ringer's Solution	Isotonic	0	147	4	4.5	0	155	0
50% Dextrose	Hypertonic	1700	0	0	0	0	0	0

not calculate the exact amount of various ions necessary for therapy. Table 2 illustrates normal body fluids and electrolytes. When electrolyte determinations cannot be made, a balanced electrolyte solution is usually used. This is especially important, since giving excessive amounts of ions such as potassium can affect cardiac function and even produce cardiac arrest. Potassium should not be given faster than 5 to 10 mEq/hr. The contents of some of the commonly used electrolyte solutions are shown in Table 1 and may be selected according to the needs of individual subjects. In certain disease states such as diabetes, diarrhea, and chronic renal disease, one needs water, sodium, potassium, and bicarbonate, and proper evaluation is critical. In cases of chronic vomiting, chloride, sodium, potassium, and bicarbonate are need-ed, whereas in acute vomiting, chloride, sodium, and potassium are adequate. With a high serum sodium level, one should correct the dehydration with hypotonic solutions. With a low serum sodium, correct hydration is achieved with hypertonic solutions. If there are normal serum sodium levels, dehydration can be corrected with isotonic solutions. Intravenous fluids should be administered at body temperature when possible, especially if the rate is to be rapid.

RATE OF ADMINISTRATION

Fluids can be given rather rapidly by oral means in most instances. However, when fluids are administered intravenously, the rate is very important. The usual rate of 10 to 16 ml/kg/hr for intravenous fluids during the first hour is usually adequate. In hemorrhagic shock, whole fresh warm blood can be administered as rapidly as possible to correct the vascular volume deficit.

Caloric maintenance of debilitated subjects is frequently overlooked. The patient may have an adequate supply of fluid, but during the process of extensive nursing care, it can receive inadequate supplementation of its caloric needs. If an animal will consume appropriate food orally, this is the best route. However, this is not always possible. It requires approximately 7 calories/kg daily to prevent most body protein catabolism and 25 calories/kg daily to prevent both body protein and fat catabolism. Dextrose is the most commonly used substance for caloric supplementation by intravenous means. Preferably, dextrose should be used in 2.5 to 5 percent solutions. The 5 percent solution supplies ap-

Table 2. *Distribution of Body Electrolytes and Fluids**

	SERUM (DOG) mEq	SERUM (CAT) MEQ
Na$^+$	141.0–157.0	152.0–161.0
K$^+$	4.3–5.6	4.0–5.3
Ca^{++}	9.8–11.4	8.9–10.6
Mg^{++}	1.8–2.4	2.0–3.0
Cl$^-$	98.0–116.0	115.0–123.0
HCO$_3^-$	17.0–24.0	17.0–24.0

	ADULT DOG	PUPPY	ADULT CAT
Total Body Water	60% of body weight	75–85%	60%
Extracellular Water	20% of body weight	40%	25%
Intracellular Water	40% of body weight	40%	35%
Plasma Volume	5% of body weight		5%
Daily Water Intake	50 cc/kg body weight		64 cc/kg
Daily Urine Output	22 cc/kg body weight		22–33 cc/kg

*Laboratory values from N.Y.S.C.V.M. Values may vary geographically or in other laboratories.

proximately 0.2 calories/cc. When administering 5 percent dextrose, one should give no more than 10 ml/kg/hr to allow maximal utilization of the dextrose.

Monitoring fluid therapy

During the administration of fluids, one should constantly monitor the flow rates. The animal is usually not motionless and thus mechanical problems are inherent during the administration of fluids. In addition to the technical requirements for administration of fluids, the following are of benefit in determining appropriate fluid therapy.

1. The return of outward signs of alertness, elasticity to the skin, and other signs determined from gross physical examination are indications that hydration is improving.

2. The capillary refill time, mucous membrane color, pulse pressure, heart rate, heart sounds, and lung sounds are valuable physical signs that help determine if excessive fluids are being administered relative to cardiovascular and renal function.

3. The blood pressure (arterial and/or central venous) serves as a valuable index of fluid therapy. In reasonably healthy subjects in which there is good cardiovascular and renal function, there will be little need to monitor central venous pressure. However, in a shock-like state, if volumes of 40 to 100 ml/kg are administered rapidly, utilization of central venous pressure is of value to avoid excessive fluid volumes. When fluids are administered rapidly, there is a greater chance of producing pulmonary and cerebral edema.

4. Monitoring urinary output is valuable in long-term therapy, especially if high volumes are utilized or if renal dysfunction is suspected. Renal dysfunction may occur with normal kidneys if the animal is hypotensive. The hypotension may be pathologic or drug-induced, as when alpha blocking agents such as acetylpromazine are used. When peripheral resistance is reduced with the alpha blockade, extra fluids are sometimes necessary to maintain blood pressure. However, during this process, renal output may be decreased and the tendencies toward cerebral or pulmonary edema may be accentuated.

Special considerations

In animals with cardiovascular disorders, special care should include slower administration of intravenous fluids, and careful monitoring of central venous pressure, arterial pressure, heart rate, EKG, and fluid electrolyte balances. A separate catheter and infusion set should be used to administer cardiac medications for the control of heart rates, heart rhythms, or contractable force in congestive failure patients. Fluid therapy should be maintained through a second intravenous administration set that is not used for cardiac medications. This avoids the possibility of interfering with the dosage rate of cardiovascular medications.

Renal function is of special concern in fluid therapy. In patients suffering from renal disease, urinary blockage, or other obstructive and non-functional renal or urinary tract disease, fluid therapy should give consideration to renal function as well as to overall hydration needs. Excessive fluid therapy in patients in renal shutdown will contribute to edema, whereas diuretics in dehydrated animals will counteract the attempts at hydration. Giving excessive fluids to an animal with an obstructive urinary problem, a non-patent ureter, or a ruptured bladder can only contribute to increasing the amount of urine in the abdomen. Controlled fluid therapy is indicated until appropriate surgical procedures can be completed to assure restoration of a normal urinary tract.

The rate of administration of fluids and the total amount given to neonates is important. In most neonatal situations, the guideline of 4 ml/kg/hr for basic fluid therapy is appropriate, but additional fluids can be added for excessive losses. Small-sized adult animals and very young or very old individuals with renal or cardiac disease may be especially susceptible to pulmonary and cerebral edema if fluid therapy is not managed properly.

After fluid therapy

After fluid administration has been completed, the intravenous catheters should be removed and attention should be given to the condition of the catheter and whether there is any need for care of the skin site or for antibiotic therapy in cases of phlebitis. One should remove the catheter with care, making sure that the entire catheter has been removed and that the area has not been traumatized excessively. A local reaction or edema should be expected when there is extensive trauma to the catheter site or peripheral vein. In rare instances, one will observe slight degrees of edema in the paws due to obstruction of venous return.

SUMMARY

The appropriate utilization of fluids is frequently overlooked in small animal medicine.

Balanced salt solutions, with or without dextrose for the supply of caloric needs, in many instances will markedly improve the physiologic function of the debilitated animal. This improves the intravascular volume and supplies needed electrolytes and calories to reduce the need for the liver to convert fats and proteins to dextrose. By administering appropriate fluids, one may adequately maintain blood pressure and obtain a functional balance between interstitial and extracellular electrolytes. Fluid therapy does not involve expensive or impossible procedures. It can be monitored adequately in the average veterinary hospital. Following the guidelines given, fluids may be safely administered, even when serial electrolyte determinations cannot be made. Patients selected for fluid therapy should include those in which there is debilitating disease, dehydration, or other conditions in which fluids and/or metabolic needs are not being supplied by oral intake, or those animals that will be submitted to anesthesia and surgery.

SUPPLEMENTAL READING

Osborne, C. A., and Polzin, D. J.: Strategy in the Diagnosis, Prognosis and Management of Renal Disease, Renal Failure, and Uremia. Proceedings AAHA, 1979, pp. 559–619.
Wong, K. C.: Electrolyte Disturbance and Anesthetic Considerations. A.S.A. Refresher Course. Am. Soc. Anesthesiologists' Annual Meeting, October 1977.

PHYSICAL FITNESS AND TRAINING FOR DOGS

ROSS STAADEN, B.V.Sc.
Perth, Australia

Since training dogs and keeping them physically fit has become a basic concern to many owners, this article addresses itself to the etiology, signs, treatment, and prevention of clinical syndromes often associated with training and racing. Particular reference is made to greyhounds, sled dogs, and the gun-field-trial-hunting-retrieving-herding group.

BASIC PRINCIPLES OF TRAINING

When the body's systems are stressed by physical work, they respond in order to increase the capacity for that work and thus reduce the stress. By continuously stressing certain systems with a particular type of work, improvement in work capacity is obtained. This is the *training response*.

TRAINING RESPONSE RATES

Some anatomic components improve in performance much more rapidly than others. The slowest ones are the structural aspects of the cardiovascular and skeletal systems. Muscles exposed to frequent prolonged work show a steady increase in the number of capillaries per mm². After several months, the number increases over 100 percent, and it continues to do so at a lesser rate, probably for years. The capillary supply to the heart also increases, as does the size of the heart. The diameters of the aorta and major vessels increase, involving complete remodelling. The trabeculae in bones must remodel to cope with the new stresses and strains. Ligaments and tendons must become thicker, tighter, and stronger. All these slower components show great improvement in a matter of two to six months, with continued lesser improvement over an even longer period.

Muscle bulk might also be considered a slow component, but detailed work shows it has a much more rapid initial response than do the skeletal and cardiovascular systems, although it will go on increasing as they do if the work is severe. Size does not continue to increase in endurance training.

The rapid response component consists of the enzymes in the pathways that provide energy for the work of the muscle fiber. These enzymes show a dramatic response within hours and days and can be brought to a peak of activity in the human in about two to six weeks.

It should be remembered that these components tend to fall back at about the same rate that they increase. The dog being trained for the first time must be given several months of slower work to allow the slow structural components to build up; otherwise, the muscle strength and enzymic systems outstrip the "wind" development and also cause injuries to bones and ligaments not given enough time to strengthen. After a one-month spell from about six months of training, the dog will have the "wind" and structural strength but its muscles will have lost much of their strength and endurance. The rapidity of the response of the muscles, however, will allow the dog to be brought back, in about one month, to the level of fitness it had at the end of the first six months. After a three- to six-month spell, there will be a significant but not complete fall-off in the "wind" and skeletal systems as well, and the return to peak fitness will take two to three months, again beginning with one to two months of slow work to avoid injury.

SPECIFICITY OF THE TRAINING RESPONSE

The response to training is specific for the structure and its particular function and the rate and duration of its use.

Structural specificity is direct: exercising the legs will not strengthen the arms. Similarly, a particular muscle and indeed a particular fiber must be worked in order for it to respond. Most muscles consist of several fiber types, and whereas one type may be used for posture maintenance and low rates of work, others may be used only at high rates of work.

Functional specificity really refers to training the nervous system. It has been shown that a limb performing a particular task improves its efficiency and accuracy as the nervous control "learns" which fibers, how hard, and in what sequence to "fire." One need only watch the hind legs of some young dogs as they learn to gallop to see the improvement in proprioception and control. Electromyograms reveal great differences in the sequence and extent of fiber and muscle use in different individuals performing the same action.

Rate specificity can be explained in terms of two components, the structural and the enzymic. Stresses on bones and joints at a flat gallop are much greater than those at a walk. Range of movement is also greater. The necessary structural remodelling will not occur unless a small but increasing "dose" of this severe stress is applied. The enzymic component is related to the different energy sources used for different rates of running. At the fastest speeds, energy is derived from local concentrations of high energy phosphate bonds. Adenosine triphosphate (ATP) is broken down to adenosine diphosphate (ADP), which is immediately reconverted to ATP by reaction with creatine phosphate (CP). This CP supply runs low in a matter of perhaps five or ten seconds (precise figures are not known). The contracting muscle needs ATP. Energy for further conversion of ADP to ATP must now come from the breakdown of glycogen. If the rate is still as fast as possible, the mitochondria cannot handle all the pyruvate generated from glycogen. Much of it is converted to lactic acid, which in turn limits the extent to which the fiber can rely on this energy source. Running as fast as it can, a greyhound generates near the maximum tolerable amounts of lactic acid in a matter of 10 to 20 seconds. While it continues to produce lactic acid in small amounts, it is then forced to slow its running rate and breathe in more oxygen. This oxygen allows the mitochondria to take the pyruvate produced from glycogen and break it down to CO_2 and H_2O, both of which are easily disposed of, unlike lactic acid. In addition, large amounts of energy are produced for converting ADP back to ATP, allowing continued muscular work. At low running speeds (15 to 25 Km/hr^{-1} for greyhounds), sufficient energy can be derived almost solely from the use of oxygen by mitochondria. Such aerobic (derived from oxygen) energy pathways are improved by training at exercise rates below those speeds. They are also trained by higher speeds but less so because of the shorter duration of higher speeds. They are also trained by the recovery process after high-speed runs, although again, this is of short duration.

At high running speeds, the ATP and CP reserves and the breakdown of glycogen to lactic acid — none of which require oxygen (hence, they are anaerobic) — provide a proportion of the total energy, which increases with increasing speed. At maximal speeds over short distances (e.g., 530 M in 32 seconds in greyhounds = 59.6 Km/hr^{-1} *average* speed), aerobic energy probably provides less than 5 percent of the total energy during the race. It is very important to realize that the anaerobic pathways receive training for maximal rates only at maximal speeds and virtually no training at low speeds.

Duration specificity is harder to explain. If a sled dog is trained to run for 10 minutes at a rate within its aerobic limits, why can it not run for 1 hour or 10 hours at the same rate? At first, the factor might seem to be depletion of glycogen, but, in fact, fatigue sets in well before significant glycogen depletion occurs. In the endurance-trained muscle, fatty acid combustion increases as glycogen stores decrease; therefore, substrate depletion in the fiber is not the cause. It has been demonstrated in laboratory animals by various means that transmission fatigue at the neuromuscular junction, adrenal medulla depletion of epinephrine and norepinephrine, adrenal cortical depletion of steroid hormones, and anterior pituitary depletion of adrenocorticotrophic hormone (ACTH) are *not* at fault either. Certainly, there can be no build-up of excess waste products as in anaerobic exercise. Increased cell membrane permeability with loss of intracellular K^+ and phosphorus compounds are not limiting. The two main possibilities are summarized as the "sum total theories" and the "yet-undiscovered-weak-link theories." The sum total theories hold that the brain is affected by lowered levels of glucose, increased blood levels of K^+ and CO_2, and sensations from the muscles and joints, and eventually these add up to a feeling of exhaustion. Training resets the threshold for the feeling and minimizes the changes for a given amount of work. The yet-undiscovered-weak-link theories use as an example the demonstrated depletion of neurosecretory material in the hypothalamus of truly exhausted rats — this in turn means no ACTH release and no steroid release. It remains to be demonstrated as a factor in less exhausted animals, but the possibility remains and indeed would seem logical that some link in the brain's stress coping system gives out a signal to stop *before* serious depletion occurs. *Suffice to say that if you want a dog to run for minutes, hours, or days, it must be built up to training sessions of the same order.*

Overlap of specificity is an important point for trainers to understand. The oxygen transport system — lungs, respiratory muscles, heart, blood vessels, red blood cells — is fairly nonspecific. It can be trained to a high pitch (e.g., with swimming) and still make an equally good contribution to running, but the link between it and the different set of muscles used must be sufficient to allow full use of that oxygen uptake. If the capillaries of these muscles and their aerobic enzyme systems are not developed enough, the oxygen transport system's capacity will be only partially used. Perhaps the most important comparison would be walking and trotting as training for galloping. Certainly, the cardiovascular fitness can be increased greatly by prolonged walking or trotting, and this will carry over to galloping and the recovery from galloping. Electromyograms on dogs at the walk, trot, and very slow gallop indicate that the principal muscles used are the same in each, so that increased muscle tone and bulk will be in the right places. However, the high-rate anaerobic energy paths receive little training, and this

bears out the experience that trainers relying heavily on walking or trotting greyhounds have to give them a few slips, trials, or races to bring them to a peak. It is not known if slow work trains all or only some muscle fibers used at competition speeds in the sled dog or greyhound.

TYPES OF TRAINING

Many of the training methods discussed here are ideally suited to one type of dog but detrimental to others. Training schemes thus must be selected carefully (Table 1).

ASSESSMENT OF TRAINING METHODS

The usefulness of training must be assessed by consideration of many factors including (1) the stage of the dog's program, (2) specificity for the competition event, (3) jading/freshening effect on the dog, (4) cost in training time, (5) convenience, (6) feasibility in bad weather, (7) risk of injuries, and (8) past experience and results.

Walking is the most universal starter for dog conditioning. When the muscles, bones, and ligaments are ready, faster rates of work are applied. When the dog has been preconditioned by self-training in long pens or on a running lead, the walk stage may be shortened to

Table 1. Types of Training

Paced walking/running with or without a leash
    walking
    running
    cycling
    horse riding
    car/tractor or other vehicle.

Free running—beach, bush, golf course, etc.
Hunting
Slip without lure ⎫
Slip with lure   ⎬ *Greyhounds*
Short trial/race   ⎪
Long trial/race   ⎭

Walking machines
    treadmill type
    rotary clothesline type

Sledding—runners on snow ⎫ *Sled dogs*
    wheels   ⎭

Swimming

Young dogs
    long wire runs
    long lead running on long wire
    lure on pulley system ⎫
    lure on rod or rope   ⎬ *Greyhounds*
    retrieving stick or ball ⎭

two weeks, but a solitary dog should be walked for periods increasing from about 15 minutes by 15 minutes per week; i.e. 30 minutes/walk in second week, 45 minutes in third, etc. Although a dog can respond at this rate, novice trainers often cannot, and the program has to be slowed. The faster the walk, the greater and more specific the training effect. Most people can walk a dog at 5 Km/hr^{-1} (3 m.p.h.), but a dog trainer should strive for 8 Km/hr^{-1} (5 m.p.h.). People fit enough to jog or run should achieve better results, and the use of bicycles, horses, or cars can provide startling results if the dog is willing to run alongside. Care should be taken to stay well within the dog's aerobic running speed for prolonged work.

Free running and hunting allow dogs to exercise at a good rate, not being limited by a human. They will seldom over-train, unless they chase something too hard for too long. However, many dogs either fail to return to the owner or injure themselves in this type of training. It is too risky for proven money-winners.

A "slip" is a greyhound racing term referring to a short sprint. One person restrains the dog while another moves away some distance — 50 to 500 meters (usually about 200). The dog is released and it gallops to the second person, who may wave something to attract its attention or use a lure or squeaker. A squeaker is a child's rubber squeeze toy that makes a high pitched whistle not unlike that of a terrified rabbit. The sound is very stimulating to most greyhounds. As the greyhound progresses from slips to trials and races of greater distance, there is a pronounced hypertrophy of the longissimus group, so that the dorsal spines of the lumbar vertebrae appear to shorten and disappear and the posterior ribs appear to go up under a solid ridge of muscle. The development of these muscles, therefore, is structurally specific for the galloping action and can only be trained fully by galloping. A slip has high rate specificity, but because of its severity, it has a jading effect on the dog if used too often. Greyhounds are usually only slipped or raced two or at most three times per week, and injuries are frequent.

Treadmill-type walking machines allow large numbers of dogs to be trained even in very crowded suburban areas and in any kind of weather. Most greyhounds will only walk at 5 to 8 Km/hr^{-1} on a walking machine. The training effect can be increased by increasing the angle. Too much angle alters the pattern of muscle use as well as the angulation of the limbs, so that there is loss of many aspects of specificity. The optimal angle is not known, but 0 to 8 degrees (approximately 0 to 16 percent grade) appears to be the best range.

The ideal duration of treadmill walking and its training effect relative to those of walking are controversial. Some consider treadmill exercise to be equivalent to two, three, or four times that of walking, even with the treadmill level, at speeds and duration comparable to those for walking. This is hard to understand. Heart rate, recovery time, and oxygen uptake are almost identical in human studies, with significant difference only at high speeds when air resistance or drag becomes a factor in track running but not in treadmill running. Drag is proportional to the velocity squared. The author's observations are that walking is more stressful (1) in hot weather, (2) when the dog pulls hard on the lead (it rarely pulls when on a treadmill), and (3) when smells or sightings keep the dog excited. Treadmill work is more stressful (but not in multiples) when the angle is more than or equal to 3° (6 percent grade). However, there does appear to be a lower psychologic tolerance to treadmill walking, and many dogs can only be given one or two short spells per day of 5 to 20 minutes without becoming sour and dejected. One trainer has had dogs on the treadmill for 40 minutes twice daily without achieving success on the racetrack, although this lack of success could have been due to other factors.

Rotary walking machines with a central revolving upright and a number of "arms" to which the dogs are attached have not been extensively used because of space and hence expense of housing for all-weather use. The machines may or may not be driven. The radius varies tremendously, as they are usually custom built.

Sledding for sled dogs is ideally conducted on land similar to the competition routes. Runners are used in winter, but sleds with wheels are used for summer training. This sport is fairly demanding of the physical fitness of the driver, so it is important that he be trained too. Sledding, of course, is highly specific, and the entire team of 3 to 16 dogs can be trained at once, which is fortunate because of the long duration often required. Sled dog races vary from 10 miles, completed in approximately 31.5 minutes, through 20 miles in 65 minutes, 100 miles in 16 hours, and 1069 miles in 12 to 14 days. The season progresses with shorter races early and longer races later so that the actual races are an important part of the build-up in endurance (duration specificity).

Swimming is used in greyhounds and many of the "field-trial-gun" group to improve stamina and to act as a specific competition activity for many of the latter. The duration is controversial in greyhounds. Most successful trainers swim the dog for a maximum of four to seven minutes. However, one very successful bitch swam for 20 minutes, 5 mornings per week. All agree that it must be introduced gradually; e.g., one-minute sessions the first week, two minutes the second week, etc. Most agree that it slows a greyhound's racetimes for several weeks, and this must be kept in mind. It would be foolish to introduce swimming into a winning dog's program other than during a spell, although it can then be continued when the dog resumes racing. Relative value is put very high; 5 minutes swimming is equal to 20 to 45 minutes walking. Its greatest value lies in maintaining the aerobic fitness of dogs with leg injuries. In the breeds of the "field-trial-gun" group, many are prone to ear infections, and swimming in fresh water is often a causal or exacerbating factor.

Young dogs should be encouraged to play and exercise as much as possible within the limits of their maturity. One should be particularly concerned for the softer bones with grown plates close on either side of each joint. Long wire runs are good, and these are often arranged in "banks." Some breeders deliberately put them on a slope or across a gully or hollow. Lengths and widths vary, but most are in the range of 10 to 100 M long by 2 to 10 M wide. With perhaps two pups or a whole litter per pen, and 2 to 10 runs alongside each other, there is much running up and down. Each pup is self-paced. The partitioning helps avoid injuries, bullying, and unequal food distribution, especially when pups' ages vary. Running young hunting dog kennelmates together, especially if they are of unequal ages, is thought to encourage "hooking" and should be avoided. "Hooking" is chasing the other dogs rather than seeking game independently. The solitary pup in a rural homestead situation can be allowed a lot of exercise by attaching its lead to a loop that runs on a wire stretched between uprights. Severe neck injuries are a possible problem but can be avoided by using a roading harness rather than a collar. Greyhound owners often have line training systems that build up the pup's endurance and strength. The best are pulley systems (sometimes geared) whereby the lure is dragged to and fro from an overhead wire of perhaps 20 M length. The easiest are lures on the end of a fishing rod and line that the trainer flicks about with the pups dashing in pursuit. This is particularly good for teaching balance and developing joints to take awkward strains. Bird wings on a fly rod and line make excellent lures for hunting dogs.

Retrieving is commonly used in the training of the field-trial-gun group and domestic pet dogs. A ball or stick is thrown (sometimes into water) and retrieved until tiredness or boredom strikes the dog or owner. Some greyhound trainers believe it risks making the greyhound "people oriented" instead of "lure oriented" and therefore should not be used in the greyhound pup.

MANAGEMENT OF TRAINING

STARTING OFF

Training begins as soon as the dog can walk. The more exercise it gets while young, the better the development of its oxygen transport system. Young animals show a more rapid response than do older animals. The owner of one or several puppies can do a lot to encourage free running and can take them for long walks so that by the traditional or "commercial" starting age (12 to 18 months for greyhounds, 4 to 6 months for field dogs, 6 to 12 months for sled dogs), his dogs are better developed and appear to have more natural talent than those that have not yet begun training.

Trainers and breeders with large numbers of pups have to rely on long pens or paddocks. The dogs are virtually self-paced in their development. Prior to breaking in, the young dog begins training in earnest. All dogs should be walked on a lead, starting with 2 to 4 Km (1.2 to 2.4 M) depending on the fitness of dog and handlers. The pace should be around 5 Km/hr^{-1} (3 m.p.h.) for the first week. The distance is built up to 3 to 8 Km (1.8 to 5 M) and the pace to 6.5 to 8 Km/hr^{-1} (4 to 5 m.p.h.). This build-up should take six weeks in a dog that has been totally unexercised (e.g., reared by itself in a family backyard). Some youngsters are almost up to this at the outset and have no trouble completing the program in two weeks. Sled dogs and trial, hunt, field, and retrieving dogs are then "hard enough" for breaking in. The gallopers (greyhounds, whippets, Afghans, salukis) require a steady program of high-speed running after initial handling by walking. The dog should preferably be given the chance to gallop freely. This usually means pre-dawn expeditions to golf courses, football ovals, beaches, or parks. The dog is set free, and after a prescribed time, it is recalled and taken home. Hazards include the disappearance of the dogs in full cry after some object of interest. However, free galloping is excellent as preparation for track sprinting and as regular training if the situation permits. When track sprinting begins, the dog should be slipped between two handlers twice per week, beginning at 50 to 100 meters. It progresses to two slips of 100 M and one of 300 M per week and eventually to the trial track. At this stage, a greyhound's recovery should be watched very carefully. Some dogs chase so hard they can only be used as sprinters; i.e., for runs of up to 450 M. Others chase hard but can run up to 600 M without taking more than three or four days for recovery. Dogs that can race over 600 to 1000 M without prolonged recovery are not common, and many dogs must be watched very carefully after their first attempts at an increased distance. It is in this beginning phase of training that most failures are weeded out. The most common cause for culling greyhounds is failure to chase the lure. Some have no instinct to kill or to chase a small, fast-moving object. Some have one trait only; e.g., it will kill but not chase or vice versa. Some accomplished winners will chase keenly but show little interest in the lure when it stops; i.e., they are non-killers.

Sled dogs, because they can be controlled to some extent (rate control is a matter of degree and sometimes impossible) build up from 3.6 to 4.8 Km (2 to 3 M) to perhaps 16 to 32 Km (10 to 20 M) of harness work per day.

INCREMENTS

Increments in workload can be small daily increases or larger weekly or fortnightly increases. The rate of increase can be decided by a predetermined plan from past experience or by the dog's recovery time. These have been described respectively as the "trainer leads" approach and the "dog leads" approach. Usually, the latter is slower but does not risk jading the dog. Problems arise when large numbers of dogs are involved. If ten greyhounds are walked from the back of a tractor, some may be limited by slower dogs that are probably not going to be the kennel's breadwinners anyway. Does the trainer step up to a higher speed and leave the slower ones at home? Does he split them into two groups and double his time load? Very similar problems arise in sled dog training and racing where teams consist of 3, 5, 7, or 12 to 16 dogs. In this case, slower dogs can "welch" a little, but nevertheless, they cannot be forgotten, as can slower greyhounds, because greyhounds race individually. With sled dogs, the poorer performers may "go down" in the harness, bringing the team to a standstill.

DURATION AND INTERMITTENCY

Duration of training should be as long as possible at low speeds to improve the oxygen transport system. Duration at high stressful speeds should be as short as possible to obtain the desired training effect. At race speed, some people use a rule of thumb fraction (two-thirds).

That is, a dog racing over 300 M will be slipped over no more than 200 M, whereas a dog running 750 M will be slipped over no more than 500 M. Some say that no dog needs to be slipped more than 300 M and that the only differences should be in the duration of slow work. Studies of duration specificity and highly anaerobic work do not at present discount or support either theory, probably because what one group gains in duration specificity, it loses in jading effects.

Intermittency refers to break-up of work and recovery in one session. Does 5 Km in one hour have the same or stronger effect than two lots of 2.5 Km in one half hour with a ten-minute rest in between? More importantly, does a 300 M slip have greater value than three 100 M slips with rest periods? The aim is to maximize the animal's rate for the enzyme systems involved without reaching a distressing level of hypoxia or lactic acid. For this reason, the minimum "slip" must deplete higher energy phosphate stores and force the lactic acid rate to its maximum. Total lactic acid production is kept low. Blood sampling after runs of 10, 15, 30, 45, and 60 seconds of running indicates that in a greyhound that runs really hard, 300 M is an adequate slip (this dog will be a natural sprinter). Greyhounds that run well but more like a natural distance dog require 400 M. Some very poor triers simply do not maximize lactate production at all, but these would not reach the racetrack.

Aerobic work in humans has been shown to require a minimum of 12 minutes to have a significant training effect. Break-up of aerobic work for greyhounds probably does not detract too much, provided each session is greater than 20 minutes. However, in sled dogs, it would cause a loss of duration specificity to break up the sessions into periods shorter than the event. Gun, trial, bird, hunting, and retrieving dogs perform intermittent work, and so intermittency may even help — i.e., it can be more specific.

FREQUENCY

Frequency refers to the number of training sessions per week. The week is the most convenient period because the minimal frequency for a training effect appears to be more than once per week. One training session per week is useless, perhaps detrimental. Most of the training effect is lost by the next session. The more frequent the training, the greater the response, provided there is no structural break-down or mental fatiguing. In man, the minimal frequency for progress is three times per week for aerobic work; preferably (and possibly optimally) five to seven times per week. Such studies have not been done in the dog but experience shows that aerobic work in walking can be beneficial in greyhounds up to any human limit. The standard of five miles at 5 m.p.h. (8 Km at 8 Km/hr⁻¹) morning and night is beyond most trainers who must rely on walking machines. Some trainers of distance greyhounds will walk them a considerable distance at a slower rate the morning of and morning after a race. Sled dogs also benefit from increased frequency of sessions.

The frequency of anaerobic work is determined by the animal's recovery time. Severity should be cut down to bring the animal's full recovery (alertness and keeness) to some fractional cycle of its racing program. A greyhound that recovers fully in two days can be slipped twice during the week between races. Others take four days, so that only a very short slip can be used midweek. A few barely recover in time to be raced once per week. The ideal is a dog that recovers quickly enough to be raced two or even three times per week, in which case only walking is necessary.

In Florida and several other parts of the world, the track is privately owned and has contracts with a small number of trainers who have 20 to 200 dogs in their care. These are the only trainers allowed to race dogs, but their contract stipulates the approximate number of starters they must contribute to each race, meeting, and season. Because of the number of dogs per trainer, even allowing for helpers, they rely on frequent racing and slips to keep the dog fit. Once the dog is fit enough to be slipped, walking is dropped from its preparation. These dogs have successfully met the other extreme of preparation, that of the Irish dogs, many of which receive five or ten miles of walking morning and night, five to seven days per week with minimal fast work. Between these extremes, the successful preparations are many and varied.

ADJUSTMENTS DUE TO JADING, ILLNESS, SORENESS, AND INJURY

Adjustments depend to some degree on the overall situation, although jading, illness, and severe injury always require rest. Soreness and mild injuries are approached in a variety of ways. Some dogs receive frequent treatment from veterinarians or from manipulators ("musclemen" or dog chiropractors). Others are treated at home with a variety of massage, hydrobath, ultrasound, faradic, and heat treatments. Trainers with many dogs frequently cannot afford too much time per dog, and the dog often has to race itself sound or fall by the wayside. This approach can be surprisingly successful but is not advisable with any dog showing potential. The lesson, however, is that with many injuries, the dog needs to perform at maximal speed before the healing scar tissue has hardened. Dogs confined during healing of a muscle tear are apt to be unable to move the adjacent joint(s) or the muscle through its full range. The training program setback can often be minimized by a change to swimming which, in the case of jaded, sore, or injured dogs, makes a change and is virtually non–weight-bearing. While in the water, the legs can be manipulated through their full range to minimize restriction by scar tissue.

Hunting dogs running on ice, rocks, or heavy stubble may develop sore or ulcerated foot pads. Many trainers toughen the pads with tannic acid preparations and protect the feet with plastic agents.

Severe illness can result in the loss of a considerable part of previous training results. Loss of muscle mass, demineralization, and restructuring of bone can mean starting again from the beginning. Where illness is not a factor, the return to peak should take about the same or a little less time than the dog's time out. The maximal time to return to peak should be two to three months; there is only a slow drop-off after the first two to three months out of training.

VARIATION VERSUS REGULARITY

Theories differ as to the contribution of a regular routine to the mental well being of the animal. Some individual animals achieve their best on a rock-rigid routine, whereas others quickly lose interest. Some very talented dogs have required a lot of ingenuity to keep them keen. The simplest approach for convenience is to train by routine and to introduce variety if the dog loses interest. Failure to respond to this probably indicates a sour type of dog that is best culled. A word should be said about the adverse or slowing effects of changes. When first introduced to swimming or belt-type treadmills, dogs often perform poorly on the track for several weeks. Changes should therefore be made in blocks of time of three or more weeks. Attempts to do something different every day of the week have not had good results. Swimming and treadmilling should probably be used three or four times per week minimum or not at all.

TYPICAL TRAINING PROGRAMS FOR GREYHOUNDS

"Slow work" means 5 to 9 Km (3 to 5.4 m.p.h.) for greyhounds. Dogs should be walked about 10 minutes to empty the bowel and bladder when the dogs are not worked.

Sprinter racing (up to 450 M) once a week:

Day	Slow Work	Fast Work
1	None	Race
2	None	
3	1 × 3 Km (1.8 M)	300 M
4	1 × 3 Km (1.8 M)	
5	1 × 3 Km (1.8 M)	200 M
6	1 × 3 Km (1.8 M)	
7	None	

Middle distance (450 to 650 M) dog racing once a week:

Day	Slow Work	Fast Work
1	None	Race
2	2 × 5 Km (3 M)	
3	2 × 5 Km (3 M)	
4	1 × 5 Km (3 M)	400 M
5	2 × 5 Km (3 M)	
6	1 × 5 Km (3 M)	200 M
7	2 × 5 Km (3 M)	

Distance (650 to 1000 M) dog racing once a week:

Day	Slow Work	Fast Work
1	None	Race
2	2 × 8 Km (4.8 M)	
3	2 × 8 Km (4.8 M)	
4	1 × 8 Km (4.8 M)	400 M
5	2 × 8 Km (4.8 M)	
6	1 × 8 Km (4.8 M)	300 M
7	2 × 8 Km (4.8 M)	

For a distance dog using swimming, substitute a 4 to 7 minute swim for one of the walks on each day that it walks twice. For a distance dog using a treadmill, substitute 20 minutes on the treadmill for one of the walks on each day that it walks twice. For training without slow work, use fast work as in the schedules given with an extra 50 to 100 M in each case.

CLINICAL SYNDROMES ASSOCIATED WITH TRAINING (OTHER THAN MUSCULOSKELETAL)

PHYSIOLOGY AND BIOCHEMISTRY OF RECOVERY

At the completion of a 15 to 60 second race, a greyhound has generated a considerable oxygen debt. In shorter races, that debt is mainly due to high energy phosphate depletion. Very heavy breathing in the first two or three minutes of recovery allows sufficient oxidation of gly-cogen and lactic acid to repay this debt, called the alactacid debt. The lactacid debt, however, is a much more complex and serious component of the oxygen debt. During very high rates of exercise, lactic acid production within the muscle cells plunges the pH downward while chemical reactions and mechanical work raise the temperature and osmotic pressure. These changes threaten the integrity of the enzymes and structures of the cell. Lactic acid diffuses out of the cell into the bloodstream, which also helps dissipate the localized heat. The blood pH falls, despite a rapid breathing off of CO_2. After a 30 second run, a very keen greyhound may reduce its venous blood pH to 6.8 to 6.9, which is considered the lower limit for proper body functions. The base excess may be −25 to −30 mEq/L. Lactic acid rises from under 20 mg percent pre-race to up to 270 mg percent five minutes post-race.

It is worth noting that it takes three to seven minutes after a 30 second run for the blood lactic acid to peak. Immediately after the run, the dog breathes very hard, and by one to two minutes, it has paid back most of the alactacid debt and may appear as though it could not blow out a candle. Then, as the lactic acid pours out of the muscle, the dog begins to breathe very heavily, more to blow off CO_2 than to take up oxygen. Blowing off CO_2 helps to minimize the fall in pH. The lactic acid may take one half to several hours to be cleared from the body. Most is converted back to glycogen in the muscle. Some is converted to glycogen in the liver, thence to glucose in the blood stream, and back to the muscle to become glycogen once more. The energy for these processes comes from combustion of part of the lactic acid (5 to 15 percent) to CO_2 and H_2O. Suffice to say that the muscle cell and to a lesser extent the whole body are subjected to a severe stress by lactic acid, heat production, and osmotic changes.

The critical factors in recovery from sled dog racing are probably more related to the central nervous system and its links to the pituitary, ACTH, and the adrenal glands. Depletion of glycogen may be a factor as it is in man after prolonged running, although as will be discussed in the diet section, it may be that man and dog differ considerably in this regard.

Selection has produced many dogs in which the will to win exceeds the dog's ability to withstand the stresses. Many greyhounds will run themselves into a suicidal condition, particularly over the longer distances. Conversely, there are dogs that have ability but are "programmed" to run at less stressful speeds. (These probably represent a type that would and did survive in the wild.)

CLINICAL SIGNS OF OVER-TRAINING/RACING

The clinical signs of over-training/racing are a matter of degree. Slight over-training — excessive long distance aerobic work or too many short slips — will cause anorexia, disinterest, and very slight dehydration. Severe overtraining will cause anorexia, depression, diarrhea, and moderate dehydration. Acute overracing will cause syndromes that vary from normal quietness for one or two days afterward through anorexia, diarrhea, and dehydration to the disastrous dehydration-acidosis-myoglobinuria complex.

"CLINICAL SIGNS" OF UNDER-TRAINING

"Clinical signs" of under-training are difficult to detect on examination unless they are gross. The animal is happy, healthy, and alert because it has been under-stressed. In the case of a greyhound with insufficient fast work, the lack of bulk in the longissimus muscles may be an indication. However, during the race, the under-trained dog usually (but not always) fails to keep up with the other dogs. After the race, the dog may be extremely distressed and its recovery may be slow. The symptoms after a race are the same as those for over-training/racing. The difference is that they were brought on by a speed, distance, and conditions with which a properly prepared dog would cope. Sometimes, dogs have had plenty of training but of an inappropriate type. Examples of inappropriate training would be programs with slow work only prior to a full-length race.

SYNDROMES ASSOCIATED WITH TRAINING

Many dogs, particularly the greyhound, Afghan, saluki, Irish setter, and great Dane, show an inability to maintain or gain weight when in training. Blanket treatment for worms or fecal worm float and tapeworm treatment (since they do not show on flotation) are rarely successful. Trypsin tests on feces will be negative in a few cases, as in pancreatic insufficiency. A few cases are borderline, and these may or may not respond to digestive enzyme supplements. One is usually left with a skinny dog that is also a little bit listless — with no obvious cause for its condition. (Irish setters may be quite hyperactive with a tendency toward yellowing and drying of the coat and fracture of the longer hairs so that color, gloss, and length are unsatisfactory.) Occasionally, the diet has been lacking in caloric density and/or the environment has been too cold. Cold housing leads to other complications, notably diarrhea — as the quantity of food is increased to try to put on weight — and sores and ulcers on the elbows, hocks, and carpi due to prolonged peripheral vasoconstriction in order to conserve heat. The diagnostic feature is the onset of the problem in autumn, and its disappearance in spring. It is worth noting that the dogs do not necessarily shiver a lot. Shivering is a short-term reaction replaced by heat generation by other means. The major source of extra heat is believed at present to come from "futile" cycling of the ATPase Na^+ transport system in cell membranes, induced by the thyroid gland. Other than with heating, the only success the author has had with any of the dogs in this group stemmed from the use of anabolic steroids such as laurabolin or vebenol (CIBA-GEIGY), 10 to 50 mg in the greyhound intramuscularly every two to six weeks. The response can be dramatic. Demeanor, coat, condition, and performance improve within one or two weeks.

Persistent or frequent diarrhea can be a problem. Gastrointestinal upsets are a recognized sign of over-training in man. In dogs, it appears more frequent when the caloric density is low — i.e., the bulk required to give sufficient calories is too great. This is particularly a problem of rations with high cereal content. Kennel routine can also be at fault, especially if commercial dry foods are used. Over-feeding by only 20 to 50 percent will produce a very watery movement that sometimes persists when proper feeding is continued, and only corrects with 12 to 24 hours of fasting.

Persistent or frequent anorexia can be a problem with dogs that are winning or performing well. They lose condition and disrupt training and racing. Appetite stimulants are largely unsuccessful. Anabolic steroids may help, but in highly motivated dogs, they sometimes decrease track speed. Anabolics have their greatest success in the lightly built, "sooky" type of dog. Vitamin B-12 injections have been used by some trainers for race conditioning. Stimulation of appetite may explain its claimed success.

Dehydration is an interesting facet of training. It is easily "guesstimated" by the time taken for the skin to return 90 percent to normal position after it has been pinched up from the body. A stopwatch makes the measurement quantifiable. In healthy dogs not in training, the return is less than one second; in healthy dogs in training, one to two seconds. If return takes two to four seconds, the dog should receive special treatment or a spell. If it takes more than four seconds, the animal is usually obviously ill. Severe dehydration is a major component of the dehydration-acidosis-myoglobinuria complex.

Dehydration-acidosis-myoglobinuria complex is generally agreed to be one group of disorders with slight clinical variations but similar basic causes. (See also page 783.) In all these conditions, a single run precipitates a steady decline, which may end in death in one to seven days or a prolonged recovery. Causal factors include (1) under-training (especially with novice trainers), (2) hot and/or humid conditions, (3) excessive pre-race excitement, and (4) a better than usual effort by the dog.

A typical severe case would be a dog that runs a race under one or several of these conditions and within half an hour exhibits hunching and soreness when touched. By 12 hours, the dog is dehydrated, depressed, and hunched in pain, and is passing dark brown, greenish, black, or reddish brown urine. By 24 to 48 hours, it has lost 2 to 5 kilos, owing partly to "melting" of the longissimus muscles and partly to dehydration. The eyes have sunken in and the coat is harsh. Less severe cases show severe dehydration and weight loss over two to seven days without the pain, myoglobinuria, and longissimus muscle loss. SGPT, SGOT, CPK, and LDH are extremely elevated and decline slowly over one to two weeks. To distinguish between myoglobinuria and hemoglobinuria (both give positive benzidine tests), one examines the plasma. If a carefully drawn and centrifuged (i.e., unhemolyzed) sample is clear, the urine pigment is myoglobin. If the plasma is pink, the urine contains hemoglobin. Treatment is basically that for hypovolemic shock. Large amounts of intravenous fluids are given to correct dehydration and help perfuse the myoglobin through the kidneys. Alternating Hartman's solution with $NaHCO_3$ solution has been the most commonly used regimen. Some dogs will not rehydrate in spite of large volumes, and plasma or serum transfusions can be used if such dogs show low plasma proteins.

The use of glucocorticoids is controversial; some authorities claim better results with and others without. The already severe catabolic breakdown of muscle cell proteins would seem to contraindicate steroids. However, in massive intravenous doses—e.g., dexamethasone* 40 to 60 mg—steroids have an alpha-blocking (vasodilator) effect on the vasculature and stabilizing effects on the damaged cell membranes. Anabolics (e.g., laurabolin) should be given to halt the catabolism, especially if glucocorticoids are given. Broad spectrum antibiotics should be given, as death has been attributed to overwhelming bacterial septicemia. Good results

have been claimed with oxygen and muscle relaxants in the early acute case and with vitamin E during recovery.

When the animal is not eating (the food and water should be raised because of neck pain in severe cases), the IV fluids should include glucose/dextrose, amino acids, and vitamins. Alternatively, one of the balanced standard maintenance fluids can be used.

The polydipsia-polyuria or water diabetes syndrome has also been a problem. This has much in common with the dehydration-acidosis-myoglobinuria syndrome. The causes are similar—a high speed run with greater than usual stress or inadequate preparation. Many dogs are believed to have been given glucocorticoids to improve race performance.

The dog's appearance is similar to that in the mild acidosis-dehydration case, showing anorexia, weight loss, dehydration, and poor coat. The main differences in this instance are the excessive water consumption (9 to 20 L/day) and the copious low SG urine, free of dark coloring. Urine SG varies from below 1.01 up to 1.02. Cooper has divided cases into those that are: (1) pitressin responsive, (2) ACTH responsive, and (3) DOCA responsive. (2 and 3 may also respond to anabolics.)

Cramping or tying up can have a wide variety of claimed causes. These include (1) diet too high in carbohydrate, (2) salt deficiency, (3) vitamin C deficiency, (4) vitamin E deficiency, (5) vitamin B group deficiency, (6) insufficient training, and (7) too much training. Cramping or tying up has appeared with changes in diet or training programs and disappeared with a return to the previous regimen or after further alteration. Some trainers have had cramp problems in the same or other dogs at the same time as they have had problems with acidosis-dehydration-myoglobinuria complex, and they regard cramping as a warning sign of that syndrome. The standard approach to cramp is to step up all the vitamins in the diet, to add or increase the alkaline salt fed in food or water, and to prepare the dog more slowly, but more soundly.

DIET AND PERFORMANCE

MINERALS AND VITAMINS: MINIMUM VERSUS MEGADOSE

There are two basic schools of thought on vitamins and minerals. One group believes that a certain minimal amount of each vitamin is required and the extra is totally wasted. The other believes that performance is improved in

---

*Dexsolone, V. R. Laboratories, Sydney, Australia.

some proportion, however small, by increasing amounts of each vitamin (particularly certain B group vitamins).

In racing, the difference between the winner and third place is usually less than 1 to 3 percent in power output (speed), so even a tiny improvement can have dramatic results. Unfortunately, controlled trials under race conditions are rare and measure only 5 to 10 percent differences. Since these large differences cannot be found, speculation follows. One group points out that most athletes (human and animal) receive increased vitamins and minerals before stepping onto a track. The second group agrees but maintains that they are given as "make-sure" placebos. Without controlled, race-condition experiments the debate will not be resolved.

PROTEINS

The turnover of amino acids in muscle is dramatically increased with work. Physical work increases the requirement for protein. The minimum for dogs is put at 22 percent of dry weight. Successful greyhound rations are usually 24 to 32 percent protein, sometimes more. In sled dogs, Kronfeld et al. (1977) found that performance improved with protein levels up to 53 percent without any sign of renal or hepatic problems.

ENERGY: CARBOHYDRATES VERSUS FATS

It was generally presumed that there was a minimal requirement for carbohydrates in dogs to maintain blood glucose and liver and muscle glycogen. However, Kronfeld et al. (1977) and Hammel et al. (1977) have demonstrated that huskies can not only survive without carbohydrate but perform better without it. Humans become ketotic and die without some carbohydrate. Ketosis was not seen in the dogs, even though the only carbohydrate was glycogen in the meat (less than 1 percent).

Kronfeld's group raced sled dogs on a variety of diets. Initially, a high carbohydrate diet was tried because of its success in human athletes. Performance was worse in dogs, however, and the dogs showed fasting hypoglycemia, tying up (rhabdomyolysis), and coprophagia. Eventually, a ration with less than 1 percent carbohydrate, 53 percent protein, and 46 percent fat proved superior. It approximates the huskies' historic staple diet — seal meat.

Greyhounds, on the other hand, have traditionally been fed little or no fat, except that present in lean meat. The rationale is that fat makes fat, which is weight to be carried. Pre-sumably, experience showed slower times on high fat diets, because otherwise, its cheapness and high caloric density would make it almost obligatory.

Possible explanations for the empirically derived success of high fat, low carbohydrate diets in sled dogs and the reverse in greyhounds include the following:

Dietary form affects the form stored in the body. Since greyhounds probably rely on glycogen for almost 100 percent of race energy, they need it stored as glycogen, which can easily be formed from carbohydrate and proteins but only from a small fraction of ingested fats. Ingested fat becomes stored fat, which is extra weight only.

Sled dogs presumably rely on metabolism of free fatty acids, but to what extent is unknown. Human endurance runners begin using predominantly glycogen, but after perhaps two to six hours, they are using mainly fats. As carbohydrates are readily converted to fat, it would not seem necessary for them to be ingested as fat.

High dietary levels increase the body's use of fat or carbohydrate and thus prepare the appropriate enzyme pathways used in exercise.

Evolutionary adaption. The prey available to the husky (fish, seals, birds) are all rich in oils, fats, and proteins and have little carbohydrate. In the regions in which greyhounds evolved, there would be less fat on the prey because the climate is hot rather than cold. However, they would not have been very high in carbohydrate unless the intestines were eaten. It would be interesting to test the tolerance (and performance) of greyhounds on a diet of 46 percent fat.

Caloric density. The caloric intake of sled dogs living in a very cold climate (a factor between races) and running for prolonged periods would have to be very high. The volume required to produce satiety would not contain enough calories unless it was high in fat.

Fat is appetizing. Sled dogs can burn fat during racing so they can eat it with impunity, and it may be that whatever will tempt an exhausted dog to eat between runs is what will keep it going and give the best results.

What is the ideal energy source for the dogs between these extremes? Dogs used for hunting, retrieving, and herding are probably using both glycogen and fats. They may not be adapted to the high protein and fat diet. Recommended approximate levels for these dogs are:

Protein	25–50% (preferably 30–40%)
Fat	10–40% (preferably 25–35%)
Carbohydrate	10–30% (preferably 10–20%)

Glycogen rebound. In man, it has been demonstrated that after extreme glycogen depletion of a muscle fiber (by exercise), if a diet rich in carbohydrates is fed, the fiber's glycogen level rises appreciably above the pre-exercise level. Diets low in carbohydrate greatly slow repletion even to pre-exercise levels. High glycogen levels in muscle have been shown to stave off fatigue. This is applicable to middle- and long-distance runners only. Glycogen is stored as a granule complete with the enzymes that break it down so the number of granules may be more significant than total concentrations. Sprinters produce little or no depletion of glycogen, so it is not a factor. The role of glycogen in sled dogs is uncertain, but if glycogen depletion occurs, it would be interesting to study repletion on the high protein, high fat, no carbohydrate diet. Presumably, gluconeogenesis (production of glucose and hence glycogen from proteins) would be the major contributor.

SALTS IN THE DIET

Replacement of Losses. During exercise, horses and man control their temperature by secreting a fluid for evaporation. The fluid carries sodium with it, resulting in sodium depletion if only water is being replaced. When sodium depletion reaches certain levels, the animal ceases sweating freely, its temperature rises, and it either stops exercising or becomes overheated and may die. Feeding extra salt for extra work or exercise has thus become a widely accepted maxim. The need for extra NaCl in dogs has not been demonstrated. However, in dogs, as in humans and horses subjected to prolonged exercise, there is a marked drop in serum phosphates and magnesium. Calcium drops to a lesser extent. The extent to which these are lost to the system — e.g., in urine — rather than simply shifted into another fluid compartment is uncertain. It would be wise to include these in any supplement.

Pre-race Base Excess. Exercise, particularly exhaustive exercise, creates an acid load. The creation of a base excess prior to the beginning of exercise has been shown to decrease fatigue and allow a greater rate or longer duration of exercise. This is usually done by oral dosing with "alkaline salts" such as $NaHCO_3$. In addition, such salts have been shown to hasten the recovery process. Most of this work has been done with humans as subjects, and unfortunately, the roles of body sodium, sweating, and body temperature were not considered at the same time. Nevertheless, serial blood pH measurements clearly indicate a marked effect on body acid-base balance as the main cause of the beneficial results.

Typical Electrolyte Powders. Powders fed to greyhounds:

Mixture No. 1

NaCl	40 gm
KCl	5 gm
$NaHCO_3$	30 gm
$MgCl_2$	5 gm
Ca gluconate	5 gm
Dextrose monohydrate	15 gm

Mixture No. 2

NaCl	25 gm
Na citrate	20 gm
$NaHCO_3$	20 gm
KCl	10 gm
$MgCl_2$	5 gm
Ca gluconate	5 gm
Dextrose monohydrate	15 gm

N.B. Both mixtures lack phosphates, but presumably the dietary supply is sufficient. These mixtures are given mostly in drinking water but also as an oral drench or on food at rates varying from 15 to 100 gm/day. Given with food, they would tend to neutralize stomach acid, be lost in the acid-base fluxes of digestion and metabolism, and lose their effect in the time between the last meal and the race. Administered in the drinking water or in divided doses as a pre- and post-race drench would seem to be optimal.

Possible Deleterious Effects. Some veterinarians believe large amounts of NaCl can cause a diuresis sufficient to cause dehydration, while alkaline salts are described as "leaching electrolytes from the body." Major problems in resolving questions in this area are the lack of detailed research and the impossibility of obtaining the formulas of common proprietary electrolyte mixtures.

SUPPLEMENTAL READING

Greyhounds. Proceedings No. 34, 1977, Postgraduate Committee in Veterinary Science, University of Sydney, Australia.

Hammel, E. P., Kronfeld, D. S., Ganjam, V. K., and Dunlap, H. L. Jr.: Metabolic responses to exhaustive exercise in racing sled dogs fed diets containing medium, low or zero carbohydrate. Am. J. Clin. Nutr. 30:409–418, 1977.

Kronfeld, D. S., Hammel, E. P., Ramberg, C. F. Jr., and Dunlap, H. L. Jr.: Haematological and metabolic responses to training in racing sled dogs fed diets containing medium, low or zero carbohydrate. Am. J. Clin. Nutr. 30:419–430, 1977.

CRYOTHERAPY

R. E. HOFFER, D.V.M.

Park City, Utah

Cryotherapy or cryosurgery are terms that refer to the controlled application of cold to living tissue in order to produce necrosis of specific tissue. The resulting tissue death is referred to as cryonecrosis. Cryotherapy is relatively new to the veterinary profession but has been utilized in human medicine for a number of years. Cryosurgery is becoming more popular within the veterinary profession as newer and less expensive units appear.

ACTIONS OF CRYOTHERAPY

The object of cryotherapy is to kill all the cells of a given lesion while producing only minimal damage to the healthy tissue. Tissues are killed by both direct cellular destruction and anoxia secondary to alteration of the microcirculation. Tissue susceptibility to freezing depends upon the density of the tissue and its blood supply. The degree of cellular destruction depends upon the rate of cooling, the final temperature, and the rate of thaw. The mechanisms producing cellular damage are:

1. Extracellular ice crystal formation. This draws water out of the cell into the extracellular space, producing a higher concentration of electrolytes within the cell resulting in electrolyte shifts, cellular dehydration, and collapse of the cellular membrane.
2. Intracellular ice crystal formation. After rapid freezing, during the slow thawing period, these minute crystals fuse into larger crystals resulting in damage to cellular organelles.
3. Denaturation of lipid protein complexes. The complexes that exist in cell membranes are damaged by the increased electrolyte concentrations resulting in loss of integrity of these cell membranes.
4. Thermal shock. This is cellular damage produced by temperatures below 0°C but not the result of crystal formation.
5. Microcirculation destruction. After the tissue has thawed, there is a brief period of vasoconstriction that is followed by vasodilatation. Embolic and thrombus formation occurs within a few hours after thawing. Arterioles and capillaries are permanently damaged, but larger vessels continue to function.

The most efficient way to produce the most cellular destruction is a rapid freeze with the temperature reaching −25°C followed by a slow thaw. Some cells will survive the initial freeze, and for this reason, a second freeze is necessary to obtain maximal cryonecrosis. Even with two freeze-thaw cycles, some cells at the periphery of the lesion may survive.

EQUIPMENT

The type of equipment utilized is dependent upon the cryogens that will be utilized. The two most common cryogens used in veterinary practice are liquid nitrogen (−195.6°C) and nitrous oxide (−89.5°C). Liquid nitrogen is the more effective cryogen, producing more rapid freezing and greater tissue penetration, and it permits spray freezing of a lesion. However, nitrous oxide is effective with small lesions. Machines are available that utilize these cryogens, ranging in price from $125.00 to $10,000.00. The cost of the machines dictates what cryogen is utilized and the capabilities of the equipment. The author prefers the large liquid nitrogen units in that they are more versatile and permit treatment of larger lesions by either probe or spray freezing.

Most nitrogen units come with a variety of probes and spray attachments to be used with different lesions, species, or areas being frozen. A good unit should be versatile and able to handle small or large lesions.

A pyrometer is also necessary. This measures temperature within the tissues and allows the operator to determine accurately the width and depth of the cryolesion. Pyrometers are available with up to four thermocouple channels. For most cryosurgical procedures, a two-channel pyrometer is adequate.

TECHNIQUES

Probe freezing and spray freezing are the two most common techniques. A third method that has been used is to pour liquid nitrogen directly into the lesion. This is used mainly for bony lesions. The disadvantage is that there is very little control of the freeze with this method. Before beginning the freeze, the lesion should be biopsied. In some cases, debulking of

65

large neoplasms is indicated to reduce the amount of time necessary to complete the procedure. When debulking the lesion or taking a biopsy, some neoplastic tissue should always be left at the site. Although not proven, there is an indication that cryotherapy of certain neoplasms has some immunologic effects, especially in relation to recurrence of the neoplasm.

PROBE FREEZING

Probe freezing is indicated with smaller neoplasms or fistulas. If the lesion is too large for a single probe freeze and is not amenable to spray freezing, the probes may be used at two or three sites, to be sure the entire lesion is frozen. Remember that multiple probe freezing requires more time.

Prior to freezing, the thermocouples are placed at the periphery of the lesion and at the deepest part of the lesion. The cryolesion should extend for 5 mm into normal tissue. If freezing visually, only about two-thirds of the visible ice ball will slough. The probe may be touched to the surface of the lesion or inserted in the center of the lesion, usually in the area from which the biopsy was taken. A freezing bond should occur between the probe and the tissue being frozen. The area is frozen to −25°C at the periphery and at the deepest part of the lesion, allowed to thaw, and refrozen to the same temperature. Remember that the area closest to the probe will be colder than the periphery of the lesion.

SPRAY FREEZING

Spray freezing is most effective for lesions that are not thick but have a wide surface area. Debulking will often permit more efficient spray freezing. Again, the thermocouples are placed at the periphery and at the deepest part of the lesion. The area not being frozen is protected by a thick covering of vaseline gauze. While spraying an area with liquid nitrogen, run-off will occur and can adversely freeze normal tissues below the lesion. The area is frozen to −25°C, allowed to thaw, and refrozen. If the area is larger than the spray generated, the operator has to move the sprayer evenly over the lesion. It is important to do this with a circular motion in order to cover the lesion evenly. Since the thermocouples are only measuring two sites, if even motion is not maintained, one area on the lesion could be −25°C and the other −10°C.

The area begins to swell after the first thaw and continues to be edematous and red for the first 48 hours. Dogs may be more prone than other animals to lick and bite the area during that period. Later, large masses undergo necrosis with an unpleasant odor. Owners should be told of this before the animal is discharged. Usually, a clean granulating tissue bed will be present by the tenth day. Complete healing depends upon the size of the original lesion. During the healing phase, the dog will lick the lesion; however, if this is not excessive, it is of no consequence. Owners are instructed to keep the area clean. Antibiotics are usually not necessary during the postoperative period unless a body cavity was invaded or there are other problems of infection.

INDICATIONS

Cryosurgery is utilized in situations in which excisional surgery will not produce a good result. Cryosurgery with closure by third intention produces more of a scar than does primary healing following a clean incision. Also, hair that grows back at the site may be a different color.

Cryosurgery can be utilized where excessive hemorrhage may be anticipated, as in capillary hemangioma. It is also effective when there are lesions on the lower leg that obviously will not close following excision. Skin grafting, especially pinch grafting, may be used to increase the speed of epithelization of a cryolesion. Cryosurgery has been employed for treatment of the following conditions in veterinary medicine:

1. Oral and pharyngeal neoplasia. Often it is used for palliation rather than cure.
2. Skin neoplasia. Cryosurgery is used for benign and malignant lesions. It seems to be very effective in treating squamous cell carcinomas.
3. Nasal tumors. It is utilized after the masses have been removed and is applied by spraying into the nasal cavity.
4. Rectal neoplasia. Probe freezing is best for these tumors.
5. Perianal fistulas.

Cryotherapy is similar to any other surgical procedure. It requires the operator to be completely familiar with the equipment, the lesion, and the effects of the cryogen on the lesion. This requires practice on the part of the operator in order to obtain the best end result.

SUPPLEMENTAL READING

Greiner, T.P., Lisha, W.D., and Withrow, S.J.: Cryosurgery. Vet. Clin. North Am. 3:565–581, 1975.
Withrow, S.J., Greiner, T.R., and Lisha, W.D.: Cryosurgery: veterinary considerations. JAAHA 11:271–282, 1975.
Zacarion, S.A.: *Cryosurgery of Tumors of the Skin and Oral Cavity.* Springfield, Charles C Thomas Company, 1973.

PREVENTIVE MEDICINE IN KENNEL MANAGEMENT

LAWRENCE T. GLICKMAN, V.M.D.

Ithaca, New York

KENNEL VERSUS CLINICAL MEDICINE

Veterinarians responsible for the health of large commercial kennels must be proficient in methods of clinical medicine as well as in principles of community medicine. The practicing veterinarian is primarily concerned with the prevention, diagnosis, and treatment of diseases in individual animals, and with the psychologic relationship between pet and owner. The kennel veterinarian must also be an epidemiologist whose main interest is in the frequency and distribution of diseases or physiologic conditions in a population of animals and in the factors that influence this pattern. He should understand economics and be competent enough to perform benefit-cost analysis for any preventive or therapeutic programs that he recommends to his clients.

Astute observation and rational medical decision making are the keys to successful kennel management. The veterinarian, or in his absence the kennel manager, must observe and record on a regular basis any abnormal clinical behavior and laboratory findings. Dynamics of disease processes in kennel populations can be monitored by noting dates of onset of clinical signs; number, age, sex, and location of affected animals; and any changes in management practices. This data can often be used to determine incubation time, mechanism of transmission, and possible source of the problem, and it may enable identification of specific etiologic agents.

Dependable and quality laboratory support is essential for accurate diagnosis. Arrangements should be made to insure access to routine diagnostic services for hematology, serum chemistry, clinical immunology, parasitology, bacteriology, virology, serology, gross pathology, histology, and special services such as electron microscopy. Both private and state diagnostic laboratories are often willing to enter into contractual agreements at a nominal cost.

The objective of surveillance is to identify specific disease problems in order to determine their cause, or if this is not possible, to define important environmental and host risk factors. The ultimate goal must be control or prevention of disease rather than treatment thereof. In general, because of economic factors, the role of therapy in kennel management is inversely proportional to the size of the colony.

DISEASE PREVENTION IN KENNELS

Preventive medicine is the dominant theme in kennel management and may be divided into two major categories: primary prevention and secondary prevention. Primary prevention refers to reducing the incidence of disease by altering susceptibility or by decreasing exposure for susceptible animals; secondary prevention is the early detection and treatment of a disease in order to reduce its severity. Secondary prevention should ideally be applied in the preclinical stages of disease and is clearly less desirable than primary prevention in kennel situations.

Approaches to primary prevention in the kennel can be directed toward the infected animal, the mode of transmission, or the potential recipient of infection. The rationale for isolating and treating animals showing clinical disease is obvious, but the reasons these fail to contain the spread of infection are often overlooked. For most infectious agents, the spectrum of host response is wide, and some animals do not develop clinical disease following infection (inapparent infection). These animals, however, are an important source of infection for other dogs and may shed large numbers of organisms into the environment. Also, for many infectious diseases, the period of maximal shedding and communicability precedes the clinical signs. In both situations, isolation procedures are ineffective in preventing transmission.

Recognition and interruption of the mechanism of transfer of disease organisms plays an important role in kennel programs. Many vector-borne or fecal-oral transmitted diseases can be prevented or controlled by changes in cage design or improvements in sanitation and hygiene. In contrast, for respiratory diseases spread by aerosol, environmental intervention is often unrewarding.

Finally, and perhaps most important, prevention can be directed toward the potential recipient of infection. These methods can be either specific — where efforts are made to decrease the animal's susceptibility to a particular disease by immunization (i.e., distemper, hepatitis) or by genetic selection (i.e., hip dysplasia, collie eye) — or non-specific — where the objective is to enhance the general resistance of all animals by an improvement in nutrition or by a decrease in environmental stress.

These principles of preventive medicine will be discussed with regard to specific management practices and to the diseases of major importance in commercial colonies of dogs for research. They are equally applicable to the professional breeder of registered stock for show purposes or for resale to pet shops and private owners.

GENERAL MANAGEMENT

Day-to-day management decisions and personnel problems are the responsibility of the kennel owner, but the veterinarian should actively participate in long-range planning and in the orientation and training of new employees. This is essential for persons who will be involved in the daily monitoring of animal health, record keeping, using laboratory procedures, or treating sick animals. The increasing availability of trained animal techicians provides an excellent resource that has proven to be cost-efficient. Routine preventive visits, at least monthly, are required to review health records, to observe the animals, and to discuss specific problems. More frequent visits, however, are often the rule.

The ideal situation is to maintain the kennel as a closed colony in which all breeding stock is selected from within the colony and in which dogs that leave the premises are not allowed to return. Selection factors for breeders will depend upon specific desirable breed characteristics and on the intended use of the offspring. Culling of breeders due to unsatisfactory performance or medical problems should be a regular practice. If it is absolutely necessary to introduce outside dogs into the kennel, they should be vaccinated, thoroughly examined, checked for internal and external parasites, and quarantined in separate facilities for a minimum of three weeks. Before release from quarantine, they should be reexamined and determined to be healthy.

Prior to transport from the kennel, all animals should be screened by rectal temperature measurement and receive a thorough physical examination, including auscultation of the heart and lungs. Appetite and feces must be noted, and any "suspect" animal should be observed for several days prior to shipment. It is not unusual for apparently healthy animals to be shipped and to arrive sick, only because they were incubating a disease that could have been detected upon departure.

ENVIRONMENTAL CONSIDERATIONS

Environmental factors are a major contributing cause to skin, respiratory, and gastrointestinal diseases. Unfortunately, environmental conditions vary widely from kennel to kennel, and it is often economically unfeasible to suggest radical changes in cage construction and ventilation systems. It is, however, the veterinarian's responsibility to see that cage size meets the space recommendations for domestic species proposed by the Department of Health, Education and Welfare in the "Guide for Care and Use of Laboratory Animals" (Table 1). For the prevention of fecal-oral transmitted infections, cages should be suspended and floors should be constructed of woven wire mesh to allow droppings and urine to pass freely. Whelping cages require a partially solid floor and a supplementary heat source, such as a heat lamp, to keep the temperature at cage level above 85°F.

Often, simple improvements in ventilation and sanitation can produce a dramatic reduction in morbidity. Ambient temperature in dog houses must be kept above freezing to guarantee availability of drinking water, although mature dogs can be successfully housed in outside pens year-round if water is provided regularly. Concrete floors are preferable to dirt or gravel floors and should be cleansed daily. Automatic watering systems obviate the need for daily cleaning and sanitizing of water bowls, but even these systems should be flushed weekly with an appropriate disinfectant, and the nipples should be checked to insure that they are functioning. Fans are necessary in dog houses for adequate exhausting of inside air and mixing of outside air. The number of complete air turnovers required per hour is dependent upon population density. If there is an odor problem or if the relative humidity is greater than 70 per cent, the ventilation is probably unsatisfactory. Manufacturers

Table 1.   *Space Recommendations for Dogs*

WEIGHT	TYPE OF HOUSING	FLOOR AREA/ANIMAL (SQUARE FEET)	HEIGHT (IN.)
Up to 15 kg	Pen or run	8.0	—
15 to 30 kg	Pen or run	12.0	—
over 30 kg	Pen or run	24.0	—
up to 15 kg	Cage	8.0	32
15 to 30 kg	Cage	12.0	36
over 30 kg	Cage	°	°

°These recommendations may require modifications according to the body conformation of particular breeds. As a general guide, the height of a dog cage should be equal to the height of the dog at the withers, plus at least 6 inches, and the width of the cage should be equal to the length of the dog from the tip of the nose to the base of the tail, plus at least 6 inches. (Guide for Care and Use of Laboratory Animals, DHEW Publication No. (NIH) 74–23, (1974):37.)

of ventilation equipment should be consulted for exact specifications.

As a general rule, several different areas or buildings are required. These include a whelping house, which can be combined with a weaning area, a holding area for bitches and studs not currently being used, a quarantine facility for new dogs entering the kennel, an area for dogs awaiting shipment, and an isolation ward for sick and potentially infectious animals.

Often neglected in planning the environment are the social and psychologic requirements of the animals. Even germ-free animals require regular human contact for normal social development and well being. It is important, therefore, that some personal attention be given to individual dogs on a regular basis if they are to be useful for research or as pets. Dogs should be culled for antisocial behavior as well as for health problems.

NUTRITION

Good nutrition is an essential component of any preventive medicine program. Nutrient requirements differ from breed to breed and vary with age, activity level, environmental conditions, and physiologic state (i.e., pregnancy, lactation, weaning). This information has been summarized by the National Academy of Sciences-National Research Council (NAS-NRC) in its Publication 989, "Nutrient Requirements of Dogs." Often overlooked, however, by zealous breeders is that overnutrition and obesity can reduce resistance to viral and bacterial infections and can lead to osteochondral changes in growing dogs. Therefore, over-supplementation is to be avoided.

Nutrition of the puppy begins *in utero* and reaches a critical stage at birth. Adequate colostral intake is perhaps the single most important measure in protecting the health of the neonate. All puppies should be observed immediately after whelping, and non-nursing puppies should be assisted. If litter size is large, smaller puppies should be transferred to foster mothers. Following weaning at six to seven weeks, puppies are again segregated by size and sex to minimize competition for food.

Most commercial dog foods are manufactured using the NAS-NRC recommended allowances as guidelines, and they are avilable in three forms: dry, semi-moist, and canned. The main difference among these is their water content, texture, palatability, and cost. We recommend a good quality commercial dry food, either alone or mixed with canned food as a maintenance diet. The evaluation of total nutrient content can be made from the manufacturer's complete chemical analysis, and it should be matched to the NAS-NRC recommendations. All-meat canned diets should be avoided. Since cost is an important factor, breeders often add chicken or meat supplements obtained from slaughterhouses. These are good sources of animal protein, and we prefer that all such foods be thoroughly cooked. Puppies can be started on moistened dry puppy chow at three to four weeks and weaned at six to seven weeks on the standard diet. All dogs are fed at least twice daily, and any leftover food is removed from the bowls. Puppies should be fed more frequently if weight gains are unsatisfactory.

At four weeks of gestation, feeding of the bitch is increased by 20 per cent compared with maintenance requirements, and at six weeks, it is increased by 75 per cent. During lactation, the bitch is fed *ad lib* with total food consumption often increasing by two to three times. Sick animals are fed more palatable rations of higher caloric density, and cooked rice is added to the diet of dogs with diarrhea. Dietary changes are kept to a minimum, and each diet is evaluated by dog acceptance and performance.

RECORD KEEPING

Systematic recording of medical information is an often overlooked component of kennel management. Essential to any record system is the early identification of individual animals by either eartag or tattoo. Information is recorded on cards attached by clipboard to each cage and includes (1) physical characteristics (both normal and abnormal); (2) behavioral traits such as barking and submissiveness, (3) breeding performance including litter size, stillbirths, number of puppies weaned per litter, sperm counts, heat periods, growth rate (weight), and (4) other characteristics that vary by breed. All vaccinations, medications, and treatments are noted by date and type. Laboratory data can be kept separately in log books with the animal identification, date, test procedure, and results.

The method of data storage will depend on the size of the kennel. Mini-computers have been decreasing in price, and some manufacturers offer software packages for billing and inventory control that can be adapted for processing medical information. Regardless of method, some mechanism must exist for collating data from individual animals.

Animal records provide information on baseline or "normal" values for laboratory measurements, growth rates, and breeding performance; and they are used to establish expected patterns of morbidity and mortality for individual kennels. Any deviation from baseline is considered to be a cause for concern. For example, in most kennels, mortality is highest during the first two weeks of age and shortly after weaning (Fig. 1). A change from this normal pattern would indicate introduction and spread of a new disease or an environmental problem. Breeding records have been used to trace genetic problems back to individual dams or sires and to evaluate changes in management or nutrition.

Vaccination is the best example of disease-specific primary prevention. The recommended program includes routine vaccination for distemper, hepatitis, leptospirosis, and parainfluenza virus (Table 2), all of which are available as a combined vaccine. While some people recommend vaccination with measles virus in puppies less than six weeks of age because it is not as sensitive to the blocking effects of colostral canine distemper virus antibody as is canine distemper vaccine virus, it is not required in kennels in which bitches are vaccinated annually for distemper and transfer significant levels of antibody to their puppies. It is a good policy not to administer any modified live virus vaccines to pregnant bitches.

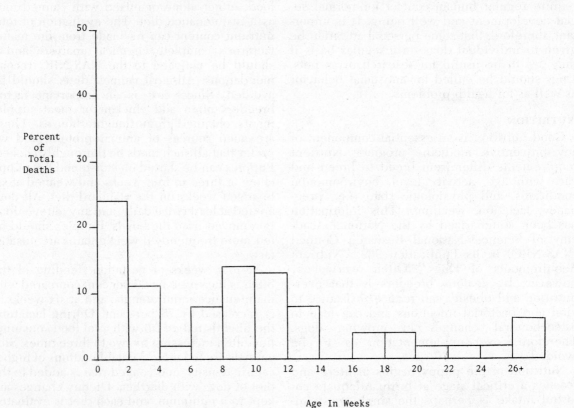

Figure 1.   Age Distribution of 71 Deaths in a Kennel—January, 1979 (Excludes Stillbirths)

Table 2. *Recommended Vaccination Schedule In Commercial Kennel*

VACCINE	TYPE OF VACCINE	SCHEDULE		
Routine		*First*	*Second*	*Booster*
Canine Distemper Virus (CDV)	Modified Live	8–9 wks.	12 wks.	Annual
Infectious Canine Hepatitis (CAV-1)	Modified Live	Given with CDV combined vaccine		
Canine Parainfluenza Virus (SV-5)	Modified Live	Given with CDV in combined vaccine		
Canine Leptospirosis	Bacterin	Given with CDV in combined vaccine		
Optional				
Rabies Virus	Modified Live	3–4 mos.	1 yr.	3 yrs.
Bordatella	Autogenous Bacterin	2 wks.	5 wks.	6 mos.

Rabies vaccination should be routine in open colonies, in kennels in which dogs are housed outside, or when specifically requested by the purchaser. Autogenous *Bordatella* bacterin, when administered at two and five weeks of age, has significantly reduced the mortality and morbidity associated with tracheobronchitis. The use of autogenous bacterins is especially effective in closed colonies for skin, gastrointestinal, and other respiratory problems in which the same bacterial pathogen is isolated consistently.

In general, approximately 90 per cent of all puppies at eight weeks of age will have sufficient levels of maternal antibody to protect against a challenge. However, since this level will vary from kennel to kennel, we recommend establishing nomograms on a yearly basis or before a new vaccination program is introduced. These serum samples, if deep frozen, also provide an excellent resource for monitoring the introduction of new infectious agents into the colony.

PARASITES

Ectoparasites. Fleas, ticks, and mites are common in large dog colonies, but these external parasites are not a problem once they are brought under control. The preventive program consists of twice-yearly dipping (spring and summer) of all dogs older than three months of age with a lindane solution (Para Dip®) and spraying of the dog houses. The kennel help routinely observe dogs for ear scratching or wax buildup or discharge, and if ear mites are found microscopically, the ears are flushed with hydrogen peroxide and treated twice, ten days apart, with a solution of three parts mineral oil to one part Canex.®

Demodectic mange is caused by a facultative pathogen that is present on a significant percentage of apparently healthy animals. If nutrition is adequate, demodectic mange is not a serious clinical problem. In closed colonies, clinical mange may indicate an underlying cell-mediated immune deficiency or other disorder and, if this is so our recommendation is usually euthanasia.

Endoparasites. The goal of endoparasite control depends on the ultimate use of the dog, and this in turn dictates the intensity of control efforts. Subclinical parasitism may be acceptable in animals for sale to pet shops, whereas migrating parasites that cause permanent tissue pathology are unacceptable in animals for research or toxicity studies. Since antihelminthics are of doubtful efficacy against the tissue stages of most parasites, the emphasis should be on elimination of adult worms from the gut and interruption of the life cycle. The latter is best accomplished by using wire mesh cages that allow feces to pass through and by frequent waste removal. Any commercial kennel should have its own laboratory with personnel trained to perform both direct fecal smears and fecal flotation techniques. The former is essential for accurate detection of protozoan parasites and tapeworm ova. The feces of all puppies starting at three weeks of age and a random sample of adult dogs should be examined by both methods. The design of a specific parasite control program will depend on the prevalence and type of endoparasites that are observed.

Toxocara canis, Strongyloides stercoralis, Ancylostoma caninum, and *Filaroides hirthi* are rarely the cause of clinical disease in closed colonies, but they can produce lung damage. *T. canis* is effectively controlled by the administration of piperazine to all breeding stock four times a year and to puppies at ten-day intervals from three to twelve weeks of age. Despite using this regimen for many years and finding negative fecals in bitches prior to breeding, an occasional litter of puppies is still infected with *T. canis* and a majority of bitches have detectable antibody to *Toxocara*.

With adaquate cage design and sanitation, hookworms and whipworms can be eliminated; the treatment for ancylostomiasis or trichuriasis is dichlorvos. Identification of *S. stercoralis* is by the appearance of larvae in the feces, and thiabendazole appears to be the treatment of choice. *F. hirthi* is endemic in some closed breeding colonies in which the adults cause extensive granulomatous reaction in the lung parenchyma. Since larvae passed in the feces are immediately infective, sanitation alone is not sufficient to prevent transmission. Either dogs must be housed individually or bitches must be treated; albendazole is effective but not yet available commercially in the United States.

Tapeworms are not a problem in well managed colonies and can be prevented by routine dipping for ectoparasites and by rodent control. In kennels in the North, or where dogs are housed indoors, heartworm prophylaxis is not required, but blood samples should be examined by the Knott's technique for microfilaria at least once a year.

The most common protozoan parasites are the *Coccidia* and *Giardia sp;* these are best identified on direct fecal smears. *Giardia sp.* may be found in 25 per cent of all dogs in a closed colony, but giardiasis rarely is a recognizable disease entity. If *Giardia sp.* is found in a dog with diarrhea, we reommend treatment with Flagyl® at a dose of 25 mg/kg B.I.D. per os for five days. Coccidia infection is not uncommon in asymptomatic puppies, but it may cause clinical disease if animals are stressed by transport, weaning, or other infectious agents. Treatment of coccidiosis with Furadex® or the sulfonamides usually results in termination of oocyst shedding and uneventful recovery. Amprolium in the drinking water (one or two tablespoons of a 9.6 per cent solution per gallon of water) and in the feed of puppies for seven days has been recommended as a preventive measure prior to shipping, but this is usually not necessary in kennels in which sanitation and waste management are adequate.

Symptomatic and supportive fluid therapy are indicated for severe diarrhea regardless of cause.

DISEASES OF KENNEL DOGS

A necropsy examination should be performed on all animals that die, including those that are stillborn, and the findings should be recorded in a log book. The gross pathologic examination should be supported by histopathology, bacterial cultures, and virus isolation when indicated. Despite adherence to such a program, as many as 50 per cent of all deaths may still remain unexplained.

As a general rule, puppy mortality before weaning can be expected to range from 5 to 30 per cent. During the first week after birth, most deaths are attributable to stillbirths, physiologic immaturity, congenital abnormalities, and trauma. After the first week, the major causes are gastrointestinal disease and pneumonia. Morbidity is highest around weaning, with respiratory and gastrointestinal disease most common. Anorexia and dehydration resulting from these illnesses are life threatening and present the greatest challenge, especially when many dogs are simultaneously affected. Trauma and reproductive problems are the major concern in mature dogs.

DISEASES OF THE NEONATE (<3 weeks of age)

FADING PUPPY SYNDROME (TOXEMIA, SEPTICEMIA)

Deaths that occur during the first three days of life are not typically associated with viral diseases. The terms *acid milk syndrome, toxic milk syndrome,* and *puppy septicemia* have been used to describe clinical syndromes during this period, but most often the cause is unknown. Toxic milk syndrome is characterized by bloating, greenish diarrhea and a red, swollen anus. The condition is attributed to incompatibility of neonatal puppies to bitch's milk. The bitch is apparently healthy and milk supply is adequate. Treatment consists of placing the puppies in an incubator at 90° F and giving 5 per cent dextrose in Lactated Ringer's orally until the bloat has subsided. The puppy is then returned to a foster mother or is handfed a commercial formula (Esbilac). This condition has been associated with uterine subinvolution in the bitch, and routine administration of oxytocin following whelping appears effective in reducing the incidence.

Puppy septicemia is characterized by crying, bloating, hypothermia, cyanosis, weakness, failure to nurse, and death within 48 hours after birth. The signs are often insidious, but once apparent, they are rapidly progressive. Frequently, the whole litter is involved. Postmortem findings include intestinal distension and congestion. Careful examination of the bitch often reveals a fever, metritis, vaginitis, or mastatis. The bitch and the intestinal tract of the puppy are cultured and treated accordingly with systemic antibiotics. The organisms most frequently isolated are *E. coli, Streptococcus, Staphylococcus,* and *Klebsiella.* Prevention consists of culling the bitch or initiating treatment with antibiotics at the time of breeding and prior to whelping.

PUSTULAR DERMATITIS

This condition can occur in puppies any time before weaning and may affect the entire litter. Pustules develop on the head, face, and neck, but any area can be involved. High humidity and poor sanitation are contributing factors. The causative organism is a *Staphylococcus,* and treatment with an iodine shampoo (Betadine®) followed by topical Furacin® ointment is effective.

TRAUMA

Poor mothering by an inexperienced bitch is the major cause of trauma in neonates. When fetal membranes are improperly removed, evisceration, umbilical herniation, hemorrhage, or cannibalism may result. Hemmorhage is further complicated by the fact that newborn puppies are borderline hypoprothrombinemic. Salvageable puppies are treated by clamping and suturing of the umbilicus, application of a pressure dressing, and parenteral administration of vitamin K (Synkavite®).

PUPPY VIREMIA (HERPESVIRUS)

Several viruses have been implicated in puppy viremia, but only canine herpesvirus is a recognized cause of neonatal illness and death. The disease is most common in puppies one to three weeks of age, but occasionally it occurs in puppies up to five weeks. Viremia is associated with the period during which the puppy's temperature is optimal for herpesvirus replication (95° F to 96° F). Healthy puppies become acutely ill, stop nursing, and cry continuously; death occurs within several hours following onset of signs. In puppies that recover, the virus may remain latent for several months, and shedding can recur following corticosteroid therapy. Diagnosis is based on clinical signs and by the pathognomonic hemorrhagic foci on the kidneys

at postmortem. Treatment consists of placing affected puppies in an incubator at 100° F and 60 per cent relative humidity for several hours, followed by incubation at 95° F for 24 hours and the administration of oral fluids. The entire litter is usually infected at birth by maternal secretions, but infected bitches may give birth to normal puppies on subsequent whelping. Culling of herpes-infected bitches is not routinely done, and the problem tends to be sporadic.

CONGENITAL ANOMALIES

Stillbirths, physiologic immaturity (runting), and physical abnormalities may account for up to 40 per cent of all early neonatal deaths in kennels. Congenital defects can be either inherited or acquired as the result of exposure to infectious or toxic agents *in utero.* When such defects are noted, breeding records are examined to determine if a particular bitch or sire is implicated, or whether there is an association with drugs administered to the bitch during pregnancy. Prevention is by removal of the offending agent. Cleft palate and hydrocephalus are common congenital defects, but this will vary by breed and management practices.

THERAPY IN THE NEONATE

Regardless of cause, most neonatal diseases are characterized by hypothermia, dehydration, and hypoglycemia. Therefore, standard procedures that require a minimum amount of effort and cost should be established for the treatment of neonatal puppies. A human infant incubator is relatively inexpensive and can accommodate several litters. Temperature should be maintained at 85 to 90° F, relative humidity at 55 to 60 per cent, and oxygen concentration at 30 to 40 per cent. Dehydration is corrected by the oral administration of 5 per cent glucose at hourly intervals and with subcutaneous Lactated Ringer's solution at a rate of 150 ml/kg of body weight per day. Once the rectal temperature reaches 95° F, hypoglycemia is treated by providing caloric intake with a milk replacer (Esbilac) at frequent intervals.

DISEASES OF THE PUPPY

GASTROINTESTINAL

Vomiting and diarrhea are commonly observed in kennel dogs during the weaning period and tend to be self-limiting. The signs may be related to dietary factors or environmental stress. Of the infectious causes of gastrointestinal disease in puppies, viruses (e.g., coronavirus and parvovirus), bacteria, and intestinal parasites should be considered. Parasites are not an important factor in well managed kennels, and bacteria are often a secondary problem.

Our initial approach to any gastrointestinal illness consists of direct fecal smears, fecal flotation for ova and parasites, and dietary management. Cooked rice is added to the feed (1:1 vol/vol), and a neomycin-anticholinergic (Neochol®) is given daily in divided doses for three days. Treatment of individual animals is preferable to the addition of bulk medication to the feed, especially when appetite is depressed. Also, the person administering the drug should check each animal for signs of dehydration. If these measures are ineffective after three days, we obtain feces or vomitus for bacterial culture and virus isolation and paired sera for viral serology. Electron microscopy performed on fecal samples has proved to be diagnostic for parvovirus and coronavirus enteritis.

Parvovirus is currently an important cause of severe enteritis in kennels and has been reported from any states. Dogs of all ages are affected, but a majority of cases occur in young dogs. Mortality is highest in dogs from five to twelve weeks of age. The route of transmission is not known but is presumed to be fecal-oral. Clinical signs include diarrhea, vomiting, lethargy, anorexia, and rapid dehydration. The feces are often pink or yellow-orange in color and may contain blood. Hematologic changes are characterized by panleukopenia or lymphopenia when blood is collected early in the disease. At necropsy, lesions vary from mild intestinal congestion and dilation to frank mucosal hemorrhages, and the thymus is often atrophied. Definitive diagnosis is based on the histologic appearance of intestinal lesions — which are similar to those in feline panleukopenia, identification of parvovirus in feces by electron microscopy, and rising antibody titers. Treatment is symptomatic as described for diarrhea, but vigorous efforts must be made to maintain fluid and electrolyte balance. We are currently testing a killed feline panleukopenia vaccine and a killed canine parvovirus vaccine in a kennel in which parvovirus enteritis has been a serious problem.

Coronavirus enteritis is difficult to distinguish clinically from diarrhea caused by parvovirus. Leukopenia is not a prominent feature of this disease, and the feces have a particularly foul, offensive odor. It is a highly contagious disease that can spread rapidly through kennels of susceptible dogs. Diagnosis and treatment would be similar to that for parvovirus.

RESPIRATORY

Tracheobronchitis, kennel cough, and contagious respiratory complex are familiar synonyms to all dog breeders. It rarely occurs in neonates, and in adult dogs, it is more a nuisance than a serious medical problem. However, in young puppies, both morbidity and mortality are high, and recovery may be accompanied by permanent lung damage. As with the diarrheal diseases, symptomatic treatment plays a limited role, and efforts should be made to identify the etiologic agents. This is important not only in planning therapy, but also in evaluating the effectiveness of the vaccination program. Under general anesthesia, deep tracheal swabs are obtained for bacterial and virus isolation. The lungs of all dogs that die with respiratory signs are similarly cultured. Initial therapy is with broad spectrum antibiotics such as tetracycline, Chloromycetin®, or trimethoprim-sulfadiazine (Tribrissen®) and antibiotic ophthalmic ointments when necessary. Nebulization with a mucolytic (Mucomyst®) and gentamicin is used for severe cases, and several animals are treated simultaneously.

Tracheobronchitis due to parainfluenza virus or canine distemper are preventable by routine immunization, though these are rarely a problem. Canine adenovirus-2 (CAV-2) is occasionally isolated from the lungs of dogs with respiratory disease, but the cross protection provided by immunization against infectious canine hepatitis (CAV-1) appears sufficient to prevent lung lesions although it may not prevent infection. A CAV-2 vaccine is available and would be useful in some situations.

Bordatella bronchiseptica is isolated from the lungs of a majority of our dogs with kennel cough, and it appears to be a primary pathogen. Other bacteria such as *Pasteurella, Streptococcus, Staphylococcus, Klebsiella, Proteus, E. coli,* and *Hemophilus* are also frequently isolated. Conflicting results are reported following vaccination for *Bordatella,* but we have found that administration of 2 ml of an autogenous *Bordatella* bacterin at two and five weeks of age has markedly reduced both the severity of clinical signs and the case fatality. In this respect, an autogenous bacterin appears preferable to commerciallly available products.

DISEASES OF THE ADULT

With few exceptions, most diseases in the adult dog are associated with reproduction. Trauma is usually the result of faulty cage construction that allows the dog's foot to become entangled in the wire mesh, overcrowding, or unsupervised mating. Each of these problems is preventable. Periodontal disease is a nuisance in older dogs that can be prevented by providing a diet with lower moisture content (e.g., dry dog food) and by routine scaling of teeth by hand to remove calculus and plaque buildup. This procedure can usually be accomplished without sedation or anesthesia.

BRUCELLA CANIS

Every kennel should have some regular serologic screening program for the detection and elimination of infected animals. Initial screening can be conducted with the highly sensitive slide agglutination test, and positive reactors should be retested by the more specific tube agglutination procedures, immunodiffusion, and blood culture. Once a clean kennel is established, reinfection is prevented by quarantine of new dogs until two monthly serologic tests are negative. Treatment of infected animals is not recommended. Clinical suspicion of brucellosis should be aroused by third trimester abortion in bitches, testicular atrophy, epididymitis or infertility in males, or by generalized lymphadenopathy in either sex. Transmission results from contact with aborted fetuses, placentae, uterine discharges, or from coitus with an infected dog.

MASTITIS

Mastitis is rarely a problem unless the entire litter dies or is suddenly removed from a lactating bitch. When mastitis occurs spontaneously, it poses a serious threat to the puppies. The puppies should be removed and the bitch should be placed on broad spectrum antibiotics such as ampicillin or Chloromycetin. Hot packs are applied to the breasts, and milk is removed manually. If the bitch is febrile and non-responsive to this therapy, a bacterial milk culture is indicated. Dogs that develop mastitis on successive whelpings are culled.

METRITIS

Metritis can best be prevented by the routine injection of oxytocin within several hours after whelping. Bitches showing an excessive or abnormal discharge on the third day post-whelping are given an injection of 0.2 to 0.5 mg of ergonovine maleate (Ergonil®) daily for three days, and the uterus is infused with furacin solution. Any dog with a temperature above 103° F also receives systemic antibiotics. Metritis will not necessarily recur on subsequent whelpings.

PARAPHIMOSIS

Paraphimosis occurs when an engorged penis cannot be retracted into the preputial cavity. It is a medical emergency, since trauma induced by the dog's licking or by cold temperatures can produce permanent damage. This is particularly a problem in young studs. When the paraphimosis is of short duration, correction is by the application of petroleum jelly to the penis and manual reduction. In advanced cases, the dog is anesthetized with Surital®, cold hypertonic dextrose is applied to the penis for several minutes to reduce the edema, and the penis is manually replaced, aided by the use of a lubricant. When this fails, the preputial orifice is enlarged by a ventral incision. Prevention of this condition in breeding males is by culling those with mild phimosis and by trimming the preputial hair prior to mating.

MISCELLANEOUS DISEASES

Eclampsia is rarely observed in kennel situations, and the low incidence may reflect good nutrition or selection for other desirable breeding traits. Pseudocyesis has not been recognized as a kennel problem.

REPRODUCTIVE CONSIDERATIONS

BREEDING STOCK

Breeding stock can be purchased from reputable sources or, ideally, can be chosen from within the kennel. Outside stock should be selected at 10 to 12 weeks of age, and a thorough history, should be obtained regarding the pedigree of the sire and dam, size of the litter from which the pups came, physical conformation and disposition of the bitch, and any congenital abnormalities in the breeding line. Pups are then examined for parasites and health problems, quarantined for three weeks, and allowed to mature in the kennel environment.

The ratio of sires in the kennel relative to dams is variable, but it tends to fall between 1:10 and 1:15. Bitches are generally bred on their first heat, and males are used starting at about one year of age. There is no exact time to cull breeders; this should be based primarily on performance. However, litter size tends to drop off as a bitch gets older, and the incidence of congenital deformities and weak puppies increase. Studs can be replaced if they yield three consecutive litters of below average size. The optimal breeding age will vary by breed.

HEAT DETECTION AND MATING

Routine use of vaginal smears to detect proestrus is unnecessary. Clinical recognition of proestrus by turgidity of the vulva and a sanguinous discharge is possible in a high percentage of dogs, especially if careful records are kept of previous estrus cycles for individual bitches. Natural breeding is attempted several times during the first five days of estrus or until the bitch refuses the stud. Several large pens in a quiet corner are reserved for mating. If dogs refuse to mate, from whatever reason, artifical insemination is used. The conception rate from artificial insemination is as high as that for natural breeding. All equipment used for artificial breeding should be sterlized to prevent metritis. Studs are limited to an average of one to two services per week, but they may be used more frequently for short periods. The semen is examined microscopically each month for sperm number, motility, and morphology. A decrease in sperm counts or the appearance of proximal droplets are indicators of overuse or a more serious problem. These dogs are rested for several weeks and retested.

PREGNANCY DIAGNOSIS

Manual palpation at 21 to 28 days postmating is an efficient method to detect pregnancy in most breeds. Careful records are kept of dogs that fail to conceive, since this may reflect fetal resorption or early abortion rather than misconception. It is not unusual, however, to find studs that have high misconception rates despite normal sperm counts; these males should be culled. Infectious agents and hormonal causes should be pursued for any mating that fails to result in a successful pregnancy.

GESTATION AND WHELPING

The length of gestation varies from dog to dog, but the average is approximately 63 days. Therefore, the bitch is moved to the whelping house after around 50 days of gestation to allow sufficient time to adapt to the new setting. Behavior is a more reliable indicator of impending labor than is a drop in temperature. Even experienced bitches become restless, pant, and show signs of nesting. Kennel workers are instructed to note on the cage cards all events relating to labor and whelping so that persons not present have a record of the process. The length of labor is variable and tends to be longer for first litters and larger breeds. A clear vaginal discharge is rarely cause for concern during labor, and a green discharge signifies rupture of the membranes.

Small breeds generally whelp their litter in two hours, whereas large breeds may whelp over 12 hours. If there is a prolonged green vaginal discharge and no puppies are delivered, or if the time interval between deliverance of puppies is excessive, a vaginal examination is performed to determine if there is a fetal dystocia. Manual manipulation is attempted, and if this fails, a cesarian section is planned. Uterine inertia, on the other hand, is treated by administration of 5 to 30 units of oxytocin at 20-minute intervals for three injections. Following whelping, the bitch is examined and palpated to be certain that no puppies remain. Oxytocin is given routinely following whelping to contract the uterus and stimulate milk letdown.

The bitch should never be allowed to labor to the point of exhaustion before surgical intervention is considered. Cesarian section is done under Surital[R] anesthesia or using Innovar[R] and a local anesthetic. We use a midline abdominal approach and aseptic procedures when possible. In large kennels, the cesarian is frequently performed by the kennel manager, who has been instructed by the veterinarian. Complications rarely result, and the success rate is high' if intervention is properly timed. The puppies are placed in an incubator until the bitch has recovered from anesthesia. It is a good practice to examine all puppies individually shortly after whelping and to apply iodine to the umbilicus. Orphaned puppies can be fed Esbilac until a foster mother is available.

SUPPLEMENTAL READING

Appel, M., and Beamis, D. A.: V, The canine contagious respiratory disease complex (kennel cough). Cornell Vet. 68 (Suppl. 7):70–75, 1978.

Appel, M. J., Cooper, B J., Greisen, H. G., and Carmichael, L. E.: Status report: canine viral enteritis. JAVMA 173:1516–1518, 1978.

Cornell Research Laboratory for Diseases of Dogs: Neonatal puppy mortality. Laboratory Report Series 2, No. 4, 1974.

Edney, A. T. B.: Small animal nutrition — the present state. Vet. Annual 18:285–289, 1978.

PEDIATRICS

ERWIN SMALL, D.V.M.
Urbana, Illinois

Pediatrics is the discipline of medicine that relates to growth, development, and disease of children. The author has applied the term to cover the canine and feline species from their prenatal and postnatal periods until weaning age.

Preventive medicine programs have been developed for many species in the animal kingdom. Prior to breeding, both the male and female should receive a complete physical examination, including routine vaccinations as well as hematologic and fecal evaluations. Any correctible abnormalities should be overcome. One must assume that both individuals have been chosen because they have the proper vigorous physical and mental health and generally meet typical characteristics proposed for their individual breed.

NUTRITION

CANINE

The size and weight of a fetus is directly dependent on the age and size of the bitch, the quantity of food provided, and proper absorption. Nutrient requirements are increased substantially during gestation to meet the needs for the lactation period and insure normal formation of the fetus and placenta. An average postpartum weight increase of from 5 to 10 percent above the pre-breeding weight is considered reasonable for adequate lactation.

Animal proteins are the best source of all essential amino acids, and a food that will provide 25 to 30 percent protein on a dry weight basis will meet the bitch's needs for gestation and lactation.

A reasonable balance of fats, proteins, carbohydrates, trace factors, vitamins, and minerals is essential to the developing fetus. Deficiency of vitamin A or a low energy diet or both may result in abortion and a weak or dead fetus. Inadequate supplies of energy, protein, and minerals, specifically during the last trimester, may stunt the growth of the fetus. The neonate will be undersized at birth and survival will be jeopardized. Muscle mass and liver, spleen, and pituitary function will be affected by inadequate nutrition. Neonates easily become ineffectual nursers, hypothermic, and hypoglycemic and die in 6 to 36 hours after birth.

The ability to nurse effectively is dependent on the maturity and the body temperature of the newborn and adequate pulmonary functioning. Undersized neonates are less likely to survive than are normal sized ones. Failure of the lungs to expand fully will reduce the respiratory capacity and contribute to hypoxia. Lack of subcutaneous fat and ineffectual nursing renders the neonate susceptible to chilling and hypoglycemia. Weekly monitoring of the weight of the newborn is an excellent method of assessing its chances of survival. One can classify litters into three categories: those with adequate weight gain, those losing 10 percent of birth weight, and those losing more than 10 percent. The third group will die early unless nursing is supplemented and care is taken to avoid chilling. A rule of thumb suggests that a daily gain of one gram for each pound of adult weight for that breed is consistent with good nutrition and normal growth. Attempts by the breeder to oversupplement should be strongly discouraged.

FELINE

The subject of feline nutrition continues to generate confusion and controversy. Available information on nutritional requirements of normal healthy cats is limited, although many experts agree that a varied diet of meat, milk, fish, and vegetables should be adequate. One must also be cognizant that a cat eats food, not requirements. Special features of feline nutrition are (1) the cat is a desert-type animal originating in sub-tropical areas, (2) under natural conditions, the cat is a true and complete carnivore, and (3) in nature, the cat is an occasional as opposed to a continuous feeder. These features have become obscured by domestication and close association with man, and today, many cats are frequent nibblers.

Protein. The cat's protein requirement is uniquely high (Table 1). The excessive protein requirement is essential for energy production.*

---

*Scott, P. P.: Dietary Requirements of Cat in Relation to Practical Feeding Problems, Small Animal Nutrition Workshop, Gaines Symposium, March 1971, Urbana, Illinois.

Table 1. *Daily Food Requirements of Cats According to Age**

AGE	EXPECTED (KG)	WT. (LB)	DAILY CALORIE/BODY WT. (KCAL/KG)	(KCAL/LB)	DAILY RATION (G)	(OZ)
Newborn	0.12	0.25	380	190	30	1
5 weeks	0.5	1	250	125	85	3
10 weeks	1.0	2	200	100	140	5
20 weeks	2.0	4.5	130	65	175	6
30 weeks	3.0	6.5	100	50	200	7
Adult ♂	4.5	10	80	40	250	8.5
Adult ♀ (pregnant)	3.5	7.5	100	50	240	8.5
Adult ♀ (lactating)	2.5	5.5	250	125	415	14

*Scott, P. P.: Dietary Requirements of the Cat in Relation to Practical Feeding Problems. Small Animal Nutrition Workshop, Gaines Symposium, Urbana Ill., March 1971.

The diet of growing kittens should contain about 40 percent protein of high biologic value in a mixed diet. The diet of adult cats should have more than 30 percent (on a dry weight basis). Proteins derived from connective tissue do not support growth adequately unless supplemented by amino acids or high quality protein. The domestic cat is penalized because it requires relatively large amounts of quality protein of high biologic value. These are scarce and expensive, so substitutes of vegetable protein may be utilized for part of the requirement.

Calories, Carbohydrates and Fats. Cats must have a high caloric density diet and under natural conditions should obtain about 60 percent of their calories from fat.

Increased animal fats and oils improve the diet's palatability. Essential fatty acid content should be at least 1 percent. Carbohydrates are not essential but they provide a cheaper source of calories than do other foods.

Vitamins and Minerals. Additional vitamins are necessary to insure against losses owing to processing or storage. Minerals in the form of crushed raw bone are preferable to chemicals that do not contain trace elements.

GENETICS

The pedigree is very important in determining the mode of inheritance of a specific trait. The mode of inheritance may involve one or more genes or the environment or a combination of these factors.

If the gene is located on the X chromosome (female), it is called "sex-linked recessive" or "sex-linked dominant." The Y chromosome (male) carries few if any genes. Sex-linked recessive traits are expressed more often in the male, since the Y chromosome has no genes to counteract a particular trait. A female must be homozygous at the locus in order to express the trait.

If the gene is not on either the X or the Y chromosome, it is called "autosomal," which indicates non–sex-related genetic factors. Polygenic traits involve more than one gene. Some traits are influenced by secondary sex characteristics, and these are called "sex-limited."

Dominant traits do not skip a generation if animals that are both homozygous dominant for that trait are mated. A large percentage of the offspring from each mating has a dominant trait, even if the parents are heterozygous for that trait. An animal will seldom pass on a dominant, undesirable trait because the breeder will identify it from its phenotype. Recessive traits, however, may skip one or more generations unless two parents with the recessive trait(s) are mated. An affected animal must be homozygous for the trait, so that trait comes from both sides of the parental generation. Since the recessive allele can be hidden in the heterozygote, the potential for transmitting the trait unknowingly is great. Therefore, an outstanding pedigree does not guarantee an outstanding dog because undesirable traits can be hidden on heterozygous loci. Purebreds are not homozygous at each locus, so littermates can be totally different from each other.

Examples of hereditary disorders found in either dog or cat that are sex-linked recessives are hemophilia A, hemophilia B (Christmas disease), carpal subluxations, cystine calculi, and deafness. Disorders that are probably autosomally dominant include cutaneous asthenia, persistent pupillary membranes, and polydactyly (excessive numbers of toes). Common autosomal recessive expressions are retinal dysplasia, Factor VII deficiency, chondrodysplasia, "Collie eye," and urinary calculi.

Polygenic problems include hip dysplasia, persistent right aortic arch, patent ductus arteriosus, and pulmonic or aortic stenosis. The mode of inheritance of these polygenic traits is complicated because multiple factors are involved. Cryptorchidism is recessive autosomal, but it is sex-limited in the male. Monogenic traits (i.e., those originating from a single gene) may be lethal. Hairlessness is a dominant lethal trait, and the hairless dog (Chinese Crested) must be heterozygous at that locus; homozygous genes for hairlessness cause death. Examples of recessive lethals are cleft palate and ataxia. Retinal atrophy is a semilethal and of a recessive nature.

Other disorders that are thought to be hereditary but whose mode of inheritance is not clear include epilepsy, cataracts, inguinal hernia, glaucoma, over- and undershot jaws, and certain skin diseases. These disorders are complex because of the impact of environmental factors.

Greater emphasis is placed on behavioral characteristics in hunting and guide dog breeds, although they are probably just as important in show and family breeds. They are not acquired through environmental influences but are instinctive. Behavioral traits are independent of training and to some degree are measurable. Some contrasting pairs of behavioral patterns are timidity and aggressiveness, active and lethargic temperament, shyness and non-shyness, passive defense reaction and active defense reaction, pugnaciousness and docility, and retrieving and non-retrieving desire.

Genetic crosses should not be made to produce one desirable characteristic, or to eliminate one undesirable characteristic, at the expense of the animal's physical and/or emotional well being. For example, brachycephalic breeds that have been bred concurrently for achondroplasia, or dwarfism of the skeleton, invariably have respiratory problems. The dachshund, also bred for achondroplasia, has lumbar disc problems. In summation, a critical awareness of pertinent hereditary principles and characteristics is a responsibility of the companion animal practitioner.

NEONATAL PERIOD

Keeping a litter of newborn puppies alive involves a spectrum of genetic, environmental, physiologic, and nutritional concerns. However, the causes of many puppy deaths are seldom determined.

Mortality rates reported from birth to weaning age range from 13 to 34 percent in various breeds. The Besenji has an unusually low rate of 3.5 percent. Studies of mixed breeds in England over a five-year period revealed 4.6 per-

Table 2. *Normal Physiologic Values for Young Puppies**

Weight Gain	Two-fold increase at 8–10 days; about 1 gram per pound expected adult weight per day.
Body Temperature	Weeks 1–2: 94–99° F.
	Weeks 2–4: 97–100° F
Water Requirement	2–3 oz/pound/day; turnover about 2 times that of adults.
Caloric Requirement	60–100 Kcal/pound/day.
	Newborn pups, especially toy breeds, become hypoglycemic if not fed for 24 hours.
Respiratory Rate	15–35/min.
Heart Rate	Approximately 220/min.
Urine Specific Gravity	1.006–1.017.
Kidney Function	Glomerular filtration increases from 21% at birth to 53% at 8 weeks of age.
	Tubular secretion rate matures at 8 weeks of age.
Sucking Reflex	Usually strong at birth. Weak in physically immature, abnormal, or chilled puppies.
Shivering Reflex	Develops 6–8 days after birth.
Muscle Tone	Firm; pups stand upright at 3 weeks with normal tone and postural reflexes. Walking and running by 4 weeks.
Eyes Open	10–16 days.
Visual Perception (owner recognition)	Absent until 3 weeks; evident at 4 weeks.
Hyperkinesia (body twitching)	Normal at 1–3 weeks; disappears after 4 weeks.

*Neonatal Puppy Mortality: Laboratory Report 2, No. 4, Cornell Research Laboratory, Veterinary Virus Research Institute, New York.

cent of pups were stillborn and 34 percent died during the first eight weeks of life. Eighty-two percent of the mortalities occurred during the second week and 5.5 percent occurred during the remaining six weeks. The investigators reported the following pattern: the percentage of puppy losses was highest among the litters of young bitches and gradually diminished as the bitches reached three years of age; however, it increased after the bitches reached four years. Most puppy deaths (12.5 percent) occurred during the first week of life; the data indicated that inbreeding was related to increased neonatal mortality, whereas hybrids of inbred breeds had significantly greater survival rates. A comparison of survival rates among 400 male and female English setter pups revealed little statistical difference during the initial week of life; however, at three and four weeks of age, the male survival rate was greater.*

Physiologic immaturity is seen in puppies during the first three weeks of life. Table 2 lists selected normal physiologic values. There is a relative underdevelopment of most physiologic and behavioral functions and activities of puppies during their first few weeks of life. Puppies

*Neonatal Puppy Mortality: Laboratory Report 2, No. 4, Cornell Research Laboratory, Veterinary Virus Research Institute, New York.

are also immunologically immature at this time, although certain elements of the immune system are functioning.

NON-INFECTIOUS DISEASES

Non-infectious diseases account for a large percentage of neonatal deaths. Table 3 lists some of the major causes.

It is significant that infectious diseases play a relatively small role when compared with stillbirths, dystocia, and management problems. Dystocia with either difficult or prolonged labor has been identified as a major cause of stillbirth. (It accounts for approximately 8 percent.) Uterine inertia is considered to be a major cause of most dystocias. Other factors appear related to excessive weight of the bitch, obstruction of the birth canal by healed fractures or fibrous bands, excessive puppy size, large calvaria of the brachycephalic breed fetuses, abnormal presentations, and fetal anomalies.

Intensive selection by breeders has resulted in an increased number of congenital abnormalities. Congenital defects can be defined as abnormalities of structure or function seen at birth. Some defects occur as single disturbances of body structure, whereas others occur as syndromes resulting from several structural defects.

The role of the bitch is a major one among the causes of neonatal deaths. A nervous, inexperienced female may traumatize her newborn puppies. In overzealous attempts to remove fetal membranes, she may accidentally induce evisceration and umbilical herniation or even become cannibalistic. Such problems may be prevented by providing an adequate whelping box and paying closer attention to the bitch during the whelping process.

Starvation can result from the inability of

Table 3. *Causes of Deaths by Percentage of Neonatal Puppies**

Stillbirth	15.0
Dystocia	11.0
Trauma of crushing	13.0
Exposure	16.0
Unidentified Disease	10.0
Undetermined	9.0
Accidents	6.0
Weakness	5.0
Cannibalism	3.0
Lactation failure	4.0
Parasites	3.0
Excessive licking	3.0
Deformity	2.0

*Mosier, J. F.: Canine Pediatric Seminar, Delaware Valley Forum, Moorestown, New Jersey, January 21, 1976.

puppies to suckle, especially if they are premature, weak, or chilled. Edema of the mammary gland may make milk unavailable. Agalactia due to underdeveloped mammae, uterine infections, septicemia, or mastitis (due to staphylococcic, streptococcic, or mixed infections with coliform bacteria) may also contribute to the pup's inability to obtain milk.

INFECTIOUS DISEASES AND THE FADING PUP SYNDROME

Infectious diseases involve a variety of bacterial and viral agents. The more common bacterial problems include umbilical infections, *ophthalmia neonatorum*, pyodermas, and septicemia. Puppies with umbilical infection have distended abdomens, discomfort, and loss of vigor. The umbilicus may be edematous and the abdominal muscles may be rigid. Treatment includes administering antibiotics and keeping the patient warm and adequately nourished. *Ophthalmia neonatorum* is characterized by an acute purulent conjunctivitis with swelling and protrusion of lids. Treatment includes lid separation and application of topical antibiotics.

Pyodermas are seen as crusted lesions primarily involving the head and neck. Bacterial cultures frequently grow hemolytic staphylococci. There is a definite relationship between contamination of pups with placental fluids and failure of the bitch to cleanse the pups adequately. Routine treatment consists of systemic antibiotics and cleansing shampoos with tame iodines, and a review should be made of kennel sanitation.

The herpesvirus and a group of organisms including *E. coli,* beta hemolytic streptococci, staphylococci, proteus, and pseudomonas may be responsible for septicemias and one aspect of the "fading pup syndrome." Puppies that are afflicted are usually vigorous and healthy at birth but within a few days show discomfort, a distended abdomen, increased respiration, and weakness, and eventually they die. Treatment consists of antibiotics, increased environmental temperature of 85° and supportive therapy. Autopsy reveals gas-distended intestines, petechial hemorrhages of serosal surfaces, lung congestion, and enteritis of the anterior segment of the small bowel.

Brucellosis is not generally considered a disease of the neonate but may cause abortion, usually between the seventh and ninth week of pregnancy. However, some pups may be stillborn or weak. Infected bitches may have enlarged lymph nodes. Prolonged vaginal discharges that are viscous, bloody, or greenish-gray suggest infectious abortion, and samples should be taken for culture. Resident male dogs may have lymphadenitis, epididymitis, and prostatitis as well as edema and dermatitis of the scrotum.

The "toxic milk syndrome" has been associated with the pup's incompatibility to the bitch's milk. Some researchers suggest that this is related to toxins in the milk, subinvolution of the uterus, or metritis. Puppies cry, become bloated, and have greenish diarrhea and red, swollen ani. Corrective measures include placing the puppies in an incubator and feeding them a formula. The affected bitch may be given ergonovine (0.2 mg three times daily) plus antibiotics. Intrauterine flushing with antiseptic solutions has also been useful.

Viral infections of the neonate are usually related to the canine herpesvirus or to the canine adenoviruses or distemper. Canine herpesvirus has a worldwide distribution. It occurs in puppies generally one to three weeks of age. Healthy, vigorous pups suddenly become dull, cry continuously, cease suckling, and die within a few hours. Fever is seldom present. The older puppies may have slight nasal discharges. Affected bitches may have nodular vaginitis. Puppies that have recovered from herpes infections may carry and spread the agent for several months. Autopsies reveal generalized necrotizing and hemorrhagic involvement of many organs. The kidneys have subserosal petechia, and other findings include fibrinonecrotic pneumonia and an enlarged spleen.

There have been recent field reports of significant outbreaks of the canine coronarvirus and the parvovirus infections in young puppies. These agents are generally considered to affect older pups (see Section 13).

FADING KITTEN SYNDROME AND KITTEN MORTALITY COMPLEX (KMC)

Scott and co-workers* recently completed a survey of selected catteries representing a total of 790 litters from 24 breeds. The Persian and Siamese breeds in this study included more than 100 litters. There were 3468 kittens born in 790 litters, of which 352 (10.2 percent) were stillborn. Males represented 65 percent and females 35 percent of the litters in numbers.

Kitten mortality reported in the same survey revealed that 209 of 3116 kittens born alive died in 24 hours, and by the second day an additional 120 kittens had died. One week after birth, 475 had died. The dramatic significance of kitten

mortality is evident when one considers that 27.1 percent of kittens born alive failed to reach one year of age; combining deaths and stillbirths, the mortality rate reached 34.5 percent by one year of age.

The survey indicated that the Manx breed had the largest percentage (19) of malformations and the Colorpoint shorthair was in second place with 17 percent. The greatest number of abortions occurred during the seventh and eighth week of gestation; there were six instances of fetal resorptions. Thus, of the 813 total reported pregnancies, abortion ended 2.1 percent and fetal resorption ended 0.7 percent. Scott's survey emphasized the significance of neonatal mortality and the need for further research in neonatal problems. A second survey emphasized the reproductive performance of 189 pedigreed female cats belonging to 29 breeders in Canada and the United States. According to this survey, the typical breeding cat produced only one litter per year with an average 3.59 kittens per litter. Stillbirths accounted for 11.6 percent of kittens born, and 27.3 percent of kittens born lived less than eight weeks. Average litter size was smaller and mortality during the first week of life was higher for Persian, Himalayan, and Manx than for Siamese, Burmese, and other short-haired breeds. Of the 29 breeders, 18 had consulted veterinarians about reproductive problems in their catteries. Some commonly reported diseases were respiratory infection (19 catteries), urologic disease (16), and enteritidis (11).*

The significance of Kitten Mortality Complex (KMC) is more compelling when one considers the unusually high rate of reproductive failures, including endometritis and pyometritis, fetal resorption, repeat breeders, abortions, stillbirths, and congenital malformations. The causes of kitten deaths include unusually small size, ineffectual nursing, fading kittens, acute congestive myopathies, feline infectious peritonitis (FIP), and mild to moderate chronic respiratory disease. The role of adult carriers of infectious peritonitis (FIP) was also stressed by Scott, since all colonies or catteries surveyed had either lost cats with clinical FIP or had a high incidence of FIP antibody-positive cats.

Breeders report an unusually high rate of reproductive failures and early deaths of young kittens. Queens involved in KMC usually experienced repeated problems with subsequent litters. The disease complex has been reported in Himalayan, Persian, Siamese, domestic shorthair, and Burmese breeds. Himalayans account-

*Scott, F., Weiss, R. C., Post, J. E., Gilmartin, J. E., and Hoshino, Y.: Kitten mortality complex. Feline Practice, 9(2):44–56, 1979.

*Povey, R. C.: Reproduction in the pedigree female cat, A Survey of Breeders. Can. Vet. J., 19 (Aug. 78):207.

ed for the highest kitten losses, 40 percent, as compared with 27 percent for other breeds. The categories identified by Scott include reproductive failures (repeat breeders, fetal resorption, abortion, stillbirths, and congenital birth defects), kitten mortality (fading kittens, acute congestive cardiomyopathies, and feline infectious peritonitis), and adult diseases (chronic respiratory disease, endometritis, intermittent fever of unknown origin, and acute congestive cardiomyopathies and cardiovascular disease).

Scott is inclined to incriminate a viral agent(s) as one of the possible causes. Two specific agents, FIP and endogenous C-type virus, have been isolated. FIP's significance was further demonstrated when 35 consecutive catteries studied were positive. He further speculates that early FIP infection may occur as either a subclinical or mild respiratory disease. Weeks or months may pass before the typical effusive or granulomatous types are obvious. The high incidence of FIP antibody-positive cats suggests that the infected cats may be shedders of the virus. Other diseases that are responsible for abortion or fetal resorption or both include feline leukemia, toxoplasmosis, and rhinotracheitis, as well as calicivirus, reovirus, and bacterial infections, with hemolytic *E. coli*, pseudomonas, or staphylococci. Certain chemical agents — e.g., griseofulvin — nutritional deficiencies, and genetic aberrations may also cause reproductive problems.

One segment of the problem that needs further emphasis relates to management of the cattery. Infectious diseases may spread through direct contact via aerosol, community food and water dishes and cages, and carrier animals, as well as through indirect contact via fomites, contaminated equipment, and food. The breeder should seek advice on cage types, air flow, traffic patterns, facilities for decontamination, and control of rodents and insects. Further emphasis should be placed on types of isolation or quarantine facilities, education of personnel, and vaccination and deworming programs.

In conclusion, neonatal animal deaths represent a major problem for the veterinary medical profession. Ill defined causes and inadequate information are two reasons for the dearth of knowledge about this issue. It is apparent from published studies that the majority of deaths of neonates are attributable to non-infectious causes. Factors that must be continually monitored are physiologic immaturity, litter size, numbers of litters per queen or bitch, age of queen or bitch, normal birth versus cesarean section, and genetic makeup of the animal. Further research must be directed toward an understanding of the immune response of newborn puppies and kittens. More attention should also be placed on management of kennels and catteries, on better understanding of the genetic implications, and on the role of nutrition if we hope to eradicate the high mortality rate of neonates.

SUPPLEMENTAL READING

Fox, M. W.: *Canine Pediatrics.* Springfield, Illinois, Charles C Thomas, 1966.

Mosier, J. E.: Canine Pediatrics. Vet. Clin. North Am. Philadelphia, W. B. Saunders Co., 1978.

National Research Council: Nutrition of Cats. Washington, D.C., 1978.

Srb, A. M., Owen, R. D., and Edgar, R. S.: *General Genetics,* 2nd ed. San Francisco, W. H. Freeman and Co., 1966.

A CATALOG OF GENETIC DISORDERS OF THE DOG

DONALD F. PATTERSON, D.V.M.

Philadelphia, Pennsylvania

With the increasing sophistication of diagnostic procedures and the declining importance of infectious, parasitic, and nutritional diseases has come a growing awareness that many disease conditions in the dog have a genetic cause. Although individual genetic diseases may be rare in the general population, they often occur with a high frequency within individual kennels or even in entire breeds. For those concerned, the economic and emotional impact may be great. The ability of the veterinarian to deal effectively with such problems depends upon a general knowledge of genetics and specific information regarding the diagnostic and genetic features of the disease in question. The latter information tends to be widely scattered and not readily available to the practitioner. As a partial solution to this problem, the author has compiled this catalog, listing disorders for which there is evidence of a significant genetic component. For ease of reference, disorders are listed in a series of tables according to the organ or system most prominently involved. The breeds known to be affected are given, along with the mode of inheritance when known.* The reader is directed to selected references for further details. No attempt has been made to include all references on a given condition.

It will be recognized that in many of the disorders listed, there is ample evidence of a genetic cause, but the lack of definitive genetic studies precludes the listing of the mode of inheritance. Family studies and breeding experiments will be needed to clarify these questions, and it is hoped that practicing veterinarians who have the opportunity to see these and as yet unidentified genetic disorders will be stimulated to undertake such observations.

*Throughout the catalog, modes of inheritance will be designated according to the following key: R, autosomal recessive; D, autosomal dominant; ID, incomplete dominant; XR, X-linked recessive; XD, X-linked dominant; P, polygenic; and ?, unknown or in question.

Table 1.   *The Blood**

CONDITION	BREED(S)	MODE	SELECTED REFERENCES
Afibrinogenemia	St. Bernard	D	Kammermann et al. (1971)
Blood group incompatibility (mainly A system)	All breeds	D*	Dewit et al. (1969) Swisher et al. (1962) Young et al. (1951)
Chondrodysplasia-anemia syndrome	Alaskan malamute	R	Fletch et al.(1975)
Cyclic neutropenia (gray collie syndrome)	Collie	R	Ford (1969) Lund et al. (1967, 1970, 1970) Cheville (1968) Cheville et al. (1970) Dale et al. (1971)
Factor VII deficiency	Beagle Alaskan malamute	R	Rowsell (1963) Spurling et al. (1972) Dodds (1974a)
Hemophilia A (factor VIII deficiency)	Irish setter	XR	Hutt et al. (1948) Field et al. (1946) Graham et al.(1949)
	German shepherd, collie	XR	Rowsell (1963)
	Labrador retriever	XR	Archer and Bowden (1959)
	Beagle	XR	Brock et al.(1963)
	Shetland sheepdog	XR	Wurzel and Lawrence (1961)
	Greyhound	XR	Sharp and Dike (1963)
	Weimaraner	XR	Kaneko et al. (1967)
	Chihuahua	XR	Kaneko et al. (1967)
	Antarctic sledge dog	XR	Bellars (1969)
	Vizsla	XR	Buckner et al. (1967)
	Miniature and standard poodles	XR	Gentry et al. (1977); Dodds (1977a)
	French bulldog	XR	Slappendell (1975)
	Other purebreeds and mongrels	XR	Dodds (1977a; 1978)
Hemophilia B (Christmas disease, factor IX deficiency)	Cairn terrier	XR	Rowsell et al. (1960)
	Black and tan coonhound, St. Bernard, parti-color cocker spaniel	XR	Dodds (1974a; 1974b; 1975; 1977, 1977a; 1978)
	Alaskan malamute	XR	Peterson and Dodds (1979)
	French bulldog	XR	Slappendel (1975)

Continued on next page

*Genes determining blood group substances are inherited as dominants in that one dose of the gene resulting in the presence of the antigen is sufficient to give a detectable reaction. For example A+ blood transfused into an A− dog elicits anti-A antibodies whether the donor is homozygous or heterozygous for the A+ allele. Natural isoantibodies against the blood group antigens are absent or weak in dogs. Hemolytic disease of newborn pups and transfusion reactions usually depend on prior immunization of A− individuals with A+ blood by transfusion.

Table 1.   *The Blood (Continued)*

CONDITION	BREED(S)	MODE	SELECTED REFERENCES
Factor X deficiency	Cocker spaniel	ID	Dodds (1973)
Factor XI deficiency	Springer spaniel	ID	Dodds and Kull (1971)
	Great Pyrenees	ID	Dodds (1977, 1977a, 1978)
Hyperlipoproteinemia	Miniature schnauzer	?	Rogers et al. (1975)
Methemoglobinemia	Borzoi, English setter	?	Letchworth et al. (1977)
Nonspherocytic hemolytic anemia (pyruvate kinase deficiency)	Basenji	R	Tasker et al. (1969) Ewing (1969) Searcy et al. (1971) Standerfer et al. (1974) Andresen (1977) Hogg et al (1978)
	Beagle	?	Prasse et al. (1975)
Platelet function defects	Otterhound, basset hound, foxhound	ID	Dodds (1967, 1974a, 1977, 1977a, 1978)
Von Willebrand's disease	German shepherd, miniature schnauzer, golden retriever, Doberman pinscher, Scottish terrier, Pembroke Welsh corgi, isolated cases in other breeds	ID	Dodds (1974b, 1975, 1977, 1977a, 1978)

Table 2. *Bones and Joints**

CONDITION	BREED(S)	MODE	SELECTED REFERENCES
Achondroplasia, limbs	Dachshund, basset	ID	Stockard (1941)
Anury (tail-less)	Cocker spaniel	R?	Pullig (1953)
Brachydactyly		R?	Green (1957)
Brachyury (short tail)	Cocker spaniel, beagle, English bulldog	R?	Pullig (1957), Curtis et al. (1964)
Carpal subluxation	Irish setter	XR	Pick et al. (1967)
Cartilaginous exostoses	Mixed	?	Gee and Doige (1970), Chester (1971)
Cervical vertebral deformity	Basset hound, Great Dane	?	Palmer and Wallace (1967), Wright et al. (1973), Selcer and Oliver (1975)
	Doberman pinscher	?	Trotter et al. (1976)
Cervical calcinosis	Great Dane	?	Flo and Tvedten (1975)
Craniomandibular osteopathy	West Highland white, Scottish terrier, Cairn terrier, Labrador retriever	?	Jubb and Kennedy (1964), Riser et al. (1967)
Cranioschisis (skull fissures)	Cocker spaniel	R?	Pullig (1952)
Dwarfism (chondrodysplasia with anemia)	Alaskan malamute	R	Smart and Fletch (1971), Subden et al. (1972), Fletch et al. (1973), Fletch and Pinkerton (1973), Fletch et al. (1975)
Elbow joint malformation	Afghan hound	?	Grøndalen (1973)
Ectromelia	——	R	Ladrat et al. (1969)
Epiphyseal dysplasia	Beagle	R?	Rasmussen (1971, 1972)
Epiphyseal dysplasia (pseudoachondroplastic)	Miniature poodle	R	Gardner (1959), Amlöf (1961), Lodge (1966), Riser et al. (1979)
Foramen magnum enlargement		?	Bardens (1965)
Hip dysplasia	Most breeds, notably German shepherds	P	Schales (1957, 1959), Riser (1964), Riser et al. (1964, 1967), Henricson et al. (1965, 1966), Henricson and Olsson (1959), Hutt (1967), Riser (1975), Leighton et al. (1977), Lust and Farrell (1977)
Intervertebral disc degeneration	Chondrodystrophoid breeds: cocker spaniel, dachshund, Pekingese, beagle	?	Hansen (1952, 1964), Vaughan (1958), Ghosh et al. (1975)

Continued on next page

*Skeletal conformation, generally. Aside from crossing strongly contrasting breeds, little definitive analysis of the genetic basis for skeletal variation has been attempted. The most extensive studies are those of Stockard (1941), who performed standard mendelian crosses, including F_2 and back-crosses, between different breeds. In these studies, there was a tendency for the F_1 to be intermediate between the parental types, and a single back-cross of the F_1 to either parental breed produced pups which closely resembled that breed.

While single gene defects, in some instances, can have marked effects on the form of the skeleton (as in achondroplasia), reports that minor variations in skeletal conformation are determined by single genes should be viewed with skepticism. Variations from the ideal type in purebred dogs are more likely to represent the influence of polygenic inheritance, "abnormal" individuals merely representing the extremes of variation possible under a polygenic system of determinants.

From a practical point of view, selection for body conformation, as important to the dog breeder, may be regarded as a problem of selecting for polygenic traits. A further discussion of this may be found in the book by Burns and Fraser (1966).

Table 2.   *Bones and Joints (Continued)*

CONDITION	BREED(S)	MODE	SELECTED REFERENCES
Legg-Calvé-Perthes disease	Small breeds	?	Moltzen-Nielsen (1937), Wamberg (1961), Lee and Fry (1969)
	Toy poodle	?	Pidduck and Webbon (1978)
Lumbosacral malarticulation	German shepherd	?	Oliver et al. (1978)
Odontoid process dysplasia	Miniature poodle, Pomeranian, Yorkshire terrier	?	Geary et al. (1967), Parker and Park (1973)
Osteogenesis imperfecta	Bedlington terrier, elkhound, poodle	?	Jubb and Kennedy (1964), Calkins et al. (1956), Lettow and Dammrich (1960)
Otocephaly (partial agnathia, hydrocephaly, parietal fontanelle defects)	Beagle	P?	Fox (1963, 1964)
Over- and undershot jaw	Cocker spaniel, long-haired dachshund	?	Phillips (1945), Grüneberg and Lea (1940), Ritter (1933), Stockard (1941)
Patellar luxation	Toy breeds	?	Hodgman (1963), Kodituwakku (1962), Loeffler and Meyer (1961), Knight (1963), Hutt (1968), Priester (1972)
Polydactyly (rear dew claws)	Many breeds	D?	Keeler and Trimble (1938), Whitney (1947)
Polyostotic fibrous dysplasia	Doberman	?	Carrig and Seawright (1969) Carrig et al. 1975
Short skull	Bulldogs, Pekingese, Brussels griffin, other breeds	?	Stockard (1941)
Short spine	Shiba-Inu (Japan), greyhound	R	deBoom (1965), Hansen (1968), Suu (1956, 1957)
Skeletal–ocular dysplasia syndrome	Labrador retriever	?	Carrig et al. (1977)
Spina bifida	English bulldog	?	Curtis et al. (1964)
Spondylosis deformans	Boxer	?	Zimmer and Stähli (1960)
Tibial metaphyseal dysplasia	Dachshund	?	Mayrhofer (1977)
Ulnar growth abnormality	Basset hound	?	Rasmussen and Reimann (1977)
	Skye terrier	?	Lau (1977)
Ununited anconeal process	German shepherd, cocker spaniel, Labrador retriever	P?	Cawley and Archibald (1959), Vaughan (1962), Loeffler (1964), Bradley (1967), Carlson and Severin (1961), Corley and Carlson (1965)
Vertebral osteochondrosis	Foxhound	P	Hime (1963), Hime and Drake (1965)

Table 3. Cardiovascular and Lymphatic Systems

CONDITION	BREED(S)[*]	MODE	SELECTED REFERENCES
Patent ductus arteriosus	Poodle (collie, Pomeranian, cocker spaniel)	P	Patterson (1968), Patterson and Pyle (1971), Patterson et al. (1971, 1972), Mulvihill (1971)
Subaortic stenosis	Newfoundland (boxer, German shepherd)	P	Patterson (1968), Patterson and Pyle (1971), Patterson et al. (1971, 1972), Mulvihill (1971), Pyle et al. (1976)
Conotruncal septum defects, including tetralogy of Fallot	Keeshond	P	Patterson et al. (1974), Van Mierop et al. (1977, 1978)
Valvular pulmonic stenosis	Beagle (English bulldog, fox terrier, Chihuahua)	P	Patterson (1968), Patterson and Pyle (1971), Patterson et al. (1972)
Persistent right aortic arch	German shepherd (Irish setter)	P	Naylor (1957), Patterson (1968), Patterson and Pyle (1971), Mulvihill (1971), Patterson et al. (1972)
Atrial septal defect and other cardiac defects	Boxer	?	Pyle and Patterson (1972)
Cardiac standstill (sinoatrial arrhythmia)	Pug	?	Branch et al. (1977)
Congenital lymphedema	Labrador-poodle cross	D	Patterson et al. (1967), Luginbuhl et al. (1967)
Congenital anasarca	English bulldog	?	Ladds et al. (1971)
Incomplete right bundle branch block (focal right ventricular hypertrophy)	Beagle	?	Moore et al. (1971)
His bundle degeneration (suspected cause of sudden death)	Doberman	?	James and Drake (1965, 1968)

[*]Parentheses indicate breeds in which definitive genetic studies have not been made but in which epidemiologic evidence suggests a genetic cause.

Table 4. Chromosomal Abnormalities[*]

ABNORMALITY	BREED AND PHENOTYPE	SELECTED REFERENCES
Autosomal centric fusion	77 chromosomes, no phenotypic defects	Ma and Gilmore (1971) Larsen et al. (1978)
Semibalanced autosomal translocation	Mongrel, male, cleft lip and maxilla, congenital heart disease, 77 chromosomes including large submetacentric translocation chromosome	Shive et al. (1965), Patterson et al. (1966)
Semibalanced autosomal translocation	Miniature poodle, female, chondrodysplastic dwarfism, 77 chromosomes including a large subtelocentric translocation chromosome	Hare et al. (1967)
Extra minute chromosome	Male cocker spaniel, congenital heart disease, 79 chromosomes including extra minute chromosome	Shive et al. (1965), Patterson et al. (1966)
XXY	German short-haired pointer, male, with testicular hypoplasia and congenital heart disease; XXY sex chromosome constitution	Clough et al. (1970)

[*]For a general discussion of cytogenetics in the dog and cat, see Hare et al. (1966). Studies of the karyotype of various breeds, including the Malayan telomian dog, have not shown any apparent differences between breeds (Borgaonkar et al., 1968). Giemsa banding studies by Selden et al. (1975) have recently further defined the canine karyotype.

Table 5. *Digestive System*

CONDITION	BREED(S)	MODE	SELECTED REFERENCES
Cleft lip and palate	Staffordshire terrier, dachshund, cocker spaniel	P?	Jurkiewicz (1965), Jurkiewicz and Bryant (1968)
	English bulldog		Gardner (1954), Pearce (1969)
	Beagle		Horowitz and Chase (1970)
	Shih-Tzu		Cooper and Mattern (1970)
Dentition abnormal	Boxer, English bulldog	?	Aitchison (1964)
Esophageal achalasia	Wire-haired fox terrier	?	Osborne et al. (1967)
	Greyhound		Spy (1963)
	German shepherd		Earlam et al. (1967)
	Miniature schnauzer	?	Clifford et al. (1972)
Esophageal deviation	English bulldog	?	Woods et al. (1978)
Gingival hyperplasia	Boxer	?	Burstone et al. (1952)
Glossopharyngeal defect (bird tongue)	Not given	R	Hutt and deLahunta (1971)
Hepatitis (copper storage)	Bedlington terrier	R?	Hardy et al. (1975) Hardy and Stevens (1977, 1978)
Pancreatic exocrine insufficiency (juvenile)	German shepherd	R?	Weber and Freudiger (1977)

Table 6. *The Ear**

CONDITION	BREED(S)	MODE	SELECTED REFERENCES
Deafness (cochlear degeneration)	Dalmatian	?	Hudson and Ruben (1962), Anderson et al. (1968)
	Collie	?	Lurie (1948)
	Foxhound	?	Adams (1956)
	White dogs of various breeds	?	Young (1955)

*These represent instances of hereditary deafness other than that produced by the merle gene. As in other animals, deafness often is associated with depigmentation. In none of the above reports was the mode of inheritance well defined. Deaf dogs are usually born of normal parents. The studies of Anderson et al. (1968) in Dalmatians are the most extensive. They yielded results which are not consistent with any simple genetic hypothesis. Although the anatomic defect in all of the above examples appears to be an abnormal development or early degeneration of the cochlea, the defect occurs in varying degrees, and may involve one or both sides. This wide range of variation in the phenotype, plus a lack of accurate means of determining minor degrees of hearing loss in the dog, make genetic analysis difficult.

Table 7. *Endocrine and Metabolic Disorders*

CONDITION	BREED(S)	MODE	SELECTED REFERENCES
Copper storage	Bedlington terrier	R?	Hardy et al. (1975) Hardy and Stevens (1977, 1978)
Cystinuria	(See Table 13, Urogenital System.)		
Diabetes mellitus°	Dachshund Miniature poodle	? ?	Wilkinson (1960) Gershwin (1975)
Goiter	Fox terrier	?	Brouwers (1950)
High uric acid excretion	(See Table 13, Urogenital System.)		
Hyperlipoproteinemia and hypothyroidism	Beagle	?	Manning et al. (1973)
Glycogen storage disease	"Toy breeds,"† Lapland dog	?	Bardens et al. (1961), Bardens (1966), Mostafa (1970)
Glycogenosis type III (debranching enzyme defect)	German shepherd	R	Ceh et al. (1976), Rafiquazzaman et al. (1976)
Methylmalonic aciduria	Basset hound	?	Jezyk (1979)
Pituitary dwarfism	German shepherd Carelian bear dog	R	Andresen et al. (1974), Allen (1978) Willeberg et al. (1975) Andresen and Willeberg (1976, 1976a) Nicholas (1978)
Hyperlipoproteinemia	Miniature schnauzer	?	Rogers et al. (1975)
GM₁ gangliosidosis (β-galactosidase deficiency)	Beagle mix	R?	Read et al. (1976)
Gaucher's disease	Sidney Silkie	?	Hartley and Blakemore (1973)
Hyperammonemia due to urea cycle enzyme deficiency (arginosuccinate synthetase deficiency)	Golden retriever Beagle	?	Strombeck et al. (1975)

°The large number of cases of diabetes mellitus in dachshunds in one study suggested a genetic influence. However, the population base was poorly defined (actual prevalence rates in dachshunds unknown) and no direct genetic studies have been made.

†Poorly defined syndrome supposedly characterized by hypoglycemia in pups 6 to 12 weeks old. There is reputed to be glycogen infiltration of liver, kidney and myocardium in some cases.

Table 8. The Eye

CONDITION	BREED(S)	MODE	SELECTED REFERENCES
Cataract	Boston and Staffordshire terrier	R?	Barnett (1972)
	Afghan hound	R?	Roberts and Helper (1972)
	Pointer	D?	Host and Sreison (1936)
	Beagle	D?	Andersen and Shultz (1958), Heywood (1971)
	Cocker spaniel	R?	Olesen et al. (1974), Yakely (1978)
	German shepherd	D	von Hippel (1930)
	Golden and Labrador retriever	D?	Barnett (1972), Rubin (1974)
	Old English sheepdog	R?	Koch (1972)
	Miniature schnauzer	R?	Rubin et al. (1969)
	Standard poodle	R?	Rubin and Flowers (1972)
Collie eye anomaly (chorioretinal dysplasia, posterior scleral ectasia)	Collie (all color varieties)	R°	Roberts and Dellaporta (1965), Donovan and Wyman (1965), Yakely et al. (1968, 1972) (See also Symposium on Collie Eye Anomaly. J. Am. Vet. Med. Assn., 155:859–878, 1969)
	Shetland sheepdog	?	Aguirre (1973)
Conjunctival dermoid cyst	German shepherd	?	Szczudlowska (1967)
Corneal cyst	St. Bernard	?	Kittel (1931)
Corneal ulceration	Boxer	?	Roberts (1965)
Entropion	Various breeds	?	Burns and Fraser (1966), Hodgman (1963)
Everted membrana nictitans	German short-haired pointer	?	Martin and Leach (1970)
Glaucoma	Basset hound	?	Martin and Wyman (1968), Wyman and Ketring (1976)
	Wire-haired fox terrier, cocker spaniel	?	Lovekin (1964), Lovekin and Bellhorn (1968), Formston (1945)
	English cocker spaniel	?	Bedford (1975)
	Beagle	?	Gelatt et al. (1977)
Hemeralopia (day blindness)	Alaskan malamute	R	Rubin et al. (1967), Aguirre and Rubin (1974), Rubin (1976)
Heterochromia iridis ("walleye")	Collie, Shetland sheepdog, dachshund, Great Dane, Australian shepherd, other breeds with merle gene	ID†	Sorsby and Davey (1954), Gelatt and McGill (1973)

Continued on next page

°It is reasonable to believe that the varied stigmata are the result of a pleiotropic single gene with variable expressivity, depending on the genetic background. It has been postulated, however, that staphyloma is inherited as a single autosomal dominant which is expressed only in the presence of recessively inherited chorioretinal change (Donovan and Macpherson, 1968).

†Merled or dappled dogs are heterozygous for M, an incompletely dominant gene with pleiotropic effects. In heterozygotes (Mm), there is often heterochromia of the iris, or both irises may be blue. Homozygotes (MM) frequently have severe eye anomalies, including microphthalmia and colobomas of the iris and choroid, and are often blind and deaf.

Table 8.*   *The Eye (Continued)

CONDITION	BREED(S)	MODE	SELECTED REFERENCES
Lens luxation	Sealyham terrier	?	Lawson (1969)
	Fox terrier	?	Formston (1945)
Optic nerve hypoplasia	Collie	?	Saunders (1952), Magrane (1953)
Persistent pupillary membrane	Basenji	D?	Roberts (1967), Barnett and Knight (1969)
Progressive retinal atrophy‡ (generalized)	Irish setter, Gordon setter	R	Magnusson (1911), Hodgman et al. (1949), Parry (1953), Aguirre et al. (1978)
	Miniature and toy poodle, English cocker spaniel	R	Barnett (1965)
	Norwegian elkhound	R	Cogan and Kuwabara (1965), Aguirre and Rubin (1971), Aguirre (1978)
	Cardigan Welsh corgi	?	Barnett (1969), Keep (1972)
	Collie	R?	Wolf et al. (1978)
	Tibetan terrier	R?	Garmer et al. (1974), Barnett and Curtis (1978)
Progressive retinal atrophy (central)	Labrador retriever	?	Parry (1954)
	Border collie	?	Barnett (1969)
	Golden retriever	?	
	English springer spaniel	?	
Retinal dysplasia§	Sealyham terrier	R?	Ashton et al. (1968)
	Bedlington terrier	R	Rubin (1963, 1968)
	Australian shepherd	?	Gelatt and McGill (1973)
	Labrador retriever	R	Barnett et al. (1970), Kock (1974)
	American cocker spaniel	R?	MacMillan and Lipton (1978)
	English Springer spaniel	R?	Lavach et al. (1978)
	Yorkshire terrier	R?	Stades (1978)
Retinal and skeletal dysplasia syndrome	Labrador retriever	?	Carrig et al. (1977)
Tapetal defect	Beagle		Bellhorn et al. (1975)

‡There is no evidence that PRA in different breeds results from gene mutations at the same locus. As has been recently pointed out by Aquirre (1976), PRA in different breeds consists of different clinical and pathologic entities.

§Consists of a number of different clinical and pathologic entities.

Table 9.   Neuromuscular System

CONDITION	BREED(S)	MODE	SELECTED REFERENCES
Ataxia	Fox terrier (Sweden)	R?	Björck et al. (1957)
	Jack Russell terrier	R?	Hartley and Palmer (1973)
Behavioral abnormalities*	Several breeds, including poodle, cocker spaniel, German shepherd	P?	Stockard (1941), Thorne (1944), Freak (1948), Krushinskii (1962), Hodgman (1963), Burns and Fraser (1966), Thompson and Melzack (1956), Dykman et al. (1969), Lane and Holmes (1972)
	Pointer	P	Brown et al. (1978)
Cavitating leukodystrophy	Dalmatian	R	Bjerkås (1977)
Cerebellar hypoplasia	Airedale	?	Cordy and Snelbaker (1952)
Cerebellar and extrapyramidal abiotrophy	Kerry Blue terrier	R	de Lahunta and Averill (1976)
Cerebrospinal demyelination	Miniature poodle	?	McGrath (1960), Douglas and Palmer (1961), Steinberg (1963)
Epilepsy	Keeshond, poodle	R?	Croft and Stockman (1964), Eberhart (1959), Wallace (1975)
	Beagle	?	Bielfelt et al. (1971) Hegreberg and Padgett (1976)
	Tervueren shepherd (Netherlands)	?	Van der Velden (1968)
	German shepherd	?	Lawler (1971), Falco et al. (1974)
	Horak's laboratory dog	?	Martínek and Horak (1970), Martinek and Dahme (1977)
Familial amaurotic idiocy† (GM$_2$ gangliosidosis)	German short-haired pointer	R?	Karbe and Schiefer (1967), McGrath et al. (1968), Bernheimer and Karbe (1970), Gambetti et al. (1970)

Continued on next page

---

*Interbreed differences in behavior. The extensive studies by Scott and Fuller (1965) on the genetic basis of interbreed differences in behavioral characteristics leave little doubt that behavior is, to a large degree, genetically determined. Genetic analysis showed, however, that the differences in such traits as aggressiveness, trailing ability, vocalization and ability to learn certain tasks are usually not determined by single genes. There is no evidence to support a conclusion that certain behavioral characteristics are "linked" or in some other way causally related to body type. The fact that breeds of a certain body type have a certain form of behavior appears more likely to be the result of the simultaneous artificial selection for two independent hereditary characteristics.

†Reported by Karbe and Schiefer (1967) to be X-linked, but evidence is insufficient. Probably autosomal recessive, based on data from McGrath et al. (1968).

Table 9. *Neuromuscular System (Continued)*

CONDITION	BREED(S)	MODE	SELECTED REFERENCES
GM$_1$ gangliosidosis	Mixed beagle	R?	Read et al. (1976)
Globoid leukodystrophy	Cairn terrier, West Highland white terrier	R	Fankhauser et al. (1963), Fletcher et al. (1966), Suzuki et al. (1970, 1974)
	Beagle		Johnson et al. (1975)
	Miniature poodle		Zaki and Kay (1973)
Hydrocephalus	English bulldog	?	Stockard (1941)
	Cocker spaniel	?	Scott and Fuller (1965)
Lissencephaly	Lhasa apso	?	Greene et al. (1976), Zaki (1973)
Muscular dystrophy	Irish terrier	XR?	Wentink et al. (1972, 1974)
Myopathy	Labrador retriever	R?	Kramer et al. (1976)
Myotonia	Chow	?	Wentink et al. (1974)
Narcolepsy	Miniature poodle	?	Mitler et al. (1976)
	Doberman pinscher	?	Mitler (1977)
Necrotizing myelopathy	Afghan hound	R	Averill and Bronson (1977)
Neurogenic muscular atrophy	Pointer	R?	Inada et al. (1978)
Neuronal abiotrophy	Swedish Lapland dog	R	Sandefeldt et al. (1973, 1976)
Neuronal ceroidlipofuscinosis	English setter	R	Hagen (1953), Koppang (1963, 1966, 1970), Patel et al. (1974)
Neuropathic necrosis, digits	Pointer	R?	Sanda and Pivnik (1964, 1966)
Quadriplegia–amblyopia	Irish Setter	R	Palmer et al. (1973)
Scottie cramp	Scottish terrier	R	Meyers et al. (1970) Meyers and Schaub (1974)
Syringomyelia	Weimaraner	?	McGrath (1965)
Trembling	Airedale	?	Kollarits (1924)

Table 10. *Other Structural Malformations*

CONDITION	BREED(S)	MODE	SELECTED REFERENCES
Elongated soft palate	Brachycephalic breeds	?	Hodgman (1963)
Inguinal and umbilical hernias	Collie, cocker spaniel, bull terrier, basenji	?	Phillips and Felton (1939), Fox (1963)
	Airedale, Pekingese, Weimaraner, Cairn terrier, Basset hound, West Highland white terrier	?	Hayes (1974)
Laryngeal malformations	Skye terrier	?	Koch (1935), Leonard (1960)
Tracheal collapse	Toy breeds, especially toy poodle, Pomeranian	?	Leonard (1960, 1971)
Tracheal hypoplasia	English bulldog	?	Suter et al. (1972)

Table 11. *The Skin*

CONDITION	BREED(S)	MODE	SELECTED REFERENCES
Atopic dermatitis	Beagle, Dalmatian, Scottish terrier, wire-haired fox terrier	?	Schwartzman et al. (1971)
Black hair follicular dysplasia	Mongrel	R?	Selmanowitz et al. (1972, 1977)
	Bearded collie	R?	Harper (1978)
Cutaneous asthenia (hyperelasticity, fragility)	Springer spaniel	D	Hegreberg et al. (1966, 1969, 1970, 1970a)
Dermoid sinus	Rhodesian ridgeback	?	Hofmeyer (1963), Mann and Stratton (1966)
	Boxer	?	Burgisser and Hinterman (1961)
Ectodermal dysplasia	Miniature poodle	XR?	Selmanowitz et al. (1970, 1977)
Focal loss of pigment (vitiligo)	Belgian Tervueren	?	Mahaffey et al. (1978)
Hairlessness	Mexican hairless, other hairless breeds	D[o]	Editorial (1917), Gaspar (1930), Hutt (1934), Kohn (1911), Thomsett (1961), Zulueta (1945)

[o]The Mexican hairless and other hairless breeds are reported to be heterozygous for a dominant gene for hairlessness. Reportedly, in the homozygous state, the gene is lethal, producing complete occlusion of the lower esophagus. Recessive forms of hairlessness probably occur occasionally in other breeds.

Table 12. *Susceptibility to Disease*

CONDITION	BREED(S)	MODE	SELECTED REFERENCES
Colibacillosis	Basenji		Fox (1965)
Distemper	Beagle, bloodhound, pointers		Whitney (1948), Baker et al. (1962)
Eosinophilic panostitis	Beagle, bloodhound, pointers		Cotter et al. (1968)
Lupus erythematosus	German shepherd		Lewis and Schwartz (1971)
Neonatal death, generally*	Purebred vs. mixed		Scott and Fuller (1965)
Neoplasms†			
Melanoma	Breeds with red or black coat color		Cotchin (1955), Brodey (1970)
Osteosarcoma	Giant breeds		Owen (1962), Tjalma (1966), Brodey (1970), Bech–Nielsen et al. (1978)
Pituitary tumors	Boston terrier		Luginbühl (1963)
Hair follicle tumors	Kerry blue terrier		Brodey (1970)
Mast cell tumors	Boxer, Boston terrier		Peters (1969)
Skin neoplasms, generally	Cocker spaniel		Brodey (1970)
Aortic and carotid body tumors	Boxer, Boston terrier		Brodey (1970), Hayes (1975)
Neoplasia, generally	Boxer		Cohen et al. (1974)
Oral fibrosarcomas and melanomas	German short–haired pointer, Weimaraner, Boxer, Cocker spaniel		Dorn and Priester (1976)
Bladder cancer	Scottish terrier, Shetland sheepdog Beagle, Collie		Hayes (1976)
Thyroiditis	Beagle		Bierwaltes and Nishiyama (1968) Manning et al. (1973)

*The much higher neonatal death rate in the offspring of purebred dogs than in the offspring of crosses between breeds suggests that deleterious recessive genes in the homozygous state are involved.

†As in other species, the high incidence of certain neoplasms in certain strains or breeds may be the result of vertical transmission of oncogenic viruses. Their expression, however, probably depends upon the genotype of the host.

Table 13.　*Urogenital System*

CONDITION	BREED(S)	MODE	SELECTED REFERENCES
Cryptorchidism	Most breeds	R?	Willis (1963), Pendergrass and Hayes (1975), Osterhoff (1977)
Cystine stones (cystinuria)	Dachshund, Irish terrier, poodle, Welsh corgi, Labrador retriever, Great Dane, German shepherd, Cairn terrier, Scottish terrier	XR?	Brand and Cahill (1936), Brand et al. (1940), Holtzapple et al. (1969), Bovée and Segal (1971), Tsan et al. (1972)
Ectopic ureter	Siberian husky	?	Johnston et al. (1977)
Intersexuality	Cocker spaniel	?	Hare (1976) Selden et al. (1978)
Nephritis	Samoyed	?	Bernard and Valli (1977)
Renal aplasia (unilateral)	Beagle	R?	Fox (1964), Vymetal (1965)
Renal cortical hypoplasia	Cocker spaniel, dachshund, Doberman pinscher, Norwegian elkhound, malamute	R?	Murti (1965), Krook (1957), Persson et al. (1961), Kaufman et al. (1969), Finco et al. (1970)
Renal tubular dysfunction (Fanconi syndrome)	Basenji	?	Easly and Breitschwerdt (1976) Bovée et al. (1978)
Uric acid stones (high uric acid excretion)	Dalmatian	R	Trimble and Keeler (1938), Keeler (1940), Harvey, and Christensen (1964), Ts'Ai-Fan Yu et al. (1971)

SELECTED REFERENCES:

The Blood

Andresen, E.: Haemolytic anemia in Basenji dogs. II, Partial deficiency of erythrocyte pyruvate kinase (PK; EC 2.7.1.40) in heterozygous carriers. Anim. Blood Groups Biochem. Genet. 8:149–156, 1977.

Archer, R.K., and Bowden, R.S.T.: A case of true hemophilia in a Labrador dog. Vet. Rec. 71:560–561, 1959.

Bellars, A.R.M.: Hereditary disease in British antarctic sledge dogs. Vet. Rec., 85:600–607, 1969.

Benn, D.M., Gentry, P.A., and Johnstone, I.B.: Classic hemophilia (hemophilia A) in a family of collies. Can. Vet. J., 19:221–225, 1978.

Brock, W.E., et al.: Canine hemophila. Arch. Path. 76:464–469, 1963.

Buckner, R.G., et al.: Hemophilia in the Vizsla. J. Small Anim. Pract. 8:511–519, 1967.

Cheville, N.F.: The gray collie syndrome. J. Am. Vet. Med. Assoc. 152:620–630, 1968.

Cheville, N.F., Cutlip, R.C., and Moon, H.W.: Microscopic pathology of the gray collie syndrome. Path. Vet. 7:225–245, 1970.

Dale, D.C., et al.: Cyclic urinary leukopoietic activity in gray collie dogs. Science, 173:152–153, 1971.

Dale, D.C., Alling, D.W., Wolff, S.M.: Cyclic hematopoiesis: The mechanism of cyclic neutropenia in gray collie dogs. J. Clin. Invest. 51:2197–2204, 1972.

Dale, D.C., and Graw, R.G.: Transplantation of allogeneic bone marrow in canine cyclic neutropenia. Science 183:83–84, 1974.

Dewit, C.D., et al.: The practical importance of blood groups in dogs. J. Small Anim. Pract. 8:285–289, 1969.

Dodds, W.J.: Familial canine thrombocytopathy. Thromb. Diath. Haemorrh. (Suppl. 26):241–248, 1967.

Dodds, W.J.: Canine factor X (Stuart-Prower factor) deficiency. J. Lab. Clin. Med. 52:560–566, 1973.

Dodds, W.J.: Hereditary and acquired hemorrhagic disorders in animals. In Spaet, T.H. (ed.): *Progress in Hemostasis and Thrombosis,* Vol. II. New York, Grune and Stratton, 1974a, pp. 215–247.

Dodds, W.J.: Blood coagulation, hemostasis and thrombosis. In Melby, E.C., and Altman, N.H. (eds.): *Handbook of Laboratory Animal Science,* Vol. II. Cleveland, CRC Press, 1974b.

Dodds, W.J.: Bleeding disorders. In Ettinger, S.J.: *Textbook of Veterinary Internal Medicine,* Vol. II. Philadelphia, W.B. Saunders Co., 1975.

Dodds, W.J.: First international registry of animal models of thrombosis and hemorrhagic diseases. ILAR News 21:A1–A23, 1977.

Dodds, W.J.: Inherited bleeding disorders. Canine Pract. 5:49–58, 1978.

Dodds, W.J.: Hemorrhagic disorders. In Kirk, R.W. (ed.): *Current Veterinary Therapy,* VI. Philadelphia, W.B. Saunders Co., 1977.

Dodds, W.J., and Kaneko, J.J.: Hemostasis and blood coagulation. In Kaneko, J.J., and Cornelius, C.E. (eds.): *Clinical Biochemistry of Domestic Animals.* New York, Academic Press, 1971.

Dodds, W.J., and Kull, J.E.: Canine factor XI (plasma thromboplastin antecedent) deficiency. J. Lab. Clin. Med., 78:746–752, 1971.

Ewing, G.O.: Familial nonspherocytic hemolytic anemia of basenji dogs. J. Am. Vet. Med. Assoc. 154:503–507, 1969.

Field, R.A., Richard, C.G., and Hutt, S.B.: Hemophilia in a family of dogs. Cornell Vet. 36:285–300, 1946.

Fletch, S.M., Pinkerton, P.H., Brueckner, P.J.: The Alaskan malamute chondrodysplasia (dwarfism-anemia) syndrome. JAAHA (review) 11:353–361, 1975.

Ford, L.: Hereditary aspects of human and canine cyclic neutropenia. J. Hered. 60:293–299, 1969.

Gentry, P.A., Johnstone, I.B., and Sanford, S.E.: Diagnosis of classic hemophilia (hemophilia A) in a standard poodle. Can. Vet. J., 18:79–81, 1977.

Graham, J.B., et al.: Canine hemophilia, observations on the course, the clotting anomaly and the effects of blood transfusion. J. Exper. Med. 29:98–111, 1949.

Hogg, G.G., Horton, B.J., and Brown, H.: Inherited pyruvate kinase deficiency and normal haematologic values in Australian basenji dogs. Australian Vet. J. 54:367–370, 1978.

Hutt, F.B., Richard, C.G., and Field, R.A.: Sex-linked hemophilia in dogs. J. Hered. 39:2–9, 1948.

Kammermann, B., Gmur, J., and Stünzi, H.: Afibrinogenämie beim Hund. Zentralbl. Vet. Med. 18A:192–205, 1971.

Kaneko, J.J., Cordy, D.R., and Carlson, G.: Canine hemophilia resembling classic hemophilia A. J. Am. Vet. Med. Assn. 150:15–21, 1967.

Letchworth, G.J., Bentinck-Smith, J., Bolton, G.R., Wootton, J.F., and Family, L.: Cyanosis and methemoglobinemia in two dogs due to a NADH methemoglobin reductase deficiency. JAAHA 13:75–79, 1977.

Lund, J.E., Padgett, G.A., and Ott, R.L.: Cyclic neutropenia in grey collie dogs. Blood 29:452–461, 1967.

Lund, J.E., Gorham, J.R., and Padgett, G.A.: Canine cyclic neutropenia: diagnosis and treatment. Vet. Med. Rev. 1:33–42, 1970.

Lund, J.E., Padgett, G.A., and Gorham, J.R.: Additional evidence on the inheritance of cyclic neutropenia in the dog. J. Hered. 61:47–49, 1970.

Peterson, M.E., and Dodds, W.J.: Factor IX deficiency in an Alaskan malamute. J. Am. Vet. Med. Assoc. (in press, 1979).

Prasse, K.W., Crouser, D., Beutler, E., Walker, M., and Schall, W.D.: Pyruvate kinase deficiency anemia with terminal myelofibrosis and osteosclerosis in a beagle. J. Am. Vet. Med. Assn. 166:1170–1175, 1975.

Rogers, W.A., Donovan, E.F., and Kociba, G.J.: Idiopathic hyperlipoproteinemia in dogs. J. Am. Vet. Med. Assoc. 166:1087–1100, 1975.

Rowsell, H.C.: Hemorrhagic disorders in dogs: their recognition, treatment and importance. "The newer knowledge about dogs." 12th Gaines Veterinary Symposium, East Lansing, Michigan, January 23, 1963.

Rowsell, H.C., et al.: A disorder resembling hemophilia B (Christmas disease) in dogs. J. Am. Vet. Med. Assoc. 137:247–250, 1960.

Searcy, G.P., Miller, D.R., and Tasker, J.B.: Congenital hemolytic anemia in the basenji dog due to erythrocyte pyruvate kinase deficiency. Canad. J. Comp. Med. 35:67–70, 1971.

Sharp, A.A., and Dike, G.W.R.: Hemophilia in the dog: treatment with heterologous antihaemophilic globulin. Thromb. Diathes. Haemorrhagica 10:494–501, 1963.

Slappendel, R.J.: Hemophilia A and Hemophilia B in a family of French bulldogs. Tijdschr. Diergeneesk. 100:1075–1088, 1975.

Spurling, N.W., Burton, L.K., Peacock, R., and Pilling, T.: Hereditary Factor–VII deficiency in the beagle. British J. of Haematology 23:59–67, 1972.

Standerfer, R.J., Templeton, J.W., and Black, J.A.: Anomalous pyruvate kinase deficiency in the basenji dog. Am. J. Vet. Res. 35:1541–1543, 1974.

Swisher, S.N., Young, L.E., and Trabold, N.: *In vitro* and *in vivo* studies of the behavior of canine erythrocyte-isoantibody systems. Ann. New York Acad. Sci. 97:15–25, 1962.

Tasker, J.B., et al.:Familial anemia in the basenji dog. J. Am. Vet. Med. Assoc. 154:158–165, 1969.

Wurzel, H.A., and Lawrence, W.C.: Canine hemophilia. Thromb. Diathes. Haemorrhagica 6:98–103, 1961.

Young, L.E., et al.: Hemolytic disease in newborn dogs. Blood 6:291, 1951.

Bones and Joints

Amlöf, J.: On achondroplasia in the dog. Zentralbl. Vet. Med., 8:43–56, 1961.

Bardens, J.W.: Congenital malformation of the foramen magnum in dogs. S. West. Vet., 18:295–298, 1965.

Bradley, I.W.: Non-union of the anconeal process in the dog. Aust. Vet. J., 43:215–216, 1967.

Burns, M., and Fraser, M.N.: *Genetics of the Dog: The Basis of Successful Breeding.* Philadelphia, J.B. Lippincott Co., 1966.

Calkins, E., Kahn, D., and Diner, W.C.: Idiopathic familial osteoporosis in dogs: "osteogenesis imperfecta." Ann. New York Acad. Sci., 64:410–423, 1956.

Carlson, W.D., and Severin, G.A.: Elbow dysplasia in the dog. J. Am. Vet. Med. Assn:, 138:295–297, 1961.

Carrig, C.B., and Seawright, A.A.: A familial canine polyostotic fibrous dysplasia with subperiosteal cortical defects. J. Small Anim. Pract., 10:397–405, 1969.

Carrig, C.B., Pool, R.R., and McElroy, J.M.: Polyostotic cystic bone lesions in a dog. J. Small Anim. Pract., 16:495–513, 1975.

Carrig, C.B., MacMillan, A., Brundage, S., Pool, R.R., and Morgan, J.P.: Retinal dysplasia associated with skeletal abnormalities in Labrador retrievers. J. Am. Vet. Med. Assn. 170:49–60, 1977.

Cawley, A.J., and Archibald, J.: Ununited anconeal processes of the dog. J. Am. Vet. Med. Assoc., 136:454–458, 1959.

Chester, D.K.: Multiple cartilaginous exostoses in two generations of dogs. J. Am. Vet. Med. Assn., 159:895–897, 1971.

Corley, E.A., and Carlson, W.D.: Radiographic, Genetic, and Pathologic Aspects of Elbow Dysplasia. Proceedings of the American Veterinary Medical Association, 102nd Annual Meeting, 1965.

Curtis, R.L., English, D., and Kim, Y.J.: Spina bifida in a "stub" dog stock, selectively bred for short tails. Anat. Rec., 148:365, 1964.

deBoom, H.P.A.: Anomalous animals. S. Afr. J. Sci., 61:159–171, 1965.

Fletch, S.M., and Pinkerton, P.H.: Animal model: inherited hemolytic anemia with stomatocytosis in the Alaskan malamute dog. Am. J. Path., 71:477–480, 1973.

Fletch, S.M., et al.: Clinical and pathologic features of chondrodysplasia in the Alaskan malamute. J. Am. Vet. Med. Assoc., 162:357–361, 1973.

Fletch, S.M., Pinkerton, P.H., and Brueckner, P.J.: The Alaskan malamute chondrodysplasia (dwarfism-anemia) syndrome. J.A.A.H.A. (review), 11:353–361, 1975.

Flo, G.L., Tvedten, H.: Cervical calcinosis circumscripta in three related Great Dane dogs. J. Am. Anim. Hosp. Assoc., 11:507–510, 1975.

Fox, M.W.: Abnormalities of the canine skull. Canad. J. Comp. Med. Vet. Sci., 9:219–222, 1963.

Fox, M.W.: The otocephalic syndrome in the dog. Cornell Vet., 54:250–259, 1964.

Gardner, D.L.: Familial canine chondrodystrophia foetalis (achondroplasia). J. Path. Bact., 77:243–247, 1959.

Geary, J.C., Oliver, J.E., and Hoerlein, B.F.: Atlanto-axial subluxation in the canine. J. Small Anim. Pract., 8:577–582, 1967.

Gee, B.R., and Doige, C.E.: Multiple cartilaginous exostoses in a litter of dogs. J. Am. Vet. Med. Assoc., 156:53–59, 1970.

Ghosh, P., Taylor, T.K.F., Varoll, J.M., Braund, K.G., and Larsen, L.H.: Genetic factors in the maturation of the canine intervertebral disc. Res. Vet. Sci. 19:304–311, 1975.

Green, E.L.: Mutant stocks of cats and dogs offered for research. J. Hered., 48:56–57, 1957.

Grøndalen, J.: Malformation of the elbow joint in an Afghan hound litter. J. Small Anim. Pract., 14:83–89, 1973.

Grüneberg, H., and Lea, A.J.: An inherited jaw anomaly in long-haired dachshunds. J. Genet., 39:285–296, 1940.

Hansen, H.J.: A pathologic-anatomical study on disc degeneration in the dog. Acta Orthopaed. Scand., 11:117, 1952.

Hansen, H.J.: The body constitution of dogs and its importance for the occurrence of disease. Nord. Vet. Med., 16:977–987, 1964.

Hansen, H.J.: Historical evidence of an unusual deformity in dogs ("short-spine dog"). J. Small Anim. Pract., 9:103–108, 1968.

Henricson, B., and Olsson, S.E.: Hereditary acetabular dysplasia in German shepherd dogs. J. Am. Vet. Med. Assoc., 135:207–210, 1959.

Henricson, B., Norberg, I., and Olsson, S.E.: Huftgelenksdysplasie beim Hund. Nord. Vet. Med., 17:118–131, 1965.

Henricson, B., Norberg, I., and Olsson, S.E.: On the etiology and pathogenesis of hip dysplasia: a comparative review. J. Small Anim. Pract., 7:673–688, 1966.

Hime, J.M.: An unusual spinal condition in foxhounds. Vet. Rec., 75:644, 1963.

Hime, J.M., and Drake, J.C.: Osteochrondrosis of the spine in the foxhound. Vet. Rec., 77:445–449, 1965.

Hodgman, S.F.J.: Abnormalities and defects in pedigree dogs. I. An investigation into the existence of abnormalities in pedigree dogs in the British Isles. J. Small Anim. Pract., 4:447–456, 1963.

Hutt, F.B.: Genetic selection to reduce the incidence of hip dysplasia in dogs. J. Am. Vet. Med. Assoc., 151:1041–1048, 1967.

Hutt, F.B.: Genetic defects of bones and joints in domestic animals. Cornell Vet., 58:104–113, 1968.

Jubb, K.V.F., and Kennedy, P.C.: *Pathology of Domestic Animals.* New York, Academic Press, 1964.

Keeler, C.E., and Trimble, H.C.: The inheritance of dew claws in the dog. J. Hered., 29:145–148, 1938.

Knight, G.C.: Abnormalities and defects in pedigree dogs. III. Tibiofemoral joint deformity and patella luxation. J. Small Anim. Pract., 4:463–464, 1963.

Kodituwakku, G.E.: Luxation of the patella in the dog. Vet. Med., 74:1499–1508, 1962.

Ladrat, J., Blin, J.C., and Lauvergne, J.J.: Ectomélie bithoracique Héréditaire chez le chien. Ann. Génét. Sél. Anim., 1:119–130, 1969.

Lau, R.E.: Inherited premature closure of the distal ulnar physis. J.A.A.H.A., 13:609–612, 1977.

Lee, R., and Fry, P.D.: Some observations on the occurrence of Legg-Calvé-Perthes disease (coxaplana) in the dog, and an eval-uation of excision arthroplasty as a method of treatment. J. Small Anim. Pract., 10:309–317, 1969.

Leighton, E.A., Linn, J.M., Willham, R.L., and Castleberry, M.W.: A genetic study of canine hip dysplasia. Am. J. Vet. Res., 38:241–244, 1977.

Lettow, E., and Dammrich, K.: Beitrag zur Klinit und Pathologie der Osteogenesis Imperfecta bei Junghunden. Zentralbl. Vet. Med., 7:936–966, 1960.

Lodge, D.: Two cases of epiphyseal dysplasia. Vet. Rec., 79:136–138, 1966.

Loeffler, K.: Glenkanomalien als Problem in der Hundezucht. Dtsch. Tieraerztl. Wochenschr., 71:291–297, 1964.

Leffler, K., and Meyer, H.: Erbliche Patellarluxation bei Toy-Spaniels. Dtsch. Tieraerztl. Wochenschr., 68:619–622, 1961.

Lust, G., and Farrell, P.W.: Hip dysplasia in dogs: The interplay of genotype and environment (an editorial). Cornell Vet., May, 1977: pp. 447–466.

Mayrhofer, E.: Metaphysäre Tibiadysplasie beim Dachshund. Kleintier-Praxis, 22:223–228, 1977.

Moltzen–Nielsen, H.:Calvé-Perthes Krankheit, Malum Deformans Juvenilis Coxae bei Hunden. Arch. Wiss. Prakt. Tierheilk, 72:91, 1937.

Oliver, J.E., Selcer, R.R., and Simpson, S.: Cauda equina compression from lumbosacral malarticulation and malformation in the dog. J. Am. Vet. Med. Assn. 173:207–214, 1978.

Palmer, A.C., and Wallace, M.S.: Deformation of cervical vertebrae in Basset hounds. Vet. Rec., 80:430–433, 1967.

Parker, A.J., and Park, R.D.: Atlanto-axial subluxation in small breeds of dogs. Diagnosis and pathogenesis. Vet. Med./Small Anim. Clin., 68:1133–1137, 1973.

Phillips, J.M.: "Pig jaw" in cocker spaniels. Retrognathia of the mandible in the cocker spaniel and its relationship to other deformities of the jaw. J. Hered., 36:177–181, 1945.

Pick, J.R., et al.: Subluxation of the carpus in dogs. An X chromosomal defect closely linked with the locus for hemophilia A. Lab. Invest., 17:243–248, 1967.

Pidduck, H., and Webbon, P.M.: The genetic control of Perthes' disease in toy poodles — a working hypothesis. J. Small Anim. Pract., 19:729–733, 1978.

Priester, W.A.: Sex, size and breed as risk factors in canine patella dislocation. J. Am. Vet. Med. Assoc., 160:740–742, 1972.

Pullig, T.: Inheritance of a skull defect in cocker spnaiels. J. Hered., 44:97–99, 1952.

Pullig, T.: Anury in cocker spaniels. J. Hered., 44:105–107, 1953.

Pullig, T.: Brachyury in cocker spaniels. J. Hered., 48:75–76, 1957.

Rasmussen, P.G.: Multiple epiphyseal dysplasia in a litter of beagle puppies. J. Small Anim. Pract., 12:91–96, 1971.

Rasmussen, P.G.: Multiple epiphyseal dysplasia in beagle puppies. Acta Radiol. (Suppl. 319):251–254, 1972.

Rasmussen, P.G., Reimann, I.: Dysostosis enchondralis of the ulnar bone in the Basset hound. Acta Vet. Scand., 18:31–39, 1977.

Riser, W.H.: An analysis of the current status of hip dysplasia in the dog. J. Am. Vet. Med. Assoc., 144:709–721, 1964.

Riser, W.H.: The dog as a model for the study of hip dysplasia: Growth, form, and development of the normal and dysplastic hip joint. Vet. Path. 12:229–334, 1975.

Riser, W.H., and Shirer, J.F.: Correlation between canine hip dysplasia and pelvic muscle mass: a study of 95 dogs. Am. J. Vet. Res., 28:769–777, 1967.

Riser, W.H., Parkes, L.J., and Shirer, J.F.: Canine craniomandibular osteopathy. J. Am. Rad. Soc., VIII:23–31, 1967.

Riser, W.H., et al.: Influence of early rapid growth and weight gain on hip dysplasia in the German shepherd dog. J. Am. Vet. Med. Assoc., 145:661–668, 1964.

Riser, W.H., Haskins, M.E., Jesyk, P.F., and Patterson, D.F.: Pseudoachondroplastic dysplasia in the miniature poodle. J. Am. Vet. Med. Assn., 1979 (in press).

Ritter, R.: Konnen Anomalien des Gebisses Gezuchtet Werden? Dtsch. Zahn Mund. Kieferheilk., 4:235–257, 1933.

Schales, O.: Heredity patterns in dysplasia of the hip. N. Am. Vet., 38:152–155, 1957.

Schales, O.: Congenital hip dysplasia in dogs. Vet. Med., 57:143–148, 1959.

Selcer, R.R., and Oliver, J.E., Jr.: Cervical spondylopathy — wobbler syndrome in dogs. JAAHA 11:175–179, 1975.

Smart, M.E., and Fletch, S.: A hereditary skeletal growth defect in purebred Alaskan malamutes. (Letter to the Editor.) Canad. Vet. J., 12:31–32, 1971.

Stockard, C.R.: The Genetic and Endocrinic Basis for Differences in Form and Behavior as Elucidated by Studies of Contrasted Pure-line Dog Breeds and Hybrids. American Anatomical Memoirs. Philadelphia, Wistar Institute of Anatomy and Biology, 1941.

Subden, R.E., et al.: Genetics of the Alaskan malamute chondrodysplasia syndrome. J. Hered., 63:149–152, 1972.

Suu, S.: Studies on the short-spine dogs. I. Their origin and occurrence. Res. Bull. Fac. Agric. Gifu. Univ., 7:127–134, 1956.

Suu, S., and Ueshima, T.J.: Studies on the short-spine dogs. II. Somatological observation. Res. Bull. Fac. Agric. Gifu. Univ., 8:112–28, 1957.

Trotter, E.J., deLahunta, A., Geary, J.C., and Brasmer, T.H.: Caudal cervical vertebral malformation–malarticulation in great Danes and doberman pinschers. J. Am. Vet. Med. Assn. 168:917–930, 1976.

Vaughan, L.C.: Studies on intervertebral disc protrusion in the dog. I. Aetiology and Pathogenesis. Brit. Vet. J., 114:105–112, 1958.

Vaughan, L.C.: Congenital detachment of the processus anconeus in the dog. Vet. Rec., 74:309–311, 1962.

Wamberg, K.: Huftgelenksleiden des Hundes. Mh. Vet. Med., 16:884–891, 1961.

Whitney, L.F.: How to Breed Dogs. New York, Orange Judd Publishing Co., Inc., 1947.

Wright, F., Rest, J.R., and Palmer, A.C.: Ataxia of the Great Dane caused by stenosis of the vertebral canal: comparison with similar conditions in the Basset Hound, Doberman Pinscher, Ridgeback and the thoroughbred horse. Vet. Rec., 92:1–6, 1973.

Zimmer, E.A., and Stähli, W.: Erbbedingte Versteifung der Wirbelsaule in einer Familie deutsche Boxer. Schweiz. Arch. Tierheilk., 102:254–264, 1960.

Cardiovascular and Lymphatic Systems

Branch, C.E., Robertson, B.T., Beckett, S.D., Waldo, A.L., and James, T.N.: An animal model of spontaneous syncope and sudden death. J. Lab. Clin. Med., 90:592–603, 1977.

Buchanan, J.W.: Morphology of the ductus arteriosus in fetal and neonatal dogs genetically predisposed to patent ductus arteriosus. Birth Defects, Original Article Series. Vol. XIV, No. 7, National Foundation, pp. 349–360, 1978.

James, T.N., and Drake, E.H.: Sudden death in Doberman pinschers. Henry Ford Hosp. Med. Bull., 13:183–190, 1965.

James, T.N., and Drake, E.H.: Sudden death in Doberman pinschers. Ann. Intern. Med., 68:821–829, 1968.

Ladds, P.W., Dennis, S.M., and Leipold, H.W.: Lethal congenital edema in bulldog pups. J. Am. Vet. Med. Assoc., 159:81–86, 1971.

Lüginbuhl, H., et al.: Congenital hereditary lymphoedema in the dog. Part II. Pathological studies. J. Med. Genet., 4:153–165, 1967.

Moore, E.N., Boineau, J.P., and Patterson, D.F.: Incomplete right bundle branch block. An electrocardiographic enigma and possible misnomer. Circulation, 44:678–687, 1971.

Mulvihill, J.J.: Comments on the epidemiology of congenital heart disease in dogs. Birth Defects: Original Article Series, Vol. XV, Cardiovascular System. National Foundation, pp. 175–177, 1972.

Naylor, R.J.: Regurgitation in pups. I. Persistent aortic arches. J. Am. Vet. Med. Assoc., 130:283–284, 1957.

Patterson, D.F.: Epidemiologic and genetic studies of congenital heart disease in the dog. Circ. Res., 23:171–202, 1968.

Patterson, D.F., and Pyle, R.L.: Genetic aspects of congenital heart disease in the dog. "The newer knowledge about dogs." 21st Annual Gaines Veterinary Symposium, Ames, Iowa, 1971.

Patterson, D.F., Pyle, R.L., and Buchanan, J.W.: Hereditary cardiovascular malformations of the dog. Birth Defects: Original Article Series, Vol. XV, Cardiovascular System. National Foundation, pp. 100–174, 1972.

Patterson, D.F., et al.: Congenital hereditary lymphoedema in the dog. Part I. Clinical and genetic studies. J. Med. Genet., 4:145–152, 1967.

Patterson, D.F., et al.: Hereditary patent ductus arteriosus and its sequelae in the dog. Circ. Res., 39:1–13, 1971.

Patterson, D.F., et al.: Hereditary defects of the conotruncal septum in keeshond dogs. Pathologic and genetic studies. Am. J. Cardiol., 34:187–205, 1974.

Pyle, R.L., and Patterson, D.F.: Multiple cardiovascular malformations in a family of boxer dogs. J. Am. Vet. Med. Assoc., 160:965–976, 1972.

Pyle, R.L., Patterson, D.F., and Chacko, S.: The genetics and pathology of discrete subaortic stenosis in the Newfoundland dog. American Heart Journal, 92:324–334, 1976.

Van Mierop, L.H.S., Patterson, D.F., and Schnarr, W.R.: Hereditary conotruncal septal defects in Keeshond dogs: Embryologic studies. Am. J. of Cardiology, 40:936–950, 1977.

Van Mierop, L.H.S., Patterson, D.F., and Schnarr, W.R.: Pathogenesis of persistent truncus arteriosus in light of observations made in a dog embryo with the anomaly. Am. J. of Cardiology, 41:755–762, 1978.

Chromosomal Abnormalities

Borgaonkar, D.S., et al.: Chromosome study of four breeds of dogs. J. Hered., 59:157–160, 1968.

Clough, E., et al.: An XXY sex-chromosome constitution in a dog with testicular hypoplasia and congenital heart disease. Cytogenetics, 9:71–77, 1970.

Hare, W.C.D., et al.: Cytogenetics in the dog and cat. J. Small Anim. Pract. 7:575–592, 1966.

Hare, W.C.D., et al.: Bone chondroplasia and a chromosomal anomaly in the same dog. Am. J. Vet. Res., 28:583–587, 1967.

Larsen, R.E., Dias, E., Cervenka, J.: Centric fusion of autosomal chromosomes in a bitch and offspring. Am. J. Vet. Res., 39:861–864, 1978.

Ma, N.S.F., and Gilmore, C.E.: Chromosomal abnormality in a phenotypically and clinically normal dog. Cytogenetics, 10:254–258, 1971.

Patterson, D.F., et al.: Congenital malformations of the cardiovascular system associated with chromosomal abnormalities: a report of the clinical, pathologic, and cytogenetic findings in 2 dogs. Zentralbl. Vet. Med., 13:669–686, 1966.

Selden, J.R., et al.: The Giemsa banding pattern of the canine karyotype. Cytogenet. Cell Genet., 15:380–387, 1975.

Shive, R.J., Hare, W.C.D, and Patterson, D.F.: Chromosome studies in dogs with congenital cardiac defects. Cytogenetics, 4:340–348, 1965.

Digestive System

Aitchison, J.: Incisor dentition in short muzzled dogs. Vet. Rec., 76:165–169, 1964.

Burstone, M.S., Bond, E., and Litt, R.: Familial gingival hypertrophy in the dog (boxer breed). Arch. Path., 54:208–212, 1952.

Clifford, D.H., Waddell, E.D., Patterson, D.R., Wilson, C.F., and Thompson, H.L.: Management of esophageal achalasia in miniature schnauzers. J. Am. Vet. Med. Assn. 161:1012–1021, 1972.

Cooper, H.K., Jr., and Mattern, G.W.: Genetic studies of cleft lip and palate in dogs (a preliminary report). Carnivore Genetics Newsletter No. 9:204–209, 1970.

Earlam, R.J., Zollman, P.E., and Ellis, F.H., Jr.: Congenital oesophageal achalasia in the dog. Thorax, 22:466–472, 1967.

Gardner, J.E., Jr.: Report of a survey on cleft palates in the English bulldog. Bulletin of the Bulldog Club of New Jersey, September, 1954.

Hardy, R.M., and Stevens, J.B.: Chronic progressive hepatitis in Bedlington terriers (Bedlington Liver Disease). In Kirk, R.W.: *Current Veterinary Therapy VI*. Philadelphia, W.B. Saunders, 1977.

Hardy, R.M., and Stevens, J.B.: Chronic progressive hepatitis in Bedlington terriers. Proc. 45th Annual Meeting, AAHA, pp. 187–190, 1978.

Hardy, R.M., Stevens, J.B., and Stowe, C.M.: Chronic progressive hepatitis in Bedlington terriers associated with elevated liver copper concentrations. Minn. Vet., 15:13–24, 1975.

Horowitz, S.L., and Chase, H.B.: A microform of cleft palate in dogs. J. Dent. Res., 49:892, 1970.

Hutt, F.B., and deLahunta, A.: A lethal glossopharyngeal defect in the dog. J. Hered., 62:291–293, 1971.

Jurkiewicz, M.J.: A genetic study of cleft lip and palate in dogs, S. Forum, 16:472–473, 1965.

Jurkiewicz, M.J., and Bryant, D.L.: Cleft lip and palate in dogs: a progress report. Cleft Palate J., 5:30–36, 1968.

Osborne, C.A., Clifford, D.H., and Jessen, C.: Hereditary esophageal achalasia in dogs. J. Am. Vet. Med. Assn., 151:572–581, 1967.

Pearce, R.G.: Anomalies of the English bulldog. Southwest Vet. J., 22:218–220, 1969.

Spy, G.M.: Megaesophagus in greyhounds. Vet. Rec., 75:853, 1963.

Weber, W., and Freudiger, U.: Investigations on the heritability of chronic exocrine insufficiency of the pancreas in the German shepherd dog. Schweizer Arch. Tierheilkd., 119:257–263, 1977.

Woods, C.B., Rawlings, C., Barber, D., and Walker, M.: Esophageal deviation in four English bulldogs. J. Am. Vet. Med. Assn. 172:934–939, 1978.

The Ear

Adams, E.W.: Hereditary deafness in a family of foxhounds. J. Am. Vet. Med. Assoc., 128:302, 1956.

Anderson, R., et al.: Genetic hearing impairment in the Dalmation dog. Acta Otolaryngologica (Suppl. 232), 1968.

Hudson, W.R., and Ruben, R.J.: Hereditary deafness in Dalmations. Arch. Otolaryngol, 75:213, 1962.

Lurie, M.H.: The membranous labyrinth in the congenitally deaf collie and Dalmation dog. Laryngoscope, 58:279, 1948.

Young, G.B.: Inherited defects in dogs. Vet. Rec., 67:15–19, 1955.

Endocrine and Metabolic Disorders

Allan, G.S., Huxtable, C.R.R., Howlett, C.R., Baxter, R.C., Duff, B., and Farrow, B.R.H.: Pituitary dwarfism in German shepherd dogs. J. Small Anim. Pract., 19:711–727, 1978.

Andresen, E., and Willeberg, P.: Pituitary dwarfism in German shepherd dogs: additional evidence of simple, autosomal recessive inheritance. Nord. Vet. Med., 28:481–486, 1976.

Andresen, E., Willeberg, P.: Pituitary dwarfism in Carelian bear dogs: evidence of a simple, autosomal recessive inheritance. Hereditas, 84:232–234, 1976a.

Andresen, E., Willeberg, P., and Rasmussen, P.G.: Pituitary dwarfism in German shepherd dogs: genetic investigations. Nord. Vet. Med., 26:692–701, 1974.

Bardens, J.W.: Glycogen storage disease in puppies. Vet. Med. Small Anim. Clin., 61:1174–1176, 1966.

Bardens, J.W., Bardens, G., and Bardens, B.: A Von Gierke-like syndrome. Allied Vet., 32:4–7, 1961.

Brouwers, J.: Goitre et heredite chez le chien. Ann. Med. Vet., 94:173–174, 1950.

Ceh, L., Hauge, J.G., Svenkerud, R., and Strande, A.: Glycogenosis type III in the dog. Acta Vet. Scand., 17:210–222, 1976.

Gershwin, L.J.: Familial canine diabetes mellitus. J. Am. Vet. Med. Assn., 167:479–480, 1975.

Hardy, R.M., and Stevens, J.B.: Chronic progressive hepatitis in Bedlington terriers. Proceedings 45th Annual AAHA Meeting, pp. 187–190, 1978.

Hardy, R.M., and Stevens, J.B.: Chronic progressive hepatitis in Bedlington terriers (Bedlington Liver Disease). In Kirk, R.W.,: *Current Veterinary Therapy.* VI. Philadelphia, W.B. Saunders Company, 1977.

Hardy, R.M., Stevens, J.B., and Stowe, C.M.: Chronic progressive hepatitis in Bedlington terriers associated with elevated liver copper concentrations. Minn. Vet., 15:13–24, 1975.

Hartley, W.J., and Blakemore, W.F.: Neurovisceral glucocerebroside storage (Gaucher's Disease) in a dog. Vet Path., 10:191–201, 1973.

Jezyk, P.F.: Screening for inborn errors of metabolism in dogs and cats. In Hommes, F.A. (ed.): *Models for the Study of Inborn Errors of Metabolism.* Holland, Elsevier/North-Holland Biomedical Press, pp. 11–18, 1979.

Manning, P.J., Corwin, L.A., and Middleton, C.C.: Familial hyperlipoproteinemia and thyroid dysfunction of beagles. Exp. & Molecular Path., 19:378–388, 1973.

Mostafa, I.E.: A case of glycogenic cardiomegaly in a dog. Acta Vet. Scand., 11:197–208, 1970.

Nicholas, F.: Pituitary dwarfism in German shepherd dogs: a genetic analysis of some Australian data. J. Small Anim. Pract., 19:167–174, 1978.

Rafiquzzaman, M., Svenkerud, R., Strande, A., and Hauge, J.G.: Glycogenosis in the dog. Acta Vet. Scand., 17:196–209, 1976.

Read, D.H., Harrington, D.D., Keenan, T.W., and Hinsman, E.J.: Neuronal–visceral GM₁ gangliosidosis in a dog with B–galactosidase deficiency. Science, 194:442–445, 1976.

Rogers, W.A., Donovan, E.F., and Kociba, G.J.: Idiopathic hyperlipoproteinemia in dogs. J. Am. Vet. Med. Assn., 166:1087–1091, 1975.

Strombeck, D.R., Meyer, D.J., and Freedland, R.A.: Hyperammonemia due to a urea cycle enzyme deficiency in two dogs. J. Am. Vet. Med. Assn., 166:1109–1111, 1975.

Wilkinson, J.S.: Spontaneous diabetes mellitus. Vet. Rec., 72:548–558, 1960.

Willeberg, P., Kastrup, K.W., and Andresen, E.: Pituitary dwarfism in German shepherd dogs: studies on somatomedin activity. Nord. Vet. Med., 27:448–454, 1975.

The Eye

Aguirre, G.D.: Hereditary retinal disease in small animals. Vet. Clin. N. Am., 3:515–528, 1973.

Aguirre, G.: Inherited retinal degenerations in the dog. Tr. Am. Acad. Ophth. Otol., 81:667–676, 1976.

Aguirre, G.: Retinal degenerations in the dog. I. Rod dysplasia. Exp. Eye Res., 26:233–253, 1978.

Aguirre, G.D., and Rubin, L.F.: Progressive retinal atrophy (rod dysplasia) in the Norwegian elkhound. J. Am. Vet. Med. Assn., 158:208–218, 1971.

Aguirre, G.D., and Rubin, L.F.: Pathology of hemeralopia in the Alaskan malamute. Investigative Ophthalmology, 13:231–235, 1974.

Aguirre, G., Farber, D., Lolley, R., Fletcher, R.T., and Chader, G.J.: Rod-cone dysplasia in Irish Setters: A defect in cyclic GMP metabolism in visual cells. Science, 201:1133–1134, 1978.

Andersen, A.C., and Shultz, F.T.: Inherited (congenital) cataract in the dog. Am. J. Path., 34:965–975, 1958.

Ashton, N., Barnett, K.C., and Sachs, D.D.: Retinal dysplasia in the Sealyham terrier. J. Path. Bact., 96:269–272, 1968.

Barnett, K.C.: Canine retinopathies. II. The miniature and toy poodle. J. Small Anim. Pract., 6:93–109, 1965.

Barnett, K.C.: Primary retinal dystrophies in the dog. J. Am. Vet. Med. Assn., 154:804–808, 1969.

Barnett, K.C.: Types of cataract in the dog. J.A.A.H.A., 8:2–9, 1972.

Barnett, K.C. and Curtis, R.: Lens luxation and progressive retinal atrophy in the Tibetan terrier. Vet. Rec. 103:160, 1978.

Barnett, K.C., and Knight, G.C.: Persistent pupillary membrane in the basenji. Vet. Rec., 85:242, 1969.

Barnett, K.C., et al.: Hereditary retinal dysplasia in Labrador retrievers in England and Sweden. J. Small Animal Pract., 10:753–759, 1970.

Bedford, P.G.C.: The aetiology of primary glaucoma in the dog. J. Small Animal Pract., 16:217–239, 1975.

Bellhorn, R.W., Bellhorn, M.B., Swarm, R.L., Impellizzeri, C.W.: Hereditary tapetal abnormality in the Beagle. Ophthalmic Res., 7:250–260, 1975.

Black, L.: Progressive retinal atrophy. A review of the genetics and an appraisal of the eradication scheme. J. Small Animal Pract., 13:295–314, 1972.

Burns, M., and Fraser, M.N.: The Genetics of the Dog: The Basis of Successful Breeding. Philadelphia, J.B. Lippincott Co., 1966.

Carrig, C.B., MacMillan, A., Brundage, S., Pool, R.R., and Morgan, J.P.: Retinal dysplasia associated with skeletal abnormalities in Labrador retrievers. J. Am. Vet. Med. Assn., 170:49–60, 1977.

Cogan, D.G., and Kuwabara, T.: Photoreceptive abiotrophy of the retina in the elkhound. Path., Vet., 2:101–128, 1965.

Donovan, E.R., and Wyman, M.: Ocular fundus anomaly in the collie. Proceedings of the 102nd Annual Meeting. J. Am. Vet. Med. Assn., 147:1465–1469, 1965.

Donovan, R.H., and Macpherson, A.M.: The inheritance of chorioretinal change and staphyloma in the collie. Carnivore Genetics Newsletter, 5:85–89, 1968.

Formston, C.: Observations on subluxation and luxation of the crystalline lens in the dog. J. Comp. Path., 55:168–184, 1945.

Garmer, L., Lagerman-Pekkari, M., Schauman, P., and Tigerschiöld, A.: Progressiv Retinal Atrofi hes Tibetansk terrier. Svensk. Vet., 26:158–160, 1974.

Gelatt, K.N., and McGill, L.D.: Clinical characteristics of microphthalmia with colobomas of the Australian shepherd dog. J. Am. Vet. Med. Assn., 167:393–396, 1973.

Gelatt, K.N., Peiffer, R.L., Gwin, R.M., Gwin, G.G. and Williams, L.W.: Clinical manifestations of inherited glaucoma in the beagle. Invest. Ophthal. 16:1135, 1977.

Heywood, R.: Juvenile cataracts in the beagle dog. J. Small Animal Pract., 12:171–177, 1971.

Hodgman, S.F.J.: Abnormalities and defects in pedigree dogs. I. An investigation into the existence of abnormalities in pedigree dogs in the British Isles. J. Small Animal Pract., 4:447–456, 1963.

Hodgman, S.F.J., et al.: Progressive retinal atrophy in dogs. I. The disease in Irish setters (red). Vet. Rec., 61:185–189, 1949.

Host, P., and Sreison, S.: Hereditary cataract in the dog. Norsk, Vet. Tidsskv., 48:244–270, 1936.

Keep, J.M.: Clinical aspects of progressive retinal atrophy in the cardigan Welsh corgi. Aust. Vet. J., 48:197–199, 1972.

Kittel, H.: Uber Dermoide der Kornea am Spaltbildungen der Lider am Ange von Bernhardinerhunden. Dtsch. Tierearztl. Wochenschr., 52:793–797, 1931.

Koch, S.A.: Cataracts in interrelated old English sheepdogs. J. Am. Vet. Med. Assn., 160:299–301, 1972.

Kock, E.: *Retinal Dysplasia: A Comparative Study in Human Beings and Dogs.* Dept. of Pathology, Karolinska Inst. Stockholm, Sweden, 1974.

LaVach, J.D., Murphy, J.M., and Severin, G.A.: Retinal dysplasia in the English springer spaniel. JAAHA, 14:192–199, 1978.

Lawson, D.D.: Luxation of the crystalline lens in the dog. J. Small Animal Pract., 10:461–463, 1969.

Lovekin, L.G.: Primary glaucoma in dogs. J. Am. Vet. Med. Assn., 145:1081–1091, 1964.

Lovekin, L.G., and Bellhorn, R.W.: Clinicopathologic changes in primary glaucoma in the cocker spaniel. Am. J. Vet. Res., 29:375–385, 1968.

MacMillan, A.D., Lipton, D.E.: Heritability of multifocal retinal dysplasia in American Cocker spaniels. J. Am. Vet. Med. Assn. 172:568–572, 1978.

Magnusson, H.: About retinitis pigmentosa and consanguinity in dogs. Arch. Verhg. Ophthal., 2:147–163, 1911.

Magrane, W.G.: Congenital anomaly of the optic disc in collies. N. Am. Vet., 34:646, 1953.

Martin, C.L., and Leach, R.: Everted membrana nictitans, in German shorthaired pointers. J. Am. Vet. Med. Assn., 157:1229–1232, 1970.

Martin, C.L., and Wyman, M.: Glaucoma in the Basset hound. J. Am. Vet. Med. Assn., 153:1320–1327, 1968.

Olesen, H.P., Jensen, O.A., Norn, M.S.: Congenital hereditary cataract in Cocker spaniels. J. Small Anim. Pract., 15:741–750, 1974.

Parry, H.B.: Degenerations of the dog retina. II. General progressive atrophy of hereditary aetiology. Brit. J. Ophthalmol., 37:487–502, 1953.

Parry, H.B.: Degenerations of the dog retina. VI. Central progressive atrophy with pigment epithelial dystrophy. Brit. J. Ophthalmol., 38:653–668, 1954.

Roberts, S.R.: Superficial indolent ulcer of the cornea in boxer dogs. J. Small Animal Pract., 6:111–115, 1965.

Roberts, S.R.: Three inherited ocular defects in the dog. Mod. Vet. Pract., 48:30–34, 1967.

Roberts, S.R., and Dellaporta, A.: Congenital posterior ectasia of the sclera in Collie dogs. Am. J. Ophth., 59:180–186, 1965.

Roberts, S.R., and Helper, L.C.: Cataracts in Afghan hounds. J. Am. Vet. Med. Assn., 160:427–432, 1972.

Rubin, L.F.: Hereditary retinal detachment in Bedlington terriers. A preliminary report. Small Animal Clin., 3:387–389, 1963.

Rubin, L.F.: Heredity of retinal dysplasia in Bedlington terriers. J. Am. Vet. Med. Assn., 152:260–262, 1968.

Rubin, L.F.: Cataract in golden retrievers. J. Am. Vet. Med. Assn., 165:457–458, 1974.

Rubin, L.F.: Hemeralopia in dogs. Trans. Am. Acad. Ophthalmol. Otolaryngol., 81:677–682, 1976.

Rubin, L.F., and Flowers, R.D.: Inherited cataract in a family of standard poodles. J. Am. Vet. Med. Assn., 161:207–208, 1972.

Rubin, L.F., Bourns, T.K.R., and Lord, L.H.: Hemeralopia in dogs: heredity of hemeralopia in Alaskan malamutes. Am. J. Vet. Res., 28:355–357, 1967.

Rubin, L.F., Koch, S.A., and Huber, R.J.: Hereditary cataracts in miniature schnauzers. J. Am. Vet. Med. Assn., 154:1456–1458, 1969.

Saunders, L.Z.: Congenital optic nerve hypoplasia in collie dogs. Cornell Vet., 42:67–80, 1952.

Sorsby, A., and Davey, J.B.: Ocular associations of dappling (or merling) in the coat colour of dogs. I. Clinical and genetical data. J. Genet., 52:425–440, 1954.

Stades, F.C.: Hereditary retinal dysplasia in a family of Yorkshire terriers, Tijdschr. Diergeneesk. 103:1087–1090, 1978.

Szczudlowska, M.: Dermoid cyst of the eye in relation to heredity and overfeeding. Med. Vet., 23:567–569, 1967.

von Hippel, E.: Embryologische Untersuchungen über Verebung angeborener Kataract, über Schicter des Hundes sowie über eine besondere Form von Kapelkarakt. Graefes Arch., 124:300–324, 1930.

Wolf, E.D., Vainisi, S.J., and Santos-Anderson, R.: Rod-cone dysplasia in the Collie. J. Am. Vet. Med. Assn., 173:1331–1333, 1978.

Wyman, M., and Ketring, K.: Congenital glaucoma in the bassett hound: A biological model. Trans. Am. Acad. Ophthalmol. Otolaryngol., 81:645–652, 1976.

Yakely, W.L.: Collie eye anomaly: Decreased prevalence through selective breeding. J. Am. Vet. Med. Assn., 161:1103–1107, 1972.

Yakely, W.L.: A study of heritability of cataracts in the American cocker spaniel. J. Am. Vet. Med. Assn. 172:814–817, 1978.

Yakely, W.L., et al.: Genetic transmission of an ocular fundus anomaly in collies. J. Am. Vet. Med. Assn., 152:457–461, 1968.

Neuromuscular System

Averill, D.R., and Bronson, R.T. Inherited necrotizing myelopathy of Afghan hounds. J. Neuropath Exp. Neurol. 36:739–747, 1972.

Bernheimer, H., and Karbe, E.: Morphologische und neurochemische Untersuchungen von 2 Formen der amaurotischen Idiotie des Hundes: Nachweis einer G_{m2}-Gangliosidose. Acta Neuropathologia (Berlin), 16:243–261, 1970.

Bielfelt, S.W., Redman, H.C., and McClellan, P.O.: Size and sex-related differences in rates of epileptiform seizures in a purebred beagle colony. Am. J. Vet. Res., 32:2039–2048, 1971.

Bjerkås, I.: Hereditary "Cavitating" leucodystrophy in Dalmatian dogs. Acta Neuropath. (Berlin), 40:163–169, 1977.

Björck, G., Dyrendahl, S., and Olsson, S.E.: Hereditary ataxia in smooth-haired fox terriers. Vet. Rec., 69:871–876, 1957.

Brown, C.J., Murphree, O.D., and Newton, J.E.O.: The effect of inbreeding on human aversion in pointer dogs. Journal of Heredity, 69:362–365, 1978.

Burns, M., and Fraser, M.N.: Genetics of the Dog. The Basis of Successful Breeding. Philadelphia, J.B. Lippincott Co., 1966.

Cordy, D.R., and Snelbaker, H.A.: Cerebellar hypoplasia and degeneration in a family of airedale dogs. J. Neuropath. Exp. Neurol., 11:324–328, 1952.

Croft, P.G., and Stockman, M.H.R.: Inherited defects in dogs. Vet. Rec., 76:260–261, 1964.

deLahunta, A., and Averill, D.R.: Hereditary cerebellar cortical and extra-pyramidal nuclear abiotrophy in Kerry Blue terriers. J. Am. Vet. Med. Assoc., 168:1119–1124, 1976.

Douglas, S.W., and Palmer, A.C.: Idiopathic demyelination of brain-stem and spinal cord in a miniature poodle puppy. J. Path. Bact., 82:67–71, 1961.

Dykman, R.A., Murphree, O.D., and Peters, J.E.: Like begets like: behavioral tests, classical autonomic and motor conditioning and operant conditioning in two strains of pointer dogs. Ann. New York Acad. Sci., 159:976–1007, 1969.

Eberhart, G.W.: Epilepsy in the dog. Gaines Vet. Symp., 18:20, 1959.

Falco, M.J., Barker, J., and Wallace, M.E.: The genetics of epilepsy in the British Alsatian. J. Small Anim. Pract., 15:685–692, 1974.

Fankhauser, R., Luginbühl, H., and Hartley, W.: Leukodystrophie vom typus Krabbe beim Hund. Schweiz. Arch. Tierheilk, 105:198–207, 1963.

Fletcher, T., Kurtz, H., and Low D.: Globoid cell leukodystrophy (Krabbe type) in the dog. J. Am. Vet. Med. Assn., 149:165–172, 1966.

Freak, M.J.: The whelping bitch. Vet. Rec., 60:295–301, 306, 1948.

Gambetti, L.A., Kelly, A.M., and Steinberg, S.A.: Biochemical studies in a canine gangliosidosis. J. Neuropath. Exper. Neurol., 29:137, 1970.

Greene, C.E., Vandevelde, M., and Braund, K.: Lissencephaly in two Lhasa Apso dogs. J. Am. Vet. Med. Assn., 169:405–410, 1976.

Hagen, L.O.: Lipid dystrophic changes in the central nervous system in dogs. Acta Path. Microbiol. Scand., 33:22–35, 1953.

Hartley, W.J.: Ataxia in Jack Russell terriers. Acta Neuropathologica (Berlin), 26:71–74, 1973.

Hegreberg, G.A., and Padgett, G.A.: Inherited progressive epilepsy of the dog with comparisons to Lafora's disease of man. Fed. Proc., 35:1202–1205, 1976.

Hodgman, S.F.J.: Abnormalities and defects in pedigree dogs. I. An investigation into the existence of abnormalities in pedigree dogs in the British Isles. J. Small Animal Pract., 6:447–456, 1963.

Inada, S., Sakamoto, H., Haruta, K., Miyazono, Y., Sasaki, M., Yamguchi, C., Igata, A., Osame, M., and Fukunaga, H.: A clinical study on hereditary progressive neurogenic muscular atrophy in pointer dogs. Jap. J. Vet. Sci. 40:539–547, 1978.

Johnson, G.R., Oliver, J.E., and Selcer, R.: Globoid leukodystrophy in a Beagle. J. Am. Vet. Med. Assn., 167:380–384, 1975.

Karbe, E., and Schiefer, B.: Familial amaurotic idiocy in male German shorthair pointers. Path. Vet., 4:223–232, 1967.

Kollarits, J.: Permanent trembling in some dog breeds as hereditary degeneration (in German). Schweiz. Med. Wochenschr., 54:431–432, 1924.

Koppang, N.: Lipodystrophia cerebri hos engelskette. Beretn. Nord. Vet. Med., 2:862–867, 1963.

Koppang, N.: Familiare Glykospingolipoidose des Hundes Juvenile Amaurotische Idiotie. Ergebn. Allg. Path. Anat., 47:1–43, 1966.

Koppang, N.: Neuronal ceroid-lipofuscinosis in English setters. J. Small Animal Pract., 10:639–644, 1970.

Kramer, J.W., Hegreberg, G.A., Bryan, G.M., Meyers, K., and Ott, R.L.: A muscle disorder of Labrador Retrievers characterized by deficiency of type II muscle fibers. J. Am. Vet. Med. Assn. 169:817–820, 1976.

Krushinskii, L.V.: Animal Behavior: Its Normal and Abnormal Development. New York Consultants Bureau, 1962.

Lane, J.G., and Holmes, R.J.: Fly catching: Hallucinatory behavior by Cavalier King Charles Spaniels. Grunsell, C.S.G., and Hill, F.W.G. (eds.): Vet Annual. Bristol, England, J. Wright and Sons, Ltd., 1972.

Lawler, D.C.: Epilepsy in dogs. New Zealand Vet. J., 19:53, 1971.

McGrath, J.T.: Neurologic Examination of the Dog with Clinicopathologic Observations, 2nd ed. Philadelphia, Lea and Febiger, 1960.

McGrath, J.T.: Spinal dysraphism in the dog. Path. Vet., 2(Suppl.):1–36, 1965.

McGrath, J.T., Kelly, A.M., and Steinberg, S.A.: Cerebral lipidosis in the dog. J. Neuropath. Exper. Neurol., 27:141, 1968 (Abstr.).

Martínek, Z., and Dahme, E.: Spontanepilepsie bei Hunden: Langzeituntersuchungen an einer Gruppe genetisch verwandter Tiere. Zbl. Vet. Med. A, 24:353–371, 1977.

Martínek, Z., and Horak, F.: Development of so-called "genuine" epileptic seizures in dogs during emotional excitement. Physiologia Bohemoslovaca, 19:185–195, 1970.

Meyers, K.M., Padgett, G.A., and Dickson, W.M.: The genetic basis of a kinetic disorder of Scottish terrier dogs. J. Hered., 61:189–192, 1970.

Meyers, K.M., and Schaub, R.G.: The relationship of serotonin to a motor disorder of Scottish Terrier dogs. Life Sci., 14:1895–1906, 1974.

Mitler, M.M., Soave, O., and Dement, W.C.: Narcolepsy in seven dogs. J. Am. Vet. Med. Assn., 168:1036–1038, 1976.

Mitler, M.M.: J. Am. Vet. Med. Assn., 170:575, 1977 (Letter to Editor).

Palmer, A.C., Payne, J.E., and Wallace, M.E.: Hereditary quadriplegia and amblyopia in the Irish Setter. J. Small Anim. Pract., 14:343–352, 1973.

Patel, V., Koppang, N., Patel, B., and Zeman, W.: p-Phenylenediamine-mediated peroxidase deficiency in English Setters with neuronal seroid lipofuscinosis. Lab. Invest., 30:366–368, 1974.

Read, D.H., Harrington, D.D., Keenan, T.W., and Hinsman, E.J.: Neuronal-visceral GM$_1$ gangliosidosis in a dog with B-galactosidase deficiency. Science, 194:442–445, 1976.

Sanda, A., and Krizenecky, J.: Genetic basis of necrosis of digits in shortcoated setters. Vet. Bull., 36:2764, 1960.

Sanda, A., and Pivnik, L.: Necrosis of the toes in Pointers. Vet. Bull, 34:2283, 1964.

Sandefeldt, E., Cummings, J.F., de Lahunta, A., Björck, G., and Krook, L.: Hereditary neuronal abiotrophy in the Swedish Lapland Dog. Cornell Vet., 63(Suppl. 3):1–71, 1973.

Sandefeldt, E., Cummings, J.F., de Lahunta, A., Björck, G., and Krook, L.P.: Animal Model: Hereditary neuronal abiotrophy in Swedish Lapland Dogs. Am. J. of Path., 82:649–652, 1976.

Scott, J.P., and Fuller, J.L.: Genetics and the Social Behavior of the Dog. Chicago and London, University of Chicago Press, 1965.

Steinberg, S.A.: Clinicopathologic conference. J. Am. Vet. Med. Assn., 143:404–410, 1963.

Stockard, C.: An hereditary lethal for localized motor and preganglionic neurones with a resulting paralysis in the dog. Am. J. Anat., 59:1–53, 1936.

Stockard, C.R.: The Genetic and Endocrinic Basis for Differences in Form and Behavior as Elucidated by Studies of Contrasted Pure-Line Dog Breeds and Hybrids. American Anatomical Memoirs. Philadelphia, Wistar Institute of Anatomy and Biology, 1941.

Suzuki, Y., et al.: Studies in globoid leukodystrophy: enzymatic and lipid findings in the canine form. Exper. Neurol., 29:65–75, 1970.

Suzuki, Y., Miyatake, T., Fletcher, J.F., and Suzuki, K.: Glycosphingolipid B galactosidases. J. Biol. Chem., 249:2109–2112, 1974.

Thompson, W.R., and Melzack, R.: Early environment. Sci. Am., 194:38–42, 1956.

Thorne, F.C.: The inheritance of shyness in dogs. J. Gen. Psychol., 65:275–279, 1944.

Van der Velden, N.A.: "Fits" in tervueren shepherd dogs: a presumed hereditary trait. J. Small Animal Pract. 9:63–70, 1968.

Wallace, M.E.: Keeshonds: A genetic study of epilepsy and EEG readings. J. Small Anim. Pract., 16:1–10, 1975.

Wentink, G.H., et al.: Myopathy with a possible recessive X-linked inheritance in a litter of Irish terriers. Vet. Path. 9:328–349, 1972.

Wentink, G.H., Hartman, W., and Koeman, J.P.: Three cases of myotonia in a family of Chows. Tijdschr., Diergeneesk., 99:729–731, 1974.

Wentink, G.H., Meijer, A.E.F.H., van der Linde-Sipman, J.S., and Hendriks, H.J.: Myopathy in an Irish Terrier with a metabolic defect of the isolated mitochondria. Zbl. Vet. Med., 21:62–74, 1974.

Zaki, F.A., and Kay, W.J.: Globoid cell leukodystrophy in a miniature poodle. J. Am. Vet. Med. Assn., 163:248–250, 1973.

Zaki, F. A.: J. Am. Vet. Med. Assn., 169:1165, 1976 (Letter to Editor).

Other Structural Malformations

Fox, M.W.: Inherited inguinal hernia and midline defects in the dog. J. Am. Vet. Med. Assn., 143:602–604, 1963.

Hayes, H.M.: Congenital umbilical and inguinal hernias in cattle, horses, swine, dogs, and cats: risk by breed and sex among hospital patients. Am. J. Vet. Res., 35:839–842, 1974.

Hodgman, S.F.: An investigation into the existence of abnormalities in pedigree dogs in the British Isles. J. Small Animal Pract., 6:447–456, 1963.

Koch, W.: New pathological hereditary characters in the dog. Z. Iwdukt. Abstamm. Vererb. L., 70:503–506, 1935.

Leonard, H.C.: Collapse of the larynx and adjacent structures in the dog. J. Am. Vet. Med. Assn., 137:360–364, 1960.

Leonard, H.C.: Surgical correction of collapsed trachea in dogs. J. Am. Vet. Med. Assn., 158:598–600, 1971.

Phillips, J.M., and Felton, T.M.: Hereditary umbilical hernia. J. Hered., 30:433–435, 1939.

Suter, P.F., Colgrove, D.J., and Ewing, G.O.: Congenital hypoplasia of the canine trachea. JAAHA 8:120–127, 1972.

Willis, M.B.: Abnormalities in pedigree dogs. V. Cryptorchidism. J. Small Animal Pract., 4:469–474, 1963.

The Skin

Burgisser, H., and Hinterman, J.: Kystes dermoides de la tête chez le boxer. Schweiz. Arch. Tierheilk., 103:309–312, 1961.

Editorial. The hairless dog. J. Hered., 8:519–520, 1917.

Gaspar, J.: Analyse der erbfaktoren des schadels bei einer Paarung von Ceylon-Nackthund X Dackel. Jena Z. Naturw., 65:245–274, 1930.

Harper, R.C.: Congenital black hair follicular dysplasia in bearded collie puppies. Vet. Rec., 102:87, 1978.

Hegreberg, G.A., et al.: Cutaneous asthenia in dogs. Newer knowledge about dogs. 16th Gaines Vet. Symp.:3–5, 1966.

Hegreberg, G.A., et al.: A connective tissue disease of dogs and mink resembling the Ehlers-Danlos syndrome of man. II. Mode of inheritance. J. Hered., 60:249–254, 1969.

Hegreberg, G.A., Padgett, G.A., and Henson, J.B.: Connective tissue disease of dogs and mink resembling Ehlers-Danlos syndrome of man. III. Histopathological changes of the skin. Arch. Path., 90:159–166, 1970.

Hegreberg, G.A., Padgett, G.A., Ott, R.L., and Henson, J.B.: A heritable connective tissue disease of dogs and mink resembling Ehlers-Danlos syndrome of man. I. Skin tensile strength properties. J. Invest. Derm., 54:377–380, 1970a.

Hofmeyer, C.F.B.: Dermoid sinus in the ridgeback dog. J. Small Animal Pract., 4:5–8, 1963.

Hutt, F.B.: Inherited lethal characters in domestic animals. Cornell Vet., 24:1–25, 1934.

Kohn, F.G.: Beitrag zur Kenntnis der Haut des Nackthundes. Zool. Jb. Anat., 31:427–438, 1911.

Mahaffey, M.B., Yarbrough, K.M., and Munnell, J.F.: Focal loss of pigment in the Belgian Tervueren Dog. J. Am. Vet. Med. Assn., 173:390–396, 1978.

Mann, G.E., and Stratton, J.: Dermoid sinus in the Rhodesian ridgeback. J. Small Anim. Pract., 7:631–642, 1966.

Schwartzman, R.M., Rockey, J.H., and Halliwell, R. E.: Canine reaginic antibody: characterization of the spontaneous anti-ragweed and induced antidinitrophenyl reaginic antibodies of the atopic dog. Clin. Exper. Immunol., 9:549–569, 1971.

Selmanowitz, V.J., Kramer, K.M., and Orentreich, N.: Congenital ectodermal defect in miniature poodles. J. Hered., 61:196–199, 1970.

Selmanowitz, V.J., Kramer, K.M., and Orentreich, N.: Canine hereditary black hair follicular dysplasia. J. Hered., 63:43–44, 1972.

Selmanowitz, V.J., Markofsky, J., and Orentreich, N.: Black hair follicular dysplasia in dogs. J. Am. Vet. Med. Assn., 171:1079–1081, 1977.

Selmanowitz, V.J., Markofsky, J., Orentreich, N.: Heritability of an ectodermal defect: A study of affected dogs. J. Dermatol. Surg. Oncol. 3:623–626, 1977.

Thomsett, L.R.: Congenital hypotrichia in the dog. Vet. Rec., 73:915–917, 1961.

Zulueta, A. de: The hairless dogs of Madrid. Proc. VIII Int. Cong. Genet.: 687–688, 1945.

Susceptibility to Disease

Baker, J.A., et al.: Breed response to distemper vaccination. Proc. Animal Care Panel, 12:157–162, 1962.

Bech-Nielsen, S., Haskins, M.E., Reif, J.S., Brodey, R.S., Patterson, D.F., and Spielman, R.: Frequency of osteosarcoma among first-degree relatives of St. Bernard dogs. J. Natl. Cancer Inst., 60:349–353, 1978.

Bierwaltes, W.H., and Nishiyama, R.H.: Dog thyroiditis: occurrence and similarity to Hashimoto's struma. Endocrinology, 83:501–508, 1968.

Brodey, R.S.: Canine and feline neoplasia. In *Advances in Veterinary Science*. Vol. 14. New York, Academic Press, 1970.

Cohen, D., Reif, J.S., Brodey, R.S., and Keiser, H.: Epidemiological analysis of the most prevalent sites and types of canine neoplasia observed in a veterinary hospital. Cancer Research, 34:2859–2868, 1974.

Cotchin, E.: Melanotic tumours of dogs. J. Comp. Path., 2:115–129, 1955.

Cotter, S.M., Griffiths, R.C., and Leav, I.: Enostosis in young dogs. J. Am. Vet. Med. Assn. 153:401–410, 1968.

Dorn, C.R., Priester, W.A.: Epidemiologic analysis of oral and pharyngeal cancer in dogs, cats, horses, and cattle. J. Am. Vet. Med. Assn. 169:1202–1206, 1976.

Fox, M.W., Hoag, W.G., and Strout, J.: The epidemiology, pathogenicity, and breed susceptibility of endemic coliform enteritis in the dog. J. Lab. Animal Care, 15:194–200, 1965.

Hayes, H.M.: An hypothesis for the aetiology of canine chemoreceptor system neoplasms, based upon an epidemiological study of 73 cases among hospital patients. J. Small Anim. Pract., 16:337–343, 1975.

Hayes, H.M.: Canine bladder cancer: Epidemiologic features. Am. J. Epidemiol. 104:673–677, 1976.

Lewis, R.M., and Schwartz, R.S.: Canine systemic lupus erythematosus. Genetic analysis of an established breeding colony. J. Exp. Med., 134:417–438, 1971.

Luginbühl, H.: Comparative aspects of tumors of the nervous system. Ann. New York Acad. Sci., 108:702–721, 1963.

Manning, P.J., Corwin, L.A., and Middleton, C.C.: Familial hyperlipoproteinemia and thyroid dysfunction of beagles. Exp. & Molecular Path., 19:378–388, 1973.

Owen, L.N.: The differential diagnosis of bone tumors in the dog. Vet. Rec., 74:439–446, 1962.

Peters, J.A.: Canine mastocytoma: excess risk related to ancestry. J. Natl. Cancer Inst., 42:435–443, 1969.

Scott, J.P., and Fuller, J.L.: *Genetics and the Social Behavior of the Dog*. Chicago, University of Chicago Press, 1965.

Tjalma, R.A.: Canine bone sarcoma: Estimation of relative risk as a function of body size. J. Natl. Cancer Inst., 36:1137–1150, 1966.

Whitney, L.F.: *How to Breed Dogs*. New York, Orange Judd Publishing Co., 1948.

Urogenital System

Bernard, M.A., and Valli, V.E.: Familial renal disease in Samoyed dogs. Can. Vet. J., 18:181–189, 1977.

Bovée, K.C., Joyce, T., Reynolds, R., and Segal, S.: Spontaneous Fanconi syndrome in the dog. Metabolism, 27:45–52, 1978.

Bovée, K.C., and Segal, S.: Canine cystinuria and cystine calculi. The newer knowledge about dogs. Proceedings of the 21st Gaines Veterinary Symposium. 1971.

Brand, E., and Cahill, G.F.: Canine cystinuria. III. J. Biol. Chem., 15:114, 1936.

Brand, E., Cahill, G.F., and Kassell, B.: Canine cystinuria. V. Family history of two cystinuric dogs and cystine determinations in dog urine. J. Biol. Chem., 133:431–436, 1940.

Easley, J.R., and Breitschwerdt, E.B.: Glucosuria associated with renal tubular dysfunction in three basenji dogs. J. Am. Vet. Med. Assn., 168:938–943, 1976.

Finco, D.R., et al.: Familial renal disease in Norwegian elkhound dogs. J. Am. Vet. Med. Assn., 156:747–760, 1970.

Fox, M.W.: Inherited polycystic mononephrosis in the dog. J. Hered., 55:29–30, 1964.

Hare, W.C.D.: Intersexuality in the dog. Can. Vet. J., 17:7–15, 1976.

Harvey, A.M., and Christensen, H.N.: Uric acid transport system: apparent absence in erythrocytes of the Dalmatian coach hound. Science, 145:826–827, 1964.

Holtzapple, P.G., et al.: Amino acid uptake by kidney and jejunal tissue from dogs with cystine stones. Science, 166:1525–1527, 1969.

Johnston, G.R., Osborne, C.A., Wilson, J.W., and Yano, B.L.: Familial ureteral ectopia in the dog. J. Am. Anim. Hosp. Assoc., 13:168–170, 1977.

Kaufman, C.F., Soirez, R.F., and Tasker, J.P.: Renal cortical hypoplasia with secondary hyperparathyroidism in the dog. J. Am. Vet. Med. Assn., 155:1679–1685, 1969.

Keeler, C.F.: The inheritance of predisposition to renal calculi in the Dalmatian. J. Am. Vet. Med. Assn., 96:507–510, 1940.

Krook, L.: The pathology of renal cortical hypoplasia in the dog. Nord. Vet. Med., 9:161–176, 1957.

Murti, G.S.: Agenesis and dysgenesis of the canine kidneys. J. Am. Vet. Med. Assn., 146:1120–1124, 1965.

Osterhoff, D.R.: Hereditary basis of cryptorchidism in dogs. J.S. Afr. Vet. Assoc., 48:145, 1977.

Pendergrass, T.W., and Hayes, H.M.: Cryptorchidism and related defects in dogs: Epidemiology comparisons with man. Teratology, 12:51–56, 1975.

Persson, F., Persson, S., and Asheim, A.: Renal cortical hypoplasia in dogs. A clinical study on uraemia and secondary hypoparathyroidism. Acta Vet. Scand., 2:68–84, 1961.

Selden, J.R., Wachtel, S.S., Koo, G.C., Haskins, M.E., and Patterson, D.F.: Genetic basis of XX male syndrome and XX true hermaphroditism: Evidence in the dog. Science, 201:644–646, 1978.

Trimble, H.D., and Keeler, C.E.: The inheritance of high uric acid excretion in dogs. J. Hered., 29:280–289, 1938.

Ts' Ai-Fan Yu, et al.: Low uricase activity in Dalmatian dogs simulated in mongrels given uronic acid. Am. J. Physiol., 220:973–979, 1971.

Tsan, M., et al.: Canine cystinuria: Its urinary amino acid pattern and genetic analysis. Am. J. Vet. Res., 33:2455–2461, 1972.

Vymetal, F.: Renal aplasia in beagles. Vet. Rec., 77:1344–1345, 1965.

Willis, M.B.: Abnormalities in pedigree dogs. V. Cryptorchidism. J. Small Anim. Pract., 4:469–474, 1963.

Section
2

CHEMICAL
AND
PHYSICAL
DISORDERS

FREDERICK W. OEHME, D.V.M.
Consulting Editor

Emergency and General Treatment of Poisonings 105
Use of Laboratories for the Chemical Analysis of Tissues 115
Common Poisonings in Small Animal Practice 122
Strychnine Poisoning 129
Warfarin and Other Anticoagulant Poisonings 131
Metaldehyde Poisoning 135
Lead Poisoning 136
Lead Poisoning in New Zealand 141
Antifreeze (Ethylene Glycol) Poisoning 144
Organophosphate and Carbamate Insecticide Poisoning 147
Common Potential Sources of Small Animal Poisonings 149
Adverse Drug Reactions 155
Teratogenesis and Mutagenesis 161
Carcinogenesis 172
Bites and Stings of Venomous Animals 174
Snakebite in Australia and New Guinea 179
Near-Drowning (Water Inhalation) 182
Inhalation Injury 186
Thermal Injury 191
Heat Stroke (Heat Stress, Hyperpyrexia) 195
Accidental Hypothermia 197
Cold Injury (Hypothermia, Frostbite, Freezing) 199
Emergency Kit for Treatment of Small Animal Poisoning 201

Additional Pertinent Information found in **Current Veterinary Therapy VI:**

Aronson, Carl E., Ph.D.: Thallium Intoxication, p. 124.

Bailey, E. Murl, D.V.M.: Herbicide and Fungicide Poisoning, p. 143.

Clay, Billy R., D.V.M.: Poisoning and Injury by Plants, p. 179.

Eberhart, George W., D.V.M.: Garbage- and Food-Borne Intoxications, p. 176.

Edwards, William C., D.V.M.: Sodium Fluoroacetate (Compound 1080) Poisoning, p. 119.

Furr, Allan, D.V.M.: Arsenic Poisoning, p. 134.

Harris, William F., D.V.M.: Antu Poisoning, p. 117.

Hobbs, Charles H., D.V.M.: Radiation Toxicity, p. 184.

Oehme, Frederick W., D.V.M.: Poisoning from Phenolic Chemicals, p. 145.

Palumbo, N.E., D.V.M., and Perri, S., B.A.: Toad Poisoning, p. 173.

Van Gelder, Gary A., D.V.M.: Chlorinated Hydrocarbon Insecticide Toxicosis, p. 141.

104

EMERGENCY AND GENERAL TREATMENT OF POISONINGS*

E. MURL BAILEY, D.V.M.
College Station, Texas

Many acutely ill animals are diagnosed as poisoned when no other diagnosis can be readily ascertained. For this reason, the treatment and management of acutely ill animals should be directed toward preserving the life of the animal regardless of the etiology(ies).

The veterinary clinician should direct his efforts toward treating the signs exhibited by the affected animal unless the correct diagnosis is obvious. Preexisting conditions and the diagnosis should be determined following stabilization of the patient.

Special goals of therapy in cases of intoxication are:

1. Emergency intervention and prevention of further exposure.
2. Delaying further absorption.
3. Application of specific antidotes.
4. Hastening elimination of the absorbed toxicant.
5. Supportive therapy.
6. Client education.

PRELIMINARY INSTRUCTIONS TO CLIENTS

Veterinarians are frequently contacted by telephone concerning an intoxicated animal. Preliminary instructions given at this time can be important to the success of subsequent therapeutic measures.

The client should be instructed to protect the animal as well as the people in contact with the affected animal. This may include keeping the animal warm and avoiding any other stress phenomena. Onlookers should be warned about the condition of the animal, and it may be desirable to place a muzzle on the animal.

If the animal's exposure was topical, the client should be instructed to cleanse the animal's skin or eye with copious amounts of water. The client should also be instructed to be careful to avoid exposure to the toxicant and to use some type of protective clothing if available.

In many instances, the client will be concerned about inducing emesis in the animal. The clinician should cite the contraindications to emesis — i.e., CNS depression and ingestion of petroleum distillates, acids, or alkalis. Emetic preparations and techniques easily available to the public such as syrup of ipecac, hydrogen peroxide, and table salt, or sticking the finger in the back of the animal's mouth, are generally ineffective and sometimes dangerous.

If the client is very insistent about administering medication, he should be advised to allow the animal to drink as much water as it wants. This will act as a diluent. In most cases, one may also suggest the administration of milk or egg whites. The client should be cautioned not to administer anything by mouth if the animal is convulsing, depressed, or unconscious.

It is imperative that the client not waste time. The animal should be brought to the veterinarian as soon as possible (or the veterinarian should be summoned). The owner should be instructed to bring vomitus and/or suspected materials or their containers with the animal. The client should be advised to bring the specimens in clean plastic containers or glass jars and cautioned not to contaminate the material. In many instances, valuable time can be saved by applying the proper therapeutic measures if the suspected intoxicant is known. This suspected material may also be valuable from a medicolegal aspect.

EMERGENCY INTERVENTION

The most important aspect of emergency treatment of intoxications is to insure ade-

*Supported in part by Texas Agricultural Experiment Station, Project No. H-6255.

quate physiologic function. All the antidotal procedures available to the clinician will be to no avail if the animal has lost one or all of the vital functions. Restoring essential function may include establishment of a patent airway, artificial respiration, cardiac massage (external or internal), and, perhaps, defibrillation. Following stabilization of the vital signs, the emergency clinician may proceed with subsequent therapeutic measures.

DELAYING ABSORPTION

Preventing the animal from absorbing additional intoxicant is a major factor in treating cases of poisoning. In many instances, intoxication may be prevented in this manner if the animal was actually observed ingesting or being in contact with suspected material. Removal of the animal from the affected environment is a necessary first step to prevent further absorption. Ideally, bringing the animal to the veterinary clinic or hospital will suit this purpose. It also may entail washing the animal's skin to remove the noxious agent. If an external toxicant is involved, caution must be exercised to avoid contamination of all persons handling the case. In addition, the judicious use of emetics, gastric lavage techniques, adsorbents, and cathartics will aid in the prevention of further absorption of toxic materials.

INDUCTION OF EMESIS

Emesis may be considered as a method of emptying the stomach of toxic materials. Some commonly available agents are not very reliable, and emesis may be of little value after one to two hours following exposure to a toxicant.

Syrup of ipecac is a general emetic. Its mechanism is gastric irritation rather than central stimulation. The dose of ipecac for small animals is 1 to 2 ml/kg, but it is only about 50 percent effective. This agent should never be used when activated charcoal is part of the therapeutic regimen, since it markedly reduces the effectiveness of the charcoal.

Other agents such as copper sulfate, table salt, or hydrogen peroxide have been advocated as locally acting emetics. However, the effectiveness of these agents is questionable.

Apomorphine is the most effective and most reliable emetic available. The effective dose in most small animals is 0.04 mg/kg IV or 0.08 mg/kg IM or SC. Apomorphine may cause respiratory depression, and protracted emesis may develop following its use. These signs may be effectively controlled with appropriate narcotic antagonists injected IV (naloxone, Narcan®: 0.04 mg/kg; levallorphan, Lorfan®, 0.02 mg/kg; or nalorphine, Nalline®; 0.1 mg/kg). In addition to the general contraindications of emetics, apomorphine may be further contraindicated for cases in which additional CNS depression must be avoided.

Contraindications for induction of emesis are unconsciousness, severe depression, and intoxication by petroleum distillates, tranquilizers, or other antiemetics. If the time interval following exposure to the toxicant is greater than one to two hours, most of the toxicant will have passed the duodenum, and emesis will not be effective.

Intoxication with acids or alkalis may be diagnosed when corrosive changes are present in and around the mouth, forepaws, and other areas on the cranial portions of the body. If emesis is induced, caustic agents can cause additional damage to the esophagus and oral cavity. In addition, these agents generally weaken the gastric wall, which could easily be ruptured during forceful emesis.

Activated charcoal may increase the efficacy of emesis. If charcoal is to be utilized, the clinician should first induce emesis with apomorphine, administer the charcoal, and reinduce emesis with a subsequent IV dose of apomorphine.

Any vomitus should be saved for analysis, especially if there are any medicolegal considerations. The clinician should consider any intoxication as grounds for a possible court case and should conduct treatment accordingly.

GASTRIC LAVAGE

Gastric lavage is an emergency procedure that has at times been maligned as being relatively inefficient. Changes in technique (e.g., using a larger tube, more volume, and more frequent lavages) have made this a very reliable procedure when undertaken within two hours of exposure to an ingested toxicant.

The animal should be unconscious or under light anesthesia. A cuffed endotracheal tube should be placed within the trachea. The distal end of the tube should protrude two inches beyond the teeth. This will increase the animal's dead space but is required to prevent any inhalation of lavage fluid. The head and thorax should be lowered slightly but not enough to compromise respiration due to the weight of the abdominal viscera. The veterinarian should premeasure the stomach tube from the tip of the animal's node to the xiphoid cartilage. In all cases, as large a stomach tube as possible should be used. A good rule is to use the same size stomach tube as cuffed endotracheal tube (1 mm=3 French). The volume of water or lavage solution to be used for each washing is 5 to 10 ml/kg of body weight. Following the infusion of the solution, the fluid should be aspirated from the stomach via the stomach tube with either a large aspirator bulb or a 50-ml syringe. The infusion and aspiration cycle of the lavage solution should be repeated 10 to 15 times. Activated charcoal in the solution will enhance the effectiveness of this procedure.

Some precautions to be taken with this technique are (1) use low pressure to prevent the forcing of the toxicant into the duodenum, (2) reduce the infused volume in obviously weakened stomachs, and (3) make sure not to force the stomach tube through either the esophagus or the stomach wall.

ADSORBENTS

Activated charcoal is probably the best adsorbing agent available to the practitioner. Although it does not detoxify toxicants, it will effectively prevent absorption of a toxicant if properly utilized. Activated charcoal can be effectively utilized with emetic and gastric lavage techniques.

The proper type of activated charcoal for treatment in toxications is of vegetable, not mineral or animal, origin. Several commercial types of activated charcoal are available: Norit® (American Norit), Nuchar C® (West Virginia Pulp and Paper), and Darco G-60® (Atlas Chemical). Compressed activated charcoal tablets are also available. These tablets are easier to handle than the powdered charcoal and are apparently almost as effective.

A bathtub or some other easily cleansed area is the best place to administer activated charcoal to small animals. The proper technique for utilizing activated charcoal is as follows: (1) make a slurry of the charcoal using water — the proper dose is 2 to 8 gm/kg body weight in a concentration of 1 gm charcoal/5 to 10 ml water; (2) administer the charcoal by a stomach tube using either a funnel or a large syringe; (3) thirty minutes following administration of the charcoal, administer a cathartic of sodium sulfate. This technique may be modified if the charcoal is used in conjunction with emetic or lavage techniques. However, with either technique, some charcoal should remain in the stomach and a cathartic should be given to prevent desorption of the toxicant.

Activated charcoal is highly adsorptive for many toxicants, including mercuric chloride,

strychnine, other alkaloids including morphine and atropine, barbiturates, and ethylene glycol. It is ineffective against cyanide.

Syrup of ipecac will negate some of the adsorptive characteristics of the activated charcoal. The "universal antidote," consisting of two parts activated charcoal, one part MgO, and one part tannic acid, is very inefficient, since the MgO and tannic acid decrease the adsorptive capability of the charcoal. Burned or charred toast as described in some emergency texts is highly ineffective as an adsorbing agent.

CATHARTICS

Sodium sulfate is a more efficient agent for evacuation of the bowel than is magnesium sulfate and is the preferable agent to use, especially with activated charcoal. There is also some danger of CNS depression due to the magnesium ion. However, either agent may be used in an emergency. The oral dose of sodium sulfate is 1 gm/kg.

Mineral oil or vegetable oils are of value if lipid-soluble toxicants are involved. Mineral oil (liquid petrolatum) is inert and unlikely to be absorbed. Vegetable oil, however, is more likely to be absorbed and therefore may be contraindicated. Regardless of the type of oil utilized, it should be followed by a saline cathartic in 30 to 40 minutes.

A colonic lavage or high enema may be of value to hasten the elimination of toxicants from the gastrointestinal tract. Warm water with castile soap makes an excellent enema solution. Hexachlorophene soaps should be avoided. There are several commercial enema preparations available that act as osmotic agents.

LOCALLY ACTING ANTIDOTES

Numerous locally acting antidotes and therapeutic regimens are reported to prevent the absorption of toxicants. Non-specific antidotal procedures for some of the more common toxicants are described in Table 1.

SPECIFIC ANTIDOTES

A few specific antidotal agents are available for some of the more common animal toxicants. A list of these specific antidotal procedures in presented in Table 2.

Caution should be exercised with the use of some of the more specific antidotes, since many of these agents are themselves toxic. In certain chronic metallic intoxications such as

Table 1. *Locally Acting Antidotes Against Unabsorbed Poisons and Principles of Treatment**

POISON	ANTIDOTE AND DOSE OR CONCENTRATION
Acids, corrosive	Weak alkali – Magnesium oxide solution (1:25 warm water) internally. *Never give sodium bicarbonate!* Milk of magnesia – 1 to 15 ml. Flush externally with water. Apply paste of sodium bicarbonate.
Alkali, caustic	Weak acid – Vinegar (diluted 1:4), 1%. Acetic acid or lemon juice given orally. Diluted albumin (4 to 6 egg whites to 1 qt. tepid water) followed by an emetic and then a cathartic, because some compounds are soluble in excess albumin. Local – flush with copious amounts of water and apply vinegar.
Alkaloids	Potassium permanganate (1:5000 to 1:10,000) for lavage and/or oral administration. Tannic acid or strong tea (200 to 500 mg. in 30 to 60 ml of water) except in cases of poisoning by cocaine, nicotine, physostigmine, atropine, and morphine. Emetic or purgative should be used for prompt removal of tannates.
Arsenic	Sodium thiosulfate – 10% solution given orally (0.5 to 3.0 gm for small animals). Protein – evaporated milk, egg whites, etc. Tannic acid or strong tea.
Barium salts	Sodium sulfate and magnesium sulfate (20% solution given orally). Dosage: 2 to 25 gm.
Bismuth salts	Acacia or gum arabic as mucilage.
Carbon tetrachloride	Empty stomach, give high protein and carbohydrate diet, maintain fluid and electrolyte balance. Hemodialysis is indicated in anuria. Epinephrine is contra-indicated (ventricular fibrillation!).
Copper	Albumin (as for Alkali above). Sodium ferrocyanide in water (0.3 to 3.5 gm for small animals). Magnesium oxide (as for Acids above).
Detergents, anionic (Na, K, NH$^+_4$-salts)	Milk or water followed by demulcent (oils, acacia, gelatin, starch, egg white, etc.).
Detergents, cationic (chlorides, iodides, etc.)	Soap (castile, etc.) dissolved in 4 times its bulk of hot water. Albumin (as for Alkali above).
Fluoride	Calcium (milk, lime water or powdered chalk mixed with water) given orally.
Formaldehyde	Ammonia water (0.2% orally) or ammonium acetate (1% for lavage). Starch – 1 part to 15 parts hot water added gradually. Gelatin soaked in water for one half hour. Albumin (as for Alkali above). Sodium thiosulfate (as for Arsenic above).
Iron	Sodium bicarbonate – 1% for lavage.
Lead	Sodium or magnesium sulfate given orally. Sodium ferrocyanide (as for Copper above). Tannic acid (as for Alkaloids above). Albumin (as for Alkali above).
Mercury	Protein – Milk, egg whites (as for Alkali above). Magnesium oxide (as for Acids above). Sodium formaldehyde sulfoxylate – 5% solution for lavage. Starch (as for Formaldehyde above). Activated charcoal – 5 to 50 gm.

*Modified from Szabuniewicz et al. (1971).

Table 1.   *Locally Acting Antidotes Against Unabsorbed Poisons and Principles of Treatment* * (Continued)*

POISON	ANTIDOTE AND DOSE OR CONCENTRATION
Oxalic acid	Calcium—Calcium hydroxide as 0.15% solution. Other alkalis are contraindicated because their salts are more soluble. Chalk or other calcium salts. Magnesium sulfate as cathartic. Maintain diuresis to prevent calcium oxalate deposition in kidney.
Petroleum distillates (aliphatic hydrocarbons)	Olive oil, other vegetable oils, or mineral oil given orally. After one half hour, sodium sulfate as cathartic. Both emesis and lavage are contraindicated.
Phenol and cresols	Soap-and-water or alcohol lavage of skin. Sodium bicarbonate (0.5%) dressings. Activated charcoal and/or mineral oil given orally.
Phosphorus	Copper sulfate (0.2 to 0.4% solution) or potassium permanganate (1:5000 solution) for lavage. Turpentine (preferably old oxidized) in gelatin capsules or floated on hot water. Give 2 ml 4 times at 15-minute intervals. Activated charcoal. Do not give vegetable oil cathartic. Remove all fat from diet.
Silver nitrate	Normal saline for lavage. Albumin (as for Alkali above).
Unknown	Activated charcoal (replaces universal antidote). For small animals—5 to 50 gm in gelatin capsules or, via stomach pump, as a slurry in water. Follow by emetic or cathartic and repeat dosage.

Table 2.   *Systemic Antidotes and Dosages* *

TOXIC AGENT	SYSTEMIC ANTIDOTES	DOSAGE AND METHOD FOR TREATMENT
Amphetamines	Chlorpromazine	1 mg/kg IM, IP, IV; administer only half dose if barbiturates have been given; blocks excitation.
Arsenic, mercury and other heavy metals except silver, selenium, and thallium	Dimercaprol (BAL)	10% solution in oil; give small animals 2.5 to 5.0 mg/kg IM every 4 hours for 2 days, 3 times a day for the next 10 days or until recovery NOTE: In severe acute poisoning, 5 mg/kg dosage should be given only first day
	N-Acetyl-*d,l*-penicillamine (only for mercury poisoning)	Developed for chronic mercury poisoning, now seems most promising drug; no reports on dosage in animals. Dosage for man is 250 mg orally, every 6 hours for 10 days (3 to 4 mg/kg).
Atropine—Belladonna alkaloids	Physostigmine salicylate	0.01 to 0.6 mg/kg.
Barbiturates	Pentylenetetrazol	10% solution; give small animals 10 to 20 mg/kg IV or IM, repeated at 15 to 30 minute intervals as needed.
	Doxapram	2% solution; give small animals 3 to 5 mg/kg IV only, repeated as necessary.
	Bemegride	3% solution; give small animals 5 to 10 mg/kg IV only, by slow infusion or in intermittent doses.
	NOTE: All the above are reliable only when depression is mild; in deeper levels of depression, artificial respiration (and oxygen) is preferable.	
Bromides	Chlorides (sodium or ammonium salts)	0.5 to 1.0 gm. daily for several days; hasten excretion.

Continued on next page

*Modified from Szabuniewicz et al. (1971).

Table 2. *Systemic Antidotes and Dosages** (Continued)*

TOXIC AGENT	SYSTEMIC ANTIDOTES	DOSAGE AND METHOD FOR TREATMENT
Carbon monoxide	Oxygen	Pure oxygen at normal or high pressure, or oxygen with 5% carbon dioxide; artificial respiration; blood transfusion.
Cholinergic agents	Atropine sulfate	0.02 to 0.04 mg/kg, as needed.
Cholinesterase inhibitors	Atropine sulfate	Dosage is 0.2 mg/kg, repeated as needed for atropinization. Treat cyanosis (if present) first. Blocks only muscarinic effects. Atropine in oil may be injected for prolonged effect during the night. *Avoid atropine intoxication!*
Cholinergic agents and cholinesterase inhibitors (organophosphates, some carbamates; but not carbaryl, dimethan or carbam piloxime, etc.)	Pralidoxime chloride (2-PAM)	2% solution; give 20 to 50 mg/kg IM or by slow IV injection (maximum dose is 500 mg/min.), repeat as needed. 2-PAM alleviates nicotinic effect and regenerates cholinesterase. Morphine, succinylcholine, and phenothiazine tranquilizers are contraindicated.
Copper	D-Penicillamine	Dose for animals not established. Dose for man is 1 to 4 gm daily in divided doses (250 mg tablets).
Coumarin-derivative anticoagulants	Vitamin K_1 Whole blood or plasma	5% stable emulsion. Give 5 mg/kg IM for 3 days. Blood transfusion, 25 mg/kg.
Curare (tubocurarine)	Neostigmine methylsulfate Edrophonium chloride Artificial respiration	Solution: 1:5000 or 1:2000 (1 ml=2 mg or 0.5 mg). Dose is 0.005 mg/5 kg, SC. Follow with IV injection of a 1% solution of atropine (0.04 mg/kg). 1% solution; give 0.05 to 1.0 mg/kg IV.
Cyanide	Methemoglobin (sodium nitrite is used to form methemoglobin) Sodium thiosulfate	1% solution of sodium nitrite, dosage is 16 mg/kg IV Follow with: 20% solution at dosage of 30 to 40 mg/kg IV. If treatment is repeated, use only sodium thiosulfate. NOTE: Both of the above may be given simultaneously as follows: 0.5 ml/kg of combination consisting of 10 mg sodium nitrite, 15 gm sodium thiosulfate, distilled water q.s. 250 ml. Dosage may be repeated once. If further treatment is required, give only 20% solution of sodium thiosulfate at level of 1 ml/kg.
Digitalis glycosides, oleander, and Bufo toads	Potassium chloride Phenytoin Propranolol (beta blocker) Atropine sulfate	Dog: 0.5 to 2.0 gm, orally in divided doses, or in serious cases, as diluted solution given IV by slow drip (ECG control is essential). 25 mg/min IV until control is established. 0.5 to 1.0 mg/kg IV or IM as needed to control cardiac arrhythmias. 0.02 to 0.04 mg/kg as needed for cholinergic control.
Fluoride	Calcium borogluconate	3 to 10 ml of 5 to 10% solution.
Fluoroacetate (compound 1080)	Glyceryl monoacetin Acetamide Phenobarbital or pentobarbital	0.1 to 0.5 mg/kg IM hourly for several hours (total 2 to 4 mg/kg); or diluted (0.5 to 1.0%) IV (danger of hemolysis). Monoacetin is available only from chemical supply houses. Animal may be protected if acetamide is given prior to or simultaneously with 1080 (experimental). May protect against lethal dose (experimental).
Hallucinogens (LSD, phencyclidine-PCP)	Phenothiazine tranquilizers or pentobarbital	Follow with symptomatic treatment.

Continued on opposite page

Table 2. Systemic Antidotes and Dosages* (Continued)

TOXIC AGENT	SYSTEMIC ANTIDOTES	DOSAGE AND METHOD FOR TREATMENT
Heparin	Protamine sulfate	1% solution; give 1.0 to 1.5 mg to antagonize each 1 mg of heparin; slow IV injection. Reduce dose as time increases between heparin injection and start of treatment. (After 30 minutes give only 0.5 mg.)
	Hexadimethrine	1 mg for each 1 mg heparin, by slow IV injection. Hexadimethrine is a synthetic product and causes fewer side effects than protamine.
Iron salts	Desferrioxamine (deferoxamine)	Dose for animals not yet established. Dose for man is 5 gm of 5% solution given orally, then 20 mg/kg IM every 4 hours. In case of shock, dose is 40 mg/kg by IV drip over 4-hour period; may be repeated in 6 hours, then 20 mg/kg by drip every 12 hours.
Lead	Calcium disodium edate (EDTA) EDTA and BAL	Dosage: Maximum safe dose is 75 mg/kg/24 hours (only for severe case). EDTA is available in 20% solution; for IV drip, dilute in 5% glucose to 0.5%; for IM, add procaine to 20% solution to give 0.5% concentration of procaine. BAL is given as 10% solution in oil. Treatment: (1) In severe case (CNS involvement of >100 mg. Pb/100 gm whole blood), give 4 mg/kg. BAL only as initial dose; follow after 4 hours, and every 4 hours for 3 to 4 days, with BAL and EDTA at separate IM sites; skip 2 or 3 days and then treat again for 3 to 4 days. (2) In subacute case or <100 mg Pb/100 gm whole blood, give only 50 mg EDTA/kg/24 hours for 3 to 5 days.
Methanol and ethylene glycol	Ethanol	Give IV, 1.1 gm/kg of 25% solution, then give 0.5 gm/kg every 4 hours for 4 days. To prevent or correct acidosis, use sodium bicarbonate IV. Sodium bicarbonate: 0.4 gm/kg Activated charcoal: 5 gm/kg orally if soon after ingestion
Methemoglobinemia-producing agents (nitrites, chlorates, etc.)	Methylene blue	1% solution (maximum concentration), give by *slow* IV injection, 8.8 mg/kg; repeat if necessary. To prevent fall in blood pressure in cases of nitrite poisoning, use a sympathomimetic drug (ephedrine, epinephrine, etc.)
Morphine and related drugs	Nalorphine hydrochloride Levallorphan tartrate	Give IV, 1.0 to 2.5 ml of solution containing 5 mg nalorphine per ml. Do not repeat if respiration is not satisfactory. Give IV, 0.1 to 0.5 ml of solution containing 1 mg/ml. NOTE: Use either of the above antidotes only in acute poisoning. Artificial respiration may be indicated. Activated charcoal is also indicated.
Oxalates	Calcium	Treatment: 23% solution of calcium gluconate IV. Give 3 to 20 ml (to control hypocalcemia).
Phenothiazine derivatives	Methylamphetamine Diphenhydramine HCl	0.1 to 0.2 mg/kg IV; also transfusion. For CNS depression, 2 to 5 mg/kg
Phytotoxins and botulin	Antitoxins	IV for extrapyramidal signs. As indicated for specific antitoxins. Examples of phytotoxins: ricin, abrin, robin, crotin.
Red squill	Atropine sulfate, propranolol	As for digitalis glycosides poisoning on opposite page.
Strontium	Calcium salts Ammonium chloride	Usual dose of calcium borogluconate. 0.2 to 0.5 gm. orally 3 to 4 times daily.
Strychnine and brucine	Pentobarbital	Give IP or IV to effect; higher dose is usually required than that required for anesthesia. Place animal in warm, quiet room.

Continued on next page

Table 2. *Systemic Antidotes and Dosages* (Continued)

TOXIC AGENT	SYSTEMIC ANTIDOTES	DOSAGE AND METHOD FOR TREATMENT
Strychnine and brucine	Pentobarbital	Give IP or IV to effect; higher dose is usually required than that required for anesthesia. Place animal in warm, quiet room.
	Amobarbital	Give by slow IV injection to effect. Duration of sedation is usually 4 to 6 hrs.
	Methocarbamol	10% solution; average first dose is 149 mg/kg IV (range: 40 to 300 mg), repeat half dose as needed.
	Glyceryl guaiacolate	110 mg/kg IV, 5% solution. Repeat as necessary.
Thallium	Diphenylthiocarbazone	Dog: 60 mg/kg orally, 3 times a day for 6 days. Hastens elimination, but is partially toxic.
	Prussian blue	0.2 mg/kg in 3 divided doses daily.
	Potassium chloride	Give simultaneously with thiocarbazone or Prussian blue, 2 to 6 gm orally daily in divided doses.

lead poisoning, the use of chelating agents has precipitated acute metallic intoxication. Consequently, the dosage of chelating agents should be reduced in some chronic metal intoxications.

ELIMINATION OF ABSORBED TOXICANTS

Absorbed toxicants are generally excreted via the kidneys. Some toxicants may be excreted by other routes (bile-feces, lung, other body secretions). Renal excretion can be manipulated in many instances. Urinary excretion of toxicants may be enhanced by the use of diuretics or altering the pH of the urine.

The use of diuretics to enhance urinary excretion of toxicants requires adequate renal function and hydration of the affected animal. Once these requisites are established, diuretics are indicated. Monitoring of urinary output is essential in these animals, and a minimum urinary flow of 0.1 ml/kg/min is necessary. The diuretics of choice are mannitol and furosemide (Lasix®). Both these agents are very potent diuretics. Dosage for mannitol is 2 mg/kg/hr; for furosemide it is 4 mg/kg.

Alteration of urinary pH to expedite the excretion of toxicants and foreign chemicals is a classic pharmacologic technique. The techniques relies on the physiochemical phenomenon that ionized compounds do not readily traverse cell membranes and hence are not reabsorbed by the renal tubules. Consequently, acid compounds such as acetylsalicylic acid (aspirin) and some barbiturates remain ionized in alkaline urine, and alkaline compounds such as amphetamines remain ionized in acidic urine. As a result, urinary excretion of many toxic compounds may be enhanced by modifying the urine pH. Urinary acidifying agents include ammonium chloride (200 mg/kg/day in divided doses) and ethylenediamine dihydrochloride (Chlorethamine®, 1 to 2 tablets 3 times a day for the average sized dog). Sodium bicarbonate (5 mEq/kg/hr) may be used as an alkalinizing agent.

Peritoneal dialysis is indicated when an intoxicated animal exhibits oliguria or anuria. It is a rather time-consuming but effective technique in many conditions. The procedure requires the use of two separate solutions that must be exchanged every 30 to 60 minutes. Two dialyzing solutions that may be used are 5 percent dextrose in 0.45 percent NaCl with 15 mEq/l of potassium as potassium chloride, and 5 percent dextrose in water with 44.6 mEq of bicarbonate and 15 mEq of potassium added. Other dialyzing solutions may be utilized.

The process of peritoneal dialysis involves (1) infusing 10 to 20 ml/kg of one dialyzing solution into the peritoneal cavity, (2) waiting the prescribed length of time, (3) withdrawing the first dialyzing solution, and (4) infusing the second solution. The infusion and withdrawal cycles with alternating solutions should be maintained for 12 to 24 hours or until normal renal function is restored. The pH of the dialyzing solutions may be altered to maintain the ionized state of the offending compound.

SUPPORTIVE MEASURES

Supportive measures are very important in intoxications. These include control of body temperature, maintenance of respiratory and cardiovascular function, control of acid-base imbalances, alleviation of pain, and control of central nervous system disorders.

BODY TEMPERATURE CONTROL

Hypothermia may be controlled by using blankets and by keeping the animal in a warm, draft-free cage. Infrared lamps or heating pads should be used with caution and with constant observation. A pad with circulating warm water may be of greater value and less dangerous than lamps or conventional heating pads. This type of pad is convenient for both emergency and surgical use (Aquamatic K Pad®, American Hospital Supply).

Hyperthermia is controlled through the use of ice bags, cold water baths, cold water enemas, or cold peritoneal dialysis solution. Regardless of the type of temperature control required, it is vitally important that the animal's body temperature be constantly monitored to insure that over-correction does not occur.

RESPIRATORY SUPPORT MEASURES

Adequate respiratory support requires the presence of a patent airway, which may be obtained by using a cuffed endotracheal tube in an unconscious animal or by performing a tracheostomy under local anesthesia. An emergency tracheostomy tube may be made from a cuffed endotracheal tube that has been shortened to reduce the dead space.

A respirator such as a Bird Respirator® or Ohio® ventilator is of greater value in cases of respiratory depression; however, an anesthetic machine may be utilized with manual compression of the bag. A mixture of 50 percent oxygen and 50 percent room air is generally adequate, unless there is a thickened respiratory membrane, in which case 100 percent oxygen is necessary.

The use of analeptic drugs in cases of severe respiratory depression or apnea is questionable owing to the short duration of their effects and to undesirable side effects. Positive pressure ventilatory support is of greater value.

CARDIOVASCULAR SUPPORT

Cardiovascular support requires the presence of an adequate circulating volume, adequate cardiac function, adequate tissue perfusion, and adequate acid-base balance. Volume and cardiac activity are of immediate concern; perfusion and acid-balance, although of no lesser importance, are not of immediate concern.

In the presence of hypovolemia due to loss of both cells and volume, whole blood is the necessary agent. A good rule is to give a sufficient quantity of whole blood to raise the packed cell volume to 75 percent of the animal's estimated normal level (minimum — 20 ml/kg).

Hypovolemia due to fluid loss alone can be treated with the administration of Lactated Ringer's solution or plasma expanders. Central venous pressures should be monitored in these cases to prevent overloading the heart with too much volume too rapidly.

Tissue perfusion should also be monitored periodically to determine the adequacy of the replacement therapy. In some cases, it may be necessary to administer massive doses of corticosteroids intravenously to restore adequate tissue perfusion (dexamethasone, Azium®, 2 to 10 mg/kg).

Cardiac activity can be aided by the application of closed-chest cardiac massage for immediate requirements, but the administration of pharmaceutical agents that can stimulate ionotropic and chronotropic activity must also be undertaken in most instances. One of these agents is calcium gluconate, infused very slowly IV. This agent is also reported to be a good non-specific measure in many toxicities. Other agents include glucagon, 25 to 50 μg/kg IV, and digoxin, 0.2 to 0.6 mg/kg IV. Care must be taken to avoid overdose with cardioactive agents, since they are highly toxic to the myocardium. The electrical activity of the heart should be closely monitored during administration of cardioactive agents.

ACID-BASE IMBALANCE

Control of acid-base balance problems is primarily a matter of maintaining an animal in a homeostatic condition physiologically. The most common acid-base disturbance seen in animals is acidosis that is mainly of metabolic origin. However, acidosis or alkalosis may occur in cases of intoxication.

In correcting acidosis not of respiratory origin, sodium bicarbonate, administered IV at a dosage rate of 2 to 4 mEq/kg every 15 minutes, is the drug of choice. Other alkalinizing solutions including 1/6 molar sodium lactate, 16 to 32 ml/kg; Lactated Ringer's solution, 120 ml/kg; or THAM buffer, 300 mg/kg. Bicarbonate is generally the easiest to administer with respect to volume and requires no metabolic conversion. Caution must be exercised with all alkalinizing agents against the induction of alkalosis.

Alkalosis, unless drug-induced, does not generally occur in animals. However, if alkalosis is present, the IV administration of 0.9 percent NaCl (physiologic saline), 10 ml/kg, is usually sufficient for initial therapy. This should be followed by the oral administration of ammonium chloride, 200 mg/kg/day in divided doses. As in the case of acidosis, the clinician should be cautioned about the overtreatment of the alkalotic patient.

PAIN

Another important supportive measure in cases of intoxication is the control of pain. A minimal dose of morphine (dogs, 1 to 2 mg/kg; cats, 0.1 to 0.2 mg/kg) or meperidine (Demerol®) (dogs, 5 to 10 mg/kg; cats, 1 to 2 mg/kg) is indicated in animals showing pain as a result of intoxications.

CENTRAL NERVOUS SYSTEM DISORDERS

Management of central nervous system disorders in cases of intoxication is simple in appearance but complex in actuality. The type of therapy will depend upon the presence of depression or hyperactivity. Either disorder can easily be turned into the opposite problem by overzealous therapeutic measures.

CNS Depression. CNS depression can also be considered respiratory depression, since the management of the two conditions is very similar. Although the IV administration of analeptic agents such as doxapram (Dopram®), 3 to 5 mg/kg; bemegride (Mikedimide®), 10 to 20 mg/kg; or pentylenetetrazol (Metrazol®), 6 to 10 mg/kg, is reported to be efficacious in these conditions, their actions are short lived, and CNS depression can return if the animals are not monitored continuously. Another disadvantage is that analeptics can also induce convulsions. Artificial respiration or respiratory support is of greater value in animals exhibiting CNS depression and may be the treatment of choice for most CNS depression syndromes.

CNS Hyperactivity. Cases of CNS hyperactivity including convulsions can be managed by the administration of CNS depressants or tranquilizers. Pentobarbital sodium is generally the agent of choice for convulsions and hyperactivity. Care must be taken, however, since in many cases, a respiratory depressing dose may be required to alleviate the signs. In these cases, respiratory support is mandatory. Inhalant anesthetics have been reported as excellent for long-term management of CNS hyperactivity, but this removes the anesthetic machine from surgery-room use for extended periods. Central-acting skeletal muscle relaxants and minor tranquilizers have been reported for use with convulsant intoxicants. Some of these include methocarbamol (Robaxin®), 110 mg/kg, IV; glyceryl guaiacolate (Gecolate®), 110 mg/kg IV; and diazepam (Valium®), 0.5 to 1.5 mg/kg IV or IM. In other cases of CNS stimulation due to amphetamines and some hallucinogens such as LSD and phencyclidine, phenothiazine tranquilizers have produced adequate control. Regardless of the therapeutic regimen for CNS hyperactivity, the animals should be placed in a quiet, dark room to prevent additional stimulation due to auditory or visual stimuli.

POISON CONTROL CENTERS AND DIAGNOSTIC LABORATORIES

Poison Control Centers and/or Animal Diagnostic Laboratories can be of great value to the clinician in cases of suspected intoxications, especially when labels or containers are presented with the acutely ill animal. When the suspected compound and the signs exhibited by the animal do not concur, the signs should be treated and the label should be disregarded.

Diagnosis should be confirmed by chemical analysis, although this may occur after the fact. An accurate diagnosis, as well as detailed records, may help the veterinarian faced with subsequent cases from the same intoxicant. Detailed records will also be invaluable considerations in any medicolegal proceedings. (See also the following chapter, "Use of Laboratories for the Chemical Analysis of Tissue".)

SUPPLEMENTAL READING

Aronson, A.L.: Chemical poisonings in small animal practice. Vet. Clin. North Am. 2(2):379–395, 1972.

Szabuniewicz, M., Bailey, E.M., and Wiersig, D.O.: Treatment of some common poisonings in animals. VMSAC 66:1197–1205, 1971.

Thienes, C.H., and Haley, T.J.: *Clinical Toxicology.* Philadelphia, Lea & Febiger, 1972.

USE OF LABORATORIES FOR THE CHEMICAL ANALYSIS OF TISSUES

WILLIAM B. BUCK, D.V.M.
Urbana, Illinois

An accurate diagnosis is the single most important factor in dealing with animal toxicoses. Once the cause of a problem is known, specific treatment and prevention can be initiated. Prior to that time, however, the veterinarian is limited to supportive and symptomatic therapeutic measures. The toxicologic diagnosis is based upon a knowledge of pertinent criteria in the case, qualified laboratory evaluation of proper specimens, and intelligent interpretation of laboratory results in light of the circumstances associated with the problem.

When the practicing veterinarian desires to consult with a diagnostic laboratory or another colleague in an effort to establish a diagnosis, certain fundamental information should be given: veterinarian's name and address; owner's name and address; and species, breed, sex, age, and weight of animal. Certain specific factors should be included: (1) type of area in which the animal lives, whether city or farm; (2) whether the animal roamed at will or was tied or maintained in the house; (3) the distance to the nearest dump, grain elevator, or other source of poison; (4) history of rodenticide or other pesticide use on the home premises; and (5) history of treatment for parasites and immunizations within the past two or three weeks.

CHEMICAL ANALYSES

Chemical evidence is often an indispensable aid in diagnosing toxicologic problems. Used properly and in the right perspective, chemical analyses provide the single most important diagnostic criterion. There are limitations, however, to the value of chemical analyses. Rarely should chemical results be used alone in making a diagnosis. Positive chemical data plus history, clinical signs, and postmortem findings may provide evidence to arrive at an accurate diagnosis. One should never request a chemistry laboratory simply to "analyze for poisons" because an animal died of unknown causes. There are thousands of toxic chemicals and plants, and performing analyses for all of them would be impossible not only because of the limited amount of sample available but also because the cost would be prohibitive. Also, there are many toxic plants and even some chemical agents for which no chemical analytical procedures are available.

Although there are some toxicologic tests suitable for the veterinary hospital or clinical laboratory, many procedures for toxicologic analyses are complicated, time consuming, and require expensive equipment. Unfortunately, many of the screening qualitative tests for toxicants are not worth the time it takes to perform them. An example is the Reinsch test for arsenic and mercury. When performed by an inexperienced individual, this test is worse than no test at all. Several metals such as arsenic, mercury, and antimony will give a positive reaction to this test. Also, sulfur and other elements found in biologic specimens will give false positives with the Reinsch test. Thus, unless a laboratory is adequately staffed and equipped for analytical chemistry procedures, little significance can be placed on toxicologic screening tests. False-positive or false-negative results can be disastrous, especially when one considers that a majority of toxicoses involve potential litigations. One can find himself in an embarrassing position when he is unable to rely upon his analytical procedures in making a toxicologic diagnosis. Perhaps a certain amount of screening and preliminary tests can be performed by a veterinary clinic for the sole purpose of aiding in treatment rationale, but the clinic should rely upon subsequent chemical confirmation by a qualified toxicology laboratory.

The minimum equipment necessary for an analytic chemistry-toxicology laboratory includes an atomic absorption spectrophotometer, a colorimeter or ultraviolet spectrophotometer, and a gas-liquid chromatograph or thin-layer chromatographic equipment. Facilities for ashing or digesting specimens, such as a perchloric

115

acid hood and a muffle furnace, should be available, as well as analytical balances, specialized glassware, and other routine analytic chemistry laboratory equipment. The cost of equipping such a laboratory would be prohibitive to all except a large group practice or hospital.

SUBMITTING SPECIMENS FOR LABORATORY EVALUATION

When submitting specimens to a diagnostic laboratory, certain considerations should be made. The importance of supplying a complete account of history, signs, and lesions with specimens submitted for laboratory evaluation cannot be overemphasized. Such information will enable the toxicologist to select toxicants intelligently for which to make analyses. This is especially important when a test for the toxicant originally suspected proves negative. A chemist still has the opportunity to test for other poisons if adequate specimens have been submitted.

The choice of specimen is important in making a chemical analysis. Specimens should be taken free of chemical contamination and debris and should not be washed because of the possibility of removing residues of the toxic agent or of contaminating the specimen with the water. Keep in mind that one is often dealing with trace amounts of a particular chemical, and even the slightest contamination may produce erroneous results. Tissue specimens should be frozen and packaged to arrive at the laboratory while still frozen. Serum and blood should not be frozen but kept refrigerated. Always package specimens of various organs separately. Use clean glass or plastic containers that can be tightly sealed. Always label each specimen with the owner's name, animal name or number, and tissue or specimen in the container. Never add preservatives such as formalin to specimens unless there is a specific reason for doing so and such information is included along with the specimen. Always send more material than you think is necessary. It is easier to throw away excess specimen than to obtain more specimen after the carcass has been discarded.

Serum cations and enzymes may be very helpful in the diagnosis of certain toxic and metabolic conditions. To obtain meaningful results, several general rules for collection and preservation of serum should be followed. Always collect blood with clean equipment and transfer it to clean vials or tubes. Avoid excessive aspiration pressure, splashing, or time lag during collection to minimize hemolysis. Make every effort to avoid trauma to the unclotted or clotted sample. Allow sufficient time for the blood to clot and begin to retract, usually about one hour. Always try to remove serum from the clot within two hours. This may be done by carefully pouring off serum from the retracted clot or by centrifugation. After the serum is separated from the clot, it can be frozen and transported with ice.

Specimens that should be submitted from a live animal include: 5 ml of serum with clot removed, 10 ml of whole blood, 50 ml of urine, and 200 gm of bait, vomitus, or other such materials.

Specimens that should be submitted from a dead animal include: 5 and 10 ml of serum and whole blood, respectively, if available, 50 ml of urine, and 100 gm each of liver, kidney, spleen, and body fat. The entire brain should be submitted. Many disorders resembling poisons can be differentiated by brain lesions. If an infectious or inflammatory process is suspected, separate the brain longitudinally, fix half in 10 percent buffered formalin and freeze the other half. Up to 500 gm of stomach contents should be included.

Plastic bags, newspaper, canned ice, and cardboard are good materials to use for transporting specimens to a laboratory for examination. Liquids such as blood, urine, stomach contents, and water should be shipped in a glass or heavy plastic container that can be sealed. Wrap each labelled specimen well in newspaper and package for mailing unless it can be delivered in person which, of course, is most desirable. Always wrap the specimens individually for mailing so that the contents cannot leak and contaminate other mail or other specimens.

If one is in doubt about proper tissues for analysis or the availability of confirmatory tests, much time, effort, and confusion can be avoided by placing a telephone call to the laboratory.

SPECIMENS FOR DIAGNOSIS OF SPECIFIC TOXICANTS

The procedures for sending in specimens as outlined under the heading, "Submitting Specimens for Laboratory Evaluation," are suitable for the detection of most toxicants. There are instances, however, in which special considerations regarding chemical analysis and pathologic evaluation are required. Some examples for specific toxicants are given in Table 1.

INTERPRETATION OF LABORATORY RESULTS

Interpretation of the significance of chemical data should be done carefully, taking into con-

Table 1. *Specimens Required for Specific Tests*

POISON OR ANALYSIS REQUESTED	SPECIMEN REQUIRED	AMOUNT OF SPECIMEN DESIRED	COMMENTS
Ammonia°	Whole blood or serum	5 ml.	Frozen (1–2 drops of saturated HgCl₂ may be used instead of freezing rumen contents)
	Stomach contents (composite)	100 gm.	
	Urine	5 ml.	
ANTU	Stomach and intestine contents	200 gm.	Can be detected only within 12–24 hours after ingestion
	Liver	200 gm.	
Arsenic	Liver	50 gm.	
	Kidney	50 gm.	
	Feed	100 gm.	
	Stomach contents	100 gm.	
	Urine	50 ml.	
Calcium	Serum	2 ml.	Serum must *not* be hemolyzed; separate clot before transit
	Feed	25 gm.	
Carbon monoxide	Whole blood	15 ml.	
Chloride	See Sodium		
Chlorinated hydrocarbon insecticides	Brain	½ cerebrum	Must not be contaminated with hairs or stomach contents; preferable to use chemically clean glass jars; avoid plastic containers
	Body fat	100 gm.	
	Stomach contents	100 gm.	
	Liver	50 gm.	
	Kidney	50 gm.	
	Whole blood	10 ml.	
Copper	Kidney	50 gm.	
	Liver	50 gm.	
	Whole blood or serum	10 ml.	
	Feces	100 gm.	
Cyanide	Whole blood	10 ml.	Freeze specimen promptly in air-tight container
	Liver	50 gm.	
	Forage, silage	100 gm.	
	Other materials	100 gm.	
Ethylene glycol	Serum	10 ml.	
	Kidney (in formalin)	Whole organ	One kidney, both in small animals
	Urine	10 ml.	
Fluoroacetate	Stomach contents	All available	Frozen
	Kidney	One whole	
	Urine	50 gm.	
	Liver	50 gm.	
	Other materials	100 gm.	
Nitrates	Water	50 ml.	
	Forage, silage	100 gm.	
	Whole blood (methemoglobin)	10 ml.	
	Other materials	100 gm.	
	Whole eyeball or aqueous humor	1 ml.	
Organophosphorous insecticides	Brain	50 gm. (cerebrum)	
	Body fat	50 gm.	
	Stomach contents (composite)	50 gm.	
	Blood (heparinized)	10 ml.	
	Urine	50 ml.	
	Feed	100 gm.	
Oxalates	Fresh forage	6–8 plants	Do *not* chop plants; freeze promptly
	Kidney (in formalin)	Whole organ	One kidney, both in small animals (qualitative test only)
Phenols	Stomach contents	500 gm.	Pack in air-tight container
	Other materials	200 gm.	
Phenothiazines	Feed or other materials	50 gm.	

°A total of 5 ml. of nonhemolyzed serum is sufficient to conduct several clinical tests.

Continued on next page

Table 1. *Specimens Required for Specific Tests (Continued)*

POISON OR ANALYSIS REQUESTED	SPECIMEN REQUIRED	AMOUNT OF SPECIMEN DESIRED	COMMENTS
Phosphates	Serum	5 ml.	
	Bone	25 gm.	
	Other materials	100 gm.	
Thallium	Urine	10 ml.	
	Kidney	50 gm.	
	Liver	50 gm.	
Urea	Feed	100 gm.	
	Other materials	500 gm.	
	See also Ammonia		
Warfarin and other anticoagulants	Whole blood	10 ml.	
	Liver	100 gm.	
	Feed	100 gm.	
	Other materials	100 gm.	
Zinc	Liver	50 gm.	
	Kidney	50 gm.	
	Other materials	100 gm.	

sideration other evidence presented with the case. Positive chemical findings are not always evidence of intoxication, nor do negative findings always indicate that a toxicosis did not occur. For example, finding chlorinated hydrocarbon insecticides in the fatty tissues of an animal only indicates that the animal was exposed to the pesticide, not that the insecticide produced a toxicosis. On the other hand, failure to find certain organophosphorous insecticides in the body tissues would not guarantee that the animal had not been poisoned by such a chemical. In the case of most chlorinated hydrocarbon insecticides, the animal may store a considerable amount of the chemical in its tissues without apparent harmful effects. With organophosphorous compounds, the body may metabolize them so rapidly that they are not detectable by chemical analysis.

LABORATORIES OFFERING TOXICOLOGY-CHEMICAL ANALYTIC SERVICE

In 1977, the Veterinary Services Laboratory, Animal and Plant Inspection Services, USDA, Ames, Iowa, made a survey of public and private veterinary diagnostic laboratories in the United States. The following is a list of those laboratories reporting capabilities for general toxicology-chemical analyses. For a more complete listing, refer to the Directory of Animal Disease Diagnostic Laboratories, August, 1977, U.S. Government Printing Office, Washington, D.C., Publ. No. 720–023/9645/1–3.

Alaska

Alaska State-Federal
   Laboratory
P.O. Box 720
Palmer, Alaska 99645
907–745–3236

Arizona

Arizona State Department
   of Health
1520 West Adams Street
Phoenix, Arizona 85007
602–765–4551

Department of Veterinary
   Science
University of Arizona
Tucson, Arizona 85721
602–884–2355

California

California Department of
   Agriculture Veterinary
   Laboratory Services
P.O. Box 255
San Gabriel, California
   91778
213–282–6127

County of Los Angeles
   Department of Health
   Services Division
12824 Horton Avenue
Downey, California
   90242
213–923–0641

Intermountain Laboratories
   Incorporated
   Veterinary Reference
   Laboratory, Inc.
800 Charcot Ave
San Jose, California
   95131
415–845–8844

Intermountain Laboratories
Incorporated
Veterinary Reference
Laboratory, Inc.
1111 E. Commonwealth
Fullerton, California
92631
714–870–0743

Wildlife Investigations
Laboratory
987 Jedsmith Drive
Sacramento, California
95819
916–465–0157

Colorado

Colorado State University
Diagnostic Laboratory
Fort Collins, Colorado
80521
303–491–6128

Connecticut

Department of
Pathobiology
Box U-89
University of Connecticut
Storrs, Connecticut 06268
203–486–4000

Delaware

Eastern Shore
Laboratories, Inc.
P.O. Box 657
Laurel, Delaware 19956
302–749–2284

Florida

Jackson County Animal
Disease Diagnostic
Laboratory
P.O. Box 37
37 E. Hwy. 90
Cottondale, Florida 32431
904–352–4461

Kissimmee Animal Disease
Diagnostic Laboratory
P.O. Box 460
Kissimmee, Florida 32741
305–847–3185

Georgia

Diagnostic and
Investigational
Laboratories
Route 2 Brighton Road
Tifton, Georgia 31794
912–386–3340

Diagnostic Assistance
Laboratory
College of Veterinary
Medicine
University of Georgia
Athens, Georgia 30601
404–542–5568

Hawaii

Department of
Agriculture Veterinary
Laboratory Branch
1428 South King Street
Honolulu, Hawaii 96814
808–941–3071 (ext. 158)

Idaho

Livestock Disease
Control Laboratory
P.O. Box 7249
Boise, Idaho 83707
208–384–3111

Illinois

Laboratories of
Veterinary Diagnostic
Medicine
University of Illinois
Urbana, Illinois 61801
217–333–1620

Regional Diagnostic
Laboratory
235 North Walnut Street
Centralia, Illinois 62801
618–532–6701

Indiana

Animal Disease
Diagnostic Laboratory
School of Veterinary
Medicine
Purdue University
West Lafayette, Indiana
47907
317–749–2496

Iowa

Veterinary Diagnostic
Laboratory
College of Veterinary
Medicine
Iowa State University
Ames, Iowa 50010
515–294–1950

Kansas

Comparative Toxicology
Laboratory
College of Veterinary
Medicine
Kansas State University
Manhattan, Kansas 66506
913–532–5679

Kentucky

Central Kentucky Animal
Disease Diagnostic
Laboratory
Rural Route 6 Newton
Pike
Lexington, Kentucky
40505
606–253–0571

Kentucky Department of
Agriculture Animal
Diagnostic Laboratory
North Drive
Hopkinsville, Kentucky
44240
502–886–3959

Louisiana

Central Louisiana
Livestock Diagnostic
Laboratory
Route 2, Box 51-F
Le compte, Louisiana
71346
318–443–6993

Northwest Louisiana
Livestock Diagnostic
and Research
Laboratory
P.O. Box 2156
N.S.U.
Natchitoches, Louisiana
71457
318–352–6272

Ruston Diagnostic
Laboratory

P.O. Box 811
Ag. Drive
Ruston, Louisiana 71270
318–255–1933

Maine

Maine Poultry
  Consultants
Box 262
Waterville, Maine 04901
207–873–3405

Massachusetts

Large Animal Diagnostic
  Laboratory
Paige Laboratory
University of
  Massachusetts
Amherst, Massachusetts
  01002
413–545–2427

Michigan

Michigan Department of
  Agriculture Laboratory
  Division
1615 South Harrison
  Road
East Lansing, Michigan
  48823
517–373–6410

Veterinary Diagnostic
  Laboratory
Michigan State
  University
East Lansing, Michigan
  48823
517–353–1683

Wildlife Pathology
  Laboratory
Michigan Department of
  Natural Resources
8562 E. Stoll Rd. R1
East Lansing, Michigan
  48823
517–339–8638

Minnesota

Veterinary Diagnostic
  Laboratories
E220 Diagnostic
  Research Bldg

College of Veterinary
  Medicine
University of Minnesota
St. Paul, Minnesota 55101
612–373–0774

Mississippi

Mississippi Veterinary
  Diagnostic Laboratory
P.O. Box 4389
Jackson, Mississippi
  39216
601–354–6091

Missouri

Bureau of Laboratory
  Services
Missouri Division of
  Health
Broadway State Building
Jefferson City, Missouri
  65101
314–751–3334

Fish-Pesticide Research
  Laboratory
Bureau of Sport Fisheries
  and Wildlife
Columbia, Missouri
  65201
314–442–2271 (ext. 3101)

Ralston Purina Veterinary
  Laboratories
Checkerboard Square
St. Louis, Missouri 63188
314–982–2611

Veterinary Medical
  Diagnostic Laboratory
School of Veterinary
  Medicine
University of Missouri
Columbia, Missouri
  65201
314–882–6811

Montana

State of Montana Animal
  Health Division
  Diagnostic Laboratory
P.O. Box 997
Bozeman, Montana 59715
406–586–5952

Nebraska

Harris Laboratories, Inc.
P.O. Box 80837
Lincoln, Nebraska 68501
402–432–2811

Veterinary Science
  Laboratory
University of Nebraska
North Platte, Nebraska
  69101
308–532–3611

North Carolina

Rollins Animal Disease
  Diagnostic Laboratory
P.O. Box 12223 Cameron
  Village Station
Raleigh, North Carolina
  27606
919–733–3986

North Dakota

North Dakota State
  University Veterinary
  Diagnostic Laboratory
Fargo, North Dakota
  58102
701–237–7511

Ohio

Ohio Department of
  Agriculture Animal
  Disease Diagnostic
  Laboratory
Reynoldsburg, Ohio
  43068
614–866–6362

Oklahoma

Oklahoma Animal
  Disease Diagnostic
  Laboratory
College of Veterinary
  Medicine
Oklahoma State
  University
Stillwater, Oklahoma
  74074
405–624–6623

Oregon

Oregon State Veterinary
  Diagnostic Laboratory
Oregon State University
Corvallis, Oregon 97331
503–424–3261

Pennsylvania

Pennsylvania Department
  of Agriculture
Bureau of Animal
  Industry Laboratory
Summerdale,
  Pennsylvania 17093
717–637–8808

South Dakota

Animal Disease Research
  and Diagnostic
  Laboratory
South Dakota State
  University
Brookings, South Dakota
  57006
605–688–5171

Tennessee

C. E. Kord Animal
  Disease Laboratory
P.O. Box 40627 Mel.
  Station
Nashville, Tennessee
  37204
615–853–1559

Texas

Texas Veterinary Medical
  Diagnostic Laboratory
Drawer 3040
College Station, Texas
  77840
713–845–3414

Utah

Branch Veterinary
  Laboratory, Utah
  Agricultural
  Experiment Station
P.O. Box 1068
Provo, Utah 84601
801–373–6383

Intermountain
  Laboratories, Inc.
870E 7145 South
Midvale, Utah 84047
801–561–2244

State Chemists Office and
  State-Federal
  Cooperative Laboratory
412 Capitol Building
Salt Lake City, Utah
  84114
801–533–5421

Utah State University
  Veterinary Diagnostic
  Laboratory
Logan, Utah 84321
801–752–4100 (ext. 7584)

Virginia

Division of Animal
  Health and Dairies
  Research Laboratory
116 Reservoir Street
Harrisonburg, Virginia
  22801
703–434–3897

Division of Animal
  Health and Dairies
  Regulatory Laboratory
Box 4191
Lynchburg, Virginia
  24502
804–846–8860

Division of Animal
  Health and Dairies
  Regulatory Laboratory
234 West Shirley Avenue
Warrenton, Virginia
  22186
703–347–3131

Washington

Poultry Diagnostic
  Laboratory, Western
  Washington Research &
  Extension Center
Washington State
  University
Puyallup, Washington
  98371
206–845–6613

Western Fish Disease
  Laboratory
Building 204 — Sand
  Point Naval Support
  Activity
Seattle, Washington
  98115
206–442–5960

West Virginia

State Federal
  Cooperative Animal
  Health Laboratory
Room B-86 Capitol
  Building
Charleston, West Virginia
  25305
304–885–2231

Wisconsin

Central Animal Health
  Laboratory
6101 Mineral Point Road
Madison, Wisconsin
  53705
608–266–2465

Wyoming

Wyoming State
  Veterinary Laboratory
Box 950
Laramie, Wyoming 82070
307–742–6638

SUPPLEMENTAL READING

Buck, W.B.: Laboratory toxicologic tests and their interpretation. J. Am. Vet. Med. Assn. *155*:1928–1941, 1969.
Buck, W.B., Osweiler, G.D., and Van Gelder, G.A.: *Clinical and Diagnostic Veterinary Toxicology.* Dubuque, Iowa, Kendall-Hunt Publishing Co., 1973.
Radeleff, R.D.: *Veterinary Toxicology,* 2nd ed. Philadelphia, Lea & Febiger, 1970, pp. 25–28.

COMMON POISONINGS IN SMALL ANIMAL PRACTICE

GARY D. OSWEILER, D.V.M.
Columbia, Missouri

Small animal poisoning is often associated with acute or peracute onset of severe clinical signs that progress rapidly to death or recovery. Many times, an animal's owner is not aware of access to foreign materials that could be toxic. In other instances, the client is firmly convinced that malicious poisoning has occurred. Dogs and cats previously in apparent good health may be found dead, and this situation frequently gives rise to suspicions of poisoning in the minds of client and veterinarian alike. There is also some tendency to consider as poisoning disease states that cannot be explained by other means. Perhaps the most common toxicologic diagnosis made is "poisoning" due to undetermined etiology.

The actual confirmed incidents of intoxication by specific materials constitute a very small portion of small animal medicine diagnoses. The topics covered in this section on chemical and physical disorders constitute the "common" specific poisonings — i.e., those intoxications most often diagnosed clinically and/or confirmed chemically. The purposes of this chapter are (1) to review some of the limitations that prevent better diagnosis of poisoning and (2) to classify the sources and situations from which poisonings commonly arise with some perspective on their importance.

To complete the goals of establishing a tentative clinical diagnosis, determining the source, and educating the client in avoidance of further problems, one must rely primarily upon clinical assessment of the patient and upon careful and thorough questioning of the client regarding possible or probable sources of toxicants. The history and clinical exam are inseparable in toxicology and must be evaluated in light of one another. As with all diagnostic medicine, several tentative diagnoses may come to mind in poisoning cases. These must then be systematically eliminated or confirmed, using all possible or available factors as aids in the process.

All pertinent facts and statements should be recorded in writing. This will serve later to review the facts and point out any inconsistencies or trends in the history. It may aid in invalidating indications of poisoning. Conversely, in the occasional malicious or negligent poisoning, written details are invaluable corroboration of the diagnostic procedure.

Animal and environmental factors that may modify responses to various poisons should be carefully noted. Was the animal young? Old? Chronically ill? Recently medicated? Changed in location? As Clarke and Clarke (1967) state with particular emphasis, almost any food or drug can be toxic if administered in too high a dosage, too frequently, too rapidly, or to a highly susceptible animal. Thus, a poison source is a hazard only when the conditions of exposure exceed the tolerance of the animal for that material.

A knowledge of the circumstances associated with poisoning is very useful and may provide a key for making a proper diagnosis. Most of the history may have no bearing on intoxication, but important points may be gleaned from it. The presence of poisons such as rodenticides, insecticides, drugs, paints, fertilizers, petroleum products, and other chemicals on the premises, or a history of their use or availability for animal exposure, should be ascertained. One should be prepared to estimate the amount or degree of possible exposure to these chemicals. The food and water supply should be checked carefully for the presence of toxic plants, molds, algae, fungi, or other toxicants. Other important facts that should be obtained include the course of events in hours or days as well as the breed, sex, feeding program, history of past illnesses, and immunization record of the animal.

Circumstantial evidence has greater value if one can determine that animals have consumed or were definitely exposed to a particular toxic agent. One should guard against diagnosing lead poisoning simply because lead paint is found on the premises, or plant poisoning(s) unless there is evidence that the suspected plant was consumed in sufficient quantity to produce toxicosis. Circumstantial evidence should be viewed as just one factor; other types of evidence must be present to reach an accurate diagnosis that could be used as input to determine which are the "common" confirmed poisonings. The veterinarian must decide, on the merits of each case, how much effort goes into reviewing the factors in a potential poisoning. When surveys or summaries are made concerning frequency of poisoning (or other diseases), one should always question the degree of surety with which diagnoses were made.

In addition to lack of circumstantial or clinical evidence (the clinician's part), lack of chemical or analytical data may be a problem. For some toxicants, such as plant toxins or animal venoms, diagnostic chemical analyses are not available or are not practical. In other cases, the cost of analyzing for many poisons is prohibitive.

Thus, our view of what is a common poison is limited by the effort expended in gathering accurate and detailed history, the thoroughness of the clinical and clinicopathologic exam, and the availability of confirmatory chemical analyses.

CLASSIFICATION OF POISONS

Toxic materials may be classified in several ways. In many cases, it is useful to group them according to where they occur or why they are used. Thus, insecticides would be potential toxicants if the owner had just sprayed extensively for roaches, and plant poisoning is more likely if the season is spring and flowers, shrubs, and vines are abundant around the home.

Toxins may be grouped according to the following general headings:

A. Natural Hazards
  1. Plants, seeds
  2. Fungi, algae
  3. Mycotoxins
  4. Zootoxins (snakes, toads, insects, etc.)
  5. Poisonous minerals in food or water
B. Man-made Hazards
  1. Industrial contamination
  2. Pesticides and economic poisons
  3. Domestic materials
  4. Drugs
  5. Food and water

NATURAL TOXINS

Toxic plants and seeds are found in many homes and places of business. While the dog and cat are not foragers, both species have been known to consume various plants or portions thereof (e.g., grass-eating dogs and catnip-loving cats). Poisoning by oleander, dumb cane, castor bean, chokecherry, jimsonweed, morning-glory, and mushrooms has been recorded to occur in small animals.

Fungi, mycotoxins, and blue-green algae have caused poisoning in pets. Most notable of the fungi are the *Amanita* spp. *A. phalloides* produces a fatal gastroenteric and hepatotoxic reaction, and *A. muscaria* causes signs that mimic cholinergic drugs and that are alleviated by atropine. Mycotoxins of *Aspergillus flavus* (aflatoxin) and *Penicillium* sp. are toxic to dogs, and outbreaks of aflatoxicosis from contaminated dog food have been observed. Most effects of the aflatoxins are recorded in dogs and are exerted on the liver, kidney, and blood-vascular system. Diagnosis of mycotoxicosis is difficult, since effects may be delayed, and a source of toxin may no longer be available. Algal blooms in late summer are associated with gastroenteritis, hepatotoxicity, and "fast-death" in many species including dogs.

Certain toxic animals, insects, and snakes are a hazard to pets in some locations of North America. Most problems are reported from the southern and southwestern United States. Snake bites (rattlesnake, copperhead, and coral snake) and toad poisoning from *Bufo* spp. are the most frequently reported problems. Animal venoms and toxins characteristically affect the nervous system, cause tissue necrosis, induce hemorrhage or hemolysis, or induce an allergic response.

Mineral poisoning in food or water is rare in small animals. Arsenical contamination of grain or availability of rodent baits containing toxins such as phosphorus, arsenic, inorganic fluorides, or barium may occasionally occur. Cured meat or the water from cooked cured meats may be high in nitrites and result in methemoglobinemia. Since pets generally consume from the same water supply as man, acute water-borne poisoning is relatively rare.

MAN-MADE SOURCES OF POISONS FOR PET ANIMALS

Sources of potential poisons are legion and are exceeded in number only by the toxicants themselves. Some 2000 chemicals and drugs are considered dangerously toxic, and new chemicals with potential toxicity are being introduced at the rate of 1500 or more each year.

In order to consider even the broadest possibilities, one must be equipped with at least some ready reference works that give detailed information about the more common poisoning problems. In addition, it is helpful to know the areas in which the more toxic chemicals, plants, and venoms are found. Furthermore, the general clinical effects associated with toxic substances should be kept as a cross reference.

INDUSTRIAL CONTAMINATION

The gases, vapors, dusts, and water pollutants that plague man are available to the companion animals that share his environment. Carbon monoxide, oxides of nitrogen and sulfur, and various pneumoconioses should be considered when evaluating respiratory problems in small animals. Water pollutants such as nitrates have been associated experimentally with hydrocephalus in young dogs. However, little work has been done specifically relating pollutants to disease problems in the small animal population.

PESTICIDES AND ECONOMIC POISONS

These materials, especially the rodenticides and insecticides, appear most often as accidental and malicious poisons in small animals. This comes from the fact that they are designed to be toxic to similar biologic mechanisms and that they are used largely by laymen in areas frequented by pets. Proper use and storage of such products would eliminate most of these problems.

The important economic poisons in small animal toxicology are discussed in individual chapters in this section.

DOMESTIC MATERIALS

A great number of products used in homes or businesses contain toxic materials. Many of these are listed in the article on "Common Potential Sources of Small Animal Poisoning." These materials are usually packaged and should not be available to pets if properly used and stored. Since most pets (perhaps primates excepted) do not remove caps or lids, and since they can be effectively locked away from these materials when in use, there is little excuse other than negligence for poisoning by these products. Many of these chemicals are volatile or corrosive, and often they are able to penetrate intact skin.

Clarke (1975) reports that overheated frying pans coated with non-stick materials emit a vapor toxic to birds. The fluorinated propellants (freons) may cause acute respiratory and cardiovascular abnormalities, with fatal consequences in pets.

Cats are peculiarly susceptible to many domestic products, and a good review of this subject has been written (Atkins and Johnson, 1975).

DRUGS

Pets occasionally gain access to drugs of abuse through living with an owner who is in-

clined to their use. Most common is the consumption of marijuana, generally with resultant non-fatal hallucination for one or two days.

Certain therapeutic agents intended for man may inadvertently or intentionally be given to pets. Excessive amounts of vitamin A, vitamin D, and aspirin may cause toxicosis, especially in cats, when given by well meaning owners. Acetaminophen pain killers may cause toxicosis in cats from one or two of the 325 mg tablets. Barbiturates ("sleeping pills") or stimulants such as caffeine tablets have been carelessly left where pets could consume toxic amounts. A part of the anamnesis of any uncharacterized potential toxicosis in pets should include some determination of drug preparations used or kept in the household.

Generally, the side effects and therapeutic incompatibilities of veterinary drugs are known prior to their release. Individuals prescribing or using therapeutic agents should be familiar with the side effects, adverse reactions, and contraindications of all such drugs. A discussion of drug-induced and adverse reactions will be found in a separate chapter within this section.

FOOD AND WATER

Food poisoning or garbage intoxication is more frequently diagnosed than any other intoxication. Mold toxins, bacterial exotoxins, bacterial endotoxins, and toxic products from putrefaction may be involved separately or in concert with one another. Much more work is needed in studying the physiologic response of small animals to contaminated or tainted foods. This subject is treated more fully elsewhere in this section.

FREQUENCY OF SMALL ANIMAL POISONING

From the foregoing plethora of potential poisons, the clinician must judge which are most likely to cause toxicosis in animals. In addition, those toxins most probably encountered should be well understood and dealt with as specifically and thoroughly as possible. To this end, it is sometimes helpful to know what one's colleagues have encountered as problems.

In 1969, a survey was conducted of the American Animal Hospital Association membership and of veterinary college teaching hospitals. Results are presented in Table 1. One must remember that such surveys are only as good as the input data. In many cases, the diagnoses were not confirmed by chemical analyses, nor

Table 1. *Reported Clinical Diagnoses of Small Animal Toxicoses in the United States*

	NORTHEAST	SOUTHEAST	SOUTHWEST	WEST	MIDWEST	NATIONAL TOTAL
Rodenticides						
ANTU	2	5	1	7	6	21
Thallium	45	19	8	3	49	124
Warfarin	60	27	35	39	118	279
Strychnine	78	60	57	66	154	415
Compound 1080						
Zinc phosphide	3	1			2	6
Pesticides						
Arsenic	11	21	12	43	58	145
Chlorinated hydrocarbons	19	38	28	21	66	172
Organophosphates	48	69	33	20	99	269
Metaldehyde		2		117		119
Glycols						
Antifreeze	6	2	4		20	32
Heavy Metals						
Lead	17	3	1	3	43	67
Mercury					2	2
Miscellaneous						
Acid		3	3	3	12	21
Alkali	3	2	1	3	12	21
Phenols			2	1	13	16
Quaternary ammonia	2					2
Food intoxication	118	111	85	219	394	927
Phosphorus			1		2	3
Toxic plants	5		5	5	10	25
Fungi	122	15		11		148
Snakes	16	85	58	46	9	214
Toads	4	35	53	3	5	100
Totals	559	498	387	610	1074	3128

was a source determined. However, the information does reflect the cases that appeared clinically to be caused by specific compounds.

The data presented in Table 1 are a composite of both canine and feline poisoning. By far, the greater number of diagnosed toxicoses occurs in dogs. The peculiar sensitivity of cats to phenolics and chlorinated aryl hydrocarbons, however, results in more frequent poisoning of cats by such compounds with ring structures, which they are unable to metabolize.

The author has recently rechecked with selected practices and institutions. In general, the same diagnoses are being made. However, certain differences appear to be developing. Some of these are as follows:

1. Poisoning by ANTU rodenticide is diagnosed only rarely and is usually based on the lesion rather than determination of the source. Organophosphate insecti-

cides and the herbicide paraquat may cause similar pulmonary lesions.

2. Thallium poisoning is almost never reported. The few cases that are found have been from metropolitan areas of Chicago and the eastern seaboard. Thallium is no longer available as a pest control agent.

3. Sodium fluoroacetate (Compound 1080) poisoning is reported with increasing frequency among the rodenticides — especially in the Midwest. It is most often associated with commercial or governmental pest control. Compound 1080 is one of the few agents toxic enough to cause secondary intoxication in *Canidae* that consume poisoned animal pests. Part of the increased incidence is probably due to greater awareness of the effects of 1080 and to greatly improved detection methods for the toxin.

4. Organophosphate and carbamate toxicoses continue to result in almost the entire number of reported insecticide poisonings. Most chlorinated hydrocarbon insecticides have been severely curtailed for both home and agricultural use. Although some chlordane and lindane products may be found on retail shelves, the registration of chlordane may soon be deleted. Young animals are more susceptible than adults to poisoning by chlorinated hydrocarbon insecticides. As a species, the cat is more susceptible to at least some of the chlorinated hydrocarbons. The dog, however, is peculiarly sensitive to toxaphene, and this chemical is one of the few chlorinated hydrocarbons still approved and in widespread use.

5. An insecticide-related problem, flea-collar dermatitis, continues to be a problem, especially for dogs. Keeping the collar dry, properly sized, and loosely fitted prevents the majority of problems.

6. Antifreeze (ethylene glycol) poisoning is a persistent and perennial problem and increasingly is recognized in cats as well as in dogs. Ethylene glycol is a season-related toxicant, with an increased incidence being seen in fall and early winter.

7. Strychnine poisoning continues to be a leading cause of chemical poisoning in dogs and is commonly implicated in malicious poisoning. It is readily recognized clinically and chemically and is of high toxicity to dogs.

8. Many of the animals seen with anticoagulant poisoning are treated and saved. Large amounts of the commonly used 0.025 percent baits must be consumed for exposure to result in fatality.

9. In the author's opinion, more poisoning from the rodenticide zinc phosphide may occur than is reported. Clinical signs of zinc phosphide toxicosis are variable, and death may be acute after a latent period. Furthermore, there is no good chemical test in routine use for zinc phosphide.

10. Metaldehyde poisoning from commercial snail baits occurs in warm, damp climates and is associated with the method of snail or slug baiting. If small piles are carelessly left accessible in the garden, dogs in particular may consume the bait.

11. Lead poisoning, in addition to the encephalitic form, may go unrecognized as a syndrome of anorexia, weakness, mild colic, and occasional vomiting. These signs often occur prior to neurologic involvement.

12. The herbicide 2,4-D, commonly used for lawn weed control, is relatively more toxic to the dog than to other species. However, based on toxicity data and applicable rates to lawns, direct contact with treated lawns is not likely to cause poisoning. However, improperly disposed spray mixtures or pools of diluted spray could be a hazard to dogs.

13. Poisonous toads and venomous animals are mainly geographic problems of the southern states. They are discussed in separate chapters of this section.

14. Acutal poisoning by plants is, in the author's opinion, rare in small animals. The most frequent response to ingested plants is nausea, vomition, and salivation. While certain seeds, bulbs, and leaves are highly toxic, only the occasional young inquisitive animal or pets with depraved appetites or insufficient food are likely to consume plants.

15. The rodenticide N-3-pyridylmethyl N^1-p-nitrophenyl urea (Vacor), while relatively safe for dogs, has been consumed under field conditions in sufficient amounts to cause toxicosis. Although cats are more susceptible to this toxicosis, they appear not to prefer the bait and are rarely intoxicated therefrom.

Recently, several studies have contributed to knowledge about frequency of toxicoses in small companion animals. Humphreys (1978) reviewed veterinary literature over a 20-year period. Lead was cited as a commonly reported intoxication of dogs. Other canine intoxications of note were carbon monoxide, organophosphate and chlorinated hydrocarbon insecticides, paraquat, ethylene glycol, and theobromine. Caged pet birds were reported highly sensitive to polytetrafluoroethylene (PTFE) fumes from overheated Teflon fry pans.

Maddy et al. (1977) reviewed poison exposure incidents involving 169 dogs in California during a 12-month period. Results of the study may be summarized as follows:

Toxicant group	Number of exposures
Anticoagulant rodenticides	27
Arsenicals	5
Carbamate insecticides	53
Chlorinated hydrocarbon insecticides	11
Metaldehyde (molluscicide)	24
Organosphosphate insecticides	15
Phosphorus	2
Pyrethroids	8
Strychnine	3
Thiocarbamates	2
Miscellaneous	35

The results recorded do not indicate if clinical toxicosis always occurs, but they do depict exposure patterns, many of which involve highly toxic chemicals.

Stowe et al. (1978) reviewed the clinical intoxications of dogs and cats at the University of Minnesota College of Veterinary Medicine over a four-year period (this work for large and small animals has been presented in detail in several publications). A total of 288 intoxications in dogs and 31 in cats were recorded. For dogs, individual toxicants diagnosed were as follows: arsenic — 12, lead — 15, thallium — 5, strychnine — 125, warfarin — 4, Vacor — 14, zinc phosphide — 7, fluoroacetate — 2, organophosphate insecticide — 11, carbamates — 2, chlorinated hydrocarbons — 2, 2,4-D herbicide — 2, abuse drugs — 22, poisonous plants — 16, ethylene glycol — 21, nicotine — 4, and other miscellaneous drugs and chemicals — 22. Of the abuse drugs, 12 involved amphetamines and 6 involved marijuana. Within the plant diagnoses, most involved from one to three poisonings per plant. When poisoning involved cats the results were: arsenic — 4, lead — 2, warfarin — 3, Vacor — 3, insecticides — 3, ethylene glycol — 6, miscellaneous — 10.

Stowe et al. observed some trends in Minnesota. Lead, strychnine, and arsenic were frequently diagnosed. Rodenticide poisoning was common in dogs, especially due to strychnine. Greatest frequency of poisoning was reported in the spring and early summer. Poisonous plants accounted for 6 percent of canine intoxications; abuse drugs caused 8 percent of diagnosed poisonings. Ethylene glycol accounted for almost 8 percent of canine intoxications, and most of those occurred from October through May.

Webber and Acha (1978) studied case records of the University of Missouri Veterinary Clinic for the period 1965–1976. From 39,260 dogs examined, 458 diagnoses of intoxication (1.2 percent) were made. Approximately 30.6 percent of all intoxications diagnosed were classified as non-specific gastrointestinal intoxications. There were no marked seasonal variations in incidence, although a seasonal peak was noted for arsenic, lead, snake-bites, and insect stings. Insecticide and rodenticide poisoning appeared to peak in winter, and ethylene glycol in this study had a higher incidence in summer.

BREED

For various breeds of dogs, Webber and Acha (1978) found that pointers, dachshunds, and beagles had more than a two-fold greater risk of being poisoned compared with other breeds.

AGE

Dogs between 6 months and 2 years of age had a significantly higher attack rate for poisoning than any other age group.

MORTALITY

Only 12 percent of the 458 toxicoses diagnosed resulted in mortality for dogs. Ethylene glycol alone, by contrast, had a mortality rate of 71 percent. Mortality was 18.5 percent for arsenic, lead, and heavy metals, whereas the figure was 11 percent for insecticides and 9 percent for rodenticides.

Case records of the University of Missouri Veterinary Medical Diagnostic Laboratory for a two-year period (1975–76) indicate 43 confirmed cases of intoxication in small animals. Individual diagnoses were as follows:

Toxicant	*Species*	*Number*
Strychnine	Canine	21
Chlorinated Hydrocarbon	Canine	1
Insecticides	Bird	1
Insecticides	Fish	1
Organophosphates or Carbamates	Canine	1
Lead	Canine	4
Arsenic	Canine	1
Arsenic	Feline	1
Fluoroacetate (1080)	Canine	3
Caffeine	Feline	2
Mercury	Canine	1
Mercury	Feline	1
2,4-D	Canine	1
Anticoagulant	Canine	1
Ethylene glycol	Canine	1

Records of one diagnostic laboratory may be at odds with one of another area. For example, the preceding data relate only to chemically confirmed diagnoses. Ethylene glycol toxicosis is commonly detected upon histopathologic examination, and chemical analysis is not requested.

Aside from the few generalizations made here, there is no definitive evidence of any one overwhelming toxicology problem. Certainly, clinical toxicoses of small animals pose a formidable diagnostic challenge. They must be dealt with clinically but can only be defined by a well organized, coordinated gathering of evidence made in light of the potential hazards available and confirmed by chemical and clinical corroboration. The final task is to educate the client to avoid such hazards or to keep and use hazardous materials in their proper place.

SUPPLEMENTAL READING

Arena, J.M.: *Poisoning. Toxicology, Symptoms, Treatment*, 3rd ed. Springfield, Illinois, Charles C Thomas, 1974.

Atkins, C.E., and Johnson, R.K.: Clinical toxicities of cats. Vet. Clin. North Am. 5:623–652, 1975.

Buck, W.B., Osweiler, G.D., and Van Gelder, G.A.: *Clinical and Diagnostic Veterinary Toxicology*. Dubuque, Iowa, Kendall-Hunt Publishing Co., 1973.

Clarke, E.G.C.: Pets and poisons. J. Small Anim. Pract. 16:375–380, 1975.

Clarke, E.G.C., and Clarke, M.L.: *Garner's Veterinary Toxicology*, 3rd ed. Baltimore, The Williams & Wilkins Co., 1967.

Kirk, R.W. (ed.): *Current Veterinary Therapy*, VII, Philadelphia, W.B. Saunders Co., 1977.

Kirk, R.W., and Bistner, S.I.: *Handbood of Veterinary Procedures and Emergency Treatment*, 2nd ed. Philadelphia, W.B. Saunders Co., 1975.

Maddy, K.T., Peoples, S.A., and Riddle, L.C.: Poisoning in dogs in California with pesticides. Calif. Vet. 31:9–15, 1977.

Malone, J.C.: Diagnosis and treatment of poisoning in dogs and cats. Vet. Rec. 84:161–166, 1969.

Osweiler, G.D.: Incidence and diagnostic considerations of major small animal toxicoses. J. Am. Med. Assoc. 155:2011–2015, 1969.

Stowe, C.M., Fangmann, G., Arendt, T.D., et al.: The Frequency of Animal Intoxications in Minnesota. Paper Presented to the 4th Biennial Toxicology Conference, Logan, Utah. June 19–23, 1978.

Szabuniewicz, M.: Treatment of some common animal poisonings. Vet. Med. Small Animal Clin. December 1971, pp. 1197–1205.

Webber, J.J., and Acha, S.M.; Poisonings, UMC Veterinary Clinic (1965–1976). Columbia, Missouri, 1978. Unpublished data.

STRYCHNINE POISONING

GARY D. OSWEILER, D.V.M.
Columbia, Missouri

SOURCE

Strychnine is an indole alkaloid. Commercial sources of strychnine are found primarily in Southeast Asia, as it is derived from seeds of plants *Strychnos nux-vomica* and *Strychnos ignatti*. It was first used in medicine in about 1540 and has been used in Europe as an animal poison since the 16th century.

Current usage of strychnine is primarily as a ruminatoric (tartar emetic), stimulant, and pesticide. However, there is no modern rational basis for the use of strychnine in therapy. Its principal pesticidal applications are for rat, gopher, mole, and coyote control. Many commercial forms are pelleted and dyed either bright green or red. It is one of the most commonly recognized causes of accidental and malicious poisoning in the dog. Strychnine has recently been classified as a restricted use pesticide. This includes its use both as a rodenticide and an avicide. This should result in increased awareness of the hazards of strychnine, and may alter the total amount dispersed to the public.

Brucine is a structurally close relative of strychnine and has physiologic effects similar to those of strychnine (although less potent). The morphone alkaloids thebaine, morphine, and codeine are structurally similar to strychnine in many respects but have obvious depressant activity rather than the excitatory properties of strychnine.

TOXICITY

Strychnine is a highly toxic compound to most domestic animals. The approximate oral lethal toxicity to various animals is as follows:

bovine	0.5 mg/kg
equine	0.5 mg/kg
porcine	0.5–1.0 mg/kg
canine	0.75 mg/kg
feline	2.0 mg/kg
fowl	5.0 mg/kg
rat	3.0 mg/kg

Parenteral strychnine is 2 to 10 times more toxic than is oral strychnine.

The hazard of poisoning from strychnine is apparent when the commercial formulations containing 0.3 percent strychnine are considered versus the toxicity values. At the 0.3 percent level, each gram of bait contains 3 mg strychnine. Thus, 3 gm of bait could be lethal to a 12 kg dog. Strychnine has also been considered a secondary toxicant, killing pets that consume poisoned rodents or birds.

MECHANISM OF ACTION

The physiologic effect of strychnine is to allow uncontrolled and relatively diffuse spinal reflex activity to proceed basically unchecked. All striated muscle groups are affected, but the relatively more powerful extensors predominate to produce symmetrical and generalized rigidity to tonic seizures. Gross or microscopic changes in the neurons, axons, and myelin sheath have not been observed.

Strychnine appears to affect the central nervous system directly by selectively antagonizing certain types of spinal inhibition. It interferes with postsynaptic inhibition in the spinal cord and medulla. Thus, the moderating and controlling effects in the reflex are eliminated. Examples of postsynaptic inhibition are the inhibitory influences between motoneurons of antagonistic muscle groups and the recurrent spinal inhibition mediated by Renshaw cells.

The amino acid glycine is an accepted inhibitory transmitter in the spinal cord and medulla. Strychnine reversibly and selectively antagonizes glycine in the spinal cord and medulla, possibly by a competitive type of antagonism. Postsynaptic membrane permeability is changed, and the net effect is that strychnine reduces the inhibitory postsynaptic potential normally controlled by glycine.

CLINICAL SIGNS

Clinical signs of strychnine poisoning appear within ten minutes to two hours after ingestion of the poison. Early signs are apprehension, nervousness, tenseness, and stiffness. Palpation in early stages reveals tense abdomen and rigid cervical musculature. Violent tetanic seizures may appear spontaneously or be initiated by stimuli such as touch, sound, or sudden bright light. There is extreme and overpowering extensor rigidity causing the animal to assume a "sawhorse" stance. The strength of the tetanic spasm may throw the animal off its feet. The legs and body are stiff, the neck is arched, the ears are erect, and the lips are pulled back from the teeth. Breathing may cease momentarily. Duration of a tetanic convulsion may vary from a few seconds to a minute or more. Intermittent periods of relaxation are observed but become less frequent as the clinical course progresses. During convulsions, the pupils are dilated, and cyanotic mucous membranes are evidence of anoxia. Convulsive seizures become more frequent and death eventually occurs from exhaustion or anoxia during a tetanic seizure. The entire course of the syndrome, if untreated, is often less than one to two hours.

Physiopathology

Rigor mortis occurs rapidly after death from strychnine poisoning. Relaxation of body musculature also follows in more rapid than normal succession. No gross or microscopic lesions characteristic of strychnine poisoning can be consistently detected. Cyanosis, petechial or ecchymotic hemorrhages, and traumatic lesions are evidence of a violent and hypoxic state. Characteristically, the stomach of strychnine-poisoned animals is filled with food or bait that has not been completely digested.

Absorbed strychnine is transported in the blood by both plasma and erythrocytes but is rapidly passed from blood to tissue. It does not appear to concentrate in nervous tissue.

Excretion is accomplished in urine and via secretion into the stomach. The ionization of strychnine, a basic drug, is influenced by pH. Thus, ion-trapping of strychnine occurs in the acid conditions of the stomach, and urinary excretion may be enhanced by acidification of the urine.

Diagnosis

Tentative diagnosis is usually based on history of ingestion, characteristic clinical signs, and lack of lesions. Similar clinical signs may be caused by chlorinated hydrocarbons, zinc phosphide, metaldehyde, lead, hypocalcemia, and acute hepatic necrosis.

Samples for analysis should include stomach contents, liver, kidney, urine, and central nervous system. In addition, baits or vomitus should be kept for analysis. Most chemical confirmations of strychnine poisoning are from stomach contents or liver. In many cases, animals die so rapidly that urinary excretion has been insignificant.

In some field cases suspected to be strychnine poisoning, pentobarbital is administered to control the convulsions. Since pentobarbital is metabolized in the liver and has amine properties like alkaloids, it may react with iodoplatinate to give a spot on thin-layer chromatography (TLC), which might be confused with strychnine. Cases in which pentobarbital might occur and give false positives are those that give negative results for stomach contents but positive results for the liver.

Biologic verification of strychnine poisoning may be accomplished by the following procedure:

1. Extract stomach contents or urine mixing with equal volume of acid.
2. Centrifuge or filter the acid extract.
3. Neutralize the supernate with ammonium hydroxide to a range of pH 7.0 to 8.0.
4. Inject 0.5 ml in the dorsal sac of a frog or intraperitoneally in a mouse.
5. Typical strychnine convulsive seizures usually occur within two to four minutes.

Treatment

Of prime concern in strychnine poisoning is the maintenance of relaxation and prevention of asphyxia. In emergency situations, pentobarbital in doses just sufficient to maintain relaxation is acceptable. However, more prolonged maintenance of relaxation may be accomplished by inhalation anesthesia or by administration of methocarbamol (150 mg/kg) and continued maintenance as needed. Because respiratory paralysis and repeated hypoxia of the CNS may occur in strychnine poisoning, facilities for artificial ventilation and administration of oxygen should be readily available.

Other successful therapeutic regimens for strychnine toxicosis have included use of diazepam or glyceryl guaiacolate ether, both of which have central muscle relaxant properties. Glyceryl guaiacolate has been employed at 110 mg/kg intravenously with repeated maintenance doses as needed. In man, 10 mg of diazepam has been utilized intravenously and repeated as needed. The animal dosage for diazepam is 2.5 to 20 mg intravenously or orally.

The advantage of combination therapy is primarily the reduction of exposure to high levels of barbiturates for prolonged periods.

Early induction of vomiting with apomorphine is recommended, provided the animal is not in a hyperesthetic or convulsive state. Rapid recovery from strychnine toxicosis may be enhanced by prompt application of the enterogastric lavage technique described by Frye (1974).

If anesthesia must be maintained, gastric lavage can be employed using 1 to 2 percent tannic acid or 1:2000 potassium permanganate. Following this, activated charcoal and sodium sulfate may be left in the stomach to aid adsorption and more rapid elimination of the alkaloid.

Forced diuresis with 5 percent mannitol in 0.9 percent sodium chloride administered at a rate of 7 ml/kg/hour and acidification of the urine with 150 mg/kg body weight of ammonium chloride orally will enhance excretion of strychnine. This must be subsequent to establishment of adequate urine flow.

Toxic doses of strychnine will be depleted from the body with 24 to 48 hours. One must expect to continue maintenance relaxation and sedation for 12 to 48 hours. It should be emphasized that the sedation time can be considerably shortened if prompt and aggressive action is taken to clear the gastrointestinal tract, inactivate unabsorbed strychnine, and hasten elimination of alkaloid via diuresis and ion trapping.

When prompt and thorough action is taken, recovery of a high proportion of strychnine poisoning cases can be expected.

SUPPLEMENTAL READING

Bailey, E.M., and Szabuniewicz, M.: The use of glyceryl guaiacolate ether in the treatment of strychnine poisoning in the dog. Vet. Med. Small Anim. Clin. 70:170–174, 1975.
Clark, E.G.C., and Clarke, M.L.: Garner's Veterinary Toxicology, 3rd ed. Baltimore, The Williams & Wilkins Co., 1967.
Curtis, D.R., and Johnston, G.A.R.: Convulsant alkaloids. In Simpson, L.L., and Curtis, D.R. (eds.): Neuropoisons, Vol. 2. New York, Plenum Press, 1974.
Franz, D.: Central nervous system stimulants. In Goodman, L.S., and Gilman, A. (eds.): The Pharmacologic Basis of Therapeutics, 5th ed. New York, Macmillan Co., 1975.
Frye, F.L.: Enterogastric lavage in small animal practice. Vet. Med. Small Anim. Clin. 69:835–836, 1974.
McConnell, E.E., van Rensburg, I.B.S., and Minnie, J.A.: A rapid test for the diagnosis of strychnine poisoning. J. S. Afr. Vet. Assoc. 42(1):81–84, 1971.
MacKinnon, J., Waite, P.R., and Hilbery, A.D.R.: Accidental poisoning in animals. Vet. Rec. 92:489, 1973.
Maron, B.J., Krupp, J.R., and Tune, B.: Strychnine poisoning successfully treated with diazepam. J. Ped. 78:697–699, 1971.
Osweiler, G.D.: Strychnine poisoning. In Kirk, R.W.: Current Veterinary Therapy V. Philadelphia, W.B. Saunders Co., 1973.
Radeleff, R.D.: Veterinary Toxicology. Philadelphia, Lea & Febiger, 1964.

WARFARIN AND OTHER ANTICOAGULANT POISONINGS

ROBERT A. GREEN, D.V.M.
College Station, Texas

and WILLIAM B. BUCK, D.V.M.
Urbana, Illinois

Accidental ingestion of anticoagulant rodenticides produces a coagulopathy due to vitamin K antagonism. A 1969 survey indicated that warfarin toxicosis was the third most common intoxication reported in small animals in the United States.

The anticoagulant rodenticides are structurally related to coumarin. All have the basic coumarin or indandione nucleus (Fig. 1).

Four common rodenticides used extensively by professional exterminators and laymen are: Warfarin, 3-(alpha-phenyl-beta-acetylethyl)-4-hydroxycoumarin (D-Con); Pindone, 2-pivalyl-1,3-indandione (Pival); Diphacinone, 2-diphenylacetyl-1,3-indandione (Diphacine); and Fumarin, 3-(alpha-acetonylfuryl)-4-hydroxycoumarin. A variety of analogues that vary in their solubility, biologic half-life, and toxicity are available.

Sulfaquinoxaline, a coccidiostat used in

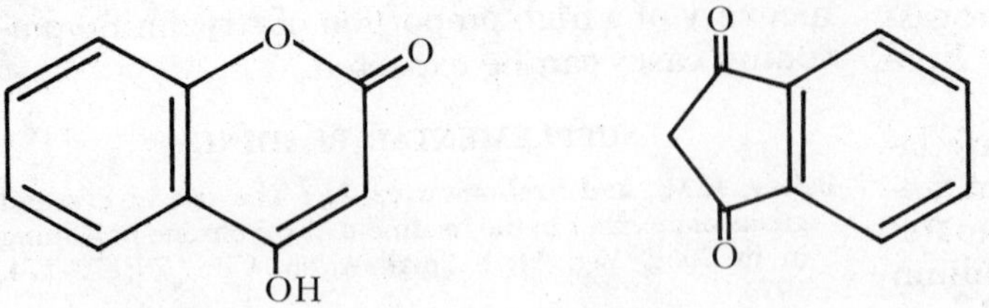

4-Hydroxycoumarin

Indane-1,3-dione

Figure 1. Chemical structures of common rodenticides.

poultry and livestock, is a potent vitamin K antagonist that has occasionally been associated with hemorrhage in dogs when administered to this species as a coccidiostat. Some commercial rodenticides contain both warfarin and sulfaquinoxaline (Prolin).

TOXICITY

The anticoagulant rodenticides are a potential hazard to all mammals and birds. Dogs appear to be most frequently affected, and swine and cats are occasionally poisoned by warfarin. The toxicity of these compounds varies widely from one to another. Susceptibility also varies among individuals in a given species. Despite the low concentration in most rodenticides, a single ingestion of 5 mg/kg warfarin can induce moderate coagulopathy in dogs. Table 1 gives some values for warfarin toxicity in various species.

The toxicity of the indandione products varies among compounds, but toxicity generally ranges from 50 to 100 mg/kg (single dose) in dogs.

MECHANISM OF ACTION

Ingested warfarin is completely absorbed from the small intestine and transported in the plasma loosely bound to albumin. The plasma warfarin half-life is 20 to 24 hours in the dog. The liver degrades warfarin, and its metabo-

lites are excreted in the urine. It is well known that vitamin K is required for hepatic synthesis of coagulation factors VII, IX, X, and II. More specifically, vitamin K is essential for the post-ribosomal carboxylation of glutamyl residues of factors VII, IX, X, and II. In this carboxylation reaction, vitamin K is transformed to an epoxide form, which must be retransformed to the K_1 form by an NADH-dependent "epoxidase" reaction to allow further carboxylation. The coumarin compounds specifically inhibit the "epoxidase" reaction and thereby deplete active vitamin K_1. Thus, in the presence of inhibitory concentrations of coumarins, the liver continues to produce physiologically inactive forms of vitamin K-dependent coagulation factors that can be recognized by immunologic studies. As inhibition is sustained, the factor activities diminish in accordance with their half-lives. The mean half-lives for factors VII, IX, X, and II in the dog are 6.2, 13.9, 16.5, and 41 hours respectively. Following hepatic metabolism of the antagonist, the inhibition gradually diminishes, allowing normal production of the vitamin K-dependent coagulation factors to be restored. Unfortunately, the *in vivo* half-lives of most antagonists as opposed to the half-lives of the vitamin K-dependent coagulation factors favor the antagonists. It follows, however, that if the liver has a large, continuous supply of vitamin K_1 throughout the duration of antagonism, synthesis of vitamin K-dependent factors can continue normally.

Table 1. *Values for Warfarin Toxicity*

SPECIES	SINGLE DOSE	REPEATED DOSES
Rats	50 to 100 mg/kg	1 mg/kg for 5 days
Dogs	5 to 50 mg/kg	5 mg/kg for 5 to 15 days
Cats	5 to 50 mg/kg	1 mg/kg for 5 days
Swine	3 mg/kg	0.05 mg/kg for 7 days
Ruminants		200 mg/kg for 12 days
Poultry	50 percent of body weight of feed containing 0.1 mg/kg	

Buck and Osweiler, 1976

LABORATORY EVALUATION AND DIFFERENTIAL DIAGNOSIS

Our understanding of the hemostatic mechanism and its laboratory evaluation has rapidly advanced during the past decade. The availability of more exacting laboratory tests allows recognition of both atypical cases of vitamin K antagonism and concurrent problems, which may modify the "classic" laboratory features of coumarin toxicity. In general, the decreased levels of vitamin K-dependent factors is eventually manifested by prolongation of coagulation tests assaying both intrinsic and extrinsic pathways. The relationship between the vitamin K-dependent coagulation factors and the common laboratory coagulation tests is given in Figure 2. Early in the course of warfarin toxicosis, only prothrombin time is prolonged due to more rapid disappearance of factor VII as related to factors IX, X, and II. After the third day of toxicosis, bleeding problems become more frequent as the intrinsic pathway also becomes moderately abnormal. Therefore, when an intoxicated patient is presented to the veterinarian, typical laboratory findings include marked prolongation of prothrombin time with moderate prolongation of activated partial thromboplastin time and activated coagulation time* (ACT). Fibrinogen, platelet count, fibrin/fibrinogen degradation products, and thrombin time are usually within normal limits although exceptions occur, as indicated below. Hemogram findings vary with the duration of toxicity and severity of blood loss but often include anemia, hypoproteinemia, and reticulocytosis. It should be kept in mind that equivalent losses of plasma and erythrocytes tend to make the hematocrit underestimate the severity of hypovolemia in acute blood loss. The poor reproducibility of Lee-White whole blood clotting time has caused most authorities to discard this test. In contrast, the simple inexpensive ACT test appears to be reliable for veterinary practices with limited laboratory expertise. As the ACT is very temperature-sensitive, it is important that the test be performed at 37° C. Early cases characterized primarily by factor VII deficiency will not be detected by ACT.

Internal bleeding into body tissues or cavities can result in moderate depletion of non-vitamin K-dependent factors and platelets. Under these circumstances, activation of fibrinolysis can result in increased fibrin/fibrinogen degradation products. Some confusion with disseminated intravascular coagulation (DIC) is possible when this occurs. Hypofibrinogenemia and thrombocytopenia are usually not as severe in Coumadin toxicosis as in DIC syndromes. In equivocal cases, finding severe depletion of factor VII may be useful to confirm suspected antagonism. Such cases may not show the "typical" rapid response to vitamin K₁ therapy.

Other vitamin K-responsive coagulopathies need to be considered in differential diagnosis. Both chronic cholestasis and malabsorption syndromes have poor intestinal absorp-

---

*Activated Coagulation Time, Vacutainer® 3206XF534, Becton-Dickinson and Co., Rutherford, New Jersey 07070.

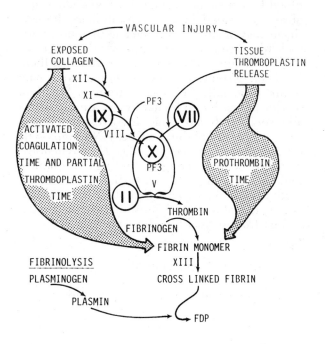

Figure 2. Relationship between vitamin K-dependent coagulation factors and common laboratory coagulation tests. Circled factors are Vitamin K-dependent. PF3 = platelet factor 3; FDP = fibrin/fibrinogen degradation products.

tion of fat-soluble vitamins, and a vitamin K-deficient coagulopathy may ultimately be induced. Nutritional vitamin K deficiency is virtually non-existent in small animals on modern commercial diets. Gut sterilization due to high levels of oral antibiotics over several weeks may markedly reduce bacterial vitamin K production and has been reported as a cause of coagulopathy in rare instances. The presence of icterus does not necessarily exclude vitamin K antagonism, since occasionally rapid lysis of sequestered erythrocytes results in mild hyperbilirubinemia. Liver function tests are of value in differentiating this hemolytic jaundice from cholestatic jaundice — e.g., serum alkaline phosphatase.

Qualitative assays for warfarin in blood (plasma), urine, or liver are available through most veterinary diagnostic laboratories. Specimens must be obtained within one to three days after the last exposure to the warfarin.

CLINICAL AND PATHOLOGIC SIGNS

The spectrum of problems encountered in clinical cases is broad and generally relates to the degree of organ dysfunction induced by either hemorrhage or hypovolemic shock. Onset may be acute, and occasionally animals are found dead with no previous signs of illness. This occurs following hemorrhage into the brain, pericardial sac, mediastinum, or thorax. In subacute cases, animals are anemic and weak, and pale mucous membranes, dyspnea, hematemesis, epistaxis, and bloody feces are common signs. Scleral, conjunctival, and intraocular hemorrhage may be seen. With severe blood loss, weakness, staggering, and ataxia are observed. Blood loss and pulmonary hemorrhage may result in dyspnea with moist rales and blood-tinged froth around the nose or mouth. Cardiac rate is irregular and heartbeat is weak. Extensive external hematomas may occur, especially in areas of trauma. Swollen, tender joints due to hemarthrosis are occasionally seen. If hemorrhage involves the brain, spinal cord, or subdural space, CNS signs will be manifested as paresis, ataxia, convulsions, or acute death. Necropsy findings frequently include anemia, subendocardial hemorrhage, mediastinal hematoma, hemothorax, subcutaneous hematoma, intramuscular hemorrhage, and gastrointestinal bleeding.

TREATMENT

The three major treatment priorities are to correct (1) the hypovolemia, (2) the coagulopathy, and (3) the organ dysfunction due to accumulation of extravascular blood. Animals should be handled with care and possibly sedated when undergoing treatment. When clinical signs of severe hypovolemia are present (prolonged capillary refill time, weak pulse, severe anemia), transfusion with fresh whole blood at 20 ml/kg intravenously may be critical to survival. Administer 50 percent of this dose rapidly and the remainder slowly by intravenous drip. Stored blood is a less satisfactory source of volume replacement. Vitamin K_1 (Aquamephyton) should be administered intravenously at a dose of 10 mg for dogs and 2 to 5 mg for cats at 12-hour intervals. In less acute cases without hypovolemia, vitamin K therapy alone results in rapid clinical improvement, and coagulation tests approach normal values within 12 hours. Oral vitamin K therapy should be maintained for five days in animals making satisfactory progress. Some coumarin analogues have considerably longer half-lives than does warfarin, and duration of therapy would need to be extended in these cases. Vitamin K_3 (Menadione) is not satisfactory in treatment of acute warfarin toxicosis. Acute cases may benefit from O_2 therapy when severe dyspnea is present. Continuing dyspnea may suggest the presence of a hemorrhagic pleural effusion. After coagulation tests have normalized, thoracentesis to remove excess blood may be indicated. However, in the presence of abnormal coagulation tests, centesis of hemorrhagic effusions may reinitiate bleeding and further complicate the hypovolemia. Hematomas and most hemorrhagic effusions in the convalescent animal resolve without medical intervention.

SUPPLEMENTAL READINGS

Buck, W.B., and Osweiler, G.D.: Warfarin and other anticoagulant rodenticides. In Van Gelder, G.A. (ed.): *Clinical and Diagnostic Veterinary Toxicology*, 2nd ed. Dubuque, Iowa, Kendall-Hunt Publishing Co., 1976.

Carson, T.L.: Diagnostic problems of anticoagulant rodenticide toxicoses. Am. Assoc. Vet. Lab. Diag. 20th Annual Proc., pp. 139–142, 1977.

Dodds, W.J.: The diagnosis, management and treatment of bleeding disorders, Parts I and II. M.V.P. 58:680–684, 756–762, 1977.

Forbes, C.D., Thompson, C., Prentice, C.R.M., McNicol, G.P., and McEwan, A.D.: Experimental warfarin poisoning in the dog. J. Comp. Path. 83:173–180, 1973.

O'Reilly, R.A.: Vitamin K and the oral anticoagulant drugs. Ann. Rev. Med. 27:245–261, 1976.

METALDEHYDE POISONING

RONALD L. MULL, D.V.M.

Pearl River, New York

Metaldehyde, a polymer of acetaldehyde, has been responsible for poisonings in children, livestock, horses, and dogs. Although cats are quite susceptible, metaldehyde poisoning has not been reported to be a problem in them. The toxic oral dose for most animals is in the range of 100 to 500 mg/kg. Although it has in the past been used as a solid fuel, the primary current use of metaldehyde is as a molluscicide in bait formulations. This is the usual form of exposure (snail and slug bait) encountered by the pet animal, and severe poisoning may follow ingestion of a few ounces of the bait. Metaldehyde is commonly used around vegetable crops, berries, and ornamentals. It seems likely that the increase in urban home gardens in recent years has resulted in increased pet exposure and subsequently more cases of poisoning.

Metaldehyde is apparently an attractant as well as a toxicant to snails and slugs. Bait formulators, however, have sought to make the baits more attractive to the mollusca by the addition of various food processing byproducts (e.g., bran, molasses). Unfortunately, these additives also make the baits more attractive to dogs. A positive change is that the baits usually now contain only metaldehyde, generally in the range of 3.5 percent concentration. In the recent past, the baits commonly contained metaldehyde in combination with calcium arsenate. Some baits now contain an organophosphorous or carbamate insecticide rather than the metaldehyde.

In the spring of 1973, there was an unusually large increase in cases of metaldehyde poisonings in dogs in California. This resulted in the California regulatory officials' requirement that the bait formulators demonstrate that their baits were not attractive to dogs prior to being marketed in that state in 1974. Research efforts generated by this requirement were soon underway at the University of California at Davis. Studies showed that the baits could be made unattractive to dogs and that the unattractiveness could be quantitated. Regulatory officials developed testing standards for baits to be sold in California. These testing procedures were subsequently put into effect at the federal level by the Environmental Protection Agency. One hopes that when supplies of the older formulations have been exhausted, the occurrence of metaldehyde poisoning in dogs will diminish to a low level.

CLINICAL SIGNS

Depending on the amount of bait ingested and absorbed, the animal may be presented showing signs ranging from incoordination and anxiety with muscle fasciculations to continuous muscle spasms and prostration. Toxic effects are thought to be due primarily to absorption of acetaldehyde released by hydrolysis of the metaldehyde in the acidic stomach, although some of the effects may be from the metaldehyde itself. Salivation, hyperesthesia, and muscle tremors are signs similar to those seen in strychnine poisoning (as well as anticholinesterase insecticide poisoning). However, the muscle spasms cannot be initiated by external stimuli as with strychnine. Marked hyperthermia also is common, with temperatures as high as 108°F reported. Severe acidosis may be an accompanying feature.

DIAGNOSIS AND TREATMENT

Goals of the clinician are to (1) stop absorption of the toxicant, (2) control the muscle tremors, and (3) provide supportive therapy to combat acidosis and dehydration. Emesis may be obtained by use of apomorphine, 0.04 mg/kg IV if the patient is ambulatory. This may be followed by (or may be supplanted by) light anesthesia that allows gastric lavage and controls muscle tremors. Care must be exercised to prevent aspiration of any vomitus.

The tremors can often be controlled by diazepam, 2 to 5 mg/kg IV, or triflupromazine, 0.2 to 2.0 mg/kg IV. In severe cases, prolonged maintenance of light anesthesia with barbiturates in combination with muscle relaxants may be necessary. Lactated Ringer's may be given to combat dehydration and acidosis. Intensive care may be required for up to 24 hours.

Necropsy of dogs that die acutely generally only shows slight to moderate inflammation of the gastric mucosa with hyperemia of the lungs, liver, and kidneys. If death is delayed for a few days, degenerative changes may be observed in the liver and brain.

As many as 50 percent of cases presented may die if signs of poisoning are severe upon admission or if a large amount of bait has been consumed. Successful therapy is sometimes frustrated by the fact that some dogs appear to develop a liking for the baits; dogs have been poisoned again following discharge from the hospital.

Diagnosis usually depends on history of exposure to the baits or finding some of the pellets in the vomitus or stomach contents. Confirmation could be done by analysis of the stomach content. The odor of acetaldehyde may also be detected. Baits are available in both pelleted and meal formulations. The pellets seem to be far more hazardous than the meal to the dogs. Poisoning may be expected to occur most often during periods conducive to gardening activity — e.g., late afternoons, weekends, and holidays. Owners can minimize the hazard by confining their pets, using the meal formulations, and dispersing the bait well.

SUPPLEMENTAL READING

Harris, W.F.: Clinical toxicities of dogs. Vet. Clin. North Am. 5 (4):605–622, 1975.

Kitchell, R.L., et al.: Palatability studies of snail and slug bait poisons using dogs. JAVMA 173 (1):85, 1978.

Maddy, K.T.: Poisoning of dogs with metaldehyde in snail and slug poison bait. Calif. Vet. pp. 27–28, March 1955.

Udall, N.D.: The toxicity of the molluscicides metaldehyde and methiocarb to dogs. Vet. Rec. 93(15):420–22, 1978.

LEAD POISONING

DAVID F. KOWALCZYK, V.M.D.
Philadelphia, Pennsylvania

Lead poisoning in man has been recognized for thousands of years and has been implicated in such historical events as the decline of ancient Rome. The association of lead with clinical disease has been extremely difficult in the past due to the ubiquitous nature of lead in the environment.

Lead poisoning in animals has probably occurred since its recognition in man, but only in the last 30 years have cases been well documented. Many of these cases were diagnosed postmortem. It wasn't until 1969 that the significance of lead poisoning in dogs was clearly recognized. Zook reported that one of every 25 dogs under six months of age, hospitalized at the Angell Memorial Animal Hospital (Boston), had been poisoned by lead. In 1970, the hospital diagnosed 107 canine cases of lead toxicity! At the School of Veterinary Medicine in Philadelphia, lead poisoning was rarely diagnosed until the availability of an in-house blood lead testing service in 1973. It is now the most common toxicity reported in dogs and cats.

The increased incidence of lead poisoning in dogs in the last few years has been the result of intensive screening programs and not due to an actual increase in exposure to lead. The fault is not with the clinician's ability but with the nonspecific signs displayed during the early stages of lead poisoning (i.e., vomiting and anorexia). The most difficult aspect of lead poisoning is establishing the diagnosis.

ABSORPTION, DISTRIBUTION, AND EXCRETION OF LEAD

The most common route of entry of lead is through the gastrointestinal tract. Inhaled lead particles are cleared by ciliary action and swallowed. In adult dogs and man, approximately 10 per cent of ingested lead is absorbed. However, in young animals, up to 90 per cent can be absorbed. The interaction of many nutritional factors with the bioavailability of lead has been well documented. An enhancement of lead absorption has been demonstrated with dietary deficiencies of calcium, zinc, iron, and protein. Lead dissolves at a much faster rate in an acid environment, such as the stomach, and thus enhances absorption. In bottom feeding waterfowl, the ingestion of one to three shotgun pellets (which tend to remain in the gizzard) can be lethal.

Once the lead has been absorbed, it is carried by the red blood cells and distributed in the soft tissue. Over 90 per cent of the circulating lead is in the red blood cells. The presence of lead in the liver, kidney, central nervous system, and bone marrow causes the major signs of lead toxicity. Eventually, the lead redistributes to the bone, where it is biologically inert. However, this stored pool of lead may be mobilized if bone demineralization occurs (e.g., in acidosis or calcium deficiency) and can cause toxicity. The penetration of lead across the blood-brain barrier occurs more readily in the immature organism, accounting for the higher incidence of severe neurologic signs in the young animal. Lead can also cross the placenta and enter into the milk.

Lead is excreted very slowly from the whole body, predominantly via bile. The enterohepatic circulation of lead can occur, but its significance in lead poisoning is not known. The elimination of lead through urine is minor unless chelating agents are being used (e.g., CaEDTA).

The measurement of blood lead can fluctuate greatly, depending on time of exposure, and it may not reflect tissue lead concentrations or the extent of lead toxicity. This is probably the reason for the poor correlation between blood lead and severity of clinical signs in dogs. Therefore, blood lead should not be the sole criterion in screening animals for lead exposure.

SOURCES OF LEAD

The sources of lead are varied and numerous, the most common being lead-containing paint. Interiors of dwellings painted before 1940 often contain layers of lead-based paint. Leaded paints are sometimes mistakenly used indoors and thus may be accessible to dogs in new as well as old dwellings. Exteriors of buildings (including dog houses) are frequently covered with lead paint, as are fences and painting materials. The lead salts in paint impart a sweet taste; thus their attractiveness to animals. Soil and vegetation may be contaminated with lead as a result of the weathering of lead pigments from painted structures.

Other sources of lead include linoleum, batteries, plumbing materials, putty, lead foil, solder, golf balls, certain roof coverings, lubricants, rug pads, acid (soft) drinking water from lead pipes or improperly glazed ceramic water bowls, and lead weights or objects such as fishing sinkers, drapery weights, and toys. Soil along streets and roadways may contain small amounts of lead from automobile exhaust fumes. Soil contaminated with lead from paint or auto exhausts is not a likely source of poisoning, but it may contribute somewhat to the total body burden of lead. Lead shot present subcutaneously or in muscle tissue usually becomes encapsulated and biologically inert.

The history may or may not suggest exposure to lead. Recent remodeling of dwellings, especially old dilapidated houses, including removal of old paint, plaster, or linoleum, or application of new lead-based paints, is a common history. Remember that in cases displaying only mild gastrointestinal signs, the history may be the sole clue.

AGE

Lead poisoning may occur at any age, but most affected dogs are between two and eight months of age. Teething and the bizarre appetites of young dogs result in the gnawing on and ingestion of strange substances.

CLINICAL SIGNS

Clinical signs of lead poisoning in dogs are associated with the gastrointestinal and nervous systems. Usually both systems are clinically involved, but sometimes only one is. Very often, gastrointestinal signs are present for several days before the dog is examined, and they usually precede the neurologic signs. Such clinical signs in young dogs have led to erroneous diagnoses of canine distemper.

The most common gastrointestinal signs are vomiting, abdominal pain, and anorexia. Diarrhea or constipation are less frequently observed. The presence of abdominal pain or so-called "lead colic" is manifest by whining, restlessness, tensing of abdominal muscles, and crying when the abdomen is palpated. Many gastrointestinal upsets display the foregoing signs, but one should suspect lead toxicity if they persist for more than three days. Occasionally, megaesophagus has been associated with lead poisoning and is probably the result of esophageal paralysis.

The most common neurologic signs in order of frequency are convulsions, hysteria (characterized by barking and crying continuously, running in every direction, and indiscriminately biting at animate and inanimate objects), and other behavioral changes. Other neurologic signs are ataxia, blindness, and chomping of the jaws. Many dogs with hysteria or convulsions have increased rectal temperatures that decrease after the episode subsides.

The need for recognition of subtle neurologic deficits such as learning impairments, hyperactivity, and loss of visual discrimination during and after exposure to lead has only recently been appreciated. One investigation demonstrated residual neurologic deficits in sheep that were exposed to low levels of lead that never produced so-called "toxic blood levels."

Differential diagnoses, based on history and clinical signs, include canine distemper, epilepsy, intestinal parasitism, non-specific gastrointestinal disturbance, acute pancreatitis, encephalitis, vertebral problems, rabies, and other poisonings. Because of the high incidence of canine distemper in young dogs, the occurrence of convulsions with or without typical signs is usually attributed to canine distemper. However, recent investigations have found many of these cases to be the result of lead poisoning.

LABORATORY FINDINGS

One of the most helpful screening tests for the diagnosis of lead poisoning, without resorting to a quantitative test for lead, is examination of a stained blood smear. Of prime importance is the finding of large numbers of nucleated erythrocytes (5 to 40/100 white blood cells) without evidence of severe anemia — packed cell volume less than 30 per cent. This is considered to be nearly pathognomonic of lead poisoning. The nucleated erythrocytes are a relatively easy cell type to identify regardless of the staining procedure.

Other common abnormalities in red blood cell morphology are anisocytosis, polychromasia, poikilocytosis, target cells, and hypochromasia. The presence of basophilic stippling in red blood cells is another common feature, but detection depends upon the staining procedure. One investigation at Angell Memorial Animal Hospital reported basophilic stippling in 94 per cent of lead poisoned dogs; however, stippling was found in 42 per cent of dogs with other problems.

Red blood cell abnormalities usually precede clinical signs except in the very acute poisoning. Once chelation therapy has been started, these changes disappear quickly.

Moderate numbers of nucleated red blood cells and a few stippled red blood cells may be found in some dogs with marked and prolonged anemias — e.g., autoimmune hemolytic anemia. Older dogs that have visceral hemangiosarcomas are usually anemic and have numerous nucleated red blood cells but few or no stippled red blood cells.

The leukocyte counts are usually elevated because of a neutrophilic leukocytosis. It is important to correct the white blood cell count for the presence of nucleated erythrocytes; otherwise, exaggerated white blood cell counts will result.

Results of other laboratory tests, such as blood urea nitrogen, creatinine, transaminase, amylase, blood glucose, sedimentation rate, and Coomb's test, are normal. Bone marrow examination discloses an increase of erythroid elements. Elevated reticulocyte counts and the finding of many immature red blood cells in peripheral blood smears indicate early release of erythroid cells from the hyperplastic bone marrow. The urine usually contains granular casts. Often, mild proteinuria and sometimes glycosuria are found. The cerebrospinal fluid may have a normal pressure, protein, and cell content.

Other tests that have become very useful in human lead poisoning are related to detection of abnormalities in heme synthesis. The interference of lead at several enzymatic steps has proved to be a most sensitive indicator of biologic change. The accumulation of various substrates such as aminolevulinic acid (urine) and zinc protoporphyrin (red blood cell) is commonly used as a screening test in high-risk children and lead-exposed workers. These tests reflect the presence and severity of lead poisoning. The substrates stay elevated despite fluctuations in blood lead. It is hoped that these tests will prove as valuable in veterinary medicine.

RADIOGRAPHIC FINDINGS

The most helpful radiographic finding is the presence of diffuse radiopaque material in the gastrointestinal tract. This material was found in over 60 per cent of the cases at the University of Pennsylvania. However, it should be emphasized that it is impossible to differentiate these radiodensities from bone chips or gravel. It is important to radiograph the animal, since chelation therapy has been shown to enhance intestinal absorption of lead.

The metaphyses of long bones may develop lead lines (metaphyseal sclerosis) in immature dogs. These radiopaque bands are best seen just proximal to the open epiphyses of the distal radius, ulna, and metacarpal bones. This is due to the incorporation of lead at the site of endochondral ossification, which stimulates active bone formation, causing a dense zone of mineralized cartilage. The lead lines are mainly the result of new bone formation and not the deposition of lead. Similar radiographic changes are reported in phosphorus and vitamin D intoxication.

The presence of lead lines is a difficult interpretation to make, even for radiologists and, as a diagnostic tool, has not been useful at our hospital.

DIAGNOSIS

Since the clinical signs of lead poisoning are not pathognomonic, a history detailing likelihood of exposure or the finding of many nucleated erythrocytes without anemia may be the first clue. Blood may be taken for lead analysis to confirm the diagnosis, but treatment for lead poisoning should be started.

The analysis of whole blood is the best single index for establishing a definitive diagnosis. Most laboratories require 10 ml of whole, oxalated, or heparinized blood in a clean, lead-free vial. Versenate (EDTA) anticoagulant interferes with some methods. The finding of $60\mu g$ or more of lead/100 ml of blood (0.6 ppm) is virtually diagnostic of lead poisoning in dogs. Blood lead values of 30 to 50 μg/100 ml. (0.3 to 0.5 ppm) are abnormally high and indicate lead poisoning if associated with typical signs and hematologic findings. Baseline levels for lead range between 5 and 25 μg/100 ml (0.05 and 0.25 ppm). The small difference between background and toxic blood levels makes interpretation of this test difficult at the lower levels. The severity of clinical signs is usually not correlated with blood-lead content.

For postmortem confirmation, analysis of liver for lead is the best diagnostic test. The upper limit of normal is 3.5 ppm (wet weight); 5 ppm or more is virtually diagnostic. Samples of hair, feces, or single specimens of urine for lead analysis are not recommended. Urine specimens taken just before and 24 hours after starting chelation therapy (calcium disodium edetate, CaEDTA, at the dosage administered for regular treatment) disclose a ten-fold to sixty-fold increase in urine lead output in dogs with lead poisoning. Although this test is reliable, it is difficult to obtain the specimens and is expensive and time consuming.

TREATMENT

The purpose of therapy in lead poisoning is (1) to remove lead, if present, from the gastrointestinal tract so that further absorption is prevented, (2) to remove lead from the blood and body tissues rapidly, and (3) to alleviate marked neurologic signs.

Lead should be removed from the gastrointestinal tract prior to chelation therapy with enemas and emetics, as chelating agents can enhance the absorption of lead from the intestines. Lead-containing substances are often found in the large intestine. Large objects in the stomach may require surgery.

Chelating agents effectively remove heavy metals such as lead by forming nontoxic complexes with the metals that are rapidly excreted via the bile or urine. The chelating agent of choice is CaEDTA (calcium ethylenediaminetetraacetate), which has been shown to be effec-

tive in treating lead poisoning in a wide variety of animals. CaEDTA must be administered as the calcium chelate in order to prevent hypocalcemia. Renal damage has occurred in man due to excessive CaEDTA; however, we have found no evidence of any side effects in dogs. Nonetheless, the daily dose should not exceed 2 gm, and therapy should not be continued for more than five consecutive days.

CaEDTA is given at the rate of 100 mg/kg of body weight daily for two to five days. The daily dose is divided into four equal portions and administered subcutaneously after dilution to a concentration of about 10 mg CaEDTA/ml of 5 per cent dextrose solution. Higher concentrations of CaEDTA can cause painful reactions at injection sites.

The use of CaEDTA has been extremely effective, with clinical improvement within 24 to 48 hours. Dogs that respond slowly or have a pretreatment blood level of more than 100 μg/100 ml (1.0 ppm) may need a second five-day treatment five days after completion of the first series. This second treatment prevents recurrence of clinical signs, provided the dog is not allowed to consume more lead after discharge from the hospital. Monitoring blood lead during treatment is not valuable, as the concentration of lead does not correlate with alleviation of clinical signs. This is probably due to CaEDTA's inability to cross cell membranes.

Penicillamine, an oral chelating agent of proven value in treating lead-poisoned children, offers promise for dogs. Penicillamine, given orally, has a distinct advantage over CaEDTA, which must be repeatedly injected subcutaneously, requiring hospitalization. Clinical trials to date indicate that pencillamine is effective in promoting urinary excretion of lead and alleviating clinical signs.

Penicillamine, given in a dose of 100 mg/kg body weight daily for one to two weeks, has some undesirable effects such as vomiting, listlessness, and partial anorexia. To decrease the side effects, penicillamine should be given on an empty stomach in divided doses. Antiemetics have also proved useful (e.g., phenothiazines, antihistamines). The capsules may be dissolved in fruit juice (acidic) for ease of administration. At present, penicillamine can be recommended for dogs that are not seriously ill or do not have marked neurologic disorders or persistent vomiting. If an owner refuses to hospitalize his dog, penicillamine can be prescribed; however, the owner should be warned that side effects may occur and that lead ingested while on treatment is apt to be absorbed more completely than it would be without treatment.

It seems that penicillamine might also be beneficial in combination with CaEDTA. It may be that CaEDTA needs to be given for only a few days, followed by penicillamine. This regimen should assure adequate hydration, promote renal function, and help reduce the care and cost of treatment. Pencillamine might also be useful in treating dogs that recovered slowly from a five-day course of CaEDTA or had an initial blood lead level of more than 100 μg/100 ml (1.0 ppm) and therefore should be treated again.

Dimercaprol (BAL) has been used successfully in combination with CaEDTA in children. It has seldom been used in lead poisoned animals. However, it does offer the advantages of removing lead directly from red blood cells and excreting lead primarily via the bile (important if renal function is compromised).

SUPPORTIVE TREATMENT

The gastrointestinal signs (e.g., vomiting, diarrhea, anorexia) do not usually require specific drug therapy because they subside quickly after chelation therapy. However, the severe neurologic signs (e.g., convulsions) are due to cerebral edema and thus require immediate attention. Mannitol and dexamethasone are the agents of choice. Seizures and hysteria can be controlled with diazepam and/or pentobarbital intravenously. Permanent mental deficiencies and recurrent seizures are common sequelae of lead poisoning in children. Thus, it seems appropriate to treat lead encephalopathy in dogs as well, because these drugs not only appear to speed clinical recovery but may also prevent permanent brain damage.

PROGNOSIS

The prognosis in the majority of lead poisoning cases that undergo chelation therapy is favorable, with a dramatic improvement in 24 to 48 hours. Chelation therapy may thus be used as a diagnostic tool in cases of high suspicion when a blood lead determination is impractical or delayed. Prognoses in cases treated promptly and adequately depend upon the degree and duration of neurologic involvement, and, to a lesser extent, upon the amount of lead found in the blood. Continuous or uncontrolled convulsions warrant an unfavorable prognosis. Dogs with 100 μg or more of lead/100 ml of blood tend to recover slowly, and signs may recur if a second course of therapy is not given. If there are no neurologic signs, or if they are mild or readily controlled by ancillary treatment, the prognosis is favorable.

The prognosis in untreated cases that are only displaying gastrointestinal signs may be favorable if further exposure to lead is prevented. If the economic situation dictates the above, a course of oral penicillamine may be advantageous.

PATHOLOGIC FINDINGS

Gross necropsic findings are generally not remarkable; however, careful examination may reveal chips of paint or other lead-containing substances in the gastrointestinal tract. White bands are sometimes found in transversely sectioned metaphyses of immature dogs. Microscopic study may disclose acid-fast intranuclear inclusion bodies in renal proximal tubular cells and less often in hepatocytes. These inclusions are essentially pathognomonic of lead poisoning but are not found in all cases. Lesions in the brain include degenerative changes in small vessels, hemorrhages, laminar necrosis, and proliferation of capillaries and gliosis in chronic encephalopathies.

VETERINARIAN OBLIGATION

Animals may manifest signs of toxicity before man when they are sharing the same environment. Birds have been used for years in mines as sensitive indicators of toxic gas accumulation. In the 1953 mercury poisoning outbreak in Japan, cats were dying a year before the disease was recognized in man. For lead poisoning, the young dog seems the most appropriate species because it shares the same environment and has eating habits (e.g., pica) similar to those of children. A recent study from Illinois indicated that an abnormally high blood lead in a family dog increased the probability six-fold of finding a child in the same family with an increased blood lead. At the University of Pennsylvania Veterinary School, owners with lead poisoned dogs were advised to have children between one and five years of age checked for lead poisoning. A few children had blood levels in the toxic range, even though they were not showing gross clinical signs.

When diagnosing canine lead poisoning to owners with small children, I strongly urge veterinarians to warn the family and/or family physician adequately. Most urban centers have free clinics for lead testing in children.

LEAD POISONING IN OTHER PETS

Cats are rarely poisoned by lead beçause, unlike dogs, they are very selective eaters and seldom gnaw on or ingest non-food substances.

Therefore, they are not subject to most sources of lead. Because of their fastidious fur-cleaning habits, however, they may ingest lead-containing dusts or other substances that contaminate their coat.

Parrots may pick at and ingest peeling paint or, if the bars of their cages are painted, they may ingest the paint while clambering about or trimming their beaks. At least two pet parrots and numerous zoo parrots are known to have died of lead poisoning. No hematologic changes were seen in the parrots studied. Any curious pet with indiscriminate eating habits and exposure to lead is a likely candidate for lead intoxication.

SUPPLEMENTAL READING

Buck, W.B., Osweiler, G.D., and Van Gelder, G.A.: *Clinical and Diagnostic Veterinary Toxicology,* 2nd ed. Dubuque, Iowa, Kendal-Hunt Publishing Co., 1976.

Carson, T. L., Van Gelder, G.A., Buck, W.B., and Hoffman, L.J.: Effects of low level lead ingestion in sheep. Clin. Tox. 6:389–403, 1973.

Clarke, E.G.C.: Lead poisoning in small animals. J. Small Anim. Pract. 14:183–193, 1973.

Finley, M.T., Dieter, M.P., and Locke, L.N.: Lead in tissues of mallard ducks dosed with two types of lead shot. Bull. of Environ. Contamin. Toxicol. 16:261–269, 1976.

Grandjean, P., and Lintrup, J.: Erythrocyte-Zn-protoporphyrin as an indicator of lead exposure. Scan. J. Clin. Invest. 38:669–675, 1978.

Kowalczyk, D.F.: Lead poisoning in dogs at the University of Pennsylvania Veterinary Hospital. J. Am. Vet. Med. Assoc., 168:428–432, 1976.

Mylroie, A.A., Moore, L., Olyai, B.S., and Anderson, M.: Increased susceptibility to lead toxicity in rats fed semipurified diets. Environ. Res. 15:57–64, 1978.

Schunk, K.L.: Lead poisoning in dogs. Small Animal Vet. Med. Update 8:2–7, 1978.

Thomas, C.W., Rising, J.L., and Moore, J.K.: Blood lead concentrations of children and dogs from 83 Illinois families. J. Am. Vet. Med. Assoc., 169:1237–1240, 1976.

Van Gelder, G.A., Carson, T.L., Smith, R.M., Buck, W.B., and Karas, G.G.: Neurophysiologic and behavioral toxicologic testing to detect subclinical neurologic alterations induced by environmental toxicants. J. Am. Vet. Med. Assoc., 163:1033–1035, 1973.

Zook, B.C., Carpenter, J.L., and Kirk, R.W. (ed.): Current Veterinary Therapy VI. Philadelphia, W. B. Saunders Co., 1977.

Zook, B. C., Carpenter, J.L., and Leeds, E.B.: Lead poisoning in dogs. J. Am. Vet. Med. Assoc. 155:1329–1342, 1969.

Zook, B.C., Kopito, L., Carpenter, J.L., Cramer, D.V., and Shwachman, H.: Lead poisoning in dogs: analysis of blood, urine, hair, and liver for lead. Am. J. Vet. Res. 33:903–909, 1972.

Zook, B.C., McConnell, G., and Gilmore, C.E.: Basophilic stippling of erythrocytes in dogs with special reference to lead poisoning. J. Am. Vet. Med. Assoc. 157:2092–2099, 1970.

LEAD POISONING IN NEW ZEALAND

BRIAN J. McLEAVEY, B.V.Sc.
Christchurch, New Zealand

DOGS

Lead poisoning is an insidious condition occurring mainly in young dogs under one year of age, with most cases being seen in the two to six-month age group. It is difficult to diagnose, and despite being one of the commonest causes of poisoning in dogs, it is frequently overlooked in the differential diagnosis. The number of cases diagnosed in any practice will vary, depending upon the awareness of this condition by the consulting veterinarian, and it is also directly related to the type of environment in which the practice is situated.

SIGNS

The signs of lead poisoning are not specific but can be divided into two main categories — abdominal and nervous. There is, however, considerable variation within the categories and much overlap between them. In general, the more severe the signs, the higher the circulating blood lead level. On occasion, the clinical picture is complicated by other conditions such as salmonellosis and distemper. Despite the variation in signs, lead poisoning should always be considered in any dog with abdominal or nervous symptoms, especially if no other cause can be found or response to other treatment is poor.

Dogs with abdominal signs in the mildest form often present with a history of poor weight gain or weight loss, poor appetite, and a dry coat with excessive shedding. More severe cases may have persistent vomiting or diarrhea and/or attacks of severe abdominal pain. These attacks of colic can often be mistaken for an intussusception or other abdominal catastrophe but tend to recur with increasing frequency in succeeding days and may eventually lead to convulsions if untreated.

Nervous signs also vary considerably. Young puppies may be excessively timid or aggressive. These signs may be accepted as normal by some owners, but they can often be observed when the dog is presented for routine vaccination or de-sexing. The author regularly blood tests any young dog that is difficult to handle, and a large number have been positive for lead poisoning. Change of temperament, such as a normally placid dog becoming aggressive, is often a sign of lead poisoning, especially in older dogs. Excessive scratching for no obvious reason can occasionally be a sign in young dogs. The most severe case is the dog throwing convulsions. These convulsions resemble epileptiform seizures but usually last much longer and are often fatal* without treatment. They are sudden in onset and usually have no premonitory signs. In many cases, the convulsions occur while the dog is being exercised, since the acidosis associated with exercise precipitates an increase in the circulating blood levels of lead. These cases are very distressing to the owner and unless prompt treatment is instituted, the dog will die. For many years, it has been the author's practice to test all dogs with nervous signs, no matter how mild, for lead poisoning, and over 30 percent have had elevated levels.

DIAGNOSIS

A final diagnosis of lead poisoning is arrived at only after consideration of the history, signs, environment, and laboratory tests. The most reliable test is the estimation of blood lead levels. Urine levels are unreliable, and many dogs with high blood levels will have no lead present in their urine. Urine levels taken before and after treatment will show substantial increases in the amount of lead present and may be used for diagnosis if blood is unable to be collected. Levels of 0.4 mg/l blood, 0.75 mg/l urine, and 5 mg/kg liver are the minimal levels consistent with a diagnosis of lead poisoning. Dogs with positive lead analysis below 0.4 mg/l blood obviously have had access to lead, and owners should be advised to find and eliminate the source thereof. It is not unusual for dogs with sub-toxic levels to return some weeks later with toxic levels due to continued exposure. In the clinic, fresh blood smears stained with Jenner-Giemsa stain will often show increased levels of nucleated red blood cells and basophilic stippling. More than 10 nucleated RBCs per 100 WBCs suggests lead poisoning, although not all positive cases show these changes.

TREATMENT

The best and most effective drug in the treatment of lead poisoning is CaEDTA. This drug combines with the lead, rendering it highly soluble so it can be excreted through the kidneys. CaEDTA may be administered as a 10 per cent solution intravenously or diluted to a 4 per cent solution for subcutaneous use, as it is very painful when given by this route. The dose is 75 mg/kg per day, which is achieved by giving 2 ml/kg of a 4 per cent solution. This dose is given daily for three days and the course is repeated in two weeks. In mild cases in which access to lead has been stopped, no further treatment is necessary. In severe cases, further blood tests are recommended so that treatment is continued until normal blood levels are maintained. In cases in which the diagnosis is uncertain, it is advisable to give one dose of CaEDTA and to limit exercise until the laboratory test results are received. It is most important that exercise be limited in dogs with lead poisoning, as two cases in this clinic in which this advice was ignored developed convulsions. If the dogs are hospitalized for treatment, this danger is eliminated, but hospitalization is not always possible.

Severe convulsive cases are carefully anesthetized using acetylpromazine IV followed by thiamylal sodium or some other short-acting barbiturate given IV. It is important to give only small doses of barbiturate, administered very slowly, as it is very easy to overdose a convulsing dog in trying to quiet it quickly. The end result may be fatal. Once the dog is anesthetized, samples should be collected for analysis, and the dog should be connected to an intravenous drip using 10 per cent dextrose in lactated Ringer's solution. Because dogs in this state are uremic, and CaEDTA can cause nephrosis, it is important to establish a good urine flow before CaEDTA is given. This generally takes 30 to 60 minutes. Anesthesia is maintained with small doses of sodium pentobarbitone repeated until the dog can wake up free of convulsions — generally about four hours later. The 10 per cent dextrose helps reduce any cerebral edema. Once a good urine flow is established, CaEDTA is given as one dose IV and the drip is then slowed but continued for about another half hour. The author also gives dimercaprol (BAL) at a dose rate of 8 mg/kg IM at the same time as CaEDTA in these cases. This drug is not as good a chelating agent as CaEDTA but does help reduce the toxicity of CaEDTA.

This method produces an initial dilution of the blood levels, followed by the rapid removal of the lead by CaEDTA. In one dog with a blood level of 1.0 mg/l and a urine level of 0.9 mg/l, the blood level dropped to 0.2 mg/l in three hours after admission and the urine level rose to 1.9 mg/l. It should be stressed that no short cuts should be taken, as dogs in convulsions given CaEDTA without establishing a urine flow may die from kidney failure.

The response to treatment for lead poisoning is very good, with a rapid return to normal so long as further access to lead is stopped. The only exception is in the case of dogs with severe nervous symptoms. These dogs often remain timid and may throw regular fits. In these cases, further anticonvulsive treatment is required. This situation is to be expected, as the small capillaries in the brain are damaged by lead with subsequent death of the surrounding neurons.

SOURCES

Most dogs acquire lead levels in their own home environment and therefore, if the owner is unable to suggest a source, the property should be visited by a health official or other qualified person. In most cases, the source is readily apparent. The commonest sources in the author's experience have been flaking paint (especially when falling over the feeding area), old linoleum, and contaminated soil and water. Other sources have been associated with the owner's occupation — e.g., lead licked off a compositor's hands, access to a carpenter's or painter's red lead priming paint and putty, and access to a plumber's lead off-cuts. It is essential that the source be identified and the dog be prohibited from further access to it.

ENVIRONMENTAL CONSIDERATIONS

Christchurch is a coastal city of about 350,000 population in the South Island of New Zealand. It is built mainly on flat land that was originally a peat-type swamp drained by the early settlers. The older houses are all timber, all of which were originally painted with lead-based paints. Because of the soil type, there is very slow leeching of soil lead levels. In some parts of the city, soil lead levels close to the houses are as high as 3000 ppm compared with the normal acceptable level of 40 ppm. Our practice is situated close to one of the older city areas, and, until recently, a large number of cases of lead poisoning were seen annually. Over 60 per cent

of these cases were seen in the fall and winter months. The winters in Christchurch are not so severe that dogs cannot spend a reasonable amount of time outdoors. They will, however, tend to stay closer to the house at this time of year. Due to the high levels of lead in the soil and water close to these old houses, a dog does not have to ingest much soil or water on a daily basis to reach toxic levels of lead. Even licking contaminated soil off their own feet or eating bones previously buried in the soil may lead to eventual poisoning in dogs. In the summer months, dogs tend to move further away from the house, where soil lead levels are much lower.

It is interesting that over the last three years, a very large number of these older houses have been demolished for residential and commercial redevelopment, and a new motorway has been constructed. The result has been a dramatic reduction in the number of cases of lead poisoning. This proves that the dog's immediate environment can be a good indication of the likelihood of its suffering from lead poisoning.

CATS

Compared with dogs, very few cats are seen with lead poisoning. Our records show only eight cats and one tiger seen with lead poisoning over a ten-year period. Considering the high soil levels in our area, and the toilet and washing habits of cats, we would have expected more cases. It is also noticeable that the blood levels in affected cats are much lower than those in dogs; usually only 0.2 to 0.3 mg/l. Even the tiger, which was in severe convulsions and whose cage was painted throughout with red lead, only had a level of 0.56 mg/l, which is unlikely to cause convulsions in a dog. The tiger also took longer to recover than did the average dog. It may be that cats do not absorb lead as readily as dogs, but when they do, smaller amounts will produce signs of poisoning. The signs seen have included anorexia leading to nervous symptoms and death. Cats with lead poisoning are often over-excitable, hypersensitive to touch, crying with dilation of the pupils, and circling to one side. This is followed by severe convulsions. Treatment as described for dogs is successful in most cases for cats.

CAGED BIRDS

Lead poisoning is not uncommon in birds and in particular in parrots who tend to be destructive.

Small budgerigars are often suddenly found dead. Sources of lead have been paints and linoleum used in the aviary and lead-glazed pottery used for drinking utensils.

One kea, a large native New Zealand parrot, was seen with a history of acute diarrhea and continuous vomiting, leading rapidly to death. Lead poisoning was diagnosed on autopsy. Later, a large Australian cockatoo was seen that had stopped talking, was depressed, and also had continuous vomiting. It showed a dramatic response when given CaEDTA IM in the pectoral muscles. This bird used to lick the solder on its cage consistently.

Two rosella parakeets were seen recently with incoordination, inability to perch, falling to one side, hyperexcitability, and excessive squawking. CaEDTA given IM produced an improvement within one half hour, and both birds made a full recovery. Lead paint had been used on their pen.

The final consideration in all cases of lead poisoning is the possibility of children in the same household acquiring the condition. This should always be brought to the attention of clients.

SUPPLEMENTAL READING

Chisholm, J. Julian Jr.: Treatment of lead poisoning. Mod. Treatment 8: 593–611, 1971.
Clarke, E.C.G.: Lead poisoning in small animals. J. Small Anim. Pract. 14:183–193, 1973.
McLeavey, B.J.: Lead poisoning in dogs. N.Z. Vet. J. 12:359–396, 1977.
Zook, B.C., Carpenter, J.L., and Leeds, E.B.: Lead poisoning in dogs. JAVMA 155:1329–1342, 1969.

ANTIFREEZE (ETHYLENE GLYCOL) POISONING

FREDERICK W. OEHME, D.V.M.
Manhattan, Kansas

Antifreeze toxicity is a common poisoning in small domestic animals. The major toxic component is ethylene glycol, which constitutes 95 percent or more of most commercial antifreeze preparations. Dogs and cats have frequently consumed radiator drainage containing antifreeze, probably due to its sweet taste. The incidence of antifreeze poisoning increases significantly in the fall of the year, when radiators are being drained and new antifreeze is being incorporated into automobile and other machinery-cooling systems. The toxic dose that has been reported in dogs varies from 4.2 to 6.6 ml of ethylene glycol/kg of body weight. Interestingly, the fatal dose of ethylene glycol in cats has been given as only 1.5 ml/kg.

CLINICAL SYNDROMES

The clinical diagnosis and treatment of ethylene glycol poisoning are difficult, since animals progress through varying stages of signs, and the clinician may be presented with the patient at any phase of the syndrome. The basis of ethylene glycol toxicity is twofold: (1) acute toxicity and acidosis due to rapid absorption of a large dose from the digestive tract, or, if the amount of ethylene glycol absorbed is small and time permits, (2) the metabolism of ethylene glycol through a series of metabolites to oxalic acid, which then combines with calcium to form a calcium oxalate complex that is deposited in the renal tubules, causing tubular epithelial damage, renal failure, and death due to uremia. Thus the clinician may be presented with dogs or cats in the acute acidotic phase or in the more chronic uremic syndrome resulting from renal failure.

ACUTE ETHYLENE GLYCOL POISONING

Absorbed ethylene glycol doses in excess of approximately 6 ml/kg of body weight characteristically produce an acute depression and death within 12 to 36 hours after ingestion. If observed, initial clinical signs of apprehension, moderate depression, and mild ataxia are seen 30 to 60 minutes after ethylene glycol ingestion. Vomiting frequently occurs, and progressive depression, incoordination, and ataxia are followed by paresis and coma. Coma usually occurs 6 to 12 hours after ingestion and progresses to death. Although convulsions are not common, some patients may display involuntary forced muscular activity ("paddling") in the terminal phases of poisoning.

Postmortem examination predominantly reveals various degrees of digestive tract hyperemia. In addition, acute congestion of body tissues and swelling of the kidneys may be observed, but the latter is more common with animals surviving longer periods. Examination of urine sediments will show increasing numbers of oxalate crystals beginning approximately six hours after ingestion. Such crystals in the urinary sediment or those observed in kidney impression smears or upon histopathologic examination of kidney tissue are useful diagnostic aids. However, the clinician should realize that small numbers of oxalate crystals may be observed in the urinary sediment of normal dogs.

CHRONIC ETHYLENE GLYCOL POISONING AND UREMIA

Dogs and cats surviving more than 24 hours exhibit increasing levels of blood urea nitrogen. The clinical signs described for the acute syndrome are present but in milder degrees. Vomiting and progressive depression with ataxia and eventual paresis may occur three to ten days following ingestion of ethylene glycol. Such animals have ingested smaller amounts of ethylene glycol or may have vomited significant portions of the compound prior to absorption from the stomach. Increasing thirst is initially apparent, but renal failure results in small amounts of dark-colored urine being voided and eventual anuria. Blood urea nitrogen levels are often in excess of 200 mg/100 ml when coma develops. Muscle fasciculations, paddling of the limbs in slow running movements, occasional periods of diffuse and general muscle contractions, and neuromuscular manifestations of uremia may be seen. Terminal uremia leads to death.

Postmortem examination of these animals reveals cachexia, dehydration, oral ulcerations, and a hemorrhagic gastritis. The kidneys may be swollen. Impression smears of the kidneys reveal abundant numbers of oxalate crystals; these are readily observed primarily in the proximal tubules when histopathologic examination utilizing polarized light is performed. In addition to the presence of oxalate crystals, cystic tubules, congestion, proteinaceous casts, and varying degrees of tubular epithelial damage are observed.

DIAGNOSIS

The clinical signs of ethylene glycol poisoning are predominantly vomiting, progressive depression, and coma with or without neuromuscular activity. These are extremely difficult to differentiate from other causes of similar signs during the acute syndrome, but the presence of numerous oxalate crystals in urinary sediment may be of value in making the diagnosis. Other intoxications, acute metabolic acidoses and neuromuscular injuries and diseases must also be differentiated from ethylene glycol poisoning. Animals with rising blood urea nitrogen levels and the presence of abundant oxalate crystals in urinary sediment should be suspected of having ethylene glycol poisoning.

Commercial laboratores are capable of determining ethylene glycol or oxalate levels in whole blood samples. Practitioners with such facilities available may utilize them for diagnostic benefit. On histopathologic examination of kidney sections, the observation of abundant calcium oxalate crystals in the tubular lumen under polarizing light is characteristic.

TREATMENT

Successful therapy of antifreeze poisoning is based upon a favorable combination of several factors: (1) limited ingestion and absorption of ethylene glycol, (2) rapid diagnosis and initiation of treatment following poisoning, and (3) faithful application of a systematic therapeutic regimen of ethanol and sodium bicarbonate.

Animals receiving unusually large dosages of ethylene glycol (in excess of 10 ml/kg of body weight in dogs; in excess of 8 ml/kg of body weight in cats) are incapable of responding to any therapy. The rapid absorption and metabolic conversion of the ethylene glycol to a series of acids results in an acute acidosis and prompt death. Animals ingesting such large quantities of ethylene glycol are rarely seen except in a comatose condition, at which time diagnosis is extremely difficult and biologic response to antidotal therapy is improbable.

Animals receiving lethal amounts of ethylene glycol respond to therapy in direct relation to the promptness with which therapy is instituted. In general, dogs will recover from twice the lethal dose of ethylene glycol if treatment is instituted within 12 hours following ingestion. Cats respond to therapy for three times the lethal dose of ethylene glycol if therapy is instituted at least eight hours following ingestion. This observation is logical when one realizes that the ethylene glycol, in itself, is relatively non-toxic;

it is the metabolites that induce the toxicosis. Hence, the longer the time allowed for metabolism to occur before therapy is instituted, the less the chance of successful treatment and recovery.

Successful therapy of ethylene glycol poisoning in dogs and cats depends upon the repeated systemic administration of solutions of 20 percent ethanol and 5 percent sodium bicarbonate. In dogs, the optimal dosage levels are 5.5 ml of 20 percent ethanol/kg of body weight given intravenously and 8 ml of 5 percent sodium bicarbonate/kg of body weight given intraperitoneally. This treatment level must be repeated every four hours for a total of five treatments, and then every six hours for four additional treatments. In cats, lower enzyme levels require that the dosage be altered. Five milliliters of 20 percent ethanol and 6 ml of 5 percent sodium bicarbonate are given per kilogram of body weight, both intraperitoneally. This is administered every six hours for a total of five treatments, and then given four more times at eight-hour intervals.

The treatment rationale is based upon ethanol blocking the enzymes responsible for metabolizing the ethylene glycol to the more toxic end-products. Hence, only limited oxalic acid is produced, and reduced calcium oxalate formation and renal deposition of crystals occur. The administration of sodium bicarbonate prevents and reverses the acidosis, favors increased excretion of the unmetabolized ethylene glycol, and reduces calcium oxalate formation by altering urinary pH. Renal excretion of unchanged ethylene glycol is further enhanced by the volume of fluids being administered and the availability of frequent small amounts of drinking water to animals undergoing therapy.

Even though the amount of ethylene glycol ingested by spontaneously poisoned animals is often impossible to determine, clinical evaluation and prognosis is possible approximately 12 to 16 hours into the therapeutic regimen. Animals regaining consciousness, drinking water, and perhaps walking with difficulty after the third or fourth treatments may reasonably be estimated to have absorbed limited amounts of ethylene glycol. The prognosis for recovery with completion of the entire treatment schedule is fair to good. Animals undergoing therapy that do not regain consciousness between treatments have a poor potential for recovery. Likewise, dogs presented in coma with suspected ethylene glycol ingestion must be given poor prognoses. Such animals are frequently in a terminal state of either acute intoxication or in the more chronic renal syndrome with uremia. Such animals will not respond to ethanol-bicarbonate therapy.

While not readily available under most clinical circumstances, hemodialysis and fluid therapy would be useful in comatose ethylene glycol-poisoned animals. Peritoneal dialysis is a practical compromise for hemodialysis, but it does not provide the effective cleansing of biologic fluids achieved by the latter. Until the current experimental resins and other techniques are further developed for practical "cage-side" use in dialyzing whole blood of foreign compounds, the prompt and conscientious application of ethanol and sodium bicarbonate remains the most effective treatment for antifreeze (ethylene glycol) poisoning in dogs and cats.

SUPPLEMENTAL READING

Beckett, S.D., and Shields, R.P.: Treatment of acute ethylene glycol (antifreeze) toxicosis in the dog. J. Am. Vet. Med. Assoc. *158*:472–476, 1971.

Kersting, E.J., and Nielsen, S.W.: Ethylene glycol poisoning in small animals. J. Am. Vet. Med. Assoc. *146*:113–118, 1965.

Kersting, E.J., and Nielsen, S.W.: Experimental ethylene glycol poisoning in the dog. Am. J. Vet. Res. *27*:574–582, 1966.

Nunamaker, D.M., Medway, W., and Berg, P.: Treatment of ethylene glycol poisoning in the dog. J. Am. Vet. Med. Assoc. *159*:310–314, 1971.

Penumarthy, L., and Oehme, F.W.: Treatment of ethylene glycol toxicosis in cats. Am. J. Vet. Res. *36*:209–212, 1975.

Sanyer, J.L., Oehme, F.W., and McGavin, M.D.: Systematic treatment of ethylene glycol toxicosis in dogs. Am. J. Vet. Res. *34*:527–534, 1973.

ORGANOPHOSPHATE AND CARBAMATE INSECTICIDE POISONING

THOMAS L. CARSON, D.V.M.
Ames, Iowa

The organophosphate (OP) and carbamate insecticides have been widely employed for control of external parasites on companion animals and livestock, and insect pests in the home and garden, as well as agricultural insecticides for crop production.

Usage of these insecticides has increased dramatically over the last few years as the more environmentally persistent chlorinated hydrocarbon insecticides have been restricted in usage.

Spilled or improperly stored insecticides, whether in the basement, in the garage, or on the farmstead, present a hazard of poisoning to companion animals. Dogs and cats have lapped up liquid concentrates and diluted sprays as well as dry powders intended for home and garden applications. Farm dogs have eaten granules of these insecticides that have been spilled on the ground or in farm vehicles. Leftover or improperly discarded insecticide preparations have also caused poisoning.

Miscalculation of insecticide concentrations in spraying, dipping, or shampooing procedures has also resulted in toxicosis. Re-treating animals with OP or carbamate preparations within a few days may result in poisoning of these animals. In addition, some animals may be predisposed to poisoning because of concurrent or previous treatment with some anthelmintics or tranquilizers.

MECHANISM OF ACTION

The OP and carbamate insecticides are discussed together because their mechanisms of action are similar.

Cholinergic nerves utilize acetylcholine as a neurotransmitter substance. Under normal conditions, acetylcholine released at the synapses of parasympathetic nerves and myoneural junctions are quickly hydrolyzed by cholinesterase enzymes. When the hydrolyzing enzymes are inhibited, the continued presence of acetylcholine maintains a state of nerve stimulation and accounts for the clinical signs observed with poisoning from these insecticides. In general, inhibition of these enzymes by the OP insecticides tends to be irreversible, whereas inhibition by the carbamates is reversible.

CLINICAL SIGNS

The clinical syndrome produced by the OP and carbamate insecticides is similar in all species of animals and in general is characterized by overstimulation of the parasympathetic nervous system and skeletal muscles. Earliest clinical signs of acute poisoning frequently include mildly progressing to profuse salivation, defecation, urination, emesis, a stiff-legged or "saw horse" gait, and general uneasiness. As the syndrome progresses, profuse salivation, gastrointestinal hypermotility resulting in severe colic and abdominal cramps, diarrhea, excessive lacrimation, sweating, miosis, dyspnea, cyanosis, urinary incontinence, and muscle tremors of the face, eyelids, and general body musculature can be observed. Hyperactivity of the skeletal muscles is generally followed by muscular paralysis, as the muscles are unable to respond to continued stimulation.

Dogs and cats may exhibit increased central nervous system stimulation, which in some circumstances may lead to tonoclonic convulsive seizures. Many times, however, marked central nervous system depression can be observed.

Death usually results from hypoxia due to excessive respiratory tract secretions, bronchoconstriction, and erratic slowed heartbeat. The onset of clinical signs in cases of acute poisoning may occur as soon as a few minutes or as late as several hours after exposure. Death can occur in severe poisoning at any time from a few minutes to several hours after the first clinical signs are observed.

NECROPSY LESIONS

Postmortem lesions associated with acute OP

or carbamate toxicosis are usually non-specific. Excessive fluids in the mouth and respiratory tract as well as pulmonary edema may be observed.

DIAGNOSIS

A history of exposure to OP or carbamate insecticides associated with clinical signs of parasympathetic stimulation warrants a tentative diagnosis of poisoning with these compounds.

Chemical analyses of animal tissues for the presence of insecticides are usually unrewarding because of the rapid degradation of the OP and carbamate insecticides resulting in low tissue residue levels. However, finding the insecticide in the stomach contents and in the suspect source material can be quite valuable in establishing a diagnosis.

The best method of confirming a diagnosis is to assess the degree of inhibition of cholinesterase enzyme activity in the whole blood and tissue of the suspected animal. A reduction of whole blood cholinesterase activity to less than 25 percent of the normal is indicative of excessive exposure to these insecticides. Depending upon the specific insecticide involved, blood cholinesterase activity in dogs may remain depressed for several days to several weeks following OP exposure. The variability of cholinesterase enzyme activity levels in clinically normal dogs may make interpretation of laboratory values difficult. In addition, it must be remembered that depletion of whole blood cholinesterase activity may not necessarily correlate with inhibition of cholinesterase at the parasympathetic synapses and myoneural junctions. Therefore, whole blood cholinesterase activity should be viewed as only an indication of the status of the cholinesterase enzymes in the body.

The cholinesterase activity can also be measured in brain tissue. The enzyme activity in brain tissue, especially the caudate nucleus, in animals dying from these insecticides will generally be less than 10 per cent of normal brain activity.

Whole blood and brain samples should be well chilled but not frozen for best laboratory results. Samples of stomach contents as well as any suspect material should be submitted to a laboratory for chemical analyses.

TREATMENT

The treatment of animals poisoned by organ-ophosphates and carbamate insecticides should be considered on an emergency basis because of the rapid progression of the clinical syndrome.

Initial treatment for poisoned animals should involve administration of atropine sulfate at approximately 0.2 mg/kg of body weight. This initial dose should be divided, and about one-fourth of the dose should be given intravenously and the balance subcutaneously or intramuscularly. Further treatment or handling should be withheld for several minutes or until respiratory distress has been alleviated. Atropine sulfate does not counteract the insecticide-enzyme bond but rather blocks the effects of accumulated acetylcholine at the nerve endings. Although a dramatic cessation of parasympathetic signs is generally observed within a few minutes after administration of atropine, it will not affect the skeletal muscle tremors. Repeated doses of atropine at approximately half the initial dose may be required but should be used only to counteract parasympathetic signs. Over-atropinization should be avoided.

The oximes, such as 2-PAM (Protopam Chloride[R]), are human drugs that act specifically on the organophosphate-enzyme complex, freeing the enzyme. The oximes may supplement atropine therapy when used relatively early in the course of treatment. 2-PAM is recommended at the rate of 20 mg/kg of body weight. The oximes are of no benefit in treating carbamate toxicosis.

Dermally exposed animals should be washed with soap and water to prevent continued absorption of these compounds. Orally administered activated charcoal in a water slurry is helpful in reducing absorption following ingestion of these insecticides.

Morphine, succinylcholine, and phenothiazine tranquilizers should be avoided in treating OP or carbamate insecticide poisoning.

SUPPLEMENTAL READING

Buck, W., Osweiler, G.D., and Van Gelder, G.A.: *Clinical and Diagnostic Veterinary Toxicology*. Dubuque, Iowa, Kendall-Hunt Publishing Co., 1976.

Clarke, E.G.C., and Clarke, M.L.: *Garner's Veterinary Toxicology*. Baltimore, The Williams & Wilkins Co., 1967.

Radeleff, R.D.: *Veterinary Toxicology*, 2nd ed. Philadelphia, Lea & Febiger, 1979.

Vestweber, J.G., and Krukenberg, S.M. The effect of selected organophosphorous compounds on plasma and red blood cell cholinesterase in the dog. Vet. Med. Small Anim. Clin. 67:803–806, 1972.

COMMON POTENTIAL SOURCES OF SMALL ANIMAL POISONINGS

GARY D. OSWEILER, D.V.M.

Columbia, Missouri

When a case of potential intoxication is presented, the first concerns are usually the accurate assessment of the clinical status of the animal and the prompt incorporation of procedures to support life and control clinical signs. Immediately thereafter, or concurrent with emergency management, a tentative diagnosis should be made.

Part of the input to determine that diagnosis is a review of potential toxicants to which an animal may have been exposed. Appropriate questioning of the owner may aid in establishing potential sources. From among the thousands of potentially toxic chemicals in the world, one usually attempts to consider those that are (1) in the animal's environment, (2) toxic enough to constitute a hazard if exposure occurs, (3) available to the animal, and (4) generally capable of causing the signs being manifested.

From the article "Common Poisonings in Small Animal Practice," it may be seen that the number of intoxications diagnosed is rather small and involves mainly natural toxins and economic poisons. Those toxins in the animal's environment generally include products in and around the home, those involved in pest control, and those that are available in the natural or altered environment. Key questions should be directed to the owner to establish what products, plants, or animals are kept or are available in or near the home. Recent use of such materials, where they are stored, and recollection of spillage should be reviewed with the client. The species, age, eating habits, and freedom of the affected animal should be known. For example, it is important to remember that the dog that roams the neighborhood nightly is exposed to "common sources" different from those of the constantly housed animal.

Each geographic area of North America has its own peculiar common sources, as detailed in the article on common poisonings (cited above). Indigenous plants, venomous reptiles, snail baits, rust inhibitors, and antifreeze solutions are but a few examples of toxicants that may be more prevalent in particular geographic areas.

This chapter covers in some detail the common sources generally associated with frequently diagnosed intoxications. However, Tables 1, 2, and 3 are presented here to offer a broad review of the scope of commonly available substances that may occasionally be toxic. These tables should be used to suggest specific potentially toxic agents found in many homes and businesses. Table 4 enumerates some data valuable in establishing exposure to various sources.

When access or potential exposure to the materials listed is established, additional details may be found in this section or in the references listed at the end of this article.

Knowledge of sources and the pattern of exposure that occurred (e.g., accidental, malicious) can serve as a focus for education of the client in safe use of toxic materials to prevent further danger to either animals or man.

SUPPLEMENTAL READING

Arena, J.M.: *Poisoning. Toxicology, Symptoms, Treatments*, 3rd ed. Springfield, Illinois, Charles C Thomas, 1974.

Atkins, C.E., and Johnson, R.K.: Clinical toxicities of cats. Vet. Clin. North Am. 5:623–652, 1975.

Buck, W.B., Osweiler, G.D., and Van Gelder, G.A.: *Clinical and Diagnostic Veterinary Toxicology*. Dubuque, Iowa, Kendall-Hunt Publishing Co., 1973.

Bureau of Veterinary Medicine: Memo. Summary of Adverse Reactions to Animal Drugs. BVMM-20, Rockville, Maryland, August, 1975.

Catcott, E.J. (ed.): *Canine Medicine*. Wheaton, Illinois, American Veterinary Publications, 1968.

Clarke, E.G.C.: Pets and poisons, J. Small Anim. Pract. 16:375–380, 1975.

Clarke, E.G.C., and Clarke, M.L.: *Garner's Veterinary Toxicology*, 3rd ed. Baltimore, The Williams & Wilkins Co., 1967.

Diechman, W.B., and Gerarde, H.W.: *Toxicology of Drugs and Chemicals*, 4th ed. New York, Academic Press, 1969.

Gleason, M.N., Gosselin, R.E., and Hodge, H.C.: *Clinical Toxicology of Commercial Products*. Baltimore, The Williams & Wilkins Co., 1971.

Text continued on page 154

Table 1.   Sources of Poisonous Plants

LOCATION	EXAMPLES
House Plants	Daffodil, oleander, poinsettia, dumb cane, mistletoe, philodendron
Flower Garden	Delphinium, monkshood, foxglove, iris, lily-of-the-valley
Vegetable Garden	Rhubarb, spinach, tomato vine, sunburned potatoes
Ornamentals	Oleander, castor bean, daphne, golden chain, rhododendron, lantana
Trees and Shrubs	Cherries, peach, oak, elderberry, black locust
Woodland Plants	Jack-in-the-pulpit, moonseed, May apple, Dutchman's-breeches
Swamp Plants	Water hemlock, mushrooms
Field Plants	Buttercup, nightshade, poison hemlock, jimsonweed, pigweed
Range Plants	Locoweed, lupine, halogeton
Grain Contaminants	Crotalaria, corn cockle, ergot
Cultural Changes	Nitrate, cyanide, herbicides, insecticides

Table 2.   Some Toxins of Zoologic Origin

ORGANISMS	LOCATIONS	GENERAL PROBLEMS ENCOUNTERED
Snakes		
Pit vipers	Terrestrial; Eastern U.S.A.	Necrosis, inflammation,
Rattlesnake	through South Central,	anaphylaxis
Copperhead	Midwest and Southwest	
Water moccasin		
Coral snake	Southeast U.S.A., mainly Florida	Neuroparalytic, loss of sensation
Lizards		
Gila monster	Terrestrial; primarily	Inflammation, vomition, shock
Mexican beaded lizard	Southwest U.S.A.	
Toads		
Bufo sp.	Terrestrial-aquatic; Southern and	Parotid glands exude a cardio-
	Southwestern U.S.A.	toxic and cholinergic toxin
Spiders		
Black widow	Terrestrial	Neuromuscular;
Brown recluse		wound heals with difficulty;
Tarantula		infection from the bite
Insects		
Fire ant	Terrestrial; Southern and	Painful, necrotizing bite;
Wasps	Southwestern U.S.A.	inflammation and anaphylaxis
Bees		
Invertebrates		
Jellyfish	Aquatic-marine	Pain, swelling, cramps, nausea,
Coral		CNS derangement
Sea anemone		
Sea urchin		Burning sensation, inflammation,
		paralysis
Vertebrates		
Fish	Aquatic-marine	Sharp pain, inflammation
Stingray		
Catfish		
Scorpion fish		

Table 3.   *Some Chemical Products Hazardous to Pets*

ARTS AND CRAFTS SUPPLIES

Antiquing Agents
Methyl ethyl ketone
Turpentine

Oil Paints and Tempera Paints
Pigment salts of lead, arsenic, copper and cadmium

Pencils, Indelible
Crystal violet

PHOTOGRAPHIC SUPPLIES

Developers
Borates
Bromides
Iodides
Thiocyanates

Fixatives
Sodium thiosulfate

Hardeners
Aluminum chloride
Formaldehyde

AUTOMOTIVE AND MACHINERY PRODUCTS

Antifreeze, Fuel System De-icer
Ethylene glycol
Isopropyl alcohol
Methanol
Rust inhibitors
  a. Borates
  b. Chromates
  c. Zinc chloride

Brake Fluids
Butyl ethers of ethylene glycol and related glycols
Ethyl ethers of ethylene glycol and related glycols
Methyl ethers of ethylene glycol and related glycols

Carburetor Cleaners
Cresol
Ethylene dichloride

Corrosion Inhibitors
Borates
Sodium chromate
Sodium nitrate

Engine and Motor Cleaners
Cresol
Ethylene dichloride
Methylene chloride

Frost Removers
Ethylene glycol
Isopropyl alcohol

Lubricants
Barium compounds
Isopropyl alcohol
Kerosene
Lead compounds
Stoddard solvent

Motor Fuel
Gasoline
Kerosene
Tetraethyl lead

Radiator Cleaners
Boric acid
Oxalic acid
Sodium chromate

Shock Absorber Fluids
Petroleum ether

Tire Repair
Benzene

Windshield Washer
Ethylene glycol
Isopropyl alcohol
Methyl alcohol

CLEANERS, DISINFECTANTS, SANITIZERS

Cleaners, Bleaches, Polishes
Ammonium hydroxide
Benzene
Carbon tetrachloride
Hydrochloric acid
Methyl alcohol
Naphtha
Nitrobenzene
Oxalic acid
Phosphoric acid
Sodium fluoride
Sodium or potassium hydroxide
Sodium hypochlorite
Sodium perborate
Sulfuric acid
Trichloroethane
Turpentine

Disinfectants, Sanitizers
Acids
Alkalis
Hypochlorites
Iodophors
Paradichlorobenzene
Phenol, Cresols
Phenyl mercuric acetate
Pine oil
Quaternary ammonium

HEALTH AND BEAUTY AIDS

Athlete's Foot
Caprylic acid
Copper
Propionic acid
Sodium
Undecylenic acid
Zinc salts

Bath Preparations
Bath oils
Perfume
Sodium lauryl sulfate
Trisodium phosphate

Continued on next page

Table 3. *Some Chemical Products Hazardous to Pets (Continued)*

Corn Removers
  Phenoxyacetic acid
  Salicylic acid
Deodorants and Antiperspirants
  Alcohol
  Aluminum chloride
Diet Pills
  Amphetamines
  Diuretics
  Thyroid hormone
Eye Make-up
  Boric acid
  Peach kernel oil, q.s.
Hair Preparations
  Cadmium chloride
  Cupric chloride
  Dyes, tints
  Ferric chloride
  Lead acetate
  Permanent wave lotions
  Pyrogallol
  Silver nitrate
  Thioglycolic acid
Headache
  Aspirin
  Phenacetin
Laxatives
  IRRITANT OR STIMULANT LAXATIVES
    Aloes
    Aloin
    Cascara sagrada
Liniments
  Camphor
  Chloroform
  Oil of wintergreen (methyl salicylate)
  Pine oil
  Turpentine
Nailetics
  Acetone
  Alcohol
  Benzene
  Ethyl acetate
  Nail enamel
  Nail polish
  Nail polish remover
  Toluene
  Tricresyl phosphate
Ointments
  Benzoic acid
  Borates
  Caprylic acid
  Menthol
  Mercury compounds
  Oil of wintergreen (methyl salicylate)
  Phenols
  Salicylic acid
Perfumes, Toilet Waters and Colognes
  Alcohol
  Essential oils
  Floral oils
  Perfume essence
Shampoos
  Sodium lauryl sulfate
  Triethanolamine dodecyl sulfate
Shaving Lotions
  Alcohol
  Boric acid

Somnolents (Sleeping Pills)
  Barbiturates
  Bromides
Stimulants
  Amphetamine
  Caffeine
Suntan Lotions
  Alcohol
  Tannic acid and derivatives

PAINTS AND RELATED PRODUCTS
Caulking Compounds
  Barium
  Chlorinated biphenyl
  Chromium
  Lead
  Mineral spirits
  Petroleum distillate
  Xylene
Driers
  Cobalt compounds
  Iron compounds
  Manganese compounds
  Vanadium compounds
  Zinc compounds
Lacquer Thinners
  Aliphatic hydrocarbons
  Butyl acetate
  Butyl alcohol
  Toluene
Paint
  Arsenic oxide
  Coal tar
  Cuprous oxide
  Lead chromate
  Petroleum ether
  Pine oil
  Red lead oxide
  Zinc chromate
Paint Brush Cleaners
  Benzene
  Kerosene
  Naphthas
Paint and Varnish Cleaners
  Ethylene dichloride
  Kerosene
  Naphthalene
  Trisodium phosphate
Paint and Varnish Removers
  FLAMMABLE
    Benzene
    Cresols
    Phenols
    Toluene
  NONFLAMMABLE
    Methylene chloride
    Toluene
Preservatives
  BRUSH
    Kerosene
    Turpentine
  CANVAS
    2-Chlorophenylphenol
    Pentachlorophenol

Continued on opposite page

Table 3.   *Some Chemical Products Hazardous to Pets (Continued)*

FLOOR
   Magnesium fluorosilicate
WOOD
   Copper naphthenate
   Copper oleate
   Mineral spirits
   Pentachlorophenol
   Zinc naphthenate

PEST CONTROL

Birds
   Endrin
   Toluidine
Fungicides
   Captan
   Copper compounds
   Maneb
   Mercurials
   Pentachlorophenol
   Thiram
   Zineb
Insects and Spiders
   Baygon
   Carbaryl
   Chlordane
   Diazinon
   Dichlorvos
   Kelthane
   Mirex
   Paradichlorobenzene
   Pyrethrins
   Rotenone
   Toxaphene
Lawn and Garden Weeds
   Arsenic
   Chlordane
   Dacthal
   Pentachlorophenol
   Trifluralin
   2,4-D
Rats, Mice, Gophers, Moles
   Arsenic
   Barium carbonate
   Dicoumarol
   Phosphorus
   Sodium fluoroacetate

   Strychnine
   Thallium (rare)
   Warfarin
   Zinc phosphide
Snails, Slugs
   Metaldehyde

SAFETY PRODUCTS

Fire Extinguishers
   LIQUID FIRE EXTINGUISHERS
      Carbon tetrachloride
   MISCELLANEOUS FIRE EXTINGUISHERS
      Methylbromide
   POWDER EXTINGUISHERS
      Borax compounds
Nonskid Products
   Stoddard solvent
   Methyl ethyl ketone

SOLVENTS

Alcohols
Chlorinated Solvents
   Carbon tetrachloride
   Methylene chloride
   Orthodichlorobenzene
   Trichloroethylene
Esters
   Amyl acetate
   Ethyl acetate
   Isopropyl acetate
   Methyl acetate
Hydrocarbons
   Aromatics, chiefly benzene, toluene and xylene
   Naphthenes
Ketones
   Acetone
   Methyl ethyl ketone
Other Common Solvents
   Aniline
   Carbon disulphide
   Cresylic acid
   Kerosene
   Mineral spirits
   Phenols
   Turpentine

Table 4.* *Small Animal Toxicology History

Date: _____ Case: _____ Owner: _____
D.V.M.: _____ Name: _____ Address: _____
Address: _____ Species: _____ _____
_____ Breed: _____ _____
_____ Weight: _____ Phone: _____
Phone: _____ Age:_____ Sex:_____ Delivered by: _____

Illnesses within the past 6 months _____
Vaccinations within the past year _____ rabies _____leptospirosis
_____distemper _____hepatitis _____other
Medications, sprays, dips, wormers, etc., given within the past month (type and date) _____
When was this animal last seen by a veterinarian? _____

How long was this animal sick?_____days _____months _____hours
If found dead, how long since last seen alive and healthy? _____days _____hours

History of confinement: _____roamed occasionally (supervised) _____roamed at will
_____roamed occasionally (unsupervised) _____always housed
_____always penned or tied _____other
Animal lived near or on (check more than one if applicable):
_____industrial buildings _____garbage dump _____small town _____city
_____commercial buildings _____railroad _____suburb _____other
_____automotive garage _____grain elevator _____farm

Has the patient always lived in this locality? _____yes _____no
If no, please explain: _____
Have there been any changes in food, water or location in recent days? _____yes _____no
If yes, please explain: _____
What is the patient normally fed? _____
When was this animal last fed? _____

What types of mouse or rat poisons, insecticides, weed killers, etc., are used on or near your property? _____

Have other animals in your home or neighborhood had similar problems? _____

Clinical signs:
_____convulsions _____depression _____weakness
_____difficult urination _____blindness _____stiffness _____diarrhea
_____difficult breathing _____salivation _____bleeding _____thirst
_____vocalization _____excitement _____vomiting _____other

Tentative diagnoses:

Use back of sheet for additional history and comments.

SUPPLEMENTAL READING (*Continued*)

Kirk, R.W. (ed.): *Current Veterinary Therapy* V. Philadelphia, W. B. Saunders Co., 1974.
Kirk, R.W., and Bistner, S.I.: *Handbook of Veterinary Procedures and Emergency Treatment*, 2nd ed. Philadelphia, W. B. Saunders Co., 1975.
Malone, J.C.: Diagnosis and treatment of poisoning in dogs and cats. Vet. Rec. 84:161–166, 1969.
Osweiler, G.D.: Incidence and diagnostic considerations of major small animal toxicoses. J. Am. Vet. Med. Assoc., 155:2011–2015, 1969.
Radeleff, R.D.: *Veterinary Toxicology*, 2nd ed. Philadelphia, Lea & Febiger, 1970.
Robens, J.F.: Animal drug toxicities. Veterinary Toxicology Training and Review Workshop. Ames, Iowa, February 21–26, 1972.
Szabuniewicz, M.: Treatment of some common animal poisonings. Vet. Med. Small Anim. Clin. December, 1971, pp. 1197–1205.

ADVERSE DRUG REACTIONS

ARTHUR L. ARONSON, D.V.M.,
and WAYNE S. SCHWARK, D.V.M.

Ithaca, New York

The value and benefit of drugs in modern therapeutics is unquestioned. Yet every pharmacologic substance has the potential to affect some individual patient adversely. While there is no drug that is completely safe, the justification of using a given drug lies in the favorable ratio of anticipated benefits as compared with potential risks.

A veterinarian ideally should be able to make a quantitative benefit-risk assessment for each drug that is used clinically. Although adverse drug reactions (ADRs) have been reported for drugs used clinically in veterinary practice, currently there is no detailed information available on their incidence. Thus it is not possible to make a quantitative benefit-risk assessment.

A brief consideration of ADRs will be made in this review, together with listings of selected ADRs in cats and dogs that have been reported to the Bureau of Veterinary Medicine (BVM) Drug Surveillance Program (Tables 1 and 2). These reports were obtained from BVM memos published since 1975.

WHAT IS AN ADR?

Several definitions of ADRs have been advanced by various groups studying these reactions. It may be useful to consider some of these definitions.

An operational definition used by the Massachusetts General Hospital (Koch-Weser et al., 1969) is "Any noxious change in a patient's condition which a physician believes to be due to a drug, which occurs at dosages normally used in man, and which (1) requires treatment, (2) indicates decrease or cessation of therapy with the drug, or (3) suggests that future therapy with the drug carries an unusual risk in this patient." This definition does not include as ADRs any trivial or expected side effects that do not require any change in therapy, or noxious events owing to deliberate or accidental overdosage.

The World Health Organization definition is similar (Venulet, 1977): "An ADR is one which is noxious and unintended and which occurs at doses used in man for prophylaxis, diagnosis, therapy, or modification of physiological functions."

The Bureau of Veterinary Medicine definition includes lack of drug efficacy as an ADR: "An unintended change in the structure, function and chemistry of the body including injury, toxicity, sensitivity reaction, or lack of efficacy associated with the clinical use of a drug."

Causes of ADRs. ADRs associated with specific drugs are listed in Tables 1 and 2. Two basic causes of ADRs are *excessive drug use* and *failure to establish a therapeutic endpoint*. Several studies have shown that the frequency of ADRs increases as the number of drugs used concurrently in a patient increases. These ADRs may or may not be due to drug interactions. Also, a toxic endpoint, if not predefined, may occur when toxicity is an extension of the pharmacologic action of a drug. For example, the maximal contractile force obtainable with digitalis glycosides occurs before alterations in cardiac conduction. ADRs to digitalis glycosides could be minimized by selecting improvement in hemodynamics or in renal function as the therapeutic endpoint rather than changes in cardiac conduction or the onset of emesis. Failure to establish a therapeutic endpoint also may render it difficult to recognize lack of efficacy, and a useless but potentially toxic drug will continue to be given.

Recognition of ADRs. There are no unique clinical or laboratory findings that distinguish ADRs from the manifestations of concurrent disease. Thus, an accurate identification of an ADR often is difficult. An alert and suspicious clinician is of utmost importance. It may be difficult to think of one's treatment as being responsible for the patient's disability. One should expect the unexpected. A suspicious reaction should not be dismissed because it is not described in a pharmacology textbook or on a drug package insert.

Comparisons of ADR evaluations among experienced observers reveal that the clinical identification of ADRs is complex and subjective. It is difficult to prove a cause-and-effect relationship, and there are differences in the subjective evaluations among individual investigators. The difficulties are compounded when

Text continued on page 159

155

Table 1. Adverse Drug Reactions Reported in Cats

DRUG	CLINICAL SIGNS AND LESIONS
Analgesics	
Acetaminophen	depression, death
Acetaminophen/codeine	restlessness, excitement, fear, mydriasis, death
Aspirin	depression or excitability, ataxia, nystagmus, anorexia, emesis, weight loss, hyperpnea, hepatitis, bone marrow depression, anemia, gastric lesions, death
Phenylbutazone	inappetence, weight loss, alopecia, dehydration, emesis, severe depression, death
CNS Depressants	
Acetyl promazine	prolonged effect, cardiac arrest, convulsions, death
Ketamine, ketamine/acetyl promazine	prolonged recovery, tremors, convulsions, excitement, hyperpyrexia, cardiac arrest, bladder and renal hemorrhage, nephrosis, fatty liver, deafness, death
Halothane	cardiac arrest
Methoxyflurane	ataxia, death
Thiamylal	cardiac arrest, respiratory arrest, prolonged anesthesia, ataxia, death
Xylazine	prolonged anesthesia, apnea, convulsions
Proparacaine	mydriasis
Antiparasitics	
Bunamidine	sudden death
Dichlorophene/toluene	ataxia, twitching, death
Dichlorvos	death
Glycobiarsol	emesis, icterus, death
Levamisole	salivation, excitement, diarrhea, mydriasis
Piperazine	emesis, dementia, ataxia, hypermetria
Hormone	
Megestrol acetate	polyphagia, hydrometra, uterine rupture
Antimicrobials	
Amphotericin B	marked elevation of BUN following single dose
Chloramphenicol	anaphylactoid-type reaction, anorexia, ataxia, emesis, depression, neutropenia, death
Tetracycline	malignant hyperthermia, emesis, dehydration
Tylosin	irritation at injection site
Gentamicin	pruritus, alopecia, erythema
Hexachlorophene	anorexia, ataxia
Miconazole	erythema, alopecia
Procaine penicillin/dihydrostreptomycin	ataxia
Trimethoprim/sulfadiazine	emesis

156

Table 2. Adverse Drug Reactions Reported in Dogs

DRUG	CLINICAL SIGNS AND LESIONS
Analgesics	
Aspirin	bleeding disorders
Phenylbutazone	anemia, leukopenia, thrombocytopenia, emesis
CNS Depressants	
Acetyl promazine	atypical behavior, aggression, apprehension, lameness of injected leg, prolonged effect, respiratory distress
Fentanyl/droperidol	behavior change, lameness, hyperthermia, aggression, seizures, bradycardia, tachycardia, hyperpnea, apnea, tremors, hyperventilation, hyperexcitability
Halothane	cardiac arrhythmia, malignant hyperthermia, nystagmus, torticollis, cardiac arrest, death
Ketamine	convulsions
Lidocaine	laryngeal and facial edema
Methoxyflurane	cardiac arrest, hepatitis after 2 weeks, death
Prochlorperazine/isopropamide	tachycardia
Promazine	depression, hypotension, hyperthermia, death
Thiamylal	cardiac arrest, respiratory arrest, prolonged anesthesia, cyanosis, death
Thiopental	cardiac arrest, prolonged recovery, pulmonary edema, slough at injection site, death
Xylazine	viciousness, bradycardia, death
Anticonvulsants	
Phenytoin	ataxia, hepatotoxicity, leukopenia, emesis, death
Primidone	liver failure, icterus, emesis, alopecia, death
Antiparasitics	
Arecoline/tetrachlorethylene	mydriasis, ataxia, diarrhea, severe colic, unable to walk
Bunamidine	dyspnea, ataxia, sudden death
Dichlorophene/toluene	incoordination, convulsions, death
Dichlorvos	diarrhea, emesis, ataxia, tremors, weakness, death
Diethylcarbamazine	pruritus, weakness, emesis, diarrhea, icterus, anaphylactoid reaction, death
Diethylcarbamazine/styrylpyridinium	diarrhea, emesis, sterilization, teratogenesis, death
Disophenol	hyperthermia, hyperventilation, ataxia, collapse, dyspnea, swelling at injection site, death
Dithiazine iodide	emesis, diarrhea, depression, apprehension, hyperpyrexia
Levamisole	dyspnea, pulmonary edema
Piperazine	paralysis, death
Phthalofyne	hepatitis, splenitis, death

Continued on next page

Table 2. *Adverse Drug Reactions Reported in Dogs (Continued)*

DRUG	CLINICAL SIGNS AND LESIONS
Ronnel	emesis, twitching, depression
Thenium closylate	enteritis, anaphylaxis, death
Thiacetarsamide	emesis, icterus, depression, anorexia, cough, renal failure, swelling at injection site, alopecia, dermatitis, bleeding disorders, death
Toluene	collapse
Trichlorfon	anorexia, weakness, lethargy
Hormones	
Dexamethasone	polydipsia, emesis, diarrhea, panting
Prednisolone	anorexia, polyphagia, pica, anemia, lethargy, diarrhea
Triamcinolone	Cushing's syndrome, emesis, depression
Estradiol cypionate	pain at injection site
Megestrol acetate	polyphagia, hydrometra, uterine inertia, uterine rupture, anorexia, depression, death
Antimicrobials	
Ampicillin	wheals
Bacitracin/polymyxin B/ neomycin (ophthalmic)	eye irritation
Cephalexin	panting, salivation, hyperexcitability
Chloramphenicol	emesis, depression, ataxia, diarrhea, death
Lincomycin	emesis, diarrhea
Nitrofurantoin	emesis
Procaine penicillin G	ataxia, edema, dyspnea
Procaine and benzathine penicillin G	sterile abscess, anaphylaxis
Sulfachlorpyridazine	ataxia, hyperirritability
Sulfaguanidine	keratoconjunctivitis
Sulfamerazine/sulfapyridine	emesis, dyspnea
Tetracycline	emesis
Miscellaneous	
Aminophylline	emesis, anorexia, polyphagia, polydipsia, polyuria, hyperexcitability
Asparaginase	ataxia, muscle weakness, lethargy
Atropine	paradoxical bradycardia, heart block
Calcium edetate	emesis, diarrhea, anorexia, depression
Epinephrine/pilocarpine (ophthalmic)	conjunctivitis
Ibuprofen	depression, emesis, gastric ulcers, death
Neostigmine/physostigmine (ophthalmic)	emesis, diarrhea, bradycardia, pannus

combinations of drugs are administered to a patient.

Nevertheless, everyone does agree that ADRs do occur. The following guidelines may be helpful in identifying an ADR.

1. There is a plausible temporal relationship between administration of the drug and the ADR. Clinical signs develop while the drug is being taken. For example, if a patient goes into anaphylactic shock ten minutes following the injection of penicillin G, there is a strong likelihood that an ADR occurred. It must be remembered that some ADRs may occur long after the drug is administered. The occurrence of cervical cancer in teenaged girls whose mothers took diethylstilbestrol during pregnancy is a case in point.
2. There is improvement in the clinical syndrome when the drug is discontinued.
3. The ADR recurs if the patient is reexposed to the drug.

Minimizing ADRs. Information relating to the frequency with which ADRs occur with drugs in clinical use would be most helpful. This would require a drug monitoring and reporting system that would document the frequency, kinds, and causes of ADRs to a specific drug in relation to the total use of the drug. A clinician then would have a basis for determining the possible benefits of a drug as compared with its possible harmful effects under a given set of conditions. It is worthwhile to emphasize that all drugs possess the potential for producing an ADR and that a drug should not be used unless there is a clearly defined therapeutic objective.

CLASSES OF ADRs

Side Effects. Side effects of drugs may be considered to be ADRs in that they lead to actions that are undesirable but are an inherent part of the drug's action. For example, mydriasis produced when atropine is used as a preanesthetic is undesirable, but it must be accepted along with the desired tachycardia and decreased salivation, since atropine blocks muscarinic receptors non-selectively throughout the body. Similarly, anti-cancer drugs, by virtue of their ability to affect rapidly proliferating neoplastic tissues, also adversely affect normal tissues with rapid cell turnover such as the gastrointestinal mucosa and hematopoietic tissues. For the most part, ADRs related to side effects are predictable and expected, unlike the following classes of ADRs.

Disruption of Control Mechanisms. Two classes of drugs have a clearly established potential for disrupting control mechanisms in the body. Suprainfection has been associated with intensive antibacterial drug therapy, particularly when broad spectrum drugs or combinations of antibacterial drugs are used. Reduced resistance to infection and activation of latent infection have been associated with adrenocorticosteroids, especially during prolonged administration.

Drug Allergy. Certain ADRs have an immunologic basis. These types of reactions require previous exposure and sensitization to the drug. These drugs combine with protein, and antibodies are formed to the drug-protein complex. Subsequent exposure to the drug leads to a typical antigen-antibody reaction with the release of pathologic mediators (histamine, serotonin, bradykinin, etc.), which are responsible for inducing the pathologic effects. Although virtually any body system may be affected, ADRs of this type usually are manifested as abnormalities of the respiratory tract (rhinitis, asthma) and the skin (urticaria, hives) or as generalized systemic reactions (anaphylactic shock). Penicillin and aspirin are examples of drugs that have been implicated in inducing these types of ADRs in man. Drug allergies, although they undoubtedly occur, are not well documented in domestic animals.

Predisposition Due to Patient Status. Age, species, and concurrent disease can predispose a patient to an ADR.

Very young as well as aged animals are more susceptible to ADRs than are middle-aged animals. Several weeks are required for a neonate to approach the capability of a young adult in drug biotransformation. The dosage schedule for drugs requiring drug biotransformation must be reduced in neonates, particularly if the drug has a high potential for producing toxicity. Chloramphenicol is an example of a drug requiring biotransformation, and it has the potential for producing bone marrow depression. The "grey baby syndrome" has been the consequence of chloramphenicol use in neonatal humans when appropriate reductions in the adult dosage schedule were not made.

There is very little information available on drug disposition in neonatal dogs and cats. As a consequence, drugs should be used sparingly and with caution in this age group. Another factor predisposing neonates to adverse effects of drugs is undeveloped renal and hepatic excretory mechanisms. As with drug biotransformation, several weeks are required for excretory mechanisms to become fully functional. Degeneration of organ function resulting in excessive drug accumulation may make older animals predisposed to ADRs. In humans, the risk of ADRs in patients over 60 years of age is about double that in young adults.

Veterinarians have long recognized that cats are more sensitive to many drugs than are other species. Some reasons for this include:

1. A slower rate of biotransformation for many drugs. Cats also cannot conjugate drugs with glucuronic acid because they lack glucuronyl transferase, a critical enzyme in this reaction.
2. Cats exhibit unusual receptor-site sensitivity to many drugs. For example, reserpine produces sedation, which persists for a week in cats, whereas a two-day period of tranquilization is characteristic of other species. Morphine, in high doses, produces excitation in cats, whereas sedation is characteristic in most other species.
3. The grooming habits of cats facilitate the ingestion of any substance falling on their fur. Thus, cats are likely to receive a larger internal dose than would other species of any substance being used in the area in the form of an aerosol or dust.

Concurrent disease can enhance the possibility of ADRs in several ways. Disease conditions characterized by depressed renal and/or liver function, dehydration, or acidosis may result in higher concentrations of drug in the body than would be expected following conventional drug doses.

Drug Interactions. An ADR may stem from the concurrent use of another drug. These ADRs may occur either outside or within the body.

The practice of mixing drugs together in the same syringe or infusion solution prior to injection is risky, as the resultant mixture may be incompatible. Some drug incompatibilities include the inactivation of aminoglycoside antibiotics (e.g., gentamicin, kanamycin) by semisynthetic penicillins and the inactivation of penicillin G by solutions of high or low pH or those that contain vitamin B complex vitamins with vitamin C. It should be kept in mind that many drugs can alter the results of laboratory tests. Specimens should be taken for laboratory analysis before drugs are given to the patient.

A number of drug interactions can occur that involve the pharmacokinetic phase of drug action (e.g., absorption, distribution, biotransformation, and excretion) as well as the action at drug receptor sites. Some illustrative examples follow.

Tetracycline reacts with divalent metals to form insoluble complexes. The coadministration of Kaopectate, milk, or iron preparations has been shown to reduce markedly the intestinal absorption of tetracycline. When tetracycline and metal-containing preparations are administered orally, they should be given at least two hours apart.

Some drugs are potent inhibitors of the biotransformation of other drugs, including pentobarbital and phenytoin (Dilantin) in several species. Dogs remained anesthetized two times and cats three times longer when a therapeutic dose of chloramphenicol was given at the same time as pentobarbital. Signs of phenytoin toxicity (including ataxia, tremors, and incoordination) have been precipitated in dogs when chloramphenicol therapy was instituted to treat a concurrent infection. Signs of toxicity abated when the dosage of phenytoin was reduced by half.

Some drugs are potent stimulators of the biotransformation of other drugs. Phenobarbital has been shown to enhance the biotransformation of many drugs in several species. Phenobarbital has been reported to enhance the rate of biotransformation of digoxin in dogs. If these drugs are given together, more digoxin may be required to digitalize the dog. An ADR from digoxin could arise if the administration of phenobarbital ceased and the dosage of digoxin remained the same.

Human Errors. An adverse response resulting from human error perhaps should not be considered an ADR because the reaction may be expected to occur under the circumstances. Nevertheless, some human errors that can result in adverse responses include (1) dosage error due to miscalculation, (2) inappropriate route of administration — for example, a suspension designed for intramuscular or subcutaneous administration may produce a fatal embolism if administered intravenously, and (3) excessive rate of administration by the intravenous route — for example, meperidine can produce a fatal hypotensive collapse if a therapeutic dose is given by rapid intravenous administration. Meperidine, as is the case with many drugs that are organic bases, is capable of effecting a rapid release of histamine in the body.

SUPPLEMENTAL READING

Koch-Weser, J., Sidel, V.W., Sweet, R.H., Kanarek, P., and Eaton, A.E.: Factors determining physician reporting of adverse drug reactions. Comparison of 2000 spontaneous reports with surveillance studies at the Massachusetts General Hospital. New Engl. J. Med. 280:20–26, 1969.

Miller, R.R., and Greenblatt, D.J. (eds.): *Drug Effects in Hospitalized Patients*. New York, John Wiley & Sons, 1976.

Venulet, J.: Methods of monitoring adverse reactions to drugs. Prog. Drug Res. 21:231–292, 1977.

TERATOGENESIS AND MUTAGENESIS

NORMAN R. SCHNEIDER, D.V.M.

Lincoln, Nebraska

Birth defects are a very real, unavoidable fact of life for both the physician and the practicing veterinarian. In the human community, birth defects have disastrous consequences for involved families and profound implications for society in general in terms of the treatment and maintenance of afflicted individuals. This fact was thrust into worldwide awareness two decades ago when the drug thalidomide, introduced as a treatment for anxiety in pregnant women, led to the birth of approximately 10,000 severely malformed children. Chemical agents are not unique in their ability to induce birth defects. The atomic explosions that successfully brought World War II to an end also exposed a large civilian population in Japan to high levels of intensely ionizing radiation. The toll of the genetic damages caused by this radiation was great and continues to grow. Another important cause of human birth defects is exposure of the pregnant mother to certain viral agents. In this regard, rubella infections in the first trimester of pregnancy have been responsible for a variety of congenital defects, frequently including blindness, deafness, and valvular heart lesions.

The same factors that adversely affect the unborn offspring in the human population can potentially induce similar genetic damage in the young of the family pet, whatever species it may be. It is hoped that birth defects in the offspring of pets will not be due to inappropriate prenatal care, whether accidental or intentional. With normal precautions, it is unlikely that an animal could be exposed to and subsequently affected by the vast majority of potentially harmful agents, yet the hazard still exists. Every precaution should be taken to minimize the potential for inducing damaged offspring, since these can impose a difficult moral and ethical quandary on both the clinician and the owner. It is much easier to prevent developmental defects than to treat them post-parturition. Consequently, veterinary practitioners need to be aware of the etiologies and sequelae of abnormal development. It is the express goal of this chapter to provide a review of teratogenic and mutagenic agents affecting small animals frequently seen

in clinical situations. The emphasis here is on information pertinent to dogs and cats. However, since laboratory animals are frequently maintained as pets, especially in urban areas where maintenance of larger animals is not feasible, data regarding rodents, lagomorphs, and primates are also included. Interspecies and intraspecies differences in metabolism and physiology make it highly unlikely that effects observed in one species can be presumed to occur in an untested species. Interspecies extrapolation of observed congenital deformities should be avoided, while bearing in mind that the possibility that an agent teratogenic in one species can be teratogenic in other species as well.

CURRENT CONCEPTS OF TERATOGENESIS AND MUTAGENESIS

Teratology is the study of prenatal developmental abnormalities in structure or function that are related to the effects of intrinsic or extrinsic factors. Teratogens are those agents that can induce or increase the incidence of congenital maldevelopment when administered to or acting on the pregnant animal. These factors can be physical, nutritional, hereditary, chemical (including drugs and environmental pollutants), infectious or metabolic (physiologic). Each of these factors will be discussed in this chapter.

Teratogenic changes are defined by some traditionalists to be only *generative* changes in development that are limited to the period of organogenesis. Developmental changes that occur during other periods of gestation are defined as toxicologic (rather than teratogenic) changes and are considered *degenerative*, since they affect biologic systems that are already partially or completely formed. Additionally, *in utero* deaths and resorptions are not regarded as specific teratogenic effects. Other experts in this field have promoted the broader concept of *developmental toxicology* and contend that exposure to potentially deleterious agents during the complete span of development can produce several different toxic effects on the developing

161

conceptuses, such as embryonic or perinatal death, structural malformations, growth retardation, post-natal functional or behavioral abnormality, and congenital neoplasia. This total concept of *embryotoxicity* includes, but is not limited to, teratogenic effects. It encompasses all the various toxic effects mentioned previously.

A mutation is any heritable macromolecular or micromolecular change of genetic material. The mutation may be due to the chemical alteration of an individual gene and is called a gene or *point mutation*. The change may also involve a rearrangement, gain, or loss of parts of a chromosome, which may be microscopically visualized and which is termed a *chromosomal mutation*. Mutations may occur in any somatic or germ cell. If the capacity for cellular division is unimpaired, the mutation may be transmitted to descendant cells. Mutagenic changes may be so severe that the cell involved dies. Results of mutations are usually undesirable and may include embryonic death, abortion, congenital anomaly, genetic disease, lowered resistance to disease, decreased life span, infertility, behavioral aberration, and carcinogenesis.

Very few agents, and only a very limited number of the many therapeutic substances, have been demonstrated to be mutagenic in animals. However, it behooves us as veterinarians to be aware of how heritable change in genetic material occurs, the agents that have the potential to induce mutagenesis, and the possible consequences of mutations on animal health and breed characteristics. High neonatal mortality may result from inbreeding and may be caused by a recessive gene in homozygous offspring. The lethal factor may be perpetuated by the heterozygote. The X-chromosome of dogs is thought to be the transmission site of familial amaurotic idiocy, hemophilia A and B, subluxation of the carpus, and cystinuria. In dogs, malformation of the mouth involving abnormal dentition usually occurs in toy breeds, especially those that are brachycephalic. Miniature poodles extensively inbred for color selection produced litters in which all the puppies had severely undershot mandibles.

Some agents that are mutagens are also potential teratogens. However, there is not a high degree of correlation between teratogenic and mutagenic activity. This may be related to the way these events are initiated in the biologic system. Mutagenicity implies action on a single cell, whereas teratogenesis requires the interference with differentiation of many cells during organogenesis. However, teratogenic expression can result from, or be accentuated by, mutagenic events. For example, the urinary system is most frequently involved in autosomal chromosomal disorders in man. All known malformations of the urinary system in humans are observed in children with chromosomal diseases, except for infantile polycystic kidney and medullary sponge kidney.

There are a number of considerations in the teratogen-conceptus interaction that affect the actual production of terata in animals. Primary among these is that susceptibility of the unborn to teratogens or embryotoxic agents varies with (and depends on) gestational age at time of exposure. There are roughly three critical periods of development between conception and parturition: (1) the predifferentiation period prior to germ layer formation (pregastrulation stage), (2) the period of early differentiation and organogenesis (embryonic stage), and (3) the period of advanced organogenesis (fetal stage).

During the pregastrulation period, the mammalian conceptus is relatively refractory to teratogenesis. At this stage, all undifferentiated cells would be expected to react to a teratogenic agent in a similar fashion. If the exposure affects a large enough portion of the cellular population, embryotoxicity rather than overt teratogenicity would be manifested either as embryolethality or growth retardation. Prior to implantation, high concentrations of teratogenic or embryotoxic agents may also inhibit placentation, thus resulting in resorption of the zygote and cessation of pregnancy. Expulsion of the developing organism from the uterus may simulate pseudopregnancy. A 5 percent fetal resorption after implantation is normal in dogs, but the causes of intrauterine deaths are not usually determined. Embryotoxic agents may not interfere with formation of the placenta, but they can still exert their effects.

Embryonic development is the period of greatest prenatal vulnerability to teratogenic agents. This embryonic stage begins with implantation and germ layer differentiation, and it continues through organogenesis and the beginning of histogenesis. Organogenesis occurs at varying times during gestation, depending on the animal species (Table 1). Early in this period, the greater the teratogenic insult, the more likely that the effect will be manifested as embryolethality and resorption of the conceptus rather than by overt teratogenesis, especially if occurring soon after implantation and placentation. Embryos surviving the teratogenic insult are easily deformed and have the highest frequency of structural defects. Susceptibility to both teratogenicity and embryolethality decline as organogenesis advances. However, both types of responses can still occur if the insult is severe. Critical periods of increased sensitivity to harmful influences are also known to occur

Table 1. *Organogenesis and Gestation in Various Mammals*

SPECIES	APPROXIMATE PERIOD OF ORGANOGENESIS (DAYS)°	AVERAGE DURATION OF GESTATION (DAYS)
Hamster	6–14	16–17
Mouse	7–16	19–21
Rat	8–17	21–23
Rabbit	6–20	30–32
Guinea Pig	10–25	67–68
Cat	13–30	63–65
Dog	14–30	58–63
Monkey (rhesus)	18–45	164–170

°Implantation is considered the start of organogenesis for this compilation.

during relatively late stages of organ system development, and repeated exposure over the entire period of organogenesis may result in multiple malformations.

During the fetal stage of development, resistance to teratogens and embryotoxic agents increases. Histogenesis, which began late in the embryonic stage, continues in the fetal stage to convert primordial organs into definitive ones through cellular and tissue differentiation. Functional activity and maturation continually progress throughout the fetal period. As embryos differentiate into fetuses, maldevelopment manifested by gross structural defects is less likely to occur, except in those structures undergoing growth and maturation, such as the palate, cerebellum, and some cardiovascular and urogenital structures. Effects of maldevelopment on structure may only be detectable at the microscopic level and may not be recognized in surviving young until well into the juvenile period, when behavioral and functional abnormalities such as learning and reproductive difficulties arise. The etiology of the functional or behavioral aberrations may be due to the interference with ongoing histogenesis or to the prevention of final functional maturation. However, it is not always possible to determine which pathway was responsible.

A dose-response relationship prevails for teratogenic and embryotoxic effects just as it does for other toxic effects. Usually, there exists a relatively limited dose range in which terata are produced. Exposure above this teratogenic zone may result in embryolethality rather than congenital anomalies, and dosages below this zone are without detectable effect. The greater the dosage range over which terata are observed without death occuring, the more likely it is that a clearly graded response to the insult will result. If an agent is teratogenic only over a very limited dosage range and embryolethal above it, the teratogenic response may even appear all-or-none in character. The dosage below which no adverse effects are apparent is called the *no-effect dosage* or the *threshold dosage*. Even though no discernible effects occur at sub-threshold dosages, this may mean that damage has occurred but has subsequently been repaired. It may also mean that the biologic system can maintain homeostasis without repair. As long as the final product does not differ appreciably from the usual product, no effects from the insult will be detected. Dosages of 1/10 to 1/100 of the threshold dosage are a generally acceptable safety limit for exposure.

Teratogenic agents are thought to act via specific mechanisms on developing cells to cause abnormal development. A mechanism includes the entire series of events between a cause and an effect. Not all mechanisms that act to produce an abnormal offspring are clearly understood. However, mutation, metabolic changes, enzymatic inhibition, and other biochemical alterations are some of the cellular reactions thought to initiate events that culminate in developmental abnormalities. Death, malformation, growth retardation, and functional disorders are the final manifestations of abnormal development.

Susceptibility to teratogenesis also depends on the animal genotype and the nature of the influencing agent. The same determinants that differentiate individuals, strains, and species in normal structure and function may also give varying degrees of sensitivity to deleterious influences. These factors include differences in metabolism, placentation, and morphology. They are related to both the host and to the nature of the agent itself. There are only two basic ways an extrinsic factor can reach a developing conceptus to exert its influence: it can either traverse the maternal body directly (such as ionizing radiation) or it can be transmitted through it indirectly (such as chemicals or infectious agents). Agents indirectly transmitted through the maternal body generally reach the conceptus in some fraction of the original concentration, of which the exact value is dependent on its route of administration, absorption, and resultant pharmacokinetics.

POTENTIAL CAUSES OF CONGENITAL MALDEVELOPMENT

GENERAL CONSIDERATIONS

The understanding of teratogenesis and mutagenesis should be related to one common goal — that of completing the gestational period with a minimum of risk to both the mother and her offspring, culminating with the delivery of normal, healthy neonates. This is true of both the veterinary practitioner and the clients served. Relatively few agents are known to cause maldevelopment in dogs and cats, especially under other than experimental conditions. Agents shown to produce mammalian maldevelopment are usually administered at higher dosages or exposures than would be normally expected, and species most often utilized are rodents and lagomorphs. Although the mutagenic, teratogenic, and embryotoxic effects of many of these agents have not been demonstrated beyond reasonable doubt, neither has adequate proof of their safety been shown. Whereas predictive extrapolation between mammalian species is difficult at best and impossible at worst, these agents still have demonstrated the potential to produce congenital defects in at least one species, and they should be managed accordingly.

HEREDITY

Since dogs, cats, and other companion animals inhabit an environment similar to that of their owners, they also share similar threats to their genetic health. Impaired genetic health can be caused by inheritance of genetic and chromosomal aberrations resulting from mutagenic effects. Ionizing radiation is a potent mammalian mutagen, but a great number of suspected mutagens are found in the environment in addition to ionizing radiation.

The following agents have been tested for mutagenicity and are referenced in the files of the Environmental Mutagen Information Center (EMIC) at the Oak Ridge National Laboratory. The presence of agents in this listing indicates *suspected*, not confirmed, mutagenicity. Although agents may belong to more than one category, they are listed only once for convenience.

SUSPECTED MUTAGENS

1. **Agricultural chemicals.** This category is subdivided into various types of pesticides currently in use that are suspected of having mutagenic potential.

Herbicide	Fungicide	Insecticide	Chemosterilant	Rodenticide
2,4-D	cycloheximide	formaldehyde	triethylenemelamine	aminopterin
2,4,5-T	ethylene oxide	DDT	TEPA	
	captan	dieldrin	metepa	
	ethylene bromide	endrin	apholate	
			hempa	

2. **Industrial compounds and environmental pollutants.** These compounds have industrial application and are also released during the processing and combustion of fossil fuels.

dimethylnitrosamine	methylcholanthrene	Hg, Pb and Cd-
ethylenimine	benzene	containing compounds
benzo(a)pyrene	1,2-benzanthracene	pounds

3. **Food additives.** These substances are intentionally added to foods during processing. However, residues (non-intentional additives) from other categories may also be present in animal diets.

sodium nitrite (nitrous acid)	EDTA
sodium cyclamate	sodium bisulfite

4. **Naturally occurring substances.** Coumarin is a plant alkaloid found in sweet clover that has anticoagulant properties. Aflatoxin B_1 is an extremely potent mycotoxin that is the metabolite of *Aspergillus flavus*, which is found as a contaminant of cereal grains and other foodstuffs.

5. **Drugs.** Compounds having a known use in veterinary medicine that were tested for mutagenic effects are listed below. Many of these are antibiotics and antineoplastic agents that have the ability to interfere with or suppress cellular function.

Drug	*Use*
caffeine	stimulant
colchicine	mammary tumors in dogs
actinomycin D	antibiotic
cyclophosphamide	antineoplastic agent
ethidium bromide	antiparasitic agent
urethane	anesthetic
hydrogen peroxide	topical antiseptic
cytosine arabinoside	antineoplastic agent
ethylene oxide	sterilizing surgical instruments
streptomycin	antibiotic
vincristine	antineoplastic agent
theophylline	muscle relaxant, diuretic, myocardial stimulant
hexachlorophene	bacteriocidal soap, anti-trematodal agent
methylene blue	diagnostic dye, cyanide antidote
dichlorvos	antiparasitic agent
adriamycin	antileukemic agent
chlorpromazine	tranquilizer, antiemetic
carbaryl	antiparasitic agent
mercury chloride	disinfectant
griseofulvin	antifungal, antibiotic
phenylbutazone	analgesic, antipyretic
urea	antiseptic
lead acetate	astringent
erythromycin	antibiotic
gamma-lindane	scabicide, antiparasitic agent
dieldrin	antiparasitic agent
phenobarbital	sedative, anticonvulsant
mustard oil	counterirritant

6. **Biologic agents.** Viruses are capable of inducing genetic injury as well as potentiating damage induced by other agents. A large number of viral agents of importance to human medicine have been suspected of having mutagenic potential. Of these, the measles virus may be of some concern in veterinary medicine, since it is utilized in the immunization of dogs against canine distemper. The use of measles vaccine is contraindicated in breeding bitches.

RADIATION AND OTHER PHYSICAL AGENTS

Radiation can be either ionizing or nonionizing. Ionizing radiation is one of the most potent teratogenic agents known. Sources of ionizing radiation commonly utilized in veterinary medicine are X-rays and radioisotopes. The classic triad of radiation embryologic syndromes includes (1) intrauterine or extrauterine growth retardation, (2) embryonic, fetal, or neonatal death, and (3) congenital malformations. The central nervous system is the structure most commonly affected in mammals. The veterinary practitioner should limit elective radiologic examinations or treatments of the pregnant bitch or queen until immediately prior to delivery.

Mammalian fetuses can also be malformed by microwave radiation, a non-ionizing radiation used therapeutically in human medicine to raise the temperature of the pelvic organs. Hyperthermia is thought to be the primary effect of microwave radiation. The mammalian embryo, like the mammalian eye, is exquisitely sensitive to hyperthermia because of its relative inability to dissipate heat from its fluid compartments to the maternal circulation. Although microwave radiation is not routinely used in therapeutic regimens in veterinary medicine, it is mentioned here as a precautionary measure.

Hyperthermia can also result from other causes. Environmental causes, such as exposure to hot summer temperatures in conjunction with exercise or inadvertently locking a pregnant animal in a closed automobile in warm climates, can elevate deep-core body temperatures significantly. Febrile illnesses during pregnancy might also pose significant risk of potential embryotoxicity due to hyperthermia. The CNS is the primary target organ of hyperthermia effects, but brain growth retardation may be the only major manifestation. At the other end of the temperature scale, hypothermia during gestation in rats, mice, and hamsters caused increased embryonic mortality and developmental defects, which include skeletal and CNS abnormalities.

Ultrasound radiation is another form of non-ionizing radiation that has application in veterinary medicine. Not only is ultrasonography used in obstetric procedures to determine size and number of fetuses but also in echocardiography and ocular examinations. Although diagnostic ultrasound in the milliwatt range has not been shown to be harmful to the mammalian embryo, it is suspected that ultrasonic radiation can produce tissue or cellular damage at any level of exposure. Therefore, the quantitative aspects are extremely important in considering its embryotoxic effects on the developing conceptus. It is not certain what relationship the quantitative and qualitative aspects of ultrasonic radiation have on its interaction with the mammalian embryo, so the decision involving its elective use with pregnant animals should be made judiciously.

Hypoxia (anoxia) is one of the oldest known environmental teratogens and can produce a significant frequency of structural and functional abnormalities in several species of animals including the cat. A number of conditions can lead to the hypoxic state: (1) inadequate oxygen in inspired air, such as from unaccustomed high altitude exposure or during anesthesia, (2) maternal or fetal anemia, or (3) chemically caused conditions such as methemoglobinemia, carboxyhemoglobinemia, or cyanide-induced inhibition of cellular respiration. *Excess* oxygen was also found to cause gross congenital abnormalities in mammals when pregnant females were exposed to hyperbaric conditions. This could occur during anesthesia. Common atmospheric pollutants that are also pulmonary irritants (ozone, nitrogen oxides, and sulfur dioxide) can have a physiologic effect by interfering with maternal breathing, and they are suspected of increasing prenatal mortality.

Trauma, such as a bad fall, cannot be overlooked as having possible deleterious effects during gestation, especially if severe. Osteogenic defects occurred following a traumatic incident with a resulting two-day coma in a pregnant bitch nearing the period of implantation. Abortions have also occurred in pregnant dogs following involvement in minor automobile accidents at days 32 to 35 of gestation.

INFECTIONS

Viruses are the most important etiologic agents in malformations caused by infectious agents, especially during the early stages of development (Table 2). The rubella (measles) virus, Venezuelan equine encephalitis virus, and mumps virus have been shown to cause congenital defects in the human fetus. Terata produced by viruses may resemble classic defects of embryogenesis, such as cerebellar degeneration and hypoplasia caused by the feline panleukopenia virus in cats. This virus has an affinity for dividing cells, making the CNS especially vulnerable to *in utero* infections. In fact, the CNS is the organ system in which lesions and malformations due to viruses are most frequently described. The feline viral rhinotracheitis (FVR) virus, also referred to as feline herpesvirus I, is implicated in abortion and embryolethality in natural or experimental infection in the pregnant queen. Pregnant bitches or queens should not be vaccinated with modified live virus vaccines until the effects on the developing young have been adequately determined.

Infectious agents other than viruses can be teratogenic or embryotoxic. *Brucella canis* has been shown to cause early embryonic deaths in dogs. The protozoan agent causing toxoplasmosis, *Toxoplasma gondii*, has been responsible for structural and functional abnormalities of the CNS in human fetuses, but it is not known whether similar effects result from congenital

Table 2. *Viral Teratology of Mammalian Species — Naturally Occurring and Experimentally Induced*

VIRAL AGENT	TERATA	ANIMAL SPECIES
Arenavirus		
Lymphocytic choriomeningitis	Cerebellar hypoplasia, ataxia	Mouse, rat
Myxovirus		
Influenza	Hydrocephalus	Monkey, hamster
Oncornavirus		
Feline leukemia virus	Thymic atrophy	Cat
Orbivirus		
Bluetongue	Hydraencephaly, porencephaly	Lamb, mouse, hamster
Paramyxovirus		
Mumps virus	Hydrocephalus	Hamster
Parainfluenza virus type 2	Hydrocephalus	Hamster
Parvovirus		
Feline panleukopenia virus	Cerebellar hypoplasia	Cat, ferret
Rat virus	Cerebellar hypoplasia	Rat, hamster, cat, ferret
Minute virus	Cerebellar hypoplasia	Mouse
Reovirus		
Reovirus type 1	Hydrocephalus	Hamster, mouse, rat, ferret
Togavirus		
Bovine diarrhea-mucosal disease virus	Cerebellar hypoplasia, hydrocephalus, blindness, cerebral destruction	Calf, lamb
Hog cholera virus	Cerebellar hypoplasia, hypomyelinogenesis, microcephaly, hydrocephalus, small cerebral gyri, cerebellar agenesis, skeletal and urogenital defects	Swine
Venezuelan equine encephalitis virus	Cerebral cysts, microcephaly, cataracts, hydrocephalus	Monkey

Modified from Wilson and Fraser, 1977

infections in dogs and cats. Another infectious agent that is a human teratogen is *Treponema pallidum*, the human syphilis spirochete, which has caused CNS and skeletal developmental abnormalities in human neonates.

NUTRITION-RELATED DISORDERS

Maternal nutrition has an important effect on prenatal development. Although problems in nutrition are usually considered to be deficiency-related, excesses of certain nutritional components can also have deleterious effects, especially concerning congenital abnormalities.

In dogs, long-term maternal malnutrition can be one of the primary causes of puppy mortality in the neonate. Experimentally, malnutrition in pregnant rats produced no structural malformations in the young, but possible metabolic changes and less rapid development were the sequelae. Maternal undernutrition in pregnant queens caused abnormal brain development (decreased brain weights) and behavioral abnormalities in the kittens, but no gross defects were observed. Fasting for long periods during pregnancy was reported to have teratogenic effects in mice, but similar results have not been described in other species.

Improper dietary levels of nutritional factors can be deleterious to the developing young. Fat-soluble vitamins such as vitamin A can induce teratogenesis at either greater or lesser than dietary requirements. Congenital malformations due to vitamin A deficiency were initially reported in swine and later in rats and rabbits. The terata observed were ocular defects and anomalies of the urogenital and cardiovascular systems. Hypervitaminosis A also produces congenital malformations in various animal species — rat, guinea pig, hamster, rabbit, and swine. In pregnant bitches, vitamin A administration of 1250-fold greater than the recommended daily intake of 100 IU/lb, when dosed from days 17 to 22 of gestation, produced abnormalities such as cleft palate, accessory auricles, and kinked tails in puppies that survived the embryotoxic effects. The minimal dosage of vitamin A known to produce teratogenic effects has not yet been identified.

Normal dietary levels of other fat-soluble vitamins are essential for normal mammalian prenatal development. Vitamin D deficiency results in skeletal defects and abnormal dentition, whereas hypervitaminosis D in rats and rabbits impairs fetal osteogenesis. Dicoumarol, a vitamin K analog used in the prevention and treatment of thromboembolic disease, has been shown to cause decreased prothrombin levels in neonatal dogs and rabbits when administered at therapeutic dosages to pregnant females.

Experimentally induced deficiencies of B-complex vitamins in diets of pregnant rats have produced developmental abnormalities in their offspring. These effects ranged from increased embryotoxicity and low birth weight to skeletal and dental anomalies, CNS abnormalities, and soft tissue defects in the cardiovascular and urogenital systems.

Major mineral elements play an important role in proper fetal development and normal gestation. With a calcium-deficient maternal diet, fetal calcification and ossification can be normal at the expense of calcium removal from the maternal skeleton. Excess dietary calcium, however, has caused abnormal offspring in rats. Dietary magnesium deficiency in pregnant rats was more deleterious to developing fetuses, with embryonic death and malformations resulting. Pregnant rats maintained on a low-sodium diet produced young not significantly different from controls with no abnormalities. However, hypernatremia in pregnant mice injected with high dosages of sodium chloride (2g/kg) contributed to increased fetal death and malformations.

Proper dietary levels of other minerals (trace elements) are important to the prenatal development. Iron, copper, iodine, manganese, and zinc deficiencies in maternal diets have all been implicated in developmental anomalies. Pregnant rats maintained on an iron-deficient diet had offspring that were severely anemic and nonviable. Copper deficiency in pregnant sheep produces a disease in their lambs called enzootic ataxia ("swayback"), characterized by abnormalities in development of the CNS. The guinea pig exhibits a similar syndrome, with marked agenesis of the cerebellum in the neo-

nate. Rats on a copper-deficient diet produce offspring with skeletal anomalies and abdominal hernias. A characteristic ataxia in offspring of manganese-deficient animals due to failure of otolith development in the inner ear has also been reported. This syndrome has been described in the rat, pig, guinea pig, and mouse. Iodine deficiency in maternal diets is manifested as hypothyroidism in the fetus, producing a condition known as cretinism in humans. Excessive iodine in the mothers' diet also produces cretinous children, and a cretinism-like condition has been produced experimentally in dogs with excess iodine in the diet of the dams. Malformations resulting from zinc deficiency in the pregnant rat affected every organ system, with a high incidence of CNS anomalies and hyperplasia of the esophageal mucosa.

METABOLIC AND ENDOCRINE FACTORS

Of the various syndromes (diabetes, phenylketonuria, virilizing tumors) that have the potential to induce teratogenic effects in the human fetus, none are reported to produce abnormalities in pets as a result of naturally occurring conditions. Diabetic animals may become pregnant, but deliberate breeding obviously would be discouraged.

CHEMICAL AGENTS

This is by far the largest group of potential teratogens and includes both therapeutic agents and environmental chemicals. Many types of drugs and environmental chemicals have been reported as teratogenic in one or more species of mammals (Table 3). Few chemical agents are proven teratogens in dogs and cats, and teratogenic effects in experimental animals have usually been seen at dosages higher than recommended levels for therapeutic agents, or far above the usual exposure levels for the environmental chemicals. Embryotoxicity other than teratogenesis is sometimes more subtle and difficult to detect or predict. Interactions with other compounds and other complicating factors may also be involved.

Many pesticides have been shown to be teratogenic in various species of animals. Carbaryl, a widely used insecticide that reversibly inhibits cholinesterase, caused multiple developmental abnormalities in 21 of 181 beagle pups when administered in the diet to pregnant bitches throughout gestation. The teratogenic effects occurred at dosages as low as 3.125 mg/kg/day and were manifested as brachygnathia, ecaudate pups, failure of skeletal formation, superfluous phalanges, and abdominal-thoracic

Table 3. Potential Mammalian Teratogens

TYPE OF COMPOUND	SPECIFIC EXAMPLES
Anticonvulsants	Diphenylhydantoin, phenobarbital, primidone
Analgesics	Aspirin (salicylates)
Tranquilizers	Chlorpromazine, thalidomide, reserpine, meprobamate, diazepam
Certain alkaloids	Caffeine, nicotine, colchicine
Antihistamines	Buclizine, meclizine, cyclizine, hydroxyzine
Antibiotics	Chloramphenacol, streptonigrin, penicillin, tetracycline
Hypoglycemics	Carbutamide, tolbutamide, hypoglycins
Corticosteroids	Cortisone, triamcinolone, dexamethasone
Alkylating agents	Busulfan, chlorambucil, cyclophosphamide
Antimalarials	Chloroquine, quinacrine, pyrimethamine
Anesthetics	Halothane, urethane, nitrous oxide, pentobarbital
Antimetabolites	Methotrexate and aminopterin (folic acid analogs), purine and pyrimidine analogs
Sulfonamides	Acetazolamide, sulfanilamide
Plants	*Astragulus* spp., *Lupinus* spp., *Datura stramonium, Lathyrus* spp., *Veratrum californicum*
Mycotoxins	Aflatoxin, ochratoxin, cytochalasin B
Insecticides	Carbaryl, diazinon, lindane, aldrin, dieldrin, dichlorvos
Herbicides	MCPA (ethylester), paraquat
Fungicides	Griseofulvin, captan, methyl mercuric chloride, tetrachlorophenol
Hormonal agents	Progesterone plus norethindrone, testosterone
Industrial effluents	Certain compounds containing As, Cd, Hg, Li, Ni, Pb
Solvents	Dimethylsulfoxide
Miscellaneous	Trypan blue, fd&c red dye no. 2, penicillamine, ethyl alcohol, opiates, mescaline

fissures with varying degrees of intestinal agenesis and displacement. Dystocia from uterine atony also occurred frequently.

The insecticides diazinon and dichlorvos have been shown experimentally to be teratogenic, and other insecticides have demonstrated embryotoxicity. In beagle dogs, diazinon-exposed pups had enlarged, pronounced fontanelles and dental agenesis. Dichlorvos, the active ingredient in flea collars and fly strips, was reported to have produced malformations in the offspring of pregnant rats dosed on a single day of gestation with 15 mg/kg intraperitoneally. DDT was initially incriminated as the etiologic agent responsible for a number of biologically deleterious effects, including teratogenesis, but extensive research recently conducted in a number of mammalian species has shown no conclusive teratogenic effects. Beagle dogs were chronically exposed to 1, 5, and 10 mg of technical DDT/kg/day with no effect on reproduction and no gross or histologic findings in any of the 650 pups examined.

The phenoxy herbicide 2,4,5-T (and its related compound 2,4-D) also were incriminated as mammalian teratogens, especially as related to human exposure due to the utilization of 2,4,5-T as a defoliant ("Agent Orange") in Vietnam. However, more recent works have shown that the teratogenic effects were due to dioxins, which were contaminants associated with the manufacturing process. A change in manufacturing methods has reduced dioxin content in 2,4,5-T to the ppb (parts per billion) range, but some experts feel this herbicide formation may still be hazardous. By itself, 2,4,5-T is embryotoxic and fetotoxic at very high dosages. Other herbicides reported to cause mammalian malformations are paraquat and MCPA (ethylester).

A number of fungicides have been shown experimentally to be teratogenic in dogs and cats, as well as in other mammals. Pups from pregnant bitches receiving captan during gestation had crooked tails, gastroschisis, open fontanelles, and hydrocephalus. Offspring of pregnant bitches exposed to methyl mercury chloride (MeHgCl — a fungicide that is also an environmental contaminant) for 129 days at a dosage of 0.1 mg/kg developed congenital anomalies in one of ten litters, and these included cleft palate, patent fontanelles, superfluous phalanges, enlarged kidneys, and omphalocele. Fetal resorptions and perinatal death were observed. Pregnant cats given MeHgCl at a dosage of 0.25 mg/kg/day had increased incidence of abortions, and increased cerebellar developmental defects in the surviving neonates. Pets should not be fed meat or fish suspected of containing excessive mercury residues not only because of the teratogenic potential but also because it may cause irreversible neuropathy and blindness in the dam.

Griseofulvin, a systemic antifungal agent, is teratogenic in dogs, cats, and laboratory rodents. Cleft palate was present in six of seven pups from a golden retriever bitch treated with 750 mg griseofulvin/day for four weeks prior to pregnancy and throughout gestation. There was no history of abnormal litters from previous or subsequent matings. Pregnant beagles given 35 mg/kg/day for periods as short as one week to as long as the entire gestation period delivered puppies that were small, weak, and short-haired, with hemorrhages in the lumbar, cranial, and mandibular areas and in the extremities and abdomen. A large number of resorptions also occurred in the prenatal period.

Kittens from a pregnant cat receiving griseofulvin therapeutically have shown developmental anomalies such as shortened tails and hindlimbs, absence of phalanges, and fused phalanges of the posterior limbs. Cleft palate was observed in one out of three kittens from an experimental queen given 35 mg/kg/day throughout pregnancy. Increased teratogenic effects of larger dosages (500 to 1000 mg/animal), given at weekly intervals to three pregnant queens, included multiple congenital malformations of the brain and skeleton, specifically exencephaly, malformed prosencephalon, hydrocephalus, cranium bifidum, spina bifida, abnormal atlantooccipital articulation, cleft palate, absence of maxillae, and lack of tail vertebrae. Cyclopia and anophthalmia with absence of optic nerves and rudimentary optic tracts were also reported. Other abnormalities present were atresia ani, atresia coli, lack of AV valves in the heart, and absence of external nares and soft palate.

Administration of hormonal agents to pregnant animals should be avoided, even late in gestation. Testosterone propionate, injected subcutaneously into a pregnant bitch between days 35 and 42 of gestation, is thought to have caused ovarian hermaphroditism in two pups and abnormal clitoral development in the third. Progesterone and norethindrone therapy, administered during the period of gestation when the external genitalia were being formed, resulted in the masculinization of the external genitalia (abnormal fusion of the labia) in female pups from a pregnant boxer.

Administration of corticosteroids during gestation results in congenital anomalies in laboratory rodents, especially certain strains of mice. Dogs are also affected, and clinical evidence indicates that the increase in anasarcous pups in the brachycephalic breed may be related to corticosteroid therapy in the pregnant animal. Deformed forelegs, phocomelia, and ankylosed forelegs were observed in an entire litter of cocker spaniel pups after the dam had been treated with dexamethasone during the terminal half of gestation.

Thalidomide, the notorious human teratogen, does not have the same teratogenic response of phocomelia in other mammals except for the simian primate. The dog is not a good model for thalidomide teratogenesis, but at high maternal dosages, the surviving neonates were weak, short-haired, and had crooked tails, renal agenesis, patent fontanelles, and testicles attached near the kidneys. In cats, thalidomide teratogenesis was manifested primarily as cardiovascular defects such as ventricular septal defect, right atrial distention involving the coronary sinus, malpositioned great vessels, and narrowed left ventricular chamber with hypertrophied walls.

Other drugs shown to produce experimental teratogenesis in dogs are aminopterin, hydroxyurea, and hydroxyzine (Atarax®). Atarax®, in addition to being embryotoxic, produced pups with hooked, curved, and screw tails. Hydroxyurea, an anti-leukemia agent in humans, caused a wide variety of defects in pups of pregnant bitches given the drug. These developmental abnormalities included tail variants ranging from hooked tails to taillessness, hairlessness, hemorrhage in the muscles of the rear limbs, and agenesis; double cleft lip and palate; gastroschisis; scoliosis; patent fontanelles; and microphthalmia. In dogs, aminopterin caused early fetal deaths as well as teratism, and surviving pups were small and hairless with skeletal defects involving the tail and gastroschisis. In cats, aminopterin caused no conclusive teratogenic response, but methotrexate, a similar compound that is also a folic acid antagonist, produced high frequencies of malformations in kittens when given to pregnant queens on days 11 to 14 and 14 to 17 at a dosage of 0.5 mg/kg. Reported defects included umbilical hernia and retarded ossification of the cranium.

Although salicylates such as aspirin are not routinely considered to cause teratogenesis in dogs and cats, they are potent teratogens in the rat, effecting resorptions and malformations such as cleft lip, spina bifida, and other anomalies of the skeletal and vascular systems. Aspirin in dosages five to six times greater (500 mg/kg) than those effective in rats was found to be embryotoxic in monkeys.

The teratogenicity of diphenylhydantoin (phenytoin), an anticonvulsant, has been repeatedly demonstrated in mice and rats and is associated with a maternal plasma level of unbound drug that is only two to three times greater than normal therapeutic levels. Phenobarbital and primidone are suspected human teratogens, and the teratogenic potential of oxyzolidinedione anticonvulsants (trimethadione and paramethadione) must be considered before being used electively in the pregnant female.

Several antibiotics are teratogenic in rodents, whereas others are embryolethal. Tetracycline, streptonigrin, penicillin-streptomycin mixtures, and actinomycin D have been reported to cause malformations. Embryolethal antibiotics include those acting primarily by inhibiting protein synthesis, such as puromycin, lincomycin, and streptomycin. Other antimicrobial agents, such as sulfonamides, would seem to be potentially deleterious to mammalian development due to their mechanism of action. Yet, except for acetazolamide and sulfanilamide, these compounds have been reported to have little effect on development. Acetazolamide, a potent carbonic anhydrase inhibitor, caused uniquely localized malformation of the forelimbs in rodents.

Many agents affect the prenatal development of "experimental" animal species, but few are undisputed teratogens or mutagens for domestic animals. Expression of embryotoxicity involves many factors, some of which are known and some of which are as yet unresolved. The veterinary practitioner should establish a policy of minimizing the exposure of pregnant animals to potentially harmful agents during all phases of gestation.

In animals used for breeding, elective therapeutic, prophylactic, and diagnostic procedures are contraindicated during pregnancy and should be avoided unless medical requirements dictate otherwise. However, one should not hesitate to risk potential prenatal damage to the unborn if the pregnant patient is in immediate need of medical attention, as long as the client is advised of the possibilities and agrees to the proposed treatment. Birth defects in animals do not involve the same magnitude of moral and legal implications for society as they do in humans. However, developmental defects in any mammalian species are far more easily prevented than they are corrected postpartum, since by this time the response is irreversible.

Drugs, biologics, and other injectables should not be routinely administered to the pregnant female, nor should pregnancy be diagnosed radiographically until immediately prior to parturition. The nutritional requirements of gestation should be met with an adequately fortified and properly balanced diet, but the client should be cautioned about excessive home-prescribed vitamin-mineral supplementation, however well intentioned. Immunization should be accomplished prior to breeding, and care should be taken to avoid exposure of pregnant females to infectious diseases during gestation. Extreme environmental temperatures, either heat or cold, should be avoided over prolonged periods, as should strenuous exercise or traumatic insult.

The veterinary practitioner will likely see terata in various species of animals. Clients should be asked for a careful history of treatments, illnesses, or unusual happenings during gestation, since causes may not be readily apparent. A breeding history of both sire and dam for three generations should also be obtained to determine the incidence of previous developmental defects. Animals with defects of genetic origin should not be permitted to reproduce, but other anomalies may be surgically corrected if feasible. Even with all the scientific data at one's disposal, the etiology may be difficult to determine, requiring a judgmental decision to be rendered.

SUPPLEMENTAL READING

Becker, B.A.: Teratogens. In Casarett, L.J., and Doull, J. (eds.): *Toxicology — The Basic Science of Poisons.* New York, Macmillan Publishing Co., Inc., 1975.

Earl, F.L.: Teratogenesis. In Kirk, R.W. (ed.): *Current Veterinary Therapy VI.* Philadelphia, W.B. Saunders Co., 1977.

Robens, J.F.: Teratogenesis. In Kirk, R.W. (ed.): *Current Veterinary Therapy V.* Philadelphia, W.B. Saunders Co., 1974.

Wilson, J.G.: *Environmental and Birth Defects.* New York, Academic Press, 1973.

Wilson, J.G., and Fraser, F.C. (eds.): *Handbook of Teratology.* Vols. 1–4. New York, Plenum Press, 1977.

CARCINOGENESIS

T. GOPAL, M.V.Sc.

Hebbal, Bangalore, India

The normal behavior of a cell in the biologic system can be changed into neoplasia by the influence of various factors. Such a transformed cell is capable of further multiplication without any restraint on its growth and hence is designated as *cancerous*. The initiation process, *carcinogenesis*, comprises a complex of sequential events within the cell that eventually lead to *cancer*. Agents or factors responsible for initiating cancer are termed *carcinogens*. The study of carcinogens and carcinogenesis broadly includes the study of cancer and its pathogenesis.

INCIDENCE

Despite the fact that cancer can be induced by various etiologic agents, as evidenced by controlled experimentation in animals and circumstantial evidence in humans, the question remains unanswered as to the specific cause of some naturally and spontaneously occurring neoplasms in animals. The incidence of cancer in animals is mostly recognized by clinical signs, and many times it is encountered as an incidental finding during necropsy. The effect is seen, but not the cause.

MODIFYING FACTORS

The commonly observed spontaneously occurring neoplasms in animals suggest that genetic composition of the host is the most important intrinsic factor determining individual susceptibility and resistance. The genetic component can be modified by various endogenous factors such as heredity, age, sex, species, and breed. Other individual physiologic variations of hormonal, metabolic, and biochemical activities, which upset the normal homeostatic restraint on cell growth, also contribute to the initiation of carcinogenesis.

Animal neoplasms probably result from favorable host genetic composition acted upon by one or more interacting exogenous factors, such as various physical, chemical, or biologic agents, in combination. The information on the incidence of animal cancer suggests that many etiologic agents associated with human cancer may also be responsible for animal cancer. This is probably true, since domestic animals often share the same environment as man.

SOURCES

Most of the environmental carcinogens are found naturally, but some of them find their way into the environment intentionally or accidentally. The increasing incidence of human cancer and the experimental induction of cancer using newly synthesized chemicals support the fact that man-made environmental carcinogens will result in a continued distinct hazard to human and animal health.

The effect of slow-growing viruses in the environment combined with low-grade exposure to various chemical pollutants has increased the risk of cancer. The possibility that many dormant viruses are capable of triggering carcinogenesis has been suspected for many years, and the evidence accumulated by recent studies supports this concept.

ETIOLOGIC AGENTS

Physical Agents. Many of the physical agents carcinogenic in man are also carcinogenic in animals. Ultraviolet rays and ionizing radiation are major initiators of malignancy in experimental animals. Radioactive fallout from nuclear reactions has the potential for carcinogenic effects in animals.

Experimental studies in different species of animals with various radioactive substances have confirmed the carcinogenic effects of ionizing radiation. Whole-body radiation in dogs has produced cancer of the thyroid and has caused leukemias. Inhalation and ingestion of radioactive compounds have resulted in cancer.

Chronic irritation, as in some horn cancers in East Indian cattle, and the presence of certain parasites, like *Spirocerca lupi* in dogs and *Gasterophilus* spp. in horses, have been incriminated as initiators of cancer.

Chemical Agents. Owing to the increased use of synthetic chemicals in agriculture, medicine, and industry, chemical carcinogens have

172

received considerable attention. The frequency with which these substances appear and their potential properties of carcinogenic activity in man and animals have gained much importance. Some of them are intentionally included in foods as additives and preservatives, and others are included as drugs for therapy and increased food production. Others unintentionally find their way into the environment as synthetic fertilizers, insecticides, growth promoters, and industrial and automobile effluents.

Some of the known animal carcinogens are 2-naphthalamine, benzidine, 4-amino-biphenyl, 2-acetylaminofluorene, N-methyl-4-aminoazobenzene, dimethylnitrosamine, diethylstilbestrol, and polycyclic aromatic hydrocarbons. Among the naturally occurring carcinogens are aflatoxins, cycasins, and pyrrolizidine alkaloids.

The mechanism of chemical carcinogenesis varies with the chemical and its biologic behavior in a given species of animal. There is wide individual variation. Many theories have been suggested concerning the actual mechanism. In general, a common mechanism is suggested in which the chemical carcinogen acts by altering or destroying the preexisting genetic information in the normal host cell. In a simple way, a chemical carcinogen behaves by "hitting and running," leaving behind an altered cell. This is probably true for many chemicals, since they are often not present in the system during the actual growth of the cancer.

This suggests that the initial reaction between carcinogen and target cell may be of short duration and is most likely irreversible. In other instances, the chemical undergoes activation by various enzymatic systems to an ultimate carcinogen, which is highly reactive with cellular components, particularly those involved with genetic control of cell growth — i.e., DNA, RNA, and proteins.

Virtually all chemical carcinogens interact with DNA to produce alkylation, acylation, and depurination reactions. Recent evidence suggests that DNA is the genetic material that plays a key role in maintaining the functional integrity of the cell; after DNA's interaction with a chemical carcinogen, faulty information will be transferred during DNA replication. If the interaction occurs when DNA is replicating, the effect is immediate and permanent. However, if the carcinogen interacts with other macromolecular components of the cell, like RNA or other proteins, the change has to be incorporated into DNA at a later stage. This will lead to slow carcinogenesis. Whether interaction with the genetic component of the cell produces sponta-

neous transformation or a slow transformation, the ultimate effect is the same. In immediate transformation, the affected cell produces cancerous cells directly; the slow transformation process is successively transmitted through several generations until a population of completely transformed cells results.

Biologic Agents. Biologic carcinogens include a broad group of viruses of the RNA and DNA type. Studies of virus-induced neoplasms in birds and mammals indicate that the genetic material contained in the virus results in altered genetic control of the host cell, with subsequent transfer of information to successive generations. The DNA or RNA component of the virus is incorporated in the DNA or RNA of the cell and initiates cancer. Virus-induced malignancies include avian leukosis, sarcomas, and cutaneous papillomas in a wide range of animals. Leukemia and lymphosarcomas are frequently encountered in cats.

Certain parasites are associated with cancer of animals. *Spirocerca lupi*-induced sarcomas in dogs and cancer associated with *Ganglionema neoplasticum* in rats are some of the examples. The initiation of cancer by these agents has been attributed to chronic irritation rather than to chemical factors. Although the occurrence of carcinogenic metabolites has not been established, the possibility should not be overlooked.

The incidence of transmissible venereal lymphogranuloma in dogs is rare in the United States, but isolated cases are reported. The neoplastic cell is not the somatic component of the host but rather is mechanically transmitted by coitus. Under favorable conditions of susceptibility, the transplanted cell gives rise to successive neoplastic generations. Since there is no involvement of the host cell material, it appears that the host is used for the *in vivo* propagation of the neoplastic cell.

SUPPLEMENTAL READING

Farber, E.: Mechanisms by which chemicals initiate cancer. J. Clin. Pharmacol. *15*:24–28, 1975.

Heidelberger, C.: Chemical carcinogenesis. Ann. Rev. Biochem. *44*:79–121, 1975.

Meier, H.: Epizootiology of cancer in animals. Ann. N. Y. Acad. Sci. *108*:617–1325, 1963.

Moulton, J. E.: *Tumors in Domestic Animals.* Berkeley, California, University of California Press, 1961.

Temin, H. M.: On the origin of the genes for neoplasia. Cancer Res. *34*:2835–2841, 1974.

Wolff, A. H., and Oehme, F. W.: Carcinogenic chemicals in food as an environmental health issue. J. Am. Vet. Med. Assn. *164*:623–629, 1974.

BITES AND STINGS OF VENOMOUS ANIMALS

G. L. MEERDINK, D.V.M.
East Lansing, Michigan

In the 1970's, our society has become increasingly aware and often alarmed by poisonous substances in our environment. With few exceptions, however, man has not yet formulated substances to match the potency of many of the naturally occurring toxins. Many members of the animal kingdom produce toxins that are used offensively in the procurement of food by killing prey and occasionally to aid in digestion, and defensively for self-protection or protection of the colony. Venomous animals exist in essentially all parts of North America, although there is much variation in the venomous species that occur in specific regions of the country. The veterinarian should become familiar with the poisonous species of snakes and spiders in his area, since he will seldom know the identity of the perpetrator when presented with the bitten victim.

The therapeutic approach is stressed here through organization of the recommendations made by experts in the various areas. If more material regarding the toxic characteristics of a species or other information is desired, an additional reading list is supplied for referral.

POISONOUS SNAKES

Many species of snakes exist in North America, only a few of which are poisonous. But these few are important, as an estimated 15,000 domestic animals are bitten annually in the United States, and rattlesnakes account for approximately 80 per cent of the deaths (Knowles, Snyder, et al., 1974). The poisonous snakes of the United States are the rattlesnake (*Crotalus* spp. and *Sistrurus* spp.), copperhead (*Agkistrodon* spp.), water moccasin or cottonmouth (*Agkistrodon piscivorous*), and coral snake (*Micrurus euryxanthus*). The California lyre snake (*Trimorphodon vandenburghi*) and mangrove snake (*Boiga dendrophila*) are also venomous but are of minor importance to domestic animals. The pit viper venoms (rattlesnake, copperhead, and water moccasin) are primarily necrotizing and hemolyzing; however, other body systems can certainly be affected. The venoms primarily contain proteinaceous and enzymatic toxins. Phospholipase A is a strong hemolytic agent; L-amino-oxidase and other homologous enzymes may be responsible for the activation of tissue peptidases. Hyaluronidase, or "spreading factor," enhances tissue penetration. Numerous other protein and nonprotein constituents have been detected that may produce deleterious biologic effects. The coral snake is a member of the elapid or cobra family and shares the venom characteristic of being primarily neurotoxic. Cholinesterase is present in high concentrations in some species; however, this enzyme has been shown not to be the neurotoxic factor and does not contribute significantly to the neuromuscular block produced by these venoms.

FACTORS THAT CONTRIBUTE TO THE SEVERITY OF THE BITE

The severity of the bite first depends on the type and size of the snake and the toxicity of the venom. Besides a species variation in venom potency, a wide variation in the volume of venom injected exists. The snake may be able to regulate the amount of venom injected (in fact, many bites may not be venomizing); more venom may be available if the snake has not eaten for some time.

The number of strikes and the degree of fang penetration are important considerations. When lost, fangs are replaced, and more than one fang may be present on each side. Thus, fang marks from pit viper bites may vary from one to as many as six from one bite. The coral snake, with relatively short fixed fangs, must strike its victim squarely and securely to gain sufficient penetration for envenomation. On the other hand, the Eastern diamondback rattlesnake, with fangs of up to 2.4 cm, can readily penetrate into deeper, more vascular tissues. Fang length, overall size and strength, and the high yield of venom give the Eastern diamondback rattlesnake the dubious honor of being one of the most dangerous snakes in the United States.

Temperament as well as the local population of the species may affect the incidence of bites seen by the practitioner. The water moccasin is reputed to be quite aggressive and may attack with little provocation. Coral snakes are secretive and remain undercover and usually strike only if disturbed. Rattlesnakes, on the other hand, cause the majority of snakebites even though they sound due warning to the intruder. (They may not always "sound off" with rattle vibration if suddenly disturbed.) The copperhead has the least potent venom of the North American viperine snakes.

As would be expected, many host factors play a role in determining the severity of the bite, including the site of the bite. Unfortunately, most snakebites in domestic animals occur around the head or neck area, increasing the chances of direct damage to vital structures and problems with treatment. Because of a lower venom/body weight ratio, increased severity would be expected in smaller animals, although cats are not often bitten and apparently have some increased resistance (Clarke and Clarke, 1975). Physical activity (which increases the uptake of venom into the circulation) and the length of time following the bite are also factors that the clinician must assess in his approach to treatment.

Clinical signs and diagnosis

Snakebite is not always easy to diagnose, particularly if heavy hair and swelling obscure fang marks. Other puncture-type wounds from objects, fish spines, or other animal bites are usually more ragged and do not have the same progressive clinical signs. Wounds from arthropods are usually smaller and do not bleed as freely. Bites of non-poisonous snakes cannot be differentiated reliably from those of poisonous snakes on the basis of puncture wound pattern. Any pattern may be observed with non-poisonous snakes, from single punctures to rows of multiple punctures; palatine and molar teeth may cause puncture wounds in addition to the one or more venom fangs of the poisonous species. However, less pain, little swelling, and absence of the progressive clinical signs will aid in differentiating non-poisonous from poisonous bites (Minton, 1974).

If venom is injected directly into the blood (vascular) system, severe systemic signs and sometimes death occur rapidly. Generally, however, the venom injected into tissues is transported via the lymphatics. Particularly with the pit vipers, the early signs are caused by the direct effects of the toxins on the local tissues. Pain, erythema, and edema develop as a result of the activation of histamine, bradykinin, and other tissue inflammatory agents. The swelling may become extensive and be accompanied by petechiae, ecchymoses, and hematomas. Secondly, in the clinical course, indirect effects from substances released from tissues because of the venom serve to enhance the local necrosis and promote the systemic effects of hypotension with tachycardia, pulmonary edema, salivation, diarrhea, and shock. After a few hours, hemolytic anemia, hemoglobinuria, and renal failure follow. In advanced cases, lethargy and paralysis develop; death is caused by respiratory and circulatory collapse (Knowles, Snyder, et al., 1974). If strikes occur in the head or neck area, swelling may rapidly cause respiratory distress.

Coral snake venom causes little local pain or swelling. Often, within a half hour, early neurotoxic effects can be observed, although a lag phase of several hours may elapse before the onset of signs. Difficulty in swallowing, depression, insensitivity of the limbs, and skeletal paralysis develop, leading to death by respiratory paralysis (Oehme et al., 1975).

TREATMENT

The bitten animal should be subdued and immobilized as much as possible to slow the uptake of venom. Basically, the objectives in the treatment of snakebite are: (1) to prevent spread of the venom, (2) to remove the venom, (3) to neutralize the venom, (4) to prevent shock, and (5) to prevent infection. Knowles, Snyder, et al. (1974) proposed the following courses of treatment after performing animal experimentation studies.

Incarcerate the venom. In cases of wounds of the extremity, a flat tourniquet should immediately be applied proximal to the fang mark area. It should not be applied so tightly that the limb becomes ischemic, but tight enough to impede superficial venous and lymphatic flow. Tourniquets of this sort may be left in place for as long as two hours without removal. A good rule to follow is to test the tightness by inserting a finger under the tourniquet band, and if this can be done easily it is applied properly. The tourniquet should *not* be removed at intervals because this will pump the venom from the initial site.

Remove the venom. A continuous linear incision should be made through both fang mark perforations and extend in depth to the fascia covering the muscle. Do not sever vital structures, such as tendons, motor nerves and major blood vessels. Do not use cruciate incisions because the tips of the incision are subject to necrosis, and such a wound is receptive to anaerobic contaminants and clostridial complications. Applying suction to the incision retrieves some of the venom and is advocated, although mouth suction is not recommended because two lives may be lost as a result of this procedure. Elliptical excision of the fang marks, including skin and subdermal fat, is more efficacious than incision and suction in removing the venom in severe envenomization. The size of the area involved in the elliptical excision is dependent upon the fang marks, but must extend at least 1/2 inch (1 cm) equidistant around the puncture wounds. This type of wound may be closed primarily at a later date.

Neutralize the venom. Polyvalent antivenin should be used in every subject suspected of serpent envenomization (Antivenin,® Fort Dodge Laboratories). The sooner the venom is neutralized, the better the therapeutic result. Because more time is required for the antivenin to reach the poisonous venom when given intramuscularly or into the bite area, we administer the antivenin intra-arterially or intravenously. We believe that the arterial route produces a faster and more potent effect than the venous route because the drug is more concentrated and acts upon the venom longer; antivenin given intravenously must traverse the cardiac-hepatic pulmonary circulation before reaching the bite area.

The method of intra-arterial perfusion should be performed only by veterinarians and is as follows: Mix the contents of one vial of polyvalent antivenin into 100 ml of normal saline and using a sphygmomanometer bulb, pump it into the regional artery with a tight tourniquet proximal to the arterial injection site. The tourniquet keeps the antivenin localized in the bite area, and direct neutralization of the venom takes effect. It requires about 20 minutes to pump the mixture into the area. If the patient has a history of allergic manifestations, 100 ml of hydrocortisone sodium succinate (Solu-Cortef®) should be added to the intra-arterial therapy. The regional arteries for infusion are the femoral artery for snakebites of the hind legs, the brachial artery for the forelegs and the carotid artery for the head and neck. We are aware that complications can ensue from intra-arterial injection, but we have not observed any in our experience; on the other hand we have observed death due to envenomization.

An antivenin is now available specifically for bites of coral snakes and may be ordered through the State Boards of Health.

Prevent shock. When less than a 100 percent lethal dose of moccasin venom is injected, pain is a significant factor in the onset of shock and in the longevity of the otherwise non-treated animal. Because morphine is excessively depressing to the respiratory mechanism, meperidine (Demerol®) appears to be the drug of choice for pain control in snakebite. Dosage should be 1 mg/lb (2 mg/kg) of body weight initially, and it should be given as needed to alleviate pain. Meperidine administration should be continued until the pain has subsided.

Prevent infection. Because snakes' mouths are frequently contaminated with pathogens, the skin in the bite area is not clean and massive tissue destruction with blood extravasation enhances bacterial activity, the administration of a broad-spectrum antibiotic is mandatory. We scrupulously follow the procedure of intramuscular or intravenous administration of cephaloridine (Loridine®) initially every 12 hours, followed by oral administration of doxycycline (Vibramycin®) every 12 hours.

Anaphylactoid Reactions. Specific anaphylactoid reactions, to either the venom or the antivenin, are rare in the dog. Corticosteroids should be given in ample dosage during the acute phase of this condition. Although they are not life-saving, corticosteroids significantly increase longevity and may therefore enable other medicaments to exert their beneficial effects. They minimize pain, improve the patient's sense of well-being, promote the even distribution of edema and hence minimize the possibility of slough. The snakebite victim that receives corticoids (prednisone, 1 mg/lb [2 mg/kg] of body weight initially and then 0.5 mg/lb [1 mg/kg] of body weight every 12 hours) is more likely to aid in the maintenance of normal fluid balance by consuming larger quantities of water and a reasonable amount of food as compared to the noncorticoid-treated patient that usually will neither eat nor drink.

Lactated Ringer's solution or blood may be indicated to bolster fluid volume and electrolyte levels. The animal should be kept warm and quiet. Immobilization is the most effective mechanical means of combating envenomization. In our opinion, immobilization can best be accomplished under these circumstances by a judicious use of the meperidine and quiet, comfortable quarters.

Ancillary Treatment. Calcium gluconate has been suggested to combat hemolysis and muscular twitching. Tetanus antitoxin is also indicated.

LIZARDS

The only species of poisonous lizards can be found in the Southwest — the Gila monster (*Heloderma suspectum*) and the Mexican beaded lizard (*H. horridum*). These lizards are lethargic and non-aggressive, and thus animal poisonings are rare. They do not have fangs per se but are armed with grooved teeth that are bathed in venom from modified salivary glands. Lizards hold on to the victim and, with chewing movements, increase the quantity of envenomation.

Initially, pain and swelling occur around the wound site and may progress toward the body. Vomition followed by shock and central nervous system depression may occur in severe cases. Treatment is primarily symptomatic and can be managed clinically in a manner similar to that for snakebite therapy. Meperidine HCl should not be used, however, as it has been reported to have some synergistic activities with the lizard venom (Fry, 1977; Oehme et al., 1976; Minton, 1974).

BEES, WASPS, HORNETS, AND ANTS

The order *Hymenoptera* contains the important stinging insects — the bees, wasps, hornets, and ants. Many species of this order are more dangerous because of the colony's aggressive reaction to disturbance and its ability to inflict a multitude of stings within a few minutes. The venom apparatus is located on the terminal portion of the abdomen. In a few species including the honey bee, the sting is barbed and the entire venom apparatus is torn from the insect's body and left attached to the victim. The venoms within this order vary among species but characteristically include proteinaceous compounds with histamine, hyaluronidase, and hemolyzing components. Insect stings are the leading cause of human deaths from venomous animals in the United States, primarily because of the hypersensitization properties of the venoms and anaphylactic deaths from subsequent exposure.

Stings of these insects cause painful local inflammation. The intensity of the reaction can be increased by multiple stings to the extent that shock becomes an important clinical problem. If the victim has been previously exposed to the venom and hypersensitized, anaphylaxis can result from only one sting.

The first consideration in clinical management is the possibility of anaphylaxis or shock from multiple stings. The site of the bite(s) can be very important; asphyxiation may result from swelling of the buccal or pharyngeal area. If needed, 1 to 5 ml of a 1:10,000 aqueous solution of epinephrine should be injected subcutaneously in dogs and cats, as well as corticosteroids and antihistamines. (Antihistaminics are of little value in fire ant stings.) The clinician must be alert to the fact that in some cases, anaphylaxis may be delayed. Oxygen may be necessary if dyspnea is evident. Pain and swelling of local reactions can be reduced by cold packs (Minton, 1975; Oehme et al., 1976).

SPIDERS

Practically all spiders are venomous; however, severe reactions are limited to two genera: *Lactrodectus* spp. (black widow and red widow, female) and *Loxosceles* spp. (brown recluse and common brown). The infamous tarantula (*Eurytelma* sp.) is capable of a venomous bite, but serious reactions from natural bites in domestic animals have not been reported.

Spiders subsist on the body fluids of their prey and thus use their venom to immobilize the victim. Venom is injected through channeled bilateral head appendage fangs called *chelicerae*. Considering the inconspicuous size of the bite marks and animal hair cover, diagnosis of spider bites is difficult for the veterinarian unless, perhaps, the spider is located. The black widow is black (other species are brown to reddish) with red or red-yellow spots, the most constant being an hourglass shape on the ventral aspect of the abdomen. Brown recluse spiders are tawny to brown with a darker (often violin-shaped) mark on the dorsal cephalothorax. Because of its relatively long legs, the brown recluse is capable of quick movement.

Lactrodectus spp. venoms are highly toxic to mammals. The severity of the black widow bite may vary, but it is usually characterized by short-lived local pain. Neurotoxic manifestations soon follow and are characterized by muscle spasms, evidence of abdominal pain, ataxia, excessive salivation, tonic and clonic convulsions, and flaccid paralysis. Weakness with dyspnea followed by paralysis may occur within six hours in an acute case or not until several days later in a less severe envenomation. Increases in blood pressure and ECG abnormalities may be observed. Antivenin is available and, if used, should be administered as soon as possible. Corticosteroids, intravenous fluids, and prophylactic antibiotics should be administered. Methocarbamol, calcium gluconate, meperidine, and atropine may be used to control muscle spasms, pain, and excessive secretions. The prognosis is uncertain for several days (Minton, 1974; Clarke, 1975; Oehme et al., 1975).

Loxosceles spp. are primarily found in the southern half of the U.S. and are best known for the potent enduring dermonecrotic effects of their toxin. The spider is often found in basements, storage areas, and other darkened areas and will not bite unless provoked. The initial reaction from the bite is evidently not painful. However, within a few hours, the hemolytic and necrotizing toxins cause local pruritus and swelling, which develops into focal erythema and the formation of a blister. Necrosis follows as a result of ischemia, and by 7 to 14 days, the focal ulceration is evident. The lesion requires 8 weeks or longer to heal. Depending on the particular *Loxosceles* species and the susceptibility of the animal, systemic signs of fever, weakness, vomition, convulsions, hemolysis, and thrombocytopenia may also occur. Latest recommendations have advocated early excision of the affected tissue with primary repair. If not removed, the lesion has a tendency to spread, particularly into dependent areas. Corticosteroids and antibiotics should be administered, particularly if signs of systemic effects are detected (Oehme et al., 1975; Wasserman et al., 1977).

SCORPIONS

Several genera of scorpions exist in North America, but the most dangerous species live in the arid climates of Mexico and Arizona. The last segment of the highly mobile tail of this eight-legged arthropod contains a hollow curved stinging apparatus through which venom is injected. Scorpion bites are not uncommon in humans and do produce fatalities; however, the incidence of bites in domestic animals is not known. Difficulty in recognition of the condition may account for its relatively low recorded incidence in veterinary medicine. Scorpion stings usually produce more severe immediate pain than do spiders. The puncture is single, bleeds little if at all, and may be very difficult to differentiate from insect stings in the early stages.

Generally, the earliest sign of envenomization is intense local pain associated with erythema and edema. Although the stings of most species cause only local reactions that subside within a few hours, the more toxic varieties may cause systemic neurotoxic effects. Parasympathomimetic signs include excessive salivation, muscle fasciculations, and weakness. Generalized weakness and paralysis may lead to respiratory distress. The clinical condition generally improves within 24 hours.

If little time has elapsed, the severity of the local reaction and the spread of the toxin can be partially prevented by prompt application of cold packs (without freezing of tissue) for up to two hours. Antivenins are available; one specific for the genus involved is best, although evidence exists of some cross protection. Atropine can be used to block the parasympathomimetic effects; and corticosteroids can decrease shock and edema. Meperidine and morphine derivatives are contraindicated, and intravenous fluids should be administered carefully because of the risk of pulmonary edema. Respiratory assistance may become necessary (Russel and Saunders, 1966; Minton, 1974; Oehme et al., 1975).

TICK PARALYSIS

Tick paralysis is an ascending afebrile motor paralysis that appears most commonly in children, cattle, sheep, and dogs. The offending ticks from paralyzed victims in North America are usually females of the *Dermacentor* or *Amblyomma* genera; their saliva contains hemorrhagic-neurotoxic elements that produce lesions of the central nervous system resulting in the clinical signs. Evidently, the tick must be attached for several days. Ataxia is first observed, which soon develops into an ascending motor paralysis. Within 36 hours from onset, the animal may become completely immobile, and death may follow if paralysis proceeds to the respiratory center. Removal of the ticks results in rapid recovery within hours, and the victim is usually completely asymptomatic within 48 hours. All ticks must be removed, as only one can cause the condition; the use of organophosphorus insecticide dips or sprays will aid in the removal process. Absence of fever, lack of abnormal spinal fluid findings, and evidence of normal sensory function will help differentiate this condition from central nervous system infections and other similar conditions.

SUPPLEMENTAL READING

Arnold, R. E.: *What to Do About Bites and Stings of Venomous Animals.* New York, The Macmillan Co., 1973.

Brown, J. H.: *Toxicology and Pharmacology of Venoms from Poisonous Snakes.* Springfield, Illinois, Charles C Thomas Publishing Co., 1973.

Clarke, E. G. C., and Clarke, M. L.: *Veterinary Toxicology.* Baltimore, The Williams and Wilkins Co., 1975.

Frye, F. L.: Bites and stings of venomous animals. In Kirk, R. W. (ed.): *Current Veterinary Therapy VI.* Philadelphia, W. B. Saunders Co., 1977.

Knowles, R. P., Snyder, C. C., Glenn, J. L., Straight, R. C.: Bites of venomous snakes. In Kirk, R. W. (ed.): *Current Veterinary Therapy V.* Philadelphia, W. B. Saunders Co., 1974.

Minton, S. A.: *Venom Diseases.* Springfield, Illinois, Charles C Thomas Publishing Co., 1974.

Oehme, F. W., Brown, J. F., and Fowler, M. E.: Toxins of animal origin. In Casarett, L. J., and Donll, J. (eds.): *Toxicology.* New York, Macmillan Publishing Co., Inc., 1975.

Russel, F. E., and Saunders, P. R. (eds.): *Animal Toxins.* New York, Pergamon Press, 1966.

Tu, A. T.: *Venoms: Chemistry and Molecular Biology.* John Wiley & Sons, 1977.

Wasserman, G. S., and Siegel, C.: Loxoscelism (brown recluse spider bites): a review of literature. Vet. Hum. Toxicol. 19:256–258, 1977.

SNAKEBITE IN AUSTRALIA AND NEW GUINEA

HENRY L. HIRSCHHORN, B.V.Sc.

Warriewood, N.S.W., Australia

With the exception of a few species of mildly venomous, rear-fanged Colubrid snakes, the venomous snakes of Australia and Papua-New Guinea belong to the family *Elapidae*.

Approximately 65 species of venomous snakes are known from Australia, and of these, about 20 species are known to be dangerous. The dangerous species, some of which rank as the most lethal land snakes in the world, belong to the genera *Acanthophis* (Death adders), *Notechis* (Tiger snakes), *Austrelaps* (Copperhead), *Pseudechis* (Black snakes), *Pseudonaja* (Brown snakes), *Oxyuranus* (Taipan), *Parademansia* (Fierce snake), *Hoplocephalus* (Broad-headed snakes), *Tropedechis* (Rough-scaled snake), *Cryptophis* (Small-eyed snakes), *Demansia* (Whip snakes), and *Denisonia*.

The dangerous snakes of Papua-New Guinea are the Taipan, Death adder, Papuan black snake and King Brown snake (both *Pseudechis* spp.), Whip snake, and Papuan small-eyed snake (*Micropechis* sp.).

PATHOGENESIS OF AUSTRALIAN ELAPID VENOMS

Snake venom is a complex mixture of toxic and non-toxic substances, mainly proteinaceous, consisting of enzymes and toxins that vary in quality and quantity from species to species. The venoms of dangerous Australian snakes contain neurotoxins, hemolysins, coagulants, cytotoxins, and enzymes such as hyaluronidase, cholinesterase, L-amino-oxidase, phosphodiesterase, and phospholipase A.

NEUROTOXINS

Neurotoxins are the main lethal factors in Australian elapid venoms. There are a number of distinct neurotoxins, with either pre-synaptic or post-synaptic (curare-like) effects. Post-synaptic effects are rapidly reversible; pre-synaptic effects are irreversible. Pre-synaptic neurotoxins of the Tiger snakes (*Notechis* spp.) and the Eastern small-eyed snake (*Cryptophis* sp.) are also severe myotoxins.

The neurotoxin of Brown snakes (*Pseudonaja* spp.) is antigenically distinct from other neurotoxins, and there is little cross neutralization of Brown snake venom by antivenins to other venoms.

COAGULANTS

The effect of the coagulant component of venom is not always to cause massive intravascular coagulation but rather to defibrinate the blood so that within a short period, it becomes incoagulable. Clinically, this may show up as continued bleeding from fang or needle punctures, hematemesis, hematuria, or fecal blood.

Brown snake and Taipan venoms activate the clotting mechanism directly by converting prothrombin to thrombin, which then acts on fibrinogen to form fibrin. Tiger snake venom is similar except that it requires the presence of factor V before prothrombin is converted to thrombin.

Copperhead, King Brown or Mulga snake, and Death adder venoms do not contain coagulants.

HEMOLYSINS

Hemolysins may be direct or indirect in their activity. Phospholipase A is an indirect hemolysin, the activity of which is greatly enhanced by the presence of lecithin.

The venoms of the Taipan and Black snakes (*Pseudechis* spp.) are strongly hemolytic, whereas the venom of the Brown snakes has little hemolytic activity.

Clinical signs of hemolysin activity are jaundice and hemoglobinuria.

CYTOTOXINS

Cytotoxins may cause a number of pathologic changes. Platelet lysis can occur, resulting in disseminated intravascular coagulopathy. Some venoms have direct myotoxic effects and others appear to be nephrotoxic. Cytotoxic effects on vascular endothelium result in hemorrhage into various tissues.

OTHER ENZYMES

Hyaluronidase is thought to be responsible for the very rapid spread of Australian elapid venoms from the site of injection. Australian snake venoms are very low in proteolytic enzymes and thus there is very little reaction at the site of the bite.

CLINICAL SIGNS

Animals suffering from snakebite may present with a diversity of clinical signs, the severity of which vary greatly from animal to animal. This diversity is caused by variations in the species, size, age, and health of the offending snake, and the amount of venom injected.

The predominant signs of envenomation are neurologic. However, any or all of the following signs may be observed: sudden collapse, ataxia, trembling, vomiting, salivation, defecation, dilated pupils, slow or absent pupillary light reflex, respiratory distress, "abdominal" respiration, pallor, jaundice, hematuria, hemoglobinuria, myoglobinuria, hematemesis, continuous bleeding from fang punctures, flaccid paralysis progressing to coma, or respiratory failure (Table 1).

DIFFERENTIAL DIAGNOSIS

Diagnosis presents no problem when the patient has been observed being bitten by a snake or when it shows signs of envenomation and fang punctures can be found.

Where the cause is doubtful, the following are some of the conditions that should be considered in the differential diagnosis:
1. Envenomation by the tick, *Ixodes holocyclus,* is characterized by ataxia, ascending paralysis, changes in vocalization, salivation, vomiting, and (in felines) pupillary dilatation.
2. Ingestion of organophosphates causes salivation, vomiting, defecation, and trembling and prostration.
3. Acute hemorrhagic gastroenteritis.
4. Acute cystitis with hematuria.

TREATMENT

If it is possible, the offending snake should be identified. If the snake has been killed, it should be brought to the doctor with the patient. Identification of the offending snake will enable the most effective treatment to be given.

Table 1. *Comparative Frequency of Commonly Observed Signs of Snakebite in Animals*

| | SNAKE SPECIFIED — ALL ANIMALS: | | | | ANIMAL SPECIFIED — ALL SNAKES: | | | |
	TIGER	BROWN	BLACK	COPPERHEAD	DOGS	CATS	HORSES	CATTLE
Sudden collapse soon after bite, temporary recover, then relapse	+	++	+	−	++	+	−	−
Neurologic signs: weakness, ataxia, flaccid paralysis	++++	++++	++++	++++	++++	++++	++++	++++
Excitement: trembling, salivation, vomiting, defecation, muscle spasm	+++	+++	+++	+++	+++°	++	+++°	+
Pupils dilated: pupillary light reflex slow or absent	++++	+++	+++	+++	+++	++++	+++	+++
Local swelling	+	+	+++	++	++	++	+	−
Hemoglobinuria, myoglobinuria, or jaundice	++	+	+	−	++	+	−	−
Non-clotting blood: extended coagulation time, continuous hemorrhage from wounds. Hematemesis/hematuria.	++	++	++	−	++	++	++	++

Key: += 1 to 10%, ++= 11 to 30%, +++= 31 to 75%, ++++= 76 to 100% of cases reported.
°Vomiting is a common sign in the dog; trembling and sweating are common in the horse. From Lewis, 1978.

Table 2. *Snake Venoms and Antivenins*

SNAKE	AVERAGE VENOM YIELD	TYPE AND INITIAL DOSE OF ANTIVENIN°
Tiger snake Tasmanian Tiger snake Chappell Is. Black Tiger snake	35 mg	3000 U Tiger snake antivenin 6000 U Tiger snake antivenin 12000 U Tiger snake antivenin
Death adder	40 mg	6000 U Death Adder antivenin
Taipan	120 mg	12000 U Taipan antivenin
Copperhead	25 mg	3000 U Tiger snake antivenin
Brown snake Dugite Gwarda	2 mg	1000 U Brown snake antivenin
Black snake	40 mg	3000 U Tiger snake antivenin or 6000 U Black snake antivenin
King Brown or Mulga snake	180 mg	9000 U Tiger snake antivenin or 18000 U Black snake antivenin
Papuan Black snake	200 mg	12000 U Tiger snake antivenin or 24000 U Black snake antivenin

°Antivenins to the bites of Australian and Papuan snakes are prepared by Commonwealth Serum Laboratories, Parksville, Victoria, Australia. Adapted from Lewis, 1978.

If the snake has not been positively identified, precise knowledge of the species found in the locality is essential. Common names are of little value, as they vary from area to area. It is impossible, in practice, to identify the snake from the symptoms of envenomation exhibited by the patient.

As Australian snake venoms are disseminated rapidly from the site of envenomation, incision or excision of the fang punctures should not be attempted. If the bite is on a limb, tightly bandaging the limb may slow absorption of venom from the site of injection. In the majority of cases, the animal is presented for treatment when signs of envenomation are already present. In these cases, treatment is instituted by the administration of antivenin. The shorter the period between the snakebite and the administration of antivenin, the better the prognosis and the faster the recovery. Whenever the identity of the snake is known, the appropriate monovalent antivenin should be used (Table 2).

If the snake is unknown, a combination of monovalent antivenins should be given to cover all possible dangerous species in the area. If the animal is very valuable, the use of polyvalent antivenin should be considered. The quantity of antivenin that is required will depend on the clinical response to treatment in each case. One unit of antivenin (Commonwealth Serum La-

boratories) will neutralize 0.01 mg of the corresponding dried venom.

Antivenins are standardized and dispensed so that one ampule of antivenin is sufficient to neutralize the average venom yield of the corresponding species of snake. Nevertheless, more than one ampule may be necessary, as the amount of venom injected can vary widely. If an animal responds to antivenin but then relapses, more antivenin should be administered. Bites of snakes for which there is no specific antivenin should be treated with Tiger snake antivenin.

With the possible exception of bites by *Cryptophis nigrescens* (Eastern small-eyed snake), antivenin should not be administered unless signs of envenomation are present. Because antivenins are prepared in horses and therefore are of heterologous origin to all animals except horses, there is a risk that anaphylactic reaction might occur during administration, particularly if the animal has received antivenin or tetanus antitoxin (also of equine origin) on a previous occasion. Anaphylactic-like reactions sometimes occur in animals that have had no prior contact with horse serum. It is believed that this is due to a complement-binding effect of antivenin. If antivenin is to be administered, it should be by slow intravenous infusion, preceded by a small dose of epinephrine given subcutaneously and a corticosteroid given intravenously.

Supportive therapy is important. Whole blood may be necessary in cases of severe hemolysis, hemorrhage, or defibrination. Lactated Ringer's solution should be given intravenously to maintain fluid volume and assist kidney function. Respiratory distress should be alleviated with oxygen and, if necessary, artificial respiration. Envenomated animals should be kept warm and quiet, and sedated, if necessary. However, the use of morphine is contraindicated. It may be advisable to give tetanus prophylaxis and/or antibiotic therapy, and any hemorrhage from fang or needle punctures must be controlled.

SUPPLEMENTAL READING

Cogger, H. G.: *Reptiles and Amphibians of Australia*. Sydney, Australia, A. H. & A. W. Reed Pty., Ltd., 1975.
Garnet, J. R. (ed.): *Venomous Australian Animals Dangerous to Man*. Victoria, Australia, Commonwealth Serum Laboratories, Parkville, 1968.
Lewis, P. F.: in Proceedings No. 36. The Post-graduate Committee in Veterinary Science. University of Sydney, pp. 287–309, 1978.
Slater, K.: A Guide to the Dangerous Snakes of Papua. W. S. Nicholas, Government Printer Port Moresby, Papua-New Guinea, 1956.
Winter, H., and Pollitt, C. C.: On the Pathology of Small-Eyed Snake (Cryptophis nigrescens) Poisoning. *Australian Advances in Veterinary Science*. Australian Veterinary Association, Sydney, Australia, 1978.

NEAR-DROWNING
(Water Inhalation)

CHARLES S. FARROW, D.V.M.
Saskatoon, Canada

Near-drowning is defined as survival, at least temporarily, following submersion in a fluid medium. Resultant pathophysiologic alterations may arise as a consequence of asphyxia due to reflex laryngospasm or more commonly as a result of aspiration of the drowning fluid.

Experimental drowning of dogs has described four distinct phases: (1) initial breath-holding and automatic swimming movements, (2) aspiration of large amounts of water with associated choking and increasingly violent struggling, (3) explosive vomiting, and (4) cessation of all movement shortly followed by death (Loughkeed et al., 1939). Similar observations have been made in cats, rats, and guinea pigs. Although controlled observations are understandably lacking in man, reconstruction of the events closely parallel the animal data (Modell et al., 1976).

PATHOPHYSIOLOGY

From a pathophysiologic standpoint, it appears that hypoxia is the most serious, as well as the most consistent, finding following near-drowning (Farrow, 1977; Modell et al., 1976). Although many factors play a role in the development of hypoxemia, its magnitude is more severe following aspiration of sea water than following aspiration of an equal quantity of fresh water. This suggests a difference in causes.

It appears that the initial cause of hypoxemia after near-drowning is shunting of blood through perfused but non-ventilated alveoli. The underlying mechanism for non-ventilation of alveoli after aspiration of fresh water is an alteration of the normal surface tension properties of pulmonary surfactant with a collapse of the alveoli. Unless the surface active material is regenerated, uneven ventilation and recurrent collapse of alveoli occur, even after they have been forcibly reinflated. After aspiration of sea water, fluid in the alveoli prevents ventilation. In addition, a decrease in compliance and an increase in airway resistance also contribute to the hypoxemia seen.

Once a true or absolute intrapulmonary shunt can no longer be demonstrated, when patients are allowed to breathe 100 percent oxygen, hypoxemia frequently persists when the patient is returned to normal atmospheric con-

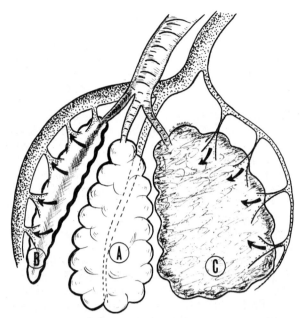

Figure 1. Pathologic changes in alveolae caused by near-drowning. A. Normal. B. Fresh-water changes. C. Sea-water changes.

ditions. This suggests that a delayed defect exists due to abnormal ventilation-perfusion ratios and/or a diffusion deficit. Very likely, this delayed lesion is the result of aspiration pneumonitis and its concomitant pulmonary edema, damage to the alveolar capillary membrane from the hyper- or hypotonicity of the water, and secondary infection (Modell et al., 1976). The pathologic sequence is illustrated in Figure 1.

Additional biologic derangements stemming from near-drowning include alterations in blood volume, hemoglobin concentration, and serum electrolytes. These changes primarily involve increased dilution or concentration, depending on the quality and quantity of the drowning fluid that is aspirated. Cardiovascular, renal, and neurologic complications secondary to hypoxia should also be anticipated in the near-drowning patient. Based upon the human experience, these factors rarely have a major bearing on the case outcome.

Water temperature is also an important consideration in cases of near-drowning. At temperatures much below 15° C, there is a rapid loss of body heat and a commensurate acceleration of fatigue. The ability to swim is greatly impaired. There is also a strong tendency to hyperventilate immediately upon entering the water. This reflex, which is mediated by widespread cutaneous receptors, will often result in the inhalation of water in the event of an unexpected submersion. The same afferent

impulses that cause the hyperventilation also result in a sensation of profound dyspnea. This often leads to a state of panic in the first moments of very cold immersions (Farrow, 1977).

ON-SITE TREATMENT

With the advent of numerous paraprofessional rescue units operating within or around most major population centers, it is entirely conceivable that a veterinary practitioner may be called upon to function as a remote medical advisor in a case of near-drowning involving a pet animal. Furthermore, it may be necessary to instruct a client directly in a similar situation.

Human cardiopulmonary resuscitation (CPR) techniques may easily be modified for veterinary field use. Clamping the animal's muzzle with both hands as one exhales intermittently via an oro-nasal seal results in an effective substitute for standard mouth to mouth methods employed in man. Specific patient positions are determined largely on the basis of individual circumstances.

Prior to initiating CPR, the animal's throat must first be cleared of any obstructive material such as vomitus, plant material, clay, sand, or gravel. The tongue should then be drawn forward and the airways should be drained. The latter maneuver is best accomplished by holding the patient in the inverted erect position for approximately 30 seconds. Postural drainage is apt to be more productive in instances of salt water immersion for the reasons mentioned earlier. Drainage should not be dwelt upon! If it is not initially successful, halt the attempt and begin the CPR. If oro-nasal fluids are forthcoming or if the animal vomits, postural maneuvers may be reinitiated. Transport to the nearest veterinary facility should be undertaken as soon as possible, with CPR being maintained if feasible.

DIAGNOSIS

History is extremely important in evaluating the condition of a near-drowning patient. Every possible detail of the immersion incident and subsequent rescue should be considered. This must include prior hyperventilation or drug ingestion, duration of immersion, loss of consciousness (however brief), presence or absence of pulse and respiration, and color and temperature of the skin. A detailed report of rescue and resuscitation must be made.

A thorough physical examination must be done, and one should be sure to check body temperature. Arterial blood-gas determinations are the most important laboratory examinations. A thoracic radiograph is important but less urgent than are blood gases. Findings may range from completely normal to mild perihilar or basilar infiltrates to diffuse pulmonary edema. *The radiologic appearance of the lungs will not necessarily reflect the severity of the patient's condition, and there may be a delay of 48 hours before the appearance of roentgenographic evidence of pulmonary edema.* A severely affected patient should have arterial and central venous lines for continuous monitoring. Hemoglobin, hematocrit, and electrolyte determinations should be made and plasma hemoglobin should be measured.

RADIOLOGIC EVALUATION

The radiographic appearance of near-drowning in the dog is basically one of terminal air space disease. The alveolar pattern predominates during the early stages of the disorder, and it is usually accompanied by strong, although less obvious, interstitial and bronchial components. Increased ventilatory effort is often inferred based upon an enlargement of the tracheal caliber and a commensurate pulmonary hyperinflation. A reduction in cardiovascular dimensions may reflect hypovolemic phenomena.

This initial radiographic display is the result of a pathologic montage composed of the fluid of near-drowning and its attending hemorrhagic, desquamative, and exudative components.

In the event that initial therapy is successful, the alveolar pattern will rapidly dissipate and leave in its stead a mixed interstitial-bronchial pattern. Continued patient improvement is reflected by continued clearing of the abnormal lung densities with marked resolution expected by the end of seven to ten days.

If, on the other hand, treatment is unsuccessful, worsening of the terminal air space disorder is to be anticipated in the form of increased intensity and dissemination of the alveolar density pattern. This radiographic picture strongly suggests the development of pneumonia, usually of a fulminant nature. Lung abscesses represent an additional potential complication, which unfortunately may be difficult to recognize in the context of widespread pneumonic disease.

On occasion, the radiographic picture may appear comparatively unchanged in the context of a precipitous patient deterioration. In this somewhat sinister situation, particularly when accompanied by severe dyspnea and cyanosis, one should be alert to the possibility of an acute onset adult *respiratory distress syndrome*.

As with any inflammatory lung disorder, intermediate and long-term progress examination may indicate the persistence of abnormal lung densities. In the case of the completely recovered patient, the likelihood is greatest that these abnormal densities represent pulmonary scar formation. Specific radiographic appearances vary, depending on the degree and extent of the inflammatory process. The most commonly encountered scar pattern is one of heightened interstitial density, as indicated by blurring of the pulmonary vasculature. Pulmonary scar may also appear as a thin linear density resembling Kerley lines in man (Farrow, 1977).

On occasion, the initial thoracic radiographs may be entirely normal. Assuming the patient has indeed suffered a submersion accident, this finding likely indicates that laryngospasm rather than inhalation has precipitated the acute asphyxia associated with near-drowning.

The presence of a "sand bronchogram" in the initial film series is a dire prognostic sign, and it indicates aspiration of clay, sand, or gravel into the tracheobronchial tree. The presence of such a sign is often associated with non-survival (Bonilla-Santiago and Fill, 1978).

The radiologic variants of near-drowning have been illustrated (Farrow, 1977).

HOSPITAL MANAGEMENT

Since hypoxia and acidosis are the cause of death, the veterinarian should direct treatment towards the correction of these biochemical lesions while awaiting the animal's recovery from the underlying pulmonary lesion. In an animal that is unconscious, has had an altered sensorium, or is suffering from acute respiratory distress, it is probably prudent to administer bicarbonate (1 to 2 mg/kg) immediately on admission without awaiting the results of blood-gas determinations. Asphyxia leads to the rapid development of severe metabolic acidosis, and the need for prompt correction justifies this empirical treatment. Supplementary oxygen alone may be enough to achieve adequate oxygenation, or severe edema and pulmonary insufficiency may cause the patient to require intubation and either positive end-expiratory pressure (PEEP) alone or intermittent positive-pressure ventilation (IPPV) with PEEP. PEEP may be started at 4 to 5 cm H_2O and adjusted according to blood gases. If IPPV is needed, a volume ventilator should be used. In cases of salt water aspiration, PEEP alone may accomplish adequate oxygenation;

mechanical ventilation may be needed in cases of fresh water aspiration. Arterial blood gases and the patient's clinical condition, however, are the determinants in each case. The veterinarian must give careful attention to details of respiratory care, including the administration of bronchodilators if there is wheezing, indicating an element of small airway obstruction. Weaning from ventilation should not be markedly different from the procedures followed in other cases of pulmonary insufficiency. *Steroids are ineffective in the treatment of aspiration* (Calderwood et al., 1975), *and antibiotics should be reserved until the development of secondary infection.* Treatment of the sequelae of cerebral hypoxia may include the use of dexamethasone, mannitol, fluid restriction, and hypothermia.

Fluid and electrolyte management is entirely a matter of following the clinical condition and laboratory findings in the individual case. Under no circumstance should hypo- or hypertonic fluids be administered on the basis of purely theoretical electrolyte changes. Administration of diuretics should be based on careful monitoring of urinary output and other clinical findings.

COMPLICATIONS OF THERAPY

In man, there is a relatively high incidence of barotrauma (pneumothorax/pneumomediastinum) associated with the use of mechanical ventilation systems. This potential problem can be eliminated or minimized by constant patient supervision and periodic thoracic radiographs.

Gastrointestinal bleeding is also seen in a third of all patients maintained on ventilation systems and has been attributed to the presence of stress ulcers. The author has not encountered this complication in the dog.

NEUROLOGIC SEQUELAE

Neurologic sequelae may be predicted with a moderate degree of accuracy on the basis of one or more of the following presenting signs: the animal (1) arrived at the hospital unconscious or obtunded, (2) required prolonged CPR, (3) had an initial pH less than 7, and required mechanical ventilation in order to maintain minimal pO_2 levels. The more of these indicators present, the greater the likelihood that permanent neurologic deficit will result.

PROGNOSIS

The outcome as far as survival is concerned seems to be directly related to the patient's condition at the time of admission. Coma, pH of less than 7.0, need for cardiopulmonary resuscitation on admission, and need for mechanical ventilation are all grim indicators. Subsequently, the same indicators point to severe neurologic sequelae, although need for mechanical ventilation is a weaker indicator than the others.

Attention to oxygenation and correction of acidosis at all stages following the immersion incident will lead to a favorable outcome in patients who have not sustained irreversible hypoxic damage.

PSYCHOSOCIAL CONSIDERATIONS

In the majority of near-drownings, the owner either rescues the dog or is usually near the scene of the accident. In cases in which there is a prolonged period during which survival is questionable or there are severe neurologic sequelae, a significant psychologic burden is placed on the owner and other family members. Usually, the involved party experiences a tremendous feeling of guilt about the condition of the dog, which is not usually seen in other illnesses. The owner often expresses sentiments of remorse and negligence to the veterinarian, as well as a profound sense of guilt for the near-drowning episode. "If only I had . . . " is a phrase repeated frequently during the clinician-client dialogue. These highly intense guilt feelings may also be expressed as criticism of the veterinarian involved in the care of the patient. Such psychologic "striking out" should be anticipated and countered with a controlled and uncomplicated explanation of the situation. Additional enlightenment of family members and friends may assist in palliating the involved party. It should be expected, however, that the majority of clients will bear their tragedy with resolution, and will require no more (or less) than basic human concern and understanding.

PREVENTION

Drowning accounts for approximately 7 per cent of accidental deaths in the U.S. and Canada annually, and it is the third most common cause of accidental death in children. Although comparable records are not maintained for pet animals, the figure is probably much lower due to the reduced interaction between these animals and the aquatic components of their environment. Formal surveys conducted among both Canadian and U.S. veterinarians by the author have indicated that drownings and near-drownings do occur and most frequently involve dogs. Home swimming pools and recreational waters constitute the most common sites of involvement. It is therefore apparent that these accidents are preventable. Unsupervised poolside activity particularly by young, aquatically inexperienced pups sets the stage for an immersion accident. The older dog, although wiser to poolside perils, may also meet an untimely end if encouraged to enter the pool by family members, thereby setting the scene for future tragedy. Small-breed dogs with relatively poor swimming skills, as well as short-legged dogs of any size, tire rapidly while in the water and require a relatively higher water level to accomplish escape.

The hunting dog, on the contrary, is usually an excellent swimmer gifted with amazing endurance and strength. An injudicious challenge in the form of a ball or stick hurled from the shoreline of a rapidly flowing river or stream may also result in a fatal misadventure. It is well to remember that the stamina of even the heartiest of dogs is quickly quenched in frigid waters even over comparatively brief time spans.

Client counseling is therefore considered to be highly advisable in cases in which aquatic activities are anticipated. Owners of retriever breeds appear especially deserving of such advice, particularly if they are inexperienced in the training of such animals.

SUPPLEMENTAL READING

Bonilla-Santiago, J., and Fill, W. L.: Sand aspiration in drowning and near drowning. Radiology 128:301, 1978.
Calderwood, H. W., Modell, J. H., and Rwiz, B. C.: The ineffectiveness of steroid therapy for treatment of fresh-water near-drowning. Anesthesiology 43:642, 1975.
Farrow, C. S.: Near-drowning in the dog. JAVRS 18:6, 1977.
Loughkeed, D. W., Janes, J. M., and Hall, G. E.: Physiological studies in experimental asphyxia and drowning. Can. Med. Assoc. J. 40:423, 1939.
Modell, J. H., Graves, S. A., and Ketover, N.: Clinical course of 91 consecutive near-drowning victims. Chest 70:231, 1976.

INHALATION INJURY

CHARLES S. FARROW, D.V.M.
Saskatoon, Canada

The care and treatment of pet animals suffering from acute inhalation injury has progressed only slightly since the author's previous review of this subject in *Current Veterinary Therapy VI.* However, methods of initial clinical evaluation (and accordingly, provisional prognosis) have become considerably more polished. This refinement can be attributed to at least three major factors: (1) increased clinical experience, (2) heightened understanding as regards the pathophysiologic composition of inhalation injury, and (3) augmented availability of sophisticated oxygen support systems to a growing number of veterinary facilities. Consequently, the clinical emphasis in this chapter will be placed upon the early evaluation and care of the acute inhalation injury patient. A classification scheme is proposed to facilitate this process.

DEFINITION AND PATHOPHYSIOLOGY

Inhalation injury may be defined as the pathologic process that arises directly or indirectly subsequent to the exposure of one or more elements of the respiratory tract to the irritating or toxic constituents of a given gas or noxious fumes.

Pathogenetically, inhalation injury may be the result of thermal as well as chemical influences, and its onset may be acute, delayed, or late.

Thermal injury affects mainly the upper respiratory tract and invariably results in some degree of pharyngolaryngeal inflammation. Commonly, the trachea and lobar bronchi are also involved, although often to a lesser extent, especially if laryngospasm is present.

In rare instances, inhalation of steam or still burning oxygen or other combustibles may also damage the more distal branches of the bronchial tree. Edema, erosions, ulcers, sloughs, and abnormal luminal secretions usually follow. These destructive events usually produce a significant degree of upper and middle airway obstruction. This in turn results in varying degrees of hypoxemia and generalized respiration-oriented patient distress. Moreover, the associated increased work of breathing will promote an increase in energy expenditure, thereby creating a concomitant demand for accelerated respiration. Thus, a self-sustaining pathophysiologic mechanism is created.

Chemical injury, in contrast to thermal injury, tends to damage the lower respiratory tract and lungs. Specific injury forms vary with the degree and duration of exposure, the extent of the entrapment, and the nature of the involved combustibles. Modern home furnishings incorporate numerous synthetics that, when pyrolyzed, produce highly toxic fumes containing not only carbon monoxide and irritant carbon particles but such substances as nitric, hydrochloric and hydrocyanic acid. Even simple wood smoke contains comparatively high levels of toxic aldehydes.

These substances, singularly or in concert, produce a spectrum of pathologic changes incorporating some or all of the following elements: (1) bronchospasm, (2) ciliary paralysis (and, therefore, a retardation or complete loss of the mucociliary clearance mechanism), (3) mucosal damage with sloughing, (4) luminal mucoid plugging, (5) atelectasis, (6) surfactant disturbance and/or loss, (7) capillary instability, and (8) pulmonary edema. Further damage to the alveolar membrane resulting in additional air space compromise may occur under the influence of circulating "burn factor." The likelihood of this complication is directly related to whether or not there is an associated cutaneous burn injury.*

CLINICAL EVALUATION AND INITIAL TREATMENT

CLINICAL EVALUATION

Obviously, many degrees of inhalation injury may exist in a given patient. It therefore becomes imperative to determine the extent of respiratory tract injury before devising a specific therapeutic plan. Once treatment is underway, the patient's early response should be observed closely, with the intent of possible plan modification. Additionally, one must be constantly alert to the possible life-threatening sequelae that may develop, often in the face of an apparent recovery. Most importantly these include post-inhalation pneumonia and the adult respiratory distress syndrome.

Table 1 indicates the author's preferred physical/biochemical/radiographic examination protocol for the inhalation injury patient. It is meant to serve as both a general guide and checklist. Expediency is advised, although not

---

*The reader is advised to read further on the subject of thermal injuries, particularly with regard to how they may adversely effect the management of the inhalation injury patient. See *Current Veterinary Therapy VI,* article on "Thermal Injuries."

Table 1. *Recommended Physical Examination in Cases of Inhalation Therapy*

PATIENT PRESENTED UNCONSCIOUS
1. Establish airway.
2. Begin breathing assistance using humidified high concentration oxygen.
3. Cardiac massage as required.
4. Drugs as needed (e.g., bicarbonate, epinephrine).
    Note: the mnemonic device "ABCD" is useful remembering this vital resuscitative sequence.
5. Begin fluids.
    Note: central venous pressure monitoring aids in preventing pulmonary flooding.
6. Continue with the steps below.

PATIENT PRESENTED CONSCIOUS
1. Evaluate mental status (may range from unconscious to hyperactive).
    Note: a rapid evaluation of cerebral function should be included if patient was unconscious at time of rescue.
2. Evaluate respiratory status (consider rate, rhythm, character).
3. If present, evaluate extent and degree of associated burn injury (be particularly cognizant of orofacial burns, singed facial hair coat and whiskers).
4. Evaluate circulatory status: mucous membranes relative to color and perfusion (capillary refill time), heart and pulse (rate, rhythm, character).
5. Evaluate oral and pharyngeal cavities as much as possible for edema and swelling.
6. Obtain saliva or cough sample via laryngeal swab and microscopically examine for presence of: carbonaceous particles, cellular debris and frank tissue sloughs, red blood cells, neutrophils.
7. If CPR or respiratory assistance is required, bronchoscopy should be performed concomitantly.
    Note: flexible, "soft-headed" scope is advisable; use extreme caution not to rake tracheal lining.
8. Evaluate for presence of naso-ocular discharge and examine microscopically as in step 6 above. Take temperature and record body weight.
9. Obtain blood and urine sample for CBC, BUN, and urinalysis; obtain blood gases if available.
10. Make thoracic radiographs.

Table 2. *Classification of Inhalation Injury*
(BASED ON PRESENTING SIGNS)

CLASSIFICATION	CLASS I	CLASS II	CLASS III	CLASS IV
Extent of pulmonary injury (estimated)	Minimal	Slight	Moderate	Severe
State of consciousness	Alert, fully conscious	Distressed	Highly distressed	Unconscious
Respiratory rate	Normal or slightly increased	Mildly increased to moderately	Accelerated	Decreased or absent
Orofacial burns, singed whiskers, hair	Rarely present	Occasionally present	Often present	Usually present
Mucous membranes cherry-red (COHgb)	Not present	Rarely present	Occasionally present	Often but not necessarily present
pale (hypovolemia)	Rarely present	Occasionally present	Often present	Usually present
Carbonaceous particles present in cough products identified microscopically	Not present	Often present	Often present	Usually present
Naso-ocular discharge	Occasionally present	Usually present	Usually present	Usually present
Radiology	Normal	Usually normal	Variable – normal to consolidation	Variable – normal to consolidation
Bronchoscopy	Usually normal	Mild edema, increased mucus	Edema, mucous tissue sloughs, obvious luminal plugging	Usually as class III, except in flash fires where these may be normal to minimal findings
CBC, Chemistries, Urine	Usually normal	Highly variable depending largely on circulatory status of patient		
Hair coat smells of smoke	←————————————NOT RELIABLE INDICATION————————————→			

at the cost of inadequate data acquisition. Flexibility is acceptable as regards the sequence of the individual examination components.

Following the initial physical examination, it is recommended that the patient be relegated to one of four major categories of inhalation injury according to the classification scheme proposed in Table 2.

Once this is accomplished, the patient may be treated in accordance with the recommendations presented in Table 3. A provisional prognosis may also be developed at this time, which should include a probability analysis relative to the development of delayed or late onset pulmonary distress syndrome. This information is provided in a following section dealing with sequelae to inhalation injury.

RADIOGRAPHIC DISPLAYS IN INHALATION INJURY

The radiographic display of an inhalation injury may change considerably not only patho-physiologically but temporally as well. The author has found no strict correlation to exist between the extent of abnormal thoracic signs (radiographic abnormalities) and the patient's respiratory status. This is not to say the radiographic examination is insensitive. On the contrary, radiographs may directly reveal pulmonary atelectasis, consolidation, effusion, and inflationary (volume) irregularities. Numerous *inferential* data may be obtained from the static roentgen image, including information on respiratory and cardiovascular dynamics. Sequential films often prove invaluable in determining trends of disease *activity, progression, resolution,* and *complication.* As a general rule, however, the greater the number of radiographic abnormalities encountered in the initial study, particularily consolidative alterations, the more guarded the early prognosis. For reasons to be described later, an initially clean lung does not preclude delayed sequelae.

The author has encountered four comparatively common radiographic displays in canine and feline patients that were suffering from acute inhalation injury at the time of initial examination. These include, in order of decreasing observed frequency, (1) diffuse bronchial-peribronchial line-on-ring densities, (2) diffuse patchy consolidation, (3) generalized hyperlucency and hyperinflation, and (4) diffuse (often massive) coalescive consolidation involving primarily the dorsal half of the thorax. Less frequently seen abnormalities include localized or regional consolidation, moderate to marked mediastinal shift, and pleural effusion. The last is somewhat more common in the cat. As indicated earlier, these appearances need not and often do not correlate with the degree of existing pulmonary injury.

Hyperinflation is a radiographic feature of most inhalation injuries, although it may easily be missed if it coexists with a significant volume loss. This is especially true if there is an adjacent consolidation on the ipsilateral side. The trachea is often dilated, as are the primary con-

Table 3. *Initial Treatment of Inhalation Injuries*
(BASED UPON CLASSIFICATION PRESENTED IN TABLE 2)

CLASS I	CLASS II	CLASS III	CLASS IV
1. Symptomatically treat any minor burns and oculonasal discharge.	Inhalation injuries within these classifications are best managed on the basis of serial blood gas determinations. If unavailable, one must then rely more heavily on serial radiography and close clinical observation.		
2. Advise owner: complications unlikely, but phone back in 24–48 hours with progress report. Act on this information accordingly.	1. Place patient in low concentration (5–15%), humidified oxygen atmosphere for 4–6 hours and re-evaluate.	1. Place patient in intermediate concentration (15–30%) humidified oxygen atmosphere and re-evaluate every hour. Repeat blood gases frequently if available. Increase oxygen concentration if pO_2 continues to drop in the face of increasing oxygen concentration.	As in Class III, *note:* increase oxygen concentrations as necessary.
	2. Start fluids as circulatory status indicates but be extremely careful not to overload. If suspect the latter, repeat thoracic radiographs.		
	3. Start steroids: methylprednisolone, 2–4 mg/lb/BW initially; follow with longer acting drug such as dexamethasone, 4 mg/kg/BW, QID (non-divided) for 24–48 hours and re-evaluate.	2. Consider: suctioning upper airway if secretions become excessive.	
		3. Establish superficial and deep fluid lines to provide fluid routes and simultaneously monitor central venous pressure. CAUTION: avoid fluid overload.	
	4. Consider: use of morphine sulfate (0.1 mg/kg/BW given S.Q. to alleviate pain and to decrease respiratory rate.	4. Start steroids as in Class II (#3).	
		5. Start morphine sulphate (0.2 mg/kg/BW) S.Q.	
	5. Withhold antibiotics until a proven need arises (e.g., pneumonia). Present evidence indicates little or no prophylactic capability.	6. Withhold antibiotics as in Class II (#5).	
		7. Consider: central antitussives if cough severe; discontinue as soon as possible.	
	6. Advise owner recovery likely (if no associated major cutaneous burn), although some degree of pneumonia will probably occur.	8. Advise owner recovery (if no associated burns) questionable. Complications likely. Play it day by day.	Advise owner recovery extremely questionable. Consider patient condition critical. Complications almost a certainty. If improving trend develops, exercise very cautious optimism.

ducting airways. Associated dyspnea often produces motion unsharpness, unless short exposure times are employed. This is a particularly critical point to appreciate, since motion blur closely mimics abnormal bronchial-peribronchial density.

The radiographic appearances of delayed and late respiratory distress syndromes will be considered next.

INHALATION INJURIES AND THEIR SEQUELAE

As many as four distinct inhalation syndromes have been described in man and experimentally reproduced in mice. In the latter instance, experimental variables included duration of smoke exposure, smoke temperature presence or absence, severity of cutaneous burn, airway infection *(Pseudomonas),* and treatment method. All were shown to influence recovery, although associated cutaneous burns appeared to be the most critical feature relative to both the development of complicating syndromes and, in many subjects, subsequent death.

In pet animals, there appear to be at least four separate presentation forms of inhalation injury. These were described in Table 2.

Table 2 describes these potential patient profiles qualitatively. Attendant to any of these injury classifications, one may expect to encounter subsequent complications. These sequelae may be of greater or lesser clinical consequence, and may develop early or late relative to the time of original injury. Average onset times are presented in Figure 1.

FIGURE 1

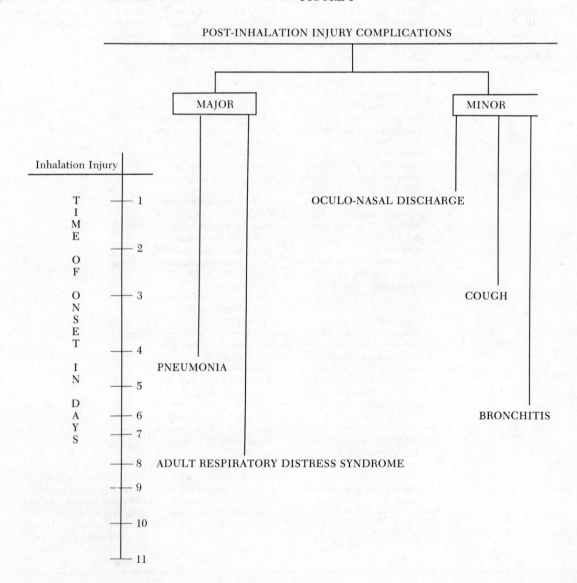

POST-INHALATION INJURY COMPLICATIONS

Radiographically, it may be difficult to differentiate pneumonia from respiratory distress syndrome. Both are often characterized by a diffuse pulmonary disease pattern that has a strong tendency to undergo a rapid transition from the peribronchial-interstitial to the alveolar compartments of the lung. In the latter stages of either disease, the air space pattern worsens precipitously, as evidenced by a marked tendency to coalesce and the development of numerous bronchogram signs.

When such radiographic alterations are viewed in the context of a patient whose clinical course is deteriorating swiftly as a result of an inability to maintain normal blood gas levels, adult respiratory distress syndrome should be strongly considered. Differential and sometimes concomitant conditions in addition to pneumonia include pulmonary infiltrates with eosinophilia and disseminated intravascular coagulation.

Management of pneumonic complications presents no specific problems, except in patients who have previously been debilitated and probably immuno-compromised. Tracheal wash combined with cultures, and a sensitive approach, are strongly advocated.

Management of respiratory distress syndrome, on the other hand, is difficult without the proper equipment and monitoring capacity. The reader is referred to the supplemental reading list for access to further information on this subject.

SUPPLEMENTAL READING

Farrow, C. S.: Smoke inhalation in the dog: current concepts of pathophysiology and management. Vet. Med. Small Anim. Clin. 70:404–422, 1975.
Farrow, C. S.: Smoke inhalation. In Kirk, R. W. (ed.): *Current Veterinary Therapy VI*. Philadelphia, W. B. Saunders Co., 1977.
Farrow, C. S.: Thermal injuries. In Kirk, R. W. (ed.): *Current Veterinary Therapy VI*. Philadelphia, W. B. Saunders Co., 1977.

THERMAL INJURY

PATRICK J. McKEEVER
St. Paul, Minnesota

Successful burn therapy is developed from the knowledge and understanding that tissue destruction due to thermal injury, if severe enough, results in a burn disease syndrome characterized by recognizable metabolic and clinical disorders.

THE BURN WOUND

ETIOLOGY

Thermal burns to the skin of animals may be due to friction, electric current, direct heat, and flame. Frictional burns usually result from the animal being hurled or dragged over the pavement after being struck by an automobile. Electrical burns are generally seen in and around the oral cavity. They occur when a young dog chews an electrical cord. The most frequent direct heat burn is the "clipper burn," which occurs from holding a hot hair clipper in contact with the skin too long. Less frequently, direct heat burns develop from situations such as cats walking over hot stove burners, poor supervision of paralytic animals on heating pads, hot liquids spilled on animals, and malfunction of hair drying equipment. Flame burns may result from fires in homes, apartments, or automobile accidents.

EXTENT OF TISSUE DAMAGE

The extent of a burn depends on the size of the area exposed to the heat source. The severity of a burn depends on the maximum temperature the tissue attains and the duration of overheating. These are dependent on such variables as the temperature and mass of the burning agent; the mass, specific heat, and thermal conductivity of the burned body; the temperature of the environment in which post-burn cooling takes place; and the amount of heat convection in the surrounding medium. Water, and tissues of which water is the main component, are characterized by high specific heat and low thermal conductivity. The term *high specific heat* implies that a large amount of heat is required to raise the temperature of tissue, and *low thermal conductivity* means the heat will be slow to dissipate. Accordingly, tissues become overheated slowly but are also slow in cooling. Therefore, the duration of tissue overheating extends beyond the contact time with the burning agent. Immediate cooling of the burned area can shorten the duration of tissue overheating, thereby decreasing tissue damage.

Tissue damage from overheating proceeds in a graduated manner. Threshold overheating of tissue causes inapparent, reversible cell damage. Further overheating will produce foci of irreversibly damaged cells scattered among reversibly damaged and non-injured cells. Finally, when a critical threshold is exceeded, necrosis of the entire tissue occurs.

Because transition from completely necrotic skin to completely healthy skin is gradual, regeneration of skin defects proceeds not from healthy but from partly damaged tissue. This is thought to be one of the reasons why burn healing takes longer than mechanical injuries of the same depth.

BURN CLASSIFICATION

Burns in people have been classified as (1) first degree, with erythema and some damage to cells of the epidermis but no blistering; (2) second degree, with blistering and complete necrosis of epidermis with varying degrees of damage to the dermis; and (3) third degree, with total loss of all elements of the skin.

Application of this classification to dogs and cats in clinical situations is difficult because the thin skin of dogs and cats does not blister as easily as does the skin of man. Accurate evaluation may not occur until after separation of necrotic tissue is complete and the wound is healing. However, early assessment of burn depth is often required because of the need to excise necrotic tissue. For this determination, it is more practical to use a simplified classification that differentiates burns into two types. *Partial-thickness burns* are characterized by incomplete destruction of the skin. Re-epithelization would be expected to occur from local epidermal elements with this kind of burn. *Full-thickness burns* are characterized by complete destruction of all elements of the skin, including skin adenexa and nerves. Re-epithelization would be expected to occur through migration of epidermal cells from the edges of the defect. Clinically, partial-thickness burns are distinguished by erythema, local edema, small vesicles, evidence of persistent capillary circulation, and partial sensation to touch.

Full-thickness burns are distinguished by lack of superficial blood flow, insensitivity of the skin to touch, and easy epilation of hair.

BACTERIA

Acute infectious diseases that develop in previously healthy individuals usually are caused by microorganisms not normally present in the environment. In contrast, infections present in burn wounds are caused by microorganisms found in the normal microflora of the skin. They are opportunists in the burn wound because damaged tissue acts as a medium to support bacterial growth, and in severe burns, the immunologic competency of the animal is impaired.

Bacteria most frequently reported to be found in burn wounds of man are *Staphylococcus, Streptococcus, Proteus, Pseudomonas, Escherichia coli,* and *Klebsiella.* Too few cases of burn wounds in dogs and cats have been cultured and reported to confirm that these same bacteria are found. However, a small number of cases have been cultured and provide confirmatory evidence.

Systemic complications due to infection are rare in small- and medium-sized burns. In extensive burns, where 15 to 30 percent of the body is involved, septicemia and invasive spread of local infection are frequent complications. Septicemia results from extensive proliferation of microorganisms in the necrotic tissues of the burn wound and penetration of these microorganisms or their toxins into the circulation. Spread of local infection may convert superficial skin necrosis into a full-thickness defect.

Qualitative bacteriologic analysis in man has shown that neither systemic nor topical antibacterial treatment can sterilize a burn wound. However, quantitative methods show that topical antibacterial treatment, but not systemic antibacterial treatment, can significantly reduce the number of microorganisms in the burn wound. Systemically administered drugs apparently have no or limited access to necrotic tissues. Therefore, to minimize the complications of invasive spread and septicemia, topical antibacterial treatment is the more appropriate.

PATHOPHYSIOLOGY OF BURNS

SHOCK

In accordance with current views, burn shock is defined as a set of signs occurring when the autoregulative mechanisms of the body are unable to insure normal blood flow in vitally important tissues and organs. These organs include the heart, brain, lungs, liver, and kidneys. Hypovolemia begins very soon after infliction of the burn and is typically most severe after several hours. The main eliciting factor is dilatation of capillaries and increased capillary permeability in the area of the burn. In extensive burns, this phenomenon occurs not only in the area of the burn but throughout the body. The reason for this acute increase in permeability of capillaries and loss of their physiologic responsiveness has not been satisfactorily explained. Histamine release seems to be involved, but this does not provide a full explanation. Experiments in dogs indicate that the central nervous system may play a dominant role. Despite the lack of knowledge concerning the exact mechanisms, it is clear that burn shock is a form of hypovolemic shock and all ramifications of hypovolemia on other organs must be considered. (For a complete discussion of shock, see the article "Shock: Pathophysiology and Management," page 32.)

If over 15 percent of the body surface area is burned, hypovolemic shock can be a serious problem in dogs and cats. It is probably not as severe as it is in man, because less fluid and plasma protein are lost due to lack of development of vesicles and bullae in these species.

HEMOSTATIC DISORDERS

Capillary damage from burns results in aggregation of blood platelets on the damaged endothelium and exposed tissue. Adenosine diphosphate (ADP) released in the course of this process causes further recruitment and aggregation of platelets. Simultaneously, exposed collagen fibers activate the intrinsic coagulation system leading to thrombin generation. Thrombin converts fibrinogen to fibrin strands, which stabilize the aggregated platelets. If damage is extensive, an initial phase of hypercoagulability passes into a phase of hypocoagulability due to exhaustion of clotting factors. This may lead to hemorrhagic diathesis.

LIVER DISORDERS

The central portion of the liver lobule is especially sensitive to anoxia. Hypovolemic shock leads to central lobular necrosis and depletion of glycogen stores. If hypovolemia persists, a state of systemic anoxia develops, manifested by metabolic disorders. These include elevated levels of ammonia, amino acids, phosphates, sulfates, and lipids.

KIDNEY DISORDERS

Abnormalities in kidney function occur partially because of the hypovolemia and partially because of vasomotor-induced changes in intrarenal blood flow. Secretion of urine ceases when systolic blood pressure drops below 60 mm Hg. Therefore, oliguria and anuria may be early sequelae. Primary ischemic renal failure may develop if hypovolemia persists.

ERYTHRON DISORDERS

Evaluation of human burn patients and animals with experimentally produced burns reveals anemia to be an early phenomenon. However, anemia is often masked by hemoconcentration. The reduction in numbers of circulating erythrocytes parallels the severity of the burn. At first, anemia is a direct effect of the destruction of erythrocytes. The cause of anemia, which occurs later in the syndrome, has not been definitively elucidated.

RESPIRATORY DISORDERS

Severely burned patients often suffer from poor pulmonary ventilation. Ventilation is affected by inspiration of hot air and gases that may burn the upper respiratory tract and cause laryngeal and pharyngeal edema and bronchospasm. This may be followed by hypersecretion of the bronchi and plasma exudation, which obstructs respiration and reduces the vital capacity of the lungs. Later (5 to 6 days), infectious pulmonary complications, focal atelectasis, and edema may appear.

IMMUNOLOGIC DISORDERS

Severely burned animals are also more prone to develop infection because of decreased immunologic capabilities. Immunoglobulin levels are decreased and cell-mediated immunity is impaired.

TREATMENT

MINOR BURNS

Experimental studies in animals and clinical studies in man have not demonstrated a particular treatment for minor burns that has distinct advantages. Accordingly, standard principles for the treatment of other small traumatic lesions of the skin may be applied to minor burns.

SEVERE BURNS

First Aid. If the burn has occurred within two hours and if the animal permits, ice-water packs (ice and water in a plastic sack) may be applied to the burned areas. Exposed tissue, if present, may be gently overlaid or loosely wrapped with strips of old sheets or pillow cases. Owners should be instructed to spend minimal time on these endeavors, as they are not as critical as veterinary management of possible shock.

Shock. Initial evaluation and treatment of the burned patient should be similar to that used in animals treated for other severe trauma. Airways should be examined to make sure they are patent, and any serious hemorrhage should be controlled; evaluation and, if necessary, treatment for shock can then be started according to the principles outlined in the aforementioned article on shock. If shock is not present, or once the animal is stabilized, evaluation and treatment of devitalized skin may be started.

Cooling. If the burn occurred within two hours, cooling of the affected areas should be the initial treatment. Cooling reduces pain, depth of the burn wound, edema, and mortality rate. The affected area may be immersed in cold water, and cold compresses can be applied. Skin should be cooled for at least 30 minutes. In dogs, the optimal temperature for the water or compresses is 3 to 17° C.

Cleaning and Débridement. Contamination and debris may be removed from the burn wound by flushing with saline or washing with povidone-iodine soap.

To facilitate evaluation of the wound, hair should be clipped from all affected areas. As indicated previously, determining the extent of burn wounds in dogs and cats is difficult, and in general, the area of damaged skin is underestimated. Final confirmation of the extent of a burn may not be possible until about 10 days post-burn, when separation of normal and necrotic skin starts to occur. All tissue that is determined to be devitalized should be excised. Devitalized tissue and exudate provide a good growth medium for bacteria. Baths are also helpful to remove necrotic tissues and surface exudates. Immersion of the affected areas in a whirlpool bath 15 to 20 minutes, twice daily, is especially effective.

Topical Antibacterial Treatment. Silver sulfadiazine cream* is one of the most effective

antibacterial drugs for topical therapy. Besides having antibacterial properties, it is non-irritating to exposed tissues, has no systemic side effects, and is easily applied to the wound. The exact technique for its use is as follows. After initial cleaning and débridement of burned skin, silver sulfadiazine cream is applied liberally to affected areas with a gloved hand or tongue depressor. Next, the area is bandaged with loose mesh gauze. Dressings are changed twice daily. During changes, necessary débridement is performed, old medication is removed, and the lesion is cleansed by irrigation with saline or immersion in a whirlpool bath.

Systemic   Antibacterial   Treatment. Although systemic antibiotics are used in the treatment of severe burns, their effectiveness is questionable. Studies on animals and human burn patients show that systemic antibiotic therapy does not favorably influence mortality, fever, or rate of healing. Their use should probably be limited to confirmed cases of bacterial septicemia. In these cases, antibiotic selection should be determined by sensitivity tests.

Skin Grafts. Severe burn wounds in dogs and cats should be treated as described previously until all necrotic tissue has been separated from the viable tissue, infection is controlled, and granulation tissue has developed. At this time, surgical procedures to decrease the wound size may be considered. Skin of dogs and cats is very elastic and has loose subcutaneous tissue that allows a marked amount of stretching. In many instances, skin defects can either be closed by direct apposition or one of several reconstructive techniques utilizing skin flaps. If the defect is too large for these techniques, a free autogenous graft of either full thickness or partial thickness may be utilized.

SUPPLEMENTAL READING

Fox, C.L.: Silver sulfadiazine — a new topical therapy for *Pseudomonas* in burns. Arch. Surg. 96:184–188, 1968.
McKeever, P.J., and Braden, T.O.: Comparison of full- and partial-thickness autogenous skin transplantation in dogs: a pilot study. JAVMA Res. 39:1706–1709, 1978.
Ofeigsson, O.J.: Water cooling: first aid treatment for scalds and burns. Surgery 57:391–400, 1965.
Rudowski, W., Nasitowski, W., Zietkiewicz, W., Ziemkiewiez, K.: Burn therapy and research. Baltimore, the Johns Hopkins University Press, 1976.

---

*Silvadene® cream, Marion Laboratories Inc., Kansas City, Missouri 64137.

HEAT STROKE
(Heat Stress, Hyperpyrexia)

WILLIAM D. SCHALL, D.V.M.

East Lansing, Michigan

Heat stroke is encountered sporadically and is characterized by hyperthermia. Rectal temperature is usually 41 to 44°C (105 to 111°F). Heat stroke is often complicated by alterations in acid-base homeostasis, disseminated intravascular coagulation, and/or cerebral edema.

Several factors are necessary for or may contribute to the induction of heat stroke. A prerequisite is high ambient temperature that may be as low as 32°C (90°F) but is more often 38 to 46°C (100 to 115°F). Virtually all dogs in which the condition occurs are confined in some manner. In most instances, dogs are confined to an enclosure with poor ventilation, such as an automobile or transporting crate. The condition can also occur in dogs confined by a chain outdoors. In these cases, excitement and exercise associated with animal fights appear to have precipitated heat stroke. Although exercise and excitement can significantly contribute to the induction of heat stroke in confined dogs, the condition is rare in dogs that run free, regardless of air temperature and exercise. High humidity contributes to the likelihood of heat stroke because evaporation of water from the oral and nasal cavities is reduced, despite maximal panting. Other predisposing factors are lack of available water, brachiocephalic anatomy, obesity, and decreased heat tolerance associated with young and old age.

Cats apparently can tolerate higher temperatures better than dogs. Heat stroke occurs rarely in this species.

PATHOPHYSIOLOGY

The initial compensatory response to increased ambient temperature is panting. This mechanism of dissipating body heat is efficient and involves the unidirectional flow of air into the nasal passages and out the oral cavity. This flow maximizes evaporation and heat loss because air is exposed to the greater evaporative surface area of the nasal turbinates. The process of panting, however, is not devoid of serious consequence. Significant pulmonary exchange takes place during panting that results in respiratory alkalosis. In dogs anesthetized with pentobarbital and subjected to an environment of 114°F at 80 percent relative humidity, respiratory alkalosis was documented 30 minutes after initiation of the experiment. Inasmuch as blood gas determinations were not done between the time the dogs were subjected to the hot environment and 30 minutes later, the precise time of onset of respiratory alkalosis is not known. The magnitude of respiratory alkalosis in our experimental hyperthermic dogs was profound. Typically, one hour after entrance into the hot environment, experimental dogs had an arterial blood pH of about 7.75 and a PCO_2 of less than 10 torr.

The respiratory alkalosis induced in pentobarbital-anesthetized dogs subjected to high temperature, however, eventually was modified by metabolic acidosis presumably due to muscle activity associated with panting. Most dogs had an arterial blood pH less than 7.30 three to four hours after experimental hyperthermia. The combination of respiratory alkalosis and metabolic acidosis was associated with cessation of panting and cerebral edema and was followed by death. Although the experimental hyperthermia that we induced may not be identical to naturally occurring heat stroke, it seems likely that dogs with heat stroke, when examined by the clinician, may have respiratory alkalosis or a combination of respiratory alkalosis and metabolic acidosis. The acid-base status of the individual patient can be known only if blood gas determinations are done.

Although serum electrolyte concentrations have not been done routinely on dogs with heat stroke, serum potassium concentration is known to increase in experimental canine and feline hyperthermia. The highest serum potassium concentrations coincide with the severest respiratory alkalosis. The increase in serum potassium concentration associated with experimental hyperthermia, however, is

195

mild and may not be clinically significant. Typical serum potassium concentrations are about 5.0 mEq/l.

Hypophosphatemia occurred in our experimental hyperthermic dogs approximately at the time of peak hyperkalemia and respiratory alkalosis. Most dogs had serum inorganic phosphorus concentrations of about 2.0 mg/dl compared with control values of 3.5 to 4.5 mg/dl. The mechanism of the hypophosphatemia is unknown.

Other alterations in serum electrolyte concentration known to be associated with experimental hyperthermia, and hence presumed to be typical of heat stroke, have been minor and probably are the result of hemoconcentration.

The degree of hemoconcentration that occurs in heat stroke may be severe. Packed cell volumes (PCV) of 75 percent have been reported. Whether hemoconcentration is mild, moderate, or severe is probably determined by environmental humidity and duration of the animal's exposure to the environment. In pentobarbital-anesthetized dogs subjected to 114°F at 80 percent relative humidity until rectal temperature reached 109°F, the PCV typically increased by 30 percent and the serum osmolality increased by 10 percent.

Disseminated intravascular coagulation (DIC) is known to occur as a result of heat stroke in man and dog. Experimental canine hyperthermia is also known to cause DIC and has been proposed as an experimental DIC model. The precise mechanism by which hyperthermia causes DIC is unknown but is characterized by progressive thrombocytopenia, increased activated clotting time, increased partial thromboplastin time, and the presence of fibrin (fibrinogen) degradation products in serum. The historical observation that some dogs with heat stroke die of a shock-like syndrome accompanied by hemorrhagic diathesis hours after seemingly complete recovery from heat stroke probably reflects the occurrence of DIC.

Another complication of heat stroke is cerebral edema. Although the mechanism by which hyperthermia induces cerebral edema is unknown, this complication is commonly present in heat stroke and experimental hyperthermia. Dogs with heat stroke-induced cerebral edema are initially stuporous. Involuntary paddling movements and coarse tremors are often present, and the dogs appear to be unaware of their surroundings. If the edema progresses, the menace reflex is lost, and the dogs lapse into a coma. The panting reflex is abolished, the respiratory rate markedly decreases, and the dogs die of respiratory arrest.

CLINICAL FINDINGS

The physical findings in dogs with heat stroke vary depending on the duration and severity of the disease. Initially, panting, tachycardia, bright red oral mucosa, and hyperthermia are the only findings. As the disease progresses, dogs become stuporous. The extremities become hot to the touch and the bright red oral mucosa becomes pale because of decreased circulating blood volume and/or peripheral vasoconstriction. At this stage, dogs may involuntarily void watery diarrhea. If the diarrhea becomes bloody or if petechiae are present, DIC may be a complication. Finally, coma and respiratory arrest follow unless spontaneous recovery or medical intervention interrupts the pathophysiologic sequence.

Laboratory findings relate to the stage and severity of the disease and are considered in detail in the discussion of pathophysiology.

THERAPY

Our understanding of heat stroke pathophysiology remains incomplete, and the direct relevance of some experimental hyperthermia observations remains uncertain. For these reasons, some of the therapeutic recommendations are quasi-scientific and based on inference.

The first objective of therapy is to lower body temperature. Experimental work supports the clinical observation that the chief determinants of survival are duration and degree of hyperthermia. An efficient method of lowering the rectal temperature is to submerge the trunk and limbs in a tub of cold or iced water. The rectal temperature should be taken at 10-minute intervals and the dog should be removed when rectal temperature reaches 39.5°C (103°F), because further cooling may result in hypothermia. Since recurrence of hyperthermia is also possible, the rectal temperature should be determined at 10-minute intervals for at least 30 minutes after the dog is removed from the tub. Cold-water enemas have been suggested as a method of cooling but have the disadvantage of interfering with the temperature monitoring. Evaporative methods of cooling that are commonly used in man are ineffective in the dog because of the hair coat. During the period of cooling, friction may be applied to the extremities to promote superficial circulation. Occasionally, severe shivering may hinder cooling. The intravenous administration of a phenothiazine tranquilizer such as chlorpromazine (1.0 mg/kg body weight) may be used to counteract shivering.

The second objective of therapy is to prevent cerebral edema. Dexamethasone should be administered intravenously in an antiedema dose (1.0 to 2.0 mg/kg body weight). This may also be helpful in preventing shock. Intravenous infusions of mannitol (2.0 gm/kg body weight as a 20 percent solution over a 10-minute period) may be used if the patient is stuporous or comatose or if these develop during therapy. Mannitol should not be administered if serious blood loss complicates heat stroke. Mannitol should be administered cautiously if DIC is documented or suspected.

Intravenous fluids are indicated if hemoconcentration is documented or if peripheral circulation failure is suspected. Fluids are of potential benefit in preventing DIC and shock but must be administered with caution because of possible induction of pulmonary edema and aggravation of cerebral edema. In the absence of specific serum electrolyte determinations, individual electrolyte replacement is contraindicated; a balanced electrolyte solution such as lactated Ringer's is the fluid of choice. Similarly, fluids that have little effect on acid-base balance should be administered, unless blood gas determinations are available.

If hemorrhagic diarrhea, excessive bleeding from venipuncture sites, or hemorrhage elsewhere is present, DIC may be a complication of heat stroke. Coagulation studies may help verify the presence of DIC and ideally should include one-stage promthrombin time, active partial thromboplastin time, activated clotting time, platelet count, and the detection of increased serum concentration of fibrin (fibrinogen) degradation products. If no facilities are available for these studies, the clinician should assume that DIC is present if bleeding tendencies are noted. Therapy for DIC should be initiated with the intravenous bolus administration of 100 to 200 I.U. of heparin/kg body weight followed by the continuous intravenous infusion of 600 units/kg day.

SUPPLEMENTAL READING

Barry, M. E., and King, B. A.: Heatstroke. S. Afr. Med. J. 36:455, 1962.
Malamud, N., Haymaker, W., and Custer, R. P.: Heatstroke. Milit. Surg. 99:397, 1946.
Perchick, J. S., Winkelstein, A., and Shadduck, R. K.: Disseminated intravascular coagulation in heatstroke. JAMA 231:480, 1975.
Shapiro, Y., Rosenthal, T., and Sohar, E.: Experimental heatstroke. Arch. Intern. Med. 131:688, 1973.
Spurr, G. B., and Barlow, G.: Tissue electrolytes in hyperthermic dogs. J. Appl. Physiol. 28:13, 1970.

ACCIDENTAL HYPOTHERMIA

R. D. ZENOBLE, D.V.M.
Ames, Iowa

There are numerous clinical settings in which hypothermia may be a consequence. Accidental hypothermia may be defined as a spontaneous decrease in core temperature, usually in a cold environment, associated with an acute problem without primary pathology of the temperature regulatory center. This is most commonly seen in old or unconscious animals, immobile animals (caught in leg traps), injured animals, and animals suffering from disease. Seldom will a healthy animal become hypothermic if it can seek shelter.

The physical findings of a patient with severe accidental hypothermia may be altered consciousness, unmeasurable blood pressure, a slow or absent pulse, and shallow, infrequent respirations. Heart sounds may be absent, the pupils may be dilated, and reflexes may be delayed or absent. At temperatures less than 32°C (90°F), shivering will be absent and the patient may appear to be in rigor mortis because of increased muscle tone.

Management of the hypothermic patient presents the clinician with unique therapeutic challenges. Therapy may be divided into two categories: general supportive measures and specific rewarming techniques.

GENERAL SUPPORT

The first principle in dealing with hypothermia is recognition that it exists. This may seem self-evident, but many patients have presented with hypothermia in which the diagnosis was not made until a complication supervened. This problem is partly due to the fact that standard thermometers record only to 34.4°C (94°F). If the thermometer has not been shaken down to begin with, a hypothermic patient may not be identified as such at all. Glass thermometers recording to 27.8°C (82°F) are available for this purpose (Heart Thermometer, Becton-Dickinson Co., Rutherford, New Jersey) in addition to sophisticated thermocouple units with rectal probes. Handling of the patient should be minimal to avoid precipitation of ventricular fibrillation in the cold heart.

Continuous electrocardiographic monitoring is important for the severely hypothermic patient because of the frequency of rhythm disturbances. Atrial fibrillation and ventricular tachycardia are commonly seen with severe hypothermia but usually revert to normal as the patient is rewarmed. The hypothermic heart is relatively unresponsive to atropine or countershock. If ventricular fibrillation occurs, an attempt to reverse it with countershock is worthwhile. If this is unsuccessful, cardiopulmonary resuscitation should be instituted and continued until core temperature is raised. Most drugs will have little effect on the cold heart and may cause serious problems once the patient is rewarmed, underscoring the hazard of overmedication of these patients due to delayed metabolism of the drugs. Fluid replacement is essential because chronic hypothermia may lead to profound volume depletion. Intravenous fluids should be warmed by passage through a hot-water bath or warmed prior to administration by using a bacteriologic incubator. Fluid and electrolyte requirements for each patient must be assessed individually because of the effects of other associated diseases, such as heart failure or diabetic ketoacidosis. If a central venous pressure line is to be used, it is important to avoid entrance into the heart so as to minimize myocardial irritability. Areas of frostbite should be treated separately once rewarming has been instituted. Close attention should be paid to chest radiographs both during and after the rewarming period for signs of pneumonia, the most common sequela of hypothermia.

SPECIFIC REWARMING TECHNIQUES

In conjunction with general resuscitative maneuvers, a mechanism for rewarming should be instituted. Rewarming methods remain a controversial area in hypothermia management (Table 1).

The choice of method to be used should take

Table 1. *Rewarming Methods for Hypothermia*

PASSIVE REWARMING
1. Remove from environmental exposure.
2. Apply insulating material (blankets).

ACTIVE EXTERNAL REWARMING
1. Apply heated objects (water bottle).
2. Apply electric heating pads.
3. Immerse in heated water.

ACTIVE CORE REWARMING
1. Peritoneal dialysis
2. Colonic irrigation
3. Mediastinal irrigation via thoracotomy
4. Hemodialysis
5. Intragastric lavage
6. Extracorporeal blood rewarming
7. Inhalation rewarming.

into account the duration and degree of hypothermia and the available resources and time involved to mobilize them. Methods of rewarming can be either external (surface) or internal (core). Passive rewarming relies upon removing the patient from a cold environment and maximizing basal heat retention by use of insulating material such as a blanket. Many experts consider this to be the safest method of rewarming a mild to moderate hypothermic patient.

Active external rewarming techniques are readily available and advocated by some authors. Concern has been raised about actively rewarming the body surface because of inherent physiologic changes that may aggravate the effect of hypothermia on core tissues. The well described "afterdrop" of core temperature after removal of chronic cold stress may be exaggerated by the peripheral vasodilation associated with active external rewarming. This can cause paradoxic central cooling by shunting stagnant, cold blood to the core, thus further chilling the myocardium and increasing the animal's vulnerability to ventricular fibrillation. Active external rewarming by immersion of the body in warm water may interfere with adequate monitoring of the patient and precipitate ventricular fibrillation due to the excessive movement of the patient. Heating blankets carry a risk of causing thermal burns in underperfused areas.

Core rewarming techniques should be reserved for patients with severe [core temperature less than 32°C (90°F)] or prolonged hypothermia (> 12 hours.). Core rewarming reduces the hazards of "afterdrop" and cardiac arrhythmias. Techniques for core rewarming useful for animals include high colonic lavage, administration of warmed intravenous fluids, direct mediastinal irrigation via thoracotomy, and peritoneal dialysis. Peritoneal dialysis has a high degree of success with a minimum of cost and required special equipment. This makes it an excellent means of core rewarming in veterinary medicine. The dialysate is warmed to 43°C (109°F) and instilled into the peritoneal cavity. Rapid instillation and immediate removal are preferable, and normothermia usually is attained within six to eight exchanges. Other methods for core rewarming are used in human medicine but are impractical for veterinary medicine at the present time. These techniques include intragastric lavage with warm saline, extracorporeal blood rewarming, and inhalation of warmed oxygen.

In summary, passive external rewarming is the safest and easiest method of rewarming the mild to moderate hypothermic patient. Active external heat is favored by some clinicians, but the rewarming must be slow to prevent "afterdrop" of the core temperature and precipitation of cardiac arrhythmias. Core rewarming should be reserved for severe or prolonged hypothermia. Peritoneal dialysis is the treatment of choice in veterinary medicine for severe hypothermia.

SUPPLEMENTAL READING

Reuler, J.B.: Hypothermia: pathophysiology, clinical settings, and management. Ann. Int. Med. 89:579, 1978.
Reuler, J.B., and Parker, R.A.: Peritoneal dialysis in the management of hypothermia. JAMA 240:2289, 1978.

COLD INJURY

(Hypothermia, Frostbite, Freezing)

ROBERT A. DIETERICH, D.V.M.
Fairbanks, Alaska

Hypothermia or freezing of tissues in domestic animals as a result of environmental exposure occurs more commonly in areas located in the northern latitudes but is seen occasionally in other areas as a result of accidental cooling or freezing of a pet held captive in household refrigerators or freezers. Another frequently encountered cause of hypothermia is interference with thermoregulatory centers during surgery by anesthetics or sedatives. Hypothermia will be considered separately from freezing, even though both may be present in a patient at the same time. Treatment for each condition involves different principles and they should be considered different entities.

HYPOTHERMIA

Hypothermia is defined as the condition produced by deep cooling from external cold, drugs, or failure of the temperature-regulating mechanisms, which results in a profound decrease in body temperature. This definition does not include normal cooling due to circadian rhythms, which produce changes in body temperature of from 1° to 2° C. Mild hypothermia is characterized by body temperatures of 30° to 32° C, moderate hypothermia by temperatures of 22° to 25° C, and profound hypothermia by temperatures of 0° to 8° C. The physiologic changes of hypothermia depend on the extent and duration of exposure. The duration of hypothermia can be characterized as acute (few hours), prolonged (several hours), or chronic (days).

Survival of animals suffering from hypothermia depends on the degree of cooling to which they are subjected. Moderate hypothermia allows survival for approximately 24 hours, whereas body temperatures of 15° C shorten survival time to five or six hours. Profound hypothermia narrows survival time still further to one or two hours.

TREATMENT

Treatment of hypothermia is directed toward rewarming and maintenance of vital body functions. Rewarming may be accomplished by external (surface) means or by internal (core) methods. External rewarming results in the body surface or shell being warmed first with the aid of warm water immersion, water or electric heating blankets, hot-water bottles, or simply a warm room and blankets. Oxygen and appropriate intravenous fluid therapy may also be needed, depending on the degree of hypothermia being treated.

Internal rewarming is accomplished using peritoneal dialysis. The dialysate is heated to 50° to 55° C and is allowed to flow into the peritoneal cavity as fast as gravity permits. After flowing through the administration tubing, the dialysate fluid will reach the abdominal cavity at a temperature of approximately 45° C. Dialysis is continued until normal body temperature is reached. Methods of procedure to carry out peritoneal dialysis are described in the article on "Peritoneal Dialysis" in this text.

The advantages of internal rewarming are several. Sometimes, when external rewarming is attempted, there will be vasodilatation of surface vessels and a transfer of cooled blood to the body core, bringing about a further drop in internal temperature that results in "rewarming shock." Normothermia can be achieved faster with peritoneal dialysis than with external rewarming methods. Cardiac output and electrocardiogram readings return to normal rapidly after rewarming by internal methods. When using either the external or the internal rewarming method, it is important to avoid overheating and resultant hyperthermia.

After a hypothermic patient is returned to normothermia, a complete examination should be carried out to determine whether another disorder led to the lowered body temperature. Renal failure, pneumonia or malnutrition can easily lower an animal's resistance to cold exposure, and the resulting hypothermia may be only a secondary symptom.

FROSTBITE OR FREEZING

Frostbite or freezing of tissue is rare in animals that are healthy and well nourished. Well acclimatized long-haired animals can remain exposed to temperatures of −50° C for indefinite periods with no ill effects. It is critical that animals exposed to very low environmental temperatures be fed adequate amounts of food to enable them to produce enough body heat to maintain normothermia. In cold regions, frostbite of the tips of the ears or tails of cats is perhaps the most common cold injury seen. This usually requires no treatment unless secondary infection is encountered. A bland ointment may be applied if needed. The scrotum of male dogs will sometimes be injured by cold from repeated contact with cold surfaces or deep snow. Erythema and scaliness or even minor sloughing of surface scrotal tissue can occur and is treated with ointments and reduced cold exposure. Continued contact with snow or cold surfaces will delay healing.

The deep-freezing of tissues is seen in animals that have been physically injured or caught in various types of wildlife traps or other circulation-inhibiting situations. Recently, major advances have been made in the treatment of severe frostbite. The owner of the frostbite patient should be encouraged to bring the injured animal directly to a veterinarian and should attempt no home treatment unless an extended period would pass before the animal could reach a veterinary hospital. Tissue damage and tissue necrosis are increased greatly if thawing and subsequent refreezing occur (freeze-thaw-freeze-thaw syndrome). The frozen part should be kept frozen and protected to avoid trauma during transport or handling.

TREATMENT

Frozen tissue should be thawed rapidly in warm water (38° to 44° C) as soon as possible after it is known that refreezing can be prevented. The frozen part should not be massaged during warming. Previously thawed parts should not be subjected to rapid rewarming. The thawed part will soon become erythematous and edematous. Large blebs usually occur, and self-mutilation by the patient should be avoided. It is best to leave the injured tissue exposed rather than to use occlusive wet dressings or petrolatum gauze. Premature debridement or other surgical intervention should not be undertaken. Treatment should be confined to protection of the part from trauma and prevention of infection. Systemic antibiotics should be administered in severe cases.

Unnecessary debridement of necrotic tissue or amputation should be delayed as healing occurs. Irreversibly damaged tissues begin to demarcate in four to seven days. Often, 15 to 20 days are required for the injured tissue to reach a point at which there is a clear demarcation of the tissue to be lost, and therefore removed, and the tissue that is viable. Pads of frostbitten feet should be preserved if at all possible.

Fractures, dislocations, and extensive trauma of frozen tissue should not be repaired until after thawing is complete. Fracture treatment should be conservative. A high-protein, high-caloric diet with vitamin supplements is helpful, particularly in the malnourished patient that has suffered both hypothermia and frostbite.

SUPPLEMENTAL READING

Mills, W.: Frostbite and hypothermia, current concepts. Alaska Med. Vol. 15, No. 2, March, 1973.

Petajan, J.: Prevention and treatment of frostbite. Report No. 103, Arctic Health Research Center, Fairbanks, Alaska 99701, 1969.

Popovic, V., and Popovic, P.: *Hypothermia in Biology and in Medicine.* New York, Grune and Stratton, 1974.

EMERGENCY KIT FOR TREATMENT OF SMALL ANIMAL POISONING

(Antidotes, Drugs, Equipment)

FREDERICK W. OEHME, D.V.M.
Manhattan, Kansas

PARENTERAL SOLUTION
Amphetamine
Apomorphine
Atropine sulfate
Barbiturates (phenobarbital, pentobarbital)
3% Bemigride (MIKEDIMIDE)
Calcium borogluconate
Calcium disodium edetate
Calcium disodium edetate in 5% dextrose
5% Dextrose
Diazepam (VALIUM)
Dimercaprol (BAL)
2% Doxapram (DOPRAM)
20% Ethanol
Glyceryl guaiacolate (GEOCOLATE)
Glyceryl monoacetate
Lactated Ringer's
10% Methocarbamol (ROBAXIN)
Neosynephrine
Nicotinamide (nicotinic acid, niacin)
Normal saline
10% Pentylenetetrazol (METRAZOL)
Pralidoxine chloride (2-PAM, PROTOPAM CHLORIDE)
Propranolol
Sedatives, tranquilizers
5% Sodium bicarbonate
Vitamin K_1
Whole blood, citrated (fresh within 2 weeks)

ORAL MEDICATIONS
Activated charcoal
0.2–0.4% Copper sulfate solution
Diphenylthiocarbazone
Egg whites, diluted
Hydrogen peroxide
Ipecac syrup
20% Magnesium sulfate solution
Milk of magnesia
Mineral oil
D-Penicillamine
Potassium chloride
1:10,000 Potassium permanganate solution
Prussian blue
Sodium chloride
Sodium ferrocyanide
20% Sodium sulfate solution
Tannic acid

MISCELLANEOUS ITEMS
Mild detergent
Oxygen
Sodium bicarbonate paste

EQUIPMENT
Aspirator bulb
Blankets
Endotracheal tubes, several sizes
Enema kit
Gauze rolls and tape
Intravenous catheters and stylets
Mechanical respirator or compression bag
Needles (hypodermic)
Stethoscope
Stomach tubes, several sizes
Syringes
Thermometers
Urinary catheters, various sizes
Venostomy kit

Section
3

RESPIRATORY DISEASES

N. EDWARD ROBINSON, D.V.M.
Consulting Editor

A Diagnostic Approach to Respiratory Disease.............................. 203
Clinical Pharmacology of the Respiratory System........................... 208
Canine Upper Respiratory Disease 214
Feline Upper Respiratory Disease.. 224
Diseases of the Canine and Feline Tracheobronchial Tree............ 229
Canine and Feline Pneumonia.. 235
Pulmonary Edema.. 243
Neoplasms of the Respiratory Tract.. 249
Pleural Effusions... 253
Parasitic Diseases of the Respiratory Tract................................. 262
Thoracic Trauma.. 268
Therapy for Respiratory Emergencies... 277
Interpretation of Pulmonary Radiographs 279
Laryngeal Paralysis in Young Bouviers 290

A DIAGNOSTIC APPROACH
TO RESPIRATORY DISEASE

JOAN A. O'BRIEN, V.M.D.
Philadelphia, Pennsylvania

HISTORY

Specific assessment of respiratory disease cannot be made without a complete history and thorough physical examination. Many disease processes can mimic and/or contribute to respiratory illness (anemia, ascites, extreme obesity). The clinician must therefore be aware of species, breed, sex, and age incidence in the occurrence of respiratory disease.

The history of the animal should be obtained in an orderly fashion and should include the presenting signs; past as well as present geographic, socioeconomic, and environmental conditions; the health status of litter mates; an inventory of other household animals and people in the household; previous surgery or illness and the response to therapy; medications being given at present; and the history of the current illness.

In detailing the history of the illness, it is often necessary to question the owner closely and repetitively to obtain a sequential picture of the disease process. The clinician must be alert for a description of signs (e.g., vomiting, diarrhea, lameness) that can suggest a multisystem disease in which the respiratory component is the client's dominant complaint. It is also important to determine whether the onset of signs was sudden or gradual, whether the signs are intermittent or constant, and whether the course of the disease seems static or progressive. Information must be obtained for each of the signs of respiratory disease described by the client.

The cardinal signs of respiratory disease are cough, dyspnea, abnormal secretions, noisy breathing, sneezing, and change in sound production. Coughing is perhaps the most common complaint in respiratory disease. Most owners do not realize that animals swallow most of their coughed-up secretions and will report that the cough is non-productive. Inquiries as to whether the cough is tight and harsh or discontinuous and bubbly followed by swallowing will often help to differentiate the type of cough.

Time of cough can also be helpful. A productive cough followed by swallowing upon rising after rest is often found in chronic bronchitis. A cough that wakes the animal from sleeping is more often a sign of left congestive heart failure, whereas paroxysms of harsh, tight coughing of recent onset are more typical of acute viral disease. A cough that gradually becomes more productive so that secretions are coughed out of the mouth is seen in pneumonia or bronchiectasis. Laryngeal incompetence or esophageal disease may be indicated if coughing after eating or drinking is noted.

It is necessary to determine how much coughing actually occurs — e.g., if it is one or two short episodes a day or a week, several short episodes a day or a week, or paroxysms lasting several minutes many times a day. Many owners do not realize that coughing is a protective mechanism against any irritation, and that minor scattered episodes may simply represent reaction to pull on a choke chain or collar or to inhaled irritants (dust, smoke).

Dyspnea is usually a sign of severe respiratory disease. Dyspnea in an open-mouthed cyanotic animal is obvious, but evaluation may be more difficult if signs are less pronounced. An increase in the normal rate of breathing for the size of the animal is often the earliest sign of dyspnea; however, it must be distinguished from panting. This information may not be obtained unless specific inquiries are made. Subtle dyspnea may become more marked after exertion or excitement. Sudden onset of dyspnea usually suggests a more acute process (trauma, aspiration, pneumonia), but this determination depends, to a great extent, on the owner's observation and the patient's activity level. The prime example is in cats with empyema, where the disease process is chronic but the dyspnea appears to be of sudden onset. Dyspnea associated with noisy breathing suggests airway obstruction, whereas short, shallow, rapid breathing may indicate a restriction of lung expansion as in pleural effusion, rib fracture, or pneumonia. Dyspnea must further be differentiated from the deep sighing respiration associated with metabolic acidosis.

Abnormal production of secretions may be the consequence of either upper or lower respiratory disease. Nasal discharge is a common presenting complaint reported by owners. Whether the discharge is at present, or was at one time, unilateral is important. Unilateral discharge of sudden onset may suggest a foreign body, whereas that of a more insidious onset may be indicative of a nasal tumor. The type and amount of discharge should be ascertained; serous or seromucoid discharges are common in viral infections and irritant or allergic responses, whereas purulent material suggests a chronic infection. Discharges that gradually become mixed with blood or are frankly bloody may indicate a destructive lesion such as a tumor or fungal involvement.

Abnormal secretions from the tracheobronchial tree are often swallowed. In animals with chronic bronchitis, mucoid sputum in small amounts may be expectorated after a coughing paroxysm. In some cases, swallowed secretions will be vomited after coughing and will appear as a mucoid watery material. Production of regularly noticeable amounts of purulent sputum is common in pneumonia and particularly so in bronchiectasis. Hemoptysis is usually a grave sign of respiratory disease and is most often associated with heartworm disease or lung tumors. Occasionally, it may be seen with foreign body aspiration and bronchiectasis.

Noisy breathing is a common presenting complaint of the client. Stertorous nasal breathing, more marked during sleep, may indicate a progressive nasal obstruction. The onset of or an increase in the amount of snoring is often seen in nasal and pharyngeal disease. Inspiratory wheezing or stridor is a sign of laryngeal or upper airway obstruction. The sound in tracheal collapse is often described by clients as honking or rattling. It is often helpful to ask the client to describe the sound and to imitate it if possible and attempt to locate it anatomically as if he were affected. Tape recordings of classic upper airway sounds that include honking, snoring, and reverse sneezing may also be helpful.

Sneezing is a very common sign in nasal disease. Since it is a very effective mechanism for ridding the nasal passages of irritants, it is important that the owner be reassured that occasional minor episodes of sneezing do not indicate disease and are common, especially in toy hairy-faced breeds such as Bichons, Lhasas, and Maltese terriers. Prolonged repetitive sneezing of sudden onset may indicate a nasal foreign body, whereas sneezing after exposure to weeds or grasses may suggest an allergy. Episodes of sneezing are very common in viral respiratory disease, especially in the cat. Sneezing associated with significant amounts of bleeding may be associated with head trauma or a destructive nasal disease. Occasionally, severe paroxysms of sneezing will result in blood-streaked mucus owing to the rupture of tiny superficial blood vessels by turbulent air flow.

Laryngeal disease is often characterized by a change in voice or sound production. Since owners do not associate this sign with disease in animals, specific questions must be asked concerning change in bark, meow, or purr.

PHYSICAL EXAMINATION

The specific approach to a respiratory problem should be initiated only after a careful general examination. Signs of systemic involvement may include fever, emaciation, inappropriate behavior or gait, pale or inflamed mucous membranes, or alterations in the skin or hair coat. The legs should be examined for signs of pain or heat suggestive of hypertrophic osteoarthropathy, and mammary tissue should be examined for possible malignancies. Funduscopic examination should be performed to determine whether viral, fungal, or lymphoid infiltrations of the retina are present. The abdomen should be examined for evidence of ascites or masses that may be responsible for pulmonary metastasis or restriction of diaphragmatic movement.

The classic parameters of physical examination of the respiratory system include observation, palpation, percussion, and auscultation. In practice, these examinations are often carried out jointly and continuously rather than as isolated procedures. This is certainly so in the case of observation or inspection, which is initiated upon first sight of the patient and continues throughout the examination.

The eyes should be inspected for deviation of gaze or proptosis and should be palpated for resilience. Likewise, the muzzle should be examined for swelling or fistula, and the nasal passages should be observed for normal conformation and patency of air passages. A clean glass slide held in front of the nares will help permit evaluation. In a cooperative patient, it is helpful to close the animal's mouth and have it breathe on the examiner's cheek while the latter gently holds off one nostril at a time to estimate nasal air flow. The type of secretion should be noted. An idea of air exchange can be obtained by holding the palm of the head in front of the nares and mouth.

The oral and pharyngeal cavity should be examined for evidence of secretions, ulceration, masses, or dental disease. In a recalcitrant patient, this examination is best deferred to the very end of the physical examination or performed under anesthesia. In a cooperative patient, the dental arcade, hard and soft palates, sublingual area, and pharyngeal wall can be palpated for signs of pain or changes in normal tissue. In a very few animals, the larynx may be visualized but anesthesia is usually required for this examination.

The larynx and trachea should be palpated for normal position and form. The consistency of these cartilaginous structures can vary greatly among breeds, but complete compressibility, areas of narrowing, and excessive coughing after palpation are abnormal.

The bony thorax should be palpated; this is especially helpful in heavily coated animals in which the hair coat may mask emaciation, masses, abnormal rib conformation, or compliance. Observations on the rate, depth, and ease of respiration are often augmented by palpation during breathing. Increased tactile fremitus can be palpated in pneumonia and other diseases characterized by bronchial fluid.

The art of percussion requires practice in order to be effective. It is most useful in detecting extreme variation from normal (e.g., hyporesonance in pleural effusion) and in following the resolution of these processes. Unless lesions of the lung parenchyma are massive, they often cannot be detected by percussion. In all instances, percussion notes in one area should be compared with those on the opposite side of the chest. Coughing after percussion often signals an area of abnormal lung underlying the percussed area, and particular attention should be paid to that area during auscultation.

In ausculting respiratory sounds, the clinician should always use the same stethoscope, since breath sounds are transmitted differently through different stethoscopes. It is necessary to auscult the entire respiratory system, first listening for noisy breathing at the mouth and nares and then using the stethoscope to evaluate laryngeal, tracheal, and bronchovesicular sounds. Obstructive upper airway noises are transmitted through the chest wall, but an orderly pattern of auscultation will permit evaluation of sites of maximal intensity. In order to evaluate breath sounds, it is necessary, at least

initially, for the student consciously to screen out cardiac sounds. Normal breath sounds are usually louder and somewhat harsher in very young and very small dogs and are of a harsh bronchovesicular to bronchial character in a panting dog. Blowing sounds are normally heard over the trachea. In most cases, true vesicular breathing in which the expiratory component is almost silent can be heard only in a quiet, unexcited animal; thus clinicians must often evaluate whether the bronchovesicular breathing of the typical excited patient is within normal limits. It must be remembered that breath sounds may sound distant and far off in the obese, heavily coated animal.

There is no area of greater confusion than that of the definitions assigned to abnormal lung sounds — e.g., rales and rhonchi. Rales have been defined as discontinuous, bubbling, moist, short sounds that are heard most easily on inspiration as air bubbles through fluid in the lung. Rales may be fine, medium, or coarse, depending on the size of the airway involved, with fine rales implying fluid in small bronchioles and medium and coarse rales in proportionately larger airways. Coarse rales are often palpable through the chest wall. Rhonchi are more musical, whistling notes produced by air moving past an obstruction in the tracheobronchial tree. They are better heard on expiration. Tumor, bronchospasm, or secretions may cause further narrowing on expiration and produce rhonchi. Localized persistent rhonchi should suggest an obstruction by tumor or foreign body, whereas diffuse rhonchi are more typical of bronchospasm. Rhonchi can often be further classified by pitch — low-pitch and sonorous in larger bronchi, high-pitch and sibilant in smaller airways.

It is much more difficult to demonstrate abnormal auscultatory findings in the dog and cat than in a cooperative human. Deep breathing is essential to proper auscultation; therefore, every effort must be made to evaluate the patient during full respiratory efforts. Listening during panting respiration is not sufficient. Although deep breaths will follow breath-holding or exertion, they also occur with coughing. This serves the multiple purpose of allowing the type of cough to be documented, permitting breath sounds to be evaluated, and demonstrating post-tusive rales, if present. A cough may usually be produced by laryngeal or tracheal palpation and, in some cases, by chest percussion. The duration and type of cough produced should be noted, and the owner should be questioned as to its similarity to the presenting complaint.

SPECIAL DIAGNOSTIC PROCEDURES

RADIOGRAPHY

Thoracic radiographs are such an essential diagnostic tool that they should represent an integral part of the work-up in the diagnosis of any severe, recurrent, or chronic respiratory problem. Fluoroscopic examination is very useful in demonstrating abnormalities of the airways or diaphragm (See "Interpretation of Pulmonary Radiographs.")

Radiographs should include lateral and dorsoventral views of the thorax, occlusal or open-mouth films of the nasal passages, and views of the frontal sinus, so that the full extent of nasal disease can be determined. (See the articles on Rhinitis and Sinusitis in the Dog and in the Cat.)

ENDOSCOPY

Rhinoscopy. Indications for rhinoscopy are chronic non-responsive unilateral or bilateral nasal discharge and obstructed air flow. This procedure requires anesthesia.

Endoscopic evaluation of the nasal passages in the dog and cat is severely limited by the well developed and convoluted turbinate pattern. It is possible, however, to visualize the rhinarium and the rostral aspects of the turbinates by using an otoscopic speculum suited to the size of the animal. The choanae and nasopharynx can be visualized by pulling the soft palate forward with tissue forceps and then using a curved, lighted, rotating laryngeal mirror* that will fit a conventional otoscopic light handle. In large breed dogs, a flexible bronchoscope, 4 mm in diameter, can be used to examine the common meatus from the nose to the pharynx. Large areas of the nasal passages, however, can be directly visualized only through surgical exploration.

The nasal mucosa is extremely sensitive, and general anesthesia is necessary to allow examination and prevent trauma. The examiner should note the condition of mucosa, the type of secretions, any deviation of turbinates, the presence of abnormal tissue, ulcerations, bleeding sources, foreign bodies, and the equality of air flow. Secretions should be gently suctioned for culture and cytologic examination. Nasal washings have been useful in documenting the presence of tumor when small pieces of tissue are examined histologically.

Laryngoscopy. This procedure requires anesthesia and is performed in a position of ventral recumbency. Indications are stridor or change in voice.

The conventional intubating laryngoscope is adequate for visualizing the larynx. The examiner should look for deviations in normal form, color, and motility. Light anesthesia is required for the accurate assessment of normal motility.

Bronchoscopy. This procedure requires anesthesia and is performed in a position of ventral recumbency. Indications are unexplained chronic or recurrent cough or dyspnea. Bronchoscopy is also used for therapeutic removal of obstructing secretions or foreign bodies (O'Brien and Roszel, 1974).

Bronchoscopy may be performed either with standard rigid bronchoscopes* of adequate length and diameter or with the flexible fiberoptic endoscope. A flexible fiberoptic pediatric gastroduodenoscope† is an excellent, though expensive, instrument for this purpose. Its small diameter and great length permit its use in animals of various sizes.

Bronchoscopic examination should include the aspiration of secretions for bacteriologic and cytologic examination. The examiner should also note any evidence of ulceration, edema, infiltration, growth, or change in color in the mucosa. The normal tracheobronchial tree expands with inspiration and constricts with expiration, narrowing to approximately one half its diameter with coughing. Any abnormal compliance, rigidity, immobility, fixation, or deviation of the trachea, the carina, or the main stem bronchi should be noted, as well as the type and source of secretions. Additional information may be afforded by cytologic and histologic examination of bronchial brushings or endoscopic biopsy specimens.

Esophagoscopy. This procedure requires anesthesia and is performed in a position of left lateral recumbency. Indications are repeated episodes of aspiration pneumonia and expectorated blood of unknown origin.

The same instruments utilized in bronchoscopy are employed in esophagoscopy. Any change in mucosal characteristics and any evidence of dilation, stricture, or bleeding should be noted.

---

*Geo. Pilling & Sons, Fort Washington, PA 19034; ACMI, 300 Stillwater Avenue, Stamford, Connecticut 06902.

†Olympus Corp. of America, New Hyde Park, New York 11040; ACMI, 300 Stillwater Avenue, Stamford, Connecticut 06902.

---

*Welch-Allyn laryngeal mirror.

Mediastinoscopy and Thoracoscopy. These techniques have not been developed as diagnostic procedures in animal medicine. In human medicine, they are utilized for the visualization and biopsy of either mediastinal or intrathoracic abnormalities.

COLLECTION OF SPECIMENS FOR CYTOLOGIC EXAMINATION AND CULTURE

Sputum. Generally, sputum samples are not valuable sources for culture, since expectoration cannot be induced in the dog or cat. Contamination with oropharyngeal microorganisms makes the evaluation of isolates difficult. In viral outbreaks, however, culture of nasal and pharyngeal mucosa can be useful in confirming the presence of a virus. In pulmonary malignancies characterized by the production of excess secretions, sputum samples can be useful in demonstrating the presence of malignant cells.

Bronchial Washings. Samples of bronchial secretions may be obtained directly after instillation of sterile saline by means of a sterile aspirator inserted through a sterile bronchoscope. Self-contained prepacked sterile specimen traps* are available for collection of the aspirate. Samples may be divided into aliquots for culture and cytologic examination. Direct smears of aspirate should also be made at the time of collection. Aspirate collection under direct visualization makes possible selective and repetitive aspiration of abnormal areas, but this procedure requires general anesthesia.

Transtracheal Aspiration. Tracheobronchial secretions may be collected by instilling aliquots of saline through an intracath.† This procedure usually requires only light sedation and infiltration with local anesthesia. After sterile preparation, a stab incision is made in the skin, the needle is passed through the cricothyroid or intertracheal membrane, and the plastic intracath is carefully guided into the trachea. Nine to 10 cc of saline are then inserted, and secretions are suctioned. If the animal coughs, secretions that coat the distal end of the catheter can also be cultured if the amount of aspirated material in the syringe is marginal.

Pleural Effusion. (See article "Pleural Effusions.")

CYTOLOGIC EVALUATION

Stains used for cytologic evaluation are:
1. New methylene blue — not permanent
2. Wright-Giemsa or Diff-Quik* — air dry; permanent
3. Papanicolaou or Sano trichrome — alcohol fix; permanent
4. Gram — permanent.

Smears from nasal exudate, tracheobronchial secretions, or pleural fluid may be examined cytologically (O'Brien and Roszel, 1974; Sano, 1949).

Whenever possible, cytologic evaluation should include examination of freshly made smears as well as of the centrifuged sediment. Smears may be useful in identifying the type of inflammation (neutrophilic or eosinophilic) and in establishing the presence of malignant cells, parasite eggs or larvae, fungal elements, and bacteria. Abnormalities of bronchial epithelium, increases in goblet cells, and bronchial casts can also be detected by cytologic examination. The presence of alveolar macrophages or "dust cells" indicates that a deep aspirate has been obtained from the bronchial tree. If a trichrome stain such as Papanicolaou is to be used, smears must be fixed while wet in alcohol or fixed in sprayed fixative.†

SKIN TESTS

Skin tests for inhalant allergens can be useful in dogs in which respiratory disease and peripheral eosinophilia suggest an allergic component. Intradermal injections of antigen plus a histamine and saline control are monitored for evidence of immediate hypersensitivity within 15 to 20 minutes or an Arthus reaction after 3 to 4 hours. These tests are most useful in confirming a clinical history suggestive of an allergic reaction.

Skin tests for systemic fungi and tuberculosis give rise to a delayed Type IV reaction observed after 24 to 48 hours. They may be negative in the presence of severe disease, and if positive, they may indicate only past exposure — therefore, their usefulness is limited.

SEROLOGY

Occult Heartworm Disease. Serum antibodies have been detected against microfilaria in dogs with suspicious evidence of heartworm disease in which circulating microfilaria cannot be detected.

---

*Clinical Products Specimen Trap, Chesebrough-Pond's Inc., Greenwich, Connecticut 06830.
†Deseret Pharmaceutical Co., Sandy, Utah 84070.

°Diff-Quik, Harleco, 480 Democrat Road, Gibbstown, New Jersey 08027.
†Spray-Cyte, Clay Adams, Parsippany, New Jersey 07054.

Nasal Aspergillus and Penicillium Disease. The agar gel immunodiffusion test has been useful in detecting serum antibodies in these diseases in the dog and cat.

Systemic Fungal Diseases. Serial samples for serology are useful in detecting active disease in histoplasmosis, blastomycosis, coccidioidomycoses, and cryptococcosis.

SUPPLEMENTAL READING

O'Brien, J. A., and Roszel, J. F.: Bronchoscopy and bronchial cytology. In Kirk, R. W. (ed.): *Current Veterinary Therapy* V. Philadelphia, W. B. Saunders Co., 1974.

Sano, M. E.: Trichrome stain for tissue section, culture or smear. Am. J. Clin. Path. Vol. 19, No. 9, September, 1949.

CLINICAL PHARMACOLOGY OF THE RESPIRATORY SYSTEM

LLOYD E. DAVIS, D.V.M.

Urbana, Illinois

Rational drug therapy consists of administering the right drug to the right patient in an appropriate dose by the correct route in order to normalize bodily functions. The decision to treat a given patient must include a careful consideration of potential benefits and risks associated with therapy. Prerequisites to rational therapy include a diagnosis, understanding of the pathophysiology of the disease and pharmacology of the drug, and the establishment of therapeutic objectives. Symptomatic treatments can be hazardous to a patient if a diagnosis has not been established. The use of any drug in any patient should be considered as an experiment because of variations in disease process, the host, and the individual's response to drugs. As with any experiment, observations should be made that will reveal efficacy or toxicity so as to set the course for continued therapy. Without such a plan, one cannot determine whether objectives have been attained.

Once an accurate diagnosis has been established, the clinician has three choices for further care of the patient. He or she can (1) perform surgery, (2) administer a drug that will restore normal function, or (3) do nothing and let nature take its course. All these alternatives are applicable to the management of various disorders of the respiratory system. For example, torsion of a lung lobe with pleural effusion requires surgical correction, a bacterial pneumonia would be treated with an antibiotic chosen on the basis of identification and susceptibility of the pathogen, and a patient with a viral infection would not be treated except by administration of good nursing care.

A conceptual framework for a rational approach to the drug therapy of various disorders of the respiratory system based on therapeutic objectives is presented here.

ESTABLISHMENT OF THERAPEUTIC OBJECTIVES

After the veterinarian has taken an adequate history, performed a complete physical examination, conducted pertinent diagnostic procedures, and established a diagnosis, he or she should consider what steps can be taken to alleviate the condition. Drug therapy is one option among many, and the decision-making process should include consideration of what is medically possible, what benefit the treatment is likely to provide the patient and client, and what the potential risks are to the patient.

Nearly all effective forms of drug therapy of the respiratory tract involve either modification of some normal occurring function or control of an infecting pathogen. Thus, the veterinarian can suppress protective reflexes, control inflammation, decrease pulmonary capillary pressure, dilate bronchioles, increase or decrease secretions, or kill bacteria with drugs. Drugs will *not* repair a tracheo-esophageal fistula, drain a pulmonary abscess, cure a viral infection, or restore to normal an emphysematous lung. The practitioner should be aware of limitations inherent in the pharmacotherapy of respiratory disorders.

BRONCHOPULMONARY CLEARANCE

Animals continually inhale particulate matter contained in air. Removal of these substances occurs by means of (1) aerodynamic filtration, (2) trapping of particles in the mucous blanket, which is moved by cilia to the pharynx from which it is swallowed, (3) phagocytosis of particles reaching the alveoli, (4) coughing, and (5) sneezing. Aerodynamic filtration occurs as a result of particle inertia, gravitation, and Brownian motion, and it is therefore not altered by therapy. Although cilia function autonomously and are not controlled by extrinsic nerves, their motility can be reduced by some noxious gases and vapors.

Phagocytosis is effective in removing particulates, including microorganisms, that have penetrated the other defenses. Glucocorticoids may interfere with this process by at least three mechanisms: (1) depression of phagocytosis, (2) inhibition of breakdown of ingested material within phagocytic vacuoles, and (3) decreased influx of monocytes from peripheral blood to the alveoli. By these actions, corticosteroids may permit the progression of an infectious process or decreased rate of clearing of alveoli. There is no known way to facilitate phagocytic activity within the lungs.

Respiratory tract fluid is secreted by glands within the epithelium and serves as (1) a vehicle for conveyance of foreign material from the bronchial tree, (2) a protectant of the underlying cells, and (3) a part of the mechanism for dissipating body heat, and it possesses anti-infective properties (IgA and lysozyme). The glands are of two types: goblet cells, which secrete mucus, and tubulo-acinar glands, which secrete a thin, non-viscid fluid. Mucus secretion occurs independent of nervous control but is increased by exposure to noxious materials; e.g., smog and tobacco smoke. The tubulo-acinar glands are under parasympathetic nervous control. Secretion is enhanced by cholinergic, anticholinesterase, and expectorant drugs. Inhalation of steam increases vascularity of the mucosa with consequent transudation of fluid.

Through stimulation of tubulo-acinar gland secretion, the therapist attempts to decrease viscosity of thick, tenacious mucus or exudate so that it can be more easily removed from the tracheobronchial tree by ciliary action and coughing. Cholinergic drugs are unsatisfactory for this purpose because of side effects on other systems of the body. A frequently overlooked therapeutic measure to decrease viscosity of mucus is to hydrate the patient. Animals with malaise and fever become dehydrated with resultant inspissation of material in the bronchial tree. Restoration of water balance will correct this problem.

Expectorants are drugs that stimulate secretion of the tubulo-acinar glands either directly or by reflex action. Three classes of compounds currently are employed in veterinary medicine: the saline expectorants, guaiafenesin (glyceryl guaiacolate), and volatile oils. The saline expectorants include ammonium chloride, ammonium carbonate, calcium or potassium iodides, and sodium or potassium citrate. These compounds and guaiafenesin stimulate receptors in the gastric mucosa, which reflexly (vagus) increase glandular secretion by the respiratory epithelium. In higher doses, these drugs produce emesis. Volatile oils such as terpine hydrate, eucalyptus, menthol, and pine oil directly stimulate the glands following absorption when administered orally or when employed in vaporizers for inhalation.

It has been difficult to evaluate the efficacy of the expectorants in patients, and controversy exists as to whether they are of value in the management of respiratory diseases. In laboratory studies, a few expectorant drugs were shown to augment the output of respiratory tract fluid, but in doses greatly in excess of those usually recommended for therapeutic use. Many of the nostrums available for the treatment of coughing are irrational combinations of drugs. Products are available that contain an expectorant to increase secretion in combination with drugs such as stramonium, hyoscine, or antihistaminics, which act to dry the epithelium. Thus, the effects are antagonistic.

COUGH SUPPRESSANTS

Although coughing is a protective reflex, a severe, non-productive cough can have harmful effects, including dissemination of infection to non-infected lobes or paranasal sinuses, rupture of lung abscesses, interference with sleep, and spread of infection to other animals. Such coughs should be controlled with central acting cough suppressants, which depress the cough center in the medulla oblongata.

The opiates (morphine and codeine) and some opioids (methadone) are potent inhibitors of the medullary cough center. They exert this effect at dosages smaller than those required for analgesia. Suggested dosage for morphine and methadone is 0.1 mg/kg. Codeine is effective at a dosage of 1 to 2 mg/kg in the dog and cat. Recently, it has been found that the antitussive effect of codeine is due to its conversion to morphine by the liver. As the opiates are subject to abuse by people, many veterinarians prefer not to prescribe them. A reasonable alternative is dextromethorphan, which is an opioid devoid of analgesic and addictive properties. It is an effective antitussive in the dog and cat at a dosage of 2 mg/kg given four times a day. The drug is not effective in rabbits. Dextromethorphan is available in various proprietary cough remedies and as 10 mg tablets (Parlam).

The veterinarian should be circumspect in his use of antitussive drugs, as symptomatic therapy can be dangerous in the absence of a diagnosis. A patient that is vomiting and has a tracheo-esophageal fistula will exhibit episodes of severe coughing owing to passage of material from the esophagus into the trachea. In such a patient, elimination of the cough reflex would have disastrous consequences. Coughing should not be suppressed in a patient with a productive cough, as this may allow the collection of fluid and exudate in the bronchial tree. Furthermore, symptomatic therapy may delay the institution of specific therapy, as in the failure to diagnose a lung worm or filaroides infection.

Sneezing is a protective reflex similar to coughing, except that the effective stimulus arises in the nasal cavity and upper pharynx. Generally, sneezing is episodic and does not require treatment. If sneezing were a problem in a given patient, it could be abolished by intranasal application of a topical anesthetic such as lidocaine or benzocaine.

MODIFICATION OF AIRWAY RESISTANCE

Effective respiration involves four interrelated mechanisms: ventilation, distribution of inspired gas, diffusion, and pulmonary capillary blood flow. Pulmonary diseases can affect all four functions, and appropriate drug therapy can effectively modify airway resistance and alter blood flow in the capillaries. Obstructive airway disease may be caused by excessive secretions, edema of the mucosa, foreign bodies or tumors, fibrosis and infiltration producing anatomic narrowing, and spasm of the bronchial musculature.

The smooth muscle of pulmonary arterioles, bronchi, bronchioles, and glands of the respiratory tract epithelium is regulated by the autonomic nervous system. An understanding of the actions of autonomic drugs and the nature of the receptors in these effector organs is essential for the rational use of drugs in the mitigation of obstructive airway disease.

Secretion by tubulo-acinar glands is controlled by parasympathetic fibers in the vagus nerves. Cholinergic and anticholinesterase drugs stimulate secretion, and anticholinergic drugs diminish secretion. Any of these classes of drugs might produce undesirable effects in patients with bronchitis, asthma, emphysema, or other conditions in which an increased resistance might compromise ventilation. Stimulation of secretion would add to the volume of respiratory tract fluid contained within the tracheobronchi, whereas inhibition of tubulo-acinar glands may increase the viscosity of mucous plugs, making it difficult for the animal to expel them. Adrenergic nerves and drugs apparently do not influence secretion of respiratory tract fluid.

Smooth muscle of arterioles and bronchioles and cardiac muscle contain adrenergic receptors that can be stimulated by drugs. Depending on the nature of the receptor in the muscle and the drug administered, adrenergic stimulation may produce excitation or inhibition. Adrenergic receptors are classified as alpha or beta types. Stimulation of an alpha receptor will induce an excitatory response (constriction), whereas stimulation of a beta receptor will cause relaxation (dilation). The exception to this classification is the myocardial beta receptor, which when stimulated by a beta agonist, will respond with an increase in rate, conduction, and force of contraction. Because of this, beta receptors are subdivided into beta 1 (heart) and beta 2 (other tisssues) types. As one generally administers an adrenergic drug in such a way that it enters the general circulation, one must know the types of receptors present in various tissues so as to be able to anticipate the overall effects of the drug. These are listed in Table 1.

Adrenergic drugs differ in their ability to stimulate the different types of receptors. Drugs such as phenylephrine are purely alpha agonists, isoproterenol is purely a beta receptor stimulant, and epinephrine will stimulate both types of receptors equally. Because of the

Table 1. *Adrenergic Effects*

SITE	RECEPTOR TYPE	EFFECT
Heart	β_1	Increase in rate, conduction, force
Bronchial muscle	β_2	Dilation
Coronary and skeletal blood vessels	β_2	Dilation
Pulmonary and cerebral blood vessels	α and β_2	Contract/relax
Cutaneous blood vessels	α	Constriction
Splanchnic blood vessels	α	Constriction

Table 2. *Adrenergic Drugs*

DRUG	PROPRIETARY NAME	RECEPTOR TYPE	CLINICAL USES°
Epinephrine	Adrenalin	α, β_1, β_2	A,P,D,B,C
Ephedrine	Many	α, β_1, β_2	P,D,B,C
Levarterenol	Levophed	strong α, weak β	P
Phenylephrine	Neosynephrine	α	P,D
Phenylpropanolamine	Many	α	D
Tuaminoheptane	Tuamine	α	D
Propylhexadrine	Benzedrex	α	D
Cyclopentamine	Clopane	α	D
Naphazoline	Privine	α	D
Tetrahydrozoline	Tyzine	α	D
Xylometazoline	Otrivin	α	D
Isoetharine	Dilabron	β_2	B
Metaproterenol	Alupent	β_2	B
Terbutaline	Bricanyl	β_2	B
Salbutamol†	Ventolin	β_2	B
Soterenol†	—	β_2	B
Quinterenol†	—	β_2	B
Isoproterenol	Isuprel	β_1, β_2	B,C

°A – allergic reactions, B – bronchodilator, C – cardiac, D – decongestant, P – pressor agent.
†Not yet commercially available in the United States.

mixed activity of the older drugs, efforts have been made to develop drugs that exert a narrower spectrum of activity so as to minimize side effects. The newer beta agonists stimulate β_2 receptors with little effect on the heart. The various types of adrenergic drugs are listed in Table 2.

The beta receptor is associated with an enzyme, adenylate cyclase, which is located in the cell membrane of the effector cell. Combination of an agonist drug with the receptor activates adenylate cyclase to catalyze the conversion of adenosine triphosphate to cyclic adenosine, 3'5' monophosphate (cyclic-AMP) within the cell. Cyclic-AMP relaxes the contractile elements within smooth muscle and inhibits histamine release from mast cells. This pathway is illustrated in Figure 1.

The important point to note is that an increase in cyclic-AMP within the cell relaxes contracted smooth muscle, such as occurs during bronchoconstriction. From an inspection of Figure 1, one can see that the concentration of cyclic-AMP can be increased either by stimulating its production (beta adrenergic drugs) or by inhibiting its rate of destruction by the enzyme phos-

phodiesterase. The xanthines, such as theophylline, inhibit phosphodiesterase and thus dilate the bronchioles. Because the xanthines and beta stimulants act through different mechanisms, it is rational to use the two groups in combination to treat a patient that might be relatively refractory to either drug alone. It is irrational to employ two different beta stimulants at the same time.

Theophylline is insoluble in water and can only be given orally. Soluble salts of theophylline such as theophylline ethylenediamine (aminophylline), theophylline sodium glycinate, and choline theophyllinate (oxtriphylline) are available in dosage forms suitable for injection. We have found the half-life of theophylline to be six hours in the dog, one to one and one-half hours in the ox, and three hours in the horse. Four times a day therapy should be appropriate for canine patients; other species would require more frequent dosage.

It has been found in recent studies that the parasympathetic nervous system is responsible for maintaining tone of the bronchiolar smooth muscle and that anticholinergic drugs such as atropine, dibenzheptropine (deptropine), and

Figure 1.   The pathway to cyclic AMP.

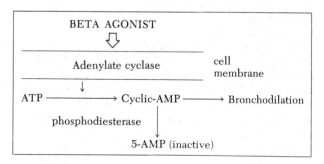

iprotropium (Sch-1000) will augment the bronchodilator effects of the beta agonists. The therapist must weigh the advantage of this effect against the possibility of drying secretions so as to increase tenacity of mucous plugs.

With this background, the veterinarian can logically choose a drug on the basis of what it is he wants to accomplish in the patient. The therapist should be aware of some problems that have been noted with bronchodilator therapy. When administered by inhalation, isoproterenol will be distributed most rapidly to well ventilated areas of the lung rather than to affected regions. Following absorption, the cardiac side effects may predominate over the desired effects on the constricted bronchioles. Following parenteral administration, it is common for the PaO_2 to drop precipitously in the asthmatic patient. This effect is due to drug-induced dilation of pulmonary vessels, which were constricted to redistribute blood flow away from poorly ventilated regions. Thus, a portion of the blood flow would perfuse areas that have not yet become well ventilated.

The principal side effects of the new beta 2 adrenergic drugs are nervousness, tremor, muscle weakness, and vomiting (with high dosage). In the case of isoproterenol and the xanthines, one should observe the cardiovascular response to the drugs.

DECONGESTION

Another factor to consider in airway resistance is edema of the mucosa of the various passages. The lining membranes become swollen in response to inflammatory mediators such as kallikrein, histamine, bradykinin, and SRS-A. Drugs that antagonize release of these mediators (corticosteroids) and drugs that directly constrict mucosal arterioles (alpha adrenergics) will reduce this edema and thereby decrease resistance to air flow. Thus, ephedrine may provide an advantage over a beta 2 agonist because its ability to stimulate alpha receptors will result in vasoconstriction of the bronchial arterioles, whereas its beta properties will dilate the bronchioles. One might combine an alpha agonist such as phenylpropanolamine with a beta 2 agonist such as isoetharine to accomplish the same purpose.

The decongestant adrenergic drugs are most commonly employed topically because of their marked pressor effects when injected. They can be sprayed into the pharynx and nasal cavity or instilled as drops.Epinephrine should not be used for this purpose because the vasoconstriction is of short duration and is followed by a reactive hyperemia. Prolonged use of the decongestants can produce ischemic necrosis and

ulceration of the mucosa. This group of drugs will relieve mucosal edema and is effective in controlling hemorrhage from accessible areas of the respiratory system. Cocaine (5 per cent solution, as a spray) is a unique drug for this purpose because it produces topical anesthesia and constricts the blood vessels of the mucosa. The author has used this technique as an adjunct to general anesthesia for performing tonsillectomies and devocalizing operations.

Corticosteroids are useful for the management of a variety of pulmonary diseases so long as they are employed in a rational manner. Thoughtful selection of patients and careful monitoring of the effects are imperative. Several actions of the glucocorticoids on the respiratory tract are noteworthy. They reduce inflammation by inhibiting release of mediators, stabilizing membranes, reducing edema, and suppressing immune reactions in allergies. They sensitize the smooth muscle of bronchioles to the action of beta adrenergic drugs, stimulate the rate of synthesis of epinephrine by the adrenal medulla, and inhibit the rate of its destruction. For these purposes, the corticosteroids can be administered parenterally, orally, or by inhalation. For chronic administration, the clinician should strive for the lowest effective dose administered by every other day therapy. The decision to institute corticosteroid therapy must be based on a balance between anticipated therapeutic benefits and the known side effects of the dose and duration of treatment. Corticosteroid therapy must not be instituted in the absence of a diagnosis, as it could activate a viral or deep fungal infection if that were the underlying problem.

A newer drug that is neither a bronchodilator nor a corticosteroid is chromolyn sodium. This drug is useful for prophylaxis of asthmatic attacks caused by allergens. It acts by inhibiting the degranulation of mast cells in the lung and thereby preventing the release of histamine and SRS-A, which are bronchoconstrictors. Chromolyn is available only as an aerosol of fine particles to be administered by inhalation. Its role in veterinary therapeutics is undefined at this time.

STIMULATION OF RESPIRATION

In patients with acute respiratory failure, intubation and mechanical ventilation is the most efficient method for resuscitation. The older drugs such as pentylenetetrazol, nikethamide, amphetamine, and picrotoxin are now regarded as obsolete. They induced convulsion and were frequently ineffective in stimulating a hypoxic respiratory center. Doxapram is a relatively safe stimulant that acts reflexly by stimulating peripheral chemoreceptors rather than the brain. It has been employed to decrease drug-induced depression of the respiratory centers, to reduce CO_2 retention in patients with obstructive airway disease that require oxygen therapy, and to stimulate respiration in neonatal asphyxia.

CONTROL OF INFECTION

General principles of antibacterial therapy were discussed in Section I. These same guidelines apply to the selection of an appropriate drug with which to control infections of the respiratory system. The cornerstone of effective, rational drug therapy is an accurate diagnosis. One should first establish that the patient has an infection and secondly should try to characterize the pathogen either by performing a Gram's stain of sediment from a transtracheal aspirate or by culture and sensitivity testing. An appropriate drug may then be selected on the basis of the therapist's knowledge of microbiology and pharmacology.

Rigorous studies of the distribution of the various antimicrobial drugs in the normal and diseased lung have not been done. There seems to be little evidence for the selection of one drug over another on the basis of penetration of tissues. The highly ionized drugs such as the aminoglycoside antibiotics are quite effective against susceptible pathogens in the lung, although they do not readily cross biologic membranes. The penicillins are hydrophilic compounds that are excluded by cellular membranes, yet they provide effective therapy against sensitive organisms infecting the lungs.

There seems to be little advantage to the practice of administering antimicrobial drugs by nebulization or by direct intratracheal instillation for the treatment of pneumonia or bronchitis. In these conditions, there will be an increased airway resistance in the affected portions of the bronchial tree. Inhaled medication will follow the pathway of least resistance and be diverted from the areas one is trying to treat.

Common pitfalls that are responsible for failure of antimicrobial therapy include:

1. Inappropriate choice of drug
2. Presence of an untreatable disease (viral or neoplastic diseases)
3. Incorrect diagnosis
4. Failure of drainage (obstruction to natural drainage or presence of a deep-seated pulmonary abscess)
5. Presence of a foreign body
6. Antagonism between simultaneously administered drugs (e.g., penicillins and tetracyclines)
7. Impairment of host defenses
8. Emergence of drug-resistant strain of organism
9. Drug interaction or incompatibility (e.g., ampicillin combined with acetylcysteine for nebulization).

ADVERSE EFFECTS OF DRUGS ON THE LUNGS

Adverse reactions to drugs may closely resemble respiratory disease, and the association may therefore be overlooked. In these cases, the veterinarian may dispense unnecessary medication rather than withdraw the offending agent.

Pulmonary disease may be induced as a result of an allergic reaction, an idiosyncrasy, or a direct toxic effect. Many of these reactions are reversible when the drug is withdrawn.

Bronchospasm may be induced by acetyl cysteine, local anesthetics, aspirin, antibiotics, cholinergic and anticholinesterase drugs, iron dextran, propranolol, vaccines, and vitamin K. Polyarteritis has been reported in response to arsenicals, phenytoin, mercurials, phenothiazines, sulfonamides, iodides, and DDT. Pulmonary eosinophilia may be associated with mephenesin, sulfonamides, penicillin, and imipramine but is most commonly associated with nitrofurantoin. Intravenous lidocaine may cause respiratory arrest. High concentrations of oxygen will produce fibrosis and hyperplasia of the alveolar epithelium accompanied by edema, hemorrhage, and congestion.

Drugs may be inhaled and produce foreign body pneumonia. The most serious is lipoid pneumonia, caused by inhalation of oily substances such as liquid petrolatum or cod liver oil.

Pulmonary embolism can be induced by inadvertent intravenous administration of insoluble suspensions — e.g., procaine penicillin, or substances in oily vehicles. A number of drugs can influence respiration through their effects on acid-base balance.

SUPPLEMENTAL READING

Carpenter, J.L.: Bronchial asthma in cats. In Kirk, R.W. (ed.): *Current Veterinary Therapy V.* Philadelphia, W.B. Saunders Co., 1974.

Costello, J.F., and Murray, J.F.: Respiratory disorders. In Melmon, K.L., and Morrelli, H.F. (eds.): *Clinical Pharamcology. Basic Principles in Therapeutics,* 2nd ed. New York, Macmillan, 1978.

Head, J.R., and Suter, P.: Approach to the patient with respiratory disease. In Ettinger, S.J. (ed.): *Textbook of Veterinary Internal Medicine, Vol. 1.* Philadelphia, W.B. Saunders Co., 1975.

CANINE UPPER RESPIRATORY DISEASE

RICHARD WALSHAW, B.V.M.S.,
East Lansing, Michigan

and RICHARD B. FORD, D.V.M.
West Lafayette, Indiana

Anatomic boundaries separating the upper and lower respiratory tract in the dog and cat are not firmly established. For this discussion, the upper respiratory tract is defined as those airways extending from the rostral aspect of the nose and mouth to the caudal larynx.

The upper airways warm, humidify, and filter the inspired air. In this capacity, the upper respiratory tract is continuously exposed to a multitude of environmental pathogens that are effectively destroyed or otherwise eliminated in the healthy animal. Sneezing, coughing, and mucociliary transport are examples of protective mechanisms necessary in maintaining the functional integrity of the upper respiratory tract. The clinician must be aware that the animal presented with overt signs of upper respiratory tract disease also has compromised the protective capacity of this "barrier" thereby increasing its susceptibility to systemic infection.

The foundation on which a diagnosis of upper respiratory tract disease (URD) is made depends on proper interpretation of the clinical history and signs of the animal presented. Clinical signs, if evident at examination, can be used to identify the site of upper respiratory tract disease (Table 1). Not uncommonly, the presenting complaint is only suggestive of URD — i.e., signs are not manifest, nor can they be elicited during the examination. Careful interpretation of information provided by the owner is essential when the diagnosis is not apparent. Frequency, duration, and character of physical signs, as well as possible exposure to infectious disease, must be considered.

Proper interpretation of the history and clinical signs is critical if the spectrum of diseases causing URD is to be narrowed. Diagnostic confirmation and successful treatment may depend on radiography and a thorough visual examination of the upper respiratory tract. These studies are best carried out in the anesthetized animal. Radiographs of upper airway structures should be made prior to a visual examination in order to avoid artifact caused by manipulation (e.g., nasal hemorrhage). Visual examination should include skull symmetry and the oral cavity, particularly the hard and soft palates, upper dental arcade, tonsils, nasal and oral pharynx, larynx, and rostral portion of the right and left nasal antrum as viewed through an otoscope speculum or rhinoscope. The clinician should be prepared to obtain biopsy samples, needle aspirates, and tissue from nasal flushings and cultures at the time of examination (Fig. 1). Interpretation of this information will be discussed in the following sections.

ACUTE UPPER RESPIRATORY DISEASE IN DOGS

EPISTAXIS

The possible causes of epistaxis are trauma, invasive intranasal lesions, and the presence of a bleeding disorder (Fig. 2).

Epistaxis can result from blunt trauma (car accident), sharp, penetrating trauma (bullet, dog fight), or severe sneezing, or it can follow nasal surgery. The bleeding, though severe initially, is usually easily controlled. A history of recent trauma will usually be obtained, and a careful physical examination will reveal evidence of trauma to the head region. The nasal bones should be carefully palpated for evidence of deformity and depression fractures. The hard palate should be inspected for a traumatic cleft or other injury as can be found in cats with the "high-rise syndrome." Radiographs will reveal the presence of fractures of the bones that make up the nasal cavity, possibly other fractures of the skull and mandible, and evidence of damage to the turbinate structures. If the epistaxis is due to penetrating trauma, presence of external wounds should be noted, and radiographs may reveal a penetrating foreign body, for example a bullet.

214

Table 1. *Localization of Clinical Signs*

SIGN	URT SEGMENT INVOLVED	COMMENT
Sneezing	Rhinarium	Commonly paroxysmal. Paranasal sinuses may or may not be involved.
Stertor	Pharynx	Characterized as a snoring sound heard during inspiration. Suggests obstructive disease—e.g., elongated soft palate.
"Reverse" Sneeze	Nasopharynx	Rapid, forced inspiratory effort made during attempts to displace material from the nasopharynx to the oropharynx. (Described in the dog only.)
Stridor	Larynx	Wheezing; inspiratory or expiratory.
Cough	Larynx	Persistent cough also warrants examination of the trachea, lower airways, lungs, and heart.
Open-mouth Breathing	Not a localizing sign	Indicative of respiratory distress secondary to obstructive disease that may involve rhinarium, pharynx, larynx, or lower airway structures.

Severe paroxysmal sneezing following inhalation of foreign material, for example grass awns, can result in epistaxis. A history of recent exposure to such material may be elicited from the owner. Radiographs of the nose will reveal fluid filling (hemorrhage) of the affected side but no evidence of bony involvement.

Bleeding disorders, for example von Willebrand's disease or hemophilia, can result in severe, uncontrollable epistaxis that can occur spontaneously or can follow minor trauma. The hemorrhage can be profuse and the poor clotting ability of the blood will be noted. Appropriate laboratory tests must be performed to confirm a diagnosis if these conditions are suspected (refer to hematology section).

Invasive intranasal lesions — e.g., aspergillosis — can cause acute epistaxis, but dogs are more likely to present with a history of chronic nasal disease that develops episodes of epistaxis later in its course. Both malignant neoplasia and fungal infections cause severe destruction of the turbinate structures within the nose, with erosion into major vessels and subsequent epistaxis. Patients presented with this history should be suspected of having these types of lesions, and suitable steps should be taken to obtain a diagnosis (see later section on nasal neoplasia and fungal infections).

Treatment. Treatment of epistaxis should control the hemorrhage, maintain a patent airway, and replenish blood and fluid loss.

Cage rest and application of ice packs to the nasal area are indicated. The animal should be placed in a slightly head down position to pre-

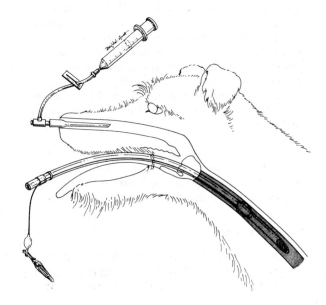

Figure 1. Method of nasal flushing in the dog.

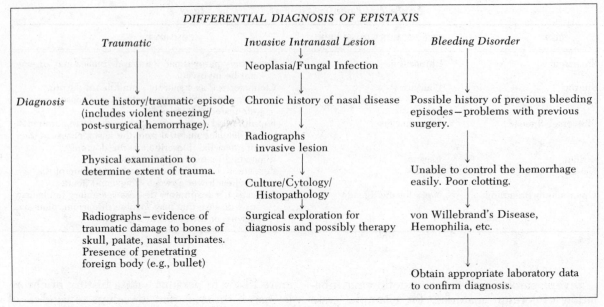

Figure 2

vent aspiration. Sedation may be required if the patient is fractious, but this should be avoided if possible, as it may compromise the patient's ability to maintain a patent airway and prevent aspiration by coughing, sneezing, and swallowing. Packing the external nares alone is of little value, as blood may continue to be lost via the internal nares. If the hemorrhage is severe, vital signs and hematocrit should be carefully monitored. A great deal of blood will be swallowed if the animal is conscious, so that the blood appearing at the external nares is not an indication of total blood loss.

If conservative treatment fails to control the hemorrhage, the patient should be anesthetized and intubated with a cuffed endotracheal tube; the pharynx, larynx, and trachea should be cleaned and both the internal and external nares should be packed with gauze sponges. Fluid and/or blood replacement will be required if hemorrhage is severe.

Rarely, surgical exploration will be required to identify and deal with the bleeding points, and the entire nasal cavity will have to be packed.

If a bleeding disorder is suspected, fresh blood transfusions will be required to replace the factors in which the patient is deficient and to enable clotting to occur temporarily.

NASAL TRAUMA

Nasal trauma results in epistaxis and/or obstruction (Fig. 3). Turbinate damage can obstruct the nasal cavity and also prevent drainage of the frontal sinuses. Trauma can be blunt (car accident), sharp, or penetrating (bullet, dog bite), or it can be the result of severe sneezing episodes or surgical intervention.

Initially, nasal obstruction results from blood clots, edema and inflammation of the nasal mucosa, displaced fragments of bones that make up the nasal cavity, and broken and displaced turbinates. If the patient is able to mouth-breathe, stabilization and conservative therapy should be instituted until the epistaxis subsides. If nasal obstruction is severe and mouth breathing does not provide adequate ventilation, a tracheotomy tube should be inserted to provide a patent airway. Conservative treatment for a few days to allow the blood clots and other secretions to clear should include keeping the external nares clear and patent, placing the patient on antibiotics systemically, and, if necessary, using intranasal medication — for example, phenylephrine hydrochloride — to help clear the nasal secretions and decrease the inflammatory reaction. If obstruction is still present and there are badly displaced fractures of the bones of the nasal cavity, the fragments must be realigned and fixed with pins and wire. Fragments depressed into the cavity must be elevated. During fixation, correct alignment of the teeth must be maintained. Fragments devoid of their blood supply should be removed as they form sequestra and cause chronic problems. Exploration and curettage of the nasal turbinates may be indicated if damage is severe. Removal of severely damaged turbinates allows the formation of a patent nasal airway and prevents subsequent frontal sinus obstruction.

Traumatic cleft palates, which are more often seen in cats with associated mandibular symphyseal fractures, need not be treated if they are less than 3 mm wide. A wider cleft requires fixation with wire.

Chronic nasal disease and obstruction are possible sequelae to nasal trauma owing to displaced bone and turbinate fragments or bone sequestra. Osteomyelitis can develop in these damaged bone fragments, and these plus the bone sequestra lead to chronic inflammatory nasal disease. Specific infections — for example, fungal infections — can become established in these areas of damaged tissue and pose serious sequelae to nasal trauma. Blockage of the opening to the frontal sinuses can lead to the development of a frontal sinus mucocele. These chronic nasal problems will be discussed in a later section.

TRAUMA OF THE PHARYNX, LARYNX, AND TRACHEA

The most common injuries to the pharynx, larynx, and trachea result from sharp, penetrating trauma (dog bite wounds, gunshot wounds) and the overzealous use of choke chains. Acute respiratory problems arise from hematoma or edema formation and displacement of portions of the hyoid apparatus or laryngeal cartilages. Besides cartilage displacement, laryngotracheal or tracheal separation may occur, particularly with the tearing forces involved in dog fight injuries. This results in loss of continuity of the airway and possibly severe respiratory embarrassment.

Diagnosis should be made based on the history of the traumatic incident and clinical findings localizing the site of dyspnea to the laryngotracheal region. Inspection for the presence of external wounds; external palpation of the structures of the hyoid, larynx, and trachea; plus the detection of cervical subcutaneous emphysema indicate the extent of injury. If severe dyspnea is present, an immediate tracheotomy may be required to maintain a patent airway. If tracheal damage is present, the tracheotomy must be performed caudal to the site of injury. Following stabilization of the patient, radiographs should be obtained of the cervical region and the thorax to determine the extent of injury. Pneumomediastinum may be present due to air tracking down the neck from the area of cervical injury. The possibility of this leading to respiratory embarrassment and pneumothorax must be considered, and therefore the patient should be monitored carefully. Treatment of the external wounds should be performed in a routine manner, and the patient should be placed on systemic antibiotics and steroids to help prevent infection and to reduce inflammatory swelling of the larynx.

Laryngoscopy and tracheoscopy should be performed as soon as the patient is stable. This is indicated in cases in which it has been determined that laryngeal and/or tracheal damage is sufficient to cause continued airway obstruction owing to displaced bony or cartilaginous structures. Portions of the hyoid apparatus penetrating the pharynx can be removed, as can avulsed or displaced laryngeal tissue. Severe pharyngeal lacerations should be sutured. If pharyngeal or laryngeal damage is extensive, a pharyngostomy tube should be inserted, as dysphagia during the recovery period may be a problem.

A possible sequela to trauma of the laryn-

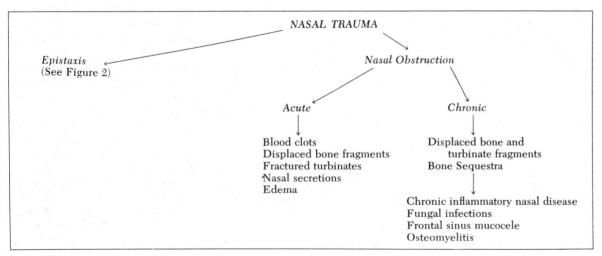

Figure 3

geal and tracheal areas is recurrent laryngeal nerve damage leading to laryngeal paralysis. This is more of a problem in working dogs that are constantly pulling on choke chains. The problem will be discussed in a later section.

Tracheal tears that result in airway obstruction and tracheal separations require surgical repair. This can be performed as a primary procedure or can follow patient stabilization, should other problems be present that preclude prolonged anesthesia. These patients usually require a tracheotomy until tracheal continuity can be reestablished. When the patient with a tracheal tear or separation is anesthetized, care should be taken to guide the endotracheal tube carefully across the damaged segment to insure correct placement and patient ventilation. If intubation is impossible, a tracheotomy should be performed, if not already done, caudal to this site. The tracheal segments are sutured together using fine nonabsorable suture material — for example, 4–0 polypropylene — in a horizontal mattress suture pattern. Care should be taken to avoid having suture material enter the tracheal lumen (to prevent granuloma formation) and to avoid further damage to the tracheal cartilages.

With penetrating trauma to the cervical region, damage to other vital structures apart from the airway should also be considered. The integrity of the esophagus should be established and, if necessary, esophagoscopy should be performed.

NASAL FOREIGN BODIES

Nasal foreign bodies are most commonly of plant material — for example, grass awns or foxtails — that enter the nose by inhalation. More rarely, other types of foreign bodies are encountered, such as bullets and other penetrating objects or foreign materials that enter by sadistic placement.

Inhaled plant material typically causes sudden onset paroxysmal sneezing. The patient may have been playing in a grassy area and will frequently be pawing at its muzzle. Clinical examination may reveal the presence of plant material around the animal's head and in its coat. The sneezing may well blow out the foreign material, leaving an area of turbinate damage and acute inflammation. Epistaxis may be present due to the severe sneezing. This foreign material is not radiodense, and radiographs of the nose will only reveal an area of increased fluid density on the affected side owing to the accumulation of secretions and blood.

The diagnosis is suspected from the history and clinical findings. Rhinoscopy may reveal the foreign material or an area of acute inflammation. When the foreign material can be seen, removal with suitable forceps is possible. If the foreign material cannot be seen, vigorous nasal flushing should be attempted. The material flushed out of the nose should be carefully examined for the presence of plant material, and the nasal cavity should be flushed until no more material is removed. Following nasal flushing, the patient should be placed on systemic antibiotic therapy. If no foreign material is obtained, it may be that it had already been sneezed out or that the nasal flushing was unsuccessful in removing it. These cases should, therefore, be followed carefully to observe for signs of continued nasal problems.

A possible sequela to this problem is chronic inflammatory nasal disease owing either to the continued presence of foreign material within the nasal cavity or to damage that occurred to turbinates in the acute phase of the problem. Surgical exploration of these cases is usually indicated, and this will be discussed in a later section.

Large foreign bodies — for example, bullets — must be surgically removed, and the extent of damage within the nasal cavity must be carefully assessed. With penetrating objects like bullets, damage to the palate must also be considered. If holes are present in the palate, plastic surgical procedures will be required to close them.

Small foreign objects such as pins, small stones, and ball bearings can become sucked into the larynx and trachea. These can cause acute airway obstruction, cyanosis, and collapse, particularly if the object lodges in the larynx. If the object is in the trachea, the animal is usually able to ventilate adequately. Oxygen should be administered and radiographs should be rapidly obtained of the larynx and trachea to localize the position of the foreign body. Endotracheal intubation or an emergency tracheotomy may be required to provide a patent airway and ventilation until the foreign body can be removed.

Laryngeal foreign bodies can be removed by laryngoscopy and forceps removal. Tracheoscopy plus forceps removal should be attempted for foreign bodies in the trachea. However, if the patient is too small or too large, of if the object is embedded in the wall of the trachea, appropriate surgical intervention may be required for certain cases. A cervical tracheotomy or a thoracic approach may be required. If the object is lodged at the carina, removal of a cranial lung lobe will allow access through the bronchus.

CHRONIC NASAL DISEASE IN DOGS

CHRONIC INFLAMMATORY PROBLEMS

Chronic inflammatory problems of the nose are sequelae of acute rhinitis, intranasal foreign bodies, and nasal trauma. Chronic rhinitis is due to chronic irritation, destruction of nasal turbinate structures, and subsequent obstruction of the nasal passages.

Patients are presented with a chronic nasal discharge that may be mucoid, serous, purulent, or bloody. The discharge can be unilateral or bilateral and is associated with frequent sneezing. These patients often gag or retch and have a chronic pharyngitis due to postnasal drip. A conjunctival discharge may be present, owing to nasolacrimal duct obstruction.

A clinical history might elicit the initiating cause of the problem, but this is frequently not so. Physical examination of the patient may reveal the presence of previous trauma to the nasal area. In these cases, nasal radiographs may reveal the presence of old, healed fractures, displaced or destroyed turbinates, bone sequestration, or areas of new bone formation. Culture and cytology from the nasal secretions is frequently unremarkable. If the problem is a result of intranasal foreign bodies, radiographs will reveal areas of increased density with possible turbinate destruction. The differentiation of this from a neoplastic or fungal lesion is difficult because of similar radiographic signs, and it can often only be made at the time of surgical exploration.

Because of their unresponsiveness to conservative medical management, a more aggressive approach to these cases is required. Providing changes in the turbinate system are miminal, vigorous nasal flushing may be attempted as a therapeutic regimen. The aims of this are to cleanse the nasal cavity thoroughly and to convert a chronic inflammatory process into an acute one that will resolve. Following nasal flushing, therapy should be continued with a broad spectrum antibiotic such as chloramphenicol. The external nares should be kept free of discharge. Corticosteriod therapy using prednisolone may also be of benefit. Careful case follow-up is required to insure resolution of the problem. Some of these cases, however, will progress and require surgical exploration.

If radiographs show extensive changes, cases of chronic rhinitis require surgical exploration of the nasal cavity and turbinate removal. Exploration confirms the diagnosis and also allows removal of the chronically irritated and destroyed turbinate structures. Cleansing of the nasal cavity in this fashion relieves the obstruction within the turbinates and within the frontal sinuses, allows good drainage, and provides a patent airway. At the time of surgery, a drain tube can be placed in the region of the frontal sinus so that the nasal cavity can be flushed postoperatively with an antiseptic solution such as 1 percent Lugol's iodine.

The surgical technique for nasal exploration and turbinate curettage has been well described. Postoperative care of these patients consists of administering systemic antibiotic therapy, keeping the external nares free of discharge and blood clots, and flushing the nose.

Occasionally, progression of dental disease of the upper arcade of teeth can result in chronic rhinitis due to erosion into the nasal cavity. The teeth most commonly associated with this condition are the canines, the premolars, and the molars, particularly the carnassial teeth. The abscessed teeth must be removed to establish drainage. Occasionally, the involvement of the nasal cavity is severe enough to warrant specific treatment. The authors have seen a case of severe actinomycotic rhinitis secondary to root abscesses of the carnassial tooth in a poodle. Extensive nasal surgery was necessary to resolve the severe turbinate damage.

In cases of chronic rhinitis of unknown etiology immunopotentiation may be of help, using drugs like thiabendazole* or levamisole†. The authors have successfully treated a number of dogs with thiabendazole at a dose of 10 mg/kg b.i.d. orally for six weeks.

MYCOTIC INFECTIONS

Mycotic infections of the canine nose can be primary, or they can be secondary to chronic rhinitis and nasal trauma. The most common fungus in canine mycotic rhinitis is *Aspergillus* spp. This is usually a secondary invader. *Penicillium* spp. and, very rarely, systemic mycoses — for example *Cryptococcus* spp. — may be encountered.

Patients with nasal fungal infections present with a chronic nasal discharge that can be unilateral or bilateral, mucopurulent or bloody. Owing to the invasive nature of this infection,

*Mintezol, Merck, Sharp & Dohme, West Point, PA.
†Levasole, Pitman Moore, Washington Crossing, N.J.

epistaxis may be a presenting sign. A history of previous nasal trauma or an acute rhinitis problem that has subsequently become chronic may be elicited from the owner. Dogs of any age can be affected, which may help differentiate this from nasal neoplasia. Apart from this age difference, the presenting signs for the two problems can be very similar and therefore difficult to discern. Case work-up should include nasal radiographs, nasal flushing, and cultures and cytologic examination of the material obtained. Radiographically, turbinate destruction, bone lysis, and generalized opacity of the nasal cavity and frontal sinuses are seen. These signs are similar to those found with neoplastic disease and therefore offer no help in the differentiation. Culture and cytologic examination of nasal flushing will often confirm the diagnosis. Rhinoscopy may reveal fungal plaques and areas of turbinate destruction. The success of this, however, depends generally upon the size of the dog and the site of the lesions. Diagnosis is frequently only confirmed at the time of exploratory surgery.

Treatment depends upon the degree of turbinate destruction evident upon radiographic examination. In cases presented early in the course of the disease, often with acute epistaxis and minimal radiographic changes within the nasal cavity, medical treatment can be attempted. Nasal flushing with 1 percent Lugol's iodine should be performed under anesthesia. Treatment should continue with 1 percent Lugol's iodine nose drops for 10 days. The dog should be placed on systemic antibiotic therapy, for example with chloramphenicol for three weeks, and thiabendazole, at a dosage of 10 mg/kg orally B.I.D. for 6 weeks. Thiabendazole has a direct antifungal action for aspergillus, but it also is a potent immunopotentiator. Dogs with nasal aspergillus infections are significantly immunodeficient, as demonstrated by mitogen stimulation studies using the dog's lymphocytes. Following treatment with thiabendazole, the immune status of the patient returns to normal. These dogs should be checked in six weeks, and culture and cytologic evaluation of nasal flushings should again be performed to determine if therapy has been successful.

Patients with significant radiographic changes within their nasal cavities require surgical exploration. Medical therapy alone is insufficient because of the walled off areas of destroyed tissue harboring the fungal infection. Surgical exploration can either be unilateral or bilateral, depending upon the extent of the disease. Thorough turbinate curettage, removal of bone destroyed by fungal invasion, and establishment of good frontal sinus drainage are essential. Prior to replacing the bone flap and closing the incision, a drainage tube is placed in the frontal sinus on the affected side(s) and the nasal cavity is thoroughly flushed with an iodine solution. Postoperative care consists of flushing the nasal cavity three times daily with 1 per cent Lugol's iodine, keeping the external nares free of discharge, and placing the dog on systemic antibiotic therapy for three weeks. The Lugol's iodine flushes are continued for ten days, after which the tube is removed.

A six-week course of thiabendazole is instituted. Patients should be rechecked at the end of this period to determine if therapy has been successful.

Providing there has not been extensive destruction of the surrounding bones that make up the nasal chamber, treatment is usually successful.

NEOPLASTIC DISEASES

Neoplasia of the nasal cavity and frontal sinus occurs most frequently in medium- to large-sized dogs, long-nosed breeds being more often affected than other breeds. Average age incidence is nine to ten years, and there is no epidemiologic difference in incidence between urban and rural dogs.

Cases of nasal neoplasia usually present with a long history of chronic nasal discharge that is progressively worsening. Frequently, these cases have been treated for chronic rhinitis symptomatically without improvement. The nasal discharge is unilateral, but it can become bilateral as the disease progresses and the tumor crosses the nasal septum. Discharge is mucoid to mucopurulent in nature, becoming bloody as the tumor erodes vessels. Severe epistaxis occurs if vessels of significant size are involved. The patient will sneeze and may paw at the nose. As the neoplasm progresses, facial distortion occurs. An ocular discharge may be seen owing to blockage of the nasolacrimal duct on the affected side. Invasion of the neoplasm through the medial wall of the orbit results in varying degrees of exophthalmos. Occasionally, the neoplasm may ulcerate through the skin. Destruction of the hard palate can also occur.

Diagnosis is based upon radiographic, cytologic, and histopathologic examination. History and clinical signs do not necessarily differentiate a neoplastic condition from an invasive fungal lesion. Radiographs of the nasal cavity and frontal sinuses reveal areas of turbinate destruction and possible nasal septal deviation or destruction. Specific areas of increased density may indicate a neoplastic mass, this being more common with sarcomas. Opacification of the frontal sinus results from either filling with tumor mass or trapping of mucous exudate. The nasal cavity has a generalized increased density caused by fluid and hemorrhage. If the neoplastic process has progressed sufficiently, there may be radiographic evidence of destruction of the surrounding bones. Cytologic examination of nasal flushings may help confirm the diagnosis, and any solid pieces of tissues that are obtained should be sent for histopathologic examination.

Laryngeal neoplasia in the dog is extremely rare. However, various neoplasms including adenoma, adenocarcinoma, squamous cell carcinoma, lymphosarcoma, and osteosarcoma have been reported. These patients present with a history of a progressive change in their bark and increasing respiratory difficulty. Diagnosis is made by using direct laryngoscopy to visualize the mass and biopsy for histopathologic confirmation. Benign lesions can be removed surgically. For malignant lesions, partial laryngectomy may be indicated to reduce the tumor mass, followed by adjunct radiation or chemotherapy depending upon the tumor type. Total laryngectomy is not a feasible or practical procedure in the dog because of the problems of permanent tracheostomy care.

Benign inflammatory polyps of the vocal cords can be treated by local removal or ventriculocordectomy. (For further details on neoplasia, see the article "Neoplasms of the Respiratory Tract.")

UPPER RESPIRATORY DISEASE IN BRACHYCEPHALIC DOGS

Selective breeding of certain breeds, for example the boxer, bulldog, Boston terrier, pug, Pekingese, and Shih Tzu, has resulted in a shortened upper jaw, leading to a severe decrease in the distance from the external nares to the trachea. This brachycephalic head shape has resulted in severe overcrowding of the nasopharyngeal and laryngeal airways, causing varying degrees of upper respiratory obstruction. Airway obstruction is not due to a single factor but to a combination of problems including stenotic external nares, misshapen nasal chamber and turbinate structure, misshapen pharynx often with folds of excess tissue, and an elongated and thickened soft palate. The reduced airway space requires greater negative pressure to be developed in

the laryngeal area during inspiration. Over time, this increased negative pressure leads to secondary changes in the pharyngeal and laryngeal areas, namely infolding of the pharyngeal wall with eversion of the laryngeal saccules and eventual laryngeal collapse. In the English bulldog, an added complication is hypoplastic trachea, which severely adds to the respiratory difficulty.

Brachycephalic dogs are always noisy breathers, and their clinical signs can vary from snuffling, snorting respirations to mild or severe dyspnea. Clinical signs of inspiratory dyspnea become worse when the patient is stressed or excited or when weather is hot or humid. Mouth breathing does not help these patients because of the elongated soft palate or if the pharyngeal and laryngeal problems are severe. Some patients present when they are only a few months old, but more usually, the syndrome becomes progressively worse over several years. There may be failure to thrive owing to respiratory difficulty. Respiratory difficulties can be localized to the upper respiratory tract by signs of inspiratory dyspnea, by physical examination, and by auscultation where the loudest respiratory sounds are audible over the pharyngeal/laryngeal area.

Treatment. Management of these cases depends upon the severity of the clinical signs and the frequency and severity of the dyspneic episodes. All brachycephalic dogs are noisy breathers, and it is sometimes hard to differentiate normal noisy respirations from abnormal ones. Patients that present with noisy respirations but no dyspnea do not require treatment. These patients should avoid stress situations and be kept cool and calm, especially in hot, humid weather. Owners should be aware of the possibility of progression of these signs and should seek veterinary help as necessary should episodes of dyspnea develop. If the patient is having dyspneic episodes, it should be calmed or sedated and placed in a cool environment. The use of corticosteroids such as prednisolone is indicated to reduce the inflammatory swelling of the palate and larynx. This treatment is only temporarily effective, and it is likely that other dyspneic episodes will develop.

Surgical treatment to help these patients is indicated in (1) dogs with repeated dyspneic episodes, (2) dogs with progressively severe dyspnea, and (3) dogs already having problems at an early age.

The patient in respiratory distress at the time of presentation should be stabilized before surgery. An emergency tracheotomy may be necessary, oxygen therapy will be required, and high doses of corticosteroids should be administered. Prior to surgical intervention, lateral radiographs of the head and neck should be obtained to evaluate the nasopharyngeal and laryngeal airways. The size of the palate should be assessed and the trachea should be evaluated for hypoplasia. Thoracic radiographs should also be obtained because these patients frequently have chronic small airway disease. Before surgery is performed, the upper respiratory tract must be thoroughly evaluated under light anesthesia. Nares should be examined for stenosis. The length and thickness of the soft palate should be assessed with the dog in a normal dorsal-ventral position. The palate normally just overlaps the epiglottis, and it is important to determine how much should be resected to achieve a normal anatomic relationship without shortening it too much and thereby encountering problems with nasal regurgitation. The tonsils and lateral pharyngeal walls should also be evaluated. Direct laryngoscopy will assess the functional ability of the larynx and the presence of everted saccules and/or laryngeal collapse.

All patients undergoing corrective upper respiratory tract surgery should be given corticosteroids preoperatively to reduce the edema and inflammation that are invariably present, plus that which will result from surgical intervention. Broad spectrum antibiotics — for example, ampicillin — should also be started. A tracheotomy tube should be placed in all dogs undergoing any type of laryngeal surgery, allowing easier visualization of the surgical site and preventing postoperative airway obstruction owing to swelling and hemorrhage. It is always better to preplace a tracheotomy tube than to try to insert it when the patient is in respiratory distress. Dogs with pharyngeal collapse — e.g., bulldogs undergoing soft palate surgery — will benefit greatly from a tracheotomy tube during the postoperative period. Surgical techniques for correction of stenotic nares, overelongated soft palate, everted laryngeal saccules, and laryngeal collapse are well described elsewhere.

Postoperative care of these patients depends upon the degree of surgical intervention. Patients undergoing external nares and soft palate surgery should be monitored carefully for 24 hours for signs of respiratory obstruction and maintained on corticosteroids and antibiotics for seven to ten days. If a tracheotomy tube has been inserted, the patient should be monitored constantly and the tube should be aseptically aspirated as frequently as required to keep it clear. The tube can usually be re-

moved after 24 to 48 hours once it has been determined that there is no postoperative hemorrhage and that the initial soft tissue swelling has subsided.

Prognosis is directly related to the degree of surgical intervention. Small dogs with advanced problems of laryngeal collapse and bulldogs with hypoplastic tracheas will have the poorest postoperative results.

LARYNGEAL PARALYSIS

Laryngeal paralysis is seen in two forms in dogs. Paralysis following trauma to the neck is usually unilateral and due to direct damage to the recurrent laryngeal nerves. It is seen in hunting and guard dogs that pull hard on leashes or chains, and also as an iatrogenic complication following neck surgery. Congenital or acquired neurogenic atrophy of the laryngeal muscles results in bilateral laryngeal paralysis. Congenital laryngeal paralysis is reported in Bouviers, bull terriers, and sled dogs. The acquired form occurs in older large- or giant-breed dogs.

Presenting history and clinical signs vary depending upon the rate of onset and the degree of airway obstruction. Unilateral paralysis is not usually associated with clinical signs apart from some change in the quality of the bark. In working dogs, however, the condition will affect work performance, and treatment may be required. With bilateral congenital neurogenic atropy of the laryngeal muscles, clinical signs of severe airway obstruction and collapse can occur at a few months to one to two years of age. In the acquired form of the disease, there is typically a gradual onset of dyspnea, with hoarseness, rasping, and increased inspiratory noise. As these progress to severe obstruction, cyanosis and collapse occur, even with moderate exercise.

Diagnosis is based upon presenting history and clinical signs with localization of the respiratory problem to the laryngeal area. Definitive diagnosis is based upon direct laryngoscopy under light anesthesia. Typically, the paralysed vocal cord(s) is immobile and lies in a paramedian position. The movements are out of phase with respiration; i.e., the cord does not abduct on inspiration. The glottic lumen is therefore considerably smaller. Signs of chronic laryngitis are present with reddening and edematous thickening of the laryngeal structures. The arytenoid cartilages are displaced medially and ventrally, which causes the aryepiglottic folds to lie in a more medial position.

If there is severe respiratory obstruction at

the time of presentation, an immediate tracheotomy may be required in order to stabilize the patient. Preoperative corticosteroids and antibiotics should be administered. Two surgical methods of treatment for laryngeal paralysis are available. Partial laryngectomy (unilateral ventriculocordectomy and arytenoidectomy) is the most commonly performed procedure. Arytenoid cartilage lateralization has been described and appears to produce successful results. Both these techniques are well described elsewhere. Postoperative care consists of routine tracheotomy care, corticosteroids, and antibiotics.

Most cases of bilateral paralysis do well postoperatively with unilateral surgery. Some, however, especially if they are working dogs, may still have sufficient obstruction from the other vocal cord to warrant further surgical correction. Bilateral surgical correction greatly increases the chance of aspiration, and the owners must be warned of this problem.

The prognosis for these cases is generally good. Problem cases occur when the disease process has been present for so long that laryngeal collapse has occurred.

LARYNGEAL COLLAPSE

Laryngeal collapse occurs in two situations: either as the final event in dogs with the brachycephalic syndrome owing to prolonged severe airway obstruction or as the end stage of chronic airway obstruction in dogs with acquired laryngeal paralysis.

Obstruction of the supraglottic laryngeal airway results from medial and rostral collapse of the arytenoid cartilages and aryepiglottic folds. Cases are presented as a respiratory emergency owing to severe laryngeal airway obstruction, and history reveals a progression of laryngeal disease.

Definitive diagnosis is made by direct laryngoscopy under light anesthesia. The arytenoids and aryepiglottic folds will be tipped medially and ventrally, obstructing the glottic opening. The saccules may be everted and signs of chronic laryngitis will be present.

If the case is presented as a respiratory emergency, immediate tracheotomy is required. Oxygen therapy should be started and corticosteroids should be administered. Following stabilization, patient evaluation and surgical correction can be attempted. Nonemergency cases should be started on preoperative corticosteroid therapy. Placement of a tracheotomy tube prior to laryngeal surgery is essential in these cases because of the possibility of airway obstruction during the immediate postoperative period. Surgical treatment consists of partial laryngectomy with unilateral excision of the arytenoid cartilage and aryepiglottic fold. Bilateral excision is avoided owing to problems with aspiration.

Prognosis is good for larger dogs with laryngeal paralysis. Brachycephalic dogs with this problem will also need correction of the other upper airway obstructions. A poorer prognosis must be given to smaller dogs with multiple problems and laryngeal collapse, as attempting to create an adequate airway is extremely difficult.

SUPPLEMENTAL READING

Bradley, P.A., and Mervey, C.E.: Internal tumors in the dog: an evaluation of prognosis. JSAP 14:459, 1973.
Ettinger, S.J. (ed.): *Veterinary Internal Medicine.* Philadelphia, W.B. Saunders Co., 1975.
Harvey, C.E., and Venker-von Haagan, A.: Surgical management of pharyngeal and laryngeal airway obstruction in the dog. Vet. Clin. North Am. 5(3):515–535, 1975.
Harvey, C.E., and O'Brien, J.A.: Management of respiratory emergencies in small animals. Vet. Clin. North Am. 2(2):243–258, 1972.
Love, J.C., et al.: Diagnosis and successful treatment of Aspergillus fumigatus infection of the frontal sinuses and nasal chambers of the dog. JSAP 15:79–87, 1974.
O'Brien, J.A., et al.: Neurogenic atrophy of the laryngeal muscles of the dog. JSAP 14:521–532, 1973.
Withrow, S.J.: Diagnostic and therapeutic nasal flush in small animals. JAAHA 13:704–707, 1977.

FELINE UPPER RESPIRATORY DISEASE*

RICHARD B. FORD, D.V.M.,
West Lafayette, Indiana

and RICHARD WALSHAW, B.V.M.S.
East Lansing, Michigan

ACUTE INFECTIOUS UPPER RESPIRATORY DISEASE (URD)

The most common and perhaps the most devastating respiratory disease of the cat is viral upper respiratory infection. Since 1970, considerable new information has been compiled regarding etiology, pathogenesis, and control of this respiratory syndrome (Table 1). Although numerous etiologic agents have been recognized as being capable of causing signs of upper respiratory disease in cats, most authors agree that two virus groups — herpes (feline viral rhinotracheitis; FVR) and calici (feline caliciviral disease; FCD) — are responsible for 80 to 90 percent of infectious URD in cats. Both FVR and FCD may cause chronic as well as acute fulminant disease. These two forms will be discussed separately, since there is virtually no similarity with regard to presenting signs.

The acute forms of FVR and FCD may occur in cats of any age. The highest incidence of morbidity and mortality occurs in cats less than six months of age. Fatal cases of FVR have been diagnosed in one-week-old kittens. The distinguishing clinical features of FVR and FCD have been described in detail (Kahn, 1976); however, the many similarities between these two diseases often preclude their separation based on physical signs alone. Virus isolation, a diagnostic procedure not beyond the realm of private practice, may be used to confirm the diagnosis of viral URD, particularly when recurrent outbreaks of respiratory disease occur in multiple cat households or breeding colonies.

Fever and paroxysmal sneezing are consistent, early signs of both FVR and FCD. A serous to mucopurulent nasal discharge often accompanies the sneezing episodes. Conjunctivitis, chemosis, and a serous ocular discharge

may be present in one or both eyes. Secondary bacterial conjunctivitis is accompanied by a mucopurulent ocular discharge. Severe viral keratitis and corneal ulceration occur in advanced cases of FVR. Ulcerative stomatitis with associated hypersalivation and anorexia are most often described in cases of FCD but may also occur in FVR. Within litters, a history of rapid death of kittens with signs of respiratory distress should alert the clinician to the likelihood of viral URD. A neutrophilic leukocytosis may develop as the disease progresses. In the naturally occurring disease, these clinical signs may occur separately or in combination.

Clinical signs may develop from two to eight days following exposure and may become fulminant within ten days following the onset of signs. Respiratory arrest, secondary to airway obstruction and/or pneumonia, dehydration, and malnutrition are ultimately responsible for death in the acute onset case. Rarely, deaths will occur subsequent to systemic herpesvirus infection during which major abdominal organs become involved.

Because of the extreme variation of host response to any one etiologic agent, the prognosis for recovery from the acute disease must be considered poor until the disease is in obvious remission. Owners of infected cats should be made aware that viral URD is potentially fatal, particularly in young kittens; recovered cats may even become chronic virus shedders, thereby representing a virus reservoir capable of exposing susceptible cats.

Treatment. Successful treatment of acute infectious URD necessitates intensive supportive therapy and nursing care. Ampicillin, potassium hetacillin, and chloramphenicol, when administered at the manufacturer's recommended dosage for cats, are usually effective in controlling secondary bacterial infections. Duration of therapy is adjusted to meet the needs of the patient; a minimum of seven days of antibiotic therapy is suggested. Oral

---

*See also "Feline Respiratory Disease Complex" in Section 13.

224

Table 1. *Summary of Current Information on Feline Viral Rhinotracheitis (FVR) and Calicivirus Disease (FCD)*

	FVR	FCD
Distribution	Worldwide	Same
Host Range	*Felidae* only	Same
Virus		
Isolates	Antigenically similar	Many strains recognized
Virulence	Highly virulent	Virulence varies with strain
Stability outside host	<24 hours	8–10 days°
Immunoprophylaxis	Natural: poor	Natural: not determined
	With vaccination: good;	With vaccination: good;
	booster annually	booster annually
Predominant site of		
replication	Nasal mucosa, trachea, conjunctiva	Lung, conjunctiva, nasal and oral mucosa
Route of infection	Nasal, oral, conjunctival	Same
Susceptibility to		
disinfectants	Hypochlorite, quaternary ammonium compounds, alcohol	Same
Clinical Disease		
Incubation period	2–17 days	2–10 days
Duration of viral phase	10–20 days	5–10 days
Respiratory signs	Sneezing, nasal discharge, coughing, hypersalivation	Sneezing, nasal discharge, ulcerative stomatitis, pneumonia
Ocular signs	Conjunctivitis, ocular discharge, blepharospasm; ulcerative keratitis in advanced disease	Conjunctivitis, chemosis, ocular discharge, blepharospasm
Abortion	Shown experimentally only	No
Transmission	Direct: cat-to-cat contact	
	Indirect: via hands, utensils, etc.	Same
	Aerosol: least likely	
Chronic carrier state	Common; clinical signs usually absent. Virus shed up to 2 weeks following "stress." Highly infectious during this time. Recurrence common.	Common; virus shed continuously from oropharynx. Clinical signs mild to absent. Carrier state may persist for several years.

° May vary with strain.

hyperalimentation by nasogastric or pharyngostomy tube is preferred over intravenous or subcutaneous hyperalimentation for meeting caloric and hydration needs of anorexic cats. Although specific guidelines for oral hyperalimentation have not been established for cats, homogenates of commercial canned cat food (C/D)* in water have successfully maintained cats for several days without appreciable weight loss.

Pediatric preparations of nasal decongestants (e.g., 0.25 percent phenylephrine [Neosynephrine†], or 0.025 percent oxymethazoline HCl [Afrin‡]) will provide temporary relief in cats experiencing respiratory difficulty owing to damaged, congested mucous membranes. Long-term treatment with nasal decongestants should be avoided in order to prevent rebound congestion of the nasal epithelium. Steam or aerosol therapy will also effectively reduce inspiratory effort; however, the necessity for frequent daily treatments may preclude this form of therapy. The physical task of removing purulent exudates from the eyes, nose, and mouth remains an important part of the overall care required by these cats. Duration of treatment is determined by the extent of tissue damage caused by the virus, secondary bacterial infections, and patient responsiveness to therapy.

Immunoprophylaxis of susceptible cats is of primary importance in the control of infectious URD. Several vaccines are currently available for immunization of cats against FVR and FCD. The parenterally administered vaccines will stimulate "protective" levels of circulating antibody; however, they do not appear to be effective in stimulating protective levels of immunoglobulin (secretory IgA) at the level of the natural routes for infection — i.e., conjunctiva and nasal and oral mucosa. Consequently, mild infections may still occur in cats naturally challenged with a virulent virus, despite having an adequate vaccination history.

*Hills, Div. of Riviana Foods, Topeka, Kansas 66601
†Winthrop Laboratories, New York, N.Y. 10016
‡Schering Corp., Kenilworth, N.J. 07033

CHRONIC INFECTIOUS UPPER RESPIRATORY DISEASE

Viral URD can no longer be viewed as an acute disease only. Cats that do recover from the acute viral disease are likely to become chronic virus carriers capable of infecting susceptible cats (Povey, 1976). Eighty percent or more of FVR-recovered cats become chronic virus carriers (Gaskell, 1977); affected cats may or may not manifest mild clinical signs of upper respiratory disease while shedding virus. FVR-carrier cats have been shown to shed virulent virus under circumstances of induced "stress" — e.g., corticosteroid administration, acute or chronic illnesses, general anesthesia, pregnancy, and lactation. These cats must be considered highly infectious, as virus may be shed for up to two weeks once stressed. Chronic herpesvirus infection should be considered when successive litters from a particular queen develop respiratory disease before weaning.

Healthy appearing FCD-recovered cats are also likely to become chronic virus carriers. Affected cats can be identified by virus isolation, since the virus is continuously shed from the oropharynx of carriers. As with FVR-recovered chronic virus carriers, clinical signs, if present at all, are mild. Occasionally, chronic periodontal disease or bilateral conjunctivitis and sporadic sneezing are the only physical signs that might suggest chronic calicivirus infection.

The chronic virus carrier must be regarded as a major factor in recurrent outbreaks of upper respiratory disease. Since physical evidence of illness is seldom apparent, chronic carriers are infrequently presented for examination. Yet it is the chronic carrier that represents perhaps the greatest reservoir for infection of susceptible cats.

The chronic virus carrier is difficult to identify. Since virus infection is much more likely to occur following direct contact with oral, nasal, or ocular secretions of infected cats than by the aerosol route, outbreaks may be controlled in part by limiting unnecessary contact between susceptible cats and suspected adult carriers. Elimination of identified (virus isolation) carriers and a rigid vaccination program are equally important in the control of outbreaks. Since FVR carriers are most likely to shed virus during the two-week period following stress, a three-week quarantine of all cats entering the colony is recommended. However, the carrier must be regarded as potentially infectious at all times.

ACUTE NON-INFECTIOUS UPPER RESPIRATORY DISEASE

Distinguishing infectious from non-infectious URD in cats is not an empirical task since fever, rhinitis, paroxysmal sneezing, nasal discharge, and anorexia may be clinical features of both. Acute onset non-infectious URD occurs more often in mature cats; the opposite is true of acute viral URD. With non-infectious disease, there is seldom historical evidence suggesting exposure to infected cats. Furthermore, respiratory disease existing in only one cat from a household of cats is suggestive of a non-infectious condition. Signs of ulcerative keratitis, conjunctivitis, ulcerative stomatitis, and lower respiratory disease would not be expected in non-infectious upper respiratory disease. Determination of serum neutralizing antibody titers for FVR or FCD will not reliably distinguish between infectious and non-infectious URD, since "protective" levels of circulating antibody may be present in either.

Traumatic rhinitis/sinusitis, occasionally seen in cats, is not easily confused with infectious respiratory disease. Bite wounds sustained during fights may result in penetration fractures into the rhinarium or a paranasal sinus. Puncture wounds through the skin of the face and head deserve careful attention, particularly when sneezing or a mucopurulent nasal discharge develops. Radiographs of the skull, preferably with the patient anesthetized, should be evaluated for asymmetry, fractures, and subcutaneous emphysema. Successful treatment depends more on thorough cleansing and flushing of the wound through the fracture site than on broad spectrum antibiotic therapy alone. Wounds may be flushed twice daily with a solution of Betadine* in addition to the administration of oral antibiotics. Treatment should be continued for a minimum of five days. Surgical reduction of fractures is seldom necessary and is only recommended after medical treatment has been tried and found unsuccessful.

Acute, paroxysmal episodes of sneezing associated with minimal serous or serosanguinous nasal discharge are characteristic signs of foreign body rhinitis. Affected cats are otherwise normal. The most commonly reported nasal foreign body of cats is parasitic; *Cuterebra* larvae that lodge between the wall of the nasal cavity and the turbinates will cause the cat to sneeze violently. To facilitate examina-

---

*The Purdue Fredrick Co., Norwalk, CT 06856.

tion, the nasal mucosa can be effectively anesthetized with topical administration of an ophthalmic anesthetic. Contrast rhinography may be of some value in identifying a nasal foreign body. Treatment is limited to forceps extraction of the offending material. Follow-up treatment with antibacterials or anti-inflammatories is seldom necessary.

Acute, spontaneous laryngeal spasm occurs infrequently in cats. The associated clinical signs, although short-lived, resemble those of acute respiratory distress and may prompt a request for immediate medical attention. The owner describes sporadic paroxysms of expiratory effort, lasting from a few seconds to a few minutes during which stridor (wheezing) occurs. Throughout the episode, the cat assumes a hunched stance with legs tucked under the body, head extended and low to the floor. However, during physical exam, the cat typically appears normal, and the signs described by the owner cannot be elicited. The disorder is not life-threatening and recovery is spontaneous, yet frequent "attacks" may become disconcerting to owners.

The etiology of laryngeal spasm is presumed to be local irritation by hair or mucus contacting the arytenoid cartilages. Initiating a swallowing reflex usually terminates the episode. Clients are instructed to introduce 2 or 3 ml of cold water into the cat's mouth with a plastic dropper or syringe at the onset of clinical signs. If the signs persist, the cat should be examined for evidence of laryngeal or tracheal injury.

CHRONIC NON-INFECTIOUS UPPER RESPIRATORY DISEASE

Damage to the upper airways subsequent to acute respiratory disease, whether infectious or non-infectious, may lead to the development of chronic rhinitis or sinusitis. Clinical signs, usually restricted to episodic sneezing and mucopurulent nasal discharges, may persist for several months or years depending on the extent of damage. Many owners are tolerant of the sneezing, nasal discharges, and repeated attempts by veterinarians to treat the condition, since the cat is normal in all other respects.

Overt signs of illness are not apparent at the time of examination, although dried mucus may remain around the nostrils. If paroxysms of sneezing occur spontaneously or can be elicited by instilling a few drops of 0.5 percent phenylephrine into the nostrils, cytologic examination of the nasal discharge with Wright's or new methylene blue stain reveals numerous mature neutrophils, some macrophages, and chains of bacteria. The response to oral antibiotics is initially impressive in ameliorating the clinical signs. However, signs typically recur within 48 hours following withdrawal of antibiotics. Attempts to treat chronic, non-infectious rhinitis with daily nasal flushings using antibiotics, saline, and enzymes (streptodornase-streptokinase) have not been significantly helpful. Surgical curettage of the nasal cavity with removal of the nasal septum and turbinates has been used successfully. The efficacy of autotransplanting fat into the frontal sinus as a means of treating chronic rhinitis/sinusitis has not been established in veterinary medicine. Chronic rhinitis in cats that are herpesvirus and calicivirus negative gradually improves without medical treatment, but the long duration of time needed for recovery (up to three years) may not be acceptable to owners.

Evaluation of any cat with a clinical history and signs consistent with chronic rhinitis should include an attempt to rule out neoplasia and mycotic rhinitis (cryptococcosis) in addition to chronic viral rhinitis (FVR or FCD).

Chronic URD may be caused by localization of *Cryptococcus neoformans* in the nasal mucosa of the cat. The primary route of infection and mode of dissemination have not been firmly established for the cat (Jungerman and Schwartzman, 1972). Respiratory signs of nasal cryptococcosis, subsequent to destruction of the nasal epithelium, include occasional sneezing, sonorous breathing, and a copious, mucoid nasal discharge. The clinician must be aware that cryptococcosis may become systemic; regional lymphadenopathy, skin lesions, and signs consistent with central nervous system involvement may be present in addition to signs of upper respiratory disease. Diagnosis may be confirmed by microscopic identification of the organisms in an India ink, wet-mount preparation of the nasal exudate. *C. neoformans* grows well on cyclohexamide-free, Sabouraud dextrose agar; yeast-like colonies develop in three to five days. Characteristic cream-colored mucoid colonies are apparent after five to seven days of additional incubation at 20°C.

Treatment of *C. neoformans* rhinitis must be considered in light of other possible organ involvement. Infections localized to the rhinarium are best treated by surgical ablation of the involved tissue followed by daily flushing with Betadine solution. Medical therapy has not been shown to be consistently effective.

The public health significance of feline cryptococcosis has not been firmly established, but the lack of reported cases of cat-to-animal and cat-to-human transmission suggests that cryptococcosis is not an infectious disease. The risk of transmitting the disease to immunosuppressed humans or animals is not known.

Although reports of solid tumor development within the upper respiratory tract of the cat are few, chronic rhinitis may be the result of intranasal neoplasia. Carcinomas and lymphoid neoplasia constitute the majority of reported nasal neoplasms in cats and are found most commonly in animals five years of age or older (Legendre, 1975; Bright, 1976). Clinical signs are inconsistent. Affected cats are usually presented for sonorous or open-mouth breathing caused by obstruction of the rhinarium, sneezing, or a blood-tinged mucopurulent nasal discharge. Hypersalivation may accompany the sneezing episodes. Diffuse facial swelling over the nasal cavity or a paranasal sinus is highly suggestive of neoplasia. Radiographic examination of the nasal passages will demonstrate the obstructive lesion and characterize the structural damage caused by the neoplastic tissue. In many cases, this is sufficient evidence to make a diagnosis of neoplasia. Diagnostic confirmation is best obtained from histopathologic studies on a core biopsy taken from the mass. Tissue specimens obtained with alligator forceps and nasal flushings are less likely to yield diagnostic cytology. There are no published reports that document successful medical therapy of nasal neoplasia in either dogs or cats. Treatment, therefore, entails radical surgical curettage of the nasal turbinates and other involved structures. Radiation therapy may be combined with surgery in selected cases. Prognosis for recovery from intranasal neoplasia must be regarded as poor, despite the use of appropriate treatment protocols. Although metastasis is unlikely in primary nasal neoplasia, local invasion is usually extensive and tumor regrowth is not uncommon following surgery.

Healthy appearing cats presented for sporadic sneezing episodes should be examined for gross and radiographic evidence of dental disease. Although more commonly recognized in the dog, chronic periodontal disease may cause osteolysis and eventual formation of alveolar-nasal fistulae. Examination of the oral cavity in the anesthetized cat may reveal what appears to be normal gingiva; however, bluntly probing the hard palate at its junction with the medial aspect of the upper dental arcade may reveal a communication between the oral and nasal cavities. Empirical treatment is accomplished by removing the affected teeth. As an alternative, the fistulae may be vigorously flushed in an attempt to debride the affected tissues. Oral antibiotics are given for seven to ten days afterward. If the periodontal tissues have not been severely damaged, loose teeth may again become firmly seated within the alveolus and the fistulae will close.

SUPPLEMENTAL READING

Bright, R.M., and Bojrab, M.J.: Intranasal neoplasia in the dog and cat. JAAHA 12:806–812, 1976.

Gaskell, R.M., and Wardley, R.C.: Feline viral respiratory disease: a review with particular reference to its epizootiology and control. J. Small Anim. Pract. 19:1–16, 1977.

Jungerman, P.F., and Schwartzman, R.M.: *Veterinary Medical Mycology*. Philadelphia, Lea & Febiger, 1972.

Kahn, D.E., and Hoover, E.A.: Infectious respiratory diseases of cats. Vet. Clin. North Am. 6:399–413, 1976.

Lagendre, A.M., et al.: Nasal tumor in a cat. JAVMA 167:481–483, 1975.

Povey, R.C.: Feline respiratory infections — a clinical review. Can. Vet. J. 17:93–100, 1976.

Winstanley, E.W.: Trephining frontal sinuses in the treatment of rhinitis and sinusitis in the cat. Vet. Rec. 95:289–292, 1974.

DISEASES OF THE CANINE AND FELINE TRACHEOBRONCHIAL TREE

BRENDAN McKIERNAN, D.V.M.

Urbana, Illinois

Irritation of the trachea and major bronchi may result in a clinical situation familiar to all clinicians — the coughing animal. Irritant receptors located just beneath the epithelial surface of these airways initiate the cough reflex. A wide variety of factors (Table 1) may stimulate this reflex, yet the presence of a cough by itself is not diagnostic of any specific disease. It is important to remember that a cough is a normal reflex and one of the basic defense mechanisms of the airways. When treating a coughing animal, one should not be too hasty in trying to suppress this reflex.

It is only when a cough becomes excessive (e.g., in frequency, duration, or severity) that a problem may exist. It is at this point that the veterinarian should strive for an etiologic diagnosis so that therapy may be directed toward a specific problem rather than at a symptom of that problem.

TRACHEITIS AND BRONCHITIS

Inflammation of the epithelial lining of the trachea and bronchi results in clinical conditions referred to as either tracheitis or bronchitis. Often, the irritating factor(s) involve both the trachea and the bronchi and the terms are combined — i.e., tracheobronchitis. These terms by themselves do not imply an etiology (although they are frequently used as if they do) — rather, they localize the affected area. If the specific etiology of the tracheitis or bronchitis is known, it should be used — e.g., allergic bronchitis. Some of these terms — e.g., chronic bronchitis — not only localize the affected area but also imply certain pathologic changes.

ETIOLOGIES

Infectious agents are the most frequent cause of feline and canine tracheobronchial diseases. Although symptoms in the cat relate more to viral agents and are more obvious in the upper respiratory tract, clinical involvement of the trachea, bronchi, and even lungs may occur. Common feline agents that may produce symptoms related to the tracheobronchial tree include the feline viral rhinotracheitis (FVR), feline calicivirus (FCV), and feline pneumonitis (FPN) organisms. Recently, the feline infectious peritonitis (FIP) virus has been shown to be capable of producing mild upper respiratory symptoms and should be considered as a possible etiology. Bacterial involvement may also occur and may be either a primary cause of disease or secondary to the viral disease.

Infectious canine tracheobronchitis, "kennel cough," is generally thought to be a combination of viral and bacterial agents. Symptoms observed depend on the animal's age and vaccination history but usually are confined to the tracheobronchial tree unless extension into the lungs occurs, — e.g., bronchopneumonia. The viruses of canine distemper (CD), parainfluenza (CPI or Simian 5 virus; SV-5), and the adenoviruses 1 and 2 (CAV-1, CAV-2) are the most common viral agents isolated. *Bordetella bronchiseptica* infection may occur secondarily to these viruses. Recent information suggests that *B. bronchiseptica* can act as a primary pathogen in the dog (Bemis and Appel, 1977). The role that *Mycoplasma* spp. play in canine respiratory disease, if any, remains to be evaluated. Other bacterial species may affect animals secondarily to the viral agents or during chronic respiratory problems. (The reader is referred to the articles on canine and feline infectious diseases for further information.)

Parasitic larval migration of many of the common canine and feline nematodes can cause sufficient inflammation and irritation in the tracheobronchial tree to elicit the cough reflex. *Filaroides osleri*, a specific parasitic tracheobronchial disease, produces granulomatous nodules near the carina. It is possible that at least some of the symptoms observed in this disease are results of airway obstruction and secretion retention as much as of tissue irritation caused by the larvae and nodules. (For a complete review, the reader is referred to the

229

Table 1.   *Common Causes for the Cough Reflex*

MECHANICAL
   Inhaled particulate matter—e.g., dusts
   Foreign bodies—e.g., endotracheal tubes, catheters, plant material, etc.
   Excessive secretions
   External compression—e.g., tumors, abscesses, lymphadenopathy, enlarged left atrium
   Tracheal collapse
INFLAMMATORY
   Bacterial
   Viral
   Fungal
   Parasitic
CHEMICAL
   Noxious fumes
   Smoke inhalation
   Intratracheal injections
   Gastric secretions
   Aerosols—e.g., perfumes
COMBINATIONS

article "Parasitic Diseases of the Respiratory Tract.")

Allergic tracheobronchial conditions may occur in association with parasitic migrations or as the result of an external allergen. Allergic bronchitis occurs in cats and is often referred to as "feline asthma." These cats appear to be much more affected by the associated airway narrowing (bronchospasms, secretions) than are dogs with allergic bronchitis. This may be explained in part by species and size differences. The musculature in the feline bronchial wall is heavier by comparison and is presumably more capable of constricting the bronchial lumen. Any decrease in lumen size (and therefore an increase in airway resistance) will be more prominent in a smaller airway (cat) versus a larger airway (dog). Other factors such as differences in responsiveness to chemical mediators of airway regulation and neural control may be important differences between species. Additional work remains to be done to delineate the pathophysiologic changes in each species. Pulmonary infiltrates with eosinophils, the PIE syndrome, may be seen in both the cat and the dog and is discussed elsewhere (see article "Pneumonia in the Dog and Cat").

Chronic bronchitis in man is a specific disease of the airways that is characterized by "chronic recurrent excess mucus secretion in the bronchial tree occurring on most days for at least three months of the year during at least two years. . . . the excess secretion should not be brought about by other diseases [such as tuberculosis, bronchiestasis, tumors]" (Wheeldon et al., 1974). Wheeldon et al. also proposed adopting "a tentative minimum requirement of coughing for two consecutive months in the preceding year" as the definition of chronic bronchitis in the dog (1974). Although no mention of excess mucus production is made in this definition, similar morphologic changes are reported in the airway of the dog when compared with man — i.e., goblet cell proliferation, bronchial gland hypertrophy, and squamous metaplasia. Since many factors may be responsible for the development of chronic bronchitis, it becomes imperative to arrive at an etiologic diagnosis for a coughing dog so as to prevent recurrences and to avoid the morbid anatomic changes that occur with chronicity. Once these changes occur, a vicious cycle is triggered (Fig. 1) that can be therapeutically slowed but never completely broken. It is the goal of clinicians to prevent this cycle from starting.

Irritation of the submucosal receptors of the tracheobronchial epithelium may result from many miscellaneous causes. External compression of the trachea or bronchi may be a cause of coughing in the dog. Examples of external compression commonly seen include abscesses, tumors, megaesophagus, lymphadenopathies, and cardiac enlargement — especially left atrial enlargement. Hilar lymphadenopathy associated with fungal disease, and tracheal collapse are two very frustrating causes of chronic coughing and are discussed in separate sections. Other causes such as noxious fumes, dusts, and (passive) cigarette smoke may be important irritants in certain dogs or over long periods in specific regions of the country.

Most of these etiologies produce diseases that are acute but with inadequate or improper therapy or lack of treatment can become chronic. It is much more rewarding to treat these diseases while they are acute than to have to try to manage their successor — chronic tracheobronchial disease.

DIAGNOSIS

Information regarding many of the causes of tracheitis and bronchitis may only be gained by taking a careful history. Although this may require valuable time, the interview should be conducted by the clinician and not delegated to non-professional employees. History of vaccination and of any exposure to other animals (e.g., in kennels and animal shelters) is helpful in diagnosing suspected cases of an infectious etiology in cats and dogs. Factors that initiate or "trigger" the animal's cough may relate directly to the underlying etiology or disease. Examples of "trigger" factors include scented litter in asthmatic cats, excitement in the dog with tracheal collapse, aerosol sprays, dusty air, and exposure to cigarette smoke.

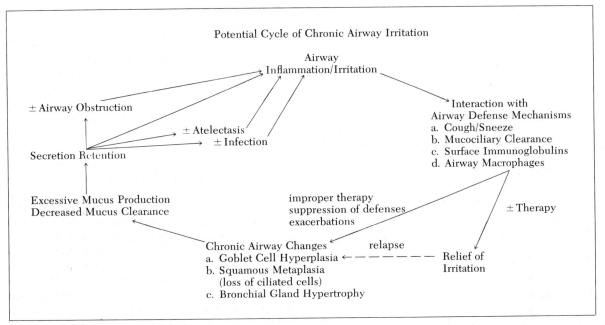

Figure 1

Since the cough is the hallmark of tracheobronchial disease, attempts should be made to qualify and quantify it. The character (moist or dry) of the cough often parallels systemic or chronic involvement. Tracheobronchial disease usually causes a dry, "hacking" type of cough, whereas systemic involvement (pneumonia) or chronic disease (bronchiectasis and possibly chronic bronchitis) most often results in a moist, productive cough. Retching is often described following a coughing episode, but owners sometimes confuse this with vomiting. As excessive secretions are cleared from the respiratory tract by coughing and the action of the mucociliary tree, they are presented to the caudal aspect of the larynx. Since there are no ciliated cells in the larynx to aid in clearing these secretions, animals and humans often will make forceful expiratory effects to "clear their throats," bringing these secretions through the larynx into the pharynx where they are either swallowed or occasionally projected out of the mouth. This is commonly called retching in veterinary medicine.

Physical examinations should include measurement of temperature, pulse, and respiratory rate in the resting animal. Additional diagnostic effort and time are warranted in chronic or recurrent coughing problems, both to prevent the development of "chronic bronchitis" if possible and to try to alleviate the animal's and the owner's discomfort.

The most frequent physical finding in cases of tracheitis and bronchitis is the presence of either a spontaneous, paroxysmal cough or an irritable trachea upon palpation. The cough is usually dry and non-productive and may be followed by a retching episode. In the author's experience, a moist cough is present more often in chronic conditions in which mucus production has increased or parenchymal involvement has occurred. Although the remainder of the physical examination is frequently non-diagnostic, it should be completed in a systematic way so no abnormalities are missed. Careful attention should be given to the cardiac examination, since murmurs may be found frequently in older dogs (valvular disease) but may not be the source of the animal's cough. Auscultation of the respiratory system is reviewed in the article "Pneumonia in the Dog and Cat."

Radiographs are usually unremarkable, or they may show a mild to severe increase in bronchial markings. Radiographs are important and useful in ruling out the presence of other causes of a cough, and they may serve as a point of reference for future examinations. Lateral and ventrodorsal (VD) views should be taken in all cases.

Laboratory evaluation is used in a similar manner. The total WBC count and differential are usually within normal limits in most cases of tracheobronchitis. Allergic bronchitis in dogs and cats may show either an absolute or a relative eosinophilia, although this is not required to make the diagnosis. Eosinophils are frequently found on cytologic specimens from these cases and can confirm a suspected allergic diagnosis. Fecal and microfilaria examinations should be performed on coughing animals, especially in heavily infested regions of the country.

Endoscopic examination is warranted only when the aforementioned tests are inconclusive or when therapy is not successful — i.e., primarily in the chronic cases. Gross changes in the tracheobronchial tree are minimal and usually consist of increased vascularity (hyperemia) and mucus accumulation. Airway compression, nodules, and foreign bodies are easily visualized by either rigid or flexible endoscopy. Specimens may be obtained for both cytology and culture by endoscopy, transtracheal aspiration (TTA), or simply via a long-guarded culture swab* passed through the larynx of an anesthetized animal.

TREATMENT

Therapy in all cases of tracheobronchitis should be as specific as possible. This necessitates that efforts be made to achieve an etiologic diagnosis. This is especially true in the case that does not respond to initial symptomatic treatment and is being presented for a second time. Parenteral antibiotic therapy should be based on sensitivity testing; when this is not available, an antibiotic with a good gram-negative spectrum should be selected. Cultures done here and at other institutions show that gram-negative organisms are the pathogens most often cultured from the respiratory tract of infected dogs. *E. coli*, *Klebsiella*, *Pseudomonas*, *Pasturella*, and *Bordetella* spp. are examples of frequently isolated organisms. With the exception of *Bordetella* infections, aerosol antibiotic therapy is not warranted for treatment of respiratory infection. Recent work on antibiotic treatment of *Bordetella* infections in dogs (Bemis and Appel, 1977) has shown a significant reduction in tracheal bacterial populations following aerosol as opposed to parenteral or oral administration of antibiotics. Further evaluation by this author is currently underway in this area. Many cases of bronchitis, especially the chronic cases, will have recurring airway infections and often are treated symptomatically and successfully with an antibiotic. Skin testing in attempts to identify external allergens in the allergic bronchitic or feline asthmatic has met with poor results to date, although work continues in this area. Aerosol challenge (provocation testing) is not utilized at present, al-

*Sterile Culture Swab, Sherwood Medical Co., St. Louis, MO 63103.

Table 2. *Antitussives for Small Animals*

Hycodan	2.5–10 mg	BID-TID (depending on body size)
Codeine	1–2 mg/kg	BID-QID
Dextromethorphan	2 mg/kg	TID-QID
Morphine°	0.1 mg/kg	BID-QID

°Caution in cats.

though frequently a detailed history will alert the clinician to the possible existence of an inhaled allergen. In these cases, removal of the suspected allergen from the animal's environment can be tried as a diagnostic tool. The majority of cases, however, will require symptomatic therapy in the form of corticosteroids.

The glucocorticoids are in fact the current drug of choice in the allergic and most of the other etiologies of tracheobronchitis. They are contraindicated in cases of bacterial, viral, and fungal etiology but are used with success in other cases to decrease tracheal irritation and inflammation. Prednisolone in doses of 1.0 to 2.0 mg/kg of body weight on a decreasing dosage regimen is used in both cats and dogs. Alternate-day therapy may be used if maintenance therapy is necessary. In cases that require long-term therapy, it is important to stress that the owners use "the least amount as infrequently as possible" just to control the problem when using these steroids. Long-lasting (e.g., dexamethasone) and repositol forms of steroids should not be used because of their pituitary-adrenal axis suppression.

Antitussives are indicated when there is a non-productive cough that has become irritating to the animal and/or the owners. Since the cough is a normal protective reflex, care should be exercised in suppressing it. Examples of commonly used antitussives are listed in Table 2.

BRONCHIECTASIS

Bronchiectasis is the permanent dilation and destruction of the walls of the bronchi or bronchioles as the result of long-standing inflammation in these airways. As the result of this dilation and destruction, mucociliary clearance is impaired, secretions accumulate, and the animal becomes prone to infection. The actual etiology is probably multifactorial, although the following conditions have been mentioned as possible factors: chronic or recurrent infections, allergic bronchitis, chronic bronchitis, bronchial obstruction (foreign bodies, stenosis, mucoid impaction), and anatomic abnormalities. Bronchiectasis is described as either cylindrical or saccular, the cylindrical form being more frequent in small animals. Cases involving both dogs and cats have been reported, although most cases are seen in the dog. Typically, these cases involve middle-aged to older animals that have a history of a chronic, often productive cough. Frequently, symptoms of systemic involvement such as fever, anorexia, and purulent sputum are present. In the author's experience, most cases have responded well to previous antibiotic therapies only to relapse a few weeks or months after treatment is stopped.

Physical examination may indicate a relatively normal animal or a debilitated, febrile animal that has an irritable trachea, productive cough, and crackles upon auscultation. Laboratory findings will likewise vary, depending upon systemic involvement. The diagnosis of bronchiectasis is based on typical (chronic) history, physical, and laboratory findings but is confirmed by radiography. Advanced cases will show dilated bronchi (usually in dependent lobes) and bronchial thickening. Mild cases may be confirmed by bronchography, using a micronized barium sulfate suspension.* Bronchographic examination is important since therapy, either medical or surgical, is selected depending upon the degree of involvement. If a single lobe is involved, lobectomy is the treatment of choice and the prognosis is favorable. With multiple lobe involvement, however, the prognosis is poor, and chronic recurring infections are likely. With either the single or multiple lobe involvement, a culture and sensitivity of the secretion present in the airways must be taken in order to choose the most appropriate antibacterial agent. Cough suppressants, steroids, and diuretics should be avoided in most cases of bronchiectasis. Bland aerosol therapy coupled with physiotherapy have been described for use in the dog (McKiernan, 1978) and may aid in the removal of secretions from the airways.

TRACHEAL COLLAPSE

Tracheal collapse, a condition seen almost exclusively in toy and miniature breeds of dogs, is one of the more frustrating problems the veterinary practitioner may encounter. Synonyms in human medicine — tracheomalacia and excessive dynamic airway compression — provide an insight to the problem as seen in veterinary medicine. Although airway caliber normally decreases during expiration — dynamic compression owing to increased intrathoracic pressures — the airways still remain open. If there are increased intrathoracic pressures and a weakening of the cartilaginous skeleton of the airways, excessive dynamic airway compression and collapse may occur. This collapse produces a mechical mucosal surface irritation. This in turn starts the cycle described in Figure 1 into motion — i.e., inflammation, coughing, anatomic changes, and secretion production and retention.

ETIOLOGY

The proposed etiologies for tracheal collapse are extremely varied (Table 3). At this time, the true cause is unknown but it is probably multifactorial in nature. Since the majority (80 to 90 per cent) of cases of tracheal collapse diagnosed at the University of Illinois (Urbana) are of the intrathoracic variety, small airway disease would seem to be a reasonable explanation for the collapse. If small airways in the lungs either close early during expiration or are partially obstructed, there will be an increase in transtracheal pressure craniad to this point. As mentioned above, this increased pressure may lead to actual collapse, especially if there is a coexistent cartilaginous demineralization. Early airway closure may be caused by such things as inflammation and mucus or secretion retention e.g., bronchiolitis. A recent review of the pathology seen in dogs with tracheal collapse (Done and Drew, 1976) noted changes in the matrix of the cartilage, glandular hyperplasia, squamous metaplasia, submucosal inflammation, and retention of secretions. Although most of these changes and the gross collapse were seen in the middle portion of the trachea, it remains to be seen whether and what type of pathologic changes are present in the small bronchi and bronchioles. Unfortunately, most cases of tracheal collapse are ignored until moderate to severe symptoms appear, and therefore it is difficult to establish the pathologic progression seen with this disease.

*Table 3.   Proposed Etiologies of
Tracheal Collapse*

Hereditary predisposition — small breeds
Dietary — both obesity and mineralization defects
Demineralization of the cartilage — congenital or acquired
Deep tracheitis with relaxation of dorsal ligament
Neurologic (CNS) deficiency similar to megaesophagus
Small airways closure — e.g., bronchiolitis

---

*Redi-Flow, Flow Pharmaceuticals, Inc., Palo Alto, CA 94303.

CERVICAL VS. THORACIC COLLAPSE

Tracheal collapse may occur either inside or outside the thoracic cavity; i.e., intrathoracic or cervical collapse. Most cases described in the literature are of the cervical type (including those at the thoracic inlet). Collapses involving the intrathoracic trachea and/or the lobar bronchi have been observed previously (Spaulding et al., 1978) and in the author's experience they represent the majority of cases. A spectrum may exist in these cases of which cervical collapse is one extreme end. Complete evaluation of cases of cervical collapse and long-term follow-up of the intrathoracic cases will be required to prove or disprove this theory.

DIAGNOSIS

Diagnosis of tracheal collapse is usually based on the history and physical examination. Laboratory evaluation is often used to rule out other causes for coughing but is rarely if ever diagnostic for tracheal collapse. The typical tracheal collapse case is seen in toy and miniature breeds, middle to older ages (ranges of 1 to 16 years are reported), and frequently overweight dogs. The history often includes a chronic intermittent cough that is induced by such factors as excitment, exercise, leash pulling, and drinking. The cough is usually paroxysmal and dry in nature. In some cases, the flattened cervical cartilage rings may be palpated. In the intrathoracic tracheal collapse cases, the cervical trachea is usually of normal shape when palpated. Auscultation may reveal an increase in bronchovesicular sounds (an increased intensity and duration of expiration when compared with inspiration), crackles (especially ventrally where secretions may accumulate), or normal lung sounds. A markedly prolonged expiratory phase and increased expiratory effort are usually present when coughing is induced in cases of intrathoracic collapse.

An almost pathognomic auscultatory finding for intrathoracic tracheal collapse is the soft end-expiratory snapping together of the tracheal walls that occurs as the dog coughs. This sound, often heard without a stethoscope, has been confirmed as originating from the collapse by simultaneously listening and observing the tracheal collapse under fluoroscopy. The "honking" cough is seen when a longer section of trachea collapses and actually vibrates or resonates with the passage of air. This is the "classical" tracheal collapse cough but is observed less frequently than the "end-expiratory snap."

Owing to the increased incidence of cardiac valvular insufficiency with increasing age, a thorough examination of the heart should be conducted. Often, a middle-aged dog with a cough and mild mitral insufficiency is automatically placed on cardiac glycosides when the murmur is actually not a problem and the cough is due to a tracheal collapse or other problem. This is especially true when crackles (secretions or pulmonary edema?) are auscultated or when a radiograph reveals a large heart (pericardial fat or true cardiac enlargement?). These cases can present a challenging diagnostic problem for the clinician.

Confirmation of the collapse may be obtained by radiographing the trachea at the time it collapses. This is a problem in routine practice, since the collapse only lasts for a fraction of a second in most cases and the radiographic exposure must be made at this exact time. In an attempt to maximize the chance of seeing the collapse, lateral chest radiographs may be made during inspiration and when the dog coughs (during peak expiration). Cervical collapse should occur during inspiration due to changing transtracheal pressures, whereas a weakened thoracic trachea will often balloon open and may appear limp and "wavy." During a cough (forced expiration), the increased transtracheal pressure is in the thoracic trachea and the cervical trachea may balloon open. Caution must be taken not to flex the neck, as excessive dorsal flexion may artificially narrow the trachea at the thoracic inlet.

When available, fluoroscopy will document the dynamic airway changes that occur during quiet breathing and coughing. Using this technique, a high degree of correlation was established between auscultatory and fluoroscopic changes. Often, a case suspected of having an intrathoracic tracheal collapse by auscultation would have non-diagnostic flat films but could be confirmed by fluoroscopy. Changes that may be seen in the EKG in conjunction with tracheal collapse relate to the chronic respiratory problem — i.e., a cor pulmonale. Although right axis deviation is not usually seen, prominent P-waves (P-pulmonale) are often present but are not by themselves diagnostic for tracheal collapse.

TREATMENT

Treatment for tracheal collapse is not curative by any means but is an attempt to control the chronic coughing symptom. Weight control is crucial as mediastinal, cervical, chest wall, and abdominal fat accumulations may either impinge on the trachea directly or add to the work of breathing. This increased work (effort) of breathing often promotes collapse. Antitussives may be used on a short-term basis when no systemic signs are present. Similarly, corticosteroids are often of benefit in quieting or soothing the irritated tracheal lining but should be used sparingly. As retained secretions may become infected, antibiotics and antibiotic-steroid combinations are frequently used in these cases with good results. If systemic symptoms are present — e.g., fever, crackles, or purulent sputum — additional diagnostic work-up should be considered. When a source of stimulation has been identified (e.g., leash pulling), attempts to remove the irritation may prove beneficial. Using harnesses rather than collars and avoiding excessive exercise and excitement are a few examples in which a change in management may help the dog's problem.

Cases that are presented cyanotic and extremely dyspneic should be handled very carefully. Cooled, humidified oxygen therapy, steroids, and often a low (0.05 to 0.1 mg/kg) dose of morphine without atropine should be administered. Stress must be avoided; diagnostic tests such as radiographs, EKGs, and blood work should be delayed until the animal is out of danger.

Surgical treatments for severe cervical tracheal collapse cases have been proposed. Intratracheal tubular prosthesis and various external chondrotomy procedures have been used with varying degrees of success. Prior to any surgical intervention in the cervical region, a thorough — preferably fluoroscopic — examination of the intrathoracic trachea should be made to rule out a simultaneous collapse in this area.

SUPPLEMENTAL READING

Bemis, D.A., and Appel, M.J.: Aerosol, parenteral, and oral antibiotic treatment of *Bordetella bronchiseptica* infections in dogs. JAVMA 170:1082–1086, 1977.
Done, S.H., and Drew, R.A.: Observations on the pathology of tracheal collapse in dogs. J. Small Anim. Pract. 17:783–791, 1976.
McKiernan, B.: Principles of Aerosol Therapy — Applications in the Canine. Proceedings of the Illinois Veterinary Respiratory Symposium, 1978.
Spaulding, G.L., Ryan, G., and Rendano, V.: The Clinical and Fluoroscopic Manifestation of Intrathoracic Collapse of the Trachea and Mainstem Bronchi. Proceedings of the Illinois Veterinary Respiratory Symposium, 1978.
Wheeldon, E.B., Pirie, H.M., Fisher, E.W., and Lee, R.: Chronic bronchitis in the dog. Vet. Rec. 94:466–471, 1974.

CANINE AND FELINE PNEUMONIA

BRENDAN McKIERNAN, D.V.M.
Urbana, Illinois

Pneumonia is a frequent primary or secondary problem in small animals, and it may prove life threatening if not diagnosed and treated promptly. The veterinary clinician must be prepared to identify the etiologic agents involved rapidly and administer both symptomatic and specific therapy as indicated.

ETIOLOGIES

The simple diagnosis of "pneumonia" should be considered unacceptable to veterinary clinicians. Although pneumonia usually implies a bacterial etiology, it is preferable to use a specific term to describe the actual cause whenever it is possible. The rationale is immediately apparent when the prognosis and treatment are considered. For example, compare the mycotic pneumonia case with the allergic pneumonia case. The prognosis for the latter is favorable; that for the former is guarded to poor. Steroids constitute the treatment of choice for an allergic pneumonia but are contraindicated in a mycotic case.

Radiographically, pneumonias may be classified as interstitial, alveolar, or bronchial, or a combination of any two or even all three of these (Suter and Chan, 1968). Most cases are of mixed origin, but even when there is only a single pattern present, it is rarely, if ever, pathognomonic for a specific etiology. Each of the etiologies that are mentioned here have a "classical" radiographic pattern but may also present with an unexpected or unusual appearance. It is important that the final diagnosis be specific so that a rational prognosis and therapy can be given. Specific pneumonias that will be discussed include (1) bacterial, (2) mycotic or fungal, (3) allergic, (4) aspiration, and (5) inhalation. Viral and parasitic pneumonias occur frequently in veterinary medicine and are discussed in separate chapters. Finally, it should be mentioned that more than one of these etiologies may be present at any given time. A bacterial pneumonia, for example, may often develop as a sequela to one of the other pneumonias.

AUSCULTATION

Auscultation of the chest must be conducted in a quiet area, in a systematic manner, and with a comfortably fitting stethoscope. Nothing is less conducive to proper auscultation than rushing to finish because of an uncomfortable stethescope. Noting the presence of adventitious (abnormal) breath sounds is obviously important. However, attention must also be given to the absence of normal sounds (i.e., a silent area) or the presence of normal sounds in an abnormal location (e.g., bronchial breath sounds where vesicular sounds should be heard). A classification scheme of breath sounds is given in Table 1.

Terminology used to describe auscultatory findings is not well defined. It is important that

Table 1. Classification of Breath Sounds*

NORMAL BREATH SOUNDS

   A. Vesicular—quiet, rustling sounds heard over peripheral lung regions. Inspiration (I) and early expiration (E) normally audible. I louder and longer than E.

   B. Bronchial—harsher blowing or tubular sounds heard over the trachea and anterior thorax. E usually louder and longer than I. Presence in an abnormal location usually indicates consolidation.

   C. Bronchovesicular—a combination of the above sounds heard where these areas overlap or in early disease.

ADVENTITIOUS (ABNORMAL) BREATH SOUNDS

   A. Discontinuous sounds—crackles—distinct, intermittent snapping sound of very short duration. May indicate fluid accumulation or fibrosis. More frequent during I.

      (1) Fine crackles ⎫
      (2) Medium crackles ⎬ depending upon loudness and duration
      (3) Coarse crackles ⎭

   B. Continuous sounds—rhonchi and wheezes—slightly longer duration, yet still only a fraction of the respiratory cycle. May have a musical quality. Indicates airway narrowing. More frequent during E.

      (1) Wheeze—high pitch
      (2) Rhonchus—low pitch
      (3) Stridor—an inspiratory, high-pitched wheeze. Originates in the laryngeal area.

   C. Pleural friction rub—a combination of continuous and discontinuous sounds. Described as a creaky leather sound. Produced when inflamed pleural surfaces rub together. May occur on I or E.

---

*Modified from Murphy, R. L. H. Jr.: *A Simplified Introduction to Lung Sounds.* Wellesley Hills, Mass., Stethophonics, 1977.

it be standardized so that all communication, verbal and written, will carry the same meaning to everyone. The terms in the following discussion have been generally accepted by the medical community and are recommended for adoption by veterinary clinicians and students alike.

Normal lung sounds are divided into three types: bronchial, vesicular, and bronchovesicular. The major differences are in location of normal sounds and in the amount and loudness of the expiratory sounds. Normally, air-filled alveoli have a dampening or filtering effect on the transmission of sound — i.e., the lung acts as a selective filter to sound transmission. Sound, then, is normally filtered (dampened) as it travels from within the lung outwardly toward the chest wall and the listener's stethoscope. The result is a quiet, soft ("rustling leaves") sound heard during inspiration and early expiration over the peripheral areas of the lungs. These are vesicular breath sounds. Bronchial breath sounds, on the other hand, are both louder and longer during expiration than are vesicular sounds. They normally occur over the large airways (trachea and anterior thorax) and have a "tubular" sound. Bronchial breathing may also be heard if the normal sound "filtering" action of underlying alveoli is altered. A good example is the difference in sound (loudness), produced when two rocks are struck together first in air and then under water. Since sound waves are transmitted better in water than in air, the sound will be louder under water. If the normally air-filled alveoli are filled with a fluid, sound will be transmitted better to the chest wall. The result is louder sounds — i.e., bronchial breath sounds — than should occur in that region of the chest. Bronchial breathing heard where vesicular breathing should be heard usually represents consolidation or filling of the underlying alveoli. Finally, bronchovesicular breath sounds may be thought of as a combination or blending of both vesicular and bronchial sounds. They may be heard where these two regions overlap on the chest or when early disease is present. The sound produced during expiration in bronchovesicular breathing is louder and longer than with vesicular sounds but shorter and more quiet than with bronchial sounds. In the author's experience, most people who use the terms "harsh lung sounds" or "dry rales" are actually describing bronchovesicular breath sounds, which is the preferable term.

Adventitious (abnormal) breath sounds are divided into continuous and discontinuous sounds. Discontinuous sounds, called rales or crackles, occur intermittently during the respiratory cycle. Continuous sounds, termed "rhonchi" or "wheezes" are slightly longer in duration but still occupy only a short portion of the respiratory cycle. Continuous sounds are indicative of an airway narrowing and are usually more pronounced during expiration as the result of the normal dynamic airway compression. High-pitched continuous sounds are termed wheezes and low-pitched sounds are called rhonchi. Stridor is usually used to describe a specific, inspiratory, high-pitched wheeze and normally is indicative of airway narrowing in the laryngeal area.

Crackles are made up of distinct, discontinuous, and intermittent sounds closely resembling the crackling noise made by a fire or the sound produced by rubbing the hairs near your ear together. The origin of crackles is still disputed, but they are usually considered to arise as the result of fluid movement within or around airways or as the result of airways snapping open. Crackles may also be heard in cases of pulmonary fibrosis. Crackles are most frequently heard during inspiration and are classified as fine, medium, and coarse, depending on their loudness and duration.

Information concerning a disease process may be gained by localizing adventitious sounds. The point at which a sound is the loudest is usually nearest the diseased area (stridor is a good example), and the listener should move the stethescope around to locate this point. Crackles heard in dependent locations usually indicate fluid accumulation, whereas crackles heard only dorsally may be indicative of fibrosis. Although there is not yet a consensus, evidence suggests that the timing within the respiratory cycle when adventitious sounds occur may reflect the size of the airway(s) that are affected. Sounds occurring early in either inspiration or expiration may reflect large airway involvement, whereas sounds late in the cycle may indicate that small airways are involved. Pulmonary edema, for example, typically auscultates as fine, end-inspiratory crackles and is thought to reflect fluid accumulating in or around the smaller airways. Coarse crackles heard during the first portion of expiration frequently indicate fluid in the large airways — often in the trachea.

Pleural friction rubs are best considered a combination of both continuous and discontinuous sounds and may be heard either during inspiration or expiration but usually recur at the same time within the respiratory cycle. This sound is described as a "creaky leather" sound and is produced when roughened pleural surfaces rub together — i.e., pleuritis. If adhesions develop or fluid accumulation separates the pleural surfaces, no friction rub will occur.

Breath sounds are affected by a variety of physical factors. Tidal volume, respiratory rate, open versus closed mouth breathing, chest wall thickness (e.g., heavy musculature, obesity), purring, mucle tremors, and hair noises can interfere with an individual's ability to auscultate effectively. These factors must be kept in mind, and the auscultatory findings must be interpreted accordingly.

BACTERIAL PNEUMONIA

Diagnosis. Bacteria are among the most frequent causes of pneumonia in the dog and cat. Certain patients are at risk for developing a bacterial pneumonia: animals that are debilitated or immunosuppressed, animals with anatomic problems (e.g., cleft palates or megaesophagus), and animals with chronic tracheobronchial disease. Bacterial pneumonia is also seen as a secondary complication of other pneumonias.

The symptoms observed in the animal with a bacterial pneumonia are often just an extension of those seen in cases of acute bronchitis. Indeed, the differentiation is usually based solely on degree of involvement. Vaccination history, exposure to other animals, and response to previous therapy are helpful in determining the underlying cause and in selecting the treatment required. Typically, an animal with a bacterial pneumonia is febrile, depressed, and inappetent, and it has a productive cough. Severely affected animals will be dyspneic and show a restrictive pattern of breathing, — i.e., rapid and shallow respirations. Orthopnea and cyanosis (with or without exertion) may also be present. Auscultation usually will reveal the presence of crackles in the ventral lung regions and may vary from fine to coarse depending on the extent of involvement. Occasionally, rhonchi may be heard as the secretions accumulate and cause a narrowing of the airways. If an area of lung is completely filled with exudate or the bronchus is plugged, there will be a silent area detected with the stethescope. When the bronchus remains open but the rest of that lung region is filled, bronchial breath sounds will be heard. Chest percussion will reveal a dull area in these cases as well. With less severe involvement, auscultation may only reveal the presence of bronchovesicular sounds.

Routine laboratory evaluation for all pneumonias (i.e., the data base) should include a complete blood count and differential, urinalysis, and depending on the geographic location, a heartworm and fecal check. An elevated white blood cell (WBC) count (often with a left shift) is usually found in cases of bacterial pneumonia. The leukocytosis may vary from near normal to greater than 35,000 WBC/cmm and, if chronic in nature, it may be accompanied by an anemia of inflammation. Arterial blood gases (ABG) correlate well with the degree of physiologic disruption the disease has produced and are a sensitive monitor of the patient's progress during treatment. A decrease in P_aO_2, the first change to occur, is a direct result of the ventilation-perfusion $(\dot{V}/\dot{Q})$ abnormalities seen in moderate to severe pneumonia cases. The change in the partial pressure of O_2 is usually followed by a small decrease in pH and finally by an increase in P_aCO_2.

Radiographically, a bacterial pneumonia case can vary from severe alveolar disease with air bronchograms ("lobar pneumonia") to a more mild mixed pattern of alveolar-bronchial-interstitial involvement. Radiographs are also an excellent means of documenting the disease state of the lungs and monitoring the response to therapy.

Although many articles have shown that the majority of organisms in bacterial pneumonias are Gram negative, cultures and sensitivities should not be overlooked. This is especially true in the per-acute case or the case that has suffered a relapse. Specimens may be obtained by using transtracheal aspiration, during bronchoscopy using suction, or simply by using a long-guarded culture swab* passed carefully (to avoid contamination) through the larynx of a lightly anesthetized animal. This last procedure is preferred in very small animals and works well with halothane gas anesthesia. When samples are obtained, routine cytology and Gram stain should be done in addition to the culture and sensitivity tests.

Prognosis. Many factors determine the prognosis in cases of bacterial pneumonia. First to be considered is whether the disease is primary or secondary. If it is secondary, the primary problem must be determined and considered before a prognosis can be made. The duration and degree of involvement are also important, as morbid anatomic changes (bronchiectasis, adhesions, atelectasis) may occur in chronic cases. Finally, the type of bacteria present and its sensitivity pattern will often predict the ease with which the pneumonia can be treated. In the author's experience, an increase in the P_aCO_2 is often an ominous and terminal sign and, if present, should warrant a guarded to poor prognosis.

Treatment. The treatment of choice for bacterial pneumonias is obviously antibiotics. Selection of an antibiotic should be based on the culture and sensitivity results. As mentioned earlier, most bacterial pneumonias involve Gram-negative organisms, frequently *E. coli*, *Klebsiella, Pseudomonas, Pasturella*, and *Bordetella* spp. If a culture cannot be taken, a Gram stain should be done to guide the clinician when selecting an antibiotic. Systemic therapy using either ampicillin, chloramphenicol, Tribrissen®, a cephalosporin, or an aminoglycoside will normally be a good choice.

Hydration is very important when treating respiratory diseases. Since tracheobronchial secretions are about 95 per cent water, dehydration will tend to thicken secretions and lead to their retention. Retained secretions may lead to further $\dot{V}/\dot{Q}$ abnormalities and deterioration of the patient. Adequate fluid intake must be insured and, if doubtful, it must be supplemented.

Aerosol therapy has received a moderate amount of attention in veterinary medicine during the past few years. It was not until 1978 that a comprehensive review of the subject was published (McKiernan, 1978). Although there still is a great deal of controversy regarding efficacy, favorable clinical results have been achieved in cases having increased airway secretions — especially the bronchopneumonia case. Additional clinical and laboratory studies are needed to answer many questions in this area of therapeutics.

In the author's opinion, the ultrasonic type of nebulizer* provides the best particle size for aerosol therapy. Sterile, normal saline is a good nebulizing fluid. The animal is "misted" in a small cage for 30 to 45 minutes, 3 or 4 times each day. Because of the high volume output of these nebulizers, small patients (less than 4 to 5 kg) must be watched for signs of overhydration. Other hazards that must be avoided are overheating in febrile animals (unable to cool themselves by panting while in 100 per cent relative humidity) and contamination. The latter is potentially the more serious problem, but it can be avoided if equipment is sterilized between patients and changed routinely if prolonged use is needed. *Pseudomonas* is most frequently incriminated.

The use of antibiotics, mucolytics, or other drugs by this form of nebulization is not recommended. With the exception of *Bordetella* infections in dogs (see "Diseases of the Canine and Feline Tracheobronchial Tree"), there is no work that shows any increased efficacy with aerosol as opposed to systemic antibiotics. Mucolytics are very irritating and should only be used via direct instillation, for instance, to help dislodge a bronchial mucous plug.

---

*Sterile Culture Swab, Sherwood Medical Co., St. Louis, MO 63103.

*Monaghan model 675; Hospal Medical Corporation, Littleton, Colo. 80122

Physiotherapy is helpful in removing retained secretions in man. Postural drainage is not practical in veterinary medicine, but chest percussion and mild exercise are of benefit in loosening and mobilizing secretions. Physiotherapy should be carried out after each aerosol treatment.

More exotic methods of removing secretions have been used experimentally in the dog (e.g., lung lavage) but require special equipment and are impractical in a clinical setting at this point.

MYCOTIC PNEUMONIA

Diagnosis. The geographic distribution of the fungal agents makes the travel history (exposure) a key point when considering the diagnosis of mycotic pneumonia. Cases have been diagnosed up to years after exposure to the agent. Agents endemic to the Mississippi and Ohio River Valey region include *Histoplasma capsulatum* and *Blastomyces dermatitidis*. *Coccidioides immitis* is endemic to arid regions of California and the southwestern part of the country. *Nocardia asteroides* and *Aspergillus fumigatus* are widespread in nature but are involved less frequently in mycotic lung disease. Although they present interesting and challenging clinical cases, they will not be discussed here.

Histoplasmosis, blastomycosis, and coccidioidomycosis are systemic fungal diseases caused by dimorphic fungi that live in a yeast form in tissue and a mycelial form in the environment. Only the mycelial form is infective, with spores entering the host via the respiratory system. In man, the majority of infections with these agents are sub-clinical and self-limiting. On occasion, however, a severe pulmonary form will develop and even less frequently may become disseminated to other organs in the body. Although the sub-clinical involvement has not been well documented in veterinary medicine, it is assumed to occur.

The dog with blastomycosis usually presents with a history of a high, non-responsive fever, weight loss, lethargy, anorexia, and a chronic, dry cough. Skin involvement (draining tracts or pustules), generalized lymphadenopathy, and ocular changes (detached retinas, anterior uveitis) are often present. Other organs that are involved less frequently include bones, prostate, and testicles. Auscultation is not diagnostic, and findings may range from near normal to increased bronchovesicular or even bronchial breath sounds. Severely affected animals are usually dyspneic and may become cyanotic if

stressed. The common radiographic appearance of canine blastomycosis is a generalized interstitial pattern (the "snow storm" or "lace curtain" pattern), yet cases of single lobe, alveolar disease have been seen. Hilar lymph node involvement is usually minimal in blastomycosis. Laboratory evaluation, except for cytology, merely reflects the degree of involvement — e.g., leukocytosis. In the author's experience, monocytosis has not been observed as often as it has been described. Cytologic data may be obtained directly from a draining tract or via lung or lymph node aspiration, and they are usually diagnostic. Multiple, thick-walled budding organisms of 8 to 15 μ diameter are usually found. Cytologic slides may be prepared with either new methylene blue or Wright's stain.

Histoplasmosis has been reported to produce at least five clinically distinct syndromes or diseases in man (Johnson, 1978). At least four of these occur in the dog, including inapparent infections, acute pulmonary histoplasmosis, chronic pulmonary histoplasmosis, and the disseminated form. The fifth form, isolated organ involvement, has not been seen by the author. The respiratory system is involved to some degree in all four forms of histoplasmosis. Symptoms referable to respiratory involvement will therefore vary considerably but may include dyspnea, coughing (mild to very severe), and airway obstruction secondary to hilar lymphadenopathy. General symptoms of fever, weight loss, anorexia, and diarrhea (with intestinal involvement) may occur. Radiographs of classical histoplasmosis cases reveal a hilar lymphadenopathy and small miliary granulomas throughout the lungs. This probably represents the chronic pulmonary form of histoplasmosis. Radiographs of the lungs in either acute cases or in disseminated cases usually only show an interstitial pattern with minimal hilar lymphadenopathy. Laboratory evaluation is rarely diagnostic, although buffy coat blood smears have shown intracellular *Histoplasma* organisms, primarily in cases of disseminated histoplasmosis.

Serology, both agar gel diffusion and complement fixation, has been used to aid in diagnosing histoplasmosis. Based on a limited number of case studies, it appears that the CF titer is often extremely high with the chronic cases and very low with the acute pulmonary and disseminated forms. Bronchoscopically, airway compression (and even obstruction) secondary to hilar lymphadenopathy is characteristic of the chronic pulmonary form of histoplasmosis. This fact alone can cause most of the severe coughing observed in these chronic cases. Auscultation in cases having this tremendous hilar lymph-adenopathy has routinely revealed rhonchi, usually more pronounced on the left side. More acute pulmonary forms only have an increase in bronchovesicular breath sounds when auscult-ed.

Coccidioidomycosis also occurs as a subclini-cal or inapparent infection in most of the human cases, and residents of endemic areas frequent-ly show a positive coccidioidin skin test (John-son, 1978). The disease as seen in dogs is usual-ly the chronic pulmonary or disseminated form, although a self-limiting form does occur. Exten-sion or dissemination has been reported to the skin, bone, liver, spleen, kidney, bladder, peri-cardium, and (in a recent case at Illinois) tes-ticles. Pulmonary forms of coccidioidomycosis usually present with a history of a dry, non-productive cough, non-responsive fever, an-orexia, depression, and weight loss. Dyspnea and severe coughing secondary to airway ob-struction from hilar lymphadenopathy may be seen. Auscultation may reveal an increase in bronchovesicular sounds or rhonchi if the air-way compression at the carina is extensive. The most characteristic radiographic appearance of a coccidioidomycosis case is hilar lymphadenopa-thy and perihilar interstitial densities. Other changes have been described (alveolar infil-trates, pleural thickening, miliary nodules, den-sities in the peripheral lung fields) but are less common (Head et al., 1975).

Samples for fungal cultures may be obtained from any of these fungal diseases but should only be cultured by special laboratories. It should be remembered that the cultured fungal organism is in the infective (mycelial) phase and must be handled with caution!

Prognosis. The prognosis for histoplasmo-sis, blastomycosis, or coccidioidomycosis is generally guarded. If dissemination to other organs has occurred, a poor prognosis should be given. Involvement of the eye is often seen with blastomycosis and warrants a poor prognosis, regardless of the animal's general condition, since organisms may remain viable within the eye despite systemic amphotericin B therapy. The cost and potential renal toxicity of ampho-tericin B therapy is of real concern and must be discussed with the owners prior to starting treatment. The public health aspect of these mycoses has been reviewed recently (Kelley and Mosier, 1977).

Treatment. Amphotericin B remains the pri-mary therapeutic agent for the deep mycoses. A variety of dosage regimes have been advocated in the past in attempts to avoid the renal toxicity that frequently occurs with therapy. The treat-ment schedule currently used at the University of Illinois is given in Table 2. An excellent

article was published recently that reviews methods of circumventing the toxicity of am-photericin B therapy and the new approaches in the treatment of systemic mycoses (Codish et al., 1979). An exciting area that is developing is the combination of amphotericin B with other antifungal drugs (notably 5-fluorocytosine and rifampicin) that seems to have synergistic ef-fects. A frustrating problem of phlebitis often develops with intravenous amphotericin B ther-apy. The review by Codish et al. suggests that the addition of heparin to the infusions may help reduce this problem. Although this has not been used to date at the author's hospital, it may prove to be a valuable addition to the ampho-tericin B therapy regime.

ALLERGIC PNEUMONIA (PULMONARY INFILTRATES WITH EOSINOPHILS)

"Allergic pneumonia" cases are occasionally seen by the veterinary practioner. Although the dog is more frequently affected, cases in the cat are also seen. In both species, the parenchymal involvement may be an extension of an existing allergic bronchitis (see "Diseases of the Canine and Feline Tracheobronchial Tree"). "Pulmo-nary infiltrates with eosinophils" (PIE) is a pref-erable term for this syndrome, as it does not imply an actual etiology. In man, the PIE com-plex is broken down into five categories accord-ing to severity of symptoms, percent eosino-philia, duration, other organ involvement, ra-diographic appearance, and specific etiology. Until such information can be obtained on ca-

---

Table 2.   *Amphotericin B Therapy Regime*

PRE-TREATMENT	Establish baseline renal function data and serum electrolytes.
DAY 1	0.5 mg/kg IV over 4–6 hours diluted in 250–1000 ml D5W depending on ani-mal's weight. Supplement with oral K+, 5–20 mEq/day in drinking water.
SUCCESSIVE ALTERNATE DAYS	Recheck BUN and/or creati-nine and serum K+, stop therapy if BUN > 60–70 mg %. Adjust oral K+ as needed. 1.0 mg/kg IV diluted as above. Fluid diuresis if uremia develops.

Total *cumulative* dose required depends upon the fungal agent involved but ranges from as little as 4.0 mg/kg to 8–10 mg/kg. Single monthly follow-up treatments for about six months are suggested.

nine and feline cases, the non-specific PIE term should be used.

Coughing is the most frequent symptom observed in cases of PIE. The cough may be sporadic and dry or severe and somewhat productive. Dyspnea, anorexia, fever, and other systemic symptoms are less commonly observed. Auscultatory findings also vary with severity, and breath sounds may range from bronchovesicular to coarse crackles, depending on the amount of secretions present and their viscoelastic characteristics. Radiographically, pulmonary alveolar infiltrates are observed (as the name PIE implies). Often, these infiltrates may "shift" and can be fairly patchy in appearance or involve entire lung lobes. A relative eosinophilia is frequently found on routine blood counts but is not required to make the diagnosis. If an eosinophilia is present, other explanations must be ruled out (e.g., parasites, heartworms, etc.) before the eosinophilia can be assumed to be associated with the pulmonary infiltrates observed on the radiographs. Samples obtained at bronchoscopy or via transtracheal aspiration are the best way to confirm a case of PIE. These samples are usually sterile when cultured and full of eosinophils on cytologic examination. An interesting endoscopic appearance observed in man and seen by the author in a few canine cases is the gross appearance of the bronchial secretions. Because of the high concentration of eosinophils, these secretions tend to take on a greenish-yellow color. Occasionally, an observant owner may describe this color change to the practicioner.

Prognosis. Treatment of the PIE case is rewarding and a favorable prognosis may be given. Recurrences will occur, however, and affected animals may have to remain on long-term (alternate-day) steroid therapy.

Treatment. Corticosteroids constitute the treatment in PIE cases. Prednisolone is the drug of choice; long-acting and respiratory forms of steroids should not be used. Dosages of 0.5 to 2.0 mg/kg are used as a starting point and are decreased after a few days when clinical improvement is noted. Alternate-day therapy is recommended when long-term maintenance therapy is required. Progress may be monitored by clinical improvement or by radiographic clearing of the infiltrates. Owners should be instructed to adjust the steroid dose continually (e.g., on a seasonal basis) so as to use the minimal dose necessary to control the symptoms.

ASPIRATION PNEUMONIA

Aspiration pneumonia was first described by Mendelson in 1946 as either an obstructive or asthmatic phenomena depending on whether solid food materials or gastric secretions were actually aspirated. Aspiration pneumonia in veterinary medicine may occur acutely owing to one of these etiologies or as the result of a chronic aspiration of saliva or small amounts of food — i.e., the megaesophagus case. Aspiration pneumonia is usually associated with an underlying disease. Animals that are severely depressed or have a reduced state of consciousness (e.g., sedated, postoperative, or comatose patients), are particularly at risk. Dysphagic animals and those that have esophageal incompetence (megaesophagus or pharyngostomy tubes) are also predisposed to aspiration. Studies in man have indicated that routine aspiration of gastric and oral secretions commonly occurs with no sequelae. Apparently, problems develop only as the result of frequent aspirations, large volumes, or caustic (gastric) secretions of low pH. Typically, the case of aspiration pneumonia goes unobserved. Symptoms that may appear include tachypnea, dyspnea, bronchospasm, tachycardia, cyanosis, and shock. If the aspirated material was infected, a fever may develop shortly after the event. Auscultation of affected animals frequently reveals rhonchi or wheezes due to the bronchospasms, and crackles, especially over the area that was dependent when the aspiration occurred. Radiographically, few changes are observed immediately after aspiration occurs, but changes may develop rapidly over the ensuing 12 to 24 hours. Diffuse or localized alveolar infiltrates, especially in dependent regions, are the most frequent finding. Arterial blood gases, if available, nearly always show a moderate to severe decrease in P_aO_2 and a decrease in blood pH. Examination of the mouth for the presence of gastric contents may help confirm the diagnosis in suspected cases of aspiration pneumonia.

Prognosis. The prognosis in cases of aspiration pneumonia is totally dependent on the degree of involvement, the type and quantity of material aspirated, and the initial physical findings. Shock, hypoxemia, and apnea immediately following aspiration have been shown to be particularly ominous signs. The underlying disease that allowed the aspiration to occur must also be considered when making a prognosis.

Treatment. Unless done immediately, lung or bronchial lavage has been ineffective in the treatment of aspiration pneumonia. If it is done, only saline should be used, and no attempts should be made to "neutralize" the gastric secretions. Particulate matter may be removed via bronchoscopy; this is indicated if the aspirate is known to contain solid material. Since hypoxemia may be severe, oxygen therapy is usually indicated. Steroids and antibiotics have been used in cases of aspiration pneumonia, yet controversy still exists as to their efficacy. At this time, research data support early steroid therapy. Unless a specific bacterial pneumonia is identified, however, other data suggest that antibiotics not be used. Although aspiration will damage the mucociliary tree and allow for bacterial colonization, early "protective" use of antibiotics may only select out resistant strains.

INHALATION PNEUMONIA

Diagnosis. Smoke inhalation that results in pneumonia is fortunately a rare occurrence in veterinary medicine. Actual thermal injury to the respiratory tract is usually confined to the larynx and supralaryngeal airways. Unless live steam is involved, the efficiency of the respiratory mucosa makes it difficult to produce actual thermal trauma of the lower respiratory tract (Cohn, 1973). The major factor in trauma from smoke inhalation is chemical in nature and results from exposure to the products of incomplete combustion found in the inhaled smoke (Cohn, 1973; Welch et al., 1977). These byproducts and the amount of damage produced vary depending upon the type of material involved and the length of time the animal is exposed.

The diagnosis of inhalation pneumonia is usually made from the history (observation) of exposure and findings from the physical examination. Singed hair or skin burns, especially around the face, should alert and concern the clinician. Burns that occur from exposure while in a closed area are of particular concern, as they are frequently associated with a higher mortality in man (Welch et al., 1977). Symptoms observed in cases of smoke inhalation range from a mild cough to shock with severe dyspnea, tachypnea, cyanosis, and blood-tinged bronchial secretions. Auscultation may reveal only increased bronchovesicular sounds or the presence of crackles, rhonchi, or even stridor. Crackles or wheezing on admission is an ominous finding in man (Cohn, 1973), although they often occur a few days after exposure. Stridor, as discussed, reflects laryngeal airway narrowing (usually secondary to edema) and may indicate the need for a tracheostomy. Membrane color should be evaluated but interpreted with caution, as the presence of carbon monoxyhemoglobin often produces a "cherry red" color and can mask the presence of cyanosis. Cases described in the dog have also revealed a conjunctivitis and nasal discharge (Farrow, 1975). Radiographs taken immediately after exposure may be normal or reveal early alveolar filling associated with the developing pulmonary edema. This pulmonary edema, however, may occur up to one to two days later and therefore

necessitates frequent patient monitoring. Areas of atelectasis and often bronchopneumonia may develop with time. Arterial blood gases are critical and should be performed if possible. Samples may be stored in an air-tight, corked syringe on ice for transportation to a human hospital for processing. The major concern is the level of hypoxia that develops and frequently progresses as more and more ventilation-perfusion inequalities develop. A mild respiratory alkalosis may be observed early in the course of the disease, as the tachypnea often allows for the "blowing off" of CO_2.

Prognosis. The initial examination is often a good prognosticator in inhalation pneumonia cases. In man, the presence of cyanosis, crackles, rhonchi, blood-tinged sputum, and burns on the face are associated with a high mortality rate when present on the admitting examination. Complicating factors, including secondary bacterial pneumonia, atelectasis, and severe hypoxemia may develop and necessitate a change in prognosis.

Treatment. Humidified oxygen is the first step in treating cases of smoke inhalation. The inspired oxygen concentration achievable in a well sealed oxygen cage (about 40 per cent) is usually sufficient but must be monitored based on serial P_aO_2 measurements. If the P_aO_2 cannot be kept above 60 mm Hg on 40 per cent oxygen, it may be necessary to administer a higher concentration of oxygen via tracheal catheter, endotracheal tube, or tracheostomy with or without mechanical ventilation. Whatever the method of delivery, it is critical that adequate humidity be provided to the inspired gases to prevent inspissation of the tracheobronchial secretions. Heated humidifiers are available that provide 100 per cent humidity at body temperature. Intermittent bland aerosol (sterile saline) nebulization may also aid in keeping secretions loose and allow for easier clearance. (Aerosol therapy is described under the section on bacterial pneumonia.) Systemic hydration is probably the most efficacious method for thinning secretions and must not be overlooked.

Fluid therapy is often indicated in burn patients (for shock, hypovolemia) but must be used with caution in smoke inhalation patients that have pulmonary edema. The edema fluid that accumulates in these cases is secondary to altered capillary permeability and is easily exacerbated by simple fluid therapy. Thought should be given to plasma therapy to try to minimize the amount of interstitial fluid accumulation.

Physiotherapy is an important means of facilitating secretion clearance. Deep breathing associated with exercise has been shown to aid secretion removal and to increase lymphatic drainage from the lung. The edema fluid that accumulates in cases involving altered capillary premeability is rich in protein. Since protein is removed only via the lymphatics, physiotherapy should speed its resolution. A third effect of physiotherapy and deep breathing will be an increased tidal (alveolar) volume and therefore better oxygenation of the blood. Chest percussion and mild (patient limited) exercise are recommended to aid in secretion removal, lymphatic drainage, and alveolar ventilation.

The decision of whether or not to perform a tracheostomy is a major one. In cases of severe laryngeal edema and upper airway obstruction, tracheostomy is absolutely necessary. It requires meticulous care afterwards, and the clinician must be available for and capable of this care. There is concern that the inability to cough effectively with a tracheostomy tube in place is a serious detriment to the patient, especially since secretions will be increased in these cases. If the decision is made to tracheostomize an animal, tracheal toilet care (removal of secretions) and humidification of inspired gases are of paramount importance.

There is considerable confusion in the literature regarding the use of steroids in smoke inhalation cases. Studies on animals have revealed adverse, beneficial, and insignificant changes in exposed versus control animals. The proposed beneficial effects of steroids (membrane stability, histamine antagonism, decreased inflammatory reaction) are important enough that the drugs should probably be used during the first 36 to 72 hours following exposure. Prednisolone in doses of 2 to 4 mg/kg every 12 hours is adequate for these purposes.

Antibiotics should be used only when a bacterial problem develops, and then they should be given based on culture and sensitivity results obtained from infected secretions. Prophylactic antibiotics are *not* indicated and will only serve to select out more resistent bacterial flora should an infection develop.

The efficacy of diuretics (such as furosemide) in the treatment of pulmonary edema of the type produced in smoke inhalation (noncardiac) is debated by different authors. Since the primary problem is one of increased capillary permeability, diuretics should be reserved for cases of cardiac origin (increased pressure) and pulmonary edema.

Analgesics and bronchodilators should be used if indicated. Morphine in low doses (0.1 to 0.2 mg/kg) will avoid respiratory depression and cause a mild vasodilation as well as relieve some of the pain and apprehension seen in these cases. If rhonchi or wheezes are noted on auscultation, bronchodilators may prove beneficial and should be used on a trial basis at least. Aminophylline at 11 mg/kg should be repeated every six hours if a favorable response is obtained.

SUPPLEMENTAL READING

Codish, S.D., Tobias, J.S., and Monaco, A.P.: Recent advances in the treatment of systemic mycotic infections: Surg. Gynecol. Obstet, 148:435–447, 1979.

Cohn, A.M.: Concepts in management of burns of the respiratory tract. So. Med. J. 66:(3)297–301, 1973.

Farrow, C.S.: Smoke inhalation in the dog, current concepts of pathophysiology and management, VMSAC 70:404–414, 1975.

Head, J.R., Suter, P.F., and Ettinger, S.J.: Lower respiratory tract diseases. In Ettinger, S.J. (ed.): *Textbook of Veterinary Internal Medicine*. Philadelphia, W.B. Saunders Co., 1975.

Johnson, J.E., III: Mycotic infections: guidelines for differential diagnosis. Drug Ther. pp 33–50, August 1978.

Kelley, D.C., and Mosier, J.E.: Public health aspects of mycotic diseases. JAVMA 171:1168–1170, 1977.

McKiernan, B.: Principles of Aerosol Therapy — Applications in the Canine. Proceedings of the Illinois Veterinary Respiratory Symposium, 1978.

Murphy, R.L.H.: *A Simplified Introduction to Lung Sounds*. (Text and cassette tape), Wellesley Hills, Mass., Stethophonics, 1977.

Suter, P.F., and Chan, K.F.: Disseminated pulmonary diseases in small animals: a radiographic approach to diagnosis. JAVRS, 9:67–79, 1968.

Welch, G.W., Lull, R.J., Petroff, P.A., et al.: The use of steroids in inhalation injury. Surg. Gynecol. Obstet. 145:539–544, 1977.

PULMONARY EDEMA

JOHN D. BONAGURA, D.V.M.

Columbus, Ohio

Pulmonary edema refers to the accumulation of abnormal quantities of liquid and solute in the lung. Edema can accumulate in the pulmonary connective tissue (interstitial pulmonary edema) or in the alveoli and terminal airspaces (alveolar edema). Although small amounts of interstitial edema can accumulate without causing clinically detectable abnormalities, alveolar edema is heralded by demonstrable signs of pulmonary dysfunction. Clinical evidence of alveolar edema includes abnormalities of ventilation (hyperpnea-dyspnea), oxygenation (cyanosis), and auscultation (moist or bubbling pulmonary rales and coughing). Thoracic radiographs demonstrate increased pulmonary densities of an interstitial and alveolar nature. Arterial blood gases reveal hypoxemia and occasionally abnormalities of carbon dioxide transfer and pH.

ETIOLOGY

The numerous causes of pulmonary edema can be grouped by their prevailing pathophysiologic mechanism: elevated pulmonary capillary pressure, decreased plasma oncotic pressure, altered alveolar-capillary permeability, and reduced lymphatic drainage. For convenience, the causes can be further divided into those associated with heart disease or failure (cardiogenic) and those unassociated with heart failure (non-cardiogenic). Some clinical abnormalities cannot be readily classified, since they result in edema through multiple or, as yet, undetermined mechanisms (Table 1).

Rational therapy is predicated on the clinician's understanding of the mechanisms causing pulmonary edema. In the normal lung, the net transfer of liquid is governed by the interaction of opposing forces (Fig. 1). The pulmonary capillary hydrostatic pressure forces liquid into the interstitial space. This movement is enhanced by the interstitial oncotic and negative hydrostatic pressures but retarded by the plasma oncotic pressure. The volume of liquid entering the alveoli from the interstitium is normally very small. Although information concerning interactions of intra-alveolar forces

Table 1. Causes of Pulmonary Edema

MECHANISM — ETIOLOGY	COMMENTS
Increased pulmonary capillary pressure	
A. Cardiogenic	Multiple causes of left heart failure
B. Non-cardiogenic: pulmonary veno-occlusive disease; overinfusion of fluids or blood	Not well described in animals
Decreased plasma oncotic pressure (hypoproteinemia)	
A. Hepatic disease	Inadequate protein synthesis
B. Renal disease	Protein loss secondary to glomerulonephritis or amyloidosis
C. Protein-losing enteropathies	Caused by lymphangectasia, or inflammatory/neoplastic bowel disease
D. Nutritional disorders	
Altered alveolar-capillary permeability	
A. Infectious pulmonary disease	Protein content of edema very high
B. "Toxic" damage to membrane	
Inhaled toxins	Smoke inhalation, aspiration of gastric contents
Circulating exogenous toxins	Snake venom, ANTU, paraquat, endotoxins, monocrotaline
Circulating endogenous toxins	Uremia, vasoactive substances released from thrombosis or shock
C. Drowning and near-drowning	Direct flooding of alveolus with secondary atelectasis and edema related to tonicity of water (fresh vs salt) and damage to membrane
D. Disseminated intravascular coagulation (e.g., secondary to heat stroke)	Microembolic damage of capillary endothelial membrane
E. Immunologic reactions and anaphylaxis	Drug and blood transfusion reactions
F. Shock and non-pulmonary trauma	"Shock lung"—non-cardiogenic pulmonary edema possibly related to release of chemicals or tissue components into the circulation
G. Pulmonary contusion	
H. Aspiration of gastric contents	Increased mortality if pH < 2.5
I. Oxygen toxicity	>50% O_2 for 24–48 hours
Lymphatic insufficiency	From neoplastic infiltration
Mixed or undetermined causes	
A. Neurogenic	Seizure disorders, head trauma, electrical shock through brainstem
B. Electrocution and cardioversion	
C. Drug induced (?)	? Ketamine HCl, anesthetic agents
D. Rapid removal of pleural fluid	Expands atelectatic lung, favors pulmonary capillary ultrafiltration and alters alveolar surface tension

and surface tension is incomplete, it is believed that at points of alveolar convexity, surface tension forces draw liquid from the vascular to the alveolar space. Fluid movement also is related to the permeability of the alveolar-capillary membrane and the capacity of the pulmonary lymphatics to drain the interstitium of "excess" liquid.

Pulmonary edema is associated with a number of clinical abnormalities (see Fig. 1). An increase in pulmonary capillary pressure, as occurs with left heart failure or overinfusion of fluids, results in an increase in pulmonary interstitial and alveolar liquid. The hypoalbuminemic states accompanying certain renal and hepatic diseases, protein losing enteropathies, and nutritional disorders result in decreased capillary oncotic pressure and pulmonary edema.

Pulmonary lymphatic blockage can occur secondary to thoracic neoplasia and can result in insufficient drainage of the constantly formed interstitial fluid. Finally, an alteration in the permeability of the alveolar-capillary membrane permits excessive influx of liquid and protein into the interstitium and alveolus. This can occur in the presence of normal pulmonary capillary pressures and is the mechanism by which diverse disorders lead to pulmonary edema. Table 1 lists some of the more common causes of cardiogenic and non-cardiogenic pulmonary edema.

Some causes of pulmonary edema cannot be classified conveniently. Pulmonary edema associated with electric shock, seizures, and head trauma probably results from hypothalamic-adrenergic mediated shifts in blood volume toward the pulmonary circulation. Pulmonary edema following cardioversion probably results from a combination of direct cardiac and pulmonary injury and vascular reflexes invoked by the electrical shock. Acute pulmonary edema has been observed in a small number of cats after the administration of ketamine HCl. The mechanism for this drug-associated edema is unknown. Near-drowning results in direct flooding of alveoli Fresh-water as opposed to salt-water drowning initially causes rapid fluid movement from the alveolus to the blood, since fresh water is hypotonic. Both conditions, however, lead to secondary osmotic injury of the alveolar-capillary membrane, causing pronounced pulmonary edema. The clinician should appreciate the spectrum of disorders associated with non-cardiogenic pulmonary edema.

DIAGNOSIS

The clinical diagnosis of alveolar pulmonary edema is not difficult if the clinician is cog-

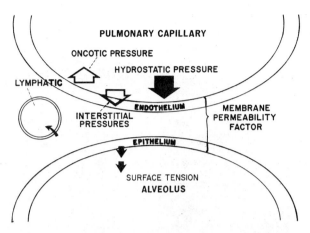

Figure 1. The terminal lung unit. The major forces responsible for normal fluid movement are shown. Factors that predispose to pulmonary edema include *increased* pulmonary *capillary hydrostatic* pressure, *decreased* pulmonary *capillary oncotic* pressure, *increased permeability* of the alveolar capillary membrane, and *inadequate lymphatic drainage* relative to net flow into the interstitial compartment (after Robin et al.).

nizant of the potential causes of this disorder. Since the onset of non-cardiogenic pulmonary edema is often delayed, the clinician should highly suspect it following seizures, electric shock, aspiration of gastric contents, uremia, thoracic trauma, shock, smoke inhalation, heat stroke, and rapid infusion of intravenous fluids. *Medical history*, therefore, is an important clue in an eventual diagnosis of pulmonary edema.

The accumulation of interstitial and early alveolar pulmonary edema often goes undetected unless thoracic radiographs are obtained. Progressive accumulation of alveolar fluid, however, results in abnormalities detectable on *physical examination*. As noted previously, dyspnea, anxiety, cyanosis, pulmonary rales, and coughing often are observed. In fulminant edema, pinkish froth can be noted exiting the nostrils. Additional physical abnormalities may reveal the underlying cause of the pulmonary disorder. For example, loud cardiac murmurs, gallops, and arrhythmias are reliable signs of heart disease and favor a diagnosis of cardiogenic edema. In the cardiomyopathic cat, aortic thromboembolism often is associated with heart failure and pulmonary edema. A necrotic oral lesion suggests an electric shock. Marked hyperthermia can be secondary to heat stroke or sepsis. Other physical abnormalities depend on the underlying etiology.

Thoracic radiographs are important in the diagnosis of pulmonary edema. They should not be obtained, however, if the procedure will decompensate the patient's pulmonary status. Properly exposed X-ray films substantiate the

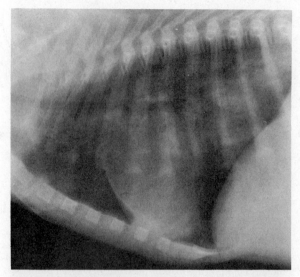
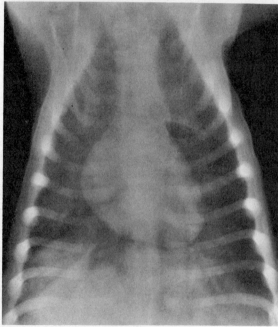

Figure 2. Radiographs from a 4½-month-old Old English sheepdog cross presented in status epilepticus. There is marked non-cardiogenic pulmonary edema (neurogenic pulmonary edema). Increased interstitial and alveolar densities may be noted in the caudal lung lobes. This pattern differs from that of typical cardiogenic pulmonary edema, since the left side of the heart is not enlarged, the pulmonary veins are not engorged, and the pulmonary infiltrates are more prominent in peripheral, as opposed to perihilar, pulmonary zones. The thymus is prominent on the ventrodorsal view.

clinical diagnosis of pulmonary edema and often illustrate its cause. Pulmonary edema accumulates initially in the perivascular and peribronchial connective tissue and results in increased linear interstitial densities with blurring of the vascular margins. Increased alveolar-capillary permeability can cause a peri-

bronchial infiltrate. As alveolar liquid increases, the abnormal densities coalesce yet maintain their indistinct borders. Air bronchoceles become prominent and are indicative of the alveolar location of the edema.

If the pulmonary edema is cardiogenic, the abnormal pulmonary densities usually are perihilar, dorsal (particularly in the dog), and bilateral. In the majority of cases, there will be left heart enlargement and dilated, dense pulmonary veins suggesting pulmonary venous congestion. Non-cardiogenic edema is not associated with cardiomegaly and often maintains a peripheral distribution in the caudal lung lobes (Fig. 2)

Aspiration of gastric contents and pulmonary infection result in edema that usually is distributed in the ventral portions of the cranial and middle lung lobes. Pulmonary neoplasia and thrombosis, thoracic trauma, and other abnormalities are associated with characteristic radiographic findings and are described in other sections of this text.

Ancillary tests are helpful in delineating the severity of pulmonary and associated disorders. This is particularly true in non-cardiogenic pulmonary edema. For example, pulmonary edema is common in uremic patients receiving moderate amounts of intravenous fluids. The clinician should be cognizant of the augmentative effects of renal insufficiency on pulmonary capillary permeability and of volume expansion on pulmonary capillary pressure. This information prompts judicious administration of fluids, which can circumvent the development of florid pulmonary edema.

If *blood gas analysis* is available, arterial samples will supply valuable information. Pulmonary edema generally results in arterial hypoxemia, hypocarbia, and respiratory alkalosis. Severe edema, however, can result in both respiratory and metabolic acidosis, since the capacity for pulmonary gas exchange is severely diminished and hypoxemia leads to anaerobic tissue metabolism.

Sometimes, an *electrocardiogram* helps to distinguish cardiogenic from non-cardiogenic edema. Detection of arrhythmias or abnormal voltages suggesting left heart enlargement or pericardial disease is valuable. The role of pulmonary capillary hydrostatic pressure in the pathogenesis of pulmonary edema is best evaluated through monitoring of pulmonary capillary-wedge pressures via a flow-directed catheter.* Pulmonary wedge pressures of 25 to 30 mm Hg are associated with formation of pul-

---

*5–7 Fr Swan-Ganz® thermodilution catheter, Edwards Laboratories.

monary edema. Lower pressures indicate treated cardiogenic edema or edema of non-cardiac origin. Unfortunately, such monitoring is not routinely available in veterinary medicine.

THERAPY

GENERAL MEASURES

Principles of therapy for pulmonary edema include reducing activity and anxiety, clearing airways, reducing alveolar hypoxia, improving blood and tissue oxygenation, and if possible, treating the underlying pathologic disorder. In cardiogenic pulmonary edema, additional therapy is directed toward improvement of left ventricular function. Although general principles of therapy are presented, it is stressed that treatment must be matched to each individual (Table 2). (Refer to page 364 for specific therapy of cardiogenic pulmonary edema.)

Animals with moderate to severe degrees of alveolar edema should be placed at rest in an oxygen-enriched environment. Intratracheal administration of oxygen with a 16 to 18 gauge catheter can be used, but this may be associated with undesirable struggling during implantation of the cannula. If oxygen therapy is not feasible, a cool (65° F), well ventilated area may suffice. Sedation of the patient is usually indicated. In general, morphine sulfate is the sedative of choice for dogs; low doses of phenothiazines are effective in cats. Diazepam (Valium) is useful in patients with a history of seizure disorders and neurogenic pulmonary edema.

MEASURES TO IMPROVE GAS EXCHANGE

Initially, administration of high levels of oxygen (40 to 60 per cent) is useful, since this increases the driving force for diffusion into the alveolar capillary. Long-term use (>24 hours) of oxygen concentrations greater than 50 per cent should be avoided, however, since this can lead to alveolar-capillary damage (oxygen toxicity) and can worsen the edema. Bronchodilators such as aminophylline are administered, as bronchial edema and bronchospasm result in luminal narrowing.

Nebulization of 40 per cent ethyl alcohol into the oxygen unit reduces surface tension and prevents foaming in the larger airways. Cases of fulminant edema require endotracheal suction to insure airway patency.

REDUCTION OF CAPILLARY HYDROSTATIC PRESSURE

With the possible exception of pulmonary edema caused by inhalation of irritant gases,

Table 2. Management of Pulmonary Edema

GENERAL MEASURES
  Reduction of activity—cage rest
  Sedation
    Morphine sulfate—0.2–0.5 mg/kg (IV,IM,SQ) (dog)
    Acepromazine—0.1–0.5 mg/kg (SQ,IM) (beware hypotension)
    Diazepam—2–5 mg IV (cat); 5–10 mg IV (dog)
    Pentobarbital—6–10 mg/kg (IM,IV)

MEASURES TO IMPROVE GAS EXCHANGE
  Oxygen therapy—40–50% or higher (avoid > 50% for >24 hours)
  Ethyl alcohol nebulization—40% solution
  Aminophylline—6–10 mg/kg (IV,SQ,Orally) Can repeat q6h
  Endotracheal suctioning
  Endotracheal intubation with positive pressure ventilation (severe cases only)
    Intravenous sedation with diazepam, pentobarbital or morphine
    Pancuronium bromide (Pavulon)—0.04 mg/kg IV if paralysis necessary
    Positive pressure ventilation (manual or mechanical ventilator)
    Positive end-expiratory pressure (PEEP)

MEASURES TO REDUCE PULMONARY CAPILLARY PRESSURE
  Furosemide (Lasix)—2–4 mg/kg (IV,IM,Oral) Can repeat q6–8h
  Positive inotropic agents—digitalis, dopamine HCl, dobutamine HCl (see section on heart failure)
  Phlebotomy—remove 6–10 cc/kg body weight
  Control cardiac arrhythmias, if present
  Vasodilator therapy afterload and preload reduction (beware hypotension)
    Na Nitroprusside—5–20 μg/kg/min
    Nitroglycerine ointment (2%)—1/4–3/4 inch topically q6h
    Alpha-adrenergic blockers—hydralazine, promazine hydrochloride

OTHER THERAPY
  Corticosteroid therapy—Prednisone 2 mg/kg BID (for permeability pulmonary edema)

---

alveolar edema regresses in response to reduction of pulmonary capillary hydrostatic pressure. This therapeutic goal is obtained by reducing blood volume, redistributing pulmonary fluid to other vascular beds, and increasing cardiac output. Furosemide (Lasix) redistributes pulmonary blood by increasing the venous capacitance, and promoting a diuresis. In addition to its sedative effect, morphine causes similar fluid shifts by increasing systemic venous capacitance. Morphine is contraindicated, however, in neurogenic pulmonary edema owing to its augmentative effect on intracranial pressure. In this type of non-cardiogenic edema, the effects of massive adrenergic stimulation can be minimized by vasodilator therapy. Suitable vasodilators include phenothiazines (contraindicated in seizure disorders), sodium nitroprusside, nitroglycerin ointment, and hydralazine, among others. These drugs achieve therapeutic benefits via peripheral vasodilatation. In neurogenic edema, they reduce the pronounced systemic vasoconstriction, allowing blood to leave the pulmonary circulation. In cardiogenic edema, they decrease resistance to outflow (afterload). The most important adverse effect of vasodilator therapy is hypotension. This deleterious consequence can be avoided through judicious drug administration, serial evaluation of blood pressure, and assessment of clinical indices of tissue perfusion — e.g., pulse pressure, capillary refill time, level of consciousness, and urinary output. In cardiogenic edema, hypotension can be circumvented by vigorous inotropic support with digitalis or catecholamine precursors (see section on acute heart failure). In fulminant cardiogenic edema, phlebotomy serves to reduce the blood volume rapidly. This procedure is not commonly performed.

ARTIFICIAL VENTILATION

Some patients do not respond adequately to these measures and demonstrate clinical or laboratory evidence of respiratory failure. Although definite criteria for respiratory failure have not been established for animals, the author has utilized the following as indications for ventilatory support: arterial PO_2 of 59 mm Hg or less while breathing at least 60 per cent oxygen; arterial PCO_2 of greater than 60 mm Hg following therapy designed to clear the airways; and persistent cyanosis, dyspnea, and tachypnea (respiratory rate greater than 70/minute) despite the therapy described previously.

Artificial ventilation is best accomplished with a volume- or pressure-cycled ventilator (e.g., Bird® ventilator), although the rebreathing bag of an anesthetic machine or a specifically designed positive pressure breathing bag (Ambu®) can be utilized for short-term therapy. Although volume-cycled ventilators are preferable, more practitioners are familiar with pressure-cycled ventilators. In either case, one should adhere to principles of artificial ventilation.

Unless unconscious or weakened from respiratory failure, the patient is sedated for endotracheal intubation and controlled ventilatory support. Pentobarbital, diazepam (Valium), and, in dogs, narcotics such as morphine or fentanyl citrate (in Innovar-Vet) are effective sedatives. Although sedated, some animals resist the ventilator. In these cases, controlled ventilation is necessary. The use of either 100 per cent inspired O_2 for 10 to 20 minutes or higher doses of sedatives can blunt the ventilatory drive. In certain cases, administration of the paralyzing drug pancuronium bromide (Pavulon®) is useful in

providing skeletal muscle paralysis for 20 to 40 minutes. The author generally administers a sedative intravenously, intubates the animal with a sterile, cuffed endotracheal tube, administers 100 per cent oxygen with positive pressure ventilation, and then injects the paralyzing agent only if needed. Needless to say, the clinician must be intimately familiar with the pharmacology of these drugs.

Once the ventilator has been attached, the animal is ventilated at a rate of 8 to 12/minute, using 40 to 60 per cent oxygen or a suitable air-oxygen mix. The tidal volume should be sufficient (approximately 7 to 10 cc/kg) to expand the chest at an end-inspiratory pressure of approximately 20 to 25 cm H_2O. In many cases, these pressure-volume guidelines are insufficient to expand the less compliant edematous lung, and higher pressures of up to 40 to 50 cm H_2O (rarely higher) are needed. The use of positive-end expiratory pressure (PEEP) of 5 to 15 cm H_2O has been advocated to decrease atelectasis and improve oxygenation. This can be accomplished with many volume-cycled ventilators but is more difficult to attain with some pressure-cycled ventilators. Practical application of PEEP requires a means for obtaining constant expiratory resistance such as an underwater seal in the expiratory line. Inspiratory time should be short (1 to 2 seconds) to minimize the reductions in venous return attending positive pressure ventilation.

Cardiac output must be monitored as accurately as possible, since reduced perfusion aggravates tissue hypoxia. An intravenous line is mandatory, although parenteral fluids must be given judiciously. If circulatory status deteriorates, decreasing inspiratory time and pressures may be necessary. In such cases, the infusion of catecholamine precursors such as dopamine HCl (Intropin) or dobutamine (Dobutrex) supports the circulation.

Fine-tuning of ventilatory parameters (tidal volume, respiratory rate, flow rate, pressures, and inspiratory-expiratory times) is guided by serial evaluation of patient parameters. These include arterial blood gases, color of the mucous membranes, character of pulmonary auscultation, volume of frank airway edema, appearance of thoracic radiographs (these can be misleading), and ability of the animal to maintain itself after discontinuing artificial ventilation. In order to wean the patient from the ventilator, it is helpful to reverse narcotic sedatives with agents like naloxone (Narcan®) and nalorphine (Nalline®). It is not always necessary to antagonize pancuronium bromide, although atropine (0.02 mg/kg) followed by neostigmine (0.02 to 0.03 mg/kg) accomplishes this reversal.

Good nursing and supportive care are essential. The animal is turned frequently and the endotracheal tube is deflated, repositioned, suctioned, and reinflated hourly. To avoid further atelectasis, the animal is deeply ventilated ("sighed") every 10 minutes. Hypothermia is avoided, particularly in the paralyzed animal unable to shiver. Prophylactic antibiotics (such as cephalosporins, ampicillin, or aminoglycosides) are administered, although their value has been questioned. The airways are hydrated by adding water to the appropriate reservoir on the ventilator apparatus. Complications such as pneumomediastinum and pneumothorax are expected if high pressures or PEEP is utilized.

OTHER MEASURES

Since many causes of non-cardiogenic pulmonary edema result from direct injury to the alveolar-capillary membrane, considerable emphasis has been directed to therapy designed to normalize membrane permeability. Corticosteroids have been advocated in non-cardiogenic pulmonary edema for their membrane and microcirculatory stabilizing effects; however, their value is equivocal based on studies in man and experimental animals. In non-cardiogenic pulmonary edema owing to aspiration of gastric contents (pH<2.5), glucocorticoid therapy achieves variable results and increases the incidence of sepsis. In the altered permeability edema associated with smoke inhalation or anaphylaxis, however, corticosteroid therapy is indicated. Anticholinergics such as atropine sulfate have been advocated in the initial therapy of edema caused by irritant gases or thermal injury. While atropine probably decreases the volume of pulmonary secretions, it also increases their viscosity, thereby inhibiting expectoration. The value of other drugs in the management of pulmonary edema depends on their ability to treat the underlying cause or complications. Antibiotics are indicated in pulmonary infections; bicarbonate is indicated if severe metabolic acidosis is present.

Symptomatic pulmonary edema often constitutes a medical emergency. This disorder is common in both heart failure and in clinical settings characterized by abnormal pulmonary fluid dynamics. Non-cardiogenic pulmonary edema is being recognized with increased frequency in veterinary medical practice. The clinician must be cognizant of the varied causes of this disorder so that both symptomatic and specific therapy can be directed for the patient's benefit.

SUPPLEMENTAL READING

Robin, E. D., Cross, C. E., and Zellis, R.: Pulmonary edema. N. Engl. J. Med. 288:239–245, 292–304, 1973.

NEOPLASMS OF THE RESPIRATORY TRACT

STEVEN E. CROW, D.V.M.
East Lansing, Michigan

Neoplasms of the respiratory tract of dogs and cats continue to present diagnostic and therapeutic difficulties for the veterinarian. Tumors of the nasal passages, paranasal sinuses, and the lungs are rarely diagnosed in small animals before the neoplastic process is advanced. Use of available diagnostic tools such as radiography, rhinoscopy, bronchoscopy, and cytology, rather than lengthy and often fruitless therapeutic trials with "panaceas" such as broad-spectrum antibiotics and corticosteroids, will allow the clinician to make an earlier diagnosis. When considering malignant disease, early detection is of paramount importance in affording the veterinarian and patient an optimal chance for cure or significant periods of remission.

NASAL AND PARANASAL SINUS TUMORS

Neoplasms of the nasal passages account for approximately 1 per cent of all canine tumors and are found prinicipally in older dogs. Long-nosed breeds may have a greater incidence of these tumors than do short-nosed breeds. Nasal tumors are usually malignant in dogs (80 per cent) but rarely metastasize, regardless of histogenetic origin. Rather, they are locally invasive, frequently causing lysis and deformity of the nasal, frontal, and maxillary bones.

Malignancies of the nasal passages include tumors of both epithelial (65 per cent) and mesenchymal (35 per cent) origin. Carcinomas may be derived from glandular (adenocarcinoma) or stratified (squamous cell carcinoma) epithelium or may be characterized by sheets of epithelial cells separated by dense connective tissue stroma (solid carcinoma). Occasionally, highly anaplastic tumors (undifferentiated carcinomas) are found. Mesenchymal tumors most frequently diagnosed are chondrosarcoma, fibrosarcoma, osteosarcoma, and undifferentiated sarcoma. In cats, 90 per cent of nasal tumors are malignant. Carcinomas are much more common than sarcomas in cats.

Regardless of histologic type, clinical presentation is fairly consistent. Signs include unilateral or bilateral mucoid or bloody discharge, intermittent sneezing, and obstruction of nasolacrimal ducts. In rapidly growing or advanced cases, swelling of nasomaxillary, frontal, or periorbital areas, exophthalmos, or neurologic abnormalities are often noted. Occasionally, erosion of the hard palate or dental alveoli may be observed.

Median duration of signs prior to diagnosis is approximately three months. Madewell et al. found that 95 per cent of dogs with nasal tumors had been given treatment prior to diagnosis. Symptomatic therapy for nasal discharge may be justified on a cost-benefit ratio for up to 14 days, but incomplete response after that time is an indication for further diagnostic efforts. Differential diagnoses should include inflammatory diseases of the nasal passages associated with bacterial or fungal infections, foreign materials, or parasitic infestations.

Following physical examination, radiographs of the nasal passages and paranasal sinuses — especially open-mouth ventrodorsal and straight lateral projections — should be made with the patient under general anesthesia. Use of high detail, non-screen radiographic films as well as oblique lateral and skyline frontal projections may facilitate differentiation of neoplasia from inflammation. Early radiographic changes including loss of nasal turbinate pattern and deviation or lysis of the nasal septum are not specific and are strong indications for biopsy. Changes suggestive of neoplasia include filling density of frontal sinuses, lysis or deviation of overlying cortical bone or hard palate, and external soft tissue mass.

Rhinoscopy with a standard otoscope some-times permits direct visualization of neoplastic tissue or foreign materials such as plant awns, allowing direct biopsy or removal. More often, however, mucoid or mucopurulent exudates and friable nasal mucous membranes preclude good visualization. Cytologic evaluation of nasal flushes may be useful in such cases, whereas fine needle aspiration may be indicated when there is lysis of facial bones.

Often, a definitive diagnosis cannot be made by non-surgical means, and exploratory rhinotomy and curettage is required to establish a diagnosis. Most surgeons prefer an aggressive approach in such cases, removing all the turbinates and mucoid material from the nasal cavity and sinuses through a dorsal nasal osteotomy. Replacement of the nasal bone flap is not necessary for good cosmetic results. A fenestrated plastic drain tube should be left in place for one to two days after surgery to facilitate flushing of the nasal cavity.

The use of cryogens such as nitrous oxide and liquid nitrogen have been recommended for treatment of residual tumor cells following nasal curettage. Published results are encouraging, but extreme care must be taken to avoid destruction of the hard palate by pooling liquid cryogens. Other shortcomings of cryosurgery for nasal tumors include capillary hemorrhage and inability to monitor with tissue temperature indicators. Controlled clinical trials are needed before cryosurgery can be recommended for use in private practice.

Topical application of triethylene thiophosphoramide (Thio-TEPA) is presently under investigation. Systemic chemotherapy with alkylating agents or anticancer antibiotics has demonstrated efficacy in some head and neck cancers in man, but it has not been investigated satisfactorily in animals.

Radiotherapy has been more thoroughly investigated than other modalities in veterinary medicine. Radiation has been used both as primary therapy and as an adjunct to surgery. Several authors have reported improved length and quality of survival following irradiation, but small numbers of cases preclude firm conclusions. Carcinomas appear to have a better response rate than do sarcomas.

At this time, it is not possible to make firm recommendations regarding the best method of treatment. It is hoped that cooperative clinical trials at veterinary cancer treatment centers will provide the answer in the next few years. Results of treatment to date regardless of type(s) used are uniformly poor, with median survivals of five to seven months. Along with surgery, radiation, and cryotherapy, earlier diagnosis should provide better results.

NASOPHARYNGEAL, LARYNGEAL, AND TRACHEAL TUMORS

Neoplasms of the upper respiratory tract organs appear to be quite rare, with single cases being reported sporadically. Consequently, little is known about the behavior or treatment of these tumors.

Tumors of the nasopharynx are usually malignant and represent extensions of the three common oropharyngeal malignancies: malignant melanoma, squamous cell carcinoma, and fibrosarcoma. Clinical features, behavior, and treatment of these tumors have been discussed elsewhere. Polyps of the soft palate or internal nares are successfully treated by surgical excision.

Tumors of the larynx include lymphosarcoma, squamous cell carcinoma, fibroma, fibrosarcoma, and thyroid carcinoma. Dogs presented for hoarseness, respiratory stridor, or voice quality change should be examined thoroughly with the aid of a laryngoscope or other instrument that permits direct visualization of the pharynx, epiglottis, aryepiglottic folds, arytenoid cartilages, vocal cords, and laryngeal saccules. Abnormal structures should be biopsied carefully with a colonic or uterine biopsy instrument. Ulcerated lesions may be gently swabbed in order to obtain cytologic specimens. Lateral and ventrodorsal radiograms of the anterior cervical region may help in identifying masses dorsal or lateral to the larynx. Treatment is dependent on histologic identification and extent of the lesion. Lymphosarcoma of the larynx is almost always an extension of the generalized form of the disease and is therefore treated by single or combination drug therapy (see discussion elsewhere). Squamous cell carcinoma, fibrosarcoma, and thyroid carcinomas are frequently too large when diagnosed to allow complete excision. Complete laryngectomy is not used in animals. Radiation of the larynx may require tem-

Table 1. *Chemotherapeutic Agents Used in the Treatment of Primary and Metastatic Malignancies of Canine and Feline Respiratory Tract*

DRUG	DOSAGE	FREQUENCY	ROUTE OF ADMINISTRATION	INDICATIONS	SPECIAL CONSIDERATIONS
Cyclophosphamide Cytoxan® (Mead, Johnson)	50 mg/M²°	Daily on 4 consecutive days each week	Oral	Carcinomas, sarcomas	Myelosuppression; hemorrhagic cystitis
	100 mg/M²	Once or twice a week	IV		
5-fluorouracil Fluorouracil® (Roche)	200 mg/M²	q 7 d	IV	Carcinomas	Neurotoxicosis, if given on consecutive days. *Do not use in cats!*
Methotrexate (Lederle)	15 mg/M² 2.5 mg/M²	q 14 d Daily on 4 consecutive days each week	IV Oral	Carcinomas, sarcomas	Myelosuppression; alkalinize urine to avoid nephrotoxicity at high doses. Gastrointestinal toxicosis. Vincristine may potentiate uptake by tumor cells.
Doxorubicin HCl Adriamycin® (Adria)	30 mg/M² DO NOT EXCEED 240 mg/M² CUMULATIVE DOSE	q 21 d	IV slowly	Carcinomas, sarcomas	Severe vesicant—do not inject perivascular. Acute toxicity—urticaria, tachycardia, vascular collapse. Chronic toxicity—cardiac insufficiency, sudden death, myelosuppression.
Vincristine Oncovin® (Eli Lilly)	0.5 mg/M²	q 7–14 d	IV	Sarcomas	Severe vesicant. Use in combination with Methotrexate. Myelosuppression.
Bleomycin Blenoxane® (Bristol)	8–10 mg/M² DO NOT EXCEED 200 mg/M² CUMULATIVE DOSE	3 times weekly	IV or SC	Squamous cell carcinoma	Cumulative toxicity—pulmonary fibrosis. Little or no myelosuppression.
Triethylene thiophosphoramide Thio-TEPA® (Lederle)	15 mg 7.5–15 mg	q 7–14 d q 7 d	intranasal intrapleural	Nasal tumors, mesothelioma, malignant pleural effusions	Give as diluted solution (up to 50 ml) to cover affected cavity.

° M² = square meters of body surface. See Appendix.

porary placement of tracheotomy and/or pharyngostomy tubes due to excessive swelling that occurs in the glottis. The use of radioisotopes such as ^{131}I for treatment of thyroid cancer in dogs deserves further investigation but is presently available only at hospitals or institutions with adequate facilities for collection and disposal of radioactive wastes. Because of these considerations, systemic chemotherapy may be the modality of choice in unresectable laryngeal cancer. Bleomycin appears to be useful in squamous cell carcinoma, whereas a combination of 5-fluorouracil and cyclophosphamide has produced regression or control of large thyroid carcinomas on several occasions (see Table 1). Further justification for the use of chemotherapy is related to the early development of metastatic disease associated with posterior pharyngeal/laryngeal carcinomas. Nodular densities are usually noted in thoracic radiograms within four months of diagnosis. Consequently, a poor prognosis is justified. Occasionally, benign tumors of the larynx such as virus-induced papilloma or fibroma are diagnosed. Surgical excision is usually curative.

The only important tumor of the trachea is the osteochondroma. Signs include respiratory stridor and persistent cough. Radiography of the trachea is often diagnostic because this tumor is frequently calcified. Recent case reports have described successful resection of lesions using overlapping end-to-end anastomosis and simple continuous closure to obliterate the defects created.

LUNG TUMORS

In both dogs and cats, primary lung tumors are uncommon, whereas secondary (metastatic) lung tumors are quite common. Differentiation between these types of tumors is often apparent following clinical and radiographic examination of the patient. Occasionally, this task may be difficult when no primary extrapulmonary tumor is found.

Primary tumors of the lung are rare in dogs less than 7 years of age and occur with an average age of 10.5 years. Histologic classification of lung tumors is based on location and cell type: bronchogenic (columnar) and bronchiolar-alveolar (cuboidal) carcinomas. Bronchogenic tumors are further divided into adenocarcinoma, squamous cell carcinoma, and undifferentiated carcinoma. These neoplasms are of variable degrees of malignancy; adenocarcinomas and bronchiolar-alveolar carcinomas are less aggressive than others. Primary lung tumors can metastasize to other portions of the lung via

transmigration of cells in alveoli and bronchioles. In addition, carcinoma cells gain access to lymphatics and blood vessels, resulting in secondary nodules in other organs or lobes of lungs. A unifocal lesion may become disseminated throughout the lung, resulting in many tumor nodules of similar size. In the case of bronchiolar-alveolar carcinomas, which tend to arise at the periphery of the lung, multiple nodules may represent multicentric origin of these tumors.

Metastatic pulmonary neoplasms result from a wide variety of malignancies in both dogs and cats. Neoplasms with a high incidence of pulmonary metastases include primary bone tumors, thyroid and mammary adenocarcinomas, oral and digital melanomas, tonsillar and digital squamous cell carcinomas, and hemangiosarcomas. Radiographic appearance of the various types of lung tumors and differentiation from other causes of radiographic density in the pulmonary parenchyma have been discussed thoroughly elsewhere (Suter, 1975).

In addition, tumors of other thoracic organs and tissues may compromise pulmonary function and should be ruled out during the diagnostic work-up. Important thoracic tumors include mediastinal lymphosarcoma (especially in the cat), thymoma, heart base tumor, mesothelioma, and sarcomas of the ribs and esophagus.

Clinical signs associated with pulmonary neoplasms are quite variable in duration but consistent in nature. A harsh, non-productive cough of increasing severity is present for one week to several months. Dyspnea is observed in advanced stages of disease.

Useful diagnostic adjuncts to survey radiographs include transtracheal washings, bronchoscopy, and bronchial brushings for collection of cytologic specimens. Thoracentesis is indicated when pleural fluid is detected. Percutaneous lung biopsy can be a rewarding and relatively safe procedure when performed by a skilled surgeon.

If no evidence of metastatic disease exists, exploratory thoracotomy is indicated, with lobectomy or pneumonectomy performed for primary or solitary secondary tumors. Whereas radiation, chemotherapy, and immunotherapy are widely used in human lung cancer, there has been little or no use of these modalities in veterinary medicine. Occasional reports of partial regression of pulmonary nodules following courses of chemotherapy or immunotherapy suggest the need for further investigation. Chemotherapeutic agents with demonstrated, though limited, success in human lung cancer include cyclophosphamide, doxorubicin HCl, methotrexate, and nitrogen mustard. Chemotherapy has been successful in palliation of symptoms, but gains in survival time have been very small.

Recent reports of adjunctive immunotherapy — e.g., intrathoracic injection of tubercle bacilli (BCG) — have indicated prolonged survival following surgery. The use of supervoltage radiotherapy has been unrewarding in human lung cancer.

Prognosis for lung tumors depends on the time of diagnosis and the biologic behavior of the neoplasm. In general, metastatic tumors warrant a grave prognosis, regardless of histologic type. For primary neoplasms, early diagnosis and treatment are essential if successful results are to be obtained. Lobectomy (or pneumonectomy) may be curative for low-grade carcinomas or may result in remission of signs for several months for more anaplastic lesions.

REMOTE EFFECTS OF RESPIRATORY TRACT TUMORS

Paraneoplastic syndromes are observed frequently in cancers of the human respiratory tract. Systemic manifestations include hypertrophic osteopathy (HPO), Cushing's syndrome, Zollinger-Ellison syndrome, syndrome of inappropriate antidiuretic hormone, carcinoid syndrome, gynecomastia, thyrotoxicosis, pseudohyperparathyroidism, hypoglycemia, fibrinolysis, cryofibrinogenemia, polycythemia, and thrombophlebitis. While only HOP is

well documented in respiratory tract tumors of dogs and cats, most of these paraneoplastic syndromes will likely be identified in small animals with more extensive staging procedures and more long-term survival. The anorexia/cachexia syndrome occurs but is not well documented in animals due to the option of euthanasia in advanced or terminal cases. In addition to these systemic effects of cancer, the veterinarian should recognize that treatment of neoplasms with multiple modality therapy can be expected to alter the biologic behavior of cancer — i.e., change sites or frequency for metastases. Referral of cases to veterinary colleges and institutions will permit accumulation of valuable data on the incidence, natural history, and treatment of small animal respiratory tract cancers.

SUPPLEMENTAL READING

MacEwen, E. G., Withrow, S. J., and Patnaik, A. K.: Nasal tumors in the dog: retrospective evaluation of diagnosis, prognosis and treatment. JAVMA 170:45–48, 1977.

Madewell, B. R., et al.: Neoplasms of the nasal passages and paranasal sinuses in domesticated animals as reported by 13 veterinary colleges. AJVR 37:851–856, 1976.

O'Brien, J. A., and Harvey, C. E.: Diseases of the upper airway. In Ettinger, S. J. (ed.): *Textbook of Veterinary Internal Medicine.* Philadelphia, W. B. Saunders Co., 1975.

Suter, P. F.: Pulmonary neoplasia. In Ettinger, S. J. (ed.): *Textbook of Veterinary Internal Medicine.* Philadelphia, W. B. Saunders Co., 1975.

Theilen, G. H., and Madewell, B. R.: *Veterinary Cancer Medicine.* Philadelphia, Lea & Febiger, 1979.

PLEURAL EFFUSIONS

STANLEY R. CREIGHTON, D.V.M.,
W. Los Angeles, California

and ROBERT J. WILKINS, B.V.Sc.
New York, New York

INTRODUCTION

Many diseases affect the pleura and result in the accumulation of abnormal volumes of fluid within the pleural space. In healthy animals, the pleural space is a potential space containing only a few milliliters of lubricating serous fluid. A constant volume of fluid is

maintained because the rate of fluid formation is equal to the rate of fluid absorption. Abnormal pleural effusions occur when an underlying disease process upsets the normal homeostatic mechanisms of the pleura and allows increased volumes of fluid to collect in the pleural space. Pleural effusion is therefore a clinical sign and not a final diagnosis, and it is the clinician's duty to determine the exact underlying etiology of the effusion.

The pleura is a serous membrane composed of a single layer of flat mesothelial cells and a strong underlying fibroelastic layer containing the pleural lymphatics, arteries, veins, and capillaries. The visceral pleura completely covers the lungs and continues onto the mediastinum and diaphragm, forming the mediastinal pleura. The thoracic wall is covered by the parietal pleura. In the normal animal, the visceral, parietal and mediastinal pleurae are separated by a thin film of normal pleural fluid which facilitates movement of the thoracic viscera during the respiratory and cardiac cycles. The mediastinum incompletely divides the pleural cavity into two compartments that communicate with each other in most dogs and cats, and therefore most effusions are bilateral. Abundant lymphatics and microscopic pores in the diaphragm allow communication between the peritoneal and pleural spaces. This feature may result in both pleural and peritoneal effusion from a single isolated lesion.

Normal fluid formation occurs through a transudative process and follows Starling's law. The majority of fluid originates from the parietal pleura, and the water and electrolytes are absorbed by capillaries and lymphatics of the visceral pleura. Absorption of protein occurs only through the lymphatics of the parietal and mediastinal pleura. Pleural lymphatics can also absorb water and electrolytes, and when abnormal quantities of fluid are present, this lymphatic reserve is mobilized to help remove fluid from the pleural cavities.

Abnormal fluids accumulate in the pleural space as a result of transudative and exudative processes. Most fluids accumulate as a result of increased fluid production rather than decreased absorption by the pleura. The increased production of fluid is usually caused by increased vascular hydrostatic pressure, decreased plasma osmotic pressure, or inflammation of the pleura. The effusion undergoes a dynamic process of continuous formation and resorption. Because the fluid is not static, the physical, biochemical, and cytologic features of the effusion change as the fluid remains in the pleural space. Results of fluid analysis will therefore vary, depending on the rate of fluid formation, the duration of the illness, and the response to treatment.

Cellular components that gain access to the pleural space through transudative processes such as increased hydrostatic pressure due to venous or lymphatic obstruction will eventually die and degenerate. This process releases cellular components that are chemotactic for neutrophils, macrophages, and other inflammatory cells. The secondary inflammatory response that occurs in fluids that entered the pleural cavities through transudative processes is very common. These effusions are called modified transudates, because an inflammatory component (exudate) has been added to the original transudate. Modified transudates have many of the traditional characteristics of exudates, and cytologic evaluation is required if the nature of the effusion is to be determined.

CLINICAL SIGNS

The history and clinical signs are variable and depend upon the etiology of the effusion, the rate of fluid formation, the quantity of fluid, and the type of fluid present. Small quantities of fluid usually do not produce signs and are difficult or impossible to detect radiographically. As the volume of fluid increases, the ability of the lungs to expand is compromised. This results in a decreased total lung capacity and tidal volume. In severe effusions, the lungs may be partially or completely collapsed. These local areas of compression atelectasis result in a mismatching of ventilation and perfusion. Clinical signs due to pleural effusion are usually a result of gas exchange abnormalities.

The most consistent sign is labored breathing. The animal's thorax may undergo a greater than normal excursion during the respiratory cycle. Abdominal breathing occurs with severe effusions, and the whole animal may move during efforts to breathe. Occasionally there is mouth-breathing, and the neck and head may be kept in an extended and elevated position. Some animals are reluctant to lie down and will stand with the elbows abducted. Others will rest only on their sternum with the head elevated. In general, animals with moderate to severe degrees of dyspnea and respiratory distress have very little remaining respiratory reserve, and even the slightest stress may result in respiratory arrest. The temperament of the animal should be considered, and minimal restraint should be used during physical examination or diagnostic procedures.

Coughing is sometimes seen and is usually non-productive. It usually occurs with inflammatory diseases of the pleura but may result from lung involvement in the underlying disease process.

Auscultation of the lungs and heart often reveals muffled heart and lung sounds. In severe effusions, the only functional lung tissue ausculted may be in the dorsal-posterior portion of the thorax. Trapped pleural fluid may result in a local area of decreased or absent lung sounds.

Non-specific extrathoracic signs are sometimes present and may be very helpful, since they usually reflect the underlying etiology of the effusion. For example, a cardiac arrhythmia may indicate that the effusion is due to cardiac failure, or subcutaneous edema may indicate that hypoalbuminemia is the etiology of the effusion. Anorexia, weight loss, depression, and dehydration may be complicating factors of a wide variety of illnesses.

RADIOGRAPHIC EVALUATION

Radiographic examination is an essential part of the medical work-up when pleural effusion is suspected. Radiographs will answer three important questions:
1. Is an effusion present?
2. Where is the most suitable site for thoracocentesis?
3. Is there any additional pathologic condition present that may indicate the source of the effusion?

Small quantities of fluid are usually not visible radiographically. When greater quantities of fluid are present, the most commonly observed changes are a loss of detail and increased density within the thorax. The cardiac silhouette may be obscured and the mediastinum may be widened. There is rounding of the lung borders at the costophrenic angles, and fluid-filled fissures may be present between lung lobes. The ventral lung lobe borders may appear scalloped. The visceral pleura may retract from the parietal pleura, making the pleural space visible.

Pleural thickening without effusion may be the result of active pleuritis or may be the sequela to prior episodes of effusion with scarring and fibrosis. Pleural thickening is sometimes an incidental finding in older animals.

Routine radiographic examination of the thorax should include both dorsoventral and lateral projections. Special techniques such as the standing lateral or lateral decubitus projections will demonstrate if the fluid is freely movable, trapped, or encapsulated within fibrin adhesions. In dyspneic animals, careful restraint should be utilized to avoid any undue stress. It is better to postpone or cancel a procedure rather than risk the life of the animal by performing diagnostic tests.

In severe pleural effusions, there is usually little doubt radiographically that an effusion is present, but much of the detail within the thorax is obscured by the fluid. In these cases, as much fluid should be removed from the thorax as possible and the radiographs should be repeated. This will allow better visualization of the thoracic viscera and may indicate the underlying etiology of the effusion.

LABORATORY EVALUATION

A routine hemogram, urinalysis, and biochemical screen is indicated for every animal with pleural effusion because of the many diseases that can cause the condition. Biochemical tests should include BUN and total protein and albumin as well as liver function tests.

THORACOCENTESIS AND CHEST DRAINAGE

In most cases of pleural effusion, complete laboratory evaluation of a fluid sample is necessary for a definitive diagnosis. Fluid can be obtained by means of thoracocentesis or closed chest tube drainage.

Thoracocentesis is a simple procedure that can also be used to drain the pleural cavity. Closed chest tube drainage is indicated (1) in severe or recurrent pleural effusions, (2) when the fluid is viscous, trapped or encapsulated, (3) following most thoracic surgery, and (4) as a route of therapy when lavage is used in the treatment of pyothorax.

The site of thoracocentesis is best determined after a careful review of the thoracic radiographs. If the fluid is diffuse, the seventh or eighth intercostal space is used. The size of the needle used will depend upon the size of the animal. An 18- to 20-gauge, 1 inch sterile needle is satisfactory for average dogs. Suitable small flexible catheters that pass over or through a needle are sometimes used, especially if very small amounts of fluid are present.* A short, flexible tube placed between the needle and syringe makes thoracocentesis safer and easier, because the needle can be controlled and the syringe can be moved without fear of lacerating the thoracic viscera. A three-way valve attached to the syringe allows drainage without repeated chest aspirations.

The area to be aspirated should be clipped and scrubbed. Infiltration with a local anesthetic occasionally makes the procedure more acceptable to the animal. The needle should be placed below the level of the effusion and midway between the ribs to prevent damage

---

*Bardic Inside Needle Catheter, C. R. Bard Inc., Murray Hill, New Jersey 07974.

to the intercostal vessels or nerves located posterior to each rib. Once the needle is under the skin, a small amount of negative pressure is placed on the syringe to prevent unnecessarily deep penetration by the needle and to allow fluid to flow into the syringe as soon as the pleural space is entered. Excessive movement of the needle or the animal should be avoided to prevent damage to the heart and lungs. Aspiration should be continued until 3 to 6 ml of fluid are collected for laboratory evaluation or until the chest is completely drained. In order to drain both pleural cavities completely, it is usually necessary to aspirate both sides of the chest. Free fluid moves under the influence of gravity, and gentle movement and lateral positioning before or during thoracocentesis sometimes increases the total fluid volume removed from each pleural cavity.

Various techniques for closed chest tube drainage have been described. In each case, a large-bore, flexible catheter is placed within the pleural cavity and attached to a gravity flow or suction device for intermittent or continuous drainage of the chest.* These tubes can be left in place for days until the effusion has stopped. Closed chest tube drainage is well tolerated by both dogs and cats. The advantages of this technique over thoracocentesis are (1) repeated needle punctures can be avoided if large volumes of fluid are continuously being formed, (2) the volume and character of the fluid can be monitored each day, and (3) it provides a route for the administration of various medications. In addition, fluid too viscous to be aspirated through a needle can sometimes be adequately removed through a large-bore chest drain.

Iatrogenic pneumothorax is a potential complication of both needle thoracocentesis and closed chest tube drainage. A small amount of air in the thorax of a normal animal is usually well tolerated. In an animal with pleural effusion, the effects of even small degrees of pneumothorax are more severe because cardiopulmonary function is already severely compromised. Needles, syringes, connectors, and tubing should be carefully examined before the pleural space is entered to avoid this unnecessary complication.

FLUID EVALUATION

Three to 6 ml of fluid should be aseptically collected by thoracocentesis or closed chest tube drainage for laboratory evaluation. About 0.5 ml of the aspirated effusion is immediately placed in a sterile container for subsequent bacteriologic evaluation. The remaining fluid is placed in an anticoagulant tube containing a small amount of EDTA. The physical appearance of the fluid is noted.

Laboratory testing should be performed as soon as possible. The total white blood cell and red blood cell counts are determined, and the myeloid:erythroid ratio is calculated. The fluid is centrifuged at 3000 RPM for five minutes to concentrate the cellular material. The supernatant is poured into a clean container, and the specific gravity and total protein are determined using a Refractometer[R].† A fluid volume equal to the approximate volume of the concentrated cellular material is left in the centrifuge tube so that the cells can be adequately resuspended. A small drop of the cell-rich fluid is placed on a glass slide and a thin smear is made. The smear is rapidly air dried and stained with a suitable stain, such as Wright's stain.

If the effusion is hemorrhagic, centrifugation will separate the red blood cells from the diagnostic inflammatory, mesothelial, or neoplastic cells that form an upper white layer (buffy coat). In these cases, a sample of the buffy coat is aspirated with a capillary pipette before the supernatant is poured off. A drop of the buffy coat is placed on a glass slide and a smear is made as before.

When milky white effusions are aspirated, the presence of chylomicrons is detected by determining the degree of clearing of the lipid fraction of the fluid in a fat solvent such as ether. The supernatant fluid is divided into two equal aliquots. One to two drops of 1N sodium hydroxide is added to each tube to make the pH greater than 8.0. To one tube, an equal volume of ether is added, and to the other, an equal volume of water is added. The tubes are then mixed. The white color of the sample containing ether will clear completely when compared with the sample containing water if the effusion contains chylomicrons. A partial or lack of clearing of the white color indicates that the effusion does not contain chylomicrons, and this is called a pseudochylous effusion. Milky white pleural effusions are not always pathognomonic of rupture of the thoracic duct, and further evaluation of these fluids is necessary if their source is to be determined.

°Brunswick Feeding Tube®, Brunswick Labs, 5836 W. 117th Place, Worth, Illinois 60482.

†American Optical Refractometer®, American Optical Co., Buffalo, New York.

PATTERNS OF PLEURAL EFFUSION

Determination of the specific gravity and total protein of the effusion is an important part in the complete analysis of the fluid, but this information alone can be misleading and many times does not determine the etiology of the effusion. Traditionally, fluids are classified as transudates or exudates, based on the specific gravity and total protein content of the fluid, but this approach does not consider the important concept of dynamic fluid modification and the formation of modified transudates. Terms such as hydrothorax, hemothorax, and pleuritis do not help in understanding the pathophysiology of the many different types of fluid formation. Cytologic evaluation of the fluid is the single most important step in fluid analysis. It is now apparent that diseases of specific organ systems produce characteristic patterns of effusion. By using the physical, biochemical, and cytologic findings to classify the pattern of effusion, it is possible to predict which organ system and, in some cases, which disease is responsible for the effusion (Table 1).

The general cytologic features of pleural fluid should be evaluated before determining the pattern of effusion. This is done by determining the following:

1. Is the fluid inflammatory or non-inflammatory? Inflammatory pleural effusions contain many neutrophils, macrophages, lymphocytes, plasma cells, mesothelial cells, and, less commonly, eosinophils and mast cells. Acute inflammation is characterized by a predominance of granulocytes, whereas chronic inflammation features a dominance of mononuclear cells. Non-inflammatory effusions have a very low cell content, specific gravity, and total protein.

2. Is the fluid septic or sterile? Septic effusions contain microorganisms and evidence of active inflammation and phagocytosis. In non-septic effusions, there is an absence of microorganisms but the fluid may be inflammatory or non-inflammatory.

3. Does the fluid contain neoplastic cells? If a tumor is responsible for the pleural effusion, the presence of neoplastic cells in the effusion will depend on the type of tumor and its location, the tendency for the tumor to exfoliate cells, and the risk of a sampling error. Normal lining mesothelial cells are very sensitive and become reactive when any type of pleural effusion is present. Reactive mesothelial cells are large and have a basophilic cytoplasm. They may appear alone or in clusters and may be incorrectly called neoplastic cells. They must be differentiated from true neoplastic conditions.

Once the general cytologic features are determined the pleural effusion should be classified into one of seven different patterns of effusion. These are pure transudative, hemorrhagic, inflammatory, obstructive, chylous, neoplastic, and pyogranulomatous.

Pure Transudates. These fluids are usually water clear and have a specific gravity of less than 1.013 and a very low total protein. The fluid usually contains very few cells. Long-standing pure transudative effusions may become modified transudates and contain more cells and protein than would be expected. A complete medical evaluation is necessary in these cases to document hypoalbuminemia. Severe hypoalbuminemia (serum albumin less than 1.0 gm per 100 ml) owing to glomerulonephritis, renal amyloidosis, protein-losing enteropathy, or hepatic failure, or following major surgery, is the most common etiology of pure transudative effusions.

Other physical findings that are sometimes seen with this type of pleural effusion include abdominal effusion and pitting edema of the limbs, face, and scrotum. Laboratory evaluation will reveal hypoalbuminemia and possible alterations in liver or renal function. A urinalysis may reveal proteinuria.

Hemorrhagic Effusions. These effusions result from free hemorrhage into the pleural cavity. The cell counts, specific gravity, total protein, myeloid:erythroid ratio, and cytologic evaluation are compatible with those in the peripheral blood. Long-standing hemorrhagic effusions may contain reactive mesothelial cells and a mild inflammatory component due to modification of the fluid. Blood-tinged fluids should not be classified as hemorrhagic effusions unless the packed cell volume approximates that of blood.

Blood within the pleural cavity undergoes rapid defibrination and does not remain clotted. It can be easily aspirated and has the same radiographic appearance as any pleural effusion. If an intercostal vessel or pulmonary vessel is accidentally tapped during thoracocentesis, the aspirated blood in this sample will clot, indicating that the blood is not from the pleural cavity. Platelets will be obvious in the latter case, a feature not seen in defibrinated effusions.

Hemorrhagic effusions occur most commonly following thoracic trauma and occasionally following thoracic surgery. Trauma can rupture

Table 1. *Classification and Etiologies of Pleural Effusions**

DETERMINANTS OF CLASSIFICATION	PURE TRANSUDATE	OBSTRUCTIVE EFFUSION	INFLAMMATORY EFFUSION	
			Septic	*Sterile*
Physical Appearance	Clear	Serous to serosanguineous	Serous, serosanguineous or purulent	
Specific Gravity	< 1.013	1.013–1.040	1.021–1.033	
Total Protein (gm./100 ml.)*	< 1.0	1.0–7.2	2.8–5.1	
Coagulation	None	May clot	None	Usually none
Common Causes	Severe hypo-albuminemia.	Heart failure; cardiomyopathy; cardiac anomalies; pulmonary atelectasis; lung torsion; dia-phragmatic hernia; thromboemboli; mediastinal tumors; other tumors.	Pyothorax; extension of infection from lungs, trachea, esophagus, mediastinum; hematogenous; foreign bodies; idiopathic.	Pleuritis; diaphragmatic hernia; thoracic surgery, chest drains; steatitis; infection; idiopathic.

*Modified from Creighton, S. R., and Wilkins, R. J.: Thoracic effusions in the cat. J. Am. Animal Hosp. Assn., *11*:66–76, 1975.

any of the systemic and pulmonary vessels near the pleural surface and allow blood to enter the pleural cavity. Rupture of a major vessel leads to significant hemothorax and systemic signs of blood loss such as tachycardia, pale mucous membranes, hypothermia, and shock. Bleeding from rupture of pulmonary vessels tends to be self-limiting as the degree of hemothorax increases, owing to reduced blood pressure and increased hydrostatic pressure. The blood pressure in these vessels is lower than the systemic pressure, and as the lungs collapse owing to the hemorrhagic effusion, the active bleeding stops.

Animals with hemorrhagic effusions must be monitored closely to determine whether the condition is remaining stable or worsening. Systemic signs of blood loss should be monitored. Progressive respiratory distress and increasing amounts of pleural effusion will require thoracocentesis or closed chest tube drainage. Blood within the pleural cavity is rapidly reabsorbed, so that complete chest drainage may not be necessary in these cases. The advantages of autotransfusion and the possibility of a moderate degree of hemorrhagic effusion causing spontaneous hemostasis due to compression must be measured against the degree of dyspnea and respiratory distress when deciding how much of the fluid to remove from the pleural cavity. Severe or progressive blood loss will require blood transfusions and possibly an emergency exploratory thoracotomy.

Clotting defects such as occur in thrombocytopenia or warfarin poisoning can cause hemorrhagic effusions. Other causes include clotting defects; parasites, such as *Dirofilaria*;

bleeding hemangiosarcomas of the heart, lungs, or pleura; other tumors that may erode blood vessels; and lung lobe torsions. Treatment in these cases is directed toward the primary lesion as well as toward control and monitoring of the hemorrhagic effusion. (See article "Thoracic Trauma.")

Inflammatory Effusions. Acute inflammatory effusions contain large numbers of neutrophils and moderate numbers of lymphocytes and macrophages. As the inflammatory component of the effusions becomes more chronic, the proportion of mononuclear inflammatory cells and reactive mesothelial cells increases. Septic inflammatory effusions contain visible microorganisms.

The severity of the inflammatory process can be estimated from the morphology of the cells present. In severe, overwhelming, suppurative pyothorax, there are large numbers of free and phagocytized bacteria, toxic necrosis, and degeneration of the neutrophils. The nuclei undergo karyolysis and karyorrhexis, which indicates rapid cell death, as opposed to nuclear pyknosis, which indicates a slower rate of death. The identity of many cells may be difficult to determine. In less severe cases, microorganisms may be absent or only within neutrophils, indicating that the infection is contained by the inflammatory response. In mild, non-septic inflammatory effusions, toxic neutrophils are absent, nuclear morphology is intact, and each cell is readily identifiable. Serial evaluation of inflammatory effusions is very helpful when assessing the animal's response to treatment. A favorable prognosis is indicated if an effusion originally containing large numbers of toxic neutrophils and many

Table 1. *Classification and Etiologies of Pleural Effusions (Continued)*

PYOGRANULOMATOUS EFFUSION	CHYLOUS EFFUSION	NEOPLASTIC EFFUSION	HEMORRHAGIC EFFUSION
Straw-colored	Milky white	Usually blood-tinged	Blood red
1.027–1.045	——	1.015–1.045	1.030–1.045
4.1–8.5	——	1.5–7.5	4.5–7.5
May clot	Usually none	May clot	None
Feline infectious peritonitis; other granulomatous diseases of the pleura.	Ruptured thoracic duct or other lymphatic abnormality; trauma; neoplasm; cardiomyopathy; chronic pleuritis.	Lymphosarcoma; metastatic carcinoma or adenocarcinoma; mesothelioma; other tumors.	Trauma; lung torsion; postoperative; thrombosis; tumors; coagulopathies.

microorganisms has changed to one containing normal intact neutrophils without microorganisms after appropriate therapy for pyothorax.

Infectious agents are the most common cause of inflammatory effusions, and the etiologic agent may be readily visible in smears of pleural fluid. Microorganisms isolated include *Pasteurella multocida, Streptococcus* spp., *E. coli, Pseudomonas* spp., *Staphylococcus* spp., *Actinomyces* spp., *Nocardia* spp., *Klebsiella* spp., *Proteus* spp., *Enterobacter* spp., *Corynebacterium* spp., *Bacterioides* spp., *Cryptococcus* spp., *Toxoplasma* spp., and *Aspergillus* spp. Many viral diseases affecting the respiratory tract of dogs and cats can, through extension of inflammation to the pleura, initiate an inflammatory effusion into the thoracic cavity.

The route of entry of the infecting agent is variable. Pleural involvement may be a result of (1) extension of infections from the lungs, mediastinum, or diaphragm, (2) penetrating wounds of the thorax, esophagus, or neck, (3) hematogenous spread of the infectious agent to the pleura (e.g., feline infectious peritonitis), (4) contaminated foreign bodies such as grass awns or sticks, and (5) secondary infection of an already established pleural effusion. Finally, pyothorax can occur with no previous history of respiratory illness or thoracic trauma.

The clinical and radiographic findings are similar to those seen with any pleural effusion. Elevation of the body temperature is not a consistent finding, and in chronically ill or debilitated animals, the temperature may be subnormal.

Needle thoracocentesis will relieve respiratory distress and obtain a sample of fluid for laboratory evaluation. Treatment programs have included the use of broad spectrum systemic and intrapleural antibiotics, intrapleural infusion of enzyme solutions containing chymotrypsin,* repeated thoracocentesis, and thoracotomy. With the use of closed chest tube drainage, the pleural cavities can be repeatedly lavaged with solutions containing saline, antibiotics, and proteolytic enzymes. This aids in sterilization of the pleural cavities by dilution and removal of infected and necrotic material and breaks down fibrinous adhesions. The volume of lavage solution administered depends on the size of the animal. A volume of 100 ml is administered twice daily in cats and small dogs. One-half the usual systemic dose of a broad spectrum antibiotic such as chloromycetin or gentamicin and 5000 NF units of chymotrypsin per 100 ml are added to the lavage solution. The same antibiotic used in the lavage solution should be used systemically at the recommended dose. Bacterial culture and sensitivity testing is essential for successful long-term management of pyothorax. For example, nocardial pyothorax is best treated with penicillin and sulfadiazine. With lavage, pyothorax carries a reasonably fair prognosis. As with other forms of serosal lavage, careful monitoring of total serum protein, electrolytes, body temperature, and cytology of the effusion is essential.

Therapy can be evaluated by progressive changes in the cytologic findings, which include a decrease in the number of white blood cells, a change in cell type from predominately neutrophils to mononuclear cells, normal morphology of the inflammatory cells, and a significant decrease in the number of bacteria. The duration of therapy is deter-

---

*Kymar Aqueous®, Armour and Co., Omaha, Nebraska 68103.

mined by the clinical response, radiographic and visual evidence of a decreasing rate of fluid formation, and progressive improvement in the cytologic picture.

Complications of pyothorax include atelectasis, constrictive pleuritis, fibrous adhesions, and sepsis.

Idiopathic inflammatory effusions are uncommon. There is no history of prior illness or trauma, and no obvious etiologic agents are seen microscopically. Treatment is symptomatic with routine broad spectrum antibiotics and good supportive care. The prognosis is fair but the pleural inflammation tends to recur.

Closed chest tube drains and other such foreign objects in the pleural cavity will, by themselves, incite a mild sterile inflammatory effusion. The volume of fluid formed each day is usually less than 50 ml in an average dog. This is a normal response of the pleura, and the fluid production will cease when the inciting agent is removed.

Obstructive Effusions. These effusions occur as a result of increased venous or lymphatic hydrostatic pressure due to obstruction, constriction, or congestion of lymph or blood vessels. Initially, these effusions contain a mixture of erythrocytes and lymphocytes with small numbers of neutrophils, eosinophils, macrophages, and mesothelial cells. As the effusion becomes modified by the secondary inflammatory response of the pleura, the proportion of neutrophils and other inflammatory cells increases. Mesothelial cells may become very reactive and must be distinguished from neoplastic cells. These effusions are distinguished from pure non-septic inflammatory effusions by the large number of erythrocytes and lymphocytes present.

The most common cause of obstructive effusions is heart failure. In the dog, this occurs when congenital anomalies or acquired heart disease results in right-sided heart failure or a combination of left- and right-sided congestive heart failure. In cats, cardiomyopathy accounts for almost 80 percent of obstructive effusions and congenital cardiac anomalies account for the remainder. Other causes include atelectasis of the lung with obstruction of blood and lymph vessels; diaphragmatic hernias, especially if the liver is herniated; constrictive pericarditis or pericardial effusion, which may occlude vessels near the heart and cause an increased hydrostatic pressure; and tumors that grow and compress vessels and lymphatics. Diagnosis depends on ruling out the various causes of obstructive effusions, and specific therapy depends upon the etiology.

Chylous Effusions. A complex network of lymphatic vessels and the thoracic duct transport intestinal lymph from the abdominal cavity to the systemic venous circulation near the heart. Any alteration in this lymphatic system that allows lymph to enter the pleural cavity results in a true chylous effusion. These effusions contain chylomicrons derived from intestinal lymph and have an opaque or translucent white, milky appearance after centrifugation. When these effusions are alkalinized and mixed with an equal volume of ether, the chylomicrons dissolve and the white color clears completely, leaving a serous, straw-colored, clear fluid.

True chylous effusions contain large numbers of normal small and large lymphocytes mixed with small numbers of erythrocytes. Smudge cells, irregularly shaped free nucleoprotein from lysed lymphocytes, are consistently found in fluids containing large amounts of lymph. Neutrophils, eosinophils, macrophages, and mesothelial cells are relatively few in number. When stained supravitally with Sudan III, the chylomicrons are easily recognized as small orange droplets.

When true chylous effusions remain in the pleural cavity for long periods, the fluid becomes modified. The relative number of neutrophils, plasma cells, macrophages, and mesothelial cells increases. Secondary bacterial infection is rare because of the bacteriostatic properties of chyle.

True chylous effusions occur most commonly following thoracic trauma. Other important etiologies include tumors that invade or obstruct the thoracic lymphatic system, thrombosis of the anterior vena cava near the termination of the thoracic duct owing to thrombophlebitis, complications of intrathoracic surgery, or congenital malformations of the thoracic duct.

The diagnosis of true chylothorax is based on the history, physical examination, radiology, and results of fluid anaylsis. Contrast lymphangiography is sometimes helpful in demonstrating the presence and location of defects in the lymphatic vessels.

A wide variety of metabolic abnormalities may occur in animals with chylous effusions. Chyle contains large amounts of lipid, lipoproteins, fat-soluble vitamins, electrolytes and lymphocytes. The thoracic duct system is the main pathway by which ingested fats and extravascular protein are transported to the general circulation. Deficiences of these important nutrients and cells may occur quickly in animals with large volumes of pleural effusion or in those in which repeated thoracocentesis is necessary to relieve respiratory distress.

Treatment of true chylothorax is initially aimed at relieving respiratory distress by closed chest tube drainage and reducing the volume of lymph formed. This allows an opportunity for spontaneous healing to occur. In normal dogs, the rate of flow in the thoracic duct is estimated to be 2 ml/kg/hr. Ninety-five percent of this volume is from the liver and intestine. The rate of formation of intestinal lymph can be reduced by restricting oral intake of food and water. Complete fasting with intravenous maintenance of fluid and electrolyte balance for four to seven days is indicated at the onset of therapy. After this period, small quantities of a diet low in fat and high in carbohydrate and protein are offered. These diets alter the fat content of chyle and reduce the rate of its formation, but they do not completely stop lymph production. Medium-chain triglyceride diets contain synthetic triglycerides that are absorbed directly into the portal circulation and bypass the lymphatic system.* Supplementation with these compounds may allow adequate ingestion of fat and energy without increasing the fat content of the chyle that is formed. In animals that become debilitated owing to removal of large volumes of chyle, parenteral hyperalimentation may offer a means of replacing essential nutrients over a long period.

If medical management fails to control the formation of true chylous effusions after 14 to 28 days, thoracotomy is indicated. The surgeon should attempt to remove any inciting agent and double-ligate the thoracic duct near the diaphragm. The procedure is at best difficult because of problems encountered in identifying the duct and successfully ligating it. A large number of animals continue to have chylous effusions after surgery, and the prognosis in these cases is poor.

Milky white effusions without chylomicrons and the typical cytologic features of true chylous effusions are called pseudochylous effusions. The white color is due to cholesterol crystals, lecithin-globulin complexes, or calcium phosphate crystals in the fluids. Cytologic examination of these fluids reveals chronic sterile inflammation, macrophages containing many fat droplets, and degenerating fragmented cells. Lymphocytes and plasma cells may be seen. This fluid will not clear completely when ether is added, and chylomicrons are not seen when Sudan III is used to stain the sample.

In cats, acquired cardiomyopathy and lymphosarcoma are the most common underlying diseases resulting in pseudochylous effusions. In dogs, most cases are idiopathic. Occasionally, tumors or infection may also be present. In idiopathic pseudochylous effusions, corticosteriods administered systemically and/or intrapleurally following chest drainage may halt the formation of fluid.

Neoplastic Effusions. These effusions may have an obstructive or inflammatory pattern but contain neoplastic cells. A diagnosis of tumor should not be made based on the cytologic evaluation alone unless confirmed by an experienced veterinary cytologist. Mesothelial cells and a wide variety of exfoliated normal cells may become reactive and undergo morphologic changes that are sometimes suggestive of neoplasia. Cytologic examination is used in conjunction with the history, physical exam, radiographic findings, and other laboratory findings only to suggest a tumor in the pleural cavity. Any primary or metastatic tumor in the thoracic cavity is potentially capable of producing a neoplastic effusion. Common examples include lymphosarcoma, metastatic carcinomas, and adenocarcinomas and hemangiosarcomas.

Pyogranulomatous Effusions. These effusions are inflammatory in nature but occur specifically in feline infectious peritonitis. A vasculitis affects all serous membranes accompained by a secondary pyogranulomatous serositis. Pyogranulomatous effusions are usually thick, viscous, and straw colored. The cytologic examination of these fluids reveals moderate numbers of neutrophils, plasma cells, lymphocytes, macrophages, and erythrocytes. A coarse, granular background material, thought to be precipitated protein, stains pink with Wright's stain. These effusions are occasionally secondarily infected with bacteria that may be visible in the fluid, resulting in an active septic pleuritis.

Other additional information helpful in confirming the diagnosis of feline infectious peritonitis includes serosal inflammation and effusion in other body parts, elevation of the total serum protein, and altered albumin:globulin ratios or ocular lesions. The same cytologic pattern also occurs in the abdominal effusion. Treatment of feline infectious peritonitis is discussed elsewhere. To date, the disease usually carries a poor prognosis.

SUPPLEMENTAL READING

Creighton, S. R., and Wilkins, R. J.: Thoracic effusions in the cat: etiology and diagnostic features. J. Am. Anim. Hosp. Assoc. *11*:66–76, 1975.

Perman, V.: Transudates and exudates. In Kaneko, J. J., and Cornelius, C. E.(eds.): *Clinical Biochemistry of Domestic Animals*, Vol. 2, 2nd ed. New York, Academic Press, 1971.

Perman, V., and Osborne, C.: Laboratory evaluation of abnormal body fluids. Vet. Clin. North Am., *4*:225–268, 1974.

Withrow, S., and Fenner, W.: Closed chest drainage and lavage in the treatment of pyothorax in the cat. J. Am. Anim. Hosp. Assoc. *11*:90–94. 1975.

---

*M.C.T. Oil, Mead Johnson Laboratories, Evansville, Indiana 47721.

PARASITIC DISEASES OF THE RESPIRATORY TRACT

J.F. WILLIAMS, M.R.C.V.S.

East Lansing, Michigan

A wide variety of clinical signs and pathologic lesions in dogs and cats results from invasion of the respiratory system by parasites. While the severity of the clinical manifestations depends largely on the number of organisms that arrive in the lungs, it is also determined by factors such as the site of predilection within the system and the nature of the host response. Further complicating the picture is the fact that not all the parasites that cause respiratory disease live as adults in the lungs or associated structures; some (e.g., *Ancylostoma caninum*) merely pass through the lungs in the normal course of their migrations, whereas others intrude on the respiratory system only as a result of aberrant migration (e.g., *Spirocerca lupi*). Finally, parasites residing primarily in other systems may cause syndromes in which respiratory difficulty is one of the foremost presenting signs (e.g., *Dirofilaria immitis*). All these considerations have an important bearing on the diagnostic and therapeutic approaches to parasitic respiratory disease.

Individual clinical entities are best discussed in terms of the causative organisms involved. These can be grouped under some general headings, but an understanding of the biology of each parasite is necessary if rational bases are to be developed for the management of clinical cases and the prevention of further infections.

PARASITES THAT RESIDE IN THE RESPIRATORY SYSTEM

Most of the nematode helminths that reside as adults in the lungs of dogs and cats are metastrongyles. Their life cycles characteristically involve invertebrates, particularly slugs and snails, which act as obligatory intermediate hosts. Rodents and birds may prey on infected invertebrates and then act as transport hosts, conveying the parasite to domestic or wild carnivores. Clinical cases in domestic animals occur infrequently, but many authors suspect that undetected infections are widespread. However, lesions caused by these organisms are generally not common incidental findings at autopsy and it seems more likely that canine or feline lungworm infections are indeed rare and result from a casual spillover from sylvatic animal cycles.

FILAROIDES OSLERI

This slender worm (up to 1 cm long) lives in granulomatous nodules extending from the bifurcation of the trachea posteriorly into the bronchi.

Clinical Signs. Clinical cases occur in dogs in the first one to two years of life; the animal is presented with a history of a chronic deep cough which is sometimes productive of a foamy mucus. As the disease progresses and the granulomatous lesions protrude further into the bronchi, severe wheezing and dyspnea develop. During the early phases, there is no effect on appetite and the dog eats well and maintains bodily condition. Later, as respiratory embarassment becomes progressively worse, the animal may become emaciated. There is usually exacerbation of the respiratory difficulty after excitement or mild exercise. There is often a history of unresponsiveness to treatment with antibiotics, although there may be temporary remission after administration of steroids or antihistamines.

Physical examination of advanced cases usually reveals dyspnea with inflammation of the pharynx and larynx associated with abnormal lung sounds, particularly prominent rales, and increased thoracic resonance. Heart sounds may be difficult to detect above the noisy respiration.

Diagnosis. There are no characteristic blood changes. Although eosinophilia may be present, this is not sufficiently characteristic to distinguish the condition from chronic allergic states that must be considered in differential diagnosis.

Radiographic examination, particularly by bronchogram, is very helpful in detecting the obstructive granulomatous lesions in the trachea and bronchi. It also serves to rule out tracheal collapse or systemic mycotic infections as potential causes of this type of clinical condition. Bronchoscopy will reveal the raised nodules at the tracheal bifurcation. However, application of these types of diagnostic tools may be limited by the fact that anesthesia may be hazardous if severe respiratory distress is present, and laryngeal edema following bronchoscopy could exacerbate the problem. Bronchial washings, if not obtainable by bronchoscopy, may be collected by puncture of the ventral trachea and aspiration through a cannula.

Washings or biopsies of bronchial nodules should be examined for the presence of embryonated eggs (80 μ long) or larvae (230 μ long). These larvae have a characteristically kinked tail. They are normally coughed up and swallowed but are hard to detect in fecal samples because they are few in number and easily distorted by flotation solutions. Microscopic examination of the sediment from fresh fecal samples diluted with a little saline is helpful. The larvae are slow in their movements. The only other larvae likely to be in fresh samples are those of *Strongyloides stercoralis*, but they are stouter and have a sharply pointed tail. Samples that are not fresh will often contain active hookworm larvae in a matter of hours.

Treatment. Temporary relief from respiratory distress can often be achieved with bronchodilators. Antihistamines are particularly appropriate, since the additional benefit of sedation may occur. Resolution of the lesions can be achieved with anthelmintic medication, but since cases are treated infrequently, it is difficult to assess the relative efficacy of drugs in clinical trials. An additional complication is that spontaneous remission may occur without anthelmintic treatment, and this also influences assessment of the value of chemotherapy.

Thioacetarsamide (Caparsolate®, Abbott Laboratories, Chicago, Ill.) at the rate of 0.22 ml of a 1 percent solution/kg body weight intravenously each day for 21 days appears to cause resolution of the nodules, beginning within 2 weeks. Bronchoscopic monitoring can be used to confirm this effect, but the clinical condition should be markedly improved by the end of the course. There is a report of successful treatment with thiabendazole (Thibenzole® Merck, Sharp and Dohme Co., N.J.) (Bennett and Beresford-Jones, 1973). The drug was given daily at an initial rate of 32 mg/kg over a 23-day period. After 9 days, viable larvae were no longer present in the feces and the nodules decreased in size over the next several weeks. Thiabendazole must be introduced gradually to avoid vomiting. Levamisole (Tramisol®, American Cyanamid, Princeton, N.J.) is effective against metastrongyles in all other domestic animals and, provided due care is taken, it is appropriate

for use in the dog. High initial doses are very poorly tolerated in dogs, and it is best to increase the dose gradually from 2 mg/kg daily per os to 8 mg/kg over a 3-week period in order to avoid toxicosis. It has a bitter taste and dogs do not like it, but the toxic side effects are less likely to occur with oral rather than parenteral dosing.

Prevention. The life cycle of *F. osleri* has not been extensively studied, and it was considered for some time to be likely to involve an invertebrate intermediate host. However, an earlier report of direct transmission by Dorrington (1968) has recently been confirmed in Australia (Dunsmore and Spratt, 1976). Dogs, and several other canids, were fed suspensions of hatched and unhatched larvae and later developed pulmonary infections. This makes *F. osleri* a very unusual metastrongyle, since other members of this group generally require development of larvae to occur in the environment or in an intermediate host. In the absence of any firm evidence for the occurrence of transport or intermediate hosts, it is difficult to identify rational preventive measures, other than those that are normally used to limit the contamination of the environment with feces that contain infective larvae.

FILAROIDES MILKSI AND FILAROIDES HIRTHI

F. osleri has been discussed at length, since many of the biologic and medical characteristics of this parasite are common to other metastrongyles of dogs and cats. *F. milksi* and *F. hirthi* both occur in the parenchyma of the lungs in dogs.

F. milksi is a natural parasite of the skunk, and only a handful of cases have been recorded in dogs. The clinical signs typically reflect the interstitial pneumonia that results from the presence of adults and larvae in alveolar spaces. Progressive respiratory difficulty unresponsive to antibiotic therapy is generally observed.

There are no lesions visible on bronchoscopy, but bronchial washings contain embryonated eggs and larvae identical to those of *F. osleri*.

There is only one record of anthelmintic treatment of *F. milksi*, and in that instance, oral levamisole was used (Corwin et al., 1975). However, the dog was extremely dyspneic, requiring oxygen for maintenance, and died within 24 hours. It is worth noting that all the worms were dead at autopsy and that the massive release of foreign antigens may have contributed to the fatal outcome. Fatalities attributed to antigen release have been seen following levamisole treatment of sheep heavily infected with small metastrongyles. It seems wise to introduce the drug at low levels in order to avoid this complication.

F. hirthi is a recently discovered parasite that has apparently become well established in research beagle colonies (Hirth and Hottendorf, 1973). Like *F. milksi*, it inhabits the alveoli and terminal bronchioles. However, no clinical signs have yet been described in infected animals, although focal granulomatous lesions occur around adult worms. These changes are important because they may confound the interpretation of experiments in which drugs are administered to dogs to determine their toxicologic or carcinogenic properties.

A great deal of work has been carried out in the last several years to establish the transmission pattern of *F. hirthi*. The worms occur with a very high frequency within dog colonies, although the intensity of infection is never great, and usually only a few dozen worms at most are present. If has now become clear that the infections are patent and that infective first stage larvae are shed in the feces (Georgi et al., 1977). However, some larvae are also believed to penetrate the gut wall and pass to the mesenteric lymph nodes before migrating to the lungs. This form of autoinfection may account for the marked increase in prevalence correlated with age of dogs in breeding establishments.

It does not appear that any of the currently available anthelmintics are effective against *F. hirthi,* and until the mode of transmission is further clarified, preventive strategies cannot be devised.

CRENOSOMA VULPIS

This small metastrongyle (up to 1.5 cm long) inhabits the bronchi and bronchioles of wild carnivores and occasionally domestic dogs. In severe cases, bronchiolar occlusion may occur acutely, owing to the arrival in the lungs of large numbers of larvae from the circulation. This may lead to emphysema and diffuse interstitial pneumonia. In the later stages of disease, the adults reside principally in the bronchi and cause a persistent deep cough and chronic bronchitis. Diagnosis is based on the detection of straight-tailed larvae (250 to 300 μ long) in bronchial washings or in fresh feces. Anthelmintic treatment should be given as described for *F. osleri.*

AELUROSTRONGYLUS ABSTRUSUS

This is the only metastrongyle of clinical importance in the domestic cat. Adult worms (up to 1 cm long) live in the terminal bronchioles, and eggs and larvae pass up the bronchial tree.

Clinical Signs. The extensive interstitial pneumonia and bronchiolitis that develop result in a progression of clinical signs from an initial deep cough to severe dyspnea, accompanied by anorexia and marked wasting.

The severity of clinical cases depends on the number of organisms and, unlike the case with other lungworms, there is evidence that many cases go undetected. In one survey in the U.S.A., about 2 percent of cats were shown to be infected. The life cycle involves snails as intermediate hosts, but mice and birds are very effective transport hosts and, given the predatory habits of cats, infection by this means is probably commonplace.

Experimental infection in cats results in marked medial hypertrophy of the pulmonary arterial system, although the mechanism whereby this comes about is unknown. However, this type of lesion is commonly observed in feline lungs, and this observation has been interpreted as an indication that lungworm infection occurs at some stage in the life of many domestic cats.

Diagnosis. After an initial phase of patency, during which larvae may be found in bronchial washings or fresh feces, infections often become latent with few adults remaining in the lungs. There is evidence that reactivation may occur later, and this intermittent characteristic complicates the diagnosis. First-stage larvae have a kinked tail that bears a terminal spine. They measure 250 to 300 μ in the lungs but may be up to 400 μ in length by the time they appear in feces. Radiographic findings in a series of 26 natural cases have recently been described by Losonskey et al. (1978). Those animals showing chronic respiratory disease had alveolar lesions, but many subclinical cases had no detectable changes on radiography.

Treatment. There is very little information regarding suitable anthelmintic treatment. Severely affected cats require supportive treatment for the emaciation and dehydration that often accompany the chronic respiratory problem. Levamisole is undoubtedly effective in killing the parasites, but care must be taken, since this drug is poorly tolerated by cats. The injectable form in particular is toxic, beside being highly irritating locally. Oral doses can be given although cats dislike the taste. However, remission of clinical signs does occur in those that survive. The drug may be given at the rate of 25 mg/kg every other day for five treatments.

There is no practical way to prevent outdoor cats from infecting themselves by hunting rodents or birds.

CAPILLARIA AEROPHILA

This slender worm (up to 4 cm long) inhabits the trachea and bronchi, and sometimes even the nasal passages, of wild carnivores and occasionally domestic dogs. It is not a metastrongyle but is closely related to the *Trichuroidea*, or whipworms. The life cycle is direct.

Clinical Signs. Clinical cases usually occur in young dogs that are presented with a chronic cough unresponsive to antibiotics. Severe bronchitis may lead to respiratory difficulty and mouth-breathing.

Diagnosis. Radiographic changes result from chronic inflammatory thickening of the bronchial mucosa. Bronchoscopic examination reveals an inflamed irregular bronchial epithelium, although the parasites themselves may be too deep in the bronchial tree to be seen with this instrument. Bronchial washings and fecal samples contain pale yellow, thick-walled unembryonated eggs (60 × 35 μ) with bipolar plugs. However, egg output may be sparse even in severe cases, and repeated sampling is necessary in order to confirm a suspected case.

Treatment. There are no records of successful anthelmintic treatment in the literature, but some promising results have been obtained in dogs treated with levamisole. Although cessation of egg production may occur and the clinical signs may become alleviated, there is a great tendency for these cases to relapse some weeks after therapy has been terminated. Albendazole, an experimental drug of the benzimidazole series, may be of value if administered daily for several weeks.

PARAGONIMUS KELLICOTTI

P. kellicotti is a digenetic fluke (up to 1 × 0.5 cm) that inhabits fibrous cysts in the lungs of wild carnivores and domestic cats and dogs. Although widely distributed in the U.S.A., the prevalence is greater in the north central region surrounding the Great Lakes. The life cycle involves two intermediate hosts, the first of which is an aquatic snail and the second a crayfish.

Clinical Signs. Although light infections may occur without clinical consequences, heavy infections result in chronic coughing that progresses to extreme respiratory difficulty accompanied by severe emaciation, especially in cats. Often, there is frequent gagging and sneezing of mucus, which may contain blood. Secondary bacterial pneumonia is often superimposed in cats. Pneumothorax may be a presenting complication in both cats and dogs, and paroxysms of coughing may occur when animals are exercised or excited.

Diagnosis. The dense, well circumscribed cysts containing the flukes are visible radiographically (Fig. 1) but must be distinguished from tumor metastases, which often assume a similar form. Radiographic changes become evident as soon as three weeks after infection, and the lesions are most common in the right caudal lobe (Dubey et al., 1978). By two months after infection, the discrete cystic forms are visible and the tracheo-bronchial lymph nodes may be markedly enlarged. Confirmation of infection can be achieved by finding the eggs that are released into the bronchial tree through small openings in the cyst wall. Eggs are brownish-yellow in color and measure approximately 100 × 50 μ. They are operculate and have a distinct shoulder at the opercular rim. On bronchoscopic examination, the bronchial and tracheal mucus contains brown streaks when eggs are plentiful. However, microscopic examination of washings or fecal flotation samples may be necessary. The eggs float well in saturated sugar or

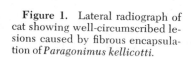

Figure 1. Lateral radiograph of cat showing well-circumscribed lesions caused by fibrous encapsulation of *Paragonimus kellicotti*.

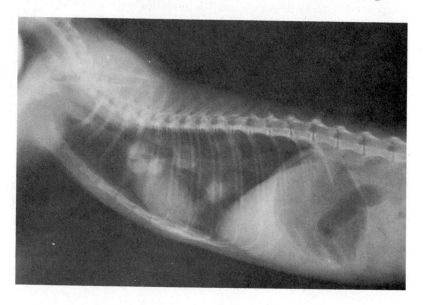

salt solutions but tend to collapse and take on a distorted crescent shape. The prepatent period is about five weeks.

Treatment. A satisfactory treatment is not currently legally available. Bithionol has been used at the rate of 500 mg/kg weight daily for seven days, but the drug is not well tolerated and may cause severe diarrhea. Experimentally, albendazole, which is not yet approved for use in the U.S.A., has shown some promise at 50 mg/kg each day for two to three weeks (Dubey et al., 1978). In natural cases, some successes have occurred at this dose, but persistence is essential and lower doses or shorter regimens lead to rapid relapse and reappearance of eggs in the feces.

Meniclopholan (Bilevon®) is a drug used overseas for fluke infections in man and probably would work in domestic animals too.

Control. Prevention of infection could only be achieved by curtailing the natural predatory habits of cats and dogs, and this is hardly feasible if the animals are allowed outdoors.

NASAL ARTHROPODS

Infections of the nasal passages of dogs with nasal mites *(Pneumonyssus caninum)* or nasal pentastomids *(Linguatula serrata)* are occasionally manifested clinically. There are no adequate records of the prevalence of these infections, since they are more often casual findings rather than primary clinical problems.

Nasal mites swarm over the mucosal surfaces of the nasal passages and sometimes cause excessive mucous discharge and frequent sneezing. Unsuspected cases are often revealed during anesthesia of dogs with gaseous agents when the mites come streaming out of the nares and out onto the operating table. Diagnosis of suspected cases depends on demonstrating mites in mucous discharges, but there are no specific treatments known. The inhalation of vaporized organophosphate from a resinous flystrip hung in the cage of hospitalized animals has been effective.

L. serrata, commonly known as the "tongue worm," also has a tendency to emerge from the nasal passages of dogs under anesthesia. The segmented adult pentastomids (up to 15 cm long) attach to the mucosal surface of the nasal passages. Eggs are either sneezed out or swallowed. Disseminated eggs are eaten by herbivores, especially rabbits, and larvae develop in viscera and lymph nodes. Larvae released from infected tissues in dogs migrate cranially up the esophagus to the nasal pharynx. Chronically infected animals may develop a foul-smelling nasal discharge in which eggs of the parasite

may present. Surgical removal of parasites may be necessary in these instances.

PARASITES THAT MIGRATE THROUGH THE RESPIRATORY SYSTEM

The larval forms of several intestinal nematodes of dogs and cats pass through the lungs as a part of their normal migratory pattern. They are coughed up and then swallowed, maturing in the small intestine.

Larvae of *Toxocara canis* and *Toxocara cati* are often present in the lungs of newborn puppies and kittens, respectively, and heavy infections result in substantial hemorrhage into the alveoli during the first days of life. This may prove fatal. Further exposure of newborn and young animals to embryonated eggs contaminating the environment can result in severe pneumonia and extensive pulmonary consolidation. Although the pathogenesis of the lesions is undoubtedly attributable in part to the physical damage caused by larvae that rupture alveolar capillaries, ascarid infections are associated with the development of marked immediate hypersensitivity and allergic inflammatory responses to the worms in pulmonary tissues form an additional pathologic component.

Acute respiratory signs may appear in puppies a few days after exposure to larvae of *Strongyloides stercoralis.* These larvae penetrate the skin and pass from the pulmonary circulation into the airway and are coughed up. During this phase, a soft cough develops and the animal becomes anorexic before the onset of the alimentary phase. Although larvae of *Ancylostoma caninum* and other hookworms travel by a similar route, the respiratory signs are much less pronounced than with *S. stercoralis.* However, extremely heavy exposure to hookworm larvae can produce massive pulmonary hemorrhage and death.

Anthelmintics are ineffective against the migrating stages of these nematodes. Attention must be given to the elimination of adult parasites in the intestine in order to prevent environmental contamination by eggs or larvae.

PARASITES THAT MIGRATE ABERRANTLY INTO THE RESPIRATORY SYSTEM

CUTEREBRA MACULATA

The larval stages of the rodent botfly quite commonly develop in the tissues of cats in rural areas. The eggs of the fly are deposited in the environment around burrows or holes made by rabbits or rodents. The larvae that hatch out can attach to the skin of many animals, including cats. They normally develop for several months in subcutaneous tissues around the face before emerging to pupate on the ground. However, the larvae quite often undergo an aberrant migration in cats and develop in the mucosa of the pharynx and occasionally even the trachea.

Clinical Signs. Signs usually occur in kittens in the late summer or fall. At this time, the larvae have reached a size sufficient to obstruct the airway, causing dyspnea. This is sometimes preceded by loud snoring and gagging. Larvae that become dislodged may be coughed or sneezed up. Bacterial infection may develop in the pharyngeal lesions, leading to systemic signs of fever, anorexia, and depression.

Diagnosis and Treatment. A thorough physical examination will reveal the obstruction, which is usually visible in the pharyngeal region and may be palpable externally. Surgical removal of the larva is necessary but care must be taken to avoid rupturing the parasite, since this may precipitate systemic anaphylactic reactions. Antibiotics should be given postoperatively.

SPIROCERCA LUPI

The esophageal worm of dogs occurs in the southern states of the U.S.A. The parasites generally inhabit granulomatous masses in the wall of the esophagus. Eggs released into the lumen through sinuses pass out in the feces. Coprophagous beetles act as intermediate hosts but rodents and birds serve as transport hosts. Larvae ingested in tissues migrate via the arterial system to the midthoracic region, where they move across to the esophagus.

Diagnosis. Respiratory signs result when aberrant larvae invade the trachea or bronchi. The resulting granulomatous mass interferes with respiration, and the severity of clinical signs depends on the size and site of the lesion. Radiographic and bronchoscopic examination will reveal the obstruction, but definitive diagnosis can be achieved only if eggs ($38 \times 12 \ \mu$) are present in bronchial washings.

Treatment. Anthelmintic therapy is unlikely to lead to complete resolution of longstanding lesions. Some success has been achieved with disophenol (D.N.P.®, American Cyanamid) at 1 ml/5 kg body weight. Prevention is difficult because of the variety of transport hosts and the reservoir of infection in sylvatic carnivores.

SYSTEMIC PARASITES THAT CAUSE RESPIRATORY SIGNS

DIROFILARIA IMMITIS

Canine heartworms, once associated only with the southern U.S. states, have become disseminated over a wide area in the eastern half of the country. This mosquito-borne filarial parasite inhabits the right heart and pulmonary artery of dogs and occasionally cats. A detailed account of the pathogenesis of heartworm disease and the associated clinical signs are presented elsewhere in this text. However, one of the cardinal signs of infection is coughing, and given the increasing frequency of *D. immitis* over such a large area, heartworm disease should always be considered in the differential diagnosis of persistent coughing and respiratory insufficiency.

ANGIOSTRONGYLUS VASORUM

This metastrongyle parasitizes the pulmonary arteries and right ventricle of dogs in many parts of the world and is occasionally imported into the U.S.A. Like most members of the lungworm group, it is transmitted in an invertebrate intermediate host. Slugs and snails serve as hosts for larvae, which are coughed up, swallowed, and appear in the feces. Dogs may become massively infected by eating intermediate hosts in which the third stage larvae have developed.

Clinical Signs. These are typically respiratory, and dyspnea and coughing result from the pulmonary congestion, extensive thrombosis, and alveolar damage caused by larvae migrating into the airways. A complicating feature of the clinical picture is the occurrence of multiple subcutaneous hemorrhages, which apparently result from the release of an anticoagulant factor from adult worms and the development of systemic bleeding tendencies. The parasite is especially associated with greyhound breeding kennels. Levamisole at 10 mg/kg daily for two days has been reported to be effective. Slug and snail control at breeding establishments is necessary for prevention.

TOXOPLASMA GONDII

Infection with cystic forms of the protozoan parasite *T. gondii* is prevalent throughout the world in almost all species of animals and man. In recent years, the complex pattern of transmission has been clarified by the identification of an intestinal coccidian phase in cats. Trophozoite and cystic stages in dogs and cats occur in a wide variety of tissues, and whereas infections are asymptomatic in the majority of cases, clinical toxoplasmosis does develop in some instances and the respiratory system is most often involved.

Clinical Signs. The clinical syndrome in both dogs and cats is variable in course but anorexia, fever, and lethargy accompanied by dyspnea are the essential features. Proliferation of the organisms in the lungs leads to focal necrotic lesions, and these coalesce to form irregularly shaped areas of coagulative necrosis that are visible radiographically. Naturally occurring cases in dogs are often complicated by the simultaneous manifestations of distemper.

Diagnosis. A protracted syndrome characterized by the above signs and unresponsive to antibiotics is suggestive of toxoplasmosis, but definitive diagnosis is difficult. Rising titers in the indirect fluorescent antibody test over the course of the disease are strongly supportive.

Treatment. No specific treatment is known, but combinations of sulfadiazine (33 mg/kg 4 times daily for one to two weeks) and pyrimethamine (2.2 mg/kg) are used in humans. This regimen has not been tested adequately in dogs and cats, but it is known to be very toxic and is at best likely only to relieve symptoms rather than eliminate infection.

SUPPLEMENTAL READING

Bennett, D., and Beresford-Jones, W. P.: Treatment of *Filaroides osleri* infestation in a 16-month-old male Yorkshire Terrier with thiabendazole. Vet. Rec. 93:226–227, 1973.

Corwin, R. M., Legendre, A. M., and Dade, A. W.: Lungworm (*Filaroides milski*) infection in a dog. J. Am. Vet. Med. Assoc., 165:180–181, 1975.

Dorrington, J. E.: Studies on *Filaroides osleri* infestation in dogs. Onderstepoort. J. Vet. Res. 35:225–286, 1968.

Dubey, J. P., Stromberg, P. C., Toussant, M. J., Hoover, E. A., and Pechman, R.: Induced paragonimiasis in cats: clinical signs and diagnosis. JAVMA 173:734–742, 1978.

Dubey, J. P., Hoover, E. A., Stromberg, P., and Toussant, M. J.: Albendazole therapy for experimentally induced *Paragonimiasis kellicotti* infection in cats. Am. J. Vet. Res. 39:1027–1031, 1978.

Dunsmore, J. D., and Stratt, D. M.: The life-cycle of *Filaroides osleri* in the dingo. Abst. presented at Ann. Mtg. Australian Soc. Parasitol., Melbourne, Australia, May, 1976.

Georgi, J. R., Georgi, M. E., and Cleveland, D J.: Patency and transmission of *Filaroides hirthi* infection. Parasitology, 75:251–257, 1977.

Hirth, R. S., and Hottendorf, G. H.: Lesions produced by a new lungworm in beagle dogs. Vet. Pathol. 10:385–407, 1973.

Losonsky, J. M., Smith, F. G., and Lewis, R. E.: Radiographic findings of *Aelurostrongylus abstrusus* infection in cats. J. Am. Anim. Hosp. Assoc. 14:348–355, 1978.

THORACIC TRAUMA

D. J. KRAHWINKEL, Jr., D.V.M.
Knoxville, Tennessee

Injury to the thoracic cage and its contents occurs commonly as a result of trauma. These injuries may be of minor significance or they may be life-threatening. Recognition of the seriousness of the injury depends on knowledge of thoracic anatomy and understanding of cardiopulmonary physiology. Because of the heart and lungs, a functional thorax is critical for proper respiration and circulation.

The thoracic cage is capable of protecting the viscera against day-to-day injury, but it is not capable of withstanding crushing or high velocity missile injury. Because of the frequency of thoracic injury, it is imperative that all trauma patients be evaluated for thoracic cage and intrathoracic damage. This is best accomplished by thorough physical examination and thoracic radiography. Evaluation of cardiopulmonary function is made clinically on the basis of color and perfusion of mucous membranes, quality and quantity of the peripheral pulse, auscultation of the heart and lung sounds, and the rate and tidal volume of respiration.

The objective of treating thoracic trauma is to restore cardiopulmonary function. Immediate treatment is aimed at the maintenance of respiration and circulation until the problem can be diagnosed and properly corrected. The following steps should be followed for the initial treatment:

1. Insure the presence of and maintain a patent airway.
2. Control any life-threatening hemorrhage.
3. Administer oxygen therapy via endotracheal tube, mask, cage, or catheter.
4. Stabilize thoracic wall so that the patient can ventilate or provide positive pressure ventilation.
5. Treat for shock by the intravenous administration of large volumes of fluids, corticosteroids, and antibiotics.

6. Seal any thoracic wound with petrolatum dressings held by loose bandages.
7. Clear the pleural space of free air or hemorrhage so that the lungs can expand.
8. Observe and monitor closely, since the patient's physical condition may change sporadically.

After emergency therapy has stabilized the patient, further diagnostic procedures should be performed. Lateral and dorsoventral thoracic radiographs are desirable if they can be taken without causing the animal stress. If this is not possible, other radiographic views such as standing laterals are substituted. Thoracocentesis may be performed if radiographs indicate the presence of fluids or free air in the thorax. Hematologic studies, especially serial hematocrits, are valuable to assess blood loss. If blood gas equipment is available, determinations of arterial Po_2, Pco_2, and pH are helpful in evaluating the ventilatory and circulatory status.

Thoracic trauma may result in a single disease condition or more commonly in a combination of conditions. These disease states may be classified physiologically as:

1. Reduction of lung volume (pneumothorax, diaphragmatic hernia)
2. Reduction of functional alveoli (pulmonary contusion, pulmonary edema)
3. Thoracic cage injury (rib fracture, sternal fracture, open wound)
4. Airway obstruction (hemorrhage, edema, tracheal rupture)
5. Hypovolemic shock (hemothorax)

These conditions will be discussed individually; however, the reader should keep in mind that this is an artificial division easier to accomplish on paper than when confronted with an injured patient. In most instances, one has to deal with a myriad of problems simultaneously.

TRACHEAL TRAUMA

The trachea may become lacerated or ruptured as a result of fight injuries, penetrating foreign bodies, or over-inflated endotracheal tube cuffs. The animal usually shows symptoms of subcutaneous emphysema and progressive dyspnea. There may or may not be a history of a traumatic episode. External wounds may not be present, although the etiology is that of a fight injury. Injury to soft tissues surrounding the trachea can result in hematomas or swelling causing external compression of the trachea (Fig. 1).

Whiplash fight injuries in cats may result in a complete separation of the trachea in the cranial mediastinum (Fig. 2). Over-inflation of endotracheal tube cuffs causes circular sloughs of the tracheal mucosa or linear rupture of the dorsal tracheal ligament.

Diagnosis. The diagnosis is made by the history of trauma to the cervical region, recent tracheal intubation, or by the presence of penetrating wounds in the cervical area. Endoscopic exam can best determine the exact nature of the injury. Radiographs usually show subcutaneous emphysema, decrease of tracheal lumen, and, occasionally, a pneumomediastinum.

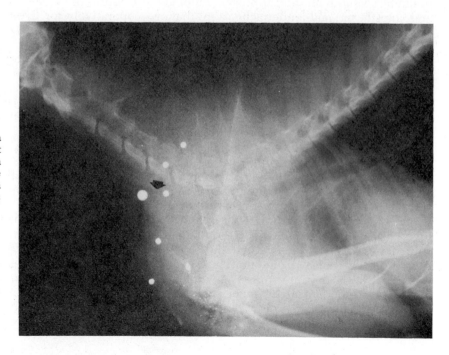

Figure 1. Radiograph of a cat with a thoracic inlet gunshot injury. The resulting hematoma and soft tissue swelling have caused a collapse of the trachea (*arrow*). The proximal humerus has been shattered.

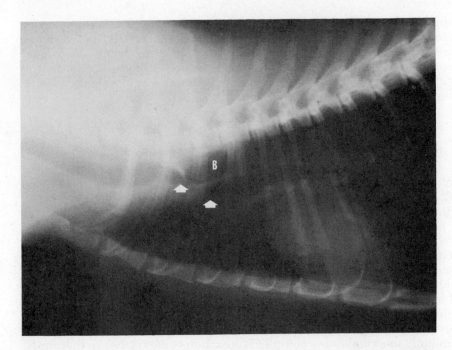

Figure 2. Thoracic radiograph of a cat with a tracheal separation as a result of a "whiplash" injury. A bulla (*B*) has formed between the separated ends of the trachea (*arrows*).

Treatment. Conservative medical treatment may in some cases be successful. If the animal can be kept quiet by sedation until the resulting wound can heal, surgery may not be necessary. Tracheal compression from hematomas or soft tissue swelling caused by trauma is best treated by oxygen therapy, corticosteroids, diuretics, and antibiotics. This therapy may also be successful in cases where there are small tracheal lacerations.

In most cases, surgery will be necessary to correct the problem. Cervical injuries are exposed by a ventral midline approach under general anesthesia and endotracheal intubation. The trachea is isolated from the larynx to the thoracic inlet, since the trauma may be anywhere along the length of the trachea. The trachea is handled gently, such as with umbilical tapes. The trachea is dissected and freed from the surrounding tissue until the injury can be identified. Once the defect in the trachea has been discovered, it is sutured with monofilament sutures placed through the adjacent tracheal rings. If it is impossible to close the tracheal defect, a trachesotomy should be performed at the site or at a more caudal site, and the tracheal wound is permitted to heal by second intention. Over-inflated endotracheal tube cuffs will commonly cause the trachea to split longitudinally, separating the tracheal rings from the dorsal ligament. These can be repaired by placing interrupted monofilament sutures from the dorsal ligament through the ends of the tracheal rings.

Complete separation of the trachea in the cra-

nial mediastinum by whiplash injury is repaired through a right cranial thoracotomy. The separated ends are located in the mediastinum and "stay" sutures are placed through each end for traction. The neck is flexed to relieve tension on the trachea and the ends are anastomosed with simple interrupted sutures of monofilament nylon. Minimal trimming of the ends should be accomplished, since shortening will cause excessive tension on the anastomosis. Despite gentle technique, postoperative stenosis is a problem.

Antibiotics should be administered postoperatively for five to seven days. Drain tubes should be left in the surgical wound for three days if significant trauma was present. The subcutaneous emphysema will be resorbed in a matter of days and should not cause any undue concern. During the recovery stage, the animal should be kept quiet, since barking or heavy exercise may cause dehiscence of the trachea.

PNEUMOTHORAX

Pneumothorax is the accumulation of free air within the pleural space (Fig. 3). This condition commonly occurs simultaneously with other traumatic injuries such as fractures of the limbs or vertebral column.

Air may gain access to the pleural space externally from a thoracic cage injury or internally from a tear of the lower respiratory tract. Traumatic causes of pneumothorax are (1) penetrating wounds of the thoracic wall, (2) laceration of tracheobronchial tree or pulmonary parenchyma, (3) blunt trauma with pulmonary contusion and alveolar rupture, (4) entry of air during thoracocentesis, and (5) alveolar rupture owing to mechanical or manual ventilation.

Signs. The signs associated with pneumothorax vary from none in mild cases to severe dyspnea in others. The more common signs include tachypnea, abduction of the forelegs, and accentuated respiratory movements. Cyanosis may be seen in severe cases. Open thoracic wounds may be present in cases of penetrating trauma. Subcutaneous emphysema is sometimes evident over the thoracic and cervical areas. Broken ribs may be palpated or observed if much displacement is present. Auscultation reveals reduced lung sounds, especially in the ventral thorax.

Diagnosis. The diagnosis is confirmed by radiography or thoracocentesis. Aspiration of free air from the pleural space is diagnostic of pneumothorax. Radiographs are a less hazardous diagnostic method if the animal is not stressed. Lateral and dorsoventral views will reveal elevation of the cardiac shadow off the sternum in recumbent lateral views, increased density of pulmonary tissue, failure of pulmonary vessels to extend to the thoracic wall, and free air between the parietal and visceral pleura. Serial radiographs are useful in ascertaining the progression of pneumothorax.

Treatment. Most cases of pneumothorax can be successfully managed by non-surgical methods. Mild cases respond to cage rest and observation. Non-narcotic sedatives may be used in active or excitable animals. If the leak has sealed, the air will be resorbed in a matter of days. Open thoracic wounds should be covered with a dressing and a bandage to prevent further aspiration of air. Supplemental oxygen should be supplied in any case of pneumothorax with respiratory difficulty or cyanosis.

Shock therapy may be required for some cases. When much air is present in the pleural space, evacuation is required by either thoracocentesis or tube drainage. Thoracocentesis is best performed with a large syringe, a three-way stopcock, and a 20-gauge needle. For best results, both sides of the thorax should be aspirated, care being taken to avoid the intercostal and internal thoracic vessels. The thorax should be sufficiently evacuated to improve respiration. Thoracocentesis in the ventral fifth intercostal space with the animal standing or in sternal recumbency will permit the removal of both air and fluid. For repeated evacuation, a thoracic drainage tube should be implanted (Fig. 4), since it is more efficient and safer than repeated thoracocentesis. Local anesthetic is injected over two to three adjacent intercostal spaces of the lateral thorax. A stab wound is made in the skin and a curved hemostat is used to make a subcutaneous tunnel cranially one to two intercostal spaces. An 18 to 24 French thoracic catheter is carried through the tunnel with the curved hemostat and bluntly inserted through the intercostal space, leaving 5 to 10 cm of the tube within the thorax. A purse-string suture is placed in the skin around the tube to prevent leakage, and a large syringe is used to evacuate the pleural space. The tube is covered with a light bandage to prevent its removal by the animal, leaving the tip exposed over the

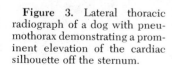

Figure 3. Lateral thoracic radiograph of a dog with pneumothorax demonstrating a prominent elevation of the cardiac silhouette off the sternum.

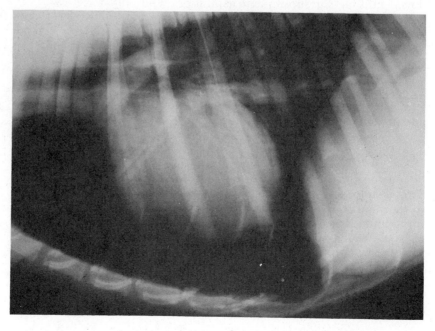

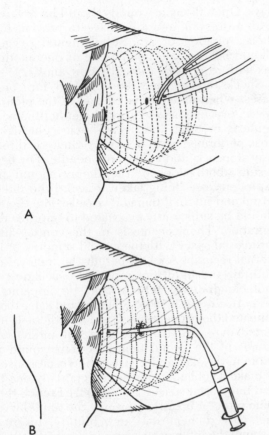

A

B

Figure 4. A thoracic drain tube is passed through a cutaneous stab wound using a curved hemostat (*A*). The tube passes through a subcutaneous tunnel for one intercostal space and enters the pleural space, leaving 5 to 10 cm of tube within the thorax (*B*). A purse-string suture is placed around the tube.

dorsal midline for subsequent aspiration. The tube can be left in place for several days if needed. When removed, the purse-string suture is used to close the skin wound.

Wounds of the pulmonary tissue will usually close spontaneously within 2 to 3 days; therefore, symptomatic treatment and thoracic drainage to maintain the cardiopulmonary system is adequate for most cases.

TENSION PNEUMOTHORAX

Tension pneumothorax can be rapidly fatal. This develops as a result of a valve-like defect in the pulmonary tissue. Air is sucked into the intrapleural space during inspiration but cannot escape during expiration. The condition is progressive, with intrapleural pressures quickly exceeding atmospheric pressures, thereby decreasing ventilation and venous return to the heart. Death results from hypoxia and reduced cardiac output.

Tension pneumothorax requires immediate thoracocentesis or tube drainage and oxygen administration. After the animal has stabilized, surgical correction may be required to repair damage to a lung lobe or tracheobronchial tree.

PULMONARY CONTUSION

Pulmonary contusion is a bruising of the lung manifested by hemorrhage and edema in the alveoli and interstitial spaces. Blunt trauma to the thorax is the usual cause of pulmonary contusion. The lungs are well protected by the rib cage; therefore, any force sufficient to bruise the lungs may simultaneously fracture ribs that penetrate the lungs, creating a hemothorax or pneumothorax. Pulmonary contusion is a frequent visceral injury but its diagnosis is neither immediate nor apparent. This disease may be present with little external evidence of trauma.

Signs. The animal is usually dyspneic with rapid respirations. Hemoptysis is not a common finding but may occur in severely traumatized patients. When present, hemoptysis warrants a guarded prognosis. Pulmonary rales may be aus-

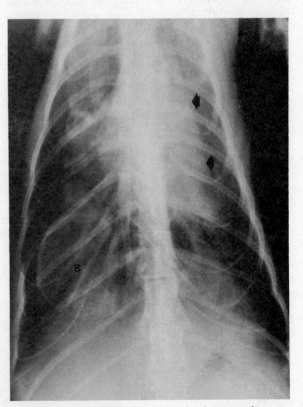

Figure 5. Dorsoventral radiograph of a cat with severe pulmonary contusion. Notice the generalized infiltration of the lung fields (*arrows*) and the formation of a traumatic pulmonary bulla (*B*).

culted. Severe pain, cyanosis, or shock may be evident when rib fractures, pneumothorax, or hemothorax is present.

Diagnosis. The diagnosis is made on the basis of a history of trauma, symptoms, physical findings, and radiographs. Lung contusions become apparent on radiographs within 2 to 12 hours following trauma. Lateral and dorsoventral radiographs reveal irregular, patchy areas of consolidation and air bronchograms within lung lobes (Fig. 5). Severe cases may be manifested by diffuse consolidation and atelectasis of an entire lobe. Some free air or blood may be present in the pleural space.

Treatment. Supportive therapy is the treatment of choice for pulmonary contusion. Enforced rest and oxygen therapy are utilized to prevent hypoxia. Antibiotics are used to preclude infection in the devitalized lung tissue. To prevent additional edema in the damaged lung, fluid therapy must be limited. One is torn between the desire to give the patient massive IV fluids to treat shock and the need to limit IV fluids in order to prevent further edema in the damaged lung. Diuretics aid in the removal of edematous fluid. Serial radiographs usually reveal much improvement in 24 to 48 hours and complete resolution in 3 to 10 days. Other concomitant disease conditions must be appropriately treated.

DIAPHRAGMATIC HERNIA

The majority of diaphragmatic hernias are acquired as a result of trauma. When the animal experiences a traumatic blow to the abdomen (e.g., motor vehicle accident, kick, or fall), there is a sudden rise in intra-abdominal pressure. Since the most flexible portion of the abdominal boundary is the diaphragm, it suddenly domes cranially. If the glottis is open, the lungs deflate, leaving no counter pressure being applied to the diaphragm, with disruption of the diaphragm and protrusion of abdominal organs into the thorax (Fig. 6).

The abdominal organs most commonly herniated are the liver, small intestines, spleen, and stomach. These organs may move freely into and out of the thorax unless adhesions or strangulation by the hernia ring develops. When the liver is involved and becomes strangulated, there is a transudation of large amounts of fluid that results in a hydrothorax as well as a diaphragmatic hernia. Obstruction of the small intestine may occur following adhesions or constriction of the hernia defect.

Signs. The signs associated with diaphragmatic hernia depend on the content and volume of the herniated organs. Signs may be intermittent as organs move in and out of the thorax. In general, the signs are related to compression of the lungs and heart by the herniated organs or to obstruction of the gastrointestinal tract when it is occluded by the hernia ring.

The history usually reveals a traumatic incident, which may be recent or long standing. Hernias of long duration are not uncommon, with symptomatology apparent only when abdominal organs "slide" into the thorax. The most common symptoms are dyspnea, hyperpnea, fa-

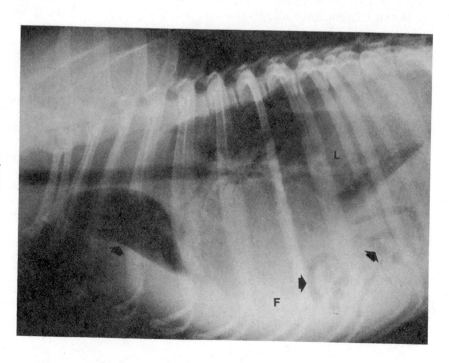

Figure 6. Diaphragmatic hernia as seen on a lateral thoracic radiograph. The silhouette of the diaphragm is not visible; the lung fields (*L*) are compressed; loops of bowel (*arrows*) are evident; and fluid (*F*) obscures the cardiac silhouette.

tigue, and lethargy. The animal usually assumes a sitting position to relieve intrathoracic pressure. Abdominal breathing is common, especially in cats. The abdomen may have a "tucked-up" appearance in chronic cases, where much of the abdominal viscera is located within the thorax. Anorexia and vomiting occur when the intestinal tract is obstructed. Gastric dilation within the thorax produces severe respiratory distress, decreased venous return, and death if not corrected immediately.

Auscultation will usually reveal the heart sounds to be displaced and muffled by the herniated abdominal viscera. Respiratory sounds are commonly heard only in the dorsal thorax. If hemothorax or hydrothorax is present, muffling of the thoracic sounds is the predominate finding. Thoracic borborygmi are not common, partially as a result of ileus of the gut within a diaphragmatic hernia. Percussion reveals a reduced thoracic resonance.

Diagnosis. The tentative diagnosis is made on the basis of the history, symptoms, and physical examination and is then confirmed by radiology. The animal should not be stressed during the examination nor held in a head-down position in an attempt to accentuate the symptoms. This may greatly increase the volume of the hernia and prove to be fatal. Lateral and dorsoventral radiographs should be taken. If these are not diagnostic, barium sulfate can be administered orally, and additional radiographs can be taken in 30 minutes. These may reveal segments of the GI tract within the thorax. In cases with associated hydrothorax or hemothorax, the fluid may have to be removed by thoracocentesis before diagnostic radiographs can be obtained.

Diaphragmatic hernias can usually be confirmed by one or more of the following radiographic signs: (1) loops of gas-filled or barium-filled intestine within the pleural space, (2) loss of an intact diaphragmatic shadow, (3) gas-filled stomach within the left hemithorax, (4) loss of the cardiac silhouette, and (5) displacement of the lung fields dorsally and laterally. The radiographic appearance of a diaphragmatic hernia can change as different abdominal organs move into and out of the thorax.

Treatment. Animals may survive with diaphragmatic hernias; however, surgical correction should be performed to return the animal to a normal physiologic status. The surgical repair may be postponed until the animal has been treated for shock and stablized, unless respiration is severely compromised. If the stomach is dilated within the thorax, an emergency thoracocentesis should be performed to deflate the stomach. If a left-sided hernia is diagnosed, surgical correction must be accomplished as soon as possible because of the possibility of intrathoracic gastric dilation. With this exception, surgery may be postponed until conditions are optimal; however, diaphragmatic herniorrhaphy is not an elective procedure and should never be unduly postponed. Preoperative oxygen and shock therapy enhance surgical success. An abdominal or sternoabdominal approach permits the surgeon to examine the abdominal organs for possible injury.

THORACIC WALL TRAUMA

The common thoracic wall injuries are rib fractures as a result of blunt trauma to the thorax and open wounds of the thoracic cage arising from fight injuries or bullet wounds. Either of these injuries may be accompanied by intrathoracic problems such as pneumothorax or hemothorax. Single rib fractures usually are not serious and do not pose treatment problems. The intact ribs on both sides provide alignment and stabilization. Multiple and segmental rib fractures result in instability of the chest wall and "paradoxic" motion (the thoracic wall is sucked in on inspiration and blown out on expiration). This condition is also termed "flail chest." Ventilation is severely impaired, resulting in hypoxia and hypercarbia.

An animal with thoracic wall injury may show few signs unless there are other associated intrathoracic problems. Painful respiration is one of the most common signs of rib fractures and results in hypoventilation in an attempt to "splint" the thorax to reduce motion. Animals with "flail chest" may have severe respiratory embarrassment as the flail section moves independently of the remainder of the thoracic cage.

Soft tissue injury to the thoracic wall is analogous to an iceberg. Small skin wounds may be all that are apparent, but underneath is massive injury to the soft tissues. Shock may be present owing to external blood loss or loss within the wound.

Diagnosis. Underlying wounds are often difficult to identify. Many trauma cases with fractured ribs are not diagnosed becaused they either are asymptomatic or have other more serious injuries, causing the rib fractures to be overlooked. Other thoracic injuries are commonly associated with rib fractures.

Diagnosis is made by palpation and radiography. In some cases, crepitation or distortion of the fracture site can be palpated, whereas in others, subcutaneous emphysema is evident. The floating section of a "flail chest" is easily observed and palpated. Dorsoventral and lateral radiographs are usually diagnostic of rib fractures.

Treatment. The animal must be treated for shock if shock is present or anticipated. Oxygen therapy is indicated when respiratory embarrassment is present. Pain should be controlled by the judicious use of analgesics.

Animals with little respiratory difficulty or minor pain may be managed with cage rest and observation. Mild tranquilization can be used to quiet nervous individuals. Supporting the thorax with a well-padded, light, elastic support bandage is helpful in some cases to reduce fracture movement and pain. Benefits gained from the use of narcotic analgesics and bandaging must be weighed against their suppression of respiration.

Positive pressure ventilation is the quickest and best way to manage immediately the patient with a "flail chest." The flail segment must be stabilized surgically for effective ventilation.

Small intramedullary pins or Kirschner wires may be used to cross-pin the fracture site, with care being taken to be sure that the pins do not penetrate the medial cortex and enter the pleural space. Fractures can also be repaired by wiring the fractured ends (Fig. 7). A thoracic drainage tube is inserted when pneumothorax or hemothorax is present. Antibiotics are administered for five to seven days and rest is enforced for two weeks. IM pins should be removed in four to six weeks.

Wounds of the thoracic wall should be immediately placed under an antibiotic dressing and bandage. After the patient's life-threatening problems have been stabilized, the wounds should be explored, debrided, and closed if pos-sible. The surgeon must remember the "iceberg" effect and not simply close minor external wounds while overlooking massive damage to the deeper layers of the thoracic wall.

HEMOTHORAX

The accumulation of blood in the pleural space results from thoracic wall or thoracic viscera bleeding. Traumatic causes include (1) missile penetration of heart, great vessels, or lung, (2) lung laceration from a fractured rib, (3) rupture of intercostal vessels by a fractured rib, (4) iatrogenic causes resulting from vascular damage during thoracic surgery, and (5) hepatic or diaphragmatic hemorrhage associated with a diaphragmatic hernia. Death is rapid when large vessels or the heart are damaged. The free blood initially coagulates but then defibrinates in a few hours and returns to a fluid state.

Hemothorax has two major consequences: (1) loss of circulating blood volume into the pleural space, leading to shock and (2) impairment of ventilation owing to lung compression by the encroaching fluid mass.

Signs. The signs are attributable to pulmonary compression and hemorrhagic shock. The animal may exhibit dyspnea, pale mucous membranes, weak thready pulse, and weakness. Auscultation of the thorax reveals muffled heart sounds and dorsally displaced lung sounds. Clinical signs may vary with the rate and amount of hemorrhage.

Diagnosis. Radiographs will reveal the presence of free fluid in the pleural space. Lateral, dorsoventral, and standing lateral views (Fig. 8) are all useful in determining the absence or presence of fluid, as well as the amount thereof. Serial radiographs are useful in ascertaining the progress of the disease. Depending on the amount of hemorrhage present, radiographs will show (1) ground-glass appearance of the thorax, (2) radiodense fluid material between visceral and parietal pleura, (3) rounding of the costophrenic angle (dorsoventral view), (4) distinct interlobar fissures, and (5) fluid line (standing lateral view).

Thoracocentesis is required to determine the type of fluid. This should be performed aseptically below the costochondral junction at the fourth and fifth intercostal space with the animal standing or in sternal recumbency. An 18-gauge 1.5 inch needle is sufficient in most animals to penetrate the parietal pleura. Care must be taken to avoid damage to the heart, the intercostal vessels caudal to the rib, and the internal thoracic vessels along the sternum. Each side of the thorax should be tapped two or three times with no aspirate obtained before

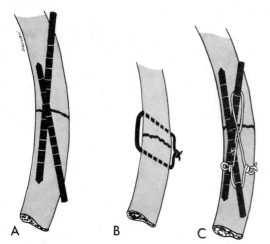

Figure 7. Rib fractures can be repaired when necessary by cross-pinning (*A*), craniocaudal wiring (*B*), or cross-pinning with a tension-band wire (*C*).

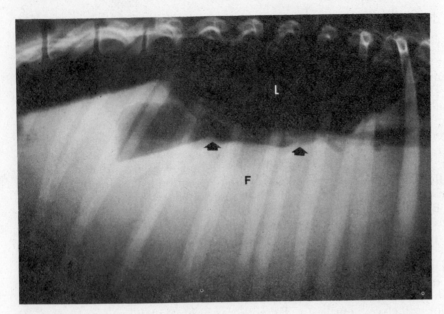

Figure 8. Horizontal beam radiograph of a dog with hemothorax. The ground-glass appearance of fluid (*F*) in the thorax obliterates the heart shadow, and the lungs (*L*) are compressed dorsally. A fluid line (*arrows*) is evident.

ruling out hemothorax. With the use of a large syringe and stopcock, as much of the blood as possible is removed. It is usually necessary to tap both sides to evacuate the pleural space adequately. Examination of the fluid is useful in determining if other disease processes are involved. Serial PCVs and sequential radiographs are helpful in evaluating whether hemorrhage is progressive or has terminated. In acute hemorrhage, the PCV will not decrease for a few hours owing to a lag phase in the shifting of body fluids.

Treatment. Treatment is aimed at the prompt replacement of circulating blood volume, expansion of the collapsed lungs, and control of the hemorrhage. Treatment for shock is the first consideration. The placement of a large-bore jugular catheter will greatly enhance subsequent treatment. Volume replacement with a balanced electrolyte solution (lactated Ringer's) is imperative along with intravenous corticosteroids, antibiotics, and oxygen. Should vital signs not improve with the above therapy and the PCV continue to decline, fresh whole blood should be administered. If subsequent radiographs and PCVs indicate continued hemorrhage, emergency exploratory surgery must

be performed. A lateral thoracotomy is preferred if the site of hemorrhage can be ascertained; otherwise, a sternotomy is used in order to explore the entire thorax.

An unevacuated hemothorax resolves in time, but it may result in fibrothorax. The sequelae of thickened pleura and adhesions decrease pulmonary compliance and restrict ventilation.

SUPPLEMENTAL READING

Archibald, J., and Harvey, C.E.: Thorax. In Archibald, J.: *Canine Surgery*, 2nd Archibald edition. Santa Barbara, American Veterinary Publications, 1974.

Berg, P.: Pneumothorax. In Kirk, R.W. (ed.): *Current Veterinary Therapy V*. Philadelphia, W.B. Saunders Co., 1974.

Carb, A.: Diaphragmatic hernia in the dog and cat. Vet. Clin. North Am. 5:477–494, 1975.

Krahwinkel, D.J.: Lower respiratory tract trauma. In Kirk, R.W. (ed.): *Current Veterinary Therapy VI*. Philadelphia, W.B. Saunders Co., 1977.

Moncure, A.C., and Scannell, J.G.: Chest injuries: chest wall, lung, esophagus, and pleural spaces. In Cave, E.F.: *Trauma Management*. Chicago, Year Book Medical Publishers, Inc., 1974.

Morris, J.D.: Patterns of thoracic trauma. In Frey, C.: *Trauma Patient*. Philadelphia, Lea and Febiger, 1976.

Ticer, J.W., and Brown, S.G.: Thoracic trauma. In Ettinger, S.J. (ed.): *Textbook of Veterinary Internal Medicine*. Philadelphia, W.B. Saunders Co., 1975.

Wilson, G.P.: The diaphragm. In Bojrab, M.J. (ed.): *Current Techniques in Small Animal Surgery*, Vol. I. Philadelphia, Lea and Febiger, 1975.

THERAPY FOR RESPIRATORY EMERGENCIES

CHARLES E. SHORT, D.V.M.
Ithaca, N.Y.

In treatment of respiratory emergencies, therapy must be undertaken with utmost speed. Fortunately, respiratory depression and arrest and the onset of the pulmonary emergency are easily diagnosed. Labored respiratory efforts, the absence of chest movements, lack of airflow, and cyanosis all indicate the need for immediate respiratory support.

Causes of acute respiratory emergencies include accidents such as trauma from moving vehicles, gunshot wounds of the thorax, fight wounds, and blunt trauma to the respiratory system. Respiratory emergencies may also arise from chronic disease problems that lead to respiratory depression, apnea, or airway obstruction. The most acute signs are produced by rapidly developing upper airway obstructions such as laryngeal edema, laryngeal paresis, elongated soft palate, and the development of extensive inflammatory responses in the upper airway. Respiratory depression and arrest may follow anesthesia and surgery or may be initiated postoperatively by medications including tranquilizers and narcotics. Primary or secondary tumors in the thoracic cavity may necessitate respiratory support because of impaired lung function owing to the space-occupying masses. Less commonly, respiratory difficulties may result from toxicity, damage to and blockage of vessels during and following heartworm therapy, congestive heart failure, parasites, and pulmonary edema resulting from inappropriate fluid therapy.

The initial phases of respiratory care may be quite similar, regardless of the etiology. The vast majority of respiratory emergencies involve either inadequate oxygen supply to the pulmonary system or inadequate uptake of oxygen within the lung. The clinician should immediately determine if the animal is obtaining adequate oxygen or air from the environment. Ventilation will obviously be inadequate when there are no respiratory movements. Less obvious but just as detrimental will be those instances in which there is an airway obstruction impeding inhalation. Oxygen uptake from the lung may be impaired by circulatory problems, lung disease, and space-occupying masses. In these cases, the clinician must determine an appropriate way to administer additional oxygen.

The delivery of oxygen via a face mask is much less effective in animal subjects than in human subjects. Facial hair and a variety of facial anatomy prevent an adequate seal between the mask and the face. Forcing gas through the nostrils into the lungs without undue flow of air into the esophagus and stomach is difficult. Oxygen therapy using a face mask, ventilator, or oxygen cage is easiest if the animal is spontaneously breathing adequate volumes. When first initiating oxygen therapy, it is desirable that the gas mixture contain at least 40 per cent oxygen. If this fails to improve blood oxygenation, higher oxygen concentrations may be necessary.

In those instances in which respiratory depression reduces ventilation, positive pressure breathing must be provided. This can be accomplished through the placement of an endotracheal tube or a tracheostomy tube. An endotracheal tube can be passed by the nares, but this is less desirable than other methods of intubation. A method of ventilation must be attached to these tubes. The simplest approach is to use a self-inflating bag, frequently referred to as an Ambu or resuscitator bag. As the bag is compressed, the lungs are inflated. Upon release of the bag in the operator's hands, the animal exhales, and at the same time the bag refills with air. A tube from an oxygen cylinder can be connected to the bag in order to supply an oxygen-enriched mixture.

Most animals may be ventilated utilizing a conventional anesthetic unit. In order to administer oxygen appropriately in this manner, the oxygen flow should provide a minimum of 15 ml/kg/minute; however, at least one liter/minute oxygen flow is needed to maintain adequate function of the anesthetic unit. Arterial carbon dioxide tension (Pa_{CO_2}) provides the best indicator of the adequacy of ventilation. Ventilators should be adjusted to maintain Pa_{CO_2} at 40 mm Hg. If a blood gas machine is not available, animals should be ventilated so as to provide obvious thoracic excursions. In lung disease, this may require the use of high inspiratory pressures. In general, respiration is assisted at a rate of 6 to 18 breaths per minute, with each breath providing an airway pressure of 15 to 30 cm of water. Smaller animals require a more rapid respiratory rate, usually with a lower airway pressure (10 to 15 cm H_2O). All animals should be given sighs every 5 to 10 minutes by inflating the lung to an airway pressure of up to 30 cm of water. The ratio of inspiratory to expiratory time should be 1:2 in order to allow for venous return to the right heart and proper pulmonary circulation. The utilization of positive end-expiratory pressure (PEEP) should be considered in those instances in which gas exchange is not improved by standard intermittent positive pressure ventilation. PEEP maintains an airway pressure of 5 to 7 cm H_2O between breaths, which increases functional residual capacity and may prevent airway closure and the consequent hypoxemia. Since PEEP also decreases cardiac output, a compromise must be found between blood oxygenation and decreased tissue perfusion.

Respiration may also be assisted mechanically. The respiratory rate and airway pressures are similar to those utilized during manual assistance to breathing. There are two main types of respirators: those with pressure control and those with volume control. The pressure-controlled ventilator recycles once a set airway pressure is obtained. The volume-controlled ventilator recycles once a given volume of gas is administered by the ventilator. Pressure-cycled ventilators may cycle without producing adequate alveolar ventilation. For example, the pressure-controlled ventilator will recycle once a given airway pressure has been reached, regardless of whether air went into the lungs. Thus, an obstruction in the airway, the endotracheal tube, or the delivery hose will cause the ventilator to recycle prematurely. Once an animal's respiration is spontaneous, it is frequently an added advantage to set the ventilator in an assist mode. In this mode, the ventilator is triggered by the subatmospheric airway pressure at the start of each inhalation. The lungs are then inflated to a preset pressure or volume. With assisted ventilation, the animal determines the respiratory rate, but ventilation is more effective because it is assisted. It is difficult to over-ventilate the animal.

Much has been said about the possibilities of oxygen toxicity and CO_2 washout during mechanical ventilation. Ophthalmic problems caused by oxygen toxicity occur during prolonged administration of 100 per cent oxygen at birth. Oxygen toxicity is not a major problem when dealing with adult dogs or cats. In most instances necessitating oxygen administration, gas exchange is impaired so that high partial pressures of oxygen are not achieved in the tissues. In addition, the tissues are protected from high partial pressures of oxygen by the shape of the oxyhemoglobin dissociation curve. However, administration of pure oxygen for over 24 hours may cause lung damage, and it is therefore advisable to use 40 to 60 per cent oxygen for therapy. Use of carbon dioxide as a respiratory stimulant is seldom if ever indicated, since carbon dioxide tension can easily be raised by reduction of tidal volume or respiratory rate. Furthermore, animals depressed by toxicity or anesthetic agents may have decreased ventilatory responses to carbon dioxide so that the added carbon dioxide causes respiratory acidosis. Even when ventilation has been utilized for 24 to 96 hours and arterial carbon dioxide partial pressure has been reduced to 15 mm Hg, spontaneous breathing rapidly develops when ventilation is stopped. If spontaneous ventilation fails to occur, respiratory stimulants such as doxapram hydrochloride (0.22 mg/kg body weight intravenously) are effective in initiating spontaneous respiration.

An oxygen cage is useful for oxygen therapy in carefully selected animals with lung disease. Improperly used, the oxygen cage can serve as a death trap. Candidates for therapy in an oxygen cage should be those that need an oxygen-enriched atmosphere and are spontaneously ventilating. The animal must not have an obstructed airway or loss of chest wall integrity. In most instances, an oxygen flow rate of 10 l/minute will maintain 37 to 40 per cent oxygen in the cage. Cage temperature must be controlled at levels that provide for adequate control of the animal's own body temperature. Utilization of an oxygen cage below 70° F might result in hypothermia. On the other hand, utilization of oxygen cages with temperatures over 80° F may result in hyperthermia and hyperventilation. Normally, the moisture content of the atmosphere in the oxygen cage should vary from 45 to 55 per cent humidity.

Control of acidosis and bicarbonate levels can only be achieved by measurement of arterial blood gases and pH. In the absence of these measurements, it can be assumed that in almost all instances of respiratory depression or arrest, there is a decrease in arterial oxygen tension and pH and an increase in arterial carbon dioxide tension. Following prolonged metabolic disease and debilitation, there will usually be a slight metabolic acidosis, but this is frequently offset by hyperventilation so that pH may be close to normal. In an animal with respiratory problems, lactated Ringer's solution will frequently be adequate to maintain pH if the animal is properly oxygenated and ventilated. Because most animals with respiratory problems are acidotic, 2.2 mEq/kg body weight sodium bicarbonate can routinely be given intravenously without detrimental effects. The use of 6 to 20 mEq/kg of sodium bicarbonate without knowing the extent of respiratory or metabolic acidosis may produce alkalosis.

When examining animals with respiratory problems, it is appropriate to consider the animal's hydration, the packed cell volume, hemoglobin values, and cardiovascular function. Respiratory problems frequently cannot be controlled unless these factors are considered. For example, it is inappropriate to expect oxygen therapy to be totally satisfactory in the accident case in which there has been extensive hemorrhage, with a decrease in circulating red cells and reduced cardiovascular function. This type of case must be given whole blood in addition to oxygen. Blood will increase oxygen carrying capacity and, by restoring vascular volume, will improve cardiovascular function.

In animals with trauma to the thoracic cavity, the lung, or the upper airway, additional steps must be taken to restore the integrity of the respiratory tract. These measures are described in the article "Thoracic Trauma."

In summary, the treatment of respiratory depression and/or arrest is dependent upon ventilation and the administration of oxygen. Although an oxygen cage or oxygen supplying mask can be used in many cases of lung disease, mechanical ventilation is necessary in cases of respiratory arrest, respiratory depression, or when there is loss of integrity of the respiratory tract and/or chest wall. It may be necessary to paralyze the animal or to use a tracheostomy tube in order to maintain this type of ventilation. Because oxygen therapy is so necessary in respiratory problems, hospitals should be equipped for oxygen therapy and preferably artificial ventilation.

INTERPRETATION OF PULMONARY RADIOGRAPHS

PETER F. SUTER, D.M.V.
Davis, California

Radiographic examination is an integral part of the diagnostic procedures in chest diseases of dogs and cats. The natural contrast provided by the pulmonary air facilitates the recognition of a large number of normal and pathologic structures of the thorax. It permits (1) exact anatomic location of a disease process at the gross and, occasionally, even at the subgross level, (2) documentation of the severity of involvement by disease, (3) screening for chest diseases in animals with obscure clinical signs or to relieve anxiety in concerned owners, (4) determination of the most likely etiologies (differential diagnoses) and sometimes determination of the final diagnosis, (5) following the progression or regression of disease over an extended period, and (6) evaluation of the effectiveness of therapy. Usually, radiography serves to confirm a tentative clinical diagnosis and supplements it with additional information. Frequently, radiographs may provide new and unexpected findings (e.g., metastatic nodules or small quantities of pleural fluid) that were not anticipated clinically or are impossible to discern by other readily available methods of clinical investigation.

Interpretation of thoracic radiographs can be difficult because of the superimposition of normal and abnormal shadows and the subtlety of many abnormal densities. The variations between breeds in normal radiographic anatomy, the substantial overlap between normal and abnormal densities, and the artifacts and density variations associated with inconsistencies in the radiographic technique and phase of respiration are substantial and require experience to interpret. This is gained by looking at large numbers of radiographs. Occasionally, technical variations, such as taking pulmonary radiographs during the expiratory pause instead of near peak inspiration (Fig. 1), may account for greater radiographic changes than the ones caused by pulmonary disease.

The accuracy of the radiographic diagnoses can be increased by adherence to the following

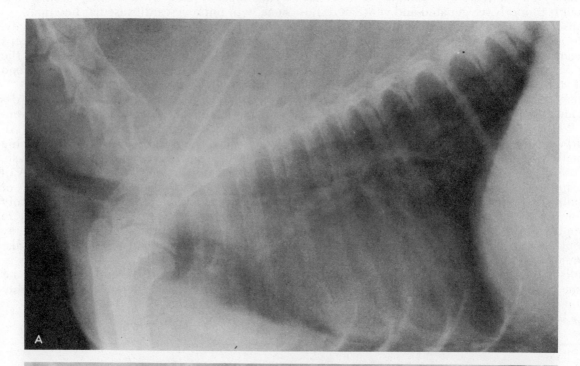

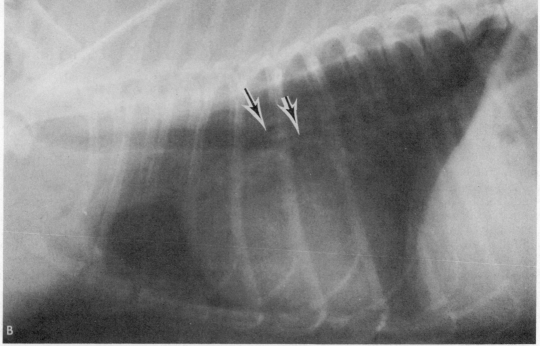

Figure 1.   Inspiratory (*A*) and expiratory (*B*) lateral recumbent radiographs of a male 7-year-old miniature poodle with a chronic non-productive cough for two years. Notice the increased radiodensity of the lung, the loss of detail, and the reduced size of the thorax in the expiratory radiograph (*A*). The trachea is smaller at expiration than at inspiration, and the lumina of the main bronchi to the caudal lobes are not visible. In the radiograph taken at inspiration (*B*), the tracheal lumen is wide and more radiotranslucent. The lumina to the main bronchi can be clearly seen (*arrows*). The increased radiodensity of the lung in the expiratory radiograph could easily lead to the erroneous diagnosis of pneumonia or lung edema. The narrowing of the trachea and bronchi at expiration was significant in this case because it was one of the ancillary dynamic factors maintaining the cough in this dog with chronic bronchitis.

suggestions. The search for abnormalities of thoracic radiographs should be done in a consistent fashion and should include (1) evaluation for proper radiographic technique, (2) a search for abnormalities in the extrathoracic areas depected on the radiograph, and (3) systematic examination of all thoracic organs and spaces. The technical evaluation should be done immediately after the radiograph has been processed. Poor quality radiographs should be repeated in order to avoid mistakes in interpretation. If the technical quality is not evaluated immediately in outpatients, the animal's owner may suffer the inconvenience of being recalled for further examination, or worse, one may base a diagnosis on a poor quality radiograph. In follow-up radiographs, the technique should be comparable with the preceding examination to permit meaningful conclusions concerning progression or regression of disease. Consistency, both in taking the radiographs and in darkroom processing, helps to avoid unnecessary repeat radiographs and equivocal results.

Thoracic radiographs should be made with short exposure times (1/30 to 1/120 sec) to reduce motion. Equipment that can deliver 200 to 300 milliamperes at 80 to 110 kilovolts is strongly recommended. The importance of having radiographs of the lung exposed while it is normally inflated cannot be overemphasized. Radiographic signs permitting the differentiation of well inflated from poorly inflated thoracic radiographs have been described. Expiratory radiographs, however, can be advantageous in visualizing small pleural effusion or pneumothorax. Grids are required only when the thoracic diameter is over 15 cm, or over 10 cm in inordinately obese cats or small dogs.

It is advantageous to begin the radiographic interpretation outside the thoracic cavity. A high-intensity light should be used to evaluate dark areas. By looking at the peripheral areas first, one can avoid forgetting to evaluate them after a significant abnormality has been found within the thorax. Extrathoracic findings such as a narrowed cervical tracheal diameter, rib fractures, hepatomegaly, abdominal fluid, subcutaneous emphysema, or masses of destructive lesions in the ribs or sternebrae often support or help to clarify intrathoracic abnormalities or provide unexpected additional information.

A disorganized search for abnormalities is often responsible for the fact that significant changes are overlooked or the search is terminated prematurely. Additional important but unexpected lesions may thus be missed. One method is to evaluate the thorax in the following order: trachea, mediastinum, esophagus, heart, lungs, pleural space, and diaphragm. An-

other method begins interpretation in the center of the thorax and works its way toward the periphery.

The abnormalities found must be screened for significance. True pathologic findings must be separated from artifactual ones or from superimposed extrathoracic shadows, such as overlying skin folds, bones (scapula), nipples, subcutaneous masses, excessive subcutaneous fat, or wet hair. Technical artifacts due to dirty or badly worn screens or poor darkroom technique can be identified by looking for comparable shadows on a second radiograph taken at a 90-degree angle to the first. Artifacts are best avoided by proper upkeep of the cassettes and darkroom. Anatomic variations must be excluded by relying on previous experience with animals of the same age range and the same breed or by consulting prior radiographs of the same animal. It is advantageous to collect representative chest radiographs of a few standard and some less common breeds for a normal reference file.

At the end of the search, the area of potential involvement, as suggested by the clinical findings and history, should be scrutinized a second time.

If there are no abnormal findings on the survey radiographs, or if the changes found are equivocal as to location or significance, additional studies may be indicated. Radiographs taken during the expiratory phase may be needed to depict collapse of the intrathoracic portion of the trachea not recognizable on an inspiratory radiograph (Fig. 2). Oblique projections may be necessary to avoid superimposition of the trachea by the spine in the dorsoventral radiograph or to bring thoracic wall lesions into profile. Ventrodorsal instead of dorsoventral radiographs, or positional radiographs made with a horizontal beam direction, may serve temporarily to visualize an area of interest obscured by pleural fluid.

Survey radiographs may have to be supplemented by special studies such as fluoroscopic examination or bronchography. Intrathoracic airway diseases such as early bronchiectasis or extramural or intraluminal bronchial obstruction may require confirmation of the suspected lesion by bronchography. Pulmonary vascular abnormalities, such as dirofilariasis, pulmonary thrombosis, or shunting with congenital heart disease, may require angiocardiography if the survey radiographs are equivocal. The nature and origin of lesions within or adjacent to the pulmonary hilus, mediastinum, or diaphragm may have to be identified by esophagography.

For radiographic diagnostic purposes, lower respiratory tract diseases may be subdivided

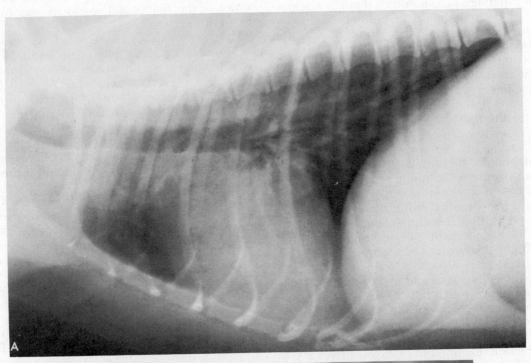

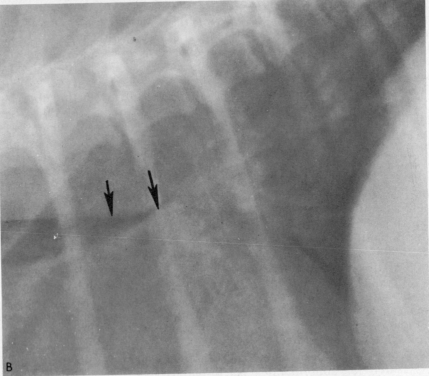

Figure 2.   Lateral recumbent radiograph of a female 7-year-old toy poodle with a dry, hacking cough and an inspiratory and expiratory wheeze. The inspiratory radiograph (*A*) contains no abnormality that would permit explanation of this animal's signs. On the expiratory radiograph (*B*), collapse of the lumen of the trachea at the bifurcation (*arrows*) is visible. The lumina of the main bronchi are also absent. A diagnosis of intrathoracic tracheal and bronchial collapse was made and confirmed by fluoroscopy. With only an inspiratory radiograph available, this dynamic type of obstructive intrathoracic disease would not have been diagnosed. This case illustrates that at times both inspiratory and expiratory radiographs are required.

into two major groups: (1) obstructive and non-obstructive lower airway disease (bronchitis, bronchiolitis, asthma) and (2) pulmonary parenchymal diseases (pneumonia, neoplasia, mass lesions).

LOWER AIRWAY DISEASE

Lower airway diseases (collapsing intrathoracic trachea, tracheobronchitis, bronchiolitis, asthma, allergic bronchitis) can be difficult to diagnose radiographically because clinical signs and radiographic findings may not correspond; severe clinical signs such as fever, dyspnea, coughing, and retching can be found in dogs or cats with normal-appearing radiographs.

Partial or total dynamic obstruction of the lower airways by collapse can be recognized only if the trachea or stem bronchi are involved. Small bronchi or bronchioli also collapse but do not cast individually recognizable shadows. A soft, poorly stabilized intrathoracic trachea or the stem bronchi collapse partially or totally during forced expiration or coughing, which can be seen as a marked narrowing of the airway lumen on expiratory radiographs (Fig. 2). On radiographs made during inspiration, the lumina of these airways appear normal or slightly dilated. In dogs with collapsing cervical trachea, the narrowing occurs during the opposite respiratory phases; namely, the trachea appears narrowed during inspiration and seems normal during expiration.

The degree of airway collapse is modified by breathing efforts and increased air flow resistance in the upper airways (nares, larynx, soft palate). These dynamic types of obstruction must be differentiated from morphologic obstructions due to hypoplastic trachea, tracheal stenosis, tracheobronchitis, intraluminal tracheal or bronchial blockage, and extramural compression of the airways by a mass. In the latter conditions, any visible tracheal and bronchial narrowing is affected only slightly or not at all by the respiratory phase.

Uncomplicated, acute tracheobronchitis in dogs or cats rarely leads to radiographically recognizable changes. Visualization of tracheobronchitis is contingent on (1) substantial inflammatory thickening of the bronchial walls by severe mucosal edema, cellular infiltration of the bronchial wall, or polypoid proliferation of the bronchial mucosa and submucosal glands; (2) extension of the inflammation into adjacent lung parenchyma; and (3) indirect or direct signs of airway obstruction. Severe inflammatory bronchial wall thickening is seen radio-graphically as an accentuation of the normal linear bronchial pattern (Fig. 3). Extension of inflammation into adjacent parenchyma makes the bronchial wall appear blurred. When looked at on-end, indistinct ring shadows, also referred to as "doughnut shadows," become visible in the central and middle portions of the lung. Concurrent inflammation in the pulmonary interstitium reduces background density of the lung and the visibility of the vascular structures. These changes are particularly severe in chronic bronchitis or bronchiectasis. A progression of bronchitis to bronchopneumonia causes blotchy parenchymal densities (Fig. 4).

Individual shadows cast by the peripheral normal or inflamed small airways (bronchioli, terminal bronchi) cannot be seen radiographically. Nonetheless, some diseases affecting the peripheral airways can be assumed, based on the resulting change in the air content of the lung parenchyma. If the inflation of the alveoli and terminal bronchioli (end-air spaces) is altered significantly by airway obstruction, atelectasis, hyperinflation, or emphysema must be expected. Mucous plugs and mucosal swelling in asthma, obstructing bronchiolitis, or microbronchitis can lead to *total obstruction* of the peripheral airways of one or more lung segments or an entire lung lobe, resulting in the resorption of the alveolar air and atelectasis. Radiographically, the collapsed lung areas become radiodense and smaller, which may induce a shifting of the mediastinum or heart toward the involved lobe(s) or may cause a substantial asymmetry of the diaphragm due to cranial displacement of the hemidiaphragm on the involved side.

Another alternative with asthma, obstructing bronchiolitis, or microbronchitis is due to *incomplete blockage* of the small airways. Mucosal swelling, cellular infiltration, mucous plugs, and bronchospasm in affected bronchioles may still allow air to enter the alveoli during inspiration. During expiration, however, the airway diameter is reduced, prolonging expiratory time and trapping air in the pulmonary periphery. Trapping of air can induce emphysema, which in severe cases may be recognized radiographically by focal or generalized hypertranslucency of the involved areas, increased thoracic size (barrel chest), flattening and caudal displacement of the diaphragm, and a small heart. Emphysematous lung lobes may displace and partially compress adjoining normal lung lobes. Openings between adjacent alveoli (pores of Kohn) or direct communications connecting bronchioles with surrounding alveoli (canals of Lambert) provide alternate ways for air to reach lung tissue distal to an obstruction of a bron-

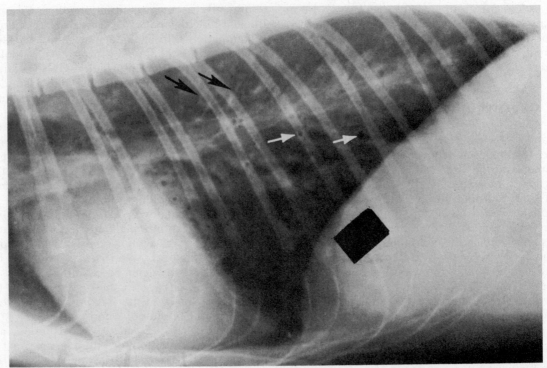

Figure 3. Lateral recumbent radiograph of an adult female domestic shorthair cat with anorexia and dyspnea of four days' duration. The radiodensity of the lung is slightly increased, and upon close inspection a large number of ill-defined linear shadows (*black arrows*) can be seen in the caudal lobes radiating toward the lung periphery. In some of the shadows small radiolucent centers (*white arrows*) representing bronchi seen end-on can be recognized. The arteries to the caudal lobe are poorly outlined. This radiograph is typical for a great many of the severe chronic bronchitis cases seen in the cat. Inflammation and thickening of bronchial walls are responsible for their increased visibility. An increased bronchial pattern of this type can be seen with allergic, parasitic or secondary bacterial bronchitis.

chus, which is called "collateral air drift," and prevent atelectasis of obstructed lung segments.

Total obstruction of a major bronchus in the hilar area by intraluminal masses, such as foreign bodies or intraluminal tumors, or by extramural compression due to enlarged lymph nodes or neoplasms results in atelectasis, which can be recognized as an increased lobar radiodensity. Often, atelectasis may be followed by edema and interstitial pneumonia resulting from hypoxia and trapping of bronchial exudates distal to the obstruction. Partial bronchial obstruction, depending on its severity, may be unnoticed radiographically or may lead to air trapping and hyperlucency of the affected lobes.

PULMONARY PARENCHYMAL DISEASE

Most *pulmonary parenchymal diseases* are recognized by an increased radiodensity of the lung. The increased radiodensity can be due to (1) replacement of the air in the end-air spaces (alveoli and terminal bronchioli) by exudates or transudates, (2) a loss of air from the end-air spaces, or (3) an increased amount of interstitial tissue and blood in the capillaries, or a combination of all three events. The majority of pulmonary parenchymal diseases induce a concurrent or consecutive change in air content, blood perfusion, interstitial tissue edema, and cellular infiltration.

A small number of pulmonary conditions can be recognized because of a diminished pulmonary radiodensity (blacker than normal), which is commonly referred to as hypertranslucency and may be caused by (1) an increased air content (hyperinflation, airway disease, emphysema) or (2) a diminished pulmonary perfusion with blood (hypovolemia, cardiac shock, Addison's disease, and right-to-left shunting of blood in congenital heart disease). Focal areas of hypertranslucency can be encountered with focal air trapping (focal emphysema), bullae, blebs, pulmonary cysts, pneumatoceles, cavitary lesions (abscesses), necrotizing neoplasms, or infarcts.

It is advantageous to discriminate among the many diseases causing increased pulmonary radiodensity by grouping them into three basic

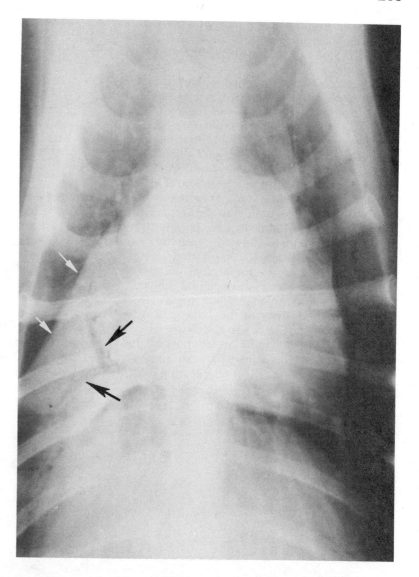

Figure 4. Dorsoventral radiograph of a male 6-year-old German shepherd dog that had sustained a fracture of the axis. The dog suffered a cardiac arrest and was resuscitated successfully. Since that event, however, the dog had a persistent fever. Contiguous with the right border of the cardiac shadow is a soft tissue–like, homogeneous radiodensity which contains two radiolucent tapering streaks (*black arrows*). The cranially well-demarcated, abnormal radiodensity represents a consolidated right middle (cardiac) lobe that contains radiolucent air bronchograms. The visualization of a lobar border (*white arrows*), the presence of air bronchograms and the absence of vascular markings within the radiodensity suggest an end–air space density (alveolar). The asymmetry of the lesion and the location are compatible with bronchopneumonia, most likely due to aspiration of vomitus during resuscitation.

categories according to easily recognizable radiographic criteria. This permits reducing the number of probable diagnoses. The three basic categories are (1) disseminated, diffuse pulmonary disease with radiodensities in one or several lobes, (2) solitary focal densities, and (3) multiple focal densities.

A disseminated pulmonary disease is characterized by radiodensity spreading diffusely across one or several lung lobes.

On the basis of radiographic appearance, disseminated pulmonary radiodensities can be classified into an end-air space (alveolar) or an interstitial, a vascular, and a mixed pattern. The radiodensities are always named after the predominant pattern. The end-air space pattern can be caused by a substantial loss of air from the end-air spaces (atelectasis) or by replacement of the alveolar air by fluid or cells (edema, pneu-

monia, hemorrhage). The resulting increased radiodensity is called alveolar density or end-air space pattern and is characterized by a confluent, mottled, or homogeneous soft tissue-like radiodensity with fluffy borders where it merges with adjoining seemingly normal lung. Air-filled first- and second-order bronchi may be visible as dark branching streaks or stripes within the radiodense areas and are referred to as air bronchograms (Fig. 4). The vascular structures are obscured by the water-dense parenchyma. Borders of consolidated lobes become visible where they are in contact with a normal or less involved lobe. Air bronchograms are a valuable localizing sign for distinguishing between pulmonary and extrapulmonary intrathoracic densities such as pleural fluid or mediastinal masses that do not contain air bronchograms. There are, however, a few diseases with end-air space patterns but without air bronchograms. Air bronchograms may be seen occasionally with severe interstitial disease.

The alveolar or end-air space pattern is compatible with diseases summarized in Table 1.

The predominant location of the radiodensities, the clinical signs, the laboratory data, and the history are helpful in differentiating among the various alveolar diseases of Table 1. Bronchopneumonias are found most often in the dependent portions of the cranial and middle lobes, whereas edemas are most often symmetrically distributed around the pulmonary hilus (Figs. 4 and 5). Hemorrhages have no local predilection but the history may provide the necessary clues for a diagnosis. Aspiration pneumonia is often seen in the dependent parts of the middle, the accessory, or the caudal lobes.

A disseminated, homogeneous (unstructured) increased radiodensity of the lung and loss of the normal contrast between the dense vascular structures and the radiolucent normal lung parenchyma can be caused by an increased amount of interstitial fluid (congestion), colla-

Table 1. *Disseminated Diseases With End-Air Space Pattern*

ACUTE DISEASES	CHRONIC DISEASES (RARE)
Alveolar edema	Disseminated neoplasia
Bronchopneumonia	Granulomatous pneumonia
Aspiration pneumonia	
Hemorrhage	
Atelectasis	

genous tissue, or cellular interstitial infiltrates. These types of radiodensities are called interstitial densities and are encountered with the diseases summarized in Table 2. The pattern is usually not radiodense enough to obscure the vascular markings totally — it merely smudges their borders. Diseases with interstitial patterns do not permit visualization of well defined air bronchograms because the amount of air in the lumina of the alveoli is reduced but not totally eliminated as with an end-air space pattern (Fig. 6). The term "diffuse infiltrative pattern" might be more appropriate than "interstitial pattern."

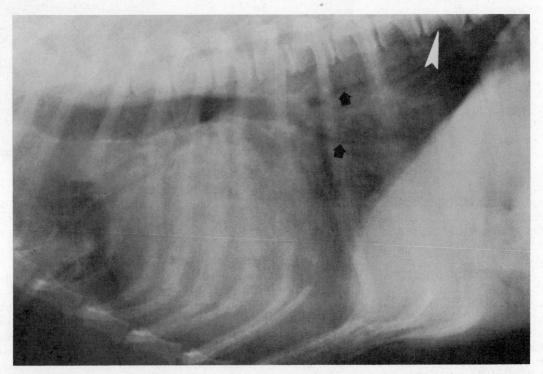

Figure 5. Lateral recumbent radiograph of a male 13-year-old miniature dachshund that was radiographed prior to anesthesia because of a loud holosystolic mitral murmur. The increased radiodensity of the lung is real and could not be compatible with an expiratory radiograph because the wide trachea and the extension of the lumbodiaphragmatic recess caudal to the level of T11 (*white arrow*) make such an assumption highly unlikely. The marked increase in the radiodensity of the caudal (diaphragmatic) lobe is thus a sign of a parenchymal pulmonary disease. The faintly visible air bronchograms within the radiodensity (*black arrows*) indicate an end-air space density. The associated cardiomegaly, the location of the lesion in the perihilar area, and the auscultatory finding make pulmonary alveolar edema due to left-sided heart failure the most likely diagnosis.

Table 2. Disseminated Diseases With Homogeneous Interstitial Pattern

Interstitial edema (congestion)
Interstitial pneumonia (pneumonitis)
Eosinophilic pneumonia
Interstitial hemorrhage
Pulmonary contusion (blunt trauma)
Fibrosis, scarring
Old age
Artifacts: expiratory radiographs, obesity

Many conditions labeled interstitial are not histologically confined to the interstitium and involve adjacent alveoli. The term "interstitial" as used by radiologists is not identical to the term "interstitial" as used by pathologists.

It is important to be aware that radiographic recognition of interstitial disease may be elusive. Animals with severe clinical signs due to interstitial disease may show little or no concurrent radiographic changes. Regardless of the underlying disease, all homogeneous interstitial patterns look very much alike. There are usually few associated radiographic characteristics, such as preferred location. Only the associated concurrent lesions in other organs, such as cardiomegaly in cases of pulmonary congestion or rib fractures in cases of traumatic contusion, may assist in radiographically differentiating diseases with interstitial pattern.

Interstitial radiographic patterns can also be structured or inhomogeneous — namely, nodular, linear, or mixed reticular and nodular (reticulonodular). It is advantageous not to use "interstitial" for these radiodensities. They should be described in simple visual terms. Nodular densities are most commonly caused by multiple pulmonary metastases. Linear and reticulonodular interstitial patterns can be found with pulmonary fibrosis, old age, granulomatous disease, chronic congestion, and disseminated pulmonary lymphosarcoma.

An abnormal vascular pattern of the lung is found with diseases that increase lung perfusion, reduce lung perfusion, or cause dilatation of arteries or veins. It can be essential to distinguish arteries from veins to made a diagnosis;

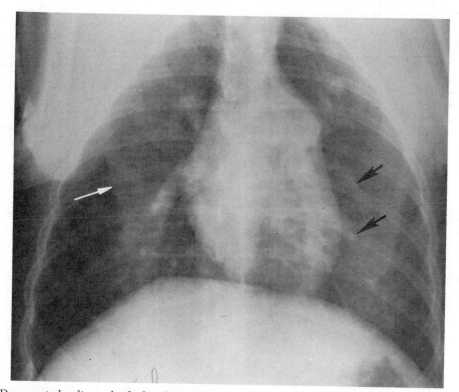

Figure 6. Dorsoventral radiograph of a female spayed 2-year-old terrier cross dog with dyspnea and gagging persisting over one year. A homogeneous, hazy, increased radiodensity of the lung markedly reduces the contrast between it and the vascular structures in the caudal lobes; in particular, the outlines of the vascular structures in the left caudal lobe (*black arrows*) are indistinct. The increased radiodensity is not intense enough to cause air bronchograms. This type of intermediate radiodensity is typical for an unstructured, disseminated interstitial type of radiodensity. Based on the clinical examination, a 23 percent blood eosinophilia, and the radiograph, the diagnosis of allergic pneumonia or pulmonary infiltrates with blood eosinophilia (PIE) was made. The dog responded favorably to the administration of corticosteroids. The white arrow points to an artifactual density caused by a skin fold that is projected into the lung.

i.e., to differentiate dirofilariasis from left heart failure. In the lateral radiograph, the vascular markings dorsal to the bronchial lumen of the cranial lobe bronchi are arteries. Pulmonary veins are located ventral to the bronchial lumen. In the dorsoventral or ventrodorsal radiograph, veins can be identified in the caudal lobes by their confluence in the area of the left atrium, whereas pulmonary arteries can be traced to their origin from the main pulmonary artery, which is located in the cranial portion of the cardiac shadow. A hypervascular pattern is characterized by increased radiodensity and size of the pulmonary vascular markings (arteries and/or veins) and extension farther into the periphery than normal. It can be associated with infection, inflammation, pulmonary congestion in left heart failure (veins enlarged), or left-to-right shunting lesions (patent ductus arteriosus, ventricular septal defect), or with peripheral arteriovenous fistulas. Enlarged vascular stuctures seen on-end appear as nodular radiodensities and can be confused with pulmonary parenchymal nodules. Dilated, distorted, and/or truncated pulmonary vascular structures are a common abnormal vascular pattern with dirofilariasis. A significant reduction in pulmonary perfusion, which can be recognized radiographically by the diminished size of the arteries and veins and a concurrent hypertranslucent lung, can be associated with hypovolemic shock, severe dehydration, Addison's disease, or reduced cardiac output due to myocardial failure (cardiac shock).

Focal pulmonary radiodensities can be of three types: (1) amorphous, blotchy densities with irregular shape, varying size, and indistinct borders; (2) round or oval radiodensities, over 4 cm (1½ inches) in diameter, with distinct borders, which are referred to as mass lesions; or (3) evenly rounded radiodensities less than 4 cm in diameter, which can be well or ill defined and are referred to as nodular lesions. All three types of densities can be solitary or multiple.

A small solitary nodule of 1 to 2 cm in diameter is called a "coin lesion." Table 3 lists diseases that should be considered in the differential diagnosis of solitary lesions. Solitary lesions quite often are incidental findings in clinically normal animals or in animals with vague clinical signs not referable to the respiratory system.

The differentiation of solitary pulmonary lesions is difficult and may require extensive clinical work-up, repeat radiographs, needle aspiration biopsy, or exploratory thoracotomy.

Multiple pulmonary, focal lesions are among the most common radiographic findings. Breaking them down into groups with a common morphologic denominator is helpful. Tables 4, 5,

Table 3.   Solitary Pulmonary Radiodensities

AMORPHOUS, BLOTCHY DENSITY	MASS LESION OR NODULE (COIN LESION)
Focal pneumonic infiltrate	Abscess
Focal lung necrosis, infarct	Granuloma
Granuloma, abscess	Primary neoplasm
Focal hemorrhage, contusion	Metastatic neoplasm
Focal atelectasis	Hematoma
Neoplasm	Fluid-filled cyst
Infarct	

and 6 can be used as a basis for differential diagnosis.

Pinpoint nodules are the smallest, barely visible size of nodules; miliary nodules are nodules less than 3 mm in diameter. Both are visible radiographically only when present in large numbers. Their great number compensates for their small size and faint tissue density, which otherwise would make them invisible radiographically. Small densities that contain calcium, such as pulmonary osteomas or calcified dystrophic nodules, can be seen individually, despite their small size. Pulmonary osteomas are small, focal pulmonary or pleural calcifications or ossifications (ectopic bone formation) commonly seen in dogs' lungs. Their significance is unknown.

Multiple nodular radiodensities can be well defined or ill defined. The probability is usually overwhelming that multiple, well to fairly well defined nodular pulmonary lesions are a manifestation of metastatic disease. Nonetheless, fungal diseases and the other diagnoses summarized in Table 5 should be carefully considered as differential diagnoses. The location of nodular lesions assists in their differentiation from vascular structures seen end-on. Nodules cast by vascular structures seen end-on are located in the central or middle portions of the lung field and are often superimposed onto another vascular structure running at approximately a 90-degree angle to the direction of the x-ray beam. These nodular shadows may be difficult to differentiate from true metastatic nodules superimposed onto a vessel. Nodular den-

Table 4.   Multifocal, Amorphous Pulmonary Radiodensities

Pneumonic infiltrates or necrosis (embolic spread of bacterial or fungal diseases; opportunistic pneumonias due to reduced host resistance)

Granulomas (fungal, parasitic, toxoplasmosis, multiple foreign bodies)

Focal hemorrhage (coagulopathies, trauma, neoplasia)

Infarcts (dirofilariasis, trauma, neoplasia, heart failure)

Neoplasms (primary multicentric neoplasia, bronchiolar alveolar carcinoma, or complications of metastatic neoplasms)

Table 5. *Disease With Well-Defined Nodular Radiodensities*

PINPOINT OR MILIARY NODULES (<3 mm.)	LARGER NODULES (3 mm to 40 mm)

Hemic spread of:
  Fungal diseases
  Bacterial diseases
  Neoplasia
	Metastatic neoplasms
	Fungal diseases
	Satellite nodules of primary neoplasia
	Hematoma
	Bacterial granuloma

Calcified, old, parasitic or fungal nodules Fibrotic nodules	Fluid-filled cysts Vascular structures projected end-on (hypervascular lung, dirofilariasis)
Alveolar microlithiasis Pulmonary osteomas	Bronchiectases filled with exudate Artifacts: nipples, subcutaneous nodules

sities seen between vascular structures or in the pulmonary periphery are highly suggestive of metastatic disease.

Radiographic recognition of metastatic pulmonary neoplasms depends on a favorable projection on the radiograph and on the number and absolute size of the nodules. The lower limit of visibility for small nodules is at 3 to 5 mm in diameter, but one or two nodules of up to 12 mm (½ inch) in diameter may often go unrecognized when located in the peripheral portions of the caudal lobes or when they are obscured by the shadows cast by the spine, vessels, or diaphragm. Thus, a negative set of radiographs does not exclude the possibility of pulmonary metastatic disease. A second or sometimes third set of radiographs at an interval of three weeks to one month is often needed to confirm a negative result.

Ill defined nodules are often mixed with well defined nodules and can occur with both interstitial and alveolar types of lung disease. When present in large numbers, ill defined nodules tend to coalesce and form amorphous, dense conglomerates of radiodensities. Poorly defined, small nodular radiodensities can also be associated with a diffusely increased background interstitial density or a reticular interstitial pattern (reticulonodular pattern). Lymphosarcoma and severe pulmonary parenchymal fibrosis are the most likely diagnoses associated with a reticulonodular pattern. Poorly defined, small nodules can also be seen owing to alveolar filling with dense aspirated material— i.e., barium.

Table 6. *Diseases With Ill-Defined Nodules*

Acute alveolar diseases (edema, hemorrhage, contusion)
Hemorrhage due to coagulopathies or severe trauma
Metastatic or disseminated primary neoplasia
Disseminated granulomatous diseases (parasitic, fungal, bacterial)
Pulmonary lymphosarcoma
Massive thromboembolic pneumonia
Aspiration pneumonia (small, 3-mm nodules, alveolarization of barium in dysphagia)

Ill defined, nodular radiodensities of 5 to 8 mm in diameter can be formed by exudates, transudates, granulation tissue, or foreign material accumulating preferentially within the alveoli of one terminal bronchiole (acinus) while leaving adjacent areas relatively unaffected. Indistinct borders of a nodule can also be caused by preferentially interstitially located disease spreading or spilling over into adjoining air spaces or extensively compressing them.

Although most pulmonary parenchymal diseases are characterized by one of the aforementioned categories of radiodensities, there are a few that defy classification. In some cases, it may be difficult to decide in which class a density fits because elements of various categories can be present simultaneously. This can be due to coexistence of two or more different disease processes within the lung, but it may also be caused by simultaneous visualization of acute and chronic phases of the same disease. The tendency to try to name the pattern in every case entails guesswork and should not be done. Associated lesions, such as cardiomegaly, pleural effusion, or mediastinal or thoracic wall masses, may obscure some of the abnormal pulmonary densities and may interfere with their proper interpretation. Conclusions from radiographs as to the cause of the underlying disease should thus always be drawn only after careful consideration of the circumstances, the history, the physical examination, and laboratory data.

SUPPLEMENTAL READING

Biery, D.N.: Differentiation of lung disease of inflammatory or neoplastic origin from lung disease in heart failure. Vet. Clin. North Am. *4*:711–721, 1974.

Silverman, S., and Suter, P.F.: Influence of inspiration and expiration on canine thoracic radiographs. J. Am. Vet. Med. Assoc. *166*:502–510, 1975.

Silverman, S., Poulos, P.W., and Suter, P.F.: Cavitary pulmonary lesions in animals, J. Am. Vet. Rad. Soc. *17*:134–146, 1976.

Suter, P.F., and Lord, P. F.: Radiographic differentiation of disseminated pulmonary parenchymal diseases in dogs and cats. Vet. Clin. North Am. *4*:687–710, 1974.

Ticer, J.W.: *Radiographic Technique in Small Animal Practice.* Philadelphia, W.B. Saunders Co., 1975, p. 285.

LARYNGEAL PARALYSIS IN YOUNG BOUVIERS

A.J. VENKER–van HAAGEN

Utrecht, The Netherlands

The Bouvier has become a very popular dog in The Netherlands as a family companion, watchdog, training-sport dog, and police dog. The recent growth in popularity of the breed resulted in a population explosion accompanied by a remarkable incidence of spontaneous laryngeal paralysis, a case of which has now also been reported in the United States. Reports on the characteristics of the disease have been based on studies in 105 affected Bouviers, and surgical intervention has now been performed in 120. Since the surgical procedure results in a permanently opened glottis, and hence loss of voice, only dogs kept as family companions are considered for surgery. There is strong evidence that the disease is transmitted hereditarily in Bouviers and thus owners are always advised not to breed affected dogs.

DIAGNOSIS

Laryngeal paralysis in young Bouviers is characterized by increasing loss of endurance, increasing laryngeal stridor, dyspnea, and cyanosis and vomiting during episodes of severe dyspnea. In most cases, the onset of clinical signs occurs at four to six months of age. Diagnosis of laryngeal abductor dysfunction can be made accurately by laryngoscopy if the examination is carried out under light anesthesia with sodium pentobarbital. Lidocaine spray can be used to control reflex swallowing. Secondary laryngitis is a consistent finding, and pharyngitis and tonsilitis are also frequently present. The vocal folds are slightly separated, as in dogs in deep anesthesia, and their movements are irregular. Occasionally, one or both folds are adducted briefly during expiration, but there is no definite wide abduction during inspiration, as should occur even under light anesthesia. The lack of abduction should be confirmed by continuous observation during several deep inspirations.

Electromyographic recordings from the individual intrinsic muscles of the larynx show denervation potentials in several but not always the same muscles. In most cases, both abductor muscles (left and right dorsal cricoarytenoid) are affected. Histologic evidence of neurogenic atrophy is found in biopsies of the affected muscles, and Wallerian degeneration has been demonstrated in the recurrent nerves obtained at autopsy.

TREATMENT

Spontaneous laryngeal paralysis in young Bouviers almost always results in severe dyspnea and is sometimes fatal without prompt surgical intervention. Clinical examination and hospital admission often constitute a severe enough stress to evoke acute dyspnea, which necessitates immediate intubation followed by tracheostomy. A small dose of sodium pentobarbital is administered intravenously to permit intubation with a normal endotracheal tube. The dog does not need supplementary oxygen (and indeed this may be contraindicated), but artificial breathing is sometimes needed for a short period. As soon as breathing is normal, surgical anesthesia is instituted and the tracheostomy is performed.

For tracheostomy, the dog is placed in dorsal recumbency with a small sand bag under the neck, which facilitates good exposure of the trachea. A 1.5 cm skin incision is made across the trachea midway between the larynx and the thoracic inlet. The left and right sternohyoideus muscles are separated to expose the trachea and a fragment of its wall (1.5 tracheal rings in length and of similar width) is removed. A Silastic cannula with an exchangeable inner cannula is inserted and fixed in place. The inner tube must be removed and cleansed every two hours after tracheostomy and every hour after laryngeal surgery. The cannula remains in place until the third day after laryngeal surgery. An antibiotic is administered systemically from the time of tracheostomy until the eighth day after laryngeal surgery. Even if laryngeal surgery cannot be performed in the clinic to which the dog is admitted initially, a tracheostomy should be performed if acute dyspnea occurs, before the dog is moved elsewhere.

The aim of laryngeal surgery is permanent abduction of one vocal fold by lateral fixation of

290

the corresponding arytenoid cartilage. Only a brief outline of the operation is given here, but a detailed and illustrated description has been presented (Harvey and Venker-van Haagen, 1975). One side of the larynx is exposed by a ventral paramedian incision in the skin. After a 1 cm long transection is made in the thyropharyngeus muscle, the dorsal edge of the thyroid cartilage is lifted and its connection to the cricoid cartilage is severed. The arytenoid cartilage is disconnected from the cricoid cartilage and the ligamental connection between the two arytenoid cartilages is also severed. The arytenoid cartilage is then fixed to the caudodorsal edge of the thyroid cartilage with stainless steel wire. The manipulation of the arytenoid cartilage and the point of its fixation must be guided by the advice of an assistant who is evaluating the effect by laryngoscopy. If histologic confirmation of the diagnosis is desired, a biopsy of the dorsal circoarytenoid muscle can be obtained by severing the muscle from the cricoid. Immediately following surgical closure, blood clots in the pharynx and nasopharynx are removed carefully.

Food is withheld until the third day after surgery. Since the operation results in a permanently opened glottis, the dog makes noisy efforts to cough up mucus and occasionally particles of food, but it learns to manage this easily within the first month.

The result of this operation is the restoration of an adequate airway for the normal activities of a companion dog. Since only one of the vocal folds is abducted, long and strenuous exercise cannot be tolerated, but both the dog and its owner soon learn the limits of comfortable exertion. It should be noted that better results are not obtained by performing lateral fixation on both sides, because the larynx is narrowed by scar tissue resulting from the more extensive surgical trauma.

SUPPLEMENTAL READING

Harvey, C.E., and Venker-van Haagen, A.J.: Surgical management of pharyngeal and laryngeal airway obstruction in the dog. Vet. Clin. North Am. 5:515–535, 1975.

Reinke, J.D., and Suter, P.F.: Laryngeal paralysis in a dog. J. Am. Vet. Med. Assoc. 172:714–716, 1978.

Venker-van Haagen, A.J., Hartman, W., and Goedegebuure, S.A.: Spontaneous laryngeal paralysis in young Bouviers. J. Am. Anim. Hosp. Assoc. 14:714–720, 1978.

Section
4

CARDIOVASCULAR DISEASES

STEPHEN J. ETTINGER, D.V.M.
Consulting Editor

Cardiopulmonary Resuscitation for People 293
Cardiac Arrest 297
Valvular Heart Disease 297
Cardiomyopathy in the Dog and Cat 307
Myocardial Disease 316
Pericardial Disease 321
Canine Heartworm Disease 326
Cor Pulmonale 335
Diseases of the Peripheral Lymphatics: Lymphedema 337
Influence of Non-cardiac Disease on the Heart 340
Cardiovascular System of the Racing Dog 347
Pharmacodynamics of Digitalis, Diuretics, and Antiarrhythmic
  Drugs 352
Acute Heart Failure 359
Long-Term Therapy of Chronic Congestive Heart Failure in
  the Dog and Cat 368
Bradycardia 376
Tachyarrhythmia 381

Additional Pertinent Information, Still Current, to be Found in Current Veterinary Therapy VI:

Breznock, E. M.: Patent ductus arteriosus, p. 400.
Buchanen, J. W.: Pulmonic stenosis, p. 403.
Ettinger, S. J.: Introduction to the diagnosis and management of heart disease, p. 313.
Fregin, G. F.: General guidelines for clinical examination of the cardiovascular system in large animals, p. 410.
Muir, W.: Anesthesia for the dog with heart disease, p. 388.
Pyle, R. L.: Common congenital heart defects: Aortic stenosis, p. 392; Atrial septal defect, p. 394; Ventricular septal defect, p. 395; Tetralogy of Fallot, p. 397; Persistent right aortic arch, p. 398.

Additional Pertinent Information, Still Current, to be Found in Current Veterinary Therapy V:

Knight, D. H.: Principles of cardiac catheterization, p. 251.
Tilley, L. P., Lord, P. F., and Wood, A.: Acquired heart disease and aortic thromboembolism in the cat, p. 305.

CARDIOPULMONARY RESUSCITATION FOR PEOPLE*

BARRY R. HORN, M.D.,
and AMY H. ANSFIELD, R.R.T.
Berkeley, California

Cardiopulmonary resuscitation, or CPR, is a first-aid procedure that includes (1) the recognition of cardiac and/or respiratory arrest and (2) the application of proper resuscitation techniques in order to provide basic life support. The primary techniques of CPR include (1) provision of an open airway and adequate ventilation and (2) circulation of oxygenated blood. Artificial circulation of unoxygenated blood will not result in a successful resuscitation, so both ventilation and circulation must be provided.

CPR techniques have been defined for the witnessed and unwitnessed arrests, and the proper sequence thereof is shown in Table 1. A witnessed arrest is one in which an individual has been seen to collapse or an arrest has been noted on a cardiac monitor. An individual who is unconscious for an unknown length of time or for more than one minute is defined as having an unwitnessed arrest. This differentiation is important because a circulatory collapse of one minute or less indicates the victim still has adequately oxygenated blood, and the proper sequence of techniques applied is different.

*Editor's note: The authors have described basic techniques in *human* cardiopulmonary resuscitation (CPR). Veterinary and paramedical personnel should learn these procedures now, since in emergencies, time is precious. Read carefully, and better yet, enroll in a full course with the Red Cross or the American Heart Association.

THE WITNESSED ARREST

The initial step to perform when confronted with an apparently unresponsive individual is to determine his or her state of consciousness. This can be done by providing both vocal and tactile stimuli. Gently shake the individual, pinch the shoulder, and shout. If the individual responds, CPR should not be administered.

If the individual is unconscious, open the airway using the head-tilt method. At times, this is the only procedure required to help the victim resume spontaneous breathing. The technique involves pushing down on the forehead with one hand and tilting up under the neck with the other (Fig. 1). When using this technique, the neck and jaw are extended, lifting the tongue from the back of the throat and allowing for a patent airway.

Next, locate the carotid pulse by placing two fingers on the larynx and then sliding them into the groove adjacent to the trachea, over the carotid artery. If there is no pulse, perform a precordial thump. First, locate the middle of the sternum, halfway between the suprasternal notch and the xiphoid process. Raise an extended arm 8 to 12 inches above the middle of the sternum and deliver one sharp blow with the fleshy portion of the fist. When delivering a precordial thump to a heart with oxygenated blood, an electrical stimulus sufficient to return the heart to a normal rhythm may be created. However, if this is

Table 1. *Techniques Used in the Witnessed and Unwitnessed Arrest*

WITNESSED ARREST	UNWITNESSED ARREST
Step 1: Determine consciousness	Step 1: Determine consciousness
Step 2: Open airway	Step 2: Open airway
Step 3: Check carotid pulse	Step 3: Check for breathing
Step 4: Give one precordial thump	Step 4: Give four quick breaths
Step 5: Open airway and give four quick breaths	Step 5: Check carotid pulse
Step 6: Check carotid pulse	Step 6: Begin cardiac compressions
Step 7: Begin cardiac compressions	

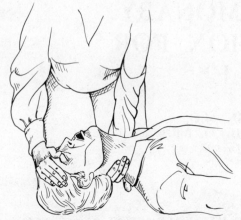

Figure 1. Note hand on forehead "pushing down" and hand under neck "lifting up"; jaw is extended upward.

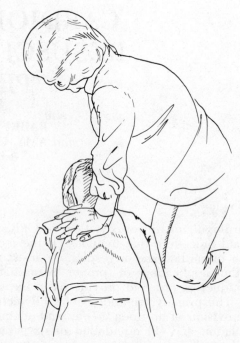

Figure 3. The heel of the hand should be 1 to 1½ inches above the xiphoid process. Pressure is directed downward over the sternum. Fingers should be off the chest, elbows locked, and arms straight.

performed on a heart with unoxygenated blood, it may lead to more severe arrhythmias. The precordial thump should be performed only once.

After doing the precordial thump, immediately open the airway with the head-tilt method and give four quick breaths. To provide adequate mouth-to-mouth resuscitation, pinch the nose with the hand performing the head-tilt, seal your mouth over the victim's mouth, and deliver four separate breaths in rapid succession without allowing for complete lung deflation between breaths. If ventilation is adequate, the chest will rise and fall (Fig. 2). Next, reopen the airway and check the carotid pulse to see if the precordial thump was effective. If there is no pulse, begin cardiac compression.

The proper position for performing cardiac compression is with the heel of the hand on the lower half of the sternum, 1 to 1.5 inches above the tip of the xiphoid process. Place the other hand on top of the first hand and bring the shoulders directly over the victim's sternum (Fig. 3). Interlock the fingers to avoid pressure on the rib cage, since this may result in rib fractures. Compression should be straight downward in a rhythmic, uninterrupted, smooth fashion with the arms straight and elbows locked. Compression depth on an adult is 1.5 to 2 inches. Contact should be maintained with the sternum at all times, but complete relaxation should occur on the upstroke of the compression cycle to allow for cardiac filling during diastole.

Proper hand placement on the sternum is critical in providing adequate CPR. Compression over the xiphoid process may lead to laceration of the liver, whereas compression higher on the sternum will produce an inadequate cardiac output.

THE UNWITNESSED ARREST

When it takes a rescuer longer than one minute to reach a victim, or if the time of collapse is unknown, the initial step is to determine unconsciousness by using vocal and tactile stimuli. Next, open the airway using the head-tilt method and check for breathing. Look, listen, and feel for the passage of air. If there is no breathing, give four quick breaths. Then check the carotid pulse. If there is no

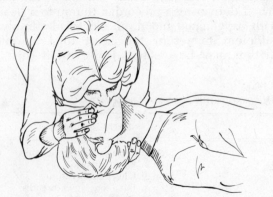

Figure 2. Maintain head tilt with hand on forehead "pushing down" and hand under neck "lifting up"; pinch nose and form a complete seal.

pulse, determine proper hand position and proceed with external cardiac compression (see Table 1).

ONE AND TWO PERSON RESCUES

CPR may be done with one or two rescuers. A single rescuer may perform both chest compressions and ventilatory maneuvers. The chest is compressed at a rate of 80 per minute. The rescuer performs 15 compressions, moves to the head, and delivers two quick deep breaths. He then returns to the chest for 15 more compressions and continues the sequence, which delivers approximately 60 compressions and 8 breaths per minute.

When there are two rescuers, CPR can be performed uninterrupted. The individual performing the cardiac compressions gives one compression per second, or 60 compressions per minute. A breath is interposed on the upstroke of every fifth compression, or once every five seconds. This achieves a rate of 60 compressions per minute and a ventilatory rate of 12 per minute. The compressions should not be interrupted to deliver a breath. Such an interruption will result in a drop of blood flow and systolic blood pressure.

When doing two-rescuer CPR, to avoid fatigue and maintain effective technique, it may be necessary to change places. After a set of five compressions and one breath, person A (doing the chest compressions) moves to the head, opens the airway, and checks for the return of breathing and a pulse. Person B (doing the ventilations) moves to the chest and locates proper hand position. If there is no pulse and no breathing, person A gives one breath and signals to person B to continue compressions. CPR by two rescuers can best be performed when they are on opposite sides of the victim.

Additional key points to remember for proper CPR are (1) the pupillary response to light should be checked periodically as an indication of adequate oxygenation of the brain, (2)

be certain that proper CPR will be maintained before transportation is initiated, and (3) CPR should not be interrupted for more than five seconds at a time except for endotracheal intubation, transportation, or defibrillation, and then for no more than 15 seconds.

THE OBSTRUCTED AIRWAY

Obstruction of the airway by a foreign body has become a relatively common cause of death. It may be caused by the tongue, food, dentures, or other objects. Recognition of an obstructed airway is the key to delivering prompt assistance. An obstructed airway may occur in a conscious or an unconscious victim. The sequence of steps to follow in clearing an obstructed airway for both the conscious and the unconscious victim is the same, with a few differences in position (Table 2).

When a conscious person appears to be choking, it is important to determine whether the obstruction is partial or complete. The easiest way to do this is to ask, "Can you speak?" If the individual can speak or move air, encourage a strong cough to clear the obstruction. If the victim cannot cough or make any significant sounds, consider it a complete obstruction. Position yourself behind and to the side of the victim. Provide physical support by placing your arm under the victim's arm and across his chest, and deliver four sharp back blows between the scapulae (Fig. 4). Next, encircle the victim with your arms and position the thumb portion of the fist between the umbilicus and the xiphoid process. Grasp this hand with the other and proceed with four firm abdominal thrusts, pulling inward and upward (Fig. 5). If the airway continues to be obstructed, repeat the sequence of four back blows and four abdominal thrusts.

When initiating resuscitation in an unwitnessed cardiac arrest, the steps are (1) determine unconsciousness, (2) open the airway, (3) check for breathing. If there is no breathing, attempt to ventilate. Failure to ventilate indi-

Table 2. Techniques Used in the Obstructed Airway

CONSCIOUS VICTIM	UNCONSCIOUS VICTIM
Step 1: Determine partial or complete obstruction; "Can you speak?"	Step 1: Reposition head and attempt to ventilate
Step 2: Deliver four back blows	Step 2: Roll the victim toward you and deliver four back blows
Step 3: Deliver four abdominal thrusts	Step 3: Roll the victim onto his back with his head to the side and deliver four abdominal thrusts
Step 4: If airway continues to be obstructed, repeat sequence	Step 4: Clear the airway (crossed-finger technique)
	Step 5: Attempt to ventilate
	Step 6: If unable to ventilate, repeat sequence

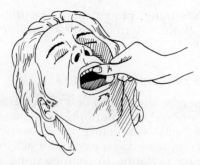

Figure 6. Cross-finger technique. Have fingers crossed with the thumb on the upper teeth and the index finger on the lower teeth. Make sure fingers are near the corner of the mouth.

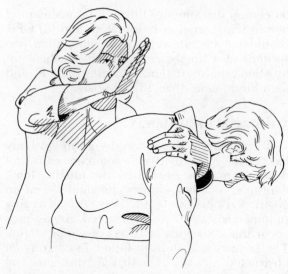

Figure 4. Back blows. These are used in the obstructed airway technique. Provide physical support by placing your arm under the victim's armpit and across his chest. Deliver four back blows between the scapulae.

cates an obstructed airway in the unconscious victim. The initial step is to reposition the head and attempt to ventilate again, because the tongue is the most common obstruction. If

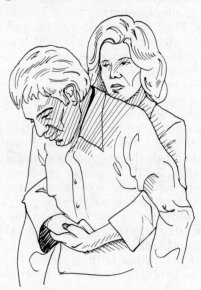

Figure 5. Abdominal thrusts. These are done after the four back blows. Using the proper hand position, pull inward and upward four times.

this is still unsuccessful, roll the victim toward you and deliver four sharp back blows between the scapulae. Next, roll the person onto his back, turn the head to the side, and deliver four abdominal thrusts. Place one hand over the heel of the other, between the xiphoid process and the umbilicus, and apply pressure inward and upward. After doing the abdominal thrusts, open the mouth and attempt to clear the airway with your fingers. The easiest way is to use the crossed-finger technique (Fig. 6). This consists of placing the index finger on the lower teeth and the thumb on the upper teeth and pushing them apart. Once the mouth is open, maintain the crossed-finger position and use two fingers of the other hand to perform a sweep of the mouth. Start at one surface of the cheek, proceed to the back of the airway, and sweep across and out. Using this maneuver avoids pushing any foreign body back into the airway. After clearing the airway, reposition the head with the head-tilt method and attempt to ventilate. If the airway is still obstructed, repeat the sequence until adequate ventilation can be given. Once ventilation is adequate, continue with CPR if necessary.

The described techniques are the basic steps in resuscitation. In order to become proficient in the application of these techniques, a course offered by the American Red Cross or the American Heart Association is strongly recommended.

CARDIAC ARREST

STEPHEN J. ETTINGER, D.V.M.
Walnut Creek, California

I. NOTE IF ANIMAL HAS:
Heart Beat
Pulse
Spontaneous Respiration
Pupils – If dilated and fixed, prognosis less favorable

II. IDENTIFY PROBLEM QUICKLY
Cardiac Arrest(?)
Brief Seizure
Syncope Only
Foreign Body in Throat
Respiratory Arrest
Terminal (Non-resuscitative)

III. STEPS TO TAKE IN ORDER OF IMPORTANCE
1. *Strong thrust to left ventral thorax:* To initiate cardiac beat.
2. *Begin external thoracic compression:* i.e., heart and lung massage.
3. *Intubate animal with endotracheal tube:* Begin artificial respiration through tube via compression of oxygen-filled bag on anesthesia breathing machine *or* blow into tube, expanding lungs at 8–12 breaths per minute.
4. *Continue external cardiac compression:* Four cardiac compressions should follow each expansion of the lungs. *Do not* compress thorax manually while expanding lungs. Attempt 40–60 compressions per minute.
   Compress thorax with animal in right lateral recumbency. Place one hand under right thorax while using base of other hand to compress left ventral thorax. Compress in direction from ventral to dorsal.
5. *Check for spontaneous respiration and/or heart beat:* If present, monitor animal and discontinue resuscitation. Check pupillary light response, pulse, and respiratory rate. Monitor ECG if rate is rapid, slow, or irregular. If no pulse or heart beat is noted, continue with Step 6.
6. *Intracardiac injection:* (Best at I.C. 4–5 near costochondral junction) Isuprel 0.2–0.5 ml or epinephrine (1:10,000– 0.2–0.5 ml). Continue to respirate artificially and massage the heart.
7. *Monitor ECG:* Watch for arrhythmias, arrest, or ventricular fibrillation.
8. *Begin IV fluids:* Place an indwelling cephalic catheter and begin rapid infusion of saline or Ringer's solution. If cardiac rate is slow but present, add Isuprel to drip and monitor response while varying infusion rate.
9. *Sodium bicarbonate:* Give 5–10 ml IV initially and continue to give IV bolus every 10–12 minutes during resuscitation.
10. *Continue artificial respiration:* Give calcium gluconate slowly IV to stimulate heart. Lidocaine if multiple ventricular arrhythmias are present. Give Isuprel to maintain adequate sinus rate.

READERS:
*Please photocopy this chart and distribute to all employees. Post in hospital and have regular drills to be prepared for such an event.

VALVULAR HEART DISEASE

KENNETH W. KNAUER, D.V.M.
College Station, Texas

Mitral valve insufficiency owing to chronic valvular endocardiosis is the most common acquired heart disease in the dog. Approximately 75 percent of dogs exhibiting signs of congestive heart failure have this syndrome. Tricuspid insufficiency, valvular endocarditis, and aortic insufficiency are acquired valvular heart diseases of the dog that occur less frequently than mitral valve insufficiency but also deserve discussion.

Congenital valvular defects of significance in the dog are pulmonic stenosis and aortic stenosis. Pulmonic stenosis is usually valvular but may be subvalvular or supravalvular, and it constitutes approximately 20 percent of all congenital heart defects seen in the dog. Aortic stenosis constitutes 15 percent of all congenital defects and tends to be subvalvular rather than valvular. Congenital mitral and tricuspid valve insufficiencies are occasionally seen but are of very low incidence.

The incidence of acquired and congenital heart diseases in the cat is much lower than that in the dog. The most prevalent acquired valvular defects in the cat are mitral and aortic valvular defects secondary to cardiomyopathy and vegetative valvular endocarditis. (Feline cardiomyopathy will be covered in a following chapter.) Valvular congenital heart anomalies in the cat of clinical importance are dysplasia of the tricuspid valve, malformation of the mitral valve complex, and aortic stenosis.

CHRONIC MITRAL VALVULAR FIBROSIS

Chronic mitral valvular fibrosis (CMVF) is the leading cause of congestive heart failure in the dog. The resulting mitral insufficiency produces slowly progressive left heart failure accounting for approximately 75 percent of dogs with congestive heart failure. The syndrome usually begins at two to five years of age, with an audible systolic mitral murmur detectable at about five to eight years of age. Signs of left ventricular failure become apparent at about eight to ten years of age, with generalized congestive heart failure occurring at ten to fourteen years of age. Chronic mitral valvular fibrosis occurs in the cat but with much less frequency than in the dog, and the sequence of progression occurs much later in life. It is seen most frequently in toy and miniature breeds, especially those of the chondrodystrophoid type. CMVF seems to lead to congestive heart failure at an earlier age in male cocker spaniels than it does in other breeds.

ETIOLOGY

Chronic mitral valvular fibrosis has been referred to as mitral insufficiency, chronic valvular myxomatosis, valvular endocardiosis, nodular valvitis, warty valve disease, chronic valvular heart disease, valvular endocarditis, and fibrous endocarditis. The etiology of the syndrome is unknown; however, an age-related increase in frequency and severity, coupled with an absence of inflammatory changes, suggests a degenerative process. The valvular lesions start with an early fragmentation of elastic fibers and fibroplasia. This is followed by an increase in acid mucopolysaccharide deposition in the subendothelial and fibroelastic layers of the valve margin. Firm nodular thickening at the free margin of the valve cusps ensues, often involving the chordae tendinae at the junction of the valve cusps. A few fibrotic nodules may be present, causing little interference with normal valve function, or there may be complete fibrosis and contracture of the valve producing an inelastic, rigid valve and profound mitral insufficiency.

Chronic mitral valve fibrosis with its resulting mitral insufficiency is actually a syndrome involving the whole mitral valve complex along with a concurrently developing microscopic intramural myocardial infarction of the left ventricular myocardium. The mitral complex refers to the septal and lateral mitral valve leaflets, the mitral valve annulus, the chordae tendinae, the papillary muscles, and the left ventricular muscle wall. The mitral complex is a finely coordinated system responsible for the closure of the mitral valve and the maintenance of its competence. The mitral insufficiency syndrome is a disease of insult to the mitral valve apparatus, and all components are usually involved as the disease progresses. Normally about half the mitral valve leaflets overlap when closed, producing a tight seal. As chronic valvular fibrosis progresses, the nodular, shortened leaflets become deformed and bulky and resist tight closure, or areas develop that do not overlap. The mitral valve annulus forms a base of attachment for the valve leaflets. In the chronic mitral valve disease syndrome, the atrioventricular support ring may dilate secondary to left ventricular dilatation, or it may lose its efficient sphincter action during systole due to inefficient contraction of a failing left ventricle. Regurgitant blood flow is further intensified by these changes. With intensification of the regurgitant flow into the left atrium, the posterior left atrial wall dilates, thereby raising the free-wall leaflet of the mitral valve dorsally and posteriorly. This further increases regurgitant volume into the left atrium. The primary and secondary chordae tendinae extend from the edge of the valve leaflets to the papillary muscles and the tertiary chordae extend from the leaflets to the ventricular wall. The same "myxomatous" process occurs in the chordae as in the valves. The chordae may shorten and thicken to prevent tight closure of the valve or may stretch, causing a portion of the valve leaflet to be everted into the left ventricle, producing the so-called "parachute" or "floppy valve syndrome."

Intramural coronary artery arteriosclerosis producing microscopic intramural myocardial infarctions is a constant, progressive finding in dogs with chronic mitral valvular fibrosis. The dysfunction produced especially in the papillary muscles but also in the left ventricular and atrial myocardium contributes to the degree of mitral complex dysfunction.

SYMPTOMS

Chronic mitral valvular disease may begin early in a dog's life, but progression is usually slow. Cardiovascular compensatory mechanisms come into effect, and many canine patients with the syndrome never show significant clinical signs. Cardiac reserve maintains normal cardiac output despite large regurgitant flows. The left atrium is very distensible and will allow a large regurgitant flow before pulmonary venous hypertension occurs, leading to pulmonary edema.

Early cases of compensated mitral insufficiency are asymptomatic. As the disease progresses, signs of mild decompensation occur. An early morning deep resonant cough usually develops first. Dogs may fluctuate between compensation and decompensation at this early stage. A small amount of white or blood-tinged foam may be expectorated or coughed up and swallowed following a coughing paroxysm. Dyspnea and/or tachypnea may also be present. Coughing becomes progressively more frequent and may be present throughout the day, or it may follow the drinking of water or exercise. The patient may then progress to restlessness at night owing to an inability to breathe while recumbent (orthopnea). Constant, diffuse pulmonary edema ensues, producing crepitant and moist rales on auscultation. Right heart failure secondary to the primary left heart failure will eventually occur, producing peripheral venous engorgement, hepatomegaly, ascites, and infrequently, subcutaneous edema. Atrial stretching and degeneration owing to microscopic intramural myocardial infarction may produce atrial premature beats or paroxysmal atrial tachycardia. These dogs are often presented because of episodes of syncope.

The general condition of affected dogs ranges from excellent to moribund, depending on the progression of the disease. The mucous membranes are usually of normal color but may be "muddy" or cyanotic in more advanced cases. Dogs may stand with the head and neck extended and elbows abducted to try to enhance air exchange. Coughing may be present and may be elicited by tracheal palpation. A precordial thrill is present when the intensity of the murmur is grade IV or V. The thrill is palpable over the left lower fifth or sixth intercostal space, which corresponds to the point of maximal auscultatory intensity of the murmur. A pronounced left apical thrust may be palpated in thin dogs in this same area. The pulse may be normal or of the pulsus alternans variety. In advanced cases, a rapid, jerky "water-hammer" pulse may palpated. Pulse deficits are present when atrial fibrillation, ventricular premature contractions, or atrial premature beats occur. The abdomen is unremarkable unless right heart failure has ensued, producing ascites and liver enlargement.

A soft, early systolic murmur is associated with early chronic mitral valvular fibrosis. The murmur becomes more intense and pansystolic as the disease progresses. Occasionally, a mid-systolic click precedes the development of a murmur. The usual murmur is a medium-frequency sound, but occasionally a high-frequency musical or "sea gull whoop" murmur may be heard. The murmur is most intense at the left apex at the sternal border and radiates cranially, dorsally, and to the right as it intensifies. It may mimic the murmur of tricuspid valve insufficiency or may be associated with concurrent tricuspid valve fibrosis.

The intensity of the first heart sound increases early in the syndrome and then decreases. If pulmonary hypertension ensues, the second heart sound becomes more intense. Low-frequency third and/or fourth heart sounds or summation gallop rhythms occur in dogs that are in congestive heart failure. These sounds are due to the rapid dumping of blood from the enlarged left atrium into the over-distended left ventricle on diastole. Normal respiratory sinus arrhythmia is the usual rhythm auscultated in most dogs with chronic mitral valvular fibrosis. As the syndrome progresses, premature contractions occur, producing early sounds, and intensity of the murmur diminishes or disappears. The second sound may be absent. The normal sinus rhythm is interrupted by bursts of rapid beats that start and end abruptly when paroxysmal tachycardias occur. Late in the syndrome, atrial fibrillation may develop. This is characterized by a very rapid irregular rate with variable intensity to the murmur and the first and second heart sounds.

DIAGNOSIS

The radiographic examination of most cardiovascular patients is the "thumb" and most important part of the "five fingers of cardiovascular diagnosis." (Others are ECG, signalment, history, auscultation, and laboratory tests.) This pertains to chronic mitral valvular fibrosis. The radiographic changes present often determine into which phase the patient has progressed, and they serve as useful guides to the effectiveness of therapy. Progress films may also be helpful for ascertaining long-term prognosis. Left atrial enlargement is the first change to occur with chronic mitral valvular fibrosis. The enlarging left atrium elevates the trachea in the lateral view, reducing the angle between the trachea and the thoracic spine. The normal ventral deviation of the trachea just cranial to the carina is eliminated. With a very large left atrium, a "bronchial Y sign" is produced on the lateral view by the left mainstem bronchus being elevated dorsally by the enlarging left atrium. The engorged pulmonary veins stand out prominently and make the left atrium appear as a "wedge" where they drain into it from the diaphragmatic lobe. The left atrium may become so enlarged that it presses on the ventral vertebral bodies and may also compress the main stem bronchi. Dilatation of the left atrium and enlargement of the left ventricle result in straightening of the left caudal cardiac silhouette on the lateral view. As the left atrium enlarges grossly, it protrudes past the left heart border at the 2 to 4 o'clock position on the dorsoventral view The left ventricle becomes more rounded and eventually the right ventricle also begins to enlarge. Pulmonary interstitial infiltrates first develop at the hilar area and spread to the periphery as progressive pulmonary edema develops. In cases with severe pulmonary edema, air bronchograms are present.

The electrocardiogram in early mitral valvular fibrosis is usually normal. Early changes associated with mitral fibrosis are a slurring and sometimes notching of the downslope of the R wave, and ST repolarization changes owing to arteriosclerosis with attendant microscopic intramural myocardial infarctions. As the left atrium enlarges, the P wave becomes wider than 0.04 seconds and may be notched. Left ventricular enlargement is noted by prolongation of the QRS complex to greater than 0.05 seconds in small and medium dogs or to more than 0.06 seconds in large breeds. The amplitude in lead II is greater than 2.5 millivolts and aVF and V_3 are larger than 3.0 millivolts. The mean electrical axis in the frontal plane usually remains normal. As the right heart beings to fail, P waves of greater than 0.4 millivolts, indicating right atrial enlargement, may appear. Right ventricular enlargement may be noted by deep Q waves in leads II, III, and aVF, an S wave in lead I, and a deep S wave in V_3, or right axis deviation in the frontal plane. The rhythm is usually a normal sinus rhythm in early mitral valve fibrosis. Compensatory sinus tachycardia develops when cardiac decompensation occurs. Atrial, atrioventricular, or junctional premature contractions may also occur. Single premature ventricular contractions may develop with progression to multifocal ventricular premature beats and paroxysmal ventricular tachycardia. Paroxysmal atrial tachycardia and atrial fibrillation may be seen also in advanced cases. The importance of more frequent serial electrocardiograms as the disease progresses is emphasized. Significant changes are often noted that directly relate to treatment and prognosis.

Laboratory findings in dogs with chronic valvular disease are not very enlightening until very late in the course of the disease. There may be a slight decrease in the PCV due to an increased total blood volume. The BUN and SGPT values are initially normal and then become slightly elevated owing to pre-renal uremia and passive venous congestion of the liver. The total protein is slightly decreased and the serum electrolytes usually remain normal. If concurrent bronchopneumonia is present, the WBC may be elevated.

TREATMENT

Management of chronic mitral valvular fibrosis must be individualized to each animal and its owner. The importance of superb initial and follow-up client education cannot be overemphasized. Client dissatisfaction can be quite high, especially in the latter stages of the syndrome when treatment needs are changing frequently. A written client information sheet is helpful in this regard. Gradually increasing the examination frequency will allow evaluation of treatment so that the primary goal of a better quality of life may be achieved.

When the murmur is first discovered early in life and the dog is asymptomatic, no treatment is needed. This is the time to use the heart murmur as a "psychologic lever" to get the client to reduce the patient to a normal, or slightly subnormal, body weight. For added emphasis, the client may be told that digoxin, which will be used to treat the heart when it starts to fail, is dosed on lean body mass and therefore is less likely to be toxic if the dog is maintained at the proper body weight. Six- to twelve-month rechecks are recommended until the patient shows mild left sided congestive heart failure. Diet education is emphasized, but only heavily salted foods such as ham and pretzels are restricted at this time.

The dog should be fed once daily, in the morning. Treats and dog biscuits should be replaced with hard vegetables. Early left heart failure animals should have severe exercise curtailed; however, moderate activity should be encouraged if possible. Low sodium diets may be instituted at this time. Distilled water can be used for drinking, but some animals can smell the difference and will not drink a normal amount. An animal with chronic compensated renal disease will be hurt more by low fluid intake than his heart will be helped by the few sodium ions in tap water excluded from the diet. By the same token, commercial low sodium diets are not palatable to some dogs If they will eat it, or if the clients are willing to fry it or flavor it with non-salty condiments such as garlic powder, they can be used satisfactorily. The client may prefer to cook a low sodium regimen as recommended for human cardiac patients. Strong emphasis need not be placed on low sodium diets, however. Mild and moderate pulmonary edema and ascites can be managed by diuretics, aminophylline or theophylline, and digoxin.

In the early pulmonary edema case, aminophylline or theophylline are good drugs to use. They are mild inotropic agents, mild diuretics, and good bronchodilators, and they promote sodium excretion by the kidneys. The theophylline elixirs work well in small dogs but some dogs do not like the taste. Because of the volume required, the tablets are a better choice for large patients Many dogs will do well for prolonged periods with this therapy, so that limited rechecks are suggested at four- to six-month intervals.

Digitalis will need to be added to the treatment regimen when the radiographs begin to show moderate cardiac enlargement and pulmonary venous congestion. If moderate or severe pulmonary edema and/or ascites are present, diuretics should also be used. Digoxin (Lanoxin®) is preferred whenever possible. About the only time it cannot be used is in the presence of severe renal impairment. Digoxin may still be used in the presence of an elevated or rising BUN, but the normal calculated maintenance dose is halved each time the normal BUN doubles. When the BUN is 80 or higher, digitoxin is preferred, as it has an enterohepatic metabolic pathway. Lanoxin® is the digoxin of choice because of its proven bioavailability. Because of poor bioavailability, "generic cardiac glycosides" should be avoided. Tablets are preferred over digoxin elixirs because clients more often administer inaccurate dosages with the elixirs than with tablets. Tablet sizes can be obtained for dogs as small as six pounds The single strength elixir (0 05 mg/ml) can be used in dogs smaller than six pounds. The usual accompanying eye dropper should be discarded and a tuberculin syringe should be dispensed for precise dosing. A child-proof cap should be on all digitalis tablets dispensed, as a recent report described the death of a young girl following ingestion of digitoxin tablets prescribed for a dog by a veterinarian. Digoxin should be dosed on lean body mass, subtracting estimated weight related to ascites and obesity. The calculated maintenance dose of 0.022 mg/kg is halved and given BID. Cats are given half of the dog dose (0.011 mg/kg) per day. Giant, very old, and very young dogs will require less digoxin. Maintenance digitalization is used on an outpatient basis in all non-emergency situations. It will take five to seven days to achieve maintenance levels. This is the time for a recheck or a phone call to ascertain if dosage adjustment is necessary. The minimum dosage that will relieve signs without producing toxicity should be used.

Digitalized animals should be rechecked frequently. Mild intermittent diuresis will need to progress to intense everyday treatment with potent diuretics such as furosemide (Lasix®) as the congestive heart failure progresses. Activity will need to be severely curtailed. Intensive diuresis may increase susceptibility to digoxin toxicity and hypokalemia. Electrolytes should be checked periodically when heavily digitalized dogs are receiving concurrent large doses of diuretics, especially if anorexia is a complication. Meat contains a significant amount of potassium, and hypokalemia is not usually a problem if dogs are eating well, but potassium supplements may be needed if appetite is poor.

Arrhythmia suppression will be indicated in the later stages of congestive heart failure. Quinidine sulfate, gluconate, or polygalacturonate is usually effective. It can be used at the rate of 11 mg/kg every six hours.

As a last resort, in refractory heart failure, use may be made of a drug that dilates the veins and arteries, thereby reducing the amount of blood presented to the heart to pump (preload) and taking the workload that it must pump against (afterload) off the left ventricle. Minipress® (prazosin HCl)° may be used as a preload and afterload reducer but must be given only to an already digitalized patient. Minipress® is given TID, and low starting doses are titrated to the individual patient's needs by clinical response.

Acute pulmonary edema emergency cases arising from ruptured chordae tendinae may require O_2, phlebotomy, rotating tourniquets, and low doses of morphine (0.44 mg/kg) SQ, in addition to intravenous diuretics, digoxin, and aminophylline.

TRICUSPID INSUFFICIENCY

Insufficiency of the tricuspid valve in the dog is usually associated with chronic tricuspid valvular fibrosis and occurs in most cases along with chronic mitral valvular fibrosis rather than as an isolated entity. Tricuspid insufficiency occurs with rupture of the tricuspid chorda tendinea, bacterial endocarditis, severe heartworm disease, and tricuspid ring dilatation in idiopathic congestive cardiomyopathy. Congenital defects that may include tricuspid insufficiency

---

°Minipress, Pfizer Laboratories, New York, N.Y.

are Ebstein's anomaly, tricuspid atresia, tricuspid stenosis with moderate orifice, severe PDA and pulmonic stenosis, and persistent A-V canals. Isolated chronic tricuspid valvular fibrosis is seen most often in chondrodystrophoid breeds, particularly the dachshund.

Most dogs with chronic tricuspid fibrosis show left heart failure owing to their concurrent and usually more prominent mitral regurgitation. Those that show isolated right heart failure or biventricular failure will have ascites, weight loss (cardiac cachexia), hepatic and splenic enlargement, possible anorexia, vomiting and diarrhea, and jugular pulsation with total peripheral venous engorgement. A holosystolic murmur is heard at the right fourth to fifth intercostal space at the costochondral junction.

The ECG is not very revealing, as left heart changes usually predominate. Occasionally, isolated right atrial enlargement may present as tall spiked P waves. Late in the syndrome, the rhythm may change to that of atrial fibrillation.

Radiography may also be confusing owing to concurrent left heart disease. When right atrial enlargement is pronounced or isolated, it is seen as a bulge on the anterior border of the cardiac silhouette in the cranial waist area (lateral view). This may elevate the trachea cranial to the carina. The caudal vena cava may be wider and more dense than normal. In the dorsoventral view, the right atrium may protrude at the 9 to 11 o'clock position.

Ascitic fluid is a modified serosanguinous transudate with increased mesothelial cells in long standing cases. Serum values for alkaline phosphatase, SGPT, and BSP retention are usually moderately elevated. Pre-renal uremia of varying degrees may also be present.

Treatment of congestive heart failure owing to tricuspid insufficiency should include diuretics and low sodium diets with emphasis on adequate maintenance digitalization without intoxication. The thin-walled, dilated right atrium may be incapable of generating enough inotropism, even with the aforementioned therapy. At this stage, total rest should be prescribed. These patients will require abdominal paracentesis, which may need to be repeated periodically. When cardiac cachexia is present, high calorie carbohydrate and fatty acid dietary supplements may be used.

PULMONIC STENOSIS

Pulmonic stenosis is the second most frequent congenital heart defect seen in the dog, ranking closely behind patent ductus arteriosus.

Together, they constitute almost 50 per cent of the congenital cardiovascular defects recognized in dogs. The cat exhibits a much lower incidence of isolated pulmonic stenosis. It is approximately the tenth most frequently recognized congenital cardiovascular defect in the cat, but it is present more frequently as a component with other defects such as tetralogy of Fallot. The defect may be hereditary in the beagle hound and is seen more frequently in the English bulldog, schnauzer, chihuahua, and terrier-type breeds.

Pulmonic stenosis may be valvular, which is the most common type in the dog, or subvalvular, as a fibrous constricted ring below the valve in the right ventricular outflow tract. Occasionally, both types are present in the same animal. Infundibular stenosis usually occurs secondarily as the right ventricular outflow tract hypertrophies in response to a distal stenosis. Supravalvular stenosis is the least frequently seen variety (the author has seen 3 such cases in 13 years).

Dogs with pulmonic stenosis are usually asymptomatic. Many will live for several years before showing signs of fatigability, syncopal episodes, ascites, and/or enlarged livers. Mild cases usually have a normal life span.

Pulmonic stenosis is usually first discovered by the incidental finding of a characteristic murmur in a puppy that has been presented for vaccination. The murmur is usually a high frequency ejection type with a point of maximal intensity at the left cranial sternal border. The murmur is a crescendo-decrescendo type and may be accompanied by a palpable thrill and splitting of the second heart sound.

DIAGNOSIS

The electrocardiogram may be normal in mild cases but shows progressive shift to the right of the mean QRS vector in the frontal plane with increasing right ventricular hypertrophy. Large S waves in leads II, aVF, and V_3 indicate the presence of right ventricular hypertrophy.

Radiographic changes include increased right-sided convexity and sometimes rightward deviation of the cardiac silhouette on the dorsoventral view. The main pulmonary artery enlargement that occurs as the result of poststenotic dilatation can be seen as a bulge at the 1 o'clock position in the dorsoventral view. The distal branches of the pulmonary arteries are usually normal, but the main branches of the main pulmonary artery will be enlarged when the stenosis is supravalvular. In the lateral view, right ventricular enlargement and main pulmonary artery poststenotic dilatation may cause loss of the cranial waist as well as elevation of the trachea cranial to its bifurcation.

A non-selective angiocardiogram can be performed to confirm the diagnosis. An iodine-based radiopaque contrast medium is injected rapidly into a jugular vein through an 18 gauge needle. One ml/kg is injected, and a lateral film is exposed at the end of the rapid injection. The thickness of the right ventricular free wall may be determined along with the approximate location of the stenosis and the degree of infundibular hypertrophy. The poststenotic dilatation of the main pulmonary artery is usually well demonstrated by this technique. A direct injection into the right ventricle avoids the superimposition of the right atrial contrast media over the outflow tract, but it carries a slight risk of tamponade or coronary artery laceration.

TREATMENT

If the client can afford to have a cardiac catheterization performed, the case should be referred for this technique. Since many cases of pulmonic stenosis in the moderate category will be asymptomatic early in life but have significant systolic gradients across the pulmonic valve area, the suspected pulmonic stenosis case should be catheterized. Pulmonic stenosis is usually an operable defect, unless the right ventricular outflow tract has become grossly affected by infundibular hypertrophy. Therefore, catheterization is indicated for early identification of cases that could be expected to benefit from surgery.

Dogs with a systolic gradient across the stenotic area less than 50 mm Hg probably do not need to be operated on. Those with gradients above 50 mm Hg will usually benefit from surgery. Sometimes, the stenosis is such that a catheter cannot be passed through the stenotic area to measure the pressure on both sides to determine if a gradient exists. In these cases, if the right ventricular systolic pressure exceeds 100 mm Hg, surgery is usually indicated.

Surgical correction of pulmonic stenosis depends on the type of lesion demonstrated by cardiac catheterization and angiocardiography. Pure valvular stenosis may be improved by inserting pediatric Carmalt forceps through a purse string suture in the right ventricle and splitting and dilating the stenotic valve. However, a case of valvular stenosis may also have a subvalvular component that has not been adequately demonstrated by catheterization and angiography. Therefore, pulmonary arteriotomy using venous inflow occlusion allows a better opportunity for effective relief of the stenosis by allowing direct visualization. If the dog is placed directly on the cold steel surgical table, the body temperature usually falls within the moderate hypothermia category.

Cooling facilitates longer periods of venous inflow occlusion (at least five minutes), allowing repair of the stenosis with a number 11 Bard-Parker scalpel blade. Satinsky forceps applied to the pulmonary artery incision allows leisurely closure when venous inflow is reinstituted. The author has repaired supravalvular stenosis using venous inflow occlusion and pulmonary arteriotomy by resuturing a longitudinal incision over the stenosis in a transverse manner, perpendicular to the flow, thereby effectively enlarging the stenotic area. Rewarming after "cold table hypothermia" may be accomplished by placing a circulating warm water blanket under the dog at circulatory inflow restart time. Severe pulmonic infundibular cases or severely complicated cases such as those of hypoplastic pulmonary arteries are best approached for surgical correction by complete cardiopulmonary bypass techniques. These cases may require time-consuming major remodeling techniques or patch grafting of the outflow tract and main pulmonary artery.

Owners who do not wish to have catheterization and work-up for possible surgery should have periodic rechecks performed on their pets with serial radiographs of the chest and serial electrocardiograms. Dogs that live to be six months of age with no progressive cardiac enlargement on radiographs or concomitant ECG changes will probably have almost normal life spans as asymptomatic individuals. In those cases where symptoms become evident but the owners do not wish to have surgery, symptomatic medical therapy should be instituted. Rest should be enforced, depending on the degree of signs present. Digitalization (preferably with digoxin) should be carried out in symptomatic individuals. If the patient has ascites, diuretics are indicated. In the severely ascitic case, abdominocentesis may be necessary to relieve the pressure on the diaphragm.

AORTIC STENOSIS

Aortic stenosis is the third most common congenital heart defect seen in the dog and the fourth most common in the cat. The site of stenosis is often supravalvular in the cat and almost always subvalvular as a fibromuscular constricted ring in the dog. Valvular aortic stenosis is infrequent in both species, but the valve is often secondarily involved with subvalvular and supravalvular stenoses.

DIAGNOSIS

The resistance to outflow from the left ventricle produced by aortic stenosis produces a small, late-rising femoral pulse. This may be difficult to detect in the cat. Cats are often stunted by this defect and may show signs of left heart failure early in life, usually before two years of age. Dogs, conversely, are often asymptomatic and may remain so for several months to years after diagnosis.

Subaortic stenosis in the dog is usually seen in moderately large breeds and more frequently in the Newfoundland, boxer, German shepherd, and Labrador retriever. Subaortic stenosis has a hereditary tendency in the Newfoundland.

The diagnosis is first suspected when an asymptomatic puppy is presented for its first routine examination. A low-pitched crescendo-decrescendo systolic murmur is heard at the left base of the heart with valvular aortic stenosis. Subvalvular aortic stenosis often is auscultated best on the right sternal border at the fourth intercostal space. The murmur may be heard over the carotid arteries and may be accompanied by a palpable thrill at the thoracic inlet and also at the point of maximal auscultatory intensity on the thorax.

If left heart failure is present, coughing and dyspnea will be evident. In the usual progression of events, the dog remains asymptomatic while profound left ventricular hypertrophy is taking place. When the thickened left ventricle is stressed by increased oxygen demand such as during exercise, arrhythmias, syncopal episodes, or sudden death may occur.

Mild and moderate degrees of aortic stenosis usually present with a relatively normal electrocardiogram in the dog. In advanced cases, left ventricular hypertrophy is evident, while the mean QRS vector in the frontal plane usually remains normal. Leads II, aVF, and V_3 are over 3 mv in amplitude, and ST segment elevation or depression indicating myocardial ischemia may be present. Many feline cases of aortic stenosis show left axis deviation on the ECG, indicating left ventricular enlargement or left anterior fascicular block. With severe left ventricular hypertrophy, arrhythmias such as ventricular premature beats or ventricular tachycardia may be present. Atrial fibrillation is an infrequent finding when secondary mitral insufficiency is present.

Plain film radiographs of the thorax in the lateral view show the poststenotic dilatation of the ascending aorta as a loss of the cranial waist owing to the anterior bulge of the aortic arch. The dorsoventral view shows a wide cranial mediastinum occupied by the enlarged ascending aorta. The left ventricle does not enlarge externally until late in the disease, but it enlarges internally because of concentric hypertrophy. In the late stage, there is left ventricular and left atrial enlargement with pulmonary venous congestion on both views.

Non-selective angiocardiography may be helpful in confirming the diagnosis by demonstrating the area of stenosis and revealing the thickness of the left ventricle and the presence of the poststenotic dilatation in the aorta. A jugular injection of radiopaque contrast media by fast bolus may be made with a lateral film exposed approximately five seconds later. A direct injection into the left ventricle with a long 20 gauge needle gives better contrast without dilution of the media, but this carries a slight risk of cardiac tamponade or direct myocardial wall injection.

Cardiac catheterization is the best method for performing selective angiocardiography via the left ventricle. In later stages, a secondary mitral insufficiency may be demonstrated. Pressure values may be confusing in mild aortic stenosis, because although a significant murmur may be heard, the pressure gradient across the area of aortic stenosis may be negligible. With moderate and severe stenosis, the pressure gradient is quite high, with left ventricular systolic pressures often remarkably elevated.

The aortic valvular and adjacent areas are located at the very center of the heart. This is a difficult area to visualize, even at the autopsy table. The diffuse nature of subaortic stenosis and the technical difficulty of bypass surgery in dogs and cats, coupled with the low percentage of success in attempted surgical corrections, cause the author to feel that for all practical purposes, this is an inoperable defect.

TREATMENT

Medical management of this condition is usually the best approach. No treatment is needed in the asymptomatic animal. Strict enforcement of mild exercise only helps delay the progression of left ventricular hypertrophy and aids in reducing the chance of precipitating fatal and non-fatal ventricular arrhythmias due to myocardial ischemia later in the syndrome. Propranolol is indicated for treatment in cases with moderate to severe left ventricular hypertrophy. Ten to forty mg TID helps the ventricle to fill completely and to empty with a smoother contraction, thereby reducing or delaying the degree of infundibular outflow restriction. This enhances coronary artery blood flow and delays the onset of arrhythmias owing to ischemia.

If left side congestive failure occurs, it should

be managed symptomatically with low salt diets, diuretics, and aminophylline. Digitalis glycosides, carefully monitored, may be used very judiciously as a last resort. Digitalis may cause the degree of infundibular secondary hypertrophy to worsen, thus decreasing coronary perfusion. This, combined with the increased oxygen demand imposed on the ventricle by the strong positive inotropic forces, along with the potential for digitalis glycosides to be arrhythmogenic in an already ischemic ventricle, makes them a last choice in the management scheme.

Antiarrhythmic therapy should be used in animals that show serious of life-threatening arrhythmias. Quinidine, procainamide, and/or disopyramide phosphate (Norpace[R]) are useful for this purpose.

CONGENITAL MITRAL INSUFFICIENCY

Congenital mitral insufficiency is a heart anomaly of relatively low incidence that occurs most often in Great Dane pups and has no sex predilection. The lesion has also been reported in German shepherds, Afghan hounds, and many other breeds. Cats with congenital mitral insufficiency usually have endocardial cushion defects such as persistent common A-V canal.

Great Dane pups have been reported to have an occasional mitral insufficiency with a near normal morphologic mitral apparatus. However, dogs with congenital mitral insufficiency usually have alterations in their mitral valve complex to include enlarged anuli, short thick leaflets with an occasional cleft, short and thick or long and thin chordae tendinae, upward malposition of atrophic or hypertrophic papillary muscles, insertion of one papillary muscle directly into one or both leaflets, and/or diffuse endocardial fibrosis, with occasional jet lesions of the left atrium.

Most dogs with congenital mitral insufficiency show clinical and radiographic evidence of moderate to severe left heart failure with or without right heart failure. Dyspnea, lethargy, intermittent coughing, and a mixed frequency holosystolic murmur at the left caudal sternal border are usually seen clinically. Sudden deaths may occur in severe cases.

Electrocardiograms usually show a biventricular enlargement pattern with deep Q waves and tall R waves in leads II and AVF. The QRS is usually wide as is the P wave, indicating left ventricular and atrial enlargment. Arrhythmias may include sinus tachycardia and atrial and ventricular premature contractions.

Moderate to severe cases show radiographic evidence of pulmonary edema as generalized or partly alveolar-type fluffy densities. Mild cases show prominent pulmonary veins with hazy perivascular patterns. The left atrium is usually enlarged in all cases and may be gigantic, touching the vertebral bodies on the lateral view.

The response to treatment varies considerably with the extent of mitral apparatus deformation. A pup that has mostly secondary annular ring dilatation may be dramatically improved by treatment and live for several months or years. The author has seen an Irish Setter puppy with a harsh left apical systolic murmur, pulmonary edema, and gigantic left atrium return to normal radiographically with disappearance of the murmur in five days, with just cage rest and maintenance digoxin therapy. At the other end of the spectrum are the severely deformed cases that require intense emergency therapy such as oxygen, cage rest, low dose morphine therapy, intravenous digoxin, furosemide, and aminophylline. Some of these respond for a short time but then expire acutely. Moderate cases that respond to initial therapy may usually be maintained at home on rest, digoxin, and diuretics as needed. Appropriate arrhythmia treatment should be used in those requiring it.

VALVULAR AND MURAL ENDOCARDITIS

Endocarditis in the dog and cat is usually a bacterial infection involving the valvular and/or mural endocardium. Mural (or parietal) endocarditis may also be the result of other systemic non-infectious diseases such as nephritis with uremia. Rarely, endocarditis may be of viral or fungal etiology.

The incidence of endocarditis in dogs has varied from 0.58 to 6.6 percent in several studies. Valvular endocarditis occurs most often in valves that sustain the highest closed pressure. The mitral valve is most commonly involved in the dog and cat, followed by the aortic, pulmonic, and tricuspid valves. Bacteremia is a prerequisite for bacterial endocarditis, and pre-existing damage to valves or the mural endocardium facilitates bacterial deposition on platelet thrombi or valvular vegetations. Dogs with acquired or congenital heart disease are predisposed to infectious endocarditis.

Gram-positive non-hemolytic streptococci are the most frequently isolated organisms, although hemolytic streptococci and staphylococci are also common. Other reported organisms include *Pseudomonas aeruginosa*, *E. coli*, and

Erysipelothrix rhusiopathiae. Bacteremia leading to endocarditis can gain entry from any infected focus. One of the most common places is the gingival tissue. The mouth usually contains all of these organisms in large quantities. When severe dental calculus causes gingival damage or when the gums are lacerated in its removal, especially during extractions, a possible portal of entry is provided for the offending organisms. Other infective foci include wound infections, soft tissue abscesses (especially in cats), and sites affected by osteomyelitis, prostatitis, metritis, pneumonia, pyelonephritis, and tonsillitis.

Valvular endocardial lesions are usually single or multiple irregular vegetations located on the valve cusps near the lines of closure. The lesions are red to orange, oval or serpentine, and superficially friable. The commonly involved mitral and aortic valves may be damaged enough to become insufficient, followed by left heart failure. Bacteria and microemboli are showered frequently from the vegetations. Metastatic embolization and abscess formation in other organs such as the kidney, spleen, brain, and myocardium are seen if the organism is of sufficient virulence and the syndrome is untreated.

DIAGNOSIS

Bacterial endocarditis unfortunately belongs to the class of syndromes referred to as the "great imitators." It would be convenient diagnostically if all the cases presented as middle-aged or older animals with a sudden onset of mitral insufficiency or aortic insufficiency and no history of previous murmur. These animals would show intermittent episodes of fever, shifting leg lameness, positive blood cultures, and a history of specific infections three to four weeks previously. One must be highly suspicious in order to diagnose endocarditis because the bacterial and emboli showers may cause multiple organ involvement and confusing or obscure symptoms. Some animals may be presented showing lethargy, chronic weight loss, lumbar tenderness, hematuria, muscle soreness, unilateral or bilateral paresis, encephalitis, myocarditis, bronchopneumonia, or gastrointestinal disturbances. Other signs include anemia, petechiation of the sclera or mucous membranes, cardiac arrhythmias, syncope, or congestive heart failure.

Electrocardiography is usually normal and not very helpful in many cases of bacterial endocarditis. However, serial electrocardiograms that show rapid progressive chamber enlargement in an animal with non-specific symptoms

of illness should suggest the possibility of endocarditis. Arrhythmias such as ventricular premature beats and ventricular tachycardia may be seen.

Radiographic changes are the same as those described for chronic mitral valvular fibrosis but the changes develop more rapidly.

Blood counts may show a leukocytosis. Neutrophilic leukocytosis may be present during bacteremic episodes and a monocytosis may be present in chronic cases. Blood cultures are often negative but are more likely to be positive if samples are taken serially during a febrile period. The vein should be surgically prepped and 5 to 10 ml samples should be collected for blood culture. To culture an animal that has been on antibiotic therapy, drugs should be withdrawn for at least seven days to facilitate the chances for positive blood culture.

TREATMENT

Positive blood cultures will indicate specific antibiotic therapy. Emphasis should be placed on intensive prolonged antibiotic therapy utilizing bacteriocidal rather than bacteriostatic antibiotics. If one is not able to obtain blood cultures, or if the cultures are negative and the diagnosis of vegetative endocarditis is suspected, the animal should receive subjective treatment for infectious endocarditis. Rapid antibiotic blood levels may be obtained by using crystalline penicillin at 1 million units per kg in an intravenous drip divided into three equal doses. Treatment may be continued using 45,000 units per kg of intramuscular procaine penicillin BID and 10 mg/kg intramuscular dihydrostreptomycin for five to seven days. Oral therapy with ampicillin at 20 mg/kg TID or other synthetic penicillin should be continued at home for at least four more weeks. The incidence of further thrombosis may be reduced by chronic aspirin administration for antiplatelet aggregation. Acute peripheral embolic episodes may cause less damage if collateral perfusion is improved by the use of a peripheral vasodilating agent such as Arlidin® (nylidin) HCl*) at 3 to 6 mg TID. Specific thrombolytic enzymes such as urokinase may be useful but presently are prohibitively expensive. Concurrent myocarditis will usually precipitate arrhythmias that may require quinidine at 11 mg/kg TID. If blood cultures allow a specific bacteriocidal antibiotic to be used, a six-day reducing dosage of corticosteroids such as prednisolone may be used in anti-inflammatory doses to aid in the treatment of myocarditis. Should

---

°Arlidin®, USV Pharmaceutical Corp., New York, N. Y.

mitral and/or aortic insufficiency cause conges-tive heart failure, digoxin and symptomatic treatment for left heart failure will be needed. If possible, blood culture should be repeated 10 days after the cessation of antibiotic therapy.

SUPPLEMENTAL READING

American Animal Hospital Association: A Manual of Clinical Cardi-ology, 1972. 3612 East Jefferson Boulevard, South Bend, Indiana 46660.

Bolton, G.R.: *Handbook of Canine Electrocardiography*. Philadel-phia, W.B. Saunders Co., 1975.
Ettinger, S.J., and Suter, P.F.: *Canine Cardiology*. Philadelphia, W.B. Saunders Co., 1970.
Ettinger, S.J.: *Textbook of Veterinary Internal Medicine*. Philadel-phia, W.B. Saunders Co. 1975.
Knauer, K.W. (ed.): Cardiology I — an Independent Study Course. American Animal Hospital Association, 3612 East Jefferson Boule-vard, South Bend, Indiana, 46660, 1976.
Tilley, L.P. (ed.): Feline Cardiology. Vet. Clin. North Am., Philadel-phia, W.B. Saunders Co., Vol. 7, No. 2, May 1977.

CARDIOMYOPATHY IN THE DOG AND CAT

BETSY BOND, D.V.M.
and LAWRENCE P. TILLEY, D.V.M.
New York, N.Y.

Cardiomyopathy and myocardial disease are terms used to describe pathology in heart mus-cle without pre-existing disease of other struc-tures such as valves or coronary vessels. Car-diomyopathy is usually classified into two main groups: primary (idiopathic) and secondary to a systemic disease. Known causes or possible as-sociations of secondary cardiomyopathy include infections (viral or bacterial), metabolic disor-ders (chronic electrolyte imbalance or uremia), infiltrative conditions (neoplasia), parasitic in-festations (trypanosomiasis), and nutritional disorders (anemia).

The two basic and most common forms of idiopathic cardiomyopathy can be further clas-sified according to the combined nature of the clinical features, the hemodynamic fault, and the accompanying pathology (Fig. 1). *Dilated (congestive) cardiomyopathy* is the dilatation of the left ventricle with resultant failure of the heart as a pump. *Hypertrophic cardiomyopathy* is cardiac hypertrophy providing a resistance to filling of the left ventricle. There may also be obstruction to the outflow tract from the left ventricle. Table 1 outlines the electrocardiogra-phic, radiologic, and clinical signs associated with myocardial disease in the dog and cat.

DIAGNOSTIC FEATURES

FELINE HYPERTROPHIC CARDIOMYOPATHY

Cats may have either symmetric hypertrophic or asymmetric septal hypertrophic cardiomyop-athy. In asymmetric hypertrophy, the septum is thicker than the left ventricular free wall. Most cats with hypertrophic cardiomyopathy have the symmetric form.

The cause of hypertrophic cardiomyopathy in cats is unknown, but evidence indicates a he-reditary component. The disease has been found in related cats, and in man, a large number of hypertrophic cardiomyopathy cases have a familial incidence.

Cats can be affected at any age, but hyper-trophic cardiomyopathy is most common in the middle-aged cat. More male than female cats are affected. Clinical signs often include the acute onset of dyspnea from pulmonary edema, lethargy, anorexia, posterior paresis from aortic thromboembolism, and sudden death.

Moist rales, cardiac murmurs, gallop rhythms, and arrhythmias are frequently auscultated. On palpation of the thorax, the point of maximal intensity over the cardiac apex is often exag-

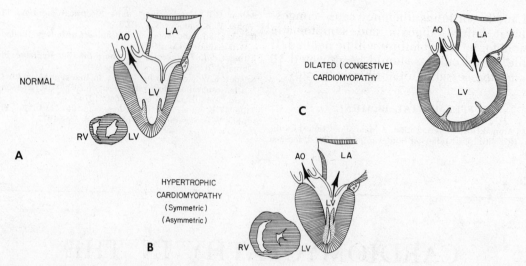

Figure 1. *A.* Normal left ventricle and a transverse section illustrating both ventricular chambers. *B.* Hypertrophic cardiomyopathy represents severe symmetric hypertrophy or asymmetric septal hypertrophy, resulting in impaired ventricular distensibility and sometimes obstruction to the outflow tract of the left ventricle. *C,* Dilated (congestive) cardiomyopathy is represented by poor myocardial contractility with dilatation of heart chambers.
LA = left atrium; LV = left ventricle; RV = right ventricle; AO = aorta.

gerated because of severe left ventricular hypertrophy. If an aortic thromboembolism is present, the femoral pulses are absent and the hind limbs are cold on palpation. The electrocardiographic abnormalities common in hypertrophic cardiomyopathy include both atrial and ventricular arrhythmias, intraventricular conduction disturbances, and increased duration and amplitude of P waves and QRS complexes.

Left anterior fascicular block is commonly seen and is compatible with an actual conduction defect and/or left ventricular hypertrophy.

Cardiomegaly is almost always evident on thoracic radiographs, with severe left atrial enlargement often seen on the dorsoventral view. Pulmonary edema, identified by generalized fluffy alveolar densities (Fig. 2), is commonly found in cats with hypertrophic cardiomyop-

Table 1.   *Common Clinical Findings in Dogs and Cats with Cardiomyopathy*

| | FELINE | | CANINE | |
	Dilated Form	*Hypertrophic Form*	*Dilated Form*	*Hypertrophic Form*[°]
Sex	Male	Male	Male	Male
Clinical Signs	Shock Hypothermia Anorexia Dyspnea Thromboembolism	Dyspnea Thromboembolism Sudden death	Cough Dyspnea Ascites Weakness Anorexia Syncope	Sudden death
Electrocardiography	Ventricular premature complexes Left ventricular enlargement Sinus bradycardia	Atrial and ventricular arrhythmias Intraventricular conduction disturbances Left ventricular and atrial enlargement	Atrial fibrillation Ventricular premature complexes Left ventricular enlargement	Third degree atrio-ventricular block
Radiology	Cardiomegaly Pleural effusion	Left atrial enlargement Cardiomegaly Pulmonary edema	Cardiomegaly Left atrial enlargement Pleural effusion Pulmonary edema	Cardiomegaly
Therapy	Cage rest Digoxin Diuretics Propranolol (?) Vasodilators (?) Grave prognosis	Diuretics Propranolol Cage rest	Digoxin Diuretics Propranolol Low sodium diet Exercise restriction	

[°] Clinical experience is limited at this time for this form of cardiomyopathy.

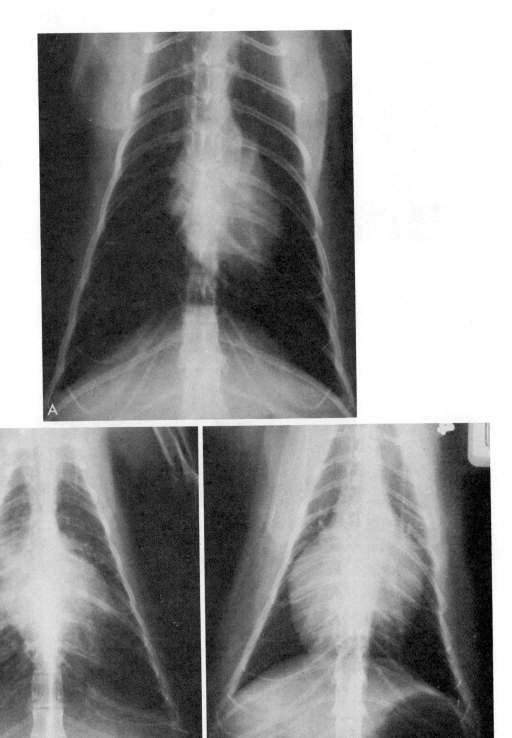

Figure 2. Dorsoventral thoracic radiographs. *A.* Normal cardiac silhouette of a cat. *B.* A five-year-old Persian cat with hypertrophic cardiomyopathy and left-sided heart failure. Pulmonary edema, regions of alveolar-type infiltration (right side), and moderate cardiomegaly are present. *C.* A nine-year-old domestic short-haired cat with dilated cardiomyopathy. Note the marked enlargement of all chambers and the lack of pulmonary congestion or edema.

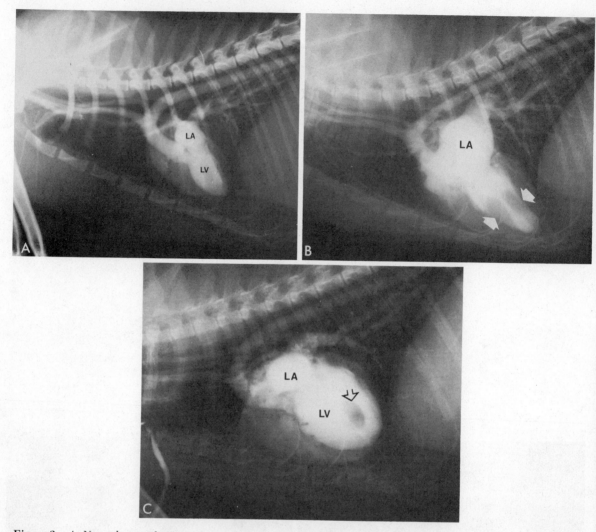

Figure 3. *A.* Normal non-selective angiocardiogram (lateral projection). This exposure was taken 8 seconds following an injection of contrast medium into the jugular vein. The left atrium (*LA*) and the left ventricle (*LV*) are of normal size. *B.* Non-selective angiocardiogram made 8 seconds after the injection of contrast medium into the jugular vein. The large left atrium (*LA*) and small left ventricular cavity with filling defects (*arrows*) caused by thickened papillary muscles are compatible with hypertrophic cardiomyopathy. *C.* Non-selective angiocardiogram made 14 seconds after an injection of contrast medium into the jugular vein. A very slow circulation time exists. The left ventricle (*LV*) is markedly dilated. A filling defect (*arrow*) represents a thrombus that was later found at necropsy.

athy. Pleural effusion, a sign of right-sided heart failure, can sometimes be seen on thoracic radiographs.

Non-selective angiograms are indicated when all clinical parameters are analyzed and the diagnosis is still questionable. Ideally, both the systolic and diastolic phases of the cardiac cycle should be represented, but this is not always possible with non-selective studies. Since the phase of the cardiac cycle cannot always be identified, measurement of left ventricular wall thickness and left ventricular volume are only approximations. Changes visualized with angiography are increased left ventricular thickness, enlarged papillary muscles, decreased left ven-

tricular volume, and an enlarged left atrium (Fig. 3).

At necropsy, there is hypertrophy of the left ventricular wall, papillary muscles, and septum. Enlargement and hypertrophy of the left atrium is also a consistent finding. In asymmetric septal hypertrophy, the septum is thicker than the left ventricular free wall. Some cats have bulging of the interventricular septum with impingement upon the lumen of the left ventricular outflow tract.

Aortic thromboembolism may occur at any stage of cardiomyopathy or may be the presenting sign. Attempts to remove the clot surgically are usually unrewarding. Platelet antiaggregates such as aspirin may be helpful in preventing formation of thromboemboli.

CANINE HYPERTROPHIC CARDIOMYOPATHY

Hypertrophic cardiomyopathy in the dog is relatively uncommon. In a review of cases of hypertrophic cardiomyopathy at The Animal Medical Center, it was found that males were affected more often than females, and the mean age at death was six years. Out of 10 dogs with hypertrophic cardiomyopathy, the German shepherd was most commonly affected (four cases).

In this study of 10 dogs, 8 had asymmetric septal hypertrophic cardiomyopathy. Four of these dogs had evidence of cardiac decompensation one week to one year prior to death, manifested by coughing, dyspnea, and radiographic evidence of cardiomegaly and pulmonary venous congestion or pulmonary edema. Three of these four dogs died unexpectedly while under anesthesia during surgical or diagnostic procedures. The fourth was euthanatized at the owner's request.

Six other dogs with hypertrophic cardiomyopathy had no evidence of cardiac disease prior to death. Two dogs died unexpectedly during operations for non-cardiac abnormalities and three died suddenly at home. The remaining dog died of causes apparently unrelated to heart disease.

Electrocardiographic recordings were obtained in five of the ten dogs with hypertrophic cardiomyopathy. Three of these dogs had evidence of complete heart block, and one also showed evidence of bifascicular block (right bundle branch block and anterior fascicular block). Of the remaining dogs with electrocardiograms, one had first degree atrioventricular block and the other was normal.

At necropsy, all the hearts of dogs with hypertrophic cardiomyopathy had hypertrophy of the left ventricular wall and septum, and most (8 of 10 in this study) showed disproportionate thickening of the ventricular septum.

FELINE DILATED CARDIOMYOPATHY

Cats with dilated cardiomyopathy often present with a sudden onset of lethargy and anorexia as the only clinical signs. They are usually in shock, depressed, dehydrated, hypothermic, and dyspneic, and some cats will have thromboemboli. Cats with dilated cardiomyopathy are usually middle aged, and more males than females are affected. Auscultation may reveal a murmur or a gallop rhythm, but heart and lung sounds are usually muffled. A mild to moderate azotemia is usually present.

The most common electrocardiographic abnormalities include ventricular premature complexes, tall and wide QRS complexes, and sinus bradycardia (Fig. 4). Radiographically, most cats have a pleural effusion, which often obscures the cardiac silhouette. After thoracocentesis or diuretic therapy, a large dilated heart can often be seen (see Fig. 2). Ascites, a common sign of right heart failure in the dog, is rarely seen in the cat.

Because of the critical condition of most cats with dilated cardiomyopathy, discretion must be used in selecting cases for angiography. Angiocardiographic abnormalities include a dilated left ventricle (see Fig. 3) and an extremely slow circulation time.

At necropsy, the heart is enlarged and globular because of extreme dilatation of the ventricles. The left and right atria are moderately enlarged. The papillary muscles and trabeculae in the ventricles are flattened and atrophic.

The long-term prognosis for cats with dilated cardiomyopathy is poor. The average survival time is often less than one month from the onset of clinical signs.

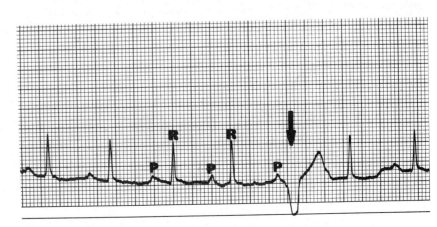

Figure 4. Lead II rhythm strip from a cat with heart failure due to dilated cardiomyopathy. The tall R waves, reflecting left ventricular enlargement, and the ventricular ectopic complex (*arrow*) are often seen with this form of cardiomyopathy. Paper speed = 50 mm/sec; 1 cm = 1 mv.

CANINE DILATED CARDIOMYOPATHY

Dilated cardiomyopathy affects mainly giant breeds of dogs, with ages ranging from three to eight years. Breeds commonly affected include the great Dane, Irish wolfhound, Doberman pinscher, Saint Bernard, German shepherd, bull mastiff, Newfoundland, and standard poodle. The disease is found more often in males than in females. Since it occurs primarily in large and fast-growing breeds, hereditary and nutritional factors should be considered. Dilated cardiomyopathy is occasionally associated with other diseases, especially the gastric dilatation/torsion complex.

Most dogs with dilated cardiomyopathy present with varying degrees of right- and left-sided heart failure. The history usually includes weight loss, general debility, weakness, and abdominal distention over a one- to three-week period. Clinically, there is coughing, dyspnea, syncope, anorexia, and ascites. A rapid irregular heart rate may be easily palpated over the left caudal sternal border. Auscultation may reveal low to moderate intensity systolic murmurs over the mitral valve region.

Electrocardiographically, almost all dogs show atrial fibrillation and left ventricular hypertrophy. The ventricular rate is usually rapid and irregular, with heart rates between 180 and 250 beats per minute. Single or multiple ventricular premature complexes may also be present (Fig. 5).

Thoracic radiographs show moderate to severe enlargement of all cardiac chambers. Signs of either right- or left-sided heart failure include pulmonary congestion, pulmonary edema, pleural effusion, and ascites.

At necropsy, the left atrium and ventricle are markedly dilated with normal mitral and tricuspid valves. The papillary muscles and trabeculae in the ventricles are flattened and atrophic.

The prognosis for dogs with dilated cardiomyopathy is very poor, the average survival time being 6 to 12 months after the onset of signs.

THERAPEUTIC PRINCIPLES

HYPERTROPHIC CARDIOMYOPATHY

Discussion of therapy will focus on the feline disease, since the majority of canine cases are diagnosed postmortem. Theoretically, therapy would be essentially the same for each species.

The principal defect in hypertrophic cardiomyopathy is pathologic hypertrophy of the left ventricle with or without left ventricular outflow obstruction. Hemodynamically, the left ventricle becomes poorly distensible during diastole owing to the hypertrophy and the accompanying high end diastolic pressure. A greater pressure is needed to fill the left ventricle, and an inflow resistance results. Outflow obstruction through asymmetric septal hypertrophy should also be considered in some cases. This increased left ventricular mass requires an increased oxygen utilization that is disparate with normal coronary blood flow.

Based on these findings, the pathogenesis of hypertrophic cardiomyopathy can be proposed. Stress and tachycardia appear to be important precipitating factors in producing dyspnea and pulmonary edema. Because of the thick hypertrophied left ventricle, there is an obstruction to left ventricular filling. Tachycardia associated with such events as stress or aortic thromboembolism shortens diastolic filling time. If the disease progresses gradually, the left atrium will enlarge to increase its reservoir capacity. It is not clear whether the hypertrophic form progresses to the dilated form of cardiomyopathy.

Left ventricular pressure studies have been performed in an effort to stimulate the hemodynamic aspects of this disease. Isoproterenol, a beta-adrenergic stimulant, has been used in cats with suspected hypertrophic cardiomyopathy and has been shown to cause a marked rise in the left ventricular end diastolic pressure. In normal animals, there should be a fall or no change in the left ventricular end diastolic pressure. The occurrence of a rise in end diastolic

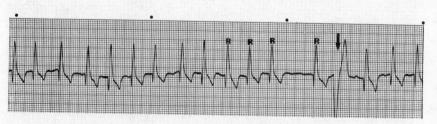

Figure 5. Lead II rhythm strip from a great Dane with heart failure due to dilated cardiomyopathy. The rapid, irregular heart rate and the absence of P waves are compatible with atrial fibrillation. A ventricular premature complex (*arrow*) is also present. Paper speed = 50 mm/sec; 1 cm = 1 mv.

pressure supports the proposed pathogenesis. Stimulation of the beta adrenergic receptors due to the endogenous catecholamine release from the stress will increase the sinoatrial discharge, the force of atrioventricular contraction, the heart rate, and myocardial oxygen utilization.

PROPRANOLOL (INDERAL, AYERST)

This drug works primarily by blocking the beta-adrenergic receptors. In doing so, it may counteract the effects of stress and the accompanying increase in the level of catecholamines. Propranolol may be an important prophylactic agent in cats and possibly in dogs. By using this drug, it is hoped that the left ventricular diastolic impediment is reduced and ventricular filling is improved. The latter should enhance ventricular performance via the Frank-Starling mechanism, particularly with stress. Because diastole is prolonged, coronary blood flow is increased, since it is during diastole that coronary blood flow is greatest.

Propranolol is being used at a dosage of 2.5 to 5.0 mg (¼ to ½ of a 10 mg tablet) every 8 to 12 hours for a 5 kg cat. Therapy must be individualized to achieve an endpoint characterized by a decreased heart rate, elimination of tachyarrhythmias, and relief of clinical signs. Propranolol also has an additive effect with digitalis in the reduction of atrioventricular conduction, especially in atrial fibrillation.

Propranolol is contraindicated in animals with asthma, sinus bradycardia, first degree heart block, and some types of cardiac failure. The drug should be used with caution in diabetic animals. Propranolol should be used in cats with hypertrophic cardiomyopathy only after pulmonary edema and other signs of heart failure have been resolved. The primary role of propranolol is prevention, as previously discussed. The drug can depress myocardial performance and accentuate cardiac failure. Signs of heart failure need to be watched closely when administering propranolol. Toxic manifestations such as gastrointestinal disturbances, weakness, visual disturbances, and thrombocytopenia are rare.

FUROSEMIDE (LASIX, HOECHST)

Diuretic therapy represents an effective method for control of cardiac failure. Diuretics are given specifically to eliminate excess fluid from the body. There is then no need to maintain a daily level. Care must be taken not to overdose diuretics in cats, as they seem to be more sensitive to diuretics and more prone to dehydration and hypokalemia than are dogs.

Diuretics act primarily by blocking resorption of filtered sodium. The two major diuretic agents used in veterinary medicine are furosemide and the thiazides. Of the two diuretics, furosemide is more effective in cats. Because of its rapid onset of action, furosemide is useful when fluid overload is imminent. In the cat with acute left ventricular failure from hypertrophic cardiomyopathy, the associated tachycardia is greatly accentuated by the pulmonary edema, and it represents serious hemodynamic consequences that require immediate therapy. In such a situation, furosemide given intravenously or intramuscularly can make a significant difference by causing diuresis within a few hours. Thus, diuretic therapy is an important adjunct to the other measures in treating this cardiac emergency.

For cats with hypertrophic cardiomyopathy that require long-term therapy, intermittent administration of furosemide (i.e., every second or third day) is effective in promoting a negative sodium balance with minimal risks of electrolyte abnormalities. Dogs usually need to be treated once to twice daily.

The usual dosage of furosemide for cats in heart failure is approximately 1 to 2 mg/kg body weight, once or twice daily. The dosage for dogs is 2 to 4 mg/kg body weight, two to three times daily. The dosage should be adjusted to the individual's response and also for the prevention of clinical signs of heart failure. The most important principle in the use of all diuretics is to administer the smallest effective dose on an intermittent schedule.

OXYGEN

Pulmonary edema may result in a decreased saturation of arterial blood for oxygen by decreasing pulmonary diffusion and increasing venous admixture. In addition, low output cardiac failure is characterized by a wide arteriovenous oxygen difference, resulting in further lowering of the partial pressure of oxygen in the tissues, especially those of the myocardium. The resulting tissue hypoxia may enhance tissue damage.

By means of inhalation of high concentrations of oxygen, the oxygen-carrying capacity of blood — and therefore, tissue oxygenation — may be significantly increased. Improved myocardial oxygenation protects the myocardium from further ischemic damage and reduces ventricular irritability.

DILATED CARDIOMYOPATHY

The non-specific therapy for congestive heart failure associated with dilated cardiomyopathy has four objectives: (1) to strengthen the function of the heart as pump, (2) to spare the pump by reducing the workload, while at the same time meeting the body's need for blood flow and perfusion pressure, (3) to prevent secondary damage to the myocardium and other organs, and (4) to promote recovery of myocardial function.

Treatment for cardiac failure associated with dilated cardiomyopathy should include rest, a low sodium diet, slowing of the heart rate with digoxin and/or propranolol, and furosemide for its diuretic effect. Patients with congestive heart failure that do not respond to digitalis and diuretics may improve after treatment with vasodilator drugs. These drugs are presently under clinical trial for cats with heart failure from dilated cardiomyopathy.

Dilated cardiomyopathy represents gross left ventricular dilatation and subsequent impaired cardiac function. The large ventricular volume results in an increased ventricular wall tension that cannot be met by adequate contractile force. The available coronary blood supply cannot meet the oxygen demand required by this increased wall tension. In the cat, progressive heart failure usually causes pleural effusion, a sign of right-sided failure. Varying degrees of right- and left-sided heart failure occur in the dog.

DIGOXIN (LANOXIN, BURROUGHS-WELLCOME)

Digoxin is the only form of digitalis that is used in the cat. It is the most common form of digitalis used in the dog, but digitoxin is also used. The major clinical effects of digoxin on the heart and circulation are a slowing of the heart rate and an increased force of cardiac contraction. Digoxin is used to control atrial tachyarrhythmias and to improve cardiac performance.

Cats are sensitive to digoxin and should almost never be rapidly digitalized. Occasionally, a cat in very severe heart failure may respond to intravenous digitalization. Dogs in severe heart failure often need to be rapidly digitalized orally. Rarely is it necessary to give a dog intravenous digoxin.

The major problem encountered in cases of dilated cardiomyopathy in the dog is the rapid, irregular ventricular rate associated with atrial fibrillation. Digoxin followed by propranolol is usually needed to slow the ventricular rate adequately to ≤ 160 beats per minute.

PROPRANOLOL (INDERAL, AYERST)

The use of beta-receptor blockade in dilated cardiomyopathy may seem paradoxic, since the heart might be dependent on increased sympathetic activity. However, reduction of a high heart rate decreases the energy demand on the myocardium and allows better diastolic filling. The stroke volume is increased, thereby improving the efficiency of the heart and possibly allowing more energy to be used for contraction.

Studies in man utilizing beta blockade with digitalis in dilated cardiomyopathy over a 2- to 12-month period resulted in increased physical activity with less exertional dyspnea. Some patients experienced a pronounced reduction in heart size. In all cases, the stroke volume was increased.

Propranolol has commonly been used in combination with digoxin in the dog, causing a further decrease in heart rate and relief of symptoms. Studies now in progress to evaluate the effect of propranolol with digoxin in cats with dilated cardiomyopathy are encouraging.

FUROSEMIDE (LASIX, HOECHST)

The dosage requirements are identical to those discussed under treatment for hypertrophic cardiomyopathy.

VASODILATORS

As a reflex response to inadequate perfusion of peripheral organs, there is increased sympathetic tone that causes peripheral vasoconstriction. If this persists, the increased peripheral resistance increases the work of the heart, and cardiac output declines. Vasodilator drugs that act on the arterial circulation decrease peripheral resistance, whereas those that act on the venous circulation decrease ventricular filling. In a failing heart, these efforts tend to improve cardiac output and decrease pulmonary congestion. Sodium nitroprusside produces venous and arterial vasodilation. This drug is given by continuous intravenous infusion and has an immediate onset and short duration of action. There are two main disadvantages to the use of nitroprusside: (1) doses higher than the optimal level cause excess arterial dilatation and a drop in systemic blood pressure and coronary blood flow to a dangerous level and (2) a reflex tachycardia is produced in response to decreased systemic arterial pressure.

Vasodilators may be effective for the acute treatment of some cases with heart failure that are unresponsive to digitalis and diuretics. However, because of the adverse side effects, their administration requires continuous monitoring of blood pressure, which, unfortunately, is not always possible.

EXERCISE RESTRICTION

The pathophysiologic and clinical manifestations of myocardial failure are precipitated by increasing the work of the heart. The increased sympathetic tone associated with congestive heart failure may raise the arterial blood pressure not only at rest but especially during exercise. Therefore, avoiding situations that produce catecholamines (such as stress and exercise) will help control or prevent the recurrence of heart failure.

DIET

The value of a low sodium diet in cardiac disease is well established. However, when potent diuretics are used, the clinician does not have to be so rigid in restricting sodium intake. Sodium restriction is helpful primarily for reducing the need for large doses of diuretics.

FELINE DILATED CARDIOMYOPATHY

Almost all cats with dilated cardiomyopathy have a pleural effusion. Thoracocentesis may relieve external pressure on the heart and lung. Because shock (a low-output heart failure state) and dehydration are common, it is usually advisable to insert a catheter intravenously and administer fluids consisting of a half-strength mixed electrolyte solution and 2.5 per cent dextrose in water. Cats that are very dyspneic are placed in oxygen. Cats in critical condition are given digoxin intravenously, at total dose of 0.02 mg/kg body weight divided in four doses over four hours or to effect. The average maintenance/dose is approximately 0.008 to 0.01 mg/kg body weight per day divided in two doses (e.g., ¼ of a 0.125 mg tablet twice a day for a 6 kg cat). Furosemide also may be given intravenously.

Renal function and electrolytes should be checked periodically. The prognosis for cats presenting with acute dilated cardiomyopathy is extremely grave, and many die within 24 to 48 hours of presentation. The cat with dilated cardiomyopathy that survives long enough to be sent home has a three-fold drug regimen: maintenance digoxin, maintenance furosemide, and propranolol. Exercise restriction and a low-sodium diet should be instituted whenever possible. The long-term use of vasodilators has not been evaluated. A re-examination in seven to ten days is advisable in order to monitor the effectiveness of therapy.

CANINE DILATED CARDIOMYOPATHY

Severely dyspneic dogs are immediately given furosemide and may need to be placed in an oxygen cage. A total dosage of 4 mg furosemide per kg body weight is calculated: half is given intravenously and the other half is given intramuscularly. Furosemide is then given at a dosage of 2 mg/kg body weight intramuscularly two to three times daily.

Thoracocentesis is generally not recommended even when a pleural effusion is present. Cage rest and diuretics are usually effective in resolving the pleural effusion.

Rapid oral digitalization should be started if the failure state is severe and the ventricular rate is extremely rapid. The digoxin is given twice daily for two days or stopped sooner if digoxin toxicity occurs. Maintenance digoxin and furosemide are then started after being withheld for at least 24 hours or until signs of digoxin toxicity have disappeared Since large breeds of dogs are mainly affected, the maintenance dosage of digoxin generally varies from 0 25 mg to 0.5 mg twice daily. For dogs not in a severe hemodynamic crisis, maintenance digoxin rather than rapid digitalization is usually satisfactory.

Once the failure state is resolved, propranolol is started at an approximate oral dose of 10 to 40 mg every 8 to 12 hours, depending on the animal's size. The dosage of propranolol should be adjusted toward specific desirable endpoints for each patient. Endpoints should be a definitive therapeutic effect and a reduction of the ventricular rate in atrial fibrillation to ≤ 160 beats per minute.

Once the dog is home, exercise restriction and a low sodium diet may be helpful. Re-evaluation in seven to ten days is advised in order to assess the effectiveness of therapy. Dogs with dilated cardiomyopathy have a better prognosis than do cats with dilated cardiomyopathy.

SUPPLEMENTAL READING

Abelmann, W.H.: Treatment of congestive cardiomyopathy. Postgrad. Med. J. 54:477–484, 1978.

Ettinger, S.J.: Diseases of the myocardium. In Ettinger, S.J. (ed.) *Textbook of Veterinary Internal Medicine.* Philadelphia, W.B. Saunders Co., 1975.

Hamlin, R.L.: New ideas in the management of heart failure in dogs. JAVMA 171:114–118, 1977.

Harpster, N.K.: Feline cardiomyopathy. Vet. Clin. North Am. 7:355–371, 1977.

Liu, S.K., Tilley, L.P., and Maron, B.J.: Canine hypertrophic cardiomyopathy. JAVMA 174:708–713, 1979.

Tilley, L.P., and Liu, S.-K.: Cardiomyopathy in the dog. Recent Adv. Cardiac Struct. Metab. 10:651–653, 1975.

Tilley, L.P., Liu, S.-K., Gilbertson, S.R., Wagner, B.M., and Lord, P.F.: Primary myocardial disease in the cat: a model for human cardiomyopathy. Am. J. Pathol. 87:493–522, 1977.

Tilley, L.P., and Weitz, J.: Pharmacologic and other forms of medical therapy in feline cardiac disease. Vet. Clin. North Am. 7:415–428, 1977.

Tilley, L.P.: *Essentials of Canine and Feline Electrocardiography.* St. Louis, C.V Mosby, 1979.

MYOCARDIAL DISEASE

DAVID B. CHURCH, B V Sc.

Sydney, Australia

Myocardial diseases may be broadly classified into congenital, primary, and secondary cardiomyopathies. The primary cardiomyopathies include a number of characteristic cardiac abnormalities of unknown etiology and are discussed in detail in the preceding article. Congenital and secondary myocardial disease will be dealt with in this chapter. Congenital abnormalities have been well described and produce relatively characteristic clinical signs. Recognition of acquired secondary myocardial disease, however, is made more difficult by the diverse and non-specific nature of so many of the signs associated with these disorders.

CONGENITAL MYOCARDIAL DISEASE

ATRIAL SEPTAL DEFECT

This congenital defect in the wall separating the left and right atria occurs in dogs and cats and is most commonly found in conjunction with other congenital cardiac abnormalities.

When present, the clinical signs associated with atrial septal defect are non-specific. Reduced exercise tolerance, weakness, and dyspnea may occur to a variable degree. Abnormalities detectable at physical examination relate to left to right shunting of blood and increased flow through the right side of the heart. There may be increased intensity or splitting of the second heart sound owing to pulmonary hypertension. A soft systolic murmur may be auscultated over the pulmonic valve region, resulting from increased blood flow to the right ventricle and consequent relative stenosis of the right ventricular outflow tract. If the defect is particularly severe, there may be extracardiac evidence of right-sided congestive heart failure such as ascites and hepatomegaly. This can develop to such a degree that right atrial pressure exceeds left atrial pressure. The resulting right to left shunting of blood may produce cyanosis.

Depending on the severity of the defect, electrocardiography and thoracic radiography may demonstrate either right atrial or right ventricular enlargement or both. Diagnostic confirmation requires the use of either angiography or

316

blood gas determinations, but preferably both. Contrast media injected into the left atrium allows radiographic visualization of left to right shunting of blood. There will be a disparity in the degree of oxygenation in blood sampled from the superior vena cava and the right atrium. The presence of either of these abnormalities supports the diagnosis.

VENTRICULAR SEPTAL DEFECTS

A ventricular septal defect (VSD) results in direct communication between the right and left ventricular chambers. Defects in the interventricular septum may occur in many locations, but they can be divided broadly into those in the region of the supraventricular crest (type I) and those located more caudally, beneath the septal cusp of the right atrioventricular valve (type II).

During embryologic development, separation of the chambers is achieved by a primitive septum growing dorsally from the apex and eventually fusing with a ventrally growing aortopulmonary septum and laterally growing endocardial cushions. Failure of the aortopulmonary and primordial septae to fuse results in type I VSD. Type II defects occur with failure of fusion between the primordial septum and the endocardial cushions. When the defect results from dextropositioning of the aortopulmonary septum, the condition is described as Eisenmenger's complex.

Because left ventricular systolic pressure is normally four to five times that of right ventricular systolic pressure, left to right shunting of blood will occur with any interventricular communication. However, when the combination of right ventricular hypertrophy and increased blood volume in the pulmonary circulation is sufficient to produce a right ventricular systolic pressure greater than left ventricular pressure, right to left shunting and cyanosis may occur. In Eisenmenger's complex, cyanosis can be present without markedly increased right ventricular pressure because of the dextropositioned aorta.

VSD is usually detected in an otherwise asymptomatic animal, although clinical signs of pulmonary hypertension (dyspnea, coughing, and reduced exercise tolerance) may be present. If signs of congestive heart failure are present, they are usually related to right sided failure (hepatomegaly and ascites). The pulse associated with VSD is described as "water-hammer" in nature, with high amplitude and a rapid fall. Auscultation reveals a harsh holosystolic murmur whose point of maximal intensity is usually on the right side of the thorax, just dorsal to the sternal border at the third to fourth intercostal space. The intensity and duration of the murmur decrease with increasing pulmonary hypertension. Splitting of the second heart sound may be heard on the left side of the thorax.

The electrocardiogram is often normal, although evidence of right ventricular hypertrophy may be present in some dogs. Increased prominence of the pulmonary vasculature and right-sided cardiac enlargement are frequently evident radiographically. The left atrium occasionally may also appear enlarged.

Diagnosis requires angiographic demonstration of contrast media moving from the left to the right ventricle. The contrast media is injected via an arterial catheter positioned in the left ventricle. Blood gas determinations provide a means of assessing the size of the defect and may be helpful prognostically.

Persistent atrioventricular canal has been reported in the cat but not in the dog. It is a confluent defect of the atrial and ventricular septae. There may also be associated atrioventricular valve abnormalities. Clinical signs are similar to those produced with VSD, although the first heart sound may be muffled or absent because of the abnormal A-V valves.

Tetralogy of Fallot is a septal defect accompanied by a stenotic pulmonary artery in which the resistance to flow is greater than the systemic vascular resistance. Other features of the syndrome are right ventricular hypertrophy and dextropositioning of the aorta.

ACQUIRED SECONDARY MYOCARDIAL DISEASE

ISCHEMIC MYOCARDIAL DISEASE

Ischemic myocardial disease in the dog is relatively common; Jonsson (1974) reported 26.4 per cent of cases necropsied for cardiac disease showed evidence of ischemic myocardial disease. The myocardial lesions are generally multifocal and microscopic and consist of various stages of myocardial degeneration and necrosis, resorption, and reparative fibrosis with associated vascular lesions. Most of the dogs studied had some form of valvular disease that resulted

in ventricular hypertrophy. It appears that the myocardial ischemia seen in animals with concurrent valvular disease is at least partly associated with altered physical and/or chemical forces brought about by myocardial hypertrophy (increased intramural tension) and perhaps alterations in the systolic pressure at the coronary ostia (resulting in reduction in coronary arterial pressure).

Ischemic myocardial disease in the dog and cat is usually insidious in onset and progressive. Associated clinical signs may vary from the subclinical to overt evidence of heart failure such as reduced exercise tolerance, coughing, and congestive heart failure. Syncope and dysrhythmias are sometimes present and are more specific indicators of myocardial disease. Not infrequently, clinical evidence of ischemic myocardial disease may be masked by the presence of a concurrent cardiac abnormality with more obvious clinical signs.

Thoracic radiography will not aid in recognizing this problem, since the radiographic changes are invariably non-specific and could be associated with any abnormality that produces myocardial hypertrophy. The electrocardiogram may demonstrate changes associated with ischemic myocardial disease. Any form of dysrhythmia or conduction disturbance, depression or elevation of the S-T segment, or changes in the T-wave pattern may be produced by ischemic heart disease.

Large myocardial infarcts or "heart attacks" are not common in either the dog or cat. Diagnosis of a large myocardial infarct requires substantial clinical, electrocardiographic, and clinicopathologic evidence for such a lesion. When it does occur, coronary thromboembolism is the usual cause. These emboli often originate from neoplastic tissue or from the fragile thrombi associated with vegetative endocarditis. Thromboemboli may, of course, also cause multiple microscopic myocardial infarcts.

INFILTRATIVE MYOCARDIAL DISEASE

Infiltrative myocardial diseases are uncommon in the dog and cat. Luginbuhl and Detweiler (1965) found postmortem evidence of cardiac neoplasia in 5.5 per cent of 509 cases necropsied for cardiovascular disease. Both primary and metastatic cardiac neoplasia have been recorded, and predictably are usually seen in middle-aged or older animals. Although cardiac amyloidosis occurs, it has been reported only rarely.

The predominant primary cardiac tumors are hemangioendotheliomas. They are found invariably in the right atrium, dorsal to the coronary vein and adjacent to the auricular opening. They appear as nodular swellings encroaching upon the lumen of the atria or as a diffuse thickening of the wall. Hemangioendotheliomas are also the most common metastatic cardiac neoplasm, usually metastasizing from primary sites in the spleen. Both primary and secondary hemangioendotheliomas occur more often in the German shepherd than in other breeds.

The incidence of cardiac tumors is increased if aortic body tumors are considered in this category. These tumors arise from chemoreceptor cells in the great vessels around the heart base. They develop in periadventitial tissue, usually between the aorta and the pulmonary artery, although other anatomically related sites have been described. In general, they are considered benign, although one report states that 22 per cent of aortic body tumors had metastasized, most commonly to the lungs (Patnaik et al., 1975). There is a significantly higher incidence of these tumors in the brachycephalic breeds, with boxers and Boston terriers being particularly over-represented. In man, the tumor appears with increased frequency in individuals with high altitude hypoxia, and it is thought that the partially obstructed airways of brachycephalic animals may result in a tendency to hypoxia, chemoreceptor hyperplasia, and increased likelihood of neoplasia.

The clinical signs associated with cardiac neoplasia vary with the type of tumor and its site and degree of invasiveness. Infiltrative neoplasms tend to produce dysrhythmias that may result in syncopal episodes or even sudden death. The site of the irritant area can be approximated electrocardiographically and appropriate symptomatic treatment can be initiated. Angiography may demonstrate filling defects in the atrium or ventricles or both if the neoplasm invades these cavities as well as myocardial tissue.

Neoplasms that invade the pericardium and epicardial surface tend to produce pericardial effusions. Congestive heart failure develops because of the consequent reduction in end diastolic volume. Pericardial effusion may be suspected when muffled or inaudible heart sounds, bilateral engorgement of the jugular veins, and decreased amplitude of the cardiac apex beat are present. Radiographically, a large globular cardiac silhouette is seen. Depending on the size and site of the tumor, deviations in the normal orientation of soft tissue structures, such as the trachea and esophagus, may also be visible. Angiography may demonstrate the tumor by revealing displacement of one of the major vessels or by opacifying the neoplasm's blood supply.

INFECTIOUS MYOCARDITIS

Infectious myocarditis can be defined histopathologically as an infiltration of the myocardial tissue by inflammatory cells in response to an infectious agent. A number of viral, bacterial, fungal, and protozoal agents have been reported to cause myocarditis in the dog and cat. In the majority of cases, the infection has a hematogenous origin with multiple organ involvement. Consequently, signs of myocarditis can be overlooked in the presence of more spectacular abnormalities associated with non-cardiac inflammation. This tendency must be guarded against, as life-threatening arrhythmias can develop rapidly from initially subtle abnormalities.

The spectrum of clinical signs associated with acute infectious myocarditis runs from the subclinical through relatively non-specific problems such as physical inactivity, weakness, inappetence, or weight loss to animals presenting in a state of collapse or even sudden death. As with any infectious disease, hyperthermia is an inconsistent finding. Examination of the cardiovascular system may reveal a number of abnormalities that will vary with the severity and chronicity of the disease.

Murmurs will usually not be present unless valvular or congenital cardiac disease, or an anemia, accompany the myocarditis. Most animals with myocarditis have a dysrhythmia. The most common abnormalities are supraventricular and ventricular premature contractions and various degrees of atrioventricular block, although the type depends on the site, severity, and multiplicity of myocardial damage. The dysrhythmia may also be influenced by other abnormalities such as electrolyte disturbances present as a consequence of the systemic disease. At physical examination, dysrhythmias manifest themselves as irregularities in the heart sounds and the arterial pulse.

Extracardiac signs of congestive heart failure are uncommon, since infectious myocarditis is usually a disease that is acute in onset. Unless other cardiopulmonary disease is present, thoracic radiography is of minimal use in further defining the problem.

A complete hematologic examination, non-discretionary serum biochemical tests, and repeated blood cultures are advisable in cases of suspected infectious myocarditis. A positive blood culture, or identification of microorganisms in an aseptically collected blood smear, supports the diagnosis and provides the opportunity for sensitivity testing and the application of appropriate antimicrobial therapy. Consequently, specimens should be collected for blood culture prior to institution of antimicrobial therapy. Myocardial complications should always be considered with any infectious or systemic disease state that is not responding adequately to treatment.

NON-INFECTIOUS MYOCARDIOPATHIES

Pericarditis and myocarditis can occur with systemic lupus erythematosus (SLE). The diagnosis is most simply made by the detection of LE cells and the demonstration of antinuclear antibodies on serial testing of an animal with one or more of the characteristic abnormalities caused by SLE. Treatment of the primary disease will usually result in resolution of the cardiac problem.

A number of other clinical syndromes may lead to impaired cardiac function. These disorders include the endometritis-pyometra complex, pancreatitis, uremia, and endotoxemias associated with gastroenteropathies. This type of myocardial disease has been termed "myocarditis," but it is probably more accurately described as inflammation secondary to myocardial degeneration. In these cases, the clinical signs associated with the primary disease usually predominate, but, as with systemic infections, the possibility of impaired cardiac function secondary to the primary illness should always be remembered.

Electrolyte disturbances secondary to extracardiac diseases may produce myocardial dysfunction. Conditions that produce hyperkalemia—such as renal failure, hypoadrenocorticism, or acidosis—can reduce cardiac output. Serum potassium concentrations of 6.5 mEq/l or more can usually be expected to produce tall, peaked T waves, flattened P waves, and a uniformly widened QRS complex on the electrocardiogram. Milder elevations in serum potassium may be suspected if serial electrocardiograms show similar but less severe changes.

Hypokalemia, hypocalcemia, and hypercalcemia are uncommon abnormalities that can result in decreased cardiac function. Severe hypokalemia (values of 2.2 mEq/l or less) will frequently result in reduction in T wave amplitude, increased amplitude and duration of the P wave, development of a U wave, and increased QRS complex duration. Less severe reduction in serum potassium concentration may be detected electrocardiographically if the animal's unaffected ECG is available for comparison. Hypocalcemia and hypercalcemia produce characteristic alterations in the electrocardiogram, but use of the ECG as a guide to disturbances in this electrolyte is less reliable.

Arterial hypertension is rarely recorded in small animals. Pheochromocytoma is an uncommon tumor that causes arterial hypertension via excessive production of catecholamines. Renal disease has been reported as causing arterial hypertension. The increased cardiac workload associated with this will result in left ventricular hypertrophy and eventually lead to left-sided congestive heart failure.

Severe chronic anemia will often produce an increase in cardiac output. This is manifested clinically by a sinus tachycardia, cardiac enlargement, and ultimately, high output congestive heart failure.

Hyperthyroidism results in a hyperdynamic circulatory state much like that associated with severe chronic anemia. Sinus tachycardia, supraventricular premature contractions, and supraventricular tachycardia are all findings consistent with this hyperkinetic state, although hyperthyroidism-induced tachyarrhythmias have not been recorded in the dog. In hypothyroidism, there is a reduction in cardiac output, probably owing to decreased myocardial contractility. In a small percentage of cases, this may be exacerbated by sinus bradycardia.

Toxic levels of certain drugs such as digitalis, quinidine, and various anesthetic agents may also produce cardiac disease.

TREATMENT OF MYOCARDIAL DISEASE

CONGENITAL MYOCARDIAL DISEASE

Treatment of congenital myocardial heart disease is not indicated in the asymptomatic animal. Surgical correction of VSD requires cardiopulmonary bypass and open heart surgery. Pulmonary artery banding can be used to increase right ventricular systolic pressure and reduce the degree of left to right shunting. Medical therapy can be instituted in animals with congestive heart failure. Digitalis, furosemide, and low sodium diets with reduced exercise help to control the problem temporarily.

ACQUIRED MYOCARDIAL DISEASE

Therapy of acquired myocardial disease should be directed against the primary disease process. Although symptomatic therapy may improve cardiac function, recognition and appropriate treatment of the primary disease is the only means by which the cardiac problem can be resolved. Not infrequently, however, initial symptomatic therapy is required to allow the clinician time for a more detailed investigation of the primary disease state. In situations in which the primary disease cannot be determined or is untreatable, symptomatic therapy is the only alternative.

Symptomatic treatment is aimed at improving cardiac output. Digitalis, by prolonging atrioventricular node conduction and increasing ventricular contractility, increases cardiac output and substantially improves coronary blood flow. However, cardiac glycosides also increase myocardial automaticity and must be used with caution in the presence of ventricular tachydysrhythmia.

Digitalization may be achieved by intravenous, "rapid oral," or "slow oral" administration (see "Pharmacodynamics of Digitalis, Diuretics, and Antiarrhythmic Drugs"). Intravenous digitalization is indicated only in the critically ill patient or in those with both congestive heart failure and ventricular tachydysrhythmia, where the cause of the increased myocardial excitability is uncertain. The response to intravenous digitalization provides a means of differentiating primary heart failure with ischemia-induced tachydysrhythmia from heart failure secondary to a dysrhythmia. If digitalis therapy exacerbates the problem, the latter situation is suggested, necessitating antidysrhythmic therapy and cessation of the cardiac glycoside. If there is no exacerbation of the dysrhythmia or the frequency of the premature beats increases, it is likely that digitalization will reduce the dysrhythmia and improve cardiac function. The advantage of intravenous digitalization is that it reduces the time required for the "therapeutic trial" and allows more rapid dissipation of any undesired effects following cessation of therapy. Rapid oral digitalization offers a temporally intermediate method of digitalization. Both methods require close electrocardiographic monitoring if iatrogenic and life-threatening dysrhythmias are to be avoided.

Antidysrhythmic therapy is indicated in all cases in which a significant dysrhythmia of nonischemic etiology is present. If the disturbance is a tachydysrhythmia and is supraventricular in origin, digitalis is the treatment of choice because it delays atrioventricular node conduction. When the tachydysrhythmia is of ventricular origin, treatment should include one of the antidysrhythmic agents such as quinidine, procainamide, phenytoin, lidocaine, or propranolol. However, these drugs reduce myocardial contractility; consequently, in patients with congestive heart failure, they should be used only if the beneficial effect of decreasing the premature contractions is more than likely to compensate for the induced reduction in myocardial contractility.

Bradydysrhythmias are most commonly caused by electrolyte disturbances or drug tox-

icities. Treatment of the underlying cause will usually resolve the dysrhythmia. Isoprenaline or atropine may be used symptomatically to increase conduction and heart rate in some types of bradydysrhythmias (see "Bradycardias").

Diuretic therapy should be used to supplement the cardiac glycosides in animals with myocardial disease and overt congestive heart failure. Of the many diuretic agents available, furosemide and the thiazides are probably the most useful. Furosemide may be given parenterally or orally. Parenteral administration results in diuresis within twenty minutes, which persists for approximately two hours. When administered orally, diuresis begins within one hour and lasts four to five hours. The thiazide diuretics are less potent than furosemide and usually are given orally. They have a more prolonged action, and their effect may last 12 to 24 hours after oral administration.

In general, furosemide is probably the diuretic of choice in dogs with myocardial congestive heart failure. In contrast to the thiazides, furosemide increases renal blood flow and glomerular filtration. This property insures that furosemide-induced diuresis will occur despite impaired renal blood flow. Furosemide also tends to redistribute fluid in the circulation, and studies in man suggest that the furosemide-induced reduction in pulmonary congestion and edema in acute congestive heart failure is at least partly associated with this redistribution effect. By virtue of their mechanism of action, persistent use of either furosemide or the thiazide diuretics tends to produce potassium depletion, which may impair cardiac output. This problem can be minimized by using intermittent therapy, but if intensive diuretic therapy is undertaken, oral potassium supplementation is advisable.

The xanthine derivatives, theophylline and aminophylline, are widely used in the treatment of congestive heart failure of any cause. They are perhaps most commonly known as bronchodilators, but their principal benefit to the cardiac patient lies in their vasodilatory and positive inotropic effects. The xanthines increase myocardial contractility and cardiac output. They also produce systemic, pulmonary, and coronary vasodilation, which lead, in the presence of increased cardiac output, to an increase in systemic blood flow. They may have a mild but inconsistent diuretic effect. Because of their effects on myocardial blood flow, the xanthines have been used for the treatment of coronary vascular disease in man, although the clinical results have been disappointing and their value is controversial. The xanthines may be given orally or parenterally. Their main value to veterinarians is as rapidly acting positive inotropic agents that can be used with relative safety in cases of acute myocardial disease and congestive heart failure to improve cardiac output and increase myocardial oxygenation.

SUPPLEMENTAL READING

Ettinger, S.J., and Suter, P.F.: Acquired and congenital heart disease. In Ettinger, S.J., and Suter, P.F. (eds): *Canine Cardiology.* Philadelphia, W.B. Saunders Co., 1970.

Ettinger, S.J.: Diseases of the myocardium. In Ettinger, S.J. (ed): *Textbook of Veterinary Internal Medicine.* Philadelphia, W.B. Saunders Co., 1975.

Jonsson, L.: Coronary arterial lesions and myocardial infarcts in the dog. Thesis. Stockholm, 1972.

Luginbuhl, H., and Detweiler, D.K.: Cardiovascular lesions in dogs. Ann. NY Acad. Sci. 127:517, 1965.

Patnaik, A.K., Liu, S.K., Hurvitz, A.I., and McClelland, A.J.: Canine chemodectoma (extra-adrenal paragangliomas) — a comparative study. J. Small Anim. Pract. 16:785, 1975.

PERICARDIAL DISEASE

REBECCA E. GOMPF, D.V.M.

Knoxville, Tennessee

Pericardial disease is not readily diagnosed since the animal often presents with signs of other underlying diseases. As the pericardial disease progresses, the animal may present with signs typical of left or right congestive heart failure. Only by further diagnostic workup can the underlying causes of these symptoms be found.

The pericardium is a membranous sac that encloses the heart and the proximal few centimeters of the great vessels. Normally, the pericardial sac contains about 1 to 2 ml of serous fluid. The functions of the pericardium are (1) to preserve the Frank-Starling mechanism by limiting the amount the heart can dilate acutely, (2) to maintain optimal heart geometry, (3) to maintain normal ventricular compliance, (4) to reduce external friction, (5) to serve as a barrier to inflammation spreading from adjacent structures, and (6) to buttress the atria and right ventricle, which have thinner muscular walls than does the left ventricle.

Diseases of the pericardium are usually secondary manifestations of a generalized problem. The pericardium has a limited manner by which it can respond to disease: it produces an exudate, fibrin, or cells or any combination of these three substances. The end result is a diminished cardiac output owing either to constrictive pericardial disease preventing the dilatation and filling of the ventricles in diastole or to pericardial effusion causing cardiac tamponade, which increases the intracardiac pressure and impedes ventricular filling.

ETIOLOGY

There are several causes of pericardial dis-

ease. Identification of the inciting factor is usually started with an analysis of the fluid in the pericardial sac.

Non-inflammatory fluids withdrawn from the pericardial sac can be transudates, modified transudates, or hemorrhage. Transudates and modified transudates can result from hypoproteinemia, peritoneopericardial diaphragmatic hernia, congestive heart failure, neoplasms obstructing the lymphatics such as a heart base tumor, acute toxemias such as *Clostridia* toxemia, or overhydration. Hemorrhagic pericardial effusions can be due to trauma, left atrial rupture in the dog and pig, ruptured intrapericardial aorta in the horse, erosive neoplasms such as hemangiosarcomas in dogs, or, rarely, coagulopathies, or they can be iatrogenic from pericardiocentesis.

Acute or subacute inflammatory processes can cause effusive or non-effusive pericarditis. Sterile effusions can result from "benign" idiopathic pericardial effusion (the most common cause of pericardial effusion in the dog), uremic pericarditis in the dog, post-traumatic pericarditis, or primary or metastatic neoplasia. Septic pericardial effusions can be caused by bacteria such as pasteurella in most species; clostridia and coliforms in cattle; salmonella and hemophilus in swine; streptococci in lambs, horses, and cats; and anaerobes in dogs and cats. Nocardia, leptospirosis, toxoplasmosis, canine distemper, coccidioidomycosis, and actinomycosis can also cause septic effusions in dogs and cats. Fungal infections of the pericardium are unusual in domestic animals.

Constrictive pericarditis can result from granulomatous reactions, pericardial scarring following inflammation, chronic effusions, or idiopathic causes. Most are idiopathic in nature. Constrictive pericarditis is uncommon and occurs in only about 1 per cent of the pericarditis cases in man, and the incidence is lower in animals.

PATHOPHYSIOLOGY

Some degree of pericardial effusion is found with all forms of acute pericarditis; however, whether the pericardial effusion causes any problems depends on the rate of formation of the fluid. If the fluid accumulates slowly, the pericardial sac can stretch slightly and the circulatory system can adjust to the changes. Therefore, it takes a greater volume of fluid in the pericardial sac to produce clinical signs. However, if the fluid accumulates rapidly, a small amount can cause clinical signs by restricting the heart's range of motion.

The fluid accumulating in the pericardial sac increases the pericardial pressure. This increased pressure affects the myocardium in systole and diastole. The increased pressure is transmitted to the cardiac chambers and increases the pressure in the chambers. This impedes ventricular and atrial filling in diastole so that the ventricles fill slowly and incompletely. Also, the increased intrapericardial pressure causes an increased resistance to coronary artery flow so myocardial necrosis can occur. The poor perfusion of the coronary arteries is aggravated by the decreased cardiac output that results from poor ventricular filling. Also, the heart rate is usually increased as a compensatory mechanism for low cardiac output; therefore, the coronary arteries have even less time to fill.

Constrictive pericarditis may be accompanied by a significant amount of pericardial effusion or there may be very little effusion. Sometimes, the parietal pericardium can become firmly adhered to the epicardium, causing an obliterative constrictive pericarditis without fluid. The result of constrictive pericarditis is a decreased compliance of the ventricles so that the ventricular diastolic filling is limited. In systole, the heart falls away from the restraining pericardium so that during early diastole, it fills rapidly until it reaches the limits of filling. This restriction of filling increases the diastolic pressure of all chambers of the heart, which further impedes the flow of blood into the atria and ventricles. Both ventricles are equally affected by the constrictive pericarditis and eventually, the diastolic pressures of both ventricles may be equal, instead of the right ventricular pressure being lower than the left ventricular pressure.

Neoplastic involvement of the pericardium produces signs only in about 10 percent of the cases. Clinical signs result from the presence of an effusion, which is usually hemorrhagic, or from constrictive pericarditis, or a combination of the two. Primary neoplasms of the pericardium are rare. Most neoplasms are secondary and result from local extension, lymphatic invasion, or hematogenous spread.

Uremic pericarditis can occur with chronic or acute renal failure. Fibrin forms in the pericardial sac and adhesions result. An effusion can also be present, which can result in clinical signs.

Regardless of whether pericardial effusion or restrictive pericarditis is the underlying problem, the signs and symptoms are going to be related to the decreased cardiac filling and the resultant venous overload. Therefore, the animal will present with signs of either right heart failure or pulmonary congestion.

DIAGNOSIS

The diagnosis of pericardial disease is readily apparent if a significant amount of effusion is present. If the fluid accumulation is slight or the restrictive disease is limited, the diagnosis can be more of a challenge. Mild forms of the disease may never be detected clinically and may resolve spontaneously or be an incidental finding at necropsy.

The history of an animal with pericardial disease can be very vague and non-specific. A concurrent illness such as decompensated mitral insufficiency, renal failure, or systemic infections can mask the pericarditis unless the pericarditis is advanced and causing signs of congestive heart failure. An animal without a concurrent illness may show no signs until congestive heart failure results from reduced filling of the heart, causing blood to back up into the pulmonic or systemic circulation.

Animals with pericardial disease may present with dyspnea or syncope owing to decreased cardiac output or pulmonary congestion, vomiting, weakness, anorexia, or signs of right heart failure such as venous engorgement, hepatomegaly or splenomegaly, and ascites. In man, pulmonary congestion occurs more frequently with cardiac tamponade than with constrictive pericarditis for unknown reasons. Symptoms can come on quickly and are more severe if the inciting factor is acute cardiac tamponade.

On physical exam, the mucous membrane may be pale and perfusion may be slow owing to decreased cardiac output. Venous distention with a prominent jugular pulse may be present. Abdominal palpation may reveal hepatomegaly and splenomegaly or ascites. On auscultation, the heart may sound muffled, depending on the amount of pericardial effusion present, the obesity of the animal, and the conformation of the chest. A thin, deep-chested dog may not have muffled heart sounds. Pericardial friction rubs may be present intermittently or continuously. The rubs are caused by the myocardial motion causing grating of the pericardial and epicardial surfaces, which have been roughened by serofibrinous exudates. Rubs can be present with large or small amounts of effusion. Usually, the rubs are louder in inspiration and do not change consistently with respiration the way murmurs do. The rubs can migrate and shift to other areas in a matter of hours and change in character and intensity, whereas a murmur has a constant location, character, intensity, and radiation of sound.

Peripheral pulses tend to be weak and rapid owing to poor cardiac output. A pulsus paradoxus, which is an alteration of pulse pressure during respiration due to changes in ventricular filling in respiratory phases, may exist. A pulsus alternans may be present, wherein every other pulse is stronger than the previous one.

Differential diagnosis should include pericardial disease plus cardiomyopathy, hypoproteinemic states, congenital heart defects such as severe pulmonic stenosis or atrial-ventricular canal, heartworms, tricuspid insufficiency, neoplastic invasion of the lymph nodes and lymphatics causing obstructive disease, and bacterial endocarditis with severe A-V valve insufficiency.

An electrocardiogram taken on an animal with pericardial disease may be normal. If a large amount of effusion is present, the QRS complexes may be dampened (R wave less than 0.7 mv in height). Non-specific ST-T changes may be present, and sometimes arrhythmias such as atrial fibrillation or ventricular premature beats may occur due to myocardial irritation. Electrical alternans, which is a smaller than normal beat appearing at every alternate QRS complex, may occur in cardiac tamponade and reflects the abnormal pendular motion of the myocardium in the pericardial sac filled with fluid (Spodick, 1976).

Radiographic changes are only evident if a significant amount of fluid is present in the pericardial sac. The cardiac silhouette takes on a globular appearance with scalloping on the dorsal ventral view where the pericardium becomes indented by touching the ribs or the thoracic wall. In constrictive pericarditis, the only radiographic change may be an increased postcaval size.

Fluoroscopy may be done on an enlarged heart to help differentiate pericardial effusions from cardiomyopathy. In pericardial effusion, there is a decreased amount of movement ventrally while the dorsal borders may appear to move normally. In cardiomyopathy, all borders of the heart appear to contract, but the movement may appear to be weaker than normal. A non-selective injection of contrast media into a vein followed by a radiograph of the thorax will show the increased distance between the cardiac chambers and the pericardial shadow in pericardial effusions. Non-selective angiography of congestive cardiomyopathy shows large, dilated chambers with thin muscle walls.

To help diagnose pericardial disease, a central venous pressure can be taken. It may be elevated greater than 15 cm of water (normal is 0 to 6 cm of water). The wave form of the CVP can be recorded; it shows characteristic changes with constrictive pericarditis (steep X and Y descent) and cardiac tamponade (loss of Y descent). As the use of echocardiography becomes more widespread in veterinary medicine, it will be used non-invasively to diagnose pericardial effusion.

Hepatic congestion secondary to right heart failure can cause increases in the SGPT, SGOT, and alkaline phosphatase while decreased cardiac output causes a pre-renal azotemia. The CBC can reflect (1) a generalized sepsis, (2) leukocytosis if the inflammation is at its peak, or (3) nucleated RBCs if a hemangiosarcoma is present.

TREATMENT

The treatment of pericardial disease is based on establishing the specific cause of the problem and treating the cause. Also, the symptoms of the pericardial disease are relieved by removing the pericardial effusion or the restricting pericardium.

Pericardiocentesis should be done to relieve cardiac tamponade as well as to have the fluid analyzed in an attempt to find the primary cause of the effusion. The method described by Tilley in *Current Veterinary Therapy V* is used with a few modifications. The catheter selected for the procedure is opened according to sterile technique and the plastic catheter is extended so that additional openings can be made along the first few inches of the catheter to permit more effective drainage of the pericardial sac. To prevent weakening of the catheter, holes are not placed right across from one another. The plastic catheter is then withdrawn back into the needle and its protective cover. The size of the catheter selected depends on the size of the animal. For larger animals, a 16 or 18 gauge needle with its catheter can be used. In a smaller animal, an 18 or 20 gauge needle should be used. The smaller catheters are tolerated well by the animal so that a local anesthetic in the area is not always necessary. Local anesthetic infiltration of the area is necessary with the larger catheters.

The animal is placed in left lateral recumbency or sternal recumbency, or it is allowed to remain standing. The right side of the chest is shaved at about the third to fifth intercostal space at the costal chondral junction or at the point at which the cardiac impulse can best be felt. It is preferable to penetrate the right side of the dog's chest because there is a cardiac notch in the lungs in that area and thus perforation of a lung lobe will be less likely. Also, there is less danger of hitting a major coronary artery on the right side than on the left side. A thorough surgical prep should be done before the pericardiocentesis is attempted. (The rest of the procedure follows that described by Tilley.) If the pericardium cannot be drained effectively from the right side owing to pericardial adhesions pulling the heart to the left or unsuccessful tapping of the pericardium, the left side should be tapped.

While the animal's pericardium is being tapped, the electrocardiogram should be watched for any signs of the needle encountering the myocardium. A few cases have been seen wherein the catheter has been passed right through the myocardium and into the ventricle without any changes on the electrocardiogram. Therefore, if a hemorrhagic effusion is encountered on pericardiocentesis, the clotting time should be compared with peripheral blood, as should the PCV. If the effusion turns out to be hemorrhage, additional fluid should not be removed, as either the catheter is in the ventricle or there is a source of vascular bleeding. If the hemorrhagic effusion is removed from the pericardial sac, further hemorrhage may be stimulated and the animal could bleed to death. If the fluid does not clot, as much fluid as possible should be removed. The dog's position may have to be shifted periodically in order to get most of the fluid from the pericardial sac. Fluid samples should be sent to the laboratory for fluid analysis (cytology), anaerobic and aerobic culture and sensitivity, and fungal cultures. Caution must be taken in the interpretation of cytologic results, as a long-standing pericardial effusion can have reactive mesothelial cells that look like neoplastic cells.

After the fluid is removed, air should be injected into the pericardial sac to outline the heart. About half the volume of fluid removed can be replaced by air. Radiographs should be taken in lateral recumbency, standing lateral

position, dorsal-ventral position, and oblique position in an attempt to locate any abnormalities such as tumors of the right atrium. More air can be added if necessary, and at the end of the procedure, all the air can be withdrawn or it can be left in the pericardial sac, since it will probably leak out of the needle hole in the pericardium and be reabsorbed in the pleural space. Contrast media can also be injected into the pericardial sac in an attempt to show abnormalities. About 10 cc of contrast media can be placed in a 30-pound dog. Care must be taken not to inject too much dye, as the dye can cause cardiac tamponade also.

Following pericardiocentesis, the animal should be placed on prophylactic antibiotic therapy for at least one week. The animal should be checked daily during that week for any recurrence of the fluid. Thereafter, the animal should be rechecked weekly for one month and then once very three months for the next year for the return of fluid.

Restrictive pericarditis is not as easily diagnosed and treated as is pericardial effusion. Many times the diagnosis is made by the elimination of all other diagnoses plus the finding of an elevated central venous pressure indicating a cardiac problem. Often, a cardiac catheterization is done in order to record intracardiac chamber pressures on both sides of the heart and to perform angiocardiography to rule out other problems. Pressure tracings at the time of cardiac catheterization will reveal elevated diastolic pressures in all chambers. Also, an arterial pressure tracing will have a characteristic wave form in restrictive pericarditis. The angiocardiogram is usually normal.

If the pericardial effusion recurs after a short time, if there is an indication of a possible tumor, or if constrictive pericarditis is present, surgery should be performed. For constrictive pericarditis or a benign, recurrent effusion that necessitates examination of the whole heart, splitting the sternum of the dog will give the best access to the greatest area of both sides of the heart. In both cases, as much of the pericardium as possible should be removed. Putting windows in the pericardial sac has been used for benign pericardial effusions in the past, but the windows can scar in the closed position and the examination of the heart is not as complete as when the entire pericardial sac is removed. Approximately 90 percent of the pericardial sac can be removed easily, and the remaining 10 percent does not seem to cause many problems if left in place.

If a tumor has been localized, the heart can be approached from the right or left lateral path between the ribs in order to get the best exposure of that area. Singular, nodular tumors with no signs of metastasis can be removed. If the tumor is on the right atrium, it can be removed, and the dog should probably be confined to a cage for 7 to 14 days following surgery to prevent exsanguination through the incision site.

Surgical removal of the pericardium in benign pericarditis allows any effusion to drain into the pleural space, where it is more readily absorbed, and helps to remove the inciting cause of the effusion. Removal of the pericardium in constrictive pericarditis allows the heart to return to normal function. However, it takes from two to four weeks for the hemodynamics to return completely to normal.

Other therapy for pericardial effusion and constrictive pericarditis has been tried. Antibiotics and steroids alone are not effective for either situation. Steroids will sometimes aid in inflammatory pericarditis and stop further effusion production but will not help to resolve the effusion or constriction already present. Diuretics will help the venous congestion but will not help to resolve the effusion in the pericardial sac, as there is only limited lymphatic and venous drainage from the pericardial sac. These drainage outlets are usually obstructed by the disease process to some extent, so diuretics are not effective in relieving the obstruction and stimulating the drainage of the pericardium.

Digitalis therapy will not improve the hemodynamics in pericardial effusion or constrictive pericarditis because the myocardium is normal and contracting adequately but is unable to fill. Digitalis has little effect on normal myocardium and therefore would not improve the situation, so it should not be used.

If frequent or significant ventricular arrhythmias are present, lidocaine should be used to control them. Supraventricular arrhythmias are usually transient and do not require therapy as long as the primary problem is being treated.

PROGNOSIS

The majority of animals with acute pericarditis do well during the acute episode and do not develop significant sequelae of cardiac tamponade or constriction. In animals that do develop a benign pericardial effusion, there is a tendency for the effusion to recur after it has been removed by pericardiocentesis. But with surgery, the problem is usually resolved and the prognosis is good.

Dogs with neoplasms of the pericardium or myocardium that can be removed and have no detectable sites of metastasis survive approximately one to two years. If metastases are present, the prognosis is poor and in most situations, the animal should be put to sleep on the surgery table. Only in situations in which the tumor can be removed and treated with chemotherapy should the patient with multiple metastases be allowed to recover from the anesthesia. Very few tumors of the pericardium seem to respond to current chemotherapy.

Constrictive pericarditis can have a favorable prognosis with surgery if the inflammatory process is resolved and the epicardium of the heart is not involved in the process and is not fibrotic. If the epicardium is fibrotic, the fibrotic areas should be removed at the time of surgery. Removal of this tissue is a bloody and time consuming procedure and should only be attempted if fibrosis is so extensive that myocardial contractility is impaired. In cases with fibrosis of the epicardium, regardless of whether most of the fibrotic areas were removed at surgery, the prognosis is guarded to poor, as constriction of the heart is still a problem.

The prognosis for septic pericardial effusion is guarded but not hopeless. It depends on the susceptibility of the organism to antibiotic therapy and any complications that can occur. A culture and sensitivity are important in these cases but can be negative in a long-standing process.

Hemorrhagic pericardial effusions owing to trauma or rupture of the left atrium are usually fatal but sometimes can resolve spontaneously. Effusions secondary to congestive heart failure respond well when the congestive heart failure is treated.

SUPPLEMENTAL READING

Bolton, G.R.: Pericardial diseases. In Ettinger, S.J. (ed.): *Textbook of Veterinary Internal Medicine.* Philadelphia, W.B. Saunders Company, 1975.
Bonagura, J.B.: *Clinical Cardiology Notes.* Columbus, Ohio, The Ohio State University Press, 1977.
Knauer, K.W.: Pericardial effusion. In Kirk, R.W. (ed.): *Current Veterinary Therapy VI.* Philadelphia, W.B. Saunders Company, 1977.
Spodick, D.H. (ed.): Pericardial diseases. In Brest, A.N. (ed.): *Cardiovascular Clinics.* Philadelphia, F.A. Davis Company, 1976.
Tilley, L.P., and Wilkins, R.J.: Pericardial disease. In Kirk, R.W. (ed.): *Current Veterinary Therapy V.* Philadelphia, W.B. Saunders Company, 1974.

CANINE HEARTWORM DISEASE

JOHN D. KELLY, B.V.Sc.

Bendigo, Australia

Heartworm disease in dogs results from infection by the filarioid nematode *Dirofilaria immitis*. The dog is the principal final host for this parasite, which is transmitted by mosquitoes.

Mature *D. immitis* are found in the right ventricle and pulmonary artery. Occasionally, adult or immature worms are found in the peritoneal cavity, bronchioles, brain, eyes, and other tissues. These are rare and should be viewed as biologic curiosities rather than as recurring clinical problems. One major exception is the presence of heartworms in the posterior vena cava and right atrium associated with the occurrence of the "posterior caval" syndrome (Jackson *et al.*, 1977).

Adult *D. immitis* are long, slender worms (12 to 30 cm) with a very thick cuticle and few obvious morphologic characteristics. In general, the male (12 to 18 cm) is usually smaller than the female (25 to 30 cm). The female, which is viviparous, produces vermiform larvae known as microfilariae, which are found in peripheral blood and measure 290 to 340 microns.

Although the most important host is the dog, *D. immitis* infects a wide variety of mammals. The parasite is reported in cats and man (Kelly, 1977). It has also been reported in horses and marine mammals.

Various filarioid nematodes occur in dogs (Table 1), but of these, the only one of major importance in the United States other than *D. immitis* is *Dipetalonema reconditum*. This parasite is found in the subcutaneous tissue of dogs and is not generally pathogenic. Its significance lies in the fact that it occurs in the same endemic areas as does *D. immitis*, and the presence of *D. reconditum* microfilariae in peripheral blood may confuse the diagnosis of canine heartworm disease. Adult *D. reconditum* are slender worms measuring up to 24 mm in

Table 1. *Characteristics of Various Filarioid Nematodes Known to Occur in Dogs*

SPECIES	HOST RANGE	VECTOR	TISSUE SITES (ADULTS)	GEOGRAPHIC RANGE	TISSUE SITES (MICROFILARIAE)	LENGTH OF MICROFILARIAE (MICRONS)
Dirofilaria immitis	Dog, cat, marine mammals, man	Mosquito	Heart and pulmonary artery	America, Africa, Australia, Italy, Spain	Blood	286–349 (314)
Dirofilaria repens	Dog, cat, man	Mosquito	Subcutaneous tissues	USSR, Europe, India, Far East	Blood	290
Dirofilaria conjunctivae	Considered identical to *D. repens* and may also be confused with *D. tenuis*, which is found in the subcutaneous tissues of raccoons, man					
Dipetalonema reconditum	Dog	Fleas, ticks	Connective tissues	America, Italy, Africa, Australia	Blood	258–292 (270)
Dipetalonema dracunculoides	Dog	Louse Fly (*Hippobosca longipennis*)	Peritoneal membranes	Africa	Blood	195–230
Dipetalonema grassi	Dog	Tick	Subcutaneous tissues	Italy, Kenya	Skin rarely in Blood	570
Brugia malayi	Man, cat (dog)	Mosquito	Lymphatic system	India, Africa, Far East	Blood	170–260 (220)
Brugia pahangi	Dog, cat Felidae	Mosquito	Lymphatic system	Africa, Far East	Blood	280
Brugia patei	Dog, cat	Mosquito	Lymphatic system	Africa	Blood	Similar to *B. malayi*

length. Adult worms occur in the subcutaneous and connective tissues, especially the fascial spaces of the limbs and back. Microfilariae circulate in blood and measure 258 to 292 microns.

LIFE CYCLES

Dirofilaria immitis. Adult female *D. immitis* produce first-stage larvae or microfilariae that circulate in peripheral blood. These complete development to the infective third larval stage only in a suitable mosquito vector. When microfilariae are ingested during blood meals, they migrate to the malpighian tubules where embryonic development is completed. Thereafter, first-stage larvae continue to grow and successively moult to second- and third-stage larvae over a period of 14 to 21 days. Infective third-stage larvae then migrate through the thorax to the labia and are transferred to dogs in hemolymph during feeding by infected mosquitoes. The time required for development in the intermediate host is primarily influenced by temperature and humidity.

Following inoculation of infective larvae into dogs, third-stage *D. immitis* actively migrate to a resting site in the subcutaneous or subserosal tissues or in the muscles or fat. In these sites, they moult to fourth-stage larvae (18 mm) at 9 to 12 days after infection and to fifth-stage larvae (4 to 8 cm) at 70 to 80 days after infection. At approximately three months, immature adults begin migrating to the right ventricle and adjacent vessels. Microfilariae are present in the uterus of female worms five to six months after infection and commonly appear in the peripheral blood six to seven months after initial exposure of the dog to infective third-stage larvae. Prepatent period for *D. immitis* is approximately six months.

If a bitch is inoculated with infective third-stage larvae, it is conceivable that a small proportion may migrate through the placenta to the fetus. In practical terms, one could then expect to find patent infection with *D. immitis* (accompanied by a microfilaremia) in dogs less than six months of age. Another aspect of transplacental migration of *D. immitis* concerns the passive transfer of non-infective (for the final host) microfilariae across the placental barrier. Such a case has been described (Mantovani and Jackson, 1966; Kelly, 1977) in which a bitch, with a patent *D. immitis* infection and accompanying microfilaremia (400,000 ml blood), gave birth to five pups, all of which had low numbers (5 to 30/ml) of circulating first-stage larvae or microfilariae. The significance of passive microfilarial transfer is that it may lead to an erroneous diagnosis of heartworm infection in young dogs.

Dipetalonema reconditum. The life cycle of *D. reconditum* is similar to that of *D. immitis* except that the arthropod intermediate hosts are fleas (e.g., *Ctenocephalides felis*) and lice (e.g., *Trichodectes canis*). Infections with this parasite are of little pathogenic significance. However, the microfilarial stage is similar to that of *D. immitis* and this may confuse diagnosis.

PATHOLOGY AND DIAGNOSIS OF CANINE HEARTWORM DISEASE

The diagnosis of infection with *D. immitis* depends on an integrated consideration of history and clinical signs plus the use of one or more of the following aids: radiography, angiography, electrocardiography, clinical pathology, and the detection and differentiation of microfilariae in blood.

HISTORY

The history should include information about the following factors: (1) presence of suitable intermediate host(s), (2) prevalence of canine heartworm disease (C.H.D.) in a given area or locality, (3) history of susceptible dogs being transported from a heartworm-free area to one of endemic CHD, (4) significantly greater prevalence of dirofilariasis in working dogs as opposed to house dogs, (5) presence of the disease in other animals — e.g., cats, and (6) history of weight loss, anorexia, coughing, reduced exercise tolerance, syncope, and episodic weakness and hemoptysis.

PHYSICAL EXAMINATION

Symptoms vary with the chronicity and severity of the infection and depend on the extent and nature of damage to target organs. These have been summarized as follows (Kelly, 1977):

Cardiovascular/Pulmonary. The adult parasites are found principally in the right ventricle and the main pulmonary arteries. In order of involvement, the pulmonary arteries affected are the diaphragmatic, the cardiac, and the apical lobar. Occasionally, adult parasites are found in the caudal vena cava and the hepatic and coronary veins. Pathologic changes are found principally in the pulmonary arteries and may be of two types: endarteritis or thromboemboli. Endarteritis is caused by viable *D. immitis*. The walls of the arteries become thickened, with proliferation of endothelial cells and infiltration by inflammatory cells, principally eosinophils. Nodular intimal lesions protrude into the lumen of the vessels. Thromboemboli are caused by dead parasites and secondary fibroblastic organization of the thrombi. Arterial changes are minimal.

The hemodynamic disturbance that results may produce signs of congestive, right-sided cardiac failure with ascites and lung edema occurring in advanced cases. Pulmonary damage often produces a chronic cough. Severe coughing spasms may result in hemoptysis. Auscultation of the chest may reveal (1) increased audibility and/or splitting of the second heart sound (over the pulmonic valve region), (2) systolic murmurs, especially in advanced cases, (3) tachypnea and/or dyspnea, (4) abnormal respiratory sounds, and (5) tachyarrhythmias — supraventricular and ventricular premature contractions. An excellent description of the physiologic response of the canine heart and lungs to *D. immitis* has been written (Rawlings *et al.*, 1978).

Posterior Caval Syndrome. This is variously referred to as the caval syndrome, vena caval syndrome, vena cava embolism, acute hepatic syndrome, and liver failure syndrome. The condition results from the presence of large masses of worms in the caudal vena cava and hepatic veins, resulting in passive hepatic congestion, centrilobular necrosis, and cavernomatous replacement of the central veins. Some of the changes appear to be basically allergic reactions. Phlebitis of the hepatic veins may produce fibrosis of the vessel walls and surrounding tissue, with intense infiltration by inflammatory cells, principally eosinophils. The symptoms are those of acute liver failure and disseminated intravascular coagulation; i.e., sudden onset of anorexia, bilirubinuria, hemoglobinuria, jaundice, dyspnea, and collapse. The syndrome is most commonly seen in young dogs with large numbers of worms. The condition has been described by Jackson *et al.* (1977).

Membranous Glomerulonephritis. Two pathologic conditions have been descrubed involving the kidneys: (1) physical obstruction of the renal capillary beds by microfilariae, causing vascular occlusion, and (2) membranous glomerulonephropathy, with the capillary basement membrane thickened with amorphous deposits. These lesions probably result from circulating immune complexes that are filtered out in the basement membrane. In these cases, urinalysis may reveal a moderate proteinurea and occasionally microfilariae.

It should be noted that at any stage of heartworm disease, sudden death owing to infarction of arteries and capillary beds in the lungs, central nervous system, heart, bowel, or kidney may occur, and this can result either from accumulations of microfilariae or from adult worms.

It has been suggested that the accumulation of microfilariae may also cause chronic cellular hypoxia to which the liver is particularly vulnerable. Chronic hypoxia causes greatly reduced hepatocyte protein synthesis, and decreased serum albumin levels have been reported in canine dirofilariasis.

Finally, it should be realized that aberrant tissue locations of the parasite may produce unusual pathologic lesions and associated clinical signs; e.g., ischemic myopathy in a dog with posterior limb weakness associated with thrombosis of the iliac arteries owing to the presence of aberrant adult *D. immitis*.

RADIOGRAPHY

In cases in which clinical signs are suggestive of and/or blood examination is negative for *D. immitis* microfilariae, radiography may be used to confirm heartworms Where dirofilariasis has been established by prior examination of peripheral blood, radiography is of value in assessing the degree of pathologic change and hemodynamic disturbance that has occurred in the cardiovascular and pulmonary systems. The principal radiographic alterations in established cases of dirofilariasis are as follows:

1. *Right ventricular enlargement.* In the lateral view, this is evident as increased bulging of the cranial border of the heart, with reduced retrosternal space and increased cardiosternal contact. In the dorsoventral view, the right ventricle may bulge excessively from the midline, giving the cardiac shape and inverted appearance.
2. *Pulmonary cone dilation.*
3. *Mainstem pulmonary artery dilation.* The peripheral pulmonary arteries are "pruned," and the gradual tapering and arborization are lost. The pulmonary arteries become truncated and tortuous owing to occlusion. These changes are best observed in the mainstem diaphragmatic lobar pulmonary arteries.

These three changes, when present together, are diagnostic of dirofilariasis. The challenge has now become detection of very slight alterations from normal, early in infection and/or in dogs with only a few adult heartworms (see Rawlings et al , 1978).

ANGIOGRAPHY

The dilation, tortuousity, pruning, and loss of normal arborization patterns in the pulmonary arteries are more easily visualized with a pulmonary artery angiogram. Adult heartworms may be more easily visualized as linear lucencies.

ELECTROCARDIOGRAPHY

The electrocardiographic changes seen in dirofilariasis may also be caused by a number of other congenital and acquired cardiac diseases that result in right ventricular enlargement. Electrocardiograms may be used in dogs without radiographic signs of right ventricular enlargement, and these have been described by Ettinger and Suter (1970) and Rawlings *et al.* (1978).

CLINICAL PATHOLOGY

Urinalysis is useful for assessement of degree of renal and hepatic damage.

Hematologic tests reveal that dogs become moderately anemic and exhibit eosinophilia.

Serum enzyme analysis — particularly SGPT, creatinine, and BUN — can be of critical importance in determining whether or not anthelmintic treatment should be initiated.

For serologic assay, an indirect fluorescent antibody technique has been used experimentally in the dog and for surveys of both human and canine populations. Unfortunately, *D. immitis* shares common antigenic determinants with *Toxocara canis*, and therefore the test is not entirely specific. A number of other techniques have been used and these have been summarized (Kelly, 1977).

DETECTION AND IDENTIFICATION OF MICROFILARIAE IN BLOOD

The examination of blood for the presence of microfilariae of *Dirofilaria immitis* has been previously reviewed (Kelly, 1977) and is summarized in this section. The methods available include the following.

WET BLOOD SMEAR. Place a drop of fresh blood on a slide, add a coverslip, and examine under low power. Motile microfilariae (sluggish movement) should be seen if infection is heavy. It must be emphasized that this method is useful only if microfilariae are seen. *A negative smear is meaningless.* It may be difficult at times to visualize motile microfilariae because of the erythrocytes. This can be overcome by the addition of a drop of 2 per cent saponin or 0.04 per cent ammonium hydroxide to lyse the red blood cells.

SERUM. Allow the blood samples to clot and decant the serum. Place a drop of freshly collected serum on a clean slide, add a coverslip, and examine under low power. Motile microfilariae tend to be found in greater concentration in serum and are generally easier to observe because of the absence of erythrocytes. Once again, this method is relatively insensitive and will not detect small numbers of microfilariae.

MODIFIED KNOTT TECHNIQUE. One ml of whole blood is mixed with 10 ml 2 per cent formalin, and the mixture is centrifuged for three to five minutes at 1500 r.p.m. Following removal of the supernatant, the sediment is mixed in equal parts with 1:1000 new methylene blue and the stained sediment is examined microscopically. This technique combines a number of important advantages. The microfilariae are concentrated in the small amount of sediment, which is composed mainly of leukocytes and debris of hemolysed erythrocytes. This is an important advantage in detecting light infections. The method is highly reliable, and width and length measurements of microfilariae can be made in order to identify the type of microfilariae present (Table 2).

CAPILLARY HEMATOCRIT TECHNIQUE. Examination of the intact "buffy coat" and of the plasma portion of the microhematocrit is employed to visualize microfilariae. These are observed as they emerge from the cellular "buffy coat" to enter the plasma layer within seconds of exposure to a direct light beam. The motility of microfilariae remains vigorous for about 20 minutes after blood collection.

FILTER TECHNIQUE. This is probably the most reliable concentration technique. In our modification of Wylie's technique, 2 ml of blood (either fresh or added to heparin) are mixed with 25 ml of either 2 per cent formalin or commercial lysing solution (8 grams Na_2CO_3 plus 5 ml triton concentrate in 1000 ml of distilled water) in a 30 ml syringe. Following thorough mixing, the syringe is connected to a plastic filter holder containing a 25 mm diameter polycarbonate filter (pore size = 8 μm). The lysed blood is gently forced through the filter disc and the syringe is detached. A second 20 ml syringe containing distilled water is then attached to the filter holder and approximately 15 ml is gently forced through the filter disc. The disc is then air-dried (by forcing 20 ml air through the syringe), removed from the filter holder, placed on a glass slide, stained with 2 to 3 drops of 0.2 per cent methyl green, and examined under low power for stained microfilariae. It is important to scan the entire filter disc, including the periphery, as frequently only one or two microfilariae may be present in light infections. In addition to its reliability, the filter technique is very rapid (insofar as no centrifugation is involved), and far less time is required to scan the slide compared with the modified Knott technique. This method should allow practitioners to screen multiple blood samples for microfilaraie quickly and accurately.

The author has found that polycarbonate filters ("Nucleopore" filter), either 5 or 8 μm

Table 2. *Differentiation of Microfilariae of*
D. Immitis *and* D. Reconditum[*]

CHARACTERISTIC	D. Immitis	D. Reconditum
Average width (in microns)[†] (Lindsay, 1961)	6.8 (6.1–7.2)	5.2 (4.7–5.8)
Average length (in microns) (Lindsay, 1961)	314 (286–340)	270 (258–292)
Mobility (Schalm and Jain, 1966)	Sluggish	Active
Presence of "button hook" on posterior extremity (Newton and Wright, 1956)	Absent	Present
Shape of anterior extremity	Tapered	Blunt
Presence of cephalic hook (Sawyer et al., 1965)	Absent	Present
Degree of straightness	Straight	Crescent-shaped
Dye uptake using Coriphosphine O (Rothstein and Brown, 1960)	Stained in 10 minutes	Staining in 30 minutes
Acid phosphatase activity (Chalifoux and Hunt, 1971)	Two distinct zones	Generalised

[*] Detailed references cited in Kelly (1977).
[†] Width measured at 50 or 60 microns from tip of anterior extremity.

diameter, give consistently better results than does the fiber millipore filter (Whitlock *et al.*, 1978).

PKW METHOD. This method involves two stages. Stage 1 incorporates procedures for screening and detection of microfilariae using polycarbonate filters and methyl green stain. Stage 2 involves the processing of microfilariae-positive membranes through a commercially available acid-phosphatase kit* for differential enzyme staining of *D. immitis* and *D. reconditum* (Whitlock *et al*, 1978). This method is also applicable to other filarioid nematodes (see Table 1).

The literature contains only limited quantitative data on relative blood concentrations of *D. immitis* and *Dipetalonema* sp. microfilaria, and most reports emphasize the serious limitations of using relative numbers of microfilariae as aids to definitive diagnosis. Accurate diagnosis necessitates the use of more specific criteria to differentiate between *D. immitis* and *Dipetalonema* sp. — i.e., acid-phosphatase activity (Whitlock *et al.*, 1978).

The number of circulating microfilariae of *D. immitis* is not an accurate indication of the presence or absence of a patent infection or of the numbers of adult female *D. immitis* present. The absence of microfilariae in the presence of

°APFIL® Heartworm Diagnostic Test Kit—Apex Laboratories, Christie St., St. Marys, NSW, 2760, Australia.

adult worms may be traced to (1) worms of one sex only, (2) worms that have not commenced microfilaria production, (3) treatment of the patient with a microfilaricide prior to blood sampling, (4) dead adult *D. immitis*, and (5) antibody suppression of microfilarial production in chronically infected dogs.

On the other hand, the presence of microfilariae in the absence of adult worms may be the result of loss of adult *D. immitis* owing to chemotherapy or to physiologic aging of the parasite. This is an important point, particularly as it has been shown that the microfilariae of *D. immitis* can survive in the cardiovascular system for several years.

Differentiation of Microfilariae in Blood. The morphologic and physiologic characteristics that may be used to distinguish between microfilariae of *D. immitis* and *Dipetalonema* sp. have been discussed (Kelly, 1977) and are summarized in Table 2. It is also relevant to point out that other filarioid nematodes can infect carnivores and produce microfilariae in blood. Examples of some of these species are given in Table 1.

TREATMENT OF CANINE HEARTWORM DISEASE

ADULT D. IMMITIS

The principal symptoms and lesions result

from the presence of adult worms in the heart and adjacent vessels, and treatment is therefore directed toward removal of worms from these sites. Until recently, phenylarsenoxide compounds (e.g., thiacetarsamide sodium) were the only anthelmintics commercially available that were consistently effective in killing adult *D. immitis*. Unfortunately, the use of such drugs may be associated with toxic side effects in the host. Treatment regimes for CHD are varied, and those that have been reported successful in eliminating adult and/or microfilarial infections are as follows.

Surgery.   The role of surgery for treatment of heartworms has been questioned (except for the posterior caval syndrome), and some former proponents now hesitate to recommend it. Jackson *et al.* (1977) described surgical procedures for the removal of heartworms from the right atrium and posterior vena cava via the jugular vein.

Chemotherapy.   The usual recommendation for chemotherapy is to use an adulticide (Table 3) followed later by one or more doses of microfilaricide, repeating the treatment if necessary until a series of negative blood smears is obtained. All cases must be thoroughly assessed before treatment is commenced in an attempt to reduce complications (Kelly, 1977). This information is critical since (1) asymptomatic dogs with dirofilariasis are not necessarily free from pathologic changes, (2) compromised hepatic and renal function may impair adulticide metabolism, and (3) specific adulticide therapy may result in pulmonary thromboembolism, the effects of which may be greatly exaggerated in dogs with deficient cardiopulmonary function.

Thiacetarsamide Sodium.   Animals with a negative or low microfilarial count but with obvious clinical and radiographic signs of heartworms may be started immediately on thiacetarsamide therapy. The recommended procedure is intravenous thiacetarsamide twice daily for two days at a dose rate of 2.2 mg/kg body weight. (Recently, a third day of medication has been advocated.) Vomiting occasionally follows initial administration, but if no other signs are present, treatment may be completed. Persistent vomiting, anorexia, or jaundice indicates immediate cessation of treatment.

Pulmonary thromboembolism from dead *D. immitis* may occur from 5 to 30 days after thiacetarsamide therapy. Such reactions, clinically evident as hyperthermia, increased respiratory rate, coughing, lethargy, and inappetence, may be treated with antibiotics and corticosteroids (e.g., prednisolone 2.5 mg/kg). Therefore, rigid confinement for at least three weeks after thiacetarsamide treatment is advised. It is important to remember that chemotherapy should not be instituted in heartworm patients with severe congestive heart failure until they have been compensated with digitalis and a diuretic; in other cases, anthelmintic and cardiac therapy may be commenced simultaneously. Animals with high microfilarial counts may be pretreated with a microfilaricide (e.g., dithiazinine 4.4 to 6.6 mg/kg or levamisole 10 mg/kg). This has been reported to reduce mortality rates following thiacetarsamide therapy.

Levamisole.*   This drug is claimed to be effective against both adults and microfilariae of *D. immitis* as opposed to the singular adulticide activity of thiacetarsamide (Kelly, 1977). It has been reported that levamisole is preferentially adulticidal against male *D. immitis*. Suggested treatment schedules using levamisole against adult *D. immitis* are:

1. Long-term daily dosage at 10 to 15 mg/kg (adverse side effects are a problem).
2. 2.5 mg/kg *per os* daily for 14 days, then 5 mg/kg daily for next 14 days, then 10 mg/kg daily for 14 days; i.e., a progressive dosage schedule from 2.5 to 10 mg/kg bw/day over

*This drug has not been approved in the U.S.A. for use in dogs. If used, clients should be so informed and a consent slip giving such permission should be obtained.

Table 3.   *Effect of Chemotherapeutics on Each Developmental Stage of* Dirofilaria Immitis

Developmental Stage	Location	CHEMOTHERAPEUTIC AGENTS						
		Antimonials	Diethylcarbamazine	Aresnicals	Dithiazinine	Organophosphates	Levamisole	Benzimidazoles
Microfilaria	Blood	+++	++ (L$_3$ only)	−	+++ (L$_1$ only)	++	+++ (L$_1$ only)	+++ L$_3$
Developing Larvae	Intermediate Location	+	+++ (dose dependent)	+	−	?	−/?	+++ (dose dependent)
Adult Worm	Heart and Pulmonary Artery	+	−	+++	−	−	+/−	+/−

Adapted from Kume-Proc. 1st International Symposium on Canine Heartworm Disease.
Key: +++ = highly effective; ++ = effective; + = some effect; − = no effect; ? = unknown effect.

six weeks. From the end of the second week, a marked clinical improvement is noticeable and microfilarial counts usually decrease by at least 60 to 70 per cent from pretreatment values

3. 2.5 mg/kg *per os* daily for first week; check up, then 5.0 mg/kg *per os* daily for next three weeks; check up, then 10.0 mg/kg *per os* daily for next three weeks; check up, then on to a suitable preventative microfilaricide (e.g., diethylcarbamazine).

Side effects of levamisole are minimal with the latter two schedules, and such treatment regimes are widely practiced in Queensland (Australia), where heartworm disease is endemic. The main problem that may arise is ataxia, which is temporary and completely reversible following drug withdrawal. Vomiting does not appear to be a problem, provided that levamisole is started at the low dose of 2.5 mg/kg. Levamisole does have a bitter taste, but this can be readily overcome by administering the drug in a honey base or in a gelatin capsule. Commercial preparations of levamisole* in tablet form are currently available in Australia. Preliminary results show that 10 mg/kg once daily for 10 days is highly effective in destroying circulating microfilariae (Ross and Kelly, 1978).

It is important to note that levamisole is not consistently adulticidal except at high or prolonged dosage schedules. Hematologic and biochemical effects of levamisole use include increased total white cell counts, transitory elevation of SGOT (insignificant), and significant increase in liver SGPT for the duration of treatment with similar changes in lactic dehydrogenase. Following levamisole treatment, surviving adult female *D. immitis* may be eliminated with thiacetarsamide sodium as previously described. Animals treated with levamisole can be placed directly on diethylcarbamazine prophylaxis, thus protecting recently treated animals from reinfection.

D. IMMITIS MICROFILARIAE

The only drug available on the U.S. market for destruction of *D. immitis* microfilariae is dithiazinine iodide. In Australia, levamisole is also registered for use as a microfilaricide. A list of drugs and their relative activities against microfilariae of *D. immitis* is given in Table 3. It should be noted that dithiazinine may need to be given in higher doses (up to 22 mg/kg over 10 days), as failure at the recommended dose levels has been reported.

---

*Levamisole tablets - Ethnor Pty Ltd, Khartoum Road, North Ryde, NSW, 2113, Australia.

PROPHYLAXIS FOR CANINE HEARTWORM DISEASE

Various methods of chemical prevention are available for *D. immitis*, and these have been discussed (Kelly, 1977). In summary, they are as follows.

SODIUM THIACETARSAMIDE

In endemic areas, thiacetarsamide (2.2 mg/kg IV BID for two days) administered every six months may be used. This treatment eliminates *D. immitis* before a sufficient number have developed to patency. The disadvantages of this scheme have been reported (Kelly, 1977).

DIETHYLCARBAMAZINE

Daily administration of diethylcarbamazine (DEC) beginning at the time a dog will be exposed to mosquitoes and continuing for two months after the mosquito season will prevent heartworm infection. This is the only drug that has a registered claim for activity against third-stage (or infective) larvae and, to a lesser extent, subsequent tissue migrating stages. Important points relevant to the prophylactic use of DEC are:

1. DEC must be given daily. This is because the drug is rapidly absorbed and completely excreted within 24 hours. There is obviously no residual action, and hence rigorous daily use is required.

2. The dose rate at which DEC is employed is critical. Commercial preparations of the drug are available as either the citrate or base, and it is important to remember that the amount of available DEC in the citrate formulation is usually 50 per cent of that available in the base. The minimum long-term effective dose is >5.5 mg/kg daily as a prophylactic against third-stage infective larvae, and up to 11 mg/kg may be required to kill tissue-dwelling fourth-stage *D. immitis*. (All dose rates quoted are referable to DEC citrate).

3. DEC must never be given to a microfilariae-positive dog. Several reports have described a shock-like and disseminated intravascular coagulopathy syndrome that is sometimes fatal, and this has occurred with doses as low as 4.4 mg/kg. In all cases, it is imperative that microfilariae are removed by dithiazinine or levamisole therapy before commencing DEC prophylaxis (either for heartworm or roundworm infection).

DEC may be used at three monthly intervals

by oral administration at a dose rate of 60 to 65 mg/kg. A similar scheme has been tried in Australia, where dogs were treated every two months with DEC at 45 mg/kg for three successive days. It should be noted that all treated dogs were protected against infection; however, indications of mild hepatic damage were reported.

DEC appears to interfere with nerve function in nematodes, which leads to paralysis. It is also a recognized cholinesterase inhibitor, similar to widely used pesticides such as organophosphates and carbamates. These drugs should not be administered to microfilariae-positive dogs. It has been suggested that such drug-induced reactions and mortality in microfilariae-positive dogs is due to acute liver necrosis. It has been claimed that removal of microfilariae prior to the use of such drugs is all that is required to prevent adverse side effects.

BENZIMIDAZOLE ANTHELMINTICS

Recent studies (reviewed by Kelly, 1977) have shown that dogs can be protected against artificial infection with *D. immitis* by the daily administration of methyl 5-benzoylbenzimidazole-2-carbamate,* beginning two days before infection and continuing for 28 days thereafter Dogs were treated at either 40 or 80 mg/kg, and the treatment regime was 100 per cent effective against developing heartworm larvae with no major side effects. No further work has been reported at the time of writing, but these results do indicate that some useful antifilarial activity will be found among benzimidazole-type drugs.

IMMUNITY AND *DIROFILARIA IMMITIS*

In enzootic areas, it is common to find up to 50 to 100 adult *D. immitis* in dogs no more than 18 months old. However, in general, this number does not tend to increase appreciably with age. It has also been suggested that parasite numbers gradually decrease over time, even though exposure to infection may be constant.

The simplest explanation for this observation is that this number of worms (or biomass) represents the approximate physiologic limit for establishment in the host, and in order for new infective larvae to reach patency, there must be continual turnover or "regulation" of worm numbers. An alternative explanation is that animals infected with *D. immitis* develop an acquired immunity. Conceptually, such an immune response would be triggered when the worm biomass (adults plus all larval stages) exceeds a critical threshold level (e.g., 50 to 100 worms). As a corollary, acquired immunity must be directed principally against incoming larval stages of the parasite rather than established adult infections, since mature *D. immitis* can survive for long periods in immunologically reactive hosts.

The role of antibodies in immunity to *D. immitis* infection is unclear. Passive transfer of resistance with immune sera to adult *D. immitis* infection in dogs has not been demonstrated. Nevertheless, dogs infected with *D. immitis* produce detectable antibodies (measurable by several different techniques), but whether these are functional and protective is not clear at this stage.

Cryptic or occult filariasis, which occurs in 10 to 15 per cent of heartworm-infected dogs, is a difficult diagnostic problem. Although no microfilariae are present in blood, these animals do produce detectable levels of antibodies to the microfilarial stage that appear to be species-specific. Such antibodies are not always detectable in dogs with circulating microfilariae. Apparently, sensitization or immunity to the microfilarial stage of a filarial species does not prevent a subsequent infection by infective larvae or their maturation to the adult stage. It may, however, inhibit the circulation of first-stage microfilariae, and it is therefore logical to suggest that elevated antibody titers may be functionally associated with the establishment of an amicrofilaremic state.

A simple test for investigating cases of occult dirofilariasis is as follows. Serum from an occult dog is incubated with fresh, heparin, or oxalate preserved blood containing *D. immitis* microfilariae. A control tube containing microfilariae-positive blood plus normal serum (i.e., serum from a known heartworm-negative dog) is set up and both are incubated at 37° C. Usually, after 15 to 30 minutes, microfilariae incubated with occult serum are sluggish and clumped together in a "Medusa-head" formation, whereas microfilariae incubated in normal serum are randomly dispersed and motile. A positive test should not be taken as conclusive evidence of occult heartworm infection but rather as an additional guide in helping the practitioner reach a decision in relation to treatment in these diagnostically difficult cases.

Recent investigations on the immunodiagnosis of human onchocerciasis (*Onchocerca volvulus*) have shown that serum IgE levels are significantly increased in the majority (80 per cent) of infected individuals. Somotin and Heiner (1976) adapted the radioallergosorbent

---

*Mebendazole — Telmin Dog Wormer — Ethnor Pty Ltd, Khartoum Rd, North Ryde, NSW, 2113, Australia.

technique for detection of specific IgE antibodies to *D. immitis*. This may be a useful diagnostic tool in the future.

Various studies have shown that animals develop cell-mediated (CMI) responses to infection with *D. immitis*. However, in common with a number of other parasitic infections (e.g., hookworm infection) it has been observed that some heartworm-infected dogs exhibit reduced blastogenesis of peripheral blood lymphocytes to *D. immitis* as well as to unrelated antigens (impaired T-lymphocyte function) (Kelly et al., 1977) Immunologically unresponsive states in heartworm dogs may predispose such animals to infectious diseases as well as to neoplasia.

The object of vaccination is not so much to mimic nature but to improve on it, because naturally acquired immune responses are frequently associated with immunopathologic damage and survival of parasites in the immunized host. The ideal vaccine would be an extract of a parasite consisting of the fraction that actually stimulates a protective response, and one that is chemically characterized so that it could be synthesized and used either on its own or in association with a carrier molecule.

Attempts to stimulate protective immunity against filarial infections by the inoculation of soluble and/or somatic antigens, prepared from homogenized adult or larval stages, have generally been unsuccessful. The immunogenicity of living or attenuated microfilariae has, however, been proved in several host-parasite systems by their ability to induce stage and species-specific immunity, which generally results in filarial infections without circulating microfilariae.

Recent studies by Wong *et al.* (1974) have investigated the potential usefulness of attenuated, living larval vaccines of *D. immitis*. They showed that dogs, challenged three months or more after receiving immunizing doses of irradiated (20 KR) third-stage larvae, had total worm counts at autopsy varying from 0 to 3.5 per cent of the challenge infection (approximately 200 third-stage larvae of *D. immitis*), compared with approximately 30 per cent worm recovery in "non-vaccinated" controls. It was also shown that irradiated third-stage larvae of *D. immitis* never reached the heart but could live up to the time of the final moult (i.e., between 2 and 3 months post-infection — late fourth-stage larvae).

Clinical application of such vaccination procedures is not practical at present, but the experimental results indicate that animals can be at least partially protected against *D. immitis*. The difficulties inherent in immunizing animals against helminths and the observations of diminished immunocompetence in some heartworm-infected dogs has led to a search for substances that might non-specifically stimulate ineffective host responses — e.g., Bacillus Camette-Guerin Vaccine (BCG). In the future, BCG or similar immunostimulants (e.g., levamisole or related compounds) might be used alone or in conjunction with the appropriate *D. immitis* antigen to boost natural or induced host immunity to this parasite.

ZOONOTIC DIROFILARIASIS

Animal filariod nematodes, largely of the genus *Dirofilaria*, have been reported to produce tissue lesions and eosinophilia in man. Case reports of human pulmonary dirofilariasis generally record chest pain, coughing, and peripheral eosinophilia as the main clinical symptoms observed. Obvious infections of this type probably represent a minority of the total human cases in populations at risk. More recently, Dobson and Welch (1974) showed a high correlation between the presence of antibodies to *D. immitis* and cases of eosinophilic meningitis in man.

Human infections with *D. immitis* are generally abortive and do not reach patency, as most of the infective larvae are unable to complete development and attain sexual maturity. After inoculation of third-stage infective larvae, most are destroyed in the subcutaneous tissues. However, with repeated infection, some may escape, begin to develop to immature adults, and migrate via the venous system to the heart.

Young adult *D. immitis* are apparently unable to lodge in the heart as they do in dogs and thus they pass on in the pulmonary circulation until they become arrested in an artery and give rise to an infarct. The infarcted tissue undergoes necrosis, which is followed by fibrous tissue encapsulation. Typical lesions consist of a centrally placed artery containing nematode sections, which is surrounded by a broad field of necrotic tissue, limited by a narrow circumferential band of collagen. Associated with the latter are fibroblasts, histiocytes, lymphocytes, eosinophils, and foreign body giant cells. The solid spherical lesions detected by radiography are referred to as "coin lesions" and measure 1 to 3 cm in diameter.

The occurrence of zoonotic dirofilariasis is almost always associated with the presence of endemic dirofilariasis in dogs. Prevention of the disease in man therefore depends on effective treatment and control of *D. immitis* in dogs.

SUPPLEMENTAL READING

Dobson, C., and Welch, J. S.: Dirofilariasis as a cause of eosinophiliac meningitis in man diagnosed by immunofluorescence and arthus hypersensitivity. Trans. Roy. Soc. Trop. Med. Hyg. 68:223–228, 1974.

Ettinger, J. T., and Suter, P. F. (eds.): *Canine Cardiology*. Philadelphia, W. B. Saunders Co., 1970.

Jackson, R. F., Seymour, W. G., Crowney, P. J., and Otto, G. F.: Surgical treatment of the caval syndrome of canine heartworm disease. JAVMA 171:1065–1069, 1977.

Kelly, J. D.: Canine Parasitology. Post Graduate Foundation in Veterinary Science, University of Sydney, 1977.

Kelly, J. D., Kenny, D. F., and Whitlock, H. V.: The response to phytohaemagglutinin of peripheral blood lymphocytes from dogs infected with *Ancylostoma caninum*. N. Z. Vet. J. 25:12–15, 1977.

Rawlings, C. A., McCall, J. W., and Lewis, R. E.: The response of the canine heart and lungs to *Dirofilaria immitis*. JAAHA 14:17–32, 1978.

Somotin, A. O., and Heiner, D. C.: A new immunodiagnostic test in onchocerciasis. Clin. Allerg. 6:573–576, 1976.

Whitlock, H. V., Porter, C. J., and Kelly, J. D.: The PKW acid phosphate modification for the recovery and histochemical identification of microfilariae of *Dirofilaria immitis* in blood. Aust. Vet. Pract. 8:201–207, 1979.

Wong, M. M., Guest, M. F., and Lavoirpierre, M. J.: Dirofilaria immitis: fate and immunogenicity of irradiated infective third stage larvae in Beagles. Exp. Parasit. 35:465–474, 1974.

COR PULMONALE

GLEN L. SPAULDING, D.V.M.
Ithaca, New York

Cor pulmonale, also referred to as pulmonary heart disease, is an uncommon sequel to respiratory disease in the dog and cat. It refers to alterations in the structure and/or function of the right ventricle induced by pulmonary hypertension secondary to primary diseases of the lung or the pulmonary vasculature. Right ventricular changes and pulmonary hypertension secondary to congenital cardiac defects or diseases of the left side of the heart do not constitute cor pulmonale. Cor pulmonale frequently exists undiagnosed and may complicate the diagnosis and treatment of concurrent diseases.

ETIOLOGY

Acute cor pulmonale results from embolization and/or thrombosis of the pulmonary arterial system. More than 30 to 50 per cent of the pulmonary arterial system must be occluded to create pulmonary hypertension. Heartworm disease is probably the most common cause of acute and chronic cor pulmonale (see "Canine Heartworm Disease"). Other causes of acute cor pulmonale include air, fat, septic or neoplastic emboli, and abnormalities of the clotting mechanism including disseminated intravascular coagulopathy, idiopathic thrombocytopenia, cold agglutinin, and cryoglobulins. Acute cor pulmonale has been documented in the dog owing to pulmonary thrombosis secondary to renal amyloidosis and pancreatitis and following the administration of *o,p'*-DDD (Lysodren®, Calbio Pharm).

Chronic cor pulmonale can result from intrinsic pulmonary disease or inadequate bellows function of the lungs. Intrinsic pulmonary diseases include obstructive disorders such as chronic bronchitis and restrictive lung disease such as diffuse interstitial fibrosis. Intraluminal obstruction or extraluminal compression of the pulmonary arteries can result in cor pulmonale, as can alveolar ventilation/perfusion abnormalities. Inadequate bellows function of the lung may result from obesity or thoracic deformities, as well as from neurologic dysfunctions affecting the respiratory muscles. A combination of factors is most often involved, and hypoxia-induced vasoconstriction further complicates the condition. In addition, exercise, respiratory infections, and concurrent chronic valvular heart disease often aggravate the condition.

PATHOPHYSIOLOGY

The development of pulmonary hypertension is the essential feature of cor pulmonale. Alveolar hypoxia or hypoventilation owing to respiratory disease results in hypoxemia, hypercapnia, and acidemia. These abnormalities, especially chronic hypoxia, are potent stimuli for pulmonary vasoconstriction in contrast to stimulating vasodilation elsewhere in the body. Pulmonary vasoconstriction results from the direct effects of hypoxia on pulmonary arterial smooth muscle and indirect responses mediated by vasoactive substances released by the lungs. A reduction of over 50 per cent of the cross-sectional area of the pulmonary vasculature must occur, regardless of the etiology, before pulmonary hypertension will occur. Pulmonary hypertension tends to become self-perpetuating as reversible medial hypertrophy of the pulmonary arteries develops. The right ventricle dilates, hypertrophies, or fails in response to pulmonary hypertension. Fluid retention and right-sided congestive heart failure may develop as the right heart fails. However, right ventricular failure is uncommon and is not an essential feature of cor pulmonale.

DIAGNOSIS

The presenting complaints are not directly referable to cor pulmonale unless right-sided congestive heart failure is present. More commonly, signs referable to the underlying respiratory disease such as difficult or labored breathing, tachypnea, wheezing, or chronic cough are present. Exertional dyspnea, weakness, cyanosis, and syncope may occur as the animal becomes progressively hypoxic. Further hypoxia is often induced by infection or transiently by exercise.

Physical examination may provide evidence to support the diagnosis of cor pulmonale while providing information as to the underlying etiology. Congenital conformational abnormalities, especially of the upper airways, can be detected, as can obesity. Compensatory conformation or postural changes such as barrel chest, abducted forelimbs, or reluctance to lie down as well as abdominal breathing and tachypnea may be present. The mucous membranes are occasionally cyanotic. Abnormal lung sounds associated with the underlying respiratory disease may be ausculted. A prominent second heart sound or split second heart sound may be heard, depending upon the severity of the pulmonary hypertension. As the disease progresses, gallop rhythms and a right-sided systolic murmur owing to right atrioventricular valvular insufficiency occasionally develop. If right-sided congestive heart failure occurs, physical findings often include distended jugular veins with pulses, muffled heart and lung sounds secondary to pleural and/or pericardial effusion, ascites, hepatosplenomegaly, and, rarely, peripheral edema.

There are no consistent electrocardiographic abnormalities associated with cor pulmonale. P pulmonale and a T "a" (atrial repolarization) wave may be present. Electrocardiographic evidence of right ventricular hypertrophy is usually absent, but when present, it may be indicated by a right axis deviation and S waves present in leads I, II, and III. Alterations in the size and configuration of the T wave and S-T segment

depression may reflect the hypoxic state. Arrhythmias are uncommon but include atrial premature contractions, atrial fibrillation, and ventricular premature contractions.

Radiographic evaluation of the thorax often produces important evidence supporting the diagnosis of cor pulmonale. Changes indicative of right ventricular enlargement in both the lateral and dorsoventral projections and enlargement of the pulmonary artery segment in the dorsoventral projection are suggestive of the condition. The pulmonary arteries may taper rapidly in the periphery. Radiographic evidence of the underlying pulmonary disease is not consistently found. If right-sided congestive heart failure occurs, signs indicating effusion are usually present.

Clinical pathologic evaluation may be helpful in the diagnosis of cor pulmonale. Arterial blood gas abnormalities of hypoxemia (PaO_2 <80 mm Hg), hypercapnia ($PaCO_2$ >40 mm Hg), and acidosis (pH <7.4) are frequently present. Monitoring these parameters may be helpful in determining the response to therapy and in establishing an accurate prognosis. A microfilaria check should be performed on any animal suspected of having cor pulmonale.

Direct pulmonary arterial pressure measurements have not routinely been performed in small animals. However, greater than eight-fold increases in mean arterial pressures have been recorded in cor pulmonale owing to pulmonary thrombosis secondary to amyloidosis and even higher pressures have been recorded with heartworm disease.

In summary, cor pulmonale should be suspected when right ventricular changes are present concurrently with respiratory disease, especially in the absence of primary heart disease.

TREATMENT

Correction of hypoxia to reverse the pulmonary vasoconstriction and hypertension should be the aim of therapy. Oxygen therapy and rest can provide some immediate relief. Specific or supportive therapy should be directed at the underlying respiratory disease. Bronchodilators such as aminophylline or isoproterenol are frequently helpful but have no direct effect upon correcting pulmonary hypertension. The available arterial vasodilators are not used because of undesirable systemic effects. Appropriate antibiotic administration if an infectious pulmonary process is present can result in significant rapid improvement. Corticosteroid administration is not recommended unless indicated specifically for the underlying respiratory disease. Weight loss should be encouraged for the obese animal. Conformational abnormalities — especially congenital upper respiratory defects in the brachycephalic breeds — should be corrected if they are significantly contributing to the development of hypoxia. Phlebotomy to control polycythemia may be necessary if oxygen therapy and rest are insufficient to correct this abnormality.

If right-sided congestive heart failure develops, diuretics and salt restriction are indicated. The need for diuretic therapy may be transient. The use of digitalis for treatment of cor pulmonale is controversial, and if it is used, it should be restricted to cases that have developed congestive failure. Dose should be carefully titrated, especially in the presence of hypoxemia, acidosis, and electrolyte abnormalities, because these factors predispose the animal to the arrhythmogenic effects of digitalis.

PROGNOSIS

The prognosis for cor pulmonale is usually favorable if signs of congestive right heart failure have not developed. Unfortunately, the underlying respiratory disease often cannot be treated effectively. If clinical heart disease does occur, the prognosis is guarded. Control of secondary bacterial infections of the respiratory system, exercise restriction, and supportive care are important in minimizing the effects of heart failure.

SUPPLEMENTAL READING

Ettinger, S.J., and Suter, P.A.: *Canine Cardiology*. Philadelphia, W.B. Saunders Co., 1970.
Fishman, A.P.: State of the art — chronic cor pulmonale. Am. Rev. Resp. Dis. *114(4)*:775–794, 1976.
Harpster, N.K.: Pulmonary vascular disease in the dog. In Kirk, R.W. (ed.): *Current Veterinary Therapy VI*. Philadelphia, W.B. Saunders Co., 1977.
Hurst, J.W.: *The Heart*, 3rd ed. New York, McGraw-Hill Book Co., 1974.
Smith, C.R., and Hamlin, R.L.: Pulmonary Circulation. In Swenson, M.J. (ed.): *Duke's Physiology of Domestic Animals*, 9th ed. Ithaca, Comstock Publishing Association, 1977.
Suter, P.A.: The Pathophysiologic Dimensions of the Interpretation of Pulmonary Radiographs. Illinois Veterinary Respiratory Symposium, 1978.
Wynne, J.W.: The treatment of cor pulmonale. JAMA *239(21)*:2283–2285, 1978.

DISEASES OF PERIPHERAL LYMPHATICS: LYMPHEDEMA

P. F. SUTER, D.M.V.
Davis, California

The term "lymphedema" refers to a swelling of some part of the body due to a lymph system disorder (Kinmonth, 1972). It should not be used for other forms of edema such as circulatory edema, venostasis, or hypoproteinemia.

The peripheral lymph system consists of endothelial-lined pathways that converge toward lymph nodes and major collecting trunks such as the lumbar cistern or the thoracic duct. Through its connection with the precava or one of its branches, the thoracic duct returns the lymph fluid to the blood.

Lymph drainage of peripheral tissue is indispensable for the return of fluid, proteins, and other macromolecular or particulate substances from the periphery to the blood stream. Since proteins are leaked universally from the capillary system, effective colloid osmotic pressure would rapidly deteriorate without the proteins being returned to the blood by the lymphatic system. The lymph system maintains the fluid and protein balance between extravascular and intravascular fluid pools and acts as a safety valve between them.

Subcutaneous tissue is particularly rich in lymph vessels. The musculoskeletal system as well as the organs of the body contain variable amounts of lymph vessels. Some organs such as the lung and liver have a rich lymph supply. Lymphatics contain valves that favor unidirectional, centripetal flow toward the major collecting trunks. Intrinsic rhythmic pulsation, as well as outside massage, provided by the contraction of adjacent muscles or pulsating arteries provides the energy for the propulsion of the lymph fluid.

Evaluation of the lymph system for disease processes is often difficult because lymph vessels are small and contain a colorless fluid, and abnormalities are difficult to see without the benefit of special procedures. The role of the lymph system in edema formation is often not fully appreciated. The diagnosis of lymphedema may be arrived at by excluding other possibilities.

If swelling of some part of the body, in particular part or all of one or several limbs, is noticed, the following conditions should be considered: generalized edema owing to heart failure; renal, hepatic, or intestinal disease causing hypoproteinemia; venostasis; mixed lymphovenous edema; edema owing to reactive hyperemia following licking or ischemia; cellulitis; arteriovenous fistula; and compartmental syndrome. A compartmental syndrome represents a local tissue ischemia that occurs if swelling affects a group of muscles surrounded by a restrictive fascia (Olivieri and Suter, 1978). The inability to expand compromises perfusion.

At least in the beginning, lymphedema is recognized by soft skin and subcutis that pit on pressure. The deformed swollen area is painless, is covered by intact skin, and has a normal temperature. With time and recurrent attacks of inflammation, skin and subcutis may become thickened by deposition of fibrous tissue. Ulceration is not a sign of lymphedema; it indicates circulatory stasis due to arterial and/or venous disease. Ulceration may occur only if trauma and infection damage skin or blood circulation in the edematous parts. Eczema, weeping, exudation of red cells into tissue, varices, brownish skin pigmentation, or fat necrosis (particularly in the inguinal area) are signs of venous stasis rather than lymphatic disease.

Most lymphedemas are recognized based on the clinical signs described. In doubtful cases, particularly in congenital lymphedema, lymphography may be needed. This can be done by subcutaneous or intradermal injection of a colored dye, which is preferentially absorbed by lymphatics (visual lymphography). Suitable dyes are Patent Blue Violet 10 percent or Pontamine Sky Blue (Kinmonth, 1972).

Radiographic lymphography is effected by intralymphatic or, rarely, intranodular injection of a radiographic contrast medium such as the water-soluble meglumine diatrizoates* or iodinated poppy seed oil.†

The lymphedemas are best subdivided into primary (idiopathic) and secondary. Primary lymphedemas develop without known underlying lymphatic disease and are often of congenital origin. In secondary lymphedemas, the lymph system has been damaged or obstructed by some well recognized disease process such as trauma, surgical excision of lymphatics or lymph nodes, malignant infiltration or compression, infection and inflammation, or radiation therapy (Suter, 1975).

Secondary lymphedema with lymph stasis is caused most often by mechanical interruption or obstruction of lymph flow and by mural insufficiency. Mural insufficiency is caused by a thinning of the wall and the opening up of intercellular junctions. Valvar insufficiency following severe lymph vessel dilatation and loss of lymph vessel contractility, as well as a dynamic insufficiency due to greatly increased lymph fluid production, modify the degree of lymphedema (Földi, 1977). In dynamic or relative insufficiency, lymph vessel capacity is no longer able to cope with a greatly augmented lymph production. Factors such as elevated venous pressure, augmented blood flow, or lowered total plasma protein content can increase lymphatic load beyond the system's capacity and precipitate lymphedema.

Lymphedema is often the result of a combination of venous and lymphatic obstruction. Within limits, the venous system can compensate for an impaired lymph flow. Partial or total obstruction of lymphatic trunks can lead to the opening up of lymphovenous anastomoses in the mediastinum, the lumbar area, or the popliteal nodes. Obstruction of veins augments the lymph production and lymph flow. If the lymph system is damaged concurrently with the venous system by trauma, surgery, or inflammation, lymphedema occurs. The manifestation of lymphedema can be delayed for several weeks or months following surgery (Földi, 1977). Scar formation and fibrosis compress, obstruct, or distort the lymph vessels, reducing their capacity and gradually inducing distal lymph vessel dilatation and lymph stasis.

Inflammatory and infectious lymphedemas are associated with inflammation of lymph vessels (lymphangitis) and lymph nodes (lymphadenitis). Lymphangitis can permanently damage lymph vessels and lymph nodes. Breaches in the epithelial barrier of the skin owing to scarification or licking that allow the ingress of microorganisms, in particular streptococci and staphylococci, are the most common causes of infectious lymphedema. Fungal infections are less common. Animals with chronic eczema are predisposed to recurring lymphedema.

Lymphedema, with its stagnant protein-rich subcutaneous pool of fluid, is prone to infection and inflammation that self-perpetuate the condition. Skin of swollen limbs seems to become breached more easily.

---

*Hypaque-M, 75 percent, Winthrop Laboratories, New York, NY 10016; or Renografin-76, E. R. Squibb & Sons, Inc., Princeton, NJ 08540.

†Ethiodol, Savage Laboratories, Inc., Houston, TX 77036.

A limb or region affected by inflammatory lymphedema is swollen, warm, and painful. Lameness may be present and the regional lymph nodes are enlarged. The latter sign may be obscured if the edema is so extensive that the nodes are no longer palpable. Fever and an elevated white blood cell count are common with lymphangitis. Owners are much more likely to seek professional help with infectious than with non-inflammatory edemas.

Lymphedema secondary to malignant disease is usually caused by the combined effects of impaired venous flow and lymphatic obstruction. Tumor tissue may compress or invade veins and lymph vessels. Lymph nodes become blocked by reactive and metastatic tissue. This stops lymph flow in the afferent lymphatics or may lead to lymphadenopathy with compression of adjacent veins. Head and neck edema, or edema of the front limb and ventral thoracic region, occur secondary to blocked prescapular, lower neck, and mediastinal lymph nodes. Invasive mediastinal and axillary tumors can also cause limb and neck edemas.

Sublumbar node blockage by local metastasis of mammary gland tumors, prostatic tumors, or perianal carcinomas may cause hind limb edema. In many cases, there is concurrent blockage of the inguinal nodes. By retrograde metastasis into the popliteal nodes, tendency for edema formation of the hind limbs is enhanced (personal observation).

Radiographic lymphography and venography can provide valuable added information for determining the location and extent of a neoplastic process in areas that are difficult to palpate (Suter, 1975). Normally, outlined lymph node chains may be missing and collateral lymph vessels leading around totally or partially blocked lymph nodes may be seen on lymphography studies. Metastatic foci within lymph nodes may appear as filling defects.

PRIMARY LYMPHEDEMA

Primary lymphedema is often present at birth, but in some puppies, it is present in a latent form and the edema must be initiated by some precipitating factor to become clinically manifest. These factors include minor trauma, "strenuous" exercise, or local infection, which on their own would certainly not cause damage severe enough to account for permanent edema in a normal puppy. Sometimes, edema in one limb is followed later by edema in the opposite, seemingly normal limb. The disproportionate reaction of the lymph system to a minor trauma or stress in these puppies indicates a defective morphogenesis of the lymph system (Luginbühl

et al., 1967). Congenital lymphedema in dogs has been reported repeatedly (Griffin and MacCoy, 1978; Ladds et al., 1971; Patterson et al., 1967). The severity of lymphedema ranges from a latent to mild transient or permanent limb edema to severe generalized edema that may cause death (Patterson, 1967). The hind limbs are more often affected than are the forelimbs. Usually, no other gross anomalies outside the lymph system are seen. Breeding experiments have shown the hereditary nature of congenital lymphedema in the dog, which resembled Milroy's disease in man (Patterson et al., 1967).

The lymphatic anomalies have been classified into three types according to morphologic criteria established by radiographic lymphography and histology in man (Kinmonth, 1972): aplasia, hypoplasia, and hyperplasia. The same criteria can be used in dogs (Leighton and Suter, 1979; Suter, 1975).

In aplasia, the lymph vessels are absent in the edematous limbs. In hypoplasia, the lymph vessels are deficient in size and number. Lymphatic hypoplasia can be associated with aplasia or hypoplasia of the lymph nodes. If the lymph vessels in the proximal limb are mainly hypoplastic, the distal lymph vessels become dilated. Hyperplasia of the lymph vessels signifies a diffuse increase in their size and number. Severe lymph vessel dilatation (megalolymphatics) is often associated with tortuosity (varicosity). Incompetence in moving lymph fluid owing to lymph vessel distention and insufficiency or absence of the valves rather than obstruction are the main physiologic faults in hyperplasia (Kinmonth, 1972). In all three types of lymphedema, injected dye moves distally into the skin instead of proximally (dermal backflow). In lymph vessel hyperplasia, injection of a colored dye makes the dilated vessels visible. In aplasia, injected dye may diffuse through the subcutaneous tissue rather than be taken up by lymphatics.

Regardless of the etiology of lymphedema, a pool of leaked protein accumulates in the subcutaneous and interstitial tissue. This protein retains water and perpetuates edema formation that defies successful therapy. Removal of this pool of proteinaceous fluid, which stimulates fibroblast activity and fibrous tissue transformation, is an important step in the therapy of lymphedema.

Therapy of lymphedema must take into account the etiology of the condition. In inflammatory and infectious lymphedema, moist warm local compresses or soaks are used to reduce swelling. Aggressive systemic and/or local antibiotic treatment should be based on the microorganisms involved. Diuretics and corticosteroids are of limited or questionable benefit. In secondary obstructive lymphedema and in primary lymphedema, the kind of treatment depends on the severity and stage of the condition. Chronic lymphedema usually makes for a guarded prognosis and may fail to respond to any kind of therapy. Mild lymphedema of one or two limbs can be treated successfully with dry, soft bandaging over several weeks or months (Leighton and Suter, 1979). Most owners, however, are reluctant to spend the necessary time and effort for conservative therapy. If the lymphedema is severe or complicated by recurrent secondary infections, surgery should be contemplated. It is important to advise owners of the potential hereditary nature of primary lymphedema.

Surgery is aimed at the following goals: (1) removal of the stagnant pool of proteinaceous tissue fluid, (2) increase in tissue tension to reduce filtration and force fluids back into the capillaries, (3) improvement of drainage via the deep venous system and intermuscular tissue planes, and (4) elimination of tissue spaces in which fluid can stagnate. In man, the "Thompson buried flap procedure" (Kinmonth, 1972) or a simpler modified method of the Thompson procedure has been advocated (Johnson and Pflug, 1975). The edematous tissue and deep fascia are excised and the edematous tissue is removed from the skin. By extensive drainage and bandaging, the attachment of the skin directly to the underlying muscles is facilitated and the possibility for fluid accumulation is eliminated. The surgical method described has been used successfully in the treatment of two dogs with congenital lymphedema (Leighton and Suter, 1979).

SUPPLEMENTAL READING

Földi, M.: Physiology and pathophysiology of lymph flow. In Clodius, L. (ed.): Supplement to "Lymphology." Stuttgart, G. Thieme, Publishers, 1977.

Griffin, C.E., and MacCoy, D.M.: Primary lymphedema: a case report and discussion. J. Am. Anim. Hosp. Assoc. 14:373–377, 1978.

Johnson, H.D., and Pflug, J.: The Swollen Leg — Causes and Treatment. Philadelphia, J.B. Lippincott Company, 1975.

Kinmonth, J.B.: The Lymphatics. Diseases, Lymphography and Surgery. Baltimore, The Williams and Wilkins Co., 1972.

Ladds, P.W., Dennis, S.M., and Leipold, H.W.: Lethal congenital edema in bulldog pups. J. Am. Vet. Med. Assoc. 195:81–86, 1971.

Leighton, R.L., and Suter, P.F.: Primary lymphedema of the hind limb in the dog. J. Am. Vet. Med. Assoc. 175:369–374, 1979.

Luginbühl, H., Chacko, S.K., Patterson, D.F., and Medway, W.: Congenital hereditary lymphedema in the dog. Part II. Pathological studies. J. Med. Genet. 4:153, 1967.

Olivieri, M., and Suter, P.F.: Compartmental syndrome of the front leg of a dog due to rupture of the median artery. J. Am. An. Hosp. Assoc. 14(2):210–218, 1978.

Patterson, D.F., Medway, W., Luginbühl, H., and Chacko, S.: Congenital hereditary lymphedema in the dog. Part I. Clinical and genetic studies. J. Med. Genet. 4:145, 1967.

Suter, P.F.: Diseases of the peripheral vessels. In Ettinger, S.J. (ed.): Textbook of Veterinary Internal Medicine. Philadelphia, W.B. Saunders Co., 1975.

INFLUENCE OF NON-CARDIAC DISEASE ON THE HEART

EDWARD C. FELDMAN, D.V.M.

Davis, California

ENDOCRINE DISEASE

Cushing's Syndrome. Hyperadrenocorticism is one of the more frequently diagnosed endocrine disorders in dogs. The systemic manifestations of this entity depend on the relative excess secretion of cortisol and corticosterone. One of the sequelae of these hormone increases is elevation of the blood pressure secondary to an increase in total blood volume. This results in increased workload on the myocardium and, thus, myocardial hypertrophy. Congestive heart failure may occur in dogs afflicted with Cushing's syndrome as hypertension and fluid retention become severe. Cushing's syndrome often affects dogs that are of middle and older age. The most common breeds associated with Cushing's syndrome are dachshunds, poodles, and Boston terriers. These breeds, as well as numerous others, frequently have chronic mitral and tricuspid valvular fibrosis. The combined effect of valvular insufficiency and Cushing's syndrome is a definite strain on the myocardium. Overt congestive heart failure is not unusual in such a setting. Radiographs of the thorax often reveal cardiomegaly associated with a prominent left ventricle and sometimes vascular congestion. Electrocardiographically, left ventricular hypertrophy is a common finding. These animals respond poorly to therapy consisting of digitalization and sodium restriction. Diuretic therapy, in dogs that are polydipsic and polyuric from their primary disease, should be used with caution. One can easily cause hypokalemia and/or alkalosis by using diuretics in such patients. Treatment of the congestive heart failure and hypertension is best accomplished by treating the underlying cause of these disorders. With the appropriate diagnosis and treatment, Cushing's syndrome dogs may be rendered normotensive, leading to a control of the cardiovascular complications of this disease.

Hypoadrenocorticism. This disorder usually results from a destructive process involving a major portion of the adrenal cortices. The systemic manifestations of adrenal insufficiency result from inadequate cortisol and aldosterone secretion. The deficiency in mineralocorticoid secretions leads to excessive salt and water losses resulting in hypovolemia. (Hyperkalemia, another sequela to lack of mineralocorticoid, will be discussed in the electrolyte section of this chapter.) The lack of cortisol results in a decreased vascular sensitivity to catecholamines with loss of vasoconstriction. Therefore, two of the most characteristic cardiovascular findings in hypoadrenocorticism are hypotension and small heart size radiographically. During periods of stress associated with the occurrence of infection, trauma, or surgery, the canine with hypoadrenocorticism is unable to elevate adrenocortical hormone levels rapidly. This leads to a loss of intravascular volume and vascular tone and may result in profound hypotension with the development of hypovolemic vascular shock. (Treatment for the disorder is outlined elsewhere in this text.) However, in patients with acute hypoadrenal crisis, one must rapidly replace sodium and water (saline 0.9 percent) intravenously to avoid a terminal situation. This is felt to be the intravenous fluid of choice because it will aid in correcting hypovolemia, hyponatremia, and hypochloremia. Hyperkalemia may be reduced by simple dilution, since saline contains no potassium. Any potassium-containing fluid is contraindicated.

In order to improve vascular integrity and provide glucocorticoid to the potential hypoadrenal animal, hydrocortisone sodium succinate (Solu-Cortef) should be administered intravenously over a two- to four-minute period. The dosage is 4 to 20 mg/kg of body weight and this may be repeated in two to six hours. One may then add dexamethasone to the intravenous infusion for continuous glucocorticoid supplementation. Desoxycorticosterone acetate (DOCA) in oil is the initial mineralocorticoid of choice at a dose of 2 to 4 mg/5 kg of body weight. This drug must be mixed thoroughly before being administered intramuscularly to the patient. DOCA is given once every 24 hours.

Hypothyroidism. Hypothyroidism is the state of slowed metabolic rate that results from inadequate levels of circulating thyroid hormones. The cardiovascular alterations seen in hypothyroid dogs include decreased cardiac output, diminished peripheral blood flow, slowing of the heart rate, and decreased velocity of blood while normal arterial blood pressure is maintained. Clinically, these changes have been reflected in the reports on such dogs. Hypothyroid dogs have been noted to have a weak apical heart beat, weak and slow pulse, palpably cool ear flaps and extremities, and areas of alopecia. The latter findings are suggestive of diminished or impaired peripheral circulation. The electrocardiogram in such animals may reveal low voltage in all complexes, flattened T waves, sinus bradycardia, and prolongation of the P-R and Q-T intervals. All these ECG abnormalities regress with thyroid hormone therapy, suggesting that they are directly related to lack of thyroid hormone. The diagnosis of hypothyroidism is based on the finding of additional clinical and laboratory abnormalities including depressed serum T4 levels before and after administration of TSH. It is important to remember that most of the animals with this disorder are not critically ill, and rapid replacement of full doses of thyroid medication is not recommended. Rather, one should replace thyroxin in these animals slowly, since unduly rapid correction may precipitate arrhythmias and/or congestive heart failure.

Hyperparathyroidism and hypoparathyroidism will be discussed under the headings of hypercalcemia and hypocalcemia in this chapter.

OBESITY AND THE CARDIORESPIRATORY SYSTEM

The physiologic alterations resulting from gross obesity are a rise in cardiac output and an increase in stroke volume. These changes correlate well with the degree of excess weight, as does the increase in left ventricular work. Severely obese people have been found to have pulmonary artery hypertension that is believed to occur secondary to elevated left ventricular filling pressure.

Symptoms commonly associated with cardiorespiratory dysfunction in obese dogs include hepatomegaly (secondary to fatty infiltration of the liver), easy fatigability, tachypnea, and exertional dyspnea. These animals are typically lethargic and may sleep for long periods daily. Increased abdominal pressure from adipose tissue might be expected to disturb ventilatory mechanics, but a nocturnal cough is not a common owner complaint. These signs are believed to be exaggerated by a marked reduction in expiratory reserve volume and a decreased chest wall compliance, which increase the work of breathing. If such a dog also has a collapsing trachea, the combination of expiratory distress associated with the tracheal problem and the changes seen with obesity can cause marked signs of respiratory disease. Similar problems can easily be appreciated if the obese dog also has chronic mitral and/or tricuspid valvular fibrosis. Signs become further exaggerated with the stress of excitement, exercise, and trauma. The author has seen and the veterinary literature has alluded to a syndrome of marked obesity, alveolar hypoventilation, cyanosis, secondary polycythemia, and heart failure. In man, this is called the pickwickian syndrome, and changes suggestive of this syndrome are not uncommon in the dog.

There are no specific ECG changes resulting from obesity. Left ventricular enlargement is rarely evident unless other cardiac disease is present. Low voltage occurs in some obese patients. Radiographically, an increased cardiothoracic ratio may be seen, but this is not considered to be a reliable measurement. The cardiorespiratory and many other systemic abnormalities resolve with weight loss. Having pets lose weight is much easier said than done. Veterinarians must convince the owner of the importance of weight loss and establish an individual treatment protocol for obese dogs. This method coupled with frequent check-ups by the veterinarian offers the best chance for owner compliance.

Electrolyte abnormalities

In the clinical veterinary setting, alterations in serum potassium are responsible for the vast majority of cardiac irregularities that occur with electrolyte imbalances. Although calcium, sodium, hydrogen, and magnesium imbalances may also induce variations in cardiac conductivity, clinical experience suggests that only potassium and calcium alterations are seen with enough frequency to warrant discussion.

Hypokalemia. The most frequently encountered causes for hypokalemia are (1) loss from the gastrointestinal tract during bouts of chronic and severe vomiting or diarrhea, (2) urinary loss in the diuresis phase of renal disease, (3) diuresis stimulated by the excessive use of diuretic agents such as furosemide, (4) alkalosis associated with the use of alkalinizing agents such as sodium bicarbonate, and (5) in diabetic animals, the use of insulin, which shifts potassium from the extracellular to the intracellular fluid compartment of the body.

Hypokalemia can be reflected on the electrocardiogram as a progressive sagging of the S-T segment and decreased amplitude of the T wave. The basic electrophysiologic alteration is a gradual shift of the repolarization wave from systole into diastole. Therefore, accompanying the decreased amplitude of the T wave is a repolarization wave occurring after the T wave (U wave). The merging of a flat or positive T wave with a positive U wave may erroneously be interpreted as a prolonged T wave and, therefore, a prolonged Q-T interval. In advanced hypokalemia, the amplitude and duration of the QRS complex are increased. It is believed that the QRS complex is widened diffusely secondary to a generalized slowing of conduction in the ventricular myocardium or Purkinje fibers. The amplitude and the duration of the P wave increase, and the P-R interval is slightly prolonged (Fig. 1).

Atrial and ventricular premature contractions are seen frequently in hypokalemic animals. Animals receiving digitalis and also suffering from low extracellular potassium concentrations are prone to the aforementioned arrhythmias as well as to supraventricular tachycardia with block and ventricular tachycardia.

Changes in the ECG are not easily recognized when the serum potassium concentration is above 3.0 mEq/L. However, changes are frequently recorded when the serum potassium level is between 2.5 and 3.0 mEq/L, and alterations occur in almost all dogs and cats with serum potassium levels below 2.5 mEq/L.

Treatment is directed toward correction of the underlying clinical problem and slow correction of the hypokalemia with potassium supplementation. Potassium is supplemented orally whenever possible, since this is the safest route. Oral potassium supplements, it must be remembered, can cause vomiting. When oral medication is contraindicated because of an animal's clinical condition, potassium can be administered subcutaneously or slowly intravenously after being diluted in the parenteral fluids. Generally, potassium therapy is begun with 7 mEq added to each 250 ml of intravenous

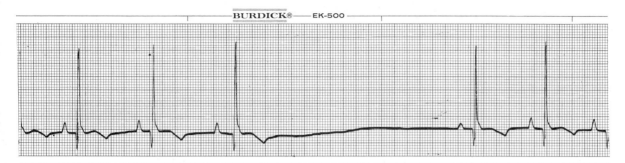

Figure 1. ECG of a dog being given insulin for ketoacidotic diabetes mellitus. The serum potassium level was 2.4 mEq/liter. This lead II example, taken at a paper speed of 50 mm/sec, illustrates the prolonged Q–T–U intervals, tall R waves, and wide QRS complexes suggestive of hypokalemia.

fluids. Adjustments in this dose are based on serial ECGs and frequent monitoring of serum electrolyte concentrations. Potassium supplementation should never be administered to an anuric patient.

Hyperkalemia. Hyperpotassemia is the most common clinically encountered electrolyte disturbance. Endocrine causes of high serum potassium concentrations include the moderate or occasionally severe elevations seen in adrenal insufficiency (Addison's disease) as well as mild elevations that may occur in untreated ketoacidotic diabetic animals. Less commonly, hyperpotassemia is attributed to patients with oliguric or anuric renal failure. Acidosis alone, which tends to shift potassium from within the cells to the extracellular fluid, may also inhibit renal potassium excretion, thereby promoting hyperkalemia. The rapid infusion of potassium-containing fluids is another cause of hyperkalemia. Potassium-sparing diuretic compounds such as triamterene and spironolactone may be responsible for a build-up of extracellular potassium levels which, if unaltered, may be critical.

The danger of hyperpotassemia involves the severe and potentially lethal cardiotoxic effects. Marked hyperkalemia can be readily diagnosed electrocardiographically, and prompt therapeutic measures, which may be life saving, will rapidly shift the imbalance to safer levels.

The clinical syndrome of hyperpotassemia is manifested by general muscle weakness, depression, lethargy, peripheral vascular collapse, and sometimes bradycardia. Effects on the heart include a decrease in excitability, an increase in the refractory period of the heart muscle, and a slowing of conduction.

The most prominent manifestations of hyperkalemia are found on the ECG, which is a vital tool for estimating its functional severity. The earliest electrocardiographic alteration is peaking of the T wave, which occurs when the serum potassium concentrations exceed 5.5 mEq/L (Fig. 2C). This change is frequently associated with shortening of the Q-T interval. The characteristic tall, steep, narrow, and pointed T waves occur before the ECG shows any measurable alteration of the QRS complex. T wave changes are not seen in all cases of mild hyperkalemia. As the serum potassium concentration continues to rise, the T wave may lose its classic "peaked" shape because the T wave abnormalities secondary to intraventricular conduction disturbances obscure the primary T wave changes.

Slowing of the intraventricular impulse conduction is responsible for the QRS complex alterations that occur as the serum potassium concentration exceeds 6.5 mEq/L. At this juncture, the T wave abnormalities and the uniformly widened QRS complex allow the presumptive diagnosis to be made (Fig. 2B). With increasing serum potassium concentrations, the QRS duration increases progressively. There is a rough correlation between duration of the QRS complex and the degree of hyperpotassemia.

As serum potassium levels rise above 7 mEq/L, the P wave amplitude decreases and its duration becomes prolonged secondary to slowing of conduction through the atria. The P-R interval also increases in duration as a result of a slower atrioventricular transmission. When serum potassium concentrations exceed 8.5 mEq/L, the P wave usually becomes invisible (Fig. 2A). When P waves are absent, an erroneous diagnosis of atrial fibrillation or atrial asystole may be made, particularly when the ventricular rate is irregular.

Continued elevation of serum potassium can be associated with deviation from the baseline of the S-T segment. With concentrations reaching the magnitude of 11 to 14 mEq/L, the electrocardiographer may see ventricular asystole or ventricular fibrillation.

Therapy in the hyperkalemic patient is three-

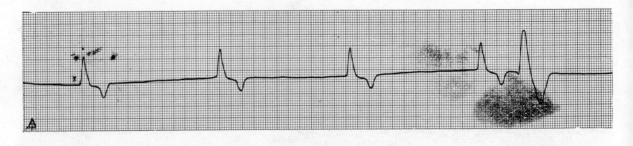

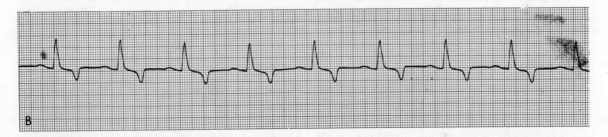

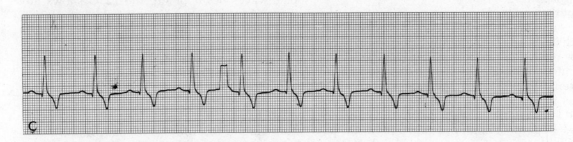

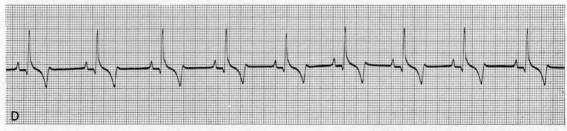

Figure 2. A. ECG segment from an addisonian dog with a serum potassium level of 9.3 mEq/liter. Note the lack of visible P waves; the short, wide QRS complexes; and the single ventricular escape beat at the far right. B. Same dog after institution of therapy. Serum potassium levels is 7.9 mEq/liter. Note the reappearance of wide P waves, prolonged P–R interval, QRS complexes that are shorter in duration than in A, and T waves that appear more "spiked." C. The serum potassium level is 6.4 mEq/liter, and the P, P–R, QRS, and T waves are of shorter duration. The R wave is taller. D. ECG of another addisonian dog, this one with a serum potassium level of 6.6 mEq/liter, illustrating "spiked" T waves.

fold: the serum potassium must be lowered, the serum sodium and/or calcium concentration must be raised, and the etiology of the electrolyte imbalance must be determined so that specific therapy may be instituted. Therapy need not be overly zealous when potassium concentrations are below 6.5 mEq/L, whereas intensive therapy must be initiated in animals with serum K^+ concentrations greater than 8.0 to 8.5 mEq/L.

For the hypoadrenal animal, the most likely to develop severe hyperkalemia, rapid infusion of normal saline (0.9 percent) intravenously has proved to be the simplest and most reliable method of lowering the serum potassium. The fluid contains no potassium, and thus it lowers the electrolyte by dilution. Saline also raises sodium and chloride levels as well as corrects the state of hypovolemia. Sodium antagonizes the cardiotoxic effects of potassium.

One may also infuse a glucose-containing solution with or without insulin to force potassium from the extracellular to the intracellular space. A 10 percent glucose solution is recommended at a dose of 5 to 10 ml/kg of body weight in the first 30 to 60 minutes. Regular insulin is dosed at 0.5 to 1.0 unit/kg subcutaneously or intravenously. One should administer at least 20 ml of 10 percent dextrose for each unit of regular insulin in order to avoid hypoglycemia.

Sodium bicarbonate also rapidly lowers serum potassium by causing a shift of the potassium ion into the cells secondary to alkalinization of the serum. Eighty to 100 mEq of sodium bicarbonate should be added to each liter of glucose-containing intravenous fluids. This procedure is especially valuable when acidosis is present, but it is also effective in animals with normal acid-base status.

In animals with extreme hyperkalemia, the intravenous infusion of 5 to 20 ml of calcium gluconate within a five-minute period and under electrocardiographic monitoring will rapidly reverse the ECG and clinical evidence of cardiac toxicity without affecting the serum level of potassium. This effect is transient and must be accompanied by other means of lowering the potassium concentration.

Hypocalcemia. Hypocalcemia is not a frequently encountered entity in veterinary practice other than in the lactating bitch. Hypocalcemia may also be attributed to idiopathic hypoparathyroidism, high intestinal fluid loss secondary to diarrhea, and chronic renal failure in association with retention of phosphorus. It may also develop in animals with paralytic ileus. Symptoms of hypocalcemia include increased nervousness, excitability, tetany, and convulsions.

The hypocalcemic dogs seen by the author have had electrocardiographic abnormalities. These include deep wide T waves, prolonged Q-T intervals, and tall R waves. There is reported to be good correlation between the severity of hypocalcemia and the duration of the S-T segment (Fig. 3).

Treatment of hypocalcemia includes intravenous calcium gluconate infusion if necessary, and determination of the underlying cause of the disturbance. We have found calcium carbonate* to be an excellent oral calcium supplement, more so than the traditional lactate tablets. Vitamin D supplementation aids in the absorption and retention of calcium by the body. Diphenylhydantoin (phenytoin) with phenobarbital reduces muscle cramps.

Hypercalcemia, Sodium, and Chloride. Numerous clinical situations exist that result in alterations of the serum sodium and chloride or in elevation of the serum calcium. Electrocardiographically, these abnormalities are of little clinical significance. Severe hypercalcemia has not been associated with changes in the ECG, aside from occasional ventricular premature contractions. The level of change in sodium or chloride necessary to alter the action potential and, thus, the ECG is usually so high that it is fatal.

TRAUMA

Alterations in the functional or structural integrity of the pericardium, myocardium, valve structures, conducting tissue, and coronary vessels may result from penetrating or blunt trauma. Injuries to the heart and great vessels are

---

*Titralac, Riker Laboratories, Inc., Northridge, California, 91324

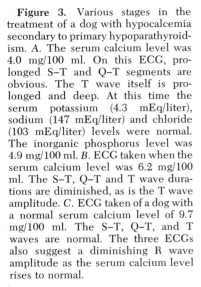

Figure 3. Various stages in the treatment of a dog with hypocalcemia secondary to primary hypoparathyroidism. *A.* The serum calcium level was 4.0 mg/100 ml. On this ECG, prolonged S-T and Q-T segments are obvious. The T wave itself is prolonged and deep. At this time the serum potassium (4.3 mEq/liter), sodium (147 mEq/liter) and chloride (103 mEq/liter) levels were normal. The inorganic phosphorus level was 4.9 mg/100 ml. *B.* ECG taken when the serum calcium level was 6.2 mg/100 ml. The S-T, Q-T and T wave durations are diminished, as is the T wave amplitude. *C.* ECG taken of a dog with a normal serum calcium level of 9.7 mg/100 ml. The S-T, Q-T, and T waves are normal. The three ECGs also suggest a diminishing R wave amplitude as the serum calcium level rises to normal.

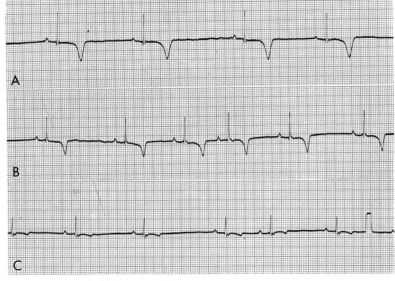

encountered frequently in small animal practice, most often arising from trauma sustained when dogs or cats are struck by automobiles. Concussive forces to the chest wall as well as sudden increases in intravascular pressure owing to compression of the abdomen or rear legs commonly produce alterations in the cardiovascular system. The jarring effect alone can lead to arrhythmias or ventricular standstill. The clinician, anxious to treat obvious injuries, must not overlook the cardiovascular system in the initial physical examination. Failure to detect evidence of cardiac injury before subjecting the animal to anesthesia may result in surgical or anesthetic death.

External signs of cardiac injury may be lacking in both penetrating and non-penetrating injuries. With non-penetrating trauma, seemingly minor forces such as a blow to the chest wall with a fist or the "Contra Coup" may produce major injury with only mild external stigmata. Cardiac injury must be suspected whenever chest trauma is obvious, as in cases with fractured ribs or pneumothorax.

Destruction of cardiac structural integrity, leading to hemopericardium and cardiac tamponade or exsanguination, is the most catastrophic event associated with cardiac injury. Intrapericardial entrapment of hemorrhage may prevent exsanguination but may rapidly lead to life-threatening cardiac tamponade. The classic clinical findings in dogs and cats with cardiac tamponade are muffled heart sounds, low voltage complexes on ECG with or without arrhythmia, and a radiographic "soccer-ball" heart.

Treatment involves feeding a jugular catheter through the chest wall into the pericardial sac, removing as much fluid as possible. Rest and proper antiarrhythmic therapy is also important. Such injuries carry a guarded to grave prognosis.

Myocardial contusion is the most common lesion associated with non-penetrating cardiac trauma. Auscultable irregularities in rhythm associated with a pulse deficit are usually the first clue of cardiac disease. Suspected arrhythmias must be confirmed by ECG to determine their nature and, thus, the proper therapy (Fig. 4). In the author's experience, arrhythmias are common after trauma. The character of the arrhythmia or conduction abnormality depends upon the site of injury. Atrial injury may precipitate atrial premature contractions or atrial fibrillation or flutter. Necrosis of the conduction systems, either through direct injury or hemorrhage, may produce intraventricular conduction defects or atrioventricular block of varying degrees. Ventricular myocardial injuries may result in unifocal or multifocal premature ventricular contractions as single abnormal beats or in pairs, runs, tachycardia, bigeminy, or trigeminy. Sudden death following chest trauma most likely results from ventricular fibrillation.

Therapy is needed only transiently in most animals with arrhythmias following trauma. Usually, after good response to medication, one can attempt to taper antiarrhythmic medication two to three weeks after initiating the drug(s). Periodic ECG tracings are mandatory to assess the success of treatment during both medication and withdrawal periods. Digitalis is used in atrial arrhythmias; quinidine, procainamide, and lidocaine are used in animals with ventricular arrhythmias. The use of disopyramide phosphate* is also being tested in such dogs with ventricular arrhythmias.

CHRONIC ANEMIA

Reduction of circulating red blood cell mass found in severe and chronic anemias of any

---

*Norpace®; G. D. Searle and Co.; Box 5110, Chicago, Illinois, 60680

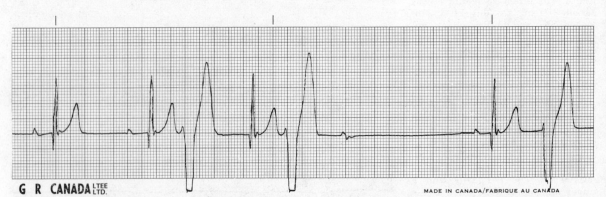

G R CANADA LTEE LTD.   MADE IN CANADA/FABRIQUE AU CANADA

Figure 4. Lead II ECG of a 5-year-old English pointer two days after being hit by a car. The abnormalities present include first-degree and second-degree heart blocks as well as unifocal ventricular premature contractions. Treatment with quinidine sulfate orally was successful in controlling all the irregularities.

etiology produces a fall in hemoglobin and, therefore, of oxygen transport to the tissues. The cardiac and peripheral circulations are called upon to compensate for this tissue anoxia. The major compensatory mechanism in correcting the relative tissue anoxia in anemic patients is an increased cardiac output. The increased cardiac output is the result of increased stroke volume brought about by increased myocardial contractility, decreased blood viscosity, and decreased peripheral resistance associated with the anemic state. Another important mechanism by which more oxygen may reach the tissues in anemic patients is by a shift of the oxyhemoglobin dissociation curve to the right.

Murmurs have long been noted to occur with anemia, the most common being a systolic murmur. Cardiomegaly is a frequent radiographic finding with severe and chronic anemia. Correction of the anemia will cause the heart to return to normal size. There are no specific ECG findings noted in anemia. However, the ECG may reflect the generalized cardiomegaly associated with chronic anemia.

THE KIDNEYS

The kidneys play a role in the pathophysiology of congestive heart failure. Changes in renal function are associated with the altered hemodynamics and fluid retention that accompany heart failure. The fall in cardiac output that accompanies heart failure is associated with a redistribution of blood flow, directed at maintaining perfusion of the heart and brain. This redistribution is accomplished primarily by regional arteriolar vasoconstriction, which in the case of the renal circulation results in a rise in renal vascular resistance occurring in the efferent arterioles of the glomerulus. Renal blood flow is thus reduced to a greater extent than is the glomerular filtration rate. This causes an increase in the filtration fraction and an increase in resorption of sodium in the proximal tubule.

As heart failure worsens, the renin-angiotensin-aldosterone system is activated, further promoting proximal tubular sodium resorption. These factors complicate the fluid retention typical of the heart failure state.

In addition, failure of the kidneys to excrete digitalis potentiates digitalis toxicity in any animals with heart failure. Thus, one must monitor renal function in patients receiving such medication and realize that doses of digitalis must be reduced as renal failure worsens. The therapeutic challenge veterinarians face with the combination of renal failure and congestive heart failure can be insurmountable.

SUPPLEMENTAL READING

Sokolow, M., and McIlroy, M.B.: *Clinical Cardiology*. Los Altos, Calif., Lange Medical Publications, 1977.
Willerson, J.T., and Sanders, C.A.: *Clinical Cardiology*. New York, Grune and Stratton, 1977.

CARDIOVASCULAR SYSTEM OF THE RACING DOG

ROSS STAADEN, B.V.Sc.
Perth, Australia

Dog racing has taken many forms over the years and is different all over the world. Today it is mainly confined to greyhound, whippet, and Afghan racing over short distances (300 to 1000 metres) and to sled dog racing from 20 to over 100 miles. Gun, field, trial, bird, cattle, sheep, and other hunting and herding dogs may perhaps be regarded as "athletes" trained for less intense intermittent exercise It should be remembered that although the modern greyhound has been genetically selected for sprinting ability for 100 to 200 years, prior to that, it was selected for some 5000 or more years for prolonged hunting on the open plains.

EXERCISE

Exercise is defined by its duration and its rate and how these relate to the animal's maximal abilities. At a rate that exhausts the animal in less than five minutes, exercise is described as supramaximal, in the sense that it uses up energy faster than it can be produced by oxygen consumption. Exercise rates that take more than five minutes to produce exhaustion are described as maximal — i.e., energy is used up at a rate approximately equal to that at which it can be produced by oxygen consumption. If the rate of use is less than the individual's maximal energy production from oxygen consumption, the exercise can be sustained for hours and is called submaximal.

Energy Sources for Exercise. ATP and creatine phosphate, high energy phosphate bonds, provide *immediate* energy at a very high rate but only for a matter of seconds. The breakdown of glycogen to lactic acid does not require oxygen. It can reach its high rate in a few seconds, but at top speeds it can only be a major source of energy for 10 to 20 seconds as lactic acid accumulates. Another energy source is the combustion of glycogen, glucose, and fats with oxygen. The longer the duration of exercise, the more important this source becomes. It is referred to as *aerobic energy* and has a lower rate than the first two sources, which are *anaerobic*.

ROLE OF THE CARDIOVASCULAR SYSTEM

Although the blood removes lactic acid from the working muscles and distributes it throughout the body (except in fat), the main role of the cardiovascular system is to transport oxygen, the determinant of maximal or aerobic running speed. The longer the race, the more important the cardiovascular system. However, even in greyhound racing, in which the anaerobic energy sources predominate, the small margin between winning and not placing renders each contribution to total energy very important. During intense bursts of speed, the work of the heart is greatly increased by the rise in blood pressure. This is presumably due to the difficulty of pumping blood into tense muscles and to the rise in PCV and hence of viscosity. Sled dogs show no significant increase in mean blood pressure during prolonged running.

To maximize oxygen transport, the animal has to optimize cardiac output — O_2/ml of blood — and efficiency of ventricular work. Cardiac output can be increased by increasing the heart rate and/or stroke volume.

Heart Rate. The basal (sleeping) heart rate of the greyhound is around 29 to 50 beats/min. During supramaximal running, the heart rate is in the range 280 to 420 (mostly 300 to 360). Beyond the optimal, increases in heart rate cause a fall in cardiac output. Limiting factors are (1) time taken to refill the ventricles and (2) blood supply to maintain coronary perfusion. Little or no blood can enter the myocardium

during contraction. For example, in one greyhound at rest (heart rate 105), the ejection phase of contraction lasted 0.16 sec or 28.5 percent of the time, whereas in the same dog running at 50 Km/hr on a treadmill tilted at a 10° angle (heart rate 306), although the ejection phase only lasted 0.10 sec, it still amounted to 50 percent of the time because of the shorter interval between beats. Flow through the myocardium is reliant upon diastolic pressure, but it is probably aided by the contraction-relaxation cycle. It is interesting to note that in the greyhound, the diastolic pressure rises during supramaximal exercise, whereas in the sled dog, during maximal-submaximal exercise, it falls. In the sled dog, coronary flow is still increased some five-fold, presumably by a more-than-compensatory fall in resistance as the myocardial vasculature dilates.

Stroke Volume. In the literature, changes in stroke volume from rest to exercise range from "non-significant" falls to increases up to 40 percent. In one sense, the greyhound has increased the stroke volume at rest compared with other dogs by virtue of its larger heart. It has been shown at rest to pump more blood/per beat/Kg than do mongrels. The greyhound heart can contract and refill 5 times/second.

Oxygen/ml Blood. The greyhound has a higher PCV (hematocrit) than do other dogs, and this increases the O_2 carried/ml of blood. It does, however, lead to an increase in the viscosity of the blood and hence of the pressure required to pump each ml. Greyhounds at rest may have a PCV as low as 45 to 50 percent. With minimal excitement, this rises to 50 to 60 percent. With pre-race excitement, it rises to 55 to 63 percent, and immediately after a run (PCV_{MAX}), it may be as high as 72 percent (more commonly 56 to 66 percent). Maximal PCV for a particular dog is very consistent while it remains healthy and falls repeatedly within a narrow range — e.g., 60 ± 1.5 percent, provided it is sampled within two to three minutes of the finish of each race. This allows trends to be determined over a period of weeks or months. The relationship of PCV and viscosity makes it difficult to determine the limits of optimal PCV_{MAX}. However, after some years of use and clinical experience, it could become much more meaningful than the "resting" PCVs.

Efficiency of Ventricular Work. The efficiency of ventricular work might be best defined as O_2 consumption of the ventricles in transporting a given amount of O_2 to the body. One way of increasing the efficiency is to increase the capacitance or elasticity of the main pulmonary and systemic arteries This distensibility allows the vessel walls to receive (from the contracting heart) a greater volume of blood per unit rise in blood pressure. In other words, the same volume can be ejected with a lesser rise in resistance or pressure. The greyhound has been shown (Cox et al., 1976) to have significantly more distensible arteries than do mongrels. There may be a further advantage in this elasticity. When the aortic and pulmonary valves have closed, the vessel contracts, maintaining the blood flow while the heart refills. A more elastic vessel presumably holds more, contracts for longer, and perhaps increases slightly the relative duration of diastole. An increase in the percent of time spent in diastole for any given cardiac output will be an advantage in oxygenating the myocardium.

THE GREYHOUND CARDIOVASCULAR SYSTEM

HEART SIZE

The greyhound has a much larger heart than do most other dogs. In general, the greyhound has a heart size in the range 0.8 to 1.7 percent of body weight (mostly 0.9 to 1.3 percent). Mongrels and a few purebreds have been reported in the range 0.55 to 1.05 percent (mostly around 0.8 percent). If the heart of a greyhound was removed from the body of a mongrel of comparable size, the ventricles would be described as grossly thickened and slightly dilated — i.e., mixed concentric-eccentric hypertrophy. This in turn would indicate severe pressure overload and slight volume overload. However, these differences are found in neonate and untrained greyhounds and would appear to be due mainly to inherited factors rather than to training.

ARTERIAL HEMODYNAMICS

Cox et al. (1976) showed that in unanesthetised, trained, chronically instrumented animals, mean arterial pressure was significantly higher in the greyhound than in the mongrel (118 vs 98 mg Hg). This was associated with a significantly higher cardiac index in the greyhound (4.3 vs 3.1 l/min/m^2) and a lower calculated peripheral resistance as compared with the mongrel.

It is interesting to speculate on the reason or reasons for the higher cardiac index and blood pressure in the greyhound. Gunn (1978) found that a greyhound's muscle mass constitutes some 57 percent of its body weight compared with 44 percent for mongrels and various breeds, and it may be that even at rest this tissue requires greater servicing. Greyhounds are comparatively poorly insulated, having almost no fat cover and a short, thin coat. Poor insulation may aid heat loss during and after running, the price being a higher heat loss at rest.

To speculate further, the enlarged (hypertrophied and dilated) heart and the high cardiac index and blood pressure, rather than being inherent, may be secondary to the inherent high proportion of muscle, poor insulation, and high PCV in the greyhound. That is, the high proportion muscle and/or poor insulation increases blood flow requirement and hence produces a high cardiac index and dilatation of the heart. The high PCV increases blood viscosity, which with the high flow leads to a high blood pressure with consequent cardiac hypertrophy.

EXAMINATION OF THE RACING DOG'S CARDIOVASCULAR SYSTEM

History. The history can eliminate or suggest various causes for a problem (see Table 1).

General Examination. Visual appraisal allows a rough approximation of the dog's state of training and fitness. An inadequately prepared dog is often presented because a novice trainer suspects it has a weak heart. The skin pinch test for dehydration is extremely useful.

Table 1. *Race Performance Problems*

PRESENTING SIGN	POSSIBLE ETIOLOGIES IN GREYHOUNDS OTHER THAN MUSCULOSKELETAL INJURIES
Does not try hard enough	illness non-chaser over-excited too long pre-race rarely the heart
Dies on his run Unable to finish Nothing left	poor aerobic ability under-trained under-raced
Pulls up choking	under-raced respiratory problem, e.g., tracheo-bronchitis
Pulls up distressed	good trier minor cardiovascular or respiratory disease
10 lengths in front in middle of the race then drops right back	tries too hard too soon for this distance
Runs with the pack for 200 to 400 metres, then collapses, stops, or slows markedly	under-trained and under-raced cardiovascular system strongly suspected if properly trained
Finishes blue in the tongue	good trier CV shunt, IA or IV septal defect, patent ductus Pulmonic stenosis
Flat, i.e., dull and/or anorexic for several days after race. May develop diarrhea and dehydrate	under-trained if after a single race too many hard runs close together unable to cope with stress; i.e., trains or races "off"

Always pull up the skin in the same area in the same way. The author pulls the skin about two or three inches out, halfway back and halfway down the rib cage. In healthy dogs not in training, return takes less than one second. In healthy dogs in training, it takes less than two seconds. Return taking more than two to four seconds signals a problem. Over four seconds, the animal is usually showing anorexia and/or depression. Time stated is for the skin to return 90 percent, and it allows some estimation of effects of training and race stress.

Cardiovascular Examination. In racing dogs, although there is occasionally some gross abnormality — e.g., a murmur or arrhythmia — the changes are mostly subtle and it is advisable to have a number of normal animals available for comparison, particularly for auscultation.

1. Heart rate must be interpreted in the light of the mental state of the dog and its fitness. It is not always useful because of wide fluctuations and ranges in normal dogs.
2. Pulse character must also be interpreted according to whether the dog is relaxed or tense. Excited dogs have variable and high heart rates, and the artery is not so soft between pulsations. If venous blood is drawn, the PCV will be high and the blood will be bright red, almost arteriolized. Excited dogs do not always jump about, and some very "uptight" dogs stand very still and may be considered by the inexperienced examiner to be unconcerned.
3. Capillary refill time and wetness of gums are useful indicators. However, some normal greyhounds have a very slow refill time — i.e., false positive.
4. Palpation of the heart is very useful but requires experience and practice. It provides an impression of the size and contractility of the heart and enables the detection of thrills. Either cup one hand under the sternum with the thumb over one ventricle and the fingers over the other, or use one hand on either side of the thorax.
5. Auscultation often provides the only clue to cardiovascular trouble, particularly straight after a run. At rest, innocent ejection murmurs may be heard, and at very low heart rates, splitting of the first heart sounds may be normal. Heart sounds are sometimes more high pitched in excited dogs, but a few greyhounds with a history of some severe illness as pups have had very "tinny" sounds of variable intensity, and both the strangeness of the sounds and the variability in loudness are exaggerated after a run. The heart sounds as though it

beats in a different part of the chest, with each beat "banging about in the chest" as in atrial fibrillation. These dogs collapse or stop after 200 to 400 meters. In one instance, the dog had to be carried from the track. (The author emphasizes auscultation, pre- and post-sprint, using normals for comparison. The practitioner usually is asked to detect heart disease at a very early stage.)

6. Electrocardiographic values for greyhounds are different from those for other breeds (see Table 2). The author has seen P waves up to 8 mV and 0.75 seconds, and R waves up to 5.4 mV in normal greyhounds. When is a greyhound's R wave too tall?

Steel et al. (1976) related QRS interval to heart size, but there have been criticisms concerning the determination of the precise endpoint of the QRS on many tracings and the statistical analysis used. Davis et al. (1977) believe there is some degree of correlation between heart score, which is the QRS duration stated in milliseconds, and performance ability.

Arrhythmias can be detected by auscultation, palpation, and pulse taking but are best characterized by ECG readings. Premature ventricular contractions are the most common sign, sometimes in dogs that are performing well. One case each of ventricular escape and premature atrial beats were shown by telemetry to lose the arrhythmia during exercise. One case of atrial fibrillation was racing below previous performance levels, particularly over long distances. Quinidine failed to reverse the fibrillation and DC shock conversion was followed by reversion within days. However, DC shock with two weeks of quinidine therapy enabled the dog to return to racing and place three times without reversion.

7. Radiography in cardiac disease in the greyhound is rarely diagnostic because performance is usually impaired at an early stage. Loss of the waist or waists occurs in more severe, advanced cases.
8. Echo, phono, and apex cardiography are all being developed for use in the dog and will eventually be applied to the greyhound. Echocardiography is useful because it provides an estimate of the size and dynamics of the ventricles. This method looks particularly promising.

Post Mortem. It has been the author's experience that at necropsy, a small percentage of otherwise normal dogs had a superficial circum-

Table 2. *ECG Values For Racing Greyhounds*

AMPLITUDE[°]	P	0.325	(0.05–0.80)	mV
	Q	0.35	(0.05–0.80)	mV
	R	2.9	(1.2 –4.0)	mV
	S	0.11	(0.0 –0.35)	mV
INTERVAL	PR	0.10	(0.05–0.14)	sec
	QRS	0.05	(0.04–0.06)	sec
	QT	0.20	(0.12–0.24)	sec
INTERVAL[†]	PR	0.12	(0.10–0.15)	sec
	QRS	0.07	(0.05–0.09)	sec
	QT	0.20	(0.17–0.23)	sec

FEMALES[‡]	H.R.	P AMP.	R WAVE AMP. L2	P WAVE DURATION	PR INT.	QRS INT.
Mean	117.2	0.301 mV	2.93 mV	0.065	0.123	0.075
SD	34.3	0.110 mV	0.65 mV	0.010	0.014	0.010

MALES	H.R.	P AMP.	R WAVE AMP. L2	P WAVE DURATION	PR INT.	QRS INT.
Mean	113.5	0.29 mV	3.05 mV	0.064	0.123	0.076
SD	31.1	0.15 mV	.71 mV	0.010	0.014	0.010

[°] Schneider, Truex, and Knowles, 1964.
[†] Davis, 1971.
[‡] Davis, 1978. A study on 103 females and 116 males. Recordings taken with left foreleg 30° in front of right foreleg. This group of 219 greyhounds included 50 percent city winners.

scribed lesion of the epicardial surface of the right auricle, close to where it is overlain by the aorta. The ECG, including the P wave, in these cases was normal.

In cases with "tinny" heart sounds, the heart was large but within the normal range. Gross and histologic signs of past inflammation were present, presumably owing to a generalized infection when they were pups.

SUPPLEMENTAL READING

Cox, R.H., Peterson, L.H., and Detweiler, D.K.: Comparison of arterial haemodynamics in the mongrel dog and the racing Greyhound. Am. J. Physiol. 230:211–218, 1976.

Davis, P.E.: Some further aspects of clinical veterinary electrocardiography. Proc. No. 12 Anaesthesia and Intensive Care Course. Postgraduate Committee in Veterinary Science, University of Sydney, 1971, pp. 130–164.

Davis, P.E.: Personal Communication, 1978.

Davis, P.E., Taylor, R.I., and Rose, R.J.: Electrocardiography and potential performance ability in the Greyhound. Proc. No. 34, Greyhounds. Postgraduate Committee in Veterinary Science, University of Sydney, 1977, pp. 223–227.

Gunn, H.M.: The proportions of muscle, bone and fat in two different types of dog. Res. in Vet. Sc. 24:277–282, 1978.

Schneider, H. P., Truex, R. C., and Knowles, J.O.: Comparative observations of the hearts of mongrel and greyhound dogs. Anat. Rec. 149:173–179, 1964.

Steel, J.D., Taylor, R.I., Davis, P.E., Stewart, G.A., and Salmon, P.W.: Relationships between heart score, heart weight and body weight in greyhound dogs. Aust. Vet. J. 52:561–564, 1976.

Van Citters, R.L., and Franklin, D.L.: Cardiovascular performance of Alaska sled dogs during exercise. Circ. Res. 24:33–42, 1969.

PHARMACODYNAMICS OF DIGITALIS, DIURETICS, AND ANTIARRHYTHMIC DRUGS

LLOYD E. DAVIS, D.V.M.,
Urbana, Illinois

Drugs are employed in cardiology primarily for increasing the strength of contraction of the failing myocardium, modifying the generation or conduction of the action potential, or decreasing hemodynamic overloading of the heart. The armamentarium of drugs available to the veterinarian comprises an array of potent, potentially dangerous substances. In order to assess benefit/risk considerations of drug therapy properly in patients with disturbances of the cardiovascular system, it is imperative that the clinician understand the pathophysiology of the disease he seeks to treat and the pharmacodynamics of the drug he selects for therapy. With this knowledge, one is prepared to establish therapeutic objectives in the patient and to assess efficacy or untoward effects in response to the treatment regimen. The pathophysiology of various cardiac disturbances in the dog and cat is discussed by other authors in this section.

DIGITALIS GLYCOSIDES

The digitalis glycosides were reviewed comprehensively by Hahn (1977). This group of drugs increases strength of contraction, decreases heart rate, and decreases size of the failing heart. The glycosides exert these effects without appreciably increasing myocardial oxygen consumption because the decreases in heart rate and intramural tension more than compensate for the increased oxygen consumption induced by their positive inotropic effect.

The exact mechanism of action of the glycosides on contractility is unknown. Digitalis enhances excitation-contraction coupling by increasing the availability of ionic calcium within the cell. This increase is believed to be related in some manner to the ability of glycosides to inhibit sodium- and potassium-activated ATP. The important clinical implication of this information is that calcium augments both the inotropic and toxic effects of digitalis, as does the

loss of intracellular potassium. Administration of calcium is contraindicated in digitalis toxicity, and administration of cardiac glycosides may be dangerous in a patient with hypercalcemia — e.g., certain patients with lymphosarcoma. Hypokalemia enhances the binding of digitalis to myocardial cells and intensifies its pharmacologic effects. Thus, it is logical to administer potassium-containing solutions intravenously in the treatment of digitalis toxicity.

Digitalis slows the heart rate by several mechanisms. In myocardial failure, sinus tachycardia is caused by increased sympathetic nervous effects on the sinoatrial node in response to baroreceptor stimulation. With improvement of myocardial function, the cardiac output increases and reflex stimulation decreases with consequent diminution of sympathetic activity. A second mechanism is to decrease the conduction velocity and increase duration of the refractory period of the atrioventricular node. This effect will be manifested in the electrocardiogram as an increase in PR interval or as varying degrees of heart block. This effect provides the basis for the use of digitalis in the treatment of supraventricular tachycardia. The third action is to increase vagal tone with consequent slowing of the sinus rate.

It should be kept in mind that the change in rate produced by digitalis can be extremely variable, owing to the influence of complicating factors. Atropine or isoproterenol may negate the effect of a glycoside on the AV node or the vagus. Hypoxemia, fever, administration of thyroid hormone, sepsis, or trauma decreases the negative chronotropic effect of digitalis. Conversely, hyperkalemia enhances the suppression of the AV node in heart block.

Once the clinician has elected to administer a glycoside to a patient, he must consider what to use, how to administer it, and what observations to make in order to assess the drug's effects. While some veterinarians still use ouabain and galenical forms of digitalis, the common practice today is to employ digoxin or digitoxin. All

Table 1. *Characteristics of Digoxin and Digitoxin**

CHARACTERISTIC	DIGOXIN	DIGITOXIN
Bioavailability of oral dosage form	Tablet 70%	90–100%
	Elixir 75%	
Protein binding	20–39%	90%
Elimination half-life	38 hr	8 hr
Therapeutic plasma concentration	1–2 ng/ml	15–35 ng/ml
Toxic plasma concentration	>2.5 ng/ml	>40 ng/ml
Maintenance dosage regimen	0.011 mg/kg, bid	0.033 mg/kg tid
Dosage forms available	0.125, 0.25, 0.5 mg tabs	0.1, 0.2, 0.5 mg tabs
	0.05, 0.15 mg/ml elixir	0.1, 0.25 mg caps
	0.1, 0.25 mg/ml injection	0.2 mg/ml injection
Lipid solubility	Low	High
Biotransformation	Liver	Liver
Excretion	Kidney	Bile

*From Hamlin, R. L.: Basis for Selection of a Cardiac Glycoside for Dogs. In Short, C. R. (ed.): Proc. 1st Sympos. Vet. Pharmacol. Therap. Baton Rouge, LA, March 13–15, 1978. V. T. Scialli and L. P. Tilley: Digitalis – Its Clinical Indication and Practical Usage. Burroughs Wellcome Co., Research Triangle Park, N.C. 1979.

the cardioactive glycosides have the same qualitative pharmacologic effects. The major differences among them are quantitative and are related to drug disposition factors such as absorption, protein binding, biotransformation, and excretion. These factors are primary determinants of rational dosage regimens. Hence, it is important for the veterinarian to appreciate differences between the dispositions of digitoxin and digoxin.

Digitoxin differs from digoxin in that the latter compound possesses a hydroxyl group at the 12 position of the steroid nucleus. Otherwise, the two molecules are identical. The hydroxyl group increases the polarity of the molecule, thereby modifying its ability to traverse cellular membranes and to interact with macromolecules. The implications of the physicochemical differences between digitoxin and digoxin are summarized in Table 1.

Equal quantities of the two glycosides within the myocardium produce approximately equivalent responses. Their differences, however, markedly influence delivery of the respective drugs to their site of action. In most cases, the oral route of administration is preferred. The oral dose of digitoxin is the same as its intravenous dose, whereas the oral dose of digoxin is greater than its intravenous dose because of incomplete absorption from the intestine. The dosage of digoxin given as the elixir will be slightly less than that for the tablet because of better absorption. The glycosides should not be administered intramuscularly or subcutaneously because of erratic absorption and the fact that they elicit severe pain at the injection site. (The pain is associated with the glycoside itself and not to any constituent of the vehicle.) Another factor to be considered relative to absorption is

the bioequivalence of various products. In the past, it was observed that different generic preparations of digoxin did not have the same bioavailability, even though they contained the same amounts of active glycoside. This resulted in patients being either underdigitalized or intoxicated following administration of recommended doses. Subsequently, it was discovered that *in vitro* tests of tablet dissolution rate correlated with bioavailability. Since 1974, the Food and Drug Administration (FDA) has required that all dosage forms of digoxin have a dissolution rate of greater than 65 percent and that any company marketing digoxin tablets must submit results of comparative bioavailability studies prior to approval of their product. These requirements should reassure the veterinarian that digoxin may be prescribed by generic name. However, because of past problems of bioequivalence and the fact that most of our knowledge is based on studies of Lanoxin brand digoxin, most veterinary cardiologists prefer Lanoxin. Based on a value for bioavailability of between 65 and 70 percent, 0.15 mg orally would be equivalent to 0.10 mg given intravenously. Drugs that are known to decrease absorption of digoxin when administered simultaneously include kaolin-pectin, anatacids, sulfasalazine (Azulfidine), and neomycin.

Both digoxin and digitoxin are metabolized in the liver, but they are excreted differently. Digoxin is excreted by the kidney and digitoxin is eliminated in the bile. The elimination half-life for digoxin is 38 hours (Breznock, 1973); that for digitoxin is 8 hours (Hamlin, 1978) in the dog. The dosage interval for the glycosides is predicated on this pharmacokinetic parameter. A daily dosage of 0.02 mg/kg of digoxin will produce steady-state concentrations in about seven days (four to five times the half-life), whereas a daily dosage of 0.1 mg/kg of digitoxin will require only 32 to 40 hours to reach a plateau concentration. Similarly, serum concentrations of digitoxin decline more rapidly than those of digoxin following cessation of therapy.

Several patient and therapeutic factors modify the rate of elimination of these glycosides and thereby necessitate the modification of the dosage regimen. Renal diseases that decrease the rate of glomerular filtration impair the excretion of digoxin and thus require the modification of the dosage regimen. Hamlin found that measurements of creatinine clearance are unreliable guides for adjustment of digoxin dosage in dogs. Scialli and Tilley recommended that the total daily dosage of digoxin be reduced by 50 percent for each 50 mg/dl increase in the BUN concentration. This reduced dosage should then be divided for q.i.d. administration. Renal insufficiency apparently does not influence the rate of elimination of digitoxin. Severe hepatic disease would be expected to influence the elimination of both glycosides if it compromised the biotransformation of these drugs.

Drugs that interact in the body to increase the rate of elimination of digoxin in the dog are microsomal enzyme inducers such as the barbiturates, primidone, phenylbutazone, and possibly others. The usual dosage regimen for digitalization of dogs may produce subtherapeutic concentrations of digoxin in patients that are receiving these drugs on a chronic basis (epileptic or arthritic patients). Conversely, drugs that inhibit microsomal enzymes (quinidine, quinine, chloramphenicol, tetracyclines) prolong the rate of elimination of digoxin causing the glycoside to accumulate to toxic concentrations. The author has seen four cases of acute digoxin intoxication in dogs receiving chloramphenicol at the time of digitalization. It is not known whether chloramphenicol interacts with digitoxin in a similar manner. The effects of enzyme-inducers on the liver persist for weeks after cessation of therapy, whereas the inhibition produced by chloramphenicol or quinidine occurs only for as long as the drug is present in the body. It should be safe to digitalize a dog the day after withdrawal of such drugs.

The major determinants of the effective dose of digoxin or digitoxin are lipid solubility and extent of binding to serum albumin. Digitoxin is approximately 90 percent and digoxin is 20 to 30 percent protein bound in the plasma of the dog. As only the unbound fraction of the glycoside is free to diffuse into the myocardium, this feature explains the need for a higher dosage of digitoxin and the larger values observed for therapeutic and toxic plasma concentrations of digitoxin in comparison to digoxin. The habitus of the patient must be considered when calculating dosage because of differences in lipid solubility of the two drugs. Digoxin is poorly lipid soluble, so dosage should be reduced in an obese animal to that appropriate for the lean body mass of the animal. As a rule of thumb, Tilley and Scialli suggested that a value for the lean body mass can be approximated by deducting 15 percent from the measured body weight of an obese animal. On the other hand, digitoxin dosage should be based on total body weight (to include fat) because the depot fat is included in the distribution of the drug. Reduction of dosage of both drugs should be made on the basis of estimates of weight of edematous fluid contained in the patient. Also, giant breeds of dogs require a smaller dosage of the glycosides per unit of body weight than do smaller breeds.

Another factor to be considered in the patient is its age and physiologic state. Both digitoxin and digoxin cross the placenta to the fetuses. Concentrations of digitoxin in the heart of the fetus may be twice those found in the maternal heart, whereas digoxin was observed to attain concentrations in fetal blood equivalent to those found in the blood of the bitch. This factor should be taken into account when treating a bitch that is late in pregnancy. Fouron observed digitalis effects on the fetal electrocardiogram at the same time that the bitch showed ectopic beats consistent with digitalis intoxication.

The disposition and pharmacologic effects of digoxin are different in the neonate than in the adult dog. Owing to immaturity of the microsomal enzyme system and renal function in puppies, the half-life would be expected to be longer and thereby would decrease the dosage requirement of digoxin. On the other hand, the volume of distribution of digoxin in the neonate is greater than that in the adult, which would result in lower serum concentrations of digoxin for a given dosage rate. Another factor that would tend to minimize the need for reducing the dose is that the myocardium of the newborn puppy is less sensitive to the action of digitalis. Considering the net effect of all these factors, it probably is unnecessary to revise the digitalization regimen during the neonatal period (first one or two months of life). It should be recognized, however, that it will probably require longer than one week to attain steady-state concentrations of digoxin in the neonate, owing to the longer half-life. Similar information is not available concerning digitoxin.

Dosage regimens for geriatric patients may require modification because of two factors: (1) the aged dog frequently has a decrease in renal function, which would increase the half-life of digoxin, and (2) the volume of distribution is decreased owing to loss of muscle mass. These changes would have the effect of increasing steady-state serum concentrations as compared with those occurring in younger dogs given the same dosage. The maintenance dose should be reduced to about half that used in a younger adult animal in order to avoid toxicity.

The digitalis glycosides have a low therapeutic index. The minimum effective plasma concentration has been estimated to be about 70 percent of the minimum toxic plasma concentration in healthy animals or patients with heart disease of short duration. Factors that were discussed previously can decrease this margin of safety — e.g., hypercalcemia, hypokalemia, and thyroid disease increase the sensitivity of the heart to the actions of digitalis. The longer the duration of heart disease in a particular animal, the smaller the therapeutic index will become. It is not uncommon to encounter a patient in which the effective dose of a glycoside may be 90 percent of the toxic dose.

The principal signs of digitalis intoxication are referable to the gastrointestinal tract, the cardiovascular system, and the central nervous system. The earliest signs of toxicity in the dog and cat are generally anorexia, vomiting, and diarrhea, and these are particularly pronounced with digoxin. The appearance of such clinical signs should suggest to the veterinarian the need to reassess his dosage regimen. Such signs are not an indication of serious toxicity, but they herald the development of serious cardiac toxicity if the dosage regimen were continued without modification. Anorexia and vomition are probably mediated by the action of toxic concentrations of the glycoside on the central nervous system. Vomiting is due to stimulation of the chemoreceptor trigger zone in the medulla. Other signs of CNS toxicity include depression, stupor, muscle weakness, and visual disturbances. Nearly any cardiac arrhythmia can be associated with digitalis toxicity. Commonly seen are varying degrees of heart block, ventricular premature contractions, ventricular tachycardia, and eventual ventricular fibrillation. *It is dangerous to continue digitalis therapy in the presence of any of these signs.*

The most important thing to do in case of intoxication is to withdraw digitalis and evaluate the patient's serum electrolytes. Both digoxin and digitoxin concentrations should decline to safe levels within one half-life (38 hours for digoxin and 8 hours for digitoxin) if renal and hepatic functions are normal. If possible (at local hospital or regional veterinary college), a determination of plasma concentration of the

glycoside in question should be done to resolve the matter of whether the toxicity is due to overdosage or to increased myocardial sensitivity.*
Of 75 dogs receiving digoxin that were studied by Hamlin, plasma concentrations were subtherapeutic in 24 percent, therapeutic in 29 percent, and toxic in 25 percent of the animals (21 percent were excluded from the study). In the same study, 43 dogs had received digitoxin. Of these, 19 percent had subtherapeutic concentrations, 60 percent had therapeutic ranges, and 5 percent had concentrations that were toxic. It is indicated by these data that the risk of digitalis toxicity is of real significance in a practice setting and not merely a matter of academic interest. If the patient were hypokalemic and heart block were not present, consideration should be given to the restoration of normal potassium concentrations in the plasma. A daily dose of up to one gram of potassium chloride (in solution) may be given orally in divided doses. In an emergency, potassium chloride in 5 percent dextrose solution may be administered slowly by intravenous infusion with electrocardiographic monitoring. Other drugs that may be useful in the control of ventricular arrhythmias include lidocaine, propranolol and phenytoin.

Cardiac glycosides are exceedingly toxic substances if misused. Sixty ml of triple strength elixir contains over nine times the lethal dose of digoxin for a child, and the drug is contained in a pleasantly flavored vehicle. As little as one milligram of digoxin or digitoxin in tablets can kill a small child. On the basis of these considerations, it is inexcusable to dispense these products in anything but child-proof containers. We are not legally bound to do so but our good conscience should direct us to observe this precaution. These containers should be properly labeled with the name of the drug and size of the dosage form to facilitate emergency treatment in case of accidental ingestion. Dosage regimens and clinical use of the glycosides are discussed by other authors in this section.

THEOPHYLLINE

Theophylline is a xanthine derivative that has been employed in the management of cardiac diseases. Like other xanthines, which include caffeine and theobromine, theophylline stimulates the cerebral cortex, dilates coronary arteries and bronchioles, induces diuresis, increases heart rate, and increases strength of contraction of the myocardium. By virtue of

*To be meaningful, samples must be taken at least 6 to 8 hours following the last dose of digitalis.

these pharmacologic effects, the use of theophylline has been advocated in the clinical management of congestive heart failure, acute pulmonary edema, cardiac asthma, and pulmonary diseases characterized by an increase in airway resistance.

The actions of theophylline resemble those of beta adrenergic drugs because both groups increase the concentration of cyclic adenosine-monophosphate (C-AMP), which in turn enhances the response of the effector tissue. The adrenergic drugs do this by stimulating the production of C-AMP within the cell, whereas theophylline, by inhibiting the enzyme phosphodiesterase, decreases the rate of destruction of C-AMP. Unlike digitalis, the beta adrenergic drugs and theophylline increase strength of contraction while at the same time increasing oxygen consumption by the myocardium. Because of this action on sympathetic nervous mechanisms, theophylline is arrhythmogenic and may induce serious ventricular arrhythmias in a hypoxic myocardium. Theophylline should not be regarded as an inotropic drug of choice in patients with acute cardiac decompensation.

The theophylline base is insoluble in water and can only be given orally. Double salts of theophylline are available that are water soluble and can be administered intravenously. These include theophylline ethylenediamine (Aminophylline), theophylline sodium glycinate (Synophylate), and choline theophyllinate (Oxtriphylline). These preparations should not be administered intramuscularly or subcutaneously because they produce severe pain at the injection site.*

The principal toxic effects of theophylline are dose related. Gastritis with nausea and vomiting may be a persistent side effect in some patients. More serious toxic effects associated with overdosage include CNS stimulation, convulsive seizures, and serious cardiac arrhythmias. In human patients, plasma concentrations of theophylline in excess of 20 μg/ml are generally associated with signs of serious toxicity.

A recent study of Aminophylline (Searle) in dogs showed that at a dosage rate of 10 mg/kg, plasma concentrations were obtained in the range of 5 to 15 μg/ml, which was reported to be effective in human subjects (Ziment, 1978). The elimination half-life was 5.7 hours, and the apparent specific volume of distribution was 0.75 liter/kg. The theophylline in the Searle tablets that were studied was 92 percent bioavailable. Following oral administration, therapeutic concentrations of theophylline were observed in the plasma within 30 minutes. It was concluded from these experimental findings that intravenous administration of Aminophylline is seldom necessary except in acute emergencies because of the rapid and complete absorption of the drug following oral administration. A dosage regimen for the dog of 10 mg/kg, given orally every eight hours, should be adequate in situations in which theophylline therapy is indicated. Because of reported differences in bioavailability of various theophylline preparations, these conclusions apply only to the Searle brand of Aminophylline that we studied.

DIURETICS

Diuretic drugs are useful adjuncts to the cardiac glycosides in that they reduce pre-load on the heart and mobilize excessive sodium and water accumulations in the tissues. It should be kept in mind that early in the course of congestive heart failure, sodium and water retention is a compensatory mechanism that acts to maintain cardiac output by increasing volume loading. In many cases, digitalization and restriction of dietary sodium will remove the excess fluid by restoring renal blood flow. This seems to be the more rational approach if the therapeutic objective is to restore normal perfusion to the tissues. Diuretic drugs do not increase the cardiac output and, if used unwisely, they can cause a deterioration in the patient's condition by decreasing blood volume and cardiac output. Such signs as pre-renal azotemia, hypotension, alkalosis, lassitude, and confusion then dominate the clinical picture.

Diuretic drugs are valuable adjuncts to digitalis in patients with advanced heart disease in which digitalis alone will not relieve tissue edema and in patients that are relatively refractory to cardiac glycosides (as in certain cases of cardiomyopathy). It is wise to reassess such patients and establish an objective for further therapy. Occasional patients with restrictive pericarditis or cardiac tamponade present with signs of congestive heart failure and will not benefit from either glycosides or diuretics; yet, proper diagnosis immediately suggests appropriate measures to be taken to relieve the problem.

Diuretics that deserve a place in the veterinarian's armamentarium are a high-ceiling diuretic (such as furosemide or ethacrynic acid), a thiazide diuretic (chlorothiazide, hydrochlorothiazide, or bendroflumethiazide), and a mercurial diuretic (meralluride or mersalyl). Each of these groups possesses attributes that are useful in specific situations.

---

*Given IV, these are also dangerous. Slow administration is recommended. The editor frequently gives aminophylline without problems in the lumbar muscles.

The high-ceiling diuretics are potent drugs that have a rapid onset and brief duration of action. These are reserved for emergency situations in which the objective is to remove considerable quantities of water and sodium as quickly as possible. Furosemide inhibits the active resorption of chloride and passive resorption of sodium by the ascending limb of the loop of Henle. This interferes with the concentrating ability of the kidney and causes intense water diuresis. Diuresis persists in response to this drug, even in the presence of dehydration, and such usage is capable of inducing cardiovascular collapse. Continuous use depletes the body of potassium by stimulating release of renin by the juxtaglomerular apparatus and by increasing delivery of sodium to the distal tubule. Furosemide also enhances the excretion of calcium and magnesium, with variable effects on phosphate excretion.

Furosemide probably should not be used in patients receiving cephaloridine, polymixins, or aminoglycoside antibiotics, as any of these drugs may interact with furosemide to damage the renal tubules. The aminoglycosides may also interact with furosemide to produce hearing loss.

The maximal effect of furosemide occurs within 30 minutes of intravenous administration and persists for two to three hours. The drug is excreted in the urine by a process of active tubular secretion by the proximal convoluted tubule. Furosemide is extensively (98 percent) protein bound in canine plasma, suggesting the possibility for drug interaction with drugs that have a high affinity for protein binding (such as phenylbutazone). The usual intravenous dosage for furosemide in the dog is 1 to 2 mg/kg.

The thiazide diuretics have a lesser maximal effect than does furosemide but produce a more sustained diuretic and natriuretic effect. For these reasons, thiazide diuretics are preferred for routine management of cardiac patients needing diuretic therapy. The main difference among the various thiazides is potency. In most cases, this offers little clinical advantage, and the newer, more potent drugs are more expensive. This group of compounds increases excretion of sodium, chloride, potassium, and water by inhibiting the active resorption of sodium in the proximal and distal convoluted tubules. Like furosemide, the thiazide diuretics can produce hypokalemia, hypochloremic alkalosis, and hyperuricemia, and they can decrease glucose tolerance. The thiazides are excreted in the urine by active transport via the proximal tubular epithelium. Drugs that compete for this active transport mechanism can inhibit the efficacy of the thiazides (penicillins, Diodrast,

PAH). The duration of action of this group is between 12 and 24 hours. The usual canine dosages are as follows: chlorothiazide (Diuril) 20 to 45 mg/kg; hydrochlorothiazide (Hydrodiuril) 2 to 4 mg/kg; and bendroflumethiazide (Naturetin) 0.2 to 0.4 mg/kg. It is probably wise to supplement potassium in the diet of cardiac patients receiving digitalis and continuous diuretic therapy.

The mercurial diuretics are, for the most part, obsolete. They must be given by intramuscular injection, are potentially toxic, and are less effective in the presence of alkalosis. Their use is reserved for the occasional patient that is unresponsive to furosemide or the thiazides. The mercurials inhibit the resorption of sodium and chloride via the proximal convoluted tubules. Chloride is excreted in excess of sodium because some sodium will exchange for potassium or hydrogen ions in the distal tubule. After several days, hypochloremic alkalosis develops, which decreases the diuretic effect of the mercurial. The diuretic action can be restored by the administration of ammonium chloride to correct the alkalosis. The usual dose of meralluride or mersalyl in the dog is 5 to 10 mg/kg, intramuscularly.

ANTIARRHYTHMIC DRUGS

A number of factors can act to increase the rate of depolarization of myocardial cells either by increasing the slope of phase 4 (spontaneous depolarization) or by altering the maximal resting potential of the membrane. These effects produce an increase in automaticity of latent pacemakers with the development of arrhythmias. Conditions that favor rapid depolarization include ischemia, acidosis, hypocalcemia, chest trauma, hypokalemia, catecholamines, heat stroke, digitalis, atropine, and stretching of the myocardium (as in atrial enlargement).

Quinidine is the dextrorotary isomer of quinine and is the oldest of the antiarrhythmic drugs. It acts to increase the duration of the effective refractory period, decrease excitability, and slow the rate of conduction of the action potential in myocardial cells. In the normal heart, quinidine produces slowing by increasing the refractory period of the SA node by depressing the slope of phase 4 depolarization. In atrial fibrillation, quinidine may either abolish fibrillation and restore a normal rhythm or slow the rate, converting the fibrillation to flutter without restoring a sinus rhythm. The latter is undesirable because as the atrial rate decreases, A-V conduction improves, allowing more impulses to reach the ventricles, thus causing a dangerous tachycardia. This sequence can be prevented by pretreatment with digitalis, which will depress A-V conduction more efficiently than the quinidine. In the author's experience, quinidine generally is not effective in converting atrial fibrillation to a sinus rhythm in the dog. However, Pyle reported that he successfully employed quinidine for this purpose (1967).

Quinidine is well absorbed following oral administration with peak plasma concentrations occurring in from 60 to 90 minutes. The half-life of quinidine in the dog is 5.6 hours and in the cat is 1.9 hours. It is approximately 90 percent bound in canine and feline plasma, and the apparent specific volume of distribution is 2.9 liter/kg in the dog and 2.2 liter/kg in the cat. Quinidine undergoes biotransformation in the liver. The usual dosage is 10 mg/kg.

Overdosage with quinidine can produce toxicity. Most common are gastrointestinal disturbances with vomiting and diarrhea. More serious dose-related toxicity is manifested by incoordination, convulsions, A-V block, atrial standstill, and ventricular fibrillation. Allergic manifestations may occur that are not dose related; these include fixed eruptions of the skin and thrombocytopenic purpura. Particular attention must be paid to the possibility of drug interactions. Quinidine is one of the most potent inhibitors of microsomal enzymes so far identified (Boulos et al., 1970). Thus, it can accentuate the pharmacologic effects and increase the duration of action of other drugs that require biotransformation by the liver to terminate their action — e.g., barbiturates, tranquilizers, opiates, and many others. Quinidine is contraindicated in patients with complete heart block, as it may extinguish ectopic pacemakers with resultant cardiac standstill.

Procainamide is a procaine derivative that is effective by oral administration. Its effects are similar to those of quinidine except that it has less negative chronotropic activity. Its primary use is to abolish ventricular premature beats and to treat ventricular tachycardia. The toxic effects are similar to those reported for quinidine. Intravenous overdosages may produce profound hypotension. The usual dosage for life-threatening ventricular tachycardia is an intravenous infusion at a rate of 100 mg/minute until conversion takes place. This must be done with continuous electrocardiographic monitoring. Ettinger (1975) recommended oral doses of from 250 to 500 mg in large dogs and 125 mg in smaller dogs given every four to six hours. The pharmacokinetics have not been studied in dogs and cats.

Lidocaine differs from quinidine and procainamide in that it depresses automaticity without affecting conduction velocity or the refractory period. It is of no value for the long-term control of atrial or ventricular arrhythmias. It is employed for the rapid and short-term control of ventricular arrhythmias. The half-life of lidocaine in the dog is about 11 minutes and the specific volume of distribution is 0.66 liter/kg (Boyes et al., 1970). Effective antiarrhythmic concentrations of lidocaine in the plasma are between 2 and 4 μg/ml. Concentrations greater than 5 μg/ml were observed to be toxic. On the basis of these parameters, one may calculate an appropriate intravenous regimen for the dog. A loading dose of lidocaine of 2 mg/kg can be given as a bolus injection, to be followed by a constant rate infusion of 120 μg/kg/min. The principal sign of toxicity observed is vomiting, although gross overdosage may produce convulsions.

Phenytoin possesses unique antiarrhythmic properties. It reduces automaticity of ectopic pacemakers by depressing the slope of phase 4 depolarization and by increasing the resting membrane potential toward normal in fibers having an abnormally low diastolic resting potential. Yet, unlike quinidine and procainamide, phenytoin decreases the refractory period and facilitates conduction in cardiac muscle. Because of these actions, phenytoin is useful in the management of arrhythmias caused by digitalis or procainamide. It is of no value in the treatment of atrial fibrillation.

In man, the therapeutic range of plasma concentrations is between 10 and 20 μg/ml. Investigations in the dog indicate that the range is similar to that in man. Sanders and Yeary (1978) observed a plasma half-life for phenytoin in the dog of three hours with a dosage of 15 mg/kg. They noted, however, that the pharmacokinetics were dose dependent. This would mean that the half-life would increase at higher doses. On the basis of their data, a dosage of about 30 mg/kg of phenytoin would be necessary to control arrhythmias. This could be repeated in six to eight hours. The principal toxic effects are ataxia, nystagmus, and gingival hyperplasia.

Propranolol is a beta adrenergic receptor antagonist. Stimulation of beta adrenergic receptors in the heart increases automaticity, heart rate, conduction rate, and strength of contraction. Beta receptor blockade prevents most of these effects. Thus, propranolol is useful in the management of various tachyarrhythmias, hypertrophic cardiomyopathy, and hypertrophic outflow tract obstructions, and in reducing myocardial oxygen consumption. In conjunction with digitalis, propranolol is useful in reducing the ventricular rate in atrial fibrillation. In addition to its beta blocking effect, propranolol exerts an independent quinidine-like effect that depresses strength of contraction and automaticity. *Propranolol should not be given in the presence of quinidine, as the effects are additive.*

The half-life of propranolol in the dog is about one hour, with an apparent specific volume of distribution of 6.5 liters/kg. The bioavailability of oral propranolol is low (2 to 17 percent) but increases considerably with multiple dosing. This was explained on the basis of saturation of extraction processes in the liver, thereby decreasing the first-pass effect. The recommended dosages for the dog are 0.5 mg/kg intravenously and 5 mg/kg orally. The oral dosage should probably be reduced for subsequent doses, given every eight hours, to prevent accumulation.

SUPPLEMENTAL READING

Baggot, J.D., and Davis, L.E.: Plasma protein binding of digitoxin and digoxin in several mammalian species. Res. Vet. Sci. 15:81, 1973.

Boulos, B.M., Short, C.R., and Davis, L.E.: Quinine and quinidine inhibition of pentobarbital metabolism. Biochem. Pharmacol. 19:723, 1970.

Breznock, E.M.: Application of canine plasma kinetics of digoxin and digitoxin to therapeutic digitalization in the dog. Am. J. Vet. Res. 34:993, 1973.

Breznock, E.M.: Effects of phenobarbital on digitoxin and digoxin elimination in the dog. Am. J. Vet. Res. 36:371, 1975.

Ettinger, S.J., and Suter, P.E.: *Canine Cardiology*. Philadelphia, W.B. Saunders Co., 1970.

Ettinger, S.J.: *Textbook of Veterinary Internal Medicine*. Philadelphia, W.B. Saunders Co., 1975.

Fouron, J.C.: Dynamics of the placental transfer of digoxin in the dog. Biol. Neonate 23:116, 1973.

Frazier, H.S., and Yager, H.: The clinical use of diuretics. N. Engl. J. Med. 288:246, 455, 1973.

Glanz, S.A., Kernoff, R., and Goldman, R.H.: Age-related changes in ouabain pharmacology. Circ. Res. 39:407, 1976.

Hahn, A.W.: Digitalis glycosides in canine medicine. In Kirk, R.W. (ed.): *Current Veterinary Therapy VI*. Philadelphia, W.B. Saunders Co., 1977.

Hamlin, R.L: Basis for selection of a cardiac glycoside for dogs. Proc. 1st Symposium on Veterinary Pharmacology and Therapeutics. Baton Rouge, Louisiana, 1978.

Juhl, R., Summers, R.W., Guillory, J.K., Blaug, S.M., Cheng, F.H., and Brown, D.D.: Effect of sulfasalazine on digoxin bioavailability. Clin. Pharmacol. Therap. 20:387, 1976.

Kates, R.E., Keene, B.W., and Hamlin, R.L.: Pharmacokinetics of propranolol in the dog. J. Vet. Pharmacol. Therap. In press, 1979.

Katz, A.M.: Congestive heart failure. Role of altered myocardial cellular control. N. Engl. J. Med. 293:1184, 1975.

Lang, T.W., Bernstein, M.D., and Barbieri, F.: Digitalis toxicity: treatment with diphenylhydantoin. Arch. Intern. Med. 116:573, 1965.

Lant, A.F., and Wilson, G.M.: Modern Diuretic Therapy in the Treatment of Cardiovascular and Renal Disease. Amsterdam, Excerpta Medica, 1973.

Lindenbaum, J., Butler, V.P., Murphy, J.E., and Cresswell, R.M.: Correlation of digoxin tablet dissolution rate with biological availability. Lancet 1:215, 1973.

Lindenbaum, J., Maulitz, R.M., and Butler, V.P.: Inhibition of digoxin absorption by neomycin. Gastroenterology 71:399, 1976.

Lindenbaum, J., Mellow, M.H., Blackstone, M.D., and Butler, V.P.: Variation in biological availability of digoxin from four preparations. N. Engl. J. Med. 285:1344, 1971.

McKiernan, B.C., Davis, L.E., Neff-Davis, C.A., and Koritz, G.D.: Pharmacokinetics of theophylline in the dog. Proc. Am. Coll. Vet. Intern. Med., July 23, 1979, p. 106.

Neff, C.A., Davis, L.E., and Baggot, J.D.: A comparative study of the pharmacokinetics of quinidine. Am. J. Vet. Res. 33:1521, 1972.

Pyle, R.L.: Conversion of atrial fibrillation with quinidine sulfate in a dog. JAVMA 151:582, 1967.

Rosen, M.R., Hordof, A.J., Hodess, A.B., Verosky, M., and Vulliemoz, Y.: Ouabain induced changes in electrophysiologic properties in neonatal, young and adult canine cardiac Purkinje fibers. J. Pharmacol. Exp. Therap. 194:255, 1975.

Sanders, J.E., and Yeary, R.A.: Serum concentrations of orally administered diphenylhydantoin in dogs. JAVMA 172:153, 1978.

Scialli, V.T., and Tilley, L.P.: Digitalis. Its Clinical Indication and Practical Usage. Burroughs Wellcome Co., Research Triangle Park, N.C. 1979.

Ziment, I.: *Respiratory Pharmacology and Therapeutics*. Philadelphia, W.B. Saunders Co., 1978, p. 192.

ACUTE HEART FAILURE

JOHN BONAGURA, D.V.M.
Columbus, Ohio

Acute heart failure refers to a sudden inability of the cardiac pump to maintain a normal circulation. This inadequacy causes decreased tissue perfusion and venous congestion, with transudation into interstitial fluid compartments (Fig. 1). These changes are heralded by clinical signs of cardiac failure. The clinician may observe evidence of inadequate tissue perfusion including weakness or syncope, pre-renal azotemia, cardiac arrhythmias secondary to reduced coronary flow, diminished arterial pulsations, and increased capillary refill time. Often, examination reveals marked circulatory venous congestion. Clinical findings of acute congestive heart failure relate to the severity of left or right ventricular failure. Typical abnormalities include marked alveolar pulmonary edema, hydrothorax, pericardial effusion, ascites, subcutaneous edema, and measurable increases in pulmonary wedge or systemic venous pressures.

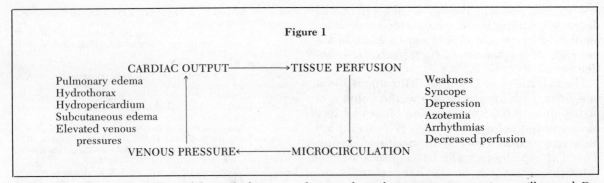

Figure 1. The potential effects of diminished tissue perfusion and circulatory venous congestion are illustrated. Decreased cardiac output can result in generalized weakness. Diminished cerebral perfusion causes depression and possibly syncope. Pre-renal azotemia results from reduced glomerular filtration, while diminished coronary perfusion is a potent mechanism for ventricular arrhythmias. When the left ventricle fails, elevated pulmonary capillary hydrostatic (wedge) pressure leads to the formation of pulmonary edema. Pleural effusion usually accompanies biventricular failure. Ascites, subcutaneous edema, hydropericardium, and elevated central venous pressure are evidence for right-sided congestive heart failure.

CAUSES OF ACUTE HEART FAILURE

To a certain extent, the description of heart failure as "acute" is a misnomer. Unlike man, animals infrequently develop true acute heart failure. Many cases of acute failure are late manifestations of chronic heart disease that have been unnoticed or disregarded by the client. This is particularly true of the fastidious cat. Some cardiac abnormalities do result in sudden cardiac decompensation. For example, both pericardial tamponade and ventricular tachycardia can cause acute heart failure.

Table 1 lists some of the causes of heart failure in small animal patients. The majority of listed abnormalities are chronic processes that require months to years to induce cardiac decompensation. A chronic disease can quickly deteriorate, however, with the development of another cardiac abnormality. This often is observed following the establishment of atrial fibrillation in giant-breed dogs with congestive cardiomyopathy. Acute cardiac arrhythmias are deleterious in other clinical settings. For example, in gastric dilatation-torsion, the combined effects of shock, anesthetics, surgery, and acute ventricular arrhythmias lead to rapid deterioration of the patient from acute circulatory failure. Often, vigorous treatment of the ventricular tachyarrhythmia is the key to successful management.

Other chronic processes can deteriorate suddenly. In chronic compensated mitral valve disease, acute heart failure develops secondary to ruptured chordae tendinae. Slowly forming pericardial effusions usually are tolerated until a critical intrapericardial pressure results in cardiac tamponade with attendant signs of heart failure. Clients aggravate compensated heart failure by using cardiac medications injudiciously or by exposing their pets to hostile en-

Table 1. Causes of Heart Failure in Dogs and Cats

ENDOCARDIAL DISEASES
Bacterial endocarditis
Chronic valvular-myocardial heart disease in dogs (endocardiosis)
Congenital endocardial fibroelastosis

MYOCARDIAL DISEASES
Myocardial disease, degeneration, or failure secondary to another disorder (e.g., myocardial depressant factor in shock, endotoxemia, sepsis, direct myocardial trauma, anemia, drugs, viruses)
Primary myocardial diseases (idiopathic cardiomyopathies)
Feline cardiomyopathies
Canine cardiomyopathies
Acute myocardial infarction (rare)

PERICARDIAL DISEASES
Constrictive pericardial diseases
Pericardial tamponade (effusions) – e.g., "benign" idiopathic pericardial effusion in the dog
Pericardial neoplasia – e.g., hemangiosarcoma (dog), lymphosarcoma, aortic body tumor

CONGENITAL HEART DISEASE
Intracardiac and extracardiac shunts – patent ductus arteriosus, atrial septal and ventricular septal defects, endocardial cushion defect
Semilunar valvular stenosis – aortic and pulmonic stenosis
Abnormal development of the tricuspid and mitral valves (dysplasia)

CARDIAC ARRHYTHMIAS

COR PULMONALE
Dirofilariasis
Other causes of cor pulmonale (e.g., pulmonary embolus)

MISCELLANEOUS CAUSES
Peripheral arteriovenous fistula
Drug overdosages (e.g., anesthetics, propranolol HCl, etc.)

vironmental situations such as excessive heat. Other non-cardiac problems can induce decompensation. These include anemia, primary pulmonary disease, disorders of fluid and electrolyte balance, renal failure, and infections. The clinician should be cognizant of the causes of sudden heart failure and complicating factors that acutely decompensate chronic heart disease.

DIAGNOSIS OF ACUTE HEART FAILURE

CLINICAL SIGNS

Acute heart failure constitutes a medical emergency. The veterinarian must efficiently evaluate the patient and its history, and then promptly initiate therapy. The clinical signs of acute heart failure are related to the development of edema or effusions and reduction of tissue perfusion (see Fig. 1). The most dramatic signs include dyspnea, weakness, and collapse. These abnormalities generally can be correlated to the development of pulmonary edema, pleural effusion, diminished cardiac output, or a malignant cardiac arrhythmia.

The medical history is helpful, particularly if it demonstrates previous signs of heart disease or reveals that the animal currently is receiving cardiac medication. This information may indicate sudden decompensation of chronic heart disease. The patient history also is explored for information that might explain a non-cardiac basis for acute dyspnea or sudden collapse. Pulmonary edema can result from a number of non-cardiac abnormalities including seizures, trauma, electrocution, and heat stroke. Sudden collapse is noted in disorders such as hypoadrenalcorticism, hemolytic crisis, and sepsis. The veterinarian should anticipate circulatory collapse in conditions that predispose to malignant arrhythmias, including gastric dilatation, traumatic shock, and systemic bacterial infections.

The physical examination is important in establishing a diagnosis of acute cardiac failure. Of particular consequence are signs that indicate probable cardiac failure and the presence of reliable signs of heart disease. Reliable signs of heart disease include loud cardiac murmurs, gallop rhythms, arrhythmias, and cardiomegaly. Equally important is the observation of physical signs that negate a diagnosis of heart failure. Therefore, electrical burns in the mouth, marked pallor of the mucous membranes, or obvious evidence of patient trauma all suggest a non-cardiac basis of sudden edema, dyspnea, or collapse.

The typical patient with acute congestive heart failure is presented with signs of pulmonary edema or pleural effusion. The animal is anxious, orthopneic, and reluctant to move. Pleural effusion causes inspiratory dyspnea; pulmonary edema results in both inspiratory and expiratory dyspnea. Cyanosis is noted if there is marked compression atelectasis of the lung or interruption in the diffusion of gases. Pleural effusion leads to muffling of the cardiac and pulmonary sounds. Pulmonary edema is associated with moist or bubbling pulmonary rales and paroxysms of coughing.

Cardiac auscultation usually is abnormal in sudden heart failure. Auscultation of a bradyarrhythmia or tachyarrhythmia may explain the presence of weak arterial pulsations, prolonged capillary refill time, decreased urinary output, weakness, syncope, or collapse. Loud cardiac murmurs usually indicate heart disease, and they lend support to a diagnosis of cardiogenic edema or effusion. Muffling of the heart sounds occurs in pericardial tamponade. The presence of ventricular (S_3) and atrial (S_4) gallops indicate ventricular decompensation. These diastolic sounds are heard commonly in the cardiomyopathies and in chronic valvular heart disease.

Typical auscultatory findings in association with characteristic signalments often suggest a definitive diagnosis. For example, the presence of a murmur of mitral insufficiency in a miniature-breed dog usually is adequate to incriminate chronic valvular-myocardial disease (endocardiosis) as the etiology of heart failure. In a giant-breed dog with a soft apical systolic murmur, gallop rhythm, and auscultatory evidence of atrial fibrillation, congestive cardiomyopathy is the usual diagnosis.

The clinician should not overinterpret potential or probable signs of cardiac dysfunction, since abnormal cardiac findings occur incidentally or secondary to other disorders. It is helpful, however, to formulate a tentative diagnosis based on the history and physical examination. The signs associated with acute heart failure are dramatic. Frequently, the need to manage acute pulmonary edema or to remove a large pleural effusion supersedes the importance of an immediate diagnosis. After patient stabilization, however, the clinician is obliged to pursue the definitive diagnosis in order to provide an accurate prognosis and proper therapy. Additional evaluations, therefore, are indicated for a complete work-up.

RADIOGRAPHY

Thoracic radiographs are particularly valuable for evaluating cardiovascular status. Properly exposed X-ray films allow the clinician to discern cardiac enlargement, pulmonary vascular dynamics, and extracardiac signs of heart failure. Most cases of acute heart failure are associated with significant cardiomegaly. Some patients with acute pulmonary edema, however, reveal unimpressive cardiac silhouettes. Normal cardiac dimensions can occur in heart failure associated with acute cardiac arrhythmias. Non-cardiogenic pulmonary edema also must be considered if the left heart is not enlarged. The clinical features of non-cardiogenic pulmonary edema are discussed on pages 243–249.

Typical radiographic signs of cardiogenic pulmonary edema are cardiomegaly, pulmonary venous distension, and increased interstitial and alveolar pulmonary densities. The intrapulmonary infiltrates are usually perihilar, dorsal, and bilateral. Radiographic features of pleural effusion include increased thoracic densities with silhouetting of the heart, blunting of the costophrenic angles, and retraction of the pulmonary lobar borders from the chest wall and adjacent lung lobes. Since large pleural effusions obscure the cardiac silhouette, the clinician initially must depend on other indices of cardiac function to evaluate the heart. Following the removal of pleural fluid, thoracic radiographs are repeated to permit critical evaluation of the cardiac silhouette.

ANCILLARY TESTS

Other diagnostic tests are helpful in the evaluation and differential diagnosis of acute heart failure. An electrocardiogram defines cardiac arrhythmias and furnishes information about the state of the myocardium. Direct measurement of the central venous and pulmonary capillary wedge pressures provides insight into right and left heart dynamics, respectively. An echocardiographic study offers useful information concerning cardiac structure and function. Echograms are particularly helpful in confirming the presence of pericardial tamponade. Once stabilized, some patients should be studied via non-selective or selective angiocardiography. In selected cases, these additional procedures are helpful. Unfortunately, with the exception of ECG and non-selective angiograms, these studies cannot be obtained routinely in most veterinary clinics.

Laboratory tests including serum biochemistries, blood counts, and blood gases are helpful in evaluating the cause and consequences of cardiac and noncardiac diseases. Exfoliative cytology and analysis of pericardial, pleural, and abdominal effusions are especially helpful in the differential diagnosis of heart failure. In contrast to some other causes of pleural and peritoneal effusions, heart failure results in fluids classified as transudates and modified transudates. Serologic testing for feline leukemia virus and feline infectious peritonitis are helpful in evaluating the cat with thoracic effusion. Pleural effusion is common in these and other disorders, as well as in feline cardiomyopathy.

Table 2. *Causes of Dyspnea in Small Animals*

INTRALUMINAL OBSTRUCTION OR EXTERNAL COMPRESSION OF UPPER AIRWAYS
1. Edematous soft palate
2. Laryngeal edema, paralysis, collapse, or spasm
3. Intraluminal tracheal-bronchial obstruction (foreign body, neoplasm)
4. Extraluminal tracheal-bronchial obstruction
 Mediastinal mass
 Mainstem bronchus collapse from enlarged left atrium
 Hilar lymphadenopathy (neoplasm, systemic mycosis)
5. Aspiration
6. Traumatic rupture of airway

DISEASE OF THE LOWER AIRWAYS OR PULMONARY PARENCHYMA
1. Bronchial disease
2. Pulmonary edema (cardiogenic and non-cardiogenic)
3. Pulmonary infection
4. Allergic or immunologic pulmonary disease
5. Pulmonary neoplasia
6. Pulmonary embolism (heartworm disease, pulmonary embolus)
7. Pulmonary hemorrhage
8. Restrictive lung disease (fibrosis)

DISEASE OF THE PLEURAL SPACE
1. Pneumothorax
2. Pleural effusions
 a. hydrothorax (heart failure, neoplasm, lymphosarcoma)
 b. hemothorax (trauma, coagulopathy)
 c. pyothorax
 d. non-septic effusion (neoplasms, infectious feline peritonitis)
 e. chylothorax
3. Diaphragmatic hernia

ALTERED HEMOGLOBIN
1. Anemia
2. Methemoglobinemia

MISCELLANEOUS CAUSES OF DYSPNEA-HYPERPNEA
1. Head trauma
2. Neuromuscular weakness or denervation of muscles of respiration
3. Abdominal masses—restrictive diaphragm
4. Pain
5. Fever
6. Shock

Table 3. *Evaluation of the Dyspneic Patient*

CLINICAL PARAMETER	COMMENTS
Patient Medical History	May give clue to etiology
Observation of Patient	
1. Psychic component	Determine level of anxiety, ability to handle
2. Degree of dyspnea	Necessity for immediate therapy, ability to obtain diagnostic information
3. Pattern of ventilation	Helps demonstrate origin of dyspnea
a. Chest excursion	r/o °Rib fractures, flail chest, tension pneumothorax
b. Inspiratory dyspnea	r/o Pleural effusion, pneumothorax, pulmonary edema, upper airway obstruction
c. Expiratory dyspnea	r/o Lower airway diseases, pulmonary edema
4. Mucous membranes	
a. Cyanosis	r/o Airway obstruction, diffusion barrier (edema), ventilation/perfusion mismatch (atelectasis, shunt)
b. Pallor	r/o Anemia, decreased cardiac output, shock
c. Brownish	r/o Methemaglobinemia
Physical Examination	
1. Body temperature	r/o Infection, sepsis, heatstroke, ↑ work of breathing
2. Oral examination (Sedation may be needed)	r/o Pharyngeal-laryngeal obstruction (dyspnea relieved by tracheal intubation)
3. Cardiac ausculation	r/o Murmurs, gallops, arrhythmias, muffled sounds (may be obscured by respiratory noises)
4. Pulmonary ausculation	Evaluate level of abnormality
a. Increased sounds (obstructive noises, rales, and rhonchi)	r/o Obstruction of large airways, pulmonary infection, bronchitis, asthma, pulmonary edema
b. Decreased sounds	r/o Pleural effusion, pneumothorax, mass lesions
5. Other findings	r/o Other signs of heart failure and other abnormalities that accompany disorders causing acute dyspnea
Thoracic Radiographs	
1. Cardiac chambers and great vessels	r/o Heart disease—congenital and acquired
2. Pulmonary vasculature and parenchyma	r/o Extracardiac signs of heart failure and other primary or secondary pulmonary disorders
3. Pleural space	r/o Pleural effusion, pneumothorax, diaphragmatic hernia
Electrocardiogram	
1. Cardiac rhythm	r/o Cardiac arrhythmias, define their significance
2. Voltage criteria	r/o Cardiac chamber enlargement
3. Other criteria	r/o Evidence for pericardial disease, myocardial disease or ischemia
Other Tests	
1. Routine laboratory tests	Important in the differential and definitive diagnosis; demonstrate effect of heart failure on other systems.
2. Serologies	
3. Fluid analysis and exfoliative cytology	
4. Special cardiac examinations	

°(r/o = rule out)

DIFFERENTIAL DIAGNOSIS

A definitive diagnosis of acute heart failure is accomplished by correlating abnormalities of fluid accumulation or diminished cardiac output with reliable signs of heart disease. This decision is based on physical, radiographic, electrocardiographic, and laboratory data. When acute heart failure is characterized by sudden reduction in cardiac output, it is usually associated with a cardiac arrhythmia, severe myocardial disease, or a non-cardiac lesion leading to volume depletion or shock.

The majority of acute congestive heart failure patients are presented for dyspnea, the causes of which are listed in Table 2. Since dyspnea is common to many non-cardiac diseases, the initial differentiation can be misleading if a cursory examination is performed. In almost every case, however, the cause of dyspnea can be determined through a careful physical examination, thoracic radiographs, and selected ancillary tests. Table 3 illustrates a simple chart for

Table 4. *Management of Acute Heart Failure*

GENERAL MEASURES

    Reduction of activity—cage rest
    Sedation
        Morphine sulfate—0.2–0.5 mg/kg (IV, IM, SQ) (canine)
        Acepromazine—0.1–0.5 mg/kg (SQ) (feline)

MEASURES TO IMPROVE GAS EXCHANGE

    Oxygen therapy—40–60% (avoid > 50% for > 24 hours)
    Ethyl alcohol nebulization—40% solution
    Aminophylline—6–10 mg/kg (IV, SQ); can repeat q6h
    Endotracheal suctioning

MEASURES TO REDUCE CAPILLARY PRESSURE

    Furosemide (Lasix)—2–4 mg/kg (IV, IM, SQ); can repeat q6–8h
    Phlebotomy—remove 6–10 cc/kg bodyweight
    Positive inotropes and vasodilators

MEASURES TO IMPROVE CARDIAC OUPUT

    Digitalis glycosides:
        Digoxin
            IV: 0.01–0.02 mg/kg. Administer ½ calculated dose IV, wait 30–60 minutes and administer ¼ of dose; wait
                30–60 minutes and administer remaining dose, if necessary.
            Oral: 0.02–0.06 mg/kg. Administer ½ dose; give remainder 12 hours later.
        Digitoxin
            IV: 0.01–0.03 mg/kg. Administer as per digoxin.
            Oral: 0.06–0.1 mg/kg. Administer ⅓ dose q. 8 h.
    Dobutamine (Dobutrex)—2–5 μg/kg/minute, constant rate infusion°
    Dopamine HCl (Intropin)—2–8 μg/kg/minute, constant rate infusion
    Vasodilator therapy:
        Na Nitroprusside (Nipride)—5–20 μg/kg/minute, constant rate infusion
        Nitroglycerine ointment (Nitrol 2%)—1/4–3/4 inch cutaneously, q6–8h
    Antiarrhythmic therapy:
        Digitalis glycosides—as above
        Propranolol (Inderal)—0.04–0.06 mg/kg IV (*with caution* if diseased myocardium!)
        Lidocaine (Xylocaine)—2–6 mg/kg IV bolus; 25–80 μg/kg/minute constant rate infusion
        Procainamide (Pronestyl)—6 mg/kg IV, IM (hypotensive IV), 10–35 μg/kg/minute constant rate infusion

OTHER THERAPY

    Aspiration of pleural effusion
    Aspiration of pericardial effusion

°Formula for CRI: $\left(\dfrac{\dfrac{\text{Infusion dose in mg}}{\text{kg}}}{\text{minute}} = \text{bodyweight in kg} \right) \left(\dfrac{360}{\text{minutes}} \right) = \begin{array}{l}\text{Total dosage in}\\ \text{mg given for a}\\ \text{6-hour period}\end{array}$

1 μg = 0.001 mg

evaluating the acutely dyspneic patient. An accurate diagnosis of acute congestive heart failure is not difficult if the clinician methodically rules out other possible reasons for this dramatic sign.

THERAPY

Treatment of acute heart failure is divided into symptomatic and specific therapy (Table 4). Symptomatic therapy includes reducing activity and anxiety, improving blood and tissue oxygenation, decreasing edema, and increasing cardiac output. Specific treatment includes measures that definitively correct the underlying disorder. Such therapy includes surgical repair of patent ductus arteriosus or pulmonic stenosis, surgical removal of a constrictive pericardium, and specific therapy of malignant ventricular arrhythmias. In veterinary medicine, only some cardiac disorders can be managed with specific therapy. More common causes of heart failure such as chronic valvular disease and cardiomyopathy cannot be definitively corrected. In these situations, only signs of heart failure can be controlled.

Animals in acute congestive heart failure are

placed at rest in an oxygen-enriched environment (40 to 60 per cent O_2). If oxygen therapy is not available, a cool, well ventilated area may suffice. Sedation of the patient generally is indicated, since this reduces activity and anxiety and allows further therapy to be administered with a minimum of stress. Morphine sulfate is administered to dogs; phenothiazine tranquilizers are given in low doses to cats. These sedatives also decentralize blood volume, which partially relieves pulmonary edema. Promazine tranquilizers are peripheral vasodilators; therefore, possible hypotension should be minimized through concurrent administration of positive inotropic drugs.

MEASURES TO IMPROVE GAS EXCHANGE

Concurrent with sedation and increasing inspired oxygen concentration, other measures are taken to improve pulmonary gas exchange. In patients with pulmonary edema, nebulization of 40 per cent ethyl alcohol serves to reduce the surface tension of froth in larger airways, thereby improving gas exchange. In fulminant pulmonary edema, endotracheal suction is necessary to maintain airway patency. Bronchodilators are administered to retard the luminal narrowing and bronchospasm that attend pulmonary edema. Aminophylline, a bronchodilator with positive inotropic effects, is administered at six- to eight-hour intervals.

Animals with large pleural effusions benefit from thoracocentesis. Removal of intrapleural fluid permits re-expansion of atelectatic lungs. In dyspneic patients with extensive effusions, immediate removal is preferable to attempts to reduce pleural fluid by diuresis only. Thoracocentesis is best done after the patient is sedated and has stabilized in oxygen for a short period. The chest wall (one or both sides) is prepared surgically, and the effusion is drained. An intravenous catheter (Intrafuser* or Venocath†) is used to facilitate fluid removal yet minimize the risk of pulmonary trauma caused by implanting a needle in the thorax. The catheter is introduced ventrally, at the seventh or eighth intercostal space midway between the ribs while the animal is restrained gently in sternal recumbency. Once the catheter is placed, fluid is removed using a three-way stopcock and a large syringe. A fluid sample is saved for analysis. One advantage of the catheter system is the ability to retrieve additional fluid volumes by gently repositioning the patient. It should be noted that re-expansion of atelectatic lungs can

be associated with the formation of pulmonary edema secondary to alterations in alveolar forces.

MEASURES TO REDUCE CAPILLARY HYDROSTATIC PRESSURE

Both pulmonary edema and pleural effusion respond to the administration of agents that reduce capillary hydrostatic pressure. These drugs include morphine, furosemide, vasodilators, digitalis glycosides, and catecholamines. The hemodynamic effects of these agents depend on a number of factors, some of which are noted in Figures 2 and 3.

Figure 2 illustrates some of the factors responsible for cardiac output. This figure demonstrates that cardiac output is decreased by (1) decreases in contractility, (2) increases in total peripheral resistance, and (3) disorders of cardiac rate and rhythm. These abnormalities commonly are present in congestive heart failure. One of the major compensatory responses noted in acute heart failure involves retention of fluid and increases in venous hydrostatic pressure. While this compensatory change helps to maintain normal stroke volume, it results in elevation of capillary hydrostatic pressures causing edema or effusions (Fig. 3).

One method of decreasing capillary hydrostatic pressure is to decrease the blood volume acutely through potent diuretics or phlebotomy. Most clinicians prefer to administer the diuretic furosemide (Lasix^R) intravenously. In addition to its diuretic action, furosemide exerts a direct vascular effect resulting in increased venous capacitance and decreased pulmonary hydrostatic pressure. Morphine sulfate has a similar vascular effect. Administration of these agents frequently results in a marked reduction in dyspnea.

MEASURES TO INCREASE CARDIAC OUTPUT

Digitalis Glycosides. A deleterious effect of diuretics results if the reduction in blood volume markedly diminishes preload and stroke volume. In order to counter this effect partially, positive inotropes such as digitalis glycosides are administered (Fig. 3, *D, E*). Both digoxin and digitoxin are effective in the treatment of acute heart failure. These agents are administered intravenously in acute heart failure, although oral loading doses also can be used. Digitalis glycosides are discussed in detail in other parts of this text.

Catecholamines. Recently, catecholamines have been used in the management of both

*Sorenson Research Co., Salt Lake City, Utah
†Abbott Laboratories, N. Chicago, Illinois

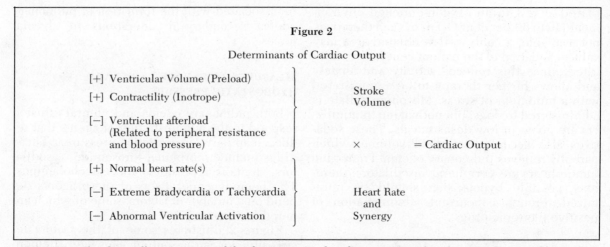

Figure 2

Determinants of Cardiac Output

[+] Ventricular Volume (Preload)

[+] Contractility (Inotrope)   } Stroke Volume

[−] Ventricular afterload
     (Related to peripheral resistance
     and blood pressure)   ] ×   = Cardiac Output

[+] Normal heart rate(s)

[−] Extreme Bradycardia or Tachycardia   } Heart Rate and Synergy

[−] Abnormal Ventricular Activation

Figure 2. This figure illustrates some of the determinants of cardiac output. Within the normal range of heart rates, the cardiac output will depend on ventricular contractility, ventricular end-diastolic volume (which is related to venous volume and pressure and diastolic properties of the ventricle), and ventricular afterload, which is the ventricular tension that must be developed to eject blood into the arterial system. Increases in peripheral resistance will increase ventricular afterload. Severe bradyarrhythmias or tachyarrhythmias result in decreased cardiac output secondary to the diminished rate, or an inadequate time for ventricular filling. Abnormal ventricular activation, as might occur in ventricular tachycardia, can result in hypodynamic ventricular contractions. The [+] and [−] signs denote the effect of amplification of that variable on cardiac output.

acute and chronic refractory heart failure. Dopamine HCl (Intropin^R) and dobutamine HCl (Dobutrex^R) have proved to be efficacious in both experimental and clinical use. Since chronic heart failure often is associated with myocardial catecholamine depletion, intravenous infusion of these agents serves to stimulate the myocardium at the cellular level. Both agents can be used in the management of severe heart failure in dogs and cats. They are administered by constant infusion over 24 to 48 hours. Since peripheral vasoconstriction and tachyarrhythmias result from rapid infusion (especially with dopamine), the drugs are administered judiciously.

Vasodilators. Vascular resistance frequently is increased in heart failure secondary to reflex sympathetic stimulation. The total peripheral resistance correlates with the ventricular afterload, the arterial pressure against which the ventricle must pump. From Figure 2, it can be seen that reducing ventricular afterload through vasodilator therapy may increase cardiac output if other determinants remain constant. In practice, vasodilator therapy usually decreases both afterload and preload, thereby "unloading" the ventricle. Since the severely failing left ventricle is believed to operate on the flattened portion of the ventricular function curve, reduction in ventricular preload need not reduce cardiac output significantly (Figure 3, *E, F*).

Both nitroglycerin ointment (2 percent) and sodium nitroprusside have been administered to dogs in acute congestive heart failure. Nitro-

glycerin is applied to the skin in the inguinal region, where it is absorbed transcutaneously. This drug exerts its greatest systemic effects on veins, causing direct vasodilatation. It is dosed

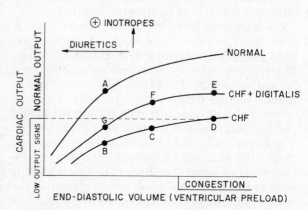

Figure 3. Ventricular function curves in heart failure. The ventricular volume (preload) determines in part the cardiac output. If other factors are constant, an increase in ventricular preload results in increased cardiac output. In acute heart failure caused by ventricular failure, cardiac output declines (from point *A* to *B*), resulting in signs of low output. Compensatory mechanisms may lead to accumulation of fluid, which increases output (point *D*) but results in edema. Positive inotropic agents like digitalis improve cardiac output (point *E*). Diuretics, phlebotomy, and venodilators decrease ventricular volume, thereby reducing clinical signs of congestive heart failure. In the digitalized patient, reduction in ventricular volume may not be associated with low output (point *E→F* vs. *D→C*). If reduction of ventricular preload is excessive, however, cardiac output will decline, although signs of congestion can be minimal (*F→G*).

by using the applicator ruler supplied with the medication. The clinician should wear gloves to avoid contacting the medication.

Sodium nitroprusside, administered as a constant intravenous infusion, dilates both arterioles and venules. Since it is a potent arterial vasodilator, it is both efficacious and hazardous. If administered too rapidly, marked hypotension occurs resulting in decreased tissue perfusion. In the author's practice, nitroprusside is administered concurrently with a constant rate infusion of dopamine or dobutamine. Clinical indices of arterial pressures are monitored, including indirect blood pressure if possible, pulse pressure, membrane refill time, level of consciousness, and urinary output. The use of combination infusions of catecholamines and vasodilators is an important advancement in the therapy of acute congestive heart failure.

MANAGEMENT OF LOW-OUTPUT HEART FAILURE

Acute heart failure in small animal practice typically is characterized by signs of congestive heart failure. The clinician should be aware, however, that acute reduction in blood flow, particularly to the myocardium or brain, can constitute a medical emergency. Such low-output states occur simultaneously with, and independent from, states of congestive failure. While most clinicians are aware that dehydration and shock result in decreased cardiac output, the incidence of low output secondary to heart disease is not well appreciated. Cardiac lesions leading to low-output failure include congestive cardiomyopathies, cardiac arrhythmias, cor pulmonale, and pericardial tamponade, among others.

The principles of therapy for low-output states are similar to those for acute congestive heart failure; however, emphasis is placed on restoration of normal cardiac output. In this situation, digitalis glycosides, catecholamine infusions, arterial vasodilators, and antiarrhythmic drugs constitute the foundation of therapy.

The rationale for giving digitalis glycosides and catecholamine precursors has been discussed. Of particular interest is their use in the management of pericardial tamponade and constrictive pericarditis. In these disorders, digitalis glycosides are ineffective, and their use is contraindicated. It has been demonstrated, however, that agents like isoproterenol, which increase inotrope and decrease ventricular afterload, significantly increase cardiac output. Similar effects are expected from infusions of dobutamine and nitroprusside. Additional therapy for acute heart failure caused by pericardial tamponade includes medical management of congestive heart failure and pericardiocentesis to reduce intrapericardial pressure. This procedure is discussed elsewhere in this volume.

Cardiac arrhythmias often accompany other cardiac lesions and contribute to the state of cardiac decompensation. Acute arrhythmias, particularly if they result in extreme tachycardia or bradycardia, cause sudden reductions in cardiac output leading to coronary hypoperfusion and possibly sudden death. This type of situation is encountered in dogs with ventricular tachycardias at rapid rates (>140/minute) and intractable supraventricular tachyarrhythmias. Rhythm disturbances like these require prompt therapy and close monitoring. For example, in the case of ventricular tachycardia, intravenous boluses of lidocaine, followed by constant intravenous infusions of this agent, usually restore sinus rhythm and improve cardiac output. Supraventricular tachyarrhythmias usually respond to vagotonic maneuvers (carotid massage), digitalis glycosides, or propranolol HCl (Inderal). Specific therapy of acute cardiac arrhythmias is discussed elsewhere in Section 4.

TRANSITION FROM ACUTE TO CHRONIC THERAPY

Most pharmacologic agents used in the treatment of acute heart failure are effective in the management of chronic heart failure. Once the patient has been stabilized, digitalis, diuretics, bronchodilators, and occasionally vasodilators are prescribed on a daily basis to control signs of heart failure. In selected cases, after appropriate diagnostic testing, specific therapy such as surgery can be administered.

Successful management of the patient with acute heart failure requires that the clinician be intimately familiar with the pathophysiology of heart failure and the beneficial and adverse effects obtained from the administration of available therapeutics. Since acute heart failure constitutes a medical emergency, the veterinarian must be an efficient diagnostician and deliver accurate and prompt therapy. The ultimate success of treatment depends upon the severity of the condition and the skill of the veterinarian.

SUPPLEMENTAL READING

Forrester, J.S., Diamond, G., Chatterjee, K., and Swan, H.J.C.: Medical therapy of acute myocardial infarction by application of hemodynamic subsets. *N. Engl. J. Med.* 295:1356–1362 and 1404–1413, 1976.

LONG-TERM THERAPY OF CHRONIC CONGESTIVE HEART FAILURE IN THE DOG AND CAT

WILLIAM P. THOMAS, D.V.M.
Davis, California

Dogs and cats suffer from a wide variety of primary and secondary cardiovascular disorders. Clinical signs of these disorders may result from inadequate cardiac output, systemic hypoxemia, thromboembolism, and systemic or pulmonary venous congestion and edema. The most frequently encountered clinical cardiac syndrome in small animal practice is congestive heart failure. The complex nature of this syndrome and the variety of therapeutic and management approaches available to prolong useful life demand a thorough understanding of the pathophysiology of heart failure and the mechanisms by which each therapeutic modality acts.

Congestive heart failure is a final common pathway or endpoint for numerous individual cardiac disease entitites. Although the clinical presentation of these cases is often similar, therapy must be individually designed for each patient depending on (1) the nature of the underlying cardiac disease, (2) the presence of any concurrent diseases, (3) the stage of cardiac failure, (4) the patient's temperament, and (5) the client's temperament, desires, and reliability. No single approach is universally applicable. Since the medical therapy and management of congestive heart failure usually focuses on the symptoms of cardiac disease rather than the cause, the palliative nature of the therapy should be understood by both client and veterinarian. A rational approach to therapy that gives the patient the greatest continuous symptomatic relief and is acceptable to both client and patient should be the ultimate therapeutic objective.

ETIOLOGY OF CONGESTIVE HEART FAILURE IN DOGS AND CATS

The heart diseases of small animals may be classified into three categories according to their primary functional effect on cardiac performance.

Primary Failure of Contractility. Primary myocardial disease (idiopathic congestive cardiomyopathy) is a common cause of congestive heart failure in both dogs and cats. In addition to causing failure of the heart as a pump, secondary AV valvular insufficiency often contributes to the ventricular overload in these conditions.

Systolic Mechanical Ventricular Overloading. These conditions primarily produce a chronic pressure overload (increased resistance to ejection) or a chronic volume overload on the affected ventricle. Secondarily, however, they also result in decreased ventricular contractility, which is greatest when congestive heart failure develops. In dogs, pressure overload occurs with congenital heart diseases (pulmonic stenosis, aortic stenosis) and in chronic heartworm disease. Volume overload occurs frequently with chronic AV valvular fibrosis and insufficiency, aortic or mitral valvular infectious endocarditis, and in congenital heart diseases (patent ductus arteriosus, ventricular septal defect, mitral and tricuspid valve dysplasia). In cats, these conditions are less common.

Diastolic Mechanical Interference. These conditions primarily inhibit ventricular filling in diastole. The most frequent cause in dogs is pericardial effusion (see "Pericardial Disease"), which limits the diastolic expansion of the ventricles. Decreased diastolic ventricular compliance and filling also occur with marked ventricular hypertrophy, particularly in cats with hypertrophic cardiomyopathy (see "Cardiomyopathy in the Dog and Cat"). Of considerable therapeutic importance is that these conditions usually cause little or no reduction in ventricular contractility and systolic performance. Therapy must therefore be directed at improving diastolic filling; attempts to improve ventricular contractile performance are usually unnecessary.

PATHOPHYSIOLOGY OF CONGESTIVE HEART FAILURE

Congestive heart failure is the syndrome of venous hypertension (congestion), abnormal sodium and water retention, and extracellular fluid accumulation secondary to inadequate cardiac output. The clinical manifestations of heart failure result primarily from excess interstitial fluid accumulation (edema) proximal to the failing ventricle. Left ventricular failure results in pulmonary venous congestion and pulmonary interstitial and alveolar edema in both dogs and cats. Right ventricular failure results in systemic venous congestion and edema. In the dog, this usually results in ascites, with pleural effusion (hydrothorax) occurring somewhat less frequently. In the cat, right heart failure most often results in pleural effusion, with ascites occurring less frequently. Peripheral (subcutaneous) edema is an infrequent manifestation of right heart failure in the dog and cat. Reduction of forward cardiac output may also be partially responsible for clinical signs of depression, fatigue, weakness, and hypotension, which may occur in advanced cases.

The pathophysiology of edema formation and the resulting clinical manifestations of congestive heart failure are best understood in terms of the compensatory (reserve) mechanisms used by the body to maintain systemic blood pressure and cardiac output when cardiac performance is impaired by any of the aforementioned problems. These reserve mechanisms are (1) increased sympathetic nervous tone, (2) Frank-Starling mechanism (ventricular dilatation), (3) renal sodium and water retention, and (4) ventricular hypertrophy. (Excellent discussions of these mechanisms can be found in the references.) Reduction of effective cardiac output results in increased sympathetic tone, which increases heart rate and contractility and causes arterial and venous vasoconstriction to maintain blood pressure and improve venous return. Decreased renal perfusion stimulates renal sodium and water retention to augment plasma volume and venous return. The resulting increase in ventricular preload (i.e., increased ventricular end-diastolic volume) increases contractility by the Frank-Starling mechanism and allows ejection of a larger stroke volume with less fiber shortening. Cardiac output is maintained, but at an elevated venous pressure. As cardiac disease progresses and contractility further decreases, the ventricular response to increasing preload is reduced (Fig. 1), requiring higher venous and ventricular diastolic pressures to maintain basal cardiac output. Ultimately, the elevated venous pressure results in the development of edema. Continued sodium and water retention provides the large volumes of extracellular fluid that may accumulate. Ventricular hypertrophy in response to increased myocardial tension partially compensates for the reduction in contractility but ultimately fails to maintain normal output without excessive venous pressure and edema.

The interaction of these reserve mechanisms is outlined in Figure 2. The fundamental abnormality in most cardiac diseases that result in congestive heart failure (except those that inhibit diastolic filling) is a reduction of contractile performance as illustrated by a depressed Frank-Starling function curve (Fig. 1). The compensatory mechanisms attempt to maintain basal cardiac output. Ultimately, these same mechanisms either fail to maintain a cardiac output sufficient for basic life support (resulting in cardiogenic shock) or result in excessive rise in venous pressure and edema formation (congestive heart failure). The principal causes of the clinical signs seen with congestive heart failure from all causes are (1) inadequate cardiac output and (2) excessive venous pressure and

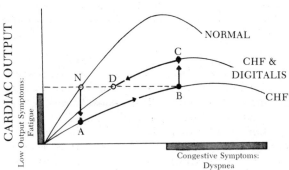

VENTRICULAR END-DIASTOLIC PRESSURE

Figure 1. Ventricular function curves in congestive heart failure (CHF) and in heart failure treated with digitalis, compared with the normal curve. When contractility is reduced (N→A), compensatory mechanisms restore basal cardiac output but at a greatly elevated diastolic pressure (A→B), resulting in venous congestion and edema. Increased contractility from digitalis therapy (B→C) allows the basal cardiac output to be maintained at a lower diastolic pressure (C→D), reducing venous congestion and edema.

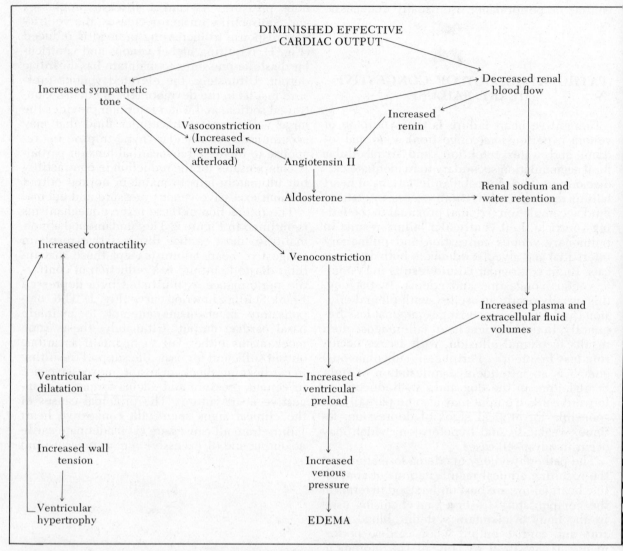

Figure 2. Interaction of the cardiovascular compensatory (reserve) mechanisms in heart failure and the pathogenesis of cardiogenic edema.

the resulting edema. Therapy in congestive heart failure is therefore primarily designed to (1) improve cardiac output and (2) reduce venous pressure and eliminate edema.

There is considerable variation in the onset and progression of cardiac dysfunction in dogs and cats with the common etiologic forms of heart disease. In those conditions where progression is relatively slow, several phases of heart disease can be distinguished. In man, four functional classes of heart disease (New York Heart Association Classification) are distinguished based upon the level of physical activity required to elicit symptoms of heart failure (fatigue, dyspnea, etc.). Class I patients exhibit signs of cardiac disease but remain asymptomatic with all normal activity. Class II patients have symptoms with moderate, ordinary activi-

ty. Class III patients have symptoms with minimal activity. Class IV patients have symptoms even at rest. Classes I through III are termed "compensated"; Class IV is termed "decompensated" (i.e., congestive heart failure at rest). A similar system has been applied to some dogs and cats with heart disease, principally to dogs with progressive mitral valvular fibrosis and insufficiency and chronic heartworm disease (Ettinger and Suter, 1970). Many small animal patients, however, are first presented in Class IV congestive heart failure. This occurs for two reasons. First, some of the common cardiac diseases, particularly the primary myocardial and pericardial diseases, are rapid in onset and progress quickly to heart failure. Second, the sedentary nature of some dogs and most cats and lack of critical daily observation by many owners result in a failure to recognize the early signs of cardiac dysfunction until the patient is in Class IV with obvious signs of congestive heart failure at rest.

CLINICAL RECOGNITION OF CONGESTIVE HEART FAILURE

There is no single clinical sign or physical or laboratory finding that always indicates heart failure. Rather, the diagnosis is based on a constellation of findings in a patient with evidence of heart disease. The clinician must be able to distinguish between signs of heart *disease* (murmurs, arrhythmias, etc.) and heart *failure* (venous congestion, edema, etc.). Differential diagnoses and concurrent conditions must also be ruled out (see "Influence of Non-Cardiac Diseases on the Heart").

The principal signs of left heart failure are coughing and dyspnea owing to pulmonary edema. The principal signs of right heart failure are systemic venous congestion, ascites, and/or pleural effusion. The diagnosis of heart failure is based on the association of these signs with other specific signs of cardiac disease or dysfunction. On physical examination, a resting tachycardia, diminished pulse amplitude, systemic venous engorgement, moist pulmonary rales, ascites, or hepatomegaly may accompany heart failure. The presence of a diastolic gallop is highly suggestive of heart failure in dogs and cats.

Radiographic signs accompanying congestive heart failure often include cardiomegaly, enlargement of the pulmonary veins and/or caudal vena cava, pleural effusion, ascites, hepatomegaly, and centrally located interstitial and/or alveolar pulmonary infiltrates (edema).

Electrocardiographic signs accompanying congestive heart failure depend on the underlying disease and may include evidence of atrial and/or ventricular enlargement, diminished amplitudes (commonly found with pleural or pericardial effusion), and cardiac arrhythmias. Atrial fibrillation is common in both dogs and cats in heart failure and is highly suggestive of serious cardiac disease.

The more signs that are present on these examinations, the more likely the diagnosis of heart failure. Absolute confirmation requires the demonstration of elevated venous, atrial, and ventricular end-diastolic pressures by cardiac catheterization. This not only is impractical but is unnecessary in most cases. The diagnosis of congestive heart failure can usually be made with confidence based on a careful history, physical examination, thoracic radiography, and electrocardiography, and therapy can be pre-scribed and progress can be assessed from these few examinations.

THERAPY AND MANAGEMENT OF CHRONIC HEART FAILURE

Based on the types of heart disease that commonly affect dogs and cats and the pathophysiology of the signs of congestive heart failure, long-term therapy and management consists of one or more of the following: (1) client education, (2) correction or modification of the primary disease, (3) prevention of heart failure, (4) reduction of the cardiac workload, (5) improvement of myocardial contractile performance, (6) reduction of sodium and water retention, (7) control of arrhythmias, and (8) symptomatic and adjunctive therapy.

Client Education. The client must understand the nature of the patient's heart disease, the prognosis with and without therapy, the rationale for therapy, and the potential costs involved in order to make an informed decision about continuing long-term therapy. The veterinarian, on the other hand, must understand the relationship between the pet and the client, the home environment, the use and the temperament of the animal, the reliability of the client, and any financial constraints in prescribing therapy. The client should understand that, in most cases, therapy must continue for the remaining life of the patient, therapy is primarily supportive and symptomatic, and complete control of all signs may not be possible.

Once therapy is initiated, the client should understand the signs that indicate disease progression, effectiveness of therapy, and side effects of the therapy, and what to do in each situation. The necessity for close observation, continuous, uninterrupted therapy in most cases, and periodic re-evaluation should be emphasized. The client must feel that he or she is responsible for the comfort of the patient and prepared for potential problems and their management.

Class I patients (i.e., those with signs of heart disease but without any functional limitations) usually require no specific management beyond client education, unless the heart disease is correctable or progression is preventable (e.g., heartworm disease). *The presence of heart disease is not an automatic indication for cardiac therapy!* The nature of the disease, the signs to watch for, and some reassurance are often sufficient management for such cases.

Correction or Modification of the Primary Disease. Every patient with heart disease with or without heart failure should be carefully examined for signs of a surgically or medically correctable etiology. Certain congenital heart diseases (PDA, pulmonic stenosis, atrial and ventricular septal defects) and some pericardial diseases (cysts, hernias, etc.) may be surgically correctable. Simple pericardiocentesis reverses heart failure in most cases of pericardial effusion and tamponade, and it is curative in some. Specific pharmacologic therapy can be used in most cases of heartworm disease and in some cases of infectious endocarditis. Early intervention may prevent the development of heart failure and halt progression of the disease. In cases that have already progressed to heart failure, medical management is indicated and may allow time for specific therapy to be initiated. Successful correction may allow subsequent withdrawal of the therapy for heart failure (e.g., PDA with heart failure and some heartworm cases). In other cases, heart failure may persist after the underlying disease has been arrested (e.g., valvular infectious endocarditis and some heartworm cases), necessitating continuous medical therapy and management.

Prevention of Heart Failure. At present, the onset and progression of many heart diseases cannot be appreciably altered. Exceptions include heartworm disease, certain congenital defects, and some pericardial diseases. In dogs and cats with existing compensated heart disease, prevention of the development of the clinical signs of heart failure can be attempted in several ways, including correction of the primary disease, enforced rest, and control of precipitating or aggravating factors. The latter involves careful evaluation of the patient's environment, activity, and diet, and the detection and correction or control of any concurrent diseases that may contribute to the pathogenesis of heart failure and edema formation. Such stresses as unusual heat or humidity, excessive exertion, or a sudden large increase in sodium intake may be sufficient to produce edema in an animal that was previously marginally compensated. Concurrent conditions such as obesity, anemia, renal or endocrine diseases, infections, pulmonary diseases, or those that produce fever place extra demands on the heart and should be identified and corrected or controlled where possible. Every cardiac patient should have a routine screening laboratory work-up to identify such conditions, which may significantly affect the nature of cardiac therapy. For example, the simultaneous treatment of chronic renal disease and chronic heart failure is particularly difficult. Fluid administration and therapy with sodium-retaining steroid hormones should be approached with caution.

Signs of heart failure may also be prevented or delayed by appropriate cardiac therapy in patients with compensated heart disease by identifying the patient at risk of heart failure. This includes patients with heart disease and subtle, early signs of dysfunction (such as fatigue with moderate to marked exertion — Class II) or those compensated patients that must undergo an unusual stress such as surgery. While there is no convincing evidence that cardiac glycoside and diuretic therapy alter the nature or progression of the underlying disease, they can improve the reduction in contractility and increased venous pressure that occurs in most cardiac diseases prior to the occurrence of frank clinical congestive heart failure and restore some of the lost cardiac reserve that may be needed during an unusual stress. This justifies the use of digitalis and/or diuretics in certain patients with heart disease but without evidence of heart failure.

Reduction of the Cardiac Workload. Decreasing the demand for cardiac output is accomplished by restricting the patient's physical activity. The amount of restriction depends on the severity of the heart failure, the animal's temperament, and the home environment. There is no evidence that exercise per se hastens the progression of most cardiac diseases, although it can induce signs of heart failure in an otherwise marginally compensated patient. A common-sense approach is indicated that will minimize clinical signs (fatigue, dyspnea, coughing) yet allow sufficient freedom to disrupt the lifestyle of the patient or client only minimally. Many animals, particularly cats, restrict themselves to activities that do not induce clinical signs, and further restriction may be unnecessary. With early signs of heart failure (Class II or III), only moderate to marked exertion (hunting or vigorous playing) should be eliminated. As the patient progresses to late Class III or Class IV, severe limitation to short walks, restriction to a house or room, or complete cage rest may be necessary to avoid excessive fatigue, dyspnea, or coughing. The client should observe the animal during various activities and avoid those that produce clinical signs. Sedation is rarely necessary, even in nervous animals, and it is usually objectionable to the client.

Vasodilator therapy is a promising new development in human cardiac therapy that has yet to be evaluated either for short- or long-term use in dogs and cats. Vasodilators may reduce peripheral resistance and improve cardiac output or reduce venous pressure and edema formation or both. They are commonly used in people hospitalized with acute myocardial failure, and the prospect of their use for long-term out-patient therapy of chronic heart failure is promising. As experience is gained in animals, this mode of "ventricular unloading" may become a useful additional therapeutic tool in dogs and cats.

Improvement of Myocardial Contractility. Since a reduction of ventricular contractile performance underlies congestive heart failure caused by primary myocardial failure or ventricular pressure and volume overload, the most direct approach in treating heart failure from these causes (other than surgical correction) is to attempt to restore myocardial contractility toward normal with the cardioactive glycosides (digitalis and related compounds). (The pharmacology of digitalis is discussed elsewhere in this text.) Essentially, digitalis increases the rate and force of myocardial contraction at any end-diastolic fiber length (preload), allowing a greater stroke volume (and cardiac output) to be produced at a given end-diastolic pressure (middle curve in Fig. 1), thereby reducing venous pressure and the tendency for edema formation. In addition, improvement in forward cardiac output increases renal perfusion — resulting in diuresis and reduced sodium and water retention — and decreases sympathetic tone — resulting in a decreased heart rate and ventricular preload and afterload. This single action thereby reverses the mechanisms of heart failure and thus attempts to treat the cause of heart failure rather than just its effects. Digitalis is also used for its antiarrhythmic effects.

The main disadvantage of digitalis glycosides is their narrow therapeutic index. While the useful inotropic effect of the drug is directly related to the administered dose, the toxic dose is often low, overlapping the therapeutic dose. It may sometimes be difficult to find an effective dose that avoids toxicity. It is a mistake, however, to abandon digitalis therapy in a sensitive patient. Some inotropic effect occurs even at dosages below the average recommended dose. It is stressed that recommended doses are average starting doses for the species. Some patients tolerate more than this average dose, and some tolerate considerably less. Attention to the signs of effectiveness and toxicity and dosage adjustments are the keys to finding the proper dose for each patient.

While digitalis affects both the non-failing and the failing heart, there is no evidence that administration in the early phases of heart disease (Class I, asymptomatic patient) is beneficial or protective in affecting the natural course of the underlying disease. It is indicated in all patients with historical, physical, or radiographic signs of heart failure associated with reduced myocardial contractility. This includes patients with obvious physical or radiographic

signs of cardiogenic pulmonary or systemic edema (Class IV). It also extends to patients with no physical signs of edema but with radiographic signs of early or impending heart failure (i.e., pulmonary venous congestion, significant cardiomegaly). The appropriate time to initiate digitalis therapy is probably in the Class III patient prior to the development of obvious clinical signs and edema at rest. Considerable clinical judgment is required in each individual case. To re-emphasize, *the mere presence of a heart murmur is not, by itself, an indication for digitalis therapy.* However, it is justified to digitalize some patients with heart disease prophylactically prior to unusual stress such as surgery. As a general rule, the author feels that preoperative digitalization is indicated only in patients with moderate to advanced heart disease that is marginally compensated. The well compensated patient without clinical or radiographic evidence of venous congestion appears to suffer minimal increased risk with carefully controlled anesthesia.

The recommended cardiac glycoside for long-term use in dogs and cats, based on current clinical experience, is digoxin. Parenteral administration is usually reserved for patients in acute heart failure (see "Acute Heart Failure"). Long-term therapy is achieved with oral administration. Based on the pharmacology of the drug, oral digoxin is usually administered on one of two schedules.

ORAL LOADING METHOD. A calculated total digitalizing dose is calculated and administered in four to six divided doses over 24–48 hours, until the desired effect is achieved or signs of toxicity occur. A daily maintenance dose, calculated as ¼ to ⅛ of the administered loading dose and given in one to two daily doses, is then continued. The recommended oral loading dose for digoxin in the dog is 0.06–0.2 mg/Kg. In general, smaller breeds require a higher dose per Kg than do larger breeds, so that the upper dose range is used for smaller breeds, the lower dose range is used for larger breeds. A loading dose has not been established for the cat, which is considered to be more sensitive to the effects of digoxin than the dog and is usually digitalized by the oral maintenance method. A loading dose of two to three times the calculated maintenance dose can be given the first day in some cats if closely observed for signs of toxicity.

ORAL MAINTENANCE METHOD. In patients with mild heart failure or in marginally compensated patients (Class II to III) with radiographic evidence of pulmonary venous congestion, slow oral digitalization on an out-patient basis is frequently preferred to minimize the stress and expense of hospital therapy. Since it takes seven to ten days for equilibration of body stores to occur, the owner must understand that signs of toxicity may not appear for one to two weeks. In the dog, the recommended average maintenance dose for digoxin is 0.02 mg/kg/day given in one or two doses. Cats are most often digitalized in this manner with the recommended dose of 0.01–0.016 mg/kg/day. If the desired effect (i.e., decreased clinical signs) does not occur within 10 to 14 days, this dose may be gradually increased, usually in about 25 percent increments every 7–14 days until a satisfactory response or toxicity occur.

Whichever method is used to digitalize the patient initially, long-term therapy involves continuous administration of the daily maintenance dose. Although it is not necessary to approach toxic doses to get an inotropic response, a maximal response is usually desirable, particularly in the later stages of heart failure. This is obtained by gradually increasing the daily dose until mild signs of toxicity occur, then maintaining the patient on the maximal tolerated dose. This remains the only practical method for maximizing the inotropic effect of digoxin.

Digitalis intoxication is common, particularly when a maximal response is sought. Clinical signs of digitalis intoxication are consistent, starting with depression and anorexia and followed by vomiting. Diarrhea may occur, but it is usually not severe. These signs are not dangerous but may aggravate any weight loss, fluid or electrolyte disturbances, or other concurrent conditions present. Fortunately, despite the arrhythmogenic potential of digitalis, ventricular arrhythmias are an uncommon manifestation of digitalis intoxication in dogs and cats on oral therapy. Rather, the more common electrocardiographic signs of digitalis effects are varying degrees of atrioventricular (AV) block, usually limited to prolongation of the PR interval (first degree block), or low-grade second degree block with dropped beats. Occasionally, higher grades of second degree block may occur; third degree block is extremely rare. There is no consistent correlation between the development of clinical signs and electrocardiographic signs of digitalis toxicity. Many patients show a slight prolongation (0.02–0.03 second) of the PR interval during digitalization, whereas others may develop clinical signs of toxicity without any changes in the ECG. The signs that require a reduction in digitalis dose include clinical signs of anorexia and vomiting and ECG evidence of advanced degrees of AV block or significant ventricular arrhythmias. The development of first- or low-grade second degree AV block, in the absence of clinical signs of toxicity, is not an indication to reduce digitalis dosage.

When digitalis intoxication is suspected, the drug is withdrawn for 24 to 48 hours (or until clinical or electrocardiographic signs regress), then it is reinstituted at a lower dose. If serum potassium is low, oral supplementation may help reverse the toxicity. Similarly, reduced renal function decreases the excretion rate of digoxin, such that a lower dose is required. It is particularly important to check renal function and serum electrolytes when signs of digitalis toxicity occur in a patient on a previously well tolerated dosage, especially when the patient is also on diuretic therapy.

Reduction of Sodium and Water Retention. Reduction of plasma volume, venous pressure, and edema formation can be achieved by reducing the excess accumulation of extracellular sodium and water that occurs in heart failure. There are two major ways to accomplish this.

DIETARY SODIUM RESTRICTION. Since the heart failure patient is unable to balance sodium excretion with intake, reducing oral sodium intake helps reduce total body sodium and water. The low sodium diet is a valuable adjunct to other therapy. The degree of sodium restriction advisable depends on the severity of the heart failure, adequacy of response to other therapy, and the acceptability of the diet by both patient and client. Many small animal patients are older, have strong dietary preferences, and do not readily accept a low sodium diet. The cost may also be prohibitive for the owners of large-breed dogs. These factors, coupled with the availability of effective diuretics, has resulted in decreased emphasis on strict sodium restriction except in more advanced cases.

In mild, early heart failure, mild sodium restriction should simply consist of avoiding high sodium treats and salt in preparation of meals. As heart failure progresses, sodium restriction should be more severe. In chronic recurrent and severe failure, maximal restriction (no more than 6 to 8 mg/Kg/day) may be necessary to help control edema. Either commercially prepared or homemade diets are satisfactory. Recommended and restricted foods are available in lists in the references, as well as from local heart associations.

DIURETIC THERAPY. The other major way to reduce total body sodium and water is to enhance their excretion. Modern diuretics are very effective inhibitors of sodium resorption by the kidney, resulting in a sodium diuresis. (The pharmacology of these drugs is covered elsewhere in the text.) The most frequently used diuretics in dogs and cats are the thiazides and the so-called "loop" diuretic furosemide. The potassium-sparing diuretic spironolactone is also used under certain circumstances. The veterinarian need only be familiar with two or three of these compounds to treat most patients.

Parenteral use is usually reserved for acute or severe heart failure. In general, diuretic therapy is indicated in patients that respond inadequately to exercise restriction, mild sodium restriction, and oral digoxin therapy. It is also indicated to achieve initial reduction of edema while digitalization is being carried out. In such patients, the maintenance dose of the diuretic can often be reduced after the patient is stabilized. Unlike digoxin, the diuretics are safe over a wide dose range. Whereas the goal of digoxin therapy should be to achieve a maximal effect without toxicity, the goal of diuretic therapy should be to use the minimal dose necessary to control clinical signs. In mild, early heart failure, a diuretic may be unnecessary (if the response to digoxin is adequate) or may only need to be given once a day or once every other day. As heart failure becomes more severe, the diuretic can be increased to two, three, or even four times a day. When such administration is still inadequate, diuretic combinations (furosemide and spironolactone; furosemide and a thiazide) should be considered.

The recommended dose for furosemide in small animals is 2 to 4 mg/Kg as required one to four times a day. Higher doses are occasionally used. The prototype thiazide is chlorothiazide (Diuril[R]). The recommended dose is 20 to 40 mg/Kg once or twice a day as needed. Once a patient is adequately digitalized and stabilized at home, adjustment of the diuretic dosage to the minimal effective amount is advisable.

There are two main side effects of diuretic therapy (besides the obvious increase in rate and volume of urine produced). Aggressive diuresis can lead to dehydration, particularly with parenteral administration. This is more likely in a patient that, because of concurrent disease or drug therapy, is anorexic or vomiting. Attention to hydration will usually prevent this problem. The second side effect is electrolyte depletion during aggressive or prolonged diuresis. The individual susceptibility to this effect is extremely variable in dogs and cats. The thiazides can result in hypokalemia, which enhances the effects of digoxin and can precipitate toxicity in a previously stable patient. Furosemide appears to cause significant hypokalemia less frequently, even at higher doses over prolonged periods. An occasional patient on oral furosemide may develop severe combined hypokalemia, hyponatremia, and hypochloremia, requiring cessation of therapy and electrolyte replacement. Whenever diuretic therapy is employed, periodic evaluation of serum sodium, potassium, and chloride is recommended, particularly when a patient develops unexplained lethargy and weakness or shows signs of digitalis toxicity on a previously well tolerated dose. Oral potassium supplementation is usually reserved for patients developing hypokalemia; it is not routinely given to all patients on diuretics.

Control of Cardiac Arrhythmias. Arrhythmias may contribute to the reduced cardiac output in heart failure, primarily when they result in an excessive heart rate. Since most antiarrhythmic agents have negative inotropic effects, their use in the heart failure patient should be limited to significant tachyarrhythmias not adequately controlled by digoxin therapy. In general, tachyarrhythmias associated with heart failure are best treated initially by digitalization (ventricular tachycardia is an exception). In particular, atrial fibrillation, a common arrhythmia in dogs and cats, is usually treated with oral digoxin until the ventricular rate is adequately controlled or signs of toxicity occur. Oral propranolol therapy (10 to 80 mg TID) is reserved for patients whose heart rate response to digitalization is inadequate. Tachyarrhythmias that develop or persist after digitalization may require other antiarrhythmic therapy. Ventricular arrhythmias due to digitalis have responded best (in humans) to parenteral lidocaine, oral propranolol, or phenytoin, along with oral potassium supplementation. Occasional supraventricular or ventricular premature beats usually require no specific therapy.

Symptomatic and Adjunctive Therapy. Although the major mechanisms of heart failure and edema formation are treated with exercise restriction, dietary sodium restriction, oral digoxin, and diuretic therapy, some patients continue to have clinical signs, even when their heart failure is well controlled. For the comfort of the patient and the peace of mind of the client, symptomatic therapy can be very important.

The most frequent persistent problem reported by clients is coughing and mild dyspnea, especially in small dogs with chronic mitral insufficiency and left atrial and ventricular enlargement. This problem is often the earliest sign of heart disease in such patients, and it often persists despite digoxin and diuretic therapy. Patients with compensated mitral insufficiency without clinical or radiographic signs of heart failure, and those in heart failure whose signs persist after adequate digoxin and diuretic therapy, may respond to therapy with oral bronchodilators or may require narcotic cough suppressants. The xanthine derivative aminophylline has weak inotropic and diuretic effects, but its major action is direct bronchodilation. Administered orally at a dose of 10 mg/Kg two or three times a day in dogs, it may help relieve such signs. Its continued use should be restricted to those cases in which the client reports a noticeable improvement when the drug is used. The persistent dry cough of the dog with cardiomegaly owing to chronic mitral insufficiency is probably caused by bronchial irritation by the enlarged left atrium. Adequate digitalis and diuretic therapy may diminish heart size and control such coughing, but it frequently persists, limiting the patient's activity and annoying the client. Such a cough is often impossible to eliminate, but it seems to be controlled best by narcotic cough suppression. Dihydrocodeinone (Hycodan[R]) 2.5 to 5 mg one to three times a day will often reduce coughing to a tolerable level, making both the patient and client more comfortable. Both aminophylline and dihydrocodeinone may cause vomiting, which must be distinguished from that caused by digitalis intoxication.

Patients with advanced, chronic right heart failure may develop recurrent ascites and/or pleural effusion despite vigorous medical therapy. When such effusions cause dyspnea or discomfort, they should be drained by paracentesis. Pleural effusion should be completely removed, if possible, and ascites should be reduced enough to relieve discomfort.

SUPPLEMENTAL READING

Detweiler, D.K., and Knight, D.H.: Congestive heart failure in dogs: therapeutic concepts. JAVMA 171(1):106–114, July 1, 1977.

Ettinger, S.J., and Suter, P.F.: *Canine Cardiology.* Philadelphia, W.B. Saunders Co., 1970.

Hurst, J.W. (ed): *The Heart,* 4th ed., part VI. New York, McGraw Hill Book Co., 1978.

Mason, D.T. (ed): *Congestive Heart Failure.* New York, Yorke Medical Books, Dun-Donnelley Publishing Corp. 1976.

Ross, J.N.: Heart failure and shock. *In:* Ettinger, S.J. (ed.):: *Textbook of Veterinary Internal Medicine.* Philadelphia, W.B. Saunders Co., 1977.

Tilley, L.P. (ed): Feline cardiology. Vet. Clin. North Am. 7(2), May 1977.

BRADYCARDIA

G. R. BOLTON, D.V.M.
Ithaca, N.Y.

Bradycardia is present when heart rates are less than 70 beats per minute for the dog or 90 beats per minute for the cat. Tachycardia is more common than bradycardia in the dog, and bradycardia is rare in the cat. Clinically significant bradycardia causes signs of weakness, exercise intolerance, shortness of breath, wobbliness, and syncope with or without seizures. Collapse and recovery are typically rapid, and postictal signs are usually absent. Syncopal episodes associated with slow heart rates are referred to as the Stokes-Adams Syndrome.

Cardiac output tends to be fixed at low levels when bradycardia occurs. Blood pressure must fall to very low levels for syncope to occur. In man, a mean arterial blood pressure of only 25 mm Hg maintains cerebral perfusion. In general, with asystole of 1.5 to 2 seconds duration, weakness occurs. Loss of consciousness occurs at 3 to 4 seconds, and seizures develop after 10 seconds or more. Under resting conditions, signs may not occur for as many as 6 seconds after asystole begins.

Clinically, most animals with bradycardia are comfortable at rest but develop clinical signs with varying degrees of exertion. Normal animals also have slow heart rates at rest. Second degree heart block is common both in adult dogs and in puppies when they are resting. The difference between a normal animal and one with a pathologic bradycardia is that the normal animal can increase its heart rate on demand, but the animal with symptomatic bradycardia cannot increase its heart rate in response to increased demand. Bradycardias likely to cause clinical signs are (1) sinus bradycardia, (2) sinus arrest, (3) sick sinus syndrome, (4) sinoventricular rhythm (atrial standstill), (5) advanced second degree heart block, and (6) complete heart block.

DIAGNOSIS

Bradycardia is easily recognized during physical examination. The clinician must first decide whether the slow heart beat is clinically significant. Secondly, the etiology must be considered.

Bradycardia in a clinically normal animal is probably insignificant. Bradycardia in an animal having signs of weakness, exercise intolerance, syncope, or seizures should be critically evaluated.

Several etiologic categories must be kept in mind. Vagal dysrhythmias, atrioventricular heart block, sick sinus syndrome, and serum potassium abnormalities are the general categories to be considered.

Vagal Dysrhythmias. Exaggerated vagal tone can cause sinus bradycardia (Fig. 1), sinus arrest (Fig. 2), and atrioventricular heart block (Fig. 3). Young animals, athletic animals, brachiocephalics, and animals with pharyngeal irritation, cervical or thoracic masses, gastrointestinal diseases, or increased intracranial pressure may have hyperactive vagal reflexes.

These vagally mediated bradycardias are often irregular and are typically associated with the respiratory cycle — the heart rate increasing with inspiration and decreasing with expiration. The hallmark of the vagal bradycardias is that they are responsive to atropine.

Atrioventricular Heart Block. Advanced heart blocks (Figs. 3 and 4) tend to slow the heart enough to cause clinical signs. Lesser degrees of block tend not to cause bradycardia. Clinical signs develop when the sympathetic stimulation of exercise or excitement cannot override the conduction block at the atrioventricular node or bundle of His. Vagal tone is capable of producing advanced heart block, but organic heart disease is the usual etiology. Digitalis toxicity is another frequent cause of these bradycardias.

The physical examination is characteristic in that soft, low-pitched atrial contractions can be auscultated between the louder slower ventricular contractions. With the atria and ventricles out of synchronization, as happens with complete heart block, an occasional jugular pulse may be seen if an atrial contraction occurs after the ventricular contraction has already closed the atrioventricular valves. These bradycardias may or may not be responsive to atropine.

Sick Sinus Syndrome. A number of names have been given to this syndrome, including lazy sinus syndrome, sluggish sinus syndrome, bradycardia-tachycardia syndrome, and sinoatrial syncope. It is best described in middle-aged female silver miniature schnauzers, although it occurs in other breeds and in mongrels as well. It is a primary disease of the sinoatrial node, as well as of the atrioventricular node and the atrial and junctional myocardium. The chief complaint is syncope. It is characterized by a variety of dysrhythmias including sinus bradycardia (see Fig. 1), sinus arrest with or without escape beats (Fig. 5), and second degree atrioventricular heart block. Periods of bradycardia often alternate with bursts of supraventricular tachycardia. Syncope tends to occur during asystolic episodes of four to six seconds or more. There are also times when the heart rate and rhythm may return to normal. A characteristic of the disease is that it responds poorly to any medication, including atropine.

Serum Potassium Abnormalities. Sinus bradycardia may be caused by either hyperkalemia or hypokalemia. In addition, hyperkalemia may cause complete heart block, ventricular tachycardia, or more commonly, sinoventricular rhythm, also called atrial standstill (Fig. 6). Hyperkalemic animals are often critically ill with weakness, vomiting, diarrhea, azotemia, dehydration, oliguria, and bradycardia. Adrenocortical insufficiency and end stage renal disease are the most common causes of hyperkalemia in the dog, whereas feline urologic syndrome with urethral obstruction of 24 to 48 hours or more is the usual etiology in the cat.

Bradycardias are recognized on physical examination. The electrocardiogram identifies the type of bradycardia, and it is also important to know whether the slow heart rate is atropine responsive and whether there are any serum potassium abnormalities.

TREATMENT

Clinically normal animals with bradycardia do not need treatment. An atropine response test is indicated when sinus bradycardia, sinus arrest with prolonged pauses and escape beats, or atrioventricular heart block is diagnosed in a symptomatic patient. A lead II electrocardiogram is recorded while 0.044 mg/kg of atropine is given intravenously. Within the first one to two minutes, atropine actually stimulates the vagus nerve centrally, and vagal dysrhythmias may be exaggerated. A positive response to atropine consists of a 60 to 100 percent increase in heart rate within two to three minutes after injection, with maximal heart rates usually 160 to 190 beats per minute or more.

Atropine-Responsive Bradycardia. A positive response to atropine suggests a vagal mechanism for the bradycardia. Initially, a search is made to identify an underlying cause for the vagotonia. Underlying factors such as everted lateral ventricles, pharyngitis, tonsillitis, cervical masses, or gastrointestinal disease should be treated. If no cause is found and clinical signs require long-term treatment, few oral drugs can be used without undesirable side effects (Table 1). Long-term atropine tends to cause dry mouth, constipation, and urine retention, and it

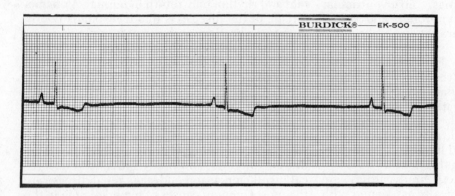

Figure 1. Sinus bradycardia. The heart rate is about 45 beats per minute. Lead II, paper speed = 50 mm/sec, 1 cm = 1 mv.

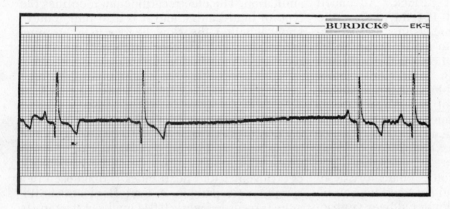

Figure 2. Sinus arrest (prolonged sinus pause). The pause in this sinus rhythm is longer than twice the normal R–R interval. Lead II, paper speed = 50 mm/sec, 1 cm = 1 mv.

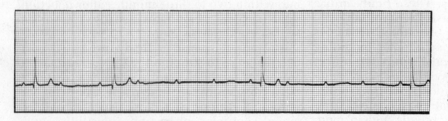

Figure 3. Advanced second-degree heart block. After the first two beats, every fourth P wave is conducted to the ventricles. The other P waves are blocked. Lead II, paper speed = 50 mm/sec, 1 cm = 1 mv.

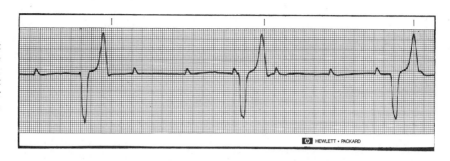

Figure 4. Complete heart block. None of the P waves are conducted to the ventricles. Notice the lack of a consistent P–R interval. Lead II, paper speed = 50 mm/sec, 1 cm = 1 mv.

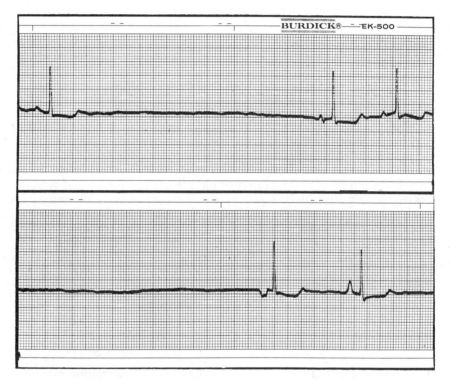

Figure 5. Sinus arrest, wandering pacemaker, junctional escape beat (first complex in lower tracing). This 11-year-old male miniature schnauzer had sick sinus syndrome (see Fig. 7). Lead II continuous strip, paper speed = 50 mm/sec, 1 cm = 1 mv.

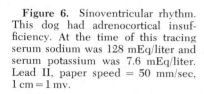
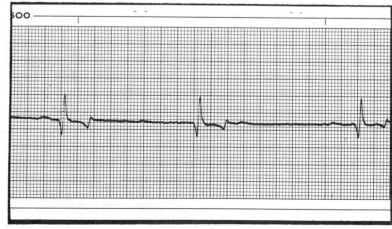

Figure 6. Sinoventricular rhythm. This dog had adrenocortical insufficiency. At the time of this tracing serum sodium was 128 mEq/liter and serum potassium was 7.6 mEq/liter. Lead II, paper speed = 50 mm/sec, 1 cm = 1 mv.

Table 1. *Oral Positive Chronotropic Drugs*

ANTICHOLINERGIC AGENTS
Atropine Sulfate—0.4 mg tablets, 0.044 mg/kg q. 6 hours.
°Darbazine® (Norden)—#1 and #3 capsules, 1–3 caps
  bid, according to body weight.
°Pro-Banthine® (Searle) — 7.5 and 15 mg tablets, 7.5–30
  mg tid

SYMPATHOMIMETIC AGENTS
Proternol® (Key)—15 and 30 mg tablets, 15–30 mg
  q. 6 hours.
Ephedrine Sulfate—4 mg/ml elixir, 5–10 mg tid

PHENOTHIAZINE DERIVATIVE TRANQUILIZERS
Prochlorperazine—5 and 10 mg tablets, 1 mg/ml syrup,
  2.5–10 mg bid.
Chlorpromazine—10 and 25 mg tablets, 1.2–2.2 mg/kg tid.

°Drugs of choice for long-term management of atropine
responsive bradycardia.

may aggravate chronic lung disease. Darbazine®
or Pro-Banthine® may be used orally with fewer
side effects than atropine, but large doses may
be required for heart rate control. Isoproterenol
may be tried, but oral absorption is unreliable.
Most of the orally effective sympathomimetic
agents increase blood pressure, which reflexly
counteracts their positive chronotropic effects.
Phenothiazine derivative tranquilizers have a
weak atropine-like effect, and they also decrease blood pressure, which reflexly inhibits
vagal tone.

Atropine Non-Responsive Bradycardia. Sinus bradycardia and sinus arrest unresponsive to
atropine in a fainting dog suggest sick sinus
syndrome, with a primary dysfunction of the
sinoatrial node. These animals may respond to
atropine in a number of ways. They may show
no response, partial response, or transient good
response, or atropine may make the condition
worse (Fig. 7). Partial response is an increase in
heart rate of only 25 to 50 percent. Transient
good response is an adequate heart rate response that lasts only 10 to 20 minutes.

Medical treatment is a pharmacologic dilemma. Since these animals have alternating
periods of bradycardia and tachycardia, treatment of one condition tends to aggravate the
other. Isoproterenol, anticholinergics, digitalis,

and antiarrhythmic agents have all been tried
with little success. Treatment of choice for sick
sinus syndrome is a surgically implanted electronic demand-type pacemaker. Used pacemakers are generally available at most veterinary
institutions, since new pacemakers are often
economically unfeasible. Digitalis is not advised prior to pacemaker insertion, as it further
suppresses sinoatrial and atrioventricular nodal
function. If tachyarrhythmias continue after
pacemaker implantation, digitalis or propranolol may be needed to control them. Another
option for the owner is to live with the syncopal
episodes, since most dogs do not die from them,
but this is a gamble.

Advanced second degree or complete heart
block unresponsive to atropine, with normal
serum potassium, should be treated with a pacemaker. Medication is of no value in this situation.

**Sinoventricular Rhythm (Atrial Stand-
still).** Hyperkalemia is the cause of this
rhythm, and treatment is directed at reversing
the electrolyte imbalance. General objectives
include support of renal function with fluid
therapy, reversal of acidosis with sodium bicarbonate, and reduction of potassium cardiotoxicity with sodium and calcium ions (Table 2).
Replacement of adrenal steroids is essential
when adrenocortical insufficiency is the cause
of the hyperkalemia (see treatment of adrenocortical insufficiency).

Rapid reversal of hyperkalemia is achieved in
obstructed cats by relieving the obstruction and
treating with intravenous fluids and sodium bicarbonate.

PROGNOSIS

Atropine-responsive bradycardias have a favorable prognosis. The main difficulty lies in
finding an oral drug that can be used long term
without unacceptable side effects. The syncopal episodes are rarely fatal even when control
is inadequate, but the animal may have limited
physical capacity.

Sick sinus syndrome in dogs is rarely controlled medically. The dog may survive without

Figure 7. Sinus arrest lasting
for almost 3½ seconds, punc-
tuated by junctional escape
beats. This is the same dog as in
Figure 5, almost 5 minutes after
receiving intravenous atropine.
Atropine has aggravated the
arrhythmia. Lead II, paper
speed=50 mm/sec, 1 cm = 1 mv.

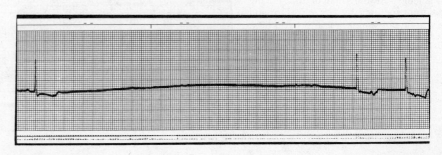

Table 2. *Treatment Rationale for Hyperkalemia*

PHYSIOLOGIC SALINE WITH 5% DEXTROSE
Maintains renal function.
Dextrose draws K^+ ion intracellularly.
Na^+ ion protects against cardiotoxic effects of
hyperkalemia.

SODIUM BICARBONATE
Reverse acidosis, shift K^+ ion intracellularly.
Protective effect of Na^+ ion against hyperkalemic
cardiotoxicity.
Give 3 mEq/kg intravenously, add 3–6 mEq/kg to the
intravenous fluids.

CALCIUM GLUCONATE
Calcium has immediate protective effect against
cardiotoxic effects of hyperkalemia.
Used when dysrhythmia is life threatening.
Give 1–10 cc intravenously to effect, with
ECG monitoring.

---

a pacemaker, but syncopal episodes are often as frequent as four or five times daily and there is a chance that these can be fatal. A pacemaker should be recommended, as the prognosis is favorable once it is in place.

The etiology of the hyperkalemia determines the outcome of these animals. End stage renal disease carries an obvious prognosis, but long-term management of adrenocortical insufficiency or urethral obstruction is optimistic if the animal survives the initial critical dysrhythmia.

SUPPLEMENTAL READING

Bolton, G.R.: *Handbook of Canine Electrocardiography.* Philadelphia, W.B. Saunders Co., 1975.
Branch, C.E., Robertson, B.T., and Williams, J.C.: Frequency of second-degree atrioventricular heart block in dogs. Am. J. Vet. Res. 36:925, 1975.
Buchanan, J.W., Dear, M.G., Pyle, R.L., and Berg, P.: Medical and pacemaker therapy of complete heart block and congestive heart failure in a dog. JAVMA 152:1099, 1968.
Clark, D.R., Knauer, K.W., Hobson, H.P., Gross, D.R., and Humphries, J.P.: Artificial pacemaker implantation for control of sinoatrial syncope in a miniature schnauzer. Southwest. Vet. 28:101, 1975.
Eraut, D., and Shaw, D.B.: Sinus bradycardia. Br. Heart J. 33:742, 1971.
Friedberg, C.K.: Syncope: Pathological physiology: differential diagnosis and treatment (1). Modern Concepts of Cardiovascular Disease XL(11):55, 1971.
Hamlin, R.L., Smetzer, D.L., and Breznock, E.M.: Sinoatrial syncope in miniature schnauzers. JAVMA 161(1):1022, 1972.
Hilwig, R.W.: Cardiac arrhythmias in the dog: detection and treatment. JAVMA 169:789, 1976.
Kaplan, B.M., Langendorf, R., Lev, M., and Pick, A.: Tachycardia-bradycardia syndrome (so-called "sick sinus syndrome"). Pathology, mechanisms and treatment. Am. J. Cardiol. 31:497, 1973.
Mandel, W.J., Hyakawa, H., Allen, H.N., Danzid, R., and Kermaier, A.I.: Assessment of sinus node function in patients with the sick sinus syndrome. Circulation XLVI:761, 1972.
Tilley, L.P.: Feline cardiac arrhythmias. Vet. Clin. North Am. 7(2):273. Philadelphia, W.B. Saunders Co., 1977.

TACHYARRHYTHMIA

R. LEE PYLE, V.M.D.
Mississippi State, Mississippi

Tachyarrhythmia refers to a rapid and often irregular heart rate. In small animal practice, there are only a few important tachyarrhythmias and antiarrhythmic drugs with which the practitioner must be familiar. Accurate diagnosis and proper drug selection markedly increases the chance for a favorable outcome in nearly all patients with a tachyarrhythmia.

The most critical information regarding any tachyarrhythmia is that contained in an electrocardiogram (ECG). Failure to make a specific ECG diagnosis can lead to disastrous therapeutic results. Lead II is considered ideal for analyzing disturbances of rate and rhythm; however, under certain circumstances, additional leads may be necessary in order to characterize a tachyarrhythmia fully.

An important clinical rule of thumb is that digitalis, particularly in toxic doses, can cause any arrhythmia or conduction disturbance. If the tachyarrhythmia in a patient is thought to be digitalis related, the most important step is to reduce the dose or to stop administration of the drug completely. In severely toxic animals, it may take three to seven days for the toxic ECG signs to disappear. If drug intervention is deemed necessary to control a life-threatening tachyarrhythmia such as ventricular tachycardia (to be discussed later), phenytoin (diphenylhydantoin; DPH) is the drug of choice.

DPH is considered the best agent for the pharmacologic management of digitalis-induced arrhythmias of atrial and particularly of ventricular origin. DPH is unusual in that it reverses the glycoside-induced depression of atrioventricular conduction as well as decreases the ventricular automaticity owing to digitalis excess. The recommended oral dose for DPH in the dog is 5 mg/kg, qid. The second choice drug would be propranolol (oral, 10 to 80 mg qid).

The therapeutic objective in administering any antiarrhythmic drug is to control the arrhythmia without rendering the patient toxic. The practitioner must remember that the recommended dosages given in this section are only approximations. Each patient must be titrated against an antiarrhythmic drug to determine if the therapeutic objective can be achieved. Occasionally, the therapeutic objective is not achieved with the drug of choice. The practitioner should not hesitate to administer another antiarrhythmic drug(s) in this situation.

Tachyarrhythmias are divided into two basic types: the supraventricular and the ventricular. By definition, supraventricular tachyarrhythmias are those whose site of impulse formation or re-entry circuit is above the bifurcation of the common bundle. The ventricular tachyarrhythmias are those originating below the bifurcation of the common bundle in the ventricular septum or ventricles.

SUPRAVENTRICULAR TACHYARRHYTHMIAS

The clinically important supraventricular tachyarrhythmias include: (1) sinus tachycardia, (2) atrial premature beats, (3) atrial tachycardia, and (4) atrial fibrillation.

Sinus Tachycardia (ST).   This refers to control of the heart by the normal pacemaker — the sinoatrial (SA) node. However, owing to physiologic, pharmacologic or pathologic influences, the rate is increased over normal. Physiologic influences include exercise and excitement; pharmacologic influences can be the administration of drugs such as atropine, epinephrine, isoproterenol, and thyroid extract. Pathologic ST occurs with abnormal states such as fever, hypoxia, hemorrhage, hypotension, shock, infection, and heart failure. In the dog, a heart rate over 160/minute is considered abnormal; however, to some extent this is breed dependent.

Clinical signs of ST are generally referable to the primary problem. For example, a dog with heat stroke and an elevated body temperature will have a rapid, regular heart rate and pulse as determined by palpation and auscultation. The ECG (Fig. 1) is characterized by rapid and regular electrical events with normal PQRST complexes. If the rate is extremely fast, the P waves may be obscured by the preceeding T waves.

The basic approach in the treatment or management of ST is to understand the physiologic, pharmacologic, or pathologic basis and to direct efforts toward correcting the underlying problem. If ST is related to congestive heart failure, the heart rate will be slowed by correcting the sodium and water load as well as using digitalis to slow conduction through the atrioventricular node.

Atrial Premature Beats (APBs).   Premature beats arising in ectopic foci in the atria are relatively common. The underlying problem in the dog, for the most part, is atrioventricular valvular insufficiency with atrial enlargement and stretching of myocardial fibers. APBs can be as-

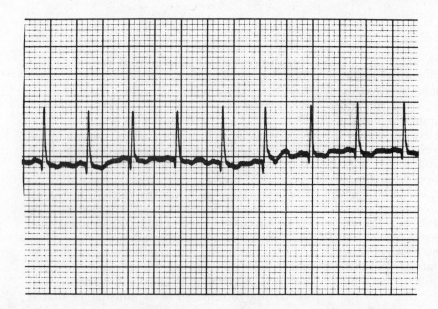

Figure 1. Sinus tachycardia. Rapidly occurring but otherwise normal appearing P, QRS, and T complexes. Heart rate = 180/min. Paper speed = 25 mm/sec. Sensitivity: 1 mv = 1 cm. Lead II.

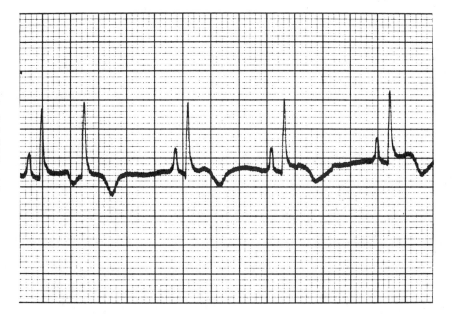

Figure 2. Atrial premature beat. The second beat from the left is a typical APB. The P wave is obscured by the preceding T wave. The QRS complex and T wave of the APB appear normal. Paper speed = 25 mm/sec. Sensitivity: 1 cm = 1 mv. Lead II.

sociated with other problems including excitement, toxic states, and tumors involving the atria.

On auscultation, premature beats are recognized because they occur earlier than expected and are followed by a short pause. They break the normal heart rhythm. It is not possible to distinguish atrial from ventricular premature beats without the aid of an ECG.

The ECG (Fig. 2) is characterized by one or more premature PQRST complexes followed by a pause. The P wave is often obscured by the T wave of the preceeding normal beat. If the P wave is visible, the shape is often abnormal because of the ectopic origin of the impulse and abnormal depolarization of the atria. One of the most important characteristics in the identification of APBs is that QRS retains a normal shape. This is because the sequence of ventricular depolarization, in contrast to that of atrial depolarization, is normal.

APBs generally require no treatment. However, if they are occurring with excessive frequency, treatment may be indicated. (See section on the treatment of atrial tachycardia for details.)

Atrial Tachycardia (AT). Atrial tachycardia is simply three or more APBs in succession. It is a considerably more severe arrhythmia and is usually a manifestation of advanced atrioventricular valvular disease in the dog. AT is recognized in other diseases including heart base tumor and toxic states such as uremia.

The physical findings vary depending on whether the AT is paroxysmal or continuous. If it is paroxysmal, there are intermittent bursts of a rapid and regular heart rate and pulse. In continuous AT, the rate remains consistently elevated and regular, usually in the range of 200/minute or faster. Occasionally, the animal becomes weak and collapses during an AT episode.

The ECG (Fig. 3) is characterized by rapid and regular electrical events with the P wave often hidden in the T wave of the preceeding beat. If the P waves can be identified, they usually have a different shape than do normal ones. One of the key features in AT is that the QRS complex appears normal in duration and contour. This feature is particularly important in distinguishing AT from ventricular tachycardia.

Most dogs with AT have underlying mitral and/or tricuspid insufficiency and frequently have left/right or generalized congestive heart failure. The preferred drug for control of AT is digitalis. The primary effect is slowing of conduction through the atrioventricular node, which results in slowing of the heart rate. In addition, the beneficial effects of digitalis on myocardial function tend to correct underlying problems that have predisposed the patient to AT.

The digitalis preparation of choice is digoxin. A patient with AT and congestive heart failure should receive an intravenous digitalizing dose during the first 24 hours followed by an oral maintenance dose. For example, if a 15 kg cocker spaniel is presented with acquired mitral insufficiency, left heart failure, and AT, the intravenous digitalizing dose would be calculated as 15 kg × 0.044 mg/kg, or 0.66 mg digoxin for the first 24 hours. One half the digitalizing dose, 0.33 mg, would be given immediately by the intravenous route. The remaining half of the

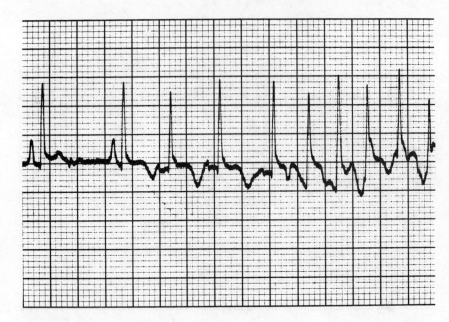

Figure 3. Atrial tachycardia. The first two beats from the left are normal. The third beat is premature, with the P wave partially obscured by the preceding T wave. The last six complexes are part of a paroxysmal atrial tachycardia with a rate of approximately 300/minute. Paper speed = 25 mm/sec. Sensitivity: 1 cm = 1 mv. Lead II.

digitalizing dose is given 6 to 12 hours later, depending upon the response of the patient. After the initial 24 hours, the digoxin is reduced to an oral maintenance level of 0.022 mg/kg. The animal in this example would receive a daily total of 15 kg × 0.022 mg/kg, or 0.33 mg given sid or divided bid. Toxic signs owing to digoxin include anorexia, vomiting, and diarrhea.

Other drugs can be employed in the treatment of AT. Quinidine and procainamide have generally similar antiarrhythmic actions. However, both drugs depress cardiovascular function and may worsen or precipitate congestive heart failure. It is generally unwise to use quinidine or procainamide without having first digitalized the patient.

Cholinergic drugs such as neostigmine or edrophonium can be used to promote a vagal effect with slowing of the heart rate. However, these drugs should not be considered of primary importance in the treatment of AT, since the mode of action is not directed at the underlying cause in most patients.

Carotid sinus massage can elicit a vagal effect that may slow the heart and perhaps convert the AT to normal sinus rhythm. In animals without underlying signs of atrioventricular disease and congestive heart failure, this maneuver may prove beneficial. Gentle eyeball pressure has the same vagal effect.

Atrial Fibrillation (AF). AF is characterized by chaotic and disorganized electrical activity in the atria. This arrhythmia exacts two hemodynamic penalties: the absence of atrial systole deprives the heart of its "atrial transport function," and the incessant and irregular bombardment of the atrioventricular junction with numerous impulses promotes rapid and irregular ventricular responses.

In the dog, AF is a serious supraventricular arrhythmia and is most commonly associated with acquired mitral and/or tricuspid insufficiency and congestive heart failure. Other causes include heartworms, idiopathic myocardiopathy, and congenital heart disease.

AF is recognized primarily in dogs more than 10 kg in weight. Palpation and auscultation of the heart reveals a rapid (usually greater than 200/minute) and absolutely irregular heart rate and rhythm. Frequently, a systolic murmur is heard with the point of maximum intensity (PMI) in the lower left fifth and sixth intercostal spaces. Owing to ineffective ventricular contractions, the pulse rate is slower than the heart rate (pulse deficit).

The ECG (Fig. 4) is characterized by rapid and irregularly spaced QRS complexes, absence of P waves, and presence of fibrillation (f) waves. The QRS complex retains a relatively normal appearance.

Considerations for the treatment of AF are similar to those discussed under AT. Digoxin is the drug of choice. The therapeutic goal is to slow conduction through the AV node so that heart rate can be decreased to as low a level as possible without making the patient toxic. Generally, a ventricular rate below 140/minute is considered desirable. Since many patients with AF have untreated ventricular rates over 200/minute, considerable slowing of the rate is necessary. Intravenous digitalization is usually preferred in the same program outlined under AT.

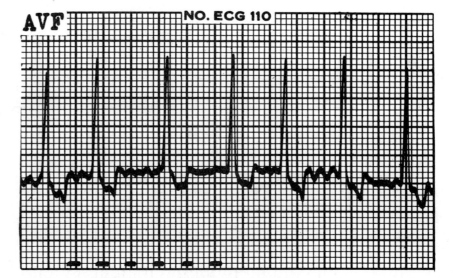

Figure 4. Atrial fibrillation. The ECG is characterized by a rapid and irregular R–R interval, absence of P waves, and presence of fibrillation (f) waves. Heart rate = 140/minute. Paper speed = 25 mm/sec. Sensitivity: 1 cm = 1 mv. Lead II.

The slower, oral, one-day digitalization program can be used in some patients depending on the severity of the clinical problem. Given the same 15 kg dog, the oral loading dose is calculated as 0.066 × 15 kg = 0.99 mg digoxin. This total dose is given immediately. Beginning the second day, the oral maintenance dose is calculated as discussed under AT. As with all antiarrhythmic drugs, the digoxin level may have to be increased or decreased to achieve the therapeutic objective.

Quinidine and direct current cardioversion have been used to convert AT to normal sinus rhythm. In rare cases, the conversion to sinus rhythm has been long lasting. Most patients fail to convert to normal rhythm or convert only transiently. Indeed, AT is associated with such severe cardiac disease that conversion is not effective and should probably not be attempted. Quinidine has a depressant effect on the cardiovascular system and can exacerbate congestive heart failure.

Ventricular tachyarrhythmias

The clinically important ventricular tachyarrhythmias include ventricular premature beats (VPBs) and ventricular tachycardia.

Ventricular Premature Beats. VPBs are the most common type of abnormal rhythm disturbances in the dog. They are caused by a variety of conditions including anxiety, stress, anesthesia, electrolyte disturbances, toxic states, trauma, pancreatitis, pyometra, subaortic stenosis, and a number of acquired diseases of the heart. The most common cause of VPBs is chronic mitral valvular disease with concomitant myocardial disease. Irritable foci of inflammation and degeneration of the ventricular myocardium promote VPBs.

On physical examination, VPBs cannot be distinguished from APBs. In each, there is a rhythm disturbance characterized by beats that occur earlier than expected and are followed by a pause. Frequently, reliable signs of heart disease are detected such as a loud mitral insufficiency murmur and/or manifestations of left/right or generalized heart failure.

The ECG (Fig. 5) is characterized by occasional bizarre QRST complexes that are not associated with P waves. These abnormal complexes are easy to differentiate from APBs because APBs are associated with P waves and have relatively normal QRST complexes. When VPBs alternate with normal PQRST complexes, it is termed "ventricular bigeminy" (Fig. 6). This arrhythmia is frequently associated with the administration of thiobarbiturates. It is reported to occur in more than 60 per cent of dogs anesthetized with thiamylal sodium and 40 per cent of dogs anesthetized with thiopental sodium. The arrhythmia is transient and usually subsides with resumption of normal ventilatory effort following induction.

If the VPBs are not occuring at a rate of more than 5/minute, specific therapy for VPBs is not indicated and attention should be directed to the underlying cause. For example, if the animal is toxic and in shock owing to the gastric dilatation-torsion syndrome or is in congestive heart failure owing to chronic valvular disease, the underlying disease should be treated and the VPBs will subside if therapy for the primary problem is successful.

Occasionally, VPBs will persist and be so numerous that treatment is desirable. For short-term control, intravenous lidocaine (to be discussed under ventricular tachycardia) is the preferred drug. Long-term treatment is best accomplished by using oral quinidine sulfate (6 to

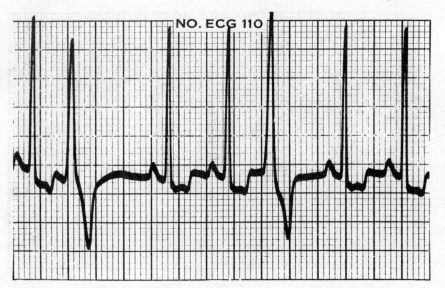

Figure 5. Ventricular premature beats. Beats two and five from the left are abnormal. They occur prematurely and are followed by a pause. The QRST complexes appear bizarre when compared with the beats originating in the sinoatrial node. In the normal beats there is P wave prolongation (P mitrale), S–T segment depression, and high-amplitude T waves. Paper speed = 25 mm/sec. Sensitivity: ½ cm = 1 mv. Lead II.

20 mg/kg every six hours) or oral procainamide (125 to 500 mg every six hours). The decision to use either quinidine or procainamide is often a matter of personal preference, since both drugs belong to the same class of antiarrhythmic compounds and have a similar mode of action. If VPBs are noted to be refractory to quinidine, it is unlikely they will be controlled by an agent from the same class. It would be wiser to select a drug from another group such as diphenylhydantoin.

Quinidine and procainamide have similar toxic effects. Some of the effects include depression of the cardiovascular system, intraven-

tricular block, and ventricular fibrillation. It is risky to use either of these drugs in congestive heart failure without previously digitalizing the patient.

Ventricular Tachycardia (VT). VT is a true medical emergency, since this arrhythmia can lead directly to ventricular fibrillation and death. There are many cardiac and extra-cardiac causes of VT that are listed under VPBs. The most common underlying problem is chronic mitral valvular disease.

The physical findings are often dramatic in patients with VT. During a VT episode, the patient frequently collapses or faints because of

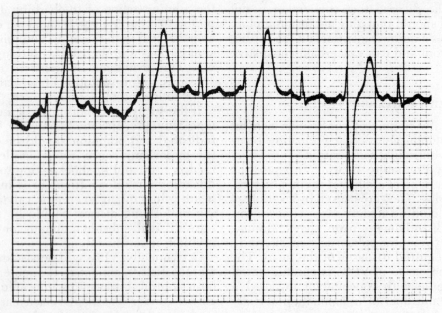

Figure 6. Ventricular bigeminy. VPBs alternate with normal PQRST complexes. Paper speed = 25 mm/sec. Sensitivity: 1 cm = 1 mv. Lead II.

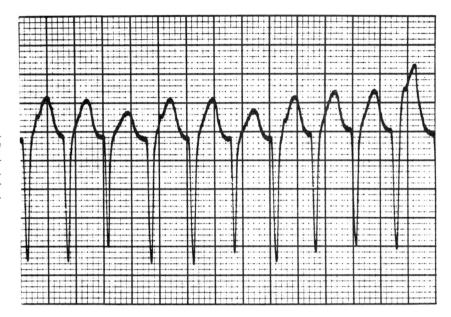

Figure 7. Ventricular tachycardia. There are rapid (200/minute), regular, and bizarre-appearing QRST complexes. Paper speed = 25 mm/sec. Sensitivity: 1 cm = 1 mv. Lead II.

the sudden decrease in cardiac output. Other signs include weakness, exercise intolerance, lethargy, seizure, coma, and sudden death. On auscultation, there is a rapid and regular heart rate. If the VT is paroxysmal, the rate varies between a rapid, regular rhythm and a slower, regular rhythm. The femoral pulse is rapid and weak during an episode of VT.

The ECG (Fig. 7) is characterized by three or more VPBs in succession, and the characteristics of the various waves are the same as outlined under VPBs.

The treatment of choice is intravenous 2 per cent lidocaine without epinephrine. If lidocaine with epinephrine is used, the chance of developing ventricular fibrillation is enhanced. Initially, lidocaine is given rapidly over a one- to two-minute period at a dose of 2 to 6 mg/kg. The therapeutic objective is to control this life-threatening arrhythmia without promoting toxic effects. Since lidocaine acts rapidly (within one to two minutes), the therapeutic effects can be immediately determined using a cardiac monitor. After controlling the VT with the rapid intravenous injection of lidocaine, an intravenous drip of lidocaine and 5 per cent dextrose at a concentration of 2 mg/ml is used to maintain normal sinus rhythm. The drip is used at whatever rate is necessary to control the VT. If the patient is in congestive heart failure, caution must be used in administering fluids. In these patients, repeated intravenous injections of 2 per cent lidocaine may be more desirable than a drip.

Every two hours, the administration of lidocaine is suspended to determine if the patient will maintain sinus rhythm. If there is a return of the VT, the antiarrhythmic agent is reinstituted. Lidocaine can be dripped for 24 to 48 hours or more. However, the longer the therapy, the greater the chances for producing the toxic triad of depression, muscle tremors, and convulsions. In most cases, the underlying problem can be corrected or controlled, and chronic lidocaine therapy is not required.

If therapy of extremely long duration (weeks or months) is needed, quinidine or procainamide is the drug of choice. Withdrawal from such a drug should be tapered over several weeks.

Direct current countershock can be used to treat VT. However, since special equipment is needed and lidocaine is very effective in treating VT, it has not been widely used in veterinary medicine.

NEWER ANTIARRHYTHMIC DRUGS

There are some newer antiarrhythmic drugs that have not yet received widespread clinical use. Bretylium tosylate is a beta blocker with potent antiarrhythmic action. It appears to be particularly useful in the treatment of ventricular tachycardia. Verapamil was originally introduced for the treatment of myocardial ischemia. The predominant antiarrhythmic effect of this agent is the slowing of ventricular rate in atrial fibrillation. Potassium canrenoate is primarily a diuretic agent; however, it appears to have a dramatic effect on digitalis-induced arrhythmias.

Caution: Although the foregoing discussion was directed at the dog, the same arrhythmias may be seen in the cat. The therapeutic principles are essentially the same; however, the reader is cautioned to refer to specific feline literature before administering potentially toxic drugs.

SUPPLEMENTAL READING

Bolton, G. R.: *Handbook of Canine Electrocardiography.* Philadelphia, W.B. Saunders Co., 1975. pp. 89–171.

Dreifus, L.S., De Azevedo, I. and Katz, M.R.: New antiarrhythmic drugs. In Donoso, E.: *Current Cardiovascular Topics — Drugs in Cardiology.* New York, Stratton Intercontinental Medical Book Corp. Vol. 1, Part 1, 1975.

Engle, M.A., Morrison, C.L., Levi, R., and Ehlers, K.H.: Antidysrhythmic therapy in children. In Donoso, E.: *Current Cardiovascular Topics — Drugs in Cardiology.* New York, Stratton Intercontinental Medical Book Corp. Vol. 1, Part 2, 1975.

Ettinger, S.J.: Cardiac arrhythmias. In Ettinger, S.J.: *Textbook of Veterinary Internal Medicine.* Philadelphia, W.B. Saunders Co., 1975.

Harris, S.G., and Ogburn, P.N.: Cardiovascular system. In Catcott, E.J.: *Feline Medicine and Surgery.* Santa Barbara, American Veterinary Publications, 1975.

Hilwig, R.W.: Tachyarrhythmias. In Kirk, R.W. (Ed): *Current Veterinary Therapy VI.* Philadelphia, W.B. Saunders Co., 1977.

Lucchesi, B.R.: Antiarrhythmic drugs. In Antonaccio, M.J.: *Cardiovascular Pharmacology.* New York, Raven Press, 1977.

Silber, E.N., and Katz, L.N.: *Heart Disease.* New York, MacMillan Publishing Co., Inc. 1975. pp. 1195–1228.

Section
5

HEMOLYMPHATIC DISORDERS AND ONCOLOGY

VICTOR PERMAN
Consulting Editor

Laboratory Diagnosis of Immunologic Disorders 390
Feline Leukemia Virus Disease Complex 404
Feline Hemobartonellosis 410
Bone Marrow Failure in the Dog and Cat 413
Heinz Body Hemolytic Anemias and Methemoglobinemias 417
Canine Lymphosarcoma 419
Cancer Chemotherapy 423
Immunotherapy of Malignant Disease 426

Additional Pertinent Information, Still Current, Found in
Current Veterinary Therapy VI:

Bull, R. W.: Autoimmune hemolytic anemia, p. 431.

Dodds, W. J.: Inherited hemorrhagic defects, p. 438.

Hurvitz, A. I.: Gammopathies, p. 451.

Kociba, G. J.: Disseminated intravascular coagulation, p. 448.

Lewis, H. B.: Management of anemia in the dog and cat, p. 421.

Lewis, R. M.: Canine systemic lupus erythematosus, p. 463.

Wilkins, R. J.: Thrombocytopenic purpura, p. 445.

LABORATORY DIAGNOSIS OF IMMUNOLOGIC DISORDERS

RONALD D. SCHULTZ, Ph.D.

Auburn, Alabama

An increased awareness of immunology and the rapid progress in immunologic technology during the past decade have led to the development of clinical immunology in veterinary medicine. As a result, immunologic methods of laboratory diagnoses have become increasingly important in all aspects of veterinary clinical medicine. In considering any animal whose condition presents a diagnostic problem, or one that has a recognized disease but of an as yet unknown etiology (e.g., granulomatous colitis of boxers, generalized demodectic mange), an immunologic aspect should be considered. To test the patient for an immunologic disorder — allergic, autoimmune, immunodeficient, or immunoproliferative — a minimal understanding of the laboratory tests available and the samples required for these tests is essential. It is the purpose of this article to provide the basic information of methods in use by immunologists that may be applicable to clinical diagnosis. For the challenges of modern veterinary medicine to be met, it will be necessary for the clinician to come into the laboratory and for the laboratory scientist to go into the clinic; when this happens, progress is inevitable.

A possible approach to the clinical and laboratory evaluation of an animal suspected of having a disease or disorder in which at least some of the signs are immunologically based is presented in Figure 1.

IMMUNE-MEDIATED DISORDERS

AUTOIMMUNE HEMOLYTIC ANEMIA (AIHA)

Autoimmune hemolytic anemia is a hemolytic state in which antibody can be demonstrated on erythrocytes (Fig. 2). These antibodies are most often warm, either agglutinating or hemolytic antibodies that can be detected by the antiglobulin (Coombs') test. However, on rare occasions, these antibodies may be cold antibodies; that is, they can only be identified if the test is performed in the cold.

The laboratory procedure used to detect warm antibodies is as follows. Blood is allowed to clot (preferred for shipment by mail) or collected in EDTA. Cells from the clot or from the EDTA tube are washed four times to insure that plasma protein is not coating cells non-specifically. The washed erythrocytes are suspended in saline to a final concentration of 2 percent. The antiglobulin (Coombs') reagents are diluted in a microtiter U plate and equal volumes (0.025 ml) of erythrocytes are added to the antiglobulin reagent and the patient's serum, followed by incubation of the plate for 30 minutes at 37° C and an additional 30 minutes at room temperature. The plate is read microscopically and macroscopically for evidence of agglutination. It is essential that the antiglobulin reagent has, as a minimum, antibody activity to IgG and C3 and that it does not react with normal red blood cells. A positive test would be diagnostic of antibody-coated red cells, a phenomenon most often associated with autoimmune hemolytic anemia but also recognized in dogs with multiple myeloma and some cats with hemobartonella infections and leukemia.

Special precautions should be used in interpreting results from feline antiglobulin test, since a common cause of anemia is hemobartonella, and a less common cause of an antiglobulin-positive test is feline leukemia virus infection.

Cold agglutinin disease in man is the most common type of cold antibody autoimmune hemolytic anemia. It can occur as an acute or chronic condition, the former being associated with *Mycoplasma pneumonia* infections and the latter seen often in older patients, sometimes associated with Raynaud's phenomenon (blue appearance in skin) and hemoglobinuria, particularly in cold weather. Blood samples collected in EDTA should be incubated

390

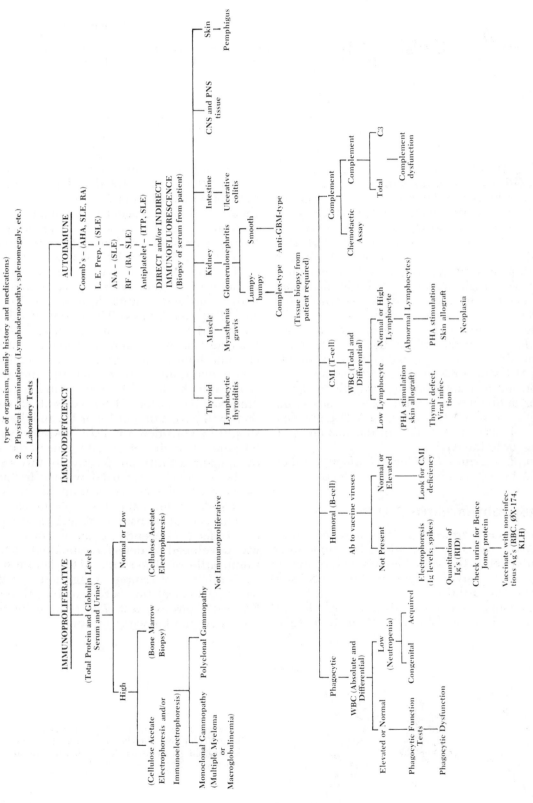

Figure 1. Approaches to Laboratory Evaluation

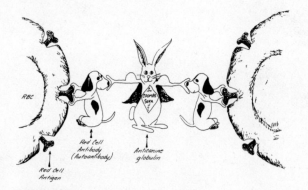

Figure 2. Schematic representation of the antiglobulin (Coombs') test for the detection of antibody-coated red blood cells in autoimmune hemolytic anemia of the dog.

at 37° C to elute the IgM antibody. Complement will remain on the surface, which can be detected by the antiglobulin test. The plasma from patients with cold agglutinin disease is then diluted and tested against the washed red blood cells. The test is incubated at 4° C in saline as a diluent and 30 percent albumin as a diluent. Cold agglutinins are usually present at very high titers (i.e., > 1:100) if the animal has the disease. Titers of less than 1:100 can be found in sera of certain normal dogs and cats. A few cases of cold agglutinin disease have been reported in the dog. (A canine Coombs' reagent is commercially available from Miles Laboratories, Elkhart, Indiana.)

The indirect antiglobulin test, which determines antibodies to erythrocytes in the serum of a patient suspected of having AIHA, appears to be of little or no value in the diagnosis of canine or feline AIHA.

Sample required: clotted blood and/or EDTA tube (lavender stopper) of blood.

RHEUMATOID ARTHRITIS (RA)

Rheumatoid arthritis is often a severe, progressive polyarthritis affecting numerous organ systems, the most frequent site of injury being the synovial lining of the joints (see "Canine Polyarthritis").

Laboratory diagnosis always includes a rheumatoid factor (RF) test. RF is IgM, IgG, or IgA with antibody activity to altered IgG. Most of the tests for RF detect predominantly IgM rather than IgG or IgA. A canine or feline rheumatoid latex reagent is not available commercially, and the human reagent is unsatisfactory. The most satisfactory test for detection of RF is the Rose-Waaler test (Fig. 3).

The Rose-Waaler test is similar to the antiglobulin test. Sheep red blood cells are coated with a subagglutinating dose of rabbit or dog anti-SRBC antibodies. These sensitized cells are added to dilutions of the patient's serum. Incubation is for a minimum of one hour at 37° C and one hour at room temperature. Agglutination is determined microscopically and macroscopically. A titer of 1:16 or greater is considered positive, a titer of 1:8 is suspect; almost all dogs will have a titer of 1:4 or 1:2 and therefore should be considered negative. Approximately 60 percent of the dogs with other criteria of rheumatoid arthritis are positive in this test.

The screening test used widely in human medicine to detect rheumatoid factor is the latex slide agglutination test. The human latex reagent cannot be used to detect canine rheumatoid factor. Recently, a canine latex reagent was developed to detect rheumatoid factor in canine arthritis. The results of the latex test on a large number of samples suggested that there was a poor correlation between clinical signs of RA and a positive test. The reasons for these results are not known at present.

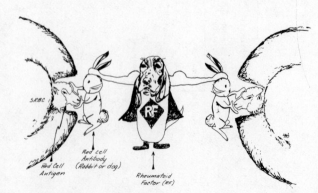

Figure 3. Schematic representation of the Rose-Waaler test for the detection of canine rheumatoid factor associated with rheumatoid arthritis.

Poor mucin precipitation of synovial fluid can also be used as a diagnostic aid for RA. The test is performed as follows. Glacial acetic acid is added dropwise to a test tube containing synovial fluid from the patient and one from a control dog (if available). In dogs with RA or septic arthritis, loose and friable clots or only a flocculent precipitate will form, whereas in normal dogs or dogs with SLE or degenerative joint disease, a firm, hard, ropy, non-friable clot will form. Complement, particularly the C3 component, is low or depleted in the synovial fluid of many human patients with RA. Similar tests for reduction or depletion of C3 in canine RA have not been reported; therefore, these tests are currently not used routinely.

Sample required: serum and synovial fluid (if available). The author is currently studying canine rheumatoid arthritis and would appreciate receiving serum samples, synovial fluid, and history from dogs in which at least five of the following nine criteria are positive:

Criteria for RA

1. Stiffness after resting
2. Pain on motion or tenderness of joints
3. Soft tissue swelling
4. Similar swelling within past 3 months
5. Symmetrical onset of joint symptoms and swelling
6. Radiographic changes consistent with RA
7. Poor mucin precipitate
8. Histologic changes consistent with RA
9. Rheumatoid factor positive

IMMUNOLOGIC THROMBOCYTOPENIC PURPURA (IMTP)

Immunologic thrombocytopenic purpura occurs when antibody and/or sensitized T cells cause the number of platelets to fall below that number essential for maintenance of vascular integrity and normal hemostasis.

Laboratory diagnosis would include a CBC and an assay for antiplatelet antibody (e.g., platelet factor 3 test). (See Wilkins, 1977.)

Sample required: CBC and blood collected for serum.

SYSTEMIC LUPUS ERYTHEMATOSUS (SLE)

Systemic lupus erythematosus is a generalized disorder that involves many organ systems. It is frequently characterized by the presence of antinuclear antibody (ANA) and lupus erythematosus (LE) cells and the simul-taneous occurrence of two or more of the following disorders: AIHA, IMTP, polyarthritis, or immune-complex glomerulonephritis (see Lewis, 1977).

The LE cell test is the most reliable indicator of SLE; however, it is only positive in about 60 to 75 percent of dogs with SLE. The antinuclear antibody (ANA) immunofluorescence test is a reliable screening test, being positive in >90 per cent of dogs with SLE, but it is not specific for SLE. The ANA test would be the test of choice for screening samples from animals suspected of having an autoimmune disease.

Antinuclear Antibody Test. This is one of the most commonly used immunofluorescence tests. A variety of substrates including mouse and rat liver and kidney sections, tissue culture cells, and homologous white blood cells have been used as substrates for the antinuclear antibody test. The two substrates most commonly used for canine and feline serum are tissue culture cells and liver sections. The procedure used in the author's laboratory is as follows.

1. Serum from the patient diluted 1:5 is placed on Vero cells and incubated for 30 minutes. *Note:* the Vero cells are grown on 8-chamber slides (Lab-Tek) until 50 percent of the cell layer is grown in. The cells are then fixed for 25 minutes with cold (4° C) methanol or acetone.
2. The cells are washed in phosphate-buffered saline (PBS) for 10 minutes with at least three changes of buffer.
3. The slides are flipped to remove as much buffer as possible, and anticanine IgG or antifeline IgG labeled with fluorescein isothiocyanate (FITC) is placed on the sections of the slide and incubated for 30 minutes.
4. Step 2 is repeated. The slides are dipped in distilled water and then air dried.
5. A counterstain (e.g., Evans Blue) is used if desired.
6. A suitable solution such as phosphate-buffered glycerol or elvanol is placed on the slide, a coverslip is applied, and the slides are viewed for fluorescence with a microscope equipped for fluorescence microscopy.

The procedure is essentially the same for the other substrates. Antibody from the patient is serially diluted or screened at a specific dilution calculated by the particular laboratory to be significant if a positive reaction is obtained. Interpretation is not always simple, and results from inexperienced personnel or laboratories not familiar with the domestic species should always be questioned. Occasionally submitting normal or known positive sample to the laboratory is a measure the practicing veterinarian can employ to test the reliability or at best the reproducibility of results from the laboratory testing the samples. Practicing veterinarians should also understand that laboratory results will not always confirm the clinical diagnosis. Certainly in rare instances, the clinical diagnosis will be incorrect and the laboratory results will unfortunately help confirm that misdiagnosis. It is not known what percentage of dogs with systemic lupus erythematosus will test positive. Furthermore, it is not known what diseases other than systemic lupus erythematosus will present with a positive antinuclear antibody test. It can be estimated from results that approximately 90 percent of dogs with systemic lupus erythematosus will have antinuclear antibody at some time during the course of disease. With the criteria for considering a sample positive, antinuclear antibody has been found in a few cases of polymyositis with no evidence of systemic lupus erythematosus. A few dogs with rheumatoid arthritis have been found to have antinuclear antibody (1:5 titer), and a few dogs with systemic lupus erythematosus have been found to have rheumatoid factor (see Table 2). The correlation between systemic lupus erythematosus cells and antinuclear antibody would suggest that approximately 60 percent of animals with a positive antinuclear antibody test have systemic lupus erythematosus cells. The presence of SLE cells can be considered to be a positive diagnosis of systemic lupus erythematosus; however, their absence should not be considered to be diagnostic for the absence of systemic lupus erythematosus, since only 60 percent of animals with SLE might be expected to be positive on any one sample, with possibly as many as 75 to 80 percent being positive if multiple samples are tested during the course of disease. The antinuclear antibody test is preferred for screening animals suspected of having systemic lupus erythematosus.

The FITC-labeled anticanine IgG is available from Miles Laboratories, Elkhart, Indiana, and substrate slides can be obtained from Zeus Scientific, Inc., Raritan, N.J. or Microbiological Associates, Walkersville, Md.

LE Cell Test. The direct LE cell test can be performed as follows. The clot from a 5 ml blood sample is incubated for two hours at 37° C strained through a fine wire mesh into a tube, and centrifuged. Smears are made from the buffy coat and are stained and examined for LE cells. LE cells are polymorphonuclear neutrophils that have phagocytized nuclear material. An indirect procedure is also available that requires serum from the patient and a blood sample from a normal dog. The technique is basically the same as that for the direct test.

Additional tests available to detect DNA antibody and antinuclear antibody include the radioimmunoassay (RIA) and the latex assay, respectively. A number of problems have been encountered with canine serum samples submitted for RIA. The diagnostic value of the RIA test for canine SLE has not been critically determined. The latex particles sensitized with calf-thymus DNA in the author's experience do not compare favorably with clinical signs, the presence of ANA by immunofluorescence or LE cells; therefore, the latex test is not recommended.

Recently, an immunofluorescence test for double-stranded DNA, using *Crithidia luciliae* as the substrate, was made available. The author tested a number of dog sera with high ANA titers using the crithidia assay, and all were negative for antibody to double-stranded DNA. The diagnostic value of this test for canine SLE requires further study.

Samples required: clotted blood sample for LE cell test and serum for ANA immunofluorescence test.

AUTOIMMUNE THYROIDITIS (LYMPHOCYTIC)

Hypothyroidism mediated by antibody and/or cells is characterized by lethargy, easy fatigability, patchy alopecia, infertility, and intolerance to cold. Antibody to thyroglobulin or microsomal antigen can be detected by the tanned red cell hemagglutination test. The indirect immunofluorescence test is also used to detect antibody to thyroid antigens.

Recently, the author used the lymphocyte blastogenesis test and a thyroid extract as antigen to detect antigen-responsive lymphocytes in dogs with autoimmune thyroiditis.

Samples required: clotted blood for serum and blood in preservative-free heparin for blastogenesis test.

IMMUNE-COMPLEX GLOMERULONEPHRITIS

(See "Glomerulonephropathy and the Nephrotic Syndrome.")

Immune-complex glomerulonephritis requires a needle or wedge biopsy of the kidneys for clinical diagnosis. The immunofluorescence test and electron microscopy are the techniques of choice. For the immunofluorescence test, an anticanine IgG and anticanine C3 labeled with FITC are used to detect immune complexes in the mesangium and/or on the glomerular basement membrane (GBM). A lumpy-bumpy pattern of fluorescence is indicative of immune-complex glomerulonephritis. A second immune-mediated, anti-GBM glomerulonephritis has not been reported to date for the dog or cat but if present would be characterized by a smooth pattern of fluorescence on the GBM.

Sample required: kidney biopsy.

Immunofluorescence (Fluorescent Antibody Technique). This technique is a histochemical or cytochemical procedure most commonly used to locate or identify antigens in tissue (direct technique) or detect specific antibody in serum or other secretions (indirect technique) of the patient.

The fluorescent compound most frequently conjugated to antibody for use in the procedure is fluorescein isothiocyanate (FITC). FITC readily binds covalently to antibody at an alkaline pH. Microscopes used for visualizing immunofluorescent specimens are simple but expensive modifications of standard transmission microscopes.

For the direct procedure, antiserum with specific antibody activity for the antigen is conjugated. If the indirect procedure is employed, antibody to the species immunoglobulins is produced in a heterologous species (e.g., antidog IgG produced in rabbits) and the anti-immunoglobulin serum is conjugated with a fluorescent compound.

The immunofluorescence technique has been applied to the diagnosis of a wide variety of diseases of dogs and cats. Antibody to a variety of tissue antigens is detected with the indirect procedure (Table 1). The critical factors in this test are the quality and specificity of the FITC-conjugated antibody and the appropriate substrate. Appropriate negative and positive controls should be included to demonstrate accuracy of the reaction. For certain tests, conjugated antiserum must have a specific fluorescein/protein (FIP) ratio for optimal results.

IMMUNOPROLIFERATIVE DISORDERS (GAMMOPATHIES)

The techniques of cellulose acetate electrophoresis, immunoelectrophoresis, radial immunodiffusion (RID), bone marrow smear, and the thermal test for Bence Jones proteins in urine are the laboratory tests most frequently used to diagnose multiple myeloma, macroglobulinemia (monoclonal gammopathies), or polyclonal gammopathies. In addition, the routine techniques to determine total protein (i.e., refractometer, biuret) and A:G ratios frequently alert the clinician to the possibility of a gammopathy.

Cellulose acetate electrophoresis is a quantitative electrophoretic technique available in most human and veterinary clinical laboratories. The Beckman Microzone® and the Corning ACI® techniques are very satisfactory. Eight samples of serum can be simultaneously separated into at least five or six fractions: albumin (most anodal), α_1, α_2, β_1, β_2, and γ globulin. IgG myeloma proteins are generally, but not always, found in the γ globulin region, and IgA myeloma and macroglobulinemia (IgM) are generally found in the β regions.

Immunoelectrophoresis differs from cellulose acetate electrophoresis in that serum is separated in an electric field, and then an agar-gel diffusion reaction with antisera to serum proteins is performed. This technique can separate serum into 20 or more fractions

Table 1. *The Indirect Immunofluorescence Test for the Detection of Autoantibody in Immunologic Disorders*

DISORDER	ANTIBODY TO	SUBSTRATE
Systemic lupus erythematosus	Nuclear proteins and nucleic acids	Tissue sections, imprints, or tissue culture cells
Autoimmune thyroiditis	Microsomal antigens, colloid antigens, other thyroid antigens	Thyroid
Pemphigus°	Intercellular cement substance	Esophagus, skin, or oral mucosa
Pemphigoid°	Epithelial basement membrane	Esophagus, skin, or oral mucosa
Primary Addison's disease	Adrenal cortical cells	Adrenal gland
Primary hyperparathyroidism	Parathyroid cell	Parathyroid
Myasthenia gravis and polymyositis	Muscle	Muscle

° Direct technique with biopsy of affected tissue is the preferred method.
From Schultz and Adams, 1978.

and is principally a qualitative technique. It is useful for demonstrating abnormalities in proteins such as myeloma globulins and Bence Jones proteins in urine. Radial immunodiffusion (RID) performed in agar containing antisera is a sensitive quantitative technique used to determine the amount of immunoglobulin or specific complement component present in serum. It requires antisera specific for the particular protein to be quantitated as well as antigens that can be used as specific for the particular protein to be quantitated as well as antigens that can be used as specific protein standards. RID kits are available commercially from Miles Laboratories for the quantitation of several canine immunoglobulins. Antisera to canine IgG and IgM are available from Cappel Laboratories, Downingtown, Pennsylvania; Pel Freez, Rogers, Arkansas; Miles Labs, Elkhart, Indiana.

The thermal solubility test for Bence Jones protein in urine is performed by adjusting the pH to 5 and heating the urine slowly to boiling. Most Bence Jones proteins will precipitate at temperatures between 50 and 60° C and will redissolve on boiling. When the urine is allowed to cool, the proteins reprecipitate. If albumin is present in the urine, the precipitate will not redissolve at high temperatures. Urostix®* is specific for albumin and will not detect the presence of Bence Jones proteins.

In certain chronic diseases (i.e., brucellosis, pyometra) and autoimmune diseases (SLE), an elevation of gamma globulin will occur that can be recognized on cellulose acetate electrophoresis as a polyclonal gammopathy (heterogenous β- and/or γ-globulin elevation). This elevation results from constant antigenic stimulation and perhaps a defect in suppressor T-cell activity.

Samples required: serum and urine.

IMMUNODEFICIENCY DISORDERS

Immunodeficiency disorders reflect an impairment in one or more of the major components of immunity: *non-specific immunity,* including (1) phagocytic cells (e.g., PMN and macrophages) and (2) effector substances (e.g., complement) and/or *specific immunity,* including (1) humoral (antibody) immunity (the B-cell system) and (2) cell-mediated immunity (CMI) (the T-cell system). Immunodeficiencies are classified as primary or secondary. The primary deficiency diseases are genetically defined inborn errors of the body's defense mechanisms and can affect non-specific as well as specific components of the immune response. Primary deficiencies are very uncommon in the dog and cat, but they do occur.

Secondary immunodeficiencies are acquired as a consequence of numerous conditions, including infectious disease, neoplasia, aging, drug therapy, failure to receive colostrum, and certain nutritional deficiencies. Secondary immunodeficiencies are more common than primary deficiencies. Reports have identified secondary immunodeficiencies or immunosuppression associated with canine distemper infections, canine generalized demodectic mange, nutritional deficiencies, feline panleukopenia, feline leukemia, and age (see "The Theory and Practice of Immunization").

Clinicians should consider immunodeficiency or immunosuppression when an animal is presented with a history of chronic infection, autoimmune disease, or neoplastic disease.

Deficiencies of the humoral immune system are most often characterized by infections with extracellular pyogenic pathogens (e.g., streptococci). Selective IgA deficiencies may be characterized by chronic respiratory or gastrointestinal infections. The presence of microbes normally not pathogenic for the animal is often a clue to immunodeficiency disorders (e.g., *Pneumocystis carinii* or streptococci isolated from the lung or *Giardia* in the gut). Deficiencies of cell-mediated immunity are associated with infections caused by facultative intracellular pyogenic pathogens (e.g., acid-fast organisms, *Brucella, Salmonella,* certain viruses and fungi).

A suggested approach to the clinical and laboratory diagnosis of an animal suspected of an immunodeficiency disease is presented in Figure 1.

NON-SPECIFIC IMMUNITY

If a deficiency in non-specific immunity is suspected, such as cyclic neutropenia or chronic granulomatous disease, the following laboratory tests may be used as an aid to diagnosis.

Phagocytic and Bactericidal Function Tests. Phagocytic index and bactericidal activity tests measure the ability of cells to phagocytize and subsequently kill bacteria, a function of the lysosomal enzymes. The test is performed by mixing a suspension of bacteria (e.g., staphylococci or *E. coli*) with a suspension of leukocytes from the patient and a normal control in the presence of fresh serum.

---

*Ames Co., Elkhart, Indiania.

After an appropriate time, the number of viable bacteria is determined for patient and control by direct bacterial plate count techniques. The inability to phagocytize and/or kill bacteria is indicative of a deficiency in neutrophil function and rarely of monocyte or macrophage function.

Nitroblue Tetrazolium Test (NBT). This test is particularly useful to detect nonfunctional neutrophils in chronic granulomatous disease (CGD). Neutrophils from normal dogs or cats rapidly reduce nitroblue tetrazolium (NBT) during *in vitro* phagocytosis. Neutrophils from animals with CGD are unable to reduce NBT. A kit for the NBT test is available from Sigma Chemical Co., St. Louis, Missouri.

Sample required: blood collected in preservative-free heparin; 50 units/ml of blood is ideal for these tests. Large quantities of heparin can affect the NBT test.

Total Hemolytic Complement. CH_{50} can be detected in dogs by adding fresh serum to sheep red blood cells sensitized with rabbit antibody. For the cat, chicken, or rabbit, red blood cells sensitized with cat antibody can be used. Sensitized cells mixed with serial dilutions of the patient's and a control animal's serum are incubated, and the highest dilution of serum giving 50 percent hemolysis is recorded. A difference of three or more dilutions from the control would suggest a complement deficiency in the patient. Total hemolytic complement assays measure all components of the complement system.

Quantitation of C3 Component by RID. The C3 component of complement as well as other individual components can be purified, and antisera to them can be made. These antisera can be used to quantitate the complement component in serum. If purified complement standards are not available for standardization, serum from normal dogs can be used to compare values with dogs suspected of having complement deficiencies. Depletion of C3 in dogs with autoimmune thyroiditis and in some dogs with immune-complex glomerulonephritis has been recognized. This assay is also used to measure C3 in joint fluid of dogs suspected of having rheumatoid arthritis.

SPECIFIC IMMUNITY

DEFICIENCIES IN THE HUMORAL IMMUNE RESPONSE (B-CELL SYSTEMS)

These deficiencies should be considered if an animal does not produce antibody to vaccine viruses after proper immunization, has very low gamma globulin levels, or suffers from chronic infection with extracellular pathogens. In dogs, antibody to canine distemper virus (CDV) and canine adenovirus 1 (CAV-1) should develop within three to four weeks after vaccination and persist for long periods. Antibody to the parainfluenza virus SV_5 could also be used as an indication of humoral immunocompetence if this virus is included in the routine vaccine schedule. In the cat, feline panleukopenia, feline herpesvirus, or calicivirus vaccine virus antibody can be used as an indication of immune responsiveness. If, after proper and repeated vaccination, antibody to these viruses is not present, a humoral immunodeficiency should be suspected.

During the early neonatal period, a humoral immunodeficiency exists in pups and kittens that do not receive colostrum, for whatever reason, since 95 to 98 percent of their immunoglobulins are obtained by means of absorption of colostrum.

Numerous other antigen preparations (e.g., foreign red blood cells, keyhole-limpet hemocyanin, ϕX-174) can be used to determine immunocompetence in the dog and cat. Tests such as cellulose acetate electrophoresis, immunoelectrophoresis, and radial immunodiffusion to quantitate the various classes of immunoglobulin can also be used to detect humoral immunodeficiencies (see previous description of techniques).

DEFICIENCIES IN CELL-MEDIATED IMMUNITY (T-CELL SYSTEM)

These disorders provide the greatest challenge to the clinician and immunologist. Recently, a number of *in vitro* correlates of CMI have been developed for clinical diagnosis; however, none of them completely correlates with CMI *in vivo*. An approach to the patient with CMI deficiency would include a CBC to determine the presence of lymphopenia. Approximately 60 to 75 percent of the peripheral blood lymphocytes are T cells; therefore, any significant reduction (less than 1000 lymphocytes/mm³) could suggest a CMI deficiency. The presence of normal numbers of lymphocytes *does not*, however, indicate that CMI is normal.

Delayed type dermal hypersensitivity (DTH) to most antigens is minimal or absent in dogs and cats; therefore, this test cannot be used routinely to determine T-cell function.

Skin allograft transplants, on the other hand, provide a reliable and simple *in vivo* method to check CMI in dogs and cats. Normal rejection time for both dogs and cats is 12 ± 2 days. Delays of one week or more from normal would be significant and would indicate impairment of T-cell function.

Skin sensitization with chemicals such as dinitrochlorobenzene (DNCB) has been suggested as a measure of CMI in man; however, DNCB sensitization in the dog and cat has proved less than satisfactory, even when biopsies are obtained for microscopic evaluation.

The Lymphocyte Blastogenesis (Transformation) Technique. This test has proved extremely helpful in the laboratory diagnosis of CMI deficiency in the dog and cat. The technique is subject to a variety of trials and tribulations; however, after optimal conditions for the test are established, it is an excellent immunodiagnostic tool in a variety of clinical conditions and promises to have wider applicability in the future.

A number of modifications of the technique are available. Optimal conditions established for mitogenic stimulation of canine and feline peripheral blood cells in the macrotest were as follows. Heparinized blood was centrifuged at $160 \times g$ for 10 minutes to obtain a buffy coat and a leukocyte-rich plasma fraction, devoid of as many erythrocytes as possible. The white cell suspension was diluted so that 0.1 ml contained between 5×10^5 to 5×10^6 leukocytes. Cells were placed into 21×70 mm screwcapped glass vials that contained 1 ml of RPMI-1640 media with 100 units of penicillin, 100 μg of streptomycin, 10 percent fetal bovine serum (FBS), and an optimal amount of mitogen. Optimal conditions for the microtest differed slightly from those for the macrotest. Heparinized blood was centrifuged on a ficollisopaque gradient for 15 minutes at 1300 g. The mononuclear cell layer was removed and the cell suspension was adjusted so that 0.1 ml contained between 5×10^4 to 5×10^5 cells. Cells were placed in wells of a flat bottom 96-well microtiter tissue culture plate that contained 0.1 ml of the media used in the macrotest. The mitogens included phytohemagglutinin (PHA), concanavalin A (Con A), pokeweek mitogen (PWM), *E. coli* lipopolysaccharide (LPS), and lipid A and streptolysin O (SLO). Culture tubes with loosened caps and microtiter plates were incubated for 72 hours at 39° C in 5 percent CO_2 and air. Two μCi of ^{3}H thymidine were added in a volume of 0.5 ml to the tubes and 1 μCi in 0.1 ml was added to the wells. For the macrotube test, the cells were centrifuged, washed, precipitated with trichloroacetic acid and dissolved in formic acid, and the radioactivity was determined by scintillation spectrophotometry. The cells in the microplate test were harvested with a MASH II (Microbiological Associates, Bethesda, Maryland).

The lymphocyte blastogenesis test was used by the author to evaluate a large number of dogs and cats admitted to the Small Animal Clinics of the New York State College of Veterinary Medicine and Auburn University as well as dogs and cats on various research experiments. The following should be used as a guideline when performing the test on clinical samples. Samples should be run in duplicate or triplicate and repeated at least one time on a second day before any conclusions are drawn from results. Lymphocytes should be cultured in autologous serum or plasma in addition to fetal bovine serum to detect immunosuppressive factors (e.g., generalized demodectic mange, vitamin E deficiency). Values should be compared with normal mean values established for a large number of control animals but more importantly should be compared with normal control samples run simultaneously with the animal being evaluated. Under the conditions outlined, the test is a very useful diagnostic tool. Clinical and experimental conditions in which significant suppression of canine lymphocyte responses to phytomitogens have been found were canine distemper, generalized demodectic mange (autologous serum or plasma present), certain nutritional deficiencies, a percentage of dogs with lymphosarcoma, a small number of dogs with aspergillosis, a percentage of dogs older than nine years, and animals treated with certain drugs. Suppression in the cat has been associated with feline leukemia virus infection, clinical leukemia, panleukopenia virus infection, and an occasional animal without specific disease. It is the author's experience that feline lymphocytes in general respond more poorly to PHA than do those of dogs or other species. The cat lymphocytes respond well to Con A and PWM. It is not currently known whether this reflects a difference in lymphocyte subpopulations of the cat as compared with other species or if it is a technical artifact. It is also of interest to note that steroid treatment of the dog does not affect the lymphocyte response to phytomitogens. Based on a number of experimental studies, numerous cell manipulations, and drug treatment of dogs and cats, the author suggests that the following populations of cells are stimulated by mitogens:

1. PHA — Predominantly T cells (this population or subpopulation may be absent in most cats)
2. Con A — T cells (perhaps more than one subpopulation or a population different from that stimulated by PHA)
3. PWM — T and B cells (early response

two and three days after stimulation predominantly T cells)

4. SLO — T and B cells
5. LPS (lipid A) — B cells (most dog and cat peripheral blood lymphocytes do not respond to *E. coli* LPS; however, their milk or splenic lymphocytes will).

Inhibition of Cell Migration (MIF). This test measures the production of the lymphokine migration inhibition factor (MIF). If this factor inhibits the migration of macrophages it is called "macrophage migration inhibition factor," and the factor that inhibits the migration of blood monocytes and neutrophils is called "leukocyte migration inhibition factor." The basic technique suitable for the dog is one in which peripheral blood cells are packed into a capillary tube or placed in a well of an agarose plate, and antigen or mitogen is added to the cells. If MIF is produced, little or no migration occurs. If the lymphocytes are unable to produce MIF, normal migration occurs. The inability to produce MIF is correlated with a lymphocyte deficiency and presumably a deficiency of CMI. There are also modifications of the technique in use for the dog and cat that utilize guinea pig peritoneal macrophages as the target cells. The author's experience with the technique as a clinical immunodiagnostic test has been unrewarding.

Cytotoxicity Tests. A number of cytotoxicity tests are available to measure lymphocyte cytotoxicity, antibody-complement cytotoxicity, or antibody-dependent K-cell cytotoxicity. The cytopathic activity of lymphocytes against target cells (e.g., tumor cells, viral infected cells, erythrocytes) in cell culture is assumed to have its *in vivo* counterpart in some of the tissue-damaging reactions associated with CMI. In the test, target cells are labeled with ^{14}C or ^{3}H thymidine, $^{125}IUDR$ or ^{51}Cr. These labeled cells are then mixed with lymphocytes and incubated for 12 to 24 hours. At the end of incubation, the amount of cell damage is expressed as a percentage of the radiolabel released. The cell damage is due to a direct cell contact or a lymphokine (T-cell product) known as a cytotoxic factor or lymphotoxin.

Antibody-dependent K-cell cytotoxicity presumably is achieved by the K cell damaging the target cell in the presence of antibody. No complement is added. Antibody with specific activity for the target cell in the presence of complement will cause cell damage. Both assays also utilize a radioisotope-labeled cell to determine the amount of cell damage.

These assays have particular application for the measurement of specific cellular or humoral activity to antigens (e.g., viral or bacterial) or tumor cells.

Specific Assay for T and B Cells. The assay currently in routine use to identify the B cell is the membrane immunofluorescence test for immunoglobulin. The test for T cells in man is the erythrocyte rosette-forming assay (E-RFC).

LYMPHOCYTE ROSETTE ASSAYS FOR T CELLS. Several years ago, it was found that human T lymphocytes spontaneously rosetted with sheep red blood cells. Investigations were initiated to determine if similar tests could be used to detect canine and feline T cells. It became immediately apparent that neither canine nor feline lymphocytes rosetted with sheep erythrocytes; however, several species of erythrocytes were found to rosette with lymphocytes from dogs and cats. It was reported that human and guinea pig erythrocytes rosette with dog cells and guinea pig erythrocytes rosette with cat cells.

Several studies have recently appeared suggesting that erythrocyte rosetting may not be specific for T cells in the canine species or the feline species. The reason for this skepticism results from the following observations: (1) in several laboratories, only 20 to 30 percent of the peripheral blood lymphocytes of dogs and cats formed rosettes as compared with 60 to 80 percent of blood lymphocytes from man, (2) approximately 3 percent of cells from the thymus of the dog rosette, whereas more than 90 percent of cells from the human thymus rosette, (3) there is a lack of appreciation for the knowledge that cells such as polymorphonuclear leukocytes and monocytes rosette, and that this is not a phenomenon restricted to lymphocytes, and (4) there was previous inability to correlate rosetting results in dog or cat with other functional tests or additional techniques to identify T and B cells.

Studies in the author's laboratory suggest that human erythrocytes are better than guinea pig erythrocytes for the demonstration of lymphocyte rosetting in the dog. Unlike results from a number of other laboratories, it was found under optimal conditions that 40 ± 10 percent of peripheral blood lymphocytes from the dog form rosettes. These results are obtained with a preparation of mononuclear cells with no polymorphonuclear leukocytes and less than 5 percent monocytes. The most important and convincing evidence that the rosetting cells are lymphocytes is that if the rosetting cells are isolated by ficoll-Hypaque density gradient, they can be demonstrated to respond to phytomitogens in the blastogenesis test, a characteristic that cannot be demonstrated for polymorphonuclear leukocytes or monocytes. However, unlike the situation in man in which all or most T lymphocytes in the blood rosette, only a certain subpopulation comprising perhaps 40 to 50 percent of the total lymphocytes of the dog rosette. This subpopulation, referred to as T_2, is made of lymphocytes that have acquired a receptor for human red blood cells after they have migrated from the thymus to the peripheral tissue. The lymphocytes of the thymus referred to here as T_1 cells have not acquired a receptor for red blood cells. A similar situation may hold for the cat, since — as with the dog — only a small percentage of cells rosette.

This finding limits to some extent the clinical usefulness of direct lymphocyte rosetting in that only a certain subpopulation rosettes and considerable variation can occur in populations presumably without significant alteration of immune function.

Specific membrane antigens have been found on the T lymphocytes in certain species. In mice, these antigens are referred to as *thy* antigens (in man as TLA) and are usually detected by immunofluorescence. Similar antigens occur on dog T cells, and antisera have been produced to thymocytes and to brain suspensions (also known to contain a similar antigen). These antisera have to date been used predominantly in canine research only. With these antisera, 60 to 75 percent of blood lymphocytes are positive — further evidence to suggest that the direct erythrocyte technique measures only a subpopulation of canine T lymphocytes.

EAC (ERYTHROCYTE-ANTIBODY-COMPLEMENT) ROSETTES FOR B CELLS. A certain percentage of lymphocytes contains surface receptors for complement (CR). These cells, known to be a subpopulation of B cells in certain species and believed to be B cells in dogs and cats, can be identified by sensitizing sheep red blood cells with antibody and complement. Complement deficiency in the C5 or C6 component or mouse complement is used so that lysis of the antibody red cell does not occur spontaneously. The rosette formed in this assay is morphologically identical to the one found in the direct erythrocyte assay described previously. The clinical value of this test is unknown at this time because of the limited application of the test with canine and feline lymphocytes.

MEMBRANE IMMUNOGLOBULIN ASSAY FOR B CELLS. Lymphocytes with readily demonstrable immunoglobulin on their surface are believed to be B cells. The procedure to detect membrane Ig-positive cells is generally direct or indirect immunofluorescence. Immu-

noglobulin will be found as a rim of fluorescence, as patches of fluorescence, or at one or both caps of the cell depending on the conditions of the assay. We find approximately 15 ± 5 percent of peripheral blood lymphocytes as membrane-Ig positive in apparently healthy dogs. The predominant membrane Ig is IgM. In a variety of diseases, the number of Ig-positive cells changes. It is essential to determine if this change is the result of an increase in the B cell population or is caused by the presence of immune-complexes or antilymphocyte antibody on T cells (usually IgG).

ADDITIONAL IMMUNODIAGNOSTIC TESTS

Radioallergosorbent Test (RAST). Immunoglobulin E, the antibody involved in the immediate hypersensitivity reaction (type I) as well as in immune responses to vermin infections, is difficult to detect with conventional tests because serum concentrations are very low. A number of laboratories interested in immediate hypersensitivity (atopy) are currently attempting to modify the RAST to measure specific IgE in dogs. In the technique, serum IgE is measured by adding the dog's serum to allergen linked cyanogen bromide–activated sepharose (dextran). After thorough washing, the absorbed IgE antibodies are measured by the uptake of radioisotope-labeled purified anticanine IgE. The reaction is extremely sensitive, as are other radioimmunoassay (RIA) procedures, but it does require a specialized laboratory. The test could be considered an *in vitro* correlate of skin testing for type I hypersensitivity.

Another RIA to measure IgE is the radioimmunosorbent test (RIST). This test is used to measure only the quantity of IgE in serum and is not a measure of the activity of IgE with regard to a specific allergen (antigen).

Total IgE levels in the serum are also measured by a radioactive single RID procedure. Rabbit anticanine IgE is incorporated into agar and standards or unknown sera are placed in wells (see discussion of RID earlier in this article). An invisible precipitin ring forms, which is visualized by incubating with ^{125}I-labeled goat antirabbit IgG followed by radioautography. The concentration of IgE is determined by measuring the diameter of the ring and comparing it with the standard preparations.

The clinical significance of quantitation of IgE is currently not known, because the range of values for normal dogs is large and because intestinal parasitic infections greatly increase the levels of IgE, making it difficult to relate values to allergic conditions. In addition, the IgE level does not identify offending allergens; therefore, skin tests or the RAST must be used for that purpose.

Histocompatibility Tests for Dog Leukocyte Antigens and Dog Erythrocyte Antigens. Two tests are currently available to type dog leukocytes. One is a serologic test that uses antisera developed in dogs by the inoculation of leukocytes from another dog. The antisera in the presence of complement kill the leukocytes of non-related (incompatible) dogs. Killing is generally detected by uptake of trypan blue by non-viable cells. A number of laboratories throughout the world have the ability to type dog leukocytes serologically. An additional test for typing leukocytes is the mixed leukocyte reaction (MLR). The test is similar to the lymphocyte blastogenesis test (described previously); however, instead of mitogen, lymphocytes from two dogs are mixed together to determine if one stimulates the other. It is possible to inhibit DNA synthesis in one animal by irradiating the cells or treating them with mitomycin C. The test is then referred to as the "one way mixed leukocyte reaction." A combination of the serologic tests and MLR can be used to determine the relative compatibility between individuals for organ transplants. Additionally, the association between certain serologically or lymphocyte-defined leukocyte antigens and disease is the subject of investigation in numerous species including the dog.

The dog erythrocyte antigens assume clinical importance in repeated blood transfusions. Although numerous blood groups have been recognized in the dog, the one with greatest importance is blood group A (A_1, A_2). Although the first transfusion with blood from an A-positive dog to an A-negative recipient will have little or no clinical consequence, additional transfusions can be fatal because of the immunologic hypersensitivity reaction that can occur. This adverse reaction can be prevented by keeping an A-negative blood donor in the clinic.

Skin Tests (Types I and III). There are several different skin tests that can be used to identify certain classes of antibody. The immediate hypersensitivity or type I reaction is commonly used to determine the offending allergen in allergic inhalant dermatitis of dogs. The reaction is characterized by a wheal and flare and appears within minutes. Normally, reaction sites would be measured at 15 and 30 minutes after intradermal administration of the antigen. Skin testing of cats is not normally done, as atopic diseases are rare in this species.

There are two passive tests to detect IgE antibodies in a number of species. They are the Prausnitz-Kustner (P-K) test and the passive cutaneous anaphylaxis (PCA) test. It has been reported that neither technique is particularly effective in the dog.

Skin tests to detect type III hypersensitivity reaction or the Arthus reaction involve the subcutaneous injection of antigen into animals that have antibody capable of precipitating the antigen (IgG) and fixing complement. An acute inflammatory reaction develops at the site of injection within several hours, starting as an erythematous-edematous swelling. As it develops, local hemorrhage and thrombosis occur and frequently progress to necrosis in a few days. Arthus reactions can be produced in both dogs and cats and may be an important mechanism in certain bacterial hypersensitivity reactions, immune complex mediated glomerulonephritis, infectious canine hepatitis uveitis (blue eye), and joint lesions in rheumatoid arthritis.

Delayed Hypersensitivity (Type IV) Skin Tests. The *in vitro* correlates of CMI assume particular significance as clinical tests for the dog and cat because typical DTH skin responses are not readily detected in these species. The author's experience, as well as that of numerous other veterinary researchers, is that DTH skin testing in dogs and cats is characterized by a predominant infiltration of polymorphonuclear neutrophils, rather than mononuclear cells, into the site, and the induration and erythema classic of DTH in other species is minimal or absent even in dogs and cats sensitized with or infected with mycobacterial species and skin tested with the classical purified protein derivatives (PPD). Poor DTH skin reactions have been particularly frustrating in clinical medicine in that the standard panel of skin test antigens commonly used to monitor cellular immunity in man cannot be duplicated in cats or dogs, employing antigens that should be useful for that purpose. Helminth antigens (*Ascaris canis*), tissue antigens, viral antigens (CDV), bacterial antigens (PPD), fungal antigens, and protein antigens have been employed experimentally and clinically in dogs and cats with limited reproducibility or irreproducible results.

Sensitization with chemicals such as dinitrochlorobenzene used successfully to demonstrate a DTH-like reaction in man and rodents was reported to be useful in the dog only if biopsies of the skin were examined micro-

Table 2. Estimated Percentage of Positive Tests for Autoimmune Responses in Immunologic Disorders

TEST	CLINIC. NORM.	SLE	AIHA	RA	MYE-LOMA	IG DEFICI-ENCY	AUTO-IMMUNE THYROID-ITIS	PEMPHI-GUS/PEMPHI-GOID	POLY-MYO-SITIS	ATOPY	GLOMERU-LONEPH-RITIS	CMI DEFI-CIENCY
Antinuclear antibody	1	90	20	10	10	0	10	0	20	10	30	10
Rheumatoid factor (Rose Waaler)	0	10	10	60	10	0	0	0	0	0	5	0
Antiglobulin (Coombs')	0	20	90	5	20	0	5	0	0	0	5	0
Thyroid antibodies or sensitized cells	5	5	0	0	10	0	50	0	0	?	10	10
Lupus erythematosus cell test	1	60	15	0	0	0	5	0	0	0	30	5
Skin-antibody	?	?	0	0	?	0	0	90	?	?	0	?
Muscle-antibody	0	0	0	0	0	0	0	0	0	0	0	0.
Immunoglobulin concentration	N	↑10	N	↑20	↑100	↓100	↑10	↑10	↑90	↑10	↓20	↓20
Complement (C₃) concentration	N	N	N	N	↓10	N	↓10	N	N	N	↓10	N
Lymphocyte blasto-genesis (mitogens)	N	N to ↓	N	N	N to ↓	N	N to ↓	N	N	N to ↓	N to ↓	↓90

N = normal; ↑ = increased; ↓ = decreased; ? = information not available.
From Schultz and Adams, 1978.

scopically. A similar technique applied to cats did not appear to be useful to measure DTH, even when biopsies were examined, in that a classic acute inflammatory response was noted rather than a DTH. This test is of limited usefulness in the dog.

Several years ago, the intradermal use of mitogens to assess the immune responsiveness of dogs immunosuppressed by canine distemper virus or in dogs with generalized demodectic mange was studied. Although the response to phytohemagglutinin and concanavalin A was found to be reduced in these two diseases, both are associated with a secondary immunosuppression. Histologic examination of biopsies from inoculated sites appear to be similar to a classic acute inflammatory reaction rather than a classic DTH reaction. Reactions to skin mitogens peak at 24 to 36 hours rather than 48 to 72 hours and are characterized by infiltration with neutrophils. Recently, a detailed comparative histologic and ultrastructural study was completed. Skin reactivity to mitogens was tested in the dog, rabbit, and guinea pig to determine if cutaneous basophil hypersensitivity (Jones-Mote) reaction, believed to be a manifestation of a T cell–mediated release of basophil chemotactic factor, was similar in these three species. The results clearly suggest that unlike the rabbit and guinea pig in which a good DTH and CBH can be demonstrated, the dog had no CBH reaction in the skin biopsies. The reason for the poor DTH and CBH in the dog is currently not known, but it should not be interpreted as a lack of CMI in this species.

The poor, delayed type skin reactivity is also manifested clinically in that there are very few documented cases of contact dermatitis in dogs and there have been no cases of contact dermatitis to the author's knowledge demonstrated to occur naturally in the cat. Many of the contact dermatitis cases demonstrated in the dog are direct contact irritants that have not been demonstrated to be due to a T cell–mediated type IV hypersensitivity.

Because of the inability to demonstrate a DTH reaction readily in dogs and cats, a greater reliance on the *in vitro* tests has required the adaptation of these techniques to the dog and cat.

CONCLUSION

Several immunologic techniques have been introduced during the past few years. Many of these are being applied to clinical specimens in an attempt to help the practicing veterinarian make a diagnosis. The introduction of new techniques requires extensive testing with clinically normal and diseased patients. It is essential for the practicing veterinarian to understand that the techniques available for the detection of immunologic disorders in the dog and cat are not routine diagnostic procedures and that adequate information has not been developed for any of the techniques described to assure the clinical significance of either positive or negative results (Table 2). This should not discourage the practitioner from submitting samples, but should encourage him or her to question the significance of those results and to attempt to correlate them with history and clinical signs before arriving at a final diagnosis.

SUPPLEMENTAL READING

Bach, F.H., and Good, R.A. (eds.): *Clinical Immunobiology*, Vol. 3. New York, Academic Press, 1976.

Bloom, B.R., and Glade, P.R. (eds.): *In Vitro Methods in Cell-Mediated Immunity*. New York, Academic Press, 1971.

Gell, P.G.H., Coombs, R.R.A., and Lachmann, P.J. (eds.): *Clinical Aspects of Immunology*. Edition 3. Oxford, England, Blackwell Scientific Publications, 1975.

Halliwell, R.E., Lavelle, R.B., and Butt, K.M.: Canine rheumatoid arthritis—a review and case report. J. Small Anim. Pract. *13*:239–243, 1972.

Hurvitz, A.I., and Halliwell, R.: Veterinary clinical immunology. Scientific proceeding. Am. Anim. Hosp. Assoc. 2:3, 1975.

Lewis, R.M.: Spontaneous autoimmune diseases of domestic animals. Int. Rev. Exp. Pathol. *13*:55, 1974.

Lewis, R.M: Canine systemic lupus erythematosus. In Kirk, R.W. (ed.): *Current Veterinary Therapy VI*. Philadelphia, W. B. Saunders Co., 1977.

Osburn, B.I., and Schultz, R.D. (eds.): *Advances in Veterinary Science and Comparative Medicine*. Vol. 23. New York, Academic Press, 1978.

Rose, N.R., and Bigazzi, P.E. (eds.): *Methods in Immunodiagnosis*. New York, John Wiley & Sons, 1973.

Rose, N.R., and Friedman, H.: *Manual of Clinical Immunology*. Washington, D.C., American Society for Microbiology, 1976.

Schultz, R.D.: Immunologic disorders in the dog and cat. Vet. Clin. North Am. *4*:153–174, 1974.

Schultz, R.D., and Adams, L.S.: Immunologic methods for the detection of humoral and cellular immunity. Vet. Clin. North Am. 8:721–753, 1978.

Tizard, I.R.: *An Introduction to Veterinary Immunology*. Philadelphia, W.B. Saunders Co., 1972.

Vyas, G.N., Sites, D.P., and Brecher, G. (eds.): *Laboratory Diagnosis of Immunologic Disorders*. New York, Grune and Stratton, 1974.

Wilkins, R.J.: Thrombocytopenic purpura. In Kirk, R.W. (ed.): *Current Veterinary Therapy VI*. Philadelphia. W. B. Saunders Co., 1977.

FELINE LEUKEMIA VIRUS
DISEASE COMPLEX

NIELS C. PEDERSEN, D.V.M.,
and BRUCE R. MADEWELL, V.M.D.

Davis, California.

EPIZOOTIOLOGY

Feline leukemia virus (FeLV) infection is widespread among cats. The overall infection rate and the proportion of cats that become chronically infected are related to the density of the cat population studied and to host and environmental factors that influence the severity of the primary disease. Epizootiologic studies indicate that about 25 to 60 percent of relatively free-roaming cats in urban and suburban populations are ultimately infected with the virus, but only 2 to 6 percent remain chronically infected. The overall infection rate in rural cat populations and in closely confined single cat households usually does not exceed 5 to 6 percent, and about 0.2 percent of these cats remain chronically infected. Mortality associated with FeLV is related to the number of infected cats that remain chronically viremic. Therefore, infection is most severe in some multiple cat households and catteries, where virtually all cats can be infected and 30 percent or more of the infected cats remain chronically viremic.

PATHOGENESIS

Feline leukemia and related diseases are caused by an oncornavirus belonging to the family *Retraviridae*. The virus is shed in the saliva, urine, and feces of infected cats, and infection occurs when susceptible cats contact any of these excretions. It is infectious by the oral route and by parenteral inoculation. Infection can occur when animals groom or bite each other or share litter and food containers. Although blood-sucking insects may theoretically transmit the virus, they are not essential for transmission. Aerosol transmission does not appear to be an important route of infection in nature. Because the virus is very unstable out of the body, a contaminated environment is probably not an important reservoir of virus. Although infected queens are usually reproductive failures, some produce kittens that carry the infection into later life.

Following continuous exposure, virus or antibody to virus cannot be detected in blood before 4 weeks; by 20 weeks, 80 percent of the cats have been infected. A small percentage of cats, especially if they are older at the time of exposure, may require up to 52 weeks of continuous exposure before they show evidence of infection.

The pathogenesis of FeLV infection can be divided into 3 stages: primary disease (apparent or inapparent); death, recovery, or apparent recovery; and recurrent or terminal illness. The primary disease is often totally inapparent, in which case most cats will eliminate the virus and become free of the infection. Cats that have inapparent primary signs either will never be detectably viremic or will be viremic for several weeks. Cats that are ill during the primary disease manifest varying degrees of fever, malaise, anorexia, lymphadenopathy, leukopenia, anemia, and thrombocytopenia. Clinical signs persist for 2 to 16 weeks, and during this time, some ill cats die. Most cats that are ill during the primary phase make an apparent recovery but will remain chronically viremic. During the next weeks, months, or years, some of these asymptomatic chronically viremic cats will develop a wide range of seemingly unrelated illnesses or suffer from recurrence of the primary myelosuppression. With proper symptomatic care and protection from undue stress, the fractional mortality rate in a group of chronically viremic cats is approximately 20 percent per year for each year that they are followed. This means that about half will be dead by the third year. Stresses that can precipitate a crisis in an infected cat include surgery, environmental changes, or other infectious diseases.

It is apparent from laboratory studies that the more severe the primary illness, the more likely the cat will become chronically viremic. The age of the cat when exposed, the severity of the exposure, and the effect of unfavorable genetic and environmental influences all contribute to the severity of the primary disease. In nature, most infected cats develop inapparent or mild

404

primary illness and recover. In catteries and multiple cat households, the primary illness is likely to be severe, and the proportion of cats developing a chronic infection is higher.

FeLV-RELATED ILLNESSES

Cats with chronic FeLV infection are at risk for a variety of disorders that are either directly or indirectly attributable to the virus. Disorders related directly to FeLV include lymphoproliferative and myeloproliferative disorders, thymic atrophy and lymphoid depletion in neonates, hypoplastic or aplastic anemia, leukopenia, thrombocytopenia, reproductive failure in queens (abortion, fetal resorption, stillbirths), production of weak unthrifty kittens, anterior uveitis, and a myriad of neurologic disorders. These neurologic disorders are frequently caused by neurolymphosarcoma; or in some cases they are caused by undefined neuropathic complications of the infection. Neurologic disorders include paralysis of ciliary nerves leading to persistent pupillary dilation, ataxia, posterior paresis, hyperesthesia along the back, or urinary incontinence.

Disorders of bone, kidney, and skin are also recognized in association with FeLV infection. Progressively developing multiple cartilaginous exostoses (osteochondromatosis) occur in cats, and FeLV has been consistently identified in blood and tissue. Glomerulonephritis has also been recognized in cats with oncornavirus infection. Glomerular lesions are of the immune complex type and may in fact be virally induced. Glomerular disease may be clinically inapparent, or it may cause overt clinical signs ranging from mild proteinuria to renal failure. The multicentric fibrosarcoma of skin and subcutaneous tissues of young cats is another disease related to FeLV. The disease is caused by the feline sarcoma virus (FeSV), a defective mutant of FeLV. FeSV infection is detected by the same tests used to detect FeLV, and all known isolates of FeSV contain a ten-fold excess amount of FeLV. More solitary fibrosarcomas in older cats are not usually associated with FeLV or FeSV infection.

Hypoplastic or aplastic anemia is a common long-term sequela of persistent FeLV infection. Unlike the transient anemia seen in some cats during the primary stage of the infection, anemia occurring in chronic FeLV-infected cats is usually progressive and fatal. In rare cases, the anemia may be intermittent. In some cases, it is a prelude to myeloproliferative disease. The anemia usually occurs from six months to three years or more after the initial infection and may

be slowly progressive for months before clinical signs occur. Erythrocytic indexes reveal that the predominant form of anemia associated with FeLV infection is normocytic-normochromic. In some cats, the hemogram may reflect pancytopenia, indicating that the entire marrow compartment is affected. Occasionally, the anemia is megaloblastic, and it may mimic vitamin B_{12} and folate deficiency. Macrocytic anemia of the hemolytic type or from blood loss has also been associated with FeLV infection. Finally, some cats may develop a low-grade depression anemia as a result of the debilitating nature of the disease itself — the so-called anemia of chronic disease or ineffective reutilization of iron.

In addition to diseases caused by virus, a large number of disorders are recognized in cats with concurrent FeLV infection. These are caused by microorganisms that are normally non-pathogenic or of a low order of pathogenicity in non FeLV-infected cats. The occurrence of these secondary diseases is presumably related to the immunosuppressive effects of the virus. Granulocytopenia, thymic atrophy, and suppression of antibody and cell-mediated immune responses have been associated with FeLV infection. Diseases potentiated by FeLV infection include hemobartonellosis, feline infectious peritonitis, upper respiratory tract infections, chronic cystitis, and chronic progressive polyarthritis. Chronic recurrent abscesses, periodontal gingivitis, tooth root abscesses, severe purulent otitis externa, intermittent enteritis, and peracute enterocolitis are other problems that often complicate FeLV infection. Given the wide range of disorders directly or indirectly related to FeLV infection, it is not surprising that 30 percent of all randomly tested chronically ill cats in some areas are infected with the virus.

It is important to remember that neoplasia accounts for only a small portion of the diseases related to FeLV. Even then, FeLV can only be isolated from 70 percent of cats with lymphoreticular neoplasms or myeloproliferative disorders. These virus-negative tumors may result from a latent effect of a previous FeLV infection, or they may be caused by other carcinogens. Many FeLV-infected cats have a normal life span without ever developing any illness, some will suffer from recurrent bouts of vague illness, and others will suffer from continuous low-grade illness for years before finally succumbing.

Treatment of FeLV-Related Diseases. There is some controversy over whether FeLV-infected cats should be treated or euthanatized. Owners must be warned that if they keep an infected cat alive, it should be confined in order to prevent infection from spreading to other cats. Although there is some expressed concern over the potential health hazard of FeLV to man, studies to date indicate that FeLV is not hazardous to humans. Ultimately, the decision to treat or euthanatize an animal is made on the basis of the type and severity of the disease, the feelings of the owner toward the animal, and the animal's potential for infecting other cats in the environment.

If an owner decides to treat an FeLV-infected cat, treatment is directed toward the disease at hand. Low-grade bacterial infections of the respiratory and intestinal tracts, abscesses, oral infections, or ear infections are treated in the same manner in which they would be treated in a non FeLV-infected cat. Anemia is managed with whole blood transfusions, low dose corticosteroids, and anabolic steroids used in combination with hematinics. Hemobartonellosis in FeLV-infected cats is treated with antimicrobial drugs; however, an underlying aplastic or hypoplastic anemia often complicates recovery. Lymphoid neoplasms are treated with chemotherapy, whereas myeloid neoplasms are less often treated because of their relative insensitivity to drugs.

Immunostimulants derived from *Corynebacterium parvum* or the bacillus of Calmette-Guerin (BCG), and synthetic agents such as levamisole, are being used by some veterinarians to treat FeLV-infected cats. Preliminary evidence suggests quite strongly that FeLV infection cannot be eliminated by such therapy. Although there are claims that immunostimulants will reduce the incidence of disease in FeLV-infected cats, this has not been substantiated in the literature at this time.

DIAGNOSIS OF FeLV INFECTION

The diagnosis of FeLV infection is made by detecting FeLV antigens in platelets and leukocytes in blood smears. This is done by an indirect fluorescent antibody procedure. Because up to 30 percent of all chronically ill cats can be infected with FeLV, not many FeLV-infected cats will be overlooked if 30 percent of the tests submitted are positive. Great deviations on either side of this figure suggest that cats are either too rigidly selected for testing or that the test is being used too indiscriminately.

PREVENTION AND CONTROL OF FeLV INFECTION

At present, the only means to control FeLV infection is by isolation or destruction of FeLV-infected cats. This approach requires constant monitoring and control of the cat population to insure that all FeLV-infected cats are eliminated. Although this method of control is practical for strictly confined cat populations, it is of limited benefit if cats are allowed to roam freely. When an infected cat is identified, all cats that are in contact with it should be tested. If the infection is endemic in the household or cattery, around 30 percent of the cats in the immediate environment will usually be infected. Negative cats in the environment are either incubating the infection or have been previously infected and are now immune. Without a determination of serum antibodies to FeLV, it is impossible to say whether a cat is susceptible, incubating the disease, or immune. When serology cannot be done, all negative cats should be retested at 12- to 20-week intervals over a period of 36 to 52 weeks. Virus-infected cats are removed from the environment after each testing. All cats in the cattery should test negative at least twice before the disease is assumed to be eliminated. At that point, all new cats should be virus negative on at least two tests done over a 12- to 20-week interval, and they should not be introduced into the cattery or household until all tests have been completed. The cat should also be kept isolated from all other cats during the quarantine period.

Although testing and removing cats are effective in eliminating the infection from confined cat populations, several factors can cause problems in rare instances. First, chronically infected cats occasionally cycle in the level of detectable viremia during the first several months of infection, so that they are negative at one testing and positive at another. This is why a negative cat should be tested several times over an extended period. Conversely, positive cats that are negative on one testing should not be assumed to be free of the virus until several more negative tests are obtained. A second problem with the test and removal procedure is caused by the long latent period between exposure and viremia that occurs in some cats. Latent periods as long as 32 to 52 weeks have been observed in a small percentage of cats. These cats could escape detection if the testing were limited to a shorter period. For these reasons, routine yearly or twice yearly testing is preferred, and new cats brought into the cattery should originate from FeLV-negative catteries that are also on a strict testing program. The prevention of feline leukemia virus infection by immunoprophylaxis is the goal of many researchers. Unfortunately, vaccines are only in developmental stages, and it is too soon to say whether they will be effective.

SEROLOGIC TESTS FOR FeLV INFECTION

Serologic tests for antibodies to FeLV or FeLV-induced antigens have been developed. The feline oncornavirus-associated cell membrane antigen (FOCMA)-antibody test detects serum antibodies to new cell surface antigens induced by the virus and not the virus itself. The virus neutralizing (VN) antibody test measures antibodies to the virus envelope antigens. The FOCMA test is commercially available; the VN test is still only a research tool. Commercially applicable tests for antibodies directed against the virus are in the development stages and should be of great aid to practitioners.

Because FOCMA is present on the surface of FeLV-transformed cells, antibodies against FOCMA are thought to protect infected cats against tumor development. Antibody to FOCMA does not react with the virus and thus does not influence viremia. Indeed, virus-infected cats with high FOCMA titers have a reduced risk of lymphosarcoma. It has not been shown to have protective value against other types of neoplasia or other FeLV-associated diseases. Because lymphosarcoma constitutes only a small proportion of FeLV-related diseases, the prognostic value of the FOCMA antibody test is limited.

Tests for virus-neutralizing antibodies, if they become commercially available, will have great value for practitioners. By utilizing tests that detect both virus and virus antibodies at the same time, it is possible to determine whether a cat is susceptible, previously infected, or viremic. A susceptible cat, or a cat incubating the disease, will be negative for both virus and virus antibodies. A previously infected cat will be negative for virus and positive for virus antibodies; an infected cat will be positive for virus and negative for virus antibodies. Precise knowledge of the cat's disease status will be valuable to catteries and multiple cat households because the emphasis of subsequent testing can be directed toward the susceptible animals and not the entire cat population. Cats that have been previously infected and have recovered can be kept in a breeding situation.

LYMPHOPROLIFERATIVE DISORDERS

Lymphoproliferative disorders include benign lymphoid hyperplasia, lymphocytosis, and overt neoplasia (lymphosarcoma). Lymphoproliferative disorders of the cat are almost always malignant and are associated with FeLV infection in 70 percent or more of the cases. There is a tendency for aged cats and cats with solitary lymphoid neoplasms to be virus negative, whereas young cats and cats with multicentric neoplasms are usually virus positive. We have not recognized tumor types that are invariably virus positive or negative. The incidence rate for lymphoid neoplasms has been estimated at 150 per 100,000 cats. There are two peaks in the age incidence, the first around two to four years and the second after eight years of age.

Lymphoproliferative disorders may be categorized anatomically, cytologically, or immunologically. Although such categorization aids in understanding disease pathogenesis and is useful in differential diagnosis, existing classification schemes have not been of great prognostic or therapeutic value. Lymphoid neoplasms are categorized anatomically into four major forms: anterior mediastinal (thymic), alimentary, multicentric, and blood (leukemia). Cytologically, lymphoid neoplasms are categorized as lymphoblastic, poorly differentiated lymphocytic, and differentiated lymphocytic. Histiocytic and mixed lymphohistiocytic forms have also been described. Immunologists have categorized lymphoid neoplasms on the basis of cell surface marker studies. Thymic lymphoid neoplasms are usually composed of T cells and alimentary lymphomas are usually composed of B-cells; multicentric lymphomas often lack B or T cell surface markers.

The anatomic classification is most widely used by clinicians. Although lymphosarcoma is usually categorized into one of the four anatomic types, it must be remembered that a given animal may have a composite disease of several forms and thus is categorized as miscellaneous. The thymic form of lymphosarcoma appears as a mass occupying the anterior thoracic cavity. The tumor involves thymus, sternal, and anterior mediastinal lymph nodes, and often causes effusion. More advanced lesions involve perihilar lymph nodes and lung parenchyma. Clinical signs include dyspnea and dysphagia. The elaboration of parathormone-like substance from an anterior mediastinal tumor causing hypercalcemia has been described in the cat.

Alimentary lymphosarcoma may involve the stomach, small or large intestine, and cecum. The terminal ileum is a frequent primary site. Tumors may arise from Peyer's patches, and local infiltration of the lamina propria and submucosa can cause segmental thickening of the gut and stricture. In other cats, the tumor infiltrates the gut wall diffusely. Mesenteric lymph nodes and the liver may also be involved. Clinical signs include intestinal obstruction, ascites, diarrhea, and melena. Malabsorption syndrome may result from diffuse bowel involvement.

The multicentric form of lymphosarcoma is

similar to the disease distribution in dogs, and virtually all peripheral and visceral lymphoid tissue is involved. Clinical signs include peripheral lymphadenopathy and symptoms relating to systemic involvement. Leukemia is the fourth anatomic form of lymphosarcoma. Discrete solid tumors are usually not present, and malignant cells are found in blood and bone marrow. Blood leukocyte counts may exceed 70,000 cells per cmm, and anemia is invariably present. Other hemogram findings frequently include thrombocytopenia and neutropenia.

In addition to the four major types, there are several miscellaneous forms. Neurolymphosarcoma is the most common of these. In this form, the neoplastic infiltrates usually occur in the extradural tissues of the spinal cord and nerve roots. Tumor infiltrates may cause individual nerve palsies, or when the spinal cord itself is involved, there may be sensory and motor deficiencies below the level of the lesion. Cutaneous lymphoma has been reported in cats. Lesions are multicentric and appear as macules or erythematous nodules. Anterior uveitis may result from infiltration of the iris and ciliary body. Solitary lymphoid neoplasms in sites such as the retrobulbar space, nasal or oral cavity, trachea, and kidney have also been described.

Myeloproliferative disorders

The myeloproliferative disorders are characterized by abnormal proliferations of hematopoietic cells. Specific myeloproliferative disorders recognized in the cat include granulocytic leukemia, monocytic leukemia, myelomonocytic leukemia, erythroleukemia, erythremic myelosis, reticuloendotheliosis, megakaryocytic myelosis, and myelofibrosis. Seventy percent or more of cats with myeloproliferative disorders are positive based on immunofluorescence for FeLV, and it is generally accepted that FeLV is the cause of the disease in these animals. Polycythemia rubra vera and eosinophilic and basophilic leukemias are rare, and the role of FeLV in these disorders is unknown. Mast cell leukemia is frequently categorized as a myeloproliferative disorder; the appearance of mast cells in blood is usually associated with a cutaneous or visceral solid tumor. Mast cell sarcomas do not appear to be related to FeLV infection.

Classification of the myeloproliferative disorders by specific cell type (e.g., granulocytic leukemia) implies that each disorder is a specific entity. There is considerable clinical and experimental evidence, however, demonstrating that simultaneous alteration of several bone marrow cell lines characterizes many of the myeloproliferative disorders. Simultaneous disturbances in granulopoiesis, erythropoiesis, and thrombocytopoiesis are often observed, and it may be more appropriate to view the myeloproliferative disorders as common stem cell disorders. Myeloproliferative disorders may change from one predominant cell type to another in blood; the progression of erythroleukemia to granulocytic leukemia has been described, blood smears may show alternating patterns of erythremic myelosis and reticuloendotheliosis, and myelofibrosis may develop ultimately in cats with myeloproliferative disorders.

The myeloproliferative disorders are characterized clinically by severe non-responsive anemia and hepatosplenomegaly. Some cats will have peripheral lymphadenopathy, reflecting extramedullary hematopoiesis. Diagnosis of the myeloproliferative disorders is dependent upon recognition of an increased number of mature and immature cells in blood and alteration of hematopoietic tissues. In some cats, abnormal cells are not recognized in blood, despite the presence of atypical or increased numbers of blast cells in marrow — a syndrome referred to as "aleukemic leukemia." Alternatively, disturbances in hematopoiesis (hemopoietic dysplasia) may precede the subsequent development of a classic myeloproliferative disorder (usually myeloid leukemia). These syndromes of preleukemia are well described in man and have been recognized in the cat. Laboratory abnormalities have dominated the clinical picture of preleukemia; anemia, leukopenia, and thrombocytopenia occurring singly or in various combinations are the most frequently recognized abnormalities. In none of these syndromes is there an excess of leukemic blast cells in either the bone marrow or the blood at the onset, and the conclusion that the condition was in fact preleukemic can only be made when the blood picture has progressed to an overt myeloproliferative disorder. Defining the onset of leukemia is difficult because the distinction between hemopoietic dysplasia and myeloid leukemia may not be clear cut.

Treatment of lymphoid neoplasms

The goals of therapy for lymphoid neoplasms are to provide palliative relief from symptoms and to prolong useful life. Currently employed methods of therapy include surgery, irradiation, and chemotherapy. The rare solitary lymphosarcoma may be managed effectively with localized forms of therapy such as surgery or irradiation. Lymphoid neoplasms are very radiosensitive, but their generalized nature

Table 1. *Induction-Remission Chemotherapy of Feline Lymphosarcoma Using a Combination of 4 Drugs*

Vincristine	0.5 mg/M² BSA° (0.1 mg)†, intravenously, once weekly for 8 weeks.
Cyclophosphamide	50 mg/M² BSA (12.5 mg), per os, every other day for 8 weeks
Cytosine arabinoside	100 mg/M² BSA (25 mg), intravenously, or subcutaneously once daily for 4 consecutive days of the first week of treatment
Prednisone	40 mg/M² BSA₂ (10.0 mg), per os, once daily for 1 week then 20 mg/M² BSA once daily every other day for 7 weeks (5.0 mg)

° M² BSA = square meters of body surface area. See appendix for conversion table of weight to surface area.
† Dose in parentheses is the approximate total dosage for a 4.8 Kg (10 lb) cat.

usually precludes this modality of treatment. Although widely used, data on the efficacy of drugs and drug schedules for treatment of feline lymphoproliferative disorders are limited. Similarly, the percentage of cats put into clinical remission and survival times from controlled studies have not been reported. Nevertheless, remission rates of 60 percent and one-year survival rates of 20 percent are commonly mentioned.

Chemotherapy has an established role in the treatment of lymphoproliferative disease in dogs and man, and the programs used for cats have been derived from favorable experience in these species. Chemotherapy is divided into three stages: induction of remission, maintenance, and relapse or recurrence therapy. All currently used methods of therapy differ somewhat in each of these stages, and undoubtedly further modifications will occur as our knowledge of existing drugs improves and as new drugs become available.

Prednisone, cyclophosphamide, cytosine arabinoside, and vincristine are drugs widely used to reduce the tumor mass and establish clinical remission. Although they may be used singly, combination therapy enhances their efficacy. All these drugs have different mechanisms of action and different toxicities, and they may in fact be synergistic in their effect. Remission is achieved when clinical signs of disease have disappeared and laboratory determinations fail to reveal the presence of tumor cell, which is usually two to six weeks. The induction-remission protocol for the treatment of feline lymphoid neoplasms used at the University of California Veterinary Medical Teaching Hospital is given in Table 1. Patient monitoring and supportive care are important. Bactericidal antibiotics are given if fever develops, and anticancer drugs are temporarily discontinued if leukopenia (less than 3500 leukocytes/ul) or thrombocytopenia (less than 50,000 platelets/ul) develops. These are detected by weekly complete blood counts. Cytotoxic drugs are not indicated if the cat is severely anemic or leukopenic. In such cases, prednisone and/or L-asparaginase are used initially until the marrow regenerates sufficiently to allow the use of the cytotoxic drugs.

If induction of remission cannot be achieved using the outlined schedule, it may be possible to induce remission with other drugs. These drugs include vinblastine, adriamycin, chlorambucil, and L-asparaginase (Table 2). Chlorambucil may be used instead of cyclophosphamide if cyclophosphamide-induced hemorrhagic cystitis develops.

Following induction of remission, maintenance chemotherapy is given. Drugs and dosages are similar to those used for induction of remission, except that drugs are given every second week, and later, if the disease is still in remission, they can be given every third week.

With time, tumor cells often become resistant to the drugs used in induction and maintenance therapy. Following relapse, a second remission may be difficult to attain. A second remission can sometimes be achieved by using the inducing drugs at the initial high dosages or by using alternative cytotoxic drugs.

Table 2. *Dosages of Alternative Cytoreductive Drugs*

L-asparaginase	8000 units/M²° BSA (2,000u)† IV daily for 5 days, then once weekly
Adriamycin	30 mg/M² BSA (8.0 mg) IV once every 21 days
Vinblastine	2.0 mg/M² BSA (0.50 mg) once weekly
Chlorambucil	2.0 mg/M² BSA (0.50 mg) per os, once daily for 4–6 days. For prolonged use, the dosage must be decreased

° M² BSA = square meters of body surface area. See appendix for conversion table of weight to surface area.
† Dose in parentheses is the approximate total dosage for a 4.8 Kg (10 lb) cat.

TREATMENT OF MYELOPROLIFERATIVE DISORDERS

The treatment of myeloproliferative disorders to date has been largely ineffectual, and few cats survive more than three months after the diagnosis has been made. Treatment is primarily supportive, and frequent fresh whole blood transfusions are often necessary to provide palliation from symptoms associated with anemia, leukopenia, and thrombocytopenia. Blast cells can be rapidly cleared from blood using drugs such as adriamycin, cytosine arabinoside, cyclophosphamide, or 6-thioguanine, singly or in combination, but severe anemia, neutropenia, and thrombocytopenia limit the long-term aggressive use of cytotoxic drugs. The authors' experience as well as the available literature on the treatment of myeloproliferative disorders suggests that chemotherapy as currently employed adds little to the life span of cats when compared with supportive therapy alone.

SUPPLEMENTAL READING

Cotter, S. M., Hardy, W. D. Jr., and Essex, M.: Association of the feline leukemia virus with lymphosarcoma and other disorders. J. Am. Vet. Med. Assoc. 166:449–454, 1975.

Essex, M., Cotter, S. M., Carpenter, J. L., Hardy, W. D., Hess, P., Jarrett, W., Schaller, J., and Yohn, D. S.: Feline oncornavirus associated cell membrane antigen. II, Antibody titers in healthy cats from pet households and laboratory colony environments. J. Natl. Cancer Inst. 54:631–635, 1975.

Essex, M., Hardy, W. D., Jr., and Cotter, S. M.: Naturally occurring persistent feline oncornavirus infections in the absence of disease. Infect. Immun. 11:470–475, 1975.

Essex, M., Sliski, A., Hardy, W. D., Jr., and Cotter, S. M.: Immune response to leukemia virus and tumor associated antigens in cats. Cancer Res. 36:640–645, 1976.

Hardy, W. D. Jr., Old, L. J., Hess, P. W., Essex, M., and Cotter, S. M.: Horizontal transmission of feline leukemia virus. Nature 244:266–267, 1973.

Hardy, W. D. Jr., Hess, P. W., MacEwen, E. G., McClelland, A. J., Zuckerman, E. E., Essex, M., Cotter, S. M., and Jarrett, O.: Biology of feline leukemia virus in the natural environment. Cancer Res. 36:582–588, 1976.

Hinshaw, V. S., and Blank, H. F.: Isolation of feline leukemia virus from clinical specimens. Am. J. Vet. Res. 38:55–57, 1977.

Hoover, E. A., Olsen, R. G., Hardy, W. D. Jr., and Schaller, J. P.: Horizontal transmission of feline leukemia virus under experimental conditions. J. Natl. Cancer Inst. 58:443–444, 1977.

Krakower, J. M., and Aaronson, S. A.: Seroepidemiologic assessment of feline leukemia virus infection risk for man. Nature 273:463–464, 1978.

Jarrett, W., Jarrett, O., Mackey, L., Laird, H., Hardy, W. Jr., and Essex, M.: Horizontal transmission of leukemia virus and leukemia in the cat. J. Natl. Cancer Inst. 51:833–841, 1973.

Mackey, L., Jarrett, W., Jarrett, O., and Laird, H.: Anemia associated with feline leukemia virus infection in cats. J. Natl. Cancer Inst. 54:209–217, 1975.

Pedersen, N. C., Theilen, G., Keane, M., Fairbanks, L., Mason, T., Orser, B., Chen, C., and Allison, C.: Studies of naturally transmitted feline leukemia virus infection. Am. J. Vet. Res. 38:1523–1531, 1977.

Pedersen, N. C.: Feline infection disease. In Proceedings of the 45th annual meeting American Animal Hospital Association, pp 125–146, 1978.

Rogerson, P., Jarrett, W., and Mackey, L.: Epidemiological studies of feline leukemia virus infection. I. Serologic survey in urban cats. Int. J. Cancer 15:781–785, 1975.

FELINE HEMOBARTONELLOSIS

JOHN W. HARVEY, D.V.M.
Gainesville, Florida

Feline hemobartonellosis or feline infectious anemia was first described as a disease entity in the United States in 1953. The disease appears to be more prevalent in certain geographic locations than others, but no scientific surveys have been conducted. The causative agent is a rickettsial epicellular parasite (Fig. 1) of erythrocytes designated *Haemobartonella felis. Haemobartonella* infections may produce clinical disease in the absence of, or concomitantly with, other diseases.

Upon microscopic examination of stained blood films, *Haemobartonella* organisms appear as basophilic coccoid, rod, or ring forms (Fig. 2). During the acute phase of the disease, organisms usually appear in the blood as discrete parasitemic entities. Although organisms often increase gradually in number over a period of one to five days, their disappearance from blood may occur in two hours or less. Cats that recover from the disease remain chronically injected. In chronically infected "carrier" cats, generally either no or only low numbers of organisms are present in blood. Strains of *H.*

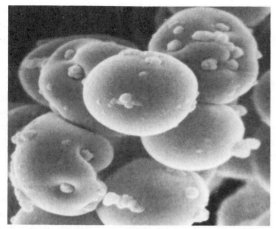

Figure 1. Scanning electron photomicrograph of erythrocytes from a cat infected with *H. felis*. (× 6,500. Photograph by Dallas Hyde.)

felis vary in pathogenicity, with some producing severe clinical disease and others producing few or no clinical signs.

TRANSMISSION

Experimentally, the infection has been transmitted by the intraperitoneal, intravenous, and oral routes. Dissemination of infection by blood-sucking arthropods such as fleas is considered by many to be the major natural mode of transmission, although such transmission has not been established experimentally. *H. felis* can be transmitted from female cats to their newborn offspring in the absence of arthropod vectors. Whether this transmission occurs *in utero,* via nursing, or by other means is not known. In addition, infections can be transmitted iatrogenically during blood transfusions. To insure that a prospective blood donor cat is not chronically infected, it is recommended that the cat be splenectomized and blood films be examined for organisms on alternate days for two weeks after splenectomy.

CLINICAL SIGNS

Acute hemobartonellosis can occur in cats of all ages but is reported to occur more frequently in males than in females. The most common clinical signs are depression, weakness, anorexia, weight loss, paleness of mucous membranes, and, at times, splenomegaly. Icteric mucous membranes are occasionally noted. Pyrexia occurs less than half of the time during parasitemias. In moribund cats, the rectal temperature is usually subnormal. Clinical signs are somewhat dependent on the rapidity with which anemia develops. If the anemia develops gradu-

ally, a cat may lose a considerable amount of weight but be bright and alert. If a precipitous drop in packed cell volume (PCV) occurs early in the disease, there may be little weight loss but marked depression occurs. Icteric mucous membranes are more likely to occur in the latter instance.

LABORATORY FINDINGS

Total and differential leukocyte counts are quite variable and of limited diagnostic assistance. Absolute monocyte counts are, however, frequently increased, and monocytes are often bizarre during the acute phase of the disease. Erythrophagocytosis by monocytes or macrophages may be observed if blood films are scanned at low magnification. The PCV is usually below 20 percent and frequently below 10 per cent before clinical signs of disease are apparent to the client.

The PCV is not always a good indicator of total erythrocyte mass in a cat with hemobartonellosis. Erythrocytes, sequestered in the spleen (primarily) and other organs when parasitized, may return to the general circulation following the disappearance of organisms from their surface. Consequently, the PCV may increase sharply after the disappearance of organisms from the blood. Repetitive parasitemias will cause progressive injury to erythrocyte membranes, however, and result in increased erythrocyte phagocytosis and destruction.

In most instances, by the time clinical signs of disease are apparent, there is peripheral blood evidence (polychromasia and reticulocytosis) of a regenerative bone marrow response to the anemia. Erythrocytes are usually macrocytic (MCV > 55 fl) and frequently hypochromic

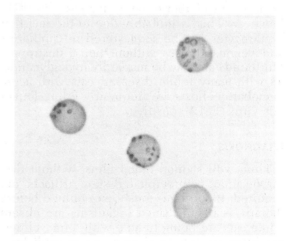

Figure 2. Peripheral blood from a cat infected with *H. felis*. Giemsa-stained film. (× 1800)

(MCHC < 30 per cent). Although nucleated erythrocytes and increased numbers of Howell-Jolly bodies are consistently observed in the circulation in feline hemobartonellosis, these findings are not reliable indicators of regenerative response in the cat. Howell-Jolly bodies are often observed in normal cats, and nucleated erythrocytes may appear in a wide variety of feline diseases.

The magnitude of the regenerative response observed in blood samples depends on the duration of the anemia. If the PCV decreases rapidly, the mean cell volume (MCV) may be normal, with little polychromasia and few reticulocytes present. Since two morphologic forms of reticulocytes have been described in cats, it is important to know what criteria a reference laboratory uses to count reticulocytes. Aggregate forms occur in a low proportion (0 to 0.4 per cent) of the erythrocytes in blood from normal cats. The percentage of aggregate reticulocytes correlates well with the percentage of polychromatophilic erythrocytes. A greater proportion (up to 10 per cent) of circulating erythrocytes in normal cats contains punctate foci of reticulum.

Autoagglutination is frequently observed in blood collection vials and capillary hematocrit tubes during early stages of acute hemobartonellosis. By the time clinical signs of disease are apparent, the direct Coombs' test will usually be positive. One must remember that only Coombs' reagents made specifically for cats can be used in this test. Plasma protein concentrations are usually in the normal range (6 to 8 gm/dl), but they may be increased. Icteric plasma is not consistently observed in feline hemobartonellosis. Icterus index values may be greater than two units within a day or two after a significant drop in PCV occurs. Icterus index values and bilirubin content are not always increased subsequent to rapid decreases in PCV, however. This is probably due to the fact that erythrocytes can be sequestered in capillaries and venous sinuses without being destroyed. Moribund cats may be markedly hypoglycemic. As with many feline diseases, cats with acute hemobartonellosis are frequently feline leukemia virus (FeLV) positive.

DIAGNOSIS

Thin, well stained blood films, without drying, fixation, or precipitated stain artifacts, are required. Blood films must be examined before therapy is begun, since organisms are absent while cats are being treated with tetracyclines. One must be able to differentiate Howell-Jolly bodies and basophilic stippling from organisms.

New methylene blue wet preparations are not recommended for demonstration of *H. felis* organisms because organisms are difficult to discern unless massive numbers are present.

H. felis organisms must also be differentiated from *Cytauxzoon* organisms, which have been recently described in cat erythrocytes. Clinically, hemobartonellosis and cytauxzoonosis may be difficult to differentiate. *Cytauxzoon* parasites are protozoa and have both a nucleus and cytoplasm. They are larger than *Haemobartonella* organisms and appear as rounded "signet rings" or oval "safety pin" bodies.

To make a clinical diagnosis of hemobartonellosis with any certainty, *H. felis* organisms must be observed in association with a regenerative anemia (in the absence of blood loss). These strict criteria have been recommended because parasites may be observed as an incidental finding in carrier cats with other diseases. The difficulty with these criteria is that although they are met during the clinical course of *Haemobartonella* infections, they may not be met in a given blood sample. If the PCV drops precipitously, a cat can be depressed and anemic for several days before a regenerative bone marrow response is evident. In addition, parasites are not constantly observed in the circulation during the acute phase of this disease. Acridine orange and direct immunofluorescent staining techniques are reported to be more sensitive than standard Romanowsky-type stains for demonstrating organisms. These tests have definite limitations, however, and are not available commercially.

THERAPY

Blood transfusions are probably not needed if the PCV is 15 per cent or greater. The necessity of a blood transfusion is related to the rapidity of onset of the hemolytic crisis. The physical appearance of the patient is an important consideration when one must decide if a transfusion is needed. If the cat is comatose, parenteral glucose may be indicated.

Cats should be treated orally for three weeks with oxytetracycline (20 mg/kg body weight, three times daily). In addition, treatment with a glucocorticoid such as prednisolone (1 to 2 mg/kg body weight, twice daily) is indicated based on evidence of immune-mediated injury to erythrocytes. The glucocorticoid dosage should be decreased gradually as desired increases in PCV are measured. Unless parasites are present in the circulation, it is impossible to differentiate hemobartonellosis from autoimmune hemolytic anemia. Consequently, the same therapeutic approach to both diseases is indicated. A majority of feline cases reported to have autoimmune hemolytic anemia in the past have, in fact, been treated with tetracyclines as well as glucocorticoids.

Thiacetarsamide sodium (1 mg/kg administered as two intravenous injections 48 hours apart) has been recommended in the past. Although thiacetarsamide is attractive as a drug for treatment of hemobartonellosis, it has not been approved for use in cats and appears to be less effective than previously reported. Chloramphenicol has also been recommended for the treatment of hemobartonellosis. Unfortunately, this drug produces significant (albeit reversible) bone marrow injury at therapeutic dosages recommended for cats. Consequently, it would not appear rational to use such a product when a regenerative erythroid response is desired. Neither tetracyclines nor thiacetarsamide appear to eliminate organisms from infected cats totally, and consequently "recovered" animals remain chronically infected.

PROGNOSIS

Without therapy, approximately one-third of cats with acute hemobartonellosis die from the disease. With proper therapy, virtually all cats recover from the acute phase but remain inapparent carriers. It has generally been accepted that chronically infected cats are prone to relapse into clinical disease following periods of "stress" when body defenses are weakened. Recent experimental studies, however, have not been able to verify this phenomenon of recrudescence.

SUPPLEMENTAL READING

Alsaker, R. D., Laber, J., Stevens, J., and Perman, V.: A comparison of polychromasia and reticulocyte counts in assessing erythrocytic regenerative response in the cat. JAVMA 170:39–41, 1977.

Harbutt, P. R.: A clinical appraisal of feline infectious anemia and its transmission under natural conditions. Aust. Vet. J. 29:401–404, 1963.

Harvey, J. W., and Gaskin, J. M.: Experimental feline haemobartonellosis. JAAHA 13:28–38, 1977.

Harvey, J. W., and Gaskin, J. M.: Feline haemobartonellosis: attempts to induce relapses of clinical disease in chronically infected cats. JAAHA 14:453–456, 1978.

Harvey, J. W., and Gaskin, J. M.: Feline haemobartonellosis. In Proceedings of the American Animal Hospital Association, 45:117–123, 1978.

Jain, N. C., and Keeton, K. S.: Scanning electron microscopic features of Haemobartonella felis. Am. J. Vet. Res. 34:697–700, 1973.

Maede, Y.: Studies on feline haemobartonellosis. IV, Lifespan of erythrocytes of cats infected with Haemobartonella felis. Jap. J. Vet. Sci. 37:269–272, 1975.

Maede, Y.: Studies on feline haemobartonellosis. V, Role of the spleen in cats infected with Haemobartonella felis. Jap. J. Vet. Sci. 40:141–146, 1978.

Maede, Y., and Hata, R.: Studies on feline haemobartonellosis. II, The mechanism of anemia produced by infection with Haemobartonella felis. Jap. J. Vet. Sci. 37:49–54, 1975.

Simpson, C. F., Gaskin, J. M., and Harvey, J. W.: Ultrastructure of erythrocytes parasitized by Haemobartonella felis. J. Parasitol. 64:504–511, 1978.

Small, E., and Ristic, M.: Haemobartonellosis. Vet. Clin. North Am. 1:225–230, 1971.

Wrightman, S. R., Kier, A. B., and Wagner, J. E.: Feline cytauxzoonosis: clinical features of newly described blood parasite disease. Feline Pract. 7:23–26, May, 1977.

BONE MARROW FAILURE IN THE DOG AND CAT

GENE P. SEARCY, D.V.M.

Saskatoon, Saskatchewan

Impaired hemopoiesis in the dog and cat is common, although illness attributable to inadequate marrow function occurs infrequently. The etiology and pathogenesis of severe marrow failure in the dog is frequently unknown and the prognosis is poor. The same is true for the cat, except in the case of the feline leukemia virus syndromes.

All marrow cells are descendents of multipotential stem cells, and differentiation toward a particular cell line — i.e., erythrocytes, granulocytes, or platelets — is a gradual process. The results of a marrow insult, therefore, depend upon the stage of differentiation of the injured cells — pancytopenia follows pluripotential stem cell injury, whereas anemia results from injury to the committed erythrocytic stem cell pool while granulocytes and megakaryocytes will be spared. The severity of hemopoietic arrest may vary, depending on the etiology; it could be slight to moderate — as in the anemia of chronic infection — or complete — as with certain chemical intoxications or irradiation injury.

Clinical findings often reflect the nature and extent of marrow injury. If depression of erythropoiesis is significant, the dog or cat will be presented with signs of anemia; e.g., poor exercise tolerance, pale mucous membranes, and tachycardia. Animals with persistent neutropenia may experience frequent infections. Thrombocytopenia results in small hemorrhages particularly evident at the gum-tooth junction and in the intestine. Detection of bleeding in these areas requires a diligent physical evaluation. Petechial hemorrhages on mucous membranes and in the subcutaneous tissue along the ventral abdomen of the patient may also be visible. Discussion of laboratory findings, pathogenesis, and therapy of the various forms of marrow failure follows.

ANEMIA

Renal Disease. Inadequate erythropoietin is probably the major cause of impaired erythropoiesis in chronic renal disease. The anemia is usually mild to moderate, but it can be more severe in younger dogs with renal disease, perhaps because they tolerate the uremic syndrome longer than do older dogs. The anemia is normocytic normochromic, and bone marrow examination reveals inadequate erythropoiesis with a high M:E ratio. Therapy should be designed to alleviate the renal disease. Little can be done to enhance erythropoiesis.

Liver Disease. Severe chronic liver disease in dogs and cats may result in mild to moderate anemia. Blood and marrow examination will be similar to that for chronic renal disease, and again, therapy must be aimed at the primary disorder.

Inflammation. Most inflammatory states result in some impairment of erythropoiesis, the significance of which varies with severity and duration of the inflammation. Blood smears reveal normocytic normochromic erythrocytes with increased numbers of leptocytes. The latter are most impressive when the smear is scanned at low magnification. The bone marrow has decreased erythropoietic activity and a high M:E ratio. Iron stores are usually increased. The pathogenic mechanisms are unclear; however, iron reutilization for erythropoiesis from destroyed erythrocytes is impaired. Since this is the principal source of iron for normal hemoglobin synthesis, and because hemosiderin iron is very slowly mobilized, the impaired iron reutilization is significant. Evidence would suggest that in chronic inflammation, iron is more readily taken up by macrophages and remains sequestered in the monocyte-macrophage system. These animals will have low serum iron levels with increased storage iron.

Therapeutic measures directed toward the anemia are usually futile until the inflammatory state has resolved. Administration of iron would be expected to have little effect, as it also will be sequestered in the monocyte-macrophage system.

Neoplasia. The debilitation resulting from neoplastic disease is usually accompanied by a mild to moderate anemia. The pathogenesis of impaired erythropoiesis may be similar to that of chronic inflammation.

Anemia Secondary to Drug Toxicity. Long-term therapy with anticonvulsant drugs such as diphenylhydantoin may result in a macrocytic normochromic anemia because of interference with folate metabolism (Lewis, 1977). Hematologic tests will reveal a mild to moderate anemia with an elevated MCV ranging from 80 to 95 fl. As anticipated, red cells are large, and some have abnormal nuclear maturation evident as increased numbers of Howell-Jolly bodies and budding metarubricyte nuclei. Folic acid is necessary for nucleic acid synthesis, and interference with this pathway results in impaired nuclear maturation. Asynchronous maturation of nucleus and cytoplasm in erythrocyte precursors is termed "megaloblastic transformation." In severe cases, these changes are visible in the peripheral blood but are always more evident in bone marrow.

Although there are reports of reversible marrow suppression and ultrastructural changes in red cell mitochondria resulting from administration of chloramphenicol to dogs and cats (Watson et al., 1978), these appear not to have significantly discouraged its use. If long-term administration of chloramphenicol is planned, red cell numbers should be monitored periodically, and if a decline is noted, the drug should be withdrawn.

NEUTROPENIA

Viral Diseases. The best example of viral-induced neutropenia is that which occurs in feline panleukopenia. The virus causes marrow necrosis but because of the short life span of neutrophils, neutropenia is the most significant finding. A recently described parvovirus-like gastroenteritis of dogs is also accompanied by marked leukopenia (Appel et al., 1978). Other viral diseases of dogs and cats are associated with variable degrees of neutropenia; however, the effects of these viruses on granulocyte kinetics are not clear. Early in the course of canine distemper, a mild to moderate leukopenia is often observed, which Schalm (1975) has attributed to generalized atrophy and necrosis of lymphatic tissue. It is likely, however, that some interference with neutrophil production or release from the bone marrow contributes to the leukopenia, especially in view of the fact that the stress experienced by these animals would be expected to induce a neutrophilia. The duration of viral neutropenia appears to be short, and superimposed bacterial infections result in neutrophilia.

Cyclic Neutropenia in Gray Collie Dogs. These dogs are usually presented because of recurring infections. Dunn et al. (1977) have shown that mitosis of the multipotential stem cell is cyclic, occurring at 12-day intervals, but because of the short neutrophil life span, neutropenia is the most significant occurrence in the peripheral blood.

THROMBOCYTOPENIA

Estrogen Toxicity. Although estrogen toxicity may result in pancytopenia, thrombocytopenia is the most common manifestation of this toxicity and is usually reversible. Dogs are usually presented because of hemorrhage typical of thrombocytopenia, and they reveal a normal PCV or mild anemia, marked neutrophilia, and profound thrombocytopenia. The dogs should be hospitalized in order to prevent trauma and to monitor the hematologic changes.

If the dose of estrogen was very high, dogs may go on to develop pancytopenia. Blood transfusions and antibiotics should then be administered as required; however, the prognosis at this stage is poor. As reported by Schall and Perman (1975), the dose of diethylstilbestrol should not exceed 0.5 mg/kg or a total dose of 20 mg. Estradiol is considered to be approximately ten times as potent as diethylstilbestrol.

PANCYTOPENIA

Pancytopenia is a useful term describing anemia, leukopenia, and thrombocytopenia. Clinical findings reflect inadequate numbers of one or more of these cells. Careful examination of blood and bone marrow is essential in these cases.

Aplastic Anemia. This condition is best defined as pancytopenia with hypocellular marrow. Examination of a blood smear will reveal normocytic normochromic anemia. In some animals, macrocytosis and reticulocytosis may be evident, but this is inadequate to compensate for the anemia. Neutropenia ranges from slight to severe and most neutrophils are mature. The degree of thrombocytopenia is variable, but usually there are fewer than 60,000 per microliter and most of the platelets are small.

Bone marrow aspiration is usually difficult, but smears should be prepared from any material aspirated into the needle. Several attempts to aspirate marrow should be made at various sites. If one obtains marrow tissue, it will contain fusiform cells resembling fibroblasts and occasionally a few macrophages. Frequently, capillaries are prominent within the stromal network. There are often increased numbers of hemosiderin-filled macrophages that can be easily observed in unstained marrow at low magnification. There is a striking paucity of hemopoietic cells, although the presence of a few recognizable erythrocyte and granulocyte precursors helps to indicate that the tissue being examined is bone marrow. The presence of pancytopenia and this type of bone marrow aspirate is consistent with a diagnosis of aplastic anemia. If marrow tissue cannot be aspirated after repeated attempts, one must resort to core biopsy or removal of a rib. Core biopsy is carried out by using large-bore needles with stylets — for example, Jamshidi needles.[1]

It is the author's impression that the incidence of canine aplastic anemia is increasing (Rich, 1979). As mentioned, estrogen toxicity may cause aplastic anemia. Another well defined etiology of this form of marrow failure is *Ehrlichia canis* infection. Demonstration of the parasite in circulating monocytes or tissue imprint, or a positive indirect fluorescent antibody test on serum, is necessary for diagnosis. When *Ehrlichia canis* suspects are leukopenic, buffy coat smears should be examined. In most cases of canine aplastic anemia, however, no etiology can be found. Observations in human medicine and work with experimental animals have incriminated various chemicals as causing marrow destruction. Despite the difficulty in associating chemical intoxication with aplastic anemia in dogs and cats, owners should be asked to investigate this possibility thoroughly. Erslev (1977), in a discussion of human aplastic anemia, noted that many of the chemicals used in the household and in the cosmetic industry contain complex benzene radicals, and the widespread use of insecticides, fertilizers, and food supplements makes even our "daily bread" suspect.

Observations on pure red cell aplasia in man have led to the hypothesis that there may be immunologic rejection of erythroid tissue. This has been supported by the positive response by some patients to adrenal steroid therapy (Erslev, 1977). Given these observations, it is tempting to suggest that some form of immune-mediated injury of less differentiated stem cells would result in pancytopenia.

---

[1]Kormed, Inc., 2510 Northland Drive, St Paul, MN 55120

Therapeutic management of aplastic anemia is as frustrating as understanding its etiology and pathogenesis. The practitioner must apply a combination of supportive and myelostimulatory therapy until remission occurs, or, more frequently, until animals succumb to infections or owners request euthanasia. Supportive therapy includes restricted exercise, (preferably cage rest), antibiotics as required to control infection, and blood transfusions. The decision to administer blood should depend on clinical evaluation of the patient as well as enumeration of red cells. In this way, transfusion requirements are reduced, since many of these animals tolerate anemia very well.

Administration of androgens is indicated in these animals despite the fact that most cases do not respond. The lack of suitable alternatives, as well as an occasionally good response to drugs such as oxymetholone, justifies this form of therapy (Fletch et al., 1975). The low success rate of androgen therapy in canine aplastic anemia may relate to the advanced state of the disease when detected. Successful therapy requires several weeks of drug administration; the suggested dosage for oxymetholone is 2 mg/kg per day (Fletch et al., 1975).

Myeloproliferative Disorders. Interference with hemopoiesis by neoplastic proliferation of one or more bone marrow cell lines is difficult to classify because the results are so variable. In the earlier stages of the disease, the peripheral blood may only reflect abnormalities in the cell line directly involved; e.g., an animal may have evidence of neoplasia in the granulocytic series without anemia or thrombocytopenia. More frequently, however, the disease has progressed to the point at which there is more generalized interference with hemopoiesis.

The feline leukemia virus-associated myelo-proliferative disorders are usually characterized by severe non-regenerative anemia. Diligent examination of blood smears may reveal a few or several poorly differentiated bone marrow cells. Sometimes these cells enable one to make a diagnosis; e.g., erythremic myelosis, granulocytic leukemia, or lymphocytic leukemia. More often, bone marrow examination is necessary to characterize the type of neoplasm and the degree of marrow involvement.

Granulocytic leukemia in dogs frequently results in anemia. Clinically significant thrombocytopenia is less common. Similar results occur with widespread marrow infiltration by lymphosarcoma. The severity of hemopoietic impairment caused by these neoplastic marrow disorders is an important factor to be considered when contemplating appropriate therapeutic measures.

SUPPLEMENTAL READING

Appel, M.J.G., Cooper, B.J., Freisen, H., and Carmichael, L.E.: Status report: canine viral enteritis. J. Am. Vet. Med. Assoc. 173:1516–1518, 1978.

Dunn, C.D.R., Jones, J.B., Jolly, J.D., and Lange, R.D.: Progenitor cells in canine cyclic hematopoiesis. Blood 50:1111–1120, 1977.

Erslev,A.J.: Aplastic anemia. In Williams, W.J., Beutler, E., Erslev, A.J., and Rundles, R.W. (eds.): *Hematology*, 2nd ed. New York. McGraw-Hill Book Co., 1977.

Fletch, S.M., De Geer, T.R., and Catherwood, J.: Impaired erythropoiesis in two dogs. Bull. Am. Soc. Vet. Clin. Path. IV. 31. 1975.

Lewis, G.E., and Huxsoll, D.L.: Canine ehrlichiosis. In Kirk, R.W. (ed.): *Current Veterinary Therapy VI*. Philadelphia, W.B. Saunders Co., 1977.

Lewis, H.B.: Management of anemia in the dog and cat. In Kirk, R.W. (ed.): *Current Veterinary Therapy VI*. Philadelphia, W.B. Saunders Co., 1977.

Rich, L.J.: Personal Communication, 1979.

Schall, W.D., and Perman, V.: Diseases of the red blood cells. In Ettinger, S.J. (ed.): *Textbook of Veterinary Internal Medicine*, Vol. 2. Philadelphia, W.B. Saunders Co., 1975.

Schalm, O.W., Jain, N.C., and Carroll, E.J.: *Veterinary Hematology*, 3rd ed. Philadelphia, Lea & Febiger, 1975.

Watson, A.D.J., and Middleton, D.J.: Chloramphenicol toxicosis in cats. Am. J. Vet. Res. 39:1199–1203, 1978.

HEINZ BODY HEMOLYTIC ANEMIAS AND METHEMOGLOBINEMIAS

GEORGE E. LEES, D.V.M.

St. Paul, Minnesota

Hemoglobin in an erythrocyte is constantly subjected to oxidative stress by the oxygen being transported. Normally, erythrocyte metabolism functions to produce reducing substances, which continually work to offset oxidative events that threaten the structure and function of hemoglobin. Excessive accumulation of oxidized forms of hemoglobin occurs when oxidative stress cannot be met by sufficient metabolic production of reducing substances. This situation may occur when certain erythrocyte enzyme deficiencies exist, thus limiting metabolic capacity. It may also occur when oxidative stress is increased, usually by the administration of drugs or chemicals that have oxidative properties. Although patients that have certain erythrocyte enzyme deficiencies are more sensitive to oxidant drugs, sufficiently potent oxidizing drugs may overwhelm even normal erythrocyte metabolism.

Oxidation of hemoglobin to an extent that exceeds the reductive capacity of erythrocyte metabolism may cause methemoglobinemia or Heinz body hemolytic anemia or both. Methemoglobin is an oxidized form of hemoglobin in which the iron atoms are in the ferric (Fe^{+3}) rather than the ferrous (Fe^{+2}) state. Although methemoglobin cannot carry oxygen, it remains soluble in the cytosol of the erythrocyte. Heinz bodies are also composed of oxidized hemoglobin; however, in this instance, the major problem is oxidation of sulfhydryl (—SH) groups. Normally, sulfhydryl groups help to maintain the protein's tertiary structure. When its sulfhydryl groups are irreversibly oxidized, hemoglobin loses its tertiary structure (becomes denatured) and loses its solubility. The insoluble hemoglobin precipitates and aggregates in the erythrocyte, forming the structure recognized morphologically as a Heinz body.

Certain kinds of hemoglobin are more easily or less reversibly oxidized. Normal cat hemoglobin forms Heinz bodies more readily than that of other species. This propensity has been attributed to the fact that cat hemoglobin molecules have more sulfhydryl groups than do hemoglobin molecules of other animals and man. Additionally, although analogous conditions have not yet been recognized in animals, many abnormal types of hemoglobin (hemoglobinopathies) that are unusually sensitive to oxidation occur in man.

There are two major divisions of erythrocyte metabolism. The Embden-Meyerhof pathway (EMP) is the more important relative to reduction of methemoglobin because it generates reduced nicotinamide adenine dinucleotide (NADH). Reduction of methemoglobin is primarily accomplished by methemoglobin reductase that is NADH dependent, which couples the reaction to the EMP. The pentose phosphate pathway (PPP) is the second major division of erythrocyte metabolism. Enzyme systems primarily responsible for protection against oxidative reactions leading to Heinz body formation are the PPP and peroxidase systems. These systems are linked because reduced nicotinamide adenine dinucleotide phosphate (NADPH), upon which the peroxidase system is dependent, is produced in the mature erythrocyte only by the PPP.

HEINZ BODY HEMOLYTIC ANEMIA

Heinz body hemolytic anemias have been recognized in both dogs and cats. In man, deficiencies of enzymes in the PPP or peroxidase system that predispose affected patients to Heinz body formation have been documented. Analogous conditions, however, have not yet been recognized in animals. All the reported cases of Heinz body hemolytic anemia in dogs and cats have been known or suspected to be caused by excess oxidative stress in the face of normal erythrocyte metabolism.

A large number of drugs and chemicals have been reported to cause Heinz body formation in man. Many cause problems only in patients with defective erythrocyte metabolisms. Relatively few agents, however, have been reported to cause Heinz body hemolytic anemia in com-

417

panion animals. These include methylene blue, acetaminophen, and phenazopyridine in cats and methylene blue and onions in dogs. Disulfide compounds appear to be the toxic agents in onions that cause Heniz body formation.

Because of their propensity for Heinz body formation, normal cats often have small Heinz bodies in their erythrocytes. Sometimes, sick cats that are not receiving oxidant drugs will have an increase in size and number of Heinz bodies observed in their red blood cells. This phenomenon has been attributed to autointoxication. Accelerated erythrocyte destruction and evidence of regenerative erythrocytic response have been observed occasionally in this clinical setting.

Clinical signs most consistently manifested by patients with Heinz body hemolytic anemia are non specific and include depression, weakness, lethargy, and anorexia. Other signs, however, may be observed depending upon the rate and mechanism of erythrocyte destruction, the severity of the resultant anemia, and concomitant abnormalities. The oral mucosa may be pale if anemia is sufficiently severe. Intravascular hemolysis may occur, producing hemoglobinemia and hemoglobinuria. The latter may be misinterpreted as hematuria. Erythrocyte destruction by reticuloendothelial cells may produce icterus. Heinz bodies, however, are not necessarily metabolized to bilirubin, and dogs with Heinz body anemia usually have normal serum bilirubin levels. Icterus has more frequently been observed in cats intoxicated with acetaminophen or phenazopyridine. In these patients, however, the toxicosis produces hepatic injury in addition to Heinz body anemia. Icterus has not been a prominent feature of methylene blue-induced Heinz body hemolytic anemia in cats. Methemoglobinemia also occurs in acetaminophen and phenazopyridine toxicoses and may cause cyanosis or brownish discoloration of the blood. Facial edema is frequently an additional clinical feature of acetaminophen toxicosis in cats. The specific cause of this change is unexplained. Two dogs with Heinz body anemia have manifested brief syncopal or seizure-like episodes.

Diagnosis of Heinz body hemolytic anemia is not difficult. Careful examination of blood smears, including use of a vital stain such as new methylene blue, will typically reveal a triad of hematologic findings: Heinz body formation, evidence of erythrocyte damage, and regenerative erythrocitic response. Heinz bodies stain intensely with new methylene blue. They vary in size, number, and location

within erythrocytes. Initially, several small aggregates form in the middle of the cell. These then coalesce, forming larger aggregates, and migrate peripherally to attach to the inner surface of the cell membrane. Heinz bodies do not always take up Romanowsky stains (e.g., Wright's stain) and may appear as pale areas within the cell, particularly when located near the cell membrane. Heinz bodies may deform cell contour, producing blunt projections that appear to bud from the cell, but these stain similarly to the remainder of the erythrocyte. In cats with Heinz body hemolytic anemia, the Heinz bodies tend to be large and single. In dogs, however, Heinz bodies are frequently multiple and of varied size.

Morphologic evidence of erythrocyte damage is more readily seen in blood smears prepared with Romanowsky stains. Numerous damaged, misshapen erythrocytes (poikilocytosis) and fragments of erythrocytes (schistocytes) are frequently seen. Cells that have lost a portion of their cell membrane may appear small and round (spherocytes) or may have a crescent-shaped piece missing ("bite cells"). Intensification of erythropoiesis (regenerative erythrocytic response) is indicated by large, polychromatophilic cells. These immature cells are reticulocytes when stained with new methylene blue. Increased numbers of nucleated red blood cells may also be seen in the peripheral blood. Evidence of intensified erythropoiesis requires some time to develop. Thus, if seen early in its course, Heinz body anemia may lack signs of regeneration. Conversely, when concomitant methemoglobinemia is severe, erythropoiesis may be stimulated before Heinz body formation and hemolysis produce a substantial reduction of the hematocrit.

Patients that have uncomplicated Heinz body anemia usually require no specific therapy, provided access to or administration of the offending oxidizing agent is stopped. Heinz body hemolytic anemia tends to be self limiting because immature erythrocytes have higher enzyme levels than do mature cells. Once the regenerative response begins, the hematocrit usually rises (often rapidly) because the new young cells are better protected against Heinz body formation. Blood transfusion, however, may be necessary for patients that develop anemia or methemoglobinemia of life-threatening severity. When Heinz body hemolytic anemia is complicated by dehydration, hepatic or renal toxicity, or concomitant unrelated disease, these entities require appropriate specific or supportive treatment as well.

METHEMOGLOBINEMIA

Methemoglobinemia caused by deficiency of NADH-dependent methemoglobin reductase has been described in several dogs. Cyanosis and exercise intolerance have been the most prominent clinical signs. In contrast to patients that have methemoglobinemia associated with anemia caused by oxidative stress, patients with methemoglobin reductase deficiency do not form Heinz bodies and may actually have compensatory polycythemia. Blood obtained from patients with methemoglobinemia is brownish in color and does not turn red upon exposure to oxygen. The degree of methemoglobinemia associated with methemoglobin reductase deficiency generally does not exceed one-third of the total hemoglobin but has occasionally been observed as high as 40 per cent. Degrees of methemoglobinemia in excess of such levels are indicative of acquired disease. In phenazopyridine toxicosis of cats, for example, methemoglobin levels approaching 50 per cent were observed.

Patients with milder degrees of methemoglobinemia caused by methemoglobin reductase deficiency may be successfully managed by restriction of exercise. More severely affected patients, however, may require treatment with methylene blue. For this purpose, methylene blue serves as an artificial electron carrier that couples an enzymatic reduction of methemoglobin to NADPH produced by the PPP. Excessive administration of methylene blue may deplete NADPH, leading to Heinz body formation. Therefore, the drug must be used cautiously, and monitoring for development of Heinz bodies is advised. Although ascorbic acid produces non-enzymatic reduction of methemoglobin, this drug is less effective than methylene blue for the treatment of methemoglobinemia.

SUPPLEMENTAL READING

Finco, D. R., Duncan, J. R., Schall, W. D., and Prassem K. W.: Acetaminophen toxicosis in the Cat. JAVMA 166:469–472, 1975.

Harvey, J. W., and Kornick, H. P.: Phenazopyridine toxicosis in the cat. JAVMA 169:327–331, 1976.

Lees, G. E., Polzin, D. J., Perman, V., Hammer, R. F., and Smith, J. A.: Idiopathic Heinz body hemolytic anemia in three dogs. J. Am. Anim. Hosp. Assoc. Accepted for Publication, 1979.

Letchworth, G. J., Bentinck-Smith, J., Bolton, G. R., Wootton, J. F., and Family, L.: Cyanosis and methemoglobinemia in two dogs due to a NADH methemoglobin reductase deficiency. J. Am. Anim. Hosp. Assoc. 13:75–79, 1977.

Schalm, O. W.: Heinz body hemolytic anemia in the cat. Feline Practice 7 (6):30–33, 1977.

Schechter, R. D., Schalm, O. W., and Kaneko, J. J.: Heinz body hemolytic anemia associated with the use of urinary antiseptics containing methylene blue in the cat. JAVMA 162:37–44, 1973.

CANINE LYMPHOSARCOMA*

E. GREGORY MacEWEN
New York, New York

Lymphosarcoma (LSA) is the most common lymphoproliferative canine neoplasm, accounting for about 5 to 7 percent of all tumors seen in the dog. The annual incidence of canine LSA is 24 cases per 100,000 dogs at risk. LSA may occur in dogs of any age but is seen most frequently in dogs over 5 years of age. There is no known sex predilection. Certain breeds such as boxers, cocker spaniels, and fox terriers develop LSA more frequently than do other breeds. In the author's clinic, German shepherds, Scottish terriers, and Golden retrievers are most commonly affected.

*This work was supported by Grant Number R01-CA-19072, awarded by the National Cancer Institute, DHEW; The Cancer Research Institute, Inc., and the Bodman Foundation.

ETIOLOGY

The etiology of canine LSA is unknown. Although viruses are known to cause LSA in several animal species, for example the cat, there is no conclusive evidence that viruses cause LSA in dogs. In humans, lymphoproliferative tumors are associated with immune deficiency syndromes and long-term immunosuppressive therapy in transplantation patients.

In the dog with LSA, it has been shown that there is a suppression of both the humoral and cellular immune response.

DIAGNOSIS

The diagnosis of LSA is usually made based on the histologic examination of a lymph node biopsy, although it may be possible to make a diagnosis from the examination of tissue from such sites as the liver, spleen, bone marrow, and skin. Gentle handling of biopsy specimens and good fixation and staining techniques are important for an accuracte diagnosis. The entire lymph node should be removed, leaving the capsule intact to maintain the architecture. Care should be taken to avoid lymph nodes from reactive areas, such as the submandibular lymph nodes. Impression smears can be made from a carefully cut lymph node to help establish a presumptive diagnosis.

The lymphomas can be histologically described as nodular or diffuse, depending upon the growth pattern of the cells as seen under low-power magnification. They can be further subdivided into two main subtypes: histiocytic — when the tumor is derived from the primitive reticulum cells — and lymphatic — when the tumor is derived from the lymphocytes. A mixed, lymphocytic-histiocytic pattern can also be seen.

Clinical features

Lymphosarcoma can develop in any organ, but there are four clinically recognized forms based on the gross distribution of disease. In order of decreasing occurrence they are (1) multicentric, (2) alimentary, (3) anterior mediastinal, and (4) the unclassified cutaneous form. The signs of LSA are variable. Dogs often present with localized or generalized lymph node enlargement and the tonsils may or may not be enlarged. Massive lymphadenopathy may be present and may result in obstruction of the lymph vessels, leading to edema of the face or extremities. Spleen and liver involvement may also occur. There may be gastrointestinal involvement; if it is diffuse, it may cause a malabsorption syndrome, and if it is nodular, it may cause vomiting or diarrhea. The lung parenchyma can also be involved. Among the patients presented to The Animal Medical Center (New York), approximately 25 percent have disease in the lung at the time of diagnosis.

The cutaneous unclassified form of LSA may take the form of non-specific erythematous patches or single to multiple raised nodules. These lesions are usually non-pruritic but may be complicated by secondary bacterial infections.

Hematologic findings are variable and frequently within the normal range. Many patients have a leukocytosis of 20,000 to 30,000 white cells per cubic millimeter, with a predominence of neutrophils. As the disease progresses, the bone marrow may become involved and neoplastic lymphocytes may be detected in the peripheral blood. Approximately 30 to 40 percent of the dogs presented to The Animal Medical Center have bone marrow involvement at the time of diagnosis. Anemia associated with marrow infiltration can also be seen. In a few cases, an autoimmune hemolytic anemia may occur.

Serum electrophoresis reveals monoclonal paraprotein spikes in 5 to 6 percent of dogs with lymphoproliferative tumors, excluding those with multiple myeloma. The monoclonal proteins may be IgG, IgA, or IgM. It is important for the management of the patient to know if a monoclonal gammopathy is present (Hurvitz, 1977).

Clinical staging

A staging system has recently been adopted by the World Health Organization (WHO) and the Veterinary Cancer Society (VCS) (Table 1). Clinical studies are needed to determine the prognostic significance of this new staging system. The extent of disease is determined by (1) the clinical history and a physical examination, (2) radiographic examination of the chest and abdomen, (3) liver and kidney function, (4) a complete blood count, and (5) a bone marrow aspiration and a lymph node biopsy.

Treatment

The aim of therapy is to control the disease process and extend the life of the dog with as few undersirable side effects as possible. LSA has a poor prognosis and is usually a rapidly fatal disease. The average survival time of dogs with multicentric LSA, without treatment, is less than one month.

A few basic concepts are important in patient management:

1. The lymphocytic cell types are more responsive to chemotherapy than are the histiocytic cell types
2. Combination chemotherapy is more effective than single agent chemotherapy
3. Dogs that achieve complete remission survive significantly longer than do dogs that have a partial remission
4. It is more beneficial to maintain a first remission than to try to attempt a second remission
5. Paraneoplastic conditions (e.g., hypercalcemia) associated with LSA must also be managed, in addition to administering chemotherapy for the neoplastic disease
6. Concurrent medical problems, liver disease, or renal insufficiency will influence

Table 1. *Lymphosarcoma and Lymphatic Leukemia in Domestic Mammals**§

CLINICAL STAGES
FINAL HISTOLOGIC DIAGNOSIS_____

Species_____
Case number_____ Date_____
Name of owner_____
Age_____ Sex_____ Breed_____
Body weight_____ lbs._____ kgs
(1 kg = 2.2 lbs)

ANATOMIC TYPE
  A. Generalized
  B. Alimentary
  C. Thymic
  D. Skin
  E. Leukemia (True)†
  F. Others (including solitary renal)

STAGE (to include anatomic type)
  I. Involvement limited to a single node or lymphoid tissue in a single organ‡
  II. Involvement of many lymph nodes in a regional area (± tonsils)
  III. Generalized lymph node involvement
  IV. Liver and/or spleen involvement (± Stage III)
  V. Manifestation in the blood and involvement of bone marrow and/or other organ systems (± Stages I–IV)

Each stage is subclassified: those without systemic signs and those with systemic signs

*Excluding myeloma
†Only blood and bone marrow involved
‡Excluding bone marrow
§Approved by World Health Organization, Geneva, April 1978

the drugs, dosage, and method of administration of chemotherapy.

A number of protocols for chemotherapy have been used to treat canine LSA (Table 2). The protocol being evaluated in the author's clinic consists of vincristine and L-asparaginase administered on day 1, cyclophosphamide on day 7, vincristine on day 14, and methotrexate on day 21. After one cycle (day 21), the cycle is repeated. If the dog is in complete remission

Table 2. *Drug Combinations Used in Canine LSA*

DRUG	DOSAGE		NO. DOGS	MEAN SURVIVAL (*Days*)	REFERENCE
Prednisone	2.0 mg/kg orally for 7 days the 1.0 mg/kg daily		19	184	Squire (1973)
Cyclophosphamide (Cytoxan®)	5.0 mg/kg/day orally for 7 days then 2.5 mg/kg daily				
Vincristine (Oncovin®)	0.03 mg/kg, IV every 14 days				
Prednisone	10 mg/m.² BSA twice daily for 7 days	} A	19	211	Madewell (1975)
Cyclophosphamide (Cytoxan®)	50 mg/m.² BSA 4 consecutive days wkly				
Vincristine (Oncovin®)	0.5 mg/m.² BSA single dose				
Cyclophosphamide (Cytoxan®)	As above	} B			
6-Mercaptopurine (Purinethol®)	50 mg/m.² BSA daily				
Methotrexate (Lederle)	2.5 mg/m.² BSA b.i.d. once wkly				
Vincristine (Oncovin®)	0.025 mg/kg I.V. Week 1	} C	59	235 (median)	MacEwen (1979)
L-asparaginase	400 IU/kg I.P. Week 1				
Cyclophosphamide	10 mg/kg I.V. Week 2				
or					
Chloramibucil (Leukeran)	1.4 mg/kg PO Week 2				
Vincristine	0.025 mg/kg I.V. Week 3				
Methotrexate	0.8 mg/kg I.V. Week 4				

A, Induction of remission. B, Maintenance therapy. C, Repeat cycle, starting on week 5.
*The usual method of expressing drug dosages is by body weight (i.e., mg/kg). Dosage based on body-surface area (BSA) in square meters (m.²) may be a more reliable method to administer chemotherapeutic agents in the dog because of the wide variation in body size. See appendix for conversion table of weight to BSA for dogs.

after one cycle, the drugs can be administered every 10 to 14 days thereafter. Orally administered prednisone (0.5 to 2mg/Kg PO) daily or on alternate days can also be added to this regime. Chlorambucil (1.4mg/Kg PO) can be given in bolus form as a substitute for the cyclophosphamide. This substitution will reduce the incidence of hemorrhagic cystitis associated with cyclophosphamide. The complete remission rate is around 80 percent. In a study of 59 dogs treated with this protocol, the median survival time was found to be 235 days; 25 percent of the dogs in remission survived one year and 10 percent of the dogs in remission survived 2 years. In this series, no dog died of drug-related causes.

Immunotherapy, using an autogenous tumor vaccine composed of lymph node cells mixed with Freund's adjuvant, in combination with chemotherapy, was reported to increase the survival time to a median of 336 days in 11 dogs versus a median survival of 196 days in 9 dogs not treated with the vaccine. Other studies using immunotherapy agents such as levamisole and BCG are also being done. At The Animal Medical Center, passive immunotherapy (the administration of blood constituents from healthy animals) was evaluated in dogs and cats with lymphoproliferative tumors (MacEwen, 1977). Studies have shown that there is a factor in normal blood that can cause destruction of malignant lymphocytes. At present, this form of therapy is experimental and cannot be routinely used in the clinical setting.

At The Animal Medical Center, a small number of patients with solitary gastrointestinal LSA involving the stomach or large bowel have been treated with the combination chemotherapy protocol, and the results have been very encouraging. Survival times have been greater than 18 months for most dogs treated. From preliminary studies done with a small number of patients, the diffuse form of gastrointestinal LSA appears to be poorly responsive to chemotherapy. Results of treating cutaneous LSA, including two cases with mycosis fungoides, have yielded poor results.

HYPERCALCEMIA

Hypercalcemia can be one of the major problems in the management of canine LSA since it can cause serious damage to the kidneys. Approximately 15 percent of dogs with LSA have elevated amounts of serum calcium (greater than 12 mg percent). The usual presenting signs of hypercalcemia are polydipsia, polyuria, muscle weakness, and renal insufficiency. Hypercalcemia is caused by the production of physiologically active substances that stimulate bone resorption. Current studies (Heath et al., 1979) have shown that this substance is not a parathyroid-like hormone or a prostaglandin derivative. The substance appears to be a factor similar to the osteoclast stimulating factor elaborated by myeloma cells.

The most critical problem associated with hypercalcemia is the effect on the kidneys. Hypercalcemia can cause degeneration and necrosis of the renal tubules and the eventual development of nephrocalcinosis. This can lead to progressive renal failure.

Therapy of hypercalcemia is directed toward (1) restoring hydration with intravenous saline; (2) maintaining urine output; (3) inducing calcium excretion with saline diuresis and diuretics (furosemide); (4) reducing the calcium intake, and (5) administering antitumor therapy (corticosteroids and chemotherapy drugs) to eradicate the malignant cells elaborating the substances causing the hypercalcemia. Cases that do not respond to the above measures can be given a cytotoxic agent, mithramycin, in single doses of $2\mu g/Kg$ for one to two days.

PROGNOSIS

Canine LSA is a fatal disease. Without treatment, it will rapidly lead to death. The response of the disease to chemotherapy varies with each individual animal. Although chemotherapy is not curative, the life of many animals can be prolonged with minimal side effects. The optimal chemotherapy protocol for canine LSA has not been determined but with appropriate chemotherapy, one can expect an average survival time of 8 months after diagnosis (with a range of 4 to 24 months). (Refer to conversion table of weight to body-surface area for dogs in the appendix.)

SUPPLEMENTAL READING

Crow, S.E., Theilen, G.H., Benjamin, E., Torten, M., Henness, A.M., and Buhles, W.C.: Chemoimmunotherapy for canine lymphosarcoma. Cancer 40:2102–2108, 1977.

Heath, H., Weller, R.E., and Mundy, G.R.: Canine lymphosarcoma: a model for study of the hypercalcemia of cancer. Endocrinology (submitted 1979).

Hurvitz, Arthur I.: Gammopathies. In Kirk, R.W. (ed.): *Current Veterinary Therapy VI.* Philadelphia, W.B. Saunders Co., 1977.

MacEwen, E.G., Patnaik, A.K., and Wilkins, R.J.: Diagnosis and treatment of canine hematopoietic neoplasma. Vet. Clin. North Am. 7:105–118, 1977.

MacEwen, E.G., Brown, N., Patnaik, A.K., et al.: Cyclical combination chemotherapy of canine lymphosarcoma. In preparation, 1979.

MacEwen, E.G.: Immunotherapy of cancer. In Kirk, R. W. (ed.): *Current Veterinary Therapy VI.* Philadelphia, W.B. Saunders Co., 1977.

Madewell, B.R.: Chemotherapy for canine lymphosarcoma. Am. J. Vet. Res. 36:1525–1528, 1975.

Squire, R.A., Bush, M., Melby, E.C., Neely, L.M., and Yarbough, B.: Clinical and pathologic study of canine lymphoma: clinical staging cell classification, and therapy. J. Nat. Cancer Inst. 51:565–572, 1973.

CANCER CHEMOTHERAPY*

E. GREGORY MacEWEN, V.M.D.

New York, New York

Since many neoplasms metastasize or are disseminated, local therapy such as surgery and radiation has limited effectiveness. Cancer chemotherapy is particularly suited to these situations. This is one reason why cytotoxic chemotherapy has evolved into a major modality of cancer management during the last 25 years.

The clinician's major problem in cancer chemotherapy is selectivity. Rapidly growing normal tissues, such as cells of the bone marrow, lymphoid system, gastrointestinal tract, and epithelial tissues, are particularly susceptible to the lethal effects of chemotherapy. When considering chemotherapy, one of the important factors is the ratio of therapeutic benefits to the toxicity. Most pet owners will not permit their pets to be treated with a form of therapy that is excessively toxic and is only minimally beneficial.

For most neoplastic conditions, chemotherapy should be thought of as a palliative and not a curative measure. Clinical studies are underway to determine how to improve the effectiveness of cancer chemotherapy in small animal oncology.

PHARMACOKINETICS

The access of the drug to the target cell is dependent on many factors. Intrinsic properties of a drug include the ionic charge, lipid solubility, and molecular size. These factors can affect absorption, volume distribution, diffusion, protein-binding effects, and, finally, excretion.

The blood brain barrier, located in the brain's capillary endothelium, is important because it limits the ability of chemotherapeutic agents to enter the central nervous system and kill malignant tumor cells. A few drugs such as corticosteroids, the lipid-soluble nitrosourea drugs (BCNU and CCNU), and, to a limited degree, cytosine arabinoside can cross the blood-brain barrier. Methotrexate is one of a few agents that can be injected directly into the central nervous system via intrathecal administration.

It is important to consider the method of drug excretion when planning treatment protocols. For example, since methotrexate is primarily excreted through the kidneys, the dose must be lowered in azotemic patients. Biliary excretion is significant for drugs such as adriamycin and vincristine, and the dose must be lowered in animals with liver disease.

Interaction between drugs is also of considerable importance in patient management. Combination chemotherapy will be discussed in a later section, but non-cytotoxic drugs can influence the effectiveness and toxicity of cytotoxic drugs. For example, phenobarbital induces the hepatic microsomal enzymes that activate cyclophosphamide, whereas chloramphenicol inhibits them.

CELL KINETICS

The patterns of cell kinetics have been studied extensively during the past two decades. Understanding the phases of proliferation of a malignant cell is important in order to plan possible therapeutic strategies (Fig. 1).

Most chemotherapeutic agents, like gamma radiation, exert their maximal lethal effect on proliferating and replicating cells. Agents can be classified according to their effects in the cell cycle:

1. Agents that kill cells, whether they are in the cell cycle or not (non–cell cycle specific). Gamma radiation and alkylating agents are examples.
2. Agents that kill cells in only one phase of the cell cycle — e.g., mitosis or S phase (cell cycle specific). This group includes vincristine and methotrexate.
3. Agents that kill cells at any stage of the cell cycle (cell cycle non-specific.) Agents such as 5-fluorouracil, adriamycin, and cyclophosphamide act in this way.

COMBINATION CHEMOTHERAPY

In general, combinations of cytotoxic agents are more effective than the same agents used in a sequential manner if the agents employed have different modes of action and different toxicities.

*This work was supported by Grant Number RO1-CA-19072, awarded by the National Cancer Institute, DHEW; The Cancer Research Institute, Inc., and the Bodman Foundation.

423

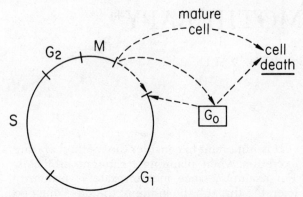

Figure 1. The mitotic cycle is illustrated on the left. Growing cells can be in cycle or out of cycle (G_0). Most chemotherapeutic agents have their maximal effects on cells in cycle. The G_1 phase represents the beginning of the mitotic cycle. S denotes the period of DNA synthesis, a period in which cells are very susceptible to chemotherapy agents, especially the antimetabolites. G_2 represents a brief postsynthetic resting phase, which is followed by the period of mitotic division (M). The time required for cells to complete one cycle is variable. The cell cycle generation time for most leukemic cells is between 50 and 70 hours.

Certain drug combinations appear to be antagonistic; for example, L-asparaginase given before methotrexate may reduce the effectiveness of methotrexate. The L-asparaginase causes impairment of DNA synthesis and thus the cells are less susceptible to methotrexate.

Cells in the G_0 phase (resting) are most resistant to the cytotoxic effects of chemotherapy. Combination chemotherapy protocols are designed to include drugs that act at different stages of the cell cycle. For example, cyclophosphamide is effective during the G_1 and G_2 phases, methotrexate is most effective on cells in the S phase, and vincristine blocks cells during mitosis (M phase). This combination of three drugs is commonly used in multiple chemotherapy protocols.

There are two basic approaches to the design of combination drug protocols. One is based on the biochemical or cell kinetics approach. That is, drugs that have different mechanisms of action attack the cell at multiple sites in the biosynthetic pathways and do not have similar or additive toxic effects. The second approach is mainly empirical and is based on the clinical observation that certain neoplastic conditions are "sensitive" to various drugs, and using them in combination has increased their effectiveness.

RATIONALE FOR ADJUVANT CHEMOTHERAPY

Many solid tumors must be considered to be a systemic disease at the time of diagnosis. These include osteosarcomas, malignant melanomas, malignant mast cell sarcomas, and breast cancer in some patients. Adjuvant chemotherapy is directed toward killing cells that have already metastasized from the original tumor.

It is hypothesized that reduction in the tumor burden by surgery or radiation will increase the effectiveness of adjuvant chemotherapy since (1) a reduced tumor burden will stimulate more cells to undergo cell division and thus become more sensitive to the chemotherapy agents and (2) smaller tumors, because of anatomic relationships (e.g., blood supply), have a greater chance of coming into contact with the chemical agents. As a result of these factors, the reduced tumor burden is more likely to be curative.

DRUG RESISTANCE

One of the major problems of clinical cancer chemotherapy is the resistance of cancer cells to chemotherapy drugs. There are two major causes of drug resistance — natural and acquired. Natural resistance is defined as "no objective response despite sufficient treatment to evoke toxicity." Acquired resistance occurs when an initial response is evoked followed by progressive disease despite continuation of treatment. Possible factors in acquired resistance include:

1. *Biochemical mechanisms:* impaired drug transport into cells; alternative enzymatic pathways may develop, a decreased requirement for the product that is inhibited by the agent and increased DNA repair.
2. *Cell kinetics:* cells with long doubling times and cells in the "resting" phase (G_0) tend to be resistant.
3. *Pharmacokinetics:* the chemotherapeutic agents may not be able to reach the cancer cells. A classic example is the blood-brain barrier, which tends to prevent the vast majority of drugs from entering the brain and cerebral spinal fluid.
4. Miscellaneous factors such as inadequate duration of therapy, suboptimal doses, etc. can all lead to resistance.

TOXICITY

Since most chemotherapeutic agents kill cells in a non-selective manner, rapidly growing cells will also be killed, and this gives rise to toxic side effects. The toxic effects most commonly encountered are mild alopecia, anorexia, vomiting, and diarrhea. Life-threatening toxic effects include bone marrow depression (leucopenia, thrombocytopenia, and anemia) and gastrointestinal ulceration. Most chemotherapy protocols must therefore allow for a "rest" inter-

Table 1. *Specific Agents Used in Cancer Treatment*

AGENT	PRINCIPAL ROUTE OF ADMINISTRATION	USUAL DOSE	MAJOR TOXIC EFFECTS
Alkylating Agents Cyclophosphamide	Oral	50 mg/m² daily	Bone marrow depression
(Cytoxan)	IV	10 mg/Kg weekly	Cystitis
Chlorambucil (Leukeran)	Oral	3–6 mg/m² daily 0.1–0.2 mg/Kg daily	Bone marrow depression
Melphalan (Alkeran)	Oral	3.0 mg/m² daily for 7–10 days, repeat 7– 10 day cycle every 2–3 weeks; 0.05–0.1 mg/Kg daily	Bone marrow depression
Busulfan (Myleran)	Oral	4.0 mg/m² daily 0.1 mg/Kg daily	Bone marrow depression Pulmonary fibrosis
Thiotepa®	IV or Intracavitary	0.2–0.5 mg/m² single dose— repeat weekly or 0.2– 0.5 mg/Kg daily for 5 days — repeat cycle every 3 weeks.	Bone marrow depression
Antimetabolites Methotrexate	Oral	2.5 mg/m² daily	Vomiting, Bone marrow depression
	IV	0.8 mg/Kg weekly	
	IV (high dose)	5 gm/m² q 3 wks with 15 mg Leucovorin q 6 hr for 3 days	Renal failure
6-Mercaptopurine (6-MP, Purinethol)	Oral	50 mg/m² daily 2 mg/Kg daily	Bone marrow depression
5-Fluorouracil (5-FU)	IV	100 mg/m² weekly 2–5 mg/Kg weekly	CNS signs Do Not Use in Cats
6-Thioguanine (6-TG)	Oral	1 mg/Kg daily	Vomiting Bone marrow depression
Cytosine arabinoside (Ara-C, Cytosar)	IV SQ	100 mg/m² daily for 4 days repeat cycle at 3 week intervals 30 mg/Kg weekly	Bone marrow depression
Antibiotics Bleomycin (Blenoxane)	IV or SQ	10 mg/m² daily for 4 days then 10 mg/m² weekly to max. dose 200 mg/m²	Pulmonary fibrosis
Doxorubicin (Adriamycin)	IV	30 mg/m² IV q 3 wks.	Bone marrow depression cardiomyopathy at cumulative doses of >250 mg
Plant Alkaloids Vincristine (Oncovin)	IV	0.5–0.8 mg/m² weekly 0.0125–0.025 mg/Kg weekly	Locally irritating Peripheral neuropathy
Vinblastine (Velban)	IV	3 mg/m² weekly or 0.1– 0.5 mg/Kg weekly	Bone marrow depression Peripheral neuropathy

Continued on next page

Table 1.   *Specific Agents Used in Cancer Treatment* (Continued)

AGENT	PRINCIPAL ROUTE OF ADMINISTRATION	USUAL DOSE	MAJOR TOXIC EFFECTS
Miscellaneous Agents o,p'-DDD (Mitotane)	Oral	50 mg/Kg daily to effect	Diarrhea
L-asparaginase	Intraperitoneal	10,000–20,000 I.U./m² weekly or 400 IU/Kg weekly	Anaphylaxis
Imidazole Carboxamide (DTIC)	IV	200 mg/m² for 5 days repeat for 5 days every 3 weeks	Bone marrow depression
Hydroxyurea (Hydrea)	Oral	40 mg/Kg daily	Bone marrow depression

val between drugs to allow for bone marrow and immunologic recovery; drugs should be given cyclically and intermittently.

No chemotherapeutic drug should be used until the veterinarian fully understands the mode of action, type of toxicity, and method of administration of the drug.

SPECIFIC AGENTS USED IN CANCER CHEMOTHERAPY

A large number of agents with anti-tumor effects are available. Those presently being used for the management of neoplasms in the dog and cat are listed in Table 1.

SUPPLEMENTAL READING

Chabner, B. A., Myers, C. E., Coleman, E. N., and Johns, D. G.: The clinical pharmacology of antineoplastic agents. N. Engl. J. Med. 292:1102–1112; 1159–1168, 1975.

Greenspan, E. M. (ed.): *Clinical Cancer Chemotherapy.* N.Y., Raven Press, 1975.

Hess, P. W., MacEwen, E. G., and McClelland, A. J.: Chemotherapy of canine and feline tumors. J. Am. Anim. Hosp. 12:350–358, 1968.

Mauer, A. M.: Cell kinetics and practical consequences for therapy of acute leukemia. N. Engl. J. Med. 293:389–393, 1975.

IMMUNOTHERAPY OF MALIGNANT DISEASE*

E. GREGORY MacEWEN, V.M.D.

New York, New York

The role of the immune system in oncogenesis and in the defense against neoplastic cell growth is an area of intensive study in current cancer research. There has been much controversy over the role of the immune system in the control of cancer, as it can prevent development in some instances and stimulate cell growth in others.

*This work was supported by Grant Number R01-CA-19072, awarded by the National Cancer Institute, DHEW; The Cancer Research Institute, Inc., and the Bodman Foundation.

IMMUNOLOGIC SURVEILLANCE

As cells undergo malignant transformation, certain alterations can occur on the cell surface that distinguish these cells from normal, nontransformed cells. The changes are called "tumor specific antigens (TSA)" when they occur in the surface membrane. It has been shown that tumors induced by chemical carcinogens possess unique individual antigens, whereas virally induced tumors carry shared or common antigens. Tumor-associated antigens have been identified in a number of spontaneous tumors, and in human and a few canine and feline tumors. In man, tumor antigens have been identified in bladder carcinomas, malignant melanomas, osteogenic sarcomas, renal carcinomas, and nasopharyngeal carcinomas. In the cat, cells transformed by the feline leukemia virus (FeLV) have a TSA termed "FOCMA" — feline oncornavirus cell membrane–associated antigen. Antibodies can be produced that will react with FOCMA and prevent lymphosarcoma/leukemia development in cats. There is suggestive evidence of a TSA in canine osteosarcomas.

The concept of immunosurveillance states that malignant cells, which possess TSA, can elicit an immune response that leads to their destruction in much the same manner as that by which a homograft is destroyed. Evidence both supports and contradicts this concept.

EVIDENCE IN FAVOR OF IMMUNE SURVEILLANCE

Aging is associated with a decline or decay of both humoral and cell-mediated immune functions, and there is an increased incidence of cancer in old animals. There is an increase in the incidence of carcinogen-induced tumors in mice experimentally immunosuppressed with antilymphocyte serum. Clinical observations in man also support the concept of immune surveillance: (1) spontaneous regression of malignant disease occurs and (2) tumors infiltrated by lymphocytes usually have a more favorable prognosis than tumors without such infiltration. Women with breast cancer who have a predominance of lymphocytes in the regional lymph node have a better prognosis than those with a lymphocyte depletion pattern. Patients who are able to mount a vigorous cutaneous delayed hypersensitivity reaction to recall antigens or to newly encountered antigens have a better prognosis than patients with no reactions.

Malignancy is associated with the degree of immunodeficiency, either primary or acquired. In people with a primary immunodeficiency, the expected incidence of cancer may be 100 to 1000 times that of people with no immunodeficiency. Acquired immunodeficiency or suppression, such as is seen in organ transplantation patients, increases the risk of malignancy 25 times.

EVIDENCE THAT CONTRADICTS IMMUNE SURVEILLANCE

The increase in the incidence of cancer associated with aging may be associated with longer exposure to exogenous carcinogens or changes in the target cells that make them more suscep-

tible to carcinogens. Mice born without thymus-dependent immune functions do not have an unusually high incidence of either spontaneous or chemically induced tumors. These animals do possess naturally occurring cytotoxic antibody, which can afford them protection from tumor development.

The increase in neoplasia associated with immunodeficiency may be associated with the damage to the reticuloendothelial system following chronic antigenic stimulation rather than with impaired surveillance. The increase in cancer associated with chronic immunosuppression may be due to the carcinogenic effects of the immunosuppressive drug or activation of a latent oncogenic virus.

ANTITUMOR IMMUNE MECHANISMS

Sensitized lymphocytes can make direct contact with tumor cells, attach to them, and directly induce damage resulting in cell death. Cell damage is enhanced by the release of soluble mediators called lymphokines. These include lymphotoxins and migration inhibitory factors (MIF). MIF can attract macrophages, and once "activated," the macrophages can release factors causing tumor cell destruction. These include enzymes and a soluble mediator called tumor necrosis factor (TNF). Macrophages can also cause direct destruction of tumor cells by phagocytosis. B-lymphocytes can produce cytotoxic antibodies (IgM) that act directly on the tumor cell, or tumor cells may be killed by another antibody-dependent mechanism. Antibody (IgG) may attach to the specific antigen on the tumor cell, and B-lymphocytes with a receptor for the Fc fragment of the IgG immunoglobulin are then activated to kill the cell. This has been termed "antibody-dependent lymphocytotoxicity."

ESCAPE MECHANISMS

A variety of mechanisms have been proposed to explain how tumor cells can escape the recognition and destruction of a normal functional immune system. Certain physical factors, such as a stromal layer around the tumor, may prevent access of immune lymphocytes to a tumor. Certain areas of the body, particularly the brain, spinal cord, and anterior chamber of the eye, are considered to be "immune sanctuaries." Neoplastic cells may produce a substance (sialomucins) that can coat the antigens on the surface to prevent recognition. Exposure to small amounts of antigens may induce tolerance, thus allowing the tumor non-recognition as foreign by the immune system. This phenomenon has been termed "sneaking through."

A possible escape mechanism that has been characterized in a mouse leukemia antigen system called the TL system has been termed "antigenic modulation." When antibody becomes bound to the TL antigens on the leukemia cell surface, it suppresses the expression of these antigens. This prevents immunologic recognition.

The intensity of the antitumor response is also very important. The immune response can be "biphasic," in which low levels of antibody tend to stimulate, while a higher level can be inhibitory to tumor growth.

One of the most effective escape mechanisms is mediated by antibody (IgG)-antigen (tumor-associated) complexes. These complexes can cover the antigenic sites on the tumor cell and block its recognition by T-lymphocytes as a result of steric hindrance. These complexes are termed "blocking factors." They can also circulate and flood the immune system to block further antitumor responses. These blocking factors can act locally, associated with the tumor, or they can have systemic immunosuppressive effects.

Certain substances produced by the tumor cells have been identified in patients with Hodgkin's disease, multiple myeloma, and various solid tumors. These factors have been shown to be antibody-like polypeptides and prostaglandins, and they can be directly suppressive to lymphocytes, whereas others can stimulate T-suppressor cells, which then suppress other lymphocytes.

Finally, certain secondary factors can affect the immune response and thus allow tumor cells to escape. It has been shown in a spontaneous leukemia in mice (AKR) that despite the presence of specific antibody, no tumor cell destruction occurs because the mice are complement deficient. Tumor cell destruction can be achieved by exogenous administration of complement (C5). A similar situation has been documented in cats that have a protective level of FOCMA antibody, but because of low complement levels, the cats develop lymphosarcoma/leukemia. One method of immunotherapy is to supply exogenous sources of complement and other blood constituents.

IMMUNOTHERAPY

Immunotherapy is an attempt to modulate or stimulate the immune system to a specific antitumor response aimed at the destruction of tumor cells or an alteration in the behavior of the growing tumor. Certain factors are thought to be necessary for the most effective response to immunotherapy. These include (1) minimal-residual disease (since it is usually easier to control), (2) immunogenic tumor, (3) immunologically competent patient, (4) tumor accessible to immune substances such as antibodies or cells (lymphocytes), and, ideally, (5) appropriate facilities and techniques available to monitor the effects of immunotherapy on the immune system.

There are two main types of immunotherapy: active and passive.

ACTIVE IMMUNOTHERAPY

Active immunotherapy involves the use of agents or vaccines that can specifically or non-specifically stimulate the immune system. Specific tumor vaccines can be killed tumor-cell preparations, fragments of tumor cells, or isolated tumor-specific or tumor-associated antigens. Recent efforts have been directed at mixing tumor cell preparations with non-specific adjuvants such as Freund's adjuvant, bacille Calmette-Guerin (BCG), and viruses. The vaccines can be administered intradermally, subcutaneously, and by intralymphatic infusions. Tumor vaccines have shown benefit in humans with lung cancer and acute myelogenous leukemia. In dogs, positive results have been reported in canine lymphosarcoma.

Non-specific immunotherapy has been studied more than other forms of immunotherapy. The two major classes of non-specific immune stimulators or modulators are the biologic agents and the chemical agents. (See Table 1 for details on the commonly available agents, clinical uses, dosages, and toxicity). Most biologic agents are either living or killed bacteria that are highly antigenic. They can have both local and systemic effects on the immune system. The disadvantage of biologic agents includes local irritating effects such as ulceration, abscessation, and inflammation. Systemic effects can include fevers, nausea, vomiting, and shock. It is difficult to control and standardize the quality of biologic agents, and thus variation in effectiveness is common. Because of this diversity in quality control, there have been efforts to develop synthetic chemical immunomodulators

Levamisole is a chemical immunomodulating agent that has been used widely as an anthelmintic in animals and man. Levamisole is known to restore cell-mediated immune responses in compromised hosts. It does not stimulate the immune response above normal levels. Levamisole improves T cell– or macrophage-dependent functions such as delayed-type hypersensitivity, graft-versus-host

Table 1.   *Non–Specific Immunomodulators*

AGENT	MECHANISM OF ACTION	POTENTIAL CLINICAL USES	UNIQUE FEATURES
Biologic Modulators			
Bacille Calmette-Guerin (BCG)°	Stimulates macrophages and lymphocytes Delayed hypersensitivity reaction (T cell)	Melanoma (man) Lymphosarcoma (with chemotherapy) Osteosarcoma (with amputations)	Living, attenuated *Mycobacterium bovis* organism
Corynebacterium parvum†	Stimulates macrophages and phagocytosis Acts primarily through B cells	Lung carcinoma (man) Wide variety of tumors in experimental animals	Formalin killed No exotoxins or endotoxins Safe Dose: 0.1 mg–1 mg/Kg IV weekly
Mixed bacterial vaccine (MBV)	Stimulates macrophages and T cells Endotoxic effect	Wide variety of solid tumors, sarcomas and feline mammary carcinomas	Mixture of *Serratia marcescens* and *Streptococcus pyogenes*
Methanol extraction residue of BCG (MER)	Stimulates macrophages, T and B cells	Lung cancer (man) Osteosarcoma (dog)?	BCG skeletal wall Intradermal (1.25 mg)
Chemical Modulators			
Imidothiazoles (Levamisole) (TBZ)‡	Immune modulator Normalizes T cell function	In leukemia, may have some anti-tumor effects May augment chemotherapy in treated leukemia patients Immune recovery after chemotherapy Granulomatous disease (feline eosinophilic granulomas) Chronic pyodermas	Oral administration safe at 5 mg/Kg body weight (3 times/week)

°BCG. Tice Strain, Research Foundation, 70 West Hubbarb Street, Chicago, Illinois 60610.
†*C. parvum.* Burroughs Wellcome (7 mg/cc.), 3030 Cornwallis Road, Research Triangle Park, North Carolina 27709
MBV. Farberfabriken Bayer, Wuppertal, Germany
   Levamisole HCl — Pitman-Moore, Inc., Washington's Crossing, New Jersey 08560
‡Thiabendazole-Mintezol—Merck Sharp & Dohme, West Point, Pennsylvania 19486

reaction, and clearing of blood colloidal particles. It has several advantages over the biologic immunoadjuvants: oral administration, known pharmacology, and good tolerance by animals.

PASSIVE IMMUNOTHERAPY

Passive immunotherapy involves the administration of the mediators of immunity. These include immune lymphocytes, specific antibody, and serum factors such as complement, interferon, transfer factor, and immune RNA preparations. (It is not the scope of this article to discuss all the current approaches to passive immunotherapy. A few selected references have been given at the end of this chapter.)

One form of passive immunotherapy that has been extensively studied in the author's clinic is termed "blood constituent therapy (BCT)." BCT is the administration of normal blood constituents (plasma, serum, whole blood, and an eluate of fresh plasma) to treat dogs and cats with lymphoproliferative diseases (Kassel et al., 1977). The salient features of this therapy are that (1) large amounts of normal blood components are necessary (15–20 mg/Kg) and they must be administered frequently every two to three days and (2) the infusion must be given within four hours of blood collection. To date, this method of immunotherapy must be considered investigational, and studies are underway to isolate and purify the appropriate antitumor factors in normal blood.

IMMUNE RESTORATION

Replacement of the patient's immune system can be achieved by bone marrow transportation. This technique is being used to treat various types of primary immunodeficiency conditions, aplastic anemias, and leukemias. Bone marrow transplants have been performed in dogs but the technique is too experimental for clinical use.

Immunotherapy is a new and potentially promising aspect of cancer therapy. Its effectiveness has not been fully evaluated and it still must be considered experimental. Caution must be exercised because immune modulation or immune potentiation could, under some circumstances, stimulate rather than retard tumor growth. A number of clinical trials are underway in human and veterinary patients, and those results must be fully analyzed before immunotherapy can be considered as an accepted form of cancer therapy.

SUPPLEMENTAL READINGS

Kassel, R.L., Old, L.J., Day, K.K., MacEwen, E.G., and Hardy, W.D., Jr.: Plasma-mediated leukemia cell distruction: current status. Blood Cells 3:605–621, 1977.
MacEwen, E.G.: An immunologic approach to the treatment of cancer. Vet. Clin. North Am. 7:65–75, 1977.
Old, L.J.: Cancer immunology. Scient. Amer. 236:62–79, 1977.
Terry, W.D., and Windhorst, D. (eds.): *Immunotherapy of Cancer: Present Status of Trials in Man.* New York, Raven Press, 1978.

Section
6

DERMATOLOGIC DISEASES

R. E. W. HALLIWELL
Consulting Editor

Autoimmune Skin Diseases 432
The Differential Diagnosis of Facial Dermatitis 436
Canine Nasal Solar Dermatitis 440
Subcorneal Pustular Dermatosis and Dermatitis Herpetiformis 443
The Management of Flea Allergy Dermatitis 446
The Diagnosis of Canine Atopic Disease 450
The Treatment of Canine Atopic Disease 453
Drug Eruption 458
Otitis Externa 461
Canine Pododermatitis 467
Crusting Dermatoses in Cats 469
Zinc-Responsive Dermatoses in Dogs 472
Subcutaneous and Opportunistic Mycoses, the Deep Mycoses,
    and the Actinomycetes 477
Hereditary Hair and Pigment Abnormalities 487
Feline Alopecias 490
Canine Cutaneous Lymphomas 493
Cryotherapy in Small Animal Dermatology 495
Pharmacology of Antipruritic Drugs 497

AUTOIMMUNE SKIN DISEASES

R. E. W. HALLIWELL, M.R.C.V.S.
Gainesville, Florida

Within the past five years, a number of autoimmune skin diseases have been described for the first time, owing to improved diagnostic techniques that have enabled full characterization. These diseases are a fascinating aspect of dermatology and in addition are important models for the appropriate human diseases.

A full work-up including history and histopathology, and the use of specialized immunologic techniques, are required to establish a definitive diagnosis of skin disorders. It is of the utmost importance that this be made precisely, as the prognosis differs for the various autoimmune diseases. Furthermore, autoimmune diseases can mimic other dermatologic entities such as deep pyoderma and mucocutaneous candidiasis. Therapy for the latter two diseases is diametrically opposed to that for autoimmune processes, and inappropriate therapy can be life threatening. Diagnostic techniques can be divided into the following two categories.

HISTOPATHOLOGIC. It is important that early lesions be selected and biopsied at the junction of normal and abnormal skin with a sharp, 6 mm punch using subcutaneous analgesia. Biopsies from old and contaminated lesions are nonproductive. Ideally, a number of biopsies should be submitted from different sites, and the services of a dedicated and competent dermatopathologist must be sought, as many sections through these biopsy specimens are often required before the diagnostic lesions are encountered.

IMMUNOLOGIC. These techniques include direct immunofluorescence — looking for deposits of immunoglobulin, indirect immunofluorescence — looking for circulating autoantibodies against skin elements, and, finally, detection of other serologic abnormalities such as antinuclear antibody, which may be found in systemic lupus erythematosus (SLE).

Biopsies for direct immunofluorescence should be frozen in isopentane (2-methyl butane) cooled to −70°C within 30 minutes, or held in Michel's medium for transportation to the laboratory. Routine histopathology can also be undertaken on specimens stored in Michel's medium, but formalin-fixed tissue is not suitable for immunofluorescent studies.

Fresh frozen buccal mucosa is a good substrate for indirect immunofluorescence, but this is generally a less sensitive technique than is direct immunofluorescence, as much of the circulating autoantibody may be bound to the substrate *in vivo*.

The major distinguishing features of the autoimmune skin diseases are recorded in Table 1.

THE PEMPHIGUS GROUP

This group, which is composed of pemphigus vulgaris, foliaceus, erythematosus, and vegetans, was the first to be clearly delineated in the dog. Pemphigus vulgaris has also been recorded in the cat. These are examples of bullous diseases, but because of the very thin epidermis in the dog, the bullous phase is transitory and the disease usually manifests as ulcerative lesions that crust over and may become secondarily infected.

Clinical Signs. Pemphigus vulgaris affects the mucocutaneous junctions, oral mucosa, and nail beds, and occasionally it becomes generalized. The onset may be sudden or gradual, and the patient is usually systemically ill and febrile and has obvious secondary bacterial infection. The deeply located bulla, which is intraepidermal but suprabasilar, implies that the animal is in effect suffering from the equivalent of second degree burns.

Pemphigus foliaceus has less predilection for mucocutaneous junctions, and the mucosal surfaces are rarely if ever involved. The bulla is more superficial, being located just under the stratum corneum, and so the disease often appears as a scaling and crusting dermatitis with hair loss. The condition is often pruritic but the patient is not severely affected constitutionally.

Reports of pemphigus erythematosus and pemphigus vegetans are few. The latter, as its name implies, is a more proliferative disease with granulomatous verrucoid lesions following the initial bulla and ulceration. Pemphigus ery-

Table 1. Important Features of Autoimmune Skin Diseases in Dogs

DISEASE	CLINICAL SIGNS	HISTOPATHOLOGIC CHANGES	DIRECT IMMUNOFLUORESCENCE	INDIRECT IMMUNOFLUORESCENCE	OTHER FINDINGS
Pemphigus vulgaris	Bullae leading to ulceration involving the oral mucosa, mucocutaneous junctions, and nail beds	Acantholysis prominent with a suprabasilar cleft	Epidermal intercellular deposits of IgG and C3 usually demonstrable	Circulating autoantibodies against intercellular cement substance usually demonstrable	Negative
Pemphigus foliaceus	Erythematous, crusty lesions often involving the head and nose; may generalize	Acantholysis with subcorneal bulla formation	As pemphigus vulgaris	As pemphigus vulgaris	Negative
Pemphigus vegetans	As for pemphigus vulgaris with proliferative chronic lesions	Suprabasilar cleft with chronic lesions showing verrucoid proliferation	As pemphigus vulgaris	As pemphigus vulgaris	*
Pemphigus erythematosus	*	Similar to pemphigus foliaceus	As pemphigus vulgaris with subepidermal deposits in addition	As pemphigus vulgaris	Positive ANA
Bullous pemphigoid	(a) Acute—as for pemphigus vulgaris without nail bed involvement (b) Chronic—ulcerative crusting lesions with no particular distribution	Linear or globular deposits of IgG at dermoepidermal junction	Circulating autoantibodies against "basement zone substance" (unlikely to be seen in chronic form)	Negative	Negative
Systemic lupus erythematosus	Scaling, crusting, and alopecic lesions sometimes unremarkable, especially involving head and ears	Hydropic degeneration of the basal cells; thinning or hyperkeratosis of the epidermis; periadnexal and periarterial mononuclear infiltrate and corrective tissue degeneration	Deposits of IgG at dermoepidermal junction of involved and normal skin	Negative	ANA usually positive, greater than 1:100; LE preparation usually positive
Discoid lupus erythematosus	*	Hyperkeratosis; hydropic degeneration of basal cells; atrophy of stratum malpighii; patchy periadnexal lymphoid infiltrate; dermal edema and vasodilation	Deposits of IgG at dermoepidermal junction of involved skin only	Negative	None—ANA and LE preparations are negative
Nodular panniculitis	Ulcerative draining skin lesions following focal swelling of dermal or subcutaneous fat	Mononuclear infiltrate of deep dermal fat tissues	*	*	*

*Sufficient documentation does not exist to enable statements to be made.

thematosus is a variant of pemphigus foliaceus with a predisposition for the facial area.

A definitive diagnosis can be made if either the histopathology or the immunofluorescence is unequivocally positive. However, as positives in confirmed cases are often not achieved by individual or multiple biopsies, it is recommended that both approaches be attempted.

Diagnosis

HISTOPATHOLOGY. The classical lesion in pemphigus is acantholysis, which can be defined as a loss of cohesion among the individual epidermal cells and the grouping thereof as more darkly staining isolated cells. This leads to a cleft that is subcorneal in the cases of pemphigus foliaceus and erythematosus and suprabasal in the cases of pemphigus vulgaris and vegetans. The subcorneal cleft in pemphigus foliaceus may resemble subcorneal pustular dermatosis except that the lesions in the latter disease are usually somewhat smaller. The pemphigus group is readily distinguished histopathologically from bullous pemphigoid, where the cleft is subepidermal.

IMMUNOFLUORESCENCE. In the case of the pemphigus group, intercellular autoantibody deposits should be demonstrable within the epidermis. As in the case of the histopathology, a definitive diagnosis is hard to achieve, and in many instances the deposits are minimal and located only in small regions in any one biopsy. Circulating autoantibodies against the intercellular cement substance of the epidermis are often demonstrable using buccal mucosa. In the case of pemphigus erythematosus, subepidermal deposits and a positive antinuclear antibody test are often evident.

Therapy.

Pemphigus is a severe disease, and before the advent of corticosteroids, it was usually fatal — particularly pemphigus vulgaris. Immediate immunosuppression is required, and high doses of corticosteroids (e.g., 1.0–2.0 mg/kg of prednisone or prednisolone) should be instituted without delay together with concomitant broad-spectrum antibiotic therapy if secondary infection is evident. Despite the use of modern drugs, prognosis with these diseases is still poor, and it is extremely difficult to get animals on alternate day corticosteroid therapy. Likewise, it is rare for the disease to go into spontaneous remission. Concomitant use of lower doses of corticosteroids together with other immunosuppressive agents such as cyclophosphamide (Cytoxan®, Mead Johnson) or azathioprine (Imuran®, Burroughs Wellcome) may give better results. The usual recommended dose of the former is 2 mg/kg daily for four consecutive days each week, and the latter is usually given at around 2 mg/kg daily. Hemor-

rhagic cystitis is a not infrequent and sometimes severe complication of cyclophosphamide use.

Dosages for long-term use, particularly when in combination with corticosteroids, are usually lower than average. It has recently been suggested that use of cyclophosphamide as initial therapy in combination with corticosteroids is more likely to lead to remission, enabling withdrawal from therapy.

BULLOUS PEMPHIGOID

Clinical Signs. Like the pemphigus group, bullous pemphigoid may be sudden or gradual in onset, and it may furthermore be acute or chronic in nature. The acute form is indistinguishable from pemphigus vulgaris, with the exception that owing to the subepidermal position of the bulla, it is more likely to be seen intact. The distribution is usually mucocutaneous and particularly affects the oral mucosa, the perioral and periocular tissues, and the ears. Some cases of rather generalized eruptions have also been recorded. Secondary infection is often present, and the animal is usually febrile and obviously sick.

The chronic form may affect almost any part on the body and is far more benign than the acute form. In distinction to the acute form, the patient is rarely systemically ill. A number of cases of corticosteroid-responsive, fairly benign oral ulcerations have been documented, with many if not all the features of benign mucosal pemphigoid of man.

Diagnosis. Again, because of the difficulties of establishing a precise diagnosis, it is recommended that biopsies be processed for both routine histopathology and immunofluorescence.

HISTOPATHOLOGY. Appropriately taken biopsies should reveal a subepidermal cleft that becomes colonized by inflammatory cells.

IMMUNOFLUORESCENCE. Direct immunofluorescence should show deposits of immunoglobulin around the basement membrane zone. This may be either narrow or broad, linear or globular in distribution. Indirect immunofluorescence may show circulating autoantibodies against antigens present in the basement membrane zone that have yet to be defined.

Therapy. Therapy involves immediate immunosuppression in the case of the acute form together with concomitant antibiotic therapy if indicated. The chronic form will usually also require corticosteroids, but in the localized forms, topical steroid therapy may be all that is required.

It appears that the prognosis for bullous pemphigoid is better than that for the pemphigus group, and the response to therapy is brisk. The chronic form is quite benign, and the acute form is more likely to go into a remission that may be very long lasting. It is usually fairly easy to get the animals on alternate day therapy, and it is seldom necessary to resort to a more potent immunosuppressive agent.

LUPUS ERYTHEMATOSUS

Systemic lupus erythematosus (SLE) is a multisystem disease, but approximately 50 percent of cases have cutaneous manifestations. There have been a number of tentative reports of discoid lupus erythematosus (DLE) in the dog, but to date, none have really filled all the classical criteria applicable in man. Thus, its existence in the dog has yet to be unequivocally shown. Both diseases in man can be exacerbated by sunlight and often occur on the exposed areas.

Clinical Signs. Cutaneous manifestations of systemic lupus erythematosus vary and are rarely dramatic. They are usually of chronic onset, tend to involve the head and ears, and consist of alopectic scarred and crusted lesions, but ulceration is rarely a feature. Cases have been noticed in which the feet and mucocutaneous junctions have also been involved, but oral lesions are apparently uncommon in the dog. It is thus safe to say that there is no such thing as a classical canine lupus dermatitis.

Discoid lupus erythematosus in man is characterized by a symmetrical butterfly-like rash on the face. The clinical appearance in man is somewhat reminiscent of the crusting, scarring alopectic dermatitis that is often seen in Shetland sheepdogs. However, it seems likely that many of these cases, particularly if there is a tendency to become generalized, are in fact epidermolysis bullosa simplex.

Diagnosis

HISTOPATHOLOGY. The histopathology of dermatitic changes in canine SLE is often somewhat unremarkable. There is a thinning or a thickening of the epidermis and often hydropic degeneration of the basal cell layer. Fibrinoid degeneration of dermal connective tissue occurs, and there may be a periadenexal infiltration with mononuclear cells. The classical histopathology of discoid lupus should include many of these features, but hyperkeratosis and follicular plugging are constant.

IMMUNOLOGY. Direct immunofluorescence in canine SLE with dermatologic involvement should show linear deposits of immunoglobins at the dermoepidermal junction. This is apparent not only in the involved skin but also in the surrounding, apparently normal skin. Other immunologic findings to be expected include a positive antinuclear antibody (ANA) test (in a

titer greater than 1:100 if a cell culture lines are used) and evidence of immune complex glomerulonephritis if there is renal involvement. In the case of DLE, the deposits of immunoglobins in the skin are limited to the involved area, and the ANA test is ordinarily negative.

Therapy. Therapy of SLE involves immunosuppression, and corticosteroids probably represent the initial therapy of choice. The prognosis is variable, but quite a number of cases can be maintained on alternate day corticosteroid therapy. However, in some instances, concomitant immunosuppression with azathioprine or cyclophosphamide is required. Occasionally, cases go into fairly long-term remission, but relapses are to be expected.

Corticosteroids are also of value in DLE, but here also the antimalarial drug chloroquin and its derivatives (e.g., hydroxychloroquine sulfate, Plaquenil®, Winthrop) are of some benefit. Indeed, chloroquin can be used to aid in the retrospective diagnosis based on response to therapy, so long as all other parameters are supported, in a dosage of around 0.5 mg/kg. The clinician should be alert to the possible side effects, which include blood dyscrasias.

NODULAR PANNICULITIS

Although immunologic parameters in this condition are not well documented, histologic evidence suggests that the condition results from an autoimmune reaction against dermal fat tissues.

Clinical Signs. There is usually a sudden onset of subcutaneous nodule formation, which liquefies and leads to abscessation. Secondary infection may ensue, and the animals are often systemically ill. There is usually a serosanguinous brownish discharge. Dachshunds and collies seem to be predisposed.

Diagnosis. Nodular panniculitis can mimic both a deep mycotic infection and a deep pyoderma (cellulitis). Ideally, samples should be taken from unruptured lesions for fungal and bacterial culture. If the latter is positive, treatment should be started with appropriate antibiotics to assess whether the bacterial involvement is primary or secondary.

Histopathology reveals a mononuclear infiltrate in the deep dermal adipose tissue. Immunofluorescent studies have not been documented but would predictably be negative.

Therapy. Immunosuppressive therapy with high doses of corticosteroids represents the initial treatment of choice. Broad spectrum antibiotics would be logical to cover secondary infection.

For long-term control, it would clearly be

necessary to get the patient onto alternate day therapy or to use supplementation with other immunosuppressive agents if necessary.

SUPPLEMENTAL READING

Halliwell, R. E. W.: Autoimmune diseases in the dog. Adv. Vet. Sci. Comp. Med. 22:221–263, 1978.
Halliwell, R. E. W., and Goldschmidt, M. H.: Pemphigus foliaceus in the canine — a case report and discussion. JAAHA 13:431–435, 1977.

Hurvitz, A. I., and Feldman, E.: A disease in dogs resembling human pemphigus vulgaris: case reports. JAVMA 166:585–590, 1975.
Kunkle, G., Goldschmidt, M. H., and Halliwell, R. E. W.: Bullous pemphigoid in a dog: a case report with immunofluorescent findings. JAAHA 14:52–57, 1970.
Michel, B., Milner, Y., and David, R.: Preservation of tissue fixed immunoglobulin in skin biopsies of patients with lupus erythematosus and bullous diseases. Preliminary report. J. Invest. Derm. 59:449–452, 1971.
Stannard, A. A., Gribble, D. H., and Baker, B. B.: A mucocutaneous disease in the dog resembling pemphigus vulgaris in man. JAVMA 166:575–582, 1975.

THE DIFFERENTIAL DIAGNOSIS OF FACIAL DERMATITIS

DANNY W. SCOTT, D.V.M.
Ithaca, New York

Facial dermatitis is a common syndrome in dogs and cats. Unfortunately, the skin has a limited number of gross pathologic patterns by which to express underlying diseases. Thus, a veritable plethora of etiologic entities can result in the same facial symptoms.

It goes without saying that virtually any skin disease can involve the face. However, this article is confined to those syndromes that predominantly or exclusively involve the face or that begin on the face before spreading to other areas. A differential diagnosis of facial dermatitis is presented in Table 1.

BACTERIAL FOLLICULITIS-FURUNCULOSIS

Bacterial infections of the facial skin are common in the dog and may be primary or secondary to a number of diseases (dermatophytosis, demodicosis, atopic disease, food allergy, seborrheic dermatitis, etc.). Primary bacterial folliculitis-furunculosis has a predilection for the muzzle, chin, bridge of the nose (nasal pyoderma), and periocular region. It is characterized by follicularly oriented papules and pustules, exudation, crusting, edema, alopecia, fistulization, and ulceration. Pain and pruritus are variable. Doberman pinschers, great Danes, Dalmatians, Labrador retrievers, German short-haired pointers, and German shepherds are commonly affected, with no apparent age or sex predilections.

Diagnosis is based on history, physical examination, and laboratory testing. Gram-stained direct smears of material taken from intact pustules and furuncles reveal (1) neutrophils (many of them degenerate and toxic) and (2) bacteria, many of which are within the neutrophils (evidence of active phagocytosis). Culture and sensitivity testing on material from intact lesions should be performed on refractory or recurrent cases. *Staphylococcus aureus* is the most commonly isolated organism.

Therapy of bacterial folliculitis-furunculosis includes systemic antibiotics for three to six weeks and wet soaks (warm water, with or without aluminum acetate 1:20). Gentle handling of involved skin is mandatory, as scarring can be a prominent sequela. Ointments are contraindicated.

DERMATOPHILOSIS (STREPTOTHRICOSIS)

Dermatophilosis is a rare bacterial dermatitis of dogs and cats. It is caused by the actinomycete *Dermatophilus congolensis*. Affected dogs and cats are usually from farms that have carrier cattle and horses. *D. congolensis* is activated by moisture; thus, dermatophilosis is most commonly seen during rainy seasons.

Table 1. *Differential Diagnosis of Facial Dermatitis*

ENTITY	KEY HISTORY AND LABORATORY TESTS
Bacterial folliculitis-furunculosis	Direct smears, culture and sensitivity
Dermatophilosis	Farm animals, direct smears, culture, skin biopsy
Fungal dermatitis	Fungal culture, skin biopsy
Demodicosis	Skin scrapings, skin biopsy
Allergic dermatitis	
Atopic	Breed and age, i.d. skin testing
Food	Hypoallergenic diet
Contact	Plastic or rubber dishes and chewies
Solar dermatitis	Breed (dog) and color (cat), worse in summer
Seborrheic dermatitis	Breed, skin biopsy
Subcorneal pustular dermatosis	Direct smears, culture (negative), skin biopsy
Pemphigus foliaceus	Skin biopsy, IFT°
Pemphigus erythematosus	As Above
Systemic lupus erythematosus	LE cell test†, ANA test††, skin biopsy, IFT
Discoid lupus erythematosus	Skin biopsy, IFT
Epidermolysis bullosa simplex	Breed and age, skin biopsy, induction of lesions with frictional trauma
Zinc-responsive dermatitis	Breed, skin biopsy, improvement when zinc is given

°Immunofluorescence testing
†Lupus erythematosus cell test
††Antinuclear antibody test

Lesions consist of thick exudative crusts and alopecia. When a crust is lifted off the skin, the underlying skin is erythematous, edematous, and covered with a yellowish green purulent material. Pruritus and pain are minimal.

Diagnosis is based on history, physical examination, and laboratory testing. Wright, Giemsa, or new methylene blue-stained direct smears of the purulent material reveal many neutrophils and chains of laterally and longitudinally dividing cocci ("railroad tracks"). The organism may be cultured on blood agar and demonstrated in skin biopsy specimens.

Therapy of dermatophilosis involves wet soaks to soften and remove organism-laden crusts, topical applications of aqueous povidone-iodine or 2 percent lime sulfur until healed (10 to 21 days), and cleanliness and dryness. Refractory cases may require penicillin and dihydrostreptomycin given systemically for 7 to 10 days in addition to topical therapy.

FUNGAL DERMATITIS

Fungal agents resulting in facial dermatitis include dermatophytes and occasionally the intermediate (sporotrichosis) and deep fungi (blastomycosis, cryptococcosis).

Dermatophytosis (ringworm) is a common cause of facial dermatitis in dogs and cats. Lesions vary from the "classic" ringworm (circular areas of alopecia, stubbled hairs, scaling, crusting, with or without erythema) to severe folliculitis-furunculosis and secondary pyoderma (especially with *Trichophyton mentagrophytes* and *Microsporum gypseum*).

Diagnosis is by history, physical examination, and laboratory testing. Wood's light examination and KOH preparations are rarely helpful. The keys to diagnosis are fungal culture and skin biopsy.

Therapy includes (1) griseofulvin given orally, with fat or oil, at 60 to 120 mg/kg daily until two weeks beyond clinical cure, (2) topical antifungal agents (total body dips with 2 percent lime sulfur or povidone-iodine, once weekly until cured), (3) isolation, and (4) environmental sanitation (weekly vacuuming and disposal, fungicides where feasible).

DEMODICOSIS (DEMODECTIC MANGE)

Demodicosis is a common cause of facial dermatitis in the dog but it rarely occurs in the cat. The pathomechanism of clinical disease with the normal skin inhabitants *Demodex canis* and *D. cati* is closely tied to genetic predilection and immunodeficiency. Lesions vary from alopecia, erythema, and scaling to folliculitis-furunculosis and secondary pyoderma. Pain and pruritus are variable. Young dogs, especially Doberman pinschers, old English sheepdogs, Afghans, and English bulldogs, are commonly affected.

Diagnosis is by history, physical examination, and laboratory testing. Skin scrapings, properly made and interpreted, are diagnostic. Diagnosis may also be made (embarrassingly so) by skin biopsy.

Therapy for the young dog includes wet soaks to dry and allay pruritus and systemic antibiotics if secondary pyoderma is significant. Therapy of chronic demodicosis is difficult (Scott, 1979).

ALLERGIC DERMATITIS

The intense pruritus accompanying atopic disease (dog) and food allergy (cat and dog) may result in severely excoriated and secondarily infected dermatitides of the face. Canine atopic disease usually involves younger animals (one to three years of age), and certain breeds are at increased risk (Irish setter, Dalmatian, English bulldogs, and terriers). Food allergy has no age, breed, or sex predilections.

Diagnosis is based on history, physical examination, and laboratory testing. Intradermal skin testing is required for the specific diagnosis of atopic disease, and response to hypoallergenic diets is required for the diagnosis of food allergy.

Therapy includes symptomatic measures, hyposensitization and/or corticosteroids for atopic disease, and hypoallergenic diet and/or corticosteroids for food allergy.

A unique but rare facial dermatitis is that due to contact with plastic or rubber feed or water dishes and chewy toys. Certain plastic and rubber products contain various sensitizing and/or depigmenting agents. Lesions consist of erythema, edema, alopecia, pruritus, excoriation, and/or leukoderma. Lesions are confined to the nose, lips, and chin. Diagnosis is by history and physical examination. Therapy includes symptomatic measures and removal of the offending dishes and toys.

SOLAR DERMATITIS ("COLLIE NOSE")

Solar dermatitis may be a common cause of facial dermatitis in temperate and tropical areas. It tends to show seasonal fluctuations in many areas, and it is much worse in summer.

Canine solar dermatitis may be seen in several breeds, but it is predominant in collies and Shetland sheepdogs. It begins on the nose and anterior nares. Loss of pigment is followed by erythema, edema, exudation, ulceration, and pruritus. Unchecked, the dermatitis will progress up the bridge of the nose and may involve the lips and periocular area.

Feline solar dermatitis is seen in white or white-eared, white-faced cats. Erythema, curling of the ear margins, and scaling are followed

by edema, exudation, ulceration, and pruritus. The margins of the ears are most commonly affected, but the nasal, labial, and periocular skin may also be affected.

Diagnosis is based on history and physical examination. Severe ulceration demands skin biopsy, as squamous cell carcinoma is a sequela to solar dermatitis.

Therapy includes avoidance of sunlight, topical sunscreens, topical and systemic corticosteroids as needed, and tattooing (see p. 442). Surgical excision of affected portions of the cat's ears may be curative.

SEBORRHEIC DERMATITIS

Primary (idiopathic) seborrheic dermatitis can localize on the facial area of dogs. German short-haired pointers, Siberian huskies, and Akitas are the breeds most commonly affected. Lesions include erythema, edema, scaling, crusting, and alopecia. Pruritus is variable, and secondary pyoderma is not uncommon. The lips, periocular region, and ears are predilected.

Diagnosis is by history, physical exam, deduction, and skin biopsy.

Therapy includes topical antiseborrheic agents, especially various combinations of sulfur, coal tar, and corticosteroids, as needed.

SUBCORNEAL PUSTULAR DERMATOSIS

This is an uncommon skin disease of dogs. The etiology is unknown, and about 50 percent of the cases occur in miniature Schnauzers. Lesions consist of papules, pustules, erosions, epidermal collarettes, exudation, crusting, scaling, and alopecia. Pruritus is variable but when present tends to be severe and poorly responsive to corticosteroids.

Diagnosis is by history, physical examination, and laboratory testing. Direct smears of material from intact pustules reveal many neutrophils but no bacteria. Culture of material from intact pustules is negative, or positive for small numbers of coagulase-negative staphylococci. Skin biopsy reveals subcorneal pustule formation with variable acantholysis.

Therapy includes symptomatic topical measures and the oral administration of dapsone (Avlosulfon,® Ayerst) at 1.0 mg/kg given three times daily. Dapsone therapy is continued until all lesions have regressed (two to four weeks). Hemograms and SGPT are performed weekly to follow bone marrow and hepatic responses, since dapsone may produce toxicities. Therapy is then stopped, and 50 percent of the cases will remain in long-term remissions. For relapsing cases, maintenance doses of dapsone will be required. (See also page 445.)

PEMPHIGUS FOLIACEUS AND ERYTHEMATOSUS

These two autoimmune skin diseases are rare, characterized by a circulating and tissue-bound autoantibody directed against the intercellular substance of stratified squamous epithelium. Pemphigus foliaceus often begins on the face and then generalizes. Pemphigus erythematosus remains localized to the face.

Lesions include vesicles and bullae, erosions, epidermal collarettes, exudation, crusting, scaling, and alopecia. Pruritus is variable.

Diagnosis is by history, physical examination, and laboratory testing. Skin biopsy reveals subcorneal blister formation with acantholysis and follicular involvement. Direct and indirect immunofluorescence testing may reveal positive intercellular staining. In pemphigus erythematosus, a low titer positive ANA and basement membrane zone staining on direct immunofluorescence testing may be found.

Therapy includes lifelong administration of corticosteroids and/or other immunosuppressive drugs (cyclophosphamide, azathioprine, chlorambucil, etc.).

SYSTEMIC AND DISCOID LUPUS ERYTHEMATOSUS

Systemic lupus erythematosus (SLE) is a rare, multisystemic autoimmune disorder of dogs and cats. Skin lesions may be seen in up to 33 percent of the cases, and these may be the initial complaint. Discoid lupus erythematosus (DLE) is a more benign variant, and tends to involve only the skin. In humans, middle-aged females are commonly affected.

Skin lesions are extremely pleomorphic and may include erythema, alopecia, scaling, crusting, leukoderma, atrophy, scarring, vesicles and bullae, erosions, and ulcers. Pruritus is variable. The bridge of the nose and the periocular regions are commonly involved, forming a "butterfly" or "batwing" pattern.

Diagnosis is by history, physical examination, and laboratory testing. A positive LE cell test is helpful but very unpredictable, and it is quite labile and fairly non-specific for SLE. It is routinely negative in DLE. A positive ANA is a constant finding in SLE but is also fairly non-specific. It is usually negative in DLE. Skin biopsy may reveal the classical findings of liquefaction degeneration of the basal cell layers of the epidermis and appendagocentric accumulations of lymphohistiocytic cells. Direct immunofluorescence testing reveals positive staining at the basement membrane zone ("lupus band"). Indirect immunofluorescence testing is negative.

Therapy includes lifelong administration of corticosteroids and/or other immunosuppressive drugs. (See also page 434.)

EPIDERMOLYSIS BULLOSA SIMPLEX

Epidermolysis bullosa simplex is a rare, inherited mechanobullous disease of collies and Shetland sheepdogs. The etiology is unknown, and the disease is characterized by an excessive blistering response to frictional trauma. There is no sex predilection, and the disorder is usually recognized within the first six months of life.

Lesions include vesicles and bullae, erosions, ulcers, epidermal collarettes, erythema, erythematous-edematous plaques, alopecia, scaling, crusting, atrophy, and pigmentary changes. These lesions are most commonly found over bony prominences (digits, carpi, tarsi, elbows), ear margins, the tip of the tail, and the "butterfly" region of the face. Pruritus is mild or absent. The disease worsens in warm weather.

Diagnosis is by history, physical examination, and laboratory testing. Skin biopsy reveals liquefaction degeneration of the basal cell layer of the epidermis, subepidermal blister formation, and minimal inflammation. Normal skin can be briskly rubbed with a pencil eraser or a thumbnail for one minute, resulting in reproduction of the typical gross and histologic lesions within about five minutes.

Therapy includes corticosteroids and avoidance of trauma. Corticosteroids are palliative, but lesions continue to develop.

ZINC-RESPONSIVE DERMATITIS

This recently recognized entity affects predominantly Malamutes, Siberian huskies, and Doberman pinschers. Dogs of either sex are affected; age of onset is commonly around six months to two years of age.

Lesions include mild erythema and edema, scaling, exudation, thick crusts, and alopecia. Pain and pruritus are minimal or absent. Lesions tend to affect the butterfly region of the face, the ears, and pressure points. Mild to moderate weight loss and a dull, dry haircoat may accompany the dermatitis.

Diagnosis is based on history, physical examination, and laboratory testing. Skin biopsy reveals severe parakeratosis. Studies of serum or hair zinc levels have not been done. Whether abnormalities of zinc absorption and/or utilization are the cause of this syndrome is speculative.

Therapy includes symptomatic topical applications and the oral administration of 125 to 450 mg of zinc sulfate, once daily. Lesions usually clear in three or four weeks. Unfortunately, most of the cases relapse when therapy is stopped, necessitating long-term maintenance therapy. (See also page 472.)

AFTERMATH

Facial dermatitis is a multifactorial, challenging dermatologic syndrome. Therapeutic success is dependent on an accurate diagnosis. Rigid adherence to an exhaustive differential diagnosis and laboratory rule-out plan helps insure the accurate diagnosis.

Secondary pyoderma and leukoderma are common complications of facial dermatitis, regardless of the primary etiology. Skin scrapings and fungal culture should be done in every case. In addition, because many of these entities (1) require specific therapeutic regimes, (2) are associated with variable degrees of possible permanent disfigurement (scarring alopecia, pigmentary disturbances), and (3) may generalize to large areas of the body, early diagnosis is critical. For these reasons, skin biopsy should be employed early in the course of these diseases (within first three weeks, if initial therapies have been of minimal benefit). Skin biopsy is often the key to diagnosis and is most helpful early, before diagnostic histopathologic changes are obscured by therapy and secondary complications, and before too much time and money are wasted on inappropriate medicaments.

SUPPLEMENTAL READING

Halliwell, R. E. W.: Autoimmune disease in the dog. Adv. Vet. Sci. Comp. Med. 22:221–263, 1978.
McKeever, P. J., and Dahl, M. V.: A disease in dogs resembling human subcorneal pustular dermatosis. J. Am. Vet. Med. Assoc. 170:704–708, 1977.
Muller, G. H., and Kirk, R. W.: *Small Animal Dermatology II.* Philadelphia, W. B. Saunders Co., 1976.
Scott, D. W., and Schultz, R. D.: Epidermolysis bullosa simplex in the Collie dog. J. Am. Vet. Med. Assoc. 171:721–727, 1977.
Scott, D. W.: Immunologic skin disorders. Vet. Clin. North Am. 8: 641–664, 1978.
Scott, D. W.: Canine demodicosis. Vet. Clin. North Am. 9:in press, 1979.
Scott, D. W.: Demodicosis. In Kirk, R. W. (ed.): *Current Veterinary Therapy VI.* Philadelphia, W. B. Saunders, 1977.

CANINE NASAL SOLAR DERMATITIS

PETER J. IHRKE, V.M.D.
Davis, California

Canine nasal solar dermatitis may be defined as an actinic or photo-aggravated reaction with definite breed prevalences and a predilection for the dorsum of the nose. The syndrome has been reported to occur most commonly in collies, Shetland sheepdogs, white German shepherds, Australian shepherds, Welsh corgis, Weimaraners, and all their related crossbreeds. It is generally accepted that heredity plays an important role in solar dermatitis. However, although definite breed predilections are seen, pedigree data is not presently available. No age or sex predilection is felt to exist.

Environmental factors appear to be considerable in this syndrome. Although nationwide statistics are not available, it is generally considered that there is a higher incidence of this condition in areas of greater sun intensity such as California, Florida, Colorado, and Hawaii. The condition is uncommon in areas of low sun intensity, which supports the contention that solar dermatitis is a photo-reactive phenomenon. In addition, seasonal exacerbation during periods of intense sun exposure has been well documented. The severity of the lesions commonly increases with each year of summer exposure unless therapy is instituted.

ETIOLOGY AND PATHOGENESIS

Although there is little doubt that exposure to sunlight is of major significance in the development of this syndrome, the exact pathogenesis is not known. Canine solar dermatitis seems to be most closely analogous to indirect photosensitivity reactions in man. In these conditions, an abnormal reactivity to light is seen in association with a congenital or acquired defect. This defect then alters the individual's normal solar defense mechanisms. In man, indirect photosensitivity reactions can be seen in association with diseases as disparate as porphyria and lupus erythematosus. The classic veterinary example of indirect photosensitization is congenital porphyria in cattle. The variations in biologic behavior in canine solar dermatitis could be explained if solar dermatitis were viewed as an indirect photosensitivity reaction of multifactoral etiology. Any number of endogenous factors in combination with ultraviolet light might create this disease syndrome. In the future, it is likely that a number of different diseases may be elucidated that all have symptomatology similar to that of canine nasal solar dermatitis. Until that time, it will be absolutely essential therapeutically to set strict criteria for canine nasal solar dermatitis so that detrimental treatments are not applied. It is likely that many therapeutic failures currently are due to misdiagnosis.

CLINICAL SIGNS

The most common site for solar dermatitis is the dorsum of the nose. Depigmentation and erythema are seen initially either at the junction of the haired and non-haired areas or around the nares. Lesions are often somewhat symmetrical. It is the author's opinion that prior to the onset of the disease, the areas that will become affected are usually pigmented normally — i.e., pigmentation is probably lost as a consequence of the disease and not as a predisposing factor. Erosion and ulceration frequently develop as sequelae to the erythema and depigmentation. Alopecia usually occurs concomitantly with ulceration. Self-trauma may then become a significant secondary problem.

During times of decreased sun intensity, the involved areas heal rather tenuously with a thin, fragile, parchment-like epithelium. Normal surface architecture is completely replaced by thin abnormal epithelium devoid of adnexae. The area is usually quite sensitive and may bleed excessively after minimal trauma. Consequently, dogs with canine nasal solar dermatitis often avoid head contact.

In certain cases, excessive involvement of the lateral alar cartilage area on the planum nasale may lead to loss of soft tissue mass. Frequently, these lesions may appear to be neoplastic. The transition from canine nasal solar dermatitis to squamous cell carcinoma has been commonly cited in the literature, although such transitions are indeed quite rare.

DIFFERENTIAL DIAGNOSIS

For the purposes of this article, animals with nasal lesions compatible with canine nasal solar dermatitis are being excluded from consideration if additional, similar lesions are present periorbitally, on the pinnas of the ears, or around the commissures of the mouth. Although other methods are not available to differentiate this multifocal condition from nasal solar dermatitis, it is being excluded as it does not respond to tattooing. Only comparatively high dosages of corticosteroids seem to be effective in controlling these cases. Response to therapy seems to associate this condition more closely with immune-mediated diseases.

A number of other diseases may present with an array of clinical signs quite similar to those of canine nasal solar dermatitis. Depigmentation, ulceration, exudation, and partial facial symmetry may all be seen in immune-mediated disease. The facial scaling and crusting seen with pemphigus foleaceus has frequently been misdiagnosed as solar dermatitis. Occasionally, pemphigus vulgaris may begin with ulceration at the junction of the haired and non-haired areas around the planum nasale. A poorly understood condition termed "sheltie syndrome" may mimic solar dermatitis. In general, however, the lesions seen in this disease are usually much more diffuse and involve other areas of the body. Recently, several cases of a condition clinically resembling nasal solar dermatitis have had histopathology and cutaneous immunofluorescence compatible with the human disease, discoid lupus. In most instances, a careful history, chronology, and the presence of lesions elsewhere on the body should be sufficient to help rule out these other diseases. Biopsy may be helpful in differentiating all these diseases if a qualified veterinary dermatopathologist examines both a hematoxylin and eosin section and a frozen section with immunofluorescence.

Fibrous histiocytoma is seen primarily as infiltrative corneal or limbal masses in dogs, especially the collie breed. Occasionally, raised, plaque-like, flesh-colored masses of tissue are also seen on the planum nasale, eyelids, and commissures of the lips. The lesions may ulcerate. The condition is highly responsive to corticosteroid therapy.

Nasal pyodermas, allergic or irritant contact dermatitis, and dermatophytosis have all been listed as differential diagnosis for solar dermatitis. However, a thorough history and careful physical examination should readily differentiate these diseases.

DIAGNOSIS

For consistent therapeutic success in treating canine nasal solar dermatitis, strict criteria must be established before an animal becomes a candidate for tattooing, such as:

1. The lesions must begin either on the dorsum of the nose near the juncture of the haired and non-haired areas or on the planum nasale
2. The lesions must be depigmented
3. The lesions must be aggravated by sun exposure
4. The lesions must improve upon removal from sunlight
5. The lesions must be partially responsive to parenteral corticosteroids
6. Animals with similar lesions on any areas other than the dorsum of the nose or the planum nasale must be excluded from consideration

THERAPY

The degree of vigor of therapy required either to control or to cure this syndrome is contingent upon the duration and the severity of the lesions. All treatments except tattooing are palliative only. Even tattooed animals may require further therapy. Various methods of therapy are described here. The clinician should choose some or all of the recommended treatments and individualize the program for each case.

Confinement. The dog should be confined indoors during the hours of sunlight for a minimum of two weeks. Hospitalization is an alternative if owner confinement is not feasible. If the animal must be allowed out for urination and defecation, the time outside must be as short as possible.

Topical Suncreens. Paraminobenzoic acid derivative sunscreens such as Presun® (Westwood Pharmaceuticals) or Sundown® (Johnson and Johnson) may be used in conjunction with confinement. The medication should be applied 30 minutes before the animal is taken outside.

Topical Corticosteroids. Topical steroids may be a useful adjunct if the animal allows the medication to remain on its nose. Products such as Topicort® emollient cream (Hoechst-Roussel, Inc.), Valisone® ointment (Westwood Pharmaceuticals), or Kenalog® ointment (E. R. Squibb & Sons, Inc.) have been used successfully.

Systemic Corticosteroids. In severe chronic cases, oral corticosteroids may be necessary to prepare an animal for tattooing or for long-term maintenance therapy if tattooing is unsuccessful or not feasible. Daily corticosteroids such as prednisolone in dosages up to 1.0 mg/kg may be necessary initially. If long-term corticosteroid maintenance is necessary, drugs such as prednisolone, prednisone, or methylprednisolone should be used on an alternate day basis.

Marking Pens. In early cases, some owners may be quite successful using marking pens to blacken the nose in conjunction with using sunscreens. Marking pens may also be used as an interim therapy in preparation for tattooing. A black indelible Sharpie (Sanford Company) seems to be most effective.

Tattooing. A variety of tattooing methods are available. Considerable variation in the cosmetic results of the procedure may be due to the method of tattooing or the skill and experience of the clinician. Some methods require specialized equipment. All require either heavy sedation or general anesthesia. It is important to note that many failures occur because clinicians tattoo lesions too soon. Before tattooing is attempted, erythema should be minimal, no exudation should be present, and if possible, a confluent epithelium should cover the lesions.

Regardless of which technique is used, the selection of a proper ink is exceedingly important. This author has had best results using either human tattooing ink (Peliken Ink, Gunther Wagner) or black india ink (Carter's Drawing India Ink). Veterinary inks marketed to tattoo identification procedures have not proved as satisfactory for this use. Several methods of applying the tattoo are available.

MIZZY® JET NEEDLELESS INJECTOR GUN (MIZZY, INC.). This instrument utilizes a hand operated pressure pump that pushes the ink evenly into the dermis. The author has had excellent success with this unit. Cosmetic results are probably the best with this method. The only disadvantage is the high cost of the instrument. However, other uses may be found for this instrument in the practice of veterinary medicine.

NICHOLSEN TATTOO VIBRATOR (NICHOLSEN, INC.). Good results may be obtained with this fairly economical unit. Cosmetic results are not as good as with the needleless injector gun, and retreatment is frequently necessary. This procedure is somewhat time consuming.

SYRINGE WITH 25 GAUGE NEEDLE USING INK ONLY. In this method, a 25 gauge 5/8 inch needle is used to deposit the ink in the dermis carefully.

SYRINGE WITH 25 GAUGE NEEDLE USING INK

AND HYALURONIDASE. A number of clinicians feel that results are significantly better if hyaluronidase is used with the ink. Patterson (1978) reported the use of this method with the addition of crystalline potassium penicillin G. The addition of this antibiotic, which is rarely efficacious against canine *Staph. aureus*, is of questionable value.

POST-TATTOOING

Corticosteroid and antihistamines may be given for a week to lessen postoperative swelling. Occasionally, a serum-ink exudate may be noted, especially if a 25 gauge needle has been used in the procedure. In these cases, twice daily wet compresses may be helpful. In most animals, the nose assumes a slate gray color within 7 to 14 days after the tattooing.

Prognosis is contingent upon early treatment of lesions. Some early cases simply respond to palliative therapy; most will do very well after tattooing. No reasonable hypothesis has been suggested to explain why dermal deposition of ink is protective in a disease that primarily involves the epidermis.

SUPPLEMENTAL READING

Muller, G. H., and Kirk, R. W.: *Small Animal Dermatology*. Philadelphia, W. B. Saunders Co., 1976.
Patterson, J. M.: Nasal solar dermatitis in the dog — a method of tattooing. JAAHA 14(3):370–372, 1978.
Stannard, A.: Actinic dermatoses. In Kirk, R. W.: *Current Veterinary Therapy* V. Philadelphia, W. B. Saunders Co., 1974.
Willis, I.: Sunlight and the skin. JAMA 217:1088–1093, 1971.
Willis, I., and Kligman, A. M.: The mechanisms of photoallergic contact dermatitis. J. Invest. Derm. 51(5):378–384, 1968.

SUBCORNEAL PUSTULAR DERMATOSIS AND DERMATITIS HERPETIFORMIS

PATRICK J. McKEEVER, D.V.M.,
St. Paul, Minnesota

and MARK V. DAHL, M.D.
Minneapolis, Minnesota

Subcorneal pustular dermatosis and dermatitis herpetiformis are uncommon but similar appearing chronic skin diseases of dogs that have an unknown etiology. They are characterized by pruritus and recurrent crops of papulovesicles or pustules occurring mainly on the trunk. Affected animals respond well to dapsone therapy (Avlosulfone[R]Ayerst).

CLINICAL FINDINGS

In the limited numbers of cases studied, canine subcorneal pustular dermatosis and dermatitis herpetiformis appear to be clinically similar. Differentiation between these conditions is made by histopathologic examination of skin biopsies. For the purposes of this discussion, the clinical manifestations of subcorneal pustular dermatosis and dermatitis herpetiformis will be discussed together. However, as more cases are documented, differentiating clinical features may be found

Affected dogs range in age from 2 to 12 years, with a majority being 3 to 4 years of age at onset. No sex predisposition is found, Miniature schnauzers account for 4 of the 13 reported cases of subcorneal pustular dermatosis; however, too few cases have been diagnosed to determine if there is a breed predisposition

Lesions occur most frequently on the trunk, except in severely affected animals, where they may also occur on the legs, feet, and head (especially over the bridge of the nose). Initially, erythematous macules are noted that progress in 36 to 48 hours to vesiculopapular lesions, which may resolve or further develop into pustules. Pustules generally rupture within 48 to 72 hours, resulting in crust formation. If lesions are in close proximity, the crusts may be confluent. If lesions are separate, they may develop an erythematous, raised scaling border and enlarge to form annular lesions 2 to 3 cm in diameter. These circular scaling lesions may resemble dermatomycosis or focal seborrheic dermatitis. Lesions clear from the center out over four to six weeks, leaving temporary residual hyperpigmentation. New crops of lesions may develop while others are healing. Infrequent atypical lesions such as diffuse erythema or small 2 to 5 mm erosions and ulcers may occur. Careful examination of animals with these types of lesions may be needed to find the pustules or vesicopapules that constitute the primary lesion.

The course of the disease is characterized by remissions and exacerbations. Pruritus will range from minimal to intense but is quite severe in the majority of cases. Affected animals are afebrile, alert, and active unless secondary infection occurs. These disorders do not respond to conventional antibiotic or steroid treatments but do respond to treatment with dapsone.

HISTOLOGIC FINDINGS

Subcorneal Pustular Dermatosis. Histologic examination of a typical lesion of dogs or humans reveals a subcorneal pustule. Epidermal separation occurs at the level of the granular layer with the stratum corneum forming the roof of the pustule and the remaining granular layer forming the base. Polymorphonuclear leukocytes and occasional eosinophils and acantholytic cells are found within the pustule. Epidermis underlying the pustule is acanthotic and spongiotic. Polymorphonuclear leukocytes are seen in the stratum spinosum and are probably migrating through the epidermis toward the pustule. An upper dermal inflammatory infiltrate composed of polymorphonuclear leukocytes is present. Small numbers of mononuclear cells, plasma cells, and eosinophils may occur in the infiltrate. Focal dermal edema is frequently present. Periodic acid-Schiff stains fail to disclose yeast or fungi. Gram stains for bacteria are usually negative. However, gram positive cocci have been demonstrated in the stratum corneum and pustules in some cases.

Dermatitis Herpetiformis. Too few cases of canine dermatitis herpetiformis have been evaluated to characterize the histopathologic or immunopathologic findings in this species. In man, early lesions are represented by collections of polymorphonuclear leukocytes, leukocyte fragments, fibrin, and variable numbers of eosinophils within the papillary dermis. Separation of the papillary tips from the overlying epidermis may occur. A perivascular infiltrate composed of mononuclear cells, polymorphonuclear leukocytes, and occasionally eosinophils is also seen in early lesions. Older lesions often evidence subepidermal vesicles, which form as the rete ridges loose their coherence with the dermis.

IgA deposition occurs in man along the basement membrane zone of normal skin in all or nearly all cases of dermatitis herpetiformis. If the diseases in dog and man are analogous, similar immunofluorescence findings should be expected in the dog.

DIFFERENTIAL DIAGNOSIS

Subcorneal pustular dermatosis and dermatitis herpetiformis must be differentiated from atopic disease, impetigo, bacterial folliculitis, pemphigus foliaceus, and bullous pemphigoid.

Atopic disease, especially when superinfected with *Staphylococcus aureus*, may be difficult to differentiate from subcorneal pustular dermatosis and dermatitis herpetiformis because all these diseases are chronic, pruritic, and vesiculopapular or pustular. Clinical features suggesting atopic disease include distribution of lesions in the groin, axilla, and ventral abdomen (rather than over the trunk), seasonal occurrence, sneezing, conjunctivitis and lacrimation resulting in periocular dermatitis, and multiple positive intradermal allergen tests. In addition, *Staphylococcus aureus* can generally be cultured from pustules associated with atopic disease, whereas the pustules and vesicles of subcorneal pustular dermatosis and dermatitis herpetiformis are usually sterile. Lack of response to at least two appropriate antibiotics (supported by culture and sensitivity) will eliminate pyoderma as a diagnosis, but an unequivocal positive diagnosis of subcorneal pustular dermatosis or dermatitis herpetiformis can be made only from the response to dapsone. Owing to toxicity associated with this drug, this should only be administered after all other diagnostic criteria have been used.

Impetigo occurs most frequently in younger animals. Lesions are located almost exclusively on the ventral abdomen. Bacteria are regularly isolated from the pustules, and response to antibiotics is good.

Papules rather than pustules are more common in bacterial folliculitis. Cultures isolate bacteria, and bacterial folliculitis usually responds promptly to appropriate antibiotics.

Pemphigus foliaceus may be confused with subcorneal pustular dermatosis because it, too, may be characterized by subcorneal vesicles or pustules. However, pemphigus is not usually pruritic. Histologically, the acantholysis may be more pronounced and extend deeper into the stratum spinosum. In addition, direct immunofluorescence demonstrates deposition of IgG in the intercellular spaces of the epidermis.

Histologically, bullous pemphigoid may be confused with dermatitis herpetiformis. Differentiation in man is based on immunofluorescence studies, which show linear deposition of IgG and C_3 at the basement membrane zone in bullous pemphigoid, and stippled deposition of IgA in dermal papillae in dermatitis herpetiformis.

TREATMENT

Both subcorneal pustular dermatosis and dermatitis herpetiformis respond to dapsone at a dose of 1.1 mg/kg four times daily. Marked improvement or remission of lesions should occur in one to four weeks. Dosage may then be reduced to 0.3 mg/kg BID to 0.6 mg/kg TID. Medication may be discontinued for variable periods after complete remission of lesions in some dogs. Other dogs will require continuous daily dapsone therapy to maintain remission.

Sulfapyridine has been used infrequently to treat subcorneal pustular dermatosis and frequently to treat dermatitis herpetiformis in man. Its long-term use for the treatment of chronic diseases such as subcorneal pustular dermatosis and dermatitis herpetiformis is discouraged in the dog because it is one of the least soluble sulfonamides in the urine of this species. Poor solubility in urine may lead to crystallization of the drug in the kidney and development of nephrotoxic nephrosis, particularly in the face of strongly acidic urine.

Dapsone therapy has been associated with numerous and sometimes serious adverse reactions. Hemolytic anemia, methemoglobinemia, agranulocytosis, lymphopenia, allergic dermatitis, hepatic disorders, peripheral neuropathy, and toxic epidermal necrolysis have been reported in man following its use. Anemia, leukopenia, elevation of liver enzymes, and thrombocytopenia have been observed with dapsone administration in dogs. Elevation of serum glutamic pyruvate transaminase levels is the most frequent abnormal finding. Most hematologic and serologic side effects are reversible if therapy is stopped, although we have encountered one case of fatal canine thrombocytopenia.

Because dapsone is a toxic drug, alternative diagnoses should be ruled out before institution of dapsone therapy. Frequent laboratory evaluation — particularly of liver and hematologic status — is recommended before and during therapy.

SUPPLEMENTAL READING

Halliwell, R.E.W., Schwartzman, R.M., Ihrke, P.J., Goldschmidt, M.H. and Wood, M.G.: Dapsone for the treatment of pruritic dermatitis (dermatitis herpetiformis and subcorneal pustular dermatosis) in dogs. JAVMA 170:697–703, 1977.
Katz, S.I., and Strober, W.: The pathogenesis of dermatitis herpetiformis. J. Invest. Dermatol. 70:63–75, 1978.
McKeever, P. J., and Dahl, M.V.: A disease in dogs resembling human subcorneal pustular dermatosis. JAVMA 170:704–708, 1977.

THE MANAGEMENT OF
FLEA ALLERGY DERMATITIS

MICHAEL D. LORENZ, D.V.M.

Athens, Georgia

Although flea allergy dermatitis (FAD) is quite common in the United States, many veterinarians fail to appreciate the ramifications and complexities of its pathogenesis. The disease is well documented in both dogs and cats and is the most common cause of allergic skin diseases in these species. A common pathogenesis is shared. The antigenic substances are contained in flea saliva and are introduced into the animal's skin when the fleas feed on the host (Benjamini et al., 1963; Feingold and Benjamini, 1961). Flea saliva contains a haptenic substance that apparently combines with skin collagen to form an antigenic complex. Thymus-dependent lymphocytes (T cells) become sensitized to this antigenic complex, and upon reexposure to the flea saliva, a delayed hypersensitivity reaction is elicited. This reaction injures cells in the skin that are thought to release lysozymes and other substances that produce the clinical signs of pruritus and erythema. Histamine is not the primary mediator of pruritus, and this may account for the ineffectiveness of antihistamines in the management of FAD. This delayed hypersensitivity reaction is an important component of the pathogenesis of FAD, although immediate reactions (antigen-antibody) also occur and play some role in the development and continuation of clinical signs. The stages of fleabite-induced hypersensitivity are summarized in Table 1. Table 2 compares the pathogenesis, diagnosis, and treatment of the most common allergic skin diseases in companion animals.

Since it is well established that humoral, skin-sensitizing antibodies play an important role in the pathogenesis of FAD (Benjamini et al., 1963; Feingold and Benjamini, 1961), it is tempting to speculate that atopic dogs may be predisposed to the development of FAD. Since 1972, the author has observed many atopic dogs that subsequently developed flea allergy dermatitis after successful management of the other sensitivities. In addition, many dogs with signs of FAD (the diagnosis clinically confirmed by the effectiveness of flea control) have developed other pruritic skin diseases highly suggestive of atopy. In a recent report, 55 of 330 dogs with FAD had concurrent signs of atopy (Nesbitt and Schmitz, 1978). Although it is wise to consider FAD as a separate disease entity, owners of atopic dogs should be warned that their dogs may be predisposed to FAD and that clinical signs related to this disease may mask the effectiveness of therapy of atopy.

CLINICAL SIGNS

The clinical signs of FAD have been well described (Muller and Kirk, 1976; Nesbitt and Schmitz, 1978). Although the disease shares a common pathogenesis in dogs and cats, different clinical findings may be present in each species. Early signs in the dog include pruritus, papules, and alopecia at the base of the tail and inside the rear legs. As the disease progresses, alopecia and excoriations become prominent in these areas. Lesions may spread rostrally down the topline from the tail head, and lesions on the abdomen are prominent in chronic cases. Severe trunkal involvement may occur in chronic cases; however, facial signs are rare, an important differentiating feature from atopy.

Small military erosions of the skin covered with crusts of dried serum or blood are characteristic lesions of feline FAD (hence the commonly used term "miliary dermatitis" as a synonym for feline FAD). Lesions in the cat usually begin at the base of the head and neck and behind the ears. Lesions are also found on the back and in the tail head region, but abdominal lesions are rare.

Clinical signs occur in all breeds and no sex predisposition is known. Affected animals are usually older than six months, and hypersensitivity may occur even in very old animals. In a recent review of canine FAD, the onset of clinical signs was most common in dogs one to three years of age, with dogs less than six months of age accounting for only 2.6 percent of cases studied (Nesbitt and Schmitz, 1978). The clinical signs may be seasonal or non-seasonal, depending on the climate and flea contamination

Table 1. *Five Stages in the Pathogenesis of Flea Allergy Dermatitis*

STAGE	SIGNIFICANT FACTS
1. Sensitization	No lesions on patient No response to IDST°
2. Delayed reaction only	Signs present; seldom respond to IDST or hyposensitization techniques†
3. Immediate reaction followed by delayed reaction	Signs present; may respond to IDST but respond poorly to hyposensitization
4. Immediate reactions only	Signs present; usually respond to IDST and hyposensitization
5. Clinical hyposensitization	No clinical signs; development of this stage is rare

°IDST—intradermal skin test with aqueous whole flea extracts
†Hyposensitization—aqueous whole flea extracts
(Stages 2 and 3 are most common)

of the inside environment. In the southeastern United States, clinical incidence of FAD tends to peak during July, August, and September; however, considerable morbidity is encountered during all months. Even in cold climates, animals will have continual signs if the home environment is infested with fleas.

DIAGNOSIS

The diagnosis of FAD should not be abandoned if fleas are not present on the patient at the time of examination. Most of the flea life cycle is spent off the host, and owners given this information usually understand the paradoxical situation of a diagnosis of FAD in the absence of fleas at the time of examination. Flea excreta in the coat proves the existence of fleas on the patient and, along with the typical clinical signs, is presumptive evidence of FAD.

Reactions to intradermal test doses (0.1 ml of 1500 PNU/ml) of aqueous whole flea extracts have been unpredictable in confirming the diagnosis of FAD. Whole flea extracts,* 1500

°Whole Flea Extract, 1500 PNU/ml, Nelco Labs, 50B-Broad Street, Deer Park, New York

Table 2. *Comparison of the Pathophysiology, Diagnosis, and Therapy of Atopy, Flea Allergy Dermatitis, and Contact Allergic Dermatitis*

	ATOPY	FLEA ALLERGY DERMATITIS	CONTACT ALLERGIC DERMATITIS
Allergen	Glycoprotein with m.w. 10,000 (true antigen)	Hapten in flea saliva	Hapten
Mediator	IgE antibody fixed to mast cells	T lymphocytes—Humoral antibody of less importance	T lymphocyte
Route of Exposure	*Inhalation* ingestion, injection	Flea bites	Direct skin contact
Allergy Type	Immediate hyper-sensitivity	Primarily a delayed hypersensitivity although immediately relevant	Delayed hypersensitivity
Diagnostic Tests	Intradermal skin tests	None that are reliable	Provocative exposure Patch tests
Therapy	Corticosteroids Hyposensitization	Flea control Corticosteroids	Antigen avoidance Corticosteroids

PNU/ml, were evaluated by the author, and approximately 25 percent of the cases with signs of classical FAD had positive reactions. In a recent limited study, another aqueous flea antigen* was evaluated in dogs with classical FAD and in control dogs with no clinical signs or historical evidence of FAD (Lorenz, 1977). In this study, comparable doses of antigen B (0.1 ml of 1:100 and 1:1000) were compared with antigen A (0.1 ml of 1500 PNU/ml) along with dilent and histamine controls. Control dogs did not respond to either flea antigen or the diluent control; however, strong positive reactions developed to the histamine control. In dogs with classical FAD, antigen B was much more reactive than antigen A, and further studies with clinical patients indicate that the majority of dogs with FAD respond positively to this antigen. Delayed reactions are rare, but this should be looked for in the absence of immediate reaction. The absence of erythema and swelling in the test sites of control dogs suggests that primary irritation from this product is minimal.

In a study of atopic dogs, 90.6 percent were skin test positive for flea antigen (Nesbitt, 1978). The preparation was used as a flea extract in 0.5 percent phenol and 50 percent glycerin,† and it was concluded that the 50 percent glycerin was responsible for the positive intradermal reactions. No cross-over studies with aqueous flea extracts were reported. One must recognize that negative reactions to flea antigens do not necessarily eliminate the diagnosis of FAD, and positive reactions, although suggestive of FAD, are not confirmatory. Therefore, intradermal skin testing with flea antigen has definite clinical limitations, and one can usually make a correct diagnosis without performing this procedure.

TREATMENT

The primary objectives in the management of FAD are to break the flea life cycle and control the allergic reaction to fleabites. The single most important factor related to successful management is client education. To insure client education and cooperation, a brochure describing FAD is given to every owner with an affected animal. Specific recommendations are written in the appropriate places, and cases are closely monitored to assure that clients are following the recommendations.

---

*Flea Antigen (Aqueous) 1:1000 w/v, Greer Laboratory, Lenior, North Carolina

†Flea Antigen, Hollister-Steer Laboratories, Spokane, Washington.

Flea Control. Flea control is the mainstay of therapy for FAD. Flea control in the patient, the home environment, and other pets must be stressed. Affected dogs and cats must be treated with appropriate insecticidal compounds every five to seven days. For short- and medium-haired dogs, 10 percent carbaryl (Sevin) powder is recommended, and 5 percent carbaryl powder is recommended for cats. Ten percent carbaryl is not tolerated by cats and should not be used for dogs younger than 16 weeks of age. For long-haired dogs, 1 percent ronnel dips (or other effective insecticides) are given weekly. Regardless of claims made by various companies, we have not found a product that produces clinically effective residual flea killing over seven days in duration. Of the various products available, carbaryl appears to be the safest and most ecologically acceptable. During the past two years, 5 percent carbaryl preparations have not been as effective as in the past; therefore, 10 percent concentrations are usually recommended for mature dogs and in environmental control programs. Flea collars are usually not effective in the control of FAD and should not be advocated except in areas where flea infestations are mild. Although flea collars may help decrease the flea population on affected animals, all fleas are not totally or rapidly eliminated, and thus the signs of FAD persist in face of this treatment. Insecticidal collars may help control fleas on non-affected animals in the environment and therefore may be of some benefit in the overall control program.

Flea control in the home environment is probably best left in the hands of professional exterminators. Insecticidal foggers also work, and owners can purchase these at garden or hardware stores; however, this control program is usually inferior to the service provided by qualified professional exterminators. The outside environment (dog runs, dog house) should be regularly treated with 10 percent carbaryl powders or malathion sprays. Care must be taken to insure that all rugs and household items likely to harbor fleas are treated and that at least three treatments at two-week intervals are applied.

Corticosteroid Therapy. Corticosteroid therapy in skin disease has been thoroughly reviewed by other authors (Halliwell, 1977). Only a brief description will be presented in this article. Owners must understand that corticosteroid therapy effectively controls the clinical signs and does not cure the disease. Veterinarians, on the other hand, should not routinely employ corticosteroids as a substitute for sound diagnostic procedures. Prednisolone, 1.0 to 2.0 mg/kg, in divided doses for three to five days, is administered to severely pruritic animals. Thereafter, 0.5 to 1.0 mg/kg is given daily or every other day for seven to ten days. Cats may respond dramatically to megesterol acetate (Ovaban), 5 mg daily for 5 days, then 5 mg every other day for two weeks. Prolonged corticosteroid or megesterol therapy should be discouraged. Hydroxyzine hydrochloride (Atarax), 10 to 15 mg TID, or trimeprazine (Temaril), 2.5 to 5.0 mg q6h, may help control pruritis in some dogs and is used with corticosteroids in the management of acute self-mutilation. Except for areas of localized acute moist dermatitus, topical corticosteroids are not indicated. These medications are expensive, difficult to apply, and ineffective.

Hyposensitization Therapy. Flea antigen injections for the control of FAD are the subject of considerable controversy in veterinary medicine. Enthusiastic proponents and outspoken critics are abundant. Both sides of the argument are presented here; the reader is left to make the final decision.

THE "PROS" OF HYPOSENSITIZATION. Early studies in humans suggested that injections of whole flea body extracts were effective (McIvor and Cherney, 1943; Cherney et al., 1939; Hatoff, 1946). Good results were based upon subjective reports of the patients, and the studies were poorly controlled. Injections of large doses of a haptenic substance derived from collected oral flea secretions induced a state of non-reactivity in flea-allergic dogs (Feingold and Benjamini, 1961). This state of non-reactivity lasted from several weeks to several months. Similar results were reported in flea-allergic dogs and cats in the San Francisco Bay area (Michaeli and Goldfarb, 1968). In this study utilizing a haptenic fraction of flea saliva in 1 percent sodium alginate, 77 percent of affected animals achieved a hyposensitive state after three to four weekly injections. The hyposensitive state lasted for five to six weeks, and one or two booster injections reportedly produced improvement in animals that had recurrence of pruritus. In a recent study, 40 percent of 70 dogs that failed to respond to initial flea control programs responded better after treatment with whole flea antigen in 50 percent glycerine and 0.5 percent phenol (Nesbitt and Schmitz, 1978). However, in this study, no statistical difference in clinical response was found between groups of dogs treated with flea control only and those given simultaneous flea control and flea antigen injections. Although the author suggests that flea antigen therapy was beneficial, the design and results of the study discount this conclusion. Perhaps the most positive work supporting the concept of antigen flea injection therapy comes not from work in animals but from controlled trials of immunotherapy in human insect hypersensitivity (Hunt et al., 1978). In this study, insect hypersensitivity was tested using whole body extracts, specific venom extracts, and placebo injections. Placebo and whole body extract gave similar results and were significantly less effective than was specific venom immunotherapy. As this study proves, the use of specific purified antigen greatly improves the probability of achieving clinical hyposensitization, whereas the use of whole body insect extracts is probably of little clinical value.

THE "CONS" OF HYPOSENSITIZATION. Early investigators reported that even after many injections over a long period, whole flea extracts failed to hyposensitize patients, and in some cases, the injections actually worsened the sensitivity (Hartman, 1946; Feingold and Benjamini, 1963). Studies with various whole flea extracts in the author's hospital have yielded similar results. The majority of dogs receiving these extracts have had a rapid onset of clinical signs when reexposed to fleabites. Approximately 25 percent of these cases may have derived some benefit from this therapy; however, poor client cooperation in many cases has made long-term clinical trials difficult to achieve. Studies that support the use of whole body flea extracts have been poorly controlled and have not been designed to remove the investigator's bias. Well controlled studies of human insect hypersensitivity strongly indicate that whole body extracts are not effective, and one must suspect that a similar situation exists for whole body flea extracts used in dogs.

Based on the currently available information, it is difficult to rationalize the use of whole body flea extracts in the routine treatment of flea allergy dermatitis. To the author's knowledge, haptenic extracts of flea saliva are not commercially available, and it is this substance that affords the best possibility of achieving clinical hyposensitization in FAD. Veterinary clinicians must decide if the small chance of success is worth the expense and inconvenience of flea antigen injection therapy. Until well controlled, double blind studies are completed, the real value of this technique remains in doubt.

SUPPLEMENTAL READING

Benjamini, E., Feingold, B.F., Young, J.D., Kartman, L., and Shimizu, M.: Allergy to flea bites. IV, In vitro collection and antigenic properties of the oral secretion of the cat flea, *Clencephalides felis felis*. Exp. Para. 13:143–154, 1963.

Cherney, L.S., Wheeler, C.M., and Reed, A.C.: Flea antigen in prevention of flea bites. Am. J. Trop. Med. 83:327–332, 1939.

Feingold, B.F., and Benjamini, E.: Allergy to flea bites: clinical and experimental observations. Ann. Allergy 19:1275–1289, 1961.

Halliwell, R.E.W.: Steroid therapy in skin disease. In Kirk, R.W. (ed): *Current Veterinary Therapy VI.* Philadelphia, W.B. Saunders Co., 1977.

Hartman, M.M.: Flea bite reactions. Clinical and experimental observations and effect of histamine-azo-protein therapy. Ann. Allergy 4:131–136, 1946.

Hatoff, A.: Desensitization to insect bites. JAMA 130:850–854, 1946.

Hunt, K.J., Valentine, M.D., Sobotba, A.K., et al: A controlled trial of immunotherapy in insect hypersensitivity. N. Engl. J. Med. 299:157–161, 1978.

Lorenz, M.D.: Allergic dermatitis. Bi-weekly Sm. Anim. Vet. Med. Update Series 2:1–8, 1977.

McIvor, B.C., and Cherney, L.S.: Clinical use of flea-antigen in patients hypersensitive to flea bites. Am. J. Trop. Med. 23:377–379, 1943.

Michaeli, D., and Goldfarb, S.: Clinical studies on the hyposensitization of dogs and cats to flea bites. Aust. Vet. Journ. 44:161–165, 1968.

Muller, G.H., and Kirk, R.W.: *Small Animal Dermatology.* Philadelphia, W.B. Saunders Co., 1976.

Nesbitt, G.H., and Schmitz, J.A.: Flea bite allergic dermatitis: A review and survey of 330 cases. JAVMA 173:282–288, 1978.

THE DIAGNOSIS OF CANINE ATOPIC DISEASE

LLOYD M. REEDY, D.V.M.

Dallas, Texas

The word "atopy," which literally means strange disease, was first coined by Coca in 1922 to describe a group of three familial human allergic conditions — asthma, hay fever, and atopic dermatitis. At that time, atopy was believed to occur only in man, to be genetically determined, to be induced by spontaneous sensitization to usually innocuous antigens, and to result from the production of reaginic antibody (IgE). It was learned later that subsequent degranulation of mast cells released chemical mediators such as histamine and proteolytic enzymes, which are responsible for the clinical symptoms.

In 1941, Whittich reported on the first case of atopy in the dog. In addition to positive direct skin, nasal, ophthalmic, and serum transfer (Prausnitz-Küstner) tests to ragweed and other fall weed pollens, the dog was successfully hyposensitized with specific weed antigens.

CLINICAL SIGNS

The predominant presenting sign in canine atopic disease is pruritus. Hay fever-like signs occur occasionally, but true canine allergic asthma is exceedingly rare. The pattern of pruritus is often generalized, but it involves facial, foot, and axillary regions preferentially. A primary lesion may not occur, but a variety of dermatitic changes result from self-trauma. Seborrhea and superficial infections commonly ensue. It must be emphasized that even though pruritus is the hallmark of canine atopic disease, *not all* pruritic canines have canine atopy.

Since atopy is believed to be genetically determined, certain strains or families have a higher incidence of the disease. It is not unusual for several littermates to be affected, especially if one or both parents have atopy. The disease can occur in any breed, including mixed breeds, but it is reported to be more common in Dalmatians and the terrier breeds.

The age of onset is early, usually between one and three years, and the signs are most often initially seasonal. After a few pollen seasons, the allergy may expand and the symptoms may worsen in severity and become perennial. At first, corticosteroids temporarily relieve the symptoms, but with time they seem to become less effective.

DIAGNOSIS

After taking a careful history of the case, the clinician should perform a thorough and complete physical examination, primarily to rule out other skin diseases. Microscopic examination of skin scrapings should be routine. Skin cultures — both fungal and bacterial, skin biopsies, and other diagnostic tests may be indicated in certain cases.

The differential diagnosis should rule out scabies, cheyletiella, fleabite allergy, primary seborrhea, allergic contact dermatitis, bacterial hypersensitivity, and dietary allergy.

Intracutaneous skin testing should only be performed after careful consideration of the history, clinical signs, physical findings, and differential diagnosis. Since canine skin is less reactive than human skin, scratch or prick testing is not recommended in the dog. It is important that the patient not be given any drug that will lower blood pressure or otherwise block the diagnostic wheal — particularly tranquilizers, sedatives, anesthetics, antihistamines, and corticosteroids. The duration of blocking action of corticosteroids in skin testing is variable and may depend on the pharmacology of the corticosteroid, the vehicle, dosage, route of administration, metabolism of the patient, and duration of drug therapy. As a general rule, oral corticosteroids should be discontinued for at least a week prior to skin testing. Long-acting injectable corticosteroids should not be given for four weeks or longer. Patients that have been on long-term corticosteroid therapy should be hospitalized, withdrawn from the drug gradually, and given ACTH injections to prevent adrenal insufficiency. In some cases, it may be months before skin reactions are normal.

The patient should be held in lateral recumbency on a padded surface for comfort. The hair over the lateral thorax is clipped with a number 40 blade. No soaps, disinfectants, antiseptics, or chemicals are applied to the test area. If the skin is infected, testing should be postponed until long-term appropriate systemic antibiotic therapy has cleared the infection. Allergy testing in other sites such as the abdominal or inguinal area is not as satisfactory as it is in the lateral thorax.

After marking the injection sites with a felt-tipped pen, 0.02 to 0.03 ml of each test antigen is injected intradermally. The author prefers disposable 26 gauge $\frac{3}{8}$ inch needles attached to tuberculin syringes. It is imperative that (1) the injections are truly intradermal and not subcutaneous, (2) exactly the same amount of antigen is administered in each test site, and (3) no air is injected (Table 1).

The allergy test should be read between 15 and 30 minutes. Since some patients will traumatize the test area so that it cannot be read, leaving an animal alone in a cage or run is not advised. With the patient again restrained in lateral recumbency, the room is darkened, and an indirect light source such as a pen light is used to accentuate diagnostic wheals. Each test site is compared with the positive control —histamine (1:100,000) — and the negative control — buffered saline. Measuring each wheal is recommended. Histamine wheals are considered maximal reactions. Failure to produce a strong wheal with histamine suggests inter-

Table 1. *Reasons for Intradermal Allergy Testing Failures*

FALSE NEGATIVES
1. Subcutaneous injections rather than true intradermal injections
2. Too little antigen to cause reaction
   a. Group testing (weed, grass, or tree mixes) — each antigen too dilute
   b. Outdated extracts — lose potency with storage
   c. Improper dilution — too dilute (1000 PNU/ml except house dust 250 PNU/ml or 500 PNU/ml)
   d. Too little volume injected — 0.02–0.03 ml ideal
3. Drugs that block or inhibit skin test reaction
   a. Corticosteroids
   b. Antihistamines
   c. Tranquilizers
   d. Any drug that depresses blood pressure and thus blocks diagnostic wheal
4. Prolonged allergy — exhaustion of skin sensitizing antibodies
5. Inherent host factors
   a. Very young and very old will give smaller skin reactions
   b. Temperature of skin; integrity of autonomic innervation of cutaneous vessels
   c. Chronic diseases

FALSE POSITIVES
1. Too large volume test allergen — 0.02–0.03 ideal
2. Irritants — certain foods, house dust, feathers, glycerin preservatives in test antigen
3. Substances that cause release of histamine or contain histamine, morphine, or codeine (cheeses have high histamine content)
4. Bacterial or fungal contamination of test antigen — usually old or out of date antigen
5. Remnant of past sensitivity; clinical sensitivity has disappeared
6. Harbinger of future sensitivity
7. Dissociation of positive skin test and clinical sensitivity
   a. Food allergy — patients will react positively to undigested food but may be non-allergic to digestive breakdown products (20 percent positive skin tests for food have clinical correlation)

ference or inability to react. Buffered saline is the same as that used for diluting test antigens and is considered negative. Grades of reactions to test antigens are based on the size of each wheal as compared with histamine and buffered saline.

SELECTION OF ANTIGENS

The selection of test antigens will vary with geographic location and has a direct relation to antigens used in hyposensitization. Knowledge of seasonal area pollen counts as well as significant pollens that produce human allergies is helpful. Valuable asisstance may be obtained from local human allergists, medical schools, and health departments. In order for a pollen to be important in allergy, it must be produced in large quantities, small and light enough to be widely dispersed by wind currents, and antigenically capable of producing allergic disease. Grass, weed, and tree pollens appear to be the most significant. The author prefers to limit the number of test antigens to not more than 30 at one time (Table 2). The ideal time to test skin is shortly after the offending pollen season.

In both skin testing and hyposensitization, two different methods are used to measure concentration of antigens, protein nitrogen units (PNU), and weight/volume. One milligram of protein is defined as 100,000 protein nitrogen units (PNU). Weight/volume is a standard based upon the weight of the dried allergen being extracted in a known volume of extracting fluid and expressed as a ratio (e.g., 1:100). Only aqueous antigens should be used for skin testing, and these may be purchased from commercial allergy firms in concentrated stock solutions. Since concentrated antigens seem to be stable longer, the author prefers buying antigens in 10,000 PNU/ml for testing. Care must be taken to dilute test antigens to 1000 PNU every one to three months, discarding unused diluted antigens. House dust is a mixture of antigens and may be irritating. For this reason, it is recommended that house dust test antigen be diluted to 250 PNU/ml.

GROUP TESTING VS. SINGLE EXTRACT TESTING

The antigenic relationship existing among members of certain botanical groups, such as grasses, weeds, and trees, is important both in diagnosis and treatment of allergic disease. For a long time, it was generally believed that based on clinical and experimental observations, members of the grass family possessed a major antigen common to all. This was also accepted to be true of members of the ragweed family but not of other weed and tree pollens. However, recent observations seem to indicate that grass pollens contain two antigenic factors, one specific for the individual pollen and another common to the entire family, or that all members of the same family contain different factors.

It is the opinion of the author, after comparing group tests (grass mixes and weed mixes) with individual tests (Bermuda grass, marshelder, etc.), that individual tests are more accurate. In many cases, intracutaneous skin tests with weed mixes are negative, whereas individual tests with specific weeds revealed one or more positives. Knowledge of the specific weed or weeds causing the allergy allowed higher dosage of the exact offending allergens in hyposen-

Table 2.   Allergy Testing Sheet

```
                                                           DATE_____
OWNER'S NAME_____        BREED_____
SEX_____AGE_____      ONSET_____
SEASONAL_____PERENNIAL_____
PATTERN_____PROGRESSION_____
FLEAS_____
RESPONSE TO STEROIDS_____
LAST TIME SUCH THERAPY WAS ADMINISTERED_____
ANY OTHER THERAPY_____
GRASSES
_____Johnson                 _____Russian Thistle
_____Bermuda                 _____English Plantain
_____Rye                     _____Western Water Hemp
_____June                    _____Wingscale
_____Orchard           TREES
_____Timothy                 _____Mt. Cedar
MOLDS                           _____Pecan (Hickory)
_____Mold Mix A              _____Box Elder (Maple)
_____Mold Mix B              _____Oak
WEEDS                     OTHER
_____Ragweed                 _____House dust          _____Flea
_____Cockleburr              _____House dust mite
_____Marshelder             _____Sheep Wool
_____Careless                _____Feathers
_____Sage                    _____Staph
_____Kochia                  _____Diluent
_____Yellow dock            _____Histamine
```

Personal File

sitization at a reduced cost. The foregoing statements were also true with grass and tree pollens. Screening with pollen mixes is not recommended because of the high number of false negatives.

OTHER TESTS

The Prausnitz-Küster (PK) or passive transfer test and the radioallergosorbent test (RAST), although not used routinely in the diagnosis of atopic disease, may be indicated in special cases when skin testing is not possible. Indications would be in patients with demographism or unmanageable skin disease or who otherwise cannot be skin tested. The PK test is performed by injecting serum from the allergic patient into the skin of a non-allergic patient and then skin testing the passively transferred non-allergic patient. (For detailed information on the technique, the reader is referred to the supplemental reading list at the end of this chapter.)

The RAST (radioallergosorbent test) is an *in vitro* means of measuring antigen-specific serum IgE levels. At present, its use is restricted because of cost and the limited availability of antigens. The immediate application of RAST is in allergen standardization, but it will be used more for diagnostic purposes as purified and less expensive antigens become available.

Provocative testing in atopic disease is useful in identifying food allergy and possibly for confirming doubtful skin test results. Intracutaneous testing for food allergy is not recommended because of the large number of false positives. Provocative testing in suspected house dust, wool, feather, or animal dander allergy may be helpful. A positive test is denoted by an appreciable increase in pruritus following exposure plus a dramatic decrease in pruritus with complete avoidance.

In summary, intracutaneous testing is a useful aid in the diagnosis of canine atopic disease. Correlation of positive skin tests with the occurrence of symptoms during a specific pollen season or certain exposure is essential. The casual or occasional use of skin testing, without extensive reading, preparation, and the devotion of a great deal of time to each case, will end in disappointing results. Even in the most experienced hands, allergy testing and subsequent attempts to hyposensitize may be successful in only 70 to 80 percent of cases.

SUPPLEMENTAL READING

Anderson, W.A.: Atopic dermatitis in the dog. Cutis 15:955–960, 1975.
Baker, E.: Diagnosis and management of clinical allergy. JAVMA 157:1607–1615, 1970.
Baker, K.P.: Intradermal tests as an aid to the diagnosis of skin disease in dogs. J. Small Anim. Pract. 12:445–452, 1971.
Chamberlain, K.W.: Diagnostic methods in allergic disease. Vet. Clin. North Am. 4(1)47–56, 1974.
Halliwell, R.E.W.: The immunology of allergic skin disease. J. Small. Anim. Pract. 12:431–433, 1971.
Patterson, R.: *Allergic Disease: Diagnosis and Management.* Philadelphia, J.B. Lippincott Co., 1972.
Reedy, L.M.: Canine atopy. Compend. Cont. Educ., 1(7):550–557, 1979.
Regional Pollen Guide, Hollister-Stier Laboratories, Spokane, Washington.

THE TREATMENT OF CANINE ATOPIC DISEASE*

GAIL A. KUNKLE, D.V.M.
Philadelphia, Pennsylvania

Canine atopic disease, otherwise known as atopy or allergic inhalant dermatitis, is one of the more common allergic diseases of the dog.

Therapy for the atopic patient presents a problem-filled challenge in both man and dog. There are many questions concerning mechanisms and actions of various therapeutic and biologic agents. Successful clinical management of the atopic dog requires not only a well informed veterinarian but also an understanding owner and cooperative patient. This article presents

*The studies reported in this article were supported by a grant from the Tarrant County V.M.A. through the Morris Animal Foundation.

successful therapeutic principles for the canine atopic patient.

DIAGNOSIS

Techniques for diagnosing atopy are outlined in the preceding article, and it is not necessary to review these methods in depth. However, the importance of a correct diagnosis cannot be overemphasized.

Clinical signs are highly variable in canine atopy owing to many factors such as previous treatment and duration of the disease. Before instituting any symptomatic or biologic therapy for atopy, it is essential that the signs be consistent with the suspected disease. It is important to remember that most of the signs of atopy that are visible are the result of self-inflicted trauma. Depending on the course and the severity, signs may range from mild erythema to severe evidence of self-trauma, hyperpigmentation, lichenification, and varying degrees of alopecia.

A supportive history also is an important finding for a proper diagnosis. Such factors as seasonality and previous response to corticosteroids may aid in support of the clinical diagnosis of canine atopy.

In addition to clinical signs and suggestive history, a definitive diagnosis of inhalant allergies requires confirmation with intradermal skin tests. (The techniques for these tests have been outlined elsewhere).

The selection of testing antigens requires considerable planning. Antigens used for testing should be those that consistently cause allergic problems in human patients in the same geographic area. Consideration of cross-reactivity and dilution factors are important when using mixtures. In some clinical cases with distinct seasonal signs, the time of year that the intradermal testing is done may be important. Generally, it is best to wait until shortly after the intense pollen season to test seasonal patients. At that time, their IgE levels are quite high, yet their symptoms have subsided and therapeutic corticosteroids are not in the circulation. A negative skin test does not eliminate a diagnosis of allergy but suggests that reevaluation be done at a later date.

Finally, once a clinical diagnosis of atopic allergy has been confirmed with positive allergy tests, it is essential that the test results be consistent with the history and supportive of the diagnosis. For example, a diagnosis of ragweed allergy cannot be justified for a patient with year-round symptoms and a positive intradermal only to ragweed. Most atopic patients are multisensitive and rarely react to only one or two antigens. It is important that the diagnostic tests, the clinical signs, and the history come together to support the diagnosis of canine atopic disease.

Once a diagnosis of canine inhalant allergy has been reached, various methods of therapy may be considered.

AVOIDANCE THERAPY

Elimination of the identified allergen results in the most successful therapy for the atopic patient, but unfortunately, it is often too impractical to consider. It can be most useful when the allergy is limited to a few antigens such as feathers, wool, cottonseed, and kapok. Without excessive inconvenience, many owners can remove some of the allergens from the environment.

In addition to removing offending substances, other household controls may aid in decreasing the antigen exposure. Air conditioning or electrostatic air filtration may help by lessening airborne house dust, mold, and pollen particles.

MEDICAL THERAPY

Many different pharmacological agents are available for use in canine atopic disease. It is important to realize that no form of medical therapy "cures" the disease, although some can be very effective in controlling allergic conditions by giving symptomatic relief. Various agents may be useful as adjuncts to avoidance or biologic therapy, but in most cases the use of drugs is not the ideal approach.

Through their anti-inflammatory effects, corticosteroids are the most effective form of medical therapy in atopic dogs. Dogs with a short period of clinical symptoms may be treated with systemic corticosteroids without too much concern. The drug is given daily initially and then gradually decreased to alternate day therapy, and it is eventually discontinued. Corticosteroids may be helpful during other types of therapy when the antigen load becomes too heavy and the dog's symptoms exacerbate. A short course of steroids often can be instrumental in halting the itch-scratch cycle, which, once started, can lead to severe self-trauma even after the instigating allergen is gone.

There are several important considerations when initiating systemic steroid therapy. The side-effects of overuse and abuse with steroids should always be remembered. A short-term, low dose steroid course is always preferred if it succeeds in controlling the signs. In patients that require long-term corticosteroid therapy, early morning alternate day therapy should be attempted to minimize the suppressive effect on the hypothalamic-pituitary-adrenal axis. In these cases, it is important to use a short-acting corticosteroid such as prednisone or prednisolone.

Although daily control can be more manageable with short-acting steroids, some clients may abuse the drugs. For this reason, some clinicians prefer to use injectable steroids, as they feel they have better control over the amount given the patient and better clinical follow-ups. Some owners also feel that their dogs obtain more effective relief from the long-term injectable steroids. By limiting the number of prednisolone tablets that are dispensed, most cases can be monitored with control over the daily dose. After an explanation of the dangers and side-effects of excess, many owners are willing to give oral drugs only when the pet needs them to remain comfortable.

There are myriads of corticosteroid products available to the practitioner. Most veterinarians can manage allergy cases medically by familiarizing themselves with only two or three products — e.g., a short-acting oral drug such as prednisolone and a long-acting injectable one such as methylprednisolone acetate (Depomedrol®, UpJohn). Dosages are highly variable and guidelines are available elsewhere. It is crucial to know the drugs one uses and to use as little as necessary to complete the task. Topical corticosteroid products rarely prove helpful as a supportive therapy and serve little use in primary therapy.

Antihistamines, another form of medical therapy, have considerable use in the treatment of human atopic disease, but results in the dog are usually unrewarding. Histamine is released in the skin of the allergic canine patient, but it appears that proteolytic enzymes and other substances released during mast cell degranulation are responsible for the majority of the resulting pruritus. Thus, even with the successful action of the antihistamine, pruritus usually remains. Some clinicians report satisfactory results with antihistamines in occasional cases, so a rational approach might include an initial trial period. Others report that at doses much exceeding those used in man, antihistamines may be successful in preventing pruritus. Unfortunately at these doses, the sedative effects of the antihistamine may be so apparent that it is difficult to assess their true value in pruritus.

Other forms of medical therapy are available but are useful only in occasional cases. Tranquilizers and sedatives may be used to aid in prevention of severe self-trauma. They provide little long-term relief if the owner desires the dog as a companion. Cromolyn sodium (Intal®,

Fisons), which is often efficacious in man, acts by inhibiting mediator release. It is toxic when injected in the dog, but oral therapy may be worthy of investigation.

HYPOSENSITIZATION

Because avoidance therapy is often impossible and medical therapy is best indicated for only short season atopics, patients that have symptoms longer than four months per year or have undesirable effects from steroids may require other therapy. Hyposensitization is a biologic therapy for the atopic patient that results when a patient is given increasing doses of the implicated antigens parenterally. The patient reacts by forming IgG antibodies directed against the specific antigen. Unlike the tissue-fixed IgE antibodies, it is suggested that the IgG antibodies circulate and are protective. When the hyposensitized patient inhales the previous symptom-provoking antigen, this antigen binds with the circulating IgG antibody before it reaches the tissue-fixed IgE. In this way, the IgG acts as a blocking antibody. The entire mechanism of hyposensitization is not this simple. In more recent years, several theories have been proposed combining the theory of blocking antibody with a later decrease in cellular sensitivity and finally a long-term diminution of the reaginic antibody available to sensitize mediator releasing cells. Although the true mode of action of hyposensitization is not understood, the blocking antibody theory is widely accepted as being in part responsible.

There are two basic approaches to hyposensitization. One uses aqueous extracts, which are rapidly absorbed and require more frequent injections. The other approach uses the alum-precipitated extracts, which are more slowly absorbed and thus require fewer injections.

It is essential before undertaking hyposensitization that the process and expectations be explained to the owners. This method of therapy is frequently successful if the correct diagnosis is made and the owner is prepared to cooperate fully in the venture.

Selection of Antigens

Hyposensitization should be initiated with allergens that are selected by comparing clinical history with positive skin tests. Generally, the vaccine is restricted to 10 antigens. Using more than 10 antigens results in too much dilution of each antigen or an increased total antigenic load, and thus the program may be ineffective and dangerous. In many cases, less than 10 antigens are used to make up the vaccine. It has been shown in man that hyposensitization results in antigen-specific blocking antibody.

Therefore, it is highly undesirable to treat patients empirically with a battery of antigens common to the geographic area.

When selecting antigens for the vaccine, one should consider the size of the skin test response and its relation to the clinical history. Environmental considerations are important, and the dog that lives in the country and has symptoms from July through September should have the appropriate weed antigens to which he reacted included in his vaccine. This same patient also may have reacted to wool but has no atopic signs except during weed season. In this case, it is unnecessary to include wool in the vaccine. A dog that exhibits the same degree of pruritus year round will probably require that the majority of antigens in his vaccine be year-round inhalants such as house dust and kapok, depending on the skin test results.

Ideally, therapy should be initiated so that the maintenance dose of 1 cc (total of 10,000–20,000 PNUs) is reached at least a month before clinical signs start. This is not possible in the case of the perenially affected dog, but generally it is best to initiate therapy when the environmental allergic load is low. Owners with great expectations may become impatient with the slow response to hyposensitization therapy if it is begun in the midst of the allergy season after the symptoms have become severe.

There are many different systems for standardization of pollen extracts. The weight by volume system and the protein nitrogen unit system seem to be used most frequently. At the University of Pennsylvania, using the protein nitrogen unit system, the preparation of

aqueous extract vaccine is done as follows (Table 1). Vial number 3, also known as the maintenance vial, contains 10 cc of allergen mixture, usually 10,000 to 20,000 PNUs/cc. This is made up of a combination of allergens selected as described. If 10 antigens are used, 1 cc of 20,000 PNUs of each antigen is added to vial 3, and each cc of the final dilution would contain only 2000 PNUs of each antigen. If four antigens are used, 2.5 cc (50,000 PNUs) of each antigen are added to vial 3. In this example, each cc of the final dilution in vial 3 would contain approximately 5000 PNUs of each of the four antigens. Vial 2 is a 10-fold dilution of vial 3, and vial 1 is a 10-fold dilution of vial 2. After the mixture and the dilutions are made, the schedule is reviewed with the owners and the vaccine is dispensed to them to give injections at home. This eliminates the extra expense and time consumption of repeated office visits. The incidence of reactions with this schedule is extremely rare, and home therapy seems most safe and convenient.

The same considerations are made in selected antigens for the alum precipitated vaccine (Table 2). Because the release is slower, only one dilution bottle is made, and the initiating therapy begins with a higher strength. Table 2 shows the schedule for alum precipitated extracts used at the University of Pennsylvania. Both schedules reach maintenance levels of 1 cc injections, which contain 10,000 to 20,000 PNU mixtures of allergens.

A third method of hyposensitization uses aqueous extracts in an extremely accelerated program of injections. Initial injections are

Table 1. Aqueous Schedule For Hyposensitization

		VIAL 1 (100–200 PNU/ml)	VIAL 2 (1000–2000 PNU/ml)	VIAL 3 (10,000–20,000 PNU/ml)
(Day)	0	0.1 cc		
	2	0.2 cc		
	4	0.4 cc		
	6	0.8 cc		
	8	1.0 cc		
	10		0.1 cc	
	12		0.2 cc	
	14		0.4 cc	
	16		0.8 cc	
	18		1.0 cc	
	20			0.1 cc
	22			0.2 cc
	24			0.4 cc
	26			0.8 cc
	28			1.0 cc
	38			1.0 cc
	48°			1.0 cc

°Thereafter, repeat injections (1.0 cc.) every 20 to 40 days for the next 18 months.
Injections are given by subcutaneous administration. The extracts must be kept refrigerated.

Table 2. *Alum Precipitated Schedule*
ALLPYRAL® (DOME LABORATORIES) AND CENTERAL® (CENTER LABORATORIES)

		VIAL 1 (100–200 PNU/ml)	VIAL 2 (10,000–20,000 PNU/ml)
Week	1	0.1 cc	
	2	0.2 cc	
	3	0.4 cc	
	4	0.8 cc	
	5		0.1 cc
	6		0.2 cc
	7		0.4 cc
	8		0.8 cc
	9		1.0 cc
	12		1.0 cc
	16		1.0 cc
	20		1.0 cc
	24		1.0 cc
	28		1.0 cc
	32		1.0 cc

Injections are given by subcutaneous administration. The extracts must be kept refrigerated. Shake well.

given every three to four hours until maintenance levels are reached. Although the experience at the University of Pennsylvania with this technique has not resulted in any systemic reactions, the risk of such may be higher than that with other methods. Because the method requires considerable time and careful monitoring, it seems quite unnecessary for seasonal atopics. It might be considered for severely affected perennial atopics, as it has appeared somewhat efficacious.

Regardless of which type product and which schedule is used, it is important to recognize that the schedule may need to be altered for various patients. Owners of dogs with summer symptoms may be able to decrease injections after the first year to every 30 to 45 days during the winter months and then increase again to every 20 days during the height of the season. Some patients may need booster injections as frequently as every 10 to 14 days during the height of the pollen season. Other patients may not be able to tolerate maintenance injections of 20,000 PNUs and may have mild exacerbations of symptoms that require reduction of the maintenance dose. Most local reactions of pruritus at injection site can be eliminated by giving an antihistamine prior to injection. Generally, most patients do well on the above schedules, but each patient should be treated individually.

THRESHOLD PHENOMENON

In therapy for the atopic patient, one should always consider the importance of each patient's threshold concerning pruritus. The aller-

gy load in one atopic dog may incite severe pruritus, whereas a dog with similar skin test sensitivities in the same environment may not even itch. All factors that may lower this threshold should be considered in the atopic dog. The pruritic atopic dog with dry skin may completely stop itching with symptomatic therapy of water soaks and bath oils. Similarly, the intensely pruritic atopic dog with pyoderma may have its pruritus decreased dramatically by treatment with proper antibiotics. Fleas can be a mechanical as well as an allergic contribution to lowering of the threshold for pruritus. Thus it is important that the normal integrity of the skin in the atopic dog be maintained with good supportive care.

ASSESSMENT OF THERAPY

The majority of atopic dogs in which the diagnosis has been carefully determined do well on hyposensitization therapy. Clinical response may not be apparent for six months, and improvement is gradual rather than immediate. After six months, dogs that are not responding should be reassessed. Assessment of atopic patients started on hyposensitization during a two-year period at the University of Pennsylvania is shown in Table 3. Evaluation of the success of the program was made by the owner and the referring veterinarian. Approximately 60 percent of the aqueous patients obtained significant clinical improvement. Allpyral® (Dome Laboratories) proved to be not quite as successful. It is interesting to note that the incidence of total failure was greater with Allpyral® than with aqueous extracts.

Table 3. Assessment of Hyposensitization
PATIENTS FROM 1976 & 1977
UNIVERSITY OF PENNSYLVANIA VETERINARY SCHOOL

% IMPROVEMENT DERMATOLOGICALLY	AQUEOUS	% OF GROUP	ALLPYRAL	% OF GROUP
0–25	21 (8)°	23.0 (8.9)°	12 (9)°	35.2 (26.5)°
25–50	16	17.8	8	23.5
50–75	27	30.0	7	20.6
75–100	26	28.9	7	20.6
	90		34	

°Numbers in parentheses refer to patients who received no benefit.

Currently, the ideal length of recommended therapy is unknown. Some dogs can be taken off injections after two years and remain symptom free. Many require maintenance booster injections indefinitely.

The most valuable tool for the veterinarian in treating canine atopic disease is familiarity with a good therapeutic system. One should not attempt all types of therapy. Knowledge of the uses of one or two antihistamines and a few corticosteroids and familiarity with one program of hyposensitization in most cases will allow the practitioner to manage canine atopic patients successfully. After following a few patients through regimens of hyposensitization, slight alterations can be made in individual cases as familiarity with the technique increases. Successful therapeutic management of canine atopic disease can be very rewarding.

SUPPLEMENTAL READING

Anderson, W.A.: Canine Allergic Inhalant Dermatitis. Ralston-Purina Co., 1975.
Baker, E.: Management of allergic disease by hyposensitization. J. Am. Vet. Med. Assoc. 154:491–494, 1969.
Chamberlain, K.W. (ed.): Allergy. Vet. Clin. North Am. 4:57–77, 1974.
Patterson, R. (ed.): *Allergic Diseases — Diagnosis and Management.* Philadelphia, J.B. Lippincott, 1972.

DRUG ERUPTION

DANNY W. SCOTT, D.V.M.
Ithaca, New York

Drug eruption is defined as a cutaneous or mucocutaneous reaction to the administration of a drug. Drugs responsible for such eruptions may be administered orally, topically, or by injection or inhalation.

Any drug may cause an eruption, and there is no specific type of reaction for any one drug. Thus, drug eruption can mimic virtually any dermatosis, with the exception of most genodermatoses, nevi, and tumors.

There is no reliable information available on the incidence of drug eruption in dogs and cats. In man, drug eruption is reported to occur in 2 or 3 percent of medical in-patients. Reaction rates (reactions/1000 recipients) were highest for trimethoprim-sulfamethoxazole (59/1000), ampicillin (52/1000), semisynthetic penicillins (36/1000), and erythromycin (23/1000).

PATHOMECHANISM

Allergic (hypersensitivity) mechanisms appear to be the most common cause of drug eruption. It should be emphasized, however, that most so-called "allergic" drug reactions are judged to be allergic on clinical grounds alone.

The types of immunologic responses thought to be involved in drug eruptions include "immediate reactions" (Type I, II, and III hypersensitivities), which are associated with humoral antibodies, and "delayed reactions" (Type IV hypersensitivity), which are associated with cell-mediated immunity.

CLINICAL SIGNS

Drug eruptions may mimic virtually any cutaneous or mucocutaneous disorder. Several morphologic types of drug-induced cutaneous eruptions have been reported in man (Table 1). Table 2 contains data on 25 cases of drug eruption in dogs and cats seen by the author over a six-year period. No breed, age, or sex predilections were found. Eruptions occurred after as little as seven days or as much as several months of exposure to the offending drug. Many of these eruptions were pruritic.

DIAGNOSIS

Because drug eruption can mimic so many different dermatoses, it is imperative to have an accurate knowledge of the medications given to any patient with an obscure dermatosis.

In general, there are no specific or characteristic laboratory findings in drug eruption. Results of *in vivo* and *in vitro* immunologic tests have not been diagnostic. Examination of skin biopsies is often helpful in arriving at a diagnosis, more by excluding other possibilities than by providing a specific pathologic diagnosis. Just as the clinical morphologic eruptions vary greatly, so do the histologic patterns. Thus, no one histologic change is indicative of drug eruption.

At present, the only reliable test for the diagnosis of drug eruption is to withdraw the drug and wait for disappearance of the eruption. Drug eruptions usually clear within 7 to 14 days, although they may occasionally persist for weeks to months after the offending drug is discontinued. Purposeful readministration of the drug to determine if the eruption is reproduced is undesirable and dangerous.

Because there is no single diagnostic test for drug eruption, one must rely on clinical impressions and history. The following points may be helpful in recognizing drug eruptions.

Table 1. *Morphologic Types of Cutaneous Eruptions Caused by Drugs in Man*

Acneiform—comedones, papules, pustules, furuncles

Eczematous—erythema, papules, vesicles, edema, oozing, scales, crusts, pruritus

Erythema multiforme-like—sudden onset of symmetrical, vividly erythematous wheals, bullae, and/or purpuric lesions

Erythema nodosum-like—tender, erythematous nodules associated with pruritus and burning

Exfoliative—marked scaling and peeling

Fixed—focal area of dermatitis that reappears in the same spot every time the drug is taken

Lichenoid—discrete papules, often flat-topped and keratotic, and variable in color

Lupus-like—erythematous macules and plaques with scaling and patulous follicles, spreading peripherally and healing centrally with frequent atrophy, scarring, and leukoderma

Morbilliform—small, red to pink macules in crescentic groups, which tend to coalesce and scale

Photosensitive—acute to subacute inflammatory reactions in light-exposed areas

Pigmentary—increase (melanoderma) or decrease (leukoderma) in normal pigmentation

Purpuric—petechiae and/or ecchymoses that tend to become confluent

Toxic epidermal necrolysis-like—pain, bullae, peeling, and ulceration; usually accompanied by fever and malaise and often by mucous membrane involvement

Urticarial—wheals

Vesiculobullous—vesicles and bullae, with resultant erosions and ulcers

---

Table 2.   *Data on 25 Drug Eruptions in Dogs and Cats Seen at the*
New York State College of Veterinary Medicine 1972–1977

SPECIES	BREED	DRUG	ROUTE	ERUPTION
C	German shepherd	Triple sulfa	Oral	Eczematous (G°)
C	Collie X	Quinidine	Oral	Exfoliative (G)
C	German short-haired pointer	Griseofulvin	Oral	Eczematous (G)
C	Collie	Neomycin-triamcinolone	Topical	Eczematous (L†)
C	Poodle	Diphenylhydantoin (Phenytoin)	Oral	Vesicobullous (G)
C	German shepherd	Diethylcarbamazine	Oral	Eczematous (G)
C	Great Dane	Chloramphenicol	Oral	Purpuric (G)
C	Pug	Lime sulfur dip	Topical	Exfoliative (G)
C	Cocker spaniel	Coal tar shampoo	Topical	Eczematous (G)
C	Collie	Benzoyl peroxide shampoo	Topical	Erythroderma (G)
C	Yellow Labrador	Benzoyl peroxide gel	Topical	Erythroderma (L)
C	Scottish terrier	Benzoyl peroxide gel	Topical	Erythroderma (L)
C	Golden retriever	Tetracycline	Oral	Urticaria-Angioedema (G)
C	Afghan	Prednisolone	Oral	Alopecia (G)
C	Afghan	Prednisolone	Oral	Alopecia (G)
C	Collie X	5-fluorocytosine	Oral	Eczematous (G)
C	German shepherd	5-fluorocytosine	Oral	Eczematous (G)
C	Malamute	Thiabendazole	Oral	Pemphigus vulgaris-like (G)
C	Boston terrier	Ampicillin	Oral	Fixed (L)
C	Dachshund	Diethylcarbamazine	Oral	Pruritus (G)
F	DSH	FeLV antiserum	Subcutaneous	Toxic epidermal necrolysis (G)
F	Siamese	Chlorinated hydrocarbon, pyrethrin, mineral oil	Topical	Otitis externa
F	DSH	Sulfisoxazole	Oral	Eczematous (G)
F	DSH	Hetacillin	Oral	Multifocal alopecia (G)
F	DSH	Sulfisoxazole	Oral	Eczematous (G)

°Generalized.
†Localized.

1. Drugs tolerated well for days, months, or years may suddenly cause eruptions.
2. After an eruption has occurred once, it may recur regularly on readministration of the same drug, even in small doses
3. The cutaneous changes are different from those that would be expected on the basis of the pharmacologic effect of the drug
4. Drugs that have entirely different pharmacologic effects, but have similar chemical structures, may cause identical morphologic forms of eruptions
5. A drug can cause different cutaneous reactions in different individuals, and even in one individual at different times
6. The dose of a drug required to elicit an eruption is usually considerably smaller than that needed to induce an expected pharmacologic effect
7. Drug eruptions often respond poorly to glucocorticoid therapy until the offending drug is stopped.

THERAPY

Management of drug eruption consists of (1) stopping use of the drug, (2) evaluating hematologic, hepatic, and renal status, (3) administering glucocorticoids, (4) administering antihistamines and epinephrine in urticarial, angioedematous, or anaphylactoid reactions, and (5) avoiding chemically related drugs.

SUPPLEMENTAL READING

Arndt, K.A., and Jick, H.: Rates of cutaneous reactions to drugs. A report from the Boston Collaborative Drug Surveillance Program. JAMA 235:918–923, 1976.
Scott, D.W., Barrett, R.E., and Tangorra, L.: Drug eruption associated with sulfonamide treatment of vertebral osteomyelitis in a dog. JAVMA 168:1111–1114, 1976.

OTITIS EXTERNA

L. R. GRONO, B.V.Sc.
St. Lucia, Australia

Otitis externa is an inflammation of the epithelium of the external auditory canal but may also involve the pinna. It is characterized by erythema, increased discharge or desquamation of epithelium, and varying degrees of pain or irritation. In the dog, particularly in chronic otitis externa, edema and ulceration of the meatal epithelium may be present. Perforation of the tympanic membrane may then occur and the condition can extend to involve the middle ear.

Otitis externa is common in the dog and has a worldwide distribution. One in eight dogs attending the Small Animal Practice Teaching Unit at the Edinburgh Veterinary School was clinically affected with otitis externa. In New Zealand at the Massey University Veterinary Clinic, 7.5 per cent of dogs had otitis. At the Queensland University Veterinary School Clinic, 4.8 per cent of dogs were presented for treatment because they were suffering from otitis externa, but in sample dog populations in the same area, 16.0 and 20.4 per cent showed clinical signs of the disease.

Certain breeds of dog have a high incidence of otitis. Breeds with pendulous ears such as the Labrador and Cocker spaniel, and those with an hirsute meatus such as poodles, account for 60 to 80 per cent of cases in most surveys.

Otitis externa is less common in the cat. An incidence of 2.0 per cent has been recorded. This is due to the upright position of the pinna, permitting good ventilation and drainage. No breed susceptibility to otitis externa has been reported in the cat, which is to be expected because variations in ear conformation are minor.

Age plays little part in the incidence of otitis externa in man, but in the dog, the highest incidence is usually between five and eight years, with no sex predisposition.

In man, elevated temperature and humidity are thought to play an important role in the incidence of otitis externa. In the dog in a subtropical environment, the greatest number of cases were presented for treatment in the summer months, but seasonal difference was not statistically significant. In some areas where grass awns are a major cause of otitis externa, there may be a definite seasonal incidence.

ETIOLOGY

A number of factors are important in the etiology of otitis externa. Trauma and foreign bodies are undoubted causes.

Extension of infection from an otitis media to cause secondary otitis externa is not common, although some researchers disagree. Moltzen (1969) considered otitis media particularly important, and in another report of 180 cases of otitis externa, 42 per cent had otitis media. Otitis externa as further manifestation of an existing skin condition has been reported in 38 per cent of cases in one study and in 10.3 per cent of cases in another (Fraser; Fraser et al.).

The ear mite, *Otodectes cynotis,* can cause otitis externa in the dog and cat. How often the ear mite is a significant factor has not been defined. A number of researchers consider *Otodectes cynotis* to be an important etiologic agent. One survey found mites in 29.1 per cent

of 350 dogs examined; 24.1 per cent of these had otitis externa. The intradermal injection of whole mite extracts has caused an immediate Arthus-type reaction in the cat, and otitis externa in the dog has been produced experimentally with ear mites.

Once otitis externa is present and discharge has increased in the external ear canal, ear mites either die or leave the now unsuitable environment, making it difficult to determine how commonly they initiate otitis externa.

The breed incidence of the disease indicates that pendulous ears are a predisposing factor. The effect of the pendulous pinna in sealing off the aditus of the meatus is illustrated in Figure 1. The pendulous pinna of the spaniel or the narrow hirsute meatus of the poodle restrict ventilation and drainage from the ear canal.

The relative humidity in the dog's external ear canal is high — usually at a level that permits the epithelium to absorb increased

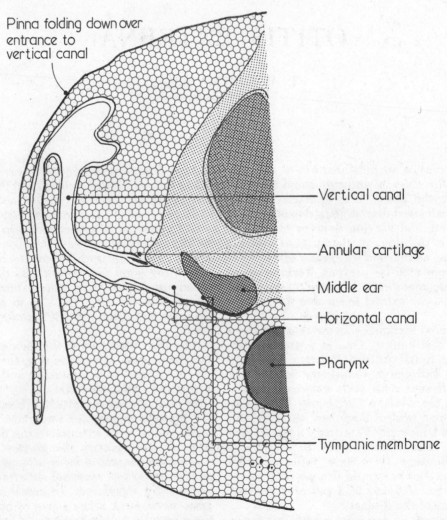

Pinna folding down over entrance to vertical canal

Vertical canal

Annular cartilage

Middle ear

Horizontal canal

Pharynx

Tympanic membrane

Figure 1.　Section of the head of a lop-eared dog at the level of the external auditory meatus.

amounts of moisture. This, together with an adequate temperature and blood supply, makes the tortuous ear canal an ideal environment for bacterial and fungal growth.

The normal flora of the canine ear canal has been studied, and there are a large number of references recording organisms isolated from ear canals with otitis externa. The findings from several centers where the flora in the normal ear and in the diseased ear canal have been investigated are presented in Table 1.

The common organisms isolated from cases of otitis externa are *Staphylococcus aureus*, yeasts (*Pityrosporum* sp.), *Streptococcus* sp., *Pseudomonas* sp., and *Proteus* sp. The gram-negative organisms (*Pseudomonas* and *Proteus* sp.) are commonly isolated from chronic cases. The sensitivities of organisms isolated at the University of Queensland Veterinary School are shown in Table 2.

CLINICAL SIGNS

The cardinal signs of otitis externa are erythema, increased discharge, pain, and pruritus. Otitis externa in the dog has been classified into a number of types, which may be several stages of a single entity. A classification, similar to that suggested in man, is clinically desirable.

Two broad primary classifications may be used: reactive and infective. The reactive group includes acute eczematous and chronic verrucose or proliferative diseases. The infective group includes inflammations that are (1) acute purulent, (2) chronic purulent, (3) chronic ulcerative, (4) parasitic, and (5) fungal (otomycosis).

Cases that are initially reactive in nature may become complicated with secondary infection. Similarly, parasitic cases previously mentioned may change in nature, and pure fungal infections are not common, so that the type of otitis externa may depend upon when the case is presented.

Acute eczematous otitis externa is rapid in onset and characterized by marked erythema, which frequently involves the pinna. Pain may be severe but discharge is scanty and serous in nature.

Chronic proliferative or hyperplastic otitis externa is characterized by marked hypertrophy of the meatal epithelium with narrowing of the lumen. The hyperplastic tissue may increase and have a "papillomatous" appearance. Little discharge is present. This type of otitis has been seen more commonly in breeds with erect ears.

Acute purulent otitis externa is sudden in onset; pain is severe and a copious yellow discharge is present.

Chronic purulent otitis externa is seen commonly in breeds with pendulous ears. Discharge is copious and foul smelling. The meatal epithelium is swollen and edematous, and it bleeds readily. Chronic purulent otitis frequently progresses to the ulcerative form. Ulcers may occur on convolutions of the pinna as well as in the meatus.

Parasitic otitis externa is commonly accompanied by increased reddish brown waxy discharge. On close examination, whitish cream-colored mites are seen.

Otomycosis in the dog is similar clinically to that in man. Irritation is severe, and the deep portion of the external meatus is packed with damp grey caseous "wet blotting paper" debris with a musty odor. The meatal epithelium beneath the debris is deep reddish or purple in color.

TREATMENT

General treatment for otitis externa involves a series of clinical steps:

1. Sedate or anesthetize the patient
2. Take a swab from affected ear for a culture and sensitivity test
3. Examine the ear with an otoscope with a 6.0 cm speculum
4. Remove debris and discharge by gently irrigating the ear canal with mild antiseptic — e.g., 0.5 per cent chlorhexidine (aqueous). Polythene tubing half the diameter of that of the meatus or a eustachian tube catheter is useful to reach the depth of the ear canal and pretympanic area
5. Gently dry the ear canal
6. Reexamine with an otoscope
7. If ears are pendulous, strap them over the head
8. Apply specific medication
9. Change treatment if necessary as indicated by laboratory findings.

Specific treatment should be based upon clinical assessment and laboratory findings. Reactive infections are treated as follows.

Acute Eczematous. Control reaction with corticosteroids systemically and topically in order to prevent secondary infection, which is mainly staphylococcal or streptococcal.

Chronic Reactive. Control reaction with steroids and restore meatal epithelium to normal. Reestablish drainage and ventilation with surgical treatment.

Infective types of otitis externa are treated somewhat differently.

Table 1. Organisms Isolated from Normal Ear Canals and from Ears Affected with Otitis Externa

ORGANISM	CLINICALLY NORMAL EAR CANALS			EARS WITH OTITIS EXTERNA			
	Grono, Frost (1969) %	Sampson et al. (1973) %	Marshall et al. (1974) %	Grono, Frost (1969) %	Boyle, Grono (data to be published) %	Sampson et al. (1973) %	Marshall et al. (1974) %
Staph. aureus	47.6	15	1.7	30.9	30.4	35.0	38
Yeast *Pityrosporum* spp.	37.9	6	28.3	35.9	44.3	23.0	86.2
Pseudomonas spp.	2.4	4	0	34.6	16.5	5.0	16.4
Proteus spp.	1.6	0	0	20.8	9.9	5.0	3.4
Streptococcus spp.	0	2	0	7.4	4.3	6.0	8.6
Aspergillus	0	—	—	0.8	1.1	—	—

Table 2. Results of Sensitivity Tests of 467 Swabs from Canine Ears Affected with Otitis Externa

		PSEUDOMONAS	PROTEUS	STAPH. AUREUS	COLIFORMS	STREPTOCOCCI	DIPHTHEROIDS	MICROCOCCI
Penicillin	S	0.0	11.8	60.9	0.0	100.0	75.0	50.0
	R	100.0	88.2	39.1	100.0	0.0	25.0	50.0
Streptomycin	S	46.2	52.9	95.4	66.7	60.0	50.0	100.0
	R	53.8	47.1	4.6	33.3	40.0	50.0	0.0
Chloramphenicol	S	3.8	58.8	97.7	55.6	100.0	100.0	100.0
	R	96.2	41.2	2.3	44.4	0.0	0.0	0.0
Tetracyclin	S	25.0	17.6	92.0	44.4	100.0	100.0	100.0
	R	75.0	82.4	8.0	55.6	0.0	0.0	0.0
Ampicillin	S	0.0	11.8	69.0	0.0	100.0	75.0	100.0
	R	100.0	88.2	31.0	100.0	0.0	25.0	0.0
Trimethoprim/Sulfadiazine	S	3.8	29.4	66.7	33.3	20.0	50.0	100.0
	R	96.2	70.6	33.3	66.7	80.0	50.0	0.0
Neomycin	S	86.5	76.5	97.7	77.8	80.0	50.0	100.0
	R	13.5	23.5	2.3	22.2	20.0	50.0	0.0
Polymyxin B	S	86.5	0.0	97.7	77.8	80.0	75.0	100.0
	R	13.5	100.0	2.3	22.2	20.0	25.0	0.0
Gentamycin	S	100.0	88.2		100.0			
	R	0.0	11.8		0.0			
Carbenicillin	S	64.7	82.4		100.0			
	R	35.3	17.6		0.0			

Table 3.   Results of Medical Treatment of 100 Canine Otitis Externa Cases

TYPE OF OTITIS EXTERNA	CURED (%)	TEMPORARY RESPONSE (%)	NO RESPONSE (%)	NO RECORD (%)
Acute (eczematous; purulent)	86.5	0	4.5	9.0
Chronic (purulent; ulcerative)	48.4	25.6	12.0	14.0
Otomycosis	77.0	14.0	5.0	4.0
Parasitic	96.1	0	0	3.9
Proliferative	0	0	100	0

Acute Purulent.   Control infection using topical treatment with chloramphenicol, neomycin, or oxytetracycline pending laboratory findings.

Parasitic.   Use topical parasiticide — e.g., benzene hexachloride preparations, monosulfiram — and treat over a three-week period (the life cycle of *Otodectes*). Other sites where *Otodectes* may be found are the head, back, and tail. Also treat any in-contact animals to prevent reinfection.

Fungal.   Treat daily with 0.5 per cent chlorhexidine in propylene glycol, nystatin, monosulfiram, or cuprimyxin (Unitop®, Hoffman-La Roche)

Chronic Purulent.   Treat twice daily with neomycin, polymyxin, bacitracin drops, or other broad spectrum preparation until laboratory findings are available, as *Pseudomonas* sp. and *Proteus* sp. are often isolated from this type of otitis externa.

Chronic Ulcerative.   Treat as for chronic purulent but cauterize ulcers with salicylic acid, tannic acid, or silver nitrate.

The results of treatment of 100 unselected cases of otitis externa are shown in Table 3. (These results were obtained before gentamycin was widely used in the treatment of *Pseudomonas*-infected cases.) The excellent *in vitro* results for gentamycin against *Pseudomonas* sp. have also been reported by others. Good to excellent response has been reported in 84 per cent of acute cases and 79 per cent of chronic cases using Gentocin Otic® (Schering), a preparation containing gentamycin sulphate (3 mg/ml) (Houdeshell and Hennessey).

Other workers have used Oterna® (Glaxo), a preparation containing 0.1 per cent betamethasone, 0.5 per cent neomycin, and 5.0 per cent monosulphiram, in the treatment of otitis externa in the dog. Marshall obtained a very good or good response in 71.0 per cent of cases. Pugh reported that 84 per cent responded satisfactorily.

Cases of otitis externa that fail to respond to medical treatment or that frequently relapse should be considered for surgical treatment, which has been widely described in the literature. Lateral resection of the cartilage of the meatus is performed to give better ventilation and drainage. The resected ear canal should have a new wide aditus opening into the horizontal canal. Zepp's method of resection performed on 70 dogs that had failed to respond to medical treatment cured 37, improved 23, and caused no improvement in 10 in the author's experience.

SUPPLEMENTAL READING

Fraser, G.: Factors predisposing to canine external otitis. Vet. Rec. 73:55, 1961.

Fraser, G.: Vet. Rec., 75:3, 1961.

Fraser, G., et al.: Canine ear disease. J. Small Anim. Pract. 10:725, 1970.

Frost, R. C., and Beresford-Jones, W. P.: Otodectic mange in the dog. Vet. Rec. 70:740, 1958.

Grono, L. R.: Studies of the ear mite, *Otodectes cyanotis*. Vet. Rec. 85:6; 34, 1969.

Grono, L. R.: Studies of the microclimate of the external auditory canal in the dog. Res. Vet. Sci. 1:307, 1970.

Houdeshell, J. W., and Hennessey, P. W.: Vet. Med. Small Anim. Clin., 67:625–629, 1972.

Marshall, M. J., et al.: The bacteriological and clinical assessment of a new preparation for the treatment of otitis externa in dogs and cats. J. Small Anim. Pract. 15:401, 1974.

Moltzen, H.: Canine ear disease. J. Small Anim. Pract. 10:589, 1969.

Pugh, K. E., et al.: Otitis externa in the dog and cat—An evaluation of a new treatment. J. Small Anim. Pract. 15:387, 1974.

Sampson, G. R., et al.: Clinical evaluation of a topical ointment. VMSAC 68:978, 1973.

Weisbroth, S. H., et al.: Immunopathology of naturally occurring otodectic otoacariasis in the domestic cat. JAVMA 165:1088, 1974.

CANINE PODODERMATITIS

DANNY W. SCOTT, D.V.M.
Ithaca, New York

Pododermatitis (interdigital dermatitis, interdigital pyoderma) is a multifaceted, occasionally frustrating dermatologic disorder of the dog. It is essential to remember that canine pododermatitis is not a single disease entity — it is a disease complex.

ETIOLOGY

The etiology of canine pododermatitis is multifactorial, and in some cases it is unknown. In no cases are these lesions "cysts."

Foreign bodies are a common cause of pododermatitis and may be exogenous or endogenous in origin. Plant awns (foxtails, spear grass, thorn apples, burdocks) are exogenous foreign bodies that are a common cause of pododermatitis in certain parts of the United States. Hair and keratin are endogenous foreign bodies that can incite pododermatitis when released into the dermis as a result of trauma and follicular rupture.

Trauma (exogenous or self-induced) may result in secondary bacterial infections and/or the introduction of hair and keratin into the dermis. This is especially common in hunting dogs and dogs housed on rough surfaces (wire, stone, wood chips), particularly if these dogs are overweight.

Contact dermatitis (primary irritant or allergic) may lead to secondary bacterial infections owing to tissue devitalization and/or excoriation. Dogs with primary irritant-induced pododermatitis usually have a history of exposure to irritating substances (salts, fertilizer, pesticide or herbicide sprays). Dogs with allergic contact pododermatitis usually have a history of pedal erythema and pruritus preceding the infected phase.

Dogs with other forms of allergic dermatitis (inhalant, food, staphylococcal) may develop pododermatitis in association with tissue devitalization and excoriation. Animals with inhalant or food allergy dermatitis often have a history of pedal pruritus, with or without involvement of other areas of the skin. Dogs with staphylococcal hypersensitivity usually have a history of prior pyogenic infection and intense pruritus, which is poorly responsive to corticosteroid therapy.

Infectious causes of pododermatitis include bacteria, fungi, and parasites. Bacterial agents are unlikely to be primary causes of canine pododermatitis. However, routinely they do secondarily infect pedal skin devitalized by other etiologic agents. Fungal agents associated with canine pododermatitis include dermatophytes and "intermediate" (mycetoma, sporotrichosis) and "deep" (blastomycosis, cryptococcosis) fungi. These fungal infections are characterized by resistance to antibiotic and/or corticosteroid therapy. Parasitic agents associated with canine pododermatitis include *Demodex canis, Pelodera strongyloides*, and hookworm (*Ancylostoma* spp., *Uncinaria* spp.) larvae. Demodectic pododermatitis is often associated with alopecia, erythema, hyperpigmentation, and lichenification of the affected feet. Pelodera and hookworm pododermatitides are usually associated with an environment containing dirt, vegetation, and filth.

Recurrent or refractory pododermatitis can be associated with various immunodeficiency states, especially those in which cell-mediated immunity or neutrophil function is compromised. Chronic pododermatitis may be the only sign of canine hypothyroidism, with secondary depression of cell-mediated immunity and/or neutrophil function.

In some cases, canine pododermatitis is due to sterile pyogranuloma formation. The cause of these sterile pyogranulomas is unknown. They are most commonly seen in boxers, dachshunds, and English bulldogs. They are refractory to antibiotic therapy.

Occasionally, canine pododermatitis will be totally self-induced and of apparent psychogenic origin. These dogs are usually high-strung and often have equally nervous owners. Poodle, small terrier, and German shepherd breeds are commonly affected.

Rarely, pododermatitis is a manifestation of an underlying local neoplastic process (squamous cell carcinoma, lymphosarcoma) or osteomyelitis. These usually involve a single foot and single digit or interdigital space.

Despite numerous possible etiologies, 20 percent of canine pododermatitis cases remain idiopathic in nature. These are recurrent and exceedingly frustrating.

467

CLINICAL SIGNS

Pododermatitis may affect dogs of either sex (males affected twice as commonly as females), any age (especially 6 to 30 months), and any breed (especially great Dane, English bulldog, dachshund, German short-haired pointer, Dalmatian, Doberman pinscher, German shepherd, and black Labrador retriever). One foot or all four feet may be affected, but the most common combination is both front feet.

Pododermatitis is characterized by varying degrees of erythema, edema, alopecia, ulceration, crusting, exudation, fistula formation, pyonychia, pain, and pruritus. The dorsal aspects of the interdigital webs and the ventral surface of the feet are usually the most severely affected areas, often containing large areas of furunculosis and nodule and/or abscess formation. Regional lymph nodes are usually enlarged. Pain may be severe enough to result in lameness or refusal to walk. Constitutional signs are usually absent, but depending on the etiologic agent(s) involved, other areas of the body may be affected.

DIAGNOSIS

The key to diagnosis is the realization that canine pododermatitis is not a single disease, and that one must adhere to a meticulous diagnostic work-up based on an exhaustive differential diagnosis.

A thorough history will often point to the diagnosis: Hunting dog? Plant awns, irritants, or sharp, hard objects in environment? Overweight (trauma, foreign bodies, contact irritants)? Pedal pruritus first (inhalant or contact allergy)? Prior pyogenic infections? Poor response to corticosteroids (food or staphylococcal allergy)? Filthy environment? Poor response to antibiotics and corticosteroids (fungi, parasites)? Chronically recurrent? Refractory or poorly responsive to therapy (immunodeficiency, sterile pyogranuloma)? Nervous patient (and owner)?

Routine laboratory tests should include skin scrapings, fungal culture, and gram-stained direct smears. Additional laboratory tests, depending on historical indications, may include fecal examination (hookworms); bacterial culture and sensitivity (resistant bacterium or sterile pyogranuloma); provocative exposure, dietary, patch, and intradermal skin testing (contact, food, inhalant, or staphylococcal allergy); hemogram, serum protein electrophoresis, *in vitro* lymphocyte blastogenesis, bactericidal assay, TSH response test (immunodeficiency states); skin biopsy (foreign bodies, microbes, cellular response, neoplasia); and radiography (foreign body, underlying bony lesion).

TREATMENT

The therapy of canine pododermatitis varies with the underlying etiology. The reader is referred to other sections of this book for specific details.

Regardless of the underlying cause, if interdigital furunculosis and fistula formation are severe, intensive medical and surgical therapy may be indicated for best results. The therapeutic plan will include most or all of the following:

1. Bacterial culture and sensitivity testing are performed on material taken aseptically from an unopened lesion. Alternatively, one can submit a lesion taken by sterile surgical techniques for culture and sensitivity.
2. The animal is put under general anesthesia, and the feet are prepared for surgery. The objective of surgery is to incise, explore, and open all fistulous tracts thoroughly, excise all nodular lesions, and debride all devitalized tissues. Presurgical broad-spectrum systemic antibiotic therapy (gentamicin, kanamycin, cephaloridine) should be instituted 12 hours prior to surgery where feasible.
3. Following surgery, the feet are packed with antibiotics (nitrofurazone, chloramphenicol, gentamicin) and bandaged for 24 hours.
4. The bandages are then removed, and antiseptic whirlpool baths or antiseptic soaks (povidone-iodine, chlorhexidine) are administered for 20 to 30 minutes twice daily, until lesions are dry and healing (usually five to seven days).
5. Systemic antibiotic therapy (based on culture and sensitivity results) is continued for a total of six to eight weeks.

Cases of canine pododermatitis associated with cell-mediated immunodeficiency may respond dramatically to oral levamisole at 2 to 4 mg/kg given once daily for three days a week. These cases do require life-long maintenance doses (2 to 4 mg/kg once or twice weekly) of levamisole, however. The drug is not licensed for this use in the dog.

The therapy of choice for the sterile pyogranuloma complex is corticosteroids. Prednisolone is administered orally at 1.0 mg/kg, given twice daily until lesions are healed (10 to 14 days). Alternate day steroid therapy is then instituted and reduced to lowest possible maintenance dose.

Canine pododermatitis associated with staphylococcal hypersensitivity and that of idiopathic origin may respond well to bacterin or toxoid therapy. These products may be of autogenous or commercial origin. The author currently uses a commercial staphylococcal bacterin-toxoid preparation (Staphoid-AB, Jen Sal) because of its better availability and cost, as compared with those of autogenous products. In addition, there is no evidence that autogenous products are any more efficacious than commercial products.

PROGNOSIS

The prognosis with canine pododermatitis varies with the underlying cause. The owners must be made aware of the complexities of the problem. In cases of idiopathic origin, the prognosis for recovery is guarded to poor. These cases repeatedly relapse during the life of the dog and result in repeated therapy, considerable financial involvement, and immense frustration for owners and veterinarians. They often are terminated by euthanasia.

SUPPLEMENTAL READING

Muller, G. H., and Kirk, R. W.: *Small Animal Dermatology II.* Philadelphia, W. B. Saunders Co., 1976.
Quadros, E.: Furunculosis in dogs. Aetiology, pathogenesis and treatment. Acta Vet. Scand. (Supp.)52:1–114, 1974.

CRUSTING DERMATOSES IN CATS

TON (A.) WILLEMSE, D.V.M.
Utrecht, The Netherlands

Crusts are formed when dried exudate, serum, pus, blood, dust, and scales adhere to the surface of the skin, often mingling with hairs. Although commonly seen as secondary lesions, sometimes it is possible to consider crusts as primary skin eruptions — particularly in association with deeper processes. The observation of crusts can be helpful in confirming a diagnosis, especially when the primary lesion is transient — for example, in cases of impetigo — owing to the fragility of the very superficial pustule.

Crusty dermatoses in cats have become synonymous with miliary dermatitis in the veterinary literature, and they are usually treated symptomatically with megesterol acetate (Ovaban,® Schering Corp.). However, crusting dermatoses represent a complex series of disease entities. Careful case history, close examination of the skin, documentation of the presence or absence of pruritus, and consideration of the age of the cat will often lead to a specific diagnosis and thus a more appropriate therapy.

DIFFERENTIAL DIAGNOSIS

The main groups of diseases causing crusty skin lesions in cats are (1) parasitic diseases, (2) allergic diseases, and (3) mycotic diseases.

PARASITIC DISEASES

Flea Infestation (Without Hypersensitivity). In this condition, the skin problems are mainly caused by the cat flea, *Ctenocephalides cati*, which is a wingless, bilaterally flattened red-brown insect with characteristic genal and pronotal ctenidia and an elongated head.

The lesions are caused by scratching due to the irritation of the fleabites. Small crusts are located mainly on the head, neck, and dorsum of the body, but papules on the abdomen may also be noticed. Scaling, crusts, and thinning hair may all be present. Cats of all ages are affected. In kittens, infestation may result in severe anemia owing to blood sucking by the fleas. Man is also incidentally affected, and bites lead to dark red papules on the legs or the skin of the abdomen.

The presence of adult fleas, flea excretions in the coat (black, irregular grains staining red-brown when placed on paper and moistened), white glistening oval-shaped flea eggs (more easily seen against a dark background), and tapeworms (*Dipylidium caninum*, of which the flea is an intermediate host) are all of diagnostic value.

THERAPEUTIC MEASURES. These include thorough vacuum cleaning of the premises and the use of dips, sprays, and antiparasitic powders containing such chemicals as bromo-cyclen, lime sulfur, rotenone, pyrethrins, carbaryl, propoxur, and methoxychlor.

Patients and their beddings, as well as the in-contact animals, must be treated once a week for at least four weeks. Powders containing bromocyclen, rotenone, or carbaryl are preferred for kittens because they are less toxic. As kittens are more sensitive to antiparasitic drugs than are adult animals, the powder must be brushed out 15 minutes after applying it to the haircoat.

Lindane must *not* be used. Toxicity is manifested by ataxia, muscle spasms, restlessness, opisthotonus, vomiting, diarrhea, piloerection, mydriasis, and even paralysis with central and peripheral respiratory depression.

In adult cats, flea collars containing 10 percent tetrachlorvinfos or 5 percent carbaryl are very beneficial. (Flea collars are apparently of less benefit in the U.S.A., particularly in the South.)

Vaporizing strips or boxes containing dichlorvos combat adult fleas as well as larvae and nymphs. Dichlorvos is toxic for birds and fish, and it must be kept away from young children. Although dichlorvos vapors may sometimes cause allergic and irritation reactions in the respiratory tract or the conjunctiva in man, they rarely cause problems in the presence of adequate ventilation.

Anthelminthic therapy in cases of tapeworm infections is useful.

Pediculosis. This rare, contagious disease caused by the non–blood-sucking lice *Felicola subrostratus* and *Trichodectes canis* gives rise to extreme pruritus.

Skin abnormalities are characterized by partial alopecia, scaling, and papulocrustous lesions. An unpleasant odor and a matted haircoat often result. Predilection sites include the skin behind the ears, at the base of the tail, and the neck, but the disease may become generalized. Kittens are most commonly involved, the predisposing factors being neglect and poor hygiene.

A magnifying lens is of great help in detecting the lice and nits that are attached to the hairs in a coccoon. Skin scrapings and subsequent microscopic examination are also helpful. Control is readily effected by simple parasiticidal therapy with concomitant environmental controls.

Notoedric Mange. This mange of cats is caused by the short-legged mite, *Notoedres cati*. It is an extremely pruritic disease affecting cats of all ages, and it frequently affects whole litters of kittens. The head, ears, and neck are primarily involved, but secondary changes are found on the medial aspect of the forelimbs (because of pawing at the head) and the perianal area (owing to licking). The disease occasionally becomes generalized. Skin changes include alopecia, scaling, and crusting. Although cats are the primary hosts, the disease may affect dogs, rabbits, and man. In man, papules on the extremities or the neck (direct contact with the affected cat) are the most common manifestations. The diagnosis is confirmed by deep skin scrapings and microscopic examination. Clearing of the scraping preparation with potassium hydroxide or chlorphenolac is often helpful (chloral hydrate, 50 g; liquified phenol, 25 cc; and 85 percent lactic acid, 25 cc). Numerous mites and oval-shaped brown eggs are found. Parasiticidal dips for the affected animals and the in-contact animals with lime sulfur or bromocyclen is the therapy of choice.

Otodectic Mange. This mange is primarily an ear problem caused by the long-legged mite *Otodectes cynotis*. It is a disease of all ages, characterized by a pruritic otitis externa with an overproduction of brownish black cerumen or a suppurative exudate. Otoscopic or microscopic examination of ear swabs will reveal the mites. Very severe infestations with mites results in involvement of the pinna and the head, and the self-trauma sometimes leads to alopecia and a crusty dermatitis.

Otodectic mange is a contagious disease that affects dogs and cats and has been reported to affect man as well. Treatment includes thorough ear cleansing with water under low pressure and subsequent applications of parasiticidal otic preparations containing lindane or carbolglycerin.

Cheyletiellosis. This is a contagious disease caused by *Cheyletiella blakei*, a long-legged mite living on the surface of the skin. There seems to be no age or sex predisposition in cats, but long-haired cats seem to be frequently affected. Pruritus may vary from minimal to extreme, regardless of the degree of infestation. Four types of clinical results can occur: (1) scaling, seborrhea, and hair loss restricted mainly to the dorsum of the body, (2) papules and erythema on the neck and/or the head, (3) focal, crusty dermatosis at the neck and the head, which may become generalized, and (4) no observable changes.

Man can also be affected, and typical primary lesions consist of papules on the abdomen and the extremities. Human involvement occurs in about 20 percent of cases.

The diagnosis may be confirmed by one of the following means.

1. A superficial skin scraping and subsequent microscopic examination. Numerous long-legged mites with characteristic hooks at

the mouth parts, larvae, nymphs, and eggs can be found.

2. Tape-method. After removing a small crust, pressing a piece of transparent adhesive tape at the underlying skin lesion will often enable detection of mites when the tape is examined microscopically. This is also useful in diagnosing lice and otodectic mange mites.

3. Vacuum the coat of the cat for 10 minutes and examine the dust-hair sample after concentrating by flotation as follows: mix dust sample with 3 cc soap solution (e.g., Extran,® flüssig, Merck, Darmstadt, W. Germany); add 50 cc of a glycerin-saturated NaCl mixture (standard solution: 400 g NaCl/l liter water + 1 liter glycerin); stir for three minutes and allow to stand for five minutes; examine the top layer microscopically.

Treatment with parasiticidal dips and attention to the environment where the mites can survive for up to 10 days will lead to satisfactory control of the disease.

ALLERGIC DISEASES

Food Allergy or Food-Induced Pruritus. This condition is particularly seen in cats less than one year of age or in older cats following an important diet change. The main symptoms are pruritus and a crusty dermatitis in well circumscribed, plaque-like lesions on the neck, head, and, less frequently, extremities. In 50 percent of cases, intestinal disorders also occur. Typical miliary dermatitis occurs less frequently.

Common offending allergens are codfish, whiting, cheese, and milk. The diagnosis has to be confirmed by administering an elimination diet containing cooked lamb or chicken for three weeks. After disappearance of the pruritus, a subsequent provocation test with the separate substances of the original diet must follow. Skin tests in the diagnosis of food allergy are not reliable.

Fleabite Allergy. The clinical picture in this type of allergy is usually a miliary dermatitis affecting mainly the dorsum, but occasionally it can become generalized. This condition differs from ordinary flea infestation by the fact that fleas and flea dirt are rarely evident.

Flea control in these cases is even more important than in uncomplicated flea infestation. Because of the difficulties associated with this, additional therapy is often required. Beside glucocorticosteroids used in an alternate day therapy regimen, megesterol acetate (Ovaban,® Schering) and hyposensitization with flea antigen are other possibilities. Megesterol acetate is more effective than prednisone in this condition. The dosage used at the University of Utrecht is 2.5 to 5 mg daily according to weight for the first week, and 2.5 to 5 mg every other day for the second week. The maintenance dose is 2.5 to 5 mg once a week.

As megesterol acetate is a progesterone derivative with slight glucocorticoid action, the development of transitory or permanent diabetes mellitus is a possible complication following long-term therapy. A tendency for weight gain is a more frequent side effect. Hyposensitization with flea antigen has given less than satisfactory results in the author's experience.

Contact Dermatitis. Although irritant contact dermatitis due to strong acids and lyes readily develops in cats, true allergic contact dermatitis is extremely rare. Initial lesions consist of pruritic erythematous and papular reactions, and later changes are characterized by crusts or an exudative dermatitis. The distribution of the lesions depends on the cause (Table 1).

A systematically taken case history and trial removal of possible antigens followed by subsequent provocation are helpful aids in confirming the diagnosis. Patch testing in cats is clearly impractical. Therapy is directed at eliminating the offending antigen.

Table 1. *Common Agents in Contact Dermatitis in Cats*
(*IRRITANT OR ALLERGENIC*)

AGENT	PRESENT IN	LOCALIZATION
Dichlorvos	Flea collars	Neck
Neomycin	Ointments	Application sites
Polyvinylpyrrolidon iodine	Shampoo	Generalized
Plasticizers	Food dish	Lips; nose
Antioxidants	Litter box	Perianal; bottom of tail

MYCOTIC DISEASE

In cats, *Microsporum canis* is the most common fungus, although *Microsporum gypseum* and *Trichophyton mentagrophytes* are occasionally seen. *Microsporum canis* is a zoophilic fungus, and its clinical manifestation is characterized by a "moth-eaten" coat. In some cases, well circumscribed crusty lesions and severe scaling is noticed all over the body but with a predilection for the head, ears, and forelimbs.

The same clinical appearance is seen in rare infections with the zoophilic fungus *T. mentagrophytes* and the geophilic fungus *M. gypseum*. Skin changes seen in the carrier state are minimal to none. All three of these fungi are transmissible to man. Diagnosis is confirmed by microscopic examination of skin scrapings, Wood's light examination, and fungus culture. Therapy consists of oral administration of griseofulvin in microcrystalline form (up to 30 mg/kg body weight daily) together with topical treatment — e.g., natamycin (1 percent) dips every third day (not available in the USA) or miconazole nitrate (2 percent) (Conofite®, Pitmann-Moore) as a topical cream. Thiadiazin must not be used because of toxicity; griseofulvin must not be given on an empty stomach. Vomiting or toxic side effects due to enhanced absorption of the griseofulvin may occur. Griseofulvin given to pregnant cats may result in increased numbers of malformed kittens — for example, kittens with palatoschizis or spina bifida. (Dosages recommended for griseofulvin in the USA are generally higher — e.g., up to 65 mg/kg — than doses in the Netherlands. Although gastric irritation may occur, it seems rare. Fat certainly enhances absorption, and indeed a certain level of fat is often recommended to insure adequate blood levels.)

In addition, isolation of infected animals; cleansing of contaminated cages, bedding, brushes, etc; detection of carriers; and wearing of special clothes while treating the affected cats are essential in combatting the disease effectively. Multiple fungus cultures on Sabouraud agar are important aids in tracing carrier cats. Hairs taken from the head, ear margins, and feet commonly yield positive cultures. It has been shown in both man and cattle that recovery from *T. mentagrophytes* infection is followed by protective immunity, but the possible role of immunity in small animals has not been investigated.

SUPPLEMENTAL READING

Jones, H. E., Reinhardt, J. H., and Renaldi, M. G.: Acquired immunity to dermatophytes. Arch. Dermat. 109:840, 1974.

Kirk, R. W.: Dermatophye infections. In Kirk, R. W. (ed.): *Current Veterinary Therapy VI*. Philadelphia, W. B. Saunders Co., 1977.

Kirkpatrick, C. H., Rich, R. R., and Bennett, J. E.: Chronic cutaneous candidiasis: model building in cellular immunity. Ann. Internal Med. 74:955, 1971.

Ottenschot, T. R. F., and Gil, D.: Cheyletiellosis in long-haired cats. Tijdschr. Diergeneesk. 103:1104, 1978.

Reedy, L.: Ectoparasites. In Kirk, R. W. (ed.): *Current Veterinary Therapy VI*. Philadelphia, W. B. Saunders Co., 1977.

ZINC-RESPONSIVE DERMATOSES IN DOGS

GAIL A. KUNKLE, D.V.M.
Philadelphia, Pennsylvania

Trends in therapy occur in human medicine as various medications come into popular use. As sulfa and penicillin once were used to treat many diseases regardless of etiology, the current "fad" among some physicians and many patients is the use of "back to nature" organic products. Vitamins and minerals are being used in megadoses for literally hundreds of symptoms and diseases with few good studies to support their use. Where vitamin C gained popularity in the past decade, the use of zinc now has become widespread, especially for dermatologic conditions such as burns and wound healing.

As treatment with zinc increases in human medicine, its usage most likely will increase in veterinary medicine. Good clinical investigations are needed to outline the therapeutic functions of zinc and to examine the effects of various disease states on the absorption, metabolism, and storage of zinc. Indiscriminate clinical use of zinc should be avoided because zinc toxicity may occur, and excess zinc can interfere with the utilization of other minerals.

Clinically, it appears that there may be a limited need for zinc therapy in the dog. Some conditions for which zinc may be useful will be described.

FUNCTION OF ZINC

Most of the work with this essential mineral has been done in other species — rats, chickens, pigs, and ruminants. Zinc has many functions in body metabolism. It is found in every human tissue and tissue fluid, although concentrations vary greatly. Zinc is present in the nuclear, mitochondrial, and supernatant fractions of cells. Among the trace elements, the concentration of zinc in the body is second only to iron. In most species, the major amount of zinc in the body resides in muscle, bone, and teeth. In animals covered with hair, fur, or wool, a considerable amount is present in these tissues. The reproductive organs, the liver, and the pancreas also contain relatively high quantities of zinc.

An extensive discussion of the functions of zinc is not necessary here. Its usages are many in maintaining a normal physiologic state. Zinc is used for muscle growth, bone growth, and food utilization, especially in the metabolism of protein and carbohydrates. Keratogenesis and wound healing are influenced by zinc. Zinc also is needed for normal reproduction, and it serves a function in hormonal development and regulation. Zinc is required for the cellular components of blood, especially the white blood cells. Zinc serves a role in taste and smell acuity in man. It also plays an active role in many enzyme systems. The specific biologic function of zinc in these metalloenzymes is currently under considerable investigation.

Only a small amount of total body zinc is carried in the blood. Serum zinc levels have been monitored in many species, and, although definite norms and variations with disease have been reported, serum zinc does not appear to be an accurate method of assessing the zinc status of the animal. Measurements of serum zinc are influenced by many factors, and different techniques of measurement produce variable results. Contamination is a major problem in collection of samples. Glass syringes, glass tubes, and rubber or cork stoppers may alter the value as well as hemolysis. Finally, many physiologic conditions significantly alter circulating zinc levels. Dogs affected by hepatic disease, infec-

tion, pregnancy, and hormonal changes may have decreased serum zinc levels.

Serum zinc assays do not assess the zinc status of the animal, since in various species one tissue level will change before another. In man, plasma may give an indication of total zinc, whereas in calves, the pancreatic tissue is the first to show a decrease with deficiency. In rats, pigs, cows, and goats, the zinc content of the hair reflects the level of zinc in the diet. Most clinical work in man and animals has been done with either blood or hair levels, and it is apparent that this too is not an adequate assessment.

Zinc is normally excreted in the urine and feces. In man, whereas there is a clear circadian variation in serum zinc, none has been observed in urinary zinc excretion. Zinc in the feces represents the major source of loss of zinc from the body.

ZINC DEFICIENCY STATES

The function of zinc cannot be discussed without an examination of the deficiency state. Zinc deficiency manifests itself differently in various species. Inappettance is one of the initial signs and may result from taste and smell abnormalities. Growth retardation may also occur. Lesions of the skin and its appendages frequently develop, as does eventual impairment of reproductive function.

Cutaneous changes have been described in several species that had zinc-deficient diets. The classic example of zinc deficiency has been parakeratosis in pigs. It has been reported that young, rapidly growing pigs develop thick crusts around the nose, ears, eyes, and scrotum. Histologically, there was excessive keratinization, retention of the nuclei, and exfoliation with exudate containing red blood cells. These lesions responded completely to oral zinc supplementation. Similar parakeratotic lesions have been described in zinc-deficient ruminants.

In zinc-deficient rats, scaling and cracking of the paws occurred with occasional deep fissures. Male rats developed hypertrophied sebaceous glands and seborrhea. In sheep, changes in the horns as well as abnormalities of the wool occurred with deficiency.

In the dog, integumentary symptoms of alopecia, hyperkeratinization, and acanthosis were reported in the zinc-deficient state. Emaciation, emesis, conjunctivitis, keratitis, general debility, and growth retardation also were reported. All the canine work was based on a single study in which a simple zinc deficiency was probably not present but rather a relative zinc deficiency induced by excessive dietary calcium had occurred.

There is a close resemblance between the symptoms of zinc deficiency in domestic and laboratory animals and those of acrodermatitis enteropathica, a disease in man which is now known to be due to an inherited defect in zinc absorption. Cutaneous lesions include alopecia and heavy scaling around the natural body orifices and the distal extremities. There is an associated enteropathy. Previously, the condition was usually fatal, but complete amelioration of clinical signs now results from zinc therapy. The lesions histologically resemble zinc deficiency of other species and include parakeratosis, hyperkeratosis, and acanthosis. Similar lesions have occurred in a human patient maintained on total parenteral nutrition in which adequate zinc was inadvertently omitted.

There seems to be a remarkable similarity between cutaneous lesions of acrodermatitis enteropathica of man and those of the dogs to be described under Syndrome I.

DIETARY ZINC REQUIREMENTS

All species have a series of minimum zinc requirements that vary with the nature of the diet and the functional activity in the animal. The end effects of the diet are reflections of amounts and proportions relative not only to actual zinc content but to factors that influence zinc absorption, utilization, and excretion. Young growing animals require more zinc than do adults. Reproducing adult animals similarly require more zinc than non-reproducing adults.

Zinc is required in the diet of all animals. It needs to be supplied continuously because there are only very small amounts of readily available zinc stored in the body. Most of the zinc present in the bones, skin, hair, and muscle cannot be quickly mobilized to meet the animal's need for zinc.

Dietary zinc requirements are affected by many factors, including the protein source in the diet as well as the content of other minerals. Interrelationships with various dietary additives may influence the zinc requirement. A mutual antagonism between zinc and copper may exist, and vitamin D may favorably influence the metabolism of zinc. Calcium plays an important role in the absorption of zinc and may inhibit the absorption of zinc from the gut. Depending on the protein source, the amount of dietary phytate may alter the availability of ingested zinc to the animal. Phytate occurs naturally in most diets in which the primary protein source is of plant origin. Soy is one protein that contains phytate.

Phytate is known to bind with zinc and decrease its absorption from the gut. Although there are interactions between calcium and zinc, calcium alone may not depress absorption of zinc from the gut. Yet, high calcium intake has been shown to potentiate the zinc deficiency syndrome in pigs, dogs, and birds. It appears that high dietary calcium is more important in decreasing zinc absorption when phytate is a significant component of the diet.

The extent to which marginal zinc deficiency occurs in animals and man is unknown. A test that will distinguish zinc deficiency from other deficiencies and is suitable for screening large populations of animals has yet to be developed. Because there is an abundance of zinc in foods, zinc deficiency has not been considered a problem of practical importance in the past. With the increased use of supplements in animal diets and of plant proteins in human diets, questions of zinc availability have been raised. Because the signs of marginal zinc deficiency are nonspecific, a valid test for zinc status is needed. Zinc levels from blood, hair, urine, and saliva give mixed results when compared with clinical symptoms and response to treatment.

Minimum zinc requirements for normal reproduction, performance, growth, and keratinization have not been given with precision, even for laboratory animals such as the rat where extensive research on zinc has been completed. The minimal daily requirements for dietary zinc in the dog have been extrapolated from work done with other species and from one study in the dog where zinc deficiency was created by increasing the calcium in the diet. Understandably, the recommended daily requirements as suggested by the National Research Council (NRC) may be far from exact, but it provides guidelines for the canine diet that maintain the normal state in the average dog. The NRC daily zinc requirement for maintenance for the adult canine is 0.11 mg/kg body weight. The requirement for growing pups is twice that of the adult recommendation. Recommendations for zinc content in various types of dog foods (dry, semi-moist, canned) also have been made by the NRC. On a dry matter basis, most commercial dog foods should contain 20 mg/kg. Many dog foods exceed this figure.

CLINICAL SYNDROMES

SYNDROME I

This condition appears primarily in Siberian huskies but has on occasion been seen in Alaskan malamutes. The onset of skin lesions frequently occurs during puberty, although older dogs may be affected. Some dogs show lesions only during times of stress such as pregnancy, lactation, or concurrent disease. There appears to be no sex predilection. Appetite may be normal or depressed.

Clinically, these dogs are presented with crusting, scaling, and underlying suppuration around the mouth, chin, eyes, and ears. The lesions that appear as thick crusts may form on the elbows or other joints on the legs. Similar crusts may appear on the scrotum, prepuce, or vulva. Hyperpigmentation may occur in some chronic cases. The dogs are usually not pruritic until the lesions have become extensively crusted, and at that time there may be some self-trauma, especially to the involved facial regions. Punch biopsies of affected skin reveal primarily parakeratosis and hyperkeratosis.

At the University of Pennsylvania, experience has indicated that many of these cases respond to oral zinc supplementation. Usually there is complete regression of signs. In one of the several cases monitored, the zinc supplementation has been halted on four occasions, once unknowingly when a pharmacist substituted another product. In all instances, there was recurrence of lesions within two to six weeks after the therapy was discontinued.

Although the response to zinc therapy alone is usually good in these dogs, other treatments sometimes have been effective. Some veterinarians have reported that moderate doses of systemic corticosteroids may result in complete clearing of lesions with recurrence once steroids are discontinued. This is an interesting observation, as negative interactions between glucocorticoids and zinc have been reported. In some instances, Siberian huskies have been found to be hypothyroid by radioimmunoassay of T4 and T3. It has been reported that in beagles with hypothyroidism, serum zinc values were significantly decreased. Results with thyroid treatment in hypothyroid huskies with the described lesions have been limited and variable.

It seems reasonable that sled dogs represent breeds that may require more dietary zinc than others. Most recently, research has revealed that the Alaskan malamutes with genetic chondrodysplasia have been found to have decreased absorption of dietary zinc from the gut (Brown, et al.). Is it not possible that a marginal zinc state exists in some individuals of these sled dog breeds? Factors that increase their daily zinc requirement only slightly — such as stresses of reproduction and higher caloric intake for winter heat maintenance — may alter the body zinc levels enough to cause clinical signs.

SYNDROME II

Puppies afflicted with this zinc-responsive syndrome are usually presented with hyperkeratotic plaques over portions of the body. Extreme thickening of the foot pads with concurrent fissuring exists. The planum nasale may be affected similarly, and puppies may seem small for their age. The degree of severity of signs within the litter seems highly variable. Most pups may appear normal, yet some may be depressed, anorexic, emaciated, and generally debilitated. Moderate lymphadenopathy may occur. Dermatologic symptoms are quite variable, with exudative crusts extending over the head, trunk, and extremities.

At the University of Pennsylvania Veterinary School, three litters of puppies with the signs of this zinc-responsive dermatosis have been seen. All puppies were pure-bred, but of various breeds (beagles, standard poodles, and German short-haired pointers). In one litter, two of the most severely affected puppies also had radiographic changes indicative of hypertrophic osteodystrophy. In all three litters, the dietary levels of calcium were greater than two times those set by NRC as requirements for the growing pup. Of the three litters seen, two litters had been treated with appropriate antibiotics for pyoderma with little response.

Response to zinc therapy has been dramatic. Within seven to ten days, marked improvement occurred in the affected pups supplemented with oral zinc, whereas the symptoms in untreated pups progressed.

THERAPY

Oral zinc supplementation is effective in rapidly relieving the dermatoses.

Zinc sulfate ($ZnSO_4$) is the only approved readily available compound for pharmacologic zinc therapy in the United States. For huskies, 100 mg $ZnSO_4$ given twice daily is usually sufficient for rapid resolution of symptoms. More may be required in some cases — on occasion, 220 mg $ZnSO_4$ BID. Zinc sulfate is available in several sizes of capsules and tablets. Zinc sulfate contains 22 per cent zinc, so that a 220 mg tablet of zinc sulfate provides approximately 50 mg of elemental zinc; a 66 mg tablet of zinc sulfate provides 15 mg of zinc.

Zinc gluconate is another oral form of zinc that is available in health food stores. Its use also may be satisfactory if equivalent levels of elemental zinc are given.

Zinc may cause emesis as a side effect. This has been uncommon, but if it occurs, halving the dose and giving it with food usually halts the emesis.

In Syndrome I, therapy with zinc may need to be continued indefinitely. Usually, supplementing the pup's diet with zinc until adulthood is all that is necessary in Syndrome II. Changing the diet alone may cause the same improvement as adding zinc. Zinc therapy alone has proved helpful in the author's experience.

It does appear that there is a specific response to zinc in the cases described in Syndromes I and II. Whether this represents a true zinc-deficient state is yet to be determined. Serum zinc levels have been measured on a few cases with mixed results. As previously stated, a good assay for body zinc states is currently not available.

OTHER POSSIBLE USES

There are conflicting reports concerning evidence as to zinc's properties in reference to healing in man. Most data appear to indicate that where marginal zinc deficiency exists, wound healing may be retarded. Most evidence suggests that patients with adequate zinc levels are not benefited by increased zinc intake for wound healing. Since levels of zinc may be marginal in some individuals, it may be postulated that zinc supplementation may benefit dogs that have slowed healing characteristics.

Zinc is an important component of sebum and cerumen. Since high calcium intake may interfere with zinc absorption, others have hypothesized that the rapidly growing giant breeds may develop seborrhea during fast-growth months. There may be a need for additional dietary zinc in these breeds at this age, especially if they have been heavily supplemented with calcium.

Finally, zinc plays an important role in taste and smell. Hypogeusia is a recognized syndrome in man that may respond to zinc. In a human with this syndrome, the primary complaint is abnormal smell and taste associated with most foods and eventual anorexia as a result of these abnormalities. Zinc used in anorex-ic huskies with Syndrome I has caused rapid improvement in appetite. Similarly, in one other case seen at the University of Pennsylvania, a dog began to eat normal quantities of food when owners had previously force fed the same dog to maintain normal weight.

Others have considered that zinc may be of benefit in the superficial folliculitis of short-haired breeds through its effect on sebum production and keratinization. Zinc also apparently plays a role in immunity; thus one may rationalize its use in deep pyodermas as well. One report of dogs with interdigital pyoderma has shown some of these dogs to have decreased serum zinc levels, but the author's experience with zinc therapy in pyoderma is too limited to comment on its efficacy.

TOXICITY

Zinc by oral ingestion is relatively non-toxic to most species. Animals are quite tolerant of high levels, and usually intake of 100 times the required dietary levels results in no signs of toxicosis.

When injected intravenously in the dog, very high levels of zinc gluconate (4 mg/kg/BW) resulted in lassitude, enteritis, paresis of hind legs, and EKG changes such as hyperkalemia. With oral ingestion, it is highly unlikely that any severe toxicosis would ever occur. Most likely, emesis would occur first.

A significant concern with using oral zinc therapy indiscriminately is its resulting interaction with other minerals and the possible upset to normal physiologic mechanisms.

SUPPLEMENTAL READING

Brown, R. G., Hoag, G. N., Smart, M. E., and Mitchell, L. H.: Alaskan malamute chondroplasia. V. Decreased gut zinc absorption. Growth 42:1–6, 1978.
Fisher, G. L.: Effects of disease on serum copper and zinc values in the beagle. Am. J. Vet. Res. 38:935–940, 1977.
National Research Council Subcommittee on Zinc: Zinc. 1979.
Nelder, K. H., and Hambridge, K. M.: Zinc therapy in acrodermatitis enteropathica. N. Engl. J. Med. 292:879–882, 1975.
Robertson, B. T., and Burns, M. J.: Zinc metabolism and the zinc-deficiency syndrome in the dog. Am. J. Vet. Res. 24:907–1002, 1963.
Underwood, E. J.: Trace elements in human and animal nutrition, 3rd ed. New York, Academic Press, 1971, pp. 208–252.

SUBCUTANEOUS AND OPPORTUNISTIC MYCOSES, THE DEEP MYCOSES, AND THE ACTINOMYCETES

MARIE H. ATTLEBERGER, D.V.M.
Auburn, Alabama

THE SUBCUTANEOUS AND OPPORTUNISTIC MYCOSES

The subcutaneous mycoses develop in the host at the site of inoculation. Entry is usually through an injury, and the fungus remains localized or may spread slowly via the lymphatics. Most of the fungi involved are soil saprophytes.

The opportunistic fungi are usually thought of as contaminants. Under certain conditions, these fungi invade the tissue and produce disease. Immunosuppressants, long-term antibiotic therapy, certain debilitating diseases, steroids, and immune deficiencies are some factors that play a role in their pathogenicity. Before these opportunistic fungi can be incriminated as the etiological agents of an infection, active tissue invasion must be demonstrated, and the fungus should be isolated from the diseased tissue two or more times. Attempts to transmit the invading fungus to other animals are usually unsuccessful.

SPOROTRICHOSIS

Definition. Sporotrichosis is a chronic infection characterized by nodules, shallow ulcers, and granulomatous lesions frequently involving the skin and often the lymphatics. It may disseminate.

Etiology and Epidemiology. The infection is caused by *Sporothrix schenckii*, a dimorphic fungus that exists in nature in the saprophytic form and in the tissue or parasitic form as an oval or elongated budding yeast. It is found in soil, on plants, and on wood and has been isolated from spaghnum moss, humus, grasses, water, horse hair, fleas, ants, and even frankfurters in cold storage. Environmental temperature may have some effect on the organism's growth in nature as well as in the host. The fungus usually enters the body through an injury to the skin, but it may be inhaled or even ingested.

Animal-to-man transmission has been known to occur, especially following the handling of infected cats. In three of these cases, there was no record of the cat biting or scratching the person. Care should be taken when handling any infected animal, especially cats, and the owner should be informed of the possibility of transmission. Fomites may transmit infection also.

Clinical Signs. In the dog with cutaneous involvement, nodules, ulcers, and granulomas may be found in a random pattern over the body or may follow along the lymphatics of the extremities. Nodules may be firm and tender and they may ulcerate or show evidence of healing. Wart-like lesions may occur. Nodules, crusty circular lesions, ulcers, abscesses, granulomas, and areas of necrosis are seen in the cat. Dissemination may occur in both the dog and cat but appears to be more frequent in the cat. It involves the lungs, liver, and possibly other organs.

Diagnosis and Culture. Direct examination of the usual stained smears or wet mounts generally is useless, as the organism is difficult to demonstrate in smears. Special fungal stains or fluorescent antibody stains will give better results. Culture (Fig. 1) is the most effective method of diagnosis; the fungus appears in five to fourteen days. (Refer to a text in medical mycology for a description of the fungus.)

Treatment. Inorganic iodides are the preferred treatment in the dog. Good results have been experienced using 1 ml of 20 percent NaI per 5 Kg body weight orally BID. Other drugs and doses are 0.5 gm KI daily for six weeks in the feed or 25 to 30 drops of saturated KI BID for four to six weeks or until all signs of the infection have disappeared. Treatment should continue for at least one month

477

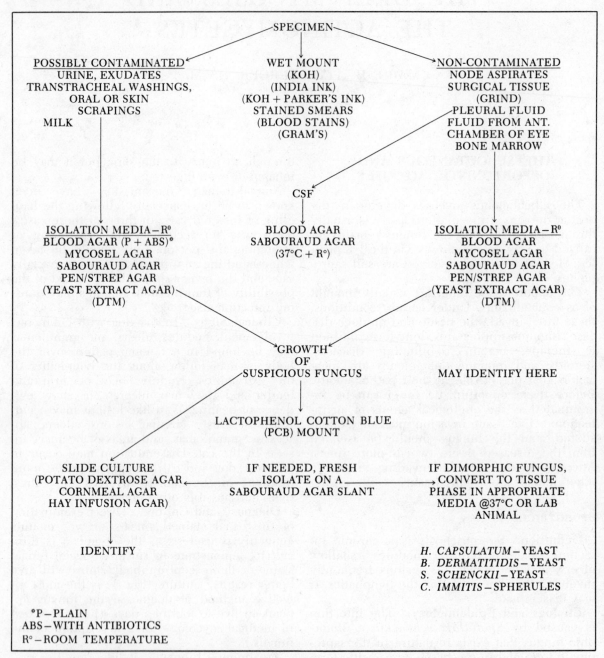

Figure 1. Processing Clinical Specimens for Systemic Fungus Infections in Veterinary Medicine

following the absence of clinical signs to avoid recurrence. Amphotericin B may be tried in the cat following the regimen for cryptococcosis.

RHINOSPORIDIOSIS

Definition. Rhinosporidiosis is characterized by polypoid growths on the mucous membranes of the nasal cavity. Occasionally, these growths appear on the conjunctiva and skin. It is chronic and benign.

Etiology and Epidemiology. *Rhinosporidium seeberi* appears in the tissue as spherical, thick-walled sporangia (up to 350μ) with endospores (9 to 7μ). The fungus has not been grown in a mycelial form. Its natural habitat is unknown and its association with water has not been documented. Trauma may be a predisposing factor in the infection, but attempts to transmit it to other animals have been unsuccessful.

Clinical Signs. The dog usually has a history of sneezing and there may be epistaxis or a mucopurulent, blood-stained discharge. The nasal passage should be examined for sessile, pedunculate, or cauliflower-like polyps. These polyps are pinkish, bleed easily, and contain white specks, which are the sporangia. Usually only one nostril is involved. The infection has not been known to disseminate in animals.

Diagnosis. Crush a small piece of polyp and examine it in water or 10 to 20 percent KOH under the 10X or 45X objective for sporangia with endospores. Culturing is not done.

Treatment. Surgical excision of the polyps is the most effective treatment. Surgery must be extensive and complete to prevent recurrence. The area may be cauterized following surgery.

ASPERGILLOSIS

Definition. Aspergillosis is a broad spectrum of diseases involving members of the genus *Aspergillus*. It involves the respiratory tract, digestive tract, skin, eyes, and other structures.

Etiology and Epidemiology. *Aspergillus fumigatus* is probably the most frequently isolated species. The aspergilli are found worldwide, are one of the most common fungi in the environment, and are frequently seen as laboratory contaminants. Because of this, their isolation on plates must be evaluated. Most are secondary invaders to some debilitating condition, but many are also the primary cause of an infection. Overexposure to large amounts of spores can stress the body's defense system and lead to infection. In some respiratory infections, it is difficult to determine if the aspergilli isolated are invading or merely colonizing. Birds are the most frequently affected species. Infection is not normally transmitted from animal to animal or animal to man. Long-term use of antibiotics, steroids, and immunosuppressants, as well as immune deficiencies and debilitating diseases, contribute to infections by the aspergilli.

Clinical Signs. Nasal aspergillosis in the dog is not infrequent, and the animal is usually presented with a history of sneezing for several weeks duration. There usually is a nasal discharge. Often only one of the nasal passages is involved, and the fungi are found growing high in the frontal sinus. In severe cases, the fungi erode through the bone and may invade the brain. Neurologic signs are evident and the temperature may rise to 104 to 105°F. Prognosis is very poor at this stage and should be guarded in the early stage of the infection. Pseudomonas infection can present an additional problem. Signs are often vague in other forms of aspergillosis, and many are diagnosed at necropsy. Some signs that may be seen in other forms of the infection are weight loss, diarrhea, eye involvement, and granulomas on the skin. In cats, aspergillosis may be secondary to infectious feline enteritis. Respiratory infections, though rare, do occur in the cat.

Diagnosis and Culture. Nasal washings, biopsies, and scrapings of infected areas should be examined in 10 to 20 percent KOH for septate hyphae and heads of the aspergilli. It should be remembered that heads frequently are not found, and other fungi show septate hyphae when invading tissue. Culture assures a positive diagnosis. Material must be collected as aseptically as possible and cultured at room temperature on Sabouraud dextrose agar with and without antibiotics. Bacterial cultures are also necessary. Nasal swabs are unsatisfactory because they do not reach the area of infection. Tissue invasion must be demonstrated either by direct smears or histopathology.

Treatment. Surgery plus a course of amphotericin B is the usual treatment for nasal aspergillosis. Other treatments that may prove effective in other forms of aspergillosis, if diagnosed in time, are potassium iodide, nystatin, and natamycin. Aerosol administration of natamycin or nystatin, as done in man, is not always possible in veterinary medicine.

PHYCOMYCOSIS (ZYGOMYCOSIS)

Definition. Phycomycosis in animals is mostly a granulomatous disease that is caused by a variety of fungi in the class *Phycomycetes*.

Etiology and Epidemiology. Members of the genus *Mucor, Rhizopus, Absidia, Hyphomyces, Entomophthora, Basidiobolus,* and others have been isolated from infections in man and animals. These organisms are associated with soil, water, and decaying vegetation. The *Mucor* and *Rhizopus* species are common laboratory contaminants. As with the aspergilli, tissue invasion and repeated isolation must be demonstrated in order to incriminate them in an infection. Attempts to transmit organisms to other animals are usually unsuccessful. Factors predisposing animals to these infections are not known.

Clinical Signs. In the dog, abdominal masses, granulomas, draining fistulous tracts, and subcutaneous nodules are some of the signs presented. Chronic vomiting is present in some cases of abdominal involvement. At necropsy, the fungi have been found invading the intestinal tract and other organs. Occasionally they may invade blood vessels.

Diagnosis and Culture. Biopsies and exudates should be examined in 10 to 20 percent KOH for wide, relatively non-septate hyphae. Specimens for culture should be obtained as aseptically as possible and cultured at room temperature on Sabouraud agar with and without antibiotics.

Treatment. Surgery is recommended where possible and can be followed with a course of amphotericin B if deemed necessary. *Basidiobolus* sp. and *Entomophthora* sp. have been treated successfully in man using 30 mg/kg of KI daily for one month or more.

PROTOTHECOSIS

Definition. Protothecosis is a cutaneous or systemic infection caused by various species of *Prototheca* that are considered to be acholric algae.

Etiology and Epidemiology. *Prototheca wickerhamii* has been isolated form gross lesions in dogs and cats and *P. zopfii* from other animals. They are found worldwide and have been isolated from soil, sewage, water, human feces in cases of sprue, lesions on potato skin, and from cases of bovine mastitis in addition to infections in man, dogs, and a cat. The infection is usually cutaneous in man and systemic in animals, although cutaneous infections in animals do occur. In the tissue, the organisms appear as hyaline, globose to oval cells 1.3 by 13.4 to 1.3 by 16.1μ in size. The cells contain two or more autospores. Budding does not occur. The colony is yeast-like in appearance and consistency. The mode of transmission to animals has not been established but ingestion, inhalation, and injury should be considered. Only a few cases of protothecosis have been reported, and there has been no evidence of transmission among individuals.

Clinical Signs. Small sores, dry crusty lesions, granulomas, and nasal exudate have been observed superficially in the dog. Pain, chronic nephritis, bloody diarrhea, polyuria, polydypsia, polyphagia, and iritis followed by blindness have occurred in the dog with systemic infection. Organisms have been isolated from heart, liver, kidneys, para-adrenal connective tissue, eyes, and brain.

The cat had a soft, fluctuant, subcutaneous mass on the plantar surface of the left tarsus.

Diagnosis. Exudates and other material should be examined microscopically in 10 to 20 percent KOH under the 45X objective for oval to globose structures containing two or more autospores. The *Prototheca* are easily cultured on blood agar or Sabouraud dextrose agar with and without antibiotics. Yeast-like colonies are visible in 48 hours. Fluorescent antibody conjugate also is available for direct smears.

Treatment. No therapeutic treatment has proved effective for protothecosis. Surgical excision is recommended for localized lesions.

PHAEOHYPHOMYCOSIS

Definition. Phaeohyphomycosis is an infection caused by dematiaceous fungi that form dark-walled septate hyphae in the host's tissue.

Etiology and Epidemiology. *Drechslera spicifera* is the fungus most frequently isolated in animals. It is widespread in the environment and has been recovered from soil and air. At present, cases have been reported only in cats and horses. The disease in animals has so far been limited to the subcutaneous tissue.

Clinical Signs. A cat at Auburn with the infection had a draining lesion on the tail and a larger, swollen area with a draining tract on the foot pad. The infection may begin as a nodule, and fistulous tracts may or may not develop.

Diagnosis and Culture. Direct examination of the exudate or pieces of tissue in 10 to 20 percent KOH reveal black, septate hyphae, some of which may show unusual dilatations. The specimen should be cultured on Sabouraud dextrose agar with and without antibiotics at room temperature.

Treatment. Complete surgical excision of the lesion has proved to be successful.

MYCETOMA

Definition. Mycetoma refers to tumefactions that have draining tracts and granules in the exudate.

Etiology and Epidemiology. There are two groups of etiologic agents: (1) actinomycotic, which include various species of *Actinomyces, Nocardia, Actinomadura* and *Streptomyces* and (2) eumycotic, which include *Allescheria boydii, Curvularia geniculata, Maduralla* spp. and others. Most are soil saprophytes or plant pathogens that gain entry to the host through injury. Most of the mycetomas in lower animals contain black granules, although white or yellow grains have been reported.

Clinical Signs. The extremities are frequently involved, but regardless of the location, the triad of signs — tumefaction, draining tracts, and granules in the exudate — is present.

Diagnosis and Culture. The granules, which are colonies of the organism, should be crushed and examined in 10 to 20 percent KOH for the presence of hyphae and chlamydospores that are seen in eumycotic mycetoma. A Gram stain also should be performed and examined under oil for gram-positive filaments found in actinomycotic mycetoma. For culture, the granules should be washed several times in sterile saline, crushed, and streaked on to Sabouraud agar without antibiotics and on blood agar. A duplicate set of plates should be incubated at room temperature and at 37°C. The group to which the etiologic agent belongs should be determined because treatment depends on which group is involved.

Treatment. Complete surgical excision of the lesion is recommended for eumycotic mycetoma. Actinomycotic mycetoma may be treated with sulfa drugs as in nocardiosis.

SUPPLEMENTAL READING

The Subcutaneous and Opportunistic Mycoses

Anderson, N. V., et al.: Cutaneous sporotrichosis in a cat: a case report. J. Am. Hosp. Assoc. 9:526–529, 1973.

Barsanti, J. A., Attleberger, M. H., and Henderson, R. A.: Phycomycosis in a dog. J. Am. Vet. Med. Assoc. 167:293–297, 1975.

Bolton, G. R., and Brown, T. T.: Mycotic colitis in a cat. Vet. Med./Sm. Anim. Clin. 67:978–981, 1972.

Brodey, R. S., et al.: Mycetoma in a dog. J. Am. Vet. Med. Assoc. 151:442–451, 1967.

Heller, R. A., et al.: Three cases of phycomycosis in dogs. Vet. Med./Sm. Anim. Clin. 66:472–476, 1971.

Jang, S. S., and Popp, J. A.: Eumycotic mycetoma in a dog caused by *Allescheria boydii*. J. Am. Vet. Med. Assoc. 157:1071–1076, 1970.

Kaplan, W., et al.: Protothecosis in a cat: first recorded case. Sabouraudia 14:281–286, 1976.

Koehne, M. A., Powell, H. S., and Hail, R. I.: Sporotrichosis in a dog. J. Am. Vet. Med. Assoc. 159:892–894, 1971.

Kurtz, H. J., Finco, D. R., and Perman, V.: Maduromycosis *Allescheria boydii* in a dog. J. Am. Vet. Med. Assoc. 157:917–921, 1970.

Muller, G. H., et al.: Phaeohyphomycosis caused by *Drechslera spicifera* in a cat. J. Am. Vet. Med. Assoc. 166:150–153, 1975.

Rippon J. W.: *Medical Mycology: The Pathogenic Fungi and the Pathogenic Actinomycetes.* Philadelphia, W. B. Saunders Co., 1974.

Scott, D. W., Bentinck-Smith, J., and Haggerty, G. F.: Sporotrichosis in three dogs. Cornell Vet. 64:416–426, 1974.

Sudman, M. S., Majka, J. A., and Kaplan, W.: Primary mucocutaneous protothecosis in a dog. J. Am. Vet. Med. Assoc. 163:1372–1374, 1973.

Werner, R. E., et al.: Sporotrichosis in a cat. J. Am. Vet. Med. Assoc. 159:407–412, 1971.

Wood, G. L., et al.: Disseminated aspergillosis in a dog. J. Am. Vet. Med. Assoc. 172:704–707, 1978.

THE SYSTEMIC MYCOSES

Excluding man, the dog appears to be the natural host for the systemic fungus infections histoplasmosis, blastomycosis, and coccidioidomycosis, whereas crytpococcosis occurs in the dog and cat. Infections in other animals are rare. Following the inhalation of spores, the infections are usually pulmonary in origin and may heal spontaneously or worsen and spread to the skin, nodes, other organs, and bone via the blood or lymphatics.

Animals with a systemic fungus infection present a wide variety of signs such as granulomatous lesions, abscesses, ulcers, fistulous tracts, enlarged and/or draining nodes, and even areas of necrosis. Most develop slowly and elicit little pain except for lameness. Usually the animal has a history of "going downhill for some time."

Rarely are these infections acute; however, when they do occur in this form, they are usually diagnosed at necropsy. Since most of these infections can be diagnosed by making direct smears of infected material, it is essential that clinicians be able to obtain correct specimens and be familiar with the organism's appearance in tissue.

With the exception of *Cryptococcus neoformans*, the other fungi causing the deep mycoses are dimorphic, growing in the mycelial or saprophytic form at 25°C and in the tissue or parasitic form at 37°C as a yeast (histoplasmosis and blastomycosis) or as a spherule with endospores (coccidioidomycosis).

Resistance to fungal infections appears to lie with cellular immunity, while humoral antibodies are useful in the diagnosis and prognosis of an infection. Any agents that suppress the immune system are contraindicated in fungus infections.

Although serologic tests aid in diagnosing fungus infections, one should not make a positive diagnosis based on serology alone. Cross reactions as well as false negatives and false positives occur in these tests. In addition to serology, there should be some clinical signs suggestive of a fungal infection or a positive direct smear or a positive culture.

Animal-to-animal, animal-to-man, and man-to-man transmission of the systemic fungi does not occur naturally. Most of the infections in animals occur in those under five years of age.

BLASTOMYCOSIS

Definition. Blastomycosis is a chronic granulomatous and suppurative infection that is primarily pulmonary in origin but may disseminate to the skin, eyes, bone, and other organs.

Etiology and Epidemiology. *Blastomyces dermatitidis*, a dimorphic fungus, appears in the tissue phase as a large, thick-walled budding yeast (8 to 20μ) and exists in nature in the mycelial or saprophytic phase, where it needs high humidity (85 to 88 percent) to grow. Although it has been isolated a few times from soil rich in organic matter during the cool wet months and from tree bark, its true habitat is still unknown. Soil microorganisms (bacilli and streptomycetes) have been shown to destroy both the mycelial and yeast forms. An association with cedar trees has been noticed with some of the dogs hospitalized in the Small Animal Clinic at Auburn University. Although infection usually occurs following inhalation of the spores, cases in man have occurred following the handling of fomites. The organism is endemic in the eastern United States and parts of southern Canada, especially in areas drained by rivers. It also has been reported from countries outside the North American continent. Blastomycosis is not contagious.

Clinical Signs. In dogs, the infection usually begins in the lung and then disseminates to other areas of the body. Dogs usually are depressed, debilitated, and thin, and they may or may not show pyrexia. A cough may or may not be present with the respiratory involvement, which may be severe or mild. Skin lesions are usually present and consist of cutaneous and subcutaneous abscesses, ulcers, draining tracts, and granulomas. These lesions may be seen in various stages of healing and breakdown. Occasionally, hair has a "greasy" feeling, which disappears following treatment. Frequently, the prescapular and/or popliteal nodes are enlarged and draining.

The eyes are very often affected by blastomycosis, and permanent blindness is not uncommon. If exophthalmia is present, it usually can be corrected with treatment and the eye becomes normal again in the socket. The eyes are especially sensitive to sunlight, but this will disappear as treatment progresses.

Lameness may occur, especially in the large breeds, and the hind legs are often swollen, probably as a result of lymphatic stasis. In male dogs, there may be an orchitis, as the prostate and testicles are often infected.

Radiographs of the lung usually reveal a dense mass at the bifurcation of the trachea due to enlargement of the bronchial and mediastinal nodes. Local or diffuse pulmonary consolidation is frequently present.

COCCIDIOIDOMYCOSIS (VALLEY FEVER)

Definition. Coccidioidomycosis (Valley Fever) is a fungus infection that is usually pulmonary in origin. It may be asymptomatic and self-limiting or it may disseminate to bone and other organs.

Etiology and Epidemiology. *Coccidioides immitis* is endemic in the arid southwestern United States, in northern Mexico, and in various areas of Central and South America. The organism is dimorphic and exists in nature in the mycelial form, and it occurs in tissue as a thick-walled spherule (20 to 60μ) with endospores (2 to 5μ). Immature spherules with no endospores may be seen.

C. immitis is frequently found in association with rodent burrows, and dogs digging in these or disturbing infected soil become infected. The organism remains viable in the soil during the hot, dry weather and appears to grow following periods of rainfall. When conditions become windy and dusty, animal infection is more prevalent. Animals inhale spores in the dust and fomite transmission can occur also. The disease is not contagious. Infection usually appears in a few days to a few weeks following exposure. Dogs are very susceptible, and it is reported that boxers and doberman pinschers are especially susceptible to the disseminated form.

Clinical Signs. Infection may be asymptomatic or benign, it may show only respiratory illness, or it may disseminate to bones and other organs. The dogs presented for treatment are usually under two years of age and have the disseminated form. There are episodes of coughing, and the temperature may be normal or rise to 106°F. Other signs include anorexia, dyspnea, listlessness, loss of weight, episodes of diarrhea, and even ascites.

Difficulty in swallowing has been observed. Nodes may be enlarged and draining.

Between the pulmonary infection and dissemination (frequently to bone), the dog may experience periods of good health, or dissemination may occur soon after the pulmonary infection. Lameness and swollen joints occur, and when bone is involved, radiographs frequently show proliferative osteomyelitis with lesions near the epiphyseal junction.

Less frequently, a meningitis manifested by incoordination or eye involvement may occur.

HISTOPLASMOSIS

Definition. Histoplasmosis is a systemic fungus infection usually contracted by inhaling spores from infected soil. Both the pulmonary form and the intestinal form are seen in the dog, but the infection is rare in cats.

Etiology, Ecology, and Epidemiology. *Histoplasma capsulatum* is a dimorphic fungus that appears in the tissue or parasitic phase as tiny, intracellular oval bodies (2 to 4μ in diameter) found in cells of the reticuloendothelial system. The mycelial or saprophytic form occurs in nature, and it is the small microaleuriospores (2 to 5μ) that, when inhaled into the alveolar spaces, transform into yeasts and begin the tissue phase.

The fungus is found in the Eastern United States, the Central Mississippi Valley, the Ohio Valley, and along the Appalachian Mountains. The highly endemic areas of the United States are in Kentucky, Tennessee, Missouri, Southern Illinois, Arkansas, Indiana, Ohio, and some parts of North Carolina, Minnesota, and Iowa. Isolated areas are also found in the St. Lawrence River Valley and Lake Champlain areas. It is also found in other parts of the world.

The organism is frequently associated with soil contaminated with chicken, bat, starling, and other bird droppings. Temperature, soil types, humidity, and other factors also influence its presence in the soil. If one wishes to disinfect contaminated soil in a confined area, a 3 percent formaldehyde or 3 percent cresol solution should be used. Nine gallons should be disseminated over a 25 square foot area daily for three days.

Although the fungus has been cultured from a dog tick allowed to feed on a dog with a known positive blood culture, the role of insects in the transmission is unknown.

Histoplasmosis is not a contagious disease.

Clinical Signs. Most dogs are seen in an advanced stage of the disease and are emaciated, lethargic, and depressed, show dyspnea and anorexia, and have an elevated tempera-

ture. A nasal or ocular discharge and a cough may or may not be present. Nodes are frequently enlarged and hepatomegaly, spenomegaly, ascites, and anemia may be present. Often there is a diarrhea of unexplained origin, which may be persistent or intermittent, resulting in dehydration. Any persistent enteritis should be cultured for fungi (*H. capsulatum*). Radiographs show a granulomatous pneumonia.

CRYPTOCOCCOSIS

Definition. Cryptococcosis is a systemic fungal infection, usually pulmonary in origin, that may remain in the respiratory tract or spread to the brain, skin, nodes, other organs, and bone, possibly via the blood and lymphatics.

Etiology and Epidemiology. *Cryptococcus neoformans* is soilborne, worldwide in distribution, and exists in nature in the yeast form. It is 4 to 7μ in diameter, and most of the yeast cells are surrounded by a polysaccharide capsule. It is found in association with pigeon nests and excreta as well as with excreta from other birds and bats. Natural infection in birds does not appear to occur. Cryptococcosis is not contagious.

Clinical Signs. These vary greatly among infected animals. Ulcerated areas may occur on the oral, pharyngeal, or nasal mucosa. The turbinates, facial sinuses, and surrounding bony structures may be invaded. Ulcerative and granulomatous skin lesions and, occasionally, abscesses may be present. These abscesses often contain a mucoid exudate. Even though the infection is usually pulmonary at first, respiratory involvement may not be seen. Lameness due to septic arthritis may occur.

If the nervous system is visibly involved, there may be incoordination, various eye lesions, or even blindness. A head tilt also occurs in advanced cases. Lymph nodes are usually enlarged, and bones and other organs may be involved.

In cats, a respiratory problem is usually evident, and granulomas occluding the nasal cavity are often seen. If no external lesions are visible, the cat's mouth should be examined for ulcerated areas. Sometimes there is no evidence of respiratory involvement and only a single lesion or abscess may be present.

DIAGNOSIS OF THE SYSTEMIC MYCOSES

DIRECT SMEARS

Exudate, node aspirates, direct scrapings from skin lesions, or granulomas are suitable for direct smears. Urine, cerebrospinal fluid, and transtracheal washings should be centrifuged and the sediment should be examined. Diagnosis by direct microscopic examination of clinical specimens in 10 to 20 percent KOH under the low and high dry objectives can be made in blastomycosis and coccidioidomycosis. Large, thick-walled budding yeasts with internal structure are seen in blastomycosis. Thick-walled spherules with endospores as well as smaller spherules devoid of spores are found in coccidioidomycosis. Parker ink added to the KOH will outline the fungi (1 drop of ink/2 drops KOH).

For cryptococcosis, the specimen is placed in a mixture of Pelican or India ink and water. Only enough ink is used to make the water dark grey in color. Typically, a small, round budding yeast surrounded by a capsule is seen under 45X. The capsule appears as a halo around the yeast because it holds back the carbon particles in the ink. Occasionally, no capsules are present and only non-encapsulated yeasts are seen. Culture and identification are then necessary.

Histoplasmosis is not easily diagnosed by direct smears. Node aspirates or biopsies may be tried and should be stained with a blood stain. Small, intracellular oval bodies (yeast cells) are found within the macrophages. Biopsies from the liver, spleen, or sternal bone marrow may be useful. Except in very advanced cases, yeasts are difficult to demonstrate in peripheral blood.

Culture. See Figure 1 for the specimens, culture media, and temperatures needed. Plates should be heavily streaked and held at least six weeks. Although most of the systemic fungi grow slowly, *Coccidioides immitis* may be visible in three to four days and mistaken for a contaminant. The mycelial phase is usually easier to recover. The mycelia of *Histoplasma capsulatum* and *Coccidioides immitis* should be wet down with sterile saline or water before removing any of the fungi for microscopic study in lactophenol cotton blue. Refer to a textbook of medical mycology for descriptions of the fungi.

Histopathology. Specimens should be submitted to pathology laboratories in 10 percent buffered formalin. In addition to the hematoxylin and eosin stains, fungal stains such as Gridley, Grocott methenamine silver, or periodic acid–Schiff also should be used.

TREATMENT AND PROGNOSIS OF THE SYSTEMIC MYCOSES

Dogs that are eating and are able to stand are most likely to benefit from treatment. Amphotericin B (Fungizone, Squibb) is the drug of choice, and each dog should be treated on an individual basis depending on the severity of the infection.

The drug should be diluted according to the manufacturer's directions, and 0.15 mg/kg is given intravenously in 25 to 30 ml of 5 percent dextrose in water over 20 to 30 minutes. Saline is avoided, as it causes the drug to precipitate. The dosage may be increased gradually over the second or third week until 0.20 to 0.25 mg/kg is reached. Only in exceptionally severe cases is a higher dose needed. Treatment is administered every other day. Because amphotericin B is nephrotoxic, the blood urea nitrogen (BUN) should be determined before treatment is begun and at least once (preferably twice) a week during treatment. It is best to keep the BUN under 30 mg/100 ml, and it should not be allowed to exceed 40 mg/100 ml. If higher, treatment should be stopped until the BUN decreases and then resumed at a slightly lower dosage so that the BUN falls into acceptable limits. No nephrotoxic effects on dogs using the above dosage have been encountered at the Auburn University Small Animal Clinic. Treatment may be given on an out-patient basis, and in most cases, it needs to be continued for six to eight weeks — 20 to 22 injections are usually sufficient but more can be given if needed. Dogs should be fed a high caloric diet and should have at least six weeks rest following treatment. Owners should be advised that dogs may become reinfected if allowed access to old areas of infection. Treatment failures, while few, may occur, and the animal may be retreated. If bone is involved, treatment should continue until there are no signs of infection as indicated by radiography or culture.

For coccidioidomycosis, 0.5 mg of amphotericin B per kg twice a week for six to eight weeks has been used with good results (Graham, 1978). Graham states that this dosage is effective in bone involvement.

For cats, the following procedure using amphotericin B has been found successful. The dry amphotericin B powder should be diluted with 20 ml of diluent (water). Each adult cat is given 0.8 mg in 10 ml of 5 percent dextrose in water every three to four days. Using a 25 guage needle, the above solution is administered intravenously as rapidly as possible. The BUN is monitored as for dogs. The BUN may reach 40 to 80 mg/100 ml following administration of the first two or three treatments and may be decreased by fluid support with lactated Ringer's solution. Treatment is continued until the cat is asymptomatic and cultures are negative. The cat may be treated as an outpatient.

The prognosis of most systemic fungus infections should be guarded. When treating bone lesions, it probably will be necessary to treat longer and possibly with higher doses of amphotericin B, so nephrotoxicity may be a problem. Prognosis is poor if the central nervous system is involved. Canine blastomycosis occurs more frequently in Alabama than do any of the other deep mycoses, and favorable results using the described therapy have been experienced. No resistance by the deep fungi to amphotericin B or any severe side effects such as those seen in man have occurred in dogs treated at the Auburn University Small Animal Clinic. Anemia may occur and should be treated symptomatically.

SUPPLEMENTAL READING

The Systemic Mycoses

Ausherman, R. J., Sutton, H. H., and Oakes, J. T.: Clinical signs of blastomycosis in dogs. J. Am. Vet. Med. Assoc. 130:541–542, 1957.

Barrett, R. E., and Scott, D. W.: Treatment of feline cryptococcosis: literature review and case report. J. Am. Anim. Hosp. Assoc. 11:511–518, 1975.

Graham, L. P.: Personal communication, 1978.

Jungerman, P. F., and Schwartzman, R. M.: *Veterinary Medical Mycology.* Philadelphia, Lea and Febiger, 1972.

Rippon, J. W.: *Medical Mycology: The Pathogenic Fungi and The Pathogenic Actinomycetes.* Philadelphia, W. B. Saunders Co., 1974.

Rhoades, H. E., Helper, L. C., and Fritz, T. E.: Canine histoplasmosis with intestinal involvements. J. Am. Vet. Med. Assoc. 136:171–173, 1960.

ACTINOMYCOSIS, NOCARDIOSIS, AND DERMATOPHILOSIS

Actinomycosis and nocardiosis are caused by bacteria that show a tendency to branch as well as to break up into coccobacillary forms. These bacteria belong to the *Actinomycetales.* Lesions are similar in both infections and animals show abscesses, draining tracts, raw ulcers, granulomas, necrosis, fibrosis, and respiratory involvement.

Dermatophilosis is included in this group, as the etiologic agent in this infection also is an actinomycete. The clinical signs consist of crusts and scabs. Infections are rare in the dog and cat.

ACTINOMYCOSIS

Definition. Actinomycosis is a localized or systemic infection characterized by suppurative and granulomatous lesions. Draining sinuses may be present.

Etiology and Epidemiology. Actinomycosis is found worldwide, and many species of actinomycetes are involved in infections. The organisms are gram positive filaments that usually show branching and break up into coccobacillary forms. They are non–acid-fast and are anaerobic and microaerophilic in their oxygen requirements. They appear to be endogenous in man and animals and seem to need the presence of other bacteria to produce infection. Injury may be a predisposing factor in their pathogenicity. Animal-to-man transmission does not occur.

Clinical Signs. Numerous clinical syndromes appear in dogs and cats infected with *Actinomyces* species, and they are very similar to those described in nocardiosis. The following signs have been observed in dogs and cats in the Auburn, Alabama area: localized abscesses with elevated temperature, deep abscesses, abdominal masses, vertebral osteomyelitis, severe respiratory conditions with pleuritis, and draining tracts.

Diagnosis. Follow the same procedure as for nocardiosis, using the Gram stain and cultural methods. Although the *Actinomyces* are non–acid-fast, this characteristic should not be used solely for diagnosis, since some nocardia are non–acid-fast. The flecks or granules present in the exudates are colonies of the organisms and should be used for staining and culture. Blood agar and brain heart infusion agar should be streaked and incubated at 37°C under aerobic, anaerobic, and microaerophilic conditions. The clubs seen in granules of *A. bovis* are not always present in exudates from dogs and cats. Culture and identification are necessary to differentiate from *Nocardia* sp. because treatment differs. *Actinomyces viscosus* and other unidentified species have been isolated from dogs.

Treatment and Prognosis. Surgery to establish drainage or to remove localized infected areas plus antibiotics and other chemotherapeutic agents is the recommended treatment. Penicillin is the drug of choice. High doses (80,000 to 100,000 units/kg intramuscularly) should be given daily. Treatment should be continued until clinical signs are absent and cultures are negative. For systemic infections, it is necessary to continue treatment for several months. For dogs allergic to penicillin, chloramphenicol may be tried. Application of topical iodine preparations to localized lesions is helpful. Prognosis is poor in systemic infections, many of which are diagnosed at necropsy. It is usually good in localized infections.

NOCARDIOSIS

Definition. The infection may be acute or chronic and may be limited to the skin and show ulcers, abscesses, or draining tracts. The lungs and possibly other organs may be involved. Mycetoma-type lesions may also occur.

Etiology and Epidemiology. *Nocardia asteroides* and *Nocardia brasiliensis* are the two species most frequently isolated from animals, and infections with *Nocardia caviae* have been reported. *N. asteroides* has often been isolated from soil; the other two have been isolated less frequently. The organisms may be inhaled or ingested but often enter through an injury. In man, they frequently disseminate to the brain. The infection is not transmitted from animal-to-animal or from animal-to-man.

Clinical Signs. In the dog or cat with the localized form, there is usually a history of some injury with a lesion developing that does not respond to treatment. There are often draining fistulous tracts and a raw, ulcerated lesion. Subcutaneous abscesses, granulomas, and enlarged nodes also occur. In the primary pulmonary form, the dog and cat show pleural effusion and empyema along with signs of respiratory distress and usually weight loss. The systemic form closely resembles distemper and is characterized by dyspnea, coughing, anorexia, pyrexia, emaciation, and possible nasal and ocular discharge. Neurologic disturbances are seen when the brain is involved.

Diagnosis and Culture. For the cutaneous form, a scraping of the ulcer or pus can be gram stained and observed under oil for grampositive, branching, beaded filaments. As many of the *Nocardia* sp. are acid fast or partially acid fast, a Hank's Acid Fast stain should also be done. When the thickened, rusty fluid is removed from the chest, it should be examined for flecks or granules, which are clumps of the organism. These granules should also be stained. The importance of the granules in making a diagnosis cannot be overstressed, as the organism often is not found in the fluid alone. These granules may be found in the fistulous tracts and in pus and may be seen in infections other than nocardiosis.

Pus, exudates, and granules should be obtained as aseptically as possible for culture. Blood agar and plain Sabouraud Dextrose agar plates should be inoculated in duplicate with the flakes or granules. One set of plates should be incubated at 37°C and the other at 25°C and held for at least two weeks. The nocardias grow as rough, adhering colonies and may show a variety of colors with age. Colonies should be examined early for filaments, as these organisms break up into coccobacillary forms, which may be mistaken for bacteria, thus resulting in an incorrect diagnosis. The Hank's Acid Fast stain should be made on colonies also.

Treatment and Prognosis. Sulfa drugs, especially sulfamerazine and sulfadiazine, are preferred. Triple Sulfa #4 (Vets Products Corp.) has been used successfully at the Auburn University Small Animal Clinic: 120 mg/kg is given intravenously as the initial dose, then 60 mg/kg bid is given for as long as needed and the dog is able to tolerate the drug. This drug may be diluted 1:10 and used to flush fistulous tracts. If preferred, oral sulfadiazine, 80 mg/kg tid may be used. Tribrissen (Burroughs-Wellcome) has proved effective in some cases. In the pulmonary and systemic forms, treatment may be needed for two to three months. Cultures and radiographs may be helpful in determining the length of treatment. In one instance, a dog in the clinic was unable to tolerate sulfa drugs and as a last resort, surgical removal of the granulomatous lesion proved effective. Chest drains are needed with empyema, and a daily lavage with physiologic saline should be carried out until the thoracic fluid is clear. Proteolytic enzymes and penicillin may be added to the lavage if needed. Prognosis is usually good and recovery is rapid in localized lesions. In the systemic and pulmonary forms, the prognosis should be guarded to poor.

DERMATOPHILOSIS

Definition. Dermatophilosis is an exudative dermatitis characterized by crusts and scabs which may be localized or spread over the entire body.

Etiology and Epidemiology. *Dermatophilus congolensis*, an actinomycete, appears as branching filaments that swell and divide longitudinally, then transversely, to form parallel rows of coccoid zoospores. Injury to the skin and excessive prolonged moisture are predisposing factors. The exact habitat of the organism is unknown, and it has not been isolated from soil. Experimentally, flies have been shown to transmit it. As healing occurs, crusts and scabs fall away and can contaminate the premises. There are a few reported cases where man has contracted the infection following the handling of infected animals. These cases are rare, and self-healing occurs.

Clinical Signs. The crusts and scabs on the dog are thickened owing to the build-up of the exudate and, when removed, they contain unbroken intact hair. The area beneath the scab may contain a yellowish pus or the skin may appear normal to slightly erythematous. Removal of the scabs leaves areas of alopecia, and some scabs are found clinging to the hair. Two cases have been reported in cats, and the lesions appeared as glossal granulomas or tumors on the tongue. The lesions resulted in dysphagia and dyspnea. An embedded feather in one case suggested entry through injury.

Diagnosis. Crush scabs in a small amount of water and prepare a heavy smear. Stain with a blood stain (Diff Quick, Harleco Co., or Camco Quick Stain, Scientific Products Co.) and examine under oil for filaments and parallel rows of spores.

Treatment and Prognosis. Daily bathing with an iodine shampoo and gently removing the loosened scabs is usually sufficient treatment. It is best not to remove tightly adhering scabs, as bleeding frequently occurs. Following bathing, the animal should be dried and kept in dry quarters until all skin lesions have healed. If secondary bacterial infection occurs, topical applications of furacin may be applied, but the furacin has no effect on the actinomycete. Spontaneous healing may occur. Prognosis is usually good in the dog. Procaine penicillin, 300,000 units daily for 5 days, was used to treat the cat in one of the reported cases.

SUPPLEMENTAL READING

Actinomycosis, Nocardiosis, and Dermatophilosis

Baker, G. J., Breeze, R. G., and Dawson, C. O.: Oral dermatophilosis in a cat: a case report. J. Small Anim. Pract. 13:649–653, 1972.

Campbell, B., and Scott, D. W.: Successful management of nocardial empyema in a dog and cat. J. Am. Anim. Hosp. Assoc. 11:769–773, 1975.

Georg, L. K., Brown, J. M., Baker, H. J., and Cassell, G. H.: *Actinomyces viscosus* as an agent of actinomycosis in the dog. J. Am. Vet. Med. Assoc. 33:1457–1470, 1972.

Jungerman, P. F., and Schwartzman, R. M.: *Veterinary Medical Mycology.* Philadelphia, Lea and Febiger, 1972.

Maderazo, E. G., and Quintilani, R.: Treatment of nocardial infection with trimethoprim and sulfamethoxazole. Am. J. Med. 57:671–675, 1974.

Rippon, J. W.: *Medical Mycology, The Pathogenic Fungi and the Pathogenic Actinomycetes.* Philadelphia, W. B. Saunders Co., 1974.

HEREDITARY HAIR AND PIGMENT ABNORMALITIES

GEORGE H. MULLER, D. V. M.

Walnut Creek, California

There are a number of hereditary abnormalities of the skin and its adnexae that occur without being influenced by environmental factors. They have also been called genodermatoses, even though non-cutaneous abnormalities are also present. Some defects are congenital (existing at birth), whereas others appear later in the individual's maturation as defective organs begin to have a damaging influence on the skin.

In domestic animals, defective young are often destroyed. Since they may not receive scientific attention, their incidence may be larger than is commonly assumed. If kept alive, they are not usually used for breeding, except for experimental genetic studies. Thus a natural selection occurs, as it would in the wild state of animals.

Genodermatoses have been extensively described and studied in man. Such conditions often include other defects in addition to those of the skin. Examples are the Rothmund-Thomson Syndrome, Bloom's Syndrome, Cockayne's Syndrome, Bird-headed dwarfism, xeroderma pigmentosa, and cartilage-hair hypoplasia.

All features of the skin are genetically determined in one way or another. Although in genodermatoses, the cutaneous defects are obvious, other skin diseases are also hereditary. Atopic disease, primary idiopathic seborrhea, and generalized demodicosis, for example, are most likely of genetic origin.

This chapter includes only those conditions in which there is an abnormality of the hair and pigment. There is a certain overlapping of hair and pigment that must be kept in mind in the descriptions. The primary pigmentary disorders will be listed first, followed by hair defects.

CONGENITAL HYPOPIGMENTATION

The most common form of congenital hypopigmentation in dogs occurs on the lips and nose. Such lack of pigment is more dramatic and more cosmetically undesirable in black or darkly pigmented breeds. In the Doberman pinscher, for example, the upper and lower lips, as well as the planum nasale, are normally deeply pigmented. When an individual dog has several pink patches on these areas, the owner is distressed by the appearance and may consult a veterinarian. The skin is otherwise healthy; there is no inflammation, itching, or scaling. The glabrous mucocutaneous junction as well as the haired skin may be involved. The cause of this lack of pigment is not known, and there is no effective treatment. In some dogs, the lack of pigment is present at birth; in others, it develops later and slowly enlarges and spreads. Usually, however, the defect is restricted to the facial area. In some individuals, only the nasal tip is involved. The normally black or brown planum nasale is either completely depigmented or affected in sharply demarcated macules and patches. Differential diagnoses include contact dermatitis of the lips from oxidizers in plastic dishes, nasal solar dermatitis, and pemphigus.

NASAL HYPOPIGMENTATION

Lack of pigment on the dorsal nasal surface occurs most commonly in white dogs or multicolored dogs with white noses. The most common breeds affected are the collie and Shetland sheepdog. Nasal solar dermatitis, in which hypopigmentation of the nose is one of the causative factors, was formerly known as "collie nose."

Nasal hypopigmentation in its classical form is characterized by a sharply demarcated patch on the dorsal nose just posterior to the planum nasale. It can vary in size from a few millimeters to 5 centimeters in diameter. Often it will start small and enlarge gradually. If the dog lives in a sunny climate, such as in Hawaii, California, Florida, and other southern states, the hypopigmented area can burn if the dog is outside during the day. Sunlight during the hours from 10 A.M. to 4 P.M. is especially damaging to the unprotected skin.

After several years of overexposure to sun, squamous cell carcinomas have developed in certain dogs. A similar condition occurs in white cats or multicolored cats with white noses.

It is beneficial to avoid direct sunshine. Sunscreens are of slight value, provided the dog does not lick them off. Some permanent improvement can be achieved in dogs by tattooing the hypopigmented areas. The sooner this is done, the better the "take" obtained with the tattoo ink. Highly inflamed noses in advanced nasal solar dermatitis are more difficult to tattoo. Successful protection by tattooing depends also on the skill and experience of the operator's technique. Intradermal injections, as well as tattoo machines, are used in the procedure.

VITILIGO (HYPOPIGMENTATION)

Hypopigmentation of this type involves lack of melanin production by the skin and hair. It can be present at birth or develop later in life. Often the cause is unknown and the lack of pigment is frequently irreversible.

A rare syndrome occurs in Newfoundlands (Muller and Kirk, 1976). The normally black hairs gradually become gray or white. Pigment is lost on the planum nasale, which turns pinkish. Skin around the nose and eyelids also loses its normal black pigment.

Black and tan Doberman pinschers can gradually develop white hairs diffusely interspersed with normal black hairs. Sometimes these hairs remain permanently white, whereas in other cases, the black hair color returns after one shedding cycle. There is no known cause and no known treatment.

Albino dogs and cats are extremely rare. The condition is recessive, and affected individuals have unpigmented (pink) irises, white hair, and no pigment in the skin. The biochemical nature of albinism is the lack of tyrosinase, which is needed for normal melanin production. Histopathologic examination shows that there are normal melanocytes in the skin, but they apparently are incapable of completing melanin synthesis.

CANINE HEREDITARY BLACK HAIR FOLLICLE DYSPLASIA

A peculiar hair defect has been reported (Selmanowitz et al., 1972) that affects only the black haircoat regions. In these areas, the hair is shorter than normal (hypotrichosis), broken at the hairshaft, and dull. The skin surface is covered with scales. Whereas the black patches have a "moth-eaten" alopecia, the white areas show a normal, lustrous haircoat. All black areas are not necessarily affected equally. In the reported cases, normal black areas were found on the lateral neck. Histopathologic findings in the affected black areas showed hair follicles to be irregularly dilated and filled with keratinous material. There is no known treatment.

FELINE ALOPECIA UNIVERSALIS

Naturally occurring congenital alopecia is rare. In recent years, cats with this defect have been bred and are called Sphinx cats. The condition can be recognized at birth. Young cats have skin that is smooth and hairless. A few hairs are sometimes found around the muzzle along with short whiskers. Since sebaceous glands are present and open directly onto the skin surface, the glabrous skin feels oily. No known treatment will produce hair growth. Owners of such cats must cleanse the cat's skin, since the cat is reluctant to lick itself. The barbed tongue apparently causes tickling and irritation. Greasy deposits are found within the nailfolds. Claws are slightly abnormal.

CANINE ALOPECIC BREEDS

The Chinese crested dog and the Mexican hairless dog are two breeds in which partial alopecia is an hereditarily established trait. Chinese crested dogs also have abnormal dentition. The skin of Chinese crested dogs is hyperpigmented (apparently to give protection from the sun) but there are some totally depigmented patches.

PINNA ALOPECIA

Hair loss on the pinnas of the ears occurs in a number of breeds, but is most commonly seen in dachshunds. The condition is not congenital, appearing instead in adult animals. Hair loss is gradual and will often progress into total absence of hairs on both surfaces of the pinnas. True alopecia of the pinna is irreversible, and this resembles the male pattern alopecia of man. The differential diagnosis includes:

1. Periodic alopecia found in poodles, dachshunds, Yorkshire terriers, and other breeds, in which the hair falls out suddenly, but regrows spontaneously in 6 to 12 months (similar to alopecia areata in man).
2. Hair loss caused by overtreatment with topical potent corticosteroids (such as

triamcinalone acetonide and flucinotlone acetonide)
3. Allergic contact dermatitis to certain topical medications, such as tetracaine and neomycin
4. Ear pinna alopecia caused by hypothyroidism.

CONGENITAL ALOPECIA

Congenital alopecia usually involves complete absence of hairs on sharply circumscribed areas. Usually such areas are bilaterally symmetrical. The condition has been observed in poodles, cocker spaniels, Belgian shepherds, whippets, and some other breeds. One study (Selmanowitz et al., 1970) in black poodles described a litter of five in which three females were normal and two males were partially alopecic. The bilaterally symmetrical alopecia was identical in both males and affected the dorsal head, legs, dorsal pelvic area, and the entire ventral trunk. The alopecic areas had no hair follicles, sebaceous glands, or apocrine sweat glands. Except for abnormal dentition, the dogs were healthy. As the puppies matured, the pinkish-gray skin on the alopecic areas developed a slate gray pigmentation. The condition seems to be of sex-linked inheritance. There is no known treatment.

COLOR MUTANT ALOPECIA

Color mutant alopecia is a congenital ectodermal defect that affects color mutants of certain breeds and is characterized by partial alopecia, dry lusterless haircoat, scaliness, and papules.

The most common color mutation associated with this skin disease is a blueish gray. Dog breeders refer to this coloration as "blue," such as in blue Doberman pinschers, but the true color is more gray. Since the blue Doberman pinschers are the most commonly seen dogs with this disease, it was once referred to as the "Blue Doberman Syndrome." However, fawn Irish setters and red Doberman pinschers also get the same disease. The fawn Irish setter actually has blonde hair and the red Doberman has chestnut or liver-colored hair. Color mutant alopecia has been observed in "blue" dachshunds, "blue" whippets, "blue" great Danes, and "gray" chow chows.

Some individuals have scaly, "moth-eaten" alopecia at birth, but in most cases the clinical symptoms appear between three to six months of age. Occasionally, an individual dog will appear normal for the first one to two years of its life.

The primary lesions are scaly, alopecic

patches on the trunk and legs. In Doberman pinschers, the elbows are severely affected. Many but not all cases show papule formation. The papules are cystic hair follicles devoid of hair. Some papules develop into pustules. Eventually, most of the body is affected, although the head is usually normal.

The disease is incurable. Treatment with antiseborrheic lotions and shampoos will improve the appearance by removing scales. The dry coat can be sprayed with oil or oil in water to give more luster to the dry haircoat. Frequent shampoos (weekly) are useful. If the cystic hair follicles become infected, systemic antibiotics are helpful. Only the skin and hairs are affected. The dogs are in good health otherwise.

ICHTHYOSIS

In canine ichthyosis, the hair loss is extensive after the disease has run a course of several years. As the skin becomes more and more hyperkeratotic, hair follicles are unable to produce normal hairs. The alopecic skin becomes pigmented until it is gray when exposed to sunlight. The skin thickens and develops deep folds. Scales and flakes adhere to the surface but are also constantly shed. Ichthyosis in dogs is always accompanied by severe hyperkeratosis of digital, carpal, and tarsal pads. The scales that tightly adhere to the affected skin surfaces are laminated and have feather-like upward projections.

One of the most characteristic histopathologic changes in canine ichthyosis is a prominent granular layer of the epidermis. Follicular plugging is seen in many hair follicles. There are dense collections of coarse keratohyaline granules, some of which infiltrate the stratum corneum.

Treatment is only partially effective. The object is to remove as many scales and crusts as possible to make the dog more comfortable. Antiseborrheic shampoos are helpful and have to be given once or twice a week. Six percent salicylic acid gel helps to loosen scales. Vitamin A acid (retinoic acid) is helpful, and the skin can be coated with an oil spray to lubricate its dry surface. Only owners who are very devoted to their afflicted dogs can tolerate such a serious skin disease.

SUPPLEMENTAL READING

Muller, G. H., and Kirk, R. W.: *Small Animal Dermatology*. Philadelphia, W. B. Saunders Co., 1976.
Selmanowitz, U. J., Kramer, K. M., and Orentreich, N.: Canine hereditary black hair follicular dysplasia. J. Hered. 63:43, 1972.
Selmanowitz, U. J., Kramer, K. M., and Orentreich, N.: Congenital ectodermal defect in poodles. J. Hered. 61:196, 1970.

FELINE ALOPECIAS

ROBERT W. KIRK, D.V.M.
Ithaca, New York

INTRODUCTION

The haircoat of cats is important for protection from trauma, irritants, temperature change, and cosmetic effects. Cat are usually concerned and fastidious and spend a great deal of time grooming their coats. The barbs on their tongues are especially formed to do this efficiently, but excessive grooming may accentuate hair and skin problems.

Cat hair is high in protein, so during periods of rapid growth (250 to 300 microns per day), the dietary protein needs may increase. Hair follicles have definite cycles of growth and rest that seem to be related to the photoperiod. In temperate zones, minimal activity occurs from winter until late spring, when intense activity begins and continues for several months. In addition to this general growth, secondary hairs often undergo periods of subsidiary growth in the fall and winter. This schedule causes the coat to be full and fluffy during winter but shed-out and thin (but growing) during the summer. This process is ideally suited to climatic needs. Seasonal changes are less marked in regions with static photoperiods (i.e., tropics or artificial environments). Replacement of hairs occurs in a mosaic pattern over the cat's body, so that hairs in adjacent follicles are at different stages of the cycle. Consequently, general alopecia or "waves of shedding" are not produced. Neutered animals have hair cycles similar to those of intact animals.

During anagen, or the growth stage of the

cycle, the hair follicles extend deeply in the skin to the region of the dermis/subcutis, and the hairs are firmly anchored. When they are extracted, the end of the root has a blunt end and is expanded, glistening, darkly pigmented, and surrounded by a root sheath.

During the resting stage, the basal layers of the follicle atrophy, and the hair moves up toward the epidermis so the base lies in the middle dermis. The hair follicle becomes fusiform and the hair root has a dry, white ball at the end, which forms a club. Hair plucked at this time epilates easily. Under conditions of ill health or generalized disease, the growing stage may be shortened or even arrested. Accordingly, a large percentage of hairs are in the resting stage and are more easily lost because they are poorly anchored. Consequently, the animal "sheds" excessively. Removal of resting hairs may actually stimulate the growth cycle, so grooming is desirable. Disease states also affect the formation of the hair cuticle, and as the hairs do not reflect light readily, the coat is "dull." Severe hair damage may produce tapered hairs, local constrictions, or multiple thickened knobs along the shaft. Affected hairs often break off or fall out. The roots or hair ends then look like spears. If the cat has been pulling or biting hair, the ends will be cut off square.

Hormone imbalances have a major but poorly understood effect on the hair cycle. Thyroid hormone stimulates growth, and a deficiency promotes resting. However, hypothyroidism has not been well documented in cats. It has been stated that cats in estrus tend to shed easily, especially in the groin region (Blakemore 1975). Hormonal changes at parturition produce anagen arrest to cause the well recognized postpartum effluvium, and rabbits have loose hair in the groin region at kindling time. Intradermal injections of depot-type formulations of progesterone or corticosteroids have caused local alopecia and atrophy of the epidermis.

Alopecia and temperature changes produce interesting pigment changes in new hair growth in several cat breeds such as the Siamese and the Himalayan. The acromelanism pattern is due to a temperature-dependent enzyme that converts melanin precursors into melanin by a process of oxidation. With high temperatures, the hair is light colored; with low temperatures, it is pigmented. Thus, kittens at birth are light and adult cats kept indoors or in tropical regions are lighter than those kept outdoors or in cold climates. Prolonged inflammation and/or hyperemia result in light-colored new growth, whereas senility, poor peripheral circulation, or shaving to remove hair (and insulation) results in darker new hair growth. These changes will be most noticeable when long-term temperature changes are present at the time of maximal hair cycle activity.

TYPES OF ALOPECIA

All diseases of the skin have the potential to cause alopecia, since the hair follicle is sensitive to many physiologic and pathologic abnormalities. Some abnormalities are especially characterized by absence of hair.

LOCAL ALOPECIAS

Causes include trauma, excessive licking, psychogenic alopecia (neurodermatitis), and physical effects from burns, freezing, sunshine, and primary (irritant) or allergic contact dermatitis. Additionally, bacterial infections, mycobacterial infections (leprosy), dermatomycosis, eosinophilic granuloma complex, and skin tumors (especially basal cell tumor, squamous cell carcinoma, and mast cell tumor) may all lead to hair loss of varying extent. Some young cats develop a localized preauricular alopecia, which is thought to be a physiologic pattern baldness.

Except for psychogenic alopecia (neurodermatitis), most of these factors can be easily diagnosed and treated.

Psychogenic Alopecia (Neurodermatitis). This disease is often an enigma. It is found in nervous or poorly adjusted cats, and approximately 30 percent of the cases occur in the Siamese, Burmese, Abyssinian, and Himalayan breeds. In the author's cases, about 60 percent of the patients were spayed females. In rare instances psychogenic alopecia may be initiated by local irritations such as infected ears or anal sacs, but it is usually seen in association with boredom, overindulgence, anxiety, or specific situations such as a new pet in the home, boarding, hospitalization, being left alone all day, or loss of a favorite companion, food dish, or bedding site.

The cat licks and/or scratches at a particular local area until the hair is removed. Some cats bite off the hair, leaving square ends on the hair stubble or on the ends of the removed hair shafts. Chronic irritation often produces lichenification of the affected skin. In other cases, the cat irritates the area enough to excoriate the epidermis, which produces denuded and ulcerated lesions. There may be extensive exudation and crusting in these areas. A major diagnostic clue is the constant attention the cat gives to the affected area. However, because the lesion is produced by the cat, and is secondary to other factors, the clinician and owner must become detectives and analyze the cat's habits in order to produce a lasting cure. Even then, some individuals will develop further anxieties and suffer relapses. The differential diagnosis includes feline endocrine alopecia, dermatomycosis, eosinophilic granuloma complex, mycotic or myobacterial granulomas, and various tumors.

Clinical management can be difficult. If licking can be stopped, the lesions heal promptly. If the teeth have tartar, cleaning them may help, and one should always look for a source of pain referred to the skin. Collars and restraint measures produce prompt but temporary responses, but they often frustrate the cat so much that when they are removed, the condition is exacerbated again. Topical medications are of little value unless the lesion can be bandaged or the cat can be restrained from disturbing the lesion. Excoriated areas respond to corticosteroids and bandaging. High doses of methyl prednisolone (e.g., 20 mg of Depomedrol,® Upjohn, weekly for several weeks followed by alternate night oral dosage with Medrol,® Upjohn, if needed) are recommended. Some form of tranquilization is usually needed too. Non-eroded lesions may respond well to tranquilization or sedation alone. Phenobarbital is particularly effective and is given in oral doses of 2 to 5 mg/kg once or twice daily. Diazepam (Valium,® Roche) in daily dosage of 1 to 2 mg/cat orally may also be useful. Although its mechanism of action is unknown, megestrol acetate (Ovaban,® Schering) is frequently a successful alternative treatment. It is given orally in daily doses of 5 mg/cat for one week or until signs abate and then continued on alternate days or once or twice weekly for several months. Once affected, cats may have a disturbing course of relapses that are triggered by any emotional upset, so owners must be reconciled to the possibility of living with the problem controlled but not cured.

GENERAL ALOPECIAS

Although notoedric mange and extensive louse and flea infestations may cause rather generalized alopecia in cats, most etiologic factors are either of internal or an unknown nature. Inheritance has produced the "Sphinx," a universally alopecic cat with only a few hairs or whiskers on the face. These cats are most difficult to manage since they do not groom themselves well and have excessive accumulations of sebum.

Thallium is a cumulative, general cell toxin that, in appropriate dosage, will produce extensive alopecia. It is no longer a commonly used rodenticide, so these cases are rare.

Telogen Effluvium. This is common in all animals and is caused by stresses such as fever, shock, pregnancy and lactation, malnutrition, and severe debilitating illness. These cause many hair follicles to synchronize in the resting stage and consequently, these hairs are shed rapidly. The resulting alopecia can be local or generalized and is somewhat controlled by mechanical factors that may pull out the club hairs.

General Allergies. Allergies to food or fleas may result in extensive areas of alopecia. These cases usually are intensely pruritic and have extensive erythema, papules, and other primary skin lesions. The hair loss is secondary and may be a considerable or only a minor part of the syndrome. In feline flea allergy, most of the lesions are along the dorsum, the neck, and occasionally the rear abdomen. While food allergies may have a general distribution of lesions, they often are especially prominent on the face, head, and along the back.

Feline Endocrine Alopecia (FEA). This produces a pattern of bilaterally symmetric hair loss affecting the posterior abdomen and hind quarters of cats. The hair loss can be patchy or relatively complete in affected areas. Usually, the primary hairs are completely lost, but some secondary hairs may remain, and these may be dry, brittle, and stubby. In some cases, they may be bitten off, and one should be concerned about a differential diagnosis of psychogenic alopecia. The skin of cats with FEA is completely normal — there are no skin lesions of any kind, no pruritus, and no hyperesthesia. Laboratory screening tests are unremarkable, and thyroid function tests are invariably normal.

In an evaluation of 34 cases seen at the New York State College of Veterinary Medicine, there were 16 males and 18 females with a relatively even distribution of FEA between intact and desexed individuals. There was only one purebred cat — a male Siamese. Most of the cats were more than two or three years old. There was a rough seasonal incidence of disease at time of presentation. Although presented throughout the year, except for a higher concentration in November, the largest number of cases was seen in the months of January through early June. This coincides with the onset and duration of the peak cat breeding season in this temperate zone.

Practitioners have known for some time that cats with this syndrome are not hypothyroid. Now, data is accumulating on other endocrine levels in affected cats. Preliminary studies[*] re-

---

[*]Hormonal assays by M. J. Becker, Immunologic Diagnostic Services, 6640 N. Western Ave., Chicago, Illinois.

vealed that one male castrate had a markedly elevated progesterone level and estradiol levels elevated above the average of eight normal male castrates. The testosterone levels were normal for male castrates. Three affected spayed female cats had slightly increased estradiol levels, but normal progesterone and testosterone levels as compared with five normal spayed females. These results are most tenuous but surprising in view of the usually favorable response of such cases to progestational or testosterone therapy.

The major differential diagnostic problem is with psychogenic alopecia, but early dermatomycosis, miliary dermatitis syndrome, flea allergy dermatitis, and physiologic causes of telogen effluvium should be considered.

Clinical management largely ignores topical therapy and concentrates on systemic treatment with various hormones. When combination testosterone-estrogen repositol injections (20:1) were available, they were highly successful. Good response is obtained now with 5 to 10 mg of repositol testosterone IM every four weeks. However, there often is a problem with excessive spraying. Excellent results are also obtained with megestrol acetate given in doses of 5 mg/cat daily for two weeks and then at de-creasing dosages three times, two times, and once weekly as needed. Beneficial results have been obtained with repositol progesterone injection at a dose of 2 to 4 mg/kg repeated in four to six weeks if needed or with Depoprovera®, Upjohn, at 20 mg/kg repeated if needed (Scott, 1979).

Feline endocrine alopecia syndrome is poorly understood. Clinical management is reasonably successful but relapses are common, and owner education to the effect that intermittent lifelong therapy may be required for a problem that is primarily cosmetic is of great importance.

SUPPLEMENTAL READING

Baker, K. P.: Hair growth and replacement in the cat. Br. Vet. J. 130:327, 1974.

Blakemore, J. C.: Personal communication, 1975.

Iljin, N. A., and Iljin, V. N.: Temperature effects on the color of the Siamese cat. J. Hered. 21:309, 1930.

Innes, D. D.: How temperature changes hair color in the Siamese. Feline Pract. 3:27–29, 1973.

Muller, G. H., and Kirk, R. W. Small Animal Dermatology, 2nd ed. Philadelphia, W. B. Saunders Company, 1976.

Ryder, M. L.: Season changes in the coat of the cat. Res. in Vet. Sci. 21(3):289–283, 1976.

Scott, D. W.: Personal communication, 1979.

Strickland, J. H., and Colhoun, M. L. The integumentary system of the cat. Am. J. Vet. Res. 24:1018, 1963.

CANINE CUTANEOUS LYMPHOMAS

WILLIAM H. MILLER, Jr., V.M.D.

Philadelphia, Pennsylvania

Neoplasia of the hematopoietic system is the third most common form of malignancy recognized in the dog, and of this group, lymphosarcoma is the most frequently recognized form. Cutaneous involvement is infrequent, and primary cutaneous lymphomas appear to be rare.

CLASSIFICATION OF LYMPHOMAS

Many schemes have been proposed to classify human lymphomas based on cytologic appearance and histologic pattern. Light microscopic evaluation is often insufficient for complete categorization. Classification of canine lymphomas is usually much less rigorous, and sophisticated categorization does not ap-pear to enable prediction of the response to therapy or survival time. When dealing with a primary cutaneous lymphoma, more rigorous attempts should be made to classify it. There appear to be two distinct forms of cutaneous lymphoma: cutaneous lymphosarcoma (LS) and mycosis fungoides (MF), each of which have different clinical courses and preferred modes of therapy.

CLINICAL PRESENTATION

A cutaneous lymphoma can present in a number of different clinical forms, which may overlap. This history may include the rapid onset of a dermatologic condition with variable pruritus. Frequently one sees multiple, alopecic, scaly, erythematous papules and plaques, which may be ulcerated (particularly in MF). Other clinical forms include discrete, firm cutaneous nodules (particularly in LS) and an exfoliative dermatitis or patches of erythematous, moist, indurated skin. Any skin surface including the mucocutaneous junctions can be involved.

Initially, the lesions are limited, but progression is sometimes rapid (especially in LS) such that the number of nodules or plaques increases or the areas of erythroderma enlarge and coalesce. Early on, the animal is constitutionally and physically normal, but as the disease progresses, the animal often becomes debilitated. In the terminal stages, a peripheral lymphadenopathy often exists either because of the inflammation in the skin (dermatopathic lymphadenopathy) or tumor invasion. Metastasis to visceral organs may occur.

DIAGNOSIS

The diagnosis and classification of lymphoma is based on histopathology, although it should be emphasized that its clinical and histologic diagnosis can be difficult in the initial stages of the disease. An inflammatory process that fails to respond to therapy or a condition that suggests neoplasia should be biopsied at several different sites, as it can be difficult to make an absolute diagnosis of a lymphoma or to categorize it on the basis of one biopsy.

Hematologic, biochemical, and immunologic parameters are initially within normal limits. If extensive epidermal damage exists, one may see a mild to moderate elevation in the serum lactate dehydrogenase. Later, one may see changes that reflect debilitation, metastasis, or infection. Cellular and/or humoral immunosuppression often can be documented.

If a lymphadenopathy is present, a biopsy should be performed to differentiate reaction from neoplasia. Systemic signs should be evaluated as required. If nodes and/or viscera are involved, the disease should be classified and treated as a systemic lymphoma with cutaneous involvement.

MYCOSIS FUNGOIDES

Mycosis fungoides is a primary cutaneous T cell lymphoma of man that is uncommon, chronic, and ultimately fatal. The classical case has a very protracted course and progresses through three clinical stages: the non-specific (premycotic), the plaque, and the tumor stage. The patient can remain in the first two stages for many years before the terminal tumor stage is reached. The type of therapy used does not appear to alter survival time. Since chemotherapy does not lengthen survival time and may shorten it, the therapy used in the premycotic and plaque stages is usually very conservative and is aimed at controlling the symptoms of the disease.

The true incidence of this type of lymphoma in the dog is unknown. Seven cases have been recognized clinically and histopathologically over a two-year period at the University of Pennsylvania, and several other cases have been reported. There is insufficient data to define the biologic behavior, but it appears that the clinical course is not as protracted as it is in man. The duration of the premycotic or the plaque stages is variable; the tumor stage is a fulminating, fatal state.

Of the cases examined at the University of Pennsylvania, four presented in the non-specific and/or plaque stage and three presented in the tumor stage. The animals in the tumor stage were euthanized shortly after the diagnosis was confirmed. Three of the remaining animals are in a state of clinical remission, which ranges from 11 to 23 months in duration. The fourth dog died of a concurrent infection during chemotherapy.

Topical nitrogen mustard (mechlorethamine*) is used to treat the first two stages of the disease in man and has proved to be effective in the dog. Ten milligrams is dissolved in 40 to 60 cc of water and applied directly to the entire skin surface after clipping. The agent is applied two to three times a week initially and then the frequency is reduced to a maintenance level, usually once weekly or bimonthly, once remission is achieved. Evidence suggests that therapy may be discontinued in certain cases. Glucocorticoids are used initially if the pruritus is intense.

No signs of toxicity have been recognized, and the drug hypersensitivity often reported in man has not occurred in the author's cases. The owner applies the medication at home, taking proper precautions to avoid contact with his skin. The dog should not be handled for the first few hours following the application of the drug.

Two dogs developed localized demodectic mange during the course of therapy, which responded rapidly to specific acaricidal therapy.

CUTANEOUS LYMPHOSARCOMA

Whereas mycosis fungoides is a primary cutaneous lymphoma, lymphosarcoma of the skin is

---

*Mustargen — Merck, Sharp & Dohme.

usually a manifestation of the multicentric nature of this neoplasm. Primary cutaneous lymphosarcoma occurs very infrequently and is a fulminating disease characterized by a sudden onset and rapid progression. The number and severity of the cutaneous lesions increases rapidly, and spread to adjacent or draining lymph nodes usually occurs early in the course of the disease. Visceral metastasis will occur if the disease is allowed to follow its natural course.

Cutaneous lymphosarcoma is usually very resistant to therapy. Chemotherapeutic regimes used successfully in other forms of lymphosarcoma often fail to induce remission, and, if remission is obtained, it is often short lived. Because of the high metastatic potential of this lymphoma, topical therapy should be used only as an adjunct to systemic therapy. Combination chemotherapy offers the best chance for remission, but even then this is usually short lived.

Cutaneous lymphomas are ultimately fatal. Cutaneous lymphosarcoma and the tumor stage of mycosis fungoides have a very poor prognosis. Although mycosis fungoides is eventually fatal, the animal's life can be prolonged for an extended period by means of a safe and relatively inexpensive mode of therapy.

SUPPLEMENTAL READING

Bostock, D. E.: Tumors of the skin and mammary glands. In Kirk, R. W. (ed.): *Current Veterinary Therapy VI.* Philadelphia, W. B. Saunders., 1977.

Kelly, D. F., Halliwell, R. E. W., and Schwartzman, R. M.: Generalized cutaneous eruption in a dog, with histological similarity to human mycosis fungoides. Br. J. Derm. 86:164–171, 1972.

MacEwen, E. G., and Hess, P. W.: Canine lymphosarcoma and leukemia. In Kirk, R. W. (ed.): *Current Veterinary Therapy VI.* Philadelphia, W. B. Saunders Co., 1977.

Reed, R. J.: Mycosis fungoides. CA — A Cancer Journal for Clinicians. 27:322–337, 1977.

Shadduck, J. A., Reedy, L., Lawton, G., and Freeman, R.: A canine cutaneous lymphoproliferative disease resembling mycosis fungoides in man. Vet. Path. 15:716–724, 1978.

CRYOTHERAPY IN SMALL ANIMAL DERMATOLOGY

TON (A.) WILLEMSE, D.V.M.
Utrecht, The Netherlands

Although in human medicine, application of cold has been employed for centuries, for example as physical therapy for inflammatory reactions or as a primitive form of anesthesia, only since 1960 has there been increased application of low temperatures for cryosurgery.

The purpose of cryosurgery is unselected but controlled destruction of live tissues containing diseased or normal cells. Two main cooling processes are known:

1. Reduction of pressure without spending energy results in a fall of temperature — the Joule-Thomson effect. Nitrous oxide will reach a temperature of −45°C and carbon dioxide will reach −70°C.
2. Alteration of phase: — during the conversion of a fluid into a gaseous phase, heat will be absorbed from the environment, resulting in a decrease of temperature. Gases that are applicable include nitrogen, freon, and nitrous oxide.

BASIC PRINCIPLES OF CRYOSURGERY

The effect of freezing is binomial: direct cell damage together with infarction as a result of blood vessel destruction. Although most tissues will freeze at −2.2°C, a temperature of at least −20°C must be reached before necrosis will occur. Cells close to the cryoprobe are quickly cooled to the lowest temperature, whereas tissue located at the periphery will remain at a higher temperature.

Slow cooling results in extracellular ice crystal formation, dehydration of cells, and subsequent increase of the intracellular concentration of electrolytes up to toxic levels. In addition, during the rapid cooling process, intracellular formation of small ice crystals occurs, causing slight damage of cell membranes but resulting in denaturation of enzymes. At the same time, small blood vessels become plugged and endothelial cells are damaged, resulting in thrombosis after thawing. Because of this blood stasis, ischemia of the frozen tissue and subsequent cell death occur.

CLINICAL EFFECT OF FREEZING

During the freezing process, an equilibrium is reached between frozen and normal tissue. During the next two hours, hyperemia and tissue swelling take place, and after 24 hours, the frozen tissue becomes dark red. Superficial necrosis occurs after three to four days, and tissue will be shed after about two weeks, leaving behind a granulating wound surface. Fast regeneration then takes place from the surrounding vital tissue.

In the skin, a residual area of hypopigmentation usually results.

METHOD OF PERFORMING CRYOSURGERY

In one procedure, a high pressure, non electric-type cryoapplicator with two round-topped, one flat-round, and one flat-oval probe was used. The shape and the size employed was chosen based on the prerequisite that the probe surface completely cover the lesion during the cryotreatment (Spembly, Ltd., Andover, England).

The freezing time varied between one and three minutes, and nitrous oxide was used as the refrigerant. Anesthetic agents used for cats were ketamine hydrochloride (Ketalar®, Substantia b.v., Mijdrecht, The Netherlands) 15 mg/kg IM, xylazine hydrochloride (Rompum®, Bayer, Nederland b.v.) 0.5 mg/kg SC, and atropine sulfate, 0.1 mg/kg SC. Dogs were sedated with methadon hydrochloride 1.0 mg/kg SC (Symoron®, Gist-Brocades b.v., Delft, The Netherlands) and atropine sulfate 0.1 mg/kg SC, and anesthetized with thiopental sodium 15 mg/kg IV (Pentothal®, Abbott).

RESULTS

Eosinophilic Ulcers in Cats. The oral form of the eosinophilic granuloma complex occurs commonly on the planum nasale, the upper lip, the hard palate, and the tongue. Morphologically, eosinophilic ulcers are well circumscribed with red-brown colored borders and central necrosis. Tissue and blood eosinophilia are rare.

The author has treated 28 cats with this condition. The average age was 3.4 years, and female cats were predisposed (65 percent). In thirteen of these animals (46.4 percent), the lesion had completely healed after three weeks, and in seven others (25 percent), a second treatment was required to effect a complete cure after five to eight weeks. In each treatment, the freezing time was two minutes. In eight cats (28.6 percent), there was little or no response to this treatment.

Papillomas. The clinical picture is characterized by white or grayish, firm hyperkeratotic masses of different sizes located in the skin.

Most of the time, the base of the nodule is narrower than the top. The surface may be smooth or slightly filiform.

Papillomas appear mainly on the head and the neck. In the majority of cases, older dogs are affected. The author's experience with cryotherapy in this condition is limited to a 12 year old male mongrel dog with multiple papillomas in the skin of the lumbosacral area. The duration of the application was two minutes, and the procedure was repeated after thawing. Visible improvement was seen after seven days, and the lesions had disappeared after fourteen days.

Epidermal Cysts. These are firm or fluctuating nodules in the dermis or hypodermis formed by a degenerative change in a hair follicle, by cystic changes in the ducts or cells of sebaceous glands, or by trauma, which displaces epidermal fragments into the hypodermis.

Kerry blue terriers, fox terriers, spaniels, and boxers are especially affected, but there is no age or sex predisposition. The cysts may fluctuate, but often they appear firm and are attached to their dermis, and they may be single or multiple. Upon rupturing, multiple hairs or a grayish cheesy material exudes.

In solitary cysts, surgical excision will be curative, but this method is impractical in the case of multiple cysts.

Cryotherapy, after incision of the cysts and curettage, was performed in three boxers with non-operable multiple cysts. The treatment time was three minutes, and it was repeated after thawing. Although initially, severe necrosis occurred, excellent results were achieved within four weeks in two of the dogs.

Basal Cell Carcinoma. This type of tumor, which arises from the basal cells of the epidermis, accounts for about 30 percent of all feline neoplasms. Basal cell tumors are most commonly seen on the head, ears, and lips. There is no breed or sex predilection, and mainly older cats are affected. Metastases are quite rare.

One case affecting the nostrils and the surrounding skin was treated by cryosurgery. Freezing was performed for one minute at each site, and the treatment was repeated after ten days and after three weeks. Healing was uneventful, and there was no recurrence by six months.

Mastocytoma. This is a common dermal tumor of mesenchymal origin consisting of accumulations of mast cells. In dogs, this neoplasm frequently involves the rear legs, the perineum, and the external genitalia. Firm, isolated nodules, which may gradually soften and may ulcerate, are characteristic.

Boxers are predisposed to mastocytoma. There is no sex predilection, but the incidence increases with age. Metastases are rare, but the infiltrative growth gives rise easily to recurrence after removal.

In cats, the nodules are yellowish in color and often ulcerated or crusted with a typical raw surface underneath, and metastases are common. Mastocytosis in cats is usually fatal. Cryosurgery was carried out under general anesthesia in one dog and one cat.

In the dog, the site was frozen for three minutes, and the procedure was repeated after thawing. After five minutes freezing, the pulse rate increased to 180 per minute and became weak but remained regular and synchronous. Mocous membranes became dark red and the capillary refill time was more than two seconds. A vasogenic shock was suspected and therefore the procedure was stopped.

Intravenous fluid therapy and corticosteroids were curative. A possible explanation is the sudden increased release of vasoactive amines, especially histamine, by the damaged mast cells.

In the cat, freezing was carried out at each site for 1.5 minutes and repeated after thawing. At the end of the freezing procedure, identical symptoms as mentioned for the dog occurred, and they responded to symptomatic therapy. A good result was, however, achieved.

SUPPLEMENTAL READING

Greiner, T. P., Liska, W. D., and Withrow, S. J.: Cryosurgery. Vet. Clin. North Am. 5:565, 1975.

Krahwinkel, D. J., Merkley, D. F., and Howard, D. R.: Cryosurgical treatment of cancerous and non-cancerous diseases of dogs, horses and cats. J. Am. Vet. Med. Assoc. 169:201, 1976.

Lane, J. G.: Practical cryosurgery — an introduction for small animal clinicians. J. Small Anim. Pract. 16:387, 1975.

Holden, H. B. (ed): Practical Cryosurgery. Pitman Medical Publ. Co. Ltd., 1975.

Willemse, A., and Lubberink, A. A. M. E.: Cryosurgery of eosinophilic ulcers in cats. Tijdschr. Diergeneesk. 103(20):1052, 1978.

PHARMACOLOGY OF ANTIPRURITIC DRUGS

PETER EYRE, M.R.C.V.S.
Guelph, Ontario, Canada

Pruritus (prurigo) is defined in the dictionary as ". . . . a disease of the skin marked by intense itching . . . . ." Pruritic dermatoses may be treated with a variety of drug preparations, the objective of which may vary from one situation to another. It may be possible to treat an animal with one specific drug in order to control an uncomplicated dermatologic condition whose etiology is easily defined. For example, the treatment of ectoparasites with specific antiparasitic drugs may be all that is necessary to remove the cause of the skin problem, which thereafter recovers "spontaneously." Frequently, however, a definitive diagnosis is difficult if not impossible to achieve and therefore the clinical use of dermatologic preparations may often serve only to provide symptomatic relief, which in itself may permit healing. Nonspecific therapy may continue indefinitely in order to control a problem of unknown etiology or may simply provide temporary relief until more specific remedies can be instituted. Topical drugs also may be used as adjuncts to systemic therapy. The success of dermatologic preparations will depend not only on the pharmacologic efficacy of ingredients but also on correct usage.

ADRENOCORTICOSTEROIDS

Anti-inflammatory preparations used in dermatologic therapy comprise mainly the corticosteroid compounds that may be applied both topically and systemically. Anti-inflammatory corticosteroids suppress inflammation at several different levels. They inhibit the early vascular events (vasodilatation, edema formation, leukocyte migration) as well as the later phenomena such as fibrin and collagen deposition, fibroblast proliferation, and scar formation. In addition, corticosteroids inhibit inflammation regardless of the underlying cause (physical, chemical, or immunologic). Not only do the corticosteroids provide symptomatic relief of inflammation, they also arrest its progress by inhibiting the fundamental biochemical mechanisms.

INDICATIONS

The clinical indications for corticosteroid treatment in skin diseases are numerous. Corticosteroids are not specifically curative for any particular syndrome, but they represent the most widely used class of drugs currently in use for symptomatic treatment of most forms of pruritic skin disorders. These include atopic disease, inflammatory reactions to ectoparasites, and autoimmune disease.

MECHANISMS OF ACTION

The adrenal cortex synthesizes corticosteroids using the cholesterol residue as an obligatory intermediary. Adrenocorticosteroids are not stored to any great extent by the adrenal gland; therefore, continuous biosynthesis is required for normal body function. The most important naturally occurring corticosteroids are aldosterone and cortisol, each of which represents a fundamentally physiologically different class of compound. Aldosterone represents the class of steroids known as mineralocorticoids, which act primarily on the distal renal tubule to facilitate the resorption of sodium and concomitantly to promote the excretion of potassium. Aldosterone is essentially devoid of anti-inflammatory actions, and its main clinical value is in treating Addison's disease, a condition characterized among other things by negative sodium balance. The other natural mineralocorticoid is desoxycorticosterone.

The anti-inflammatory corticosteroids, the so-called glucocorticoids, are exemplified by cortisol and all its synthetic analogs. The term "glucocorticoid" has evolved to describe drugs that enhance plasma glucagon concentrations, stimulate gluconeogenesis, inhibit carbohydrate catabolism, and enhance glycogen storage. Glucocorticoids are potent inhibitors of inflammation and of the immune system. One of the most important effects of the glucocorticoids is suppression of the synthesis of DNA and protein. These drugs thereby inhibit cell division and cell growth, and they interfere with the synthesis of immunoglobulins. A remarkable effect of glucocorticoids is their ability to suppress the size of lymphoid tissue and to reduce the numbers of circulating mononuclear leukocytes. At the same time, there may be an increased number of polymorphonuclear leukocytes. However, it is by no means correct to

assume that this "lympholytic" action of glucocorticoids necessarily abolishes immunity. Sufficient lymphoid tissue may remain to maintain minimal levels of immunity, and there is little evidence that corticosteroids markedly lower the titer of circulating antibodies. It is therefore most probable that these drugs act mainly by attenuating the inflammation associated with the allergic state rather than by interfering with its immunity per se.

It is now becoming very clear that glucocorticoids interfere with the actions of certain lymphocyte-derived soluble factors — lymphokines — some of which are responsible for the cytotoxic effects of lymphocytes. Other lymphokines (e.g., MIF — macrophage migration inhibitory factor) cause macrophage accumulation in inflamed tissue. Corticosteroids also inhibit the responsiveness of leukocytes to chemotactic factors and inhibit phagocytosis.

Another extremely important property is the ability of glucocorticoids to suppress acute vasodilatation and increased microvascular permeability, which leads to edema formation. The corticosteroids exert this vascular action by enhancing the intrinsic sympathetic vasoconstrictor effects of epinephrine and norepinephrine. This is achieved because the corticosteroids inhibit the catabolism of sympathomimetic catecholamines in a variety of ways.

One of the more widely quoted actions of the glucocorticoids is their ability to "stabilize" (i.e., inhibit activity of) biologic membranes. There is good evidence that corticosteroids inhibit the degranulation of tissue mast cells and circulating basophils in type I hypersensitivity, thus inhibiting the release of vasoactive agents such as histamine, slow-reacting substances, and kallikreins. In this case, it is questionable whether the critical mechanism of action is membrane/granule stabilization as such or an indirect beta-sympathomimetic action mediated through cyclic 3'5' adenosine monophosphate (cyclic AMP) in the cell. Corticosteroids also prevent the rupture of lysosomes. Lysosomal enzymes include proteases, collagenases, and lipases, among others, which are responsible for the tissue destruction so characteristic of cell-mediated immunity. Lipases in particular are responsible for catabolizing cell phospholipids and triglycerides and generating fatty acids such as arachidonic acid and bis-homo linolenic acid, both of which are immediate precursors of prostaglandins. Prostaglandin synthesis is thought to play a central role in the vascular and cellular events of inflammation, and the corticosteroids thus inhibit inflammation by inhibiting prostaglandin production.

There is good evidence that glucocorticosteroids also block the complement pathway, possibly at more than one position. This anticomplementary action is important in control of so-called Type III hypersensitivity — e.g., Arthus reactions.

TOXICITY AND CONTRAINDICATIONS

A broad indication of the relative potencies and approximate dosage ranges for adrenocorticosteroids is given in Table 1. It is most important to note that the published data about comparative potencies of the corticosteroids vary from one author to another. This is because the effectiveness of a drug may vary somewhat depending on the disease model and the species under investigation. Therefore, dosages have to to be quoted in terms of suggested ranges rather than specific quantities. It follows that it is essential to become familiar with this class of drugs under clinical conditions and to realize that considerable adjustments to corticosteroid doses must be made according to the species, the age of the animal, and the stage or state of the condition (acute or chronic, mild or severe).

In general, toxic effects of the corticosteroids may be considered under two headings: (1) undesirable manifestations resulting from continuous use and (2) acute withdrawal. Greater than normal caution should be observed in very young or very old animals and in patients suffering from impaired renal, hepatic, or cardiovascular functions. Corticosteroids, first and foremost, increase the susceptibility of tissues to infection. This applies equally to bacterial, fun-

gal, and parasitic diseases of the skin. It may be best not to use corticosteroids in demodectic mange, for example. Cases of pyoderma also may become more severe after steroid therapy. It is generally recommended that apppropriate anti-infective drug treatment be applied concurrently with the corticosteroid compound.

Other potentially serious complications of long-term corticosteroid therapy are:

1. *Hypokalemia and edema.* These phenomena are usually associated with the use of the natural corticosteroids, cortisone and cortisol, and are manifestations of their intrinsic mineralocorticoid activity, which causes sodium retention (edema) and potassium loss in man. Such mineralocorticoid effects are usually not observed with the synthetic cortisol analogs. Dexamethasone and triamcinolone are essentially devoid of effects on sodium/potassium balance.

2. *Musculoskeletal effects* are characterized by osteoporosis and myopathy, which are manifested respectively in the form of radiographic rarefaction with "spontaneous" fractures and muscular weakness. Musculoskeletal side effects are potentially serious and usually require withdrawal of treatment. Recovery is usually slow and may not be complete.

3. *Induction of parturition* has been observed in some species when high systemic doses of corticosteroids are administered late in pregnancy. It is possible that the corticosteroids either mimick the fetal adrenal or cause regression of the corpus

Table 1. *Relative Potencies and Average Systemic Dosage of Glucocorticoids*
(POTENCY BASED ARBITRARILY ON A STANDARD IN WHICH CORTISOL = 1)

	APPROXIMATE ANTI-INFLAMMATORY POTENCIES	APPROXIMATE RANGE OF DAILY DOSAGE (MG/KG/DAY)
Cortisone	0.5–1.0	2.0 –10.0
Hydrocortisone (cortisol)	1.0	2.0 – 5.0
Prednisone and Prednisolone	3.0–4.0	0.5 – 1.5
Methylprednisolone	5.0	0.5 – 1.0
Triamcinolone	5.0	0.2 – 0.5
Fluoroprednisolone	5.0–10.0	0.2 – 0.5
Dexamethasone	10.0–20.0	0.02– 0.04
Betamethasone	10.0–20.0	0.02– 0.05
Flumethasone	20+	0.01– 0.03

luteum. Although consistent induction of pregnancy by corticosteroids has been reported only in domestic herbivores, the practitioner should be cautious of administering high doses of corticosteroid to any pregnant animal.

Withdrawal of corticosteroid therapy may induce a "withdrawal syndrome" characterized by depression and malaise, fever, and arthralgia. Corticosteroid therapy induces inhibition of corticotrophin production by the hypothalamic-pituitary system (negative feedback); i.e., natural steroid production is suppressed. Therefore, when the extrinsic (therapeutic) supply of corticosteroid is suddenly withdrawn, the patient suffers acute adrenocortical insufficiency, which is potentially life-threatening. Recovery of normal pituitary-adrenal function may take many months, during which time the patient may be more sensitive to stressful situations — e.g., extremes of temperature and trauma.

The toxic effects of corticosteroids may be reduced in several ways. Administration of the hormone on alternate days allegedly provides satisfactory long-term therapy in all but the most severe dermatologic diseases. At the same time, it is said that the adrenal cortex is provided with an opportunity to "recover" on the off-treatment days. It is important to note that this technique provides relative rather than absolute insurance against long-term steroid toxicity. Withdrawal effects may be minimized by a regimen of gradual withdrawal of treatment over a period of about one month, halving the dose each week prior to final withdrawal.

It is also worth noting that prolonged therapy with topical medicaments only is unlikely to produce any of the signs of systemic toxicity because insufficient hormone will be absorbed percutaneously to induce systemic effects. It is also unlikely that high dosages for a short period — e.g., less than one week — will measurably affect the pituitary-adrenal system.

ANTIHISTAMINES

Antihistamines are not in the strict sense truly anti-inflammatory. They may, however, play a useful role in the relief of the clinical signs of allergic conditions, particularly Type I (reaginic) or atopic hypersensitivity.

The effects of histamine on the body have recently been divided into two categories. Those actions of histamine on blood vessels and on non-vascular smooth muscle are produced by a class of histamine receptors called H_1 receptors. Traditional antihistamines used in the control of allergic disorders are known as H_1 receptor antagonists or H_1 blockers (Table 2). A second class of histamine receptors, H_2 receptors, are now known to be responsible for mediating the action of gastrin in evoking gastric acid and pepsin secretion. Antihistaminic drugs that block gastric acid output are known as H_2 blockers and are exemplified by the new drug cimetidine (Tagamet®, Smith, Kline and French), which is now in clinical use in the control of gastric hypersecretory-ulceration conditions (e.g., the Zollinger-Ellison syndrome). Histamine H_2 blocking drugs like cimetidine are devoid of antiallergic/antipruritic properties. On the other hand, it has recently been shown that certain cells that are important in allergic inflammation (e.g., mast cells, basophils, and lymphocytes) carry histamine H_2 receptors. Stimulation of these H_2 receptors by endogenously released histamine operates a negative feedback mechanism which serves to inhibit the further release of chemical substances from the cells. It therefore follows that therapy of gastrointestinal hypersecretion with the H_2-blocker cimetidine may impair the natural feedback and thereby intensify the allergic state by increasing the release of chemical mediators.

Histamine H_1 receptor blocking agents inhibit the effects of histamine released immunologically during allergic reactions. They do this by competitively antagonizing histamine at the H_1 receptor sites in vascular, bronchial, and intestinal smooth muscle and by antagonizing the permeability-enhancing action of histamine in the microvasculature.

The acute flare and itch response in pruritic dermatoses may be caused in part by released histamine. Histamine directly causes vasodilatation and increased vascular endothelial permeability. Histamine also excites sensory neurons, producing reflex vasodilatation and pain or itch. H_1-type antihistaminics inhibit all these effects. They may do so by selectively blocking histamine H_1 receptors and also by their local anesthetic actions. All H_1 antihistamines have some local anesthetic properties. Promethazine has approximately the local anesthetic potency of procaine. Some H_1 antihistamines cause enhancement of the effects of sympathomimetic catecholamines such as epinephrine. This provides yet another possible antiallergic mechanism.

The therapeutic value of antihistamines in the treatment of hypersensitivities has been questioned. Certain pruritic dermatoses seem to respond well to antihistamine therapy. In the acute stages of urticaria, antihistamines may benefit the patient. There is no doubt that much

Table 2. *Examples of Classes of H_1 Antihistaminics, Dosage Ranges and Principal Pharmacologic Properties*

CHEMICAL/GENERIC NAMES	COMMON COMMERCIAL NAME	AVERAGE SINGLE DOSE (MG/KG)	PRINCIPAL PHARMACOLOGIC CHARACTERISTICS OF GROUP
PHENOTHIAZINES			
Promethazine	Phenergan® (Wyeth)	0.2–1.0 (o,s)	Highly effective antipruritics. Promethazine powerful local anesthetic.
Trimeprazine	Temaril® (Smith, Kline, French)	1.0–2.0 (o, s)	Marked sedative action
Methdilazine	Tacaryl® (Westwood)	°	Antiemetic.
ETHANOLAMINES			
Diphenhydramine	Benadryl® (Parke Davis)	1.0–2.0 (o) 0.5–1.0 (s)	Antipruritic. Anticholinergic.
Doxylamine	Bendectin® (Merril National)	°	Strong sedative action.
ETHYLENEDIAMINES			
Pyrilamine	Triaminic® (Dorsey)	1.0–2.0 (o,s)	Good antipruritics. Pyrilamine powerful local anesthetic.
Tripelennamine	Pyribenzamine® (Ciba)	1.0–1.5 (o)	Sedative at normal doses. May induce excitement/convulsions, particularly at high doses.
Methapyrilene	Histadyl® (Lilly)	°	
ALKYLAMINE			
Chlorpheniramine	Chlortrimeton® (Schering)	0.5–2.0 (o)	Antipruritic. Weakly sedative. Excitation at high doses.
PIPERAZINE			
Chlorcyclizine	Perazil® (Burroughs Wellcome)	°	Weakly antipruritic. Weakly sedative. Antiemetic.
MISCELLANEOUS			
Cyproheptadine	Periactin® (Merck Sharp & Dohme)	°	Good antipruritic. Anticholinergic. Sedative. (Antiserotonin as well as antihistamine).

(o) = oral, (s) = subcutaneous route (small animals)
° No specific veterinary information available. Dose should be calculated *pro rata* from human data.

of the improvement seen in the patient is due to the marked sedation caused by many of these drugs. Depression of the central nervous system is particularly prominent with compounds of the ethanolamine and phenothiazine classes. While it must be emphasized that all the antihistaminics of the H_1 class are fundamentally similar in their efficacy in allergic dermatoses, they differ in potency and in some of their wider pharmacologic properties. These are summarized in Table 2.

TOXICITY AND CONTRAINDICATIONS

The most obvious side effects of the antihistamines are sedative and anticholinergic actions. The former is a potentially useful property that may represent an important component in the therapeutic effectiveness of the antihistamines. Atropine-like actions may also be recognized as significant contributions to the control of allergic disease, especially smooth muscle spasm in the bronchial and digestive tracts. Acute antihistamine poisoning following

a massive overdose is principally characterized by central nervous system excitation — ataxia, convulsions, and dilated pupils.

A paradoxic side effect of antihistamines in some individual animals is dermal hypersensitivity to the drug itself. This is a clear indication for withdrawal of the preparation. Severe complications such as agranulocytosis are extremely rare. It is well known that some antihistamines are teratogenic. This has been established for the piperazine group of drugs. Systemic therapy with antihistamines should be avoided in early pregnancy.

LOCAL ANESTHETICS

Local anesthetics may be regarded as truly antipruritic in the sense that they block the sensation of pain or itch — i.e., they anesthetize the irritated area. Application of an appropriate local anesthetic preparation to pruritic skin will produce the most rapid symptomatic relief of all the antipruritic drugs available. Antihistamines are slower in onset than local anesthetics, and corticosteroids are even slower. Unlike other antipruritics used both topically and systemically, local anesthetics are used only topically as antipruritics. They are not antiinflammatory in the strict sense, nor do they antagonize the effects of chemical mediators.

INDICATIONS

As with all other antipruritics, local anesthetics act symptomatically and do not cure any particular dermatologic syndrome. These drugs have been rated highly for the general relief of acute itching associated with all forms of minor skin irritation, insect bites, and burns. Local anesthetics are likely to prove less effective in the long-term control of severe/chronic skin afflictions.

MECHANISM OF ACTION

The exact mode of action of local anesthetics is still a matter of discussion among pharmacologists. In general, it is believed that the salt of the local anesthetic — e.g., the hydrochloride — interacts with tissue buffers to release the so-called free base, which penetrates the cell membrane. It is further understood that the free base then becomes ionized to produce a free quaternary ammonium ion, which is the active form of the drug. The quaternary cationic moiety has the ability to inhibit specifically the conductance of sodium and calcium, which non-specifically stabilizes or inhibits activity in cell membranes. This applies to nerve axons and also to other cell types such as smooth muscle cells and leukocytes. Local anesthetics not only impair electrical conduction in nerve cells and thereby inhibit the sensation of pain or itch, they also arrest smooth muscle contraction and may diminish the release of some inflammatory chemicals from mast cells and leukocytes.

Local anesthetics in general are well absorbed through mucous membranes, the most notable exception being procaine. They are not well absorbed through intact skin, although percutaneous absorption is greater in the presence of fat solvents and is also enhanced when skin is abraded or markedly inflamed.

Cocaine, one of the most interesting drugs in medicine, is highly efficient in anesthetizing mucosal surfaces and produces at the same time intense local vasoconstriction. Butacaine is approximately as effective as cocaine. Proparacaine (a procaine analog) is an efficient anesthetic for mucosal surfaces. Cyclomethacaine is a popular and effective dermatologic anesthetic that has, paradoxically, proved to be of low effectiveness on mucosae.

A number of benzoate ester local anesthetics with low water solubility have been widely employed in fatty ointments, dusting powders, and suppositories. These compounds (e.g., benzocaine and butylaminobenzoate) are slowly hydrolyzed by tissue fluid and produce a prolonged anesthetic action. They are especially useful on abraded skin. Pramoxine is another effective topical local anesthetic. This drug is sometimes of value in patients that have become sensitive to the more usual benzoate-ester compounds.

The names and general pharmacologic properties of the topical local anesthetics are given

Table 3. *Principal Pharmacologic Properties of Topical Local Anesthetics*

CHEMICAL/GENERIC NAMES	COMMON COMMERCIAL NAMES	PRINCIPAL PHARMACOLOGIC PROPERTIES
Cocaine	–	Excellent topical anesthetic. Vasoconstrictor.
Cyclomethacaine	Surfacaine® (Lilly)	Good anesthetic for mucosae and abraded skin. Weak effect on eye. May be irritant.
Proparacaine	Opthaine® (Squibb)	Used almost exclusively for eye.
Butacaine	Butyn® (Abbott)	Good anesthetic for eye, nose and throat. May be irritant.
Ethyl-Aminobenzoate (Benzocaine)	–	Insoluble drugs used in powders, ointments and suppositories. May cause hypersensitivity.
Butyl-Aminobenzoate	Butesin® (Abbott)	
Pramoxine	Tronothane® (Abbott)	Good dermal anesthetic. Generally too irritant to use on the eye. Used in laryngobronchoscopy.

in Table 3. Many other local anesthetics (e.g., Procaine, Lidocaine, Carbocaine, and Dibucaine) are used mainly for infiltration or spinal anesthesia. These drugs will however, with the exception of procaine, produce effective topical anesthesia if applied locally in aqueous solution.

TOXICITY

It is highly improbable that serious toxic reactions would arise from the topical use of local anesthetics with the concentrations and methods of application recommended by manufacturers. However, local irritation is sometimes reported following the use of butacaine, cyclomethacaine, and pramoxine, in particular. Hypersensitivity reactions are potential side effects of prolonged use of any local anesthetic. Clearly, it may be very difficult to distinguish an adverse skin reaction to the local anesthetic from an exacerbation of the original dermal condition per se. Suspicion of an adverse reaction necessitates changing the anesthetic or replacing it with another class of antipruritic.

Section
7

OPHTHALMOLOGIC DISEASES

CHARLES L. MARTIN
Consulting Editor

The Ophthalmic Examination and Anamnesis 505
Neuro-ophthalmology 510
Ocular Therapeutics 517
Algorithms for Ophthalmologic Problems 528
Ocular Emergencies 542
Diseases of the Eyelids 546
Diseases of the Conjunctiva 550
Diseases of the Lacrimal Apparatus 553
Diseases of the Cornea 558
Diseases of the Lens 565
Diseases of the Anterior Uvea 570
Canine and Feline Glaucoma 576
Diseases of the Vitreous, Retina, and Choroid 579
Diseases of the Orbit 583
Intraocular and Orbital Neoplasia 585
Ophthalmic Disorders of Proven or Suspected Genetic
    Etiology in Dogs and Cats 587
The Eye and Systemic Disease 593

Additional Pertinent Information, Still Current, Found in
Current Veterinary Therapy VI:

Fischer, C. A.: Diseases of the uveal tract, uveitis and
  immunologically mediated ocular disorders, p. 638.
MacMillan, A. D.: Feline ocular disorders, p. 656.

THE OPHTHALMIC EXAMINATION AND ANAMNESIS

CHARLES L. MARTIN, D.V.M.

Athens, Georgia

ANAMNESIS

In a busy general practice, the gathering of historical data pertaining to ocular complaints is often neglected or limited to what the owner volunteers. Although most ocular diagnoses are anatomic, based on direct visual inspection and augmented by known breed, age, and species-related syndromes, the importance of the history should not be minimized. Not only should the ocular history be scrutinized, but the general medical history should be included, as many systemic states may be manifest in the eye and its adnexia.

The breed, age, and occasionally the sex are important data for the experienced clinician, as many ocular syndromes are inherited or at least have a breed predisposition. (See "Ophthalmic Disorders of Proven or Suspected Etiology in Dogs and Cats.")

The owner's complaints usually are among the following: decreased vision or blindness, ocular discharge, ocular color changes, pain, an opacity or film, pupillary changes, and bulging eye(s). These complaints form the basis for the problem-oriented approach to ophthalmology and are discussed in more detail in a subsequent chapter.

Decreased Vision or Blindness. Depending on the function of the dog, the environment, the amount of vision lost in one or both eyes, and the rapidity of development, the historical data may be accurate or misleading. Insidious loss of vision such as progressive retinal atrophy in the house dog, is notoriously late in its course when the animal is presented. Dogs that work by sight are more critically evaluated as to type (moving vs. stationary objects) and degree of deficiency. Non-leading questions should be asked regarding night vision, day vision, and ability to see moving objects as opposed to stationary objects, and near objects as opposed to far objects. This must then be interpreted in light of the animal's function and environment and the owner's ability to discriminate. Most animals are not presented with this complaint unless the condition is bilateral and relatively severe.

Ocular Discharge. Historical data regarding chronicity, progression, and modification by therapy, season, and environment should be obtained.

Ocular Color Changes. Color changes in the eye may be noted extraocularly, such as the red eye of conjunctivitis and some corneal opacities on the ocular surface, or intraocularly, such as the abnormal anterior chamber or iris color changes. The changes are usually most dramatic with unilateral involvement, as the normal eye serves as a control, and in animals with lightly pigmented irides.

Ocular Pain. Blepharospasm and rubbing the eye(s) are readily noted by owners, but ocular pain is often manifest in a more nebulous manner — e.g., general malaise, depression, excessive sleeping, and a worsening of the temperament. These signs are often not appreciated by the owners until improvement occurs and retrospective comparisons are made.

Opacities. Opacities or films over or in the eye may result from prolapse of the membrana nictitans, tenacious ocular discharges, corneal opacities, fibrin or masses in the anterior chamber, and cataracts. Historical data regarding chronicity, laterality (constant or intermittent), progression, and precipitating factors should be obtained.

Pupillary Changes. These are usually noted when unilateral extremes in size are present or when changes are accompanied by another complaint such as blindness, which draws the owner's attention to the eye. The pupil size is most easily seen in lightly pigmented irides or against the background of a white cataract.

Bulging Eye(s). The symptom is usually unilateral. It may be acute or chronic in nature and is often accompanied by another complaint such as red eye, pain, ocular discharge, or a film over the eyes.

The initial clinical appearance and its modification with time, therapy, and environmental change should be documented.

Particularly for chronic cases, information as to administration of prior "home" or professional remedies should be obtained. The disease process may have been modified, and the interpretation of the ocular examination such as pupillary light reflexes and intraocular pressures may be complicated by prior therapy. Failure of response to previously prescribed therapy should provoke questions as to the owner's compliance with instructions.

With new clients, it is obviously necessary to obtain historical data on previous ocular problems and their course of and response to therapy.

As many ocular problems are breed related, it is often desirable to establish possible inheritence, although the necessary information is often not available. In most instances, genetic syndromes are inferred by the occurrence of a known syndrome in a particular age and breed of dog.

As the eye often manifests systemic illness, it is imperative that possible extraocular ramifications be considered. In addition, topical medications may have systemic side effects, and conversely, systemic drugs may have ocular side effects. Candidates for ocular surgery need to be evaluated preoperatively for systemic disease.

Historical data pertaining to environmental factors such as animal exposure, type of housing, bedding, fenced yard, dusts, irritants such as fumes and fiberglass, and function of the dog may help establish an etiologic diagnosis for a previously unresolved problem.

OCULAR EXAMINATION

DIFFUSE ILLUMINATION WITH HEAD UNRESTRAINED

This examination is the initial step in evaluating conformation and symmetry of the eye and its adnexia. It is important to keep the head unrestrained, as simply touching the side of the head will modify lid conformation. In addition, manipulation of the head will often precipitate blepharospasms in a dog that is "eye shy" by nature, in pain, or has received prior ocular medication. Comparison of ocular and adnexial symmetry is important and should be performed from various angles of observation — i.e., frontal and dorsal. Palpebral fissure symmetry, membrana nictitans position, globe size, orbital position, iris color, and pupil size should be evaluated for symmetry. At this time, ocular discharges, lid swellings, alopecia, and erythema can be noted. The cornea is inspected for its luster, surface irregularities, and opacities. The specular light reflex off the cornea superimposed on the pupils allows accurate assessment of ocular alignment, and gross opacities in the anterior chamber and lens may be noted.

At the conclusion of the gross examination, one can usually determine whether conjunctival or corneal cultures are desired and if a Schirmer tear test is indicated. A bright light is then utilized to determine the direct and consensual pupillary light reflexes. These three determinations should be made early in the examination, as subsequent procedures that utilize topical anesthetics and add moisture to the eye will interfere with their interpretation. As it takes 10 to 15 minutes for good mydriasis, it is desirable to initiate pupil dilation early so that time is not wasted at the end by waiting. An exception to hasty mydriastic therapy would be cases in which glaucoma is suspected on initial examination because of a red eye, a large eye, a dilated pupil, or corneal edema.

MICROBIOLOGIC CULTURES OF CONJUNCTIVA/CORNEA

If the type of discharge, history of chronicity, lack of response to therapy, or severity of the problem indicates that an infectious agent is involved, cultures are obtained early in the examination, before topical anesthetics are applied, as they are bacteriocidal. Cultures of both eyes are preferred for comparative purposes, even if the problem is unilateral. *Staphylococcus* sp. and *Streptococcus* sp. are the most consistent flora of the normal and diseased conjunctiva.

The swab may be moistened with sterile nutrient broth or saline before using it, so as to make the procedure more comfortable. Calcium alginate swabs are preferred. They should be placed in a transport medium or immediately plated to prevent drying of the small samples.

EXAMINATION WITH MAGNIFICATION, BRIGHT LIGHT, FOCAL LIGHT, AND RETROILLUMINATION

Magnification in the form of a loupe or slit lamp is a critical aid in lesion recognition owing to the minute structures involved. This technique is mainly limited to the anterior ocular segment and adnexia. Various inexpensive head loupes or a magnifying lens can be utilized, but the slit lamp (biomicroscope) is the most sophisticated means of accomplishing a magnified examination. A bright light source, which can be directed at various angles, is utilized in conjunction with magnification to examine topographic surfaces of the lid margins, conjunctiva, membrana nictitans, cornea, anterior chambers, iris, and lens. In addition to direct illumination, proximal illumination (lighting the region adjacent to the object of regard) and retroillumination (lighting the "background" of the region studied) are also helpful. The lids, lid margins, and canthal regions are examined for distichiasis and trichiasis. The former may be difficult to detect without magnification. Retroillumination of the eyelids may be performed with a transilluminator in searching for foreign bodies. The conjunctival surfaces are examined for aberrant cilia (palpebral surface), foreign bodies, and degrees of pathologic changes such as follicles, hyperemia, chemosis, symblepharon, and discharges. The cornea is examined by retroillumination of the iris and fundus (dilated pupil) to detect small opacifications and then studied in more detail in direct illumination. Irregularities of the surface, opacifications, and neovascularization are searched for and characterized based on extent and depth.

The anterior chamber is examined for changes in depth and abnormal contents. The depth is increased with the loss of lens support (aphakia, microphakia, posterior luxated lens, hypermature cataract) and decreased with iris bombé, peripheral anterior synechea, intumescent lens, or a mass in or behind the iris. Abnormal contents such as leukocytes, erythrocytes, fibrin, cysts, lens, and tumors are noted. Changes in the blood-aqueous barrier can be detected by using a focused light source or thin beam of light to demonstate the Tyndall effect or "flare" produced by an increased protein content (plasmoid aqueous) and cells in the anterior chamber.

The iris is examined for texture, masses, color, vascularity, pupillary membrane strands, and stability. With loss of the lens support from a displaced lens or peripheral iris adhesions, the iris trembles on ocular movements. If the pupillary light reflexes have not already been examined, they are recorded. The iris, particularly the pupillary region, can be examined in the retroillumination of the tapetum to detect areas of atrophy or hypoplasia. If the pupillary light reflexes are incomplete or ani-socoria is present, sphincter atrophy, hypoplasia, or synechia may be responsible. The pupil is examined for irregularities in shape that may indicate atrophy or adhesions.

The lens is first examined in retroillumination from the fundus to detect opacities rapidly and then in direct and focal illumination to determine the depth of the lesion. Any noted opacities are characterized by their shape, number, color, texture, and location. Irregularities in surface (wrinkled capsule in hypermature cataracts), shape (coloboma, lenticonus), and size (microphakia, intumescent lens) may be noted.

The anterior vitreous can be examined for hyaloid artery remnants, veils, haze (usually cells), and blood.

SCHIRMER TEAR TEST

If, after the initial examination, a decrease in tear production is suspected, the commercial Schirmer tear test or Whatman #40 filter paper strips can be utilized to measure tear production objectively. This should be performed before topical drops or anesthetics are applied. The test used most often in veterinary ophthalmology is the Schirmer I test, which measures basal and reflex secretion rate. This is accomplished by bending the strip at a notch near the end of the strip and hooking the short end over the medial lower lid into the lower conjunctival cul-de-sac. The strip can be kept from falling out owing to ocular movements by closing the lids once it is in place.

The strip is removed after one minute and the amount of wetting, measured in millimeters, is immediately recorded. The norm for the dog is 19 to 21 mm of wetting and for the cat, 15 to 17 mm. Signs are usually not associated with decreased tear production until values are between 5 and 10 mm.

The Schirmer II test measures the basal tear secretion by eliminating the reflex irritative component with a topical anesthetic. After application of the topical anesthetic, the lower cul-de-sac is dried by swabbing with a cotton-tipped applicator. The basal secretion in the dog is about 12 mm of wetting.

MYDRIASIS

Before instilling the mydriatic of choice, the pupillary light reflexes are accessed. (The pathways and interpretation of the reflexes are discussed in "Neuroophthalmology.") Most mydriatics take 10 to 15 minutes to act, so to conserve time, they should be given early in the examination. Mydriasis is necessary for complete ophthalmoscopy and for a thorough examination of the lens. The mydriatic of choice should be short in action as well as effective. Atropine in the normal eye lasts for days, and thus its use is an "overkill." Tropicamide 1 percent (0.5 percent may be preferred in cats) is a short-acting mydriatic that is popular for diagnostic purposes. When licked from the nose, the bitter taste may stimulate profuse salivation. In young puppies, maximal mydriasis may not be achieved or may be very fleeting, and combining the parasympatholytic drug with a sympathomimetic drug such as 10 percent phenylephrine may be necessary.

OCULAR STAINING

Sodium fluorescein is an invaluable tool in detecting corneal epithelial defects as well as in monitoring the healing process. It is utilized mainly as single-use strips, since it was discovered that the solution is a good culture media for *Pseudomonas* sp. If used as a 1 to 2 percent solution in multiple-use bottles, care must be taken to avoid contamination. Fluorescein is water soluble and turns from orange to bright green at a pH of 7.

If a break in the corneal epithelium is present, the aqueous fluorescein gains access to the corneal stroma which is alkaline enough to turn it a bright green. The lipid nature of the epithelium prevents this when it is intact. Staining extensive ulcerations often results in the fluorescein being visible in the aqueous. The corneal staining is transient (about 15 to 30 minutes).

If the strips are used and the ocular surface is not very moist, adding one to two drops of collyrium to the strip will insure adequate fluorescein solution on the eye. The eye is rinsed thoroughly with collyrium to remove excess fluorescein and mucus, and the retention of stain is evaluated. With small defects, the use of an ultraviolet light (Wood's lamp) or cobalt-blue light in a dark room will cause fluorescence of the fluorescein, making minute stain retention visible.

Other uses for fluorescein stain in ophthalmology are (1) topically, to detect aqueous leaks in perforating wounds and patency of the lacrimal outflow system; (2) systemically, to visualize ocular fundus and iris angiography; and (3) to measure arm-to-retina circulation time.

Rose Bengal 1 percent, a supravital stain, is used to stain devitalized corneal and conjunctival epithelium red. Its main use is in staining devitalized cells in keratoconjunctivitis sicca. In these cases, it is said to be more sensitive than the Schirmer tear test.

CANNULIZATION OF THE LACRIMAL OUTFLOW SYSTEM

In problems regarding epiphora or a stubborn conjunctival infection, it is often necessary to cannulate the lacrimal outflow system in order to establish patency. This is readily performed in most dogs with topical anesthesia, using restraint, in lateral recumbency. A blunt 22 gauge needle or a commercial malleable lacrimal needle on a 6 cc syringe is passed into either the upper or lower puncta. The upper puncta is usually more accessible. Tauting the lid, threading the catheter down the cannaliculus, and keeping it parallel to the cannaliculus all help to prevent kinking and obstruction by the wall of the cannaliculus, thus avoiding a false impression of a pathologic obstruction. Resting the hand that is controlling the syringe against the animal's head minimizes traumatizing the duct as the result of minor head movement.

A fountain of fluid should emerge from the opposite puncta and the nostril. If fluid is not seen at the nostril, the puncta that has not been cannulated is occluded while flushing. Owing to imperfect nasolacrimal ducts in some dogs, the fluid may not be immediately visible, but the dog often starts to choke, sneeze, and swallow from fluid running posteriorly into the pharynx. If an obstruction is present, heavy sedation or a general anesthesia may be required, as the force necessary to unblock the obstruction is painful.

Cats are more difficult to cannulate because of the small cannaliculus size and the animal's temperament. A 25 to 27 gauge blunt needle, ketamine sedation and a loupe are used for best results.

DOUBLE EVERSION OF THE EYELIDS AND MEMBRANA NICTITANS

The palpebral conjunctiva and bulbar surface of the membrana nictitans can be examined by a process of double eversion, which is performed under topical anesthesia. Gently grasp the lid margin with forceps and lift it up caudally from the eye. Use an instrument such as a strabismus hook near the base of the lid to push toward the eye. This will cause the lid to roll back over the hook, exposing the palpebral conjunctiva. This maneuver also can be performed on the membrana nictitans to expose the lymphoid follicles and gland.

CONJUNCTIVAL AND CORNEAL CYTOLOGY

Scrapping the conjunctiva and/or the corneal surface under topical anesthesia may enable a rapid etiologic diagnosis to be made. The scraping may be performed with various instruments, but a malleable platinum spatula (Kimura) is best. The small amount of material is transferred to glass slides, air dried, fixed, and stained with Giemsa's and Gram's stains. The slides are examined for cell type, bacteria, viral and chlamydial inclusion bodies, fungi, and foreign particles.

TONOMETRY

The measurements of intraocular tensions may be made with a variety of instruments, all of which were designed for use on people. Indentation tonometry is exemplified by the Schiötz tonometer, which is one of the more applicable tonometers to veterinary use because of its low cost. This instrument measures the amount of corneal indention produced by a given weight, and this figure is converted from a scale reading to millimeters of mercury. A conversion table for the dog has been calculated that gives higher readings than comparable scale readings on the human conversion table.

After topical anesthesia is administered, the animal is placed in dorsal to dorsolateral recumbency so the eye being measured is looking vertically and the tonometer is allowed to rest with its full weight on the central cornea for one to two seconds. The scale reading is noted. This is repeated three to four times for consistency, and the nose is then tilted to bring the other eye into position. While most animals object to being placed on their sides or backs for proper ocular position, the sitting patient presents poor eye position, which often necessitates placing the tonometer near or over the limbus. Inaccurate or spurious values with the Schiötz tonometer can be produced by dried mucus and tears on the instrument, small corneal curvature (microphthalmos), large corneal curvature (buphthalmos), corneal scars, corneal edema, anterior luxated lens, and transference of pressure to the globe while holding the lids open.

Applanation tonometry measures the force necessary to flatten a given corneal area and may be measured with a variety of instruments. However, many have limited applicability to veterinary ophthalmology owing to expense and lack of patient cooperation.

The intraocular tensions may be estimated by palpating the globe through the closed eyelids alternately with the index fingers. The "give" of the globe is estimated by gentle pressure. This obviously is a crude estimate and only differentiates soft, medium, and hard tensions.

TONOGRAPHY

Tonography is a technique whereby the weight of a tonometer is allowed to rest on the globe for a given time (four minutes). The weight of the tonometer forces fluid out of the eye, and the pressure decay is recorded. With appropriate formulas and certain previously calculated constants, the coefficient of aqueous outflow can be determined. In veterinary ophthalmology, this is mainly a research tool.

GONIOSCOPY

Gonioscopy is the act of viewing the iridocorneal angle. To view the iridocorneal angle adequately, a contact lens is necessary to allow light to exit the cornea externally. This region contains the aqueous outflow pathways and thus is important in the pathogenesis of many glaucomas. The procedure can be accomplished with topical anesthesia and manual restraint in lateral recumbency. A variety of gonioscopic lenses designed for man are available, and most are applicable to veterinary ophthalmology. A strong light and a source of magnification also are necessary. In addition to investigating the pathogenesis of glaucoma, gonioscopy is useful in evaluating lesions of the peripheral anterior chamber such as iris cysts, foreign bodies, tumors of the region, and traumatic lesions.

The normal iridocorneal region is dominated by a well developed pectinate ligament with a bluish white trabecular region in the background. The pigmentation in the angle region is variable.

OPHTHALMOSCOPY

Ophthalmoscopy is one of the most difficult routine procedures that the veterinary student is asked to master. Using the traditional direct ophthalmoscope is not the technique of choice in small animal practice. The binocular or monocular indirect ophthalmoscope is preferred. The main disadvantage of the binocular indirect ophthalmoscope is its high cost. Essentially, all that is necessary for indirect ophthalmoscopy is a +14 to +28 diopter lens and a good focal beam of light. The pupil must be dilated well for a thorough examination, which includes more than just visualizing the optic nerve and posterior pole. Although the image with indirect ophthalmoscopy is reversed, the technique is easily learned.

Examination of the ocular fundus should include evaluating the optic disc for size, color, elevations, depressions, vascular pattern, and shape. The tapetum, if present, is evaluated for its reflectivity, mosaic detail, color, size, and retinal vascular pattern. The non-tapetum is evaluated for pigment density, motteling, and vascular patterns. The normal dog's ocular fundus has more normal variations than that of other domestic animals and thus can present difficulties for even an experienced examiner who is trying to differentiate mild pathology from extreme normal variations.

ELECTROPHYSIOLOGIC TESTS

Electroretinography, visually evoked responses, and electro-oculography are electrophysiologic responses that may be utilized in clinical investigations. The tests are rather simple, but the specialized electronic equipment is expensive and relegates much of the testing to institutions. The tests help to elaborate the basic etiopathogenesis of ocular and visual pathway disease at both the applied and research levels.

MISCELLANEOUS DIAGNOSTIC TESTS

Fluorescein angiography is used to study retinal and iris vasculature, whereas orbital arteries and veins can be studied radiographically by selective injection of radiopaque dyes. Radiology is also utilized to detect ocular and orbital foreign bodies (mainly metallic), and masses may be outlined by pneumo-orbitography. Injection of contrast material into the nasolacrimal duct may be utilized to study obstructive diseases.

Ultrasonography in A, B, and M modes has become routine in some centers for studying ocular lesions, particularly with opaque media. The equipment is expensive and not available in most veterinary colleges.

Aqueous and vitreous paracentesis are performed frequently for cultures and cytology. Diagnosing systemic mycoses involving the eye has been one of the most fruitful indications for vitreous paracentesis.

SUPPLEMENTAL READING

Gelatt, K., Peiffer, R.L., Erickson, J., and Gum, G.: Evaluation of tear formation in the dog, using a modification of the Schirmer tear test. JAVMA 166:368–370, 1975.
Lavach, J., Thrall, M., Benjamin, M., and Severin, G.: Cytology of normal and inflamed conjunctives in dogs and cats. JAVMA 170: 722–728, 1977.
Martin, C.L.: Slit lamp examination of the normal canine anterior ocular segment. Parts I, II, III: J. Small Anim. Pract. 10: 143–169, 1969.
Martin, C.L.: Gonioscopy and anatomical correlations fo the drainage angle of the dog. J. Small Anim. Pract. 10:171–184, 1969.
Martin, C.L.: The normal canine iridocorneal angle as viewed with scanning electron microscopy. JAAHA 11:180–184, 1975.
Rubin, L., Lynch, R., and Stockman, W.: Clinical estimation of lacrimal function in dogs. JAVMA 147:946, 1965.
Urban, M., Wyman, M., Rheins, M., and Marraro, R.: Conjunctival flora of clinically normal dogs. JAVMA 161:201–206, 1972.
Wyman, M., and Donovan, E.F.: The ocular fundus of the normal dog. JAVMA 147:17–26, 1965.

NEURO-OPHTHALMOLOGY

RANDALL H. SCAGLIOTTI, D.V.M.
Carmichael, California

Neuro-ophthalmology is a special field that seeks to link the neurosciences with ophthalmology in order to study the ophthalmic manifestations of central nervous system disorders. This article establishes a foundation for understanding the various pupillary reactions that occur under a myriad of clinical conditions based on new understandings of the anatomy and pathophysiology of pupillary reactions.

PUPILLARY REACTIONS

A complete general medical history with emphasis on prior systemic infections, metabolic disorders, and injuries to the head and neck facilitates interpretation of pupillary disorders. A thorough ocular exam should follow, especially of the iris and lens, and it should be performed with the aid of magnification (e.g., loupes or biomicroscopic slit lamp). Many dyscorias (misshapen pupils), anisocorias (unequal pupils), and other pupillary abnormalities are the result of mechanical or anatomic disturbances of the iris (e.g., iris atrophy, synechia) or are a consequence of lens problems or other ocular disease (e.g., subluxated lens or glaucoma). When primary or secondary ocular disease is not present, a disturbance of the neurologic pathways that control pupillary behavior is considered.

ANISOCORIA

Anisocoria is observed most commonly in its static state, but it also develops during a contraction. Dynamic contraction anisocoria or alternating contraction anisocoria develops when the direct response in either eye to light stimulation is more extensive than the consensual response. This is a normal physiologic reaction in cats and dogs, whereas in man or other primates it is considered pathologic. The presence of a static anisocoria while both retinas are receiving equal light indicates the presence of an underlying neurologic disturbance, provided that the structural and mechanical integrity of the iris is normal.

LIGHT REFLEX

Understanding the clinical significance of pupillary abnormalities in neurologic disorders depends on a thorough understanding of the functional neuroanatomy of the light reflex. The afferent arm of the light reflex pathway includes all those neurons relaying nerve impulses from the retina to the parasympathetic component of the oculomotor nucleus, the Edinger-Westphal nucleus. The efferent arm of the light reflex consists of those neurons conducting impulses from this nucleus to the sphincter muscle of the iris.

NORMAL FUNCTIONAL NEUROANATOMY — AFFERENT ARM

Incoming light influences the size of the pupil by activating the photoreceptors in the retina converting light energy into the electrochemical energy of nerve impulses, which are then relayed from the retina to the mesencephalon. The afferent arm is a three-neuron pathway, with the neurons linked in chain-like fashion.

The first neuron stimulated is the retinal chain neuron, which consists of the intraretinal rod and cone photoreceptors and the true first order neuron, the retinal bipolar cells, as shown in Figure 1. The second order neurons are the optic nerve fibers, which extend from their origin in the retinal ganglion cells to their synapse on cell bodies of the third order neurons in the pretectal nuclei of the midbrain. The nonmyelinated optic nerve fibers, which originate from the ganglion cells, form the nerve fiber layer that exits the globe at the lamina cribrosa, forming the optic nerve head. The second order neurons can be visually evaluated at the nerve head with the aid of an ophthalmoscope, as the fibers are myelinated here. The optic fibers then project caudally through the optic canals and partially decussate at the optic chiasm, as shown in Figure 2. In the dog, approximately 75 percent of the fibers from either eye decussate to the contralateral side, and the remaining fibers project ipsilaterally. In the cat, 65 percent of the fibers decussate as compared with 50 percent in man. The pupillomotor fibers (i.e., optic nerve fibers participating in the light reflex) that form part of the optic tract project to the midbrain via the superior brachium of the rostral colliculus and synapse on cell bodies of

Figure 1. Schematic drawing of retinal histology, illustrating the anatomic location of first order neurons (retinal chain neurons) and the intraretinal portion of second order neurons (ganglion cells and their axons).

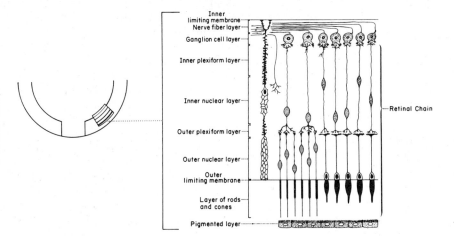

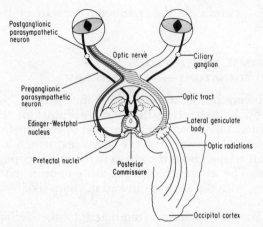

Figure 2.   Light reflex pathway. Drawing illustrates the unequal distribution of extraocular second order neurons at the chiasm and third order neurons at the posterior commissure. The majority of second order and third order neurons cross, while the minority remain uncrossed. This applies to the dog as well as the cat. (Adapted from: Lowenstein, O., Murphy, S. B., and Lowenfeld, I. E.: Functional evaluation of the pupillary light reflex pathways. Arch. Ophthalmol. *49*:565–570, 1953.)

the third order neurons of the pretectal nuclei. The remaining second order neurons composing the optic tract are visual fibers that enter the lateral geniculate body for cortical projection for vision. Therefore, lesions in the lateral geniculate body will not affect the pupillary reflexes to light stimuli.

The third order neurons originating from the pretectal nuclei deserve special attention and study because their proposed distribution to the constrictor nuclei of Edinger-Westphal departs from the anatomy as understood in man and primates. The majority of third order neurons arising from either pretectal nucleus, whether synapsed on by the crossed or uncrossed second order neurons, decussate to the contralateral Edinger-Westphal nucleus via the caudal commissure. The remaining minority of third order neurons of either pretectal nucleus arch around the central grey matter to reach the constrictor nucleus on the ipsilateral side. This species difference in third order neuron decussation and the unequal decussation at the chiasm partially accounts for the differences in functional behavior of the pupils between man and the dog and cat.

NORMAL FUNCTIONAL
NEUROANATOMY — EFFERENT ARM

The efferent arm of the light reflex is a two-neuron pathway composed of neurons from the parasympathetic division of the autonomic nervous system, which remain uncrossed during their projection to the iris as shown in Figure 2.

The preganglionic parasympathetic fibers arise from cell bodies in the Edinger-Westphal nucleus that is located in the rostral end of the larger oculomotor nucleus. There fibers leave the brain in intimate association with the somatic motor efferent fibers of oculomotor nerve (cranial nerve III), but part from the motor fibers in the orbital cone just proximal to their synapse on the ciliary ganglion, which is a collection of postganglionic parasympathetic cell bodies lateral to the optic nerve.

Anatomic differences in the short ciliary nerves between the dog and cat have important consequences to clinical interpretation when lesions develop in this segment of the efferent arm. In the dog, five to eight short ciliary nerves enter the posterior aspect of the globe and are mixed nerves composed of postganglionic parasympathetic fibers arising from cell bodies in the ciliary ganglion, postganglionic sympathetic fibers from the cranial cervical ganglion, and sensory afferent fibers from the ophthalmic branch of the trigeminal nerve. In the cat, however, only two short ciliary nerves arise from the ciliary ganglion and consist solely of postganglionic parasympathetic fibers until just before penetrating the globe, where they are joined by the sympathetic and sensory fibers of the eye via the nasociliary nerve. The short ciliary nerve innervating the lateral half of the iris sphincter muscle in the cat is referred to as the malar nerve, and that which innervates the medial half of the iris is the nasal nerve.

FACTORS MODIFYING NORMAL
PUPILLARY RESPONSES

In the alert, normal animal, pupillary size and behavior is dependent on the equilibrium level established between the sympathetic and parasympathetic systems. The sympathetic system is an active mechanism working on the iris dilator muscle and is affected by increased hypothalamic activity from psychosensory stimulation (i.e., fight or flight).

Supranuclear inhibition of the Edinger-Westphal nucleus prevents outflow of impulses from the parasympathic system, causing passive relaxation of the iris sphincter muscle. These mechanisms are responsible for the rapid dilation of the suddenly excited animal and for the extreme pupil dilation in the quiet but alert individual that is dark-adapted.

As the patient drifts toward sleep, higher brain centers cease to function, the supranuclear inhibition of the Edinger-Westphal nucleus decreases, and sympathetic activity is gradually lost. This results in increased parasympathetic outflow with consequent miosis.

Light stimuli of weak intensities lengthen the

latent period between stimulus and contraction, decrease the amplitude of contraction, and shorten the duration of response. The use of a 3.5 volt Halogen handle* with a Finoff transilluminator is advised when evaluating pupillary responses. Most new pen lights will do an adequate job but are frequently allowed to run down to an ineffective level.

All areas of the retina should be stimulated, as various regions demonstrate different pupillomotor sensitivities.

CLINICAL EVALUATION OF NORMAL PUPILLARY RESPONSES

Clinical assessment of the integrity of the light reflex pathway commences with the patient's entrance into the examination room. It is incumbent upon the clinician at this point to have an appreciation for the average pupil diameter of quiet, non-excited dogs and cats in normal room light and what factors modify the pupil size, should there be any marked deviations. Horizontal pupillary diameters vary within normal ranges among individuals owing to different levels of sympathetic-parasympathetic equilibrium. Provided that the exam room light entering each pupil is equal, however, the pupils should be equal in size in the normal animals.

Determination of pupil equality by gross observation, particularly in some dogs, is inadequate because of the lack of frontal position to the eyes (this makes simultaneous exam of both pupils nearly impossible). In cats and some brachycephalic dogs, gross assessment may be all that is required. Reliance on gross observation can be overcome with the aid of a direct ophthalmoscope. With the lenses of the direct ophthalmoscope set on O to positive diopters (black numbers), the examiner directs the scope's light source toward the center of the bridge of the nose at eye level while standing three to five feet away. This technique will outline the tapetal reflex. Although this technique is crude by pupillographic standards, a surprisingly simple and accurate clinical assessment of pupil equality can be made.

The swinging flashlight test is then performed, which assesses the integrity of the first order neuron and the prechiasmal second order neuron. In this test, a focal light source (pen light or Finoff transilluminator) is alternately swung from one eye to the other, with the direct light being maintained for two to four seconds in each eye. Occasionally, the normal pupil will redilate slightly following the initial contraction while under direct stimulation. This response is

normal and is referred to as "pupillary escape," which is the result of photoreceptor adaptation. Pupillary escape is especially noticeable when a weak light source is used.

Direct light stimulation of an eye creates a dynamic contraction or alternating contraction anisocoria in the normal cat and dog. It is dynamic because it is apparent only while the eye is under stimulation, with the more miotic pupil on the side receiving the stimulation, and it is alternating because the direct response is the same in either eye, as is apparent during the swinging flashlight test. This response is explained by the uneven distribution of crossed and uncrossed fibers of the second and third order neurons in the optic chiasm and caudal commissure, respectively.

Assessment of pupillary size and the swinging flashlight test are then repeated in the dark-adapted eye in a darkened room.

CLINICAL EVALUATION OF AFFERENT ARM LESIONS

Localization of lesions along the afferent arm is dependent upon the development of characteristic pupillary responses, and therefore the evaluation is approached systematically. The first indication of an underlying neurologic disturbance is the presence of static anisocoria or bilateral symmetrically dilated pupils. If these pupils dilate maximally and symmetrically in darkness, they qualify as having a lesion in the afferent arm of the light reflex. If they do not dilate or dilate incompletely or unequally, the lesion is somewhere other than in the afferent arm — e.g., the efferent arm or sympathetic pathway, which dilate unequally in darkness.

All unilateral lesions of the first, second, or third order neurons in the dog or cat create a static anisocoria owing to unequal input or nerve impulses into the constrictor nuclei in the midbrain.

CLINICAL FEATURES OF UNILATERAL RETINAL OR PRECHIASMAL OPTIC NERVE

As is characteristic of all afferent arm lesions, the pupils dilate maximally and symmetrically in darkness. In room light, a static anisocoria is present with the more constricted or miotic pupil on the side opposite the lesion. This is the result of differential light stimulation to the eyes created by the diminished nerve impulse transmission from the affected eye. The affected eye fails to constrict under direct light stimulation but does constrict consensually when light stimulates the normal eye.

A positive swinging flashlight test is pathog-

*Welch-Allyn Incorp., Skaneateles Falls, N.Y. 13153

nomonic for disease in either the retina or prechiasmal optic nerve. The test is positive when, as the light shifts from the normal to the abnormal, the abnormal pupil dilates instead of constricting, as would a normal eye. This dilation is also referred to as the Marcus Gunn sign. If a pupil exhibiting a Marcus Gunn sign constricts slightly before redilating, it usually indicates that not all the afferent fibers are diseased. It could also be caused by scatter illumination entering the normal eye from the light source directed into the abnormal eye, creating a consensual response in the abnormal eye.

Funduscopic examination of both eyes is necessary to determine whether retinal abnormalities are the source of the static anisocoria. If no gross retinal abnormalities are detected, an electroretinogram (ERG) should be performed to evaluate the integrity of the first order neurons of the retina. If these two test techniques do not indicate disease, the lesion has to be between the globe and chiasm in the prechiasmal second order neurons of the optic nerve.

CLINICAL FEATURES OF UNILATERAL OPTIC TRACT LESIONS

The pupils dilate maximally and symmetrically in darkness. Unilateral optic tract lesions also present with a static anisocoria; however, the constricted pupil is now on the same side as the lesion. A negative swinging flashlight test serves to eliminate a lesion in the retina or prechiasmal optic nerve as the source of this anisocoria.

CLINICAL FEATURES OF BILATERAL RETINAL, PRECHIASMAL OPTIC NERVES, OPTIC TRACTS, CHIASM, OR CAUDAL COMMISSURE

Lesions that interrupt all nerve impulses from both retinas, prechiasmal optic nerves, optic chiasm, both optic tracts, or the caudal commissure of the midbrain create widely dilated, fixed pupils in normal room light. The most frequent site of lesions that create bilateral afferent arm disease are the retinas or the chiasm; primary lesions affecting other sites are rare. When present, or if there is secondary involvement of these structures, neighborhood neurologic signs (e.g., paresis or paralysis from long tract signs) are apparent.

Lesions of the optic chiasm in the dog or cat that destroy only the crossed fibers (sparing the uncrossed fibers) produce pupils that are larger than normal yet are smaller than in total chiasmal destruction and remain equal in size in dif-

fuse room illumination. It the lesion spares the uncrossed fibers, directing a focal light source into one eye will elicit a direct and consensual response and will also produce a dynamic contraction anisocoria with the more constricted pupil on the side opposite the side stimulated, as careful study of Figure 2 reveals. Swinging the light source to the contralateral eye will reverse the response. Pupillary contraction with incomplete lesions of the optic chiasm will not be as extensive as that with an intact pathway.

CLINICAL FEATURES OF EFFERENT ARM LESIONS

Provided that the mechanical and anatomic integrity of the iris is normal, impairment of the efferent pathway can be due to the presence of atropine or atropine-like drugs in the eye or to defective parasympathetic innervation. The location of the lesion determines the clinical configuration of the signs.

The functional effect of unilateral paralysis of the efferent pupillary pathway — otherwise referred to as internal ophthalmoplegia — regardless of the location of the lesion along the pathway, is strictly unilateral, with the injured side reacting less or not at all to direct and consensual light, whereas the unaffected side retains normal pupillary responses. The widely dilated pupil, which is present ipsilaterally, creates a static anisocoria that has pupils with greater differences in size than would be present with afferent arm lesions under similar conditions.

In the dog and cat, nuclear lesions (i.e., nucleus of Edinger-Westphal) cause pupillary responses identical to those created by lesions anywhere along the preganglionic parasympathetic fibers.

Lesions of the ciliary ganglion and the short ciliary nerves in cats have the same functional effects on pupil response as do lesions of the preganglionic parasympathetic fibers or third nerve nuclei because when the ciliary ganglion or its short ciliary nerves are damaged, only postganglionic parasympathetic fibers are injured. A lesion in the cat that affects only the temporal short ciliary nerve creates a hemidilated pupil in the lateral half of the iris, thus creating a "reverse D" pupil in the patient's right eye and a "D" pupil in the left eye. Likewise, an interruption of the medial short ciliary nerve affects only the nasal half of the iris and produces a "D" pupil in the right eye and a "reverse D" in the left.

In darkness, the pupils of the cat dilate maximally and equally regardless of the site of the lesion along the efferent pathway. In contrast, injury to the ciliary ganglion or short ciliary nerves in the dog creates an anisocoria in darkness, with the smaller pupil ipsilateral to the injury. The dark-adapted response is different because the sympathetic fibers are left intact with lesions to the short ciliary nerves or ganglion in the cat, whereas they are damaged in the dog, preventing the iris dilator muscles from contracting to dilate the pupil in darkness.

Localization of a lesion site to the nuclear region or preganglionic parasympathetic axons is achieved clinically when signs of external ophthalmoplegia accompany the signs of internal ophthalmoplegia. Because of the close proximity of the oculomotor nucleus (i.e., nucleus of the third cranial nerve) to the Edinger-Westphal nucleus and the fact that the motor efferents of the third cranial nerve travel together in the same nerve trunk as the preganglionic parasympathetic fibers, lesions that affect one easily affect the other. In addition to the signs of internal ophthalmoplegia, ipsilateral ptosis, prolapse of the third eyelid, and inability to rotate the globe dorsally, ventrally, or medially exist.

PHARMACOLOGIC LOCALIZATION OF EFFERENT ARM LESIONS

In the eserine test, one drop of 0.5 percent physostigmine (Isopto-Eserine*), an indirect-acting parasympathomimetic, is instilled into the lower conjunctival sac of both eyes. The normal eye will constrict, but not until long after (40 to 60 minutes) the eye that has a central or preganglionic parasympathetic lesion. No constriction takes place with lesions in the postganglionic fibers or the ciliary ganglion. A false negative test exists if neither eye constricts.

After a lapse of 24 hours, the pilocarpine test, which uses a direct-acting parasympathomimetic, is conducted in the same manner using 2 percent pilocarpine (Isopto-Carpine†). In a positive pilocarpine test, a pupil that has been denervated anywhere along the efferent pathway will constrict more quickly, to a greater extent and for a longer period than the control eye. This test is not as localizing as the eserine test, but it unequivocally confirms the presence of a neurologic lesion in the efferent arm if it is positive. A false negative pilocarpine test occurs when neither the control nor the affected eye constricts. If the pilocarpine test is negative, primary or secondary iris disease exists or ingestion or topical instillation of atropine or atropine-like drugs has occurred.

---

*0.5 percent Isopto-Eserine, Alcon Laboratories, Dallas, Texas

†2 percent Isopto-Carpine, Alcon Laboratories, Dallas, Texas

The negative pilocarpine test, which is caused by pharmacologic blockade (e.g., the ingestion or topical instillation of atropine or atropine-like drugs), is a clinical problem. The author has tested unilateral fixed dilated pupils for "brain tumors" on four separate occasions, only to discover that staff at the referring veterinary hospital has made a medication mistake or that home treatment with "eye medication" by unsuspecting owners had created the problem. The ubiquitous presence of Jimson Weed (containing an anticholinergic agent) has probably led to a unilateral fixed, dilated pupil in hunting dogs on more than one occasion, as it has done in farm laborers who have gotten it in their eyes. A pupil dilated by pharmacologic blockade will return to normal size in one to three weeks.

If the pilocarpine test is negative and the medical history rules out the possibility of a pharmacologic blockade, primary or secondary iris disease must be eliminated from the differential diagnosis.

EFFERENT SYMPATHETIC NERVOUS PATHWAY

Interruption of the efferent sympathetic pupillomotor system anywhere along its three neuron chain creates a Horner's Syndrome.

The efferent sympathetic pathway controls the iris dilator muscle and is a three-neuron pathway. The central neuron descends primarily ipsilaterally from the caudal and lateral hypothalamus through the brain stem and lateral funiculus of the cervical spinal cord to synapse on preganglionic cell bodies located within the grey matter of the intermediolateral column of the spinal cord at levels T_1 to T_3. The preganglionic sympathetic fibers leave the spinal cord and project without synapse through the thoracic sympathetic trunk and cervicothoracic ganglion and continue uninterrupted cranially along the cervical sympathetic to synapse on the cell bodies of postganglionic sympathetic neurons of the cranial cervical ganglion, located just caudomedial to the tympanic bullae. The postganglionic pupillomotor sympathetic axons enter the middle ear, where they join the tympanic branch of the glossopharyngeal nerve (IX) to form what is collectively referred to as the caroticotympanic nerves. These are the fibers damaged with the middle ear lesions that create ipsilateral Horner's Syndrome. Leaving the middle ear, the postganglionic fibers join the ophthalmic division of the trigeminal (V) nerve, which arborizes into the long ciliary nerve that enters the globe and innervates the ciliary body and iris dilator muscle. Some postganglionic sympathetics innervate the smooth muscle fibers, the musculus orbitalis present in the orbital sheath. This muscle is under constant sympathetic tone, causing contraction of the periorbital fascial sheath that forces the globe forward.

Clinical Features of Horner's Syndrome. The location, nature, and extent of the lesion within the sympathetic pathway will determine the duration and number of clinical signs present, some of which are:

1. Miosis — ipsilateral miosis as a result of decreased stimulation to the iris dilator muscle; seen immediately following the lesion and is most pronounced with postganglionic lesions. Preganglionic fibers have a better chance for recovery than do postganglionic axons depending on the nature of the lesion.

2. Anisocoria — in bright light, the pupillary size difference decreases because of the bilaterally intact iris constrictor pathway. Lack of innervation to the iris dilator muscle causes the anisocoria to become more pronounced in darkness and therefore excludes an afferent arm lesion as the cause of this anisocoria.

3. Ptosis — ipsilateral ptosis is not always clinically apparent and is said to be due to loss of sympathetic supply to the smooth muscle of the eyelid, referred to as Müller's muscle.

4. Narrowing of the palpebral fissure — the narrowing is due to ptosis of the upper lid and elevation of the lower lid. It is present only when clinically apparent ptosis of the upper lid is present.

5. Enophthalmos — when it is present in dogs, it is in part due to denervation of the musculus orbitalis of the periorbital sheath, along with the antagonistic effect of globe retraction created by the retractor oculi muscle. The narrowed palpebral fissure gives the impression of enophthalmos, particularly in the cat, when in fact there is none. This is referred to as an *"apparent enophthalmos."*

6. Prolapse of the third eyelid — frequently made more marked by a real enophthalmos, which allows for greater passive protrusion.

DeLahunta (1973) compiled a table of disorders associated with Horner's Syndrome. Lesions of the postganglionic fibers, especially those secondary to otitis media, are probably the most frequently seen by the general practitioner.

Pharmacologic Localization of Horner's Lesions. The classically described cocaine and epinephrine tests frequently fail to allow localization of the lesion site causing Horner's Syndrome. Hydroxyamphetamine, an indirect-acting sympathomimetic, acts by releasing endogenous norepinephrine from the adrenergic nerve endings and provides a clear distinction between preganglionic and postganglionic lesions.

Instillation of one to two drops of 1 percent hydroxyamphetamine (1 percent Paredrine*) into the lower conjunctival sac of each eye results in normal mydriasis of the miotic Horner's pupil if the lesion is central or preganglionic. When the lesion is postganglionic, the stores of norepinephrine contained in the adrenergic nerve terminals are reduced or absent, and the Horner's pupil therefore dilates incompletely or not at all.

The direct-acting sympathomimetic, 10 percent phenylephrine, can be used to confirm the presence of the postganglionic lesion localized by the Paredrine test. The sympathetically innervated effector cells become supersensitive to what is ordinarily a weak and ineffective concentration of phenylephrine. The use of phenylephrine is recommended over 0.1 per cent epinephrine because epinephrine penetrates the cornea poorly, and individual differences in sensitivity to epinephrine are great (see Table 1).

Cocaine has little practical use and is highly variable in its response.

*1 percent Paredrine, Smith, Kline & French Labs, Philadelphia, Pennsylvania 19101

Table 1. Pharmacologic Localization

AGENT	CENTRAL	PREGANGLIONIC	POSTGANGLIONIC
6% Cocaine	Impaired mydriasis	No dilatation	No dilatation
10% Phenylephrine	No dilatation	No dilatation	Mydriasis
1% Hydroxyamphetamine	Normal mydriasis	Normal mydriasis	Incomplete to no mydriasis

DRUG TESTING PRECAUTIONS

In all these pharmacologic tests (pilocarpine, eserine, Paredrine), both normal and abnormal eyes should receive drugs as a basis for comparison. Since the pupillary response to many drugs is dose dependent, an equal quantity should be instilled in each eye. Proper drug absorption is dependent on an intact corneal epithelium; therefore, diagnostic procedures that might compromise the corneal surface integrity should be performed following completion of drug testing.

SPASTIC PUPIL SYNDROME

The presence of a static anisocoria in cats that remains unchanged or only slightly changed during adaptation to dark may have a condition that the author calls the "Spastic Pupil Syndrome." It has been recognized since 1974 that these cats have no iris abnormalities, their pupils do not dilate under dark conditions, and they are positive for feline leukemia virus. The owners historically describe abnormal pupillary behavior for periods of up to six months prior to presentation, often with alternating static anisocorias on daily or weekly intervals, with or without intervals of normal pupil appearance. No visual deficits are reported with this syndrome. The patient may be clinically healthy except for abnormal pupillary responses or systemically ill with abnormal pupillary reactions. Infrequently, an ill cat will present with only a history of abnormal pupillary behavior or with bilaterally fixed semi-dilated pupils with no visual deficits. Most of the spastic pupils do not dilate at all in darkness or they may dilate 1 mm or so while retaining the relative anisocoria. Any such incomplete movement is invariably slow.

In a series of 17 such FeLV-positive cats, 10 cats were clinically normal except for the presence of abnormal pupillary responses (i.e., static anisocoria) or had only a history of bizarre pupillary behavior. The remaining seven cats had associated clinical signs referable to a generalized systemic disease. Of these seven cats, five had confirmed diagnosis of lymphoreticular disease, one had FIP, and one had hematopoietic disease. Of the remaining cats, one developed systemic clinical signs diagnosed as FIP and nine had lymphoreticular disease within six months of the original presentation.

With electron microscopy or with immunofluorescence, C-type RNA virus localizing in the short ciliary nerves or the ciliary ganglion of cats has been seen. However, the author has been unable to demonstrate the presence of this virus in the same case by both techniques. The pupillary abnormality may be due to a polyneuropathy, with involvement of other nerves that influence the pupil.

SUPPLEMENTAL READING

Christensen, K.: Sympathetic and parasympathetic nerves in the orbit of the cat. J. Anat. 70:225–235, 1936.

DeLahunta, A.: Small animal neuro-ophthalmology. Vet. Clin. North Am., Sept. 1973, p. 497.

Lowenstein, O., Murphy, S. D., and Loewenfeld, I. E.: Functional evaluation of the pupillary light reflex pathways. Arch. Ophth. 49:656–670, 1953.

Lowenstein, O.: Clinical pupillary symptoms in lesions of the optic nerve, optic chiasm and optic tract. Arch. Ophth. 53:385–403, 1954.

OCULAR THERAPEUTICS

STEPHEN BISTNER, D.V.M.

St. Paul, Minnesota

Medications used in treating ocular disorders of animals may be divided into categories based on pharmacologic action. The purpose of this article is to describe drugs that the author feels are practical to maintain in a basic armamentarium of ophthalmic agents used in diagnosing and treating the common ocular disorders seen in animals. A large number of ophthalmic agents do not have to be stocked in a veterinary hospital. Many of the special products mentioned here can be prescribed and will obviate maintaining inventories of drugs.

PRINCIPLES OF OPHTHALMIC DRUG ABSORPTION AND ADMINISTRATION

Before discussing routes of administration of ophthalmic pharmaceuticals, one should understand several basic principles pertaining to the absorption of local ophthalmic drugs. The rate of delivery of an ophthalmic drug to the desired site is dependent on numerous factors.

1. The vehicle in which the drug is suspended and the nature of the drug itself, including toxicity, pH, and stability. The cornea is covered by a precorneal tear film, and the cornea itself has variable permeability, the corneal epithelium being more permeable to fat-soluble compounds and the stroma being more permeable to water-soluble compounds. If the corneal epithelium is damaged, a much higher level of drug may be achieved in the corneal stroma. Ophthalmic drugs should possess biphasic solubility to maximize corneal penetration.

2. The degree of vascularization and inflammation present in the eye can affect the level of drug present. A highly inflamed eye will carry away drugs more rapidly.

3. Drainage of ophthalmic agents through the nasolacrimal system can also influence the rate of disappearance of agents.

There are numerous ways in which ophthalmic agents can be delivered to the eye:

1. Topical solutions are easily instilled into the eye but do not remain in the eye for long periods. Therefore, if solutions are used, increased frequency of dosage is recommended. Solutions may be suspended in vehicles such as polyvinyl alcohol or methylcellulose to increase their contact time.

2. Ointments have advantages over solutions in that a longer ocular contact time is maintained and they are carried away through the nasolacrimal system less rapidly.

3. Subconjunctival injections are a very effective way of achieving high levels of medication in the anterior ocular segment. The injections can be made under topical anesthesia using a tuberculin syringe, and a 25 or 26 gauge needle.

   The route by which a subconjunctival injection enters the eye has not been clearly defined. Diffusion across the sclera and underlying tissues is one mechanism, and leakage through the needle puncture site into the conjunctival sac is another. Recent experiments using topically applied prednisolone acetate drops indicate that the frequent application of drops achieves a higher level in the aqueous than does the subconjunctival injection of prednisolone acetate.

4. Subpalpebral lavage with ocular medication can be performed by placing a poly-ethylene tube in the superior conjunctival fornix through the upper lid and delivering medication either through a continuous drip or by injecting medication into the polyethylene tube. A commercial subpalpebral lavage set is available.*

5. Retrobulbar injections can be given for local anesthetic blocks or to deliver steroids such as might be needed in retrobulbar neuritis. For dogs and cats, a 1.5 inch, 20 gauge needle is inserted at the caudal angle formed by the junction of the lateral orbital ligament and the zygomatic arch and is directed toward the lateral canthus of the opposite eye.

6. In cases of severe infection, agents may also be injected directly into the eye (intracameral injections — see Table 6).

7. New drug delivery systems have produced methods for the slow release of medication by sustained release devices (Ocusert®†). Although these devices are currently being developed and used in people, tests would indicate that they will have equally good potential for sustained drug delivery in animals.

DRUGS AFFECTING THE AUTONOMIC NERVOUS SYSTEM

Manipulation of the autonomic nervous system involves the use of agents that stimulate the adrenergic or cholinergic receptor sites.

MYDRIATIC AGENTS

Mydriasis (dilatation of the pupil) may be produced by sympathomimetic or parasympatholytic mechanisms. The parasympatholytic agents also induce cycloplegia, but the sympatholytic drugs have minimal cycloplegic action.

Clinically, mydriatics are used to dilate the pupil to permit fundus and lens examination. Tropicamide, 0.5 to 1.0 percent, is used for this purpose. The longer-acting mydriatics are used most routinely in the therapy of anterior uveitis. Because of the cycloplegic action of these agents, the ciliary body is relaxed and ciliary spasm is relieved. Mydriatics are also used when dense, central nuclear or immature cortical cataracts interfere with vision. Dilation of the pupil permits the animal to see around the obstructed direct visual axis.

Administration of bitter parasympatholytic

---

*Subpalpebral Lavage Apparatus, Becton-Dickinson, Rutherford, New Jersey.

†ALZA Pharmaceuticals, Palo Alto, California

Sympathomimetic Drugs

	PERCENT	MYDRIASIS	DURATION OF ACTION
Phenylephrine	10	20 to 30 min.	2 to 3 hours

May produce conjunctival irritation with prolonged use. Major use is in achieving maximal mydriasis when used in conjunction with a parasympatholytic drug such as atropine.

Parasympatholytic Drugs

	PERCENT	MYDRIASIS—CYCLOPLEGIA	DURATION OF ACTION
Atropine	1 to 4	30 to 40 min.	5 to 7 days or longer
Cyclopentolate HCl	0.5 to 2	30 to 45 min.	3 to 5 days

(Will produce severe chemosis if not combined with phenylephrine 10%)

Tropicamide	0.5 to 1	30 min.	4 to 6 hours

(Short-acting dilating agent—author's choice for fundus examination.)

---

agents in dogs and especially in cats induces salivation. In cats, 0.5 percent Mydriacil® (tropicamide, Alcon) drops or atropine ointment will eliminate this undesirable side effect.

Mydriatic agents are contraindicated in narrow-angle glaucoma. However, the prolonged use of atropine will not produce undesirable side effects, and it is frequently used for long periods in uveitis cases.

CHOLINERGIC DRUGS

Cholinergic agents are used for their miotic effects. They produce pupillary constriction, ciliary muscle contraction, dilatation of conjunctival and iris blood vessels, and increased aqueous outflow. Miotics can be classified into two groups based on their mechanism of action (direct or indirect).

Cholinomimetic agents act directly on muscle end plates and resemble acetylcholine. Pilocarpine, available in solution of 0.5 to 4 percent, is the agent most frequently used. Pilocarpine may be used in treating initial attacks of glaucoma (see "Canine and Feline Glaucoma"); however, prolonged use of pilocarpine in animals frequently produces ocular irritation.

Miotics of longer duration of action may be used. These agents inhibit the enzyme cholinesterase and prolong the locally produced acetylcholine at the motor end plates. Longer-acting miotics are very potent and must be used with caution to avoid cholinergic side effects. The miotic that the author uses is Phospholine Iodide® (echothiophate iodide, Ayerst) because of its low irritant properties over a prolonged period. Dosage frequency is one drop every 12 to 24 hours.

It should be emphasized that most forms of glaucoma seen in animals are of the closed angle type, with large areas of anterior synechia obstructing the drainage angle. The use of miotics in these cases will not help to alleviate the glaucoma and may make the situation worse. The miotic agents are most efficacious in open angle glaucoma, which is diagnosed infrequently in animals (Table 1).

Timolol maleate is a new antiglaucoma medication used topically in the eye in a 0.25 percent and 0.5 percent concentration. Timolol maleate is a general beta-adrenergic receptor blocking agent, and the precise mechanism of ocular hypotensive effect is not known. The drug has been evaluated in man and found to be effective in chronic open angle glaucoma. The effectiveness of the drug in narrow angle or angle closure glaucomas has not been evaluated. The role of this new drug in the types of glaucomas seen predominantly in dogs has not been evaluated.

TOPICAL ANESTHETIC AGENTS

There are numerous topical ophthalmic anesthetic agents available. The choice of agent best suited to a particular condition is left to the individual's discretion. The author prefers proparacaine hydrochloride,* 0.5 percent; however, it should be refrigerated to prevent breakdown and discoloration of the product. Topical anesthetics are used primarily for diagnostic and minor surgical procedures. Prolonged use of topical anesthetics may retard corneal healing and produce systemic toxicity.

---

*Ophthaine® drops, E.R. Squibb Co., Princeton, New Jersey.

Table 1.   *Topical Miotics for Canine Glaucoma Therapy*

	STRENGTHS USED	USUAL REGIMEN	KEEPING QUALITY OF EYE DROPS	RELATIVE DURATION OF ACTION
Parasympathomimetics—Direct acetylcholine-like action on nerve endings:				
Pilocarpine	0.5% to 4%	q. 4 to 6 hr.	Satisfactory	Short
Cholinesterase inhibitors—Indirect action by accumulation of acetylcholine:				
Eserine® ° (physostigmine)	0.25% to 1%	q. 4 to 6 hr.	Unsatisfactory	Moderate
Isoflurophate® (DFP)	0.1% (oil)	q.d. to BID	Unsatisfactory	Long
Phospholine iodide® (echothiophate iodide)	0.125 to 0.25%	q.d. to BID	Satisfactory	Long
Humorsol® † (demecarium bromide)	0.125 to 0.25%	q.d. to BID	Satisfactory	Long
Drug with both direct and indirect actions:				
Carbachol	0.75 to 3%	q. 4 to 8 hr.	Satisfactory	Short

° Abbott Laboratories, North Carolina, Illinois
† Merck Sharp and Dohme, West Point, Pennsylvania

Onset and Duration of Topical Anesthetics in Man

SINGLE ADMINISTRATION	ONSET	DURATION (minutes)
0.4% Benoxinate HCl	15 seconds	20
1.0% Butacaine sulfate	2 to 3 min.	30 to 60
1.4% Cocaine HCl	2 min.	10
0.5% Dyclonine HCl	2 to 4 min.	30 to 50
1.4% Lidocaine HCl	4 to 5 min.	30
0.5% Proparacaine HCl	15 sec.	15
0.5% Tetracaine HCl	2 to 3 min.	20 to 30

CORTICOSTEROIDS

Ocular inflammation is one of the most serious of all ocular diseases. If inflammation is not treated early and effectively, ocular function can be lost. Corticosteroids produce generalized suppression of ocular inflammatory disorders and help to maintain ocular structure and physiology.

ACTION OF ANTI-INFLAMMATORY AGENTS

The beneficial effects of corticosteroids in treating ocular disease can be summarized as follows: (1) they reduce cellular and fibrinous exudation and decrease tissue exudation, (2) they diminish the formation of scar tissue, (3) they limit neovascularization, and (4) they reduce capillary permeability.

In order to achieve maximal beneficial effects from corticosteroids in ocular disease, several very important principles of treatment must be understood.

1. Determine what route of administration will best treat the ocular disorder; i.e., topical, subconjunctival, or systemic

2. Use high levels of steroids early and long enough to suppress inflammation

3. Do not discontinue steroid therapy too

early, especially in treating the more chronic cases of uveitis.

A low dose of steroid therapy may have to be used continuously in order to maintain ocular comfort.

INDICATIONS

External Ocular Disease. Allergic blepharitis, conjunctivitis, irritant conjunctivitis, superficial punctate keratitis, infiltrative corneal disease, chronic neovascularization, deep interstitial keratitis.

Uveitis. Anterior uveitis, posterior uveitis, iritis, iridocyclytis, scleritis, episcleritis.

Orbital Disease. Optic neuritis, pseudotumor of orbit.

SELECTION OF STEROIDS

Important points to consider in choosing steroids are: (1) the ocular bioavailability of the drug (penetration of the steroid into the tissues desired), (2) the anti-inflammatory activity desired, and (3) the duration of effect.

Following topical administration of corticosteroids, the highest drug levels are found in the cornea and conjunctiva. The penetration of topically applied steroids is determined by differential solubility characteristics and tissue factors. The derivative of corticosteroid preparation is significant because it affects corneal penetration. Changing the steroid derivative from the alcohol to the acetate greatly increases the penetrative ability of prednisolone; e.g., 1 percent prednisolone acetate* provides higher

---

*Prednefrin Forte Drops® Allergan Pharmaceuticals, Irvine, California.

concentrations of corticosteroids in the aqueous and corneal stroma than do 0.1 percent dexamethasone alcohol, 0.1 percent dexamethasone phosphate, and 1.0 percent prednisolone phosphate. However, if the corneal epithelium is severely damaged, other forms of steroids, especially prednisolone phosphate, may penetrate just as well.

Knowing the anti-inflammatory activity of various steroid compounds can also be helpful in selecting agents for treating ocular disease:

STEROID	RELATIVE ANTI-INFLAMMATORY ACTIVITY
Hydrocortisone	1
Prednisolone	4
Methylprednisolone	5
Betamethasone	25
Dexamethasone	25
Fluorometholone	40

Corticosteroids have their most dramatic effect in those diseases affecting the cornea, uveal tract, and external structures of the eye. They are ineffective in degenerative diseases of the cornea, retina, and uveal tract.

The choice of steroid depends on the location and severity of the lesion. Inflammation of the deeper layers of the cornea and the anterior uveal tract requires a steroid that will penetrate the intact corneal epithelium. The drug of choice is 1 percent prednisolone acetate suspension.* In evaluating prednisolone acetate in anterior segment inflammation, no significant increase in therapeutic response was obtained by increasing the concentration greater than 1.0 percent. However, frequent use of prednisolone acetate, such as every two hours, can greatly increase the effective levels of steroid in the anterior ocular segment. Evidence indicates that as high a level of anti-inflammatory steroid can develop in the anterior ocular segment with the repeated use of drops as with subconjunctival injection of steroids.

For topical use on the cornea or conjunctiva to reduce inflammation, a wide variety of steroids are available (Table 2). In general, the author prefers to use ointments in treating animals because of the longer contact time and decreased frequency of administration. In general, topical therapy should be continued for two weeks after all signs of disease have disappeared.

Much controversy exists over the use of corticosteroids during the course of infection and inflammation in the anterior ocular segment. Corticosteroids are important in minimizing scar tissue in the cornea and reducing anterior uveal tract inflammation. Corticosteroids can be used in the face of ocular infection, provided there is simultaneous administration of effective agents that will control infection.

Injection. Local injection of corticosteroids refers to subconjunctival injections, which provide a rapid way of delivering high concentrations of drug. The repository forms of injections, such as triamcinalone (Kenalog®, 40 mg/ml) provide a source of steroid that may last for up to two weeks.

NON-STEROIDAL ANTI-INFLAMMATORY PREPARATIONS

Recent investigations into the role of prostaglandins PGE_2 and $PGF_2\alpha$ as mediators of ocular inflammation have created new interest in the possible use of aspirin in ocular inflammatory diseases. Prostaglandins in the eye play a significant role in alteration of the blood-aqueous barrier and in perpetuation of inflammation. Aspirin and aspirin-like drugs such as indomethacin can inhibit the synthesis and release of prostaglandins. Once prostaglandins have been formed and released, however, the administration of aspirin has little effect.

Aspirin can be used to help ameliorate ocular inflammation resulting from uveitis, keratoconjunctivitis, and inflammation following intraocular surgery. The author has routinely been using aspirin prior to intraocular surgery in the dog. Caution must be exercised in the administration of acetylsalicylic acid, especially to cats. Dosage of aspirin in cats can be given at 5 mg/kg twice daily, and it is recommended that the dosage not exceed 40 mg/kg per 24-hour period. In dogs, aspirin dosage should not exceed 10 mg/kg BID because gastrointestinal bleeding is evidenced at higher dosages.

ANTIBIOTICS AND SULFONAMIDES

In external ocular infections, the use of conjunctival and corneal scrapings and bacterial culture and sensitivity tests is important in guiding the therapeutic regimen.

When possible, specific antibiotics should be used to treat specific ocular disorders. Examples of such disorders are as follows.

Bacterial blepharitis is usually associated with staphylococci that may produce an external or internal hordeolum (sty) or may lead to chronic marginal blepharitis. Hordeola can be treated with frequent warm compresses fol-

---

*Pred. Forte-Allergan; Econopred plus-Alcon

Table 2. Glucocorticoid Therapy*

TOPICAL GLUCOCORTICOID OPHTHALMIC PREPARATIONS

Generic Name	Trade Name	Strengths Available
Cortisone acetate ointments	Cortone acetate	1.5%
Hydrocortisone acetate suspensions	Hydrocortone acetate	2.5%
Hydrocortisone solution	Optef drops	0.2%
Hydrocortisone acetate ointment	Hydrocortone acetate	1.5%
Hydrocortisone ointment	Cortril	0.5% and 2.5%
Hydrocortisone phosphate solution (as the disodium salt)	Corphos	0.5%
Prednisolone phosphate solution (as the disodium salt)	Hydeltrasol, Optival	0.5%
Prednisolone phosphate ointment (as the disodium salt)	Hydeltrasol	0.25%
Prednisolone alcohol solution	Prednefrin S	0.2%
Prednisolone acetate suspension	Prednefrin Forte	1.0%
Prednisolone acetate suspension	Prednefrin	0.12%
Prednisolone sodium phosphate	Inflamase	0.125%
Prednisolone sodium phosphate	Inflamase Forte	1.0%
Dexamethasone phosphate solution (as the disodium salt)	Decadron	0.1%
Dexamethasone phosphate ointment	Decadron	0.05%
Dexamethasone suspension	Maxidex	0.1%
Fludrocortisone hemisuccinate solution	Florinef hemisuccinate	0.1%
Betamethasone	Celestone	0.1%
Triamcinolone acetonide	Kenalog	0.1%
Fluorometholone	FML	0.1%
Medrysone (hydroxymesterone)	HMS	1.0%

INJECTABLE GLUCOCORTICOIDS

Generic Name	Trade Name	Strengths Available
Cortisone acetate suspension U.S.P.	Cortone acetate	25 mg and 50mg/ml
Dexamethasone phosphate (as the disodium salt)	Decadron phosphate Hexadrol phosphate	4 mg/ml 4 mg/ml
Hydrocortisone for injection (as the sodium succinate)	Solu-Cortef	100 mg, 250 mg, 500 mg and 1000 mg vials
Hydrocortisone injection	Cortef sterile solution Infusion hydrocortisone	5 mg/ml 5 mg/ml
Hydrocortisone suspension	Cortef intramuscular	50 mg/ml
Hydrocortisone acetate	Cortef acetate Hydrocortone acetate Cortril acetate	50 mg/ml 25 mg and 50 mg/ml 25 mg/ml
Hydrocortisone butylacetate suspension	Hydrocortone-TBA	25 mg/ml
Methylprednisolone acetate suspension	Depo-Medrol	20 mg, 40 mg and 80 mg/ml
Methylprednisolone sodium succinate	Solu-Medrol	40 mg, 125 mg, 500 mg and 1000 mg vials
Prednisolone acetate suspension	Meticortelone soluble Nisolone aqueous Sterane intramuscular and intra-articular	25 mg/ml 25 mg/ml 25 mg/ml
Prednisolone butylacetate suspension	Hydeltra-TBA	20 mg/ml
Prednisolone phosphate	Hydeltrasol	20 mg/ml
Triamcinolone diacetate suspension	Aristocort parenteral	25 mg/ml
Triamcinolone acetonide suspension	Kenalog parenteral	10 mg/ml 40 mg/ml
Betamethasone (acetate and disodium phosphate combination)	Celestone Soluspan	6 mg/ml

*From Ellis, P. P., and Smith, D. L.: *The Handbook of Ocular Therapeutics and Pharmacology*, 4th ed. St. Louis, The C. V. Mosby Co., 1973, pp. 22 and 23.

lowed by incision and drainage where necessary. Systemic antibiotics such as cephalosporins as well as topical antibiotic therapy may be necessary. In chronic staphylococcal infection of the lid margins, bacitracin ointment, 500 units/gm in one-eighth-ounce containers, should be applied to the lid margins TID. Erythromycin 5 mg/gm and gentamicin 3 mg/gm are available in ophthalmic ointments and can also be used.

For most non-complicated external ocular diseases, a combination of neomycin, polymyxin B, and bacitracin may be useful.

Specific conjunctival infections may require different antibiotic therapy. Ocular infections associated with chlamydial agents in cats are treated with 1 percent tetracycline ophthalmic ointment.

Erythromycin ophthalmic ointment 0.5 percent is a bactericidal/bacteriostatic antibiotic available in ointment form. It is effective against beta hemolytic streptococci, although its use against staphylococci is limited because of rapid resistance developed to it. Bacitracin ophthalmic ointment, 500 units/gm, is a bactericidal antibiotic and is very effective against gram-positive cocci.

The ocular penetration of systemically administered antibiotics is variable and depends on the penetration ratio of the drug. The penetration ratio is a measure of the intraocular concentration of an antibiotic and is expressed as a percentage of the peak serum concentration. In gram-positive ocular infection, methicillin and the cephalosporin antibiotics are the agents of choice. Both these agents have low protein binding and therefore have good ocular penetration. The tetracyclines and chloramphenicol can be used in gram-positive infections; however, they are bacteriostatic.

In gram-negative infections of the eye, it should be assumed that a *Pseudomonas* infection is present. Treatment aimed at controlling this infection will also control other gram-negative infections. Although pseudomonas may be sensitive to several antibiotics, the drugs of choice are gentamicin, tobramycin, and carbenicillin. Carbenicillin can act in a synergistic way with gentamicin and tobramycin. Following systemic administration, the intraocular penetration of gentamycin is poor. If a gram-negative endophthalmitis is suspected, carbenicillin administered systemically may be the treatment of choice.

For gram-negative corneal infections, particularly *Pseudomonas* infections, the author prefers the use of gentamicin ophthalmic ointment (Garamycin® ointment, Schering) coupled with subconjunctival gentamicin. Additional treatment for *Pseudomonas* infections should include the topical use of disodium EDTA, 10^{-2} molar solution, which serves as an antagonist for the proteolytic enzymes released by *Pseudomonas* organisms. Disodium EDTA is available from Abbott Laboratories* in the form of Endrate® solution (150 mg/ml). To formulate the solution for topical administration, add 0.4 ml of Endrate solution to 14.6 ml of Adapt® solution (Burton, Parsons). Apply the mixture to the affected cornea five to six times a day.

Topical zinc sulfate can act as an antagonist to the protease elaborated by the organism. Zinc sulfate 0.5 percent in saline solution is used every two hours for the first two days and six times a day for the next five days. The pseudomonas protease retains its activity in the cornea for at least two days after the elimination of viable bacteria.

Rapidly progressing corneal ulcers may be spreading because of the production of collagenase enzyme in the cornea. This enzyme can be inhibited by the use of acetylcysteine (Mucomyst® 10% solution, Mead Johnson). Although not approved for use in the eye, topical application of acetylcysteine drops four times a day helps to prevent further spread of corneal ulcers associated with collagenase. The penetration of various antibiotics applied topically is summarized in Table 3.

One of the best methods of delivering high concentrations of antibiotics to the eye is subconjunctival injections. Subconjunctival injections of antibiotics are useful in treating severe corneal ulcers, anterior uveitis, panophthalmitis, and endophthalmitis. Care must be taken in administering subconjunctival injections so that minimal amounts (less than 1 cc) are administered (Tables 4 and 5). Some agents used for subconjunctival injections are quite irritating and may produce pain and conjunctival sloughing. The intracameral injection of antibiotic and antibiotic-steroid preparations has been reserved for very severe cases of endophthalmitis or panophthalmitis. Anterior chamber or vitreous aspiration with small-gauge needles may precede injection of antibiotics or steroids. Aspirated material is submitted for culture and sensitivity. Intravitreal injections are usually made through the pars plana and anterior chamber injections at the limbus. Care must be taken, since excessive concentrations of antibiotics may produce damage to the corneal endothelium or to the retina (Table 6).

In preparing gentamicin for anterior chamber injection, gentamicin solution 50 mg/cc can be used. Steroid can be added to the injection by

---

*Abbott Laboratories, North Chicago, Illinois.

Table 3. *Intraocular Penetration of Antibiotics in the Normal Eye**

| | ROUTE OF ADMINISTRATION | | |
AGENT	*Systemic*	*Topical*	*Subconjunctival*
Ampicillin	Fair	Fair-Good	Good
Bacitracin	None	Fair	Good
Chloramphenicol	Good	Good	Good
Colistin	Poor	Poor	Good
Erythromycin	Poor	Poor	Fair
Gentamicin	Poor	Poor	Fair
Kanamycin	Poor	Poor	Fair-Good
Neomycin	Poor	Fair	Good
Novobiocin	None	None	Good
Penicillin	Fair (high doses necessary)	Fair-Good	Good
Polymyxin B	Poor	Fair	Good
Streptomycin	None	None if cornea is intact	Fair-Good
Tetracyclines	Poor	Poor	Poor

*These data represent only general estimations because of limited investigations in domestic animals.

Table 4. *Antibiotics and Dosages for Subconjunctival Administration*

ANTIBIOTIC	DOSAGE
Neomycin	100 to 500 mg
Bacitracin	10,000 units
Plus Polymyxin B	5 to 10 mg
Erythromycin	100 mg
Novobiocin	15 mg
Plus Polymyxin B	5 to 10 mg
Penicillin G	500,000 units
Plus Streptomycin	50 mg
Soframycin	250 to 500 mg
Other Agents	
(listed alphabetically):	
Amphotericin B	15 to 125 µg
Carbomycin	2.5 mg
Chloramphenicol	50-100 mg
sodium succinate	
Kanamycin	10 to 20 mg
Oleandomycin	1.25 mg
Spiramycin	10 to 20 mg
Tetracyclines	2.5 mg

Table 5. *Preparation of Antibiotics for Subconjunctival Injection**

PROCESS	AMPICILLIN	GENTAMICIN	PENICILLIN G	METHICILLIN
Amount in commercially prepared vial	1000 mg	80 mg./2 ml	5.0 megaunits	1000 mg
Number of vials needed	1	1	1	1
Diluent volume to be added to each vial	5.0 ml	——	2.5 ml	5.0 ml
Volume to remove for injection	0.5 mg	0.5 ml	0.5 mg	0.5 ml
Antibiotic dose in injection volume	100 mg	20 mg	1.0 megaunits	100 mg

*From Jones, D. B.: External ocular diseases: diagnosis and current therapy. Internat. Ophthalmol. Clin. *13*:21, Winter, 1973.

Table 6. *Antibiotic Treatment of Endophthalmitis**

ANTIBIOTIC	DOSAGE	USUAL SENSITIVITY SPECTRUM
Gentamicin[†]	0.4 mg	Broad spectrum of gram-positive and gram-negative organisms: especially effective against *S. aureus, Proteus, Pseudomonas* and other Enterobacteriaceae.
Lincomycin[‡]	1.5 mg	Group A strep, *D. pneumoniae S. aureus, Corynebacteria, Clostridia,* Bacteroides.
Kanamycin	0.5 mg	Includes both gram-positive and gram-negative organisms, esp. *E. coli,* Proteus species, *Salmonella, Shigella, Neisseria* and some staphylococci.
Tobramycin	0.5 mg	Similar to gentamicin; especially effective against *Pseudomonas aeruginosa* and Enterobacteriaceae.
Methicillin	2 mg	Gram-positive organisms, esp. coagulase-positive staphylococci.
Cephaloridine	0.25 mg	Broad spectrum including *S. aureus* and gram-negative organisms, but not *Pseudomonas*.
BBK-8	0.4 mg	Broad spectrum of gram-positive and gram-negative organisms, esp. *Pseudomonas*.
Carbenicillin	2 mg	Gram-negative organisms, esp. *Pseudomonas*.
Clindamycin	1 mg	Gram-positive organisms, esp. resistant coagulase-positive staphylococci
Amphotericin B	5 to 10 μg!	Fungal endophthalmitis such as *Candida albicans* and Aspergillus
Chloramphenicol	2 mg	Broad spectrum of gram-positive and gram-negative organisms: effectiveness determined by specific sensitivity data

*Dosage recommended for intravitreal injection.
†0.4 mg (400 μg) of gentamicin can be used safely in anterior chamber.
‡A mixture of 1 mg of lincomycin and 0.2 mg (200 μg) gentamicin has been used clinically and experimentally without toxic effects.

using soluble dexamethasone with a concentration of 4 mg/cc. Draw 0.1 cc of gentamicin into a tuberculin syringe, add 0.9 cc of dexamethasone to the same syringe, and allow the solutions to mix. Using a 26 gauge needle, withdraw some aqueous fluid for culture and cytologic examination, and inject 0.6 cc of the solution mixture into the anterior chamber.

TEAR SUBSTITUTES

The precorneal tear film is described in "Diseases of the Cornea." The mucous layer of the corneal tear film is equally important as the aqueous layer in maintaining health of the cornea. Numerous artificial tear preparations have been developed that have characteristics that resemble mucous secretion. Most of these preparations contain either polyvinyl alcohol or various forms of high molecular weight water-soluble polymer mucins that resemble material produced by conjunctival goblet cells. In all cases, these artificial tear film products must be used frequently to maintain their effect. Some of the products that are commercially available are listed in Table 7.

Another ocular lubricant that is marketed as a sterile ophthalmic ointment is Lacri-lube® ocular lubricant. This bland ointment is basically a white petrolatum base with mineral oil.

Table 7. *Artificial Tear Film Products*

TRADE NAME	PREPARATION	MANUFACTURER
Adapt Drops Adsorbotear	High molecular weight water-soluble polymer	Burton Parsons and Company
Isopto Tears	Hydroxypropyl methylcellulose	Alcon Labs
Liquifilm Tears	Polyvinyl alcohol	Allergan Pharmaceuticals
Tearisol	Hydroxypropyl methylcellulose	Smith, Miller, Patch
Tears Naturale	Water-soluble polymeric system	Alcon Labs
Lacri-Lube S.O.P.	Sterile white petrolatum	Allergen Pharmaceuticals

The author has administered Adapt Drops® five to seven times a day in cases of keratitis sicca. Recently, the use of Lacri-lube ointment (Allergan) has been increased because of the longer contact time that it provides. Lacri-lube ointment is especially good for evening treatments, although it is also used during the day.

ANTIVIRAL AGENTS

The use of antiviral agents has limited application in veterinary medicine. Idoxuridine ointment (0.5 percent)* at four hour intervals has been used to treat keratitis associated with feline viral rhinotracheitis-induced keratitis and conjunctivitis in cats.

ANTIFUNGAL AGENTS

Keratomycoses have proved to cause some of the most difficult medical cases. The incidence or recognition of keratomycosis has been increasing, especially in horses, although some cases are seen in dogs. Most mycotic infections of the cornea are associated with saprophytic fungal organisms that result in opportunistic infection. The use of topical antibiotic-steroid preparations in fungal infections can increase the severity of the disease problem. Diagnosis is based on scrapings of the corneal lesion that reveal mycelial elements and is confirmed by isolation in Sabouraud's agar. Organisms most frequently isolated in keratomycosis include *Aspergillus, Mucor,* and *Candida* species.

---

*Stoxil Ophthalmic Ointment®, Smith, Kline and French, Philadelphia, Pennsylvania

Various forms of treatment for mycotic keratitis are available. However, if the disease is suspected, a veterinary ophthalmologist should be consulted to assist in treatment. Cultures and sensitivity tests of mycotic organisms are important in establishing effective therapy.

The proven ocular antifungal agents are divided into three groups: the polyene antibiotics, the imidazoles, and the pyrimidines.

The Polyene Antibiotics. These are classified according to the number of double bonds they possess. Examples of classes of polyene antifungal agents are the tetrenes — consisting of nystatin and pimaricin, and the heptenes — consisting of amphotericin A and B and candimycin.

Nystatin is not formulated for the eye, and its level of action is usually not high enough to suppress anything but a very superficial corneal infection.

Amphotericin B (Fungizone) is available in a lyophilized powder and is highly insoluble in water. It is solubilized by the use of sodium desoxycholate. Unfortunately, amphotericin B is extremely irritating when used in the eye and also has poor penetrating capability. When used topically, it should not be in concentrations greater than 0.3 percent. Amphotericin B can also be administered subconjunctivally in dosages of 125 to 300 micrograms. Higher concentrations can produce tissue necrosis and ulceration at the site of injection.

Natamycin (pimaricin) is the least irritating and least toxic of all the polyene antifungal agents. It is the drug of choice in many cases of keratomycosis. Unfortunately, at this time the drug is still under an NDA. However, it will be available as a 5 percent suspension (Table 8). The recommended initial therapy is one drop

Table 8. Antifungal Therapy

ORGANISM	AVAILABLE AGENTS	INVESTIGATIONAL COMPOUNDS
No identification; diagnosis based on finding organisms in scrapings	Topical: Amphotericin B (1.0–2.5 mg/ml); Flucytosine (10 mg/ml); Thiomersal ointment (1:5,000)	Natamycin° (50 mg/ml); Clotrimazole† (10 mg/ml)
Yeast (candida)	Flucytosine (10 mg/ml); Amphotericin B (1.0–2.5 mg/ml)	Natamycin (50 mg/ml); Clotrimazole (10 mg/ml)
Filamentous organism (mold)	Amphotericin B (1.0–2.5 mg/ml); Thiomersal ointment (1:5,000)	Natamycin (50 mg/ml); Clotrimazole (10 mg/ml)
Actinomycetes; actinomyces	Topical: penicillin G 500,000 units/ml); Subconjunctival: penicillin G (1.0 million units)	
Nocardia	Topical: sulfacetamide (30%); Subconjunctival: Lincomycin (75 mg)	

° Primaricin was obtained in a 5% ophthalmic suspension from Alcon Laboratories, Ft. Worth, Texas.
† Has been obtained as an investigational drug from Dan B. Jones, M.D., Associate Professor of Ophthalmology, Baylor College of Medicine, Texas Medical Center, Houston, Texas.

instilled into the conjunctival sac at two-hour intervals for the first three days, then reduced to 6 to 8 times daily. Therapy should continue for 14 to 21 days or until there is resolution.

The Imidazoles. Of the imidazole class of antifungal agents, clotrimazole has been used in the eye as a 1 percent concentration in arachis or peanut oil. The topical form of the drug is non-irritating in both the horse and dog. Unfortunately, this drug is not yet commercially available, although it might be obtainable through an investigating institution.

CARBONIC ANHYDRASE INHIBITORS AND HYPEROSMOTIC AGENTS

Carbonic anhydrase inhibitors in the form of diuretics are used synergistically with miotics and hypertonic agents in lowering intraocular pressure. Various types of carbonic anhydrase inhibitors are available. The exact cause of the ocular hypotensive effect is not known, but carbonic anhydrase inhibitors may decrease aqueous outflow by 60 percent, thus leaving 40 percent aqueous humor formation.

If the anterior drainage angles are severely compromised, other agents such as intravenous urea or mannitol or oral glycerin (glycerol) may have to be administered.

Side effects with carbonic anhydrase agents are variable and depend on the agent being used. Some side effects are: (1) polydipsia and polyuria, (2) anorexia, (3) weakness and ataxia, (4) panting, (5) vomiting, and (6) diarrhea. If any of these signs develop, reduction in dosage of medication is indicated. Dichlorphenamide (Daranide®, Merck Sharp and Dohme) seems to cause fewer side effects in dogs than does acetazolamide (Diamox®, Lederle).

PRACTICAL DIAGNOSTIC AIDS

Fluorescein and rose bengal are two commonly used dyes that aid in the diagnosis of external ocular disorders. Fluorescein is used primarily as impregnated paper strips. Corneal epithelial lesions stain green and conjunctival lesions stain orange-yellow. Fluorescein can also be used to test nasolacrimal patency by observing the passage of dye through the nasolacrimal system and its exit at the external nares. The use of ultraviolet light can be helpful in assessing the passage of dye.

Rose bengal is a vital stain for dead and degenerating corneal or conjunctival epithelium and mucus. A topical anesthetic should be placed in the eye before the use of rose bengal because of the irritative nature of the dye. Dead and degenerating epithelial cells can be demonstrated by rose bengal in keratoconjunctivitis sicca, pannus of German shepherds, corneal lipoidosis, and pigmentary keratitis.

The Schirmer tear test is used to evaluate tear production. Prepared filter paper strips, 5 × 30 mm are used.* The notched end of the strip is placed in the inferior conjunctival cul-de-sac for one minute. No topical anesthesia is used. Normal wetting is 10 to 25 mm in one minute.

SURGICAL PREPARATION OF THE SKIN

Careful clipping of the hair around the eye is important for both plastic surgery procedures involving the lids and preparation for intraocular surgery. Care should be taken to avoid excoriating the skin with the clippers. The periocular skin can be washed with 1 percent povidone-iodine soap, and the eye should be irrigated with saline to remove any soap. Half-strength povidone-iodine solution (0.5 percent available iodine) can be used to irrigate the conjunctival cul-de-sac.

SUPPLEMENTAL READING

Bistner, Stephen, and Riis, Ronald: Clinical aspects of mycotic keratitis in the horse. Cornell Vet., 69:364–374, 1979.

Ellis, Philip P.: *Ocular Therapeutics and Pharmacology*, 5th ed. St. Louis, C. V. Mosby Company, 1977.

Havener, W.: *Ocular Pharmacology*. St. Louis, The C. V. Mosby Company, 1978.

Physician's Desk Reference for Ophthalmology, 1978/1979. Oradell, N.J., The Medical Economics Company, 1978.

Wilson, Louis A., and Schwarzmann, Stephen W.: Antibiotic use in ophthalmology: In Duane, Thomas (ed.): *Clinical Ophthalmology*, Hagerstown, Maryland, Harper and Row Publishers, 1978.

---

*Schirmer Tear Test Papers, SMP Division, Cooper Laboratories, Cedar Knolls, New Jersey.

ALGORITHMS FOR OPHTHALMOLOGIC PROBLEMS

GRETCHEN SCHMIDT, D.V.M.

East Lansing, Michigan

An algorithm is a step-by-step method of solving a problem. Algorithms do not replace the complete ophthalmic examination; they organize the diagnostic plan for a problem identified by ophthalmic examination much like a decision tree. The problem or sign can be compared with the trunk of the tree from which branches evolve as more data are gathered. The purpose of this chapter is to guide the general practitioner in a systemized approach to ophthalmologic problems. The algorithms are to be supplemented by the other chapters in this section as well as by other references and by specialists in the field. For example, the first algorithm is for the problem of a watery ocular discharge (Fig. 1). In solving this problem, one determines first if the watery discharge is due to overproduction of tears (lacrimation) or overflow of the normal amount of tears (epiphora).

The lacrimating eye is red and irritates the animal. The lids are blepharospastic or self-traumatized. Adnexal, corneal, and intraocular inflammation cause an eye to lacrimate. If the adnexa are normal, evaluate the cornea. If the cornea is normal, examine the intraocular structures for signs of inflammation. Following this step-by-step approach, one discovers the cause of the lacrimation.

The non-irritated (quiet), watery eye causes no discomfort to the animal. Obstruction of tear flow through the lacrimal passages routes the tears down the face (epiphora). Chronic drainage of tears stains the facial hair reddish brown. Instill flourescein dye into the conjunctival cul-de-sac to color the tear film. Normally, tears flow over the cornea and into the medial lacrimal lake. Blinking of the eyelids moves the tears from the lacrimal lake into the lacrimal puncta, through the nasolacrimal duct, and out the nostril. The presence of green dye-colored tears at the nostril confirms the patency of the lacrimal passages. This is a positive fluorescein dye test. Causes of epiphora with a positive fluorescein dye test are listed in the algorithm in Figure 1. Questions to answer now are: Is the blink mechanism effective? Are the eyelids placed against the cornea so as to allow proper passage of the tear film into the lacrimal lake? Is there sufficient area for a lacrimal lake? Is the assessment that the watery discharge is epiphora rather than lacrimation correct?

If the fluorescein dye test is negative, cannulate the lacrimal puncta and flush the lacrimal passages. If the puncta cannot be cannulated, a congenital or acquired defect prevents the tears from entering the lacrimal passage. If the puncta cannulate well but the entire system cannot be flushed, the blockage lies between the lacrimal sac and the nasal punctum. If both cannulating and flushing the lacrimal passages are accomplished, a temporary blockage may be released and the material will appear at the opposite ocular puncta or at the nostril. If the system flushes easily and no material is released from the passages, the fluorescein dye test was a false negative. Algorithm 1 lists possible diagnoses for each of these results. For more detailed descriptions of these diseases and their treatments, refer to standard ophthalmologic textbooks.

Other problems for which algorithms are included in this chapter are thick ocular discharge (Fig. 2), cloudy eye (Fig. 3), cataract (Fig. 4), corneal ulcer (Fig. 5), chronic superficial keratitis (Fig. 6), red eye (Fig. 7), uveitis (Fig. 8), protrusion of the third eyelid (Fig. 9), anisocoria (Fig. 10), and loss of vision (Fig. 11).

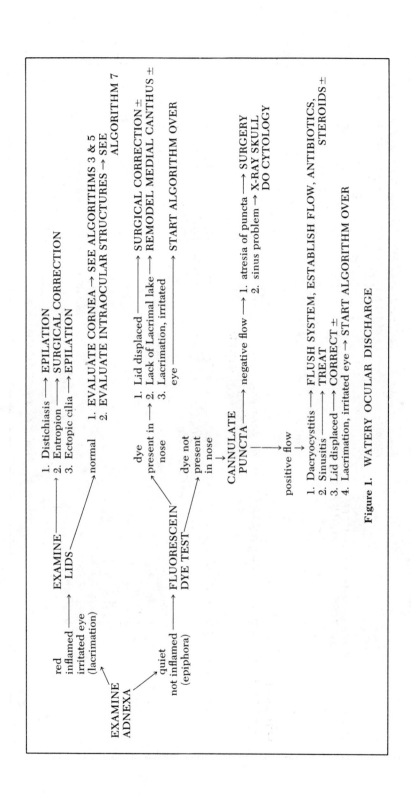

Figure 1. WATERY OCULAR DISCHARGE

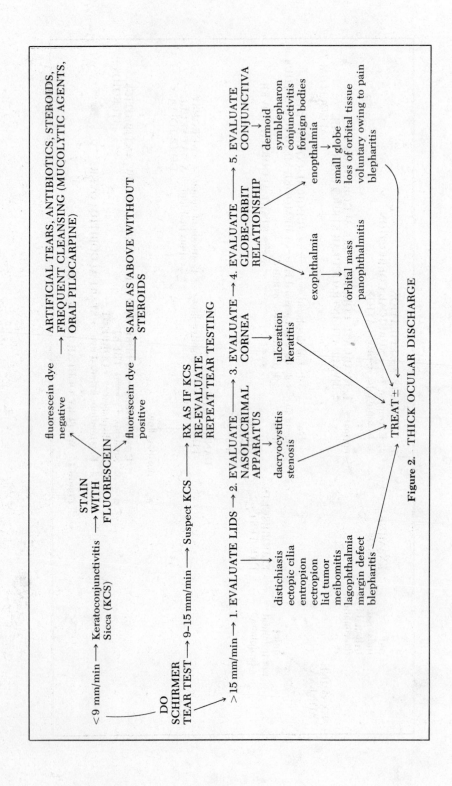

Figure 2. THICK OCULAR DISCHARGE

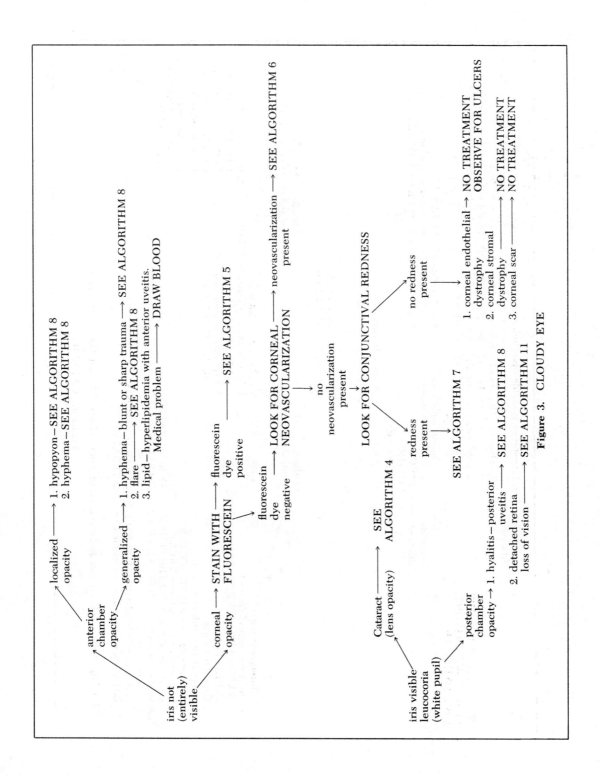

Figure 3.   CLOUDY EYE

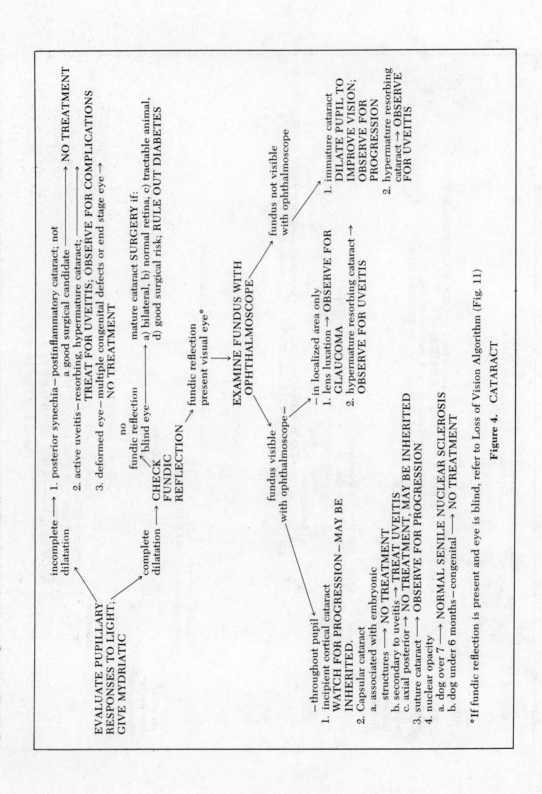

EVALUATE PUPILLARY RESPONSES TO LIGHT; GIVE MYDRIATIC

incomplete → 1. posterior synechia — postinflammatory cataract; not a good surgical candidate → NO TREATMENT
dilatation   2. active uveitis — resorbing, hypermature cataract; TREAT FOR UVEITIS; OBSERVE FOR COMPLICATIONS
              3. deformed eye — multiple congenital defects or end stage eye → NO TREATMENT

complete → CHECK FUNDIC REFLECTION
dilatation

no fundic reflection → blind eye → mature cataract SURGERY if: a) bilateral, b) normal retina, c) tractable animal, d) good surgical risk; RULE OUT DIABETES

fundic reflection present visual eye*

EXAMINE FUNDUS WITH OPHTHALMOSCOPE

fundus visible with ophthalmoscope —
  —throughout pupil
    1. incipient cortical cataract WATCH FOR PROGRESSION — MAY BE INHERITED.
    2. Capsular cataract
        a. associated with embryonic structures → NO TREATMENT
        b. secondary to uveitis → TREAT UVEITIS
        c. axial posterior → NO TREATMENT, MAY BE INHERITED
    3. suture cataract → OBSERVE FOR PROGRESSION
    4. nuclear opacity
        a. dog over 7 → NORMAL SENILE NUCLEAR SCLEROSIS
        b. dog under 6 months — congenital → NO TREATMENT
  —in localized area only
    1. lens luxation → OBSERVE FOR GLAUCOMA
    2. hypermature resorbing cataract → OBSERVE FOR UVEITIS

fundus not visible with ophthalmoscope
    1. immature cataract DILATE PUPIL TO IMPROVE VISION; OBSERVE FOR PROGRESSION
    2. hypermature resorbing cataract → OBSERVE FOR UVEITIS

*If fundic reflection is present and eye is blind, refer to Loss of Vision Algorithm (Fig. 11)

Figure 4.   CATARACT

Positive Fluorescein Retention Pattern Observed:

Punctate

Multiple Areas
1. KCS—SEE ALGORITHM 2
2. Pannus—SEE ALGORITHM 6
3. Superficial Punctate Keratitis—ANTIBIOTICS, STEROIDS, OBSERVE
4. Neuroparalytic keratitis—ANTIBIOTICS, SUPPORTIVE THERAPY. WAIT FOR RETURN OF FUNCTION

Dendritic

Herpes Keratitis—cat→IDOXURIDINE THERAPY

Oval to Round

Determine depth:

A. *Superficial*
1. Non-adherent margins
   a. indolent ulcer → DEBRIDE NON-ADHERENT EPITHELIUM, ANTIBIOTICS, ATROPINE, (SOFT CONTACT LENS, DES*)
2. Adherent margins
   a. 2° to KCS—SEE ALGORITHM 2
   b. 2° to lid defect—SURGERY, ATROPINE, ANTIBIOTICS
   c. 2° to ectopic cilia—EPILATION, ATROPINE, ANTIBIOTICS
   d. 2° to conjunctival or corneal foreign body—REMOVE, ATROPINE, ANTIBIOTICS
   e. 2° to bacterial infection—ATROPINE, ANTIBIOTIC, ANTICOLLAGENASE, OBSERVE FOR DEEPENING OF ULCER AND ANTERIOR UVEITIS

B. *Deep Stromal* ——→ DO CYTOLOGY OF ULCER: increased corneal edema; anterior uveitis usually present
1. Bacterial—gram neg.—ATROPINE, GENTAMICIN, ANTICOLLAGENASE, INTENSIVE THERAPY
2. Mycotic—DEBRIDE AREA, ATROPINE, CLOTRIMAZOLE
3. Collagenase ulcer—SAME AS BACTERIAL ULCER
4. Chronic KCS—INTENSIVE THERAPY, BE READY TO DO SURGERY

C. *Descemetocele*
clear center with only margins retaining fluorescein; uveitis present
→
RECOMMEND SURGERY—Conjunctival flap or equivalent.
1. Causes of A2 and B left untreated
2. Collagenase ulcer

D. *Staphyloma*, iris prolapse
1. Corneal laceration → SURGICAL REPAIR, TREAT ASSOCIATED ANTERIOR UVEITIS
2. Corneal perforation—intraocular foreign body → MEDICAL THERAPY ONLY DEPENDING ON SIZE AND TYPE OF F.B.
3. Untreated descemetocele which ruptured → CONJUNCTIVAL FLAP OR EQUIVALENT

Linear

A. Trauma—ATROPINE, ANTIBIOTICS, OBSERVE
B. Exposure—TARSORRHAPHY, ANTIBIOTICS

*Diethystilbesterol, low doses

Figure 5. CORNEAL ULCER

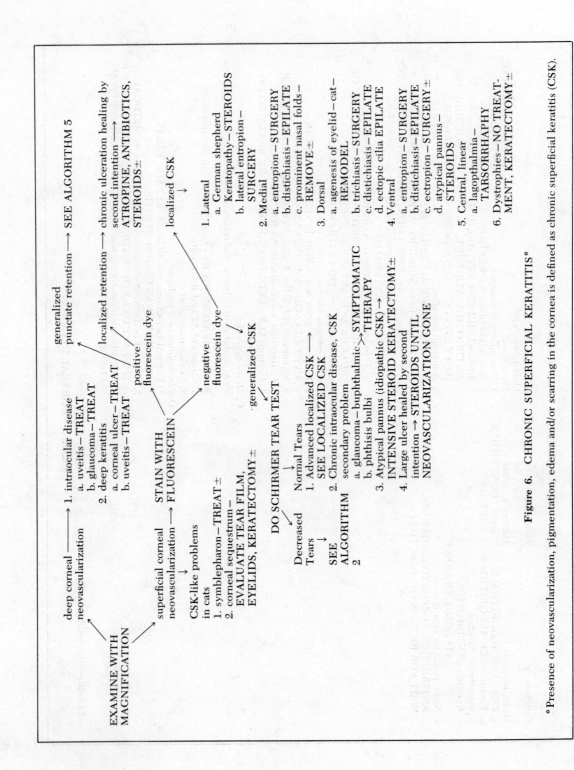

Figure 6.   CHRONIC SUPERFICIAL KERATITIS°

°Presence of neovascularization, pigmentation, edema and/or scarring in the cornea is defined as chronic superficial keratitis (CSK).

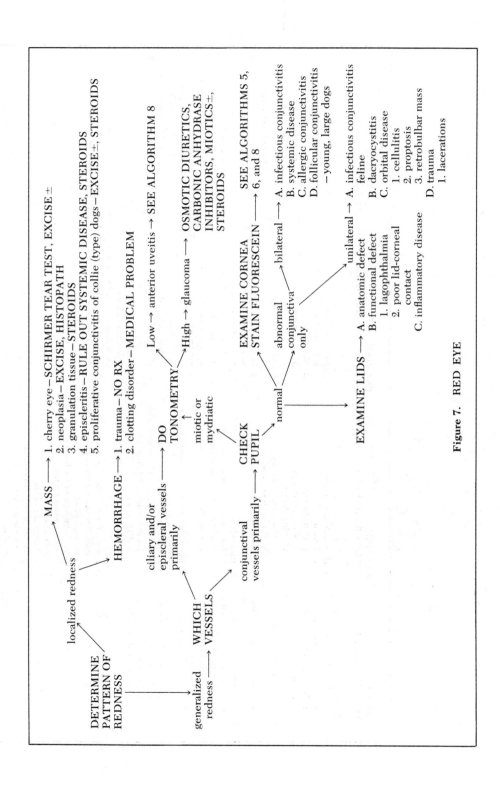

Figure 7.   RED EYE

EXAMINE
CORNEA → no edema → EXAMINE ANTERIOR CHAMBER → Clear → EXAMINE IRIS → no swelling → EXAMINE PUPIL

edema ↓

A. *Localized Edema*
1. Ulcerative keratitis
2. Necrogranulomatous sclerouveitis

B. *Generalized Edema*
1. Severe°—normal sized eye
   a. Ulcerative keratitis
   b. Hepatitis vaccination reaction
   c. Endophthalmitis
   d. Panophthalmitis
2. Severe°—abnormal sized eye
   a. small—phthisis bulbi
   b. large—chronic glaucoma
3. Mild—non-diagnostic

EXAMINE ANTERIOR CHAMBER

A. *Hemorrhage*—Hyphema
1. Trauma
   a. Perforating
   b. Non-perforating
2. Clotting defects
   a. Thrombocytopenia
   b. Factor deficiency
3. Non-diagnostic

B. *Hypopyon*
1. Infectious—bacterial, mycotic
2. Non-infectious—most common, non-diagnostic

C. *Keratitic Precipitates*—endogenous causes
1. Mutton fat—chronic (waxy or fatty appearance, lie on mid- and lower-corneal endothelium)
   a. FIP—cats
2. White—acute; non-diagnostic

D. *Flare*—Tyndall phenomenon as light passes through protein—rich aqueous humor. Non-diagnostic breakdown of blood-aqueous barrier

E. *Fibrin clot*
1. Surgical trauma
2. Acute severe iridocyclitis—non-diagnostic

F. *Parasite*
1. Filariasis—dogs, birds

G. *Lipid*
1. Hyperlipidemia with anterior uveitis

EXAMINE IRIS

A. *Diffuse swelling*
1. Edema—non-diagnostic
2. Neoplasia
   a. lymphosarcoma

B. *Localized swelling*
1. Neoplasia
   a. Melanoma
   b. Metastatic carcinoma
   c. Ciliary carcinoma
   d. Lymphosarcoma
   e. Hemangiomas
2. Granuloma
   a. FIP
   b. Cryptococcosis
   c. Blastomycosis
   d. Coccidiomycosis

C. *Dyscoria*
1. Synechia—chronic; Non-diagnostic—DO TONOMETRY
2. Lens luxation—DO TONOMETRY
3. Neoplasia—see B

EXAMINE PUPIL

A. *Dyscoria* (irregular pupil)
1. Synechia—chronic; Non-diagnostic—DO TONOMETRY
2. Lens luxation—DO TONOMETRY
3. Neoplasia—see B

B. *Pupil Absent*
1. Posterior synechiae; chronic uveitis—non-diagnostic
   a. Iris bombé—DO TONOMETRY; secondary glaucoma

Figure 8. UVEITIS

Normal or Miotic pupil → CHECK FUNDIC REFLECTION → Present → DO FUNDOSCOPIC EXAM → Normal → EXAMINE FOR SYSTEMIC DISEASE → Idiopathic

CHECK FUNDIC REFLECTION

A. Absent *Leucocoria* (white pupil)
   1. Seclusion, occlusion of pupil—chronic
      Non-diagnostic
   2. Cataract—Algorithm 4
      a. Lens-induced uveitis—resorption occurring
      b. Secondary to chronic uveitis
   3. Cyclitis membrane; chronic recurrent uveitis
      Non-diagnostic

DO FUNDOSCOPIC EXAM

A. Abnormal *Retinal detachment*
   1. Feline infectious peritonitis
   2. Cryptococcosis
   3. Blastomycosis
   4. Coccidiomycosis
   5. Hyperviscosity syndrome
   6. Other systemic disease
B. *Chorioretinitis*
   1. Acute
      a. Toxoplasmosis
      b. Septicemia
      c. Other systemic diseases
      d. FIP—cats
   2. Inactive
      a. Canine distemper
      b. Toxoplasmosis
      c. Non-diagnostic
C. *Optic neuritis*
   1. Extension of neurologic disease
   2. Acute pancreatitis
   3. Other systemic disease

EXAMINE FOR SYSTEMIC DISEASE

A. *Neurologic* Problem
   1. FIP
   2. Cryptococcosis
   3. Encephalomyopathies
B. *Gastrointestinal* Problem
   1. Diarrhea
      a. Protothecosis
   2. Dental infections
C. *Respiratory* Problem
   1. Pneumonia
      a. Mycotic
      b. Bacterial
   2. Sinusitis
D. *Multi-System* Disease
   1. Lymphosarcoma
   2. Leishmania
   3. Toxoplasmosis
   4. Leptospirosis
   5. Others
E. *Skin* problem
   1. Onchocerca—horse
F. *Musculoskeletal*
   1. Founder—horses
   2. Osteomyelitis
   3. Rheumatoid arthritis
G. *Genitourinary*
   1. Pyometra
   2. Glomerulonephritis
   3. Prostatitis
   4. Lower urinary tract infections
H. *Eosinophilia*
   1. Immune-mediated disease

Idiopathic

Most common cause.
Symptomatic
Treatment:
MYDRIATIC, ANTI-INFLAMMATORY, ANTI-PROSTAGLANDIN DRUGS. OBSERVE FOR SECONDARY CATARACTS, RETINAL DEGENERATION RECURRENT FLARE-UPS.

*unable to visualize intraocular structures.

Many of the other algorithms refer to uveitis because the clinical signs of uveitis involve all parts of the eye and include redness, corneal edema, corneal neovascularization, cloudy anterior chamber, cataracts, hyalitis, decreased intraocular pressure, miosis, abnormal iris, chorioretinitis, and retinal detachment. After defining the eye problem as uveitis, pursue the cause of the problem by systematically re-examining the eye and the whole animal. Many of the findings are non-diagnostic, leading the clinician to the idiopathic column and symptomatic therapy. Consult with area specialists and other references for detailed diagnostic and therapeutic plans.

Figure 8. UVEITIS (*Continued*)

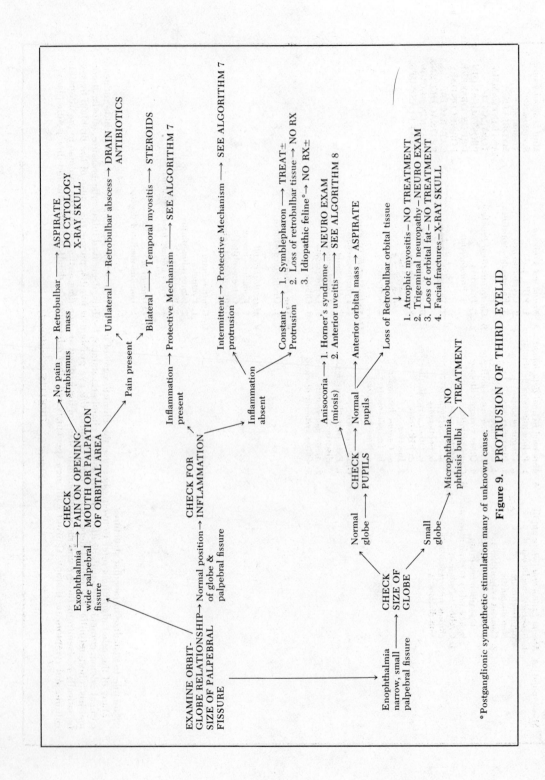

Figure 9. PROTRUSION OF THIRD EYELID

*Postganglionic sympathetic stimulation many of unknown cause.

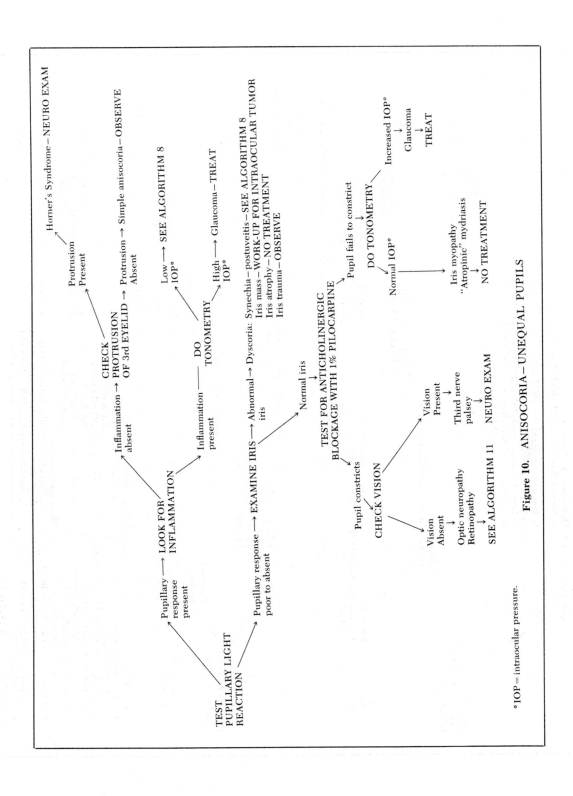

Figure 10. ANISOCORIA—UNEQUAL PUPILS

°IOP = intraocular pressure.

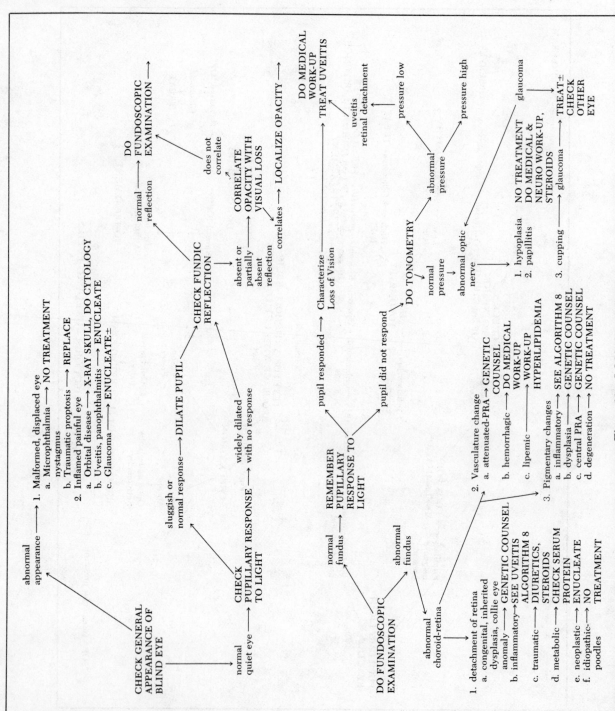

Figure 11. LOSS OF VISION

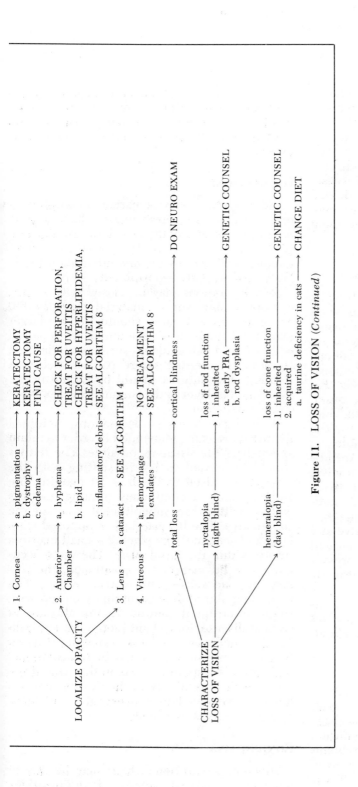

Figure 11. LOSS OF VISION (*Continued*)

OCULAR EMERGENCIES

MILTON WYMAN, D.V.M.
Columbus, Ohio

An ocular emergency is any acute ocular or adnexal disease that may cause pain, blindness, or loss of function owing to deformity. However, "presumed" emergencies must be separated from "true" emergencies. Some clients consider epiphora a very serious problem, whereas others do not consider a traumatic proptosis severe enough to be an emergency. This discussion is limited to those problems that are considered true emergencies and the management thereof.

EYELIDS

Blepharoedema (edema of the eyelids) is usually attributed to an allergic reaction when there is bilateral involvement and to insect bites and trauma when there is unilateral involvement. Urticaria causes bilateral lid edema, in addition to which there may be other edematous skin lesions elsewhere on the body. Patients are presented with signs of acute onset, discomfort, pruritus, severe swelling, and blepharospasm. It is often difficult to observe the cornea or conjunctiva. Epiphora is variable.

Therapy is generally symptomatic. Antihistamines have little beneficial effect. Prednisolone, 0.5 mg/kg or its equivalent given twice daily, is most effective. Non-steroidal, antiinflammatory drugs such as antiprostaglandins may be of value. Aspirin appears effective at a dose of 12 mg/kg three times daily for a dog and 25 mg/kg once daily for cats. Warm compresses applied to the periocular region may provide some relief.

In the absence of complications such as periorbital cellulitis, the swelling regresses within 24 hours and the prognosis is excellent.

ECCHYMOSES

Direct trauma to the eyelids may cause ecchymotic hemorrhage, larger hemorrhagic areas, and lesions as severe as proptosis. Hemorrhage within the lids is not serious but is an indicator of ocular trauma and more serious problems such as intraocular hemorrhage, anterior uveitis, or fractures of the orbital bones. These should be ruled out by a careful ocular examination and radiographs.

Initial therapy for acute ecchymoses involves cold compresses followed by warm compresses. Antibiotics and steroids are not indicated in uncomplicated ecchymoses, and the prognosis is excellent.

LACERATIONS

Lid lacerations may be partial or complete. If repaired carefully, these injuries have a good prognosis because of the excellent vascular supply to the eyelid. Even lesions of a few days duration will heal by the first intention if tissue layers are properly repositioned.

Skin lacerations may be closed with a fine, non-absorbable suture material such as 6-0 Nurolon.* Skin sutures should not be larger than 4-0. Conjunctival lacerations are repaired with a fine, biodegradable suture material in a continuous inverting suture pattern such as a Connell. The sutures should be buried in the subepithelial layer of the conjunctiva to prevent corneal irritation.

With full thickness lacerations, minimal débridement is recommended in order to retain as much viable tissue as possible. The tissues should be closed in layers, starting with the conjunctiva distal to the free lid margin. The author prefers a continuous running mattress pattern within the subepithelial layer of the conjunctiva. The lid margin is reopposed carefully and accurately by placing a small mattress suture within the tarsal plate. The more accurately the lid margin is repositioned, the less notching and subsequent scarring occurs. The remaining skin defect is routinely closed with single interrupted sutures. In the absence of corneal disease, topical antibiotics are not indicated or necessary and may cause local irritation. Systemic antibiotics may be indicated and will reach therapeutic levels in the wound because of the vascularity of the eyelid. Skin sutures are removed in approximately 10 days. The prognosis is excellent.

CONJUNCTIVA

Subconjunctival hemorrhage may be due to trauma or coagulopathies. Coagulopathies

*Ethicon Inc., Somerville, N. J. 08876

542

should be ruled out by a thorough search for other mucous membrane ecchymoses, petechia, or overt hemorrhage. Warfarin intoxication, thrombocytopenia, inherited coagulopathies such as Factor VII, VIII, or IX, and other deficiencies must be eliminated first. It is important that these serious systemic diseases and intraocular hemorrhage or inflammation be excluded from the differential diagnosis. Simple conjunctival hemorrhage is benign and treated initially by cold compresses followed by warm compresses two to four times a day.

Conjunctival Lacerations. The most frequent cause of conjunctival lacerations is trauma, most often from animal fights, foreign bodies, or gunshot wounds. The animal is frequently presented with a complaint of blood in the tears and acute blepharospasm. Penetrating or perforating injuries to the globe or orbit and intraocular disease such as hemorrhage, inflammation, and foreign bodies must be ruled out. When these important considerations are excluded, the prognosis is excellent. The size of the conjunctival defect determines whether surgical closure is necessary. Small, well opposed defects do not require sutures, whereas larger defects do. Number 6-0 or 7-0 biodegradable sutures should be used in the previously described pattern.

When topical therapy is necessary, solutions are preferred for initial therapy. Solutions must be placed in the eye more frequently than ointments in order to maintain therapeutic concentrations. Lipid inclusions may result if ointments with petrolatum bases are used for topical therapy of conjunctival defects. However, they may be used after the conjunctiva has epithelialized. A broad spectrum antibiotic (Gentamycin*) or a combination (Neosporin®†) is preferred. The use of topical steroids must be determined by professional judgment. Subconjunctival steroid injections are not recommended because they cannot be removed if complications occur, and even a small volume may complicate an already compromised lesion.

Foreign Bodies. Foreign bodies lodged in the conjunctival cul-de-sacs (including the third eyelid) are frequently overlooked, and the "signs" are treated instead. Typically, the onset of signs is acute and observed after the animal has been outdoors with access to weeds, woods, etc. These signs include blepharospasm, epiphora, and varying degrees of corneal edema. Corneal edema usually indicates epithelial erosion or anterior uveitis.

The diagnosis is based on finding the foreign

material by everting the eyelids. Treatment involves the removal of the foreign body and resolution of the secondary lesions, which usually improve rapidly. The prognosis is excellent in uncomplicated cases.

CORNEA

Ulcers and Abrasions. These lesions may be due either to mechanical injury such as from clippers, scratches, or foreign bodies or to chemical injury such as from shampoos. Regardless of the cause, ocular pain is the primary reason for presentation. The eye should be topically anesthetized to facilitate examination. It is necessary to determine the extent of the injury and to remove any foreign material present in the cul-de-sacs, the conjunctiva, or the cornea.

Superficial abrasions should be irrigated with warm sterile saline solution or other collyrium. Irrigation is most important in treating alkaline chemical injuries, but it is also valuable in the removal of particulate irritants. Fluorescein staining will delineate the extent of the lesion and monitor the progression of healing.

Treatment primarily involves prophylactic topical antibiotics to control the bacterial flora on the injured cornea. Broad spectrum antibiotic ophthalmic ointments administered four times a day are preferred because of the prolonged contact time of ointments. If anterior uveitis is present, atropine sulfate ointment (1 percent) should be used to effect. Topical anesthetics are contraindicated because of their toxic effect on epithelium. If severe pain persists despite atropine therapy, systemic analgesics may be useful.

Frequent re-evaluations are warranted, and therapy should be altered when necessary. Simple abrasions heal within four to seven days, and those that do not must be critically re-evaluated for complications such as overlooked foreign material, infection (bacteria or fungi), or collagenase-induced ulceration.

Foreign Bodies. Corneal foreign bodies may mimic corneal abrasions in their clinical signs, although the deeper corneal lesions caused by foreign bodies paradoxically often produce less pain than do superficial abrasions. Intracorneal foreign bodies may be masked by edema, neovascularization, or cellular infiltration and may require a slit lamp or magnifying loop for diagnosis and examination. The animal may require general or topical anesthesia. If a delicate or difficult extraction is anticipated, general anesthesia is preferred. Care must be taken not to push the foreign object through the cornea. An incision is made carefully over the foreign material with a #11 Bard Parker blade

---

*Schering Corp., Kenilworth, N.J. 07033

†Burroughs Wellcome Co., Research Triangle Park, N.C. 27709

until the incision is adjacent to the sliver or foreign body. A 25 or 26 gauge needle attached to a tuberculin syringe is then inserted under the foreign body, and pressure is exerted until the foreign body is disengaged from the stroma. This procedure should be done with extreme caution to prevent either pushing the foreign body into the anterior chamber or perforating the cornea with the blade or needle. The resulting lesion is irrigated and treatment similar to that described for corneal ulceration is instituted. If the foreign body is plant material, a mycotic infection could be involved and a re-evaluation should be performed within three days.

Perforated Cornea. Corneal perforations may result from deep stromal ulceration or traumatic injuries. These require immediate attention, but care must be exercised in manipulating the eye so that further damage to the intraocular structures does not result. A general anesthetic may be administered in order to facilitate examination of the eye if the animal resists opening its lids. Small perforations may not have a uveal prolapse owing to the fibrin present in the plasmoid aqueous, which may form an adequate seal. There may be variable signs of anterior uveitis including miosis, flare, hypotony, pain, and possibly some focal corneal edema. If the anterior chamber does not appear to be of normal depth, there may be a leak in the cornea that can be identified by fluorescein (fluorescein fountain). A fluorescein strip is moistened and a drop of concentrated dye is placed over the defect. If there is a leak, the aqueous exiting the defect will produce a rivulet of bright green in the orange-colored fluorescein.

When the lesion is 1 mm or less in size, it can be sealed by cauterization with trichloroacetic acid carefully applied with a sterile cotton applicator directly over the defect. The cornea and cul-de-sacs are thoroughly irrigated with warmed collyria. This treatment is applicable only to small perforations, not to gaping wounds. When the lesion is larger, a suture of 6-0 or 7-0 biodegradable material may be placed intrastromally (approximately ½ to ⅔ the depth of the cornea). Inflammation should be treated as an anterior uveitis (described elsewhere in this text). Topical antibiotic ointments are applied, and topical steroids may be indicated if the anterior uvea is severely inflamed.

LACERATIONS WITH PROLAPSE OF THE UVEA

Prolapse of the uvea warrants surgery as soon as possible. Parenteral broad spectrum antibiotics should be started promptly, even if ocular surgery must be dealyed. Ointments should not be used, since petrolatum and lanolin are extremely irritating to the uvea. Manipulation of the damaged eye should be minimal.

The eye is carefully examined to determine the extent of the injury with the animal under general anesthesia. Radiographs may be taken to rule out the presence of perforating radiopaque foreign bodies if the history is incomplete. The prolapsed uvea is examined to determine its viability.

Removal of incarcerated uveal tissue can sometimes be accomplished pharmacologically rather than mechanically. Iris tissue that is trapped in the axial cornea sometimes can be retracted into the anterior chamber by using sterile mydriatic eyedrops, — e.g., 1 percent atropine and/or 10 percent phenylephrine. The prolapsed iris usually requires excision, although if viable, it may be gently replaced with an iris repositor. The anterior chamber is gently irrigated with warmed Ringer's solution. The corneal laceration is reopposed by placing simple interrupted ⅔ depth sutures starting from either end of the laceration and continuing across the defect. All the sutures should be placed before tying any of them. When they are all placed, tension is applied to the suture ends by an assistant, and the uvea is held away from the incision with an iris repositor. The sutures are then tied. The anterior chamber is refilled with warmed Ringer's solution or Balanced Salt Solution (BSS)* and a small air bubble. The suture line should be watertight; additional sutures may be placed to repair leaks and a conjunctival flap may be used if leakage persists.

Medication following surgery includes the use of mydriatics, cycloplegics, antibiotics, and anti-inflammatory drugs. Aspirin may be used as an antiprostaglandin in dogs at a dose of 10 mg/kg QID for two days, then 10 mg/kg BID. Cats require 25 mg/kg once daily. The prognosis depends on the amount of time elapsed before treatment and the extent of uveal damage.

SCLERA

Lacerations. These wounds are often extensions of corneal lacerations that cross the limbus. The conjunctiva may still be intact and therefore it may be difficult to determine the extent of the laceration. To evaluate scleral involvement when the corneal laceration extends to the limbus, the conjunctiva can be dissected off the sclera.

---

*Alcon Laboratories, Inc. Forth Worth, TX 76101

Anterior scleral lacerations are managed similarly to corneal lacerations with 6-0 or 7-0 biodegradable sutures under a conjunctival flap. The sutures should not pass completely through the sclera. Medical treatment is similar to that described for corneal lacerations.

HYPHEMA

Hyphema refers to blood within the anterior chamber. Hyphema may be caused by perforating and non-perforating trauma, choking, neoplasia, systemic disease, and congenital defects. The amount of blood in the entire anterior chamber varies, but usually it is incomplete with cells settling inferiorly. Traumatic disinsertion of the iris (iridodialysis) is sometimes associated with contusion and frequently accompanied by continued bleeding.

The management of uncomplicated hyphemas should be conservative. In man, the patient is hospitalized and confined to bed with both eyes covered and sedated if necessary. Cage rest and sedation is usually necessary in dogs and cats. Uncomplicated hyphema is not extremely dangerous to the eye unless it is complete. Rebleeding may fill the entire anterior chamber, and if it then clots and secondary glaucoma occurs, the prognosis becomes guarded. With age, the clot may appear as a dark black color ("eight ball hyphema") and is often associated with secondary glaucoma. The latter condition is rare in animals. Some authors advocate systemic or topical steroids; however, experimental evidence suggests that steroids result in prolonged resorption. Some ophthalmologists use topical atropine; others use pilocarpine. Double blind studies in man show that neither contributes to the resolution of the blood. However, the author advocates pilocarpine 1 percent topical drops administered two to three times daily for two to three days. Daily observations should indicate whether to continue this therapy.

Evidence of anterior uveitis dictates the use of atropine and steroids supplemented by a broad spectrum antibiotic. Systemic enzymes have not proven efficacious for clot removal.

It should not be assumed that a blood clot can be aspirated easily through a hypodermic needle. This technique may cause a secondary cataract owing to injury to the lens capsule or possibly more serious injury to the retina or other intraocular structures. The clot requires a surgical technique similar to but not as extensive as a cataract extraction. This procedure should be done by an ophthalmologist. Those cases in which secondary glaucoma is present should be treated with carbonic anhydrase inhibitors or hyperosmotic solutions (described under glaucoma therapy). Neither of these drugs are efficacious if continued bleeding is present, and hyperosmotic agents are definitely contraindicated.

PROPTOSIS OF THE GLOBE (PROLAPSE OF THE EYE)

Proptosis of the globe is truly an ocular emergency. The earlier the globe is repaired, the better the prognosis, with few exceptions. Traumatic myectomies are common secondary lesions. The resultant lesions include exophthalmia, dorsal lateral strabismus, ulcerative keratoconjunctivitis owing to exposure and sicca, and avulsion of the optic nerve and ciliary arteries. The cases with the best prognosis are treated within two to three hours of proptosis and have a firmly attached globe that is tight against the eyelids, a clear cornea and anterior chamber, a miotic pupil, and little or no evidence of extrinsic myectomies. Enucleation is not necessary unless the sclera is ruptured and the eye is hanging without extrinsic muscle support.

The animal should be given any necessary therapy to combat possible shock as well as systemic, broad spectrum antibiotics. The animal is then anesthetized and the globe is irrigated with warm sterile Ringer's solution. Methylcellulose tear replacement ointments or solutions may be used as lubricants. Strabismus hooks or Allis tissue forceps are placed in the upper and lower lids to engage the free lid margin and apply tension out and away from the globe. Simultaneous counter pressure is applied carefully to the globe with care not to abrade the cornea. The lids act as a dam, and they must be repositioned anterior to the equator of the globe in order to replace the eyeball in its normal position. Orbital hemorrage or edema often produces exophthalmos after correction and necessitates a temporary tarsorrhaphy to prevent reprolapse. Care should be taken to prevent injury to the globe when placing the tarsorrhaphy sutures.

The author does not advocate injecting any drugs into the orbital space. Severe orbital inflammation may be treated with systemic steroids. Prednisolone, 2 mg/kg BID is administered for two days followed by 1.0 mg/kg BID for two additional days, and the regimen is extended if indicated. Hyperosmotic agents should not be administered when there is potential hemorrhage within the orbit.

Topical antibiotics may be placed medially through the tarsorrhaphy, especially if corneal abrasions or ulceration is present. Care must be exercised to avoid injuring the eye in the process of medication.

The tarsorrhaphy is left in place for at least a week. Evaluation can be made by gently palpating the globe through the closed lids. If the eye resists depression into the orbit, the tarsorrhaphy should remain. However, if the eye depresses easily into the orbit or is extremely soft, the tarsorrhaphy can be removed for a more complete ocular examination. (The eyes should be followed closely for corneal ulceration after removal of the tarsorrhaphy.)

ACUTE GLAUCOMA

Acute congestive glaucoma is a frequent disease in dogs, and it is definitely an emergency. When intraocular pressure acutely reaches 45 mm Hg or greater, the "cardinal signs" of glaucoma become evident. In order to restore or preserve vision, the pressure must be quickly and safely reduced. Aqueous centesis should not be attempted. The most effective method of lowering intraocular pressure is the administration of a hyperosmotic agent. Oral glycerin at 2 gms/kg or 20 percent mannitol 2 gms/kg IV dehydrates the vitreous and results in rapid reduction of intraocular pressure.

Acetozolamide, 50 mg/kg IV, may be given to decrease aqueous production. After the initial dose, oral dichloramphenamide may be given at a dose of 2 mg/kg two to three times daily.

Outflow can be improved by placing one or two drops of 2 percent pilocarpine in the eye every hour three or four times. Pressure should be decreased within one or two hours. If therapy is not effective, the hyperosmotic agent may be repeated.

The eye should be examined to identify the cause or classification of glaucoma. This is imperative in order to treat the disease effectively. Once the pressure is down and the classification is made, the eye should be treated as described elsewhere in this chapter.

SUPPLEMENTAL READING

Bistner, S.I., and Aguirre, G.D.: Management of ocular emergencies. Vet. Clin. of North Am. 2(2):359–379, 1972.
Blogg, J.R.: *The Eye in Veterinary Medicine*, 1st ed. Victoria, Australia, Medos Company PTY LTD., 1977.
Havener, W.H.: *Ocular Pharmacology*, 4th ed. St. Louis, Mo., C.V. Mosby Company, 1978.
Yeary, R., and Swanson, W.: Aspirin dosages for the cat. JAVMA 163:1177–1178, 1973.

DISEASES OF THE EYELIDS

KERRY L. KETRING, D.V.M.
Cincinnati, Ohio

Diseases of the eyelids and the sequelae to lid disease such as conjunctivitis and keratitis are the most frequent ophthalmic illnesses presented to the veterinarian. This article includes discussion of abnormal cilia, inadequate lid positioning (including entropion, ectropion, and lagophthalmus), infections and inflammations of the lid, and neoplasms.

ABNORMAL CILIA

DISTICHIASIS

Distichiasis refers to the presence of cilia arising from the orifices of the meibomian glands. These may form a complete or partial row of cilia in the upper and/or lower lid. Although canine distichiasis has been reported as a sequela to chronic inflammation of the lids, most cases are congenital or appear within the first six months of life.

Distichiasis may be found in any breed, but the incidence appears higher in the American cocker spaniel, Pekingese, Shih Tzu, Saint Bernard, poodle, pug, and golden retriever. This incidence may only reflect the popular breeds in a given geographic area.

In most cases, the extra row of cilia causes no structural or functional damage to the eye, and surgical removal is contraindicated. These cilia may confuse the diagnosis with any problem that induces blepharospasms such as corneal injury or anterior uveitis. Many veterinarians have removed the cilia from an adult dog that develops an ocular disease acutely without identifying the primary etiology.

Severe cases are found in young dogs that have a history of blepharospasms, squinting, severe epiphora, conjunctivitis, or corneal disease including ulceration. If an entire row of cilia is present, the author prefers a lid splitting procedure. Two parallel incisions are made with a #64 beaver blade on both sides of the meibomian glands along the length of the lid. The incision is extended to a depth of 3 to 5 mm, which is the extent of the meibomian glands into the lid. Tenotomy scissors are then used to remove the strip of lid containing the meibomian glands and cilia. Postoperative care involves systemic antibiotics. If only several cilia are involved, electrolysis may be used to destroy the follicle by placing the needle into the meibomian gland orifice. Simple epilation is seldom curative, and the hairs will regrow. Epilating long hairs that are not causing problems may result in regrowth of short stubby hairs that will cause severe corneal irritation.

TRICHIASIS OR ABERRANT CILIA

These cilia penetrate the palpebral conjunctiva or the surface of the lid adjacent to the globe. They may be found in the same breeds as previously mentioned but are usually not congenital. Dogs with trichiasis usually have a history of recurrent corneal ulcers that are often located in the superior half of the cornea. The ulcers may be linear in shape with the long axis extending vertically. Trichiasis will frequently cause a characteristic head jerk at the height of the blink, as the cilia comes into contact with the cornea. The cilia are found by using magnification to examine the everted lid of the tranquilized dog. They are located 3 to 5 mm from the free lid margin in a position corresponding to the corneal lesion. Often, only a small bleb will be seen on the conjunctival surface. On closer examination, it will be found to contain one or more cilia. Frequently, the hair shaft is coiled, with only a small section of the shaft penetrating the conjunctiva. Electrocautery or electrolysis may remove the shaft without destroying the follicle. In this case, the hair will regrow. Careful epilation may enable uncoiling of the shaft and removal of the follicle. In many cases, surgical resection of the lid such as a V-plasty is needed to remove the follicles. Cryosurgery, using nitrous oxide as the cryogen, has been used successfully to destroy the follicle and remove the cilia.

INADEQUATE LID POSITIONING

These abnormalities result in chronic irritation to the cornea and conjunctiva. Frequently, the veterinarian treats the sequelae to the lid disease without treating the inciting etiology. This type of treatment results in chronic conjunctivitis and keratitis, which may progress to keratoconjunctivitis sicca and/or deep stromal ulcers and eventual loss of the globe.

Owners of dogs with these lid diseases are advised that the defect may be inherited. According to the American Kennel Club, entropion and ectropion are disqualifying traits in many breeds. Dogs also are disqualified from showing if they have had corrective lid surgery.

ENTROPION

Entropion or rolling in of the free lid margin is probably the most common congenital eye disease of dogs. Anatomic or primary entropion must be differentiated from spastic entropion. The latter is usually unilateral, develops acutely in the adult dog, and is the result of severe blepharospasms owing to corneal ulcerations, foreign bodies, or anterior uveitis. As a diagnostic aid, topical anesthetics may reduce the blepharospams and allow the lid to maintain a normal position. Treatment is correction of the primary etiology. A temporary tarsorrhaphy is often needed to allow the cornea to epithelialize without irritation from the lid.

Primary entropion is usually bilateral and present in the young puppy. If it is mild and causing no corneal disease, correction is delayed until the dog reaches maturity. Primary entropion is seldom self-limiting.

Medial entropion is frequently found in the poodle, Shih Tzu, pug, Lhasa apso, and English bulldog. This is the most common cause of nasal corneal pigment in these breeds. Even mild entropion of the lower lid can occlude the inferior puncta and result in chronic epiphora. Depending on the extent of entropion, either a crescent-shaped section of skin parallel to the entropic lid is removed, or a permanent medial tarsorrhaphy is performed. The latter is preferred if both the upper and lower lids are involved. In either case, the lacrimal puncta must be identified and preserved so as not to interfere with the normal drainage of tears.

Mild entropion involving only a section of the lower lid without extension to the lateral canthus can be surgically corrected by a modification of the Hotz procedure or a Y-V plasty. If the entropion includes the lateral canthus, a modification of the Hotz procedure can be done by extending the incision and section of tissue removed around the lateral canthus. Entropion involving the lateral canthus and upper and lower lid is frequently found in enophthalmic breeds such as Irish setters, Doberman pinschers, Labrador retrievers, and golden retrievers. A permanent lateral tarsorrhaphy is performed in those cases, which removes the entropic section of lid and shortens the palpebral fissure. Saint Bernards, chows, and Chinese Shar-Peis frequently have severe entropion owing to a combination of enophthalmia, laxity of the lateral retractor muscle, and excessive facial folds of skin. Depending on the extent of the entropion, a lateral canthoplasty, a permanent lateral tarsorrhaphy, or a combination of one of these with a modification of the Hotz procedure should be performed.

ECTROPION

Ectropion can be divided into two groups — primary or anatomic ectropion and cicatricial ectropion. The rolling out or drooping of the lower eyelid is accepted and desired in such breeds as the bloodhounds and Bassett hounds. Whereas the primary clinical sign associated with entropion is corneal disease, dogs with ectropion have chronic conjunctivitis, which frequently results in decreased tear production and/or corneal disease. Ectropion does not usually cause as severe damage as does entropion. Dogs with periodic and mild conjunctivitis associated with ectropion can be successfully controlled by flushing the eyes with a collyrium to remove irritating debris such as plant material.

Ectropion is common in hounds, spaniels, and Saint Bernards. In the Saint Bernard, the central section of the lid may be ectropic and the lateral section may be entropic.

Cicatricial ectropion is corrected by a V-Y plasty. Several procedures have been described for the surgical correction of primary ectropion (Bistner et al., 1977). The author's preference is a lateral canthoplasty, or alternatively, a permanent lateral tarsorrhaphy in the Saint Bernard. In other breeds, a permanent lateral tarsorrhaphy eliminates the ectropic section of the lid and reduces the exposure of bulbar and palpebral conjunctiva. It is extremely important to accomplish both these goals in the dog with decreased tearing owing to chronic conjunctivitis.

LAGOPHTHALMUS

Lagophthalmus, or inadequate lid closure, is a common problem in the exophthalmic breeds such as the pug, Boston terrier, and Pekingese. When asked, owners frequently report that the dog sleeps with the eyelids partially opened. If the dog is observed closely, it is noted that only a forceful blink completely covers the cornea. These dogs have a history of axial, centrally located corneal ulcers. These ulcers, which develop owing to drying of the cornea, can rapidly perforate and result in iris prolapse or staphyloma. If there is no indication of medial entropion, such as nasal corneal pigment, these patients are best treated by a permanent lateral tarsorrhaphy that reduces the palpebral fissure by up to one-third its total length.

If a medial entropion is present, both a permanent medial and lateral tarsorrhaphy may be needed to reduce the palpebral fissure adequately.

A permanent lateral tarsorrhaphy is also used to protect the cornea in cases of permanent paralytic ectropion owing to facial nerve paralysis.

INFECTION AND INFLAMMATION

HORDEOLUM

A hordeolum is an acute infection and inflammation of the glands of Zeis or Moll (external hordeolum) or meibomian glands (internal hordeolum). The condition is characterized by reddening and a painful swelling on either or both sides of the lid. These small abscesses are treated by gently expressing their contents, applying warm compresses and a topical antibiotic ointment, and, if the infection is severe, using systemic antibiotics.

CHALAZION

A chalazion is a painless swelling of the meibomian gland, best visualized on the conjunctival surface of the lid. It is caused by a granulomatous reaction within the gland or by a build-up of meibomian gland secretions. This swelling, which is pale yellow in color, may cause irritation to the cornea. Treatment consists of incising the swelling from the conjunctival surface and curetting out the granulomatous material. Postoperatively, the eye is treated with a topical antibiotic and corticosteroid solution.

BLEPHARITIS

Blepharitis, or inflammation of the eyelids, is characterized by reddening and swelling of the lids. A thick, purulent, ocular discharge may be present, with dried exudate on the lid margins. In cases of chronic blepharitis, alopecia of the lid is frequently seen. If the lids are everted, one can see a long row of small abscesses involving the meibomian glands.

Treatment consists of draining the abscesses with a small gauge needle from the conjunctival surface, applying warm compresses and topical antibiotics, and using systemic antibiotics.

In puppies, blepharitis may be seen as a component of demodectic mange. The diagnosis is based on identification of the mite in skin scrapings or in the expressed content of the meibomian glands. Treatment is directed at eliminating the mite. Blepharitis is also a component of juvenile pyoderma and may be the initial sign before acute swelling of the lips and regional lymph nodes develop. This condition responds to the systemic use of broad spectrum antibiotics and low' levels of corticosteroids such as prednisolone.

Blepharitis is also a component of allergic inhalant dermatitis. Diagnosis is based on physical examination, history (which often includes pruritus), and skin testing. The preferred treatment is hyposensitization with specific allergens.

Dogs with non-responsive blepharitis, including medial canthus erosion, have been successfully treated with staphylococcal antigen.* Since this not only is a staphylococcal antigen but is believed to be a non-specific T cell stimulator, the exact mode of action in effecting a response is unknown. This treatment alone has been used successfully in several cases that failed to respond to conventional antibiotic therapy.

Autoimmune skin diseases, such as pemphigus foliaceus and pemphigus vulgaris, frequently involve the lids in addition to other areas of skin. Depending on the disease and the stage of development, the lesion of the lids may be ulcerative, exudative, and/or crusty in appearance. Definitive diagnosis is based on histologic findings and the demonstration of autoantibodies in biopsy samples by immunofluorescence. Therapy consists of continuous high level dosage of systemic corticosteroids.

Determination of the etiology of blepharitis is important, since systemic corticosteroids are indicated in cases of pemphigus but are contraindicated in demodicosis, they are of little value in cases of abscesses of the meibomian glands, and they give only temporary relief in allergic dermatitis. Although the history and clinical findings may be helpful, skin biopsies are the most informative diagnostic tool. If skin other than the lids is similarly involved, it may be preferable for biopsy. Bacterial cultures are insignificant since staphylococcus and other potential pathogens are common skin contaminants.

---

*Staphage Lysate, Delmont Lab, Swarthmore, PA 19081.

NEOPLASMS

Neoplasms involving the lids are common, especially in aging dogs. Adenomas and adenocarcinomas of the glands of Zeis and Moll or of the meibomian glands are most frequently encountered. These tumors are usually darkly pigmented and may be ulcerated, lobulated, cauliflowered, or firm and well delineated. Adenocarcinomas are usually larger, faster growing, and locally destructive.

Papillomas are found in dogs of all ages and usually have a well defined base that does not penetrate deeply into the lid. Squamous cell carcinomas of the lid are especially common in white cats. These tumors are quite destructive and frequently result in severe ulceration of the lid margin. Basal cell carcinomas have been reported in older dogs and are firm, rounded masses that have a tendency to ulcerate. Melanomas, mastocytomas, and histiocytomas have also been reported on the lids.

Lid tumors that are not on the free lid margin and are not penetrating the palpebral conjunctiva usually cause no irritation to the eye and need not be removed. Tumors that have penetrated the palpebral conjunctival surface usually cause a keratoconjunctivitis and should be removed. Proven cases of metastasis of lid tumors even to regional lymph nodes are rare.

Tumors up to one-third the length of the lid can be removed by a full thickness resection of the eyelid. Tumors involving larger areas of the lid require more extensive reconstruction to obtain cosmetic and functional repair.

Cryosurgery, using nitrous oxide as the cryogen in a closed system, is extremely useful in treating large and small lid tumors. A complete discussion of the principles and techniques of cryosurgery is beyond the scope of this chapter. The advantage of cryosurgery is that it can be completed with tranquilization and/or local infiltration around the lesion. This is particularly desirable, since many older dogs with lid tumors also may be anesthetic risks. Tumors greater than one-third the length of the lid often can be managed with cryosurgery, although it may be necessary to repeat the procedure. Regrowth of lid tumors after surgery is common, owing to the conservative manner in which perilesional tissue must be removed, but regrowth is less common after cryosurgery.

Extensive reconstruction of the lid following excision of a large lid tumor can result in pain and self-trauma, which may cause dehiscence. Animals are usually quite free of pain following cryosurgery. Circulating antibody titers and lymphocyte activity rise following cryodestruction of tumors, but their significance is unknown at this time.

The major disadvantage of cryosurgery is the unsightly appearance of the tumor during the period of initial swelling and necrosis of the frozen tissue.

SUPPLEMENTAL READING

Bistner, S.I., Aguirre, G., and Batik, G.: *Atlas of Veterinary Ophthalmic Surgery*. Philadelphia, W. B. Saunders Co., 1977.

Brightman, A.H., and Helper, L.C.: Full thickness resection of the eyelid. JAAHA 4:483–485, 1978.

Doherty, D.J.: A bridge-flap blepharorrhaphy method for eyelid reconstruction in the cat. JAAHA 9:238–241, 1973.

Goldstein, R.S.: *Handbook of Veterinary Cryosurgery*. Santa Clara, California, Spembly Inc., 1977.

Halliwell, R.E.W., and Goldschmidt, M.H.: Pemphigus foliaceus in the canine: a case report and discussion. JAAHA 13:431–436, 1977.

Hurvitz, A.I., and Feldman, E.: A disease in dogs resembling human pemphigus vulgaris: case reports. JAVMA 166:585–590, 1975.

Stannard, A.A., Gribble, D.H., Baker, B.B.: A mucocutaneous disease in the dog resembling pemphigus vulgaris in man. JAVMA 166:575–582, 1975.

Wyman, M.: Lateral canthoplasty. JAAHA 7:196–201, 1971.

DISEASES OF THE CONJUNCTIVA

LEWIS H. CAMPBELL

Los Altos, California

The conjunctiva is a thin, transparent mucous membrane that lines the posterior surface of the eyelids and covers the anterior surface of the globe. It is divided into palpebral and bulbar portions and the regions connecting these two portions, the superior and inferior fornices. Its presence is normally indicated only by the characteristic luster of its surface and by the few blood vessels that are normally apparent in it. The conjunctival epithelium is continuous with the corneal epithelium and that lining the lacrimal passages and glands.

SIGNS

Signs arising from disease involving only the conjunctiva are mainly exudation and sometimes ocular discomfort. Severe pain suggests corneal rather than conjunctival involvement. Itching is common in allergic conditions. The signs of conjunctival disease are mainly related to abnormalities of appearance such as vascular change and edema (chemosis). Both the conjunctival and ciliary vascular beds are usually injected in inflammation of the anterior segment, although one is more markedly involved than the other. The external appearance of the eye is one of dilated conjunctival vessels. Eversion of the eyelids will reveal a similar injection of the palpebral conjunctiva. In distinguishing conjunctival disease from deeper diseases of the eye, it is wiser to direct attention to signs of corneal and iris involvement and the pupillary

reaction to light. Even though the appearance of the external eye is typical of a conjunctivitis, the diagnosis should not be accepted in the absence of a characteristic history or until examination of the anterior segment of the eye has excluded coincident keratitis or uveitis. Classification is often based upon cause (bacterial, viral, fungal, chemical, or lacrimal), the age of occurrence (ophthalmia neonatorum), the type of exudate (purulent, mucopurulent), or the disease course (acute, subacute, or chronic).

EXAMINATION

Clinical examination requires good illumination and magnification. Attention should be directed to the patency of the lacrimal system, the severity and nature of the vascular injection, the occurrence of follicles or papillary hypertrophy, and the nature of the secretion. Diagnosis and etiology of conjunctivitis are based upon (1) history and clinical examination, (2) Gram's and Giemsa's stains of conjunctival scrapings, and (3) culture of the conjunctival surface. Conjunctival scrapings are obtained with a heat sterilized platinum spatula, and the material is then placed on a clean glass slide. Slides may be heat fixed and then gram stained or they may be fixed in 95 percent methanol and then stained with Giemsa solution. Cytologic study of epithelial scrapings stained with Giemsa's stain requires a familiarity with the procedure. Since the conjunctiva is an exposed surface, a number of bacteria are indigenous to the surface. Usually they are present in too few numbers to be recognized readily on Gram's stain, but they may be demonstrated on culture. When culturing, sterile swabs moistened in sterile broth or saline are utilized. (It is undesirable to use topical anesthetics.) The swab is plated on blood agar and placed in thioglycolate or tryptic soy broth. An alternative is to use prepackaged sterile culture sets supplied with transport media. These are then submitted to a local laboratory for culturing.

DISEASES OF THE CONJUNCTIVA

CHEMOSIS

Edema of the conjunctiva is seen infrequently but is often observed with underlying inflammatory disease. Causes include trauma, allergy, or drug reaction. Traumatic chemosis has a rapid and complete spontaneous resolution. If it is necessary to protect the swollen conjunctiva from exposure, topical antibiotic ointments may be used. Ulcers, if present, must be treated as a primary entity. When allergens can be incriminated, topical steroid therapy will alleviate the signs, and, upon remission, they should be discontinued.

SUBCONJUNCTIVAL HEMORRHAGE

Generally, subconjunctival hemorrhage is traumatic in origin and, for the most part, unilateral. If bilateral hemorrhage is observed with no antecedent traumatic history, systemic bleeding disorders must be considered.

Some cases of traumatic subconjunctival hemorrhage also present with anterior uveal signs. If this is the case, topical atropine and steroids are indicated to control the uveitis.

When no other ophthalmic abnormalities are present in the trauma case, treatment is not necessary and resolution is complete within ten days to two weeks. Subconjunctival hemorrhage is treated as an entity in itself if the conjunctiva is swollen and exposed.

BACTERIAL CONJUNCTIVITIS

The aerobic conjunctival flora in the normal dog is composed primarily of *Staph epidermidis*, *Staph aureus*, alpha-hemolytic streptococci, diphtheroids, *Neisseria* species, *Pseudomonas* species, non-hemolytic streptococci, and beta hemolytic streptococci. The conjunctival sac of the normal cat is relatively sterile compared with that of the dog. Either pathogenic or non-pathogenic bacteria may be involved in conjunctival infections.

The onset of primary bacterial conjunctivitis is relatively acute, and one or both eyes are involved with a mucopurulent exudate. Acute conjunctivitis of bacterial origin is readily amenable to antibiotic therapy, and corticosteroids need not be used. The instillation of an ointment at night may prevent the lids from sealing closed with exudate.

Dacryocystitis should be suspected in all cases of chronic, recurring, unilateral conjunctivitis. The cause is an obstruction of the lacrimal sac or nasolacrimal duct followed by bacterial infection. The ocular discharge ranges from purulent to mucopurulent and may be excessive.

Initial therapy should include flushing the nasolacrimal duct with saline and probing the nasolacrimal system if an obstruction that resists flushing is suspected. Once patency is obtained, the duct should be flushed with an antibiotic solution or tincture of iodine 2 percent. Threading the lacrimal passages with a fine polyethylene catheter may prevent stricture of the duct. Recurring dacryocystitis may indicate a foreign body in the lacrimal sac. Surgical exploration of the sac is indicated in this instance.

CHRONIC CONJUNCTIVITIS

This includes cases of conjunctivitis caused by exposure to a primary irritant (allergen), lid abnormalities (exposure), trichiasis or distichiasis (irritation), or keratoconjunctivitis sicca (xerosis of the ocular tissue). The typical discharge may range from tearing to thick mucoid exudation. The latter response is observed with drying or constant irritation of the ocular tissues and is an attempt by the goblet cell to protect the ocular surfaces.

Surgical correction of lid abnormalities or removal of extra cilia is advised. Although ophthalmic ointments may alleviate the signs, once the ointment is discontinued, they recur. Longterm antibiotic ointment therapy is to be avoided and therefore, if surgery is not performed, ocular lubricants (Lacri-lube)* without antibiotics and rinsing solutions are advised.

Excessive mucoid exudation — which is tenacious and often adheres to the lids, conjunctiva, and cornea — is frequently associated with keratoconjunctivitis sicca. The Schirmer tear test will usually measure 0 to 5 millimeters of

---

*Allergan Pharmaceuticals

wetting after one minute. Treatment is then directed toward this particular entity.

CHLAMYDIAL CONJUNCTIVITIS

Chlamydial conjunctivitis may be unilateral with secondary involvement of the opposite eye within a short period. Initial signs include epiphora with sneezing. The conjunctival surface is thickened and hyperemic with the development of a mucopurulent exudate. No corneal involvement has been reported in the cat.

Giemsa-stained conjunctival scrapings reveal polymorphonuclear leukocytes with basophilic intracytoplasmic inclusions about the nucleus of the epithelial cell. The inclusions are difficult to demonstrate after seven to ten days from the onset of clinical signs.

Chlamydia reproduce within the epithelial cell cytoplasm and as such they are resistant to topical antibiotic therapy. The infective forms are released as the epthelial cell ruptures, and at this time, topical tetracycline ointment is effective. Therapy should be continued for at least 28 days to cover the complete life cycle of the organism.

MYCOPLASMA-ASSOCIATED CONJUNCTIVITIS

Mycoplasma-associated conjunctivitis in cats has been reported as a unilateral conjunctivitis that may become bilateral. The initial clinical sign is epiphora with a papillary hypertrophy of the conjunctival surface manifesting clinically with a deep red, velvet appearance. If untreated, the discharge and clinical appearance change within five days to a mucoid tenacious exudate, with some cases developing a pseudomembrane. The conjunctiva becomes indurated and thickened with time. No corneal involvement has been reported. Giemsa-stained conjunctival scrapings reveal polymorphonuclear leukocytes with basophilic pleomorphic coccobacilli on the surface of the epithelial cells.

The response to antibiotic topical therapy is dramatic, with resolution of the clinical signs within three to five days. Untreated cases may persist for as long as 60 days. The organism is reported to be sensitive to most antibiotics except penicillin and neomycin. Topical steroids, either alone or in conjunction with an antibiotic, tend to prolong the course of the disease.

HERPETIC KERATOCONJUNCTIVITIS

Herpetic keratoconjunctivitis is characterized by a necrotic conjunctivitis with ulceration of the conjunctiva and cornea. The systemic dis-

ease may vary and the clinical signs are usually dependent upon the age of the cat. Usually it is associated with ocular involvement plus systemic disease (rhinotracheitis) or sneezing. Ocular signs may include mucopurulent discharge, extensive conjunctival hypermia and chemosis, formation of a pseudodiphtheritic membrane, conjunctival necrosis with ankyloblepharon or symblepharon, corneal ulceration, descemetocele, or corneal perforation.

Idoxuridine (IDU) therapy alone or combined with corneal epithelial cauterization (tincture of iodine 2 percent) is indicated in active herpesvirus infection. IDU has no therapeutic effect upon other causes of keratitis. Low concentrations of topical corticosteroids may be indicated with IDU therapy to minimize corneal and conjunctival scarring.

FOLLICULAR CONJUNCTIVITIS

Follicular conjunctivitis is evidenced by small follicle formation on the bulbar and palpebral conjunctival surfaces. The most common site is the posterior surface of the nictitans. The animal may, on occasion, exhibit epiphora and mucoid exudate. The etiology is unknown, but probably the most commonly incriminated cause is chronic antigenic stimulation.

Follicle formation is commonly observed in dogs with no clinical signs of ocular disease. If the conjunctiva is markedly engorged with tearing or exudation and the animal is in discomfort, therapy is suggested. Other clinical entities must be thoroughly explored before making a definitive diagnosis of follicular conjunctivitis.

Rupture of the follicles with or without cauterization has been the treatment most advocated. In addition, topical antibiotic-steroid combinations are used for short periods. The owner is advised that the follicles may remain but the eye will soon be free of "inflammation."

NICTITATING MEMBRANE: PROTRUSION OF THE NICTITANS

Occasionally, the membrana nictitans prolapses over the corneal surface. In most cases, this finding is secondary to some other abnormality, either orbital or ocular in origin. Some of the orbital causes include retrobulbar cellulitis, mucocele, space-occupying mass, or sinusitis. Irritative lesions of the cornea or conjunctiva are ocular causes for protrusion.

One of the cardinal signs of Horner's Syndrome or sympathetic denervation in the dog and cat, regardless of cause, is protrusion of the membrana nictitans. This is accompanied by enophthalmos, miosis, and ptosis of the involved eye.

In the cat, protrusion occurs without an observable cause. If protrusion proves to be congenital, a portion of the body of the nictitans can be resected to achieve a cosmetic result, but the entire third eyelid is never resected unless there is definitive biopsy proof of a malignancy. Temporary therapy with sympathomimetic drugs may be utilized.

PLASMA CELL INFILTRATION OF THE CONJUNCTIVA

In the German shepherd dog, a prolapsed membrana nictitans that is hyperemic and exhibits giant follicle formation is often seen. On biopsy, plasma cells and histiocytes are present, and the term "plasmoma" has been given to the condition although it should not be considered a malignancy. The membrana nictitans signs may be prodromal to the development of a degenerative pannus and may represent the conjunctival signs of this disease. Treatment may consist of a decongestant (Vasocon-A, Zincfrin) or topical steroid (Maxidex) once daily for control of the conjunctival signs. With therapy, the conjunctival signs decrease, but total remission is rarely achieved.

EVERSION OF THE CARTILAGE

The cartilage of the third eyelid may be everted, usually at the junction of the horizontal and vertical portions. In itself, the eversion is not a serious problem, but occasionally the cartilage rubs on the corneal surface, causing ulcers or acute conjunctivitis. In untreated eyes, a chronic inflammation of the conjunctiva with a mucoid discharge is frequently observed. The defective portion of the cartilage is removed surgically. The free edge of the nictitans is not altered.

TUMORS OF THE CONJUNCTIVA

Conjunctival tumors are rare, usually benign, and most frequently are encountered at the limbus, the anterior surface of the membrana nictitans, or the ventral cul-de-sac. Small tumors may be surgically removed, whereas large tumors involving the conjunctiva or corneal extension should be biopsied before deciding on enucleation or other extensive therapy.

Pseudotumors (fibrous histiocytomas) are frequently encountered at the limbus with corneal extension. This condition is most common in the collie. The histopathologic characteristics include inflammation with a stromal matrix of histiocytes and fibrocytes. The growth is responsive to intralesional and topical steroids or excision or a combination of these procedures. Prolonged topical steroid therapy may be indicated to prevent recurrences.

SUPPLEMENTAL READING

Campbell, L.H., Fox, J.G., and Snyder, S.B.: Ocular bacteria and mycoplasma in the clinically normal cat. Feline Pract. 3:10, 1973.

Campbell, L.H., Snyder, S.B., Reed, C., and Fox, J.G.: Mycoplasma Felis — associated conjunctivitis in cats. JAVMA 163:991, 1973.

Fedukowicz, H.: External Infections of the Eye. New York, Appelton-Century Crofts, 1963.

Smith, J., Bistner, S., and Riis, R.C.: Infiltrative corneal lesions resembling fibrous histiocytomas: clinical and pathological findings in six dogs and one cat. J. Am. Vet. Med. Assoc. 169:722–726, 1976.

Urban, M., Wyman, M., Rheins, M., and Marraro, R.V.: Conjunctival flora of clinically normal dogs. JAVMA 161:201–206, 1972.

DISEASES OF THE LACRIMAL APPARATUS

DAVID COVITZ, D.V.M.
White Plains, New York

The lacrimal apparatus may be divided into secretory and excretory components. Problems involving the excretory component or lacrimal drainage system manifest as obstructions and epiphora. Diseases of the secretory component include lacrimal gland tumors, which are rare in small animals, hypertrophied nictitans glands, which are fairly common and have been adequately reviewed elsewhere, and abnormalities of the tear film.

This discussion is limited to tear film abnormalities and pathology involving the lacrimal drainage system, with an emphasis on medical treatment. In one instance, a surgical technique that has not been previously described is discussed in detail. In other cases, surgical treatment is mentioned where appropriate and the supplemental reading list directs the reader to complete descriptions. The mechanical aspects of examining the lacrimal apparatus are reviewed elsewhere in this text (p. 508).

TEAR FILM

The tear film supplies most of the metabolic needs of the corneal epithelium and superficial stroma. Its other functions include carrying away debris and metabolic waste products, providing antibacterial activity by supplying lysozymes and leukocytes, correcting refractive errors associated with epithelial imperfections, and providing lubrication for proper lid function.

A satisfactory if not entirely accurate description of the tear film is as a three-layer or three-phase precorneal film composed of a superficial oily phase, a middle aqueous phase, and an inner mucin phase.

The oil phase is a product of meibomian glands and serves to prevent evaporation of the aqueous component. The oil also stabilizes the tear film and inhibits epiphora. Incomplete closure of the palpebral fissure prevents complete resurfacing with an oil layer and is important in exposure keratitis. This may be observed in brachiocephalic breeds with exophthalmic conformation and in animals with lid deformities. Hypersecretion and hyposecretion of oil has not yet been identified in veterinary ophthalmology, although the oil phase must play some role in tear film abnormalities associated with generalized seborrhea.

The mucin phase is primarily the product of conjunctival goblet cells. Mucin is a mixture of glycoproteins and forms the basis of mucus, "the free slime of the mucous membranes." By lowering surface tension and prolonging the contact time between the tears and cornea, mucin stabilizes the tear film. Excess production of mucin is a consistent sign associated with keratoconjunctivitis sicca and will be discussed as part of that topic. Mucin deficiency is rarely mentioned in veterinary literature.

Aqueous tears are primarily produced by the lacrimal gland and the nictitans gland, an accessory lacrimal gland producing up to 40 percent of the tears. Minor amounts are contributed by small accessory lacrimal glands within the conjunctiva. When they are functioning normally, the primary lacrimal gland and the nictitans gland are each capable of supplying the total tear requirement, unaided by the other glands. The aqueous component supplies most of the primary functions of the tear film. Hypersecretion of aqueous tears is a normal response to any ocular irritant. By far, the most common tear film abnormality is deficiency of the aqueous component.

KERATOCONJUNCTIVITIS SICCA

Reduction or absence of the aqueous component of tears results in keratoconjunctivitis sicca (KCS). This disorder has a significant incidence and duration in dogs. In cats, it is rarely more than a transient event.

Breed-related forms of KCS represent the largest number of cases in dogs. Clinically, there appear to be at least two distinct breed-related groups. One is breeds with a high incidence of generalized seborrhea — Cocker spaniels, English bulldogs, and perhaps pugs and dachshunds. In affected animals, seborrheic keratoconjunctivitis with excessive mucin production precedes the reduction of aqueous tears. Prior to the development of absolute sicca, vigorous treatment can often result in maintenance of adequate aqueous tear levels. This is especially fortunate when contemplating parotid duct transposition in the English bulldog, a breed with a significant incidence of parotid duct agenesis.

A second breed-related form of KCS is unassociated with seborrhea. Reduction of aqueous tears precedes or occurs simultaneous to the production of excessive mucus. These cases are generally more acute in presentation and faster in progression. Minature schnauzers and West Highland white terriers typify this group, in which maintenance of aqueous tear production is temporary if it exists at all.

Other causes of KCS are neurologic damage, iatrogenic factors, dry eyes associated with systemic disease, and chronic conjunctivitis. Idiopathic cases arise, proving that this classification system is far from complete.

Loss of efferent stimulation from the facial nerve can result in transient or permanent lack of lacrimal secretion. Central facial nerve palsy will show the classic facial muscle paralysis in addition to KCS, whereas more peripheral injuries can produce KCS without facial paralysis or facial paralysis without KCS.

Damage to the ophthalmic branch of the trigeminal nerve results in corneal anesthesia and loss of the first step in the lacrimation reflex. Lack of adequate tearing complicates the management of neurotropic ulcers.

Iatrogenic (drug-induced) KCS has been observed with sulfadiazine and phenazopyridine. Examples include Azulfidine, which contains both these drugs, and Azo Gantrisin, which contains the phenazopyridine dye. Sulfasoxazole, the sulfonamide in Gantrisin, does not seem to retard aqueous tear production. Other sulfonamides have been suspected from time to time, including Avlosulfon, a sulfone used in immune-mediated dermatoses. The tetracycline group was originally suspected but apparently does not affect tear quantity. Drug-induced KCS is usually reversible once the cause is eliminated.

Another iatrogenic cause may be related to nictitans gland removal. Although this will not produce KCS as long as the primary lacrimal gland is functioning normally, there appears to be a higher incidence of KCS in older animals whose nictitans glands previously had been removed.

Any debilitating systemic disease can result in neurogenic KCS, and lacrimal adenitis with KCS is a frequent sign of canine distemper and occasionally of feline rhinotracheitis. If these patients survive, tear secretion will usually return to normal.

Chronic conjunctivitis with scarring and obstruction of lacrimal gland ductules is usually listed as a cause of KCS. This may be significant with seborrhea; however, in other cases it seems more likely that chronic conjunctivitis is the result of tear deficiency and not the cause. The most common error made in the diagnosis of KCS is merely a failure to consider it in the differential diagnosis in any case of chronic conjunctivitis. Diagnosis is fairly straightforward once the possibility is considered.

Diagnosis is based on clinical signs and the Schirmer tear test. Low-normal Schirmer values are reported as 9 mm in one minute for dogs and 6 mm for cats. Definite cases will show less than 5 mm of wetting in one minute. The Schirmer tear test must be performed with minimal restraint and minimal patient upset. Extreme anxiety will result in diminished lacrimal secretion and false Schirmer values, especially in cats.

The clinical signs of KCS vary with the duration and extent of hyposecretion and include congested, thickened, and velvet-textured conjunctiva and signs of chronic keratitis including ulcers, vascularization, pigmentation, scarring, and keratinization. Initially, blepharospasm can be severe. This diminishes as corneal changes become more advanced. Changes in ocular secretions vary from slightly mucoid to the classic picture of a tenacious yellow or greenish yellow mucoid exudate, which clings to conjunctiva and cornea. Dryness and caking of the external nares may be another sign of KCS; however, tears are not the primary source of nasal moisture and unless there is concurrent neurologic damage affecting the nasal mucosa, the nose can appear normal.

In severe cases, the eye is distinctly dry. In milder cases, the eye may appear moist, the only signs being conjunctival congestion, excessive mucus production, and a low Schirmer value. It should be emphasized that unless KCS is remembered in a differential diagnosis of chronic or recurrent conjunctivitis, milder cases will be missed.

Topical treatment with a mixture of pilocarpine, Mucomyst,* and Adapt† ("sicca mix") has improved the medical management of KCS, especially cases associated with seborrhea. When applied topically, pilocarpine directly stimulates viable lacrimal gland tissue; Mucomyst acts as a mucolytic and improves the fluidity of the ocular discharge; and Adapt acts as a vehicle and a long-acting artificial tear. A satisfactory starting mixture is 2 cc 2 percent pilocarpine, 7 cc 10 percent Mucomyst, and 7 cc Adapt mixed to make 16 cc. A final concentration of 0.25 percent pilocarpine seems adequate and produces minimal side effects. An occasional patient will show local hypersensitivity even to dilute pilocarpine solutions.

The transient discomfort when sicca mix is applied is usually due to the Mucomyst. This seems much worse when the mixture is cold; therefore it is kept in a cool spot but it is not refrigerated. When Mucomyst is used as a respiratory mucolytic, the manufacturer advises discarding after 96 hours. That may also apply for treatment of collagenase ulcers; however, when incorporated as a mucolytic in sicca mix, it appears to remain active and shows no increase in side effects when used up to one month.

Initially, sicca mix is applied hourly when possible. The frequency is reduced as improvement is noted. If mucus accumulation ceases to be a problem, Mucomyst can be eliminated from the mixture. Some patients reach a point at which control is good with once or twice daily application of 2 cc 2 percent pilocarpine mixed with 14 cc Adapt.

---

*Acetylcysteine
†Methylcellulose, artificial tears

In the initial treatment period, an antibiotic-steroid ointment (Ophthocort*) is applied twice daily. The steroid is omitted if corneal ulceration is more than punctate. In well controlled cases, the antibiotic-steroid ointment may not be necessary.

In addition to sicca mix and Ophthocort, a vigorous trial is given to systemic stimulation of the lacrimal glands with oral pilocarpine. In establishing an effective dose for a patient, an assumption is made that the salivation stimulating dose of pilocarpine is the same as the lacrimation dose. Usually listed as an undesirable side effect, the salivation point is much easier to monitor as an endpoint. It is a fairly predictable side effect that usually occurs 45 minutes to 1 hour after ingestion, at a dose below the level that produces diarrhea or vomiting.

The dose is established at home by the owner. Starting dose for most patients is one drop 2 percent pilocarpine TID, and final levels vary from two to five drops TID for the average case. Very small patients may show fewer adverse reactions with 1 percent or even 0.5 percent concentration. Considering the possible malfunction of any dropper device, mixing the pilocarpine with a small quantity of food seems safer than direct oral administration. The owner is instructed to look for signs that precede drooling and include lip smacking, tongue flicking, and frequent swallowing. The dose is increased by one drop on the next scheduled treatment, and this is continued until the salivation point is reached. This dose is then maintained TID. If excessive drooling becomes a management problem, the dose is reduced by one drop.

Once a case has reached a fairly stable point, the owner is instructed to compare results with and without oral pilocarpine. Although there are cases maintained on oral pilocarpine for long periods, these are not common. In general, cases that stabilize quickly can usually be maintained with topical treatment alone, and cases showing no significant change in Schirmer values will rarely do well with long-term medical treatment. Within one to two months, cases with inadequate response to medical management will be obvious, and parotid duct transposition is advised. The management of lid caking with salivary precipitates has been simplified with the discovery that 3 percent hydrogen peroxide is a reasonably good solvent.

MUCIN DEFICIENCY SICCA

The corneal epithelium is hydrophobic, and mucin is essential for stability and maintenance of the tear film. In the absence of mucin, the cornea experiences dryness and there is a reflex aqueous hypersecretion. The appearance of the conjunctiva and cornea is similar to that in a case of early KCS, but there is no mucus and there is a paradoxic epiphora. Multiple punctate erosions, squinting, and hypersensitivity to even mild irritants are common signs.

At present, there is no practical method of measuring the mucin content of tears, and diagnosis is based on the appearance of the cornea, the absence of mucus, and a subjective evaluation of tear film stability. This is more difficult to evaluate than aqueous tear production, and it requires a cooperative patient. A fluoresceinized tear film is observed with the biomicroscope through a cobalt blue spot filter. The endpoint is similar to the breaking up of an oil slick on water. "Dry holes" are formed in the tear film and a baring of the corneal epithelium is noted. Break-up times have not been established in dogs, but less than 10 seconds of tear stability would probably be abnormal.

Several cases that fit these criteria have been observed in Shetland sheepdogs and in aged dogs in other small breeds. To date, mucin deficiency has not been suspected in cats.

Available mucin replacers (Adsorbotears and Adapt) seem to irritate these patients. This could be a species difference, or the hypersensitivity could relate to the erosions. It is also possible that the etiology is inaccurate or incomplete.

A lubricant-protectant ointment (Lacri-lube*) applied three to four times daily gives fair to good control. Topical antibiotic or antibiotic-steroid ointment replaces Lacri-lube when indicated.

A trial with oral diethylstilbestrol may be indicated in spayed bitches; mucin deficiency is not rare in menopausal women and is sometimes responsive to hormone replacement. An occasional spayed bitch will show a marked improvement with stilbestrol. A reasonable trial in small dogs might be 0.25 mg diethylstilbestrol per day for one week and every other day thereafter for one month. Low-level maintenance dose is gradually established in responsive cases. If response is less than dramatic during the trial period, the hormone is discontinued.

LACRIMAL DRAINAGE SYSTEM

Tears drain into the lacrimal canaliculi (lacrimal ducts) through the lacrimal puncta, slit-like

---

*Parke Davis

*Allergan Pharmaceuticals, Irvine, California

openings near the nasal canthus at the mucocutaneous junction of both upper and lower lids. The canaliculi converge deep to the canthus and join at the lacrimal sac. In dogs and cats, the sac is almost vestigial and completely encased in bone. A common nasolacrimal duct continues the passage of tears from the sac to the nasal cavity.

Epiphora is a spilling of tears beyond the lid margins onto the face. Once hypersecretion has been ruled out, obstructions in the lacrimal drainage system must be considered. Congenital obstructions are rare. Imperforate puncta are seen occasionally in Bedlington terriers and rarely in other breeds. Atresia of the puncta is observed frequently in small animals, but it is difficult to correlate the size of the openings with the presence or absence of epiphora—i.e., not all animals with small puncta have epiphora. Congenital atresia of the lacrimal or nasolacrimal ducts is rare, and an imperforate nasal opening has never been reported in dogs or cats. Correction of imperforate puncta has been adequately described elsewhere, and the creation of a new tear drainage system has recently been published.

Acquired obstructions include inflammatory closure of the puncta and/or canaliculi associated with conjunctivitis; dacryocystisis and foreign bodies; tumors involving the canaliculi, lacrimal sac, or adjacent tissues; and obliteration by trauma or surgery.

Inflammatory closure usually responds quickly to topical treatment of conjunctivitis. A notable exception is cicatricial stenosis following neonatal herpes conjunctivitis in kittens.

Dacryocystitis is not common in dogs and cats. When it occurs, it is always associated with an obstruction, and most of these are related to plant foreign bodies. External obstructions associated with tumors and nasal or dental infections are less common. Foreign body obstructions can usually be relieved by simple irrigation through the puncta. This is followed by antibiotic-steroid drops (e.g., Cortisporin* or Gentocin† durafilm) four to six times daily for ten days. When patency cannot be established, or in chronic or recurring cases, general anesthesia is advised for further evaluation and initiation of other types of treatment. This might include flat radiographs, dacryocystorhinography, culture and sensitivity, retrograde flushing via the nasal punctum, or placement of an indwelling catheter. (For detailed information consult Supplemental Reading list.)

Benign tumors, cysts, and granulomas occasionally invade from surrounding tissues or arise directly from the canaliculi or lacrimal sac. Malignant tumors of the upper portions of the drainage system and nasolacrimal duct tumors of any description are rare and have not been seen by the author.

When the lacrimal excretory system has been obliterated by surgery or trauma, conjunctivorhinostomy can be considered. This procedure has recently been described for use in dogs and cats. The result of a successful procedure is a mucous membrane-lined fistula from the medioventral conjunctival cul-de-sac (basically the lacrimal lake) to the nasal cavity.

The most common forms of epiphora are breed related. Epiphora in these cases is associated with anatomically patent but functionally inadequate drainage systems. One group in this category comprises the small and medium-sized brachiocephalic breeds such as Persian cats, Pekingese, pugs, and bulldogs. The basic defect is a shallow bony orbit resulting in an exophthalmic globe and an obscure relative position of the drainage system. This is further complicated by nasal canthus entropion, which compresses the puncta and canaliculi. In addition, the trichiasis associated with entropion and to a lesser degree the nasal fold stimulate excessive tear production, which adds to the epiphora. The role played by the nasal folds is probably overstated. The longer hairs from the nasal fold are less of an irritant than are the shorter hairs associated with the medial canthus entropion.

Another breed-related form is the characteristic tear staining seen in miniature and toy poodles, Maltese, the small terrier breeds, and a few others. The cause of epiphora is not as clear in this group. Suspected factors include increased lid tension and compression of the puncta and canaliculi associated with a large globe size, hair growing near or into the nasal canthus (ectopic dermis) acting as a wick, faulty position of the puncta, or a drainage system whose capacity is not adequate for the secretory supply. A combination of these factors is probably a more accurate pathogenesis.

On occasion, epiphora results in moisture dermatitis, but usually the problem is cosmetic and concerns the owner more than the pet. A trial therapy may be given of tetracycline administered orally at a dose of 50 mg daily or every other day. This will sometimes provide surprisingly good control as long as it is continued. Improvement is especially noticeable in white poodles and Maltese, but an equal number of cases show inadequate response. Apparently, the tetracycline group does not alter the rate of tear production, and any beneficial effect is due to the binding of porphyrins, the probable cause of staining associated with epiphora.

*Burroughs Wellcome
†Schering

Reduction of tear production by removal of the nictitans gland is a poor approach to epiphora, especially in brachiocephalic animals that are barely able to maintain an adequate tear film under normal circumstances. Conjunctivorhinostomy is probably excessive treatment for poodle epiphora, although some owners would not agree.

A procedure that may be worthy of trial is resection of the medial palpebral ligament. The purpose is to release the tight anchorage between the nasal canthus and the medial orbital wall. Resection of the ligament relaxes lid tension, improves nasal canthus entropion, and improves the position of the puncta.

The surgical technique has not been previously described. Lateral and anterior traction is placed on the nasal canthus with thumb forceps, and the taut ligament is cut with a single stab incision through the overlying conjunctiva. The conjunctival entry point is immediately below the mucocutaneous junction. Additional separation is completed with blunt or sharp dissection using a tenotomy scissors. The ligament is resected where it originates from the orbicularis muscle. By staying close to the lid margin, only a small conjunctiva opening is required, and the canaliculi will not be injured. Bleeding is usually minimal. Occasional heavy bleeding will occur if the angular vessels are injured. This can be controlled with digital pressure, and no complications have been noted to date. If indicated, hair-producing skin growing within the medial canthus may be resected at this time. Sutures are rarely necessary.

In brachiocephalic dogs, in addition to resection of the ligament, a small permanent nasal tarsorrhaphy will markedly improve the blink reflex, correct any persistent entropion, and protect the nasal aspect of the cornea from nasal fold trichiasis. This will often compromise the upper punctum; however, the improvement in function of the lower punctum and duct will more than compensate.

SUPPLEMENTAL READING

Bistner, S.J., Aquirre, G., and Batik, G.: *Atlas of Veterinary Ophthalmic Surgery.* Philadelphia, W. B. Saunders Co., 1977.

Bryan, G.M.: Diseases of the nasolacrimal system. In Kirk, R.W. (ed.): *Current Veterinary Therapy VI.* Philadelphia, W.B. Saunders Co., 1977.

Covitz, D., Hunziker, J., and Koch, S.A.: Conjunctivorhinostomy: a surgical method for the control of epiphora in the dog and cat. J. Am. Vet. Med. Assoc. 171:251–255, 1977.

Severin, G.A.: Nasolacrimal duct catheterization in the dog. J. Am. Anim. Hosp. Assoc. 8:13–16, 1972.

Severin, G.A.: *Veterinary Ophthalmology Notes,* 2nd ed. Colorado State University Press, Ft. Collins, Colorado, 1976, pp. 111–129.

Yakely, W.L., and Alexander, J.E.: Dacryocystorhinography in the dog. J. Am. Vet. Med. Assoc. 159:1417–1421, 1971.

DISEASES OF THE CORNEA

ROBERT M. GWIN, D.V.M.
Gainesville, Florida

The cornea represents the anterior portion of the outer fibrous tunic of the eyeball, which consists of opaque sclera posteriorly and transparent cornea anteriorly. The cornea in animals is somewhat larger than that of man and occupies approximately one-fifth of the total fibrous tunic. The cornea is not circular in nature but is, in general, somewhat longer in the horizontal meridian, the diameter of which will vary from species to species. The cornea may be considered a functional unit in three separate areas: (1) the cornea is the anterior part of the fibrous tunic, which holds the intraocular contents within the eye and retains the shape of the globe; (2) the cornea is a refractive lens in the ocular visual system, and (3) the cornea is a transparent structure that allows the passage of light through its medium.

The ocular visual system in higher animals contains a total of 60 diopters of refractive power. The cornea is responsible for approximately 40 diopters of the total system and is thus the main refractive lens of the eye. The lens, in fact, acts more as a fine tuning mechanism for acute vision at varying distances. The power of the cornea in the refractive system is associated with both the curvature of the cornea and the difference in refractive indexes between the surrounding medium; i.e., air anteriorly and aqueous humor posteriorly. Diseases involving abnormal refractive errors of the cornea, such as astigmatism in man, are not clinically significant disease processes in animals, although refractive errors do occur in diseases such as keratoconus.

Alterations in corneal transparency are significant clinically and may be associated with decreased vision owing to imbibed fluid in the corneal stroma, increased pigmentation, corneal vascularization, and deposition of metabolic byproducts such as calcium and lipid. Numerous disease entities are associated with loss of vision owing to deposition of these materials.

Loss of the normal supportive capacity of the cornea is frequently observed in cases of acute trauma and in cases of chronic corneal disease such as ulceration, infection, and keratitis.

ANATOMY AND PHYSIOLOGY

The cornea may be divided into four layers: the epithelium with its underlying thin basement membrane, the substantia propria or stroma, Descemet's membrane, and the corneal endothelium.

The corneal epithelium consists of several layers, (usually five to seven), of stratified squamous epithelium which rest on the very thin basement membrane. The basement membrane should not be confused with Bowman's membrane, which is a distinct structural component of the cornea in man. The size and shape of the corneal epithelial cells vary from layer to layer, with the basal layer consisting of plump, cylindrical cells while the outer layers become progressively flattened. The stratified squamous epithelium is not keratinized and is covered with an overlying layer of tear film. This tear film serves a multiple function in that it supplies nourishment and oxygen to the cornea, removes debris and infectious agents from the anterior corneal surface, and provides a more optically smooth anterior corneal surface. The underlying basement membrane is, as previously mentioned, exceedingly thin, but it may represent an important structure in maintaining normal epithelial cell adherence to the underlying corneal structures.

Beneath the corneal epithelium and its basement membrane lies the corneal stroma or substantia propria. The corneal stroma constitutes approximately 90 percent of the total thickness of the cornea. As with the other structures of the cornea, the stroma is avascular, and it consists of two elements — the corneal lamellae and the fixed corneal cells or keratocytes. The corneal lamellae are broad bands of collagenous fibrils that extend in a lamellar pattern across the cornea, parallel to the epithelial surface. The keratocytes are cells of connective tissue origin that lie within the spaces between the corneal lamellae and appear as flat cells with thin nuclei and poorly defined borders.

Deep to the corneal stroma are the remaining layers of the cornea, Descemet's membrane, and the corneal endothelium. Descemet's membrane is an eosinophilic, acellular, homogeneous membrane that separates the corneal stroma from the endothelial cell layer. Descemet's membrane is not modified stroma but appears to be a secretory product of the corneal endothelium. This membrane is a relatively inelastic structure and is also impervious to destruction from collagenase activity. Descemet's membrane represents the last functional barrier to corneal rupture.

The corneal endothelium is a monolayer of cells that extends over the entire inner surface of the cornea. This single cell layer is intimately involved in the process of corneal transparency. The corneal endothelium in animals appears as a mosaic pattern of cells lying upon the inner surface of Descemet's membrane. In some animals, particularly man, the cat, and primates, the regenerative capacity of the corneal endothelial cells is extremely limited. In cases of cellular death, the monolayer system is retained by the enlargement of individual cells and the sliding of these cells over the area deficient in endothelial cells. In the rabbit, on the other hand, mitotic activity within the endothelial cells is extremely profuse. The capacity for mitotic activity in the dog has not been definitively examined. A deficiency in corneal endothelial cells stimulates rapid hydration of the overlying stroma, resulting in corneal edema.

The transparency of the cornea appears to be dependent on several factors, some of which are poorly understood. The physical arrangement of the corneal stromal fibers and their relative state of dehydration are thought to contribute to its clarity. This relative dehydration is partially dependent upon a corneal endothelial cell pumping mechanism, which results in the removal of excessive interstitial water. The epithelium and the endothelium are semipermeable membranes that are resistant to water-soluble solutions while they are more freely permeable to fat-soluble substances. Substances that traverse the cornea must have both water and lipid solubilities to penetrate the cornea.

CONGENITAL CORNEAL DISEASES

Congenital abnormalities of corneal size include microcornea, in which the corneal diameter is smaller than normal, and megalocornea, in which the diameter of the cornea is too large. Both conditions are rare in animals. Microcornea has been observed in the collie breed and is associated with a normal-sized globe, although the cornea is congenitally small. This should not be confused with microphthalmia, which is the presence of a small globe, and which is much more common than microcornea. Megalocornea, an enlargement of the cornea with a relatively normal-sized globe, is probably more rare than microcornea. In cases of congenital glaucoma, the cornea may be enlarged owing to a generalized enlargement of the globe, producing an acquired case of megalocornea. Treatment for either microcornea or megalocornea is not possible; however, the possible inherited aspects of the congenital anomaly should be considered.

Congenital dermoids may be seen in all species of animals and in most cases are probably not inherited. A dermoid, which literally means "resembling skin," is a congenital cystic tumor that is filled with fluid or sebaceous material; the walls are of dermal origin and sometimes give rise to hair, teeth, and other dermal appendages. Congenital dermoids appear most commonly in the larger breeds of dogs and may be unilateral or bilateral. They appear as large or small masses involving the cornea and conjunctiva in the limbal region, usually temporally. Dermoids may be irritating merely by their presence and may cause some degree of visual loss. Treatment of dermoids consists of a local excision from the conjunctiva and adjacent cornea.

Persistent pupillary membranes are another cause of congenital corneal disease. They consist of strands of persisting embryonic tissue of mesodermal origin, which arise from the anterior surface of the iris; they may be found floating free in the anterior chamber or attaching to the opposite side of the iris, the lens, or the corneal endothelium. These regions of corneal attachment appear as focal areas of deep corneal opacification. On occasion, persistent pupillary membranes may stimulate a corneal reaction, which results in diffuse corneal edema. Treatment for persistent pupillary membranes is usually not indicated, and vision in all but the most severe cases is not clinically altered. A mydriatic may be used to try to dilate the pupil and break down the pupillary strands; however, this may also result in a tearing of the corneal endothelium and subsequent corneal edema.

CORNEAL DYSTROPHIES

The word "dystrophy" implies abnormal nutrition. It is used in ophthalmology to describe a number of syndromes in which there is an opacification or degeneration of the various corneal layers that is not associated with a concomitant disease process such as corneal ulceration or corneal trauma. Corneal dystrophies in general are not associated with prominent vascularization or other types of inflammatory phenomena and are often congenital in nature. They are frequently bilateral, may be slowly progressive or static, and are usually not associated with other systemic disease processes or anomalies.

A hereditary corneal dystrophy has been described in the Manx cat. This disease process is observed initially in young animals at approximately four months of age and is characterized by edema of the anterior corneal stroma. The corneal edema becomes progressively worse and produces a bullous keratopathy with resulting epithelial erosion. Preliminary studies have revealed a normal corneal endothelium, and the pathogenesis is not well understood. Treatment for this type of corneal dystrophy includes the topical use of hyperosmotic agents to reduce the amount of fluid present in the cornea. However, treatment is of extremely limited value and the corneal disease will still progress. Owing to the inherited nature of the disease process, these animals should not be bred.

A bilateral, axial corneal dystrophy has been described in the Airedale. Patients are presented with a milky appearance in their eyes that is first noticed at 10 or 11 months of age. The animals may occasionally stumble or bump into objects under darkened conditions. There is no history of previous ocular inflammation, injury, or systemic disease. The lesions appear as white, homogeneous opacities with a 4 to 5 mm area of clear cornea in the paralimbal area and no corneal vascularization. Slit lamp examination reveals sub-epithelial opacification with an apparently normal Descemet's membrane and corneal endothelium. The stromal opacification may also involve deeper stromal layers. Histochemical findings demonstrate intracellular and extracellular lipid deposition. A superficial keratectomy may prove valuable in restoring some vision in these animals; however, the depth of the opacification may preclude total removal of the involved tissue. Owing to the possible inheritance, breeding is not recommended.

A primary endothelial cell dystrophy has been described in the Boston terrier and is associated with a progressive and permanent corneal edema secondary to an abnormal corneal endothelium. The corneal stroma becomes excessively hydrated, resulting in the bluish-appearing cornea. Because of the lack of pain, in many cases these animals are not presented until the corneal edema is pronounced. There is an absence of neovascularization or ocular inflammation. Chronic stromal edema eventually results in a bullous keratopathy and associated rupture of these bullae, resulting in ulceration. Affected animals may present as mature dogs, five years old or older. It is a bilateral disease, and females may be more frequently affected than males. Supportive treatment would include the use of hyperosmotic agents to try to remove the excess fluid from the corneal stroma.

Oval corneal opacities have been observed in the beagle. The lesions are symmetrical and appear horizontally oval at the junction of the middle and lower thirds of the corneas. In this case, the corneal stroma is affected, and lesions may vary from small focal nebulae to lesions with a circular "racetrack." The central lesions are avascular and appear in the same form in different individuals. Although the inheritance pattern, natural history, and etiology are unknown, these lesions are thought to be dystrophic in nature.

CORNEAL DEGENERATIONS

In general, corneal degenerations are associated with ocular diseases or are secondary to trauma. They appear to be somewhat similar to many of the corneal dystrophies in that they are often composed of lipid depositions or mineralization of various corneal layers. However, corneal degenerations are associated with a previous disease process, are frequently unilateral, and are associated with corneal vascularization.

Corneal lipidosis typically has a crystal-like, granular consistency and is made of stromal opacities of various sizes and diameters. Corneal lipidosis may be seen secondary to a variety of corneal inflammatory conditions such as trauma, degenerative pannus in the German shepherd, severe episcleritis, and other disease conditions. Calcium deposition may be observed in dogs with similar disease processes, and its appearance is similar to that of lipid deposition. Treatment for either lipidosis or mineralization of the cornea is dependent on the amount of the cornea involved and the depth of the lesion. In most cases, treatment is not required, since the lesions are focal and the animal is visual; however, a superficial keratectomy should be performed if vision is impaired and if the deposition involves the anterior stroma or corneal epithelium. The primary inflammatory disease should be controlled prior to the corneal surgery.

KERATITIS

ULCERATIVE KERATITIS

The causes of ulcerative keratitis are numerous and include trauma, foreign bodies, exposure, infectious diseases (bacterial, viral, mycotic, chlamydial), and other disease processes (keratoconjunctivitis sicca, corneal endothelial cell degeneration, palsy of the ophthalmic branch of the trigeminal nerve). Ulcerative keratitis frequently exhibits the following signs: pain, blepharospasms, ocular discharge, corneal edema and blueing, corneal vascularization, prolapse of the third eyelid, and enophthalmia.

Diagnosis of ulcerative keratitis is made with the topical application of moistened sterile strips impregnated with fluorescein stain. Since fluorescein is water soluble, it will not penetrate the intact corneal epithelial surface; however, if there is a disruption of the corneal epithelium, the stain will readily penetrate the water-soluble stromal tissues and stain a brilliant green color. Once the presence of a corneal ulcer has been ascertained, it is equally important to determine the cause of the ulcer. Cultures for infectious agents may be taken prior to instillation of a topical anesthetic. Cultures are especially important in animals that have been treated with long-term corticosteroid and/or antibiotic therapy.

The conjunctival fornices and the membrana nictitans should be examined for the presence of a foreign object. Foreign bodies that are still present within the eye generally result in a very painful eye with marked lacrimation and blepharospasms. After instillation of the topical anesthetic, the lids should be gently retracted and the eye should be examined. Foreign bodies are frequently found behind the nictitating membrane, which should be pulled temporally and anteriorly for examination. The use of tranquilization may be necessary, especially in deep ulcers where the blepharospasms and struggling associated with examination of the eye may cause a rupture of the corneal ulcer. Entropion, which commonly involves the lower lid, frequently results in corneal ulceration. This may be difficult to ascertain owing to the secondary blepharospasms that stimulate an inward turning of the eyelid; it may be necessary to examine the dog after the pain is reduced and the ulceration is controlled before determining whether or not a lower lid entropion is truly present.

The position of a corneal ulcer is often important in determining the cause. Central ulcers are frequently associated with exposure keratitis and lack of normal tear production. Ulcers in the medial and inferior cornea may result from foreign bodies present behind the third eyelid, whereas ulcers in the superior and central area of the cornea are often secondary to ectopic cilia in the central upper eyelid, 3 to 5 mm posterior to the lid margin. Lower lid entropion, on the other hand, often presents with an inferior, lateral corneal ulcer. A linear, serpentine, tree-like ulceration that remains fairly superficial may be indicative of a herpetic viral ulceration.

Topical medical treatment is adequate for the majority of corneal ulcers. Deeper corneal ulcers and ulcers that have other complicating problems may require surgical intervention. Topical medications include drugs to control the suspected infectious agent, to relieve the ocular pain and discomfort, to prevent collagenase activity, and, in general, to produce an environment favorable to the healing of the corneal wound. If an infectious agent is not suspected, a broad spectrum antibiotic such as a neomycin-polymyxin-bacitracin ophthalmic ointment may be used four to six times daily to prevent bacterial contamination. If a viral agent is suspected, treatment with idoxuridine* or vidarabine† may be used six to eight times a day initially and then less frequently once the virus is controlled. Mycotic infections may be treated with pimaracin, clotrimazole, or topical amphotericin B. In cats with upper respiratory disease and keratitis associated with chlamydia or mycoplasma agents, the use of either a tetracycline or chloromycetin ointment is indicated six times daily.

Many cases of corneal ulcers present with severe pain and anterior uveitis. This is especially true in cases of chronic ulceration and deep corneal ulcers. The use of topical cycloplegic-mydriatic agents should be instituted. Topical atropine ointment three to four times a day initially is sufficient in the majority of cases to dilate the pupil within 24 hours. After this time, the frequency may be reduced to once or twice daily. It is important not to overtreat an eye with atropine owing to complications such as reduction in tear secretion. In cases of severe uveitis, the use of a combination cycloplegic-mydriatic is indicated. A combination of 0.1 percent scopolamine and 10 percent phenylephrine‡ is much more effective in dilating the pupil. This may be given every two to four hours initially, then less frequently after mydriasis is achieved.

The use of anticollagenase agents is indicated in the treatment of any ulcer showing evidence of "corneal melting" or necrosis. In certain corneal ulcers, either from bacterial agents present or from stimulation of the corneal tissues themselves, a collagenase enzyme is released, causing a breakdown of stromal collagen. The cornea becomes a soft, cloudy, "melting" structure that may soon produce a descemetocele ulcer or corneal rupture. Acetylcysteine should be administered in a concentration of 5 to 10 percent to be effective and non-irritating. Mucomyst* must be refrigerated or it rapidly deteriorates. A combination of topical medications that are beneficial for the treatment of corneal ulcers has been formulated (Table 1). This solution may be put into a one-ounce dropper bottle but must be refrigerated to retain efficacy. Since the cold solution may be discomforting to the animal, a smaller ophthalmic dropper bottle may also be dispensed; the medication necessary for one day may be put into the unrefrigerated smaller bottle to be used on a daily basis. This combined solution may be administered as indicated every two hours the first day and less frequently over the next four to five days, depending on the severity and resolution of the corneal ulcer.

In cases of exposure keratitis or chronic recurrent superficial ulceration, a third eyelid flap may be indicated. In cases of self-mutilation, it may be necessary to bandage the foreleg to the chest to prevent a rubbing or scraping of the paw against the eye.

With deeper corneal ulceration, the severity

---

*Mucomyst®, Mead Johnson and Co., Evansville, Ind. 47721

Table 1. Corneal Ulcer Solution

	FINAL CONCENTRATION
1. 1.2 ml 20% Chloramphenicol Succinate	1%
or	or
1.5 ml 5% Gentamycin Solution	0.3%
2. 6 ml 20% Acetylcysteine	5%
3. 6 ml 1% Atropine Ophthalmic Solution	0.25%
4. 10.8 or 10.5 ml Artificial tears	q.s. to 24 ml

TOTAL 24 ml

Corneal ulcer solution containing all of the topical medications beneficial for ulcer therapy. Must be refrigerated (from Severin, G.A.: *Veterinary Ophthalmology Notes.* 3rd printing. Ft. Collins, Colorado, Colorado State University, 1978.

---

*Stoxil®, Smith Kline and French Labs, Philadelphia, Pa.

†Vira-A®, Parke, Davis and Co., Detroit, Mich. 48232

‡Murocoll #2, Muro Pharm. Labs, 121 Liberty St., Quincy, Mass. 02169

of the disease is obviously compounded and a rupture of the cornea is more likely. A descemetocele ulcer is the deepest of corneal ulcers, since only Descemet's membrane and the corneal endothelium are left. In these cases, Descemet's membrane itself will not retain fluorescein, since it is not water-soluble. The descemetocele ulcer has a clear glassy appearance, whereas the surrounding corneal stroma is frequently edematous and may be soft and "melting." A descemetocele ulcer should be considered an ophthalmic emergency, as rupture of this thin membrane results in a loss of aqueous humor and collapse of the globe. Descemetocele ulcers may be covered surgically with a thin conjunctival flap, which is pulled over the ulcerated area and sutured directly to the adjacent cornea or sutured at either side at the limbus. A second method of surgical therapy for a descemetocele ulcer involves the transposition of adjacent corneal and scleral tissues in what has been termed a "lamellar corneal-scleral transposition." The advantages of this technique are that it immediately fills in the ulcerative defect with healthy corneal tissue and results in a clearer cornea with less scarring in the central cornea. The corneal-scleral transposition is more difficult to perform than the conjunctival flap and requires some degree of expertise.

In cases of ulcerative keratitis in which the descemetocele ulcer ruptures, the wounds must be corrected surgically. Necrotic tissue is removed from the central portion of the ruptured cornea and anterior synechiae are broken down with a cyclodialysis spatula. The cornea may be either closed directly, if the ulcer is small, or closed with a corneal scleral transposition. The anterior chamber is then reformed with air or a balanced salt solution. One of the most critical factors in corneal rupture is time; the quicker the wound can be closed, and the faster the anterior chamber can be reformed and the eye returned to a more normal physiologic state, the better the prognosis.

PANNUS

Degenerative pannus is an immune-mediated disease that stimulates the subepithelial proliferation of fibrovascular tissue in the cornea, usually in a bilateral pattern beginning in the inferior lateral quadrant. Pannus is observed most frequently in the German shepherd dog, although similar lesions may be seen in other breeds. The disease may vary greatly in the degree of corneal involvement and in the amount of fibrovascular proliferation present. In

certain instances, the membrana nictitans and the medial canthus of the eye may also be involved. A scraping or a biopsy of the affected tissue reveals a preponderance of plasma cells; hence, the term "plasmacytoma" was once used. Treatment involves controlling rather than curing the disease, and the owner should be made well aware of this fact. Corticosteroids with or without antibiotics are extremely useful in controlling degenerative pannus. One percent prednisolone acetate* or 0.1 percent dexamethazone† may be used to control the disease in the vast majority of cases. Treatment depends upon the severity of the disease, but in general, when beginning treatment, the eyes need to be medicated at least six times daily for one week and then should be re-examined. In many cases, the animal may be maintained on a once a day treatment in both eyes, but this will vary greatly. The frequency of secondary bacterial infection or mycotic infection with chronic steroid administration is low in the dog. In certain cases in which the treatment becomes refractory, other types of topical steroids may be administered.

KERATOCONJUNCTIVITIS SICCA KERATITIS

Keratoconjunctivitis sicca ("dry eye," KCS) is one of the most common causes of chronic keratitis seen in the dog. It is also seen in the cat but at a much lower frequency. Although this is discussed in other sections on the nasolacrimal system, it is important at least to remind the reader of the high incidence of cases of KCS in the dog as a cause of chronic keratitis. KCS usually presents with a history of red eyes with a thick mucoid discharge that responds poorly or incompletely to topical medications. It would be advisable for the clinician to test routinely with the Schirmer tear test strip any time an animal is presented with a thick mucoid discharge, and whenever a conjunctivitis or keratitis persists for over 30 days.

CHRONIC KERATITIS AND SEQUESTRUM

There is a rather unusual syndrome seen in the domestic cat that is believed to be observed most frequently following chronic ulcerative keratitis and other rather non-specific conditions. The syndrome is termed "corneal seques-

---

*Pred Forte®, Allergan Pharmaceuticals Inc., 2525 Dupont Drive, Irvine, Ca. 92713
†Maxitrol®, Alcon Labs, 6201 South Freeway, Fort Worth, Texas 76134

trum" and is characterized by the presence of a darkly pigmented tissue in the anterior corneal stroma and epithelium. This degenerative tissue appears to be necrotic cornea. The sequestrum may be somewhat flat, involving a large portion of the cornea, or it may be more focal and raised in appearance. The treatment of choice in these lesions is a superficial keratectomy to the depth of the sequestrum. The incidence of recurrence is small and may be associated with incomplete removal of the deeper portions of the sequestrum.

CORNEAL ENDOTHELIALITIS

Inflammation of the corneal endothelium is observed in natural cases of canine hepatitis infection or can be secondary to the first vaccination of young dogs with the modified live canine adenovirus I. This disease process is frequently termed "blue-eye" owing to the diffuse corneal edema that occurs when the corneal endothelium is damaged, giving the cornea a bluish coloration. This endotheliotropic virus may invade the corneal endothelium, resulting in marked destruction of the corneal endothelial cells. The bluish appearance of the cornea is not part of the primary disease process but is secondary to the loss of corneal endothelium and may occur in any case of corneal endothelial disease. Dogs should be treated with topical and, in severe cases, systemic corticosteroids to try to reduce the immune reaction and anterior uveitis. Topical mydriatics such as atropine sulfate may be administered initially every two to three hours until the pupil dilates, and then two to four times daily to maintain the dilated pupil. In the majority of cases, this regime of therapy to control the uveitis and keep the pupil well dilated is sufficient to control the disease process. In other instances, a persistent chronic corneal edema may involve a portion or, rarely, the whole cornea owing to the lack of corneal endothelial cells. The most common secondary complication is the development of glaucoma as a result of destruction of outflow channels.

TUMORS OF THE CORNEA

Primary tumors of the cornea are extremely rare, and the majority of tumors that are seen arise from the limbus, which is the area of epithelial transition between the cornea and conjunctiva, or invade the cornea from other adjacent structures such as the conjunctiva, sclera, or anterior uvea.

Two disease processes involving the proliferation of fibrous tissue combined with an inflammatory component have been described in small animals. These two tumor-like proliferations, nodular fasciitis and fibrous histiocytoma, frequently arise in the limbal area and invade the cornea. They are nodular, smooth, and non-pigmented with an abundant vascular supply and a variable growth rate. The lesions have several similarities and may be variations of the same general process. Fibrous histiocytoma if found almost exclusively at the limbus, is frequently bilateral, and is seen frequently in the collie. Nodular fasciitis, on the other hand, may be observed in other areas of the eye and adnexal structures. In either case, the majority of these growths may be treated by local excision. The incidence of recurrence is small, but it may occur.

Squamous cell carcinoma is customarily seen in albino or lightly pigmented animals, and it appears to be more common in the cat than in the dog. Corneal involvement is seen when the squamous cell carcinoma arises in the region of the limbus, and in the majority of cases, this non-pigmented mass remains fairly superficial. A superficial keratectomy with removal of the tumor and adjacent conjunctiva, episclera, and scleral tissues is the treatment of choice for squamous cell carcinoma.

The cornea may be invaded by neoplastic cells associated with lymphosarcoma. Corneal changes associated with this tumor invasion may include a white, cellular infiltrate, keratitis with corneal edema and vascularization, keratic precipitates, and intrastromal hemorrhages. Secondary ulceration of the cornea may also be observed.

Other processes such as an infected corneal abscess or epithelial inclusion cysts may mimic corneal tumors. These masses may be easily removed with a superficial keratectomy if indicated.

TRAUMATIC CORNEAL WOUNDS

Traumatic corneal wounds are frequently seen following automobile trauma, gunshot wounds, and cat fights. Corneal wounds, whether penetrating or non-penetrating, are usually surgical emergencies. On occasion, small wounds may be self-sealing and therefore may not require surgical intervention. In closing a corneal wound, only ophthalmic suture with a swaged-on spatula or reverse cutting needle designed specifically for suturing the cornea should be used. The use of other types of needles and suture material that are not swaged-on results in poor and inadequate closure of the cornea wound. Corneal wounds are closed most frequently with absorbable suture such as Dexon* or Vicryl.† These sutures may be used in the range of 4–0 to 7–0, are relatively non-reactive, and handle well. In non-penetrating wounds, the sutures should be placed approximately 1 to 1.5 mm apart with a 1 mm bite on either side of the corneal wound. The needle should be passed through the deepest portion of the corneal wound and brought up evenly on the opposite side. Sutures should be tied snug but not overly so, since tearing and dehiscence of the wound may result. In penetrating wounds, the margins of the cornea should be trimmed of all necrotic tissue, and any tissue extending through the wound (such as iris tissue) should either be trimmed off or replaced into the anterior chamber. Anterior synchiae, which are frequently present following corneal rupture, should be freed from their adhesions with a cyclodialysis spatula or similar instrument. The corneal wound should be sutured in a manner similar to that for a non-penetrating corneal wound, with the sutures

placed deep in the corneal stroma; this results in a primary healing of the corneal wound with good apposition and little scarring. If the corneal wound is difficult to secure with single interrupted sutures, a continuous suture pattern may then be placed over the single interrupted sutures to provide more adequate support. Sutures should remain in the cornea for two to three weeks, depending on the rate of healing of the primary wound.

---

*Dexon®, Davis and Geck, American Cyanamid Co., Pearl River, N. Y. 10965

†Vicryl®, Ethicon Inc., Somerville, N. J., 08876

SUPPLEMENTAL READING

Bistner, S.I., Aguirre, G., and Shively, J.N.: Hereditary corneal dystrophy in the Manx cat: a preliminary report. Invest. Ophthalmol. 15:15, 1976.

Dice, P., and Martin, C.L.: Corneal endothelial — epithelial dystrophy in the dog. Proceedings of the 7th Amer. Coll. of Vet. Ophthalmologists: 36, 1976.

Gelatt, K.N., Peiffer, R.L., and Stevens, J.: Chronic ulcerative keratitis and sequestrum in the domestic cat. JAAHA 9:204, 1973.

Gwin, R.M., Gelatt, K.N., and Peiffer, R.L.: Ophthalmic nodular fasciitis in the dog. JAVMA 170:611, 1977.

Parshall, C.J.: Lamellar corneal-scleral transposition. JAAHA 9:270, 1973.

Smith, J.S., bistner, S., and Riis, R.: Infiltrative corneal lesions resembling fibrous histiocytoma: clinical and pathologic findings in six dogs and one cat. J. Am. Vet. Med. Assoc. 169(7):722–726, 1976.

DISEASES OF THE LENS

R. C. RIIS
Ithaca, New York

The lens evolved in the development of the eye as an aid to image formation by virtue of its ability to change its shape under the influence of zonular tension. This range of change has yet to be evaluated for companion animals. The lens capsular accommodation depends on the original lenticular shape. The flatter lenses of primates and some birds are well adapted to accommodation. However, the almost spherical lenses of cats or rodents are hard to deform, even with full accommodation. For this reason, fish with spherical lenses have an accommodative mechanism based on lens movement rather than on changes in lens shape.

The range of accommodation in different animal groups is influenced by several factors, including the size of the eyeball, the pupil diameter, the retinal surface area, and the tapetal

characteristics. The smaller an animal's eye, the closer objects can be to the eye before the need to accommodate arises. The smaller the animal eye, the larger the relative lens volume.

LENS GROWTH

Lens growth continues after body growth is fully achieved. The lens epithelium is a monolayer of cells internal to the anterior capsule. Growth activity occurs in the equatorial region during the life of the animal, with the new fibers growing axially toward the two poles, directly beneath the epithelium anteriorly and beneath the capsule posteriorly. The continued addition of new fibers from the epithelium gradually thickens the cortex with age, and the nucleus simultaneously compacts or becomes sclerotic.

NUCLEAR SCLEROSIS

As animals age, reduced transparency of the lens is normal owing to light scattering by the nucleus. If physiologic, no opacities are visible, even with slit lamp examination. The prognostic significance is considerably different than that for cataracts, since nuclear sclerosis does not progress to blindness. Occasionally, nuclear sclerotic changes have concurrent incipient cataracts in the peripheral cortex, but most of these remain static and the animal remains visual. Classification of cataracts based on slit lamp examination is shown in Table 1.

LENS COLORATION

In lenses with a nuclear coloration (brunescence), light absorption by the brown proteins and light scatter contribute to the loss of transparency. Considerable experimental evidence has been presented showing that the brown color of lens proteins could result from the binding of colored quinones to the amino and thiol groups of lens proteins with a consequent lowering of the protein solubility in water. Brunescent cataracts, while common in man, are infrequently seen in animals. The normal cat lens is comparable to the normal human lens in coloration. Kynurenine and the fluorescent glucosides are pale yellow pigments with absorption in the 360 nm wave lengths.

Ommochromes are colored pigments derived from 3-hydroxykynurenine and are often responsible for the color of insect lenses.

LENS SUBLUXATIONS AND LUXATIONS

The lens is fixed in position behind the iris by fibers of the ciliary zonule. These fibers are aggregates of exceedingly fine fibrils. At the origin and insertion, the component fibrils fan out to attach over a wide area. Two distinct groups of fibers are recognized — the anterior fibers and the posterior fibers. The anterior fibers orig-

Table 1. Lens Classification by Slit Lamp Examination

1. Clear lens
2. Nuclear cataract—cortex relatively clear
3. Cortical cataract—spoke-like opacities and water clefts
4. Subcapsular cataract—most of the cortex remains clear
5. Opaque lenses:
   a. Intumescent cataract (swollen lens)
   b. Mature cataract
   c. Hypermature cataract (the cortex is liquefied and the capsule wrinkled)

inate near the ora serrata and follow the major ciliary processes to insert anteriorly at the equator of the lens. The posterior fibers arise from the surface of the ciliary body in front of the origin of the anterior fibers. These fibers lie on either side of the major or minor ciliary process, which they follow to their insertions on the posterior lens capsule near the equator. The two groups of fibers cross at an oblique angle near the tips of the ciliary process to hold the lens stable.

The clinical significance of abnormal lens-zonular attachments is subluxation or luxation of the lens. Displaced lenses are common and occur in a variety of breeds (basset hound, cocker spaniel, Jack Russell terrier, miniature schnauzer, Norwegian elkhound, Sealyham terrier, smooth-haired fox terrier, wire-haired fox terrier). A complete rupture results in total luxation; partial rupture leads to subluxation.

The breeds most frequently affected are the terriers, but the miniature schnauzers and Norwegian elkhounds also have been involved rather often. The breeds considered hereditarily predisposed to lens displacement usually are affected between the ages of three and seven years. In these breeds, the luxation may cause glaucoma, especially if the lens luxates completely into the anterior chamber. Even though lens displacement may initially be unilateral, it should be considered a bilateral condition. The displacement is usually downward and rarely off to one side. Clinically, this allows one to visualize a dorsal aphakic crescent. A hereditary predilection for canine lens luxation is suspected. The development of this condition is usually bilateral, but each eye may present at different times. The history may note depression, lacrimation, blepharospasm, and visual loss. If the lens is luxated or subluxated posteriorly behind the iris, iridodonesis may be evident when the eye or head moves. Iridodonesis may result in an anterior uveitis. Secondary glaucoma may occur if the iridocorneal angle is compromised by a dilated pupil and lens luxation from the posterior to the anterior chamber.

A lens luxation or subluxation may be an exciting factor, the sole contributor or the sequela of glaucoma. Anterior lens luxation that results in glaucoma may be a diagnostic challenge owing to corneal endothelial contact causing a dense stromal edema. Transillumination of the anterior chamber may be required to outline the lens and verify the diagnosis. Intraocular pressure measurements with indentation tonometry are not accurate because of the position of the lenses immediately adjacent to the cornea. Buphthalmos is characteristic of chronic anterior luxations with permanent retinal damage.

Acute anterior luxations can be manually replaced into the posterior chamber with the aid of intravenous 15 percent mannitol administered at 10 mg/kg given over 20 to 30 minutes. Gentle ocular massage through the lids usually repositions the lens into the posterior chamber after maximal osmotic affect is obtained (30 to 45 minutes post-IV therapy). The lens then can be held in the posterior chamber with a miotic agent such as Phospholine Iodide* 0.03 percent once daily.

Acute posterior luxation into the vitreous usually causes no immediate complication other than marked iridodonesis or total aphakia if the vitreous is liquefied. If the vitreous is normal and the lens is held medically in place by miotics, conservative medical control may be acceptable. A possible eventual degeneration of the vitreous and retina may develop from the lens instability. Complications of glaucoma and retinal degeneration from lens luxation may be avoided by intracapsular lens extraction.

Intracapsular extraction is much easier if the lens is entrapped in the anterior chamber. A posteriorly luxated lens may be extremely difficult to remove without creating excessive trauma. Both procedures should be performed by an experienced ophthalmic surgeon.

In the treatment of the displaced lens within breeds known to have goniodysgenesis (i.e., bassets and cocker spaniels), glaucoma therapy should be considered as well.

Lens displacement and widely dilated unresponsive pupils in primary open angle glaucoma of the beagle may be a clinical sign relative to a visual complaint. The lenses may appear to be small. Microphakia is a possibility in this breed and in several others. To establish microphakia as a contributor to lens displace-

---

*Ayerst Laboratories, 685 Third Avenue, New York, N.Y. 10017.

ment, lens measurements should be taken routinely after the removal of an acutely displaced lens. ("Canine and Feline Glaucoma" should be referred to for treatment recommendations.)

Lens displacement can occur secondary to trauma, inflammation, hypermature cataracts, and ciliary neoplasms. Lens discolorations in the cat are usually secondary to these complications.

CATARACTS

A cataract is any lens opacity and may be hereditary or non-hereditary. Congenital cataracts are present when the eyelids first open; acquired cataracts appear later in life (Table 2). A non-hereditary congenital cataract may result from fetal insults during pregnancy or postnatal nutrition-related deficiencies during the first few weeks of life.

Congenital cataracts may be inherited, secondary to other ocular developmental abnormalities, or the result of maternal influences. Breeders are especially concerned about hereditary possibilities. Essential historical information includes:

1. Dam access to toxicants during pregnancy
2. The health of the dam during pregnancy
3. Medication of the pregnant dam
4. Normality of the dam and sire
5. Known cataracts in the blood lines
6. Mortality rate in litter
7. The diet of the dam and litter
8. Normal birth and nursing
9. Previous litter history
10. Number in litter affected.

In cataract formation, the loss of transparency begins in the nucleus or cortex. Totally opaque lenses represent advanced stages of cataracts

Table 2. Cataract Heredity

BREEDS WITH UNKNOWN INHERITANCE	BREEDS WITH KNOWN INHERITANCE	INHERITANCE CHARACTERISTICS
Alaskan malamute	Afghan hound	Suspect recessive
Australian shepherd	American cocker spaniel	Suspect recessive
Basenji	Beagle	Dominant
Borzoi	Boston terrier	Simple autosomal recessive
Chesapeake Bay retriever	German shepherd	Dominant
Collie	Golden retriever	Dominant
English cocker spaniel	Labrador retriever	Dominant
English springer spaniel	Miniature poodle	Simple autosomal recessive
Irish setter	Miniature schnauzer	Simple autosomal recessive
Samoyed	Old English sheepdog	Recessive
Shetland sheepdog	Pointer	Dominant
Siberian husky	Staffordshire bull terrier	Simple autosomal recessive
	Toy poodle	Simple autosomal recessive

Table 3. Cataract Progression Based on Location

POSITION OF LENS OPACITY, CLEFT, VACUOLE, OR WEDGE	PROGNOSIS FOR PROGRESSION TO MATURITY
Anterior capsule	Usually non-progressive
Anterior subcapsule	Usually non-progressive
Anterior cortex	Progressive
Perinuclear	Usually non-progressive
Nuclear	Usually non-progressive
Posterior cortex	Progressive
Posterior subcapsule	Unpredictable
Posterior capsule	Unpredictable
"Y" suture	Usually non-progressive

that began in the cortex. In intumescent lenses and mature cataracts, the lens nucleus also opacifies. The developing or incipient cataract can progress to opacification of either the nucleus or cortex. The progression of any lens opacity is difficult to predict. Bimonthly evaluations of the opacity following diagnosis is recommended. Table 3 gives an estimate of potential cataract progression based on location of the opacity that may clarify the prognosis.

CATARACT DEVELOPMENT

Early subtle changes of the lens resulting in minimal opacities is defined as an "incipient cataract." These opacities may be fine grey striae or minute globules that appear in the lens periphery. They may be caused by physical or chemical changes in the lens fibers.

The developing cataract causes swelling of the lens fibers and forms an "intumescent cataract." Intumescence of the lens is not fully understood but is described as an increase in intracapsular osmotic pressure after proteolysis of the cataractous lens proteins. Occasionally, intumescence of the lens increases the lens volume considerably and consequently reduces the depth of the anterior chamber. Concern over compromise of the iridocorneal angle from an edematous lens is most common in diabetic dogs. The anterior lens capsule may be very prominent and the anterior chamber may be shallow when viewed from the side. Oblique illumination casts a shadow on the opaque portions of the lens. Transparent portions of the lens among opaque cortical wedges allow the fundus reflex to be observed. The animal is variably visual at this stage.

The "mature cataract" is uniformly opaque. The anterior chamber is within normal depth limits. However, the fundus reflex is no longer evident and the animal is blind at this stage. In a mature cataractous lens, a decreased lens volume is suggested when measured by ultrasonography. The depth of the anterior chamber serves as an indirect measure of lens thickness. In unilateral cataract patients, the anterior chamber depth may be deeper in the cataractous eye.

Progression to a "hypermature cataract" occurs when the lens cortex liquefies, allowing the nucleus to gravitate freely. The lens capsule wrinkles and flattens, with the absorption of cortex material especially at the periphery. Translucent areas may become transparent, depending upon residual opacities of the capsule and nucleus. Vision is partially restored if this clearing progresses slowly. Frequent examinations are recommended at this time because lens protein-induced uveitis may result. Owners should be observant for the development of the characteristic "red eye" signs of uveitis. Topical corticosteroid preparations used three times a day for two weeks usually give good control initially and should be followed by reduced dosages for prolonged periods as needed. Mydriatics are not recommended because of the possible complications of phacolytic glaucoma.

Phacolysis is the change from dense cataractous lens tissue to a fluid consistency. The fluid nature allows migration from the lens capsule, which may be recognized by the immune system as foreign protein. A severe inflammatory reaction may increase the resistance of aqueous outflow to cause a "phacolytic glaucoma." Oral carbonic anhydrase inhibitors along with topical corticosteroids (Maxidex®)* are indicated. Generally 2 mg per kg of body weight, three times daily of dichlorphenamide (Daranide®)† helps control the intraocular pressure. Ethoxzolamide (Cardrase®)‡ is an alternative diuretic that can be used at 5 mg/kg BID or TID. Over prolonged periods, dosages of these diuretics cause hypokalemia and metabolic acidosis if supplementary potassium is not prescribed.

SUGAR CATARACTS

The monosaccharides glucose, galactose, and xylose rapidly pass from the blood into the aqueous. The appearance of experimental sugar cataracts develops most rapidly in young animals. Xylose cataracts can only be produced in

*Alcon Laboratories, Inc., 6201 South Freeway, Fort Worth, Tex. 76134

†Merck, Sharp and Dohme, Division of Merck Company, Inc., West Point, Penna. 19486

‡Allergan Pharmaceuticals, 2525 Dupont Drive, Irvine, Calif. 92664

weanling rats. Glucose and galactose cataracts developed in rats made diabetic and fed a diet of 20 percent galactose. All three sugars are reduced to the corresponding sugar alcohol by aldose reductase in the lens. The reduction of glucose by aldose reductase is greatly accelerated when the concentration of glucose in the aqueous is raised. The net result is the accumulation of sorbitol within the lens.

The lens is relatively impermeable to sugar alcohols — therefore, once formed, they cannot readily diffuse from the lens. The presence of sugar alcohols upsets the osmotic equilibrium, encouraging water to be drawn into the lens. The increased water content causes the lens fibers to swell and form vacuoles and clefts. With fiber damage, the lens becomes an opaque white. Provided the lens changes are not too far advanced, galactose cataracts are reversible if the diet is discontinued. Xylose cataracts in rats regress even if the diet is continued. Glucose cataracts are permanent.

Undiagnosed diabetic dogs and cats may have a visual problem on initial presentation. The ocular examination usually identifies either a homogeneous mature cataract or a vacuolated lens with rapidly developing punctate opacities. Historically, the loss of vision is rather acute. Polydipsia and polyuria may be present.

Although a diabetic animal may have normal lenses at the time of examination, cataracts are predictable within the next six months. Regulation of the diabetic patient with insulin is of little help, since the disease in animals cannot be finely controlled. The experimental development of an aldose reductase inhibitor may some day prevent the development of diabetic cataracts in animals.

TRANSIENT LENS OPACITIES

Acute reversible lens opacity has been described in rodents. The etiology of this opacity has been explained on the basis of increased aqueous osmolarity, which encourages dehydration of the anterior superficial lens fibers and epithelium. Factors contributing to osmolarity changes are incomplete lid closure resulting in evaporation from the corneal surface, infrequent blinking, or decreased aqueous production. Decreased aqueous production has been noted following hypothermia, anesthesia, and vasoconstriction. Lens transparency returns once normal conditions are reinstated.

The effect of chronic administration of dimethyl sulfoxide (DMSO) to the eyes of laboratory animals is unique. The cortical fibers become less transparent than normal, but the deeper cortical and nuclear fibers remain normal. This change appears as a pearl-like opalescence. The effect of DMSO on the lens has been recorded following skin application to dogs (2.5 g/kg/day) and rabbits (1 g/kg/day) for extended periods of from 9 and 11 weeks, respectively. The lens changes disappear after the drug is discontinued.

CATARACT THERAPY

Cataract resolution from medical therapy using vitamin complexes, selenium, zinc, quericitin (Quertin®), and palosein (Orgotein®) is not acceptable according to the American College of Veterinary Ophthalmologists.

Surgical therapy to restore vision is worthy of consideration in animals that qualify physically for the procedure. In breeds that develop cataracts in association with either progressive retinal atrophy (PRA) or central progressive retinal atrophy (CPRA), an electroretinogram (ERG) is necessary to justify surgery (Table 4).

Surgical techniques are divided into several procedures: those that remove (1) the entire lens (intracapsular extraction), (2) the anterior lens capsule and cataract (extracapsular extraction), (3) the cataract by aspiration, or (4) the cataract by ultrasonic fragmentation and aspiration. Each procedure has indications that render it most appropriate for the individual patient and surgeon. All procedures should be performed by an experienced ophthalmic surgeon.

Table 4. Breeds with Cataracts Associated with PRA and CPRA

PRA	CPRA
American cocker spaniel	English cocker spaniel
Irish setter	English setter
Miniature poodle	Labrador retreiver
Toy poodle	
Norwegian elkhound	

SUPPLEMENTAL READING

Aquirre, G.C., and Bistner, S.I.: Microphakia with lenticular luxation and subluxation in cats. VM/SAC 498–500, 1973.
Barnett, K.C.: Hereditary cataract in the dog. J. Sm. Pract. 19:109–120, 1978.
Butenandt, A., and Schafer, W.: *Ommochromes in Chemistry of Natural and Synthetic Coloring Matters.* New York, Academic Press, 1962.

Dodt, E.: Physical factors in the correlation of ERG spectral sensitivity curves with visual pigments. Am. J. Ophthal. 46:87–91, 1958.

Formston, C.: Observations on subluxation and luxation of the crystalline lens in the dog. J. Comp. Path. 55:158–185, 1945.

Hanna, C., and Frannfelder, F.T.: Acute reversible lens opacity: Fine structure changes. Exper. Eye Res. 12:181–183, 1971.

Lawson, O.D.: Luxation of the crystalline lens in the dog. J. Sm. Anim. Pract. 10:461–463, 1969.

Martin, L.C.: Zonular defects in the dog. A clinical and scanning electron microscopic study. AAHA 14:571–579, 1978.

Playter, R.F.: The development and maturation of a cataract. AAHA 13:317–322, 1977.

Pollock, R.V.H.: The eye. In Evans, H.E., and Christensen, G.C. (eds.): *Anatomy of the Dog*, 2nd ed. Philadelphia, W.B. Saunders Co., 1979.

DISEASES OF THE ANTERIOR UVEA

KIRK N. GELATT, V.M.D.,
J. DANIEL LAVACH, D.V.M.,
and R. DAVID WHITLEY, D.V.M.
Gainesville, Florida

The anterior uvea consists of the iris and the ciliary body. Both structures are highly vascular and pigmented. The iridal aperture regulates the amount of light entering the posterior segment, and its pigmentation absorbs light, thereby preventing light-induced damage. The anterior iridal surface of the dog is more uniform than that in man, exhibiting few shallow depressions ("crypts"). A large basal arteriolar circle is situated either in the iridal root or in the anterior ciliary body. Incision of the iridal root in the dog, therefore, is apt to produce extensive hemorrhage without the use of electrocautery.

Pupil size represents a balance between the iridal sphincter and the dilator musculature. The sphincter tone predominates, with the pupil appearing miotic in the normal eye and often extremely miotic in the inflamed eye. The sphincter muscle is innervated by the parasympathetic fibers (see "Neuroophthalmology").

The light-induced pupillary reflex is subcortical; it requires the integrity of the retina, optic nerve, optic chiasm, optic tracts, Edinger-Westphal nucleus, oculomotor nerve (parasympathetic fibers), ciliary ganglion, and the iridal sphincter. Lesions of the afferent-efferent pathways and the iridal sphincter are usually extensive before detectable changes occur in the pupillary reflex. Variables in the light-induced pupillary reflex include the intensity of the light stimulus, direction of the beam, psychic state of the patient, presence of ocular and neural diseases, amount of background illumination, and drugs.

The iris is examined by illumination and magnification, preferably with a biomicroscope. A focused beam of light is directed across the anterior surface to check for aqueous humor flare and inflammatory exudate. With iridocyclitis, the aqueous protein concentration increases from 30 to 50 mg percent to several grams percent; this increased protein appears as turbidity or a "flare."

The ciliary body's pars plica or processes is the source of the aqueous humor. Formation of aqueous is by active secretion and ultrafiltration. The ciliary body musculature is poorly developed in the dog and, consequently, accommodation is limited. The predominantly longitudinal muscle fibers mainly affect aqueous humor outflow.

Examination of the ciliary body is obstructed by the iris and necessitates special procedures. Indirect ophthalmoscopy and mydriasis allow partial observation of the caudal pars plana ventrally and medially. With adequate illumination, occasional ciliary body processes can be viewed directly. The sclero-ciliary cleft in the anterior chamber angle can be observed by gonioscopy.

CONGENITAL ABNORMALITIES

The most common congenital iris abnormalities include persistent pupillary membranes, colobomas, and iridal hypoplasia. Heterochromia represents a normal color variation but may be associated with other concurrent ocular and hearing abnormalities.

PERSISTENT PUPILLARY MEMBRANES

The pupil is covered by a vascular membrane (pupillary membrane) until the last trimester of gestation and occasionally as late as two to six weeks postparturition. Persistent pupillary membranes (PPMs) refer to the incomplete atrophy of the pupillary membrane or its adherence to the lens and/or cornea. Contact between the cornea and/or lens by PPMs usually results in a focal corneal opacity (leukoma) or a capsular cataract.

The extent and involvement of PPMs are highly variable. The persistent pupillary membrane syndrome may appear sporadically in purebred dogs and cats or may be inherited as in the Basenji dog (although the mode of inheritance is uncertain). PPMs may also occur more frequently in the Shetland sheepdog.

Persistent pupillary membranes may be pigmented and/or translucent, appearing as linear to branching bands. They arise from the collarette region of the iris and thus can be differentiated from posterior synechiae, which are sequelae to iridocyclitis.

The corneal and lens opacities associated with adherent PPMs are variable. The corneal opacities are caused by alterations in the endothelium, Descemet's membrane, and the posterior stroma. Thin, translucent PPMs can touch the anterior lens capsule but do not produce cataract formation, whereas pigmented PPMs usually produce static anterior capsular-subcortical cataracts. PPMs that bridge the pupil may distort the pupil and interfere with mydriasis.

Treatment of PPMs is not usually necessary unless vision is impaired. Drug-induced mydriasis can improve vision and occasionally break the PPMs. Mydriasis with PPMs adherent to the cornea may induce corneal edema from traction on the posterior corneal structures. In patients blind from extensive PPMs and cataracts, cataract extraction and resection of PPMs can be performed by utilizing electrocautery to maintain hemostasis.

COLOBOMAS OF THE IRIS

In the dog, colobomas of the iris are rare and occur most frequently in the blue irides. Iridal colobomas are frequently associated with other uveal anomalies and are classified as typical (6 o'clock position) or atypical. Colobomas in the brown iris manifest as an irregular pupil with the affected area a light tan color or lacking in pigment entirely. Concurrent ciliary body colobomas and the absence of zonules in the defect result in an obvious flattening of the adjacent lens equator.

Colobomas of the blue iris may be partial (involving the stroma) or full thickness. Partial iridal colobomas are usually black because of the exposed pigment epithelium, and these may simulate a melanoma. Full-thickness iridal colobomas consist of holes of varied sizes and shapes (pseudopolycoria) that can be somewhat compressed by mydriasis.

Animals with colobomas of the iris may exhibit increased sensitivity to light (photophobia). Treatment is not usually necessary.

HETEROCHROMIA IRIDES

Heterochromia irides is a normal color variation in the dog that commonly occurs in the blue merle collie, Shetland sheepdog, Pembroke Welsh corgi, Australian shepherd, Siberian husky, old English sheepdog, harlequin great Dane, beagle, and Pekingese. In some breeds, the blue irides are associated with the merling gene.

In the homozygous merled Australian shepherd, collie, Shetland sheepdog, and harlequin great Dane, heterochromia irides may be associated with other anomalies. These include microphthalmia, microcornea, dyscoria, corectopia, cataracts, equatorial staphylomas, retinal dysplasia, and detachments. In the Australian shepherd, the complex is inherited as an autosomal recessive disease with variable expression.

Heterochromia irides in cats is associated with a dominantly inherited white haircoat. Deafness and blue irides are inherited as autosomal dominant traits with incomplete penetrance and incomplete dominance, respectively. The ocular fundus is subalbinoid, exhibiting limited pigmentation of the non-tapetal fundus and absence of a tapetum.

INFLAMMATIONS OF THE ANTERIOR UVEA

Anterior uveitis or iridocyclitis in dogs and cats may be restricted to the eye or may be part of a pansystemic disease. The ocular reaction may be the presenting clinical sign and often can provide useful information relative to the cause of the systemic disease.

SIGNS

The signs of anterior uveitis include miosis, ocular hypotony, aqueous flare to frank hypopyon, corneal edema, deep corneal neovascularization, and ciliary flush (bulbar conjunctival hyperemia). Other clinical signs include blepharospasm, tearing, photophobia, and increased sensitivity or tenderness about the eye.

Upon close examination, the aqueous humor appears turbid; the increased protein and inflammatory cell concentrations are evidenced as "flare." Cellular and proteinaceous precipitates may adhere to the posterior cornea, anterior lens capsule, and anterior iris. Loose iridal pigment cells can be detected with 25 to 40 × magnification on the anterior lens capsule, in the posterior cornea, and in the iridocorneal angle.

The corneal stroma is diffusely edematous. Deep corneal neovascularization occurs circumcorneally; the fine, short blood vessels are easily confused with pigmentation. The pupil is usually pinpoint. When mydriasis is induced, the shape of the pupil frequently becomes irregular owing to adhesions (posterior synechiae) between the iris and anterior lens capsule.

Hypopyon is common in severe iridocyclitis. The larger inflammatory cells — plasma cells and macrophages — are most apt to be involved. Iridal swelling is usually present, and with chronicity, marked thickening of the iris, which impedes drug-induced mydriasis, occurs.

ETIOLOGIES

The causes of iridocyclitis are summarized in Table 1. The majority of known causes are related to systemic diseases. Unfortunately, even after extensive clinicopathology work-ups, no demonstrable cause is found for many anterior uveitides. However, chronic and recurrent anterior uveitis are rare in the dog and cat.

In intense and chronic anterior uveitides in the dog, anterior chamber paracentesis and iris

Table 1. Causes of Iridocyclitis

Trauma
Pansystemic disease:
   a. Virus—Infectious canine hepatitis (ICH), postvaccinal ICH, canine distemper, herpes (dog and cat)
   b. Bacteria—Leptospirosis
   c. Fungi—Aspergillosis, Blastomycosis, Candidiasis, Coccidioidomycosis, Cryptococcosis, Histoplasmosis, Nocardiosis, Paecilomycosis
   d. Parasitic—Dirofilaria immitis, Toxocara canis
   e. Protozoa—Toxoplasmosis
   f. Neoplasia—Malignant lymphoma (dog), Feline leukemia virus, Metastatic adenocarcinomas, Metastatic hemangiosarcomas
Ocular Neoplasia—Malignant melanomas, primary ciliary body adenocarcinomas
Postsurgical/Postparacentesis
Autoimmune—Lens-induced, sclerouveitis

biopsy may be helpful. The limited aqueous humor sample (0.1 to 0.3 ml) is passed through a 8μ millipore filter for cytologic analysis, and the remaining fluid is analyzed for total protein, A/G ratio, and protein electrophoresis. A drop of aqueous humor can also be used for bacterial, viral, and fungal culture. The authors usually restore the anterior chamber volume after paracentesis with balanced salt solution (BSS — Alcon Laboratories, Ft. Worth, Tex.) to minimize intensification of the disease and the possibility of angle closure glaucoma.

Iris biopsy involves some risks; generally, a complete iridectomy is performed through a limbal incision and limbal-based conjunctival flap. The thickened, inflamed iris is externalized through the limbal incision and excised by judicious electrocautery. The biopsy is examined by an ophthalmic pathologist.

If the disease affects the entire uveal tract — i.e., panuveitis — vitreous paracentesis may be indicated. The authors have been able to diagnose metastatic intraocular neoplasms, cryptococcosis, and blastomycosis with this technique.

SPECIFIC TYPES

Two specific anterior uveitides in the dog are discussed here in further detail. Lens-induced anterior uveitis in the dog occurs as two distinct diseases: (1) lens-induced uveitis associated with traumatic perforation of the anterior lens capsule and (2) lens-induced uveitis associated with resorbing cataracts. In the former, the lens material is normal; in the latter, the lens is cataractous. All lens substance is antigenic to the body because the embryologic lens is isolated before the development of the fetal immune system.

Acute lens-induced uveitis, secondary to anterior lens capsule perforation, usually has concurrent corneal pathology such as a penetrating cornea foreign body, cat scratch, or lead shot. The anterior uvea is moderately inflamed, and a cataract rapidly develops. White flocculent material may be detected when some of the lens material is lost into the anterior chamber, and the contour of the anterior lens may be irregular or flat. Anterior chamber paracentesis and cytologic examination reveal lens material and a predominantly neutrophilic infiltration. Immediate removal of the remaining lens is recommended before further intensification of the anterior uveitis occurs.

Chronic lens-induced uveitis associated with cataract resorption is not infrequent in breeds of dogs with inherited juvenile cataracts. Typically, the cataract has been present for several months, and the reduced molecular size of its proteins allows their escape through the anterior lens capsule into the aqueous humor. Anterior chamber paracentesis and cytologic examination reveal predominating macrophages with "foamy" cytoplasm (ingested lens material).

Chronic lens-induced uveitis can usually be controlled by intensive topical and systemic corticosteroids and mydriatics. If the condition fails to respond and intraocular pressure begins to increase, removal of the intact lens is recommended.

Anterior uveitis with extensive corneal edema has been associated both with spontaneous and post-vaccinal cases of infectious canine hepatitis (adenovirus type 1). The anterior uveitis results from a delayed Arthus-type hypersensitivity response. In the early mild anterior uveitis, virus can be isolated from the aqueous humor, and viral replication occurs in the corneal endothelium. In the later stage of anterior uveitis with corneal edema, the inflammatory cells within the aqueous contain viral-antibody complexes.

Treatment for ICH-anterior uveitis is similar to that for other types of uveitis. Mydriatics and corticosteroids (topical and systemic) are administered to effect. Glaucoma, an infrequent complication, is associated with anterior uveitis, peripheral anterior synechiae, and damage to the trabeculae by the Arthus reaction. With the recent introduction of the adenovirus type II vaccine for ICH, this type of anterior uveitis should occur less frequently.

PRIMARY AND SECONDARY INTRAOCULAR NEOPLASMS

Primary and metastatic intraocular neoplasms may simulate or stimulate iridocyclitis. The iridocyclitis may result from direct tumor invasion, host rejection, tumor and normal tissue necrosis, and noxious metabolic by-products. A persistent chronic iridocyclitis with hyphema warrants additional investigation. Malignant melanomas frequently induce iridocyclitis, and the secondary inflammation can mask the primary tumor. Metastatic adenocarcinomas and hemangiosarcoma may also initiate a secondary iridocyclitis. Focal enlargements of the iris may signal the presence of an intraocular neoplasm.

Ultrasonography of these eyes with an opaque media is often useful and may define the borders, consistency, and dimensions of a mass. Therapy for most primary intraocular neoplasms is enucleation.

ANTERIOR UVEITIS IN THE CAT

Three systemic diseases — malignant lymphoma, feline infectious peritonitis, and toxoplasmosis — commonly involve the feline uvea and are often difficult to distinguish (Table 2). Malignant lymphoma predominantly affects the anterior segment; toxoplasmosis predominantly affects the posterior segment. Feline infectious peritonitis (FIP) commonly affects the entire uvea (panuveitis).

Some ophthalmologists feel that exudates from the anterior chamber are important in differentiating these diseases. Malignant lymphoma commonly exhibits hypopyon, whereas toxoplasmosis usually exhibits an aqueous flare and only infrequently shows hypopyon. FIP causes large keratitic precipitates in combination with hemorrhage.

Treatment of these systemic diseases is covered in other sections of this text. Therapy for the anterior uveitis is discussed later in this section.

Table 2. Guidelines for Anterior Uveitis in the Cat

	UVEAL INVOLVEMENT	ANTERIOR CHAMBER	AQUEOUS CYTOLOGY	SYSTEMIC TESTS
Malignant lymphoma (FeLV)	Mainly anterior, occasionally posterior	Hypopyon	Mainly neutrophils; lymphocytes—some demonstrate malignancy	+ fluorescent antibody test (±)
Toxoplasmosis	Mainly posterior, occasionally anterior	Flare	Mainly neutrophils	+ or rising Sabin-Feldman test
Feline Infectious Peritonitis	Mainly anterior,° infrequently posterior	Hypopyon, keratitic precipitates with hemorrhage	Macrophages, neutrophils, and large amounts of fibrin	Hyperproteinemia Reversed A/G ratio + FIP test + FeLV±

° Posterior involvement may be obstructed by anterior uveal involvement.
Editor's Note: FeLV and FIP produce granulomatous anterior uveitis, and the cases are indistinguishable.

COMPLICATIONS

The complications and sequelae of anterior uveitis are influenced by the cause and duration of the disease and the patient's response to therapy. Posterior synechiae (adherence of the iris to the anterior lens capsule) are the most frequent complications and are most apt to occur with a miotic pupil. Iris bombé occurs and predisposes the eye to glaucoma if annular posterior synechiae develop.

Both active and resolved iridocyclitis produce changes in iris coloration, especially in lightly pigmented irides. The blue irides of the Siamese turn tan, and green irides can become dark brown to black. In dogs, the iridal coloration becomes irregular, with some areas appearing almost white and others black.

Peripheral anterior synechiae (PAS) can occur in iridocyclitis, closing the iridocorneal angle and collapsing the sclerociliary cleft. Extensive PAS may result in the development of glaucoma.

The corneal edema involved in iridocyclitis usually resolves without scarring. However, with anterior synechiae formation or ICH reaction, endothelial damage may persist for months and is sometimes permanent.

Retrocorneal, iridal, and pupillary membranes may develop from organization of the aqueous humor exudates and may impair tissue function and vision. Phthisis bulbi can occur as a sequela to intensive and/or chronic iridocyclitis. Ocular hypotony and reduced globe size indicate extensive irreversible ciliary body damage.

Cataracts may develop as a sequela to iridocyclitis. Anterior capsular and subcapsular cataracts are usually associated with posterior synechiae and deposits of inflammatory debris. "Toxic elements" in the aqueous humor may induce equatorial, anterior, and posterior cortical cataracts in the absence of posterior synechiae. If the lens cortices are involved, progression of the cataract is likely.

THERAPY

Three objectives are important in treating iridocyclitis: (1) iridocycloplegia, (2) suppression of inflammation, and (3) elimination of the causative agent. Parasympatholytics, such as 1 to 3 percent atropine, induce mydriasis and cycloplegia and thereby minimize posterior synechiae formation and reduce pain. The combination of 10 percent phenylephrine with the parasympatholytic agents may facilitate maximal mydriasis.

Corticosteroids are administered topically, subconjunctivally, and systemically to reduce inflammation. Dexamethasone (0.1 percent) or 1 percent prednisolone acetate is preferred for topical treatment, and methylprednisolone and triaminolone acetonide are preferred for subconjunctival injections. Dexamethasone (0.025–0.075 mg/kg/day) and prednisolone (0.5–2.0 mg/kg/day divided BID) are administered orally and gradually reduced as the anterior uveitis subsides.

Antibiotics, sulfonamides, and antifungals are administered against specific organisms. Satisfactory penetration of most systemically administered antibiotics occurs when the blood-aqueous barrier is reduced in inflammation.

HYPHEMA

Hyphema (hemorrhage in the anterior chamber) results from several causes (Table 3). Whether or not the blood is clotted in the anterior chamber appears to be related to concurrent iridocyclitis and increased fibrin levels in the aqueous humor. Hyphema in dogs rarely causes an elevation in intraocular pressure.

Treatment of hyphema is directed at the primary disorder. Osmotic and carbonic anhydrase inhibitors may facilitate removal of hyphema but are infrequently indicated. Mydriatics may be necessary to control iridocyclitis, but parasympatholytic agents such as atropine or cyclopentolate may cause recurrence of hemorrhage owing to their vasodilative effects. The authors prefer 10 percent phenylephrine in the initial treatment of traumatic hyphema because of its moderate mydriatic and vasoconstrictive effects. Corticosteroids may be indicated, since fibrin tends to delay the resorption of hyphema. If intraocular pressure is elevated, the anterior chamber is lavaged with balanced salt solution (BSS) and fibrinolysin (1000–1250 units/ml) to facilitate removal of large blood clots.

DEGENERATIONS

PRIMARY IRIS ATROPHY

Iridal degeneration or atrophy occurs frequently in older dogs, especially in toy and miniature poodles. The atrophy may produce slow and incomplete light-induced pupillary reflexes. Iridal atrophy usually involves the sphincter region, which gives the pupil a scalloped appearance. The degenerative process can also affect the main substance of the iris, resulting in progressively enlarging crypts that become full-thickness holes.

Patients with iris atrophy and mature cata-

Table 3. *Manifestations of Hyphema in the Dog*

CAUSE OF HYPHEMA	APPEARANCE	RECURRENCE	BREED OR RELATED CONDITION
Traumatic	Clotted	Unlikely	Unrelated
Systemic clotting disorders	Unclotted	Likely	Warfarin poisoning
Intraocular neoplasm	Clotted	Likely	Malignant melanoma; malignant lymphoma
Iridocyclitis	Clotted	Unlikely	Chronic types with neovascularization
Congenital anomalous globes	Unclotted; multiple levels	Likely	Collie eye anomaly; Bedlington terrier retinal dysplasia; Australian shepherd; Microphthalmia with colobomas
Glaucoma with megaloglobus	Unclotted	Likely	May originate from the ciliary body or retinal detachments
Penetrating foreign body	Clotted	Unlikely	Usually associated iridocyclitis or panuveitis

racts require electroretinography for the detection of PRA before cataract surgery is performed. Dogs with iris atrophy and normal lenses may exhibit photophobia in bright illumination.

ESSENTIAL IRIS ATROPHY

Essential iris atrophy is rare in the dog and usually presents concurrently with iridocyclitis-glaucoma. Large sections of the iris are deposited on the anterior lens capsule, iridocorneal angle, and posterior cornea.

The etiology of essential iris atrophy is unknown. It may be associated with a primary vascular insufficiency of portions of the iris or it may occur secondary to iridocyclitis. Glaucoma and phthisis bulbi are common sequelae to essential iris atrophy. In glaucoma, the iridocorneal angle becomes obstructed with debris from the degenerating iris, iridocyclitis, and peripheral anterior synechiae. Treatment is directed toward the iridocyclitis, glaucoma, or a combination of both.

IRIDAL AND CILIARY CYSTS

Iridal and ciliary cysts occur frequently in older dogs. There is no breed predisposition, although Boston terriers are often affected. Iris cysts in man have been associated with chronic inflammation and topical organophosphate miotics. In dogs, etiology is usually unknown.

Iris cysts in the dog are most often black, spherical, free-floating 2 to 4 mm bodies. They may occasionally become wedged in the irido-

corneal angle, simulating a ciliary body malignant melanoma. Multiple iris cysts are usually present, and when mydriasis is induced as part of the ophthalmic examination, additional cysts may be released from the posterior chamber.

Ciliary body cysts are usually larger than those of the iris and are light brown to translucent. They are usually attached to the ciliary body but may protrude into and distort the pupil.

Both iridal and ciliary cysts rarely produce ocular signs. The cysts can be confused with anterior uveal melanomas, but they usually transilluminate and are free within the anterior chamber in contrast to melanomas. Rolling the dog during examination will cause the cysts to move. Gonioscopy may be necessary to examine cysts lodged in the iridocorneal angle.

Removal of iridal and ciliary cysts is not usually indicated unless they obstruct the pupil. The cysts can be removed by aspiration or gentle lavage of the anterior chamber through a limbal-based incision.

SUPPLEMENTAL READING

Aguirre, G., Carmichael, L., and Bistner, S.: Corneal endothelium in viral induced anterior uveitis. Arch. Ophthalmol. 93:219–224, 1975.

Bergsma, D.R., and Brown, K.S.: White fur, blue eyes and deafness in the domestic cat. J. Hered. 62:171–185, 1971.

Carmichael, L.E.: The pathogenesis of ocular lesions of infectious canine hepatitis. Path. Vet. 1:73–95, 1964.

Gelatt, K.N.: *Veterinary Ophthalmic Pharmacology and Therapeutics*, 2nd ed. Bonner Springs, Ks., Veterinary Medicine Publishing, 1978.

Gelatt, K.N.: Ophthalmic biopsy procedures. Vet. Clin. North Am. 4:437–448, 1974.

Gelatt, K.N., and McGill, L.D.: Clinical characteristics of microphthalmia with colobomas of the Australian shepherd dog. J. Am. Vet. Med. Assoc. 162:393–396, 1973.

CANINE AND FELINE GLAUCOMA

PAUL F. DICE, II, V.M.D.

Seattle, Washington

Unfortunately, glaucoma in the dog and cat is often presented and/or diagnosed in the chronic stages. Since significant irreversible retinal and optic nerve changes can occur within 24 hours, it is imperative that the patient be presented early and the clinician be astute in understanding the clinical and pathophysiologic aspects of the disease. Most imperative is the evaluation of both eyes when the patient is presented. The following is an update of aqueous dynamics and the types, diagnosis, and treatment of glaucoma.

AQUEOUS DYNAMICS

Aqueous is produced both actively and passively by the ciliary body and processes. The active process is based on secretion and is associated with the active transport of sodium ions, causing a shift in osmolality across the ciliary epithelium. Increased osmolality results also from the active transport of both chloride (Cl^-) and bicarbonate (HCO_3^-) ions. Carbonic anhydrase occurs in large amounts in ocular tissues and increases by a factor of approximately 1000-fold the reaction:

$$CO_2 + H_2O \rightleftharpoons H_2CO_3 \rightleftharpoons H^+ + HCO_3.$$

The passive processes are responsible for approximately 50 percent of the aqueous and involves diffusion, dialysis, and ultrafiltration. This will vary among species, since these processes are reflections of the blood composition.

Once produced, aqueous humor enters the posterior chamber and passes into the anterior chamber via the pupil. It then exits the anterior chamber through the trabecular meshwork (iridocorneal angle) and the adjacent scleral venous plexus. A small volume of aqueous is absorbed by the iris vessels. An alternative route for aqueous outflow is through the interstitial spaces of the ciliary body musculature into the suprachoroidal space (uveoscleral route). This route may account for 30 to 65 percent of bulk flow in subhuman primates, but this appears to be much less in cats, rabbits, and dogs. In this pathway, aqueous absorption appears to be a colloid osmotic force and is not pressure dependent.

TYPES OF GLAUCOMA

Both primary and secondary forms of glaucoma are recognized in the dog. It is important to determine the type of glaucoma in order to make the best judgment in diagnosis and therapy.

Primary Glaucoma. By definition, there is no associated ocular disease with primary glaucoma as the precipitating cause. In the dog, both primary open and narrow angle glaucoma are seen. The narrow angle cases may become closed as the patient becomes older.

Open angle glaucoma has been reported mainly in the beagle. It has been observed occasionally in multiple purebreds and mongrels. The cat also has a form of open angle glaucoma, at least at the gonioscopic level. There is, however, closure to various degrees of the ciliary cleft posterior to this. In an open angle, the distance between the base of the iris and the cornea appears normal, with a normal pectinate ligament. The outflow interference appears to be posterior to this region (ciliary cleft).

Narrow and closed angle glaucoma is found in the American cocker spaniel, basset hound, poodle, terriers (wire and smooth fox, toy, Bedlington, and Manchester), Samoyed, malamute, Norwegian elkhound, dachshund, and Dalmatian. It can occur, however, in any purebred or mongrel.

Congenital Glaucoma. This type has been described in the veterinary literature mainly in the basset hound because of a concurrent goniodysgenesis. This congenital iridocorneal angle bridging of mesodermal sheets can vary in its extent. The onset of glaucoma does not occur until after one year of age, and there appear to be more factors involved than just the appearance of solid sheets of tissue in the angle.

The author has observed an occasional congenital glaucoma as soon as the eyes open in a few dogs, and invariably there have been multiple intraocular anomalies.

Secondary Glaucoma. These cases are complicated by another intraocular disease. There are multiple variations of secondary glaucoma.

INFLAMMATORY. This may be postsurgical or secondary to hepatitis vaccine or iridocyclitis of any origin. The increased pressure may result from the iridocorneal angle becoming compromised by inflammatory cells or from the "swollen" iris base severely compromising the aqueous outflow. Clinical signs are an increased intraocular pressure and iridocyclitis with a pupil of various shapes (dyscoria) and sizes. If the patient is young, buphthalmia occurs quickly. Treatment must include drugs to decrease intraocular pressure (hyperosmotics and diuretic) and symptomatic therapy for the iridocyclitis to decrease the inflammation. Decreasing the inflammation may increase the ciliary body function and induce increased pressures in a previously soft eye with obstructive lesions in the aqueous outflow pathway.

Inflammatory glaucoma may also occur if the pupil aperture is abnormal — annular posterior synechia (seclusion) or an intrapupillary membrane formation (e.g., adherence of the pupil to itself) (occlusion). In these instances, the iris will bulge forward, particularly in the midregion, causing a shallow anterior chamber. Treatment involves the previously mentioned drugs and, in many instances, a concurrent iridectomy.

LENS-ASSOCIATED. This disorder is called "associated" rather than "induced," as glaucoma with a concurrent lens abnormality occurs frequently in the dog, but the exact relationship is controversial and probably varies from patient to patient.

LENS LUXATION. Lens luxation occurs early in the glaucoma history in many of the terrier breeds and may induce the glaucoma. Many of these cases also demonstrate a narrow angle with or without mesodermal dysgeneses. This may be one of the reasons that once the glaucoma occurs, removal of the luxated lens must be followed by continued medical therapy and/or combined antiglaucoma surgery. In breeds other than terriers and in cats, lens luxation appears to exacerbate a pre-existing glaucoma or simply to be the end result of zonular breakdown in an extremely buphthalmic globe.

The contributing factors of lens luxation vary and may be due to the anatomic location of the displacement (anterior or posterior), associated iridocyclitis with resultant debris in the anterior chamber, occlusion of the pupil in anterior displacement, forward displacement of the lens-iris diaphragm along with vitreous, or posterior luxation allowing vitreous alone to migrate into the anterior chamber.

Therapy consists of decreasing intraocular pressure medically as previously described and then deciding on removal of the lens with a combined antiglaucoma operation if the lens is forwardly displaced. If posteriorly displaced, the author strongly suggests not removing the lens unless the proper ophthalmic surgical equipment is available (including a cryostat) owing to the number of cases that have concurrent liquefied vitreous that, if lost at surgery, may result in a phthisical eye as well as retinal detachment.

TRAUMATIC. Traumatic glaucoma in the dog and cat, while not common compared with the previous categories, also has inflammation as a predominant feature. Hyphema is often a contributing factor, but usually the patient has a predisposed narrow or closed angle. Blood staining of the cornea may occur in a glaucomatous eye, making it difficult or impossible to evaluate thoroughly. Many of these cases have perforating metallic foreign bodies, and for these, skull radiographs are strongly recommended.

INTRAOCULAR TUMORS. Intraocular neoplasia is the least common cause of glaucoma observed in the author's clinic. Focal uveal tumors do not cause glaucoma unless there is massive neoplastic debris or hemorrhage in the anterior chamber, embarrassing the aqueous outflow. Without a history or clinical evidence of trauma, a neoplasm should be considered in glaucoma with a concurrent hyphema. The few cases observed with glaucoma were quite extensive and required enucleation.

TREATMENT

There is no single treatment for glaucoma that produces consistently favorable results in the dog and cat owing to the variations in etiology and associated disorders. Treatment consists of a medical and/or surgical approach. Much of the variety in response can be blamed on inadequate diagnosis of the disease, chronicity of the disease when presented, failure of consistent drug administration, and incomplete follow-ups. A method to reduce the intraocular pressure and prevent further optic nerve and retinal damage until a more precise etiology is established is as follows.

Primary glaucoma (first 24 to 48 hours):
1. Hyperosmotic — glycerin on presentation (per os) or mannitol IV
2. Diuretic — acetazolamide IV on presenta-

tion, then in 3 to 4 hours, either Daranide or Neptazane q8h.

3. Miotic — pilocarpine 2 percent q 15 to 20 minutes for one hour then q4h.

As a general rule, the author does not recommend aqueous paracentesis to decrease the intraocular pressure owing to the rapid forward displacement of the lens-iris diaphragm, which can embarrass an already compromised iridocorneal angle. There is also a possibility of causing a retinal separation with this procedure.

48 hours and later for maintenance:

1. Miotic — If narrow or closed angle glaucoma, 2 to 4 percent pilocarpine with or without epinephrine QID. If narrow angle glaucoma, Phospholine iodide should be tried if the schedule for pilocarpine cannot be followed. For open angle glaucoma, choice of Timolal, Phospholine iodide, or Epinephrine-pilocarpine.

2. Diuretic — choice of Daranide or Neptazane.

Narrow or closed angle glaucoma is seldom successfully controlled over long periods with medical therapy alone. The author recommends a combined sclerectomy, cyclodialysis, and iridectomy procedure in addition to medical therapy at the 48-hour period if vision is present. With proper technique, cyclocryotherapy appears promising for the treatment of primary glaucoma. Table 1 lists some drugs commonly used for glaucoma.

Table 1. *Drugs and Dosages for Glaucoma*

OSMOTICS
  a. glycerin—USP—1 ml/kg TID per os; Glyrol® (Mallinckrodt)—2 ml/kg TID per os

MIOTICS
  a. pilocarpine 2 to 4% TID-QID
  b. Carbachol® (Alcon) 0.75 to 3.0% TID-QID
  c. Phospholine iodide® (Ayerst) 0.06 to 0.125% SID-BID

DIURETICS
  a. acetazolamide (Diamox®-Lederle) 10 mg/kg BID per os; 5 to 10 mg/kg IV
  b. dichlorphenamide (Daranide® — Merck, Sharp and Dohme) (Oratrol®-Alcon) 5 to 10 mg/kg BID-TID in divided doses.
  c. methazolamide (Neptazane®-Lederle) 5 to 10 mg/kg BID-TID
  d. ethoxzolamide (Cardrase®-Upjohn) 5 to 7.5 mg/kg BID-TID

BETA-BLOCKER (ADRENERGIC)
  a. timolal (Timoptic®-Merck, Sharp and Dohme) 0.25 to 0.5% BID

ALPHA-BLOCKER
  a. thymoxamine 0.5%. Drug is used experimentally at present and may be drug of choice for angle closure glaucoma such as that observed in the dog. Its primary action is a blocker of alpha receptor sites; it does not shallow the anterior chamber as does pilocarpine or echothiophate. It will counteract a dilated pupil from sympathomimetics but not parasympatholytics.

ALPHA-STIMULATOR
  a. epinephrine 1 to 2%.

COMBINED
  a. Epinephrine-pilocarpine, 2 to 4% (E-Pilo®-Alcon) TID-QID.

SUPPLEMENTAL READING

Friedenwald, J.S.: Formation of intraocular fluid. Am. J. Ophthalmol. 32:9–27, 1949.

Gelatt, K.N., Peiffer, R.L., Gwin, R.M., and Sank, J.J.: Glaucoma in the beagle. Trans. Am. Acad. Ophthalmol. Otolaryngol. 81:636–644, 1976.

Gelatt, K.N., Peiffer, R.L., Gwin, R.M., Gum, G.G., and Williams, L.W.: Clinical manifestations of inherited glaucoma in the beagle. Invest. Ophthalmol. Vis. Sci., 16:1135–1142, 1977.

Gelatt, K.N.: *Veterinary Ophthalmic Pharmacology and Therapeutics,* 2nd ed. Bonner Springs, Kansas, Veterinary Medicine Publishing Co., 1978.

Henkind, P., and Friedman, A.H. (eds): *Physician's Desk Reference for Ophthalmology.* Oradell, N.J., Medical Economics Co., 1972.

Zimmerman, T.J., and Garg, L.C.: The effect of acetazolamide on the movement of anions into the posterior chamber of the dog eye. J. Pharm. Exp. Ther. 196:510–516, 1976.

DISEASES OF THE VITREOUS, RETINA, AND CHOROID

NED BUYUKMIHCI, V.M.D.

Davis, California

Because of the close association of the vitreous, retina, and choroid, conditions affecting one often involve the others as well. Generally, it is unusual to have severe vitreal disease without concurrent or associated retinal disease (although the reverse is often true).

In order to appreciate the complexities of retinal, choroidal, and vitreal disease, the reader must have a basic understanding of the normal embryology, anatomy, and physiology of these structures.

VITREAL DISEASE

Persistence of Hyaloid Vasculature. Varying degrees of persistence of the hyaloid vascular system may occur. Because vision is rarely affected, this condition does not require treatment. The most common and benign persistent hyaloid remnant is termed "Mittendorf's dot," which is a small posterior polar opacity of the lens capsule. It may also appear as a small gray circle and is the site at which the hyaloid artery attaches to the anterior condensation of vitreous adjacent to the lens. Often, a tiny remnant of artery remains behind the lens and hangs (loosely coiled) in a canal (Cloquet's) in the vitreous.

A more extensive persistent artery may terminate on the posterior lens capsule with a branched appearance. Depending on the amount of tissue remaining, vision may be disturbed, especially in conditions in which the pupil is constricted. Some of these vessels are patent and contain blood so that retrolental hemorrhage may occur.

Rarely, there may be extensive proliferation of fibrovascular tissue, often with invasion of the posterior lens, in which case the condition is termed "anterior persistent hyperplastic primary vitreous." Other ocular anomalies such as a variable degree of microphthalmia, elongated ciliary processes, and retinal dysplasia may be present. Affected eyes are usually blind owing to cataract. Lens extraction and vitrectomy may

be performed, but the prognosis is guarded. If vision is affected by central opacities, chronic mydriatic therapy (1 percent atropine weekly is best) may be utilized to improve vision.

Vitreous Floaters. White or grey opacities of various sizes may commonly be seen in the vitreous of otherwise normal eyes randomly and in certain breeds and families of dogs. These are usually in the form of strands that move with ocular movements and may increase in quantity as the animal ages. The cause and substance of these are uncertain. Their main importance is in their differentiation from inflammatory exudates (hyalitis), which represent retinal and/or posterior uveal inflammation. Inflammatory exudates are often darker and hazier than benign floaters. The presence of inflammatory exudates necessitates a search for the primary process.

Asteroid Hyalosis. This is a degenerative disease of older animals and is usually unilateral. The vitreous remains in its gel state and contains numerous, tiny, round, opaque bodies that reflect light and vibrate with ocular movement. They are calcium-lipid complexes and do not appear to interfere with sight, nor are they necessarily involved with other ocular disease. Treatment is neither feasible nor necessary.

Hyalitis. Inflammation of the vitreous (hyalitis) is usually secondary to uveitis and retinitis. Inflammatory cells, exudate, and blood enter the vitreous, giving it a diffuse, hazy appearance; the fundus cannot be seen clearly. Successful treatment of the underlying disease process is followed by restoration of vitreous clarity. However, if hemorrhage and/or fibrin form clots, traction bands can form, which may result in retinal separation and severe distortion of the globe with blindness.

RETINAL AND CHOROIDAL DISEASE

Absence or Underdevelopment of Tapetum. The tapetum is a specialized part of the choroid. Its function and significance are not clear. When it is absent or underdeveloped, clinical signs are not apparent. Frequently, albino or color-dilute animals will not have tapeta, but absence or hypoplasia can occur in pigmented animals as well. At this time it would seem that the presence or absence of a tapetum is not clinically significant.

Peripheral Cystoid Retinal Degeneration. From middle age onward, the peripheral sensory retina (adjacent to the ora ciliaris retinae) begins to show structural changes of splitting with the formation of cysts. They are best visualized with indirect ophthalmoscopy and mydriasis. The condition is considered a normal aging phenomenon, and vision appears not to be affected.

Retinal Separation (Detachment). A distinction is made here between true retinal detachment and separation. The site of discontinuity in clinically termed retinal "detachment" is almost always between the retinal epithelium (retinal pigment epithelium) and the sensory retina (neural retina). These two layers are part of the same tissue, so that the term "separation" would be more accurate and will be used throughout this section. If the retinal epithelium were to lose continuity with the choriocapillaris (an unusual occurrence), this would be a true detachment.

Retinal separation is usually secondary to intraocular inflammatory disease, especially choroidal disease. It can also be associated with renal disease and systemic hypertension, or it can occur alone (idiopathic). If the area of separation is small and flat, it is called a flat separation. If a bulla is formed, the term "bullous separation" is used. When there is complete separation so that only the attachments at the optic disk and ora ciliaris retinae are intact, this may be called funnel-shaped or morning glory separation. Dialysis refers to a tearing of the peripheral or peripapillary attachments. Rhegmatogenous separations refer to those associated with breaks, tears, or holes in the retina. Indirect ophthalmoscopy through a dilated pupil is the easiest method of diagnosis of retinal separation. If the separation is complete, the folded sensory retina is often grossly visible just behind the lens without the use of any diagnostic instruments.

Once the diagnosis of retinal separation is made, a search for the cause is imperative for successful treatment. When it is associated with ocular maldevelopment (such as the collie eye anomaly or retinal dysplasia), treatment is not feasible. If associated with choroidal, vascular, or renal disease, these entities must be treated simultaneously.

Generally, the prognosis for retinal separation is poor. If there is sufficient distance between the retinal epithelium and the sensory retina so that proper nutrition of the photoreceptor cells is lacking, there may be irreversible degenerative changes in these cells after ten days. If these two layers are reunited prior to this time, return of function may occur. For simple effusive separations, symptomatic treatment includes the use of systemic corticosteroids and diuretics in addition to definitive treatment of any primary disease. Corticosteroids should be used at anti-inflammatory levels for an extended period, sometimes as long as six weeks, before being considered ineffective. Prednisolone and dexamethasone are commonly used. Prednisolone should be used orally at 1.0 mg/kg or higher daily, tapering to the usually recommended 0.5 to 1.0 mg/kg range after 10 to 14 days. Dexamethasone can be given orally at the rate of 0.25 to 2.0 mg (depending on weight of patient) daily.

Furosemide is commonly used at 2 to 4 mg/kg orally once or twice daily. If the patient is hypertensive, oral methyldopa at approximately 5 mg/kg twice daily may be helpful, in addition to a tranquilizer such as promazine (orally at approximately 2 mg/kg twice daily).

Therapy is empirical, particularly with respect to the diuretics. However, the use of this regimen in purely idiopathic effusive cases is often helpful. These cases generally have a better prognosis simply because there are no (obvious) contributing pathologic processes. Rhegmatogenous separations or those in which there is dialysis usually do not respond to any type of therapy.

Surgical therapy is widely used in humans but is difficult to apply to animals mainly because surgical exposure is not adequate. Also, many veterinary patients are presented late in the process, so that correction would not result in vision. These animals often have rhegmatogenous separations or are dialyzed.

Retinitis and Choroiditis. Although there are some specific diseases in which there is primary retinitis or choroiditis, secondary changes usually occur in the initially uninvolved tissue. Unless this type of disease is suspected, and ophthalmoscopy is performed, most lesions will be missed in their early stages. It is not until there is diffuse bilateral involvement, anterior progression, optic nerve involvement, or secondary changes such as retinal separation that clinical signs are manifested. If the chorioretinitis is secondary to systemic disease (which it usually is), the animal may be manifesting other signs that may suggest ophthalmic examination. For example, a young dog with signs of encephalitis or gastroenteritis may have distemper, and ophthalmic examination may provide additional supportive evidence of the same.

Determination of whether a particular lesion is active or static is important, since chorioretinal scars are commonly seen throughout dog and cat populations and do not require treatment. Active lesions appear as grey or white areas with indistinct borders. These may extend into the vitreous so that visualization of other structures is obscured. These areas may be surrounded by edema, hemorrhage, or elevations of the sensory retina. Granulomatous inflammation is often more discrete than is nongranulomatous inflammation; the granulomas may appear fluffy or cotton-like and have more substance.

In the tapetal area, inactive lesions may be hyperreflective owing to retinal thinning, or there may be aberrant pigmentation. Inactive lesions in the non-tapetal area may be depigmented, hypopigmented, or hyperpigmented.

Once a lesion is determined to be active, treatment can be prescribed. One must carefully evaluate the patient to diagnose and treat the primary process. When a systemic diagnosis is not possible or if the ocular lesion is primary, symptomatic treatment should be instituted. This includes the use of systemic corticosteroids at high levels for several weeks. This is important because changes secondary to the inflammatory process itself may lead to irreversible damage, particularly to the retina. Contraction of fibrovascular tissue within the retina or vitreous may lead to further distortion of the intraocular contents. Broad spectrum antibiotics should be used simultaneously.

The prognosis must remain guarded, but ultimately it depends on the etiology. An important fact to keep in mind is that regardless of the cause of retinal and/or choroidal inflammation, the ophthalmoscopic signs are similar; one cannot determine the etiology simply on the basis of ocular fundus changes. If a lesion appears granulomatous, the possibilities are limited but there is still no specificity owing to appearance. Any time active retinitis and/or choroiditis is diagnosed, a complete physical examination must be performed. Non-granulomatous inflammation may be produced by many bacteria, viruses, and toxins. Granulomatous reactions are attributable to mycotic (such as blastomycosis, protothecosis, toxoplasmosis, coccidioidomycosis, cryptococcosis, and geotrichosis), protozoan, and helminthic (such as toxocariasis) infections.

Progressive Retinal Atrophy. Progressive retinal atrophy (PRA) comprises a group of diseases characterized by loss of outer retinal function. PRA describes only the endstage retinal disease and not the pathogenesis, although most are considered hereditary. Three canine breeds have been fairly well studied and represent a spectrum of changes with respect to the early disease. The Irish setter has been shown to have a rod-cone dysplasia in which neither photoreceptor cell matures structurally or functionally. The Norwegian elkhound has rod dysplasia with secondary cone atrophy. In the miniature and toy poodle, true rod and cone atrophy occur after apparently normal structural and functional maturation. PRA has been diagnosed in the cat, but the pathogenesis has not been determined for any particular breed.

Although there are different pathologic processes, PRA characteristically produces night blindness (nyctalopia) initially, which eventually progresses to include day blindness (hemeralopia), at which time the animal is totally blind. Ophthalmoscopic changes include early retinal vascular attenuation and tapetal granularity (owing to disturbance of the optical characteristics of the retina by degenerating photoreceptor cells). As the disease progresses, there is an increase in tapetal reflectivity (owing to a thinning retina), further vascular attenuation, and mottling of the non-tapetal area because of retinal epithelial disturbance (hyperplasia, hypertrophy, and hypopigmentation). In the late stages, the tapetum may be brilliantly hyperreflective, the optic disk may be atrophic, and the retinal vessels will be "ghost-like."

PRA occurs in virtually every breed of dog including mongrels. As mentioned before, the pathogenesis may be considerably different from breed to breed. The following is a list of a few breeds with the approximate age at which an ophthalmoscopic diagnosis can be made:

Breed	Age
Irish setter	6 months
Cardigan Welsh corgi	6 months
Cairn terrier	Under 1 year
Miniature long-haired dachshund	Under 1 year
Collie	Under 1 year
Doberman pinscher	1 to 2 years
Norwegian elkhound	2 to 3 years
Samoyed	3 years
English cocker spaniel	3 to 5 years
Miniature and toy poodles	3 to 5 years
Miniature schnauzer	4 to 6 years

Since all PRA cases seem to begin with night blindness and since vitamin A is widely known to be necessary for night vision, many people mistakenly advise using vitamin A as treatment. Regardless of this or any other type of therapy, the disease will continue to progress at its own variable rate.

With the modern level of sophistication in producing foods for domestic animals, primary nutritional deficiencies would be rare unless dietary management is not appropriate for the species in question (see taurine deficiency). Most of the patients with PRA seen by this author have been apparently healthy. It is conceivable that there *is* a nutritional deficit but on a biochemical level. Thus, although there is sufficient nutritional intake, a defective or absent enzyme, for example, would still render the animal deficient. Research into this and other facets is ongoing and intensive.

In the meantime, the only adequate method of controlling this group of diseases is selective breeding. Affected animals should not be used, and timely neutering is recommended. Unfortunately, PRA is recessive in many (if not all) breeds, so that this leaves a large number of carrier animals that are undetectable by present diagnostic methods. Conscientious breeders may want to undertake a test-breeding program to identify phenotypically normal heterozygotes in their colonies. This combined with either early histologic (for those that are dysplasias) or electroretinographic examination will be a positive step toward eliminating this devastating disease.

Central Progressive Retinal Atrophy. Unlike PRA, central progressive retinal atrophy (CPRA) is a specific retinal epithelial dystrophy. It begins in the central (posterior) retina and proceeds peripherally. The retinal epithelial cells accumulate a light brown pigment and become hypertrophied to form individual giant cells or multicellular clumps of pigmented cells. The sensory retina is normal early in the disease, but soon the photoreceptor outer segments overlying the abnormal epithelial cells degenerate, followed by further degeneration of all outer retinal layers.

The process begins in the tapetal area temporal to and above the optic disk. At this time, altered vision is not clinically detectable. As the degenerative process intensifies and spreads, central vision is compromised but peripheral vision (particularly for moving objects) is normal. Late in the disease, the ocular fundus appears similar to that of late stage PRA but with the additional presence of pigment clumps.

The pigment in the epithelial cells is a normal lipopigment, which is increased in amounts. This may signify a primary metabolic defect of the retinal epithelial cells or perhaps a deficient or abnormal enzyme in the photoreceptor-epithelial cell environment. Although this is encouraging in terms of potential treatment or prevention, there is currently no beneficial therapeutic regimen. The disease is hereditary in many breeds of dogs, possibly dominant with variable penetrance, so that selective breeding is a plausible means of control.

Taurine Deficient Retinopathy and Feline Central Retinal Degeneration. Feline central retinal degeneration (FCRD) was originally thought to be a specific disease of unknown etiology that was only moderately progressive or non-progressive. Affected animals show no visual deficits but have ophthalmoscopic and electroretinographic abnormalities. Ophthalmoscopically, the lesion can vary from a small, circular area of retinal degeneration in the area centralis, to a larger, elliptical lesion with prominent nasal extensions or satellites. These lesions appear variably hyperreflective to dark, depending on the angle of incident light. The electroretinogram of these animals demonstrates a generalized cone abnormality.

It has been shown that cats fed a diet consisting only of dog food, or having casein as the only protein, develop similar disease (ophthalmoscopically) to that seen in FCRD cats. However, in these animals, continuation of the abnormal diet results in progression of the central lesion to complete retinal atrophy. Research has revealed that taurine, an aminosulfonic acid, is deficient in these diets. Taurine is necessary for proper retinal function, at least in the cat.

A question that might be asked now is whether FCRD cats were actually nutritionally deficient at one time but recovered before retinal damage had progressed too far, or whether FCRD and nutritionally induced retinal degeneration in the cat are separate diseases. Nevertheless, three points should be considered: (1) FCRD has not yet been shown to be hereditary, (2) improper nutrition in the cat is a significant cause of retinal degeneration, and (3) cats should not be fed an all dog food diet.

Taurine is almost absent in vegetables but is rich in meat, milk, or seafood. Cats apparently cannot synthesize adequate amounts of taurine and thus require an exogenous source. Although the progression of retinal degeneration in a deficient cat can be stopped by reversion to a normal diet, degeneration that has already taken place is permanent.

SUPPLEMENTAL READING

Aguirre, G.D.: Hereditary retinal diseases in small animals. Vet. Clin. North Am. 3:515–528, 1973.

Aguirre, G.D.: Retinal degeneration associated with the feeding of dog foods to cats. J. Am. Vet. Med. Assoc. 172:791–796, 1978.

Aguirre, G.D., and Laties, A.: Pigment epithelial dystrophy in the dog. Exp. Eye Res. 23:247–256, 1976.

Barnett, K.C.: Primary retinal dystrophies in the dog. J. Am. Vet. Med. Assoc. 154:804–808, 1969.

Bellhorn, R.W., Aguirre, G.D., and Bellhorn, M.B.: Feline central retinal degeneration. Invest. Ophthalmol. 13:608–616, 1974.

Roberts, S.R.: Detachment of the retina in animals. J. Am. Vet. Med. Assoc. 135:423–431, 1959.

DISEASES OF THE ORBIT

SETH KOCH, V.M.D.
Alexandria, Virginia

Orbital disease is relatively common and yet is often overlooked as a primary diagnosis. The clinical signs associated with orbital disease are generally similar, despite the etiology. The first sign seen in most cases is conjunctivitis with nictitating membrane prolapse. The anatomic location of the orbital abnormality then causes directional changes (deviation, strabismus). Displacement of the globe in any direction indicates established orbital disease. Most commonly, exophthalmos or anterior displacement occurs. Deviations can, however, be medial, lateral, ventral or dorsal and are helpful in localizing the possible anatomic site of the orbital disease. With exophthalmos, manifestations of secondary exposure keratitis may occur. Other clinical signs associated with orbital disease are enophthalmos, keratoconjunctivitis sicca, uveitis, retinal detachment, and pupillary changes (either irritative — indicating an iritis, or neurogenic — usually evidenced by a fixed dilated pupil).

DIAGNOSTIC TECHNIQUES

In addition to a complete physical examination and palpation, radiography of the orbit and surrounding tissue is often necessary. The techniques are varied and include air contrast radiography and the injection of radiopaque dye. Sialography, sinus radiography and angiography may, in some instances, be indicated. Obviously, when one speaks of extensive radiographic work-ups, it is a "searching mission" for an explanation for orbital disease that has not otherwise been physically diagnosed. Some radiographic techniques are beyond the means of general practioners or ophthalmologists and should be referred to a radiologist for further work-up.

SPECIFIC ORBITAL DISEASES

Retro-orbital Abscess and/or Orbital Inflammation. According to published literature, the most common cause for retro-orbital abscess is a migrating foreign body. However, the author has never found a foreign body in association with an orbital abscessation. The cause is generally unknown but often there may be concurrent dental disease. Whether the root of the carnasial tooth is inflamed or there is migration of a so-called "foreign body" through the oral pharynx is academic, since the presenting signs, history, and response to treatment are usually diagnostic.

Historically, the animal has stopped eating, or has had trouble chewing the dry forms of dog food and appears to have trouble opening its mouth. Orbital swelling may have been observed. A mildly prolapsed nictitans or a sudden onset of conjunctivitis with a hyperemic conjunctiva may be the initial presenting signs with no deviation or swelling initially observed. The presence of normal pupillary reflexes should help rule out glaucoma as the cause for the "red" eye. Whereas the early signs may be non-specific, during the later course of abscess development, the orbit becomes swollen and the other systemic signs of abscessation appear.

As a diagnostic test, the author prefers passing the finger along the inner cheek to the oral mucosa in the area of the last tooth and applying dorsal pressure. If pain is elicited with this maneuver, suspicion of abscess increases.

Therapeutically, these cases respond rapidly (ten days) to high levels of injectable broad spectrum antibiotics. Once the mouth can be opened, oral broad spectrum antibiotics and anti-inflammatory drugs — ampicillin 250 mgs *B.I.D.* in the 30-pound dog for five days and prednisolone 30 mgs daily in the 30-pound dog are given for three days. Dosage is then reduced over the next ten days. If, in ten days, there has not been good response, radiography and exploratory surgery may be in order.

Cats frequently seem to have orbital disease but the impression is that an abscess is less common than chronic sinusitis or an orbital tumor. Therefore, if remission does not occur quickly with therapy, a secondary diagnosis of sinusitis or tumor should be considered.

Surgical drainage of orbital abscesses behind the last molar tooth is described fully in surgical tests. If probing is necessary, it should be aggressive. After incising the oral mucosa, the probe should be introduced until it can be felt behind the rim of the orbit from the external aspects. No damage will be done to the ocular structures by pushing the probe this way.

The Myositis Complex. The disease complex of eosinophilic myositis has sometimes been confused with that of an orbital abscess. In most cases, there is sudden anorexia and pain on opening of the mouth. The difference between the myositis complex and the abscess appears to be in the ocular signs. The myositis complex is usually bilateral and seen primarily in German shepherds, golden retrievers, and Labrador retrievers. Immune-related muscle disease cases have also been seen in the Samoyed and the Akita. Myositis cases generally respond to high levels of steroids within 72 to 96 hours and usually resolve without recurrence.

Tumors. Perhaps the most common orbital disease seen by the author in practice* is orbital tumors. The age incidence is quite variable; young adults are affected as well as aged animals. Although the clinical signs are similar to those of other space-occupying orbital diseases, a tumor mass can often be palpated or be demonstrated by contrast radiography. Older cats with orbital tumors are presented more frequently than are dogs. Dolichocephalic dogs seem prediposed to sinus tumors, and poodle-type dogs with lacrimal gland masses have been seen with some degree of regularity. Histologically, the fibrous tissue type of tumors are the most frequent.

Zygomatic gland mucoceles. Swelling of the zygomatic salivary gland or mucoceles causes the nictitating membrane to prolapse, and there may be a palpable mass below the lower lid. Occasionally, the accessory lacrimal gland is swollen, and when removed or aspirated, a mucoid-type discharge is observed. Spontaneous zygomatic gland mucoceles, most common in Pekingese and English bulldogs require surgical removal.

Enophthalmos. Enophthalmos is defined as a recession into the orbit. It occurs congenitally

---

*Since it is a referral practice, the population is biased.

with the collie breeds and in Schnauzers owing to microphthalmia. Inflammatory disease, or trauma with perforation of the cornea and a leaking wound, results in an enophthalmic globe. Degenerative enophthalmos can occur with retrobulbar fat loss because of systemic disease or as a result of muscle atrophy, senility, or Horner's syndrome.

TREATMENT

Many orbital diseases require surgery. The retro-orbital abscesses, pseudotumors, and myositis cases respond to high levels of antibiotics and corticosteroids.

Some important points concerning orbital disease are:

1. Rapid development of exophthalmos with pain should lead one to consider the possible diagnosis of abscess or retrobulbar inflammation.
2. With slow development of exophthalmos or deviation, one should consider a tumor, chronic inflammatory disease, or systemic disease, and a radiographic work-up is indicated.
3. Glaucoma may always be present with a space-occuying mass and should be treated accordingly.
4. The cause for the exophthalmos or enophthalmos may not be determined until completion of orbital exploration.
5. Exophthalmos is difficult to detect in a doliocephalic breed.
6. An exophthalmic eye must be kept moist and lubricated to prevent exposure keratitis.

SUPPLEMENTAL READING

Koch, S.: Differential diagnosis of exophthalmos in the dog. JAAHA 5:229, 1969.
Munger, R., and Ackerman, N.: Retrobulbar injections in the dog: a comparison of three techniques. JAAHA 14(4):490–499, 1978.
Rebhun, W., and Edwards, N.: Two cases of orbital adenocarcinoma of probable lacrimal gland origin. JAAHA 13:691–694, 1977.
Schoster, J., and Wyman, M.: Remission of orbital sarcoma in a dog using doxorubicin therapy. JAVMA 172:1101–1103, 1978.

INTRAOCULAR AND ORBITAL NEOPLASIA

CAROL SZYMANSKI, D.V.M.
New York, New York

Neoplasia is an important consideration in the differential diagnosis of intraocular and orbital disease. Unfortunately, most globes with intraocular tumors are presented late in the course, and their presence frequently may be masked by uveitis, hemorrhage, and secondary glaucoma. Animals with orbital tumors may be presented only after severe proptosis has occurred. Early diagnosis (i.e., before the tumor has attained a size that is destructive to the eye) may permit excision of certain localized mass lesions and preservation of vision or a cosmetically acceptable globe. Also, an underlying systemic disease (e.g., lymphosarcoma) or metastatic tumors may be recognized, and appropriate therapy, such as chemotherapy, can be initiated.

INTRAOCULAR TUMORS

PRIMARY INTRAOCULAR TUMORS

Melanomas of the anterior uvea are the most common primary intraocular tumors of dogs and cats. Melanomas arising from the posterior choroid are uncommon. Degree of malignancy is variable; the spindle cell type is the least malignant and the epithelioid type is the most anaplastic. Other features associated with a high degree of malignancy are large tumor size, high mitotic activity, and extrascleral extension. Since malignant melanoma may spread via infiltration into the orbit or via the hematogenous route to various organs, enucleation rather than local excision is recommended for most intraocular melanomas.

Local excision (iridectomy) may be carefully performed in cases of a solitary, well demarcated mass that involves less than two and one-half "clock hours" of the iris, and, on gonioscopic examination, does not extend into the drainage angle. Wide pupillary dilatation, gentle scleral depression, and examination with the binocular indirect ophthalmoscope may ascertain if the ciliary body is involved. If so, enucleation is recommended.

A wide sector iridectomy may be performed to remove a small focal pigmented iris nodule entirely without causing dissemination of tumor cells into the eye or the incision site. Histologic examination is important for prognosis. The iris specimen should be pinned flat on a tongue depressor blade to prevent anatomic distortion and then fixed in 10 percent buffered formalin.

Enucleation should be performed when large masses or secondary glaucoma are present. If extraocular extension is observed, exenteration (removal of the globe and the orbital contents) should be performed. In cases in which melanoma has extended into the orbit or along the optic nerve, the prognosis is poor and local recurrence or distant metastasis may follow. In these cases, the postoperative use of non-specific immunoadjuvants such as levamisole or BCG (Bacillus Calmette-Guerin) should be investigated. Radiation therapy or radon seed implantation may be considered.

Ciliary body adenomas and adenocarcinomas are the second most frequently reported primary intraocular tumors in the dog. Nonpigmented ciliary body neoplasms characteristically appear early in their course as white to gray or pink nodular masses behind the iris. The iris and lens may be displaced. Secondary glaucoma and intraocular hemorrhage are later sequelae. Adenocarcinomas of the ciliary body invade locally, and lung metastases have been reported.

Surgical excision of a small, localized ciliary body or process mass is feasible, and vision may be preserved. In some cases, the mass may be gently "peeled" away from the ciliary processes; in others, iridocyclectomy is necessary but may be complicated by hemorrhage.

The possibility of enucleation should be discussed prior to surgery, in the event that the mass is found to be too extensive for surgical resection. Enucleation is recommended if secondary glaucoma or scleral invasion is present.

SECONDARY INTRAOCULAR TUMORS

The vascular network of the uveal tract is the most common site of ocular metastases in dogs and cats. Metastatic mammary gland adenocarcinoma is the most frequently reported secondary intraocular tumor in the dog. Other secondary tumors include those from thyroid, renal, or pancreatic carcinomas, rhabdomyosarcoma, and hemangiosarcoma. Metastasis of a nasal adenocarcinoma to the iris of the ipsilateral eye has been reported. The author has observed bilateral ocular metastasis to the posterior choroid from a primary lung carcinoma in a cat.

Ocular metastases are generally encountered in advanced systemic diseases. However, cases may be presented in which the ocular manifestations are the primary concern of the owner. Two dogs with acute visual loss that were referred to the author were found to have splenic hemangiosarcoma. One case had intravitreal hemorrhage and exudative retinal detachment owing to ciliary body and choroidal metastases. The other case had rapidly progressing uveitis with secondary glaucoma owing to iris and ciliary body metastases.

Metastatic carcinoma may appear as solitary or multiple pale nodules on the iris surface. Growth is rapid, and secondary complications of hyphema and glaucoma ensue. Metastatic foci in the ciliary body may cause both intravitreal hemorrhage and glaucoma. A posterior choroidal metastatic lesion may be visualized as a solid, elevated retinal detachment; as the tumor grows, intravitreal hemorrhage may obscure this finding.

The presence of an intraocular tumor must be considered in cases of uveitis or glaucoma that remain intractable despite vigorous medical therapy. The value of an accurate history, thorough physical examination, and accompanying hematologic, biochemical, and radiographic evaluations cannot be overemphasized.

Ocular involvement owing to lymphosarcoma is a common finding in dogs and cats. In the dog, ocular manifestations usually occur late in the course of the disease, although rare cases may be presented in which the ocular signs precede the systemic manifestations. Uveitis, either hemorrhagic or resembling a granulomatous process, is common. Secondary glaucoma is frequently seen. Exudative retinal detachment owing to choroidal involvement with accompanying retinal hemorrhage may occur. Cases with either unilateral or bilateral papillitis owing to lymphomatous involvement of the optic nerves has been observed. Diagnosis can be made after a thorough work-up, which should include bone marrow aspiration and lymph node biopsies.

Treatment protocols for canine lymphosarcoma are discussed elsewhere. Topical atropine sulfate and topical or subconjunctival corticosteroids for anterior uveal involvement can augment systemic chemotherapy.

More diverse ocular manifestations occur with feline lymphosarcoma. The iris is the most frequent site of ocular involvement, and a raised, flesh-colored mass involving the stroma is a characteristic finding. There may be minimal accompanying inflammation, or hyphema and lymphocytic exudate may be present within the anterior chamber. Involvement may be bilateral. The posterior segment of the globe may be affected, and exudative retinal detachment, retinal hemorrhage (usually in the presence of anemia), or focal chorioretinitis can be seen. Papillitis resulting from leukemia involvement of the optic nerve has been seen in cats with spinal or epidural lymphosarcoma. Retrobulbar lymphosarcoma, producing proptosis, is occasionally seen.

The usual medical work-up, which includes feline leukemia virus test and bone marrow biopsy, may be helpful in establishing the diagnosis. A small percentage of cats with focal iris masses may be FeLV negative. Fine needle aspiration biopsy of the iris lesion is diagnostic if both immature and mature lymphocytes are present. If chemotherapy is elected, the involved eye need not be enucleated. The involved eye(s) help monitor the response to therapy.

ORBITAL NEOPLASIA

Orbital tumors are either primary or secondary owing to direct extension of a tumor from the adjacent paranasal sinuses or nasal cavity. Retrobulbar lymphosarcoma is occasionally seen in the cat. Orbital tumors owing to metastases from distant sites are rare.

Primary orbital tumors may arise from any of the tissues that compose or occupy the orbital cavity — i.e., bone, muscle, fascia, nerve, fat, vessel and lacrimal gland. Progressive, generally non-painful exophthalmos is the main clinical sign of expanding orbital neoplasia. The size and position of an orbital mass determine the extent and direction of the proptosis. Lacrimal gland neoplasia produces ventral and nasal deviation of the globe. Zygomatic gland lesions produce dorsal or dorsolateral globe deviation. Masses within the muscle cone or involving the optic nerve may produce forward displacement of the globe. Tumors of the ethmoid, maxillary sinuses, and nasal cavity may extend into the orbit and produce lateral or dorsal deviation of the globe. As exophthalmos progresses, protrusion of the nictitating membrane, exposure keratitis, and restriction of ocular motility become apparent.

Retinal striae (horizontal, parallel pressure folds owing to scleral indentation) may be an early sign of an orbital mass. Striae involving the superior temporal retina have been observed in dogs with lacrimal gland tumors.

Radiographs of the orbit are fundamental in the evaluation of orbital disease. Survey radiographs may detect osteolytic changes that are compatible with neoplasia. Orbital venography may be performed in dogs to visualize the orbital venous system and determine the extent of an orbital mass. Retrograde sialography is indicated if involvement of the zygomatic gland is suspected. As in any case of suspected neoplasia, thoracic radiographs should be obtained.

An aspiration biopsy of an orbital mass is best performed under general anesthesia following skull radiography. Sufficient material may be aspirated from the retrobulbar space by inserting an 18 gauge needle immediately posterior to the lateral orbital ligament. An aspirate of a medial orbital mass is best obtained by inserting the needle along the ventromedial bony orbit into the nasal retrobulbar space. Oropharyngeal masses may be aspirated directly.

Orbital exploratory techniques have been described. Orbital tumors in the dog and cat are frequently invasive and surgically inaccessible; exenteration generally is the treatment of choice. Limited personal experience includes excision of lacrimal gland adenomas, zygomatic gland adenocarcinoma, and fibrohistiocytoma of the orbit with preservation of functional globes.

Orbital fibrosarcomas and the highly anaplastic sarcomas in the dog have extremely poor prognoses owing to their rapid growth, local extension, and the tendency in some cases to metastasize. Remission of an orbital sarcoma in a dog with the use of a chemotherapeutic agent, doxorubicin,* has been reported. Other types of chemotherapy or combination radiation therapy and chemotherapy may be alternatives to surgery in selected cases.

---

*Adriamycin. Adria Laboratories, Inc., Wilmington, Delaware 19899.

SUPPLEMENTAL READING

Gelatt, K.N., Ladds, P.W., and Guffy, M.M.: Nasal adenocarcinoma with orbital extension and intraocular metastasis in a dog. Anim. Hosp. 6:132–142, 1970.

Reese, A.: *Tumors of the Eye*, 3rd ed. New York, Harper & Row Publishers, 1976.

Saunders, L.Z., and Barron, C.N.: Primary pigmented intraocular tumors in animals. Cancer Res. 18:234, 1958.

Saunders, L.Z., and Rubin, L.E.: *Ophthalmic Pathology of Animals*. Basel, S. Karger, 1975.

Schoster, J.V., and Wyman, M.: Remission of orbital sarcoma in a dog using doxorubicin therapy. J. Am. Vet. Med. Assoc. 172:1101–1103, 1978.

OPHTHALMIC DISORDERS OF PROVEN OR SUSPECTED GENETIC ETIOLOGY IN DOGS AND CATS

ROBERT L. PEIFFER, JR., D.V.M.
Chapel Hill, North Carolina

For reasons not well understood but almost certainly involving the complexity of its development and the unique characteristics of the tissues, the canine and feline eye and its related structures are relatively frequently affected with inherited disease. Although many of these diseases do not lend themselves to specific therapy, the clinician is obligated to recognize these problems, offer an accurate prognosis, provide breeding recommendations, and, where possible, render effective treatment.

Inherited eye disease may be congenital (present at birth) or acquired; in general, congenital defects involve structural alterations, whereas acquired diseases are metabolic in nature. Congenital lesions are not necessarily inherited, nor is acquired inherited disease always distinguishable from non-inherited conditions. This distinction frequently is a critical one for the concerned breeder who has purchased or produced an animal with non-inflammatory ocular disease. Breed, age, history, examination of parents and litter mates, and characteristics of the lesion aid the clinician in making this distinction. If doubt remains, test breedings may be recommended. If the distinction is not clear (and it seldom is), and the disease is serious in terms of its effect on functional vision, it is best to regard the condition as being inherited until controlled test breedings prove otherwise. The obligations of the clinician go beyond the individual patient to include the elimination of affected or carrier animals of significant ocular disease from the genetic pool. Unfortunately, acquired genetic disease may not appear until middle or old age, by which time genetic dispersion has already occurred.

While our understanding of Mendelian heredity is considerable, the role of external or environmental factors in the expression and transmission of genetic disease is limited. In addition, the variable nature of the patient and the specific diseases have resulted in a limited definitive knowledge of genetic eye disease in the dog and cat. Mode of inheritance may be recessive or dominant, autosomal or multisomal, and it may have variable penetrance. Expression may be influenced by genes for other somatic characteristics such as pigmentation and coat color. Sex-linked ocular disease has not been reported in the dog and cat. The majority of the documented conditions are autosomal recessive, resulting in a population of genetically normal animals, normal appearing heterozygous carrier animals, and affected dogs and cats. Carriers are usually recognizable only by test breeding the animal in question with an affected mate and observing the offspring.

A large group of inherited diseases are associated with a particular breed or characteristics of that breed, such as brachycephalic dogs. Other conditions seem to appear in certain lines within a breed but without recognized or defined genetic patterns; the term "familial" is frequently used to describe these conditions and implies a genetic condition that has not been studied adequately enough to label it more specifically.

Organization of this discussion is based on anatomy. Inherited conditions involving multiple ocular structures or the globe as a whole are presented, followed by brief descriptions of diseases of the adnexal and ocular tissue in an anterior to posterior direction.

MICROPHTHALMIA

Microphthalmia is a congenital defect that varies in extent from a slight decrease in size of the globe to near total absence of the ocular structures; it may occur as an isolated condition or in association with multiple ocular anomalies. It can occur sporadically or can result from genetic influences; the process is a breed-related phenomenon in the collie and has been observed in consecutive generations in a family of Samoyed dogs. Mild to moderate microphthalmia without associated pathology is usually compatible with functional vision. A bilateral microphthalmia-microphakia syndrome occurs in beagles as a dominant trait.

Microphthalmia with multiple colobomas is an autosomal recessive trait in the Australian shepherd linked to coat color; animals must have predominantly white coats for expression. The congenital anomalies include microphthalmia, heterochromia irides, persistent pupillary membranes, dyscoria or corectopia, iridocorneal angle dysgenesis, cataract, equatorial staphylomas, choroidal hypoplasia, retinal dysplasia and detachment, and optic nerve hypoplasia. The disease is bilateral, although the globes may be involved asymmetrically. Vision is frequently impaired.

STRABISMUS

Outward deviation (divergent strabismus or exotropia) of the ocular axes is a common breed-related condition in brachycephalic dogs, notably the Boston terrier, in which it is associated with exophthalmos. Convergent strabismus or esotropia is inherited in the Siamese cat as a simple autosomal recessive trait related to aberrant development of the visual pathways. While stereopsis and binocular fixation are undoubtedly impaired, functional vision is intact; surgical correction rarely provides satisfactory results.

NYSTAGMUS

Rapid, repetitive, involuntary movement of the eyes has a genetic basis in the Siamese cat, and the etiology may be similar to the neuroanatomic abnormalities responsible for strabismus in this breed. Vision is normal and the condition may be intermittent — disappearing when the animal fixates on an object — or it may improve with age.

OCULAR DERMOIDS

Aberrant foci of epidermal and dermal tissue may involve the eyelids, conjunctiva and nictitating membrane, or cornea alone or in combination, and they are not uncommon in the canine. Although the condition appears sporadically, dermoids appear with frequency in the Saint Bernard and German shepherd, suggesting genetic influences. Excision and blepharoplastic repair are indicated for cosmesis and to relieve irritation due to the aberrant hair.

ABNORMALITIES OF EYELID CONFORMATION

Entropion in dogs and cats may be acquired secondary to chronic inflammation and/or blepharospasm but is usually inherited and breed related. The specific mode of transmission is not known; the disease is inherited in an irregular manner suggestive of dominance with variable expressiveness. The location of the entropion is often characteristic in a particular breed; lateral lower lid entropion is commonly observed in the Norwegian elkhound and the sporting breeds, and medial lower eyelid entropion is seen in the pug and the poodle. Both upper and lower eyelids may be affected in the chow chow, sharpei, and bulldog. In the chow and Kerry blue terrier, micropalpebral fissures may be present as well.

The giant breeds, notably the Saint Bernard, are afflicted with a weakness of the lateral canthal support structures necessary for an almond-shaped palpebral fissure. The lid laxity results in medial and lateral entropion and central ectropion of both the upper and lower eyelids. Entropion is uncommon in the cat; however, the high incidence demonstrated by the Persian is suggestive of genetic factors.

Inherited entropion may appear any time prior to maturity. While mild entropion may improve spontaneously with growth of the pup, significant corneal irritation warrants prompt surgical therapy.

Ectropion is seen in breeds with excessive or loose facial skin such as spaniels, Saint Bernards, and hounds. The condition may predispose to a chronic conjunctivitis that is usually medically controllable. Severe cases may require blepharoplasty.

CILIA ABNORMALITIES

Distichiasis is an inherited disease seen in a multitude of dogs, but the American cocker spaniel (especially buff-colored members of this breed), miniature and toy poodle, pekingese, and Saint Bernard have an exceptionally high incidence. The condition is probably inherited as a dominant trait. In the majority of cases, the anomalous cilia float in the tear film with minimal irritation, and treament is unnecessary. If corneal irritation does result, a variety of manipulative procedures may be utilized to remove the offending lashes and their associated follicles; consistent satisfactory results are achieved with surgical resection of the cilia-bearing tarsoconjunctiva.

Trichomegaly, or excessively long upper eyelashes, is observed as an inherited condition in the American cocker spaniel. Mode of transmission has not been determined, and the condition does not cause clinical disease.

NASAL FOLD IRRITATION

Some brachycephalic breeds, most commonly the Pekingese, have breed standards that encourage large nasal folds. The trichiasis associated with these folds alone or in association with medial lower eyelid entropion and exophthalmia/lagophthalmia contributes to a syndrome of pigmentary keratoconjunctivitis. Ideally, the folds should be surgically removed early in life prior to the onset of extensive pathologic change if they are judged to have significant potential for corneal irritation. If the dog is a show animal, an alternative mode of therapy is the application of an ointment to the facial hair to direct it away from the globe and topical lubricants to protect the cornea.

NASOLACRIMAL SYSTEM

Epiphora related to impaired drainage of tears is common in predisposed breeds of dogs and cats. The lower punctum is primarily responsible for tear outflow, and in the American cocker spaniel, schnauzer, and Bedlington and Sealyham terrier, atresia or impatency of this structure frequently results in excessive tearing. The problem is congenital but for unknown reasons clinical signs may not be observed until one to three years of age. In the majority of cases, the canaliculi and nasolacrimal duct are normal.

Epiphora in the miniature and toy poodle is frequently related to misplacement of the lower punctum secondary to medial lower eyelid entropion; surgical correction of the entropion relieves the epiphora. Chronic medication with tetracycline or metronizadole and removal of the lacrimal gland of the nictitating membrane are not recommended to manage epiphora; in the former case, potential adverse and toxic effects of the drugs may occur, and the latter case induces a predisposition to keratoconjunctivitis sicca later in life. (While caution should be exercised in advocating excision of the gland, low dose tetracycline has had few adverse effects.)

In the Persian cat, epiphora is observed without antomic malformation and may be related to this breed's prominent eyes and flattened face, which may make the lacrimal lake shallow and hinder the passage of tears. Conjunctivorhinostomy may be performed but represents a drastic means for treatment of a usually mild problem.

The American cocker spaniel, miniature Schnauzer, and West Highland white terrier appear to have genetic predisposition to keratoconjunctivitis sicca.

NICTITATING MEMBRANE

Eversion of the cartilage of the nictitating membrane is inherited in the German shorthaired pointer, Weimaraner, Newfoundland, Chesapeake bay retriever, Saint Bernard, and great Dane and usually occurs prior to six months of age. Removal of the malformed section of the cartilage through an incision on the bulbar surface is curative.

Adenomatous hypertrophy and prolapse of the gland of the nictitating membrane occur in young beagles, Boston terriers, American cocker spaniels, and bulldogs as a result of inadequate fixation to the deeper tissues. Conservative resection leaving a portion of the secretory tissue is curative without predisposing to keratoconjunctivitis sicca. Excellent results are achieved as well by fixing the prolapsed gland to the pericanthal periosteum with a buried suture.

A pigmented encircling remnant of the nictitating membrane is seen in American cocker spaniels and beagles in the superior temporal bulbar conjunctiva and is an incidental finding.

CORNEAL DISEASE

Inherited corneal dystrophies have been observed in several breeds of dogs and Manx cats. These conditions are thought to be acquired local metabolic defects.

The Siberian husky demonstrates a stromal dystrophy that appears as an axial, doughnut-shaped opacity related to the deposition of extracellular triglycerides, neutral fats, and phospholipids. The condition develops in the first years of life and functional vision is not impaired. A familial axial dystrophy has been described in Airedales that appears at approximately one year of age owing to anterior stromal deposition of triglycerides and neutral fats. Lamellar keratectomy may be beneficial if vision

is impaired. The Boston terrier demonstrates a progressive corneal edema associated with an endothelial dystrophy; the condition is bilateral and appears in animals over five years of age. The edema first appears centrally or temporally and is slowly progressive. Topical hyperosmotics are of minimal benefit. An epithelial dystrophy is seen in boxers and is manifested as epithelial bullae and erosion; the course is usually chronic and débridement of diseased epithelium hastens resolution.

Stump-tailed Manx cats are affected by a corneal dystrophy inherited as an autosomal recessive trait. Early signs of axial anterior stromal edema are noticed at about four months of age, and the disease progresses to a diffuse bullous keratopathy.

Siamese and Persian cats exhibit a predisposition to a corneal degeneration characterized by focal stromal necrosis, pigmentation, and sequestration. Lamellar keratectomy is the treatment of choice.

The German shepherd has a breed predisposition to chronic superficial keratitis (pannus), and the condition has been reported in sibling greyhounds. Chronic administration of topical corticosteroids in titered dosage is usually effective in controlling the condition. Pannus is considered an immune-mediated disease, but the environment also plays a role.

The collie demonstrates a breed predisposition for a proliferative inflammatory process of unknown etiology, although solar irritation is suspected to play a role. Excision and/or corticosteroid therapy provide effective management.

BLUE IRIDES, HETEROCHROMIA IRIDES, AND IRIS HYPOPLASIA

Uveal pigmentation is associated with coat coloration. In complete or partial albinism, the iris may be blue or a combination of blue and brown in appearance, related to the extent of stromal and epithelial pigmentation. Iris hypoplasia may accompany these pigmentation variations. Both conditions are related to coat-color genetics and may be observed in blue merle collies, Shetland sheep dogs, Australian shepherds, Siberian huskies, malamutes, harlequin great Danes, Dalmatians, and beagles and Siamese and white cats. Concurrent deafness may occur, associated with pigment abnormalities of the cochlea. In cats and dogs, white or merle coat is inherited as an autosomal dominant trait. Heterochromia irides and deafness are autosomal dominant with incomplete penetrance. The genes for coat and iris color may be identical or closely linked. Variations in the tapetum, retinal pigmented epithelium, and choroid may accompany these conditions. Visual function is unimpaired, and nystagmus, strabismus, and photophobia are occasional associated findings.

Persistent pupillary membranes (PPMs)

Incomplete regression and differentiation of the pre-lenticular mesodermal sheet is observed sporadically in a number of breeds, and dominant inheritance with variable penetrance has been documented in the basenji. In most cases, vision is unimpaired, although extensive PPMs may cause focal non-progressive anterior capsular cataracts and/or corneal opacities. Therapy is generally not indicated. Posterior segment colobomas may be associated with PPMs. Mode of inheritance and association of these defects are complex and not well defined.

Glaucoma

Open-angle glaucoma in the beagle is inherited as an autosomal recessive trait; moderate increases in intraocular pressure occur between one and two years of age. As the disease progresses, bilateral mild megaloglobus stretching of the ciliary processes and zonular disinsertion with secondary lens luxation are observed. Degenerative changes of the retina and optic nerve occur late in the course of the disease.

The basset hound has a familial predisposition to glaucoma that may occur in the first year of life but more frequently presents as an acute congestive glaucoma in dogs older than two years of age. Megaloglobus is marked, and a luxated lens is a common associated finding. The disease is bilateral, but involvement in each eye may be sequential rather than concurrent. The iridocorneal angle may be open, narrowed, or closed, and consolidation of the pectinate ligament may or may not be present.

Acute, congestive, closed narrow-angle glaucoma occurs in middle-aged American and English cocker spaniels. Chronic open-angle and closed-angle glaucoma have been observed in miniature and toy poodles.

Siamese cats demonstrate a predisposition to a chronic open-angle glaucoma.

Glaucoma secondary to dislocation of the lens occurs in genetically predisposed terriers, presumably related to hypoplastic or dysplastic zonules. The wire-haired fox, Sealyham, Welsh, Manchester, and Boston terriers are affected in order of decreasing incidence.

Therapy of the glaucomas is the topic of detailed discussions elsewhere in this section; with the exception of an occasional open-angled glaucoma, the author regards effective long-term management of glaucoma as a surgical problem. Primary luxated or subluxated lenses should be removed, and this procedure, if performed prior to the onset or early in the course of secondary glaucoma, provides rewarding results.

Cataracts

Inherited cataracts occur in a number of breeds with a broad range of clinical characteristics (Table 1).

Congenital or developmental cataracts in young dogs are best managed by temporization if functional vision is present, as a high percentage may undergo spontaneous resorption. Cataract surgery provides rewarding results in dogs and is performed when bilateral involvement results in significant visual impairment and retinal integrity can be established by prior fundus examination or electroretinography.

Variations of fundus pigmentation

Variation in pigmentation of the retinal pigment epithelium and choroid and absence or hypoplasia of the tapetum may be associated with coat color, and, in complete or partial albinism, a spectrum of variation may be observed ophthalmoscopically. Breeds commonly affected are those mentioned in the section on variation in anterior uveal pigmentation; the two conditions are usually associated and identical genetic patterns apply.

Retinal dysplasia and degeneration

Retinal dysplasia is inherited as an autosomal recessive trait in the English springer spaniel, Sealyham terrier Labrador retriever, and Bedlington terrier. The condition is congenital and may be associated with retinal detachment or cataracts. Multifocal retinal dysplasia (retinal folds) is probably a recessive characteristic in the American cocker spaniel and is not associated with clinical disease.

Generalized progressive retinal atrophy (PRA) has been shown to be inherited as a recessive trait in the Irish setter, toy and miniature poodle, Norwegian elkhound, and Samoyed. A number of other breeds are affected, including the American cocker spaniel, Gordon setter, miniature and long-haired dachshund, English cocker spaniel, collie, miniature schnauzer, and saluki. The disease is acquired, with onset of clinical and ophthalmoscopic

Table 1. Cataracts of Proven or Suggestive Genetic Etiology in the Dog

BREED	MODE OF GENETIC TRANSMISSION	AGE OF ONSET	CHARACTERISTIC EARLY APPEARANCE	PROGRESSION
Afghan hound	simple autosomal recessive	6 mos.–2 yrs.	equatorial vacuoles	rapid°
Irish setter	?	4½ mos.–2 yrs.	cortical	rapid°
American cocker spaniel	? recessive	congenital 6 mos.–7 yrs.	nuclear and cortical posterior axial sub-capsular	slow° may remain static or progress slowly for months or years, then rapidly progress to maturity°
Boston terrier	?	4 mos.	nuclear	slowly progressive
Staffordshire terrier	?	4 mos.	nuclear	slowly progressive
Miniature schnauzer	simple autosomal recessive	congenital	nuclear and cortical	rapid
Golden retriever	dominant with variable expression	congenital ? or up to 1 yr.	posterior axial sub-capsular	non-progressive
Old English sheepdog	recessive	1–3 yrs. congenital (?) or up to 2 yrs.	cortical cortical and nuclear-associated retinal detachment	progressive progressive
Beagle	dominant (?)	4 mos.	posterior axial opacities	non-progressive
German shepherd	dominant	congenital (?)	cortical	slowly progressive
Miniature and toy poodle	?	3–10 yrs.	cortical	progressive
Standard poodle	simple autosomal recessive	prior to 2 yrs. of age	equatorial	progressive
Welsh corgi	probably recessive	prior to 2 yrs. of age	posterior sub-capsular axial or equatorial	very slowly progressive
Pointer	dominant (?)	–	–	–
Labrador retriever	dominant	–	–	–
Siberian husky	recessive	6–24 mos.	posterior sub-capsular axial	very slowly progressive

°Likelihood of spontaneous resorption in young dogs.

signs and pathogenesis variable between and characteristic of specific breeds (see "Diseases of the Vitreous, Retina, and Choroid").

Central PRA is familial, with suggestion of dominant transmission in Labrador and golden retrievers and Shetland sheepdogs; onset occurs in middle age or later.

Retinal degeneration in the borzoi is probably transmitted as a recessive trait. It appears as multifocal retinal degeneration that progresses to diffuse retinal involvement, and it may be seen as early as six months of age.

Hemeralopia (day blindness) occurs in the Alaskan malamute as a simple autosomal characteristic and is observed behaviorally in pups by eight to ten weeks of age, but no fundus lesions are seen ophthalmoscopically.

Diffuse outer segment degeneration has been described in two litters of Persian kittens born to common parents. The kittens were ophthalmoscopically and clinically normal at birth. Fundus abnormalities and visual deficits appeared during the first months of life. Simple autosomal inheritance was suggested.

OPTIC NERVE HYPOPLASIA

Optic nerve hypoplasia is usually a sporadic congenital condition with a variable effect on vision, dependent upon extent. The condition has been observed in related German shepherds and miniature poodles, suggesting that some cases may have a genetic basis.

COLLIE EYE ANOMALY

Focal choroidal hypoplasia is a hereditary bilateral congenital defect that affects collies and shetland sheep dogs and is characterized by focal choroidal hypoplasia, posterior segment coloboma and staphyloma, and retinal detachment with giant peripheral dialysis. Only choroidal hypoplasia is observed in the Shetland sheepdog. Transmission is not completely understood but is generally thought to be auto-somal recessive related to a single gene with variable expressivity.

SUPPLEMENTAL READING

Aguirre, G.D.: Hereditary retinal disease in small animals. Vet. Clin. North Am., 3:515–528, 1973.
Barnett, K.C.: Hereditary cataract in the dog. J. Small Anim. Pract. 19:109–120, 1978.
Bedford, P.G.D.: The etiology of primary glaucoma in the dog. J. Small Animal Pract. 16:217–239, 1975.

Bistner, S., Rubin, L.F., and Roberts, S.R.: A review of persistent pupillary membranes in the Basenji dog. J. Am. Anim. Hosp. Assoc. 7:143–157, 1971.
Bistner, S.I., Aguirre, G., and Shively, J.N.: Hereditary corneal dystrophy in the Manx cat: a preliminary report. Invest. Ophthalmol. 15:15–26, 1976.
Gelatt, K.N., and McGill, L.D.: Clinical characteristics of microphthalmia with colobomas of the Australian shepherd dog. J. Am. Vet. Med. Assoc. 167:393–396, 1973.
Sorsby, A., and Davey, J.B.: Ocular association of dappling (or merling) in the coat colour of dogs. I. Clinical and genetical data. J. Gent. 52:425–440, 1954.
Yakely, W.L., et al.: Genetic transmission of an ocular fundus anomaly in collies. J. Am. Vet. Med. Assoc., 152:457–461, 1968.

THE EYE AND SYSTEMIC DISEASE

CHARLES L. MARTIN, D.V.M.
Athens, Georgia

To ophthalmologists, the eye is a window into the body, but in veterinary internal medicine, it is a window that is unfortunately underutilized. In the rush to be clinically sophisticated, undue emphasis is placed on expensive technical tests and instruments, and not enough is placed on thorough histories and physical examinations. A thorough ocular examination should be part of any physical examination, and when that goal is achieved, it will be evident how our present knowledge is incomplete. A paradox exists in that the busy practitioner is perhaps most likely to neglect performing a detailed ocular examination, but he/she is also most in need of rapid, inexpensive diagnostic tests.

Ocular lesions may be classified as being either of primary or secondary importance. Primary lesions are those that impair visual function, often cause the animal to be presented for examination, and require specific therapy if available. Lesions of secondary importance are relatively mild and often easily overlooked. They usually do not require specific therapy, but they may provide diagnostic clues as to the type of disease process involved and occasionally lead to a specific diagnosis.

Table 1 summarizes the documented associations of ocular signs with systemic disease. Limitations of space preclude detailed discussions and inclusion of all the exotic reports. The section on toxic changes could be greatly expanded. However, the compounds included are those most likely to be utilized by veterinarians.

Table 1. The Eye and Systemic Disease

INFECTIOUS DISEASES	OCULAR LESIONS	SYSTEMIC SIGNS	DIAGNOSTIC FEATURES
A. Viral Distemper	Serous–mucopurulent conjunctivitis, keratoconjunctivitis sicca, chorioretinitis, optic neuritis	± Depression, anorexia, fever 102.5–103.5+, nasal discharge, dyspnea, vomiting, diarrhea, seizures, paresis, paralysis	Lymphopenia, + fluorescent antibody test on epithelial surfaces or tissues, neutralizing antibody in CSF
Infectious Canine Hepatitis	Corneal edema from endothelial damage, anterior uveitis, glaucoma	Ocular signs occur after recovery, ± recent H/O, depressed, fever (104–105), vomiting, abdominal pain, anorexia, MLV vaccination in last 2–3 weeks	Leukopenia, c̄ lymphopenia, liver enzymes elevated later; H/O no vaccination or recent vaccination
Canine Herpes	Panuveitis c̄ keratitis, cataract, retinal dysplasia and atrophy, retinoschesis, optic neuritis, cavitation	Crying, dyspnea, tender abdomen, yellow diarrhea, rapid death	Less than 2 weeks of age, pain preceding rapid death, postmortem ecchymosis on kidney, liver, lung, c̄ inclusions on histopathology
	Follicular conjunctivitis?	Vaginitis? balanoposthitis	Adult syndrome needs further investigation
Herpes felis	Neonatal and adult conjunctivitis, dendritic corneal ulcers, keratitis, occasional uveitis, optic neuritis	±Depressed, sneezing, anorexia, nasal discharge, tracheitis, oral ulcers	Viral isolation. H/O URD
Panleukopenia	Chorioretinal scars, optic nerve hypoplasia	± Cerebellar signs, ataxia, intention tremors, hypermetria	Concurrent cerebellar signs
Feline Leukemia Complex	Granulomatous anterior uveitis, secondary glaucoma, tumors in anterior uvea, chorioretinal infiltrates, pale retinal vessels c̄ hemorrhages	± Signs may not be concurrent c̄ ocular lesions and take weeks to months to manifest	FA for virus in neutrophils, leukopenia, anemia, mutton fat KP's, leukemia, masses in abdomen, chest, peripheral LN
Feline Infectious Peritonitis	Granulomatous anterior and posterior uveitis, retinal hemorrhages, vasculitis, secondary glaucoma	± CNS signs, ascites, large kidneys, dyspnea, depression, anorexia, fever, weight loss	Elevated SN titers, typical abdominal fluid, 50% viremic c̄ feline leukemia virus, mutton fat KP's
B. **Chlamydia** *Chlamydia felis*	Conjunctivitis	± Mild nasal signs	Early conjunctival scrapping have elementary bodies
C. **Rickettsia** *Ehrlichia canis*	Subconjunctival hemorrhages, hyphema, perivascular retinal infiltrates	Fever, depressed, weight loss, epistaxis, anemia	Morula (inclusions) in monocytes

Agent	Ocular Signs	Systemic Signs	Diagnosis
D. Bacteria			
Leptospira sp.	Icteric sclera, conjunctivitis, subconjunctival hemorrhages, anterior uveitis	Fever, dehydrated, vomiting, abdominal pain, stiff gait, icteric	Neutrophilia, ↑ ESR, ↑ Bilirubin, ↑ Liver Enzymes, ↑ BUN, Rising Lepto titer, Lepto in urine on darkfield, Lepto cultured in urine or blood
Brucella canis	Anterior uveitis, endophthalmitis, secondary glaucoma	± Orchitis, abortion	Aqueous titers, culture of vitreous, blood cultures and titers, placental cultures
Clostridium tetani	Prolapsed membrana nictitans, enophthalmos	Hypersensitivity to stimuli c̄ spasms, facial spasms, ears erect, opisthotonus	Clinical syndrome, H/O wound
Mycobacterium sp.	Anterior uveitis, granulomatous chorioretinitis, retinal detachment, keratitis, blepharitis	Varies c̄ organ involvement, CNS, digestive systems, chronic signs c̄ weight loss	Vitreous cultures and cytology, biopsy
Septicemia c̄ staph. sp., strep. sp.	Endophthalmitis, secondary glaucoma	Depends on source of septicemia – i.e. mouth, endocardium, etc.	Blood cultures, aqueous and vitreous cytology and cultures
E. Systemic Mycoses *Cryptococcus neoformans* *Histoplasma capsulatum* *Blastomyces dermatitidis* *Coccidioides immitis*	Granulomatous uveitis, retinal detachment, optic neuritis, secondary glaucoma	Pulmonary signs c̄ all, CNS and upper respiratory signs c̄ crypto.. blasto., and histo. (cats), skeletal signs c̄ blasto., cutaneous abscessation c̄ crypto. and blasto., weight loss, fever	Typical geographic area, chest x-rays, organisms in exudates from abscess, trachea, vitreous, lymph nodes, serologic testing, skin testing
F. Algae *Prototheca* sp.	Granulomatous chorioretinitis	Chronic hemorrhagic, diarrhea, CNS signs	Vitreous aspiration, biopsy of intestinal tract
G. Protozoan *Hemobartonella felis* and *canis*	Pale retinal vessels, retinal hemorrhages	Fever, pale mucous membranes, weak	Regenerative anemia, organisms on RBC, many cats are + FA for leukemia virus, dogs usually splenectomized or severely stressed
Toxoplasma gondi	Granulomatous anterior uveitis, retinochoroiditis, optic neuritis, myositis of extraocular muscles	± Variable, multifocal CNS signs, myositis, dyspnea, fever, hepatitis, lymphadenopathy	High or rising toxoplasma antibody titers, organ or muscle biopsy, oocysts in feces of cat, leukopenia
Leishmania donovani	Keratitis, conjunctivitis, endophthalmitis, blepharitis	Weight loss, fever, anemia, splenomegaly, hepatomegaly	H/O living in Mediterranean region, organism in peripheral and marrow monocytes or on lymph node aspiration
H. Metazoan *Dirofilaria immitus*	Worm in anterior chamber or vitreous	± ↓ Exercise tolerance, cough	± Microfilaremia, identification of worm on removal
Toxocara canis larva	Focal chorioretinal granuloma	None	Appearance, histology
Demodex canis	Blepharitis	±	Skin scraping

Table 1. The Eye and Systemic Disease—Continued

METABOLIC DISTURBANCES	OCULAR LESIONS	SYSTEMIC SIGNS	DIAGNOSTIC FEATURES
A. Diabetes mellitus (Hyperglycemia)	Cortical cataracts, occasional micro-angiopathic retinopathy	Polydipsia, polyuria, weight loss, hyperphagia, vomiting, depressed	Hyperglycemia, glycosuria, ketotic ±
B. Hypothyroidism	Corneal lipidosis, arteriosclerosis c̄ hypertensive retinopathy—i.e., papilledema and retinal hemorrhages, retinal detachments	± Cold intolerance, lethargy, dermatologic changes, infertility	Depressed T_4 after TSH stimulation, ↑ blood pressure, ↑ cholesterol
C. Hypoparathyroidism (Hypocalcemia)	Cortical punctate, cataracts	Seizures, muscle twitching	Decreased serum calcium, increased serum phosphorus
D. Hypercalcemia from hyperparathyroidism and pseudohyperparathyroidism (PHP)	Band keratopathy—i.e., superficial corneal calcium deposits	Skeletal fractures, anorexia, vomiting, weakness, calcium nephropathy, lymphosarcoma related signs c̄ PHP	Increased serum calcium, decreased serum phosphorus unless in renal failure
E. Hyperlipoproteinemias	Lipemia retinalis—i.e, lipemia visible in retinal blood vessels, lipids in anterior chamber, lipid keratopathy	±Abdominal distress, seizures	↑ Triglycerides c̄ lipemia retinalis, ↑ lipoproteins
F. Azotemia, Uremia	Enophthalmos and keratoconjunctivitis sicca from dehydration. Effusive retinal detachment, retinal hemorrhages if severely hypertensive	Polyuria, polydipsia, vomiting, depressed, dehydrated	Urinalysis, BUN, ↑ blood pressure
G. Hyperadrenocorticism	Refractive corneal ulcers, keratoconjunctivitis sicca	Polydipsia, polyuria, hyperphagia, alopecia, muscle wasting, distended abdomen	↑ Plasma cortisol response to ACTH injection
H. Mucopolysaccaridosis	Hazy cornea	Siamese cat c̄ short stature, head short and broad	↑ MPS in urine, metachromatic granules in leukocytes
I. Albinism—partial or complete	Blue irides, heterochromia ± absence of tapetum, "tigroid" fundus, microphthalmos, cataracts, colobomas, retinal dysplasia, strabismus	White haircoat, ± deaf—unilateral or bilateral	Signs
CARDIOVASCULAR DISEASES			
A. Polycythemia	Dilated, tortuous ruddy colored conjunctival and retinal vessels, retinal and vitreous hemorrhages	Usually cyanotic heart disease, weak, ↓ exercise tolerance, CNS signs	Cyanotic or brick red mucous membranes, ↑PCV with normal plasma protein level, hemoglobin, chest radiographs and cardiac auscultation
B. Anemia	Pale retinal vessels, retinal hemorrhages, icterus if intravascular hemolysis	Weak, tachycardia, polypnea, pale mucous membranes	CBC
C. Hyperviscosity syndrome c̄ macroglobinemia	Dilated, tortuous retinal vessels, retinal hemorrhages	Epistaxis, GI bleeding, renal disease, lameness, weight loss, pathologic fractures	Pleomorphic, immature solid cluster of plasma cells in bone marrow or lymphocytic leukemia
D. Thrombocytopenias and Thrombasthenia	Hemorrhages in orbit, subconjunctivally, anterior chamber, iris, vitreous, and retina	Petechia and ecchymosis on mucous membranes and skin	↓ Platelet count c̄ thrombocytopenia
E. Hypertension c̄ pheochromocytoma, renal disease, hypothyroid arteriosclerosis, hypernatremia	Papilledema, retinal hemorrhages, effusive retinal detachment	±Nervous, anxious animal, depends on associated etiology	↑ Blood pressure, + specific work-up for each disease

	Ocular Signs	Systemic Signs	Diagnosis
NUTRITION			
A. Taurine deficiency in cat	Macular degeneration, bilateral diffuse retinal atrophy	None	H/O dog food diet, typical ocular lesions
B. Vitamin A deficiency	Papilledema, blind, in the growing dog	Vestibular signs of head tilt, ataxia, circling	↓ Plasma vitamin A levels
C. Thiamin deficiency (B₁)	Dilated, non-responsive pupils	Anorexia, weight loss, ataxia, ventral-flexion when suspended	↓ Erythrocyte transketolase activity, blood thiamin levels
D. Riboflavin deficiency (B₂)	Corneal edema, corneal vascularization	Weight loss, scaly dermatitis	Poor diet?
E. Vitamin E deficiency	Dilated pupils, ↓ vision, retinal degeneration	↓ Fertility, ↑ puppy mortality, hemolytic anemia	Plasma tocopherol levels, lipofuscin accumulation in intestinal muscularis
TOXIC			
A. Phenazopyridine	Keratoconjunctivitis sicca	—	History
B. Sulfadiazine	Keratoconjunctivitis sicca	—	History
C. Atropine	Keratoconjunctivitis sicca	—	History
D. Disophenol	Temporary cataracts in pups less than 4 months of age	—	History
E. Orphan milk replacements	Cataracts	—	History
F. Griseofulvin	Cyclopia, anophthalmia	Widespread central nervous system and skeletal malformation	Teratogenic, drug given in first trimester of pregnancy
G. Warfarin	Retrobullar and subconjunctival hemorrhage	Hemorrhages elsewhere in body	↑ Prothrombin time, ↑ partial thromboptatin time, normal thrombin time
H. Soaps and caustic agents	Corneal erosions, iritis, blepharitis	±	History
NEOPLASTIC			
A. Canine lymphosarcoma	Uveal infiltration and uveitis, glaucoma, hypopyon, hyphema, corneal infiltration, retinal hemorrhages, retinal detachment	Enlarged peripheral lymph nodes, weight loss, anorexia, vomiting, diarrhea cutaneous nodules	Biopsy of affected lymph nodes, bone marrow
B. Reticulosis of CNS	Papilledema, optic atrophy, retinal detachment, anterior uveitis, secondary glaucoma	Multifocal CNS lesions	Reticulocytes in CSF, response to steroids
C. Neoplasms of diencephalon	Papilledema, optic atrophy, ±Horner's Syndrome, hemianopia, pupil dilation	±Polydipsia, polyuria, pain, endocrine disturbances	Lesion localization, Hx slowly progressive, cavernous sinus venography
D. Neoplasms of midbrain, pons and medulla	Vary c̄ location and cranial nerve involvement III, IV, V, VI, VII; pupil dilation, ptosis, paralysis of ocular movements, decreased lacrimation, anesthesia of cornea, corneal ulcers	Upper motor signs in limbs, involvement of other cranial nerve	Signalment, ↑ CSF pressure ↑ CSF protein, slowly progressive
E. Metastatic Neoplasia	Tumor in lid, anterior uvea, occasional posterior uvea, secondary glaucoma	Depends on source of primary lesion and metastatic disease elsewhere	History of tumor elsewhere, chest x-rays
F. Neoplasia from contiguous anatomic sites	Space-occupying orbital lesion c̄ exophthalmos, ocular deviations, lacrimal outflow obstruction	Extension from sinus, oral cavity, nasal cavity, skull, skin	Biopsy

Table 1. *The Eye and Systemic Disease—Continued*

MISCELLANEOUS	OCULAR LESIONS	SYSTEMIC SIGNS	DIAGNOSTIC FEATURES
A. Pancreatitis	Papilledema, lipemia retinalis	Vomiting, depressed to coma, tender abdomen	↑ Serum lipase and amylase
B. Trauma	Lacerations and contusion of lids, conjunctiva, corneal abrasion, miosis, mydriasis, hyphema, iritis, retinal hemorrhages, detachment, proptosed globe, ruptured globe, avulsion of optic nerve and/or retinal vessels	Varied	History and trauma to other areas of body
C. Atopic and allergic contact dermatitis	Blepharitis, conjunctivitis, cataract?	Pruritic dermatitis	History—seasonal ±, skin tests, negative skin scraping
D. Pemphigus vulgaris	Blepharitis	Bullous and erosive lesions in oral cavity, lips, anus, vulvar margin, or prepuce	Histopathology, direct and indirect immunofluorescent antibody testing or skin biopsies
E. Eosinophilic Myositis	Exophthalmos, conjunctival injection, exposure keratitis	Muscles of mastication swollen, difficult to open mouth	Biopsy of temporal muscle

Hx = History
H/O = History of
SN = serum neutralization titers
KP = Keratitic precipitate
FA = Fluorescent antibody
URD = Upper respiratory disease
ESR = Erythrocyte sedimentation rate
CNS = Central nervous system
T$_4$ = Thyroxine
TSH = Thyroid stimulating hormone

Section
8

DISEASES OF CAGED BIRDS AND EXOTIC PETS

MURRAY E. FOWLER, D.V.M.
Consulting Editor

Introduction 601
Veterinary Involvement in Rehabilitation Centers 601
Mycobacterial Infections in Non-domestic Animals 604
Medical Care of Tropical Fish.. 606
Amphibian Care and Diseases.. 616
Anesthesia of Reptiles... 618
Surgery in Captive Reptiles 620
Infectious Diseases of Reptiles.. 625
Respiratory Disease in Reptiles 633
Medical Care of Aquatic Turtles.. 637
Antibiotic Therapy in Reptiles 647
Avian Radiographic Technique and Interpretation....................... 649
Anesthesia of Caged Birds 653
Otoscope Technique for Sexing Birds 656
Diagnostic Laparoscopy in Birds 659
Avian Orthopedics 662
Foreign Diseases and Imported Birds 674
Psittacosis — An Ever-present Problem in Caged Birds 677
Management of Oil-soaked Birds 687
Care and Treatment of Captive Wild Birds 692
Respiratory Disease in Psittacine Birds 697
Acute Avian Herpesvirus Infections 704
Anesthesia for Rabbits and Rodents 706
Medical Care of Non-domestic Carnivores 710
Virus Diseases of Primates — Their Hazards to Human Health 733
Individual Care and Treatment of Rabbits, Mice, Rats,
    Guinea Pigs, Hamsters, and Gerbils................................. 741

Continued

Additional Pertinent Information, Still Current, Found in
Current Veterinary Therapy VI:

Altman, R. B.: Diseases of the avian urinary system, p. 703.
Altman, R. B.: Fractures of the extremities of birds, p. 717.
Altman, R. B.: Parasitic diseases of caged birds, p. 682.
Amand, W. B.: General techniques for avian surgery, p. 711.
Detrick, J. F., and Raff, M. I.: Husbandry of captive wild birds, p. 687.
Fowler, M. E.: Restraint mortality in wild animals, p. 723.
Frye, F. L.: Bacterial and fungal diseases of captive reptiles, p. 787.
Frye, F. L.: Hematology of captive reptiles (with emphasis on normal morphology), p. 792.
Harris, J. M.: Restraint and physical examination of monkeys and primates, p. 721.
Lafeber, T. J.: Feather disorders of common caged birds, p. 675.
Marcus, L. C.: Salmonellosis in reptiles, p. 799.
Silverman, S.: Exotic animal radiology, p. 756.
Soifer, F. K.: Hematology of some zoo animals and exotic pets, p. 765.
Wallach, J. D.: Management and nutritional problems in captive reptiles, p. 778.

Additional Pertinent Information, Still Current, Found in
Current Veterinary Therapy V:

Lafeber, T. J.: Physical examination, laboratory and medication techniques and hospitalization procedures for the common parakeet and canary, p. 533.
Leonard, J. L.: Clinical laboratory examination of caged birds, p. 543.
Miller, R. M.: Feeding zoo animals and exotic pets, p. 617.
Petrak, M. L.: Neoplasia in cage birds, p. 585.

INTRODUCTION

MURRAY E. FOWLER, D.V.M.
Davis, California

The American Veterinary Medical Association and many state veterinary associations have published policy statements opposing private ownership of non-domestic animals. There are many and varied reasons to support such a stance. Nonetheless, possession of wild animals is legal in most states, although special permits may be required. It is incumbent upon the veterinarian to know the legal requirements existant in his or her practice area. Refusal to care for a wild animal based on the logic that "wild animals should not be kept as pets; therefore, I won't work on them" simply condemns the animal to inferior care, no care, or death. If it becomes illegal to own wild pets then we must support the law. Until then, we should offer the wild animal–owner client all the professional medical skills we possess. It is an individual's right to decide whether or not to include wild species in a practice. However, the profession as a whole must not turn its back on wild animals because of emotionally charged, legalistic human battles involving the right of ownership.

This section of Current Veterinary Therapy is designed to assist those who are willing to deal with non-domestic pets. Many new approaches to old topics are presented. All repeated titles have been updated and revised.

Restraint is one of the most challenging aspects of dealing with wild animals. Various techniques are described by individual authors in this section. Readers desiring more detailed information on restraint and handling are referred to texts in the supplemental reading list.

SUPPLEMENTAL READING

Fowler, M. E. (ed.): Zoo and Wild Animal Medicine. Philadelphia, W. B. Saunders, 1978.
Fowler, M. E.: Restraint and Handling of Wild and Domestic Animals. Ames, Iowa, Iowa State University Press, 1978.
Harthoorn, A. M.: The Chemical Capture of Animals. London, Bailliere, Tindall, 1976.
Young, E. (ed.): The Capture and Care of Wild Animals. Capetown, South Africa, Human and Rousseau, 1973.

VETERINARY INVOLVEMENT IN REHABILITATION CENTERS

RAYMOND A. KRAY, D.V.M.
Burbank, California

Because of increased public awareness of the plight of endangered species of animals in the wild, there is growing concern for the welfare of wildlife. Rehabilitation centers that are designed to treat injured or unwanted wildlife are springing up all over the United States and in other countries as well, with the ultimate goal of rehabilitation and release of these animals back into their natural environment. An alternative to the plight of the unreleasable is to salvage the individual for possible captive reproduction, exhibition, or research.

Rehabilitation in its true sense means to restore to a condition of health or useful and constructive activity. The key phrase here is "useful and constructive." To the veterinarian involved in rehabilitation centers this concept must be weighed against the emotional desire to save every animal brought in, e.g., the hawk that is presented in perfect condition except for its feet, which were mutilated beyond saving by a steel trap.

The role of the devil's advocate is one that veterinarians often find themselves playing, and when euthanasia is the decision or recommendation, their stand is not often the popular one. Whether the veterinarian is a part-time healer or a full-time member of the board, the duties and responsibilities will be multifaceted and demand a full measure of patience and ingenuity.

The following is an attempt to describe some of the problems that will involve a veterinarian as an associate of an animal rehabilitation center.

THE CAUSE AND EFFECT OF ECONOMICS

In a realistic appraisal, economics is the one criterion that determines the future of the rehabilitation center. The facility may have a few short-lived accomplishments, acquire a large number of animals, and shortly thereafter disappear into economic ruin and oblivion. Alternatively, the center may be satisfied with less spectacular accomplishments, work with fewer animals, give them higher quality treatment, and so avoid bankruptcy. Obviously other factors can be involved, but they are more easily resolved.

Most rehabilitation centers start out small, the veterinarian being one of the principals, and as the facility grows so does the responsibility of the attending D.V.M. Soon the veterinarian is devoting more time to the center and less to the private practice that provides his or her own financial stability and independence. Money to run rehabilitation centers is almost always in short supply, and the number of animals waiting to come in seems inexhaustible. The veterinarian soon finds many of the volunteers at the center wondering why he or she is not doing more and perhaps furnishing all the drugs gratis. The veterinarian may be used to impress certain wealthy prospective donors or may be expected to go out and solicit funds personally. Unfortunately, these are not conjectures but situations that really occur. It is incumbent upon the veterinarian to establish guidelines and define the limits of his or her involvement in the center from the very beginning. The other personnel in the facility must know exactly what to expect of the veterinarian. Only by setting limits and then rigidly adhering to them can the practitioner hope to remain apart from the politics and instabilities that can develop.

VOLUNTEER AND EMPLOYEE MANAGEMENT

Urban rehabilitation centers such as those in southern California are usually staffed by part-time volunteers who have other permanent jobs, by students on vacation, or by individuals who are "fed up" with bureaucracies and corporate images and want to change their life style completely. A center's staff may also include a few retired people who wish to make a contribution to the world of living things. Wealthy individuals who donate money may also wish to participate in using it.

This array of talent from individuals with various backgrounds who all want "to work with the animals" often produces a perplexing problem for the allocator of jobs. Since many claim to have some form of previous animal-handling experience although their references are untraceable, it often falls to the veterinarian to make the final decision about who will come into direct contact with the animals. When the facility is handling small mammals or birds this decision is not as difficult as when wolves, bears, and mountain lions are being rehabilitated. Obviously this requires personal experience with these animals and their behavior on the part of the veterinarian. It also requires the ability to judge human personalities and to predict how people will react in potentially dangerous situations. It will be the veterinarian, the so-called "animal expert" in this group of principals, who must take final responsibility for any tragic accident involving animal interactions or animal and human altercations. When events flow smoothly and uneventfully the veterinarian must maintain unremitting surveillance, since more than anyone else he or she knows what can result from a simple miscalculation by an animal technician. The D.V.M. must, as it were, stand with one foot inside the cage and one outside, seeing the animal handler through the animal's eyes and the animal through the handler's.

PUBLIC RELATIONS

Public relations is a field in which most D.V.M.'s are very inexperienced, but unfortunately few will admit this. Fewer still will seek professional guidance. Veterinary doctors are often quoted, and as often as not their comments sound either very pedantic or very simple. The news media are very effective tools for educating the people or warping the way they think. Reporters, sometimes unknowingly, will twist what we have said to further or intensify the intent of their articles or broadcasts. A cute, cuddly raccoon or bear cub, a delicate fawn or a young owl is only slightly newsworthy in itself, but when coupled with a villainous or heroic act it becomes good copy on a newsless day. Often unintentionally the veterinarian becomes the spokesperson for the center when an off-the-cuff remark to a reporter is read or heard the next day by thousands of people. To guard against tarnishing veterinary brilliance I would suggest a policy of giving no verbal comments, but submitting a written press release instead. This is the official policy of most large animal theme parks and seems to create the least misunderstanding. Public relations managers of parks dealing with animals have learned through experience not to trust a verbal comment to the memory of a reporter.

When properly used, an article or broadcast about a rehabilitation center can generate much public support, and there is then no reason why the veterinarian should not be quoted. Almost every center will have in its roster of volunteers someone involved in the theatrical arts, public speaking, or advertising. Utilize that person's expertise; it will be invaluable, the volunteer will feel that he or she has contributed, and the news release will be more professional.

ADMINISTRATIVE DUTIES

Records, permits, and related paperwork are all necessary evils in a rehabilitation center. This is an area in which the veterinarian can use non-professional volunteers to their best ability. For some reason the administrator, accountant, or secretary volunteer who is disgruntled with his or her own office job will absolutely shine when asked to keep records of diet, appetite, drugs administered, and bowel movements of animals. Such workers bring a new zeal to a task that is boring to a veteran animal handler. Because they are not indoctrinated with someone else's rules they often can be very innovative with labor- and time-saving techniques adapted from commerce and industry.

Any type of wild animal rehabilitation will require special permits from interested state and federal agencies. Cooperation with the officers of these agencies is both advisable and necessary. Since regulations vary from state to state and are continually being changed, the veterinarian must be advised frequently by these officials as to the status of the animals in his or her charge. Agencies involved in wild animal regulation cooperate with each other,

and communication with one will open up lines for the exchange of information with others.

Liaison should be established between the veterinarian and local humane organizations because of the common interest and mutual assistance each can provide. With the increased concern for saving endangered species, many humane groups have formed committees that specialize in providing temporary care and housing facilities for these animals.

Universities and zoologic parks can provide a wealth of expertise and experience to the veterinarian, so establishing a working relationship with them should be the first priority. Not only can they help with free advice and laboratory assistance, but they are also a source of trained and qualified personnel because of the many people who apply to them for jobs. Their behavioral biologists will also be invaluable in readaptive training of rehabilitated animals to the wild environment.

ANIMAL COMPOUND MANAGEMENT

Within recent years a formidable number of guidelines and regulations have been established by various state and federal agencies that set standards for sizes of cages and runs for wild animals and that control conditions under which animals may be transported across state and federal boundaries. Seeing that these guidelines are adhered to is also a function of veterinarians, who must familiarize themselves with the application of these rules to their animals.

Nutrition on a tight budget is often a problem. There are many sources of palatable food available free or at reduced prices. A few examples are day-old bread from bakeries, unsold dated vegetables from grocery markets, discolored meat from butcher shops, and uneaten prepackaged items such as sandwiches from caterers. Most of this food is good and wholesome, but the veterinarian must monitor its quality and its source periodically and not leave this responsibility entirely to assistants.

Equipment and drugs necessary for a wild animal practice are becoming more and more expensive and, next to feed, usually account for the largest part of the budget. Operating within a budget can make one very resourceful. Talking to other veterinarians, drug sales representatives, and medial equipment supply houses and attending auctions of human hospital equipment often can turn up some real bargains and sometimes outright gifts. This is especially true for centers that have a tax-exempt status.

Once the veterinarian has established the contact, details are turned over to a volunteer assistant. The source often becomes a steady supplier.

CONCLUSION

Because of the scope of a veterinarian's involvement in all these areas, time limitation dictates that the D.V.M. become a manager. The veterinarian's usefulness depends to a great extent on how well he or she utilizes the time and talents of other qualified people. Knowledge is our most important tool, and in the emerging field of veterinary medicine continuing specialized education is very important. Participation in workshops at zoological parks and membership in organizations such as the American Association of Zoological Parks and Aquariums, the American Association of Zoo Veterinarians, the Wildlife Disease Association, and many others offer the rehabilitation center veterinarian a chance to meet sympathetic colleagues. These people can understand the unique problems of each practitioner and can offer practical advise on care and rehabilitation. They may suggest institutions that will accept animals not fit for release into the wild, since such animals have a way of accumulating at the center and form its largest financial burden and its biggest logistical problem.

MYCOBACTERIAL INFECTIONS IN NON-DOMESTIC ANIMALS

SUZANNE KENNEDY, D.V.M.
Knoxville, Tennessee

Mycobacteria are slightly curved or straight aerobic rods. They do not stain well by Gram's method, but all are acid-fast at some stage of growth. The Ziehl-Neelsen technique of staining is routinely used to demonstate this acid-fastness. The genus *Mycobacterium* includes obligate parasites, saprophytes, and intermediate forms. Diseases produced include tuberculosis, Johne's disease and leprosy. Growth on culture media is variable but slow, so plates should not be discarded before eight weeks.

TUBERCULOSIS

Because of extensive tuberculin testing in cattle and the rapid turnover of birds in the poultry industry, tuberculosis could be considered a disease of the past much as polio is in people. However, nothing could be further from the truth. Wherever animals are kept in close confinement with each other or with people, such as in zoos or laboratories, the potential for tuberculosis exists.

Though some species are more susceptible than others, almost any animal may become infected, including reptiles and fish. Clinical signs are non-specific. Mammals and birds may exhibit weight loss and lethargy. Primates may develop a cough or diarrhea, depending on the site of infection, and this may indicate whether the organism entered its body by inhalation or ingestion. Tuberculosis in non-human primates is a fulminating disease and is invariably fatal. Clinical signs in fish include cachexia, exophthalmia, and ulceration of the scales and fins. Primary lesions in turtles usually are cutaneous or pulmonic. The digestive system is involved in other reptiles. In most cases of tuberculosis, a diagnosis is made at necropsy.

Primates may be infected with any of the three major species of *Mycobacterium: M. tuberculosis, M. bovis,* and *M. avium,* in that order. Infections do occur with some of the atypical species, such as *M. kansasii* and *M. intracellulare.* Exotic hoofed stock and parrots are also susceptible to each of the three major species. Other birds are susceptible only to the avian types of mycobacteria. The ectotherms (reptiles, amphibians, and fish) are usually infected by the saprophytic mycobacteria such as *M. marinum, M. chelonei,* and *M. fortuitum.*

Tuberculin testing still remains the best way to monitor the prevalence of tuberculosis in mammals. Frequency of testing varies, but some laboratory facilities test primates four to six times a year. Most zoos test their primates once a year. Privately owned primates should be tested at least once a year and preferably every six months. Recommendations for tuberculin testing of primates in quarantine vary from two to six negative tests two weeks apart.

Mammalian Old tuberculin (OT)* is recommended for use in primates and other exotic mammals. In primates, a 0.1 ml suspension of OT is injected intradermally into the upper eyelid with a 25 to 27 gauge ³⁄₈-inch needle. The skin of the abdomen is an additional test site. The test site should be observed daily for three consecutive days. A positive reaction can vary from slight reddening and edema of the test site to localized necrosis. The maximum response is usually observed at 72 hours, though squirrel monkeys react strongly at 48 hours. When reactions are questionable the test should be repeated in the opposite eyelid or in another site on the abdomen.

Hoofed stock should be tested with 0.1 ml OT intradermally in the caudal fold. Positive or suspected reactors should be evaluated further by comparative cervical skin testing using avian and bovine purified protein derivatives (PPD). Unfortunately, many facilities that keep exotic hoofed stock do not test routinely because of the stress placed on the animals by restraint and because of the time consumed. Such excuses have permitted *M. bovis* to exist in zoologic collections in countries where the disease is no longer seen in domestic stock.

Controversy exists concerning the efficacy of tuberculin testing. Admittedly, false positive results do occur but, fortunately, few false negative results have been reported. Lymphocyte transformation (LT) has been used to differentiate false or questionable reactions with varying degrees of success. The LT is more sensitive than tuberculin testing in detecting early disease in primates. Chest radiographs are sometimes helpful in diagnosing advanced cases of tuberculosis in anergic primates.

Tuberculin testing is not effective in birds. Eliminating avian tuberculosis from an aviary or zoologic collection is almost impossible, since there is no reliable method of identifying infected birds. Laparoscopy has been used to check the spleen and liver for granulomas (see page 659). This is a useful technique, but a bird may be infected for several months before granulomas develop. Radiography can be helpful in those instances in which tuberculous osteomye-

litis develops in one or more long bones. In the latter stages of the disease, birds may have elevated leukocyte counts ranging from 30,000 to over 100,000/mm³. An increase in total serum protein (>6 gm/dl) is often observed. Neither the clinical pathology nor the radiographic findings, however, are diagnostic for tuberculosis. Acid-fast stains of tracheal and cloacal swabs are usually negative. There is some indication that enzyme immunoassay tests may prove to be diagnostic.

Organisms are usually abundant in tuberculous skin lesions of fish and reptiles. Thus, an antemortem diagnosis can be made relatively easily using an acid-fast stain of a skin scraping.

Treatment is not recommended for positive skin reactors. Only in cases where endangered species such as great apes are involved should therapy be considered. Isoniazid can be used at 10 to 30 mg/kg/day up to 300 mg total/day in primates. Streptomycin and rifamycin may also be used in addition to isoniazid when active disease is present. Isoniazid does not eliminate the tuberculosis organism but merely suppresses it and the animal's reaction to tuberculin.

When a mammal dies from tuberculosis, all mammals in the area should be tuberculin-tested. When possible, any positive reactors should be killed and their enclosures disinfected. Since tuberculin testing is ineffective in birds, the only way to eradicate the disease once it occurs is to eliminate the exposed birds and change the topsoil or bedding, because mycobacteria may live there for several years. Kanamycin has been recommended for treatment of fish tuberculosis. However, depopulation of the tank and improvement of husbandry are more beneficial, since the disease usually occurs where sanitation is poor.

Preventive measures include vaccination with BCG in primates. Though BCG does increase resistance to infection with tuberculosis, it can also reduce sensitivity to tuberculin, rendering testing unreliable. The best way to prevent the spread of the disease is still by routine tuberculin testing and elimination of reactors.

People who work for a zoo or a facility that houses non-human primates should be tuberculin-tested prior to employment. Testing should be repeated at six-month intervals. This rule should also apply to the occasional owner of a pet monkey. Anyone who develops a positive skin test should not work in close association with primates. Contrary to popular belief, tuberculosis is not a primary disease of non-human primates that is transmitted to people.

---

*Jenson-Salsbury Laboratories, Kansas City, Missouri

Rather, most non-human primates contract the disease when they associate closely with man.

Care should be exercised when working around aquariums. The saprophytic mycobacteria can be pathogenic for man. *M. marinum* causes swimming-pool granuloma, a chronic skin infection that often is refractory to treatment.

OTHER DISEASES CAUSED BY MYCOBACTERIA

Johne's disease, caused by *M. paratuberculosis*, has occurred in exotic hoofed stock. Clinical signs are identical to those seen in domestic cattle, i.e., emaciation and diarrhea. It is necessary to employ specific diagnostic tests to differentiate Johne's disease from other causes of diarrhea. As is true with tuberculosis, no one test is entirely satisfactory. A combination of intradermal and intravenous injections of johnin, fecal cultures, complement fixation tests, and acid-fast stains of fecal smears and biopsied lymph nodes can be used to identify infected animals. Treatment is unsatisfactory. Whenever possible, eradication of the herd, disinfection, and vacating the area of all hoofed stock for two years is necessary to eradicate the disease completely. Otherwise the risk of transmitting the disease to other ungulates in the area by water contamination is possible. One zoo placed birds (ratites and cranes) in the hoofed stock area during their two-year quarantine so that the exhibits would not stand empty.

Nine-banded armadillos have been used as an animal model for studying human leprosy (*M. leprae*). Naturally acquired leprosy, that is histopathologically compatible with the experimentally produced disease has been found in feral nine-banded armadillos.

SUPPLEMENTAL READING

Davis, J. W., Karstad, L. H., and Trainer, D. O. (eds.): *Infectious Diseases of Wild Mammals*. Ames, Iowa, Iowa State University Press, 1970.
Fowler, M. E. (ed.): *Zoo and Wild Animal Medicine*. Philadelphia, W. B. Saunders Co., 1978.
Montali, R. J. (ed.): *Mycobacterial Infections of Zoo Animals*. Washington, D.C., Smithsonian Institution Press, 1978.

MEDICAL CARE OF TROPICAL FISH

MICHAEL THOMAS COLLINS, D.V.M.
Fort Collins, Colorado

INTRODUCTION

There are more tropical fish kept as pets in the United States than there are cats, dogs, and pet birds combined, yet very few veterinarians are servicing the medical needs of these animals. The financial as well as the emotional investment of the owner often exceeds that for other pets. The average fish may cost only one to five dollars but many cost over $50, and the aquarium and accessories to maintain the fish cost from $30 to $500. Tropical fish hobbyists are certainly willing to pay for veterinary services to protect their investments and keep their fish healthy.

Veterinarians have all of the basic training necessary to handle fish disease problems. Only two elements are lacking. First is an understanding of the aquatic environment and second is experience. The quickest and surest way to gain both is to own and operate an aquarium. Putting an aquarium in the office lobby also serves to notify clients that you might offer veterinary services for tropical fish. This chapter is designed to familiarize the practitioner with ways to approach, diagnose, and treat only the most common tropical fish diseases. For more comprehensive discussions of fish diseases, the reader is referred to texts in the supplemental reading list.

There are three important elements necessary to arrive at a fish disease diagnosis: history, water quality analysis, and examination of the fish (usually post mortem).

HISTORY

A good thorough history often can lead the way to a diagnosis. The following outline lists and gives the potential significance of some of the more important information that should be gathered.

I. The aquarium and its maintenance.
  A. Equipment.
    1. Aquarium. The size of the aquarium should be appropriate for the number, kind, and size of fish.
    2. Filters.
       a. Undergravel filters are the easiest to maintain, most efficient, and least susceptible to mechanical failure. The absence of an undergravel filter can lead to water quality problems.
       b. Outside box filters containing activated carbon are good for removing particulate matter and color from the water. They also assist in aeration but generally do little for biologic filtration. Their primary role should be as an adjunct to an undergravel filter.
       c. Corner box filters are inexpensive but inefficient and a problem to maintain. Unless cleaned regularly they do not filter properly. These too should be used only as an adjunct to an undergravel filter.
    3. Aerator. This is essential for most aquaria. Without aeration, an aquarium will support one inch of fish body length for each seven square inches of water surface area.
    4. Heater. A thermostatic heater and thermometer are important, especially if the aquarium is small (e.g., ten gallons). The ideal temperature for most tropical fish is 78° F. Temperatures more than 6° F above this optimum temperature, or large daily fluctuations in temperature, can be stressful to fish and predispose them to disease.
    5. Ornaments and "aqua-scraping" materials. These are desirable not only for aesthetics but also to allow fish to hide, thereby minimizing the stress of captivity and existence in a glass cage.
       a. Wood, rocks, and plants gathered from lakes and streams are potential carriers of pathogenic agents into the aquarium. They should be disinfected or purchased from a pet store.
       b. Gravel is usually made of synthetic material or quartz and has no buffering capacity. It should be mixed with oyster shell or dolomite (calcium and magnesium carbonates) to provide a chemical buffer to the system. Without a buffer the pH will steadily decline to suboptimal levels.
  B. Fish. The size, number, and kind of fish should be appropriate for the aquarium. A sense of this can be gained only through experience. Aggressive fish often lead to social problems and stress, resulting in disease.
  C. Management practices.
    1. Length of time the aquarium has been set up. There is a well recognized condition known as the "new tank syndrome," in which most if not all the fish in an aquarium will die within two to six weeks following set-up. (See under "Water Quality Problems" for a discussion.)
    2. Frequency of water changes. One fourth to one third of the aquarium water should be changed monthly. This practice will minimize the buildup of nitrates in the aquarium.
    3. Addition of new fish. The recent addition of new fish to an aquarium could signal the possible introduction of a pathogen (usually an ectoparasite) to the aquarium.
II. The disease problem.
  A. Dead fish. Most tropical fish disease problems, especially with novice aquarists, begin with a dead fish. Examination of such specimens is usually unrewarding. A good history and water quality analysis, however, can often lead to a diagnosis.
  B. Behavior.
    1. Buoyancy. When fish float to the surface or sink to the bottom they have lost control of their swim bladders. This condition may be primary or may be secondary to a

bacterial septicemia, in which case it is usually the terminal event of a fatal infection. Fish with a primary swim bladder problem and no generalized disease may live for some time, provided they can still eat and are not harassed by other fish. This condition is most common in goldfish, is of unknown etiology, and has no known remedy.

2. Balance. Fish that tilt to one side usually have an infection involving the brain. Concentrate the postmortem examination in this area.

3. Flashing. Fish bothered by ectoparasites will scrape their bodies against the bottom or against the rocks in an aquarium in an attempt to rid themselves of the parasites. This has been termed "flashing" because the shiny scales of some fish will glint in the light during this maneuver. Fish infested with ectoparasites may also show erratic spurts of activity, jump out of the water, thrash, or swim with a jerking motion.

4. Respiratory rate. Gasping movements of the mouth, rapid moving of the opercula (gill covers), and floating at the surface indicate hypoxia. This may be due to lack of dissolved oxygen in the water or may occur secondary to ammonia poisoning, nitrite poisoning, or gill parasites.

C. Lesions.
1. White spots. This is probably one of the most common complaints. White spots generally indicate ectoparasite infection, and "ich" (*Ichthyopthirius multifiliis*, a protozoan parasite) is the most common cause. Sporozoan or lymphocystis virus infection can cause similar lesions.

2. White, cotton-wool–like lesions. These indicate fungal infection.

3. Ragged fins. The fins are the best indicator of the general health of a fish. Almost any physical, chemical, or social stress or infectious disease will cause ragged, frayed fins. The fins may then be infected secondarily by bacteria.

4. Other lesions. Reddening in the mouth or at the base of the fins, ascites (indicated by a swollen abdomen and raised scales), and exophthalmos ("pop-eye") are all common signs of bacterial septicemia.

WATER QUALITY PROBLEMS

Water quality is an integral part of the disease process in fish. When water quality is not optimal for fish they become stressed and therefore more susceptible to infectious diseases. Water quality tests are quick and simple and kits for the purpose are commercially available. Any legitimate attempt at disease prevention and control should begin with routine water quality measurements and water quality control. The most important water quality measurements are ammonia, nitrite, and nitrate concentrations and pH. Temperature and dissolved oxygen concentration are also important but less commonly a problem.

NITRIFICATION AND THE "NEW TANK SYNDROME"

Nitrification is a microbial process whereby ammonia is converted to nitrate in a two-step process. *Nitrosomonas* species bacteria oxidize ammonia (as ammonium, NH_4^+) to nitrite (NO_2^-), and *Nitrobacter* species bacteria oxidize nitrite to nitrate (NO_3^-). Nitrification is a natural process constantly occurring in soil and water as a major part of the nitrogen cycle (Fig. 1). Ammonia constitutes 80 per cent of fish nitrogenous excretory products. Nitrification is the most efficient method of removing the highly toxic ammonia from the fish's environment. In an established or "conditioned" aquarium nitrifying bacteria can oxidize ammonia through nitrite to nitrate so effectively that, even with very dense fish populations, ammonia and nitrite concentrations will remain extremely low. Nitrate concentrations, however, will rise steadily in the somewhat artificial ecosystem of an aquarium because there cannot be enough plants in an aquarium to utilize all of the nitrate produced. This is not a major concern, however, because nitrate is non-toxic to fish, and concentrations as high as 4000 parts per million will not affect them.

The "new tank syndrome" is probably responsible for killing more tropical fish every year than any single infectious disease. The "new tank syndrome" occurs when too many fish are placed into an unconditioned aquarium. The unconditioned aquarium does

NITROGEN CYCLE

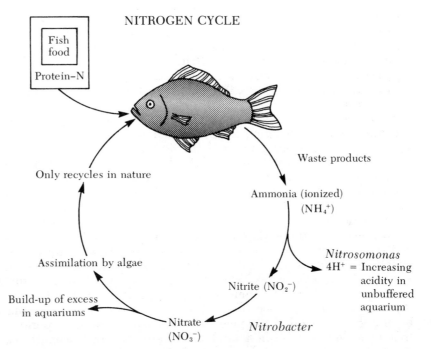

Figure 1. The nitrification process in the nitrogen cycle.

not have a sufficient complement of nitrifying bacteria to oxidize the ammonia as fast as the fish excrete it. When this happens, ammonia concentrations rapidly increase and may kill the fish. High concentrations of ammonia then stimulate the growth of *Nitrosomonas* species bacteria, which quickly oxidize the ammonia to nitrite. Nitrite is also extremely toxic to fish and is very likely to kill all the remaining fish in the aquarium. High concentrations of nitrite stimulate the growth of *Nitrobacter* species

bacteria, which then oxidize the nitrite to nitrate. At this point the aquarium has become conditioned and will easily support many fish (Fig. 2).

The time between when fish are placed into an unconditioned aquarium and when they start dying from the "new tank syndrome" varies directly with the rate of ammonia production, which is in turn determined by the number and size of fish. Generally, the average hobbyist starts losing fish from two to four

ESTABLISHING NITRIFICATION

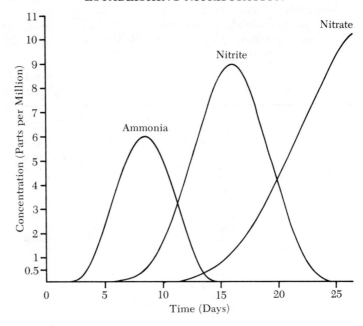

Figure 2. Ammonia, nitrite, and nitrate levels during the conditioning process of an aquarium.

weeks after setting up a new aquarium. Presumptive diagnosis of the "new tank syndrome" can be made based on a typical history and symptoms of ammonia or nitrite toxicity (see next section). Confirmation of the diagnosis can be made by doing a few simple water quality tests.

Treatment of the "new tank syndrome" is accomplished by changing 25 percent of the water in the aquarium daily until the nitrification process has become established. This will effectively dilute the offending toxicants and cause a marked improvement in the condition of the fish.

Prevention of the "new tank syndrome" can be achieved by three simple methods. First, and easiest, add fish to a new aquarium very slowly, e.g., for a ten-gallon aquarium, add two small fish each week. This will keep the peak concentrations of ammonia and nitrite low and within tolerance of the fish. Second, obtain about a handful of gravel from the bottom of a well established (and disease-free) aquarium and put it into the new tank. Nitrifying bacteria cling to the gravel surfaces, and this procedure will, in essence, inoculate the nitrifiers into the new aquarium. Fish, however, should still be added cautiously. Third, the conditioning process can be simulated artificially by adding ammonium and nitrite salts to a new aquarium. This will stimulate growth of nitrifying bacteria, and by monitoring ammonia, nitrite, and nitrate concentrations one can determine when the tank is conditioned and suitable for adding fish.

COMMON TOXICOLOGIC PROBLEMS

Ammonia. In water, ammonia exists in two forms, ionized (NH_4^+) and un-ionized (NH_3). The ionization state of ammonia is determined primarily by the pH of the water. This relationship is mathematically expressed by the equation.

$$\text{concentration of un-ionized ammonia } (NH_3) = \frac{\text{total concentration of ammonia}}{1 + \text{antilog} (pKa - pH)}$$

For the reader's convenience, the calculations have been performed for the commonly encountered ammonia concentrations and pHs (Table 1).

The concentration of un-ionized ammonia is much more important than the total concentration of ammonia because only the un-ionized ammonia is toxic to fish. Table 1 has been marked off into two areas. In the "safe" area (above the line) the concentrations of un-ionized ammonia are non-toxic to fish even for extended periods of time. The area below the line encompasses concentrations of un-ionized ammonia that are toxic. Un-ionized ammonia primarily affects the gills. It causes hyperplasia and fusion of gill lamellae, resulting in impaired respiration. Fish suffering from ammonia poisoning exhibit signs of hypoxia.

Nitrite. Nitrite is extremely toxic to all animals, including fish. As little as one part per million nitrite-nitrogen is lethal to fish. The mechanism of nitrite toxicity is similar to that of carbon monoxide. Nitrite binds to hemoglobin and, once bound, prevents it from carrying oxygen. Therefore, fish suffering from nitrite toxicity exhibit signs of oxygen starvation and ultimately die of asphyxiation.

Nitrate. As mentioned previously, nitrate is non-toxic to fish. Its presence in an aquarium in appreciable concentrations, however, does have the undesirable side effect of stimulating

Table 1. *Concentration of Un-ionized Ammonia at Various Concentrations of Total Ammonia and pHs*

pH	TOTAL AMMONIA CONCENTRATION [c]								
	1.0	2.0	3.0	4.0	5.0	6.0	7.0	8.0	
6.0	0.001	0.001	0.002	0.002	0.003	0.003	0.004	0.005	↑
6.2	0.001	0.002	0.003	0.004	0.005	0.005	0.006	0.007	Safe
6.4	0.002	0.003	0.004	0.006	0.007	0.009	0.010	0.011	
6.6	0.002	0.005	0.007	0.009	0.011	0.014	0.016	0.018	↓
6.8	0.004	0.007	0.011	0.014	0.018	0.021	0.025	0.028	
7.0	0.006	0.011	0.017	0.022	0.028	0.034	0.039	0.045	↑
7.2	0.009	0.018	0.027	0.035	0.044	0.053	0.062	0.071	
7.4	0.014	0.028	0.042	0.056	0.070	0.084	0.098	0.112	
7.6	0.022	0.044	0.066	0.088	0.110	0.131	0.153	0.175	Toxic
7.8	0.034	0.069	0.103	0.137	0.171	0.206	0.240	0.274	
8.0	0.053	0.107	0.160	0.213	0.266	0.320	0.373	0.426	↓

[c]Concentrations are given in ppm (parts per million) un-ionized ammonia nitrogen (NH_3–N).

the growth of algae. Nitrate concentrations are easily controlled by changing approximately 25 percent of the aquarium water every three to four weeks.

pH. The pH of water alone is not usually a problem in terms of direct toxicity. Most water supplies have a relatively neutral pH at which most fish can live. However, many fish from various parts of the world have adapted to living at extreme pHs; for example, many South American fish live in water of pH 3 or 4. Most fish can adapt to a wide range of pHs provided that the pH change is gradual. If a South American fish that has adapted to living in water with a pH of 4 is suddenly dropped into water with a pH of 8, it will be stressed and may even die from the shock. Therefore, the rate of pH change is the most important consideration for this particular water quality parameter.

The pH of the water in an aquarium is directly affected by the nitrification process. Oxidation of ionized ammonia (NH_4^+) to nitrate (NO_3^-) results in the release of four hydrogen ions (H^+) (see Fig. 1). This will cause a gradual decline in the pH of the water unless the system is somehow buffered. The easiest way to buffer the water is by incorporating crushed oyster shells or dolomite into the gravel in the tank. These products are composed primarily of calcium and magnesium carbonates and have excellent buffering capacity.

One additional consideration relative to pH is worth noting. As was discussed previously, pH and ammonia are intimately related. As can be seen from the table of un-ionized ammonia concentrations, ammonia is much less toxic at lower pHs. Therefore, it is advisable to maintain aquaria in a pH range of 6.5 to 7.0.

Oxygen. Aquariums set up with the usual small aerators have sufficient concentrations of oxygen. Most oxygen is absorbed at the surface and not from the bubbles produced by the aerator. The most important function of the aerator is to circulate the water from the bottom to the surface. The basic oxygen requirements of fish are listed in Table 2. Secondary lack of oxygen occurs when enough oxygen is dissolved in the water but the fish cannot absorb it. This may be due to gill parasites, blood parasites, ammonia poisoning, or nitrite poisoning.

INFECTIOUS DISEASES

A few minor procedures, such as skin scraping, can be performed on a living fish. Generally, however, examinations are performed on dead specimens. It is best to euthanize and examine a moribund fish. Specimens that have been dead for more than a couple hours are almost worthless for bacteriologic culture, and most parasites leave the fish soon after it dies. Fish that die and must await examination should be refrigerated, not frozen, in a moist condition in a plastic bag. Refrigerated specimens do not last long. The best guides to the suitability of a specimen for examination are the gills. Only when the gills are still red is there any chance of making an accurate diagnosis by necropsy.

Bacteria capable of producing disease in fish are ubiquitous in the fish's environment and on the surface of the fish. Infections seldom arise spontaneously but generally result from some insult or stress that makes the fish more susceptible. The two most common stress-inducing factors are adverse environmental conditions and parasite infections.

Table 2. Safe and Toxic Levels of Common Water Quality Parameters*

	AMMONIA (UN-IONIZED) (NH_3-N)	NITRITE (NO_2^--N)	NITRATE (NO_3^--N)	FRESHWATER pH	DISSOLVED OXYGEN (O_2)
Safe	0.000 to 0.200	0.0 to 0.5	0.0 to 4000.0	8.0 to 6.5	10.0 to 6.0
Stress	0.021 to 0.100	0.6 to 1.0	—	6.4 to 5.0	5.9 to 4.0
Deadly	0.101 to 10.000	1.1 to 4.0	—	4.9 to 3.0	3.0 to 0

*All measurements except pH in parts per million (mg/liter).

The approach to the diagnosis of a bacterial infection should be first, to exclude water quality problems that could be the cause of the mortality and second, to exclude the presence of external or internal parasites. If water quality is good, with an absence of heavy parasitism, then examine for bacteria. The liver and kidney are the best organs from which to take a culture.

STEPWISE PROCEDURE FOR EXAMINATION OF A FISH

1. Pith the fish or sever its spinal cord just behind the head.
2. Examine the fish grossly and with the aid of a hand-held magnifying lens. Many parasites are visible with little or no magnification.
3. Prepare skin scraping for microscopic examination.
   a. Scrape the sides of the fish, especially the base of the fins, with a scalpel blade or the edge of a coverslip.
   b. Place the scrapings on a microscope slide, add a drop of water, and cover with a coverslip.
4. Prepare a fin for microscopic examination.
   a. Clip approximately one square centimeter from one or more fins.
   b. Place clippings on a microscope slide, add a drop of water, and cover with a coverslip.
5. Prepare a gill section for microscopic examination.
   a. Remove the operculum (structure covering the gill) using scissors and forceps.
   b. Remove one or more gill arches and cut the gill filaments away from bony or cartilagenous parts.
   c. Place several gill filaments on a slide, add a drop of water, and cover with a coverslip.
6. Prepare internal organs for microscopic examination.
   a. Using scissors and forceps, remove the lateral body wall of the fish.
   b. For very small fish all abdominal viscera, including liver, spleen, and intestines, may be placed on a slide with a drop of water and squashed under a coverslip.
   c. For larger fish use small pieces of the liver, spleen, and intestines and mount in a similar fashion.

GROSS EXAMINATION

Details of the gross examination of fish are given in the following table.

Lesion or Sign	Possible Diagnosis
Emaciation	Many disease conditions cause emaciation; however, two agents in particular should be looked for: *Ichthyosporidium hoferi* (a fungus causing systemic infection) and *Mycobacterium* species, which causes piscine tuberculosis.
Abdominal distention ("dropsy") and/or raised scales	Bacterial septicemia, usually caused by *Aeromonas hydrophila*. (The role of a viral agent is also suspected but unconfirmed.)
Exophthalmos ("pop-eye")	A very non-specific sign associated with many diseases, most commonly with a bacterial septicemia.
Frayed fins	A very non-specific sign. Check water quality, look for ectoparasites, and examine the edges of the fins microscopically for *Flexibacter columnaris*.
White cottony lesions	Fungal infection, usually *Saprolegnia sporozoan* or *Achlys* species; examine a scraping of the lesion for mycelial elements.
White spots or nodules	Ectoparasitism. Examine a skin scraping and fins microscopically to differentiate protozoans and sporozoans.
Whitish areas under the skin	*Plistophora* or other sporozoans.
Whitish wartlike growths on the skin or fins	Lymphocystis viral infection (a pox virus causing dramatic hypertrophy of fibroblasts).
Reddish ulcers	*Aeromonas* is a secondary invader that can almost invariably be cultured; however, the primary problem may be ectoparasitism or mechanical injury.

MICROSCOPIC EXAMINATION OF SKIN SCRAPINGS, FINS, AND GILLS

Look for movement. Most parasites can be visualized using low power (5× or 10×) objectives. When parasites are encountered, switch to the high dry (40×) objective and refer to text material to assist in identification. One of the best books for identification of fish parasites is *Parasites of Freshwater Fishes* by Drs. Hoffman and Meyer (see Supplemental Reading).

EXTERNAL PROTOZOANS

External protozoan infestations are the most common parasite problem of fish. These single-cell microorganisms are usually motile by means of cilia. Heavy infestations with pathogenic protozoans irritate the skin and gills, causing the fish to produce excessive amounts of mucus as a defense mechanism. This excessive mucus production may impair respiration through the gills, leading to suffocation. In addition, protozoan infestations generally weaken the fish and may cause lesions that are subject to secondary bacterial infection.

Protozoans that are a serious problem even when present in small numbers include:

Ichthyopthirius multifiliis ("ich"): Large, spherical, motile organisms with cilia covering their surface, often having characteristic horseshoe-shaped nuclei. The white spots they commonly produce are encysted parasites that are not susceptible to antiprotozoan drugs.

Trichodina: Saucer-shaped ciliates with a conspicuous "toothed" disk in the center; they usually move in a rotary fashion.

Chilodonella: Small, oval to heart-shaped ciliates with faint bands of cilia running longitudinally along the parasite.

Costia: Minute, pear-shaped parasites often overlooked by observers. They are best observed at the margin of a fin, where their motility resembles a flickering flame.

Protozoans that are generally a problem only if abundant include

Ambiphrya (Scyphidia): Small, urn-shaped organisms that attach to the body, gills, and fins. Cilia at the top beat actively.

Epistylus: Parasites that have a long stalk attached to the fish, bell-shaped bodies at one end, and a circular ring of cilia at the top.

Tetrahymena: These pear-shaped ciliates are free-living parasites that attack debilitated fish. They have been associated with problems in guppies ("guppy killer") in which they cause a whitish ring of necrosis around the body.

SPOROZOAN PARASITES

These parasites form white cysts in the tissues of fish that are often visible without magnification. Diagnosis can be made by placing a dissected cyst on a microscope slide and squashing it with a coverslip. The structure of the zoospores will assist in the identification.

Henneguya form cysts primarily on the gills, where they interfere with respiration, and on the fins. They produce distinctive, long, twin-tailed spores.

Plistophora hyphessobryconis cause "neon tetra disease." They infect and destroy the musculature, causing whitish areas of necrosis that show through the skin. This disease occurs in other fishes as well as neon tetras. The cysts (pansporoblasts) contain numerous, characteristic oval spores.

FUNGI

Most superficial fungal infections are secondary to mechanical injury or parasite-induced lesions. The lesions are filled with hyphal elements. *Saprolegnia and Achlya* are the two most common agents. These agents cannot be differentiated unless cultured; however, treatment is the same for both types of infection.

ALGAE (DINOFLAGELLATES)

Oodinium is the only important parasite in this group. This agent causes "velvet disease." Infected fish show a white to dark coating on their surface. The gills may also be infected. The parasite is spherical to casket-shaped and usually contains highly refractile granules.

TREMATODES (MONOGENETIC)

Fish may carry a number of minute parasitic worms on their bodies, fins, and gills. Since these parasites can multiply on the fish without additional hosts, they are called monogenetic flukes and are common parasites. Heavy infections can occur and result in high mortality rates. They are easily transmitted from fish to fish by contact and through the water. Although there are many species, two are typical of this group.

Gyrodactylus: Generally found on the body and fins, but may occur on the gills. They can be identified by their lack of eyespots, by a single pair of large hooks, and by the fact that they give birth to live young. Unborn individuals can be seen within living worms.

Dactylogyrus: A species of trematode commonly found on the gills, they have four eye-spots and are egg layers.

COPEPODS (CRUSTACEANS)

Copepod parasites are common, bothersome, and difficult to control. There are freshwater and marine crustaceans. Some non-parasitic species are intermediate hosts for helminths. Some copepods bury deep in the flesh and cannot be affected by chemicals.

Achtheres: Common on the gills of fishes, where their light-colored bodies stand out in sharp contrast to the deep-red gill filaments. Legs in this form have disappeared from the body, and two mouth parts have become modified to form a pair of curved appendages that may fuse at their tips to attach the parasite to the gills. Egg sacs protrude from the posterior end of the bodies of mature females. These parasites consume blood from the gills and are a serious menace to fish.

Ergasilus: This form grossly resembles the free-living copepod *Cyclops*, but the second antennae are enlarged, terminating in large claws that serve as a means of attachment. The parasites feed on blood and body fluids. Secondary infections in wounds thus caused are common.

Argulus: Commonly referred to as "fish lice." They have a flattened, saucer-like shape and can be observed creeping rapidly about over the body of a fish. When motionless the parasite resembles a scale. Close examination of individuals will reveal the presence of jointed legs and two large sucking disks for attachment, which may give the organism the appearance of having large eyes. When attached to fish, the parasites feed on blood and body fluids. Even large fish may be killed by these organisms if they become abundant.

Lernaea ("anchor worm"): The anchor parasite is found on both scaled and scaleless fishes. Inflamed areas accompany the site of attachment, and a secondary bacterial or fungal infection frequently develops. *Lernaea* are attached so firmly to their hosts that care must be exercised in removing them. After the juvenile forms attach, the appendages of the head become modified so that the parasite resembles an anchor at its anterior end. These branching protrusions prevent release of the parasite. The parasite frequently is a primary factor in bacterial infections.

MICROSCOPIC EXAMINATION OF INTESTINES AND OTHER INTERNAL ORGANS

PROTOZOAN

Hexamita may inhabit the lumen of the intestines or be found in the gallbladder and liver. They are called debility parasites because they become a problem when fish are stressed. It is possible, however, that they are a primary pathogen, especially in angel fish. These organisms are high motile and quite small. Use a high dry (40×) objective to look for these parasites.

TREMATODES (DIGENETIC)

Flukes that use fish as intermediate hosts generally penetrate the body and encyst in the flesh, fat bodies, or mesentery. If abundant, these encysted worms give a "grubby" appearance to the fish flesh. The encysted worms are often referred to as "the yellow grub of fishes." In most cases these worms reach adulthood only if the infested fish are eaten by the proper bird host. Infections due to digenetic flukes have been known to cause death in isolated situations in which the number of penetrating larval worms was very high. In most instances a light worm burden does not cause much problem.

CESTODES

Tapeworms are common in the intestines of tropical fish. Unless excessively abundant, however, they are not a problem.

NEMATODES

Roundworms are fairly common in aquarium fish, especially those raised in open ponds or caught from the wild. Roundworms may be found inside the intestines, free in the peritoneal cavity as mature worms, or in cysts. Immature forms within cysts may be observed in the liver and visceral membranes of aquarium fish and may cause many deaths. Encysted forms develop to maturity in fish-eating birds or other larger fish.

ACANTHOCEPHALA

In nature, acanthocephala (spiny-headed worms) are found in many fish but are less common in aquarium fish. Acanthocephala are hard to remove since the hooks on the proboscis hold firmly to the intestinal wall. If removed intact, the parasites are readily recognized by the proboscis hooks. Small numbers of these parasites do not appear to cause serious injury to the fish, but inflammation occurs in the area where acanthocephala attach, and the wounds they cause may serve as foci of secondary bacterial infections. Occasionally, cysts containing immature forms of acanthocephalans may be seen in the viscera.

FISH DISEASE TREATMENTS

The following is a list of the most highly recommended fish disease treatments. Two things must be noted when treating aquarium fish: First, some medications will be adsorbed from the water by active carbon or charcoal. Therefore, filters containing these products should be turned off during treatment. Second, a few medications, especially methylene blue, will kill the nitrifying bacteria, resulting in a situation similar to the "new tank syndrome" in about 10 to 20 days following treatment. The treatments listed, however, have been proved safe for use in aquariums. Treatments are listed only for the common disease problems.

GENERAL TONIC

Sodium chloride is recommended for all freshwater aquariums. At low levels, salt will increase the vitality of the fish and inhibit the growth of many fish parasites. The recommended dose is one teaspoon per gallon, which is roughly equivalent to 10 grams per gallon or 2.5 grams per liter. Only non-iodized salt should be used.

PARASITICIDE AND FUNGICIDE

A mixture of formalin and malachite green is the best all-around parasiticide and fungicide for use on tropical fish. The recommended formulation is not commercially available but is easily prepared.

Add 1.4 grams of zinc-free malachite green to 3800 cc of formalin. Treat at the rate of 1 cc per 10 gallons. Treat on alternate days for a minimum of three treatments. Beware! This treatment is marginally toxic to fish, so watch them carefully and stop treatment at the first signs of distress.

This medication is effective for treatment of:
1. External protozoans: *Ichthyopthirius, Trichodina, Chilodonella, Costia, Ambiphrya, Epistylus, Tetrahymena.*
2. External fungi: *Saprolegnia, Achlya.*
3. Dinoflagellates: *Oodinium.*
4. Monogenetic trematodes: *Gyrodactylus, Dactylogyrus*

ANTIBACTERIAL DRUGS

Furanace®* (nifurpirinol) is the drug of choice for bacterial infections in fish. It is absorbed rapidly from the water and achieves therapeutic blood levels within minutes of administration. Few resistance problems have been witnessed to date. Most other antibacterial drugs, when added to aquarium water, are not absorbed by fish and hence treat the fish only topically instead of systemically. Therapeutic blood levels of these drugs can be achieved only by feeding or injecting them. Medicated tropical fish feeds are available commercially.

For additional treatment regimens consult the following reference list.

SUPPLEMENTAL READING

Amlacher, E.: Textbook of Fish Diseases. (Translated and updated by D. A. Conroy and R. L. Herman.) Neptune City, N. J., T.F.H. Publications, 1970.

Anderson, D. P.: Fish Immunology. Neptune City, N. J., T.F.H. Publications, 1974.

van Dujin, C.: Diseases of Fishes, third ed. Springfield, Ill., Charles C Thomas, 1973.

Hoffman, G. L., and Meyer, F. P.: Parasites of Freshwater Fishes. Neptune City, N. J., T.F.H. Publications, 1974.

Mawdesley-Thomas, L. E. (ed.): Diseases of Fish. Symposia of the Zoological Society of London, No. 30. New York, Academic Press, 1972.

Reichenback-Klinke, H. H., and Landlot, M.: Reichenback-Klinke's Fish Pathology. Neptune City, N. J., T. F. H. Publications, 1973.

Ribelin, W. E., and Migaki, G. (eds.): Symposium on Fish Pathology. Madison, University of Wisconsin Press, 1975.

Schubert, G.: Cure and Recognize Aquarium Fish Diseases. Neptune City, N. J., T. F. H. Publications, 1974.

Spotte, S. H.: Fish and Invertebrate Culture: Water management in Closed Systems. New York, John Wiley & Sons, 1970.

*Zodiac Pets, Division of Zoecon Industries, 12200 Denton Drive, Dallas, Texas 75234

AMPHIBIAN CARE AND DISEASES

GERALD E. COSGROVE, M.D.

San Diego, California

There are about 2500 species of amphibians, which include the Anura (frogs and toads), Caudata (salamanders and sirens), and Gymniphona (caecilians). Of these numerous species, few have been studied in much detail in relation to care, health, and disease. The biologic requirements vary extremely in the amphibians. Such factors as habitat, respiration, need for immersion, water quality, temperature, light, feeding requirements, seasonal variations, conditions for successful reproduction, and life cycles are among those to consider.

DISEASES

Many types of problems occur, varying considerably in importance (Table 1). The most important is the microbiologic complex called "red leg," which is a septicemic disease. When

Table 1. *Frequency of Amphibian Disease in a Necropsy Series*
(XENOPUS LAEVIS, 369 FROGS)

LOCATION	DISEASE	FREQUENCY (%)
General	Injury	1
	"Redleg"	4
	Edema	3
	TB	2
Skin	Dermatitis	2
	Ulcer	4
	Fungus	1
	Nematodes	33
GI tract	Enteritis	0.5
	Rectal prolapse	1
	Ciliates	100
	Trematodes	5
	Cestodes	5
	Nematodes	50
GI accessory	Liver necrosis	3
	Cholecystitis	1
Urinary	Cystitis	25
	Nephritis	34
	Degeneration	10
	Ciliates	17
	Trematodes	24
Hematopoietic	Hyperplasia	4
	Anemia	5
Respiratory	Pneumonia	1
	TB	1
	Nasal Mites	3
Miscellaneous	Bone deformity	3
	Tumor or hyperplasia	5
	Vascular thrombosis	1
	Larval trematode cysts	50

Table 2. *Important Environmental Considerations for Amphibians*

TEMPERATURE:	Usually 62–72°; try gradient.
CONTAINER:	Adequate space Non-traumatic, non-toxic materials Suitable resting and hiding areas Escape-proof Proper balance of water and land Proper lighting
WATER:	Depth Facilities for entry and departure Clean by filtration, flow, changes, and so on Avoid chlorine and chemicals Test all additives Proper pH for species
FEEDING:	Suitable feeding temperature Proper food for species Technique of presentation Avoid competition Remove excess food to avoid fouling

red leg starts in grouped amphibians, a high mortality rate can be expected. Alterations in the environment of the captive animals can also be devastating. Heat, dehydration, fouling, and toxicants, such as chlorine in water and others, are important. Inspection of the animals' environment is often diagnostic (Table 2). Starvation may occur because of refusal to eat, competition, or dietary deficiency. Conditions tolerated in one life stage may be suddenly or slowly lethal to amphibians in another stage. Metamorphosis is an especially stressful time.

Shipping of amphibians from supplier to user is a critical process and the animals should be introduced carefully into their new habitat, preferably after a trial period. In the colony they are subject to damage from husbandry practices or prophylactic procedures carried out without adequate pre-testing for effects.

A wide range of conditons may be encountered sporadically in individual amphibians. Among these are neoplasms, which are rare except for renal adenocarcinoma of frogs, a virus-initiated disease that is "epidemic" in certain frog populations. Tuberculosis in amphibians is transmissible but usually only slowly progressive. Mild degrees of parasitism are ubiquitous in amphibians, but lesions are usually mild (Table 1).

TREATMENT AND CARE

Methods of handling individual animals for observation and diagnosis vary and may be perfected with practice, using helpful suggestions from the literature. Diseased individuals should be removed from groups and either quarantined or killed when the disease is noted. Pathologic and microbiologic studies may reveal whether there is any danger of an epidemic. Clinical laboratory specimens such as those used for hematology, microbiology, parasitology, or other procedures are valuable adjuncts to diagnosis. Information is available about treatment of amphibian disease. In red leg, a variety of antibiotic and bacteriostatic regimens have been reported, including treatment with penicillin, tetracycline (Achromycin), nitrofurazone, or gentamicin in tank water, by stomach tube, in food, or injected (Table 3). Increasing the salinity of the tank water up to 0.6 percent is highly recommended for crowded lab tanks of certain species. Subtoxic amounts of tank additives such as fungicides, parasiticides and chemicals successfully reduce surface fungal or ectoparasitic infestations (Table 3). Visceral lesions of tuberculosis or fungal granulomas apparently have not been treated successfully by tank additives. No matter what additive treatments are used, a test for toxicity should be made on an isolated individual before the whole tank is treated. Dosage experimentation is often necessary.

More experimentation in the treatment of amphibian disease is certainly needed, and microbiologic studies for identification of pathogens and necropsies for disease study should be performed more often. At present, consultation on amphibian disease is not easily obtained. There are a few centers of amphibian research that are disease-orientated, and some pathology registries have amphibian disease experts.

Table 3. *Reported Therapeutic Regimens for Amphibian Disease*

DRUG OR CHEMICAL	DOSAGE AND ROUTE	INDICATION
Potassium permanganate	1/1000 bath or tank	Parasite Infection
Copper sulfate	1/5000 bath or tank	Parasite
Malachite green or methylene blue	1/5000 bath or tank	Parasite Fungus
Sodium chloride	0.4% solution tank	Parasites General conditioning
Thiabendazole	50 mg/kg oral	Intestinal parasites
Piperazine salts	50 mg/kg oral	Intestinal parasites
Gentamicin	5 mg/gal bath	Infection
Tetracycline HCl	5 mg/30 gm intubation	Infection

SUGGESTED READING

Balls, M., and Clothier, R. M.: Spontaneous tumors in amphibia. A review. Oncology, 29:510–519, 1974.

Cosgrove, G. E., and Jared, D. W.: Diseases and parasites of *Xenopus*, the clawed toad. *In* Amborski, R. L., Hood, M. A., and Miller, R. R. (eds.): Gulf Coast Regional Symposium on Diseases of Aquatic Animals, 1974 Proceedings. Center for Wetlands Resources, Louisiana State University, Baton Rouge, 1974, pp. 225–242.

Dawe, C. J., and Harshbarger, J. C.: A symposium on neoplasia and related disorders of invertebrate and lower vertebrate animals. National Cancer Institute Monograph, Vol. 31, 1969, 772 pp.

Frye, F. L.: General considerations in the care of captive amphibians. *In* Kirk, R. W. (ed): Current Veterinary Therapy VI. Small Animal Practice. Philadelphia, W. B. Saunders, 1977, pp. 772–778.

Gibbs, E. L., Gibbs, T. J., and Van Dyck, P. C.: *Rana pipiens*: Health and disease. Lab. Animal Care, 16:142–160, 1966.

Glorioso, J. C., Amborski, R. L., Amborski, G. F., and Culley, D. D.: Microbiological studies on septicemic bullfrogs (*Rana catesbeiana*). Am. J. Vet. Res., 35:1241–1245, 1974.

Mizell, M. (ed.): Recent Results in Cancer Research: Biology of Amphibian Tumors. New York, Springer-Verlag, 1968, 484 pp.

Nace, G. W. (ed.): Amphibians: Guidelines for the breeding, care, and management of laboratory animals. Washington, D. C., NRC/NAS, 1974, 153 pp.

Nace, G. W.: The amphibian facility of the University of Michigan. BioScience, 18:767–775, 1968.

Nace, G. W., Waage, J. K., and Richards, C. M.: Sources of amphibians for research. BioScience, 21:768–773, 1971.

Priddy, J. M., and Culley, D. D., Jr.: The frog culture industry, past and present. Proc. 25th Ann. Conf. Southeast. Assoc. Game and Fish Commission, 1971, pp. 597–601.

Reichenbach-Klinke, H., and Elkan, E.: The Principal Diseases of Lower Vertebrates. New York, Academic Press, 1965, 600 pp.

Temple, R., and Fowler, M. E.: Amphibians. *In* Fowler, M. E. (ed.): Zoo and Wild Animal Medicine. Philadelphia, W. B. Saunders Co., 1978, pp. 81–88.

ANESTHESIA OF REPTILES

CHARLES J. SEDGWICK, D.V.M.
Davis, California

The efficiency of administering anesthesia to reptiles is very closely tied to their unique metabolism. Reptiles are ectothermic, at least for most of their life cycles. (An exception is the female rock python [*Python sebae*], which may have a body temperature 3 to 4°C above certain natural environmental ambient temperatures when brooding eggs.) A large snake weighing 32 kg is estimated to have a standard metabolism of 106 kcal per day, as compared with a 32-kg mammal, which would have a standard metabolism approximating 1000 kcal. Because of this ectothermism, most reptiles must seek warm places so as to raise their body temperatures passively. Increases in metabolism occur during short periods of high activity, such as when capturing and ingesting prey. At all other times, reptiles have very low metabolic rates.

Reptiles are highly sensitive to skin incision and react as vigorously as possible to penetrating wounds. Therefore, anesthesia is required in reptiles for many surgical procedures. The effects of injectable anesthetic agents that are suitable for mammals and birds are totally unpredictable when used in reptiles because of the low metabolic rate of these animals. The intramuscular or subcutaneous injection of pentobarbital sodium (Nembutal®*) at the rate of 3 mg/100 gm body weight in common gopher snakes (*Pituophis sp.*) causes unnatural posturing, but little or no analgesia is obtained for skin incision. Intramuscular injection of 10 mg/kg phencyclidine hydrochloride (Sernylan®†) in caimans (*Caiman sp.*) produces no analgesia for skin incision. Ketamine hydrochloride (Vetalar® ‡), 4 mg/100 gm, in gopher snakes barely immobilizes them and fails to obtund the pain of skin incision. Ketamine injected intracardially provides light anesthesia at a dose of 2 mg/100 gm, but this method of administration is judged potentially too traumatic for routine practice in the administration of anesthesia to snakes.

A total dose of 5 mg of etorphine hydrocloride (M99®§) was administered to a 45-kg American alligator (*Alligator mississippiensis*), over a period of 3 hours. The first dose of 1 mg produced no visible effect after 30 minutes. A second dose of 2 mg produced no effect after another 30 minutes, and a final dose of 2 mg caused the animal to be very sluggish only after 1.5 hours. The alligator was neither anesthetized nor completely immobilized by this heavy dose of anesthetic. The animal's mobility was impaired for 8 days. (The same dosage of etorphine would anesthetize a large elephant.)

It must be questioned critically whether an injectable anesthetic is absorbed in reptiles completely enough in any given site to obtain an anesthetic concentration in the blood suitable to produce anesthesia. Merely increasing the dosages of agents until massive levels are obtained seems irrational when the final effect produced is only prolonged incapacity of the subject and not anesthesia.

The anesthetic ketamine, 4 mg/100 gm is of value when injected intramuscularly into venomous reptiles for immobilization to facilitate safer handling, for example, when removing retained eye scales. However, the handler must always control such animals as if they were fully capable of biting and causing envenomation and should not assume that they are surgically anesthetized.

Immobilization caused by profound reduction of body temperature has not proved consistently effective in reptiles in the author's practice. A large red rattlesnake (*Crotalus ruber*) contained in a cotton sack was placed in a refrigerator at a temperature of 7°C for 24 hours. When the sack was removed from the refrigerator, the animal could still rattle. It was manually restrained and the cloacal temperature was recorded by thermometer as approximately 8°C. When released into a box the animal could strike, albeit sluggishly. In a precision controlled-temperature ice-water bath, effective immobilization and possibly anesthesia could probably be achieved for reptiles. However, monitoring and maintaining consistent anesthetic levels would obviously be difficult. The tolerance to cold exposure apparently varies among species of reptiles as it does in mammals.

A small Western rattlesnake was placed in a closed quart jar with a pledget of ether-soaked cotton. The animal was watched closely for one hour. When removed from the jar, it was sluggish but retained its righting reflexes and was not considered to be anesthetized. It is felt that inducing inhalant anesthesia by closed anesthetic chamber has limitation in many reptiles because of their ability to hold breath.

Reptiles have sac-like lungs. When ventilating their lungs, such animals literally gulp in air and hold it for varying periods of time. The usual resting position for the glottis in reptiles is closed, and it opens only intermittently for breath-taking. (This is the reverse situation of that seen in mammals and birds, in which the usual position for the laryngeal orifice is open, closing only for deglutition.)

Reptiles that can be intubated endotracheally by manual restraint, without benefit of preanesthetic sedation, may be administered effective inhalent anesthetic by ventilating the agent into lung sacs mechanically. Induction of anesthesia by this method is nearly as rapid as it would be for mammals. All forms of reptiles, including snakes, lizards, turtles and crocodilians, have been surgically anesthetized by this method. The animal's mouth is held open by a suitable speculum by manual restraint, without benefit of preanesthetic sedation. The laryngeal orifice is located at the base of the tongue and intubated. The endotracheal tube is attached to an inhalant anesthesia ventilator, and positive-pressure ventilation of the animal's air sacs is commenced at a rate of 4 to 6 breaths per minute. The peak positive pressure at the end of inspiration is set at 12 cm H_2O. Halothane (Fluothane®**) is administered at 4 percent

---

*Abbott Laboratories, Chicago, Ill. 60064
†Parke-Davis, Detroit, Mich. 48232
‡Bio-Centic, Kansas City, Mo. 64502
§D-M Pharmaceuticals, Inc., Rockville, Md. 20850

**Ayerst, New York, N.Y. 10017

concentration in oxygen until struggling ceases and the muscular body tone of the reptile begins to relax. When relaxation commences, halothane concentration is reduced to between 2 and 3 percent. As anesthesia levels become light, muscular tone usually returns first to posterior body segments such as the tail in snakes and the tail and hind limbs in lizards. When full recovery is desired, halothane anesthetic is discontinued and the periods of intermittent positive-pressure lung sac ventilation are provided at a rate of once per 3 to 5 minutes.

Surgical anesthesia in all forms of reptiles, including snakes, lizards, turtles and crocodilians, has been maintained for three hours or more with full recovery obtained within eight hours of withdrawal of halothane anesthetic. It is probable that the serous surfaces of the respiratory lung sacs provide the most efficient site for administration and withdrawal of anesthetics in reptiles when using positive-pressure ventilation.

SUPPLEMENTAL READING

Dill, D. B. (ed.): *Handbook of Physiology: Adaptation to the Environment*. Washington, D.C., American Physiological Society, 1964, p. 357.

Robinson, P. T., Sedgwick, C. J., Meier, J. E., and Bacon, J. P.: Internal Fixation of a humeral fracture in a Komodo dragon lizard (*Varanus komodoensis*). Veterinary Medicine and Small Animal Clinician, 73:645–649, 1978.

Sedgwick, C. J.: Veterinary anesthesia ventilation. Modern Veterinary Practice, 60:120–126, 1979.

SURGERY IN CAPTIVE REPTILES

FREDRIC L. FRYE, D.V.M.
Davis, California

INTRODUCTION

With the ever-increasing interest and technology within the veterinary medical profession and the growing expectations and affluence of private and institutional repositories of captive reptiles has come the concomitant development of highly sophisticated surgical techniques that are fully applicable to this lower class of vertebrates. I refer specifically to the major abdominal (or for the purist, *coelomic*), orthopedic, and neurosurgical procedures more commonly performed upon man and the higher vertebrates. In the mid-1960's to mid 1970's the techniques of rigid fixation of bone fractures by employing bone plates and related devices made repair and subsequent return to normal function possible in cases that previously had been considered hopeless. Invasion of the coelmic cavity of hard-shelled chelonians became a routine procedure in private and institutional practice. With the improvement of anesthetic agents and techniques has come great advancement in methods of safe and effective restraint and clinical diagnosis. The ever-widening variety of surgical procedures can not only save lives but also totally resolve severe medical and surgical problems.

This discussion will focus upon the more frequently encountered clinical problems best dealt with by surgical intervention. Emphasis will be placed upon practicality; all the procedures can be performed by veterinary surgeons using equipment that any small animal practice routinely has on hand (or can borrow from colleagues).

In order to be successful in performing surgery upon reptiles, as in any species, strict attention must be paid to sterile technique. *There is absolutely no excuse for non-sterile surgery, and failure to observe this dictum cannot be compensated for by preoperative or postoperative antibiotic therapy.* The only logical exception to this admonition is in the incision and drainage of confirmed abscesses. Sometimes what at first appears to be an abscess is something entirely different (e.g., a tumor, fracture, luxation, cyst, or other lesion), and for the clinician to convert a non-infectious lesion into an iatrogenic abscess or osteomyelitis is unforgivable!

Many reptiles are approaching the status of endangered or threatened species, and every one that can be salvaged lessens the pressure imposed by human exploitation upon the wild population.

PRESURGICAL PREPARATION OF THE OPERATIVE SITE

Preoperative preparation of reptilian surgical patients poses few, if any, special problems. After the patient is properly anesthetized and restrained, the incisional site and the surrounding area are scrubbed thoroughly several times with an organic (povidone) iodine-containing surgical scrub (e.g., Betadine Surgical Scrub®)° and then rinsed and painted or sprayed with a povidone iodine surgical preparation (e.g., Betadine Solution®)° or a similar antiseptic solution. The operative area should be draped with sterile towels, which may have to be held in place with sterile liquid adhesive if towel clamps cannot be employed because of the nature of the patient's integument or shell.

INSTRUMENTATION

Few specialized surgical instruments are required to perform general surgery in reptilian patients. Some of the particularly useful items are (1) a variety of small dental curettes and small cerumen loops, all of which are well suited for enucleation of the contents of inspissated abscesses (the cerumen loops are especially valuable for working in or around the orbit, where sharp-edged instruments might damage the delicate orbital contents); (2) five-inch angled-wire suture scissors; (3) Rotary hand drills or saws that can be employed to cut through the plastron or carapace of turtle or tortoise patients. If a high-speed pneumatic handpiece is not available, a hobbyist's inexpensive electric motor-driven chucked drill (such as the Dremel Moto-Tool®) is a reasonable substitute. It can be sterilized by ethylene oxide gas. The drill may be partially enclosed in a lint-free, sewn bag that can be sterilized prior to surgery, or a small stockinette, which has been previously sterilized and included in the surgical pack, can be stretched over the handpiece with the electric cord doubled over and back in such a fashion as to preclude contamination of the surgical field; (4) a variety of twist drills, rotary burrs, and circular saw blades (best sterilized with ethylene oxide gas to prevent degradation of their cutting edges); and (5) a gallbladder spoon or long-handled ice-tea spoon, which is useful in helping deliver calculi or shelled ova from an incision.

Most surgical scissors, forceps, hemostatic clamps, and suture needles employed for mammalian surgery are applicable to reptilian operative procedures.

SUTURE MATERIALS

Suture materials are much the same as those employed in surgery of the higher vertebrates: chromic gut, polyglycolic acid (Dexon®), polyester (Dacron®, Mersilene®, Polydek®, Tycron®, and others), and Vetefil® have all been used with success.

In the very heavy-bodied crocodilians and chelonians, the preferred suture material is *monofilament* stainless steel wire carried upon a very stout, reverse-cutting needle. This material will withstand abrasion and tension better than other materials. This is particularly important in ventral, palmar, and plantar incisions, which may come into frequent contact with abrasive surfaces.

SUTURE PATTERNS

The suture pattern employed in most reptilian surgery is optional, in that the species and procedure may dictate the particular technique to use. For ease of removal, continuous sutures are convenient, but there is an inherent hazard of incisional disruption if any portion between the two knotted ends is divided. Simple interrupted sutures (with at least three half-knots) are probably the most secure, but in some non-surface-contact areas continous patterns are preferable, particularly when suturing the soft skin lining the anterior and posterior leg fossae in aquatic turtles.

In suturing the integument of snakes and lizards, great care must be exercised to produce a slightly *everting* skin closure, because there is a natural tendency for the skin of these animals to roll inward at the margin, thus retarding primary healing. In order to create a slightly outward-facing closure, the suture needle is directed inward and then outward as each stitch is placed.

Generally, it is preferable to begin the skin closure by placing the first sutures in the *middle* of the incision and working toward the two outer ends of the defect. This technique helps prevent puckering and therefore promotes uncomplicated, early healing. Upon the first ecdysis following suture removal, the surgical incision scar usually disappears with the old epidermis. The first molt following surgery may have to be aided but thereafter, once healing is complete, shedding is usually uneventful.

CHELONIAN SHELL REPAIR

Fractured chelonian carapaces and plastrons, or those that have been invaded surgically, are

*Purdue-Frederick, Norwalk, Conn. 06856

repaired with single or multiple overlapping patches consisting of sterilized fiberglass fabric impregnated with freshly prepared, rapidly polymerizing epoxy resin. If the shell has been fractured traumatically, the edges should be debrided and any depressed bone fragments elevated and replaced into their proper anatomic sites. With a relatively small (less than 3 cm in diameter), depressed fracture, the devascularized bone fragments may be discarded with impunity. In those instances in which the fractured bone is lost or is deemed to be useless as an autologous implant, the defect may still be bridged with epoxy-impregnated fiberglass; the distance from edge to edge may preclude complete osseous regeneration which, although not cosmetically ideal, does not interefere with normal physiologic functions. Smaller defects usually will bridge over with new bone within two years.

Respiration is unimpeded by direct communication of the coelomic cavity with the outside environment. Reptiles do not possess a functional diaphragm; their respiratory gas exchange is accomplished with the aid of intrapulmonary smooth muscle and extrapulmonary skeletal muscle contractions. Moreover, most reptiles are capable of enduring severe oxygen deficits by employing anaerobic respiration in times of stress.

In cases where the shell defects result from trauma, the patient is usually active and should be sedated or tranquilized with minimal doses of appropriate agents. A light dose of ketamine hydrochloride and atropine sulfate, with or without acepromazine maleate is an example of such mild sedation. The dosage of these drugs should be as low as possible because they are intended only to quiet the animal sufficiently to facilitate the approximation and fixation of the shell fragments.

The method for applying these patches is as follows: (1) Previously autoclaved fiberglass patches (either round or oval in shape to avoid wrinkles and puckers) are selected so that at least 1.5 to 2.0 cm will remain beyond the edge of the body defect. (2) The surface of the shell to be repaired (i.e., on which the epoxy is to be applied) is cleaned by several applications of ether or acetone and allowed to air-dry completely (3) Quantities of freshly prepared 5-Minute Epoxy Cement® are applied to the *periphery* of the defect, extending outward for a distance of approximately 2 cm, *but not actually extending into the defect.* (4) The first fabric patch is positioned over the hole so that its margins are in contact with the freshly applied epoxy cement, and the resin is worked carefully into the interstices of the patch, making certain that the fabric remains tautly stretched over the

hole. (5) As soon as the first coat of epoxy polymerizes, the central portion of the patch can receive its first light coat of cement — sufficient to moisten the fabric but not so much that it drips through into the bony defect or coelomic cavity. Several thin coats are more desirable than a single thick one (6) Once this layer has polymerized, additional patches impregnated with epoxy may be added until the desired thickness and strength have been achieved.

Although exothermic heat develops from the process of polymerization, it is dissipated over the surface of the patch and does not create any problems. Total time required for polymerization to begin is approximately four to six minutes when the two-part epoxy kit is used in a ratio of 1:1 epoxy:catalyst. Between applications of epoxy, a light wiping of the finished surface with diethyl ether will improve the bond between successive layers.

When a portion of devascularized bone is to be replaced and thus serve as an autograft, the technique is essentially identical to that just described. The implant is bonded to the central portion of the fabric first and, when fully polymerized, the bone and its fabric patch are bonded to the periphery of the hole just as was done for a simple patch. However, it is imperative that the fresh epoxy be prevented from flowing in between the autograft and the edges of the shell defect because the epoxy will act as a barrier to osteogenic bridging.

Clear epoxy resin is preferred by the author because it is inexpensive, readily available, and cosmetically acceptable, and the epoxy-fiberglass prostheses possess excellent abrasion resistance. Dental acrylic plastics and colored resins also can be used. If a totally natural repair must be made, finely ground shell substance can be added to the final layer of epoxy, and the surface can be etched with an engraving tool to simulate the natural growth rings and striae. Alternatively, a piece of natural tortoise carapace can be used to emboss a ringed pattern on the slightly soft surface of the partially polymerized epoxy resin. This piece of shell thus acts as a die or model.

Occasionally, interfragmentary wiring and plating of severely collapsed shell fractures must be done to repair massive crushing injuries. If the patient shows evidence of paralysis or posterior limb paresis the prognosis must be regarded as unfavorable, since the animal would remain crippled. Efforts to repair lesions in such animals may not be justified on humane grounds, and euthanasia would seem to be the kindest alternative. Dorsal-ventral and lateral view radiographs aid in defining the extent of spinal injury.

In juvenile or still-growing animals, patched

areas overlying growth interfaces must be removed as soon as healing is complete in order to allow unimpeded growth. This healing can be determined by periodic radiography. A rotary bur or similar instrument is used to remove the overlying fiberglass-epoxy prosthesis. *(Caution: The dust resulting from this removal procedure is highly irritating to the human ophthalmic, respiratory, and gastrointestinal epithelia and, in fact, may be carcinogenic in the same way that asbestos and gypsum fibers are. Therefore, suitable protection must be worn to avoid contamination. A simple disposable respiratory mask and eye goggles will afford protection from needless exposure).*

CELIOTOMY

Techniques for surgical invasion of the coelomic cavity depend upon the order of reptiles involved, because the anatomic features of these animals differ markedly. Once the surgeon has gained entrance into the coelomic cavity, the procedures performed are much the same as those undertaken in higher vertebrates. Removal of visceral neoplasms and intralumenal or extralumenal obstructive lesions, gastrotomy, enterotomy, intestinal anastomosis, cystotomy, and biopsy are all possible. A variety of gynecologic operations are now performed by innovative surgeons. Also, several experimental procedures calling for the surgical implantation of chronic flow probe transducers, temperature- and pressure-registering telemetric transmitters, and other electronic devices too large to be encapsulated and ingested have been accomplished. With the increasing utilization of reptiles as experimental models, undoubtedly more of these devices will be implanted.

The coelomic cavities of snakes, lizards, and crocodilians are easily approached via incision through the body wall. Generally, these incisions are created in the lateral or ventro-lateral aspect of the body wall. Care must be taken when making the incision(s) to select the skin *between* the scales or dermal plates rather than across them. Once the integument and underlying muscular layers have been divided, the relatively avascular coelomic (peritoneal) membrane may be seen. Once this tissue is incised the contents of the cavity become accessible. In some lizards and crocodilians, two parallel incisions may have to be made perpendicular to the first one to increase the exposure. This technique creates two flap-like portions; the overall appearance is that of a broad "H." Retraction of the incision's edges can be accomplished using small, self-retaining retractors. In small snakes, light-weight, self-retaining ophthalmic eyelid retractors serve this purpose well. If major non-visceral blood vessels are encountered, they should be avoided or, if that is impossible, double-ligated and transected. Pin-point electrocautery is useful and time-saving. When a hollow viscus is invaded, the recommended closure is one in which at least two layers of absorbable sutures are employed.

External wound closure is similar to that employed in mammals; the coelomic membrane is sutured with chromic gut or polyglycolic acid sutures. The subcutaneous tissues are approximated so as to reduce dead space, and the skin is closed with non-absorbable or polyglycolic acid material employing the everting pattern described earlier. The finished incisional line may be sprayed with a methylmethacrylate dressing to help protect it during the initial stages of wound repair. In smaller lizards, crocodilians and the Tuatara a protective dressing may be employed; topical antibiotic medication can be applied beneath the dressing for additional protection. Such a dressing should be examined frequently. If self-adherent bandage materials (e.g., Vetrap® or Coban®)† are used, adhesive tape is neither necessary nor desirable.

Celiotomy in the chelonians may be the most challenging yet satisfying procedure for the surgeon during his or her *first* attempt; any subsequent forays into surgical "spelunking" within these armored animals will be a familiar process.

To help guide the location of the incisional site on the plaston, a survey radiograph should be made to locate the pelvic girdle. Once this structure has been found, the turtle or tortoise is placed upon its back and prepared for aseptic surgery. In most cases, polyurethane foam bolsters are used to help maintain the inverted position during preparation and surgery.

A high-speed orthopedic or dental drill is used to cut through the plastron. Slower-speed drills or saws may also be used, but it is imperative that the cutting bur or saw blade be kept cool. The incisional site may be flushed with cooled Ringer's solution or its equivalent. The incision is usually quadrilateral in shape and approximately 6 to 15 cm on a side, depending upon the size of the animal, the location of its pelvic girdle, and the nature of the condition for which surgery is being performed. Once a generous piece of shell-covered bone has been isolated, it is elevated gently with a periosteal elevator and the underlying soft tissues are separated from the bone flap or severed with Metzenbaum scissors or a scalpel blade. The bone flap is transferred to a container of cool

---

†3-M Company, St. Paul, Minn. 55101

Ringer's solution or moistened gauze sponges to prevent desiccation. If the coelomic membrane has remained intact during elevation and removal of the bone flap, it is now incised *longitudinally* at a point midway between its two lateral margins. Two ventral venous sinuses will be found about midway between the ventral midline and lateral junction of the plastron and carapace in most species. These venous structures should be preserved if possible but, if one or both are damaged, they may be ligated without serious effect to the patient. If significant blood loss develops from either or both of them, they should be ligated.

Once the coelomic membrane is incised, the viscera will be in view. If anesthesia is deep, it is wise to have an assistant continue positive-pressure ventilation via an endotracheal catheter at a rate of 6 to 10 respirations per minute.

After surgical correction of the problem, the coelomic membrane is approximated and sutured, employing routine mammalian technique. The shell-bone flap is now retrieved from its physiologic solution or sponges, thoroughly dried on its exterior surface, and replaced and fixed with a fiberglass-epoxy patch as described previously. The patch is affixed to the flap first and then the bonded flap-patch is cemented to the plastron. The animal may be returned to its normal prone attitude once the epoxy resin has polymerized.

FRACTURE REPAIR

It is no longer rare to repair limb fractures in captive reptiles. With the advent of more sophisticated methods for internal fixation of long bone fractures, far better postoperative results may be expected than when external splinting is employed.

In the majority of cases of fractured reptilian long bones, the elasticity and toughness of the overlying skin tends to prevent compounding or skin perforation by sharp bone fragments. Experience has also shown that a reptile's long bones usually do not comminute severely after external trauma.

Surgical approaches to reptilian limb fractures are almost identical to those used in mammals. Incisions should be made between adjacent scales whenever possible. Once the major fragments have been isolated and the soft tissue damage has been assessed, fixation with appropriate intramedullary pins or bone plates may be accomplished. Occasionally, intrafragmentary compression using cortical or cancellous bone screws may be possible. The use of tension-band wires carried around a pin or bone screw is the method of choice in many fractures. Once mechanical fixation is complete and the incision is ready for closure, the soft tissues are approximated with absorbable gut or polyglycolic acid sutures.

Some of the smaller lizards will tolerate lightweight padded external splints for simple fractures, and this is the method by which these injuries should be managed. Moreover, when the fracture results in minimal displacement, cage rest will be adequate to effect spontaneous and suitable healing without further medical or surgical intervention. It should be noted that even without medical care most closed fractures in reptiles will eventually heal by themselves—with varying degrees of displacement. Most limbs regain some function.

In most cases, intramedullary pins should be left in place for about two to three months, although the skin sutures may be removed in three or four weeks.

Irrespective of the choice of internal or external stabilization of limb fractures, the animal should receive supplemental calcium and vitamins C and D_3 in its diet.

AMPUTATIONS

When individual phalanges or entire digits require surgical removal because of highly destructive lesions such as severe injury or gangrene, the amputations are best performed at the appropriate palmar or plantar junction. The patient is left with a stumpless and highly functional limb, and the cosmetic appearance is satisfactory. Two curvilinear skin flaps that join together medially and laterally are made, and the phalanx is disarticulated at a point proximal to the ends of the curved incisions. Soft tissues are preserved, brought down to cover the disarticulated bone, and then sutured together to provide a well-padded, protected surface. The two flaps of skin are joined with non-absorbable sutures, beginning in the middle and working outward to prevent puckering of the finished incisional line.

When an entire limb must be sacrificed owing to irreparable tissue loss, neoplasia, or infection, it is preferable to remove the affected forelimb or hind limb at its respective scapulohumeral or coxofemoral articulation; this will result in a totally stumpless postoperative effect. Again, two-flap method is employed.

When performing these amputations, blood loss can be controlled by sequential ligation of major vessels as they are encountered. Large nerves also are ligated and transected as in mammals; they may be folded over on themselves and ligated if the surgeon desires.

Whenever possible, viable soft tissues, especially heavy muscles, should be stripped from the bone that is to be removed; i.e., strip the area of bone insertion so that the muscle is free. This tissue is used to cover the proximal bone stump. Once this has been accomplished, the skin flaps are sutured as previously described. The result is maximally comfortable for the patient and free from additional trauma caused by contact with the substrate.

If the tail must be shortened surgically, some judgment must be exercised as to whether the stump is to be sutured. In lizards whose tail *will* regenerate, it is best not to suture the proximal stump because this will inhibit regrowth. In snakes, chelonians, crocodilians, and those species of lizards in which the tail is known not to regenerate, a ventral-dorsal or lateral-lateral flap incision is employed; adequate soft tissue coverage for the coccygeal stump is provided from salvaged coccygeal musculature. Skin closure is routine, and non-absorbable or polyglycolic acid sutures are indicated.

CRYOSURGERY

The application of cryosurgery should be considered in those cases in which excisional techniques are inappropriate. Examples of such lesions are broad-based or diffuse neoplasms and non-neoplastic disease that, if removed by more conventional methods, would result in large defects that could not be covered by primary closure.

After sufficient material is gathered for histopathologic and microbiologic processing, the lesions are deeply frozen and thawed several times by the intermittent application of liquid nitrogen-cooled cryosurgical instruments. The frozen tissues eventually undergo necrosis and are sloughed and replaced by the ingrowth of fibrocollagenous connective tissue in a more orderly fashion than would be the case following sharp excision or electrocautery.

SUPPLEMENTAL READING

Frye, F. L.: Surgical removal of a cystic calculus from a desert tortoise. J. Am. Vet. Med. Assoc., *161*:600–602, 1972.
Frye, F. L.: Clinical evaluation of a rapid-polymerizing epoxy resin for repair of shell defects in tortoises. Vet. Med. Small Animal Clin., 68:51–53, 1973a.
Frye, F. L.: *Husbandry, Medicine, and Surgery in Captive Reptiles.* Bonner Springs, Kansas, VM Publishing, 1973b.
Frye, F. L., and Schuchman, S. M.: Salpingotomy and cesarian delivery of impacted ova in a tortoise. Vet. Med. Small Animal Clin., 69:454–457, 1974.
Frye, F. L.: *Biomedical and Surgical Aspects of Captive Reptile Husbandry.* Bonner Springs, Kansas, VM Publishing, 1980.
Robinson, P. T., Sedgwick, C. J., Meier, J. E., and Bacon, J. P.: Internal fixation of a humeral fracture in a Komodo dragon lizard (*Varanus komodoensis*). Vet. Med. Small Animal Clin., 73:645–649, 1978.

INFECTIOUS DISEASES OF REPTILES

ELLIOTT R. JACOBSON, D.V.M.
Gainesville, Florida

INTRODUCTION

The class Reptilia phylogenetically represents the first truly terrestrial vertebrate group. The development of the cleidoic egg, coupled with a cornified skin and uric acid as the primary nitrogenous waste product, allowed radiation into untapped niches. Of the 17 orders of reptiles present during the Mesozoic period today four orders representing approximately 5900 species survive: Chelonia, (turtles and tortoises) 222 species; Crocodilia, 22 species; Rhynchocephalia (tuatara), 1 species; and Squamata (lizards, amphisbaenians, and snakes), 5700 species. Although present-day species show a range of ectothermy, fossil and zoogeographic evidence suggest that the ancestral dinosaur orders that resulted in the evolution of crocodilians and birds were endothermic.

It is only logical to theorize that with this terrestrial diversification there was a challenge, with many new "potential" pathogens existing as soil saprophytes or invertebrate infectious agents. Additionally, infectious agents that were brought along with their hosts from an aquatic environment must have developed specific adaptations to the "harsh" terrestrial life style. Thus, the phylogenetic vertebrate continuum seen from fishes to mammals must have resulted in a co-evolution of infectious agents.

The group of vertebrates least studied from the standpoint of pathogens, especially in wild populations, is the class Reptilia. This is unfortunate because of the evolutionary importance of the group. As the class that phylogenetically resulted in the independent evolution of birds and mammals, reptiles should offer an exciting group to the comparative virologist, microbiologist, and mycologist.

Numerous reasons, including lack of interest, unfamiliarity, and difficulty in captive maintenance, have resulted in an avoidance of reptiles by diagnosticians and medical researchers. Most important, the cost of diagnosis coupled with a lack of financial support has precluded detailed studies on reptile disease and associated infectious agents.

Most reports on disease and infectious agents in reptiles involve animals in zoologic and research collections. The public health significance of salmonellosis has resulted in numerous reports of *Salmonella* spp. shedding by pet turtles. Mismanagement accounts for many disease problems in captive reptiles, and clinical problems may be directly related to captive environmental conditions. Reptiles in captivity are seldom maintained under optimum environmental conditions. Below-optimum environmental conditions may lead to a depressed immune system,[13] with possible invasion of opportunistic pathogens.

There are numerous case reports of bacterial infections in reptiles, with gram-negative organisms being the most significant. In a recent review (Clark and Lunger, 1978) viral agents identified for reptiles have been categorized as (1) viruses circumstantially associated with reptilian disease, (2) viruses associated with reptilian tumors, (3) viruses pathogenic for reptiles, in which reptiles may play a reservoir role, and (4) viruses of unknown disease-producing potential that are restricted to reptiles. Recently a pox-like virus has been found to be associated with skin lesions in captive caimans (*Caiman sclerops*) and a herpes-like virus has been found by the author to be associated with a venom gland infection in captive Siamese cobras (*Naja naja kaouthia*). Reports of mycotic disease in reptiles are uncommon compared with those available in the literature for higher vertebrates. While most reports involve the respiratory and integumentary systems, almost any system may be affected. *Aspergillus*, *Fusarium*, *Geotrichum*, *Paecilo-*

myces, *Candida* and a variety of Phycomycetes have been identified as causative agents of mycotic disease in reptiles.

The following is a review of current information on infectious agents identified for reptiles, including viruses, bacteria, and fungi; diagnosis and treatment will be discussed at the end of this article. Infectious agents and associated disease will be discussed phylogenetically for three of the four present-day reptilian orders. There is a single report on microsporidiosis in the tuatara *Sphenodon punctatus*, with no other documentations of infectious disease.

TAXONOMIC DISTRIBUTION OF INFECTIOUS AGENTS IDENTIFIED IN REPTILES

CHELONIA—TURTLES AND TORTOISES

VIRUSES

A virus with the morphologic appearance of the herpesvirus group has been shown to be the causative agent of epizootic skin lesions termed "grey-patch disease" in young green sea turtles (*Chelonia mydas*) between 56 and 90 days after hatching in aquaculture.[42] Skin lesions consisted of either circular papular lesions or spreading patches containing epidermal cells with basophilic intranuclear inclusions. The most severe epizootic occurred under stressful environmental conditions such as crowding, organic pollutions, and high summer water temperatures of approximately 30° C.[22] The herpesvirus associated with grey-patch disease of green sea turtles represents the only reptilian virus to date that is capable of producing infectious disease under experimental conditions.

Although togaviruses are nonpathogenic in turtles, these animals may act as reservoirs for transmission of infected insects to mammals. Togaviruses have been isolated directly from turtles[24] and have also been demonstrated serologically.[24] Twenty-seven of 28 gopher tortoises (*Gopherus berlandieri*) developed viremia up to 105 days after inoculation with western equine encephalitis virus (WEEV) if maintained at an ambient temperature of at least 20° C.[5] The previremic period decreased as the environmental temperature was increased from 20° C to 30° C.

BACTERIA

Abrasions in tortoises caused by rubbing of the carapace and plastron on the forelimbs and hind limbs allow contamination with fecal and surface organisms. Several red-footed tortoises (*Geochelone carbonaria*) have been presented with streptococcal dermatitis from such abrasions. *Clostridium novyi* in chelonians has caused a fatal septicemia that was manifested clinically by a decreased appetite and lethargy.[32] "Floppy flipper" disease, a disease of green sea turtles (*Chelonia mydas*) in aquaculture, was associated with a *Clostridium botulinum* infection.[*] Turtles developed a dysequilibrium and eventually drowned.

A fatal septicemia of chelonians caused by the organism *Escherichia freundii*, later considered to be *Citrobacter freundii*, may be accompanied by skin and shell ulcerations and necrosis, with involvement of the liver, heart, blood, kidney, and spleen.[32] This disease has been designated speticemic cutaneous ulcerative dermatitis (SCUD) of turtles, may be transmissible via water, and may affect various emydine turtles. Chloramphenicol is considered the antibiotic of choice. It was reported subsequently that *Serratia* may be necessary to initiate the infection, insofar as the lipolytic, proteolytic action of *Serratia* might allow for entry of *Citrobacter*.[26] SCUD is a mismanagement problem caused by the low nutrition status of captive aquatic turtles and the high rate of contamination via filthy water. Good water quality and a good feeding schedule for turtles kept at optimum temperatures should eliminate this problem.

Middle and inner ear infections are well documented for box turtles[26] and other emydine turtles. Turtles are usually presented with unilateral or bilateral swellings below the tympanic scale that consist of caseous laminar material surrounded by a mixed inflammatory reaction. *Citrobacter*, *Enterobacter*, *Proteus morgani*, *P. rettgeri*, and *Pseudomonas* have been cultured from such lesions. This is one of the few infectious problems documented in wild populations of box turtles.

Respiratory disease is a common problem of chelonians in captivity.[25] Pure cultures of *Pseudomonas aeruginosa* have been isolated from tracheal washings of captive box turtles housed under improper environmental conditions. In captive gopher tortoises (*Gopherus polyphemus*) respiratory disease is associated with a variety of bacteria, including both gram-positive and gram-negative types. In a study of the desert tortoise (*Gopherus agassizi*), no single pathogen was implicated as a cause of respiratory disease.[16] Multiple

stresses resulting in interference of the immune system were hypothesized to be contributing factors leading to possible invasion by any one of a number of opportunistic pathogens. Hypervitaminosis A was also considered a contributing factor in this syndrome.

Salmonellosis due to a variety of *Salmonella* serotypes probably represents the most important zoonotic disease of captive turtles. Approximately 15 percent of the isolations of *Salmonella* reported by the U.S. Center for Disease Control in 1973 were obtained from reptiles, mostly turtles,[2] and it was estimated that in 1970 to 1971 some 280,000 U.S. residents acquired salmonellosis from contact with turtles or their maintenance water.[34] The public health significance of this organism has resulted in a ban on the sale of juvenile turtles (*Pseudemys scripta elegans*) by the pet industry. Although gentamicin/chlorine egg dips appear effective in eliminating the reservoir state in hatchling turtles,[44] there is evidence that stressing turtles may result in a latent *Salmonella* infection.[12]

Mycobacterial infections are uncommon in reptiles in general, and there are few documentations in turtles. *Mycobacterium chelonei* was originally described from turtles but subsequently was shown to be bacteriologically and immunologically identical to *M. abscessus*, *M. runyoni* and *M. borstalonse*. Two cases of tuberculosis have been reported in snapping turtles (*Chelydra serpentina*) from a zoologic park.[25] Mycobacteriosis with cutaneous and hepatosplenic involvement has been described[43] for a side-necked turtle (*Phrynops hilari*).

FUNGI

In one report, mycotic disease in turtles in a zoologic collection involved the respiratory system and the bony and epidermal lamina of the shell.[25] Pulmonary mycoses were responsible for 3 percent of the total number of recorded deaths, with *Aspergillus* being the causative agent. Shell necrosis was due to invasion of Mucorales beneath the plates of the epidermal laminae. Mycotic infections have been described in members of the families Chelyidae (side-necked turtles), Chelydridae (snapping turtles, musk turtles, and mud turtles), Testudinidae (tortoises and aquatic turtles), and Chelonidae (sea turtles). Mycotic pneumonias have been reported[20] on several occasions in giant tortoises (*Geochelone elephatopus* and *G. gigantea*). *Paecilomyces fumoso-roseus* and *Beuavana bassiana* were cultured individually from pulmonary abscesses in two Aldabra tortoises. Additionally, a

---

[*] James Wood, Resident Manager, Cayman Turtle Farm, Grand Cayman Island, British West Indies: Personal communication.

fatal pneumonitis due to a combined *Aspergillus amstelodami* and *Geotrichum candidum* infection was documented in a Galapagos tortoise.

Several juvenile green sea turtles (*Chelonia mydas*) that had a respiratory disease manifested by a swimming tilt to one side were found to have multifocal firm nodules that were particularly prominent in the right lung. Histopathologic studies reveal multiple granulomas containing numerous hyphae. Several agents were cultured from the lungs, including *Cladosporium* sp., *Sporotrichum* sp., and *Paecilomyces* sp.

CROCODILIA (ALLIGATORS, CROCODILES, AND CAIMANS)

VIRUSES

The only report of a virus-associated disease of crocodilians is that of a poxlike virus associated with skin lesions in captive caimans. Three captive juvenile spectacled caimans (*Caiman sclerops*) were presented with greywhite circular skin lesions scattered over the body surface and particularly prominent on the palpebrae, tympanic membranes, and integument overlying the maxillae and mandibles. Epithelial cells were found on digital biopsy to have large eosinophilic intracytoplasmic inclusions within hypertrophied cells when stained with hematoxylin and eosin. Electron microscopic evaluation of scrapings taken from lesions on the lower jaw revealed particles morphologically resembling pox virus. This represented the first poxlike virus identified for a reptile.

One American alligator (*Alligator mississippiensis*) has been demonstrated to be susceptible to eastern equine encephalomyelitis virus (EEEV), as seen by its development of neutralizing antibodies following natural exposure.[33]

BACTERIA

There are relatively few reports of bacterial infections in captive crocodilians. One report documents a death associated with *Aeromonas hydrophilia* and *A. shigelloides* in the American alligator (*Alligator mississippiensis*) in a eutrophic inland lake in Florida.[46] Cutaneous lesions due to *Erysipelothrix insidiosa* have been reported in a 100-year-old American crocodile (*Crocodilus acutus*) from a zoologic park in Florida.[30] *Pasteurella multocida* and *Staphylococcus aureus* have been cultured from several members of a herd of American alligators exhibiting a respiratory disease.[38]

Many of these alligators were coughing and sneezing and had a serous and purulent discharge from the nostrils. Chloramphenicol at 16 mg/kg (8 mg/lb) for five days resulted in a distinct improvement in most affected animals.

FUNGI

Candida albicans has been identified as the agent responsible for pneumonia in unspecified species of crocodile and caiman.[53] *Aspergillus fumigatus* and *A. ustus* have been cultured from pneumonic lesions in several captive American alligators 2 to 6 weeks of age.[30] Trevino described a fatal diffuse granulomatous pneumonia and hepatitis due to *Cephalosporium* in three *Caiman sclerops*.[49] Poor adaptation to their captive environment was considered a predisposing factor. Three species of crocodilians in a zoologic park, including a Morelet's crocodile (*C. moroleti*), an American crocodile (*C. acutus*), and a Nile crocodile (*C. niloticus*) developed a respiratory infection with lung lesions from which *Mucor* was isolated.[47] Overcrowding of animals in pools and buildup of debris in the exhibit were considered contributing factors. Several American alligators (*A. mississippiensis*) have been submitted from local alligator farms with multiple granulomatous inflammatory lesions on the foot pads and granulomatous lesions in the lungs from which a variety of fungi have been identified. Long-term housing in cement tanks results in abrasions on ventral body surfaces and invasion of opportunistic fungi. Poor diet and poor water quality are often associated and are contributing factors.

SQUAMATA: LACERTILIA (LIZARDS)

VIRUSES

Several viruses have been identified from lizards. The herpes virus of *Iguana iguana*[8] and the rhabdoviruses of *Ameiva ameiva*[6] represent viral agents of unknown disease-producing potential in their natural hosts. Several agamids and lacertids have been documented as reservoirs for Japanese encephalitis virus.[11]

A variety of other lizards, including *Eumeces laticeps*, *Anolis carolinensis*, and *Ophisaurus attenuatus*, were found to be susceptible to experimental infection with EEEV.[33] the erythrocyte virus in the gecko *Tarentola mauritanica* affected with a progressive anemia[7] and infecting numerous other reptile species was originally considered to be an intraerythrocytic protozoan. Three morphologically distinct particles resembling herpesvirus, reovirus and papovavirus have been identified[41] in papillomas from a laboratory breeding colony of European wall lizards (*Lacerta muralis*).

BACTERIA

A variety of gram-positive and gram-negative bacteria have been identified as causative agents of disease in captive lizards. Mismanagement, as evidenced by improper diet, temperature, and humidity and inappropriate cage mates, is a contributing factor. Bite wounds from combat between cage mates often become infected with surface and mouth contaminants. Anaerobic pathogens such as *Peptostreptococcus* have been cultured from such lesions. *Pseudomonas aeruginosa* is another organism commonly involved. Several American anoles (*Anolis carolinensis*) from a large research breeding colony that were presented with nuchal hematomas attributed to male-male combat were found to have a mixed *Pseudomonas/Trichosporon* infection. *Pseudomonas* may result in a septicemia that has few discernible clinical signs. Individual scales or groups of scales may be hemorrhagic, and often the animal will be presented in a lethargic anorexic state, with convulsions preceding death. Subcutaneous and internal abscesses are commonly reported in lizards. Often these represent a central core of caseated material surrounded by a fibrous capsule. Various bacteria have been isolated from these lesions, including *Serratia anolium* from *Anolis equestris*,[9] *Bacterium sauromali* from the Chukawalla (*Sauromalus varius*), and *Micrococci, Salmonella maurina,* and *Serratia marcescens* individually isolated from subcutaneous abscesses in iguanid lizards.

Dermatophilosis has been identified in agamid lizards. Two of these reports are in the Australian bearded lizard (*Amphiboluris barbatus*). One group of beared lizards had subcutaneous abscesses[48] and the other had cutaneous nodules.[40] Spontaneous dermatophilosis in a marble lizard (*Calotes mystaceus*) also was manifested by cutaneous nodules.[3]

FUNGI

Mycotic diseases have been reported in a variety of lizards, including members of Iguanidae, Agamidae, Chamaeleontidae, Teiidae, and Lacertidae. *Chrysosporium keratinophilum* has been isolated from visceral lesions in *Iguana iguana*.[53] Several *Anolis carolinesis*

submitted from a research colony were found to have nuchal hematomas from which the fungus *Trichsporon cutaneum*, the causative agent of white piedra of man, and the bacterium *Pseudomonas aeruginosa* were isolated. A *Mucor* sp. has been isolated from multiple cutaneous lesions in a beared lizard.[17] Organisms resembling *Candida albicans* have been identified[53] from multiple necrotic areas of the liver in a two-banded chameleon (*Chameleo bitaeniatus*) and Shaley reported a mycotic enteritis in an adult Jackson's chameleon (*Chameleo jacksoni*).[45] The enteritis was associated with an intussusception of the posterior portion of the colon. Aspergillosis[23] and candidiasis[53] have been identified for a black tegui (*Tupinambsis nigropunctatus*) and a crocodile lizard (*Crocodilurus lacertinus*), respectively.

SQUAMATA: SERPENTES (SNAKES)

VIRUSES

The only reported virus associated snake epizootic involved a colony of fer-de-lance (*Bothrops atrox*) housed at a snake farm.[15] Snakes initially exhibited a loss of muscle tone characterized by resting in a prostrate position, followed by the development of a terminal respiratory disease manifested by an open mouth with a discharge from the glottis. Postmortem evaluation revealed fluid-filled lungs and body cavity. Lung hemogenates injected into false water cobra eggs (*Cyclogras gigas*) resulted in egg death seven days after inoculation. Suspensions of these eggs caused cytopathic effects in gecko embryo (GE2) and rattlesnake fibroma cell cultures incubated at 30° C. This cytopathic agent recovered from the cell cultures was designed fer-de-lance virus (FDHV) and, based on electron microscopic appearance and biophysical properties, this agent was categorized as a paramyxovirus.

A herpeslike virus has been identified[39] in venoms of Indian cobras (*Naja naja*) and banded kraits (*Bungarus fasciatus*). Recently a herpeslike virus was demonstrated in intact venom glands of Siamese cobras (*Naja naja kaouthial*) that were presented with venom gland infections. The infections were manifested by a low-grade venom production characterized by an abnormal quantity of desquamated cells and pus. Histopathologic studies revealed a chronic inflammatory reaction with tubular destruction, fibrosis, and a mononuclear infiltrate. Although no inclusions were demonstrated by these studies, electron microscopic evaluation revealed particles typical of herpesvirus. Attempts to cultivate the virus have been unsuccessful owing to venom destruction of tissue cultures.

A variety of snakes have been found to be infected naturally with WEEV[19] and Japanese encephalitis virus[35] or experimentally found to be susceptible to EEEV.[33]

C-type viruses have been reported from a Russell's viper (*Vipera russelli*) diagnosed as having a precardial myxofibroma[52] and from an embryonal rhabdomyosarcoma in a corn snake.[37] Type A particles have been reported in neoplastic cells in a California king snake diagnosed as having a lymphosarcoma.[29] At present the significance of these particles accompanying the neoplasms is unknown, and any causal relationship will depend on *in vivo* challenge.

BACTERIA

Snakes are susceptible to a variety of gram-positive and gram-negative bacteria; the latter appear to predominate in captive infectious disease conditions.

Ulcerative stomatitis, also known as "mouth rot," is an infectious disease initially of the oral mucosa that may progress to an osteomyelitis of the bony structures of the head and may ultimately result in a systemic infection via the circulatory system or a bacterial pneumonia via inhalation of cellular debris into the respiratory tract. The infection is initially characterized by ulceration of the mucous membranes surrounding the maxillary, dentary, and palatine teeth, with an accumulation of caseous material within the mucous membranes. In most cases the snake's rubbing on objects in the cage or on screened tops, bites from rats or mice, poor nutrition, and improper environmental temperatures may be predisposing factors. The gram-negative opportunistic organisms (*Pseudomonas* and *Aeromonas*) that are commonly associated with this infection are normal inhabitants of the mouth cavity. The oral lesions often result in a decline in feeding behavior, which ultimately results in a decline in the overall condition of the snake.

Subcutaneous abscesses are commonly seen in snakes and are often due to puncture wounds and rodent bites or are associated with ticks. Organisms commonly cultured are *Proteus, E. coli, Pseudomonas,* and *Salmonella.* Subcutaneous migration of pentastomid larvae is often associated with such abscesses.

Eye infections in snakes are not uncommonly encountered and may be either unilateral or bilateral. The spectaculocorneal (S-C) space may become cloudy (do not confuse this with the normal bluing of the eye during ecdysis) and accumulate cellular debris and pus, with distention of the spectacle. Blockage of the lacrimal duct with cellular debris adds to the initial problems. Puncture wounds to the spectacle, bacteria ascending the lacrimal duct from a mouth infection, and periorbital masses compressing the lacrimal duct may all lead to infection and increased fluid in the S-C space.

Diseases of the respiratory system are common in reptiles and are responsible for a considerable part of the mortality rate in snake collections.[28] Sudden lower of ambient temperature, insufficient humidity, and starvation may be predisposing factors. Snakes may exhibit labored breathing, with crackling sounds heard on auscultation. Often, bubbles exude from the nares or the glottis or both. The glottis may be extended forward and the mouth held open. *Aeromonas hydrophila*, one of the agents associated with infectious stomatitis of snakes, may also cause respiratory tract infections. Although predisposing factors such as malnutrition and injury to the mouth may be involved, the organism can also be aspirated readily into the respiratory system. Invasion of the blood stream may cause septicemia. Because the snake mite (*Ophionyssus natricis*) has been shown to be involved in the transmission of *A. hydrophila*, the importance of good mite control can not be stressed too much. Various *Proteus* spp. and *Pseudomonas* spp. have also been associated with respiratory disease.

Tuberculosis is an uncommon disease in snakes. *Mycobacterium thamnopheos* was first isolated[4] from garter snakes (*Thamnophis sirtalis*). Intestinal, respiratory, and cutaneous forms of tuberculosis have been reported. Factors such as debilitation from injury, malnutrition, or other disease may be involved.

Salmonellosis is a major public health hazard associated with keeping snakes as pets. Numerous *Salmonella* and *Arizona* serotypes have been isolated from the intestinal flora of a variety of snakes. Often salmonellosis is subclinical in snakes, but septicemia resulting in anorexia, listlessness, and death has been documented. Most septicemias have been associated with parasite migrations and ulcerations of the gastrointestinal system. Amoebiasis seen as hepatoenteritis is often associated with *Salmonella* and *Arizona* septicemias. There is no documentation of total elimination of the carrier state with antibiotics.

Experimental infections of snakes with leptospires (*L. pomona*) have been reported.[1] Leptospira organisms were demonstrable in snake kidneys 6½ months after inoculation, and infections were shown to persist after a 70-day period of induced hibernation. One infected snake was found to have an interstitial nephritis. There is also serologic evidence of leptospirosis in free-ranging snakes,[51] and *L. ballum* was isolated from a hog-nosed snake, *Heterodon platyrhinos*.[14]

FUNGI

There are several reports of mycotic infections of snakes, with mycotic dermatitis being the most common. Oral candidiasis may be involved in infectious stomatitis. Clinical signs of systemic disease preceding death are often subtle and so go unrecorded.

Mycotic dermatitis is easily diagnosed by culture correlated with the histopathologic appearance of a skin biopsy. Skin lesions commence as discolored necrotic scales that may spread in a circular fashion; ventral scales appear to be more common involved. *Geotrichum candidum*, *Trichoderma* spp., and *Fusarium* spp. have been isolated. As in higher vertebrates, mycotic dermatitis may be associated with predisposing factors such as high humidity, malnutrition, overcrowding, and debris buildup in the animal's environment.

DIAGNOSIS AND TREATMENT

VIRUSES

There are relatively few reports of viruses associated with disease in captive reptiles. Viral identification depends upon electron microscopic evaluation or isolation in tissue culture, or both; several reptile cell culture products are commercially available. Even when associated with disease, the presence of a viral agent is only presumptive evidence. The fulfillment of Koch's postulates with monoclonal isolates in tissue culture is necessary to establish a causal relationship. The herpesvirus of grey-patch disease of green sea turtles comes closest to meeting these criteria.

There are no reports of treatment for reptilian viral disease. A killed vaccine for grey-patch disease of green sea turtles has had limited success.* Reptiles suspected of viral disease should receive supportive treatment with antibiotics and fluids. Housing at optimum environmental temperature is crucial for maintaining an adequate immune response.

BACTERIA

Bacteria pathogens are the most significant infectious agents associated with disease in captive reptiles. Diagnosis will depend upon isolation and identification on artifical media. With respiratory disease, bronchial washings can be obtained by inserting a sterile cannula (P.E. 50) into the respiratory system via the glottis and then instilling and aspirating 0.5 cc of sterile saline. Samples obtained can be cultured on artificial media and incubated at 30° C and 37° C.

Isolation of a single pathogen is rare, while multiple organisms are more commonly cultured. Often it is difficult to identify a primary agent, and complex synergisms and predisposing or contributing factors may be involved. Mismanagement accounts for a majority of the disease problems in captive reptiles.

Treatment will depend upon several factors, including the organisms involved, the degree of involvement, and the status of the reptile. With infectious stomatitis of snakes removal of the caseated material, irrigation of the mucous membranes with hydrogen peroxide, and topical application of povidone-iodine should be initiated and continued for a minimum of ten days. Often snakes are anorexic at this time, and force-feeding may be necessary. Administration of vitamin C has been suggested.[50] Systemic antibiotics and topical and injectable enzyme preparations are necessary in more advanced cases. Based on sensitivities of isolated pathogens, chloramphenicol and gentamicin sulfate are the antibiotics of choice. Antibiotic therapy is discussed in another section and will not be elaborated upon here. One comment that will be made in regard to gentamicin administration is this: Because of the nephrotoxic effect of this drug, reptiles should be starved during the period of treatment. Clinical signs of neophrotoxicity are generally seen nine days following initial treatment and are manifested by an accumulation of uric acid within the mucous membranes of the mouth and adjacent to the palatine vessels in the roof of the mouth.

Subcutaneous abscesses can be surgically removed with débridement and removal of the surrounding fibrous connective tissue capsule. The involved area is routinely irrigated with a betadine solution.

Eye infections in snakes are treated initially by draining the spectaculocorneal space. The lacrimal duct can be cannulated in the roof of the mouth and flushed with a gentamicin ophthalmic solution.

For bacterial respiratory disease, systemic

---

* Harold Haines, University of Miami School of Medicine, Miami, Florida: Personal communication.

treatment with a sensitive antibiotic is necessary. Nebulization with gentamicin (2 mg/10 ml of saline) and acetylcysteine has been helpful on several occasions. Maintenance at optimum environmental temperature again is crucial for an adequate immune response.

FUNGI

Diagnosis of mycotic disease will depend upon culture correlated with histopathology if a biopsy is practical. Most cases of systemic disease are diagnosed postmortem.

Many of the mycotic agents identified in reptiles are opportunistic invaders. Predisposing factors include low temperature, high humidity, malnutrition, unsanitary environmental conditions, and prior bacterial disease. The only report of treatment is that of eye enucleation in a rainbow boa diagnosed as having a *Fusarium* eye infection.[54] Two ball python (*Python regius*) cage mates diagnosed as having a *Trichoderma* sp. dermatitis were treated unsuccessfully with oral griseofulvin, 20 mg/kg body weight and 40 mg/kg body weight, respectively, every three days for five treatments. Suspected mycotic pneumonias in reptiles are treated with 5 mg of amphotericin B nebulized in 150 ml of saline twice a day (for one hour each time) for one week. Oral candidiasis resulting from bacterial infectious stomatitis has been treated orally, via stomach tube, with mycostatin at 100,000 units/kg s.i.d. for ten days.

SUPPLEMENTAL READING

1. Abdulla, P. K., and Karstad, L: Experimental infections with *Leptospira pomona* in snakes and turtles. Zoonoses Res., *1*:295–306, 1962.
2. Anon.: Salmonella surveillance. Annual Summary, 1973 Report. Atlanta, Ga., Publication No. 121. Center for Disease Control, 1974.
3. Anver, M. R., Park, J. S., and Rush, H. G.: Dermatophilosis in the marble lizard (*Calotes mystaceus*). Lab. Anim. Sci., *26*:817–823, 1976.
4. Aronson, J. D.: Spontaneous tuberculosis in snakes. J. Infect. Dis., *44*:215–223, 1929.
5. Bowen, G. S.: Prolonged western equine encephalitis viremia in the Texas tortoise (*Gopherus berlandieri*). Am. J. Trop. Med. Hyg., *26*:171–175, 1977.
6. Causey, O. R., Shope, R. E., and Bensabath, G.: Marco, Timbo and Chaco: Newly recognized rhabdoviruses from lizards of Brazil. Am. J. Trop. Med. Hyg., *15*:239–243, 1966.
7. Chatton, E., and Blanc, G.: Sur un hematozoaire nouveau, *Pirhemocyton tarentolae*, du gecko, *Tarentola mauritanica*, et sur les alterations globulaires qu'il determine. Compte Rend. Soc. Biol., 77:496, 1914.
8. Clark, H. F., and Karzon, D. T.: Iguana virus, a herpes-like virus isolated from cultured cells of a lizard, *Iguana iguana*. Infect. Immun., 5:559–569, 1937.
8a. Clark, H. F. and Lunger, P. D.: Viruses of reptiles. In Cooper, J. E., and Jackson, O. F. (eds.): *Diseases of the Reptilia*. New York, Academic Press. (In press.)
9. Claussen, H. J., and Durand-Reynolds, F.: Studies on the experimental infection of some reptiles, amphibia and fish with *Serratia anolium*. Am. J. Pathol., *13*:441–451, 1937.
10. Conti, L. F., and Crawley, J. H.: A new bacterial species isolated from the chuckwalla (*Sauromalus varius*). J. Bact., *33*:647–653, 1939.
11. Doi, R., Oya, A., and Telford, S. R., Jr.: A preliminary report on infection of the lizard, *Takydromus tachydromoides*, with Japanese encephalitis virus. Jpn. J. Med. Sc. Biol., *21*:205–207, 1968.
12. Duponte, M. W., Nakamura, R. M., and Chang, E. M. L.: Activation of latent *Salmonella* and *Arizona* organisms by dehydration in red-eared turtles (*Pseudemys scripta elegans*). Am. J. Vet. Res., *39*:529–530, 1978.
13. Evans, E. E.: Comparative immunology. Antibody response in *Dipsosaurus dorsalis* at different temperatures. Proc. Soc. Exp. Biol. Med., *112*:531–533, 1963.
14. Ferris, D. H., Rhoades, H. E., Hanson, L. E., Galton, M., and Mansfield, M. E.: Research into the nidality of *Leptospira ballum* in campestral hosts including the hog-nosed snake (*Heterodon platyrhinus*). Cornell Vet., *51*:405–419, 1961.
15. Folsch, von, D. W., and Leloup, P.: Uber eine verlustreich verlaufene infektion in einem schlangenbestand. Verhandlungsbericht des XVIII Internationalen Symposiums uber die Erkrankungen der Zootiere. Berlin, Akademie-Verlag, 1976.
16. Fowler, M. E.: Respiratory disease in desert tortoises. Annual Proceedings of the American Association of Zoo Veterinarians, 1977, pp. 79–99.
17. Frank, W.: Multiple hypkeratose bei einer Bartagame, *Amphibolurus barbatus* (Reptilia, Agamidae), hervorgerufen durch eine Pilzinfektion; zugleich ein Bertrag zur Problematik von Mykosen bei Reptilien. Salamandra, 2:6–12, 1966.
18. Frye, F. L., Oshiro, L. S., Dutra, F. R., and Carney, J. D.: Herpesvirus-like infection in two Pacific pond turtles. J. Am. Vet. Med. Assoc., *17*:882–884, 1977.
19. Gebhardt, L. P., St. Jeor, S. C., Stanton, G. J., and Stringfellow, D. A.: Ecology of western encephalitis virus. Proc. Soc. Exp. Biol. Med., *142*:731–733, 1973.
20. George, L. E., Williamson, W. M., Tilden, E. B., and Getty, R. E.: Mycotic pulmonary disease of captive giant tortoises due to *Beauveria bassiana* and *Paecilomyces fumoso-roseus*. Sabouraudi, 2:80–86, 1962.
21. Glosser, J. W., Sulzer, C. R., Eberhardt, M., and Winkler, W. G.: Cultural and serologic evidence of *Leptospira interrogans* serotype *Tarassovi* infection in turtles. J. Wildl. Dis., *10*:429–435, 1974.
22. Haines, H., and Kleese, W. C.: Effect of water temperature on a herpesvirus infection of sea turtles. Infect. Immun., *15*:756–759, 1977.
23. Hamerton, A. E.: Report on the deaths occurring in the Society's garden during the year 1933. Proc. Zool. Soc. London, *104*:389–403, 1934.
24. Hoff, G., and Trainer, D. O.: Arboviruses in reptiles: Isolation of a Bunyamwere group virus from a naturally infected turtle. J. Herp., 7:55–62, 1973.
25. Hunt, T. J.: Notes on diseases and mortality in testudines. Herpetologica, *13*:19–23, 1957.
26. Jackson, C. G., and Fulton, M.: A turtle colony epizootic apparently of microbial origin. J. Wildl. Dis., 6:446–468, 1970.
27. Jackson, C. G., Jr., Fulton, M., and Jackson, M. M.: Cranial asymmetry with massive infection in a box turtle. J. Wildl. Dis., 8:275–277, 1972.
28. Jacobson, E.: Diseases of the respiratory system in reptiles. Vet. Med. Small Anim. Clin., *1169*–1175, 1978.
29. Jacobson, E. R., and Seely, J. C.: Lymphosarcoma associated with viral-like intranuclear inclusions in a California king snake. Submitted for publication, 1978.
30. Jasmin, A. M. and Baucom, J. N.: *Erysipelothrix insidiosa* infections in the caiman (*Caiman crocodilus*) and the American crocodile (*Crocodilus acutus*). Am. J. Vet. Clin. Path., *1*:173–177, 1967.
31. Jasmin, A. M., Carroll, J. M., and Baucom, J. N.: Pulmonary aspergillosis of the American alligator (*Alligator mississippiensis*). Am. J. Vet. Clin. Path., 2:93–95, 1968.
32. Kaplan, H. M.: Septicemic cutaneous ulcerative disease of turtles. Lab. Anim. Care, 7:273–277, 1957.
33. Karstad, L.: Reptiles as possible reservoir hosts for eastern encephalitis virus. Transactions of the 26th N. Am. Wildlife and National Resources Conference, Wildlife Management Institute, Washington, D. C., 1961, pp. 186–202.
34. Lamm, S. H., Taylor, A., Gangarosa, E. J., Anderson, H. W., Young, W., Clark M. H., and Bruce, A. R.: Turtle-associated salmonellosis. I. An estimation of the magnitude of the

problem in the United States, 1970–1971. Am. J. Epidemiol., 95:511–517, 1972.

35. Lee, H. W., Min, B. W., and Lim, Y. W.: Isolation and serologic studies of Japanese encephalitis virus from snakes in Korea. J. Korean Med. Assoc., 15:69–74, 1972.

36. Lunger, P. D., and Clark, H. F.: Intracytoplasmic type-A particles in viper spleen cells, J. Nat. Cancer Inst., 58:809–811, 1977.

37. Lunger, P. D., Hardy, W. D., and Clark, H. F.: "C-type" virus particles in reptilian tumor. J. Nat. Cancer Inst., 52:1231–1235, 1974.

38. Mainster, M. E., Lynd, F. T., Cragg, P. C., and Karger, J.: Treatment of multiple cases of Pasteurella multocida and staphloccocal pneumonia in Alligator mississippiensis on a herd basis. Annual Proceedings of the American Association of Zoo Veterinarians, 1972, pp. 33–36.

39. Monroe, J. H., Shibley, G. P., Schidlovsky, G., Nakai, T., Howatson, A. F., Wivel, N. W. and O'Connor, T. E.: Action of snake venom on Rauscher virus. J. Nat. Cancer Inst., 40:135–145, 1968.

40. Montali, R. J., Smith, E. E., Davenport, M., and Bush, M: Dermatophilosis in Australian bearded lizard. J. A. Vet. Med. Assoc., 167:553–555, 1975.

41. Raynaud, A., and Adrian, M.: Lésions cutanées à structure papillomateuse associées à des virus chez le lézard vert (Lacerta viridis Laur). C. R. Acad. Sci. Paris, 283:845–847, 1976.

42. Rebell, H., Rywlin, A., and Haines, H.: A herpesvirus-type agent associated with skin lesions of green sea turtles in aquaculture. Am. J. Vet. Res., 33:1221–1224, 1975.

43. Rhodin, A. G. J., and Anver, M. R.: Mycobacteriosis in turtles: Cutaneous and hepatosplenic involvement in a Phrynops hilari. J. Wildl. Dis., 13:180–183, 1977.

44. Seale, T. J., and Ziller, H. H.: Position paper No. 1 of the National Turtle Farmers and Shippers Association, submitted to Congressional staff, Louisiana delegation. Why the F. D. A. should lift the ban on domestic turtle sales. 1977, 24 pp.

45. Shalev, M., Murphy, J. C., and Fox, J. G.: Mycotic enteritis in a chameleon and a brief review of phycomycoses of animals. J. Am. Vet. Med. Assoc., 171:872–875, 1977.

46. Shotts, E. B., Jr., Gaines, J. L., Martin, L., and Prestwood, A. K.: Aeromonas-induced deaths among fish and reptiles in an eutrophic inland lake. J. Am. Vet. Med. Assoc., 161:603–607, 1972.

47. Silberman, M. S., Blue, J., and Mahaffey, E.: Phycomycoses resulting in the death of crocodilians in a common pool. In Annual Proceedings of the American Association of Zoo Veterinarians, 1977, pp. 100–101.

48. Simmons, G. C., Sullivan, N. D., and Green, P. E.: Dermatophilosis in a lizard (Amphibolurus barbatus). Aust. Vet. J., 48:465–466, 1972.

49. Trevino, G. S.: Cephalosporiosis in three caimans. J. Wildl. Dis., 8:384–388, 1972.

50. Wallach, J. D.: Medical care of reptiles. J. Am. Vet. Med. Assoc., 155:1017–1034, 1969.

51. White, F. H.: Leptospiral agglutinins in snake serums. Am. J. Vet. Res., 24:179–182, 1963.

52. Zeigel, R. F., and Clark, H. F.: Electron microscopic observations on a C-type virus in cell cultures derived from a tumor-bearing viper. J. Nat. Cancer Inst., 43:1097, 1969.

53. Zwart, P.: Parasitare und mykotische Lungenaffektionen bei Reptilien. X International Symposium Erkr. Zootiere (Salzburg). Berlin, Akademie Verlag, 1968, pp. 45–48.

54. Zwart, P., Poelma, F. G., Strik, W. J., Peters, J. C., and Polder, J. J. W.: Report on births and deaths occurring in the Gardens of the Royal Rotterdam Zoo "Blijdorp" during the years 1961 and 1962. Tijdschr. Diergeneesk, 93:348–365, 1968.

RESPIRATORY DISEASE IN REPTILES

MURRAY E. FOWLER, D.V.M.
Davis, California

INTRODUCTION

Respiratory disease (RD) may occur in any reptilian species; however, a respiratory syndrome is rare in all species except chelonians (turtles and tortoises) and snakes. Within those groups, respiratory disease is one of the more common clinical conditions encountered.

Nutritional deficiencies, particularly hypovitaminosis A, may mimic the clinical syndrome of RD. Additionally, malnourished individuals with devitalized mucous membranes are predisposed to infectious diseases of the respiratory tract.

From a practical standpoint the diseases encountered are rhinitis, tracheobronchitis, pneumonia, and hypovitaminosis A. Etiologies include infectious agents (bacterial and fungal), noxious vapors, and nutrient deficiencies (hypovitaminosis A).

PREDISPOSING FACTORS

Reptiles are quite hardy creatures. They have adapted to many harsh environments in the world, excluding extremely cold climates, by judicious use of a microclimate within a habitat. Captive environments are frequently devoid of opportunities for a reptile to seek a microclimate suitable for optimal life. Lacking sophisticated homeostatic mechanisms, the reptile in captivity is frequently placed under constant high-level stress.

Well-meaning owners may place a reptile in a terrarium kept at a constant temperature of 75 to 80°F, frequently using incandescent light bulbs as the heat source. Reptiles have circadian rhythms like mammals and birds and need variable ambient temperatures. Furthermore, free-living reptiles seek seclusion and darkness for rest. Constant light is stressful.

Malnourishment is a major predisposing cause of RD. Exact nutrient requirements are not known for any species of reptile, but successful feeding practices are known that, if followed, can prevent nutrient disorders.[2, 3] Many privately owned reptiles are commonly fed a marginal or deficient diet.

Snakes are the easiest to feed because whole prey provides a balanced diet. Too often, herbivorous chelonians are fed only lettuce and carnivorous species are fed nothing but hamburger or beef heart. Both diets are deplorable from a nutritional standpoint.

ANATOMY AND PHYSIOLOGY

Reptiles have a simple respiratory system characterized by a short, uncomplicated nasal cavity, no functional nasal sinuses, a long trachea or paired bronchi with complete cartilaginous rings, and a sacculated lung accompanied by various types of air sacs that serve as storage depots but do not provide surfaces for oxygen exchange.[2]

The lungs of chelonians are multicompartmented and saccular (Fig. 1) and lack bronchiolar structures. The bronchi open directly into the compartments. The bronchus enters toward the dorsal surface of the lung. Oxygen exchange occurs on the reticular surface of the lung compartments. Although the mucous membrane is ciliated, drainage of exudates from the lung is inhibited by the numerous septa that allow pooling of fluids. Snakes have

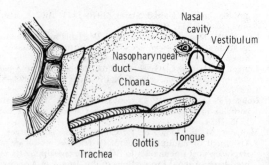

Figure 2. Diagram of a longitudinal section of the head of a tortoise illustrating the simple nasal cavity. Other reptiles have similar simple nasal cavities.

a hollow, tubular lung with a reticulated respiratory epithelial surface that continues on to become a thin, squamous epithelial-lined air sac.

Since a nasal exudate is a commonly reported sign of respiratory disease, one should understand the anatomy and physiology of the reptilian nasal area. The nasal cavity of chelonians (Fig. 2) and snakes is simple. Secretions emanating from the nose or mouth of a tortoise or snake are more likely to be mucous and serous secretions of the glandular epithelium of the mucous membranes rather than exudates, since an inflammatory response in a reptile differs from that of a mammal in that exudates tend to be more viscid. Reptiles are unable to sneeze or cough. Ciliary action is disrupted at the glottis, and there is no soft palate to provide a continuous tract for discharge from the nose. Simple mechanical drainage would dictate that liquid coming from the glottis would flow into the oral cavity and either be swallowed or exude from the mouth.

SYNDROME

Reptilian respiratory disease is usually characterized by a nasal discharge, audible breathing, and some form of dyspnea.[2] Additionally, the animal may be depressed and anorectic, experience weight loss, and have variable amounts of oral discharge. A foul odor may emanate from the nose or mouth. Aquatic species frequently lose buoyancy and are unable to float or may have a tilted posture in the water, causing them to prefer spending most of the time out of water. The presence of nasal exudate is considered a cardinal sign of pneumonia in reptiles by many lay people and some clinicians. This sign is not sufficient to support such a diagnosis. Nasal exudate in a

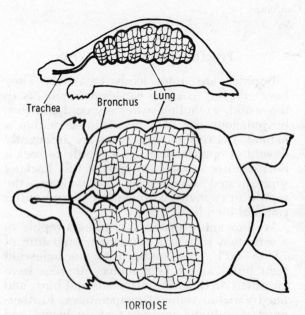

Figure 1. Diagram of the lungs of a tortoise.

Table 1. *Signs of Respiratory Disease*

	MAMMALS	BIRDS	REPTILES
Fever	+	±	?
Nasal exudate	±	±	±
Odor	±	±	±
Cough	++	+	−
Dyspnea	++	++	±
Rales	+	±	±
Pain	+	+	?
Oral exudate	±	±	±
Open-mouth breathing	±	±	±

reptile may arise from the nasal cavity, oral cavity, pharynx, glottis, trachea, bronchi, or lungs. From an anatomic and physiologic standpoint, the least likely source of the exudate would be from the lungs, bronchi, trachea, and glottis. While pneumonia is an important disease of reptiles, a nasal exudate is not likely to be the prominent sign.[2] A comparison of the signs of reptilian, mammalian, and avian respiratory diseases is found in Table 1.

DIFFERENTIAL DIAGNOSIS

None of the foregoing signs are definitive enough to assign the syndrome to a specific segment of the respiratory tract. In fact, it is difficult to do so in the living reptile. The diagnostic procedures that can be used to differentiate RD in the reptile are limited. A comparison of various aids to diagnosis in mammals, birds, and reptiles is found in Table 2.

Radiography. Radiographic techniques have been developed for examining the lungs of reptiles. Advanced pneumonia, with lung pockets of accumulated exudate, is easily diagnosed radiographically. Unfortunately, early lesions are not discernible.

Bronchoscopy. Optical examination of hollow organs and spaces has been facilitated by the use of fiberoptic instruments. Anesthetized chelonians and medium-size lizards are excellent candidates for such examinations. The fiberoptic scope cannot be inserted into the trachea of small snakes, and the trachea of larger snakes is too long for standard equipment.

Cytology. Cytology is a standard diagnostic technique of mammalian medicine. It has application in the diagnosis of reptilian pneumonia, but base-line information is lacking. More clinical experimental work must be done in this area.

Hematology. Hematology is at the same level of development as cytology.

Cultures. Cultures may be obtained by intratracheal washings or, in chelonians, by catheterization of the lung through a 2 to 4 mm hole drilled through the carapace.

In a three-year study of pneumonia in desert tortoises (*Gopherus agassizi*) the following bacteria were isolated from the trachea or lungs of healthy free-living animals: *Corynebacterium* sp., *Staphylococcus epidermidis*, *Bacillus* sp., *Streptococcus viridans*, enterococcus, *Pasteurella haemolytica* (indole-positive), and *Pasteurella ureae*.[3] The same organisms have been isolated from tortoises with pneumonia.

Table 2. *Diagnostic Methods of Respiratory Disease*

	MAMMALS	BIRDS	REPTILES
Observation	+	+	+
Auscultation	++	±	−
Percussion	+	−	−
Radiography	++	+	+
Bronchoscopy	+	−	±
Thoracocentesis	+	−	−
Hematology	+	+	±
Cytology	+	+	±
Culture	+	+	+

To date, no specific microorganism can be said to be the cause of RD in tortoises. Rather it would appear that opportunistic microorganisms invade devitalized tissue in a stressed animal. It was of some interest to note that an *Aeromonas* sp. was not isolated from tortoises but has been cultured from snakes suffering from respiratory disease.

HYPOVITAMINOSIS A

Hypovitaminosis A is most common in aquatic chelonians but may be seen in herbivorous species that are fed nothing but lettuce. The basic lesion of hypovitaminosis A is focal squamous metaplasia of respiratory and digestive tract mucous membranes. Early in the course of the disease the cilia disappear, incapacitating a prime line of defense against infectious agents. Glands are also affected by squamous metaplasia. Small epithelial glands may be totally affected, rendering them nonfunctional. The duct of a larger gland may become plugged. The resulting dryness of mucous membranes may predispose the animal to infection.

The focal distribution of the lesions of hypovitaminosis A may leave some glands unaffected. An inflammatory response incited by squamous metaplastic foci or from secondary infection may cause hypersecretion from the functioning respiratory mucous membrane, resulting in an oral or nasal discharge. The most prominent sign of hypovitaminosis A in the chelonian is swollen eyelids due to metaplasia of the orbital glands. The cornea and the epithelium of the conjunctiva may also be affected. Squamous metaplastic foci are difficult to observe in the respiratory tract of the living chelonian. However, similar lesions can be seen in the oropharynx. The lesion consists of a white plaque 2 to 6 mm in diameter.

In addition to the foregoing unique signs and lesions produced by hypovitaminosis A, all the classic signs of respiratory disease may be seen in a chelonian with uncomplicated hypovitaminosis A (Table 3).

STOMATITIS

Stomatitis, common in snakes and occasionally occurring in chelonians, may complicate the diagnosis of RD. An entirely different group of microorganisms may be isolated from oral lesions. An extension of the oral lesion into the nasal cavity may produce rhinitis, or the accumulated discharge may be forced out mechanically through the nostril.

THERAPY AND PREVENTION OF RESPIRATORY INFECTION

The fact that many reptilian respiratory infections are refractory to conventional antibiotic therapy strengthens the premise that this syndrome is a complex phenomenon, involving environmental, nutritional, mechanical, and infectious factors.

Temporary response is sometimes obtained from antibiotic therapy, but unless dietary deficiencies are overcome and other environmental stressors minimized, the condition will reappear. It is simple to inject vitamin A but more difficult to insure adequate dietary intake. Protein and energy intake and mineral balance must also be adequate. Deficiencies of any essential nutrient are devitalizing.

Alfalfa hay and dark green vegetables are excellent sources of carotenes but are only of value if eaten. Iceberg lettuce is a poor source of carotenes, calories, protein, and calcium. In short, lettuce is a poor choice of food for a tortoise.

Table 3. *A Comparison of Respiratory Disease and Hypovitaminosis A in Chelonians and Snakes*

| | CHELONIAN | | | SNAKE | | |
Condition	Nasal Discharge	Prevalence	Prognosis	Nasal Discharge	Prevalence	Prognosis
Rhinitis	+	Very common	Fair to good	+	Common	Good
Tracheobronchitis	±	Occasional	Fair	±	Rare	Fair
Pneumonia	±	Common	Poor	±	Occasional	Poor
Hypovitaminosis A	±	Common	Good if uncomplicated	±	Rare	

I routinely administer a parenteral vitamin A preparation to all reptiles suspected of having RD.* The dose is 10 international units of vitamin A per gram of total body weight.

Many antibiotic preparations are used to treat reptilian diseases. I suspect that often more harm than good is done by indiscriminate use of antibiotics in reptiles. The only definitive work on antibiotic usage in reptiles has been done by Bush and associates. (See page 647.)

Reptiles receiving antibiotic therapy, particularly with those antibiotics that have nephrotoxic propensities, should be kept well hydrated. Subcutaneous or intraperitoneal administration of physiologic saline solution may be warranted.

CONCLUSIONS

Respiratory disease is an important disease complex of reptiles. Infections do occur, but the organisms are usually opportunistic species that invade devitalized epithelial surfaces. Although a nasal discharge may be a sign of pneumonia it is more likely that the exudate originates directly from the nasal or oral cavities. The anatomy of the reptilian lung precludes easy egress of fluid from the lung. Other signs must be observed and sophisticated techniques used to arrive at a definitive diagnosis of RD.

SUPPLEMENTAL READING

1. Bush, M.: Antibiotic therapy in reptiles. In Kirk, R. (ed.): Current Veterinary Therapy VII (this volume). Philadelphia, W. B. Saunders Co., 1980.
2. Fowler, M. E.: Respiratory disease in desert tortoises. In Murphy, J. B. (ed.): Reproductive Biology of Captive Reptiles. Lawrence, Kansas, The Society for the Study of Amphibians and Reptiles, 1979.
3. Fowler, M. E.: Comparison of respiratory infection and hypovitaminosis A in desert tortoises. In Montali, R. (ed.): Comparative Pathology of Zoo Animals. Symposia of the National Zoological Park. Washington, D.C., Smithsonian Institution, 1979.
4. Frye, F. L.: Husbandry, Medicine, and Surgery in Captive Reptiles. Bonner Springs, Kansas, Veterinary Medical Publishing Co., 1973.
5. Graham-Jones, O.: Some clinical conditions affecting the North African tortoise, Testudo graeca. Veterinary Record, 73:317–320, 1961.

*Injecom (Roche Laboratories, Nutley, N.J.)

MEDICAL CARE OF AQUATIC TURTLES

W. J. ROSSKOPF, Jr., D.V.M.
Hawthorne, California

Turtles have been kept by man as pets and zoologic specimens for centuries. Their unusual appearance, quiet nature, adaptability to captive environments, and unfortunate use as dissecting specimens have made them a frequent target for human collectors.

Turtles have become popular pets in the United States. Until recently they were removed by the thousands from many of our Southern lakes, rivers, and ponds, where most originate. Current changes in the law have helped reduce chelonian exploitation, but the turtle trade still flourishes throughout the world.

As clinicians we must see that these animals receive proper care and are given the best available medical treatment. We must also fight to prevent these and other animals from becoming victims of human mismanagement.

CLINICAL PRACTICE WITH TURTLES

In practice one sees a wide variety of clients presenting aquatic turtles for treatment. They vary from beginning pet keepers to hobbyists (the latter often possessing impressive knowledge in husbandry and scientific terminology). Also seen are commercial operators, many of whom are knowledgeable and honest, but there are others who are responsible for ill-managed and overcrowded pet mills that provide thousands of sick animals to an unsuspecting public. Occasionally the clinician has the privilege of working with a zoologic director who is trained to handle turtles properly and who has their welfare in mind.

This discussion covers aquatic turtles, which we shall define as turtles that spend the majority of their time in and around water. They are to be contrasted with the land tortoises (e.g., *Gopherus agassizi*) and the terrestrial turtles (e.g., *Terrepene carolina*, *T. ornata*, and others, the so-called "box" turtles).

Examples of aquatic turtles seen in clinical practice are the eastern diamondback terrapin (*Malaclemys terrapin*), the common red-eared slider (*Chrysemys scripta elegans*), the musk turtle (*Sternotherus odoratus*), the painted turtle (*Chrysemys picta*), and the soft-shelled turtles such as *Trionyx* spp. and *Lissemys puncttata*.

Species encountered in zoologic collections are the large marine turtles such as the loggerhead (*Caretta caretta*), the Pacific Ridley (*Lepidochelys olivacea*), the green turtle (*Chelonia mydas*), and the leatherback turtle (*Dermochelys coriacea*). Also seen are snapping turtles such as the alligator snapper (*Macroclemys temminckii*), ownership of which is now illegal in many states, including California.

THE CLINICAL EXAMINATION

The initial examination is approached in the same way as an exam done on any other animal species. A complete history is necessary: Was the turtle purchased at a pet store? What were the conditions there? Was it overcrowded? Certain retail establishments always have trouble, and I try to keep a record of these. How long has the person had the turtle? What has it eaten? Has it been fed properly? Improper diet and husbandry are responsible for most of the medical problems. Subtle factors may be involved. For instance, the eastern diamondback terrapin, a frequently seen pet, requires slight salinity to maintain shell integrity. Without added salt, shell rot may develop. Certain species are particularly susceptible to parasites, wounds, diseases, and other problems. The clinician must keep these factors in mind at all times.

Only after a complete history is taken do we get to the presenting complaint, because many times the diagnosis can be made by analyzing the history alone. The physical examination then begins. I always pick the turtle up and get a feeling of its weight, then weigh it. The weight of a turtle can give an idea of the length of time a disease process has been present and help in determining prognosis. Usually the more underweight a turtle is, the poorer the outlook and the more chronic the condition. Normal "feelings" for weight come from experience. Many hobbyists are only too happy to have a veterinarian take an interest in their spe-

cies and will gladly let you handle their healthy animals.

Always look at the head and eyes. Does the skin look healthy? Are the eyes swollen? Are there signs of vitamin deficiency, wounds, parasites, and so on? Try to look in the turtle's mouth. Many pugnacious water turtles will offer to bite and can easily be scrutinized. Sometimes the mouth may be carefully pried open with forceps. Is the color good? Are there signs of mouth rot? Know what a normal turtle looks like; it should have clear eyes and be active and alert. Aquatic turtles appear to "swim" vigorously when held. The shell should be hard to the touch (except in soft-shelled turtles and the very young). If the animal is sluggish and does not react when picked up, it is usually sick. (Certain sluggish species like *Chelus fimbriata*, the mata-mata, are exceptions to this rule.)

Ask the owner if he or she has noticed any obvious clinical signs. Many times I am presented with a turtle that has not been eating but seems normal otherwise. The owner will casually mention that the turtle has been breathing with its mouth open, leading the clinician to suspect respiratory disease. Most astute hobbyists can assist the veterinarian in establishing a diagnosis because they are continually observing their charges. Sometimes the clue may be something subtle, such as an abnormal change in disposition. The practitioner should never be so self-centered that he or she will not listen to what an owner has to say.

Palpate the abdomen in front of the rear legs. Obstructions, constipation, impacted eggs, and other problems can be ascertained in this way.

Know the normal diet, habits, country of origin, habitat, physiology, and anatomy of the species with which you are dealing. Many water turtles slow down in the winter, and some eat less or not at all. There are several excellent books on normal water turtle behavior, origin and habits, (see supplemental reading list).

LABORATORY AIDS TO PROPER MEDICAL CARE

As we become more knowledgeable in the diagnosis and treatment of chelonian disease, we realize how limited the proper diagnostic procedures are. Trying to do a proper physical on a turtle is a difficult task because of its shell structure. Whenever possible, clinical ideas should be confirmed using correct laboratory procedures. Routine radiographs can outline uroliths, growths, eggs, foreign bodies (such as fishhooks), lung fields, and intestinal impaction. The slow metabolism of turtles makes them excellent subjects for radiographic study. Some reference texts that describe normal and abnormal anatomy are listed at the end of this article.

I try to perform a routine blood smear on every case possible. Clipping a nail will produce just enough blood for two slides. Our laboratory has become quite adept at estimating a white blood cell count and giving us a differential.

I do not recommend cardiac puncture on clients' animals. A hematocrit determination can easily be performed with a capillary tube. Other blood tests are available at the clinician's discretion. Using microhematocrit tubes I perform CBC, BUN, SGOT, LDH, creatinine, total protein, glucose, and uric acid tests.

Cultures and sensitivity tests are often performed, particularly in cases of persistent respiratory disease. Mouth swabs and wound cultures are routine when reasonable and necessary.

Fecal exams are performed the same way as in mammals. Many parasites can be identified in turtles and are often seen in routine blood smears. The laboratory can learn to recognize them.

Clients should be instructed to have a necropsy performed on any of their turtles that die. Many county laboratories will perform tissue sections at no charge.

TREATMENT TECHNIQUES

ENVIRONMENT

A sick turtle should be kept in a warm environment. Remember that cold-blooded animals have a metabolic rate directly proportional to the environmental temperature. Increasing the temperature to at least 26 to 32°C (80 to 90°F) will help the animal's metabolism combat the disease condition as well as provide an internal environment that is inhospitable to the pathogenic organism. Remember that many pathogens prefer a specific temperature range for proliferation. An attempt is being made to produce an environment unfavorable to the disease-causing agent. This can be done artificially with turtles by controlling and increasing the surrounding temperature. I recommend increasing the temperature at least 2 to 5°C (5 to 10°F) daily until the ideal recovery temperature of 80 to 90°F has been reached. Normal environmental temperature for healthy turtles varies with species.

One other point that is extremely important: *Do not let a sick turtle hibernate.* The body defenses are at a low ebb at this time, and the animal's condition will usually worsen. Many times in practice I have seen a turtle or tortoise that was allowed to enter hibernation with a slight "cold" either not wake up at all or progress to pneumonia or septicemia. I often tell clients not to allow a turtle or tortoise that has recently recovered from an illness to hibernate. This point can not be emphasized too much. Hibernation is not physiologically necessary in turtles and can be avoided if desired.

Many other points should be considered. A sick turtle may not be able to swim effectively and might drown, so a shallow isolation tank may be advisable. It is necessary to isolate sick turtles to prevent the spread of contagion, but some delicate, gregarious species may pine away and not eat simply because they are away from their companions. In such cases it may be advisable to provide a recovery tank next to the healthy one or to treat all the turtles prophylactically, thus leaving them together. This is always a difficult decision for the clinician and must be made individually after consultation with the owner.

Careful control of water acidity and alkalinity and of organism proliferation must be considered. Frequent water changes may be necessary in the face of disease because parasitic, bacterial, viral, and fungal pathogens can spread rapidly in an aqueous habitat. It is always a good idea to feed aquatic turtles in a feeding tank to avoid fouling the water with food particles and excrement. A good filtration and aeration system is necessary to prevent contamination.

Be sure that rocks and crawling areas are not too abrasive. Many traumatic shell rot cases could be avoided if this rule were observed. Indoor-outdoor carpeting makes an excellent padding for ponds and exercise areas.

Turtles must be given a spacious environment because they require room for health. Housing three or four five-inch red-eared sliders in a 20-gallon aquarium is inhumane.

Be sure that the turtles have a place to rest. Many can live a continuously aqueous existence, but they need to be able to climb out of the water if they so desire. I have seen many young aquatic turtles die from exhaustion and drown because they could not leave the water to rest. There should be a dry area available for them.

Water turtles need a source of ultraviolet light. Sunlight through glass is not enough. Ordinary incandescent bulbs and household fluorescent tubes are also deficient in ultraviolet light. Tubes such as Vita-Lite® are preferred for turtles and tortoises. These tubes duplicate natural sunlight very closely, including the ultraviolet portion of the spectrum. Without this aid, many water turtles may not be able to assimilate calcium because of a vitamin D deficiency, and serious problems may arise. Sunlamps can also be used but only for short periods of time (i.e., 15 minutes per day at a distance of three to five feet). Incandescent bulbs can then be left in the terrarium for heat.

In summary, it can be seen that a proper environment is an important part of turtle maintenance and rehabilitation. Know the *normal* environment for each species with which you are dealing; it varies tremendously from species to species, and a discussion such as this can only deal in generalities.

QUARANTINE MEASURES

When adding new arrivals to a collection, it is of utmost importance to isolate the animals for a minimum of two weeks to check for impending disease and abnormal behavior. Sick turtles should always be isolated.

If possible, routine blood tests and fecal examinations should be undertaken for each new arrival and appropriate treatment initiated when necessary.

Upon introduction of new animals to the established collection, observation for compatability is advisable. Pecking orders often develop, and fights and resulting wounds may occur. Certain particularly pugnacious individuals may have to be removed. Most turtles will settle into a peaceful routine once pecking order is established.

Remember that carrier states of disease can exist, and the introduction of apparently healthy animals could result in an epidemic. Avoid continual additions and constant changing of individuals once a habitat is established.

SPECIFIC TREATMENTS

The same principles apply to treating turtles as to treating other animal species. Antibiotics must be used for bacterial infections. Fluids, electrolytes, feeding solutions, ointments and vermifuges may be administered when indicated.

I find injectable treatments for most disease conditions necessary. Oral treatments are difficult to give and doses are inaccurate. Exceptions to this rule are vermifuges and solid food substitutes.

Antibiotics must be given by injection to insure proper blood levels. However, antibiotic soaks may be useful for wounds and abscesses. I instruct the client on proper injection technique for treatments that will be administered in outpatient care. Most clients are eager to learn this to save their animals, although the occasional squeamish person will object. Antibiotic injections are given subcutaneously in the loose skin along the rump or under the arms. If a particularly pugnacious species is to be injected, I try to avoid the head area. In land tortoises, the site of choice is the armpit area, after trapping the foreleg against the gular projection (see anatomy texts). The use of 25 gauge or smaller needles is recommended when possible.

Fluids such as lactated Ringer's solution, Aminoplex,®° dextrose, and Ambex,®° can be administered if care is given to alternate injection sites. Never use alcohol or other disinfectants on the skin of an aquatic species (other than on thick-skinned animals such as marine and terrestrial turtles and tortoises) because it may be absorbed, producing toxic effects.

Anesthetics can be administered intramuscularly, subcutaneously, or intraperitoneally as necessary, depending on the drug employed. I prefer ketamine hydrochloride as an anesthetic in turtles (see section on surgical conditions). Remember when calculating drug dosages that the shell size will affect the weight of a turtle. A good rule of thumb is to allow half of the turtle's weight as shell. Additional anesthetic can always be given. Injection and surgical sites in the turtle are shown in Figure 1.

I prefer Nutrical® (Evsco) as a force-feeding gel. The substance is widely available, relatively easy to administer, and high in caloric and vitamin content. Mixtures of ground-up natural food (such as whole fish) or dog or cat food with vitamins may be used, but in comparison, Nutrical is less messy and almost impossible for a turtle to expel.

When force-feeding a turtle, I try to pry the mouth open with forceps or other blunt instruments. Certain species such as land tortoises are easy to manipulate using hand and fingers only, but most aquatic species must be forced or fooled. One can try to stimulate an angry turtle to bite and then apply a mouth gag (a syringe or syringe case works well) before giving oral medication. Care must be taken not to damage or crack the beak. When force-feeding is impractical, this technique must be abandoned, and injectable amino acid solutions such as Aminoplex should be used instead.

°Professional Medical Supply, Santa Fe Springs, California

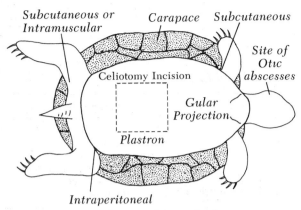

Figure 1. Ventral aspect of the turtle showing injection and surgical sites.

For administering vermifuges and sometimes for force-feeding a stomach tube is useful. I like to use a mouth gag and pass a small disposable plastic catheter that will not traumatize the turtle. The animal's head must be extended to enable smooth passing of the tube.

Frequently used drugs and topical preparations are shown in Table 1.

SPECIFIC DISEASE SYNDROMES

DIETARY DISORDERS

Most problems seen in aquatic turtles are those associated with poor feeding practices. It is imperative that any turtle kept in captivity be fed properly. As previously mentioned, the hobbyist or naturalist should thoroughly research the particular species being kept captive. Particular care must be taken to provide a diet with proper mineral balance.

All of the common water species are carnivorous. Some of them are omnivorous but all rely on animal protein for sustenance. The red-eared slider (*Chrysemys scripta elegans*), for example, feeds mainly on insects, fish, tadpoles, and dead animals. When these turtles eat, they consume the whole of their prey, not simply the meat. Balance of body calcium, minerals, and vitamins is achieved by consuming skin, fur, bone, intestinal contents, and dirt. This fact, however, is repugnant to many pet owners, who prefer to think of their pets as being better off with a "cleaner" diet. Uninformed hobbyists assume that a meat-eating animal can thrive on "clean" meats such as hamburger, beef heart, and boned and cleaned fish. While satisfying for the owner, this diet can kill the turtle. Such a diet has little calcium and so much phosphorus (1:44 ratio) that a state of nutritional hyperpara-thyroidism develops. Before long, the turtle weakens and succumbs to disease. The younger ones never develop properly and the familiar "soft shell" (hypocalcemia) syndrome appears. If the animal can be saved by injecting calcium and vitamins and correcting the diet, it usually becomes grotesquely deformed and stunted.

Other deficiency diseases are well documented. Prolonged vitamin A deficiency produces squamous metaplasia of the orbital gland, eyelid, and cornea, leading to ocular disease and swelling. Prolonged vitamin E deficiency produces steatitis, a classic oxidation of fat that produces yellow nodules throughout the adipose tissue. Many other deficiency syndromes are possible. Usually there is a combination of all of these.

My recommendations for feeding carnivorous water species are simple. First, thoroughly research the species, its natural environment, water conditions, and food sources. Try to duplicate the natural diet. Live guppies and goldfish (watch carefully for diseased feeder fish) are an excellent food source. Supplement this with dry, good-quality dog or cat food. A fish-based cat food is often very appealing to water turtles. The client may have to work with the turtles to help them adapt to this diet, but the effort is well spent. Vegetation can be added for omnivores. A calcium-mineral block kept in the aquarium or pond is always a good idea. Turtles can be fed in a separate feeding tank and afterwards returned to their living quarters, thus reducing the mess and avoiding contamination.

If turtles are fed properly, most problems can be prevented. I would estimate that at least 80 per cent of the medical problems are induced by poor nutrition.

Treatment of dietary disorders should be performed symptomatically. Injectable calcium and vitamins, and antibiotics to prevent concurrent infection, are indicated. Once the symptoms are alleviated, keeping the turtles on a proper maintenance diet usually insures good health. As previously mentioned, many will be permanently deformed.

RESPIRATORY INFECTIONS

Respiratory infections are common in turtles. Many of these are brought on by lowered resistance, stress, and improper diet or surroundings. Respiratory disease in chelonians is described in detail on pages 633 to 637 of this volume.

Occasionally surgical draining of the ears may be indicated and followup with antibiotic solutions and gels appropriate.

Table 1.   *Drugs Most Frequently Used in Turtles*°

GENERIC AND TRADE NAMES	ROUTE	FREQUENCY	SUGGESTED DOSAGE
Antibiotics			
Ampicillin trihydrate (Polyflex®, Bristol)	s.c.	s.i.d. or b.i.d.	6 mg/kg
Chloramphenicol (Mychel-S®, Rachelle Labs)	s.c.	s.i.d. b.i.d.	10–15 mg/kg in divided doses if necessary
Gentamicin sulfate† (Gentocin®, Schering)	s.c.	Every two days	10 mg/kg
Oxytetracycline hydrochloride‡ (Liquamycin®, Pfizer)	s.c. i.m.	s.i.d.	6–10 mg/kg
Penicillin§ injectable (many brands)	s.c.	s.i.d.	10,000 U/kg
Streptomycin injectable (many brands)	s.c.	s.i.d.	6 mg/kg
Vitamins and Minerals			
Vitamins A, D, and E Injectable‖ (Injacom 100®, Roche)	s.c.	Twice weekly	5,000–50,000 U
Vitamin B complex (many brands)	s.c.	Daily if necessary	0.5 cc/kg
Calphosan® (Carlton)	s.c.	Daily if necessary	1–50 mg
Steroids			
Dexamethasone (Azium®, Schering)	s.c. i.m.	Only when required, i.e., for shock	0.06–0.15 mg/kg
Fluid and Electrolyte Solutions			
Amino acid solutions such as Aminoplex®, Ambex®, etc.	s.c.	Daily or as needed	1 cc/kg
Dextrose, Ringer's®, lactated Ringer's®, etc.	s.c. i.p.	Daily or as needed to combat dehydration	Up to 10 cc/kg
Vermifuges			
Niclosamide (Yomesan®, Chemagro)	Oral	Once—repeat if necessary in one month	150 mg/kg
Piperazine citrate (many brands)	Oral	Two doses at two-week intervals	40–60 mg/kg
Thiabendazole¶ (Omnizole®, Equizole®; Merck)	Oral	Weekly if necessary	50 mg/kg
Ointments, Solutions, and Powders			
Panalog® (Squibb)			
Optisone® (Evsco)			
Betadine® (Purdue-Frederick)			
Chloromycetin® (Parke-Davis)			
Terramycin® (Pfizer)			
Gentocin® (Schering)			
Furacin® (Eaton)			
Kymar® (Burns)			
Various iodine and sulfa powders			

°Use actual weight of turtle divided by two to calculate dosage.
†Monitor kidney and liver function and force fluids if necessary.
‡May produce local irritation
§Occasional anaphylactic-type reactions
‖Overdosage can be toxic
¶Add equal amount of water to prevent expansion in stomach and intestines

SEPTICEMIC CONDITIONS

Many turtles presented for examination are lethargic and anorectic and have other non-specific symptoms. The owner may complain that the turtle is not as "responsive" or that it isolates itself from the others. A great many such animals are undergoing generalized infections caused by a variety of different bacteria. Again, the clinician must be aware of the normal habits of the species involved, since some turtles may slow down at certain times of the year (for example, during hibernation and egg-laying, when in season, and others). In cases like this I usually rely on a leukocyte count with a differential count to aid in diagnosis.

For simplicity, I group these diseases together as septicemias; many organisms can cause them. They may be a result of stress associated with lowered resistance due to improper diet or of puncture wounds leading to blood poisoning (fish bones and fishhooks are common causes), fight wounds (many water turtles such as the soft-shelled varieties are extremely pugnacious), contaminated water (warm water rapidly grows and spreads bacteria), consumption of unhealthy live food (particularly sick goldfish), or a combination of these. The result is that an infectious organism is introduced into the turtle's blood stream that overwhelms the animal and leads to involvement of the internal body tissues. The liver, attempting to filter out this organism, may in turn be overcome and damaged. For this reason, many necropsied turtles show signs of heptatitis. Most of these findings are actually secondary to septicemic conditions.

Treatment consists of the administration of antibiotics, fluids, force-feeding, and supportive care. My antibiotic of choice is ampicillin (Poly-flex,® Bristol), 100 mg/ml, which is bactericidal and well tolerated by the animal. The bactericidal nature of this drug is extremely important to a weakened animal. Prognosis depends on the organism, the duration of its presence, and the turtle's ability to fight disease. I usually monitor the course and response to treatment by blood count and may change antibiotics several times in stubborn cases. I try to continue antibiotics for several treatments after a cure has been achieved in order to prevent relapse.

BODY LUMPS AND SWELLINGS

Quite frequently the clinician will be presented with a turtle exhibiting one or more lumps or swellings. These can represent a variety of conditions. Swellings involving the ears are often abscesses from otitis secondary to respiratory infection and must be lanced. Various benign and malignant tumors, cysts, calluses, parasite cysts, abscesses, blood clots, and granulomas are also common. The only way to differentiate these swellings is by aspiration lancing, biopsy, or radiography. Treatment varies with the cause. The common abscess must be thoroughly cleaned and ointment applied by pack or gel. Abscesses can be cored out in stages to allow for localization and to minimize bleeding. In turtles abscess exudates are usually caseous. I often lance and curette an abscess, dispense antibiotics to allow localization, and finish the job a week later when the core can be removed more easily. Systemic antibiotics are often needed to prevent spreading of infection and resulting septicemia. Tumors may be surgically excised.

OCULAR DISORDERS

Eye disease frequently occurs secondary to generalized infection, but primary eye disease is also seen. Vitamin A deficiency can lower the resistance of the ocular membranes, paving the way for generalized infection of the surrounding tissue of the eye. Vitamin A deficiency can, by itself, cause swelling of the conjunctival tissue and swollen eyes but, as before mentioned, these problems are usually multiple in nature and often involve secondary infection and other deficiencies. Pure vitamin A deficiency in clinical practice is rare in my experience, but does occur. If bilaterally swollen eyes are present, I would suspect generalized debility and systemic disease, and would attempt to correct poor feeding practices and alleviate vitamin deficiencies as well as treat for systemic infection. Rarely does simple ocular therapy prove effective, although I do use ophthalmic ointments along with systemic treatment in most cases. Turtles may have to be force-fed or given injectable feedings until their eyes open. They rarely eat if they cannot see, although I have observed several exceptions to this rule.

MOUTH ROT (NECROTIC OR ULCERATIVE STOMATITIS)

This term is used for a variety of conditions, traumatic or infectious, seen in tortoises, turtles, snakes, and lizards. It is rarely seen in water turtles but may be the result of trauma or systemic disease. It is sometimes seen as a complication in respiratory infections. Injectable antibiotics, antibiotic ointments, hydrogen peroxide washings, and supportive therapy are used to treat mouth rot. The clinician should always consider the underlying causes of mouth rot in water turtles.

SHELL ROT (ULCERATIVE SHELL DISEASE, USD)

Shell rot is a term used for infections present in the shell that may have started from a trauma or as a specific disease. Shell rot can progress rapidly to septicemia, but usually limits itself to the outer skin and bone of the shell as a chronic condition. Most cases begin when the shell membrane is broken on rocks or other sharp objects.

In 1975 Wallach described a specific form of highly infectious shell rot caused by the gram-negative bacillus *Beneckea chitinovora*. This organism is a common pathogen in free-ranging shellfish and has been reported in crayfish, lobsters, shrimp, and various crabs. As a result of this discovery, it has been recommended that turtle keepers avoid feeding crayfish, shrimp, or shrimp meal to turtles and that they not house living crustaceans with turtles.

Treatment of shell rot includes careful isolation of affected individuals, improvement of tank conditions by such means as providing space and eliminating sharp rocks, curettage of active lesions and cauterization with iodine preparations, and administration of antibiotics such as ampicillin or chloramphenicol when necessary. Topical applications of appropriate antibiotics (culture and sensitivity testing may be advisable), antibiotic soaks, or treatment by allowing the antibiotic solutions to dry on the turtle, repeated several times a day may be necessary. Certain turtles (e.g., the eastern diamondback terrapin *Malaclemys terrapin*) require brackish water to promote shell integrity. Certain bottom-dwelling species such as the mata-mata (*Chelys fimbriatus*) may require special attention to prevent shell rot.

IMPACTIONS

From time to time the clinician is presented with a turtle that is not eating, is lethargic, and may be straining to defecate. Palpation anterior to the hind legs under the carapace will reveal hard swellings. A radiograph will elucidate large masses of gravel, sand, or other material impacted in the intestines. Surgery may be indicated, but often enemas and lubricants such as mineral oil will alleviate the problem. Antibiotics and supportive therapy are needed if secondary infection or intestinal damage is present.

No one knows why some turtles become "rock eaters," but needless to say they should not be fed in or around sand or gravel. This condition must be differentiated from egg binding.

EGG BINDING AND OBSTETRICS

Egg binding occurs occasionally in all female turtles and is diagnosed by clinical signs and radiographs. The turtle is usually presented in distress or may simply not pass her eggs (uterine inertia). If uterine inertia is the problem, I administer calcium (Calphosan®), 1 ml/kg, and oxytocin injections, 0.04 ml/kg, to stimulate passage of the egg. The egg may have to be repelled and repositioned. Radiography is a significant aid to this technique. Mineral oil applied in the cloaca and oviduct will often assist passage and "delivery" of the egg.

If the egg is too large to pass, it can occasionally be broken and removed by forceps (a very difficult task considering that the shell limits manipulation) or removed surgically through the shell (caesarian section). Some turtles will hold their eggs until the next laying season with no apparent problems (through hibernation).

WOUNDS

Wounds resulting from trauma, fighting, disease, and other causes are common. Pet dogs, for example, often delight in gnawing on turtles. Treatment consists of cleansing with hydrogen peroxide, application of iodine, and the use of antibiotic injections and ointments. Shell wounds may require reconstruction with epoxy resin.

Turtles may have to be kept out of water (except for daily soaking to prevent dehydration and for eating) to facilitate healing. Water turtles are slow to heal because of the aquatic environment but otherwise do respond well. Healing time is decreased by increasing the surrounding temperature.

PARASITIC CONDITIONS

A wide variety of internal and external parasites are encountered. Fecal examinations for all new arrivals are advisable. One should scrutinize the skin of all new animals for any external parasites.

Protozoa. Amebiasis caused by *Entamoeba invadens* has been seen in turtles. Intestinal damage due to tissue destruction may result in diarrhea, dehydration, septicemia, and death. The organism may invade the blood stream and lodge in various internal organs (e.g., the liver). Treatments most commonly prescribed are emetine hydrochloride (Eli Lilly) at a dosage of 0.5 mg/kg daily for ten days and metronidazole (Flagyl,® Searle), 50 mg/kg, daily for one week. The oral tetracyclines have also been used.

Routine blood films will reveal a variety of

blood-borne protozoa such as the hemogregarines, trypanosomes, malarial parasites (*Plasmodium* sp.), and others. The significance of these parasites is unknown at this time but may be elucidated as further research is undertaken. In the face of overwhelming parasitemia, chloroquine (Aralen®) treatment should be considered. Aralen dose is as follows: 10 mg base/kg first day, then 5 mg base/kg every other day for three treatments. Course may have to be repeated two weeks later.

External Parasites. Leeches are common external parasites of aquatic turtles. They can act as the intermediate hosts for blood-borne parasites such as the hemogregarines. Leeches should be removed by topical applications of alcohol or salt solutions so as to cause release of their hold and avoid damaging the turtle's skin or leaving imbedded mouth parts. Care should be exercised to avoid contaminating an environment with these parasites.

Ticks are commonly seen on newly caught turtles. They often burrow into the skin of the neck, the corners of the mouth or eye, and the base of the tail. They may appear as brown or black spots and may be quite noticeable during a close inspection of the turtle. As with leeches, care must be taken to remove the tick properly. A thick application of mineral oil, cod liver oil, or Vaseline will aid in removal of these parasites by suffocating them, causing release of their hold on the skin. After all the ticks have been removed, apply an antibiotic ointment to each sore spot and allow it to dry prior to placing the turtle in water. Watch carefully for any signs of local infection.

Myiasis is commonly seen in terrestrial turtles. Flies will lay eggs that quickly hatch on turtle wounds, with resultant tissue destruction. This is not common in water turtles but may occur if the turtle is being kept out of water. One should always protect injured turtles from flies and subsequent maggot infestation. Occasionally water turtles may be seen with bot fly myiasis (larvae of *Cuterebra*, *Sarcophaga*, and other flesh flies). This is more commonly a condition of terrestrial turtles such as box turtles. The larvae should be expelled and a suitable antibiotic cream applied to the resulting cavity.

Nematode Parasites. A wide variety of roundworms occur in water turtles. These will spread rapidly in the unnatural situation of crowding in aquariums and ponds. Nematode parasites are easily diagnosed by fecal examination, and many of them resemble mammalian roundworms such as *Strongylus*.

Careful attention must be paid to cleanliness to prevent the spread of these ubiquitous parasites. Most are passed by direct life cycle and do not require an intermediate host. For that reason they can spread rapidly and can quickly overwhelm a collection of water turtles. Treatment of choice is either thiabendazole or piperazine. Treatment should be repeated periodically until all fecal examinations are negative. I like to use thiabendazole (50 mg/kg) weekly for at least three treatments. Thiabendazole (Omnizole,® Merck) should be diluted at least half-and-half with water to prevent expansion in volume and should be administered by stomach tube. One should monitor success by periodic fecal examination.

Cestode Parasites. Cestode parasites are occasionally seen in turtles. Their life cycles are poorly understood. These parasites respond to treatment with niclosamide (Yomesan,® Chemagro), 150 mg/kg, repeated after one month.

Trematode Parasites. Fluke eggs are rarely seen in exotic turtle feces. These infestations appear to be transient and asymptomatic, and I have not attempted treatment. It is hoped that further research will elucidate their life cycles, but one can speculate about possible snail, tadpole, or other intermediate hosts.

Acanthocephala. Marcus, in *Current Veterinary Therapy* V and VI, has quite adequately described these parasites. Thorny-headed worms may be visible in the small intestines of aquatic turtles that have become infected by consuming specific snail, insect, or other intermediate hosts. Nodular granulomas of the intestinal wall with intestinal perforation have been described. The eggs resemble thorny-headed worms found in swine (thick-shelled oval, and containing rostellar hooklets). Treatment at this time has not been effectively developed. Preventive measures such as cleanliness and isolation must be stressed. Larval forms have been described in the abdomen or subcutis of terrestrial turtles. These larvae may be seen on necropsy and their clinical significance is minor.

NEUROLOGIC CONDITIONS

A variety of neurologic problems are common in turtles. Encephalitis can be the result of septicemia or trauma. Spinal cord inflammation is sometimes responsible for rear leg paralysis. This is usually a bacterial meningitis resulting from generalized infection, but I have seen cases of apparent primary spinal cord involvement. These cases may respond to injections of antibiotics (I prefer ampicillin), B vitamins, and steroids. As in most bacterial infections, care must be taken to avoid relapse by continuing antibiotics after clinical symptoms have disappeared. I monitor these cases with white blood cell counts. Varying degrees of partial paralysis may remain, and the nervous system may take two to three months or more to regenerate.

Traumatic nerve damage is common in the larger species. I frequently see turtles with signs of partial or complete paralysis after being dropped. The weight of the body is concentrated at the edge of the shell, which may crush a limb or the neck on impact. Treatment is symptomatic and consists of anti-inflammatory drugs and B-vitamin complex injections. Sometimes a limb can be rested by being taped to the shell.

Encephalitis may develop from trauma (e.g., puncture wounds) or from the spread of infection from the ear.

ORTHOPEDIC PROBLEMS

Broken limbs occur particularly in those turtles that have borderline calcium balance. A variety of techniques may be employed in repair. Bandaging techniques, intramedullary pins, bone plates, and sometimes no treatment at all are used.

Occasionally amputation of a limb is necessary. Many such patients adapt well but may have to be protected and fed and housed separately because of problems of competition with other turtles.

SKIN DISEASES

Skin disease is usually the result of generalized weakness. Wounds, contaminated water, vitamin deficiency, fungal and bacterial pathogens, and combinations of these are the common causes. So-called "fungus" is for the most part bacterial in nature. Treatment involves correcting any predisposing factors and providing appropriate antibiotics and supportive therapy.

A specific cutaneous disease, septicemic cutaneous ulcerative disease (SCUD), has been described by Frye as being characterized by cutaneous ulceration, anorexia, lethargy, and paralysis advancing to internal necrosis (e.g., of the liver). He describes the etiologic agent as *Citrobacter freundii* and suggests Chloromycetin® injections for treatment along with local applications of Betadine.®

SALMONELLOSIS

A report on medical care in turtles is not complete without some mention of salmonella infection. Before the laws were made more stringent, it was common practice to import baby turtles from the southern United States as pets. These animals were frequently housed in human waste ponds prior to shipping. As a result, many times they were contaminated with various strains of *Salmonella* spp. and *Arizona* spp. Turtles, being for the most part asymptomatic carriers, would then spread these enteric organisms to children and hobbyists.

Our laws now ban importation of turtles smaller than four inches and require testing of the water for salmonellosis. However, outbreaks of enteric diseases are still possible, and it behooves all veterinarians to instruct clients about this danger and to do cultures if possible to detect carrier animals.

SURGERY

From time to time, surgery must be performed on turtles. This may consist simply of lancing an abscess or trimming a beak or nail or may be very technical internal surgery. Sometimes an egg-bound turtle must be relieved, an impaction corrected, or a foreign body removed. One classic case was the removal of an ingested fishhook from a red-eared slider through celiotomy.

The anesthetic of choice for aquatic turtles is ketamine hydrochloride (Ketaset,® Bristol, or Vetalar,® Parke-Davis) given at the rate of 22 to 44 mg/kg (10 to 20 mg/lb). The shell weight has been accounted for in this dosage. Care must be taken to allow for dehydration and debility when using ketamine. It should always be remembered that additional anesthesia can be administered at 30-minute intervals if necessary. Attempts should be made to prepare a turtle for surgery by giving antibiotics, amino acids, or fluids, if time will permit, prior to administering the anesthetic. While on this drug, the turtle's respiratory rate will be severely depressed and the heart will slow considerably. Introduction time (15 to 60 minutes) varies with the species and environmental temperature and lasts 2 to 10 hours. I have always used the subcutaneous route of administration. Anesthesia can also be introduced by halothane chamber but may be more difficult to regulate.

Surgical technique is relatively simple. A small power saw (120 volt, 1.1 amp, 28,000 rpm motor) is used to open the plastron (lower shell). Once through the shell, the surgery is remarkably like that done on mammalian species. After suturing the pleuroperitoneum (no diaphragm is present), acrylic resin is used to cover the flap incision. (Many brands of epoxy resin are available). The turtle can heal and resume its life in the water without experiencing internal contamination. Acrylic resin is also used to repair broken or damaged shells, to solidify or reconstruct injured beaks, and to fill in scars.

Other common surgical procedures are cloacal or rectal prolapse repair (purse-string technique), amputation or replacement of prolapsed genital organs (e.g., for paraphimosis), and suturing of wounds.

TOXICOLOGY

From time to time turtles are presented suffering from symptoms of chemical poisoning. It is imperative that hobbyists exercise caution when using chemical sprays around turtles. These cases are treated symptomatically and proper supportive care is instituted.

EUTHANASIA

Occasionally one sees a turtle that is beyond repair, either medically or surgically. It is amazing how long a fatally damaged turtle can live without eating. Many of these can survive for months and should be euthanized if there is obviously no hope for recovery. Intraperitoneal barbiturates are preferred.

SUMMARY

There are many medical problems associated with the keeping of turtles in captive environ-ments. The most important point to remember is that a well-housed, well-fed turtle will rarely have problems. Incorrect management by humans usually leads to trouble. If we are to keep these animals as pets or for scientific study or display, we must do our best to maintain their health and prevent their exploitation for selfish interests.

SUPPLEMENTAL READING

Ashley, L. M.: *Laboratory Anatomy of the Turtle.* Booth Laboratory Anatomy Series. Dubuque, Iowa, Wm. C. Brown Co., 1970.
Burke, T. J. (ed.): Reptiles. *In* Fowler, M. E. (ed.): *Zoo and Wild Animal Medicine.* Philadelphia, W. B. Saunders Co., 1978, pp. 89–150.
Carr, A.: *So Excellent A Fishe: A Natural History of Sea Turtles.* Garden City, N.Y., Natural History Press (Doubleday), 1973.
Frye, F. L.: *Husbandry, Medicine and Surgery in Captive Reptiles.* Bonner Springs, Kansas, V. M. Publishing, 1973.
Jacobson, E.: Disease of the respiratory system in reptiles. Vet. Med. Small Anim. Clin. 73:1169–1175, 1978.
Marcus, L. C.: Parasitic diseases of captive reptiles. *In* Kirk, R. W. (ed.): *Current Veterinary Therapy VI.* Philadelphia, W. B. Saunders Co., 1977, pp. 801–806.
Nicol, E. B.: Personal communications, 1978.
Nicholls, R. E.: *Turtles.* Philadelphia, Running Press, 1977.
Northrup, G. A.: Personal communications, 1978.
Pritchard, P. C.: *Living Turtles of the World.* Neptune City, N.J. T. F. H. Publications, 1967.
Rosskopf, W. J.: *Tortuga Gazette.* California Turtle and Tortoise Club articles, 1972 to present.
Rosskopf, W. J.: *Turtles Magazine.* Articles on medical care of turtles. Pueblo, Colo., Quest Publications, 1978 to present.
Wallach, J. D.: Medical care of reptiles. J. Am. Vet. Med. Assoc., 155:1017–1034, 1969.
Wallach, J. D.: The pathogenesis and etiology of ulcerative shell disease in turtles. J. Zoo Anim. Med., 6:11, 1975.

ANTIBIOTIC THERAPY IN REPTILES

MITCHELL BUSH, D.V.M.
Washington, D.C.

Many medical problems of reptiles can be controlled by following an appropriate preventative medical program, including strict monitoring during quarantine periods, followed by proper management, housing, and feeding procedures upon release to a permanent collection. Since the early diagnosis and treatment of ill reptiles is often difficult due to their abilities to mask overt signs of disease, the primary aim of reptilian medicine is to prevent medical problems. The early detection of illness requires an increased awareness of the individual reptile's activities and the development and refinement of diagnostic techniques.

The most frequently encountered bacterial infections in reptiles are infectious stomatitis (mouth rot), pneumonia, and septicemia caused by gram-negative organisms (e.g., *Aeromonas* sp., *Pseudomonas* sp., and *Klebsiella* sp.), which are resistant to many antibiotics. Gentamicin*

---

*Gentocin, Schering Corp., Bloomfield, NJ

and chloramphenicol† are two broad-spectrum antibiotics with good *in vitro* activity against most of these organisms, and consequently they are the drugs of choice.

Once an infectious process is diagnosed and antibiotic therapy is indicated, another clinical question arises. What dosage of antibiotic should be given and at what interval? With many of the newer broad-spectrum antibiotics, organ toxicity is often encountered when high blood levels of the drugs are reached. For example, gentamicin will cause a dose-related nephrotoxicity in reptiles, resulting in secondary gout. Through sequential kidney biopsies, renal damage has been observed in normal snakes given mammalian doses of this drug at mammalian schedules (4.4 mg/kg/24 hr). Such renal damage could be potentiated in ill snakes because of dehydration and impaired renal blood flow.

The rational use of any antibiotic first requires basic information on the pharmacokinetics of that drug in the various reptilian species. The metabolism of an antibiotic is dependent on the patient's metabolic rate, which is related, in reptiles, to environmental temperature. This further complicates pharmacokinetic studies, since variations in environmental temperature may alter the dosage and treatment schedules appropriate for an individual. Basic studies have begun on the antibiotic gentamicin in snakes and turtles and on chloramphenicol in snakes, which have provided starting points for further study and serve as guidelines for the formulation of dosages in other species.

In normal bullsnakes (*Pituophis melanoleucus*) kept at 24° C, the average half-life of gentamicin is 82 hours. In normal turtles, western painted (*Chrysemys picta bellii*) and red-eared pond sliders (*Chrysemys scripta elegans*) kept at 26° C, the average half-life is 32 hours following gentamicin administration. The half-life in these reptiles seems prolonged when compared with a 2½-hour half-life of gentamicin in mammals (Fig. 1). The half-life of chloramphenicol at 24° C, following subcutaneous injection, is 5.2 hours in bullsnakes, compared with 1½ to 3 hours in mammals. The half-life of gentamicin in bullsnakes is about 33 times that of mammals, whereas the half-life of chloramphenicol in bullsnakes is only twice that of mammals. This indicates that the pharmacokinetics of each individual drug must be determined, since errors would occur if information on gentamicin were to be extrapolated to chloramphenicol, or vice versa.

†Chloromycetin Sodium Succinate, Parke-Davis, Detroit, MI

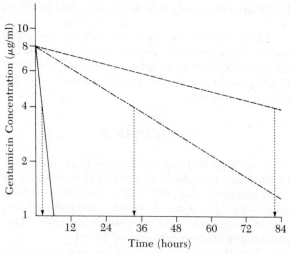

Figure 1. Comparison of gentamicin plasma concentrations in three species following the administration of doses sufficient to provide initial levels of 8 µg/ml. Humans are represented by the solid line, red-eared turtles by the dot-dashed line, and bullsnakes by the interrupted line. Note the logarithmic coordinates on the ordinate (*y*) axis. Arrows indicate the plasma half-life of gentamicin for each species.

Utilizing these half-lives, the following dosage rates and treatment schedules were developed. For gentamicin in bullsnakes at 24° C, 2.5 mg/kg every 72 hours is the recommended treatment regimen; for turtles at 26° C, 10 mg/kg/48 hr is suggested. The total body weight of the turtles is used in calculating doses. In establishing these recommendations, it was assumed that therapeutically effective blood levels in reptiles are comparable to those in man. It was assumed that if a certain antibiotic level is therapeutically adequate in man, the level will also be effective against reptilian pathogenic bacteria. These dosage and treatment schedules did not produce blood levels considered nephrotoxic, and renal damage was not observed in treated snakes that were monitored by sequential kidney biopsies and tests of uric acid levels.

When administering an antibiotic to a snake, the subcutaneous route is used. Prior to injection, the needle is advanced subcutaneously for 1 to 2 cm to minimize seepage from the injection site. Injections in turtles are given either subcutaneously or intramuscularly. When dose volumes of less than 0.1 ml are indicated, microliter syringes‡ should be used to insure accurate dosing.

In ill snakes, gentamicin is administered for 3 to 6 treatments or for 9 to 18 days. If the snake is dehydrated, subcutaneous or intracoelomic fluids may be indicated. Lactated Ringer's solution or normal saline plus 5% dextrose may be used at a rate of 10 to 15 ml/kg to insure ade-

‡Hamilton Co., Reno, NV

quate kidney function and to minimize the risks of nephrotoxicity. Monitoring of gentamicin blood levels in sick snakes treated with this regimen has shown no potentially toxic accumulation of the drug, and good clinical response has been observed.

For treatment of turtles, gentamicin is administered for 6 to 14 days in most clinical infections. It has not been necessary to give systemic fluids in conjunction with the antibiotic therapy.

For gentamicin therapy in the desert tortoise (*Gopherus* sp.) the dosage and treatment schedules for snakes should be followed, using total body weights. The use of systemic fluids to insure kidney function may be indicated. These

desert tortoises should not receive the same treatment regimens as aquatic turtles.

The administration of subcutaneous chloramphenicol in bullsnakes at 40 mg/kg every 24 hours produced and maintained adequate blood levels (as compared with mammalian levels) of the drug. The length of therapy may range from 5 to 14 days, depending on the clinical situation and the response to therapy.

These recommendations may appear limited, because specific reptiles at specific environmental temperatures have been discussed, but they are intended to be guidelines until more precise information on the pharmacokinetics of various antibiotics in reptiles can be determined.

AVIAN RADIOGRAPHIC TECHNIQUE AND INTERPRETATION

SAM SILVERMAN, D.V.M.
San Francisco, California

Radiography is a routine diagnostic procedure performed on the majority of avian patients presented to our practice with a history of trauma, internal disease, or non-specific signs such as depression. Radiography often provides information regarding the organ system involved as well as the classification of the pathologic process, i.e., traumatic or infectious. This information is necessary to formulate a diagnosis and treatment regimen. It is not uncommon to base a diagnosis primarily on radiographic changes when the clinical signs are nonspecific. Although hematology and serum chemistry analyses are being utilized more frequently in avian medicine, radiography has remained a most valuable diagnostic technique because of the availability of rapid interpretation and the ability to perform it on patients of all sizes. Sample size is not a limiting factor in radiography.

NORMAL ANATOMY

Birds are well suited for radiographic evaluation because their air sacs provide negative contrast for the abdominal and thoracic structures.

The small size of the patient makes whole-body surveys practical.

The thoracic and abdominal cavities are continuous because of the absence of a diaphragm in birds. The lungs are located in the dorsal portion of the thoracic cavity. They are best evaluated on the lateral radiographic projection and appear as a honeycombed structure. The majority of the lucent (air-filled) structures are tertiary bronchioles viewed on end in the lateral projection. The walls of the bronchioles are normally well defined and distinct on this view. In some of the smaller birds (parakeet size or smaller) it may not be possible to identify individual bronchioles distinctly. On the ventral-dorsal view the bronchioles appear as transverse, indistinct linear structures. Although the bronchioles are not as well visualized on this view, the ventral-dorsal radiographic study is needed so that laterality of lung disease can be identified.

The air sacs are identified as lucent areas in the thoracic and abdominal regions. On the ventral-dorsal view the abdominal air sacs are noted lateral to the viscera in the caudal abdomen. The right abdominal air sac usually extends somewhat caudal to the left one, both of them terminating just lateral to the cloaca. The walls of the air sacs are usually not identified. The clavicular air sacs are variably identified in the region of the shoulder joints on the ventral-dorsal views. On the lateral view the thoracic air sacs are identified as lucent areas ventral to the lungs.

The crop, a diverticulum of the esophagus, is located in the region of the thoracic inlet. It is normally distended with ingesta. The size of this structure varies with species, and in some species it is absent.

The proventriculus is the straight tubular portion of the digestive tract located between the esophagus and the ventriculus (gizzard). The proventriculus serves as a storage organ in the raptors and some of the seabirds. It can therefore vary greatly in size, depending on the volume of its contents. The proventriculus can be identified on the lateral projection in the caudal portion of the thoracic cavity and the anterior portion of the abdominal cavity, traversing toward the ventriculus. Occasionally the proventriculus may contain radiodense grit.

The ventriculus is round or oblong in shape and can easily be identified by the radiodense grit it usually contains. Not all species of birds have grit in their digestive tracts. The gizzard is identified in these species as a rounded soft-tissue density just caudal to the proventriculus. It is usually somewhat denser than the remainder of the intestinal tract. The normal location of this organ is at the level of the acetabula, slightly to the left of the midline, and two-thirds or three-fourths of the distance from the spine to the sternum. The ventriculus is mobile, and therefore its location is affected by abdominal mass lesions.

The intestines occupy the caudal portion of the abdomen. The cloaca can occasionally be identified as an air-filled round structure.

The dorsal portion of the mid- and posterior abdominal regions is occupied by the kidneys, adrenals, and gonads. The anterior poles of the kidneys protrude ventrally from the pelvic bones and can therefore be identified, whereas the major portion of the kidneys is embedded in the pelvic skeleton and so is not clearly defined radiographically. The spleen is a small, rounded soft-tissue density usually identified in the midabdominal region dorsal to the ventriculus and usually overlying the dorsal portion of the proventriculus on the lateral view. It is difficult to identify the spleen on the ventral-dorsal view unless it is severely enlarged. The spleen is an important organ to identify in cases of suspected psittacosis. It is usually not larger than 0.8 cm in normal birds the size of Amazon green parrots.

EQUIPMENT

X-ray equipment for avain radiography should be capable of producing at least 80 kvp at 100 ma, with exposure times of 1/60th of a second or faster. Ideally 200 ma is a practical minimum capacity. If the output of the machine is less than this it may be necessary to decrease the focal film distance to compensate for the decreased output of the x-ray generator. Exposure times of 1/60th of a second or faster help negate the artifacts produced by patient motion, including respiratory movements and muscle fasciculations.

Both screen film with ultradetail intensifying screens and non-screen films are used. Selection of the film type depends upon the size of the patient, the detail required to define the lesion, and the capabilities of the x-ray unit.

RESTRAINT AND POSITIONING

Most examinations of birds smaller than cockatiel size can be accomplished without sedation. The larger or more fractious psittacine patients can be sedated with ketamine hydrochloride (Vetalar, Parke-Davis) at a dose of 0.05 mg/gm of body weight intramuscularly. No adverse effects have been seen at this dosage. Adequate immobilization of adequate duration is produced, and the patient is usually ambulatory within 45 minutes.

The patient is restrained with masking tape on a plastic sheet (Plexiglas, Rohm & Haas, Philadelphia, Pa.). A sheet 1/8 × 30 × 30 inches is adequate for most birds. The plastic sheet and the masking tape are relatively radiolucent. Masking tape is preferred to other forms of adhesive tape because it is more radiolucent, is less traumatic to the skin and feathers, and can be removed more readily.

In most examinations, tape is applied at the distal portion of the wings, the tarsometatarsal regions, and the anterior cervical region. If the patient is not sedated, a piece of tape also is applied across the body. The tape should not be applied in a way that will compromise the patient's respiratory movements. Expansion of the thoracic and abdominal walls is necessary for respiration in birds.

The lateral radiograph is obtained by placing the patient in lateral recumbency and extending the wings and legs away from the body (Fig. 1). The dependent extremities are positioned anterior to the contralateral extremity. The de-

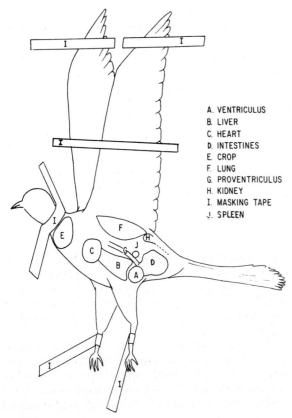

A. VENTRICULUS
B. LIVER
C. HEART
D. INTESTINES
E. CROP
F. LUNG
G. PROVENTRICULUS
H. KIDNEY
I. MASKING TAPE
J. SPLEEN

Figure 1. Positioning technique for lateral radiograph. Masking tape is used to restrain the patient. The location of some of the internal organs is indicated.

pendent side and the anteriorly positioned extremities are marked with an appropriate right or left lead marker. Full extension of the extremities will preclude their superimposition on the abdominal and thoracic organs.

The ventral-dorsal projection is most informative if the wings and legs are fully and symmetrically extended (Fig. 2). Patient rotation can be minimized by positioning the sternum parallel to the spine.

The x-ray cassette is placed under the plastic sheet after the patient is restrained and positioned. The film can be replaced easily without repositioning the patient. This is advantageous if multiple exposures are required. The patient can be taped directly to the x-ray cassette if the plastic sheet is not used.

The stress associated with radiographic examination can be minimized by the administration of supportive treatment to the patient before, during, and after the examination. A heat lamp often is focused on the patient during the study. Upon completion of the examination, the patient is placed in an incubator, where the temperature, humidity, and oxygen level can be regulated.

EXPOSURE TECHNIQUES

Table 1 lists some of the exposure factors for the species of birds commonly encountered in our practice. Standardization of the exposure factors and processing are of the utmost importance in order to obtain comparable followup radiographs. Very slight exposure variations can produce marked alterations of the radiographic image when radiographing birds. For this reason, an aluminum step-wedge is often included in the study to allow rapid comparison of the exposure techniques. This is especially important in skeletal surveys for conditions such as metabolic bone disease. The exposure will be

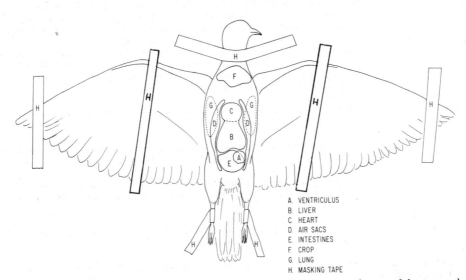

A. VENTRICULUS
B. LIVER
C. HEART
D. AIR SACS
E. INTESTINES
F. CROP
G. LUNG
H. MASKING TAPE

Figure 2. Positioning technique for ventrodorsal body radiograph. The location of some of the internal organs is indicated.

Table 1. *Avian Radiographic Techniques*

PATIENT	FILM TYPE	MA.	KVP	EXPOSURE TIME (second)	FOCAL FILM DISTANCE (inches)
Canary	Nonscreen°	100	70	1/60	30
Parakeet	Nonscreen°	100	72	1/60	27
Parrot	Nonscreen°	100	70	1/60	21
Red tail hawk	Screen†	200	70–78	1/60	40
Pigeon	Screen†	200	66	1/60	40
Macaw	Screen†	200	72	1/60	40
Parakeet	Screen†	200	58	1/60	40

°Kodak NS54T (Eastman Kodak Co.). Patient restrained on cassette.
†Cronex 6 (E. I. DuPont & Co.) with ultradetail intensifying screens.

slightly greater when acrylic sheets are used to restrain the patient.

INTERPRETATION

Basic radiographic changes such as alteration of density, size, shape, and contour are indices of pathology in the avaian as well as the mammalian species. The radiologist must be familiar with normal and abnormal radiographic anatomy in order to obtain the maximum amount of information from radiographic studies. The establishment of a cross-referenced filing system keyed to species and pathologic process is also of value. Radiographic changes seen in some of the more common avian diseases are listed in Table 2.

The ventriculus is the most sensitive indicator organ for the detection of abdominal masses. Since it is quite easily identified and mobile, certain patterns of ventricular displacement are useful in diagnosing the origin of an abdominal

Table 2. *Pathologic Radiographic Changes in Birds*

PATHOLOGIC CONDITION	RADIOGRAPHIC CHANGES
Psittacosis	Splenomegaly. The spleen will be larger than 0.8 cm in parrot-sized birds and 0.5 cm in birds the size of a cockateil. Air sacculitis and focal pulmonary consolidation are sometimes also seen. The caudal abdominal air sacs are the most sensitive area to observe for these changes.
Pyogranulomas	Well-circumscribed abscesses can be identified as focal discrete increased densities within the lung parenchyma of air sacs. Occasionally they are also seen as smooth protrusions from the contour of the liver or other internal organs.
Hepatomegaly	Ventral-dorsal projection: Liver wider and larger than normal, with possible compression of the air sacs. Possible caudal displacement of the gizzard. Lateral projection: Liver enlarged with gizzard displaced caudally and slightly dorsally. Abdomen less lucent than normal.
Air sacculitis	Increased density of air sacs, varying from very slight increased opacity to complete consolidation.
Pneumonia	Walls of the bronchioles thickened, decreased lucency of bronchioles, possible complete obliteration of the "honeycombing effect."
Peritonitis	Increased homogenous density of abdominal and thoracic activities. Distention of the caudal abdomen. Possible anterior displacement of the gizzard and/or intestines.
Gonadal or renal tumor or cyst	Increased density in the dorsal pelvic region. Ventral displacement of the gizzard and intestines. Possible free abdominal fluid.
Calcium, vitamin D deficiency or calcium-phosphorus imbalance	Decreased bone density and cortical thickness. Pathologic fractures.

mass suggested by the presence of increased abdominal density. Caudal and ventral displacement of the ventriculus suggest cranial abdominal and thoracic mass lesions such as liver tumors. Occasionally the liver will displace the gizzard dorsally if the ventral portion of the liver is involved with a mass lesion. Dorsal abdominal masses displace the gizzard ventrally; if the mass lesion is located in the left dorsal abdomen some right-sided displacement of the gizzard is also apparent. Caudal abdominal masses, e.g., in the intestines or uterus, displace the gizzard craniad.

Special procedures are infrequently performed on the avian species; however, barium sulfate is occasionally administered orally to evaluate the possibility of intestinal mass lesions or obstruction. One-half ml is adequate for parakeets; larger birds (e.g., macaws) will require as much as 8 to 10 ml. The sequence of

taking radiographs varies with the transit time of the contrast medium through the digestive tract; however, it is recommended that lateral survey radiographs be performed until the contrast material reaches the area of interest, and then ventral-dorsal views should be taken as well. I have found it best to take films immediately after the contrast medium is given and then every half hour for a total of two hours.

SUPPLEMENTAL READING

Lafeber, T. J.: Treatment of hepatopathies in budgerigars. Animal Hosp., 3:191–193, 1967.
Lafeber, T. J.: Radiography in the caged bird clinic. Animal Hosp., 4:41–48, 1968.
Morgan, J. P., Silverman, S., and Zontine, W. J.: Techniques of Veterinary Radiography. Davis, Calif., Vet. Rad. Assn., 1975, pp. 255–268.
Silverman, S.: Avian radiographic techniques. In Ticer, J. W. (ed.): Radiographic Techniques in Small Animal Practice. Philadelphia, W. B. Saunders Co., 1975.

ANESTHESIA OF CAGED BIRDS

CHARLES J. SEDGWICK

Davis, California

Few successful avian operations performed in zoos or exotic animal practices are of long duration. One reason for this is that the response of birds to anesthesia differs from that of mammals and is more difficult to monitor. Surgical procedures that can be performed quickly are routinely done because they may be achieved using short-term anesthesia. Discrete tumors are removed, limbs are amputated, long bone fractures are fixed with intramedullary rods, wounds are sutured, and indurated pus is curetted from sinuses and air sacs. Eggs lodged in the cloaca can be removed using surgical anesthesia lasting less than 1 hour. The experienced bird surgeon is familiar with the problem of having too little time to complete a procedure before difficulties with anesthesia arise. An anesthetized bird may become apneic and require resuscitation during one phase of anesthesia and a few moments later may require additional anesthetic to remain recumbent.

NARCOSIS AND ITS PARADOXIC SIGNS

Lightly anesthetized birds have been characterized as being in a state of narcosis, or drug-induced deep sleep, from which they may be aroused. The problem for the anesthetist is that the bird in this state often profoundly resembles a mammal in deep surgical anesthesia. There may be complete muscular relaxation and slow respiration. The eyelids may be closed and the feathers relaxed. Unfortunately, the bird may accept a surgical scrub and draping, and a skin incision may be completed, when suddenly the animal displays unequivocal signs of being unsuitably anesthetized for surgery. It throws itself about on the table with flopping wings and neck. The eyelids suddenly open and it may vocalize. More anesthetic is given, the animal relaxes, and the surgical preparation is repeated, but this time respiration ceases abruptly and resuscitative maneuvers must quickly be started.

Authors try in vain to characterize subtle signs of changing anesthetic depth in birds from very light anesthesia or narcosis to deep surgical anesthesia, but such descriptions are unconvincing in the operating room.

INJECTABLE ANESTHETICS

The general problems with injectable anesthetics in birds are similar to those in mammals, but they are augmented when it is necessary to administer agents intramuscularly or intraperitoneally rather than intravenously. Induction time is greatly prolonged, and any endeavor to titrate the anesthetic depth to a prescribed endpoint is difficult, particularly when it is necessary to deal with a variety of species that have differing emotional characteristics.

Ketamine hydrochloride (Vetalar®, Parke-Davis) by intramuscular injection is a very useful anesthetic in birds. Most birds respond favorably to this dissociative anesthetic, although comparable doses do not produce equivalent levels of anesthesia in all species. Small caged birds generally do well with a dose of 5 to 25 mg/kg, but pigeons may require four to six times this amount. Parakeets and lovebirds receive 1 mg/30 grams. As in mammals, ketamine increases blood pressure slightly in therapeutic dosages. Very high dosages may reduce blood pressure. Following 5 mg/kg of xylazine hydrochloride (Rompun®, Haver-Lockhart*), 10 to 20 mg/kg of ketamine may be administered to most larger species of birds to provide 20 to 30 minutes of excellent surgical anesthesia. However, this combination can result in hypotension, and if it causes profound depression the animal should be administered intravenous Ringer's solution, mechanical ventilation should be started, and surgical procedures should be suspended. Ketamine is an excellent anesthetic to facilitate minor surgical procedures or endotracheal intubation for administration of inhalation anesthesia, in most birds.

INHALATION ANESTHESIA

Many inhalation anesthetics are commonly administered to birds by means of a face cone. Highly volatile agents such as halothane (Fluothane®, Ayerst†) should never be administered by closed face cone because of the possibility of delivering lethally high concentrations of anesthetic. Most gases inhaled by birds do not initially cross the respiratory gaseous ex-

change surface but pass first to the posterior thoracic and abdominal air sacs. Too-high concentrations of inhalant anesthetic delivered to the bird's larynx will therefore be transferred to the animal's posterior air sacs before the anesthetic effect begins to occur. Respiratory gaseous exchange in birds takes place on expiration, when the posterior air sacs discharge gas into the respiratory capillaries (airways). If this gas is laden with very high concentrations of inhalant anesthetic, very deep anesthesia accompanied by respiratory arrest is likely to occur as an acute effect. If respiratory arrest occurs before the concentrated inhalant is flushed from the posterior air sacs, the bird will die unless given mechanical ventilation with oxygen.

Because it has very low volatility and does not produce lethal concentrations of vapors at normal room temperatures, methoxyflurane (Metofane®, Pitman Moore‡) may be administered by face cone for short periods of anesthesia. However, it is essential for the patient to receive adequate oxygen. An animal that is forced to breathe into a volume dead space devoid of adequate oxygen is potentially as endangered as one breathing too high a concentration of inhalant anesthetic.

Endotracheal intubation is not difficult to perform in larger birds. Many animals can be intubated during manual restraint. However, if such manipulations cause great excitement, it is better to give a basal anesthetic such as ketamine. The laryngeal structures are quite mobile in most birds and because of the elastic tissues may be manipulated from outside the throat to a position in the back of the mouth where adequate visualization and cannulation with an endotracheal tube can be accomplished. Noncuffed tubes such as infant Cole or Magill intranasal endotracheal tubes should be used. The avian trachea is very fragile, and an inflated cuff can easily damage delicate tissues.

Certain members of the order Anseriformes (swans) have a trachea that divides completely into two bronchi from the back of the laryngeal orifice. Members of the order Psittaciformes (parakeets and parrots) are often difficult to intubate because of the awkward position of the laryngeal orifice at the base of a very thick, heavy tongue. It is necessary to adapt endotracheal tubes to special problems such as these. An endotracheally intubated bird is an excellent subject for volatile anesthesia. However, a precision vaporizer should be used with any highly volatile anesthetic such as halothane.

---

*Haver-Lockhart and Co., Kansas City, Mo. 64100
†Ayerst, New York, N.Y. 10017

‡Pitman Moore, Washington Crossing, N.J. 08560

INTERMITTENT POSITIVE-PRESSURE VENTILATION (IPPV)

Surgical technology for birds can progress little if suitable anesthesia cannot be provided for all potential needs. Anesthetics that limit operative time to an hour or less also limit progress in surgical technique. It is feasible to anesthetize birds and maintain them with excellent inhalation anesthesia for periods of four hours or more. This can be accomplished by using IPPV in conjunction with inhalation anesthetics (anesthesia ventilation) such as halothane administered by precision vaporizers. The intact air sacs of the bird will accept inspiratory peak positive pressures of 12 to 24 cm H_2O. The posterior air sacs are ventilated with positive pressure on inspiration, and their elastic recoil in turn ventilates the animal's respiratory gaseous exchange membranes in the pulmonary capillaries on expiration. This supportive maneuver may be accomplished even with specimens having penetrating wounds from the outside into the air sacs. Ventilation anesthetic machines are commercially available,§ or the anesthetist may utilize a modified Ayres T-piece attached to a rebreathing bag fitted with an adjustable bleed valve. The bleed valve is adjusted so that the bag will remain partially inflated while the anesthetist intermittently compresses the bag, producing IPPV.

Depth of anesthesia during anesthetic ventilation is best monitored with an ECG electronic oscilloscope. It is possible to provide anesthesia for birds that is no less appropriate for any potential surgical procedure than that provided mammals. The additional knowledge regarding avian anatomy and respiratory physiology and the equipment needed to provide suitable avian anesthesia are readily available.

Table 1 lists some anesthetic, analgesic, and neuroleptic agents for use in birds.

----

§Bird Corporation — 3M Co., Palm Springs, Calif. 92262

Table 1.   Anesthetics, Analgesics, and Neuroleptics for Birds

GENERIC AND TRADE NAMES	ACTIONS, DOSAGES, INDICATIONS	PRECAUTIONS
Oral		
Sodium pentobarbital (Nembutal ®, Abbott)	As in mammals, this is a poor analgesic except in high dosage. Parakeets: 2 mg in 0.25 ml water given orally. May repeat in 15 minutes.	Have oxygen available. Slow recovery with struggling is frequent. Have quiet recovery site with *heat* available.
Reserpine°	Used to tame falcons and calm nervous game birds on breeding farms. Give falcon 2 mg/kg first day, 1 mg/kg second day in meat.	Tranquilization lasts 5 to 6 days, and birds may require force-feeding. Birds may vomit after first dose.
Phenothiazines	Cause convulsions in many birds.	Do not use as sole agent.
Injectable		
Ketamine hydrochloride (intramuscular) (Vetalar, Parke-Davis)	Pigeons: 25 mg/kg gives more than 15 minutes of anesthesia; 200 mg/kg gives 2 hours. Parakeet: 1 to 2 mg/30 gm Small birds in general: 5 to 25 mg/kg Large ratites: 3 mg/kg	May not produce a state of anesthesia in certain species, but can be supplemented by other anesthetic agents. Increases blood pressure in low dosages; reduces it in very high doses or in combination with other agents.
Sodium pentobarbital, 60 mg/ml, dilute standard solution 10 times with saline (Nembutal, Abbott)	Intravenous dosage may vary from 16 to 60 mg/kg; small birds, 16 to 20 mg/kg. Intramuscularly, used in solutions in strengths of 0.5 to 7.5 mg/ml at dosage of 7.5 to 50 mg/kg.	With oral use of this drug, analgesia is not satisfactory except at high dosages. Hypotensive in high doses.
Inhalation		
Ether	Induction is usually by face cone.	Concentrations are difficult to control by cone.
Methoxyflurane (Metofane)	Induction is slow when used by itself.	Much easier anesthetic to control in a face mask. Very soluble compound.
Halothane (Fluothane, Ayerst)	Highly volatile anesthetic. Induction is rapid, 0.5 to 1.5%	Should not be used in cone.

°Ciba, Summit, N.J. 07901

SUPPLEMENTAL READING

King, A.S., and McLelland, J.: *Outlines of Avian Anatomy.* New York, Macmillan Co., 1975, pp. 43–64.

Sanford, J.: Avian anesthesia, *In* Soma, R. (ed.): *Textbook of Veteri-* *nary Anesthesia,* Baltimore, Williams & Wilkins, 1971, pp. 359–368.

Sedgwick, C.J.: Veterinary anesthesia ventilation. Mod. Vet. Practice, *60*:120–126, 1979.

Sturkie, P.D.: *Avian Physiology,* 3rd ed. New York, Springer-Verlag, 1976, pp. 122–145.

OTOSCOPE TECHNIQUE FOR SEXING BIRDS

KATHRYN A. INGRAM, D.V.M.

Phoenix, Arizona

Many species of birds have no external characteristics that can be used to determine their sex. Practitioners may be asked to aid owners in determining the sex of their birds for breeding, sale, or exchange purposes. The surgical technique described here uses simple, inexpensive equipment already in use in most small animal practices. The otoscope has been used to determine the sex of hundreds of individuals of many species, including psittacines, cranes, finches, and raptors. Slight modifications adapt the technique to other diagnostic purposes, such as gross examination of other organs, biopsy of abnormal tissue, and culture of abdominal air sacs.

The bird to be examined is weighed, and ketamine hydrochloride is administered intramuscularly at a dose of 0.03 to 0.04 mg/gm body weight.

Since most female birds have only one ovary, on the left side, the bird must be positioned in right lateral recumbency so that the left side may be examined. This position is maintained on insulating material or a heating pad by manual restraint applied by an assistant or by restraint devices such as cords or rubber bands. The left wing is extended craniodorsally, and the left leg is extended posteriorly. The feathers are plucked from a small area cranial to the thigh muscles and the area is prepared with a suitable surgical preparation.

A skin incision is made dorsoventrally over the last intercostal space. In some species the sartorius muscle has to be dissected free and retracted posteriorly to expose the last intercostal space. The intercostal muscles are incised with a scalpel blade to enter the posterior thoracic air sac, and the opening is enlarged by blunt dissection to allow entry of an otoscope speculum sterilized by autoclave. A standard Welch Alyn otoscope with light and magnifying lens provides adequate visualization.

Various sizes of specula can be used, depending on the size of the bird and the purpose of the laparotomy. The ribs are flexible and will spread to accommodate a surprisingly large instrument, even in a small finch. The speculum should be of a type that can be steam-sterilized.

In all except very small birds the membrane separating the posterior thoracic and abdominal air sacs interferes with visualization of the gonad, which lies dorsal to the membrane in the abdominal air sac.

The membrane can be punctured with a needle and the puncture hole enlarged by blunt dissection to allow penetration by the otoscope speculum. Dorsal to this membrane an ovary or testis is seen at the cranial pole of the kidney, adjacent to the adrenal gland and caudal to the lung.

The incision can be closed with absorbable suture material. In many species of birds the incision can be left unsutured if the thigh muscles in their normal position lie between the skin incision and the intercostal incision. Subcutaneous emphysema originating from the posterior thoracic air sac can be a side effect of unsutured intercostal wounds.

Recovery from ketamine anesthesia is enhanced if the birds are allowed to recover in a warm environment, i.e., 27 to 32° C.

If this surgical procedure is performed carefully, risk is minimal and accuracy of sex determination is 100 percent for mature, healthy birds.

SUPPLEMENTAL READING

Ingram, K.A.: Laparotomy technique for sex determination of Psittacine birds. J. Am. Vet. Med. Assoc. *173*:1244–1246, 1978.

Riser, A.C.: A technique for performing laparotomy on small birds. The Condor, 73:376–379, 1971.

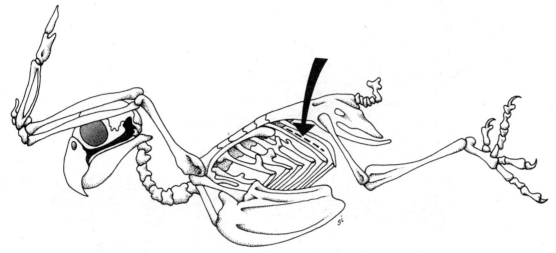

Figure 1. Incision site between last two ribs (*arrow*).

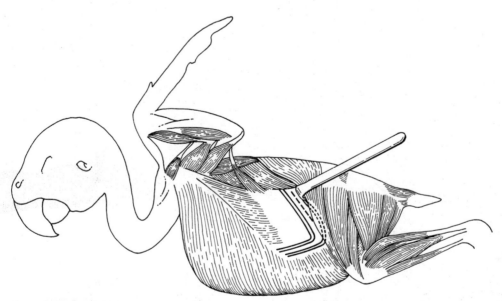

Figure 2. Posterior retraction of sartorius muscle to expose incision site.

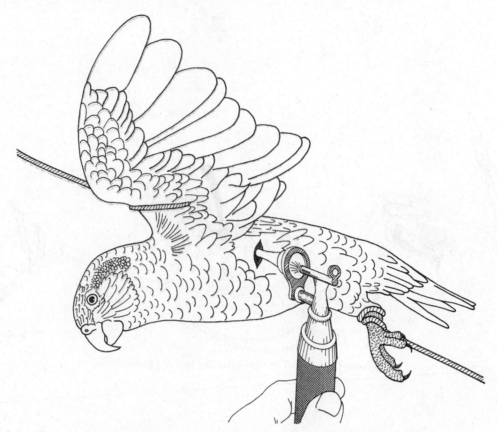

Figure 3. Otoscope in position to view gonad.

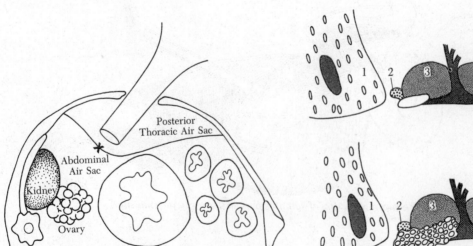

Figure 4. Transverse section of a bird's abdomen showing the air sac membrane that must be punctured at the X to allow visualization of the gonad with a speculum.

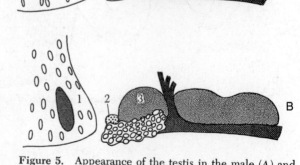

Figure 5. Appearance of the testis in the male (*A*) and of the ovary in the female (*B*) and adjacent landmarks: (*1*) lung, (*2*) adrenal gland, (*3*) kidney.

DIAGNOSTIC LAPAROSCOPY
IN BIRDS

WILLIAM C. SATTERFIELD, D.V.M.
Boston, Massachusetts

INTRODUCTION

The reasons for determining the sex of avian species are mostly those concerned with husbandry and reproduction. With the world population of all wild animals rapidly decreasing, the need to foster captive propagation programs has become paramount. This is especially true of slow-breeding avian species that lack sexual dimorphism. Laparoscopy has become an invaluable conservation and husbandry technique, as well as a diagnostic tool. Laparoscopy in addition offers a convenient method for repeated evaluation of the developing sexual condition of individuals.

SEXING TECHNIQUES

Manual vent sexing remains one of the most useful and rapid techniques for sexing newly hatched waterfowl and poultry. Most aviculturists effectively utilize this easy-to-learn method. There are many species, however, for which this technique is not effective. In such cases, aviculturists are left with the limited option of pairing birds "naturally." Unfortunately, later they are frequently found to have been paired with a member of the same sex.

Modification of the caponizing procedure has been used in various ways to allow for direct visualization of the gonads via laparotomy. It is an effective technique but is time-consuming in exotic species, is not suited to smaller specimens, and has not gained wide acceptance because of its seemingly radical nature.

Two non-invasive techniques include sex chromosomal determination and sex determination by fecal steroid analysis. Both procedures involve a unique laboratory and are time-consuming. The obvious advantage of these techniques is that they constitute virtually no risk to the bird.

MEDICAL APPLICATION OF THE RIGID ENDOSCOPE

Rigid endoscopes have been utilized only relatively recently to allow the surgeon to look into spaces in the body without gross surgical invasion of the space. This has provided a more thorough diagnostic technique that has in some cases prevented unnecessary surgical exploration. Additionally, the technique allows for specific sampling techniques not possible by any other method.

AVIAN DIAGNOSTICS

In addition to its use in the visual determination of sex in avian species, endoscopy is a versatile diagnostic tool. The gonads may be evaluated for physiologic condition by noting size, follicular development, and vascular perfusion. These data may be correlated with behavioral patterns and may be indicative of a positive response to environmental, nutritional, and husbandry techniques. Air sacs and the posterior surface of the lungs may be examined for infection or lesions. Samples may be taken for bacteriologic culture or histopathologic study. Other organs, such as the kidney, adrenal, spleen, intestines, and liver, may be rapidly evaluated visually. Much information that has previously been available only via major surgery may now be obtained in a short time.

EQUIPMENT

The combination of a unique optical material and specialized human endoscopic requirements culminated in the development of the miniaturized instrument called the Needlescope.° The instrument used routinely in avian endoscopy is 2.2 mm in diameter (14 gauge); however, it is also available in 1.7 mm (16 gauge) and 4.0 mm diameters. A 30-power magnification microscope system in the 1.7 and 2.2 diameter instruments enlarges the final viewing image. The system has the ability to form sharp images from a 1 mm focal distance to infinity. The Needlescope lens system has an internal light guide that provides illumination of the viewing area. A 6-foot flexible fiberoptic light guide brings light to the instrument from a tungsten-halogen light source. The source is

---

*Dyonics, Inc., 71 Pine Street, Woburn, Massachusetts 01801

659

provided with a brightness control with a maximum color intensity of 3500°K. Sterilization of the equipment is most conveniently accomplished either by gas sterilization (ethylene oxide) or by cold sterilization for 20 minutes in Cidex solution,† although some components may be steam-sterilized. Cidex has routinely been used satisfactorily and without adverse effects.

TECHNIQUE

For most species only one assistant is required to restrain the bird manually in right lateral recumbency by holding the wings together over the back and extending the legs slightly posteriorly (Fig. 1). When anesthesia is indicated, as it may be in certain species (i.e., psittacines), two assistants are utilized, one for positioning the bird and the other to monitor anesthesia and restrain the head if needed.

A small skin area in the subiliac area is prepared aseptically. The landmarks for locating the optimum area for introducing the cannula are the last rib, the ilium, and the proximal half of the shaft of the femur (Fig. 2). A stab incision is carefully made through the skin and muscle fascia. An attempt is made to penetrate between the sartorius and iliotibialis muscles, but the sartorius is often penetrated in the more

---

†Arbrook, Inc., Arlington, Texas 76010

muscular species with no subsequent lameness observed.

The cannula and sharp trocar are directed perpendicular to the median axis of the bird and are rotated to enter the peritoneum. Although full penetration is essential, care should be taken to prevent entering the abdomen with excessive force.

The cannula and trocar are then directed forward and dorsally toward the anterior pole of the kidney. The trocar is removed and the Needlescope is inserted in the cannula. If properly placed, the tip will be inside the abdominal air sac. If placement is in the more lateral caudal air sac then the trocar may be used to enter the abdominal air sac. The gonad may be observed and evaluated and other organs examined. For birds weighing less than 100 grams, the scope can be inserted alone through the stab incision to reduce the diameter of the entry wound.

If no complications are encountered the procedure can be completed in about one minute. The cannula is withdrawn and a topical antibiotic power is placed on the puncture wound.

COMPLICATIONS

The most frequently encountered problem is obstruction of the viewing tip of the scope. Since a small amount of blood on the lens will prohibit viewing, the procedure must be as bloodless as possible. Should minute amounts

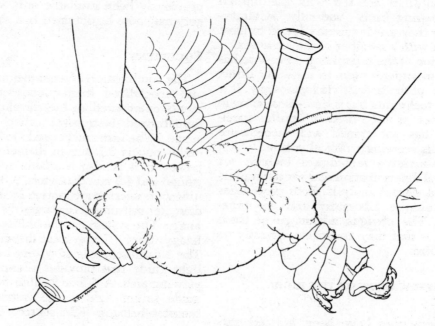

Figure 1. Positioning is accomplished by holding the wings together over the bird's back and extending its legs slightly posteriorly.

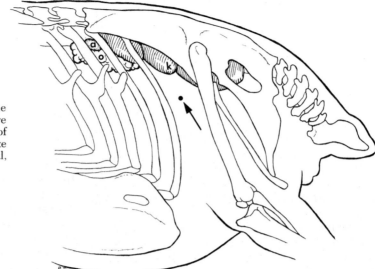

Figure 2. The landmarks for locating the optimum area for introducing the cannula are the last rib, the ilium, and the proximal half of the shaft of the femur. The approximate site is marked by the arrow and dot. *a* = adrenal, *o* = gonad, and *k* = kidney.

of blood be encountered, the tip should be touched to an intra-abdominal organ. If this fails, withdraw the tip and wipe it off with a sterile alcohol sponge, then reinsert. In the presence of significant bleeding, the cannula is withdrawn and the procedure is rescheduled. With experience and care, bleeding is not a problem in most birds. Only a single fatality due to bleeding has been experienced, and this was caused by penetration of the internal iliac vein. Other problems that prevent adequate viewing are air sacculitis, fat, and tachypnea.

PHOTOGRAPHIC TECHNIQUE

Photography is possible through all endoscopes; the limiting factor is the amount of light focused on the object to be photographed. The best illumination for photographic purposes is a "daylight" intensity light at 500 K color temperature with adjustable intensity. The more recently introduced high-speed Kodachrome ASA 400 has provided the best photographic results with good color saturation. Photographs can be taken at 1/30 to 1/15 of a second with little distortion from motion.

Adapters for the attachment of Nikkon and Minolta SLR cameras to the endoscope are available (Storz, Dyonics, Wolf). It is important to have a clear viewing screen instead of a ground-glass screen for optimum light conservation.

CONCLUSION

Laparoscopy is one of the major recent advances in avian medicine and husbandry. Its main advantages are the direct observation of the gonads and visualization and sampling of the gonads and abdominal organs via a relatively non-traumatic procedure. Used as an adjunct to other techniques, it will provide a useful tool for the management and conservation of avian species in captivity.

SUPPLEMENTAL READING

Bush, M., Wildt, D.E., Kennedy, S., and Seager, S.W.J.: Laparoscopy in zoological medicine. JAVMA, *173*:1081–1087, 1978.

Czekala, N.M., and Lasley, B.L.: A technical note of sex determination in monomorphic birds using faecal steroid analysis. Inter. Zoo Yearbook, *17*:209–211, 1977.

Harrison, G.J.: Endoscopic examination of avian gonadal tissue. Vet. Med. Small Anim. Clin., 73:479–484, 1978.

McIlwaith, C.W., and Fessler, J.F.: Arthroscopy in the diagnosis of equine joint disease. JAVMA, *172*:263–268, 1978.

Satterfield, W.C., and Altman, R.B.: Avian sex determination by endoscopy. Proc. Am. Assoc. Zoo Veterinarians, 1977, pp. 45–48.

Siemering, G.H.: Arthroscopy of dogs. JAVMA, *172*:575–577, 1978.

AVIAN ORTHOPEDICS

JAMES C. ROUSH, II, D.V.M.
Santa Cruz, California

There are four categories of birds presented to the veterinary practitioner for treatment of orthopedic disorders: cage and aviary birds, backyard poultry, "working" or performance birds, and wild birds presented for rehabilitation.

The people responsible for these various categories relate to their birds in different ways and for different purposes; therefore the treatment of orthopedic disease must be tailored to the individual patient's expected function. Obviously, a broken wing is more serious in a racing pigeon or a hunting falcon than it is in a laying hen or a bird confined to a cage. Larger psittacine birds are expected by many of their owners to fly and perform acrobatics. Wild birds must be able to function nearly perfectly in order to survive.

For these reasons it has become necessary for the veterinary profession to search for adequate methods for dealing with avian orthopedic disease. The chief aim is to return the injured part to full function as early as possible.

A bird's wing is one of Nature's most precisely engineered appendages, being both strong and lightweight and able to withstand millions of cycles of strenuous activity without breakdown. When injured it must undergo very precise repair if it is to function adequately. The legs are less important than the wings for most species, except for raptors, which depend upon their talons for apprehending prey animals. Raptors therefore need more attention to leg injuries than many other birds.

CATEGORIES OF AVIAN ORTHOPEDIC DISEASE

With a few exceptions, musculoskeletal disorders in birds fall within three categories: traumatic injuries, the most frequently encountered problem; growth disorders, which can develop in young birds; and metabolic or infectious problems, which we occasionally encounter. Most of this section will deal with trauma, but some comments about the non-traumatic syndromes are in order.

GROWTH DISORDERS

Growth disorders in young birds are most frequently associated with nutritional deficiency: calcium, phosphorus, vitamin D_3, and manganese imbalances. Perosis (slipped tendon at the tarsus) in poultry has been associated with a manganese deficiency, and it seems reasonable that other bird species could develop this syndrome. A lack of calcium or an excess of phosphorus can result in hyperparathyroidism with subsequent bone decalcification. These bones can bend or develop folding fractures. (This condition is essentially a very severe form of rickets.) Calcium deficiency can be due to a low calcium diet or to a deficiency of vitamin D_3, which results in calcium not being absorbed from the gut. Vitamin D_2 is not well utilized by birds. They can synthesize their own supply of vitamin D_3 if they are exposed to a few hours of sunlight a day; otherwise, a dietary source of D_3 is necessary. Birds of prey that are fed organ meats — heart, kidney, and liver — exclusively can develop the same disease from an excess of phosphorus. A calcium-to-phosphorus ratio of 1½ to 1 or 2 to 1 is ideal. It has been stated that, in very young birds, exposure to cold can cause muscle contractures that can bend or break their bones.

These growth disorders can be prevented easily, but the deformities are very difficult if not impossible to correct. Crooked legs can sometimes be helped with a traction apparatus if some bone growth is still taking place. I am not aware of a good traction apparatus for the wing. It is very difficult to attach anything to a growing bird's wingtip.

INFECTIONS

Birds can present with gout-induced arthritis, septic polyarthritis, tuberculosis in bones and joints, bacterial abscesses and a variety of other disorders outside the scope of this discussion. However, the principles of treating these diseases are essentially the same as for mammals. One relatively common and potentially limb-threatening infection is bumblefoot, an abscessation occurring in the ball of the foot. It is seen in all species but is especially common in birds of prey. Falcons, particularly the peregrine, are the most susceptible. In all species unsanitary surroundings are a predisposing factor. In raptors, foot injuries from improper perching substrates or self-inflicted punctures from overgrown talons can also be causes. Bumblefoot is much easier to prevent than to cure. Many cases end up as osteomyelitis of the bones of the foot and are at that point incurable. As with any disease that does not respond well, a variety of treatments have been developed. A mixture of 250 ml dimethylsulfoxide, 50 mg dexamethasone, and 1000 mg chloramphenicol sodium succinate, applied to the foot three or more times a day, is a favorite of many practitioners. I recommend applying external heat by means of hot soaks, heating wires placed under the perch, a hair dryer, or other device. This should be done three or more times a day. Systemic antibiotics may be useful. X-ray therapy has been attempted experimentally with variable results. In advanced cases without any radiographically evident osteomyelitis, it may help to open and debride the abscess cavity, attempting primary closure. Success using this technique is more the exception than the rule.

TRAUMA

Trauma to the musculoskeletal system usually results in fractures and dislocations. However, it must be remembered that injuries may also occur to muscles, tendons, nerves, and the integument (skin and feathers). The importance of the feathers is sometimes misunderstood, A functional wing is impossible without them, and the author has seen some very well-done bone and joint operations become completely nullified when the doctor plucked or cut the flight feathers. Pulling the flight feathers can damage the feather-forming organ within the follicle and result in twisted, frazzled, or deformed feathers. Cutting the flight feathers is hazardous for two reasons. First, most large birds molt once a year, so it may take a year for the patient to regain its flying ability. More important, flight feathers are molted one at a time, and a growing feather depends upon the support of its neighboring feathers for protection during the growing phase. A new feather with a pulpy shaft, sticking out of the wing without protection, is extremely susceptible to trauma. These birds molt old feather stubs, and one by one break off the new feathers as they grow. Then it will be yet another year before that bird gets a chance to regain its wing function.

Growing feathers require a rich blood supply, and a vascular injury to a portion of the wing (usually the tip) can result in permanent loss of the flight feathers.

Muscles heal very readily because of their blood supply. Tendons usually must be sutured, whether they are ruptured, cut, or avulsed from their attachments. Tendon repair will be discussed later in this section.

NON-OPERATIVE ORTHOPEDICS

Casts, splints, and slings can be very effective methods of treating certain disorders. The avian leg is anatomically similar to the mammalian leg except for the tarsometatarsus and the foot. The thigh is located almost subcutaneously, and it is difficult to immobilize femoral fractures adequately with external fixation alone. Even with tibial fractures it is difficult to follow the cardinal rule of splinting — to immobilize the joint above and below the fracture. In fact, a very common error is inadvertently placing the splint *below* the stifle, thereby creating a fulcrum that will cause more motion than if the leg were left unsplinted (Fig. 1). Some avian specialists report good results simply from confining birds with tibial fractures in a small, darkened box, reasoning that the weight of the leg provides traction. This course of action is actually better than an improper splint.

It is possible to make a splint out of materials such as Orthoplast (Johnson & Johnson) and Hexcel, which are malleable when heated but rigid at room temperature, and to shape them so that there is a "tongue" that extends laterally up the thigh and curves over the back behind the wings. This is a modification of a hip spica cast and will provide limited immobilization of the stifle, femur, and hip (Fig. 2). While a spica is not adequate for femoral fractures, it may be suitable for tibial fractures and may be a useful adjunct to pinning these bones. In very small birds, leg splints can be fabricated from x-ray film, and some other methods are described in *Current Veterinary Therapy VI.*

Splinting is the method of choice for repairing a fractured tarsometatarsus because of the proximity of the bone to the skin and the ease of immobilizing the joint above the fracture.

The toes can be immobilized best in an extended position. This is accomplished by making a large ball of soft gauze and placing it within the grasp of the foot. The toes are then bound to this ball by wrapping more gauze over and around them. The whole ball may then be taped to the foot (Fig. 3). The bird may be able

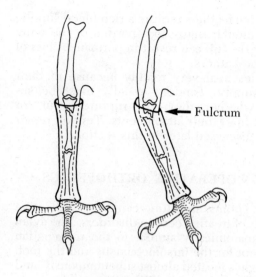

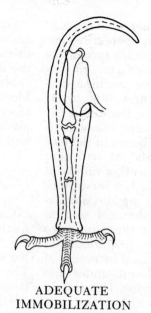

← Fulcrum

Figure 1. Proper application of leg splints.

INADEQUATE
IMMOBILIZATION

ADEQUATE
IMMOBILIZATION

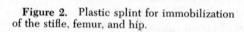

Figure 2. Plastic splint for immobilization of the stifle, femur, and hip.

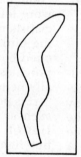

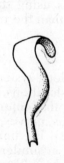

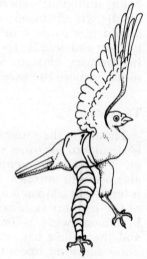

Step 1
Cut Plastic to
Proper Outline

Step 2
Mold Plastic Around
Leg and Over the Back

Step 3
Pad Leg and Body
Well and Bind Splint
to Bird

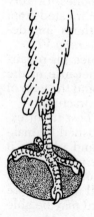

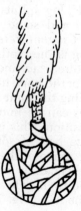

Figure 3. "Foot-ball" splint for immobilization of toes.

Step 1

Step 2

to bear weight on it. This gauze ball is also handy for holding a splint to the upper leg. Spreading of the toes prevents a splint from slipping over the foot and falling off. It is important to pad well between the bottom of the splint and the top of the toes.

Another foot splint can be made by cutting an X-shaped piece of flat plastic or cardboard and binding each toe to a portion of the X; this bandage is a little flatter than the foot-ball splint (Fig. 4). Because of the possibility of joint stiffness following immobilization, holding the toes in extension makes it easier for a bird to begin weight-bearing after immobilization is over; moreover, the strong flexor muscles are more capable of overcoming stiffness than the weaker extensors. An exception is when digital flexor tendons are under repair. Then the toe must be bandaged in extreme flexion.

The leg can be placed in an Ehmer sling like the kind placed on a dog or cat. The tarsometatarsus can be folded against the tibia, and gauze can be wrapped around both of them. If necessary, they can be bound to the body (Fig. 5).

The wing is dissimilar to the mammalian pectoral limb; therefore, the methods of immobilizing the wing are different. It is difficult but not impossible to splint a wing in extension. One method has been to fold a piece of x-ray film in half and to place the wing so that the cranial edge lies within the fold (Fig. 6). The trailing edge of the film can be trimmed to conform to the outline of the flight feathers. The wingtip is held within the film by grasping two or three of the cranial flight feathers with tape and affixing them to the distal portion of the fold. The cut edges of the film can then be stapled together, completely enclosing the

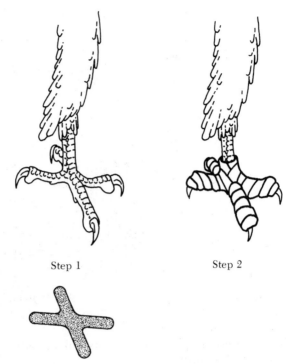

Step 1   Step 2

Figure 4. X-splint for immobilization of toes.

wing. It is best to place tape over the edges of the film that touch the bird's body so as to prevent cuts. Excessive or extended traction can cause the wingtip feathers to loosen. These splints are cumbersome, necessitating confinement to prevent further injury. When used, they should be removed as early as possible.

Many avian veterinarians will incorporate a trimmed tongue depressor or popsicle stick into the bandage to help position a wing in flexion,

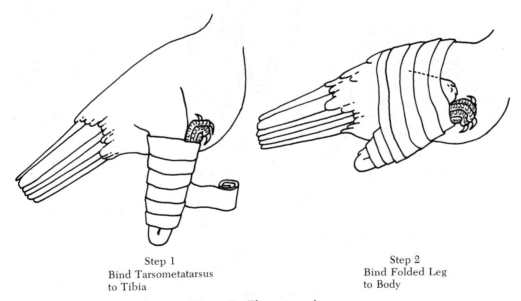

Step 1
Bind Tarsometatarsus
to Tibia

Step 2
Bind Folded Leg
to Body

Figure 5. Ehmer-type sling.

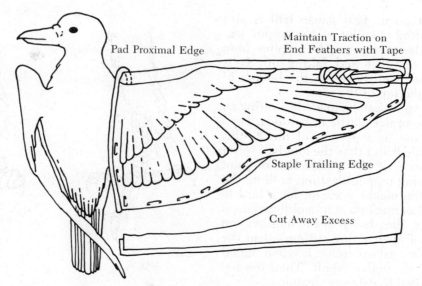

Figure 6. Extension wing splint.

thus forming a splint. This is useful in radial and ulnar fractures.

The wing can be placed in a flexion sling called a brail (Fig. 7). This is a long narrow strip of gauze, cloth, or soft leather, with a longitudinal slit cut about midway. This slit is placed over the folded carpal joint, leaving the two loose ends hanging. These loose ends are then wrapped around the folded wing and tied behind the humerus, which prevents the slit portion from coming off the folded carpus. The remainder of the loose ends can then be wrapped around the flight feathers and tied to bind them compactly.

A traction splint has been devised (Bogue) to help straighten deformed leg bones in a growing bird (Fig. 8). A cloth hammock is made for the bird to lie in. Holes are cut so that the legs may protrude comfortably beneath the hammock. Then the feet are placed in the gauze-ball bandages previously described. In this case, however, weights are also placed within the ball of gauze so as to provide traction.

Binding materials must be chosen carefully.

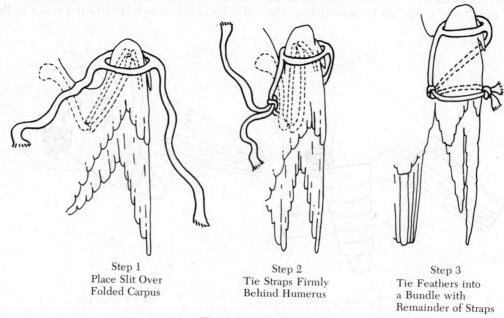

Step 1
Place Slit Over
Folded Carpus

Step 2
Tie Straps Firmly
Behind Humerus

Step 3
Tie Feathers into
a Bundle with
Remainder of Straps

Figure 7. Wing brail.

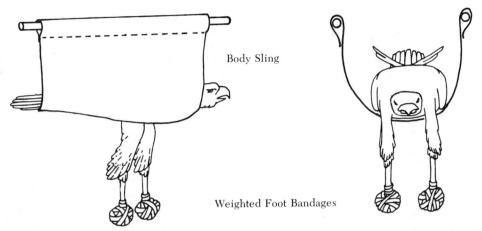

Figure 8.   Traction device for legs.

It is best not to stick adhesive tape directly onto feathers, because it is hard to remove without damaging the feathers or leaving them sticky. A product called Vet-rap is very useful because it sticks to itself and not to feathers. Birds of prey tend to pick at the red-colored Vet-rap, so when ordering tape for these birds one might specify white or flesh color.

Webril cast padding is soft and conforms well to the contour of the limb, and so it is useful when splinting. Kling gauze also conforms very nicely. Splints can be covered with Vet-rap, adhesive tape, or a product such as Elastikon (Johnson & Johnson), a tough tape similar to Ace bandage but with powerful adhesive on one side. Elastikon is good for birds that pick at their bandages. Both Elastikon and Vet-rap are stretchy and, if applied with too much traction, can constrict a limb's blood supply, causing necrosis and gangrene.

When bandaging around the body, be careful not to interfere with the bird's respiration or defecation.

OPERATIVE ORTHOPEDICS

LUXATIONS

Luxations must be treated soon after they occur, otherwise one of two complications may develop. If the luxation persists for several days, fibrosis can make reduction difficult or impossible. On the other hand, if the joint pops in and out of place frequently, permanent ligamentous laxity may occur. It is of extreme importance that a joint be held in anatomic reduction for a long enough period to allow fibrosis to repair the joint. It is equally important that joint motion resume after stabilization occurs but before joint stiffness becomes overwhelming. This judgment can be a rather criti-

cal decision, but joint motion should usually resume within one to two weeks after reduction. Sometimes physical therapy is necessary to regain a full range of motion (ROM). It has been useful to give physical therapy while the bird is under the influence of chemical immobilization (e.g., ketamine), and it is usually done every other day until full ROM is achieved. A joint will sometimes reluxate after reduction and fixation, unbeknownst to the veterinarian. If left uncorrected, it may be irreparable at the end of the healing period. In valuable birds it may be worthwhile to examine the joint radiographically every few days.

The shoulder joint is rarely dislocated, which is fortunate because it is difficult to repair. Reduction and fixation of the wing to the body is preferable. If this fails to hold, one might consider transfixing the joint with an unthreaded Steinmann pin as well as external fixation (Fig. 9). (Never span a joint with a threaded pin — such pins break before they bend.) I am not aware of an open reduction procedure for repairing a permanent ligamentous laxity of the shoulder joint.

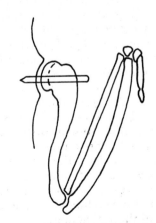

Figure 9.   Shoulder joint transfixation.

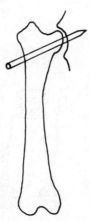

Figure 10. Coxofemoral joint transfixation.

The elbow joint can luxate with or without rupture of the ligaments that hold the proximal ends of the radius and ulna together. If these ligaments are intact, the joint can probably be reduced manually and held with a flexion bandage or a brail. If not intact, open reduction will be necessary to bind these two bones together with sutures before reduction can be accomplished. Interestingly, the avian elbow joint contains a cartilaginous meniscus.

The carpus usually responds well to closed reduction, but sometimes it is necessary to experiment with it in both extension and flexion to see which position is best.

Sometimes a bird in flight will appear to have one wingtip that is "floppy" compared with the other. This is due to a slight luxation between the metacarpal and phalangeal bones. It responds well to immobilization in a bandage or brail.

The wing joints have complex rotational as well as angular motion components; this fact has made it difficult to devise operative methods for replacing ligaments with synthetic materials.

The hip joint is occasionally luxated. Although the relationships are somewhat altered, they can be treated exactly like those in mammals. Closed reduction and slinging is preferable, but open reduction, suturing, and slinging plus transfixation with a smooth pin are possible (Fig. 10).

The stifle joint is remarkably similar to the mammalian stifle. It seems that excessive forces applied to the stifle region are more likely to cause fractures to the femur or tibia than to cause luxation. In fact, the author has never treated a cruciate or collateral ligament rupture in a bird. However, it stands to reason that standard operative techniques could be applied to ruptures of these ligaments.

In birds the tarsus and metatarsals are fused, and there is no tuber calcis to serve as a lever arm. The tibiotarsal joint is occasionally luxated, and splinting should be attempted as a primary treatment. Sometimes splinting fails to be adequate. A trained hunting hawk was presented to this hospital with a persistent ligamentous laxity of the tibiotarsal joint, unresponsive to repeated splinting. Transverse holes were drilled, one through the distal tibia and one through the proximal tarsometatarsus. Exposure was provided by both medial and lateral arthrotomy incisions. A loop of non-absorbable suture (zero tevdek-Deknatel) was threaded through these holes, tightened, and tied securely with the joint in a reduced position, thereby replacing both the medial and lateral collateral ligaments (Fig. 11). A protective splint was applied for ten days. The joint became stable, the limb returned to full function, and the hawk was able to resume hunting.

The metatarsophalangeal joints are not too susceptible to luxation, and I do not know of any prescribed procedure for fixing them. This is a case in which ingenuity becomes valuable. Luxated toes may be popped into position and held with the foot-ball bandage or the X-splint. If necessary, the aforementioned collateral liga-

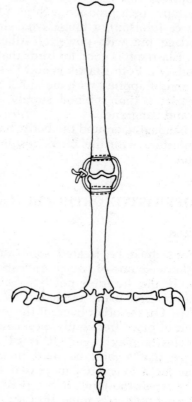

Figure 11. Collateral ligament repair at the tibiotarsal joint.

ment procedure could be applied to a toe joint.

FRACTURES

Fracture surgery presents some special problems. Because bird tissues undergo rapid scarring, damage to joints can result in stiffness, particularly when the limb has been immobilized for several weeks. Therefore fracture fixation methods that do not invade the joint and that allow the earliest possible resumption of joint motion should be used.

Steinmann pinning is the method most available to veterinarians and is effective if certain principles are followed. The advantages of pinning are simplicity, economy, and ease of implant removal. The disadvantage is that the bones can rotate around the pin, resulting in good axial alignment but torsional deformity. Preventing this necessitates either hemi-cerclage wiring or suturing at the fracture site or supplementary external fixation for the same purpose. Again, the splint must be adequate or it can do more harm than good (Figs. 12 through 16).

When using hemi-cerclage wires to prevent rotation, it is necessary to place the wire across the fracture site and, if possible, around the Steinmann pin. Including the IM pin within the cerclage places a bit of "spring-load" force on the pin within the marrow cavity, thereby adding stability. On an exactly transverse fracture, a figure-of-8 suture (perhaps incorporating the IM pin) is more effective in preventing rotation than one that simply spans the fracture line. On oblique fractures, the hemi-cerclage is placed at right angles to the fracture line, if possible. Cerclage sutures can also be used to incorporate fragments into the fracture area. Wire sutures are traditional, although polypropylene and other non-absorbable sutures may be used, and the totally absorbable glycolic acid–derived sutures are good for holding chips in place.

This author has used ASIF finger plates and small fragment plates on leg fractures with excellent results. Wing bones seem to have thinner cortices and do not hold screws as well, so plates have had a more limited application on wing fractures. The advantage of plates is that joints are not invaded, immobilization is rigid, and rotation is impossible. If solid fixation is achieved, early weight-bearing and limited use of the limb are possible. The disadvantages are expense, more difficult application, and more difficult removal. Sometimes poor bone quality can result in screws loosening, so cases for plating must be chosen with prudence. It is an effective and worthwhile technique for valuable or endangered birds with broken legs.

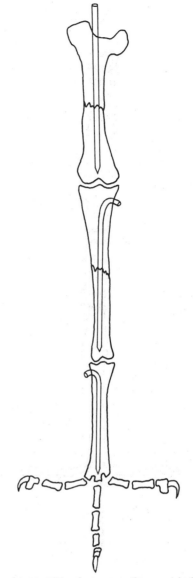

Figure 12. Pin placement – femur and tibia.

There have been fruitful attempts to use half-pin devices on avian bones, using the same principle of the Kirschner-Ehmer or Stader splint. Most techniques involve placing two pins transversely through each main bone segment at a slightly divergent angle. These four pins are then bound together, using a bar and connecting clamps in large birds and a long mass of plaster or dental acrylic in smaller birds. These methods can be very effective, providing that the limb is not subjected to excessive forces postoperatively. One case was seen in which the connecting plaster had put pressure on the underlying limb, resulting in necrosis and subsequent infection of the fracture. It is therefore important to pad adequately between the skin and the connective device.

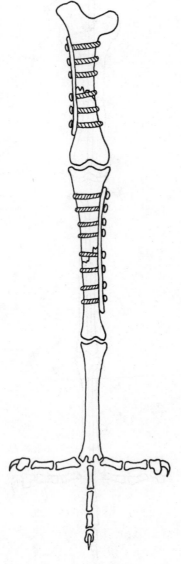

Figure 13.   Plate placement—femur and tibia.

lene from a syringe case, drilling a hole in it, tapping it, and placing it opposite the bone from the stripped-out screw hole. The screw engaging this makeshift nut will pull the plastic snugly against the medial portion of the bone, increasing purchase. This plastic piece must be flash-autoclaved or soaked 10 minutes in betadine solution. An alternative is to abandon plating and do a pinning procedure instead.

If fixation is solid and there is no rotation around a pin, it is best to confine the bird without a splint in a protected enclosure until provisional callus has formed. If there is doubt about the stability of internal fixation, it may be advisable to splint the limb temporarily.

The tibia is approached medially, separating the flexor muscles from the extensors. A pin

The femur is approached laterally, dividing the quadriceps and the biceps femoris muscles. A Steinmann pin is best placed retrograde up the proximal segment and out through the trochanteric fossa. The fracture can then be reduced and the pin driven into the distal segment. Hemi-cerclage wires or sutures are placed as needed. In larger birds (crow size and larger) a small ASIF plate can be applied to the lateral aspect of the femur. The rule is to have screw thread engagement in at least four cortices (two screws through both cortices) or, preferably, in six cortices (three screws) on either side of the fracture. If bone quality is poor and the screws keep stripping out, one can fabricate a "nut" by taking a piece of polypropy-

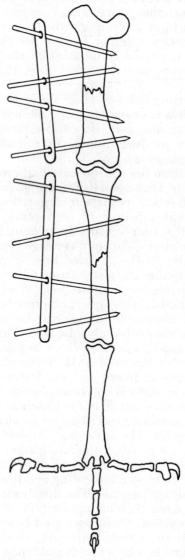

Figure 14.   Half-pin placement—femur and tibia.

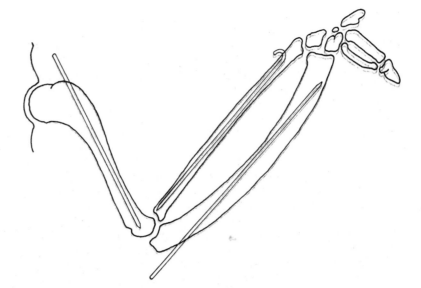

Figure 15. Pin placement — humerus, radius, and ulna.

cannot be driven retrograde through either end of the tibia without invading a joint. However, if the operator insists on doing this, the tibiotarsal joint is more forgiving than the more complex stifle joint. A much better, although slightly more difficult, method is to bend a small Steinmann pin so that it can be placed in a manner similar to that of a Rush pin; that is, it plunges through the cortex near the end of the bone and courses through the marrow cavity. This spares insult to the joint. Again, ASIF plates can be applied to the tibia with excellent results if bone quality is good. A rather long plate is best, one with four holes on either side of the fracture if feasible. Splints are applied postoperatively only if needed. The tarsometatarsus and toes

rarely require surgery, as previously stated. When necessary, the Rush-type pinning or cross-pinning is effective.

The humerus can be approached laterally (dorsally), but one must carefully protect the radial nerve, which courses laterally to the bone in the midshaft area. The humerus has a slight S curve that enables one to place a straight pin into the bone without invading a joint. It is easiest to place a pin retrograde through the proximal segment so that it protrudes through the anterior cortex just cranial to the shoulder joint. Then the fracture may be reduced and the pin seated distally.

The ulna is gently bowed, and in birds it is larger than the radius. A straight pin may be

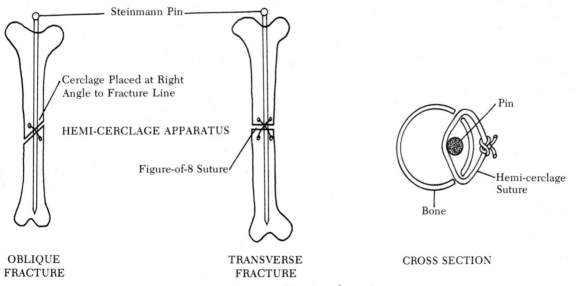

Steinmann Pin

Cerclage Placed at Right Angle to Fracture Line

HEMI-CERCLAGE APPARATUS

Figure-of-8 Suture

Pin

Hemi-cerclage Suture

Bone

OBLIQUE FRACTURE

TRANSVERSE FRACTURE

CROSS SECTION

Figure 16. Placement of hemi-cerclage wire.

drilled retrograde through the caudal cortex of the proximal segment so that it protrudes just behind the elbow joint. It then is driven past the reduced fracture line and seated distally. The radius is smaller and straighter than the ulna. An anatomic reduction of the ulna usually provides acceptable reduction of the radius, with the ulna acting as a splint. However, if the radius is lying close enough to the ulna to heal it, creating a synostosis, it should be pinned into a more normal position. Synostosis of the radius and ulna limits the pronation-supination activity of the distal wing. A pin for the radius must be somewhat flexible and should be bent similar to a Rush pin.

The metacarpals usually respond to closed reduction, but if need be they can be pinned. An important artery and vein are located between the two metacarpal bones and must be preserved to nourish the follicles of the flight feathers. The phalanges are too small to operate upon with ease.

Compound Fractures. Open, or compound, fractures are very serious and must be debrided and closed as soon as possible after occurrence — preferably within a few hours. If dirt and debris have been impacted into the marrow cavity and the bone ends have already dried out, the prognosis for healing is very guarded. Infections in birds result in a cheesy type of pus, because birds lack the enzyme to liquefy pus. These caseous masses form a foreign body that blocks bone healing. Infection is the number one cause of non-union in bird fractures, and aseptic technique is as important in bird surgery as it is in surgery for dogs, cats, and humans.

Non-union and Malunion. The classic non-infected types of non-union are uncommon in birds, but they do occur. They can be either the common "elephant's foot" type caused by excessive motion or the avascular type in which the fracture repair process simply does not get under way at all. The treatment consists of reaming out the marrow cavities to re-establish medullary circulation, freshening up the fracture ends, and achieving solid fixation.

One avascular type of non-union in the anterior metacarpal bone of a peregrine falcon was treated by opening the marrow cavities, removing the last rib on one side, grooving the metacarpus, and placing the rib into the groove. This constituted an inlay bone graft that spanned the fracture site and subsequently healed. (When removing the last rib of a bird, try to preserve the internal periosteum. If the air sac is invaded, subcutaneous emphysema can result, complicating the postoperative period.) Whole-

segment cortical bone transplants have been successful in birds.

Frequently, malunions are encountered that are so severe that limb function is compromised. These deformities can be angular and rotational in the same bone. It is entirely feasible and indeed desirable to perform osteotomies on many of these bones. Correcting the deformities realigns the bones and joints and improves limb function. Once the proper cutting and remodeling is done at the osteotomy site, the bone is handled as if it were freshly fractured.

TENDON INJURIES

Tendon injuries are usually manifested by dysfunction of a specific joint. Tendons are repaired using the Bunnel method (Fig. 17). The most critical aspect of tendon repair is immobilization of the limb in a manner that will remove tension from the tendon. For flexor tendon repair, bandage in flexion; for repair of extensor tendons, splint in extension.

IMPING

As previously stated, flight feathers are as important as the rest of the wing. It is useful to learn a technique called "imping" (Fig. 18), an ancient falconry method for repairing broken feathers. One can splice the same feather back together, or one molted previously by the same bird, or one from a different bird. A rigid pin or needle made of metal or good-quality bamboo is placed within the pulp cavity and held in place with contact cement. This re-establishes the continuity of the feather. An alternative is to enlist the aid of a local falconer who may be familiar with imping.

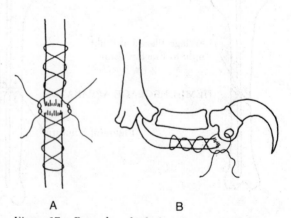

A   B

Figure 17. Bunnel method of tendon repair. *A.* Repair of ruptured tendon. *B.* Repair of avulsed tendon attachment.

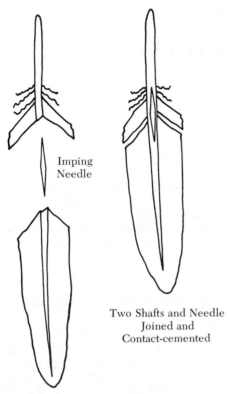

Imping
Needle

Two Shafts and Needle
Joined and
Contact-cemented

Figure 18. Imping.

BASIC PRINCIPLES — A REVIEW

I would now like to review some of the basic principles that have been discussed, which I call the Ten Suggestions (not commandments) for Avian Orthopedics:

1. Evaluate other organ systems before performing surgery.

2. Use strict aseptic technique during surgery.

3. Avoid invasion of joints with appliances.

4. Eliminate or minimize angular or torsional deformity.

5. Utilize methods that will allow early return to function.

6. Avoid long periods of limb immobilization.

7. Immobilize the joint above and below the fracture site when relying on external fixation.

8. Never span a joint with a threaded pin.

9. Operate upon open (compound) fractures within a few hours.

10. Avoid injuring flight feathers and their follicles.

FRONTIERS IN AVIAN ORTHOPEDICS

There has been considerable interest in devices that will hold fracture segments solidly from within the marrow cavity. One of the most promising methods involves filling the marrow cavity with polymethyl methacrylate resin and allowing it to harden. This substance expands its volume by 3 per cent as it sets, thus anchoring itself firmly. It is incompressible, but brittle, which suggests that it could be combined with some type of metal reinforcing rod to compensate for its brittleness (the same principle as the concrete and steel structural combination). If this technique proves to be successful on a reasonable number of patients for a long period of time, it offers the hope of immediate stability and very early use of the limb. Sterile plaster (laboratory plaster) has been used to fill bone defects in surgery of the human jaw and in repair of canine leg fractures. This plaster is eventually absorbed, and so it would be used as a temporary rather than a permanent intermedullary prosthesis. Other intermedullary devices are being developed, and it will be interesting to see what the future brings. In the past, there have been reports of the successful use of Jonas pins.

It is questionable whether joint prostheses can have an application in bird surgery, but when a joint has been totally destroyed in a valuable specimen, it would be tempting to try implanting one of the human knuckle prostheses — especially in the stifle and tibiotarsal joints. Some of the bone and whole-joint transplant techniques being studied for mammals may become applicable to birds, and there is still the challenge of developing better joint repair techniques.

Another challenge involves scaling down standard procedures to apply to tiny (20 to 100 gm) birds. Giving good medical and surgical care to hummingbirds and small finches is one of the most demanding endeavors in veterinary clinical practice. The next edition of this text will undoubtedly contain many advances in this and other aspects of avian surgery.

SUPPLEMENTAL READING

Altman, R. B.: Fractures of the extremities of birds. In Kirk, R. W. (ed.): *Current Veterinary Therapy VI.* Philadelphia, W. B. Saunders Co., 1977.

Fowler, M. E. (ed.): *Zoo and Wild Animal Medicine.* Philadelphia, W. B. Saunders Co., 1978.

Petrak, M. L.: *Diseases of Cage and Aviary Birds.* Philadelphia, Lea & Febiger, 1969.

FOREIGN DISEASES AND IMPORTED BIRDS

LINDA J. LOWENSTINE, D.V.M.
Davis, California

Every year, hundreds of thousands of birds are imported into the United States from all over the world. Most of these are passarines, especially finches and related birds (fringillids), and psittacines destined for the pet trade. Since 1973, federal trade regulations require that all birds presented for importation be quarantined in United States Department of Agriculture (USDA) approved, privately operated stations at which the birds are checked for foreign diseases that might affect our domestic poultry. From 1972 to 1973 there was a complete embargo on exotic birds because of an epiornithic of exotic Newcastle disease, which caused extensive losses in California in 1971. This outbreak was traced to imported ornamental birds (mostly psittacines) that were in contact with poultry. Prior to this time, quarantining of pet birds fell under the jurisdiction of the Public Health Service (USPHS) of the Department of Health, Education, and Welfare (HEW). Their concern was protection of the American public from ornithosis. Under HEW regulations, still in effect, birds must be treated for at least 45 days with tetracycline (incorporated into the feed) and must be free from signs of disease before entry. Before 1973, the USDA maintained quarantine stations for imported livestock and poultry that are still in existence. "Poultry" are defined as chickens, turkeys, ducks, pigeons, and related birds.

In spite of these regulations, foreign diseases and ornithosis still occur in the pet–zoo bird industry. Smuggled birds are often the culprits. Because of the increasing popularity of pet birds, the fantastic prices obtainable on the retail market, and the fact that many of the popular species do not breed well in captivity, bird smuggling is becoming big business. No one knows how many birds are smuggled into the United States annually, but the numbers may increase as the cost for quarantine confinement and testing is transferred from the taxpayers to the importers. The only assurance that a bird has been properly quarantined and is free of disease is a certificate for the lot in which the bird was imported. Since individual birds are not yet banded upon importation, the importer's word must be accepted as proof. It is not a foolproof system and, though it has prevented the legal entry of affected birds, the practicing veterinarian must still suspect foreign diseases when dealing with exotic species.

FOREIGN VIRAL DISEASES

The foreign diseases of concern to the USDA are exotic velogenic, viscerotropic Newcastle disease (VVND) and the fowl plague (FP) strain of avian influenza (AI). Another viral disease of great concern to the pet and zoo bird industry is psittacine herpesvirus infection (PHI, also called Pacheco's parrot disease).

EXOTIC NEWCASTLE DISEASE

Exotic Newcastle disease is caused by a paramyxovirus. It is thought to be indigenous to Asia but is endemic in parts of Africa, Europe, and South America as well as throughout the Orient. Nearly all orders of birds are susceptible, but the highest morbidity and mortality rates occur in gallinaceous birds (chickens, pheasants, and related birds) and psittacines. Other birds, especially fringillids and other finches (ploceids) may be asymptomatic carriers. In 1975, nearly 25 percent of the lots of birds presented for importation were positive for VVND. The number of positive lots has been decreasing, probably as a result of prequarantine holding outside the U.S.

Birds held in quarantine are tested by culturing cloacal swabs from living birds and tissues from birds that are ill or have died. The specimens are inoculated into embryonate chicken eggs. Isolates are identified and are inoculated into test chickens and turkeys to confirm pathogenicity for domestic poultry. Many viruses as well as *Chlamydia sp.* can be picked up by this method, although eggs are usually not held long enough to identify the slower-developing organisms such as *Chlamydia*. Birds are held in quarantine for at least 30 days and until all tests are completed. The presence of the VVND virus in a lot of birds results in rejection or destruction of the entire lot.

Clinical signs of VVND may be respiratory, nervous, or enteric. Diarrhea is often a feature, but death may be peracute without premonitory signs. Nervous signs occur in subacute cases and usually include clonic spasms. Gross postmortem findings, like the clinical signs, are not pathognomonic. The virus attacks vascular endothelium, causing loss of vascular integrity, which leads to congestion, edema, and hemorrhage. These changes are most apparent in the proventriculus and throughout the small intestine. Catarrhal and hemorrhagic tracheitis and opacification of the air sacs may also be present. Often, however, there are no gross lesions.

Definitive diagnosis is established by culture. If Newcastle disease is suspected, the practicing veterinarian must contact the local or regional veterinary services laboratory of the USDA. Tissues from birds suspected of having a foreign disease should not be shipped until clearance is received from the laboratory. Usually the local federal veterinarian prefers to receive the entire carcass refrigerated but not frozen. If this is not possible, a thorough postmortem examination should be performed. A complete set of tissues should be placed in 10 percent buffered formalin, except for samples of the following tissues, which should be collected in a sterile manner and frozen on dry ice in sterile plastic or cold-resistant glass containers: lung, brain, trachea, spleen, liver, and distal intestine. Once frozen, these tissues may later be shipped in insulated containers with dry ice.

A word of caution is in order when dealing with recently imported birds. Newcastle disease virus can cause severe conjunctivitis in humans. Protective goggles, gloves, and a mask should be worn when performing postmortem examinations.

AVIAN INFLUENZA — FOWL PLAGUE VARIANT

Fowl plague is caused by a type A influenza virus. Influenza viruses are of the orthomyxovirus group. There are numerous avian influenza viruses; however, FP is the only one not endemic in the U.S. The relationship between human and avian influenza viruses is unclear and, while not considered to be of public health significance, fowl plague is a threat to domestic poultry, with morbidity and mortality rates approaching 100 percent. Turkeys, ducks, chickens, and quail are most often affected. The exact host range of the FP virus is unknown, but avian influenza viruses have been isolated from gulls, terns, shearwaters, and other shore and sea birds and from herons, migratory waterfowl, mynahs, "exotic caged birds from southeast Asia," parakeets, parrots, cockatoos, and crows. Birds from Asia and Australia are most frequently involved.

Testing for FP in quarantine is the same as that for VVND. Usually, avian influenza viruses and other hemagglutinating viruses (except FP virus) isolated from quarantined birds are not pathogenic when inoculated into poultry. From October 1973, to September 1975, over 2000 viruses were isolated (not including 450 VVND isolates) and none caused disease when inoculated into poultry. Most isolates were from fringillids. To date, there has been only one pathogenic influenza isolate found in the USDA testing program. If a non-pathogenic strain is isolated, the lot is still released for entry.

Clinical signs of FP are generally referrable to the respiratory system; however, diarrhea and even nervous signs may be present. The clinical picture often resembles Newcastle disease and is not specific. The gross lesions are those of congestion, hemorrhage, and necrosis. The skin, liver, kidneys, and spleen are often affected, with red areas and necrotic grey foci. Sinusitis and fibrinous exudates on air sacs and serosal surfaces are sometimes seen. Reliable diagnosis is based only on virus isolation. Procedures are the same as for VVND; this is a reportable disease. Tissues to be submitted for culture are trachea, lung, liver, and spleen samples.

PSITTACINE HERPESVIRUS INFECTION

This disease may be present in a group of birds without disqualifying them for importation, because it is not contagious to domestic poultry or indigenous wild life. It is, however, devastating to most species of psittacines and of major importance to the pet and zoo bird industry. This disease will be dealt with in detail in another article in this section. Currently, in my experience, this is the major cause of death in recently imported birds. Death is usually peracute. The liver and spleen may appear grossly normal but are usually mottled or stippled with pale foci and somewhat swollen or enlarged. Intranuclear inclusions on impression smears or histologic sections are pathognomonic. Cultural isolation can be made from liver and spleen tissue frozen as for VVND. Although not a reportable disease per se, the USDA is interested in receiving samples from outbreaks in order to confirm the diagnosis and to compare the specimen with known serotypes.

FOREIGN CHLAMYDIAL, BACTERIAL, AND FUNGAL DISEASES

ORNITHOSIS

Although this is not truly a foreign disease, since it is probably endemic in this country, it is included here because it is often a cause of death and debility in recently imported birds, especially psittacines and columbids (pigeons and doves). It is of public health significance, and local public health officials should be notified especially if people in contact with the suspect birds are clinically ill. It is a highly pleomorphic disease, and all signs and gross and histologic postmortem findings can be mimicked by other avian diseases. Impression smears and culturing of affected tissues (liver, spleen kidney, air sacs or effusions) are necessary for definitive diagnosis. The National Veterinary Services Laboratories will accept specimens frozen on dry ice directly, or specimens may be submitted through the local federal veterinarian. This disease will be discussed more fully in another article (see page 677).

BACTERIAL DISEASES

There are no strictly foreign bacterial or fungal diseases of concern to the USDA or USPHS. Serotypes of bacteria such as *Salmonella* spp. and *Mycobacterium avium* may be foreign to the U.S. but are not regarded as health hazards to poultry or people. Foreign birds may have a multitude of bacterial diseases, and cultures should be done to document these cases. Aspergillosis and candidiasis are common in exotic birds, especially after quarantine treatment with antibiotics.

FOREIGN PARASITIC DISEASE

Protozoan and metazoan diseases may be of significance in an individual bird but are not reportable to the USDA and USPHS. Many parasites of wild birds are as yet unclassified, and their significance in any one bird must be judged on clinical and pathologic changes observed. Many of these parasites require an intermediate host not available in this country and therefore do not present a problem to other susceptible birds. Occasionally, all portions of a parasite's life cycle are imported together into a suitable zoo or aviary environment. An example of this occurred in a group of zoo waterfowl infected with the oriental eye fluke. The life cycle was completed by snails in the aquatic environment of the display area.

GENERAL COMMENTS

One of the challenges of dealing with exotic birds is the presence of clinical and pathologic entities of unknown etiology. Sometimes there are parallels in domestic poultry. Sometimes a specific virus, bacterium, or parasite can be identified. Often, however, these conditions remain a mystery because of inadequate diagnostic efforts. If we are to advance in our knowledge of diseases affecting exotic species (as well as indigenous wild life) it will require conscientious effort on the part of the veterinarians who are presented with these animals. Complete postmortem examinations, with histopathologic workup and cultures, should be performed. Tissues that should be examined routinely include brain, lung, heart, liver, kidney, spleen, small intestine, pancreas, large intestine with ceca (when present), bursa, bone marrow, and, of course, any other grossly evident lesions. Tissues can be frozen on dry ice and retained for viral or bacterial culture pending results of the postmortem examination. Impression smears of lesions stained with Giemsa, acid-fast and Gram stains may yield rapid diagnosis. Only with such documentation of clinical and pathologic lesions will we gain an understanding of the diseases affecting exotic birds.

SUPPLEMENTAL READING

Hofstad, M. S. (ed.): *Diseases of Poultry*, 7th ed. Ames, Iowa, Iowa State University Press, 1978.

Pearson, J. E., et al.: Virus isolations from exotic birds offered for importation into the United States. U.S. Anim. Hlth. Assoc., 79th annual meeting, 1975, pp. 219–225.

Pearson, J. E., et al.: Techniques for the isolation of viruses from exotic birds submitted for importation into the United States. 18th Annual Proc. of Am. Assoc. of Vet. Lab. Diagnosticians, 1975, pp. 61–68.

Petrak, M. D. (ed.): *Diseases of Cage and Aviary Birds*. Philadelphia, Lea & Febiger, 1969.

Toft, J. D., III: Philophthalmus infection in zoo waterfowls. Proc. of Symposium on the Comparative Pathology of Zoo Animals. (In press.)

PSITTACOSIS — AN EVER-PRESENT PROBLEM IN CAGED BIRDS

RALPH COOPER, D.V.M.
San Gabriel, California

INTRODUCTION

Every clinician who deals with caged birds will ultimately be presented with a bird infected with psittacosis or ornithosis. The disease is commonly called psittacosis in psittacine birds and man and is known as ornithosis in turkeys, pigeons, and other non-psittacine birds. It may be referred to as chlamydiosis after the etiologic agent, *Chlamydia psittaci*. In order to serve the client's best interests, as well as to protect themselves and their employees from illness, veterinarians must be prepared to diagnose the disease and to make definite recommendations as to its treatment and management. Because psittacosis is capable of causing death in humans, even if only rarely, it must be accorded the respect it deserves.

ETIOLOGY

Psittacosis is said to have been described first as a clinical entity in Europe by Juergensen in 1874. Following a widespread outbreak in Paris in 1892, Morange (1895) studied the illness and proposed the name *psittacosis* for the condition, because of its apparent relationship to psittacine birds. Nocard (1893) isolated a gram-negative bacillus from affected birds, and for some 38 years, Nocard's baccillus was wrongly believed to be the causative organism.

A number of notable epidemics occurred in Europe in subsequent years, and in 1929 over 100 human cases were reported from Argentina (Barros, 1929). Progress in the field of virology enabled researchers to identify the psittacosis "virus" in 1930. It was not until 1964 that Moulder summarized the evidence that the organism was an obligate, intracellular bacterium, not a virus. In 1966 Page proposed that the organism should be placed in the genus *Chlamydia* and in 1966 proposed that there should be two species designated: *C. psittaci* and *C. trachomatis*. There is still reference to the "virus" of psittacosis in the older literature, and the term may still be heard or seen from time to time.

MORPHOLOGY AND MODE OF REPRODUCTION

Chlamydiae are non-motile spheroids ranging from 0.3 to 1.5 microns in diameter. When the infectious form or elementary body is ingested by a host cell, it begins to enlarge and becomes the initial body, measuring from 0.6 to 1.5 microns in diameter. It then appears to multiply by binary fission to produce daughter organisms that shrink to a final size of about 0.3 micron in diameter.

STAINING CHARACTERISTICS

Chlamydiae may be seen in sections of infected tissues and in impression smears that have been stained by the Giemsa, Castaneda, Macchiavello, or Gimenez methods.

PROPAGATION OF THE ORGANISMS

All strains of *C. psittaci* grow and multiply readily in the yolk sac of chicken embryos. Most but not all strains will multiply in mice. All strains will multiply in secondary cell cultures derived from chicken embryos and in some of the common mammalian cell lines. Under no circumstances should culture attempts be initiated except under perfect isolation conditions by experienced personnel.

The hazards of handling dead birds at necropsy are minimal when proper precautions are observed, such as wetting the feathers with a quaternary ammonium disinfectant and preventing the carcass or organs from drying. The hazards of manipulating cultures of *Chlamydia* are extreme, and even under the best of conditions, laboratory infections are not rare.

RESISTANCE TO CHEMICAL AND PHYSICAL AGENTS

Chlamydiae are rapidly inactivated by surface-active compounds such as quarternary ammonium compounds and lipid solvents, even in the presence of organic materials. They are

677

more resistant to dilute alcohols, hydrochloric acid, sodium hydroxide, phenol, and ordinary soap and water. They are resistant to the cresol compounds and lime. In dried excrement, they may remain infectious for many months.

EPIZOOTIOLOGY

RESERVOIR HOSTS

Meyer in 1967 listed over 120 wild avian species that have been transient hosts, if not carriers, of chlamydiae. Probably any species should be viewed as a possible carrier of at least some strains of chlamydiae. A given species of bird may establish a good host-parasite relationship with its own peculiar strain of chlamydia but still be highly susceptible to a different strain. It is commonly reported that the rate of infection among pigeons is very high, but such unlikely birds as gulls, herons, and egrets also have been found to carry and excrete highly virulent strains, without themselves suffering ill effects. During a recent investigation of an outbreak in turkeys, Page found an opposum and a house cat on the premises that were carrying the same strain of chlamydia that was killing the turkeys. It has also been reported that the strain that causes polyarthritis in sheep may cause typical ornithosis in turkeys.

TRANSMISSION

Infected birds may shed enormous numbers of organisms in their feces or exudates. Intimate contact with the infected materials or inhalation of the resulting dust can readily initiate an infection in either birds or mammals, including man. Eddie in 1962 recovered chlamydiae from nest mites remaining in nest boxes of turkeys some three months after the turkeys had been removed. Whether they were true carriers or only mechanical vectors is not clear, but the possibility of this mode of transmission deserves attention. The habit of the adult bird to feed its nestling by mouth offers an excellent way to spread the infection.

HISTORY

At times, a detailed inquiry into the history of the bird will yield highly suggestive clues as to the true nature of the problem. Infrequently, the bird may have become ill or may have died rather unexpectedly in a closed flock. More commonly, there is a history of recent introductions of birds to a flock. Often the bird will have died a few days after its introduction, but the cause of death may not have been determined. Subsequently, other exposed birds become ill or die, perhaps two or three weeks later, and veterinary help is sought. At this point it is well to remember that the incubation period may be as short as three days in cases of massive artificial exposure, but more commonly it lies in the range between one and four weeks. There is one report that puts the upper limit at eleven months, but that is very rare. Usually, the complete background of the bird will be unknown or hazy. If the case shows any sign of involving a smuggled bird, for example, a young parrot that was purchased at a bargain price from a private individual who was driving an old panel truck filled with parrots, the clinician should be on guard. Unfortunately, in the absence of any uniform system of identification, one parrot looks very much like another. Realistically, it is only prudent to suspect any parrot that has recently been released from quarantine. The owner may report that the bird has been sick for weeks and has been treated by several veterinarians with all the usual antibiotics, but that the bird will neither get better nor die. If it can be determined that none of the tetracyclines were included in the treatments, then psittacosis must be given a prominent position among the differential diagnoses. If the owner or another member of the family has suffered or is suffering from an intractable case of the "flu," especially if he or she has not been treated with one of the tetracyclines, then psittacosis must be considered. It often happens that the presence of psittacosis in a flock of budgerigars is signaled by the identification of the disease in a human. The flock itself may be found to be suffering only from a marginally lowered production or some unthriftiness. Invariably, however, the flock will "bloom" with health as soon as medication is begun.

SIGNS

Psittacosis is clinically indistinguishable from several of the other febrile septicemic diseases of birds. A bird may exhibit several or many of the following signs: ruffled feathers, listlessness, loss of appetite, watery greenish feces, conjunctivitis, trembling, and unbalanced gait. In fact, there are so many possible combinations of non-specific signs that they are really not very helpful for diagnosis. The occasional bird may simply be found dead by its owner, with few or no premonitory signs. This is especially true of the rice birds, canaries, some of the other finches, and some parakeets. At the other extreme, adult pigeons usually show only a reduction of their racing ability and rarely die, although their squabs may die in the nest. It is often the case that the clinician will be reminded of psittacosis when a bird fails to respond to the usual antibiotic therapy. At this point, treatment with one of the tetracyclines may initiate a striking improvement in as little as two or three days. This phenomenon has been utilized by some clinicians to confirm their suspicions that the problem may be psittacosis. In fact, at this point they may arbitrarily make a working diagnosis of psittacosis and proceed with a complete program of medication and sanitation and a discussion of the public health implications with the owner.

DIAGNOSIS IN THE LIVE BIRD

The diagnosis of psittacosis in the living bird is difficult both technically and logistically. Isolation of chlamydiae from blood or feces may be accomplished but, because of the serious hazards to humans, must be attempted only by experienced personnel working in specially equipped laboratories. Any clinician who works with birds should seek out and establish a good working relationship with such a laboratory before assistance is needed. In some areas public health laboratories are prepared to render assistance to the practitioner, especially if there is a human involvement. In other areas, state, county, university, or private laboratories should be contacted.

BLOOD SAMPLES

Samples of blood may be submitted in accordance with the instructions of the cooperating laboratory. If sufficient blood can be obtained from the jugular or wing veins, or perhaps from a closely clipped toenail, the laboratory may choose to perform the complement fixation (C-F) test as well as to make an isolation attempt for the infectious agent. A word of caution is in order: Although most species of birds will respond to infection by producing complement-fixing antibodies, the budgerigars and the African grey parrot are known to respond irregularly. Thus, the C-F test is not dependable in these species. If at least a four-fold rise in titer can be demonstrated between acute and convalescent sera, the test may be interpreted as positive. A medicated bird may not develop this rise in titer, although it was infected. Although a very high initial titer of 1/128 tends to reinforce a tentative diagnosis, the C-F test is of limited value to the clinician.

FECAL SAMPLES

If suitable arrangements can be made with a laboratory, fecal samples or rectal swabs may be submitted for culture. If the agent is isolated and identified, a process that may require only 10 days in tissue culture systems or as long as 42 days in mice, the diagnosis is confirmed. However, the suspected bird should have been placed on medication promptly and may even have completed the entire course of medication before the report is received. If a large flock of birds is involved, or if there are legal implications, it is important to confirm the diagnosis, even if the process is time-consuming.

DIAGNOSIS IN THE DEAD BIRD

In the dead bird, a diagnosis may often be made based solely on the gross lesions and the finding of typical bodies in a stained smear of the organs and exudate. Commonly, the bird will be thin, with evidence of diarrhea. The liver may be conspicuously enlarged and yellow or grey in color, and often it will have tiny necrotic foci. The spleen will usually be enlarged, perhaps two or three fold. The air sacs may be only cloudy but more commonly are covered with a thick yellow exudate. There may be a pericarditis. It is very important to confirm any preliminary diagnosis by making smears at least of the liver, spleen, and air sac tissues, staining them with one of the common stains such as Macchiavello's, and then examining them under the oil immersion objective. The organisms may be seen in smears from any or all of these organs. Any clinician can learn to prepare, stain, and read the smears with confidence. He or she should make every effort to seek the help and advice of an experienced pathologist if this is at all possible. At least 90 per cent of the diagnoses in parrots in the author's laboratory have been made in this simple and rapid manner.

MACCHIAVELLO STAINING METHOD

Because it has proven to be helpful to many practitioners, detailed instructions for preparing, staining, and reading the smears follow:

Smears of liver, spleen, and air sac tissue may be placed on a single slide. Using thumb forceps and scissors, tiny bits of tissue, about 1 to 2 mm in diameter, are removed from the organs and smeared on a third of the slide. Ideally, the tissues should be free of excess blood and should be spread in an even, relatively thin film. This is then fixed by passing the slide over a flame, avoiding overheating.

Three stock staining solutions are necessary: basic fuchsin (0.25 gm in 100 ml distilled water), citric acid (0.5 gm in 200 ml distilled water), and methylene blue or methyl green (1.0 gm in 100 ml distilled water).

The basic fuchsin solution is dropped onto the film and left for 5 minutes, then quickly drained off. The slide is washed in tap water, and dipped quickly about ten times in the citric acid solution, which is conveniently held in a Coplin jar. Next the slide is washed thoroughly with tap water, stained with 1 percent methylene blue for 20 to 30 seconds, washed again in tap water, and dried by blotting. Exposure to the citric acid for more than about 30 seconds will decolorize the elementary bodies, and then they will all stain blue. In a properly prepared slide, most of the chlamydiae will stain red. *Note:* The citric acid solution remains usable until mold appears.

INTERPRETING THE SMEAR

The smear is first scanned under high dry magnification (450×) so as to locate a suitable area for examination under oil (1000×). The tiny red-staining bodies may be found within macrophages or scattered throughout the smear. Until the practitioner is thoroughly familiar with the appearance of chlamydiae, he or she is well advised to seek the advice of an experienced diagnostician. It is very helpful to obtain several smears of known positive cases for comparison. It is reported that mycoplasmas may be confused with chlamydiae. Certain smears may also contain non-specific particles that mimic chlamydiae and may confuse the interpretation or even render it impossible. In these cases, the practitioner may have to rely on the other facts of the case and may wish to submit the bird for isolation of the organism.

ISOLATION OF THE ORGANISM

If a diagnosis cannot be made on the basis of gross lesions and an examination of the stained smears, it may be appropriate to submit the whole carcass or selected tissues for isolation of the agent. This should be done only after prior arrangements have been made with the laboratory. Their instructions for the submission of specimens should be followed precisely. Because isolation attempts may require from 10 to 42 days, if a tentative diagnosis of psittacosis has been made, appropriate steps should be taken immediately. They may be interrupted or modified when the laboratory report is received.

CRITICALLY ILL BIRDS

If the bird is too ill to eat or drink, treatment should be initiated by the intramuscular injection of tetracycline, chlortetracycline, or oxytetracycline, at least for the first day or two. The dosage will vary with species and size, but 5 to 10 mg daily is adequate for budgerigars and 40 to 50 mg daily is adequate for pigeons and some parrots. The handling of the critically ill bird will expose the clinician and his or her employees to a very real hazard, and all appropriate precautions must be taken, including the wearing of a face mask. The birds should receive all the usual supportive measures, including the provision of a heated environment and force-feeding with a medicated mixture if necessary.

CHRONICALLY ILL OR EXPOSED BIRDS

Birds that are able to eat and drink on their own should be given a medicated feed according to specific instructions. The following information comes from the *Outline of Treatment to Eliminate Psittacosis*, prepared and distributed by the Veterinary Public Health Unit of the California Department of Health Services, Berkeley, California. It is presented almost in its entirety through their courtesy, so that the practitioner will have complete and detailed instructions readily available in the event of an emergency.

The oral administration of chlortetracycline (CTC), using food as a vehicle, provides a means of eliminating latent psittacosis in both large and small birds. The methods used are simple and direct, making possible the treatment of any number of birds, including the larger parrots, which are sometimes difficult to handle. Once the birds are properly caged, this method of treatment eliminates the need to catch and handle individual birds.

The treatment of the small psittacines (parakeets or budgerigars) has been simplified through the use of hulled millet seed impregnated with CTC (Keet Life, Hartz Mountain), which is available commercially. This preparation, provided it is not used beyond the expiration date and is stored away from direct sunlight, will eliminate psittacosis in small psittacines. Since the large psittacine parrots do not eat millet seed, the antibiotic must be incorporated in some other type of food for them.

Newly arrived shipments of psittacine birds may include a variable number infected with psittacosis. Such infection may be chronic or acute, and the infected birds may appear ill or healthy. Only through laboratory testing can it be determined whether or not the birds have psittacosis. From a control standpoint, however, it is feasible to assume that infection is present and to treat all of the birds in the group systemically.

During treatment, precautions should be taken to keep circulation of feathers and dust to a minimum. This can be done by frequent wet-mopping using a disinfectant (see the following section, Housing), liberal use of oil-impregnated sweeping compounds between moppings, and prevention of air currents and drafts. Bird droppings, sweepings, and other waste should be incinerated or sterilized, because they may contain the infective organisms.

All people who are in contact with the birds should be informed about the nature of the disease. They should be instructed to wear protective clothing, which should be laundered frequently. A physician should be consulted if illness develops in personnel so that early and specific treatment for psittacosis can be initiated if indicated.

HOUSING

Cages should provide ample room and should have a sliding screen at the bottom to keep the birds off the floor of the cage. Several layers of newspaper can be placed on the bottom of the pan under the screen. The soiled newspapers can be removed frequently and burned or dropped into a disinfectant solution. When the cage requires cleaning, the bird is transferred to a clean cage and the soiled cage is immersed in a 1 percent solution of Lysol or quaternary ammonium chloride (Roccal, Zepherin) for at least 30 minutes. It is then scrubbed thoroughly in hot soapy water and rinsed in clean running water.

TREATMENT FOR LARGE PSITTACINE BIRDS (Parrots, Macaws, and Cockatoos)

At the present time, commercially prepared medicated feeds for treating larger birds are not widely available.* There is, in the Code of Federal Regulations (par. 558.128, Chlortetracycline), authorization to add 10 mg of the drug per gram of mash for the treatment of psittacine birds suspected or known to be infected with psittacosis. In general, however, the only readily available method is through the use of a cooked mash.

COOKED MASH PREPARATION

Equipment. Vessels used for preparing the drug-feed mixture and for feeding the bird must be of non-corrosive material such as plastic, heavy glass, or stainless steel. These must be kept scrupulously clean.

Basic Mash Preparation. The best vehicle for introducing CTC has been a cooked mash prepared from rice, hen scratch feed, and water in the ratio of 2:2:3 (e.g., 2 pounds of rice, 2 pounds of scratch feed, and 3 pints (473 ml) of water). This mixture may be cooked in a pressure cooker, autoclave, or similar cooking utensil until soft but not mushy. If a 30-quart pressure cooker is available, the usual procedure is to cook the mixture for 15 minutes, or about 10 minutes after the full operating pressure of 15 pounds per square inch is reached. The heat is then turned off and the pressure released immediately. The mixture is emptied into a large mixing container and allowed to cool at room temperature.

Drug. Chlortetracycline (CTC) is the antibiotic most thoroughly tested for use against psittacosis in parrots. It effectively and quickly suppresses multiplication of the organism and almost immediately stops cage-to-cage transmission once it is adequately absorbed by the bird. However, it requires prolonged use to eliminate the infection completely. Comparative studies have not revealed a more effective antimicrobial agent for psittacosis.

The commercially available product known as Aureomycin S.F. Mix 66 contains 100 grams of pure drug per pound (22 per cent), the diluent being soybean meal. This formulation has the advantage of being readily accepted by most parrots if mixed with the cooked mash.† Final concentrations of from 4.4 to 10.0 mg of the drug per gram of mash are readily accepted by most birds. (*Note:* If S.F. Mix 66 is absolutely unobtainable, Polyotic [American Cyanamid] may be substituted, with some loss of palatability.)

Compounding. Table 1 shows the amounts of S.F. Mix 66 needed for various quantities of mash in order to get 5 mg of CTC per gram of

---

*There is at least one company that currently offers a medicated pellet for parrots: Pacific Animal Diets Corporation, 710 East Ball Road, Anaheim, Ca. 92805; telephone (714) 533-3850.

†Aureomycin S.F. Mix 66 is available from the American Cyanamid Company, Agricultural Division, P. O. Box 400, Princeton, N.J.

Table 1.　Preparation of Medicated Mash for Treatment of Psittacosis in Large Psittacines

WEIGHT OF COOKED AND COOLED MASH	AMOUNT OF S.F. MIX 66 BY MEASURE OR WEIGHT
1 lb	1½ tablespoons (11 gm)
2 lb	3 tablespoons (22 gm)
5 lb	½ cup (64 gm)
10 lb	1 cup (¼ lb)
20 lb	2 cups (½ lb)

PROCEDURE

1. Weigh out carefully the desired amount of cooked mash.

2. Weight out the drug on a sensitive balance in the amount of 2 percent of the weight of the cooked mash.

3. Sprinkle the dry S.F. Mix 66 over the surface of the mash in a large mixing vessel. Ingredients should be mixed thoroughly until the antibiotic is completely and uniformly distributed among the grains and no lumps of soybean meal are visible.

4. Weigh out brown sugar equal to the amount of the S.F. Mix 66. This improves the palatability of the mixture for the birds. It must be added after the antibiotic is thoroughly mixed into the mash, otherwise the mixture becomes too sticky for further mixing. The sugar may be discontinued after several days when the birds have become accustomed to the new mixture.

Note: It is essential to prepare fresh mash daily, because wet mixtures of this type lose substantial antibiotic potency after standing for 24 hours.

mash. If the directions in Table 1 are followed, the final concentration of pure CTC will be about 4.4 mg per gram of cooked mash. As much of the medicated mash as the bird will consume in 24 hours should be made up. A rough guide is that a bird will eat about one fourth of its weight per day once it has become accustomed to the diet. Consumption will differ and the amount offered should be varied accordingly. While receiving this formulation, birds tested have built up blood levels of 2 to 15 μg of CTC per ml of blood within a few days. Levels above 1 μg per ml appear to be adequate to suppress multiplication of chlamydiae.

Other food should not be provided during the 45-day treatment period. A small supply of grit can be given in a separate group, and fresh water should be made available at all times. No additional source of calcium should be provided. A complete multivitamin preparation should be supplied daily. Package directions provide that fruit may be included in the diet of parrots, macaws, and cockatoos, providing that the antibiotic level is raised to 10 mg per gram of complete ration instead of the 5 mg per gram level that is adequate by itself.

TREATMENT FOR SMALL PSITTACINE BIRDS

MEDICATED SEED

Millet seed impregnated with 0.5 of CTC per gram of seed is commercially available under the trade name of Keet Life (Hartz Mountain). The preparation is effective in eliminating psittacosis from parakeets and budgerigars, provided that the drug is fresh (check expiration date on the container) and the full course of treatment is completed. Keet Life is now available only in five-pound bags. The local Hartz Mountain Products dealer may be contacted or the manufacturers may be contacted directly.[‡]

TREATMENT

Birds to be treated should be held in clean cages and not overcrowded; the fewer birds per cage the better. All breeding should be stopped. Medicated seed should be the only food provided to the birds for a 30-day period, coarse sand or grit should be made available, and fresh water should be provided at all times. *Note:* The administration of antibiotics in the water will not eliminate psittacosis infection from either parakeets or parrots, although they will improve remarkably.

Treated birds are fully susceptible to reinfection with psittacosis and should be kept isolated from untreated birds or other potential sources of infection. Any new birds being introduced into a treated aviary should be isolated and placed on medicated feed for a 30-day period before being placed in contact with the main group.

TREATMENT FOR NECTAR-FEEDING PSITTACINE BIRDS

A special diet may be necessary for birds belonging to a subfamily of psittacine birds known as Loriinae (lories and lorikeets), which feed on nectar and fruit in nature. The following specially formulated liquid diet was worked out by Arnstein, Eddie, and Meyer in 1969.

The basic ration is a mixture with the proportions 4/6 (2/3) water, 1/6 honey, and 1/6 canned liquid dietary food such as Nutrament or Metrical. To this ration, pure CTC is added fresh daily in the amount of 500 mg per liter (1.05 percent). Boiled

---

[‡]Hartz Mountain Products, 700 South Fourth Street, Harrizon, N. J. 07029; telephone (201) 485-5300

rice or dry kibbled dog food, or both, can be added to increase the palatability and to provide added nutrients. This liquid medicated diet must be fed exclusively for 45 days, with no other feed being given.

TREATING PIGEONS FOR ORNITHOSIS (PSITTACOSIS)

Aureomycin S.F. Mix 66, containing 100 grams of chlortetracycline per pound, is used in the preparation of medicated feed for pigeons. Hen scratch, which is a mixture of milo, cracked corn, wheat, and kaffir, is mixed with S.F. Mix 66 according to the directions given in Table 2.

The final concentration of pure CTC in this mixture is 0.9 percent. Pigeons usually eat only 10 to 15 grams of this mix for the first few days. When they become accustomed to it, consumption will average 50 grams daily. The medicated feed must be mixed fresh each day and must be fed for 45 days.

If the flock of pigeons is large enough to consume as much as a half ton of feed or so during the course of the 45-day treatment, it should be remembered that some local feed mills will produce, by special order, mash or pelleted feed that contains 10 mg CTC per gram. In two cases it was found that feed-grade CTC containing 50 mg per pound is less expensive than S.F. 66 and yields a palatable mixture for pigeons.

The price of ready-made product should be compared with the time and labor costs of preparing the mixture for a large flock oneself.

TREATMENT FOR OTHER SPECIES OF BIRDS

Finches, canaries, ricebirds, and cockatiels

Table 2. *Preparation of Medicated Feed for Treatment of Psittacosis in Pigeons*

WEIGHT OF HEN SCRATCH	AMOUNT OF S.F. MIX 66 BY MEASURE OR WEIGHT
1/2 lb	1 1/2 tablespoons (11 gm)
1 lb	3 tablespoons (22 gm)
5 lb	1 cup (1/4 lb)

1. Weigh out the desired amount of scratch feed and add S.F. Mix in the amount of 4 percent of the weight of the hen scratch.

2. Moisten with just enough water (approximately 15 ml/100 gm of feed), light vegetable oil, or vitamin-in-oil compound to make the antibiotic powder stick to the seeds in the hen scratch feed. Mix thoroughly.

all appear to develop adequate blood levels of CTC by the consumption of Keet Life.

LOVEBIRDS

Wachendorfer in 1973 reported that lovebirds are unable to develop adequate blood levels of CTC from Keet Life. For this reason they should be fed according to the directions for large parrots. To date there is no definite evidence to suggest that grass parakeets fail to develop adequate blood levels of CTC from Keet Life, but it may be prudent to supplement their Keet Life ration with other properly medicated feeds.

For additional information on treating birds for psittacosis (ornithosis), the reader may wish to contact the Veterinary Public Health Unit of the California Department of Health Services* or, preferably, a local health department.

The preceding instructions, which were kindly supplied by the Veterinary Public Health Unit, have proved to be highly practical and effective. They represent the best information developed from controlled trials and field experience. For the rare individual bird, belonging to one of the species that has not been adequately tested, that absolutely refuses one of these prescribed diets, a special diet may be formulated by following these guidelines:

1. The diet must be both palatable and nutritious after the addition of the drug.
2. The ingredients should be of relatively small particle size so that the medication may be mixed uniformly throughout the mass and will adhere to the particles. No seeds with hulls may be used.
3. No unmedicated feed should be given.
4. No additional source of calcium should be added so as to avoid the inactivation of chlortetracycline.
5. A complete multivitamin preparation should be given daily. Wachendorfer in 1973 reported that fatal cases of enteritis with liver involvement were prevented by adequate multivitamin supplementation.
6. Prolonged medication may promote the growth of *Candida* sp., especially in birds that are deficient in vitamin A. The inclusion of a fungistat such as calcium or sodium proprionate, gentian violet, or Mold Curb should be considered.

---

*2151 Berkeley Way, Berkeley, California 94704; telephone (415) 843–7900, extension 555

PREVENTION AND CONTROL

Before antibiotics, specifically the chlortetracycline medicated feeds, were available, the only effective course was the strict enforcement of a sound isolation policy. Even today, isolation of individuals and flocks of non-infected birds from any possible source of infection deserves widespread application. All too often a real disaster, either personal or financial, is precipitated by a momentary disregard of sound isolation practices. Under no circumstances should a strange bird be assumed to be free of infection and be introduced into a new flock until it has gone through a quarantine period of not less than one month with no evidence of disease. If there is any question at all to its history, or if it should begin to exhibit any of the symptoms of psittacosis, prudence dictates that it be presented for diagnosis and then medicated in strict accordance with the instructions appropriate to the species if psittacosis is suspected. Inasmuch as a positive diagnosis in the live bird can be confirmed only if the organism can be isolated, and inasmuch as such isolation requires that advance arrangements be made with a fully qualified laboratory, it is often expedient to assume that the bird is infected and to treat it as such.

Immunization

Although an increased resistance to infection was reported as early as 1930 by Bedson and Weston, attempts to produce a bacterin that would protect birds or mammals have been frustrating and only marginally successful until recently. In the 1970's it began to appear that cell-mediated mechanisms might play a dominant role in the development of effective immunity. Pursuing that line of reasoning, Page reported in 1978 on the development of a highly effective killed bacterin for turkeys. When turkeys were given two doses of bacterin by the intratracheal route or by aerosol, at an interval of eight weeks, 90 percent were protected against condemnable lesions and 100 percent were protected against mortality. Page has just begun preliminary trials with parrots, and it may be hoped that an adequate bacterin will be available in the not-too-distant future. It is exciting to speculate on what impact the availability of an effective bacterin might have on the problem of psittacosis.

IMPORT REGULATIONS

Personal pets

At this time, requirements for the entry of personal-pet psitticine birds are quite simple.

The U.S. Department of Agriculture will permit the entry of two pets per family per year. Prior inquiry about the requirements is a good idea, but no prior arrangements need to be made. At the time of arrival at the airport, the federal port veterinarian will require the owner to sign an affidavit certifying that the birds have been in his or her personal custody for at least 90 days, during which time they have not been exposed to any other birds. The veterinarian will require that the birds be quarantined to the owner's property for at least 30 days, during which time they must be medicated properly to control psittacosis. At or near the end of the quarantine period, a USDA veterinary officer will inspect the birds and, if all is satisfactory, will release them from quarantine.

There was a proposal to change the regulations in early 1979. The new regulations would not require any statement as to the previous period of custody but would require all pets to be quarantined in government facilities at the owner's expense.

Any person planning to bring personal pets into the country should be advised to contact one of the local offices of the U.S. Department of Agriculture, Animal and Plant Health Inspection Service (APHIS), Veterinary Services. Written inquiry may be directed to the Deputy Administrator, Veterinary Services, Animal and Plant Health Inspection Services, U.S. Department of Agriculture, Federal Building, Hyattsville, Maryland 20782.

Commercial birds

The practitioner who is approached by a client for information regarding the importation of commercial birds (that is, birds for resale, research, breeding, or public display) will be in something of a dilemma. Perhaps the best course is to contact the federal authorities for the current regulations. In case the client wishes a general outline of what is required, the following topics deserve discussion (Requirements are as of November 1978.)

1. *Quarantine Stations:* All birds must be held in a privately owned, government approved and supervised facility for at least 30 days. During this period, all psittacine birds must receive treatment with chlortetracycline in order to control psittacosis. Since currently there is a moratorium on the construction of new stations, the client must either purchase an existing station or enter into an agreement with a station operator.

2. *Cooperative and Trust Fund Agreement:* This agreement must be signed between the station operator and the Veterinary Services of the U.S. Department of Agriculture, and a deposit of $10,000 must be made with them

before the import permit will be issued. Legal action has been initiated against this provision, and the client should seek information regarding the current status of the agreement at the time of his or her inquiry.

3. *Import Permits:* When the client has arranged for a quarantine station, and after the Cooperative and Trust Fund Agreement has been completed, Veterinary Services will issue an import permit that will allow the importation of a specific lot of birds. On the back of one copy of the permit will be a health certificate, which must be executed by a national veterinarian in the country of export.

These requirements may be changed at any time. The client may wish to call the Area Office of Veterinary Services by telephone for assistance. They are listed in the telephone directory under the heading, "United States Government. Agriculture, Department of, Animal and Plant Health Inspection Service, Veterinary Services." A written inquiry may be addressed to Veterinary Services, Animal and Plant Health Inspection Service, U.S. Department of Agriculture, Federal Building, 6506 Belcrest Rd., Hyattsville, Maryland 20782.

DISEASE CONTROL REGULATIONS

STATE PUBLIC HEALTH DEPARTMENTS

Two excerpts from the California Health and Safety Code will serve to exemplify the types of regulations common to many state public health departments.

Whenever the director finds that psittacosis, or any other diseases transmissible to man from pet birds, have become a public health hazard to the extent that control measures are necessary or desirable, the board shall adopt such additional regulations as it deems necessary for the public health, which regulations shall apply to all pet birds whether or not of a species otherwise regulated under this chapter.

No person, association, organization, partnership, or corporation shall raise and sell, offer for sale, trade, or barter any shell parakeet or budgerigar unless such bird is banded with traceable, seamless, closed bands of standard size, color, and material as specified by the department after consulting with the advisory committee.

In California psittacosis in humans is required to be reported by law. Psittacosis in birds is not required to be reported by the State Department of Health by law, but reporting of cases is actively encouraged and highly recommended. A practitioner should become acquainted with the veterinary public health officers at both the state and local levels. He or she will find that they are happy to offer information and support to veterinarians and their clients. In California the reporting of a case of psittacosis to either state or local officials will initiate a visit to the premises by a veterinary health officer. He or she will place the premises under quarantine and will discuss the proper treatment of the birds and the sanitation of the premises with the owner in great detail. Many officers have detailed printed or mimeographed materials for distribution that cover all aspects of the problem. Depending on the species involved, the quarantine will be applied for 30 to 60 days. In the case of wholesale or retail premises, the health officer may offer the owner the option of moving the infected birds to isolation facilities, cleaning and disinfecting the premises, and then repopulating with new birds so that the business may be back in operation for a short time. Time permitting, the officer will re-check the premises periodically and is always available to answer questions from the practitioner or the owner.

As the general public has learned the facts about psittacosis, they have begun to lose their unreasoning fear and even shame of the disease. They have learned that a diagnosis of psittacosis does not result in the destruction of their collection and even have begun to accept the idea that birds from a properly treated flock may be among the safest to own or to offer for sale. This is not the case throughout the entire country, which suggests that the informed practitioner has an important job of education to do in his or her own area.

STATE DEPARTMENT OF AGRICULTURE

The regulations of the state departments of agriculture will vary from state to state according to their past experiences and their areas of responsibility. Commonly, ornithosis in turkeys is a reportable disease by law, but psittacosis in other species may not be covered. Practitioners should contact their own state officials for the regulations in their areas.

U.S. PUBLIC HEALTH SERVICE

The U.S. Public Health Service has had regulations controlling the importation of psittacine birds since 1930. In 1967 the current Public Health Service quarantine regulations were adopted. In essence, they established a system by which psittacine birds could be imported commercially following treatment for 45 days with chlortetracycline in overseas treatment centers.

In 1973 the U.S. Department of Agriculture adopted regulations requiring that all commercially imported birds undergo a 30-day quarantine in either USDA operated or USDA supervised, privately operated domestic quarantine facilities. These regulations were adopted for the control of velogenic, viscerotropic Newcastle disease. At the same time, it was agreed that medication of these birds for psittacosis control should be done in the quarantine facilities under USDA supervision. According to the U.S. Public Health Service, compliance with these regulations has been unsatisfactory, and psittacosis has been diagnosed repeatedly in birds recently released from the quarantine facilities.

Because of dissatisfaction with the current state of affairs, the U.S. Public Health Service recently considered three options in recommending changes in quarantine regulations.

Option 1: Rescinding all restrictions on importation. This was deemed unacceptable when examined in light of the upsurge in human cases in England and Wales in the period immediately after those countries' restrictions were dropped.

Option 2: Tighter restrictions on importation. This was deemed unacceptable because of the prohibitively high annual personnel and operational costs that would be required.

Option 3: Prohibiting importation with certain exceptions. This would prohibit importation of psittacine birds except for bona fide scientific and propagation research, conservation purposes, and exhibition in zoologic parks. Exception would also be made for re-entry of birds previously taken from the United States. No more than two birds belonging to a single owner or family unit would be allowed re-entry in a calendar year.

Option 3 is still in limbo, but it is in the best interests of both practitioner and client to be aware of the regulations and the pending changes. The veterinarian may then respond to an informed and timely manner to requests by this and other agencies for comments.

PSITTACOSIS IN HUMANS

It often happens that veterinarians are the first to become aware of psittacosis in a household. For that reason, in order to alert the owners as well as to protect themselves and their employees, it is prudent that clinicians know the symptoms of psittacosis in humans.

A brief description follows, as abridged from *A Manual for the Control of Communicable Diseases in California,* compiled by the California State Department of Public Health in 1971. This or a similar book should be in the library of every veterinarian who deals with birds.

DESCRIPTION

Identification. Psittacosis is an acute, generalized infectious disease with fever, headache, and early pneumonic involvement; cough is initially absent or non-productive; sputum is mucopurulent and not copius; anorexia is extreme. Constipation is common; pulse is usually slow in relation to temperature; lethargy is present; and there are occasional relapses. Human infections may be severe but are most often mild in character, and death is rare.

Mode of Transmission. Infection is usually by inhalation of the agent from desiccated droppings of infected birds in the enclosed space. This has occured in the home, in pigeon lofts, and in poultry processing and rendering plants. Household birds have been the most frequent source.

Incubation Period. This may be from 4 to 15 days and commonly is 10 days.

Immunity. For all practical purposes, there is no immunity in humans.

Treatment. A full course of tetracycline (1 gm/day for 21 days) should be given to prevent relapse. Treatment should be under the direction of a physician.

SUPPLEMENTAL READING

Arnstein, P., and Meyer, K.F.: Psittacosis and ornithosis. In Petrak, M. (ed.): *Diseases of Cage and Aviary Birds.* Philadelphia, Lea & Febiger, 1969, pp. 384–391.

Beaudette, F.R. (ed.): Psittacosis: Diagnosis, epidemiology, and control. Proceedings of Symposium on Psittacosis. New Brunswick, N.J., Rutgers University Press, 1955.

Burkhart, R.L., and Page, L.A.: Chlamydiosis (ornithosis-psittacosis). In Davis, J.W., et al. (eds.): *Infectious and Parasitic Diseases of Wild Birds.* Ames, Iowa, Iowa State University Press, 1971, pp. 118–140.

Cooper, R. (ed.): Proceedings of the Psittacosis Roundtable. Los Angeles, California, 1976.

Page, L.A.: Chlamydiosis (ornithosis). In Hofstad, M.S., et al. (eds.): *Diseases of Poultry,* 6th ed. Ames, Iowa, Iowa State University Press, 1972, pp. 414–447.

Schrag, L.: *Healthy Pigeons.* Hengersberg, West Germany, Verlag L. Scholer, 1974, pp. 35–56.

Wachendorfer, J.G.: Epidemiology and control of psittacosis. J. Am. Vet. Med. Assoc., *162*:300, 1973.

MANAGEMENT OF
OIL-SOAKED BIRDS

JAMES M. HARRIS, D.V.M.
Oakland, California

During the last decade, veterinarians have made a significant contribution to the advancement of the art and science of wildlife medicine. Oil spills and other environmental disasters offer special challenges to veterinarians.

Whereas 20 years ago little time was spent academically and clinically in the area of wildlife medicine, today interest in the field on the part of the public, government agencies, and individual practitioners is great. Many events — natural, accidental, and deliberate — have contributed to this phenomenon. Of these, oil spills, often involving thousands of birds, seem to produce one of the greatest public responses and present a special challenge to the veterinary practitioner. Patients often are presented in large numbers. Their care, husbandry, and maintenance are somewhat different from those of the usual veterinary patient.

Oil spills are an environmental disaster. The United States Fish and Wildlife Service is given the responsibility to take charge of all aspects of cleaning, caring for, and rehabilitating all affected birds. Euthanasia may be the decision for all birds presented with signs associated with a poor prognosis for recovery. Persistent hypothermia, cachexia, and traumatic injuries are some of the criteria used to make this choice. Spills involving large numbers of birds, complicated by inaccessible location or inclement weather, or both, may yield large numbers of birds to be euthanized. The involvement of endangered species further complicates any decision making.

If cleaning and rehabilitation are to be attempted, veterinary expertise is helpful for proper patient evaluation, treatment, and care. Volunteers and other interested citizens must be selected, organized, trained and supervised. The interested veterinarian is well suited to handle this job. In addition to the obvious medical skills needed, he or she must also be able to work with people in highly charged emotional settings.

The wildlife rehabilitation center is an ideal setting for this area of practice. If equipped, staffed, and operational prior to a disaster, these centers are helpful partners in the team effort.

International Bird Rescue Research Center Inc. was founded in response to a need for an organization to deal with a massive oil spill in San Francisco Bay in January 1971. This organization can serve as a model for other rehabilitation centers. International Bird Rescue Research Center has evolved into a highly specialized organization. Technical advising and training related to caring for oil-soaked birds are its primary current activities.

Since 1971, Bird Rescue has performed most of the following functions of a rehabilitation center:

1. Screen, train, and schedule a work force.
2. Coordinate volunteers' work.
3. Act as liaison to state and federal agencies.
4. Stockpile materials, equipment, and supplies.
5. Establish, maintain, and update educational and reference library material.
6. Coordinate studies and research projects.
7. Carry on research projects.
8. Prepare, present, and distribute teaching programs on rehabilitation work.
9. Supply training teams for short courses and training sessions.
10. Supervise responses to disasters.
11. Seek, obtain, and administer funds and grants.
12. Set up and maintain an adequate facility.
13. Hire professional staff and assistants to supervise and augment the work of volunteers.
14. Present papers and reports.
15. Prepare publications.
16. Work with other established wildlife rehabilitation organizations.
17. Care for and rehabilitate wildlife.

Groups or individuals starting rehabilitation projects should consider warehouses, city or county facilities, humane societies, and private industry or individuals when looking for space. The primary needs are an adequate inside area with utilities and an outside area for pools holding pens, and other specialized equipment.

The International Bird Rescue Research

687

Center has handled thousands of birds since its inception. It has responded to many oil spills, given numerous training sessions and, in January 1978, under a grant from the American Petroleum Industry, published *Saving Oiled Seabirds — A Manual for Cleaning and Rehabilitating Oiled Waterfowl*. This publication is a must for clinicians who wish to work in this area.*

Oil-soaked birds suffer from a number of acute conditions: hypothermia, shock, stress, starvation, the toxic effects of oil, and trauma. Birds that survive the acute stages of exposure to petroleum products may subsequently succumb to the resulting chronic problems: long-term stress, malnutrition, toxicity, aspergillosis, ammonia fume irritation of mucous membranes, cloacal impaction, bumblefoot, and sternal bursitis. Prevention by good husbandry is better than treatment for these chronic conditions.

Oiled feathers do not provide insulation and so allow the bird's body heat to escape at a greatly increased rate. The bird's metabolic rate increases to as much as three times the normal rate to maintain normal body temperature. A relatively small spot of oil on the breast of a bird can result in severe heat loss. Hypothermia is almost always present in oiled birds that are brought for evaluation and treatment. In addition, the oiled bird ceases to forage for food, resulting in catabolism of subcutaneous fat stores and pectoral muscles for needed energy. It is imperative that warmth be provided so that these birds can survive long enough to be treated for their other problems. Piles of rags in the bottom of ventilated, covered cardboard boxes of fairly solid construction will help keep the birds warm. Birds should be transported one to a box. Heaters in clinics or treatment centers also are essential to reduce the chilled state of these patients. Concurrent with hypothermia are stress and shock due to exposure, handling, and transportation. Birds should not be cleaned until they are adequately rehydrated, warmed, out of shock, and nourished.

HANDLING AN OILED BIRD

INITIAL TREATMENT

The recommended precleaning treatment of oil-soaked birds is as follows:
1. Clear the mouth and nostrils of oil
2. Give 60 ml/kg warm rehydrating solution *per os* (see Table 1).

---

*It can be ordered from Distribution Services, American Petroleum Institute, 2101 L Street, N.W., Washington, D.C. 20037

Table 1. *Rehydrating Solutions for Oil-Soaked Birds*

1. 2½ percent dextrose in half-strength lactated Ringer's solution.
2. 1 level teaspoon of table salt plus 50 ml of 50 percent glucose solution in 1 quart of fresh water.
3. 100 ml of light Karo corn syrup in 1 quart of fresh water.

---

3. Check birds for signs of oil toxicity: (a) erythema, (b) epiphora, (c) hemorrhagic enteritis, and (d) ataxia or tremors.
4. Wrap the bird in a diaper or rag to prevent further preening and swallowing of oil, place it in an individual container, and transport it to the cleaning center.

LATER TREATMENT

At the cleaning center, treatment is as follows:
1. Establish individual bird records.
2. Clear remaining oil from the mouth and nostrils.
3. Take and record cloacal temperature; 39 to 41°C (102 to 106°F) is the normal range.
4. Weigh the bird and record its weight.
5. Determine the extent and type of oil and look for signs of injuries.
6. Band the bird and record its identification.
7. Give 60 ml/kg of rehydrating solution via intragastric tube (Table 1).
8. Check for oil toxicity; if epiphora is noted, treat the eyes with ophthalmic ointment and clean them as soon as possible.
9. Birds with hypothermia (body temperature below 38°C) should be warmed using ambient temperatures of 29 to 32°C (85 to 90°F) and by giving warm (26°C) rehydrating solution hourly for four to six hours. Then if the bird responds, give strained fish purée or waterfowl mix via intragastric tube.
10. Place birds in pens to await cleaning, maintain at 24 to 27°C (75 to 80°F), and give rehydrating solution via intragastric tube three times a day.

The cleaning method employed should completely eliminate the oil from the feathers but should not produce long-term reduction in the waterproofing and insulating effects of the feathers. The following information, from *Saving Oiled Seabirds*, details the current preferred cleaning and drying methods.

When the oil is aged, or known to be one of the less toxic oils, birds with temperatures of at least 39.5°C (103°F) and with adequate body weight can be cleaned immediately. The others should be kept for a few days until their condition improves, and then cleaned. However, when the oil is very toxic, such as gasoline or jet fuel, all but the very weakest birds should be cleaned as soon as possible.

Rough handling will retard waterproofing. Treating feathers roughly during handling and cleaning will destroy the arrangement of feather elements needed for waterproofing.

The cleaning agent must be appropriate and properly used. Birds are cleaned either in detergent or in light mineral oil followed by detergent. Solvents such as Shell Sol 70 have been used successfully in the past to clean oiled birds. However, solvents are both difficult to use correctly and hazardous to the health and safety of volunteers. Consequently, the U.S. Fish and Wildlife Service does not permit their use in volunteer bird treatment operations.

Fortunately some detergents, such as Lux Liquid Amber (Lever Brothers), if used correctly, can effectively remove most oils from a bird's feathers. The effective concentration of the detergent solution must be determined prior to cleaning birds by testing it on oiled feathers or carcasses. The effective concentration will vary with the detergent as well as with the kind and age of oil contaminating the bird's feathers. For example, a 12 to 15 percent concentration of Lux Liquid Amber has been found effective for removing Bunker C (No. 6) fuel oil. Too concentrated or too dilute a detergent solution will inhibit cleaning. Oils that cannot be removed with detergents can be dissolved first in warm light mineral oil (55 to 75 viscosity) and then washed off with detergent solution.

Feathers must be cleaned and rinsed very thoroughly to be waterproof. Any residue of oil or detergent that remains on feathers after cleaning will retard waterproofing. Detergent residues must be rinsed very thoroughly. When all oil or detergent residue cannot be removed in one cleaning, a second cleaning is needed later. The cleaning process and proper use of detergents are described in the following section.

THE CLEANING PROCESS

The cleaning process requires two or three workers per cleaning station. Large quantities of warm water at 40 to 45°C (104 to 113°F) will be needed for preparing detergent solutions and for rinsing birds. Each bird will require from 10 to 25 gallons of warm water; therefore, a continuous-demand water heater or other source of large quantities of hot water is necessary. A step-by-step description of the cleaning procedures follows.

1. *Fill basins with warm detergent solution.* Line up three or four light-colored plastic dishwashing basins on a narrow table and fill with a warm detergent solution.

2. *Give the bird warm rehydrating solution via intragastric tube (25 ml/lb).* Select only active birds with temperatures above 39.5°C (103°F). After giving the solution, tape the bird's bill closed to prevent it from drinking the detergent solution. Be careful not to cover or obstruct the bird's nasal openings. (Cormorants and pelicans do not have external nostrils; therefore, their beaks should be taped only loosely to permit breathing.)

3. *Begin cleaning in the first basin.* One worker should hold the bird's wings in one hand (by the humerus) and dip the bird deeply into the first basin of detergent solution. With the other hand, the same worker should loosely encircle the bird's neck to keep its head out of the cleaner. The other worker should then slosh the cleaning solution with both hands up into the plumage and press it out with a flat hand stroked in the direction the feathers lie.

4. *Squeeze out excess cleaning agent.* After one to three minutes, the cleaning agent will probably become too soiled to aid further in cleaning. At this point, lift the bird clear of the basin. Gently squeeze dirty detergent solution from the plumage by stroking downward with the edge of the hand for about 5 seconds.

5. *Continue to the other basins.* Continue cleaning the bird in the remaining basins, repeating steps 3 and 4 until the detergent solution and solution squeezed from the bird appear almost clear. Several basins of detergent solution may be required. If necessary, a bird may be cleaned by the dip-bath method for ten minutes, but cleaning must be stopped and the bird quickly rinsed and dried if it shows signs of being overstressed (e.g., shivering or lethargy).

6. *Rinse the bird.* One person should hold the bird above an empty basin or sink, while a second worker uses a flexible hose (with a shower nozzle, if possible) to spray warm water (110°F or 43°C) up into the plumage with a fair amount of force. Rinsing should begin at the neck and work back toward the tail. The bird's front, back, sides, and wings should be rinsed repeatedly, as needed, until the feathers bead water and resist wetting. (Caution: if considerable oil residues remain on the feathers, they may also bead water. Cleaning must be thorough to ensure that all oil has been removed.) When the feathers have been properly cleaned and all of the detergent wetting agents have been

thoroughly rinsed out, the feathers will appear "dry." Birds cleaned with Lux Liquid Amber should require no more than five to ten minutes of rinsing. If an alternative cleaning agent is used, as long as 30 minutes of rinsing may be required to remove surfactant residues entirely. If the bird appears overstressed (e.g., lethargic or shivering) rinsing should be halted.

7. *Dry the bird with rags.* Wipe the bird with absorbent rags for two to three minutes, taking care to wipe the feathers in the same direction in which they lie naturally. Then wrap the bird in a dry rag and carry it immediately to the drying area. Drying is described in the following section.

8. *Dispose of dirty detergent solution and set up for the next bird.* Pour the dirtiest and coldest detergent solution into a waste drum or sewage drain, if the city or county officials approve. The cleanest and warmest basins may be used as the first bath for the next bird. Fill the remaining basins with warm detergent solution.

DRYING

Birds must be dried with forced hot air to prevent chilling. Drying should be done indoors, regardless of weather, to keep the birds from being chilled. Prepare each bird for drying as follows:

1. Give the bird warm rehydrating solution (25 ml/lb).
2. Smear a fine layer of A & D Ointment (Schering) or another lanolin-base ointment on the bird's feet to prevent cracking and drying from the hot air. Wipe off excess ointment with a cloth.
3. Apply a small dab of ophthalmic ointment to the corner of the bird's eyes to keep the cornea moist during the drying process.
4. Cloth booties may be made from rags and fastened loosely around the bird's legs with tape. This protects the delicate skin of the feet and prevents blistering from the dryer heat.

Pet grooming dryers (115v, 1700W) rather than hair dryers or space heaters should be used, for the latter do not provide enough heat for rapid drying. Two pet dryers are better for drying each bird, but one will suffice. Set dryers on "high" and hold the bird about 8 inches from the hot air outlet. As the bird dries, wipe it with rags until all feathers, including the down, are thoroughly dry. Drying by this method will take 25 to 35 minutes.

If possible, a multi-unit bird dryer should be used. Such a system allows several birds to be dried safely at one time, with a minimum of handling. Drying boxes must be well ventilated. Use kitchen timers to keep track of each bird's time in the dryer. Remove the bird only when all the feathers are dry and the down is fluffy. (Check particularly under the wings and around the legs.) Drying will probably be completed after 25 minutes.

POST-DRYING TREATMENT

After drying, birds should be given more rehydrating solution and placed in clean, warm pens with food available. The room temperature should be between 24 and 30°C (75 to 80°F). Birds cleaned with detergent may initially show signs of stress from the washing and drying process. They should be left undisturbed for at least two hours, after which they may be permitted their first swim.

POST-CLEANING MANAGEMENT

Following cleaning, good husbandry and rehabilitation are instituted. The plumage of water birds will deteriorate when kept out of water owing to contamination, mechanical disruption, and diminished care by the bird. Seabirds in the wild depend upon the impeccable condition of their plumage for protection from the cold air and water, and when kept in warm and dry surroundings, they neglect their plumage to some extent.

Putting a weakened bird into a harsh environment immediately is not the answer, because exposure adds to the bird's state of exhaustion and stress. Intermediate steps, such as lightly spraying the bird occasionally or placing it into a pool that is somewhat protected from the weather but which the bird can leave easily, are needed. In practice, a properly cleaned bird may be put into a protected artificial pool eight hours after cleaning and then may be put into an unprotected environment (with plenty of food) within two or three days. Pools must have constant surface overflow, since bird droppings contain large amounts of fish oils that, in still water, will form a surface film that will re-oil birds' feathers.

CLINICAL SYNDROMES ASSOCIATED WITH OILING

In the past many medications — antibiotics, antifungals, and other drugs — have been given to these patients on a prophylactic basis. Except for specific therapy, this practice is contraindicated. Future work may determine what medications, if any, are useful prophylactically.

Many birds that have been oiled, having been at sea for a number of days, may be in a state of starvation. Palpation of the keel that reveals marked reduction in the pectoral muscle mass usually indicates starvation and dehydration. It is best not to attempt to clean birds in this state until they have been hydrated, given nourishment, and allowed to rest for one to four days.

Signs of oil toxicity may be readily apparent, especially if oil is ingested, and include respiratory distress, diarrhea in which feces are mixed with petroleum, and cutaneous inflammation. Chronic enteritis not corrected by fluids and food given by mouth may be responsive to oral neomycin, methscopolamine, kaolin and pectin, or combinations of these or to antibiotics such as ampicillin.

Trauma associated with capture and with wave and sea action should also be treated. When possible, culture and sensitivity studies should be performed. When antibiotics are required, the broad-spectrum types seem to be most useful. Ampicillin *per os* (25 mg/kg b.i.d. or t.i.d.) and chloramphenicol (50 mg/kg) by various routes are effective against a wide range of pathogens affecting wildfowl. Procedures requiring anesthesia can be handled with ketamine hydrochloride and fluothane. Ketamine is the agent of choice in almost all cases, at a dose of 30 to 65 mg/kg.

Since the feet of most water birds are particularly sensitive to drying and heat, bland ointments should be applied on a regular basis.

Accurate medical records should be kept for each patient. Weight, cloacal temperature, and clinical impressions should be noted in addition to recording treatment given.

Birds whose feathers do not regain waterproofing and insulating qualities must be kept a considerable length of time. It is during this period that many of the chronic problems develop. Long-term stress may be associated with population density, light exposure, temperature, noise, and salt. All these factors must be considered in order to reduce stress to its lowest possible level.

Malnutrition is a potential problem with birds kept for any length of time. An adequate diet is essential. Fresh or frozen fish or substitute foods such as dog food pellets and commercial duck foods can be used for some species.

Long-term oil toxicity may develop if amounts of oil are absorbed because of the bird's long exposure to petroleum products. The liver, kidneys, spleen, intestinal mucosa, and heart can be affected. The symptoms of toxicity will vary with time.

Aspergillosis is a common problem encountered in captive wildfowl. Use of bedding material that will not encourage the growth of *Aspergillus fumigatus* seems to be the most practical means of prevention. Newspaper covered with sheets, rags, and foam rubber make good bedding. Straw and hay should not be used, and all bedding should be changed frequently. Although a number of drugs have been used for the treatment of aspergillosis, none have been practical or effective.

If the bedding is not changed regularly, the ammonia fumes produced by decomposing droppings will cause irritation to the conjunctiva and nictitating membranes. Good sanitation is of primary importance at all times.

Most sea birds are used to defecating in water. Birds kept out of water will develop impactions of the cloaca. Inadequate oral fluid intake contributes to this problem. Mineral oil inserted into the vent will give relief, but for prevention birds must be adequately hydrated and encouraged to swim.

Lesions of the joints, resembling bumblefoot in domestic fowl, are frequently encountered. Treatment for these joint lesions has been uniformly unsuccessful, but prevention can be accomplished with proper bedding and walking surfaces and access to water. Sternal bursitis, similar to breast blisters in chickens, occurs when improper pen surfaces are used and poor care is given. Corrective measures should be taken and the lesions treated as open granulating wounds.

Many questions about the care of oil-soaked birds still remain unanswered. Work is needed in avian pharmacology and the dynamics of bird diseases. However, great progress has already been made in the care and treatment of these birds. Whereas eight years ago a 2 percent survival rate was considered good, present methods can, in the right circumstances, return 50 to 75 percent or more of oil-soaked birds to the wild.

SUPPLEMENTARY READING

Clark, R.B., and Kennedy, J.R.: Rehabilitation of oiled seabirds. Report to the Advisory Committee on Oil Pollution of the Sea. Newcastle, England, Department of Zoology, University of Newcastle-upon-Tyne, 1968.

Clark, R.B., and Kennedy, J.R.: How oiled seabirds are cleaned. Second annual report of the Advisory Committee on Oil Pollution of the Sea. Newcastle, England, Research Unit on the Rehabilitation of Oiled Seabirds, Department of Zoology, University of Newcastle-upon-Tyne, 1971.

Naviaux, J.L.: *Aftercare of Oil-covered Birds.* Pleasant Hill, Cal., National Wildlife Health Foundation, 1972.

Snyder, S.B., Fox, J.G., and Soave, O.A.: Mortalities in waterfowl following Bunker C fuel exposure: An examination of the pathological, microbiological, and oil hydrocarbon residue findings in birds that died after the San Francisco Bay oil spill, January 18, 1971. Stanford, Cal. Division of Laboratory Animal Medicine, Stanford Medical Center, 1971.

Stanton, P.B.: *Operation Rescue*. Washington, D.C. American Petroleum Institute, 1972.
Williams, A.S.: *Saving Oiled Seabirds: A Manual for Cleaning and*

Rehabilitating Oiled Waterfowl. Berkeley, Cal., International Bird Rescue Research Center, 1978. Sponsored by the American Petroleum Institute, Washington, D.C.

CARE AND TREATMENT OF CAPTIVE WILD BIRDS

CHARLES GALVIN, D.V.M.
Corte Madera, California

Each year more rehabilitation centers are established and more people take an active interest in providing care for orphaned and injured wildlife. Birds make up the greatest numbers of wildlife involved. As a result, veterinarians are asked or volunteer to advise in the treatment and care of many species of wild birds.

In general, successful management requires (1) a knowledge of avian medicine in general, (2) a familiarity with the habits, behavior, and requirements of the particular species of bird involved, and (3) a commitment of time to devote to the patient. If possible, it is best to seek the advice of, or refer the patient to, a local veterinarian or rehabilitation organization experienced with the care of wild birds. Many wildlife rehabilitation workers are keen observers, with much experience in the care of injured wild birds. Such people, under the guidance and assistance of veterinarians who have wildlife experience, can be part of an excellent team approach to the care of these birds. (See page 687 in *Current Veterinary Therapy VI*.

Most wild birds are protected by state and federal laws. To secure authorization to treat protected species, one should contact the local Department of Fish and Game.

The following is intended as a brief guide to the care of injured, diseased, or orphaned wild birds.

TYPES OF DISEASES ENCOUNTERED

The majority (70 to 90 per cent) of wild bird health problems are related directly or indirectly to contact with humans. A rough categorization of these problems is as follows:

1. Young birds taken from their nests. These birds are usually improperly cared for, and if kept for days or longer may suffer from nutritional deficiencies brought on by improper diet. Young birds are often brought to rehabilitation centers as orphaned birds but are not really orphaned.
2. Birds hit by cars; birds that have flown into telephone wires, windows, fences, buildings, and so on.
3. Birds attacked by domestic cats or dogs.
4. Birds that have fallen from their nests or that were pushed out by nestmates.
5. Birds shot by hunters.
6. Oil-covered birds.
7. Poisoned birds that, for example, have eaten animals that ate grain set out by local government agencies for rodent control, or have ingested lead shot, or have botulism.
8. Birds tangled in kite string or fishing lines or injured by fish hooks or other devices.
9. Miscellaneous problems: Birds heavily infested with gastrointestinal worms; birds with trichomoniasis, aspergillosis, coccidiosis, or tuberculosis; and birds with other infrequent diseases of unknown cause.

Of the traumatic injuries encountered, wing injuries are the most common, followed by injuries of the head, eye, foot, and beak.

The outcome of these disease conditions is that (1) some will die from their injuries, (2) some will receive humane euthanasia because of non-reparable injuries, (3) some may be repaired or cured partially but will be deemed non-releasable because of inability to compete in the wild. After obtaining permission from appropriate authorities, some of these birds may be placed in scientific research projects, or given for display at zoos or museums, or used in grade-school classroom demonstrations to emphasize the importance of preserving our natural wildlife. (4) Some of the healthy orphans may be re-placed in their own nest or a foster nest, where they are usually accepted. On an average, approximately one third to two thirds of the wild birds presented for rehabilitation can be effectively treated, managed, nursed back to health, prepared for release, and released into the wild again.

HISTORY AND PHYSICAL

It is important to get as much background information on each patient as possible, including where and when the bird was found and under what circumstances (e.g., hit by a car or shot). What has transpired between the time the bird was found and when it was brought for care? What treatment has it been given already? What has it been fed?

A complete physical examination should be given even if the initial injury is obvious. Take a few moments to examine the bird before actually handling it. A physical examination should include, among other things, checking the color of mucous membranes; observing for blood on the body surface, puffiness, nasal discharge, and general attitude; palpating muscles, recording accurate weights, checking for feather damage, examining bones and joints for breaks or swellings, and checking legs, feet, and body for injury. The mouth should also be checked carefully for lesions. Look for equality of pupil size and for drooped wings. Check to see that feet can grasp and wings can flap. Feel carefully for enlargements, scabs, and other abnormalities. Look for any central nervous system disturbances (e.g., convulsions, rapid blinking, loss of equilibrium, involuntary flapping, vocalization, or nystagmus). The cloacal temperature may be taken, looking primarily for hypothermia. Temperatures usually vary from 102 to 107° F, depending on the species. The color and consistency of the droppings should be observed to see how they compare with what is normal for that particular species. A thorough physical examination should be performed gently and quickly, taking just a few minutes. In severely stressed birds, it can be done in stages or after initial basic care has been provided.

The physical examination should be repeated daily, watching closely for changes in weight, in the appearance and number of droppings, in appearance (feathers ruffled, eyes closed, seeking warmth, sitting low on perch or on cage bottom), in general attitude (listless, decreased activity), in food or water consumption, and in respiratory sounds. A medical record should be kept for each individual.

LABORATORY EVALUATION

In some cases, depending upon the disease state, the species, and the resources available, laboratory tests are indicated. The most commonly performed tests are fecal flotation, radiographs, culture and sensitivity, hematocrit, plasma protein, and microscopic smears of lesions. Many other tests, such as blood chemistries, toxicologic analysis, bronchial washing, urinalysis, biopsy, and laparoscopy, are less commonly performed but have value when appropriate.

THERAPY

PROVIDING WARMTH

The bird should be kept in a dark, quiet, warm area. This will minimize stress and conserve energy needed to maintain a high body temperature. Overheating is just as detrimental as chilling, so the temperature should be monitored carefully with a room thermometer placed in or near the area of confinement. Signs of overheating are manifested by panting and holding the wings away from the body.

The suggested environmental temperature for naked nestlings is around 85 to 90° F and 80 to 85°F for feathered fledglings or adults in poor condition. Fully fledged birds that are not systemically ill and are in good condition can be maintained at normal room temperature (70 to 75° F) in a place free of drafts.

There are many methods of providing warmth. Heating pads, infrared lamps, and human infant incubators work well if used properly.

Do not force-feed solid food to a hypothermic bird.

FLUID THERAPY

The degree of dehydration is not always easy to determine, so it is often standard practice to give a rehydrating solution by means of a feeding tube. Twenty to 25 ml or more per pound of body weight is often given initially. This can be repeated three to four times per day. In some cases, subcutaneous or intravenous fluids are appropriate. For intravenous fluids in larger birds the medial tarsal veins or the wing veins may be used, being careful to hold off the vein long enough to prevent hematoma formation. If needed, 40 to 60 ml per pound of body weight may be given intravenously over a five to ten minute period without causing pulmonary edema. Dextrose (2½ per cent) in half-strength lactated Ringer's solution will provide water, electrolytes, and a small amount of readily utilizable energy. Warmed rehydrating fluids may be given to hypothermic birds.

FEEDING

If the bird is in poor condition when first presented, it is best to warm up and rehydrate it before feeding. Wild birds may be divided into categories on the basis of their eating habits: seed eaters (e.g., sparrows), insect eaters (e.g., swallows), predatory land birds (e.g., owls), fruit and nectar eaters (e.g., hummingbirds), omnivorous water birds (e.g., cranes), and predatory water birds (e.g., grebes). An excellent discussion of suggested substitute captivity diets for the various categories can be found in *Current Veterinary Therapy V* and *VI* and will not be repeated here. To the substitute diet is added a multiple vitamin and mineral supplement that contains vitamin D_3 (e.g., Vionate®,* Vet Nutri®*). Whatever the formula, the food must not be allowed to spoil and should be warmed up after being removed from the refrigerator.

Immature non–self-feeders will need force-feeding. Some of the mature adults will not eat at first and also will require force-feeding. Most will gradually eat voluntarily.

Each feeding should provide enough to fill the esophagus or the crop (if present). If regurgitation or filling of the pharynx is observed, too much has been given. Water should be given with or following food. Gaping birds should be fed until they no longer gape. For non-gaping birds, gentle palpation of the crop or esophagus is a good way to evaluate when the next feeding should be.

Nestlings (unfeathered birds or feathered birds that cannot fly) are often fed 2 to 4 more times per hour. Food the consistency of a thick paste can be placed on a rounded stick, such as the rounded end of a toothpick, and placed to the back of the throat, where the swallowing reflex is triggered. For nestlings that are reluctant to gape, try tapping on the head, wriggling the "nest," making repeated sounds or whistles, alternating shadows overhead, or putting the bird with a gaping bird. If gaping does not occur, the mouth may be opened by gently exerting equal pressure on both sides of the beak, placing a fingernail between upper and lower beak, and trying to separate them slightly. Wait until tension is released, and then the beak can be opened. Fractures and displacement of the beak can result from rough handling. The feathers and beak should be kept clean by wiping away any dropped food. As an alternative, the nestlings — as well as birds of all ages — may be tube-fed using a syringe and soft rubber feeding catheter, the size of which will vary with the size of the bird. Fledglings (feathered birds that can fly, although poorly) are fed every 30 to 60 minutes, converting to an "on-demand" schedule later. When the bird starts to fly fairly well, food should be left out so as to start the bird on self-feeding. As the bird self-feeds more, force-feeding is gradually stopped.

In sea birds, fish may be placed manually at the back of the throat and massaged down the esophagus. In raptors, smooth-tipped hemostats may be used to grip suitable food and deliver it well below the glottis.

In time and with age, most birds will convert to self-feeding. Certain species and individuals within species may not convert easily to self-feeding, and these must be force-fed throughout the entire period of captivity.

Daily weighings will measure the effectiveness of the feeding program.

DRUG THERAPY

In the majority of cases in which drugs are given, only a small number of drugs are involved. If the patient is severely depressed or stressed or appears to be in shock, injectable dexamethasone at a dose of 2 to 4 mg/kg is given IM or IV. Broad-spectrum antibiotics often are given to inhibit opportunistic bacteria. Chloramphenicol and ampicillin often are given when no culture or sensitivity test results are available as guidelines.

Birds that are debilitated and have internal parasites are given parasiticides. For suggested empirical drug dosages in avian species, consult the supplementary reading list (Galvin).

ANESTHESIA AND SURGERY

Discussions of anesthesia and surgery in birds may be found on pages 653 and 662.

HOUSING AND HUSBANDRY

The physical setup of the pens, cages, and aviaries will vary with the requirements of the species in question. If the bird requires frequent handling for therapy, the cage must allow easy access to the bird with a minimum danger to the handler. Cardboard boxes work well as temporary holding areas. They are sturdy yet soft and when damaged or soiled can be thrown away. Pine shavings make a suitable absorbent material for the bottom. Perches can be placed

---

*E. R. Squibb and Sons, Princeton, N.J.

through the boxes. Perches for raptors are best wrapped with rope to decrease the incidence of bumblefoot. The container should be large enough so that tail and wingtips do not touch the edges. Failure to protect a bird's feathers can turn a simple medical problem into a long-term holding problem. Tail sheaths made from manila envelopes work well on raptors and other groups of birds for this purpose. If the wing primaries are becoming bent, move the bird to a larger enclosure. Bent feathers can be reshaped by soaking them first in hot water. Broken feather quills can be glued together with the aid of a small wooden plug between the two pieces (see Imping, p. 673). Wooden chopsticks or toothpicks may be shaped to fit and glued with five-minute epoxy glue. Feathers from deceased birds can be banked for this purpose. Pulling out damaged feather quills and allowing a new feather to come in usually works well. However, it can take two months for the new feather replacement, and occasionally a feather follicle will be damaged permanently by quill removal.

Birds that are handled frequently may lose their waterproofing owing to disturbance of feather placement, lack of preening, and other reasons. Before being released, birds should be checked for waterproofing. Waterproofing may be regained by frequent spraying with warm water in a warm environment; this may take one to two weeks.

A bird harboring a large number of ectoparasites is probably a sick bird that has stopped bathing and preening. Such birds should be treated with carbaryl or pyrethrons.

It is important that the areas in which the bird is kept be clean. Dirty pens or cage areas can stain feathers, decrease their water-repelling capacity, harbor infection, and result in fumes that irritate the eyes and respiratory system.

It is best not to use wire cages for adult birds, unless the bird is particularly calm. Most recently acquired wild adult birds tend to become easily frightened and may damage feathers or beaks on the bars. Holding areas that have sides covered with cardboard, canvas, bamboo, or other protective material are generally better than wire cages. Wire cages are usually all right for hand-raised birds.

For nestlings a "nest" should be made from a small box lined with tissues, paper towels, or cloth that is frequently changed. When they become fledglings and older, they can be placed in cardboard boxes with perches or other appropriate holding areas.

Diving birds such as loons and grebes are not used to being out of water for long periods of time and do not adapt well to hard surfaces. Padding such as absorbent cloth or crumpled newspaper should be provided to decrease the incidence of keel, hock, and foot lesions. Some species of water birds develop impacted cloacae if not allowed to swim. Sometimes merely picking the bird up will produce droppings and so prevent impaction.

Sudden noises, loud conversation, and the sight of humans can be disturbing to wild birds. Holding areas should therefore be quiet and escape-proof, provide little visual stress, and be out of drafts and direct sunlight. Food and water containers should be cleaned, disinfected, and rinsed frequently. Sudden changes or extremes in temperature should be avoided.

Two or more young birds of the same species or compatible species often do better than those kept by themselves. The birds may be of different ages but should be of approximately the same size.

SUGGESTIONS AND PRECAUTIONS

Young birds under one week of age have a higher mortality rate than older birds. If the young bird does not appear to be injured but is merely orphaned or somehow has left the nest prematurely, an attempt should be made to return it to its nest if possible, or a substitute nest can be made from a berry box and cloth attached to a tree near the original nest. In most cases the parents will not reject a young fledgling just because it has been handled by humans. However, if the returned baby bird is rejected, it should be retrieved and cared for. An alternative is to put the bird in another nest with nestlings of similar age and species.

Identification of the wild avian species is very important so that knowledge of natural diet and eating habits, migratory patterns, and expected captivity problems of the individual species can be applied to its care. One species may be able to survive in the wild with a certain type of injury or other handicap, but another species may not. Also, knowledge of what is normal fecal and urinary excrement for that particular species is important. What would be considered diarrhea or polyuria in one species may be normal excrement for another. Identification may be difficult or impossible in nestlings and some fledglings. A local ornithologist may be able to help in these cases.

Wild birds are often easily stressed. Certain species as well as certain individuals within species are more sensitive to the stresses of captivity and handling than others. Therefore, it is important to handle all wild birds as little as possible, especially those in a weakened condition.

Avoid imprinting. These birds are beautiful,

delightful little creatures, and sometimes there is a tendency to overhandle, talk to, and "tame" them. Resist the temptation, because some birds are easily imprinted, and in the wild it is healthy for them to fear humans, dogs, and cats. In birds kept with other birds imprinting is less of a problem.

Supportive care and treatment following veterinary evaluation and care is often best accomplished at a wildlife rehabilitation center, where trained volunteers can work in shifts, providing round-the-clock feeding, cleaning, administration of drugs, and monitoring of progress, if needed. The veterinary practitioner may follow up these cases by making periodic medical rounds at the rehabilitation centers or by having patients returned to him or her for periodic checkups. Owing to limitations of veterinarians' time, the responsibility of providing veterinary care for wild birds is often best shared by more than one veterinarian in a community.

Certain rehabilitation centers have more experience and expertise in specific areas or with certain species. For example, some facilities specialize in the care of oil-soaked birds. Others deal primarily with land birds, while some specialize in the care and rehabilitation of raptors. As more and more wildlife rehabilitation organizations come into existence, it is important that they work together in a spirit of cooperation, exchanging knowledge, experiences, and ideas.

Establish a good, mutually beneficial working relationship with the rehabilitation agencies in your area.

SAFETY

Certain species of wild birds can be dangerous to work with. The most notable examples are the raptors, whose talons can inflict serious damage and whose beaks are powerful and sharp and can rip their handler's flesh. Birds with long, pointed bills, such as egrets and grebes, can easily poke out a person's eye, and even a gull's beak can break the skin easily. These birds can strike quickly and unexpectedly. It is best to hold birds at or below waist level, away from the eyes.

It is important to wash your hands after handling birds or cleaning their cages or pens and to clean and treat all cuts and scratches received. For both the animal handler's and the bird's sake, work carefully, use gloves when needed, wear protective goggles when needed,

have adequate assistance, and think out loud so that the assistant knows what to do and when.

REHABILITATION AND RELEASE

The goal should be to rehabilitate birds and prepare them for release as soon as possible. Young birds should be completely self-feeding for a minimum of two weeks before release. The bird should have daily flying practice and be good at it. It should have had sessions to familiarize it with the outdoors — sun, shade, grass, trees, outside noises, and so on. It should have had a minimum of five to seven days of 24-hour acclimatization to outdoor temperatures. The bird should be shy of dogs, cats, and humans and should not like to be held or touched. Placing the bird in an aviary with other wild birds of appropriate species and with minimal human contact helps it to become "wild." As far as it can be determined, the bird should be in good health, including good weight for age and normal stools and feathers.

The release site should be as far as possible from places where it can encounter humans. A suitable area for release will be a natural habitat for that species and there should be other birds of the same species nearby. The local Audubon Society may be consulted for advice on release sites.

CONCLUSION

In rehabilitation a great deal is still experimental, and more than one approach to a given problem may be effective. The degree of success depends upon the types of birds and their injuries as well as upon the experience of the wildlife workers and veterinarians involved.

The effort is worthwhile and contributes to the continued presence of wild birds in our countryside.

SUPPLEMENTAL READING

Cucuel, J. P. E.: Husbandry of captive wild birds. In Kirk, R. W. (ed.): *Current Veterinary Therapy* V. Philadelphia, W. B. Saunders Co., 1974.

Detrick, J. F., and Raff, M. I.: Husbandry of captive wild birds. In Kirk, R. W. (ed.): *Current Veterinary Therapy* VI. Philadelphia, W. B. Saunders Co., 1977, pp. 687–693.

Fowler, M. E. (ed.): *Zoo and Wild Animal Medicine.* Philadelphia, W. B. Saunders Co., 1978.

Petrak, M. I. (ed.): *Diseases of Cage and Aviary Birds.* Philadelphia, Lea & Febiger, 1969.

Galvin, C. E.: Avian drugs and dosages. Available from Wildlife Rehabilitation Council, P.O. Box 3007, Walnut Creek, Cal. 94598.

Bogue, G., and Garcelon, D.: Raptor care and rehabilitation. Alexander Lindsay Junior Museum, 1901 First Ave., Walnut Creek, Cal. 94596.

RESPIRATORY DISEASE IN PSITTACINE BIRDS

SCOTT E. McDONALD, D. V. M.
Davis, California

Respiratory disease is one of the most commonly encountered disorders in psittacine birds, especially the large psittacines. Newly imported or recently purchased birds are particularly prone to infections that are respiratory in origin.

Unlike mammals, birds do not have a diaphragm. Instead, a complex system of air sacs encloses and interconnects with the lungs. The avian lungs are semirigid and positioned tightly against the thoracic vertebrae and dorsal parts of the thoracic ribs. A bird breathes by the movement of its ribs and sternum. Inspired air initially fills the lungs, then the posterior air sacs, and finally the more anterior air sacs. (James, et al., 1976). The air sacs serve as "bellows" to move air in and out of the lungs. In birds, the glottis is clearly visible directly behind the tongue. The choana, or internal opening of the nasal passageway, appears as a slit that begins between the palatal folds and continues along the roof of the pharynx. For a complete anatomic review, a reference such as Petrak's book (see Supplemental Reading) should be consulted.

Differential diagnosis of respiratory disease can be difficult because presenting signs are usually the same. Diagnosis and treatment are based on clinical signs, physical examination, radiology, and clinical pathology.

CLINICAL SIGNS

Early symptoms of respiratory disease include nasal discharge and sneezing. The birds may seem clinically normal at rest but tire easily after exercise. "Tail bobbing" may indicate labored breathing. Loss of voice or change in the pitch or tone can occur. Ruffling of the feathers indicates chilling. If the condition worsens, lethargy, weight loss, decreased appetite, and varying degress of dyspnea may occur. Birds near death may exhibit cyanosis of the beak and feet.

PHYSICAL EXAMINATION

Upon presentation, each bird should be observed in the cage while a history is being taken. Handling a bird with respiratory disease involves increased risk; therefore, physical examination should be as short as possible. Owners of large psittacines that are mildly diseased can usually help to get the bird out of the cage. The bird is released on the examination table or floor, and the overhead light turned out. Then the bird is grasped with a towel and its head is held firmly through the towel while the rest of the body is gently cradled. Budgerigars are caught barehanded in the cage with the room darkened. These procedures have been found to be the least stressful for catching and handling psittacines. Some parrots are so dyspneic or depressed that they offer no resistance. These birds should be carefully removed from the cage, quickly examined, and then replaced. Oxygen therapy may be indicated if apnea or anoxia develop. Examination of the respiratory system should include the following structures:

Nares. Any amount of nasal discharge is abnormal. Exudates may accumulate and occlude the nares, causing crusting of the feathers above the cere. With chronic infection, necrosis of the turbinates or nasal septum may occur. Birds with rhinitis characteristically wheeze and breathe with their mouths open.

Eyes. Blepharitis, conjunctivitis, ocular proptosis, swelling around the eye, or partial closure of the eye can occur with upper respiratory infections. One or more of these symptoms may occur at any one time. Abnormalities within the globe itself normally are not present with respiratory disease.

Infraorbital Sinus. The sinus is located extraosseously in the area between the eye and the commissure of the mouth. Sinusitis may cause swelling, which can be soft and fluctuant, containing fluid, or hard, consisting of caseated exudate. Tumors can occur here as well.

697

Mouth. A speculum is needed to examine the mouth properly. Hemostat forceps work well for small birds and carmalt forceps can be used for larger species. The choana, tongue, pharynx, and glottis are inspected for areas of inflammation, exudates, abscesses, and other abnormalities. A tongue depressor or cotton-tipped applicator can be used to depress the tongue for better visualization of the glottis.

Lungs. In large, healthy parrots a faint, smooth, rushing sound may be auscultated. In our experience the interpretation of auscultated sounds in birds with respiratory disease has been of limited diagnostic value.

Abdomen. Because there is no clear division between the abdomen and thorax, any enlargement in the abdomen can cause severe respiratory embarrassment. Tumors or cysts of the testes, ovaries, or kidneys; hepatomegaly; retained eggs; and ascites are conditions that can cause abdominal enlargement.

Breast Muscle. Breast muscle atrophy is indicative of chronic illness. The probability of recovery is lower in birds showing significant weight loss.

An assessment of clinical signs and physical findings is important in deciding whether to hospitalize the bird for further diagnostic tests and therapy or to medicate it at home.

RADIOGRAPHY

Radiography is a valuable diagnostic tool for birds with respiratory disease. Unless extremely depressed, all birds are lightly anesthetized for this procedure. Ketamine (15 to 25 mg/kg) has been suggested for chemical restraint. However, we have found methoxyflurane anesthesia induced with an open-end cup to be extremely safe and more advantageous than ketamine. Induction and recovery are faster and smoother, and a greater control of anesthesia is possible. Birds under ketamine may often exhibit cataleptoid movements such as shivering; birds under methoxyflurane usually lie completely still. This allows for more detailed radiographs. One cotton ball, saturated with methoxyflurane and placed in a small plastic vial, works well for small birds. Several saturated cotton balls in a medium-size cup are used for larger species. The bird is held with a towel and the head is placed in the container. Small psittacines are lightly anesthetized within 15 seconds, larger species within one minute. Depth of anesthesia is kept light and is monitored by heart rate, respirations, and body movements. If the anesthesia becomes too deep, the cup is simply pulled away from the head and room air is

breathed. Sources of ketamine and the other drugs and equipment discussed in this article are given in Table 1.

Radiography is helpful in the differential diagnosis of abnormalities in the lungs, air sacs, trachea, abdomen, and sinuses. Methods and interpretation of avian radiology have been described elsewhere (Silverman, 1977). Radiographs are useful in differentiating an upper respiratory infection from air sacculitis or pneumonitis. Lack of pathologic radiographic changes in the lower respiratory tract offers a more favorable prognosis.

CLINICAL PATHOLOGY

While the bird is still anesthetized, blood is drawn for a hemogram and serum chemistry, if indicated. The brachial vein is the vein of choice. A 26 gauge needle is inserted in the vein and blood is removed with heparinized capillary tubes as it fills the hub. In large parrots, blood can be drawn into a syringe with a 26 gauge needle. It is not difficult to restrain a small unanesthetized psittacine for brachial veni puncture, but it is difficult and even dangerous to do so in large parrots. The bird may become overstressed and even fracture its humerus if it struggles too much. A clipped toenail will produce adequate amounts of blood in such cases. Aluminum chlorate is used to stop excessive bleeding. A hemogram can be run with as little as 0.1 ml of blood, and only 0.35 ml is needed for a serum chemistry panel using microtechniques.*

The packed cell volume and total protein are the most useful tests to evaluate the current status of the patient. The normal packed cell volume for all psittacines averages 45 to 50 percent. Normal total protein values range between 2.5 and 4.9 gm/dl. From our limited number of samples, high white blood cell counts and alterations in the differential count have not been consistent enough to be of any diagnostic value for respiratory disease. Normal white blood cell counts average 10,000/mm³. Normal differential counts are as follows: heterophils 75 percent, lymphocytes 13 percent, eosinophils 6 percent, monocytes 4 percent and basophils 2 percent. Blood chemistry, likewise, has not been an important tool in respiratory conditions. However, it is utilized to assess other systems, especially the liver and kidney.

Whenever possible, microbiology is used to make a specific diagnosis. Abscesses, nasal or

---

*Lazaroni Laboratories, 1500 Southgate Ave., Daly City, California 94015.

Table 1. *Drugs, Equipment, and Sources*

GENERIC NAME	TRADE NAME	SOURCE
	DRUGS	
	Alevaire	Breon Laboratories, New York, NY
Aluminum chlorate	Kwik Stop	Animal Research Co., Div. G.W. Products, Portland, OR
Amphotericin B	Fungizone	E.R. Squibb & Sons, Princeton, NJ
Chloramphenicol	Chlorasol	EVSCO Pharmaceutical Corp., Dvena, NJ
Chloramphenicol palmitate	Chloromycetin Palmitate	Parke-Davis, Detroit, MI
Chloramphenicol sodium succinate	Chloromycetin Succinate	Parke-Davis, Detroit, MI
Crotamiton	Eurax	Geigy Pharmaceuticals, Ardsley, NY
Dexamethasone	Azium	Schering Corp., Kenilworth, NJ
Dimethyl sulfoxide	DOMOSO Solution	Diamond Laboratories, Des Moines, IA
Dimetridazole	Emtryl	Ruson Laboratories, Portland, OR
Erythromycin	Gallimycin	Abbott Laboratories, No. Chicago, IL
Gentamicin	Genticin; Genticin Ophthalmic Solution	Schering Corp., Kenilworth, NJ
	Gevral Protein	Lederle Laboratories, Pearl River, NY
Ketamine	Ketalar	Parke-Davis, Detroit, MI
Methoxyflurane	Metofane	Pitman-Moore Inc., Washington Crossing, NJ
Minocycline hydrochloride	Minocin	Lederle Laboratories, Pearl River, NY
	Neo-Mull-Soy	Syntex Laboratories, Palo Alto, CA
Nystatin	Mycostatin	E.R. Squibb & Sons, Princeton, NJ
Povidone-iodine	Betadine	Purdue Frederick Co., Norwalk, CT
Spectinomysin dihydrochloride	Spectinomycin Injectable	Diamond Laboratories, Des Moines, IA
Thiabendazole	TBZ	Merck Animal Health, Rahway, N.J.
Triamcinolone acetonide	Vetalog	E.R. Squibb & Sons, Princeton, NJ
Tylosin plus vitamins	Tylan Plus Vitamins	Elanco Products Co., Indianapolis, IN
Vitamin A	Injacom	Roche Laboratories, Nutley, NJ
Vitamins (water-soluble)	Headstart Vitamins	Whitmoyer Laboratories, Horsham, PA
	EQUIPMENT	
Infant feeding tube	Cutter-Resiflex Infant Feeding Tube	Cutter Laboratories, Berkeley, CA
Microcautery unit	Accu-Temp Cautery	Concept, Inc., Clearwater, FL
Nebulizer (disposable)	Inspiron Nebulizer	C.R. Bard, Upland, CA

pharyngeal exudate, sinus aspirations, and tracheal washes are all sources for culture. Antibiotic sensitivity is essential for instituting proper therapy in bacterial infections. Smears can be stained either with Gram's stain or new methylene blue and examined microscopically. Histopathologic study becomes necessary when tumors, avian pox, or hypovitaminosis A is suspected.

When all diagnostic procedures are completed, the bird is placed in a small cardboard box in a darkened room for recovery. The mouth and pharynx should be checked first for excess mucus or fluid from passive regurgitation from the crop, which could cause asphyxiation in the sedated, recumbent bird. If present, mucus or fluid should be swabbed out. Most birds are able to perch in 15 minutes. Total anesthesia time averages less than 15 minutes.

In summary, evaluation of the results of diagnostic procedures helps determine the etiology and type of respiratory disease present and the need for specific therapy.

HOSPITALIZATION TECHNIQUES

Hospitalized birds are kept at a temperature of 80 to 90° F. Budgerigars, cockatiels, and lovebirds are transferred to small cages that are placed in an incubator. Human incubators or improvised models work well. Large psittacines are kept in standard parrot-size cages. Large-diameter perches are set up in dog cages for macaws. If the temperature of the room cannot be raised to at least 80° F, heat lamps are utilized to elevate the cage temperature.

It is important to record the weight of each bird daily. Even though a bird appears to be eating adequate amounts, if its weight is decreasing then tube feeding is necessary. A formula described by Lafeber, of Gevral Protein mixed in a ratio of three to one (weight per volume) with Neo-Mull-Soy, is fed. A no. 8 French infant feeding tube is used on all psittacines except macaws; a no. 10 French size works best on these species. Large parrots require a speculum to pass the tube, but small species do not. Accidental passage of a tube into the trachea of a large parrot, though unlikely, can occur. Birds are fed the following amounts twice daily:

budgerigars	1 ml
lovebirds	2 ml
cockatiels	2–3 ml
conures	5 ml
average parrot	10–15 ml
large parrot	15–20 ml
macaw	20–40 ml

Water-soluble vitamins are added to the drinking water of all birds.† They are given a seed diet, supplemented with vegetables and fruits.

Nebulization has become a routine part of therapy for all birds hospitalized with respiratory disease. Inexpensive plastic disposable nebulizers are commonly used at many human hospitals and are obtainable from them.‡ An adapter may be needed to connect these units to an oxygen source. If properly cleaned and cared for, a unit can last more than a year, even with heavy use.

For the past year the author has been employing for all respiratory cases an antibiotic nebulization solution that was originally formulated by Lafeber. The ingredients are as follows:

AMOUNT	INGREDIENT	ACTION
1 pint	Dimethyl sulfoxide	Vehicle
40 gm	Gallimycin (4.62 gm, active ingredient erythromycin)	Antibiotic
1 ml	Spectinomycin (injectable)	Antibiotic
14 ml	Dexamethasone	Anti-inflammatory agent

Birds are nebulized daily during hospitalization. They are placed in a covered ten-gallon aquarium, and the chamber is kept fogged for one hour. The use of other types of antibiotic solutions has been described previously. (Lafeber, 1973). Although it is difficult to assess the value of nebulization, most birds appear to benefit from it. Nebulization is almost always used in conjunction with parenteral antibiotics.

ETIOLOGIC AGENTS OF RESPIRATORY DISEASES

HYPOVITAMINOSIS

Hypovitaminosis A, accompanied by secondary bacterial infection, is a common respiratory condition of large psittacines that causes sinusitis. It does not seem to be a problem in smaller species. Stress and poor diet are predisposing factors. Birds recently moved from quarantine stations to pet stores and from there to a new owner are especially prone. The diet of many psittacines kept as pets consists wholly of seeds, especially sunflower seeds and peanuts. Parrots can become habituated to seeds, eating nothing else. Many clients have the wrong belief that this is an adequate diet for their birds. In fact, an all-seed diet is very low in vitamin 'A.

Hypovitaminosis A causes squamous metaplasia of columnar and cuboidal epithelial surfaces in the respiratory tract. The protective ciliary layer of the respiratory tract is lost as well. These changes predispose the respiratory tract to secondary infection.

Early clinical lesions include minute oropharyngeal plaques (1 mm in diameter) that coalesce to form cysts (2 to 4 mm in diameter). These cysts may become infected, forming abscesses that can be found along the border of the choana, at the base of the tongue, around the glottis and, rarely, in the soft palate. Distortions of the glottis due to swelling may cause dyspnea.

Treatment includes lancing and curettage of all abscesses and swabbing of the cavities with iodine. Light anesthesia is recommended for this procedure. For optimal therapy, the exudate should be cultured and antibiotic sensitivity determined. Birds are generally hospitalized for at least one week and treated with parenteral antibiotics and nebulization. Antibiotic therapy should be continued for at least three weeks. Vitamin A therapy is indicated. Vitamin A (100,000 units repositol vitamin A/ml) is injected at a dose of 0.01 ml/100 grams of body weight. The daily requirement in psittacines is 0.21 IU/gram. Water-soluble vitamins are supplied in the drinking water. At home, the diet should offer variety. Fresh green vegetables, fruits, and table foods are recommended to supplement parrot mix.

More than 50 percent of the cases we see require lancing and curettage a second or even a third time, at weekly intervals. Complete recovery time is often prolonged, but most cases will respond favorably.

BACTERIAL INFECTIONS

A multitude of organisms cause disease in the respiratory tract. The most frequently cultured organisms include *Pseudomonas aeruginosa*, *Escherichia coli*, and *Pasteurella* sp. Less frequently cultured organisms include *Staphylococcus aureus*, *Proteus vulgaris*, *Klebsiella* sp., and *Streptococcus* sp. Rarely, *Salmonella* sp.

---

† ½ ml vitamin powder mixed with 1 pint water.
‡ Inquire at a local hospital.

has been isolated from the lung in a septicemic patient. *Mycoplasma*, including the pleuro-pneumonia-like organisms (PPLO), has been incriminated as a primary pathogen in sinusitis in poultry, but the organism is rarely cultured from cage birds. Gram-negative organisms occur secondarily to PPLO. *Mycobacterium avian* has been cultured from the lung, but infection in psittacines primarily involves the liver and alimentary system.

Upper respiratory infections are often caused by bacteria; a clinical diagnosis of sinusitis is commonly made. Clinical signs include rhinitis, sneezing, blepharitis, and conjunctivitis. Swelling and loss of feathers may occur around the eyes or over the area of the infraorbital sinus. If symptoms are mild, such birds are often treated on an outpatient basis. Therapy includes antibiotics, which are dispensed for home use. Ideally, medication should be placed directly into the bird's mouth, but unfortunately many people are unable to do this. In such cases antibiotics must be added to the drinking water.

The initial drugs of choice include tylosin plus vitamins (400 mg of active ingredient [1 level teaspoon] added to 5 ounces of drinking water), erythromycin (450 mg of active ingredient [1 level teaspoon] added to one pint of water), and chroamphenicol palmitate (150 mg/5 ml; 20 drops added to 1 ounce of drinking water).

If the owner can medicate the bird directly, then choramphenicol palmitate (150 mg/5 ml), given orally at a dosage of 1 drop four times daily (q.i.d.) for a budgerigar and 6 to 8 drops q.i.d. for a parrot weighing 300 to 500 grams is dispensed. Minocycline hydrochloride syrup (10 mg/ml), which is a semisynthetic derivative of tetracycline, has also been used. The dosage is 30 mg/kg, twice daily.

If a favorable response to medication is not achieved within seven to ten days, or the condition worsens, the bird should be re-evaluated and appropriate diagnostic tests, including culture and sensitivity, should be performed. If the bird is hospitalized, antibiotics are given parenterally.

For birds hospitalized with respiratory disease, gentamicin (50 mg/ml) and chloramphenicol sodium succinate (100 mg/ml) are the most frequently selected drugs, based on culture and sensitivity testing. These drugs are given intramuscularly in the breast. Unless the bird's condition is extremely depressed, gentamicin is usually given while awaiting culture results. The dose is 0.5 mg (0.01 ml) per 30 grams of body weight once daily for eight days. A transitory polyuria has been observed during gentamicin therapy. If indicated, a second eight-day course of therapy can be repeated after a one-

week interval. The dosage for chloramphenicol succinate is 5 mg (0.05 ml) per 30 grams of body weight, twice daily.

Inspissated pus may collect in the infraorbital sinus, making surgical intervention necessary. Exudates may also collect in the subcutaneous tissues supraorbitally. Adequate drainage is difficult because exudate is rarely liquified. A no. 15 scalpel blade is used to incise the skin directly over the swelling; the exudate is curetted out, and the sinus is lavaged with irrigation fluid. Excessive bleeding may occur. Hemostasis is obtained by direct pressure, application of aluminum chlorate, or use of a hand-held, disposable opthalmic microcautery unit.

A technique for infusion and lancing of the infraorbital sinus that allows for drainage and facilitates lavage has been described by Lafeber. For infusion, a needle is inserted at the commissure of the beak and directed upward, parallel to the head, under the zygomatic bone, midway between the orbit and nares. The injection depth should not exceed 2 mm. From 0.1 to 0.3 ml of irrigation fluid will fill the sinus cavities of a budgerigar. Since the sinus cavities of psittacines are continuous, fluid will exit from both nostrils.

Irrigation fluids have included antibiotic solutions consisting of ophthalmic gentamicin or chloramphenicol diluted half and half with sterile water; povidone-iodine solution, 5 drops in 1 ml of sterile water; and sterile saline.

The sinus lancing site is the same as for infusion. A no. 11 scalpel blade is used to incise the skin. Iris scissors can make a blunt opening in the sinus 3 to 4 mm wide. Antibiotic solutions or ointments can be used to infuse the sinus daily, until inflammation and exudates are controlled.

For chronic rhinitis, ophthalmic antibiotic solutions used as nose drops, applied three times daily, are beneficial.

Except in cases of aspergillosis, air sacculitis is usually bacterial in origin. The normally clear, serous lining of the air sacs undergoes a marked inflammatory response, appearing cloudy upon gross examination. In some instances caseated exudate accumulates and causes consolidation within an air sac. The clinical signs of air sacculitis are not always spectacular, even when consolidation is present. The bird may seem clinically normal at rest. When stressed, however, respirations become deeper than normal, requiring more effort, and are accelerated. Rhinitis and sneezing can occur. As the disease progresses, breathing may be labored all the time. A chronically ill bird will sit with its abdomen on the perch and its head extended, breathing hard.

True pneumonic conditions often are part of

systemic involvement by a septicemic disease. Besides respiratory distress, symptoms are like those of a depressed bird that keeps nodding off to sleep. Such a bird sits huddled on the cage floor with its head drooped, rocking back and forth with each respiration.

Diagnosis of air sacculitis and pneumonitis is based on clinical signs and radiology. Culture and sensitivity testing is important so that proper therapy can be instituted. If no exudation is present, a tracheal wash should be taken for culture. Antibiotic treatment for lower respiratory tract infections should be continued for at least three weeks. Pneumonitis responds poorly to therapy, because advanced disease is usually present before a diagnosis is made.

Non-specific respiratory signs can occur in psittacines with chlamydiosis. These may include ocular or nasal discharge and dyspnea due to fibrinous air sacculitis. Gradual weight loss and green polyuria are common signs. Diagnosis and treatment are discussed elsewhere. Psittacosis is a reportable disease.

FUNGAL INFECTIONS

Aspergillus fumigatus and *Candida albicans* are the most important fungal organisms causing disease in the respiratory tract.

Aspergillus fumigatus is a ubiquitous, opportunistic organism. Seeds, chaff, musty hay, straw, and other dusty material are sources of spores. Weak, debilitated, stressed birds are highly susceptible to aspergillosis because of their decreased resistance. Lesions are usually confined to the lungs and air sacs but may occur in the sinuses and oropharynx. Grossly, aspergillus organisms can appear as a filamentous, cottony "mold" in the air sacs or as yellow, caseated masses, one to ten mm in diameter. The course of the disease is chronic. Labored breathing is a common sign, but some birds may show only weight loss and depression. Aspergillosis should always be highly suspected in newly imported or recently purchased birds showing these signs.

Ante mortem diagnosis is difficult. Radiographs may reveal plaques or small densities in the lungs or air sacs, but this is only suggestive and not specific for aspergillosis. A diagnosis can be made from culture or by visualization of fungal elements in direct smears of tracheal aspirations or pharyngeal plaques.

Treatment is usually unsuccessful, but amphotericin B in combination with broad-spectrum antibiotics has been suggested. Amphotericin B (25 mg) in 15 ml of Alevaire is nebulized into a darkened chamber for four hours daily until there is a remission of clinical signs. Additionally, amphotericin B can be given by intratracheal injection. With the bird held upright, the mouth is opened and a blunt 18 or 20 gauge needle on a 3 ml syringe is introduced into the glottis. About half of the dose is injected with the bird tipped to the right and the other half with the bird tipped to the left to insure proper distribution of the drug. The injection mixture consists of amphotericin B (1 mg/kg) and chloramphenicol (50 mg/kg) given once daily until the bird is asymptomatic for 48 hours. Total volume injected should not exceed 3 ml/kg. Saline is used as a diluent. Gentamicin (5 mg/kg) can be substituted for chloramphenicol (Redig, 1978).

Candida albicans primarily affects the crop and esophagus. Patches of whitish, dead epithelium are seen in the mouth and can be scraped from the mucous membranes. Inflammation and exudation can directly affect the glottis and cause respiratory distress. In one instance, a Candida organism was isolated from a necrotic, granulomatous focus in the lung.

The organism is easily cultured and identified in direct smears as single oval cells (5 microns in diameter) that bud. In some instances these develop into chains or hyphae. Satisfactory treatment has been achieved with nystatin. For a budgerigar or cockatiel, 0.1 to 0.3 ml of an oral suspension (100,000 units/ml) is given two to three times daily directly into the mouth or via a stomach tube into the crop.

VIRAL INFECTIONS

Avian pox has been reported in small psittacines, although it is much more likely to be seen in canaries, pigeons, and raptors. In an outbreak involving lovebirds, the presenting signs included a chronic unilateral or bilateral blepharitis. Sinusitis may occur secondarily from opportunistic bacteria. Histologic examination of necrotic eyelids or scabs will reveal epithelial cells containing granular, eosinophilic, intracytoplasmic inclusion bodies. Treatment is aimed at controlling secondary bacterial infection. There is no specific antiviral therapy.

Newcastle disease is a highly contagious, multistrain viral disease affecting most avian species. The numerous strains of Newcastle disease produce variations in pathogenicity and organ specificity. Velogenic, viscerotropic Newcastle disease (VVND) is an extremely virulent form; an outbreak in California in 1971 was traced to the importation of psittacine birds. Early clinical signs include ocular discharge, sneezing, and varying degrees of respiratory difficulty, not unlike the signs of other respiratory diseases. Within a few days, however, neurologic signs including incoordination, depression, paralysis, and torticollis occur. In epidemics of VVND, birds of nearly all orders succumb. Signs and lesions are not pathognomonic. Virus isolation by state or federal laboratories is the only acceptable diagnostic technique.

PARASITIC INFESTATIONS

Sternostoma tracheacolum is the only true pathogenic mite described as occurring in the respiratory system of canaries, budgerigars and, rarely, other psittacines. Mites occur in all parts of the respiratory system. Varying degrees of respiratory distress and loss of condition occur. Clinical descriptions include sneezing, clicking, wheezing, and gasping in an effort to clear the mouth and trachea of mucus. Secondary bacterial infections occur in light of decreased resistance. Death is the usual outcome within a month of the onset of signs. The entire life cycle of the mite is within the respiratory tract. Parents may infest nestlings while feeding via regurgitation.

A diagnosis is dependent upon visualization of mites, which appear as minute black specks with the unaided eye. In the sedated bird, a no. 3½ French tube or 20 gauge intravenous type catheter can be passed down the trachea. Aspirations for a tracheal smear may dislodge a few mites, which normally move about freely. At necropsy, mites may be seen moving about within the air sacs. According to Lafeber (1973), treatment includes nebulization of 10 percent malathion with alevaire for one hour at a rate of 40 ml/hr in an area of 1 cubic foot. Treatment is repeated five times.

Severe infestations of *Cnemidocoptes pilae* on the head may occlude the nostrils, causing open-mouth breathing. Distortions of the beak and cere are common. Mites are easily identified microscopically in scrapings. Crotamiton, applied to the affected areas every third day for three weeks, then once weekly for five to seven more weeks, is an effective treatment in light to moderate infestations. If encrustations are severe, débridement may be necessary.

The gapeworm, *Syngamus trachea,* is seen infrequently in psittacine birds. Transmission is by ingestion of snails, earthworms, or soil that contains infective eggs or larvae. The parasite migrates to the upper respiratory passages, where it breeds. The smaller male permanently attaches to the female, which is attached to the tracheal epithelium. Clinical signs include frenzied coughing, sneezing, head shaking, and gasping in an attempt to dislodge the parasite. Treatment is successful using thiabendazole at 50 to 100 mg/kg daily for seven to ten days (Greve, 1978).

Although much more common in pigeons, raptors, and song birds, trichomoniasis should be included in the differential diagnosis of upper respiratory infection in psittacines, especially smaller species. Characteristic lesions appear as sticky, creamy, diphtheritic deposits in the mouth, pharynx, choana, and esophagus, sometimes extending into the trachea. As a result, gradual weight loss due to anorexia and noisy breathing occur. The flagellate protozoan is identified in direct smears using warm saline. Dimetridazole (500 mg/kg) in a single dose is an effective treatment.

NEOPLASIA

Tumors of the beak, nasal cavity, and sinuses occur infrequently. Squamous cell carcinoma and fibrosarcoma are the most common types encountered. Primary and secondary tumors of the lung are rare. A recent report describes a case of squamous cell carcinoma of the beak in a scarlet macaw that later developed multiple metastases in both lungs.

Neoplasia of the upper respiratory tract does not lend itself readily to surgical excision. Radiation therapy and cryosurgery are alternatives, but side effects, including burns, loss of feathering, and destruction of healthy tissue, can occur.

MISCELLANEOUS CONDITIONS

Subcutaneous emphysema occurs as a result of ruptured air sacs. Potential causes include an external wound, which can puncture an air sac, and collision with some object such as a window, which can cause internal rupture. Less likely causes include wounds of the axilla or groin without air sac involvement, fracture of pneumonic bones, and clostridial infection. Common sites of emphysema include the groin, axilla, and neck, the area over the shoulders, and the thoracic inlet.

In acute cases, maintaining an open airway from the air sac to the outside will permit the air sac to collapse and seal. In some cases, exploration of an external wound may reveal the torn air sac, which can then be sutured. If air is gaining access only through the skin, complete closure of the skin will suffice. If the condition results from internal rupture of an air sac, no treatment may be possible. In chronic cases in which a permanent fistula has formed, intermittent aspiration of air is all that is possible. Bacterial or fungal air sacculitis may develop from a puncture wound through an air sac or from the fracture of a pneumonic bone.

Obesity or lipomas over the breast and sternum can cause respiratory embarrassment directly or secondarily via cardiovascular degeneration.

Enlargement of the thyroid glands in budgerigars may compress the trachea and esophagus. The prominent symptom is a chronic squeaky noise heard incessantly with each respiration. Alimentary disturbances, including emesis, regurgitation motions of the head, pendulous crop, and delayed emptying of the crop, occur secondarily. Initial treatment includes intramuscular injections of sodium iodine, 0.01 to 0.03 ml, and triamcinolone acetonide, 0.01 mg daily until symptoms regress. Two ml of Lugol's solution is added to 28 ml water, and one drop of this solution is put in 1 ounce of drinking water daily for 14 days, then once every two weeks for maintenance therapy.

SUPPLEMENTAL READING

Altman, R. B.: Palatine and lingual abscesses in large psittacine birds. Presented at the American Association of Zoo Veterinarian's annual meeting, 1976

Altman, R. B.: Respiratory diseases of psittacine birds. Biweekly Small Animal Update Series, Vol. I, no. 10, Princeton, N.J., 1977.

Altman, R. B.: Respiratory system diseases. In Fowler, M. E. (Ed): Zoo and Wild Animal Medicine. Philadelphia, W. B. Saunders Co., 1978, pp. 389–391.

Arnall, L., and Keymer, I. F.: Bird Diseases. Neptune, N.J.: T.F.H. Publications, 1975.

Greve, J. H.: Parasitic diseases. In Fowler, M. E. (ed.): Zoo and Wild Animal Medicine. Philadelphia, W. B. Saunders Co., 1978, p. 379.

James, A. E., Hutchins, G., Bush, M., and Natajao, T. K.: How birds breathe: Correlation of radiographic with anatomical and pathological studies. J. Am. Vet. Radiol. Soc., 17:77, 1976.

Lafeber, T. J.: Respiratory diseases. Vet. Clin. North Am., 3:199, 1973.

Petrak, M. L. (ed.): Diseases of Cage and Aviary Birds. Philadelphia, Lea & Febiger, 1969.

Redig, P.: Mycotic infections of birds of prey. In Fowler, M. E. (ed.): Zoo and Wild Animal Medicine. Philadelphia, W. B. Saunders Co., 1978, p. 274.

Silverman, S.: Avian radiographic technique and interpretation. In Kirk, R. W. (ed.): Current Veterinary Therapy VI. Philadelphia, W. B. Saunders Co., 1977, pp. 671–764.

ACUTE AVIAN HERPESVIRUS INFECTIONS

DAVID L. GRAHAM, D.V.M.
Ames, Iowa

Acutely fatal herpesvirus infections occur in parrots, pigeons, owls, falcons, and hawks. The clinical course of these infections is relatively short; the signs of illness are non-specific, and clinical diagnosis is thus difficult. Bacterial septicemias, acute toxicoses, Newcastle disease, and chlamydiosis should be included among the differential diagnoses. There is, at present, no effective therapy, nor are there commercially available vaccines. Prevention and control of these diseases in captive bird populations require a management rationale based upon an understanding of their epizootiology.

POSTMORTEM DIAGNOSIS

Necropsy may reveal gross evidence of hepatic and splenic degeneration and necrosis, but it is not uncommon to find no gross lesions. Although intranuclear inclusion bodies are found on microscopic examination of infected tissues, definitive diagnosis of herpesvirus infection requires identification of the virus by electron microscopy or isolation in cell culture.

PARROT HERPESVIRUS INFECTION (PACHECO'S PARROT DISEASE)

Although Pacheco's parrot disease was first described in the 1930's, it was not recognized as an economically significant disease in imported parrots until the early 1970's.

Outbreaks of parrot herpesvirus infection usually occur in recently imported birds during the quarantine period or within a few weeks of release from quarantine. Most outbreaks occur between the months of November and February. The stress of reproduction, which peaks during this period in the Southern hemisphere, and the increased availability of baby and immature birds, which presumably are less resistant to stress and infectious diseases, may account for the seasonality of outbreaks observed in the Northern hemisphere.

SPECIES DIFFERENCES

There is pronounced variation in susceptibility to fatal infection with the virus among different species of parrots. One hundred percent mortality is not uncommon in blue-fronted amazons (*Amazona aestiva*) and half-moon conures (*Aratinga canicularis*). Other highly susceptible parrots include other amazons (*Amazona* spp.), African gray parrots (*Psittacus erithacus*), Senegal parrots (*Poicephalus senegalus*), monk parakeets (*Myiopsitta monachus*), cockatoos (*Cacatua* spp.), and macaws (*Ara* spp.). Certain other species, such as the Patagonian conure (*Cyanoliseus patagonus*), maroon-bellied conure (*Pyrrhura frontalis*), Nanday conure (*Nandayus nenday*), and white-eyed conure (*Aratinga leucophthalmus*), appear to be highly resistant to fatal infection and exhibit no evidence of clinical disease in the face of severe outbreaks in other species with which they are in close contact. At least one of these, the Patagonian conure, can serve as an asymptomatic shedder of parrot herpesvirus and is undoubtedly a common source of infection for other parrot species.

INFECTION AND CLINICAL ILLNESS

The virus is shed in the feces of asymptomatic carriers and clinically ill birds. Ingestion of infective feces is the means by which the disease is spread.

The incubation period and clinical course tend to be shorter in small species and more protracted in larger species. In budgerigars and small parrots, the incubation period is approximately three to six days, and most birds are obviously weak and listless for, at most, a few hours before death. In larger parrots — amazons, cockatoos, African grays, and macaws — the incubation period may range from five days to as long as five weeks or more. These larger species become lethargic and may evidence diarrhea during one to three days of illness preceding death. Anorexia prior to agonal extremis is uncommon, and there usually is no significant weight loss.

TREATMENT, PREVENTION, AND MANAGEMENT

There is no commercially available vaccine against parrot herpesvirus infection, nor is there effective therapy for the clinical disease.

Prevention of the disease and management of outbreaks must be based upon preventing fecal contamination of the food, water, and plumage of susceptible birds. Most severe outbreaks occur under conditions of crowding; caging birds individually or in smaller groups will help minimize mortality. Food and water containers should be roofed to avoid fecal contamination and should be washed and disinfected daily. Adequate perch space should be provided so that no bird is forced to perch or roost directly beneath another; this will avoid infection transmitted by preening of feathers soiled by a bird on a higher perch. Sound sanitation practices and the avoidance of contact between susceptible and carrier or possible carrier species are currently the best defense against this disease.

The parrot herpesvirus is experimentally pathogenic in kestrels, and toucans are suspected of being susceptible to the infection. These species, as well as parrots, should be considered at risk if exposed to the parrot herpesvirus.

PIGEON HERPESVIRUS INFECTION

The pigeon herpesvirus has been isolated from wild and domestic pigeons (*Columba livia*) in North America, Europe, and Australia. Fatal disease is usually limited to young birds less than six months old. Mortality varies from 5 to 50 percent.

Adult pigeons are asymptomatic carriers. The virus can be isolated from the crops of carrier adults, and regurgitation feeding is the likely means by which squabs are infected.

Clinically affected squabs are listless and may evidence ocular and nasal discharge, anorexia, and dyspnea.

Necropsy of dead squabs reveals hepatic and splenic necrosis and, less consistently, necrosis of the bone marrow and other parenchymatous organs and diphtheritic laryngitis and esophagitis.

It should be noted that some pigeon lofts are apparently free of the infection. Should the herpesvirus be introduced to such a loft by the introduction of infected birds, the ensuing disease outbreak would be expected to cause mortality in birds of all age groups.

The pigeon herpesvirus is experimentally pathogenic for some parrots, as well as for birds of prey. The experimental infection in parrots is difficult to distinguish from that caused by the parrot herpesvirus.

HERPESVIRUS INFECTIONS IN RAPTORS

Herpesviruses have been identified as the cause of fatal disease in owls ("owl hepatosplenitis"), hawks, and falcons ("inclusion body disease"). The raptor herpesvirus infections are uniformly fatal and have a clinical course of one to three days characterized by listlessness and partial to complete anorexia. There is severe terminal leukocytopenia.

In experimental infection by the oral route the incubation period varies from four to six days in kestrels (*Falco sparverius)* and screech owls *(Otus asio)* to seven to twelve days in larger falcons, hawks, and owls.

Postmortem examination typically reveals grossly evident necrosis of the liver, spleen, and bone marrow.

The raptor herpesviruses are serologically indistinguishable from the pigeon herpesvirus and share with that virus the same spectrum of susceptible experimental hosts. It is likely that the uniformly fatal raptor herpesvirus infections are examples of accidental infection by pigeon herpesvirus, and this illustrates the hazard posed by using pigeons as food for captive raptors.

SUPPLEMENTAL READING

Cornwell, H. M. C., Weir, A. R., and Follett, E. A. C.: A herpesvirus infection of pigeons. Vet. Rec., *81*:267–268, 1967.
Graham, D. L., Maré, C. J., Ward, F. P., and Peckham, M. C.: Inclusion body disease (herpesvirus infection) of falcons. J. Wildlife Dis., *11*:83–91, 1975.
Simpson, C. F. and Hanley, J. E.: Pacheco's parrot disease of psittacine birds. Avian Dis., *21*:209–219, 1977.

ANESTHESIA FOR RABBITS AND RODENTS

CHARLES J. SEDGWICK, D.V.M.
Davis, California

All modern anesthetic technology is applicable to the amelioration of pain in surgery for rabbits and rodents. Medications, techniques, and anesthetic machines are available to provide the entire spectrum from light sedation to profound surgical anesthesia. Many anesthetic medications are currently misused in laboratory species, particularly rabbits and rodents. The reasons for this are often trivial and self-delusory. They fail to consider the fact that because of current knowledge in the field, such animals need not endure surgical pain. Tailoring technology to the peculiar anesthetic needs of these animals is a true challenge to the resourcefulness of the veterinarian.

BARBITURATE ANESTHETICS

The barbiturates have long been the workhorse anesthetics for use in rabbits and rodents. These valuable drugs are also the most misused of all anesthetics in laboratory animal practice. They have been used for anesthesia in every technique from simple restraint for venipuncture to orthopedic surgery. They have been administered intraperitoneally as the sole anesthetic agent for complicated and difficult surgery that often lasts for hours. Barbiturate anesthetics provide poor analgesia except at very high dosage, and at these high dosages barbiturates depress the respiratory centers and blood pressure. Additional doses given during surgery to prolong or increase anesthetic effect also disproportionately prolong recovery.

The best use of barbiturate anesthesia in rabbits and rodents is to facilitate minor short-term surgery, endotracheal intubation, and vascular catheterization for more profound anesthesia and physiologic support. Preferably, barbiturates should be administered to effect by venoclysis, but they may also be given intraperitoneally in appropriately modified dosages. Barbiturate anesthetics should be augmented by local and topical anesthetic agents to improve analgesia, when indicated.

Pentobarbital sodium (Nembutal®*), thiopental sodium (Pentothal®*) and thiamylal sodium (Surital®†) are the most common barbiturate anesthetics used in rabbits and rodents. Dosages are given in Table 1.

If possible, pentobarbital should be administered intravenously in rabbits (*Oryctolagus cuniculus*). The dose can range from 15 to 46 mg/kg intravenously (IV) in this species. Onset of anesthesia may require as long as 20 minutes if given intraperitoneally (IP). There is a grave possibility of either underdosage or overdosage if the drug is not given by the intravenous route.

---

*Abbott Laboratories, Chicago, Ill. 60064
†Parke-Davis, Detroit, Mich. 48232

Table 1. *Dosages of Barbiturate Anesthetics for Rabbits and Rodents (mg/kg)*

	RABBIT	GUINEA PIG	RAT	HAMSTER	MOUSE
Pentobarbital	30 IV 40 IP	40 IP	25 IV 50 IP	60 IP	35 IV 60 IP
Thiopental	15 IV		20 IV		25 IV
Thiamylal	15 IV		20 IV		25 IV

IV = intravenous; IP = intraperitoneal.

Pentobarbital is commonly administered IP to rodents. Anesthesia lasts for approximately 45 minutes in rabbits and rodents that are not subjected to extensive invasive surgery such as celiotomy. However, if surgical manipulation is extensive, the apparent anesthetic effect of pentobarbital will persist up to 3 or 4 hours. It is sobering to consider that this observed phenomenon may be the effect of hypotension and surgical shock rather than anesthesia.

The anesthetic effect of barbiturates are quite variable in rodents, possibly because of fluctuating titers of microsomal liver enzymes that are active in the metabolism or elimination of chemical agents. Microsomal enzyme production is stimulated in rodents by exogenous aromatic volatile oils, such as those from wood shavings or from the ammonia in urine. Rats maintained in urine-contaminated cages have been known to be more refractory to barbiturate anesthesia than rats maintained in clean cages.

Intraperitoneal injection of barbiturate should be made lateral to the ventral midline of the abdomen near the left or right flank fold. The hindquarters should be raised above the head and the needle should be aspirated carefully to avoid puncturing the intestine or urinary bladder. Intravenous injection of the restrained rabbit is usually done in a marginal ear vein. In mice and young rats the ventrolateral tail vein may be used, but in many other rodent species venoclysis is virtually impossible without incision of cutaneous tissues to reach underlying vessels.

The ultrashort-acting barbiturate anesthetics ideally are not administered intraperitoneally in rodents, because the effects are so variable. The practice is not recommended except in an emergency. Concentrations of barbiturate anesthetics used in intravenous injection in rodents must be very dilute, both to provide practical working volumes at the required low dosages and to facilitate their easy passage through fine needles (25 to 27 gauge). For example, the usual 6 percent pentobarbital solution is diluted to a 0.3 percent solution (2 mg/ml). This provides 1.5 mg of pentobarbital in 0.5 ml, which is an acceptable working volume for intravenous clysis in a 40-gram mouse.

It is often desirable to prevent vascular spasm in rabbits and rodents. Arteries and veins constrict alarmingly when manipulated. A femoral or carotid artery of the rabbit will virtually close down and halt blood flow if roughly handled during surgery. Vascular catheters can be difficult to insert when this happens and may be occluded completely if the spasm occurs subsequent to cannulation. Papaverine Hydrochloride injection [NF]‡ may be useful in preventing spasm in rabbits and rodents. Three drops (minims) of papaverine are placed in 5 ml of sterile distilled water, and 2 ml of the solution is injected intramuscularly into the rabbit.

DISSOCIATIVE ANESTHETICS

The dissociative anesthetics threaten to replace the barbiturates as the most abused anesthetic agents used in laboratory animals. Ketamine hydrochloride (Vetalar®, Parke-Davis) is most effective and useful in primates. All species of the order Primates characteristically respond well to this agent, which has a wide safety margin. However, in rabbits and rodents the effects of various dosages of ketamine range from ataxia with excitement to cataleptoid anesthesia. Ketamine used as the sole anesthetic agent in rabbits and rodents is not a satisfactory surgical anesthetic. It must not be used in animals used for neurologic research in which electroencephalographic studies are made (unless the study involves ketamine) because administration of the agent permanently and profoundly disorders previously established individual EEG patterns. Ketamine may be safely injected intramuscularly in all laboratory animal species. Ketamine causes an increase in

‡Eli Lilly & Co., Indianapolis, Indiana 46206

blood pressure if used alone in the rabbit and rat. However, the hypertensive effect does not offset hypotension that occurs when ketamine is combined with acetylpromazine maleate (Acepromazine®, Ayerst) or other tranquilizers. Acetylpromazine, diazepam (Valium®, Roche), and other tranquilizers may be combined with ketamine to help control cataleptoid and convulsive seizures. Anesthesia lasts 20 minutes (or less) in rabbits and various rodents; however, there may be wide variation in response to a single dosage in different individuals.

The surgical anesthetic effect of ketamine varies widely, topographically. The abdominal skin may be rendered insensitive to the stimulation of incision, while the skin of the throat remains exquisitely sensitive in an anesthetized animal. Ketamine by itself may be scarcely adequate in rabbits and rodents for minor surgical procedures such as cardiac puncture, examination of dentition, or suturing of small superficial wounds. If ketamine is used for more extensive surgical procedures, the surgeon must tolerate varying amounts of patient movement in response to surgical stimuli.

Ketamine combined with phenathiazine-derivative tranquilizers ameliorates much of the cataleptoid and convulsive seizures seen when it is used by itself. Xylazine hydrochloride (Rompun®*) may be administered 15 minutes prior to a ketamine-acetylpromazine induction. Muscular relaxation is vastly improved. The manufacturer of xylazine cautions against its use with tranquilizers. The combination anesthetic produces profound hypotension in rabbits and rats, but such patients are apparently tolerant and usually recover well. Ketamine-acetylpromazine and xylazine as a combination anesthetic in the rabbit, rat, and guinea pig facilitates endotracheal intubation with only moderate stimulation of the gag reflex (Table 2).

DROPERIDOL-FENTANYL ANESTHESIA

The droperidol-fentanyl combination (20 mg droperidol and 0.4 mg fentanyl/ml) (Innovar-Vet®†) is a neuroleptanalgesic useful in rabbits and rodents. The success of this combination anesthetic agent depends to some extent upon a low noise level in the surgery room and calmness in manipulating the patient. Sudden, sharp sounds or too-vigorous manipulation of a rabbit's limbs will cause it to struggle, even though previously it had been still and had good analgesia.

---

*Haver-Lockhart & Co. Kansas City, Missouri 64100
†Pitman-Moore, Inc., Washington Crossing, NJ 07901

Table 2. *Ketamine and Ketamine-combination Anesthetic Dosages (mg/kg IM)*

1. Recommended Dosages of Ketamine:

RABBIT	GUINEA PIG	RAT	HAMSTER	MOUSE
25–55	25–55	22–44	–	22–44

2. Addition of Acetylpromazine to Ketamine (Ketamine dosage is maintained at full strength as shown on line 1.):

RABBIT	GUINEA PIG	RAT	HAMSTER	MOUSE
0.75	0.75	0.75	–	0.75

3. Xylazine dosage used in conjunction with steps 1 and 2:

RABBIT	GUINEA PIG	RAT	HAMSTER	MOUSE
2–5	2–5	2–5	2–5	2–5

(Xylazine is best administered 10 to 15 minutes prior to giving ketamine-acetylpromazine.):

Example:
    Combination surgical anesthetic for a 4-kg rabbit:
      220 mg ketamine
        3 mg acetylpromazine
      20 mg xylazine

The anesthetic described in this example is usually suitable for a surgical procedure that has the potential to elicit deep pain. Duration of anesthesia is 20 minutes, and blood pressure is severely reduced, but the prospect for recovery is good.

Droperidol-fentanyl is useful to facilitate cardiac puncture for blood withdrawal in rabbits and guinea pigs. The droperidol-fentanyl combination is in a very acidic carrier base. Intramuscular injections of the agent can be very irritating, especially in small muscle masses, and may produce post-injection self-mutilation. This phenomenon has been observed in my practice in guinea pigs, rats, and a fox (Table 3).

INHALATION ANESTHESIA

The domestic rabbit and some rodents have pulmonary physiologic characteristics that should be considered before subjecting these animals to prolonged anesthesia of any kind. One adaptational characteristic of mammals that burrow is a very compliant rib cage. It is probable that the functional residual capacity (FRC) of some of these animals approximates the vital capacity (VC). A normal resting respiratory rate for such an animal is very rapid (60 per minute in the rabbit). However, when profoundly anesthetized, these animals breathe slowly, with little rib cage excursion. Atelectasis, with shunting and inadequate oxygenation of the erythrocytes, occurs. The length of time such animals may be maintained in deep surgical anesthesia without respiratory support is limited.

Inhalation anesthetic agents offer the easiest

Table 3. *Dosages for Droperidol-fentanyl Combination (ml/kg IM)*

RABBIT	GUINEA PIG	RAT	HAMSTER	MOUSE
0.33	0.66°	0.2	—	—

°0.08 ml/kg in the guinea pig is sufficient for cardiac puncture.

control of depth of anesthesia. With recent developments in ventilation anesthesia machines, it is practical to maintain endotracheally intubated rabbits and rodents in deep surgical anesthesia for periods in excess of 6 hours with a good prognosis for recovery.

The simplest method of administering inhalation anesthesia to rabbits and rodents is with the anesthetic chamber. Ideally, such chambers have an inlet and an outlet so that volatile anesthetics in a gaseous carrier, such as oxygen or air, may flow through the chamber at prescribed concentrations from a precision vaporizer. A chamber that is closed, containing a highly volatile agent such as halothane (Fluothane®*) may quickly develop anesthetic concentrations that may be lethal. Agents of low volatility, such as methoxyflurane (Metofane®, Pitman-Moore) are safer for closed chambers.

When administering inhalation anesthesia for prolonged periods it is desirable to intubate the animal and apply intermittent positive-pressure ventilation (IPPV). This is best accomplished with a mechanical respiratory ventilator that is integral with an inhalation anesthetic machine (anesthesia ventilator). The lungs of all animals will accept inspiratory peak positive pressures of 12 to 24 cm H_2O. In mechanically ventilating a lung it is unnecessary, and probably undesirable, to try to approximate the normal breathing rate. It is more important to endeavor to have inhalation for approximately one third and exhalation for two thirds of the breathing cycle to permit adequate time for the right heart to fill with blood. Without an anesthesia ventilator the veterinarian may utilize a modified Ayres T-piece attached to a rebreathing bag fitted with an adjustable bleed valve. The inlet side of the T-piece is filled from a precision anesthesia vaporizer. With the endotracheally intubated animal attached to the T-piece, the rebreathing bag bleed valve is adjusted so the bag will remain partially inflated. Intermittently the anesthetist compresses the bag, producing intermittent positive pressure ventilation (IPPV).

*Ayerst, New York N. Y. 10017

ENDOTRACHEAL INTUBATION OF THE RABBIT

Anatomic impediments exist with endotracheal intubation of the rabbit and certain rodents. However the technique, once learned, may be carried out routinely by many students. Unlike animals of the order Carnivora, herbivorous animals like the rabbit can not open their mouths widely. The dental interarcadial groove is narrow and filled with a large tongue. The pharynx forms a right angle with the laryngeal structures located well below the line of sight into the mouth. The soft palate is long and curtainlike, and the epiglottis fits snugly above it. The laryngeal orifice between the arytenoid cartilages is very sensitive when touched by any foreign object and quickly snaps closed. It readily becomes edematous if manipulated too roughly. The rabbit may be intubated, having been given intravenous thiamylal anesthetic or halothane previously in an anesthetic chamber. The rabbit is placed in left lateral recumbency with the neck in maximum extension held by the veterinarian's left hand. A no. 1½ Miller or Flagg laryngoscope is introduced into the oral cavity, and the tip is gently worked into the pharynx while the animal's tongue is incarcerated between the convex surface of the laryngoscope and the left dental arcades. If the head and neck of the animal are adequately extended, the laryngeal orifice can be visualized immediately in front of the tip of a no. 1½ laryngoscope when it is entirely seated in the oropharyngeal cavity. A 2-mm diameter stylet is then introduced into the larynx and advanced 1 cm down the trachea. With the position of the head maintained and the stylet carefully held in a fixed position, the laryngoscope is removed. A Cole infant endotracheal tube (no. 3.5 French for a 4-kg rabbit) is then placed on the stylet and carefully advanced to the larynx. When the beveled fore end of the endotracheal tube touches the laryngeal orifice, the animal will buck slightly, and the tube is then gently rotated on the stylet so the edge will "find" the slitlike laryngeal orifice. When this happens, the endotracheal tube will drop into the trachea and may be tied in this position to the animal's mandible. The endotracheal tube is then attached to the anesthesia ventilator. This technique is complicated, but once mastered it can be repeated infallibly and quickly. Although it is a little more difficult, the same technique is possible for rodents weighing as little as 250 grams. In this case a 1 mm stylet is passed into the animal's trachea utilizing a small (3-mm diameter) canine ear speculum as the laryngoscope. With the stylet in place and the otoscope removed, a 2-mm (outside diameter) Cole tube is placed on the stylet, which guides it into the trachea. The stylet is removed and the Cole endotracheal tube is tied to the animal's head and attached to the anesthesia ventilator. (The stylet method of endotracheal intubation is applicable to many exotic species.)

Anesthesia ventilation provides controllable levels of inhalation anesthesia for potentially long surgical procedures. Anesthetic depth is best evaluated by electronic heart monitor. However, an esophageal stethoscope may be used in the rabbit.

Anesthesia for rabbits and rodents offers the veterinarian an opportunity to practice optional anesthetic techniques that are also applicable to other species and situations.

The practice required to become familiar with techniques for rabbit and rodent anesthesia is readily acquired by purchasing animals for this purpose at reasonable cost from local vendors.

SUPPLEMENTAL READING

Beck, C. C.: Chemical restraint of exotic species, Zoo Animal Med., 3:10, 1972.

Frost, W. W.: *Analgesics, Hypnotics, Sedatives, and Anesthetics Used in Laboratory Animals.* American College of Laboratory Animal Medicine and Washington State University, Pullman, Washington, 1977, pp. 2–9.

Melby, E. C., Jr., and Altmam, N. H.: *Handbook of Laboratory Animal Practice*, Vol. 3. Cleveland, Ohio, CRC Press, 1976, pp. 566-567.

Spector, W. S.: *Handbook of Biological Data.* Philadelphia, W. B. Saunders Co., 1956, p. 267.

Sedgwick, C. J.: Veterinary anesthesia ventilation. Mod. Vet. Pract., 60:120–126, 1979.

MEDICAL CARE OF NON-DOMESTIC CARNIVORES

MARTIN R. DINNES, D.V.M.

Encino, California

INTRODUCTION

The order Carnivora comprises seven families and 101 genera (Table 1). Members of this order are generally considered to be meat eaters; however, some (Ursidae and Procyonidae) are definitely omnivorous in their quest for food, and aardwolves are insectivorous or herbivorous. Characteristics common to the order include the presence of clawed digits, rooted and carnassial teeth, and scent glands; however, the inclusion of species that are not solely terrestrial or flesh eaters influences greatly the care and husbandry of those members of the order kept as pets. The reader is referred to other literature for the detailed and diversified characteristics of the order Carnivora (Walker, 1968).

Disease susceptibility varies among the families of carnivores and also within each family. A knowledge of these diseases, species susceptibilities, and prevention is tantamount to successful management of the pet carnivore (Table 2).

The author has seen representatives of all seven families kept as pets and is of the opinion that none are suitable for that purpose, being unable to fulfill the parameters expected of a companion animal. In all cases, the keeping of exotic carnivorous pets should be discouraged and limited to professionals who are thoroughly familiar with wild animal care and husbandry as well as with the dangers involved in personal possession of these animals.

Table 1.   *The Carnivores*

ORDER: Carnivora (seven families, 101 genera)

FAMILIES

Canidae:	Dogs, dingos, jackals, wolves, coyotes, foxes
Ursidae:	Bears
Procyonidae:	Cacomistles, raccoons, coatimundis, olingas, kinkajous, lesser pandas, giant pandas
Mustelidae:	Weasles, polecats, ferrets, minks, martens, tayras, grisons, wolverines, badgers, skunks, otters
Viverridae:	Civets, mongooses, binturongs, linsangs, fossas
Hyaenidae:	Hyenas, aardwolves
Felidae:	Cats, lynxes, bobcats, pumas, jaguars, lions, tigers

Table 2. *Susceptibility of Carnivora to Diseases for Which Vaccines are Available*

FAMILY	CANINE DISTEMPER	CANINE HEPATITIS	CANINE PARAINFLUENZA VIRUS & BORDETELLA BRONCHISEPTICA	LEPTOSPIROSIS	FELINE DISTEMPER	FELINE VIRAL RHINOTRACHEITIS (CALICIVIRUS)	FELINE CHLAMYDIAL DISEASE (*C. psittaci*) PNEUMONITIS	RABIES	BOTULISM TYPES C & D	VIRAL ENTERITIS
Canidae	+	+	+	+	−	−	−	+	−	−
Felidae	−	−	−	+	+	+	+	+	−	−
Ursidae	+[a]	±[b]	±[c]	+	+[d]	−	−	+[e]	+	−

Key: + = Susceptible; ± = apparently not susceptible or data is lacking; − = not susceptible.
[a] Several species reported susceptible.
[b] Reported but unconfirmed.
[c] Resisted infection in midst of exposure in severe outbreaks.
[d] Two cases reported but not confirmed by virus isolation.
[e] Rabies is a factor in the population dynamics and control of the wild bear population.

This discussion will cover all seven families, with emphasis on the members of each family commonly seen by the veterinarian. Regardless of the veterinarian's attitude toward individual ownership of these animals, we must recognize that they are kept as pets and may be presented to us for care. It is therefore the obligation of the attending clinician either to become familiar with the general aspects of medical care and husbandry for exotic carnivores or to refer the client to a colleague who can provide the medical services necessary for preserving the animal's life.

IMMUNIZATION

GENERAL CONSIDERATIONS

Vaccination procedures for members of the order Carnivora vary considerably. There is the problem of whether to use killed or modified live virus (MLV) vaccines. Furthermore, there is marked variability in the susceptibility of various families and species to different diseases.

Table 3 summarizes my recommendations for vaccination of members of the seven carnivore families. It must be pointed out that none of the vaccines currently in use are approved for use in non-domestic animals. Taking all these factors into consideration, my rationale for the utilization of vaccines, my vaccination regimen, and my choice of brands of vaccines stem from experience, results obtained relative to "breaks," the possibility of vaccine-induced disease, and the conclusion that, based upon various studies, infant non-domestic carnivores should be considered agammaglobulinemic.

MLV vaccines should never be used on non-domestic carnivores for immunization against rabies. Vaccine-induced rabies has been reported in the coyote, skunk, and raccoon (Carpenter et al., 1976); I have seen it induced in a red fox that was given MLV-CEO vaccine. One must not rely upon the apparent closeness of some animals (i.e., the wolf and coyote) to the domestic dog when vaccinating against rabies. To prevent against accidental use of MLV rabies vaccine in the non-domestic carnivore, I have completely eliminated these vaccines from my shelves in favor of a killed vaccine.* The quantity (dosage) of killed virus vaccine required to produce an immune response in the non-domestic carnivore is unknown. I generally vaccinate small pet carnivores, all animals in petting zoos, circuses, and other places where they are in constant contact with the public, and those that are generally unprotected in rabies-endemic areas. My dosage varies from 1 to 5 ml, according to the size of the animal. Further requirements for rabies vaccination may be imposed on non-domestic carnivores destined for shipment to foreign countries, since most regulations concerning rabies vaccinations fail to recognize differences between domestic and non-domestic carnivores, antigenicity and hence dosage of a vaccine required, and vaccination intervals required to retain continuous immunity. Some countries require a quarantine period against rabies regardless of whether or not a vaccine has been given.

*Trimune, Fort Dodge Laboratories

Table 3. *Recommendations for Vaccinations for the Carnivora*

FAMILY	CANINE DISTEMPER	CANINE HEPATITIS	CANINE PARAINFLUENZA VIRUS & BORDETELLA BRONCHISEPTICA	LEPTOSPIROSIS	FELINE DISTEMPER	FELINE VIRAL RHINOTRACHEITIS (CALICIVIRUS)	FELINE CHLAMYDIAL DISEASE (C. psittaci) PNEUMONITIS	RABIES	BOTULISM	VIRAL ENTERITIS
Canidae	+	+	+	+	−	−	−	+	−	−
Felidae	−	−	−	−	+	+	+	+[a]	−	−
Ursidae	−	−	−	−	−[h]	−	−	+[a]	−	−
Procyonidae	+[b]	±	−	+	+	−	−	+[a]	−	−
Mustelidae	+[c]	±	−	+	+[f]	−	−	+[a]	+[d]	+[e]
Viverridae	+	±	−	+	+	−	−	+	−	−
Hyaenidae	[g]	[g]	−	[g]	[g]	−	−	+	−	−

Key: + = Vaccination recommended; − = vaccination not recommended at this time; ± = author vaccinates based upon known virus susceptibility amongst members of the family.

[a]Vaccination elective based upon geographic area and risk of exposure to feral animals; degree of contact with humans; handling problems; international, state and local regulations; owner's preference; and veterinarian's opinion. Only killed vaccines should be used; efficiency and dosage of killed vaccine in exotic species is unknown.

[b]MLV vaccines should not be used on lesser pandas or giant pandas.

[c]MLV vaccines should not be used in black-footed ferrets. Vaccines prepared from ferret cell culture should not be used in any species of ferret. Killed vaccines are slow to produce an immunity.

[d]Minks and ferrets. *Clostridium botulinum* type C toxoid.

[e]Minks. Autogenous or mink enteritis vaccine or killed feline distemper vaccine.

[f]Excluding the ferret.

[g]Most literature recommends vaccination of the Hyaenidae for canine distemper and leaves vaccination against hepatitis, leptospirosis, and feline distemper to the judgment of the attending veterinarian. The author does not vaccinate against any of these diseases.

[h]Vaccination may be undertaken in high-risk areas or in cases in which exposure is known to have occurred.

VACCINATION REGIMENS

Vaccination regimens vary with the age at which the animal is presented, whether or not the animal has nursed, and the risk of exposure to the various diseases to which it is susceptible.

When protection against the canine diseases (distemper, hepatitis, leptospirosis, parainfluenza) is desired, the manufacturers' recommended dosages and intervals are the ones I follow. At present, no killed canine distemper vaccines are available. I have utilized vaccines manufactured by Pitman-Moore, Norden, Dellen, and Fromm and have had good results as judged by (1) very few "breaks" following vaccination and (2) a lack of vaccine-induced disease. After the initial series, boosters are given at one year of age and then annually.

Protection against feline distemper is accomplished by giving young felines a full dose of killed vaccine every two weeks through the eighth week. Young animals that have not nursed are started at two weeks of age and are maintained in as isolated or clean an environment as possible through four weeks of age. Normal or hyperimmune serum can be used for temporary protection against bacterial and viral diseases. The animal is given MLV vaccines against feline distemper, rhinotracheitis, calicivirus, and feline chlamydial disease at 10, 12, and 16 weeks of age. After that, yearly boosters are given. The antigenicity of chick embryo–propagated *Chlamydia psittaci* is questionable, as is the duration of any immunity produced by its inclusion into the respiratory disease complex of vaccines. However, I cannot point to any side effects by including the feline penumonitis faction. Boosters are given at one year and then annually.

Members of the Procyonidae, Mustelidae, and Viverridae families are vaccinated according to the schedule just described for both canine and feline diseases. Both canine and feline vaccines are given concurrently. Killed feline distemper vaccine produced by the previously mentioned manufacturers is utilized at a unit dosage of one extra dose per 5 kg (10 lb) of body weight. The questions of dosage and duration of immunity are still largely unanswered.

Rabies vaccines (killed, in all cases) are administered at four months of age. While no side effects have been noted when canine and feline distemper and rabies vaccines are given concurrently, it would seem more logical to administer the rabies fraction separately. A combination of killed panleukopenia and killed rabies vaccines† is now available, providing a convenient method of immunizing the small felines, procyonids, and mustelids against both diseases.

Ferrets should be inoculated at weaning with type C botulism toxoid (Ryland, 1978). This will protect them for one year against *Clostridium botulinum*. Annual boosters are recommended. Mink should also be vaccinated against botulism.

Mink may be protected against "mink viral enteritis" by either autogenous or commercial mink enteritis vaccine (formalized) or by the use of killed panleukopenia vaccine. Annual boosters are recommended. Kits are first vaccinated at six to eight weeks of age, following the manufacturer's recommendations.

INFECTIOUS DISEASES

In addition to those diseases given in Table 2, for which vaccines are available, members of the carnivore family are susceptible to other infectious diseases seen in domestic animals. Table 4 lists the susceptibilities to the more common of these diseases; however, the following additional diseases have been observed: anthrax in carnivores that were fed meat from infected horses (Foster, 1974); candidiasis, especially in youngsters receiving high levels of antibiotics; systemic mycoses; *Clostridium perfringens;* pasteurellosis; brucellosis (canids); tuberculosis (procyonids and mustelids); canine and feline infectious anemia; and infectious warts (felids). Some of these diseases that are noteworthy from the standpoint of the non-domestic animal will be discussed.

---

†Panrab®, Douglas Industries.

FELINE DISTEMPER

The susceptibilities of carnivora to feline distemper are discussed in the preceding section. The disease takes the same form in the non-domestic species as it does in the domestic feline. Treatment should be the same; however, one should realize that it is the nature of the non-domestic animal to respond better in its own environment. Treatment may best be prescribed and then administered by the animal's owner, since the animal's comfort and desire to eat and drink are the most important factors in recovery. Blood transfusions are of some value; blood from one feline species may be transfused into another, with the exception of the cheetah as either donor or recipient.

The practitioner can often prevent feline distemper by administering at least the first dose of vaccine outside the hospital so as not to expose the animal to any disease that may be present in the clinic. Often the incidence of this disease is concurrent with the presence of disease in feral animals to which the patients are exposed. Isolation of newly acquired and young animals until they are 12 weeks of age is highly recommended.

FELINE LEUKEMIA

Feline leukemia is reported to occur in the non-domestic feline and has been seen by the author in mountain lions, leopards, and tigers. None of these animals survived; whether or not a diagnosis can be made via FeLV peripheral blood smears is not known.

FELINE INFECTIOUS PERITONITIS

This disease has been seen in ocelots, margays, mountain lions, and tigers. The form is similar to that seen in the domestic cat, and the

---

Table 4. *Susceptibility of Carnivora to Common Infectious Diseases For Which No Vaccines Are Available*

FAMILY	TOXOPLASMOSIS	FELINE INFECTIOUS PERITONITIS	FELINE LEUKEMIA	RINGWORM	SALMONELLOSIS	COCCIDIOSIS
Canidae	+	−	−	+	+	+
Felidae	+	+	+	+	+	+
Ursidae	+	−	−	+	+	+
Procyonidae	+	−	−	+	+	+
Mustelidae	+	−	−	+	+	+
Viverridae	±	−	−	+	+	+
Hyaenidae	±	−	−	+	+	+

Key: + = Known susceptible; ± = may be susceptible; − = not known to be susceptible.

mortality rate has been 100 percent. The drug of choice in attempting treatment is reported to be tylocine (Elanco) at 160 mg/kg per os along with oral prednisolone at 4 mg/kg per os in divided doses (Timoney, 1976). Treatment should continue for four weeks after remission at one-half the above dose for each drug.

FELINE RESPIRATORY DISEASE

All felids are susceptible to the rhinotracheitis, calici, and reo viruses and the *Chlamydia psittaci* organism. These all cause signs of the feline respiratory disease complex. Symptoms vary, as in the domestic cat, from conjunctivitis to ulcerative stomatitis and pneumonia. There is some indication that susceptibility among the various species varies, with the cheetah being most susceptible. In one outbreak where 29 cheetahs became ill and showed severe symptoms of calicivirus infection, 50 tigers, including cubs, and more than 35 adult and subadult lions remained unaffected, although these animals were housed in the same building and although only den bars served as barriers between the animals. However, these species — along with mountain lions, bobcats, ocelots, margays, leopards, and jaguars — have been observed with obvious respiratory disease. Morbidity is usually high while mortality is generally low; more than one outbreak has occurred on an almost annual, seasonal basis in several animal compounds. This last fact may suggest infection with a different respiratory virus; new animals added to a previously affected but recovered population have become ill, leading one to believe that a carrier state exists and perhaps that recurrences of the symptoms or different forms of the disease each year are caused by a stress factor.

Initial vaccination and annual boosters have been very effective in preventing annual disease outbreaks previously seen in my practice.

Treatment is palliative and supportive in the hope of preventing secondary bacterial pneumonias and of keeping the animal in a hydrated state. The antibiotic of choice is tylocine (Elanco) at 10 mg/kg intramuscularly twice daily the first day, then once daily thereafter. Vitamins, including the B complex and large doses of vitamin C, are used and seem to be of some benefit. For many years, I used a timed-disintegration capsule, Enderm (EVSCO), containing cortisone, fatty acids, and antihistamine. This product is no longer available, but the use of antihistamines appears to be of value. Symptomatic relief can be obtained utilizing steroids and antihistamines.

As mentioned previously, a syndrome similar to feline respiratory disease is seen in otters, and the treatment is the same. Oddly enough, in a large number of cases of otters whose respiratory symptoms caused the owner to present them for treatment, the pneumonia was judged to be secondary to severe nephritis with or without kidney stones.

PARAINFLUENZA–BORDETELLA BRONCHISEPTICA INFECTIONS

One should be reluctant to think that these organisms infect only members of the canine family. Outbreaks of kennel cough in wolves and coyotes have been observed, along with concurrent infection having the same signs and symptoms among members of the Felidae family in the same animal compound. While it is only conjecture at this point, it is felt that the infection also has occurred in the human handlers of these animals. Since it is known that the *Bordetella* organism is omnipresent and an opportunist, it is possible that, in several cases, Canidae, Felidae, and possibly humans are susceptible to what is commonly called kennel cough. I include at present parainfluenza-*Bordetella* vaccine in my schedule of required Canidae vaccinations. Treatment does not differ from that given to domestic canines and felines and is basically geared to relieving the cough and preventing secondary bacterial infection. Dextromethorphan, hydrocodone bitartrate (Hycodan, Endo) and trimeprazine with prednisolone (Temaril-P, Norden) have all been used at the usual domestic canine dosage without side effects.

FELINE INFECTIOUS WARTS

I first saw this disease in 1976 in a group of mountain lions in California. Eight of 34 pumas in the population were affected. The lesions were multiple in all cases and were located on the head, lips, buccal mucosa, and gums. The affected animals, while not necessarily housed together, could easily have had contact with one another. Treatment via cryosurgery of selected lesions and lesions causing mechanical problems involving the mouth was successful in causing a remission in two to three weeks. An exacerbation was observed in one animal two months after all previous lesions had disappeared.

Warts are also commonly seen in the Procyonidae around the lips and eyelids. Most of these cases have been isolated ones in which no other animals of a similar family or species were exposed; therefore, it is unknown whether or not these are of the infectious variety.

Autogenous vaccines can be made for use against warts in any species utilizing approximately 5 grams of the removed wart. A veterinary clinical laboratory should be consulted when vaccines are desired.

RINGWORM

Ringworm has been seen mainly in the canids and felids, although all carnivores are susceptible. Systemic treatment with griseofulvin (Fulvicin®) at a level of 10 to 20 mg/kg per os gives good results if the drug is administered in mass doses every seven to ten days. I do not reduce the dosage, regardless of the size of the animal; however, in order to decrease the volume and amount given at one time to a larger animal, the drug may be given every seven days instead of every ten days. Treatment should be carried out for at least one month and preferably for six weeks, since relapse of apparently inactive lesions frequently occurs. If handling does not represent a problem to the owner or the animal, topical treatment with Tresaderm Solution® (Merck), or Conofite® (Pitman-Moore) is helpful. When a ringworm lesion is discovered, once-weekly bathing using an iodine base shampoo should be undertaken. Topical treatment with tincture of iodine may cause a photosensitivity reaction if the lesion becomes exposed to sunlight.

Diagnosis of ringworm preferably is confirmed via culture (Fungassay®). Lesions are most common on the head, above and between the eyes, and on the lateral aspects of the limbs. Healthy carriers exist, especially among the Felidae.

SALMONELLOSIS

In all families of carnivora, this is a serious and not uncommon disease. The infecting bacteria of this highly contagious disease are usually found in spoiled feed but can be carried by birds, rodents, and feral mammals. By habit or nature, feed is often hidden by many of these animals, or it may become contaminated upon arrival or in storage. Improper thawing of frozen food products may also allow growth of the salmonella bacteria. The clinical signs, diagnosis, lesions, and treatment are similar in all species of animals.

TOXOPLASMOSIS

All families of the Carnivora are susceptible to toxoplasmosis; however, the incidence of the disease and probably the susceptibility to it is much greater among the Felidae. The disease is caused by *Toxoplasma gondii*.

Toxoplasmosis can be transmitted to the fetus *in utero,* easily passes from one animal to another via fecal contact, and is also seen in newly imported animals from South America, Asia, and Africa. Contaminated meat and primarily-meat food also are sources of infection.

The disease manifests itself in many forms: Anemia, ocular lesions (retinitis or iritis), hepatitis with clinical icterus, blindness, CNS signs, respiratory disease, and diarrhea all may be seen, with or without concurrent lethargy, anorexia, and fever. In some cases, combinations of these symptoms may occur.

Diagnosis in felids is made by finding oocysts in the stool or pseudocysts in granulomas (especially where liver disease is present) and by serologic studies, mouse inoculation (Frenkel, 1977), and careful history-taking. Fecal oocysts may be absent from a random sample, and several consecutive daily samples may be required to find the organism. When a serologic diagnosis is sought, one must be familiar with the method used to arrive at a titer. If the IFA (indirect fluorescent antibody) test is utilized, a diagnosis of 1:256 is diagnostic, whereas in the IHA (indirect hemagglutination antibody) studies, lower titer may be diagnostic. Two consecutive serum samples taken 7 to 14 days apart should be tested against feline antiserum. If a rising titer is observed in the face of typical signs and symptoms, then a diagnosis of toxoplasmosis can be made. Absence of antibody or an unchanging titer is inconsistent with a diagnosis of toxoplasmosis. Since the test kits used to dilute serum samples are usually equipped to conclude a titer of no greater than 1:1600, the laboratory should be requested to dilute the sample beyond this point until no further reaction is observed. I have seen titers of 1:25,000.

Treatment consists of the use of sulfonamides that are active at the intracellular level, such as sulfadiazine, sulfamethazine, and sulfamerazine. Pyrimethamine (Daraprim®, Burroughs Wellcome), which along with the sulfonamide synergistically interferes with the synthesis of dihydrofolate by the organism, is used at a level of 0.5 to 1.0 mg/kg/day. An extrinsic source of folic acid (Fero-Folic-500®, Abbott) at ¼ to 1 tablet per day, depending on the species, and bakers' yeast at 100 mg/kg/day are also recommended. The yeast and extrinsic folic acid are used to eliminate any toxic side effects of the dihydrofolate inhibitors. The organism cannot use the folic acid, but the animal can.

PEDIATRICS

The non-domestic carnivore commonly seen as a pet animal is usually presented at a young age. The appeal of the young exotic pet is great; furthermore, most people feel that if any of these animals are to be reared in a tamed state to be kept as pets, they must be weaned at an early age. This feeling is valid from the standpoint of narrowing the instinctive flight-fright distance from man with which all non-domestic animals are born. It should be noted, however, that this heritage can never be fully overcome and that it may be a significant factor in the ultimate success of keeping a non-domestic carnivore as a compatible pet.

In addition, many exotic pets are presented as orphaned animals, making pediatrics an important consideration in any discussion of exotic pet medicine. Pertinent factors influencing the success of hand-rearing these animals include (1) proper general husbandry of the young animal at various ages, (2) artificial diets, feeding intervals, and dietary requirements, (3) common pediatric problems and therapy, and (4) preventive medicine in addition to the vaccination procedures previously recommended.

All neonates in all the carnivore families lack the ability to regulate their own body temperatures. These thermoregulatory mechanisms are not present or remain reduced during the first two to three weeks of life. Optimum external environmental temperatures range from 85 to 90° F (95° F at birth). An infant incubator or a heating pad may be used to maintain this environmental temperature; however, caution should be used with the heating pad to prevent burns, since the temperature produced by these pads is not easily controlled.

The navel should be disinfected with a buffered iodine solution, and young animals should be kept as isolated as possible from other animals and from large numbers of people. However, caution should not be so great as to maintain the animals in too sterile an environment. Except for bears, all youngsters should be considered to be immunosuppressed and agammaglobulinemic. However, routine antibiotic therapy is not undertaken. Bear cubs should be given antibiotics from birth. I use kanamycin sulfate (Kantrim®, Bristol Laboratories) at the canine dosage for ten days.

Hand-reared animals should be fed a diet of either Esbilac or KMR (Borden). Many people advocate one or the other of these two preparations; however, I have noticed no difference between them from the standpoints of acceptability, digestive problems, and adequate nutrition in felids, canids, and ursids. Esbilac is my preference for the procyonids, mustelids, viverrids, and hyaenids. Both products can be fed in liquid form, undiluted. If powdered Esbilac is used, it is mixed as one volume of powder to three volumes of water. If the animal is presented as a newborn, it can be fed after 12 hours of life; the powdered Esbilac® should be mixed with either bottled or boiled water. This can gradually be replaced over a five-day period with soft tap water.

The type and size of nipple to be used depends upon the species of animal being fed, since this dictates the size and shape of the mouth, tongue, and lips. Pet nursers (NIP®) are satisfactory for very young raccoons, skunks, coyote pups, and fox kits; larger animals may require any of the wide variety of available nipples manufactured for human infants. In all cases, caution should be exercised to prevent leaking of the formula through the nipple opening. Nipple openings should be increased as the sucking reflex and size of the animal increase so that the animal can nurse easily. An animal that is nursing well will usually take in the amount of food it wants very rapidly and then fall off to sleep. An animal that is having difficulty nursing owing to the size of the nipple will take its formula slowly, in a restless manner as though it is "fighting the bottle."

In addition to the size of the nipple opening, nursing position is most important in preventing aspiration pneumonia. All the carnivores nurse the parent female in a ventral recumbent position; this, or the standing position, is the posture in which the young animal should be held when it nurses. Support of the front limbs or feet is usually required to simulate the female abdomen, against which the young knead during the nursing process.

Feeding intervals vary, but generally a feeding of every three hours beginning at 8:30 A.M. and ending at 11:30 P.M. is satisfactory. Intervals decrease with age; at six weeks of age most animals are eating four times per day at 8 A.M., 12 noon, 4 P.M., and 8 P.M. It is unnecessary to feed an animal of any age every three hours over a 24-hour period. However, as a rule of thumb I advise the client that if an animal becomes hungry during the night, it will usually become restless and will cry, at which time a feeding may be offered. As cubs, bears show the strongest tendency to require feedings beyond the schedule just described.

Food intake varies. Some people use 10 percent of the body weight as a rule of thumb. However, many carnivores take in up to 35 percent of their body weight in liquid formula. The percent of body weight figure for food intake goes down as the proportion of solid food increases. Midday food intake is usually less than the early morning feedings. The best indication of adequate food intake and nutrition is constant weight gain. Young animals should be weighed daily through five weeks of age to determine that they are gaining weight.

The rate of gain (growth rates) varies with the species as well as with the age of the animal. Skunks and raccoons have minimal growth rates compared with those of felids and canids. Bear cubs gain up to two or three ounces per day in the first few weeks of life.

Solid foods should be added to the milk formula as soon as the animal's canine teeth have come in. At this point (age 3½ to 4½ weeks), the appropriate commercial diet is added in small amounts, e.g., 1 tablespoon of canned ZuPreem per 8 ounces of formula for felids and canids and for many of the procyonids and mustelids. ZuPreem Omnivore can be used for bears and many of the procyonids and mustelids, such as raccoons, kinkajous, skunks, and badgers.

The proportion of solid food to formula is increased gradually, and the animal should begin to be bowl-trained at five weeks. Once bowl-trained, fresh water is offered and the amount of liquid formula is reduced in proportion to the amount of water consumed. Most animals should be on a diet of commercial feed and water by the time they are eight weeks old. Tidbits added to the commercial diet can be offered at six weeks of age, provided that caution is exercised to prevent the animal from favoring these foods over the commercial feeds and formulas.

The most common pediatric problems observed are usually with the digestive tract. Animals hand-raised from birth require stimulation of the anogenital area to cause them to urinate and defecate during the first week of life. This should be done after each meal, utilizing cotton soaked with warm water. Zinc oxide, vitamin A and D ointment (Desitin®), and petroleum jelly are useful for preventing irritation of the perineal and perianal areas following stimulation.

Young animals that cannot tolerate disaccharides or other complex sugars owing to a lack of disaccharidases, such as sucrase or lactase, can be fed carbohydrate-free products such as CHO-Free® (Syntex) with a simple sugar, e.g., dextrose, added as a source of digestible carbohydrate. This product, as well as other carbohydrate-free products, is complete as far as vitamins, minerals, and electrolytes are concerned. Protein supplementation with sugar-free protein sources such as Casec® (Mead-Johnson) must be added as well to provide a source of protein.*

Oral alimentation as practiced with domestic puppies and kittens can easily be performed on exotic species as long as one realizes that the size of the feeding tube to be used varies greatly from one species to the next. Generally speaking, stomach capacity is approximately 50 ml/kg, so that any amount of formula from 20 to 40 ml/kg can be administered at one time. If an animal has not eaten for a period of time prior to presentation, 5 percent dextrose in water may be given. Under no circumstances should normal amounts of formula be administered in this case.

Small amounts of formula should be given at shorter feeding intervals and the number of feedings should be increased to avoid enterotoxemia. The same recommendation should be followed when attempts are made to nourish animals presented in a hypothermic state.

An animal should be considered to be constipated if it does not defecate within 36 hours after its last stool or if signs of constipation such as straining, bloating, reduced food intake or restlessness occur. Pediatric glycerin suppositories should be tried prior to the administration of an enema. All or part of the suppository can be used. The addition of Karo® syrup to the formula in amounts up to 2 or 3 ml per 8 ounces can be useful in alleviating constipation if it becomes a chronic problem.

Diarrheas, when mild, are best given conservative therapy. I add a source of lactobacillus organisms (Lactonoc, Norden; Lactinex, Hynson, Westcott). The latter is used at a level of 80 mg/kg in the formula. Many young animals, members of the Mustelidae and Procyonidae families in particular, will accept yogurt, which is an excellent source of lactobacillus. If the duration of the diarrhea is more than 24 hours or if the stool is extremely watery, fecal cultures should be taken. Dilution of the formula to supply more water and administration of fluids and antibiotics are discretionary measures that may be undertaken.

Antibiotics given orally may cause additional gastrointestinal upset. I have found Centrine (Bristol Laboratories) very helpful in treating simple diarrheas. It can be used at the recommended canine dosage for all species of carnivores at any age from 1 to 2 days.

Aspiration pneumonia is another problem common among bottle-fed animals handled by inexperienced people and in cases in which improper nipples and bottles are utilized.

Young animals — especially the felines and notably ocelots, margays, mountain lions, and leopards — are prone to eating foreign bodies. The animal's owner should be cautioned about "toys," towels, shoes, and other chewable objects to which their animals are exposed.

---

*Alternatively, the enzyme lactase (Lact-Aid®, Sugar-Lo Co.) can be added directly to the formula.

NUTRITION

Because excellent commercially manufactured diets for exotic carnivores are now available, there is no excuse for improper nutrition or malnutrition of these pets. Lack of information or misinformation on the part of the pet owner is usually the cause of improper nutrition.

I recommend feeding all members of the canine, feline, and hyena families a commercially manufactured carnivore diet. Several are available that vary slightly in formulation, but all have produced good results. Central Nebraska Carnivore Diet* is available in a frozen sausage–style package, and the ZuPreem® Feline Diet† is available both frozen and in cans. Holiday Science Diet Exotic Feline canned cat food† (equivalent to canned ZuPreem) is available in pet shops. Food consumption levels vary according to the physiologic state of the animal (size, activity level, pregnancy, lactation) as well as between individuals of the same species that are in the same physiologic state and kept under similar conditions. Generally speaking, consumption will range from 1 to 10 percent of the animal's body weight per day.

The choice of frozen or canned products depends upon availability in a given area, storage capability, number of animals to be fed, age of the animal, acceptance of the feed, and cost. I feed all animals under three months of age canned Feline ZuPreem†. If the animal is a member of the larger species (e.g., tiger, lion, cheetah, hyena, or wolf) I will make the transition to the frozen product after three months of age. Acceptability of the canned products as opposed to the frozen seems to decrease with an increase in age beyond three months. The digestibility, palatability, and ease of handling favors feeding the canned product to younger and smaller animals (e.g., ocelots, margays, and foxes).

When recommending the use of a commercial carnivore diet to a client who is psychologically set to feed raw, red meat or who is feeding meat because it is cheaper, it should be pointed out that commercial diets have the following advantages: (1) they are a balanced, adequate diet that requires no supplementation; (2) compared with meat diets, consumption of the commercial diet may be 10 to 20 percent less because it is a complete diet; (3) digestibility (efficiency of utilization) is higher and therefore fecal output is lower; (4) fecal odor is reduced; and (5) there is less waste.

Often the practitioner is confronted with an animal that is eating meat or chicken and whose owner claims that it will not eat the less attractive, less palatable commercial diet. In this case, it may be necessary either to deprive the animal of food until it is hungry enough to eat or to add the commercial diet to the present diet in increasing amounts until the animal has been converted. Although there are some animals that will never accept these diets, the number is extremely low. The addition of rendered chicken or turkey fat (available in supermarkets) as a top dressing on the desired food substance has proved to be very helpful in persuading an animal to accept food. This technique can also be of help in inducing sick animals to eat. Sometimes heating the product will make it more acceptable.

The commercial carnivore diet can be used as the basis of diets formulated for the mustelids, viverrids, and procyonids. Since many members of these families are omnivorous, foods such as eggs, bread, vegetables, citrus fruits, nuts, and fish can be added in small amounts. Commercial dog food, preferably dry, can constitute 75 to 85 percent of a satisfactory diet. Meat is not recommended as a supplement because it may be habit-forming and may cause certain animals to bite. It should be pointed out that all food items offered in addition to a commercial dog, cat, or zoo diet should be presented in a manner that does not allow the animal to choose what it wants to eat in favor of what it should eat. This can be accomplished, for instance, by feeding produce, fruit, fish, or treats at the end of the day or as a top dressing in small amounts added to the basic diet.

For certain members of these families, such as minks, commercial feeds‡ are available. Choice of which feed to be used in this case depends upon the age of the animal. Other members of the Procyonidae (such as lesser pandas and giant pandas), Mustelidae, and Viverridae require special diets. Details of these diets are discussed elsewhere (Siegmund, 1973).

The Asian small clawed otter and, less often, the North American river otter are also seen by practitioners. Several diets are given in Table 5, since selectivity among individual pet otters appears to be high.

Bears are omnivorous in their eating habits. Commercial omnivore feed such as ZuPreem Omnivore,† Albers Omnivore,§ or pelleted dog food should be used as the basic diet, with

---

*Central Nebraska Packing Co., P.O. Box 550, North Platte, Nebraska 69101. Phone (308) 532-1250

†Hill's Division, Riviana Foods Inc., P.O. Box 148, Topeka, Kansas, 66601

‡Ralston-Purina, Checkerboard Square, St. Louis, Missouri 63188

§Albers Milling Co., Division of Carnation Co., Los Angeles, California 90036

Table 5. Otter Diets

INGREDIENT	AMOUNT
1. Frozen or canned commercial feline diet or bird-of-prey diet (ZuPreem or Central Nebraska)	50%
Kibbled dog food	25%
Ground-up whole fish: herring, mackerel, or smelt	25%
Vitamin supplement should be mixed into carnivore or bird-of-prey diet. Often the ground fish is mixed with the commercial diet.	
°2. Prescription diet c/d	60%
Bird-of-prey-diet	30%
Smelt	10%
PLUS	
Hard boiled eggs	6
Calcium gluconate	10 tablets (650 mg ea)
Desiccated liver meal	½ cup
Calf starter	1 cup
Yeast	1 cup
Tomato	1 large
3. Butterfish	2 lb (1.0 kg)
Smelt	¼ lb (125 gm)
Raw meat	½ lb (250 gm)
Mixture of chopped raw meat, dog meal, cod liver oil, and bone meal	½ lb (250 gm)

°Busch Gardens otter diet.

additives such as those mentioned for mustelids and other omnivores given in small amounts.

Prescription diets† can be used to replace the basic diet for all carnivores when a specific clinical condition is being treated. Particular attention must be given to the species being fed when vitamin and mineral supplementation is a concern.

PHYSIOLOGIC NORMS

Hematologic values from various sources, including the author's experience, for some species within the order Carnivora are presented in Table 6. The vessels from which blood can be drawn and their collection sites are presented in Table 7. Blood is drawn from the exotic animal species under more varied conditions than from domestic or laboratory animals. Often they are excited, and at times anesthesia is required to obtain the sample. Sex, type of anesthetic, site of collection, pregnancy, and other factors may influence laboratory values.

Table 8 contains pertinent data on various reproductive factors of the common pet felids, canids, mustelids, procyonids, and ursids and for hyenas. An excellent, detailed discussion of

---

† Hill's Division, Riviana Foods Inc., P.O. Box 148, Topeka, Kansas, 66601

reproduction among the carnivores is given elsewhere (Seager and Demorest, 1978). The reader is referred to it for an in-depth discussion of reproductive physiology.

Dental formulae for the carnivores are shown in Table 9.

PARASITES

Many parasites observed in the domestic dog and cat occur in members of one or more families of exotic carnivores. The usual precautions taken with dogs and cats to prevent constant reinfestation should be undertaken, and all secondary manifestations of internal or external parasitism deserve consideration.

Anthelmintics may be administered by injection or orally. However, medication given orally must be mixed with food or water to be rendered palatable and acceptable.

Table 10 lists internal parasites that have been observed and the drugs(s) that can be used to treat them. Table 11 gives sources of each product used.

External parasites can present a great problem to the practitioner, since treatment requires handling of the animal. However, fleas, ticks, and mange mites have caused very serious skin disease in a variety of species, so one cannot take a conservative approach in treatment. It is best if diagnosis and treatment can be performed at the same time, thus eliminating some handling problems and allowing immediate institution of therapy. Table 12 lists treatment for external parasites.

RESTRAINT AND ANESTHESIA

Restraint and handling procedures are a challenge to the practitioner. Details of physical and chemical restraint are found in the supplemental reading list. My recommendations for chemical restraint in various species are found in Tables 13 and 14.

To maintain anesthesia it is desirable to follow the administration of any of the immobilizing agents with an anesthetic that can be controlled easily and that has the additional benefit of providing a patent airway through intubation of the trachea. A combination of 50 percent nitrous oxide and 50 percent halothane is best. Induction should begin with 5 percent halothane administered via an anesthetic mask. Following intubation, 1.5 to 2.5 percent halothane should be sufficient for maintaining surgical anesthesia.

Barbiturates can be used; however, *only*

Text continued on page 728

Table 6. *Hematologic Data for some Exotic Species in the Order Carnivora*[*]

NO.	FAMILY	RBC (10⁶/mm³)	HB (gm/dl)	PCV (%)	WBC (10³/mm³)	PERCENT OF DIFFERENTIAL				
						Neutrophils	Lymphocytes	Monocytes	Eosinophils	Basophils
	Canidae									
42	Wolves[a]	6.1	15	45	8–13	0.5(B)† 70(S)	20	6.5	3	0
90	Wolves and foxes[b]	7–8	12–16	35–45	10–12	60	38	1	1	0
6	Silver foxes; black foxes[d]	6–12 (8.80)	8.3–14.2 (11.0)	—[c]	4.2–15.8 (9.26)					
12	Silver fox[e]	7.4–8.5 (8.0)	13.9–16.1 (15.0)	53–64 (59)						
3	Gray fox[f]	6.91 7.05	12.7 12.7	41.0 41.0	8.1 6.6	53 1(B) 52(S)	34.5 31	7.0 6.0	5.5 10.0	0 0
1	Gray fox[g]	4.76	10.8	34.0	20.1	5(B) 61.5(S)	10.0	13.5	10.0	0
	Felidae									
12	Lion[h]	7–8	8–12	35–40	10–15	63	30	5	2	0
?	Lion[i]	5.51	10.985	30	12.58	0.428(B) 80.85(S)	17.14	0	1.14	0
1	Lion[j]	7.85	11.5	36	4.5	59.5	31.0	9.0	0.0	0.5
40	Lion	(7.4)	(11.2)	(35)	(12.3)	(76)	(21.8)	(0.2)	(2)	0
1	Tiger[k]	6.18	9.8	31	16.6	78.0	17.5	2.5	1.0	0
1	Tiger[l]	6.59	12.1	37	15	84.0	9.0	3.0	4.0	1
25	Tiger[m]	(6.8)	(13.1)	(40)	12.7					
6	Tiger[m]	6–8	9–14	35–45	10–15	63	30	5	2	0
61	Tiger	(6.7)	(13.7)	(41)	(12.3)	(76.5)	(21)	(2)	(1)	(0)
11	Cheetah[n]	6.25	13.1	38.6	10.15	66.42	28.57	2.0	4.7	0
4	Cheetah[o]	6–8	8–13	35–40	10–12	63	30	5	2.0	0
22	Cheetah	7.9	12	37.9	10.1	65	27	4	4.0	0
4	Leopard[p]	6–8	8–13	35–45	10–14	63	30	5	2	0
?	Leopard[h]	7.9	14.8	50	10.5	51	47	2	0	0
36	Leopard	7.58	12.33	37.5	11.8	56	37.0	5	2	0
7	Mountain Lion[o]	7–8	10–18	35–50	8–12	63	32	2	3	0
1	Mountain Lion[n]	10.52	15.4	47	22	86	10	4	0	0

No.	Species									
34	Mountain Lion	9.16	13.6	39.8	10.6	72	24	2	2	0
3	Jaguar[a]	6–8	8–13	35–45	10–14	63	30	5	2	0
6	Jaguar	6.9	12.2	38	11.2	72	28	7	3	0
28	Ocelot[u]	7–8	10–18	35–40	8–13	65	33	0	2	0
12	Ocelot	7.6	13.8	42	10.6	65	31	2.5	1.5	0
1	Serval Cat	9.36	13.8	45	13.6	81.5	—	—	—	—
1	Serval Cat[q]	5.29[q]	10.3	34	22.5	44	49.0	5.5	1.5	0
4	Serval Cat[q]	(7.43)[q]	(14.9)	(49)	(7.9)	(74)	21	4	1	0
2	Caracal Cat	7.1	13.7	42.5	8.1	73	23	3	1	0
8	Jaguarondi[q]	7–8	10–15	35–40	8–13	65	33	0	2	0
2	Leopard-Jaguar Cross[r]	(6.15)	(10.1)	(30.7)	(13.5)	(80)	17	1	2	0
Procyonidae										
23	Coatimundi[o]	11	10–11	35–40	13–16	45	49	2	3	0
14	Kinkajou[o]	10–12	11–12	35–40	14–18	56	38	6	0	0
6	Racoon[s]	9.6–13.3 (11.2)	11–12 (11.5)	—	10.6–26.8 (17.80)	30.5–60.5 (45.3)	35.0–65.5 (49.3)	0.0–3.5 (0.8)	1.5–8.0 (4.3)	0.0–2.5 (0.8)
10	Racoon[s]	7.5–11.3 (9.72)	11.4–17.3 (15.0)	—	5.2–12.2 (7.80)	26.5–65.5 (46.3)	30.0–68.5 (47.5)	0.0–5.0 (1.5)	0.0–13.0 (4.0)	0.0–13.0 (0.8)
27	Racoon	10.6	12	38.4	12	48	46	2	4	0
18	Racoon[o]	11	10–11	35–40	13–16	45	49	2	3	0
Mustelidae										
0	Mink[1]	8.9–10.4 (9.68)	9.5–15.6 (11.9)	—	3.8–10.2 (6.38)	18.5–69.0 (47.1)	22.5–57.5 (43.5)	0.0–5.5 (1.1)	2.5–16 (7.2)	0.0–2.5 (0.8)
9	Mink[t]	7.5–11.3 (9.72)	11.4–17.3 (15.0)	—	5.2–12.2 (7.8)	26.5–65.5 (46.3)	30.0–68.5 (47.5)	0.0–5.0 (1.5)	0.0–13.0 (4.0)	0.0–13.0 (0.8)
5	Mink[v]	5.7–9.3 (7.50)	13.5–17.5 (14.7)	41–57 (48)	3.2–11.2 (6.0)	45–88 (66.0)	11–14 / 32	0.0–3.0 (1.0)	0.0–3.0 (1.0)	0.0–1.0 (0.0)
3	Skunk[w]	—	—	35–40	12–25	4	50	1	2	0
6	Ferret[aw]	—	—	35–40	9–13	65	35	0	0	0
	Ursidae									
6	Black bear[o]	8	16	45–50	11–14	70	25	3	2	0
	Black bear[x]	7.32	18.2	55	8.9	73	13.5	12.0	1.5	0.0
1	Black bear[y]	6.33–9.30	11.6–18.8	40–58	8.3–24.3	70	25	3	0–2	0–1

Table continued on following page

° Figures in parentheses are average values.

Table 6. *Hematologic Data for some Exotic Species in the Order Carnivora* * (Continued)

NO.	FAMILY	RBC (10⁶/mm³)	HB (gm/dl)	PCV (%)	WBC (10³/mm³)	Neutrophils	Lymphocytes	Monocytes	Eosinophils	Basophils
							PERCENT OF DIFFERENTIAL			
2	Grizzly bear[u]	8	22	45–50	6–8	65	20	7	7	1
2	Polar bear[o]	6	16–18	50–55	10–14	75	12	7	6	0
	Polar bear[z]	5.43–7.69	15.8–19.3	46–56	6.3–13.9	75	12	7	0–6	0–1
6	Kodiak bear[aa]	4–4	9–11	30–40	13.16	60	35	4	1	0
	Alaskan brown bear	5.20–7.05	14.9–22.4	42–65	8.3–16.6	60	35	4	0–1	0–1
	Malayan sun bear[z]	4.62–6.78	11.1–16.8	35–53	11.2–23.2	–	–	–	–	–
	Sloth bear[z]	5.86–6.55	16.4–17.4	52–54	10.7–11.1	–	–	–	–	–
	Spectacled bear[z]	6.94–7.50	13.8–14.5	41–44	5.7–6.2	–	–	–	–	–
	Viverridae									
7	Binturong[o]	11.2	22.2	55	10–14	68	30	0	2	0
11	Binturong[bb]	7.7 ±1.5	17.1 ±2.1	53±6	10.6 ±3.9	–	–	–	–	–
8	Common palm civet[bb]	10–10.9 ±4.6	16.4 ±3.5	45 ±12	9.6 ±3.8	–	–	–	–	–
3	Small spotted genet[bb]	10	15.2 ±2.8	44	5	–	–	–	–	–
4	Small Indian civet[bb]	12.7	16.5	22	7.4	–	–	–	–	–
5	Malay civet[bb]	10.2 ±4	13.8 ±5.7	32.6 ±15.9	14 ±5	–	–	–	–	–
1	Slender mongoose[cc]	9.8	13–15.4	43	5.4	62	37	1	0	0
1	Small Indian mongoose[cc]	10	13.4	44	5.2	–	–	–	–	–
2	Crab-eating mongoose[cc]	11.2–12.1	14.4–16.2	45–52	4–4.4	35–47	47–55	5–7	0–4	0
	Hyaenidae									
1	Striped Hyena[x]	–	–	43	19.3	72.0	15.0	4.0	4.0	0

1	Spotted Hyena[x]	5.65	9.0	28	17.1	—	—	—	—	—
	Striped and Brown Hyenas[cc]	7–7.5	12.5–15.0	40–45	13–16	—	—	—	—	—
	Striped Hyena[dd]	6–7 (6.5)	12–17 (14.7)	37–53 (45)	11–19	—	—	—	—	—
	Brown Hyena[dd]	5–6.1 (5.5)	8.8–13 (10.9)	29–39 (34)	6–12	—	—	—	—	—
	Spotted Hyena[dd]	6.1–7.9 (7)	12–16 (14)	35–47 (41)	9.5–14.5	—	—	—	—	—

° Figures in parentheses are average values.
† (B) = bands; (S) = segmented
[a] White, timber, black, and silver wolves.
[b] Species not given. Data from Soifer, 1977.
[c] Reported PCV value was inaccurate.
[d] 48 months old. Data from Kennedy, 1945.
[e] All animals mature. Data from Spitzer et al., 1941.
[f] Pups. Data from Schalm et al., 1975.
[g] Had abscess. Data from Schalm et al., 1975.
[h] Data from Soifer, 1977.
[i] Number of animals known to be significant. Data from Rhodes, 1975.
[j] 8 months old. Data from Schalm et al., 1975.
[k] 6 month old male. Data from Schalm et al., 1975.
[l] 3 year old male. Data from Schalm et al., 1975.
[m] Average mean value; ages assorted. Data from Soifer, 1977.
[n] Data from Rhodes, 1975.
[o] Data from Soifer, 1977.
[p] Male, 2 years old.
[q] Data from Soifer, 1977.
[r] 4 month old male.
[s] Data from Kennedy, 1935.
[t] Adult males. Reported PCV value was inaccurate.
[u] Adult females. Reported PCV value was inaccurate.
[v] Data from Rubin and Mason, 1948.
[w] Data for RBC and PCV were lacking. Data from Soifer, 1977.
[x] Data from Schalm et al., 1975.
[y] Number not reported but known to be significant. Data from Seal et al., 1967; and Soifer, 1970.
[z] Data from Seal et al., 1967; and Soifer, 1970.
[aa] All cubs.
[bb] Data from Makey and Seal, 1974.
[cc] Data from Hawkey, 1975.
[dd] Data from Divers, 1978.

Table 7. Blood Collection Sites in Carnivores*

FAMILY	VEIN	COLLECTION SITE
Canidae	Jugular vein	Neck
Hyaenidae	Cephalic vein (best)	Foreleg, dorsal aspect, radial-ulnar region
	Saphenous vein	Hind leg, medial aspect, tibia-fibula region
Felidae	Jugular vein	Neck
	Cephalic vein (in smaller species or cubs of larger species)	Foreleg, dorsal aspect, radial-ulnar region
	Saphenous vein (best)	Hind leg, medial aspect, tibia-fibula region
	Lateral saphenous vein (plantar branch)	Hind leg, lateral aspect of tarsus
Ursidae	Jugular vein	Neck
	Saphenous vein (best)	Hind leg, medial aspect of the tarsus anterodorsal to tibial tarsal bone
	Lingual vein	Tongue, ventral aspect
Procyonidae	Jugular vein	Neck
Mustelidae	Jugular vein	Neck
Viverridae	Jugular vein (usually best)	Neck
	Saphenous vein	Hind leg, medial aspect, tibia-fibula region

*In all animals toenails can be clipped to obtain blood smears and samples for PCV determination and heartworm analysis.

Table 8. Reproductive Physiology

FAMILY	BREEDING AGE (Years)[a]	CYCLE	LITTER SIZE	GESTATION PERIOD (Days)[a]	SUGGESTED WEANING AGE FOR HAND-REARING (Weeks)	NATURAL WEANING AGE
Felidae						
Bobcat	F 1½ M 2	Seasonal: Jan–July, peak March	1–6 (3.5)	59–63 (60)	3	8 wk
African lion	F 2–3 M 3	Polyestrous	1–6 (3)	98–114 (105)	3	3–4 mo
Tiger	F 2 M 3	Polyestrous	1–5	89–110	3	3–5 mo
Leopard	F 2 M 2–3	Polyestrous	1–5 (2)	98–105	3	6 wk
Cheetah	F 9 mo M 14–16 mo	Seasonally polyestrous: Jan–April	1–4	90–95	4	5 mo
Jungle cat	F 1 M 2	Polyestrous all year	1–5 (3–4)	66	3–4	?
Serval cat	F 2 M 2	Polyestrous	1–4 (2–3)	67–77 (74)	2	?
Leopard cat	F 2 M 2	Polyestrous	2–3	63–66	2	?
Mountain lion	F 3 M 3	Polyestrous	1–5 (2–3)	90–93 (91)	2–3	3 mo
Ocelot	F 2 M not known	Polyestrous	1–3	87–91	3	?
Margay	not known	Polyestrous	1–2	83	3	?
Caracal	F 1 M 1½	Polyestrous	1–6 (2–3)	69–78	3	8 wk
Canidae						
Timber wolf	F 1–2 M 1½	Seasonal: Feb–April	(6.5)	63	3–4	2 mo

Table continued on opposite page

Table 8. *Reproductive Physiology* (Continued)

FAMILY	BREEDING AGE (*Years*)[a]	CYCLE	LITTER SIZE	GESTATION PERIOD (*Days*)[a]	SUGGESTED WEANING AGE FOR HAND-REARING (*Weeks*)	NATURAL WEANING AGE
Canidae *(Continued)*						
Coyote	F 1 M 1½	Seasonal: March	3–5	63	3–4	2 mo
Red fox[c]	F 1 M 1	Seasonal: Dec–Feb	4	51–52	3	3 mo
Gray fox	F 9 mo M 9 mo	Seasonal	4	52	3	6 mo
Ursidae						
No. American black bear[d]	3	Seasonal: June–July	1–4	7 mo	8	?
Alaskan brown bear[d]	4–6	Seasonal: May–July	1–4 (2–3)	6½ mo	8	?
Malayan sun bear[e]			1–2	210		?
Mustelidae						
Skunk	F 1 M 1	Seasonal: Feb–March	6–7 (4)	62–66 (63)		
Mink[f]	F 1 M 1	Seasonal: March	1–12 (4)	75		
No. American otter		Seasonal	2–5 (3–4)	9–13 mo		
Ferret	F 1 M 1	Seasonally polyestrous: Mar–Aug	2–17 (8)	42		
Asian otter	F 1 M 2	Polyestrous	1–6	60–64		
Procyonidae						
Raccoon	F 9 mo M 9 mo	Seasonal: Jan–June	1–6	60–73 (63)		
Hyaenidae						
Spotted hyena	?	?	1–3	110	?	?
Striped hyena	?	?	1–4	90	?	?
Brown hyena	?	?	1–4	90	?	?

F = female; M = male

Figures in parentheses are average values.

[a] Except as otherwise noted.

[b] Alaskan timber wolf. Similar observations made in white, black and gray wolves.

[c] Location (range) influences breeding seasons. Usually January–February.

[d] Implantation delayed. Gestation period includes the delayed period.

[e] Implantation not known to be delayed.

[f] Implantation delayed.

Table 9. Dentition of the Carnivores

FAMILY	DENTAL FORMULA
Felidae	$I\frac{3}{3}\ C\frac{1}{1}\ P\frac{2\text{-}3}{2}\ M\frac{1}{1} = 28\ \text{or}\ 30$
Canidae	$I\frac{3}{3}\ C\frac{1}{1}\ P\frac{4}{4}\ M\frac{2}{3} = 42$
Procyonidae	$I\frac{3}{3}\ C\frac{1}{1}\ P\frac{3\text{-}4}{3\text{-}4}\ M\frac{2}{2\text{-}3} = 36\ \text{to}\ 42$
Mustelidae	$I\frac{3}{3}\ C\frac{1}{1}\ P\frac{2\text{-}4}{2\text{-}4}\ M\frac{1}{1\text{-}2} = 28\ \text{to}\ 38$
Viverridae	$I\frac{3}{3}\ C\frac{1}{1}\ P\frac{3\text{-}4}{3\text{-}4}\ M\frac{-2}{1\text{-}2} = 32\ \text{to}\ 40$
Hyaenidae	$I\frac{3}{3}\ C\frac{1}{1}\ P\frac{4}{3}\ M\frac{1}{1} = 34$
Ursidae	$I\frac{3}{3}\ C\frac{1}{1}\ P\frac{4}{4}\ M\frac{-}{3} = 42$

Table 10. Treatment of Internal Parasites in Carnivores

PARASITE	OCCURRENCE	DRUGS UTILIZED[a]	DOSAGE[b] (mg/kg)	REGIMEN[b]	EFFICIENCY	COMMENTS
Ascarids	Most common in felines, canines, bears; rare in other families	Piperazine compounds	80–100 per os	Repeat in 14 days	+++	Can be toxic to Felidae, especially cheetah and older animals. Excellent in bears.
		Mebendazole	20 per os	Canines: 5 days Felines: 4 days Bears: 2–3 days Others: 3–5 days	++	Safest of all products; palatable, easily mixed with diets currently in use. Not approved by FDA for use in exotic carnivores.
		Dichlorvos	20–30 active ingredient per os	Divide dosage over 3–5 days	++	Have had bad reaction in bears. Probably not necessary to dose for a weight above 100 lb.
		Diethyl-carbamazine	10–60 per os	One dose. Repeated as required	+++	Use low dose range in cats.
		Levamisole	11 per os	One dose. Repeated in 14–21 days	+++	High incidence of excessive salivation, incoordination, vomiting, colic. Can be injected subcutaneously; IM injection not recommended.
		Fenbendazole	–	–		Recommendations are being evaluated. Shows promise.
		Thiabendazole	50–100 per os	As one dose	+	Toxic reactions reported in felines.
Whipworm	Most common in Canidae; observed in Felidae; rare in others	Glycobiarsol (Milibis-V)	200 per os	Daily for 5 days	+++	Cannot be used in cats; acceptability low.
		Dichlorvos	See ascarids	Same as ascarid therapy	+++	As above for ascarids.
		Mebendazole	20 per os	All species 5 days	+++	Number of days of administration and dosage can be increased in difficult cases.
Hookworms	Very common in Canidae, Felidae, Ursidae; may be seen in all other families	Disophenol	7.5 (0.2 ml/kg)	Repeat in 21 days	+++	Some refractory cases noted. Have administered up to 4 ml. Must advise caution in dosing animals in excess of 50 kg.
		Dichlorvos	See ascarids	Same as ascarid therapy	+++	As above for ascarids.
		Thiabendazole	See ascarids	Same as ascarid therapy	+	Efficacy increased if used for 2 days.
		Levamisole	See ascarids	Same as ascarid therapy	+++	See ascarids.
		Mebendazole	See ascarids	Same as ascarid therapy	+++	See ascarids.

Table continued on opposite page

Table 10. *Treatment of Internal Parasites in Carnivores* (Continued)

PARASITE	OCCURRENCE	DRUGS UTILIZED[a]	DOSAGE[b] (mg/kg)	REGIMEN[b]	EFFICIENCY	COMMENTS
Stomach worms (*Physaloptera* spp.)	Canidae, Viverridae	Mebendazole	As above	–	Unknown	–
		Dichlorvos	As above	–	Unknown	–
		Levamisole	As above	–	Unknown	–
Tapeworms	All families affected by various species	Niclosamide	150 per os	As one dose	+++	Very safe.
		Mebendazole	20 per os	As for ascarids	++	Safe. Not rated against *Dipylidium caninum*.
		Niclosamide	5 per os	One dose. Repeat as required.	+++	Unavailable in U.S. at this time
Flukes	Canidae, Felidae, Ursidae, Procyonidae, Mustelidae	Mebendazole	20 per os	2–5 days	+	Further studies will probably show increased efficacy.
Thorny-headed worms	Occasionally or only rarely seen	None	–	–	–	No effective treatment.
Lungworms	Common in mustelids; rare in other families; occasionally seen in canids	Levamisole	11 per os	Repeat in 7 days	++	Injection more effective than oral route.
		Mebendazole	20 per os	Daily for 3 doses, repeat 7 days after last dose		
Pinworms	Viverridae	Piperazine salts	100 per os	Can be repeated as needed	+++	
		Diethyl-carbamazine	10–60 per os	Repeat as needed	+	
		Levamisol	11 per os	Repeat as needed	+	Side effects as above (see ascarids)
		Pyrvinium pamoate	5 per os	1–2 days	?	May cause vomiting; stains hands and clothing; feces appear red. Intestinal absorption very low.
Heartworms	Canidae most common; rare but occurs in felids, procyonids and mustelids; probably can occur in bears, hyenas, and viverrids in endemic areas	Diethyl-carbamazine	5 per os	Daily	+++	As a preventative.
		Levamisole	11 per os	Daily for 6–12 days until microfilaria are gone	++	To treat microfilaria. May have toxic side effects. Experimental—not yet approved for use.
		Dithiazine iodine	4–20 per os	Daily for 7–10 days until microfilaria are gone	++	Vomiting and diarrhea common. Can be nephrotoxic.
		Thiacetarsimide	0.2 IV	In divided daily doses b.i.d. for 2–3 days	++	As an adulticide. Arsenical. Can be very toxic. Nephrotoxic.
		Levamisole	Low doses	Long-term	?	May be used where arsenicals cannot be tolerated. Not approved for use—experimental. Toxic to CNS and liver.

Key: +++ = most efficient; ++ = efficient; + = somewhat efficient.
[a]Data from Schobert, 1973; Burkhart and Schock, 1973; and Siegmund, 1973.
[b]Data from the sources listed in footnote *a* and from Soifer, 1977.

Table 11. *Anthelmintic Agents for Carnivores*

GENERIC NAME	TRADE NAME	MANUFACTURER
Piperazine salts	Pipertabs (2)	Burns-Biotec
	Pipertabs (10)	Burns-Biotec
	Pipersol	Burns-Biotec
	Pipzine tabs	Affiliated
	Piperate tabs	Fort Dodge
	Piperazine Citrate Tabs 500	Med-Tech
	Pipcide	Haver-Lockhart
Mebendazole	Telmin	Pitman-Moore
Dichlorvos	Task	Shell
	Equigard	
	Atgard-V	
Diethylcarbamazine	Caricide	American Cyanamid
Levamisole hydrochloride	Levasole	Pitman-Moore
	Ripercol	American Cyanamid
Fenbendazole	Panacur	National
Thiabendazole	Equizole	Merck
	Omnizole	Merck
Glycobiarsol	Milibis-V	Winthrop
Disophenol	D.N.P. Parenteral	American Cyanamid
Niclosamide	Yomesan	Haver-Lockhart
Pyrvinium pamoate	Povan	Parke-Davis
Dithiazine	Dizan	Elanco
Thiacetarsamide (caparsolate)	Caparsolate	Diamond
Praziquantel	Droncit	Bayer

short-acting barbiturates should be employed. Barbiturates act so synergistically with most immobilizing drugs that the dose should be reduced to as little as one twentieth of the usual dose when used alone. They should always be given to effect. The product of choice is thiamylal sodium (Surital). As a rule of thumb the total amount, administered in aliquot doses to prolong anesthesia, should not exceed 1 mg/kg.

SURGERY

Several surgical procedures are requested frequently by the exotic pet owner and so are mentioned here. The practitioner should be responsible for carrying out these procedures selectively, since they may relate to the owner-animal relationship or have a profound effect on an animal's future. Clients who think that neutering, declawing, and defanging their pets will render the animals harmless are badly misinformed and should be advised of their misconception. The practitioner who carries out such procedures, particularly more than one on a single animal, with the goal of creating a harmless exotic pet may be doing a great disservice to an animal whose instinctive nature and species survival depend on the presence of claws, fangs, and an intact reproductive apparatus. There are very few outlets for abandoned exotic pets that cannot breed or live with cagemates

that have claws or that are of poor display value because they lack teeth. Each procedure has merits and definite indications that should be considered seriously before such operations are performed.

DECLAWING

Onychectomy is a frequently requested procedure. Indications include prevention of (1) damage to the owner's premises, (2) accidental claw wounds (instinctively or play-induced), (3) claw injury to cagemates, and (4) tree and fence climbing.

Whether or not the claws are removed from both front feet, front and rear feet, or rear feet only depends upon the species and certain special situations. Generally speaking, lions, tigers and bears are declawed only in the front, because these species use mainly their front feet to climb, fight, and play; others — such as the mountain lion, leopard, ocelot, margay, and jaguar — are declawed on all four feet. Certain performing animals belonging to arena acts are declawed on the back feet only to prevent damage to expensive costumes when jumping through the air to their owners. Cheetahs, whose claws are not retractable, should never be declawed. Such a procedure would be similar to declawing a dog. Dewclaws are often removed from the cheetah because they are virtually non-functional in captivity and can be responsible for injuries to cagemates, handlers, and owners.

The age at which onychectomy is performed also varies with the species. The procedure is more difficult in larger animals than in small ones. The larger species, such as lions, tigers, mountain lions, leopards, and jaguars, can be declawed as young as 10 to 12 weeks of age; the smaller species can also be declawed at that age. However, if the owner can tolerate his or her pet's claws for awhile, I prefer to wait until the animal is four months old. Cheetah dewclaws are best removed at a very early age. Details of this surgical procedure are similar to those for dogs and cats and are reported elsewhere (Fowler, 1978).

DE-SCENTING

Skunks and ferrets are the two members of the carnivore family that are usually de-scented routinely.

Anesthesia can be accomplished by placing the skunk in a chamber containing a pledget of cotton soaked with ether; ketamine can be used at 10 mg/kg prior to gas anesthesia, or sodium

Table 12. *Treatment of External Parasites in Carnivores*

PARASITE	TREATMENT	PREPARATIONS	COMMENTS
Flies	Spray repellants; general fly control program	Flair (Jensen-Salsbery) Sect-a-Spray (Evsco) Para Bomb M (Haver-Lockhart) Sprecto (Pitman-Moore)	Products safe for use on cats are satisfactory for all species. Products safe for dogs can be used on the canids and hyenas. Caution in species that tend to swim or otherwise get wet.
Fleas, ticks, lice	Powder	Vet-Kem Pet Spray (Vet-Kem) F-L-T Bomb (Bio-Ceutics) Diryl (Pitman-Moore) Para Powder (Haver-Lockhart) Pet Dust (Diamond) Flea and Tick Powder (Vet-Kem)	All species. Same as above. Applies to all these preparations.
	Shampoo	Mycodex Pet Shampoo (Beecham) Mycodex Pet Shampoo with Carburyl (Beecham) Fleatol Shampoo (Haver-Lockhart)	All species: Fleas and lice. All species over 4 weeks old: Fleas, lice, and ticks. Coat brightener, kills fleas and ticks.
		D-Flea (Evsco)	Fleas and lice only.
	Spray Flea and tick collars	Same as for flies	Not recommended.
Mites Sarcoptic Psorioptic Chorioptic Demodectic	Use dip or local application every 7 to 10 days; clean up environment; isolate animal; give antibiotics for secondary bacterial infection	Ectoral (Pitman-Moore) Benzyl-Hex (Evsco) Mange Lotion (Bio-Ceutics) Mycodex with Lindane (Beecham) Lime-Sulfur (L.A. City Chemical) Lym-Dyp (D.V.M. Co.)	Use only on canines, bears, hyenas. Observe cautions on package label. Same as for sarcoptic mites. Same as for sarcoptic mites. Shampoo treatment may not be sufficient. Use on all other species; every 7 days. Solution must be warm. Lym-Dyp preparation has a more desirable odor. Both preparations dilute 1 to 8 to 1 to 16 with water for local application.
Otodectic	Clean ears with D-S-S; apply preparations as directed ± treat secondary bacterial infection in ears	Tresaderm (Merck) Cerumite (Diamond) Zero-Mite (Dermavet)	Safe in all species. Treatment for mites not specifically recommended; however, results are excellent. Safe in all species. Safe in all species.
Candidiasis	Topical: Apply nystatin or miconazol preparations	Panalog (Squibb) Mycostatin (Squibb) Conofite (Pitman-Moore)	
	Systemic: (1) Feed lactobacillus organisms; (2) Oral miconazol	Lactinex (Hinson, Westcott) Lactonoc (Norden) Daktarin (Bayer)	80 mg/kg in food. 12 mg/kg. Oral form not yet available in U.S.

pentobarbital can be given IP at 20 mg/kg. If ketamine is used on the ferret, 35 mg/kg is required. Choice of anesthetic technique depends upon whether or not it is desirable to handle the animal and risk being sprayed with musk. Skunks under six weeks of age usually do not spray; since it is necessary for the young skunk to have its back legs against the ground to aid in musk ejection, the likelihood of being sprayed can be reduced by picking the animal up by the tail.

The procedure should be performed outside of the clinic to prevent any musk odor caused by ejection or gland rupture from getting into the heating and cooling system of the hospital. Protective clothing, gloves, and goggles are recommended additions to the normal apparel. Musk can be neutralized with sodium hypo-

Table 13. *Tranquilization, Immobilization, and Anesthesia of Non-domestic Carnivores*

DRUGS UTILIZED	DOSAGE (mg/kg)°	ROUTE	CANIDAE	FELIDAE	URSIDAE	PROCYONIDAE	MUSTELIDAE	VIVERRIDAE	HYAENIDAE	COMMENTS
Mixture #1 Phencyclidine Acetylpromazine Atropine	1 0.1 0.04–0.08	IM	a	a	a	a	b	b	b	May cause tonoclonic convulsions in certain individuals. These are overcome via 4% thiamylal sodium IV to effect or diazapam 0.30–0.5 mg/kg IV. The mixture is significantly synergistic with barbiturates. Phencyclidine recently (1977) became unavailable; however, it may be available at this time or in the near future. *Caution:* Avoid accidental administration to humans. May be absorbed orally by some animals.
Mixture #2 Phencyclidine Atropine	1 0.04–0.08	IM	a	b	b	b	b	b	b	Convulsions more common than with mixture No. 1. Excellent in wolves, coyotes, dingoes, and other canids.
Mixture #3 Ketamine HCL Acetylpromazine Atropine	10–20 0.1 0.04–0.08	IM	a	a	b	b	b	b	b	Advantage: shorter-acting than mixture 1. Fewer convulsions than with mixture 1. Disadvantage: Large dose volume for larger animals. Convulsions handled as with mixture 1.
Mixture #4 Ketamine Atropine	10–20 0.04–0.08	IM	a	a	b	a	a	b	b	Ketamine may be given IV alone or in combination with atropine following immobilization. Mink and ferrets require up to 34 mg/kg ketamine. Otters require less—6 mg/kg ketamine. Convulsions may occur as in mixtures 1, 2, and 3 and are treated similarly.
Mixture #5 Ketamine Xylazine Atropine	10 0.5 0.08	IM	—	—	—	—	—	—	b[1]	Followed by gas anesthesia for long procedures.
Mixture #6 Ketamine Xylazine	11–22 1.1–2.2	IM	—	—	—	—	—	b[2]	—	Ketamine given first. Xylazine added after immobilization to increase relaxation.
Mixture #7 Ketamine Xylazine	10–14 2.0–3.0	IM	—	a[3]	—	—	—	—	—	As above.
Mixture #8 Ketamine Xylazine	5 5	IM	—	—	a[4]	—	—	—	—	Doses have ranged from 2–30 mg/kg.
Mixture #9 Ketamine Xylazine	1.2–1.6 1.2–1.6	IM	—	—	a[5]	—	—	—	—	
Drug #10 Xylazine	0.5–1	IM	a[6]	—	—	—	—	—	—	Used mostly in wolves. Dopram used as an antidote to respiratory depression.
Drug #11 Xylazine	2–5	IM	b	—	—	—	—	—	—	Dose range from various sources.
Drug #12 Etorphine	0.003–0.01	IM	—	d	a	—	—	—	—	Antidote (dyprenorphine) is available. Give IV at twice the etorphine dosage.
Mixture #13 Etorphine Methotrimeprazine	7.5 μg/kg 6.0	IM or IV	a[7]	d	—	—	—	—	—	Mixture is unavailable commercially in U.S. However, it can be made utilizing etorphine and methotrimeprazine, which can be purchased separately. Antagonist diprenorphene at 30 mg/kg.
Drug #14 Diazepam	2.0–7.0	PO IM IV	b	b	b	c	c	c	c	Used as a tranquilizer and anticonvulsant (0.3–0.5 mg/kg)

Table continued on opposite page

Table 13. *Tranquilization, Immobilization, and Anesthesia of Non-domestic Carnivores* (Continued)

DRUGS UTILIZED	DOSAGE (mg/kg)[*]	ROUTE	CANIDAE	FELIDAE	URSIDAE	PROCYONIDAE	MUSTELIDAE	VIVERRIDAE	HYAENIDAE	COMMENTS
Mixture #15 Halothane Nitrous oxide	Induction: 5% halothane Maintenance: 1.5–3% halothane	Mask Endotracheal tube	a	a	b	b	b	b	b	Nitrous oxide can be mixed 50/50 with the halothane.
Drug #16 Methoxyflurane	As above for halothane	As above	a	a	b	b	b	b	a	
Drug #17 Thiamylal sodium	To effect	IV	a	a	a	a	a	a	a	See notes in text re use of barbiturates.
Drug #18 Sodium thiopental	To effect	IV	a	a	a	a	a	a	a	
Drug #19 Acetylpromazine maleate	5 mg/50 kg	IV IM	b	a	b	—	—	—	—	IM as preanesthetic or tranquilizer; IV to effect.

[*]Except where otherwise noted.
a = Excellent in these species
b = Can be used with good results
c = Results fair
d = Should never be used
— = No recommendations
[1]See Divers, 1978, p. 649.
[2]See Divers, 1978, p. 644.
[3]See Miller, 1977, p. 763.
[4]Haigh, J. C.: Personal communication, 1978.
[5]Rapley, W.: Personal communication, 1978.
[6]Foster, J. A.: Personal communication, 1978.
[7]Alford and Wozniak, 1970.

chlorite (Clorox®) diluted to 500 to 1000 ppm available chlorine or with one or more over-the-counter preparations such as Super CD®.

The ferret is descented in a similar manner; however, the papillae are replaced by a furrow into which glandular orifices open. The edge of the furrow can be grasped with an Allis forceps and ligated; then an elliptical incision can be made around it. Details of this operation are reported in the literature (Fowler, 1978).

SPAYING AND CASTRATION

These procedures are carried out similarly to those performed on domestic animals. One has a choice of incision sites in males for castration between the median raphe or over the testicles. Generally speaking, canids are best castrated through an approach on the median raphe; mustelids and procyonids are also castrated in this manner, provided an incision site is large enough. Felids are castrated through an incision over each testicle. Site choice in bears depends on the judgment of the surgeon, since both sites are suitable. Absorbable sutures are best placed subcutaneously in all cases.

Spaying is performed through a midline incision, except in large felines, for which the flank approach can be used.

STERILIZATION

Today, because of an apparent overpopulation of captive exotic species, one may be requested to sterilize an animal in a manner other than by neutering. Choices in the male are vasectomy externally via surgery (Reed and Tennant, 1975) or internally utilizing the endoscope (Seager and Demorest, 1978). Females can receive implants containing hormones that are released over a long period of time (Seal et al., 1976). This method entails making an incision on the lateral aspect of the neck anterior to the shoulder and burying the implant in the subcutaneous tissue. Strictly sterile technique must be used.

Table 14.   *Tranquilizing, Immobilizing and Anesthetic Agents*

GENERIC NAME	BRAND NAME	MANUFACTURER
Phencyclidine injection 20 and 100 mg/ml	Sernylan	Bio-Ceutics (formerly)
Acetylpromazine maleate injection 10 mg/ml	Acepromazine	Ayerst
Ketamine HCl injection 100 mg/ml	Vetalar Ketaset	Parke-Davis Bristol
Xylazine injection 20 mg/ml 100 mg/ml	Rompun	Haver-Lockhart
Etorphine HCl 1 mg/ml	M99	D-M Pharmaceuticals
Etorphine HCl plus methotrimeprazine	Immobilon	Reckett and Colman-Britain
Methotrimeprazine	Levoprome	Lederle
Diprenorphine	M50-50 Revivon	D-M Pharmaceuticals Reckett and Colman-Britain
Diazepam 2,5,10 mg tablets 5 mg/ml injection	Valium	Roche
Halothane	Fluothane	Ayerst
Methoxyflurane	Metofane	Pitman-Moore
Thiamylal sodium	Surital	Parke-Davis
Sodium thiopental	Pentothal	Abbott

FRACTURE FIXATION

Fixation of fractures, whenever possible, should entail techniques that eliminate forms of external fixation or coaptation such as casts and splints, since these forms of fixation are not well tolerated in non-domestic animals.

FOREIGN BODY REMOVAL

Foreign body removal is a common surgical procedure in exotic animal practice. Rupture of the gastrointestinal tract due to foreign body perforation is seen in many of these cases. In general, nonabsorbable sutures should be used in a case of gastrointestinal perforation with or without apparent peritonitis. Young animals that are presented off-feed, vomiting bile, and dehydrated, with otherwise normal hemograms, are those that are highly suspect for having a foreign body obstruction. Careful history-taking and radiography are helpful diagnostic aids.

DENTISTRY

Dental prophylaxis and dental extraction can be carried out utilizing techniques similar to those used for domestic canines and felines. Pulpotomy and root canal are more desirable than total extraction in nearly all cases. The reader is referred to other references for further information (Fowler, 1978).

WOUNDS

Factors that are extremely important in the treatment of wounds in exotic species include the establishment of adequate drainage and the elimination of postinjury infection. The use of Penrose drains instead of suturing and the administration of high levels of antibiotics are encouraged.

Self-mutilation of traumatic or surgical wounds is common in exotic animals and can be expected of many of the canids, especially wolves, and most of the felids. Postoperative protection of surgical wounds and post-treatment protection of traumatic wounds by means of neck collars, bitter sprays, bandaging, and even tranquilization should always be considered.

SUPPLEMENTAL READING

Alford, B.T., and Wozniak, M.S.: Neuroleptic analgesia in the dog; and reversed by antagonist. J. Am. Vet. Med. Assoc., *156*:208–212, 1970.

Burkhart, R.L., and Schock, R.C.: The use of Tramisol in zoo animals. Proc. Am. Assoc. Zoo Vet., 1973.

Carpenter, J.W., Appel, M.J.G., Erickson, R.C., and Novilla, M.N.: Fatal vaccine-induced canine distemper virus infection in black-footed ferrets. J. Am. Vet. Med. Assoc., *169*:961–963, 1976.

Divers, B.J.: Hyaenidae. In Fowler, M.E. (ed.): *Zoo and Wild Animal Medicine.* Philadelphia, W. B. Saunders Co., 1978; pp. 647–650.

Foster, J.W.: Animal anthrax associated with pack saddle bags. Morbidity and Mortality Weekly Report, 1974, p. 340.

Fowler, M.E.: (Various articles.) In Fowler, M.E. (ed.): *Zoo and Wild Animal Medicine,* Philadelphia, W. B. Saunders Co., 1978; pp. 617–625.

Frenkel, J.K.: Toxoplasmosis. In Kirk, R.W. (ed.): *Current Veterinary Therapy VI.* Philadelphia, W. B. Saunders Co., 1977; pp. 1318–1324.

Kennedy, A. H.: A graphical study of the blood of normal foxes. Can. J. Res. *12*:796, 1945.

Kennedy, A.N.: Cytology of the blood of normal mink and raccoon. I. Morphology of mink's blood. II. The numbers of the blood elements in a normal mink. III. Morphology and numbers of the blood elements in a raccoon. Can. J. Res. *12*:479–495, 1935.

Hawkey, C.M.: Comparative Mammalian Haematology: Cellular Components and Blood Coagulation in Captive Wild Animals. Philadelphia, International Ideas, Inc., 1975.

Makey, D.G., and Seal, U.S.: *International Species Inventory System.* St. Paul, Minn., Minnesota Zoological Gardens, 1974.

Miller, R.M.: Diseases of exotic felines. In Kirk, R.W. (ed.): *Current Veterinary Therapy VI.* Philadelphia, W. B. Saunders Co., 1977, pp. 762–765.

Reed, G.T., and Tennant, M.B.: Vasectomy procedures for African lions. J. Zoo Anim. Med. *6*:15, 1975.

Rhodes, J.A.: Biochemical profiles in exotic captive animals. Ann. Proc. Am. Assoc. Zoo Veterinarians. San Diego, Cal., 1975, pp. 81–111.

Rubin, R., and Mason, M.M.: Normal blood and urine values for mink. Cornell Vet. *38*:79, 1948.

Ryland, L.M., and Gorham, J.R.: The ferret and its diseases. J. Am. Vet. Med. Assoc. *173*:1154–58, 1978.

Schalm, O.W., Jain, N.C., and Carroll, E.J.: Veterinary Hematology, 3rd ed. Philadelphia, Lea & Febiger, 1975, pp. 268 and 273.

Schobert, E.E.: Parasites of carnivores and hoof stock. Proc. Am. Assoc. Zoo Veterinarians, 1973.

Seager, S.W.J., and Demorest, C.N.: Reproduction of captive wild carnivores. In Fowler, M.E. (ed.): *Zoo and Wild Animal Medicine.* Philadelphia, W. B. Saunders Co., 1978, pp. 674–706.

Seal, U.S., Svain, W.R., and Erikson, A.W.: Hematology of the Ursidae. Comp. Biochem. Physiol. *22*:451, 1967.

Seal, U.S., Barton, R., Mather, L., Olberding, K., Plotka, E.D., and Gray, C.W.: Hormonal contraception in captive female lions. J. Am. Assoc. Zoo Veterinarians 4:12, 1976.

Siegmund, O.N. (ed.): *Merck Veterinary Manual*, 4th ed. Rahway, N.J., Merck & Co., 1973.

Soifer, F.K.: In Current Veterinary Therapy VI. Philadelphia, W. B. Saunders Co., 1977, p. 761.

Soifer, F.K.: Report of physiological normals committee. Proc. Ann. Meeting Am. Assoc. Zoo Veterinarians, 1970.

Spitzer, E.M., Coombes, A.I., and Wisnickey, W.: Preliminary studies of the blood chemistry of the fox. Am. J. Vet. Res. 2:193, 1941.

Timaney, J.F.: Feline infectious peritonitis. Vet. Clin. North Am. 6:391, 1976.

Walker, E.P.: *Mammals of the World*, 2nd ed., vol. 2. Baltimore, Johns Hopkins University Press, 1968, pp. 1146–1147.

VIRUS DISEASES OF PRIMATES — THEIR HAZARDS TO HUMAN HEALTH

JANIS E. OTT, D.V.M.
Brookfield, Illinois

Non-human primates long have been popular zoo and circus attractions because of their behavioral and physical resemblance to man. They also have been popular as pets. Moreover, their close phylogenic relationship to man has made them ideal animal models in research. Unfortunately, our "relatives" share many diseases with man and thus are potential hazards to public health.

Bacterial diseases such as salmonellosis, shigellosis and tuberculosis long have been recognized as potential health hazards in handling primates. The viral diseases of non-human primates are much less well defined but frequently are more dangerous. There is extensive serologic evidence that primates, including man, interchange many viruses; fortunately, few of these cause disease.

Non-human primates can be involved in the transfer of viral disease to man in several ways (Table 1). The animal can (1) harbor a viral disease while exhibiting minor signs yet transmit it to an unsuspecting human, (2) acquire the virus from one human or animal and transfer it to another, (3) act as a dead-end host for human viruses, (4) participate in arboviral arboreal disease cycles, or (5) maintain viruses as non-pathogenic agents (although the virus may be transmitted to man by tissue transfer or vaccination material).

Animals under stress (e.g., from recent importation or illness) have an increased incidence of virus shedding although they are in what appears to be an otherwise static state. These animals should be treated with special concern because of their potential hazard to human health. Strict quarantine of newly imported monkeys for 60 to 90 days should cover the incubation period of most potential diseases.

Additional preventive procedures should be followed to decrease the possible health hazards. Monkeys and their tissues should be handled as if infected. Proper restraint techniques, either physical or chemical, should be employed to prevent animal bites. Protective clothing that can be cleaned after use (i.e., gloves, masks, and long-sleeved laboratory coats) should be worn. Proper vaccinations for the non-human primate and hospital personnel as well as for pet owners are recommended (Table 2).

Different species of monkeys should be housed in isolation from each other. Specifically, Asian species ought to be kept separate from African, Old World species from New World, and New World species from each other. Fortunately, the longer the animal is in captivity the lower the risk of viral infections.

Human viral diagnostic laboratories may be able to assist in diagnosing a suspected viral disease should it occur in a non-human primate. In addition, the Regional Reference Center for Simian Viruses has been established at the Southwest Foundation for Research and Educa-

Table 1. *Viral Diseases Affecting Man and Non-human Primates*

DISEASE	PRINCIPAL ANIMALS AFFECTED	GEOGRAPHIC DISTRIBUTION	MEANS OF TRANSMISSION TO MAN
Herpesvirus simiae (herpes B.)	Macaque spp., African green monkey? man	World-wide	Bites, scratches, handling contaminated tissues
Herpesvirus T (*H. tamarinus, H. platyrrhinae*)	Squirrel monkey, marmoset, owl monkey, man?	World-wide	Unknown
Yaba virus	Macaque, baboon, vervet, patas, mangabey, man	Unknown	Contact
Monkeypox	Macaque, langur, baboon, chimp, orang-utan, squirrel monkey, marmoset, gorilla, gibbon, man	Africa	Contact
Benign epidermal monkeypox (BEMP, Yaba-like, Tanapox, OrTeCa)	Macaque, langur, man	Unknown	Contact
Marburg disease (green monkey disease, vervet monkey disease)	African green monkey, man	Unknown	Contact with infected tissues
Infectious hepatitis (simian hepatitis)	Chimp, woolly monkey, gorilla, celebes ape, patas, marmoset, man	World-wide	Contact
Rabies	Carnivores, chiroptera, monkeys, man	World-wide, except some islands	Bites of infected animals
Molluscum contagiosum	Chimps, man	Unknown	Unknown
Human respiratory viruses (human respiratory syncytial virus, reovirus, rhinovirus, influenza)	Chimp, monkey, man	World-wide	Ingestion
Lymphocytic choriomeningitis	Mouse, guinea pig, dog, monkey, man	World-wide	Contact contaminated urine of dogs
Poliomyelitis	Chimp, gorilla, orang-utan, man	World-wide	Ingestion
Measles	Macaque, gibbon, baboon, African green, squirrel monkey, marmoset, ape, man	World-wide	Ingestion
Herpesvirus hominus H. simplex	Man, gibbon, owl monkey, tree shrew	World-wide	Unknown
SV40	Rhesus, man	World-wide	Inoculation with inactivated poliomyelitis vaccine
Arboviral arboreal disease cycle	Monkey, man, rodent, bird	World-wide	Mosquito, tick
Chickenpox	Man, monkey?	World-wide	Unknown
Smallpox	Man, monkey?	World-wide	Unknown

tion in San Antonio, Texas, to investigate simian viruses. This foundation may be of assistance in identifying the viral agent.

There have been several new natural viral infections (Marburg, monkeypox, and others) reported in non-human primates in the last 15 years. These diseases generally are confined to the country of origin of the non-human primates affected. However, because of the convenience of air travel, these diseases easily could be brought to our back door by an individual bringing in a pet monkey. Therefore, practitioners must be aware of the potential risk and should acquaint their clients with the potential zoonotic hazards.

VIRAL DISEASES WITH MINOR SYMPTOMS IN MONKEYS

HERPESVIRUS SIMIAE (HERPES B)

Herpesvirus simiae long has been the most feared of monkey viruses because of its usual fatal consequence to humans. The virus is found in numerous members of the macaca species: rhesus (*Macaca mulatta*), bonnet macaque (*M. radiata*), crab-eating macaque (*M. fascicularis*), Formosan rock macaque (*M. cyclopis*), and Japanese macaque (*M. fuscata*). Serologic evidence of viral exposure also has been identified in baboons (*Papio* spp.), chim-

Table 2. *Suggested Preventive Measures for Viral Diseases*

MAN

Vaccinations

Measles: check for titers and vaccinate if indicated (especially owners of marmosets)

Smallpox: protects against monkeypox

Polio: if not previously immunized with trivalent oral vaccine

Yellow fever: if animals are procured from endemic areas

Immunoglobulin (immune serum globulin): every 4 to 6 months, if newly imported chimps are received, to protect against hepatitis A

Rabies: for individuals in high risk areas—veterinarians, animal keepers, and others

Tetanus (repeat every 5 years): not virus-associated but a good preventive measure

Other

TB test and/or chest x-ray yearly: a good preventive measure

Serum samples: 4–6 ml of serum taken yearly and stored at 10°C

NONHUMAN PRIMATES

Vaccinations

Polio: trivalent oral vaccine for chimpanzee, gorilla, and orang-utan. Infants are vaccinated at 3, 6, and 9 months and 2 years of age. Adults are vaccinated 3 times at 2-month intervals if not previously vaccinated.

Rabies: killed vaccine only; give if animal has a lot of human contact (i.e., a chance to bite)

Smallpox: prevents against monkeypox, not highly recommended

Yellow fever: only of use for the primate's point of origin if in an endemic yellow fever area

Measles: not to be given to marmosets

Tetanus: not virus-associated but a good preventive measure

Other

TB test and/or chest x-ray yearly (minimum): a good preventive measure.

Serum samples: 2–4 ml of serum taken yearly and stored at 10°C

panzees (*Pan troglodytes*) and African green monkeys (*Cercopithecus aethiops*). The significance of the titers and the potential risk from these last three animals are unknown. However, there has been reported a case of presumed B-virus infection in a person exposed to African green monkeys only. The diagnosis was made on rising titers to herpes B in both the individual and the suspected monkey. No virus was isolated in either instance.

There have been 24 documented cases of herpes B in humans since it was first reported in 1934. Eighteen of these cases were fatal. The mode of transmission of the virus from monkey to man usually is through bite wounds (documented in two of the human cases), scratches, or improper handling of contaminated monkey tissues. The virus may be isolated from saliva, blood, kidney tissue cultures, urine, and feces of infected monkeys.

Herpes B in man is characterized by ascending myelitis and encephalitis. In addition, other symptoms (nausea, sore throat, and cough) may occur. Definitive diagnosis requires a supporting history of exposure to a macaque, rising herpes B titer, and possibly virus isolation. The incubation period in man is 10 to 21 days. There has been one case of the disease in a virologist who did not exhibit signs until several years after contact with Herpesvirus simiae.

The disease in monkeys is similar to Herpesvirus hominus type I in man. The infected monkey can be asymptomatic or have ulcers (similar in appearance to the human herpes mouth sores) on the tongue, lip, face, or muco-cutaneous junction of the lip. There may be a slight nasal discharge and mild conjunctivitis. The ulcers heal rapidly (within 14 days), followed by rising levels of serum-neutralizing antibodies. The virus may remain in the host monkey and be shed periodically without the occurrence of lesions. The virus is maintained in the gasserian ganglion of the fifth cranial nerve. Infant macaques are infected by these carrier animals shortly after their passive maternal immunity has ended and hence also become carriers. Thus, in captive colonies of macaques up to 20 percent of juveniles and 80 percent of adults can have serum titers to herpes B.

In the event that an oral ulcer is observed in a macaque, the owner of the animal should be advised of the potential risk. A tentative diagnosis may be made by examining for typical herpes intranuclear inclusion bodies in epithelial cells taken from scrapings of the ulcer margins. The smear must be stained by the Papanicolaou method (Pap stain), which can be done by most human labs. Definitive diagnosis of herpes B is made on rising serum titers and virus isolation. The animal should be placed in strict quarantine until the culture results are completed. If the saliva culture is positive for Herpesvirus simiae, the animal should be euthanized. In a laboratory situation it may be best to euthanize the animal before the definitive diagnosis is made to minimize the possibility of a human infection.

The present method of euthanizing all animals in non-human primate colonies showing herpes ulcers will not eliminate herpes B from the collection because of the problem of the latent carrier in most established colonies. By screening animals for herpes B titers and breeding herpes B–negative animals, it is possible to establish a herpes B–free colony of rhesus macaques for research use. This method may eliminate the disease, but the colony must be strictly isolated from carrier animals.

Considering the number of people who have handled monkeys and their tissues, man appears to be very resistant to infection. There are antigenic similarities between human Herpesvirus hominis and the Herpesvirus simiae, so antibodies to the former may protect against the latter. The disease in some individuals may be asymptomatic, since neutralizing antibodies to Herpesvirus simiae have been encountered in monkey handlers who exhibit no outward signs of the virus. In the future, additional protection may be available in the form of a formalized vaccine for herpes B. This vaccine has been developed but is not commercially available at present. It protects animals from experimental infection and produces antibody levels in humans.

Because of their aggressive behavior and their potential zoonotic hazard, macaques are not recommended as pets.

Herpesvirus T (Herpesvirus Tamarinus, Herpesvirus Platyrrhinae)

Herpesvirus T is a virus that naturally affects squirrel monkeys (*Saimiri sciureus*). The virus is normally latent in these monkeys, but if it infects marmosets (*Saguinus* spp.) or owl monkeys (*Aotus trivirgatus*) the outcome is inevitably fatal.

There is no clear evidence that herpes T can infect man. One case has been reported of an individual working with squirrel monkeys who developed encephalitis. He had rising neutralizing antibody titers to herpes T, but no virus was isolated.

Monkeypox

Monkeypox is a reportable disease because of its resemblance to smallpox. The disease occurs in rhesus macaques, crab-eating macaques, langurs (*Presbytis* spp.), baboons, chimps, orangutans (*Pongo pygmaeus*), squirrel monkeys, marmosets (*Callithrix jacchus*), gorillas (*Gorilla gorilla*) and gibbons (*Hylobates lar*). In one reported outbreak in a zoo the virus was introduced by a newly imported anteater (*Myrmecophaga*) with smallpox-like lesions.

Monkeypox in man is rare. Because of its close relationship to smallpox, immunity to the disease can occur subsequent to smallpox vaccination in man and monkey unless the individu-

al is incubating the disease. The majority of the reported human cases occur in unvaccinated children in Africa.

The disease in monkeys has a high morbidity rate but a low mortality rate. The lesions — cutaneous eruptions — occur mainly on the limbs and face. The lesions begin as small papules that coalesce, forming umbilicated vesicles. The vesicles become covered with reddish-brown crusts and slough in seven to ten days. Crab-eating macaques may exhibit more generalized signs — fever, lymphadenopathy, and rash — and mortality may range up to 50 percent. Histologic examination of the lesions reveals cellular proliferation, degeneration and necrosis of the epidermal cells, and eosinophilic cytoplasmic and intranuclear inclusions. Isolation of affected animals and other control measures frequently are ineffective in preventing the spread of the disease. The mode of transmission is by direct contact. The virus enters through abrasions of the skin, causing a localized lesion. Diagnosis is made on the typical progression of the lesions, histologic examination, and virus isolation. There is a low concentration of antibody produced; therefore, serologic studies are of little diagnostic use.

Yaba

Yaba virus is also a pox virus, first identified in 1958 in an outbreak of subcutaneous tumors in a rhesus colony in Yaba, Nigeria. Twenty rhesus monkeys and a baboon were affected, while other African species of primates housed in the same area were not. It appears to be a latent infection in African species that infects Asian primates and U.S.-born African primates. It is also reported in a crab-eating macaque, mangabey (*Cercocebus atys*), vervet (*Cercopithecus pygerythrus*), patas (*Erythrocebus patas*), and stumptail macaque (*M. speciosa*).

Yaba tumors, which may reach several centimeters in diameter, are benign subcutaneous histiocytomas that regress spontaneously after three to six weeks. The virus infects man, but the potential is probably of little zoonotic importance. Infection usually follows accidental contaminated puncture of an individual's skin.

Benign epidermal monkeypox (BEMP, yaba-like disease, tanapox, orteca)

Benign epidermal monkeypox (BEMP) was first isolated in 1965 from skin lesions of rhesus monkeys and man in a primate colony in California. Over the next several years, three other outbreaks of the disease occurred in other U.S. laboratories, two of which received monkeys from the same importer as the California colony. A variety of macaque species were affected: pig-tailed macaque *(M. nemestrina),* bonnet macaque, stump-tailed macaque, and crab-eating macaque. Langurs also were affected. African monkeys are believed to be the reservoir of the infection, and immunologic data suggests that the virus is not naturally present in wild Asiatic macaques.

Sixteen people have been affected in outbreaks of this disease. There exists one reported case of person-to-person transmission. The symptoms were mild; however, some people developed fever and regional lymphadenopathy, particularly when the lesion was removed. The BEMP virus is identical to an agent identified as tanapox in East Africa in 1957 and 1962. Several hundred people were affected. Both of these viruses were serologically related to yaba disease, hence the "yaba-like" designation.

Transmission of the tanapox virus is believed to be via mosquitoes. BEMP is spread via direct transmission from a common source of infection such as a tattoo needle or scratches.

In monkeys, the lesions of BEMP begin as slightly elevated areas on the face and upper portions of the limbs. The lesions become circumscribed, firm, flat elevations (1 to 3 mm high) reaching a maximum diameter of 20 to 30 mm over one to two weeks. They frequently become secondarily infected or regress spontaneously over the next six weeks and are confined to the epidermis. The infected cells contain prominent intranuclear vacuoles and intracytoplasmic eosinophilic inclusions.

Control measures such as isolation are not very effective. Vaccination with smallpox vaccine does not affect the spread of disease in either monkeys or people.

MARBURG DISEASE (AFRICAN GREEN MONKEY DISEASE, VERVET MONKEY DISEASE)

Marburg disease first occurred in laboratories in Marburg, Germany, and in Yugoslavia in 1967. African green monkeys were shipped from Uganda to Europe via London. The animals spent up to 36 hours in a London airport holding facility with 48 other species of animals and birds before being shipped to the continent. A total of 31 people were affected, seven of them fatally. Another outbreak occurred in South Africa in 1975, where three people became ill. The individuals were traveling and claimed not to have contacted monkeys.

In Europe illness appeared in people handling tissues or blood or after human patient contact. No disease occurred in people who handled intact animals. The incubation period in man was five to eight days. In both man and monkey signs were similar: fever, malaise, vomiting, petechial rash, thrombocytopenia, and death, with hemorrhages throughout the body. The diagnosis was made by rising antibody titers.

Serologic examination of African green monkeys in Uganda, where the affected animals were trapped, indicated a currently active Marburg virus infection among these animals at the time of the monkey shipment to Europe. Titers subsequently taken from feral animals indicated antibodies to Marburg virus also were present in baboons, chimps, and African green monkeys in East Africa. This would imply that the disease may be latent in naturally affected animals.

Marburg disease supports the necessity for strict quarantine of newly imported animals before handling tissues. The greatest risk to humans occurs soon after arrival, when animals are stressed and most likely to be shedding viruses.

VIRAL DISEASES ACQUIRED FROM HUMANS OR ANIMALS AND TRANSMITTED TO ANOTHER HUMAN

INFECTIOUS HEPATITIS (SIMIAN HEPATITIS)

Viral hepatitis in man is divided into three classifications: infectious hepatitis (hepatitis A), which has a short incubation period; serum hepatitis (hepatitis B), which has a longer incubation period; and non-A, non-B hepatitis. Transmission of hepatitis A takes place via fecal contamination. Hepatitis B is transmitted by contaminated needles or blood transfusions and has a specific antigen, Australia antigen. Non-A, non-B hepatitis accounts for the majority of cases of post-transfusion hepatitis in man. An association between the chimpanzee and infectious hepatitis in man was first reported in 1961 after an epidemic involving 11 people and newly imported chimps. More than 70 additional cases of hepatitis in humans transmitted from non-human primates could be traced from 1953 to 1961.

The woolly monkey *(Lagothrix lagothricha),* gorilla, celebes ape *(Cynopithecus niger),* patas, and some species of marmosets also have been incriminated in the transmission of hepatitis. The non-human primates rarely show any signs of clinical illness other than elevated liver enzyme levels (SGOT, SGPT) or abnormal liver biopsies (mild to moderate inflammatory changes). Newly imported young chimps are most often associated with the infection. It is possible that these chimps become infected with the human agent after capture and subsequently can transmit the virus to man for periods of up to two months.

Non-A, non-B hepatitis has been experimentally induced and subpassaged in chimpanzees. Non-human primates have not been involved in transmission of hepatitis B, serum hepatitis. The specific antigen, Australia antigen, associated with it and antibodies to the antigen have been found in small numbers of chimps, orangutans, gibbons, baboons, celebes apes, patas, vervets, macaques, mangabeys, langurs, and several New World monkeys. Hepatitis B has been transmitted experimentally to chimps, vervets, and rhesus macaques.

The best preventive measure against hepatitis A is to limit the number of people who have contact with newly imported non-human primates for the first 60 to 90 days. In addition, there should be passive immunization with immune gamma globulin for humans who have contact with newly imported chimps. The usual hygienic procedures to minimize fecal contamination should be followed. The late discovery (eight years after the first case) of the zoonotic aspects of this disease points to the possibility that other viral diseases may have similar zoonotic potential.

RABIES

Rabies is always a potential hazard when handling any warm-blooded animal that has a tendency to bite. Clearly, monkeys fit within this category. There have been more than a thousand people throughout the world who have received antirabies treatment as a result of exposure to rabid monkeys. Several cases of rabies in monkeys have been traced to infection from inoculation with attenuated rabies vaccines. The killed vaccines are safe but their efficacy is unknown; human vaccines are nonprotective in non-human primates.

Pet simians are often infected by bites from rabid dogs. The disease in monkeys is usually the paralytic form, and bites from monkeys only occur if they become agitated. Monkey-to-monkey or monkey-to-man transmission is very rare.

The incubation period of non-human primates is unknown, but it is likely to be similar to that for man and dog. There is one experimental infection in a rhesus that lasted over 100 days prior to the appearance of clinical signs.

Once an animal bite occurs the monkey should be isolated, routine precautions should be taken, and public health officials should be notified. Non-human primates held as pets or that possibly will have human contact should be vaccinated routinely with killed rabies vaccine.

MOLLUSCUM CONTAGIOSUM

Molluscum contagiosum is a mildly contagious skin disease of children. It also has been reported in eight young chimps with papular lesions located on the eyelids. The mode of transmission is unknown.

Histologic examination of the lesions is diagnostic for the disease. Pox-like virus particles are seen with electron microscopy; however, the virus has not yet been isolated.

COMMON COLD (HUMAN RESPIRATORY SYNCYTIAL VIRUS, REOVIRUS, RHINOVIRUS, INFLUENZA)

Numerous epidemics of the common cold that are coincident with diseases present in the local human population have occurred in non-human primate collections. One is rarely able to culture the virus involved, but several candidates are suspected.

The human respiratory syncytial virus was first isolated in captive chimpanzees and identified as chimpanzee coryza agent (CCA). The virus causes rather severe respiratory infections in children and mild colds in adults. Treatment for this and the other respiratory viruses is symptomatic, but one should remain alert to the possibility of secondary bacterial pneumonia.

Other human viruses (reovirus, rhinovirus, and influenza) have been implicated in epizootics of rhinitis in chimps and gibbons. The evidence of susceptibility of monkeys and apes to these viruses has been tenuous. However, on numerous occasions epidemics of common colds are shared by non-human primates and man, which would seem to implicate a common virus.

LYMPHOCYTIC CHORIOMENINGITIS (LCM)

Lymphocytic choriomeningitis (LCM) is a viral disease of mice, guinea pigs, dogs, monkeys, and man. The house mouse is the major reservoir, excreting the virus in feces and urine. Humans or monkeys that contact affected animals or inhale dust contaminated with urine may become infected and become temporary shedders. The disease in humans is generally mild, with short febrile episodes, but may progress to a generalized fatal infection.

Monkeys affected with LCM are usually asymptomatic or show respiratory signs. Non-human primates are of minimal importance both as human health hazards and as virus reservoirs.

VIRAL DISEASES TRANSMITTED FROM HUMANS TO MONKEYS

POLIOMYELITIS

Poliomyelitis is a viral disease of man caused by a picornavirus. It has been diagnosed in chimps, gorillas, and orang-utans. These species can become infected by the oral route. The virus localizes in the tonsils, then moves via the gastrointestinal tract to the mesenteric lymph nodes. A viremia develops and a CNS infection occurs with subsequent meningitis, encephalomyelitis, and paralysis. The great apes can become carriers for up to eight weeks. There is no evidence of infection in man as a result of contact with any simian primate.

Prevention takes place by administering oral trivalent polio vaccine to the susceptible great apes. Seroconversion rates for great apes are often lower than those observed in humans.

MEASLES (PARAMYXOVIRUS)

Measles has been reported in newly imported non-human primates (i.e., rhesus monkeys, crab-eating macaques, Formosan rock macaques, gibbons, baboons, African green monkeys, squirrel monkeys, chimpanzees, and marmosets).

Measles is a primary infection in man. It infects the highly stressed, newly imported monkey. The incubation period is six to eight days after exposure. The animals develop facial edema and erythema, which changes into a maculopapular rash that subsides in three to four days. There often is conjunctivitis, moderate nasal discharge, and a dry cough. The disease can progress to interstitial bronchitis and giant cell pneumonia. Often a secondary bacterial pneumonia due to *Diplococcus*, *Klebsiella*, *Bordetella bronchiseptica*, *Streptococcus*, or *Pasteurella* will occur. Old World monkeys often develop a facial rash, while New World monkeys develop the rash on the ventral abdomen. Once the non-human primate recovers, it develops life-long immunity.

The mortality rate in Old World monkeys is 10 percent; in New World monkeys it may reach 50 percent and is especially devastating to marmosets. Abortions and stillbirths may occur with an epidemic.

During an outbreak in non-human primates, vaccination with human gamma globulin may reduce mortality and morbidity. Vaccination of newly captured primates with measles vaccine may decrease morbidity. Vaccination of marmo-sets with live vaccines is not recommended. Since the disease is most commonly observed in newly quarantined monkeys, it should be recognized that measles infection may mask a positive intradermal tuberculin reaction.

There is little evidence that non-human primates can infect man, so the disease has little zoonotic importance. However, it is recommended that people in close association with non-human primates be vaccinated for measles.

HERPESVIRUS HOMINIS TYPE I (H. SIMPLEX)

Man is the only reported natural host of Herpesvirus hominis. Fatal infections have been reported in gibbons, owl monkeys, and tree shrews *(Tupaia glis)*. Experimental infections have occurred in marmosets and cebus monkeys. Owl monkeys infected with herpes simplex virus developed anorexia, weakness, ataxia, conjunctivitis, and buccal and lingual ulcers. The disease in gibbons is similar, and in addition they may exhibit seizures and paralysis. Diagnosis is based on virus isolation and serology.

People with active herpes fever blisters should not be allowed to have contact with susceptible animals. The non-human primate usually develops this disease shortly after importation, when it is most vulnerable.

CHICKENPOX (VARICELLA VIRUS)

Chickenpox has been reported in chimps, gorillas, and orang-utans. The animals developed a macular papular rash that healed in two to three weeks. The diagnosis is questionable, however, since serologic studies and virus isolation were not performed.

SMALLPOX (VARIOLA)

Smallpox has been reported in various species of monkeys: crab-eating macaque, pigtailed macaque, and orang-utan. The animals developed a generalized skin rash. The diagnosis is presumptive, since virologic and serologic studies were not performed. There have been no reports of smallpox transmission from monkeys to man; thus, non-human primates are not believed to present a reservoir for human smallpox.

ARBOVIRAL ARBOREAL DISEASE CYCLES

YELLOW FEVER

Yellow fever is a reportable disease occurring in Africa and Central and South America. It is a hemorrhagic disease of non-human primates and man that is transmitted by mosquito vectors of the *Aedes* sp. and *Haemagogus* sp. The mosquito, once infected, remains infectious for life and hence acts as a reservoir and vector. Owing to the presence of *Aedes aegypti* in this country, it is possible that yellow fever could be transmitted to man in the U.S.

In Africa and South America, non-human primates may aid in maintaining the virus. In the jungle form of yellow fever the virus is transmitted from monkey to mosquito and then to monkey or to man. The monkeys suffer transitory infections and after recovery are immune to the virus. African species such as guenons (*Cercopithecus* spp.) and guerezas (*Colobus* spp.) rarely show clinicial disease. South American primates, spider monkeys (*Ateles* spp.), squirrel monkeys, titi monkeys (*Callicebus* spp.), white-faced monkeys (*Cebus* spp.), howler monkeys (*Alouatta* spp.), owl monkeys, and marmosets are severely affected. South American primates with experimental infections develop signs similar to those of the disease in humans, including fever within a week, listlessness, and either recovery in two weeks or death. There may be jaundice, emesis, and albuminuria.

Control procedures at the point of origin of an animal shipment should prevent introduction of yellow fever into the United States. All monkeys shipped from a yellow fever area must be maintained in a double-screened, mosquito-proof enclosure for nine days prior to shipping or be immunized with yellow fever vaccine prior to export. They must be inspected at the quarantine station and be found healthy at the time of shipment. If an animal dies within ten days after arrival, it must be necropsied and examined for evidence of yellow fever. Humans and monkeys with exposure to newly imported simians from endemic areas should also be vaccinated for yellow fever. Although there is no evidence that the disease can be transmitted from non-human primates to humans after importation to another country, the presence of the vector in the United States makes the possibility likely.

CHIKINGUNYA, O'NYONG-NYONG FEVER, AND OTHERS

Many other arbovirus-related diseases have been recognized around the world (Table 3). Non-human primates are often implicated as reservoir hosts by their presence in areas where outbreaks arise or by serologic evidence. Often the non-human primate acts as a sentinel, and its death heralds the attack of the disease. The risk of the spread of these diseases to the United States is minor; however, it points to the need for a period of quarantine after importing non-human primates from anywhere in the world.

NON-PATHOGENIC AGENTS IN MONKEYS THAT ARE TRANSMITTED TO MAN

SV40 (SIMIAN VACUOLATING VIRUS)

SV40 is a papovavirus that is apparently host-

Table 3. *Infectious Viral Diseases Caused by Arboviruses*

DISEASE	PRINCIPAL ANIMALS AFFECTED	GEOGRAPHIC DISTRIBUTION	PROBABLE VECTOR
Kyasanur forest disease	Man, monkey (bonnet macaque, langur), rodents, birds?	India	Tick: *Haemaphysalis* spp., *Ixodes* spp., *Dermacentor* spp.
Yellow fever	Monkey (see text), man	Central and South America, Africa, Trinidad	Mosquito: *Aedes* spp., *Haemagogus* spp.
Dengue	Man, monkey?	Asia, Africa, Australia, Southern Europe, South America	Mosquito: *Aedes* spp.
Chikingunya	Man, monkey (vervet, baboon, chimpanzee, rhesus macaque), birds?	Africa, Southeast Asia, India	Mosquito: *Aedes* spp., *Culex* spp.
O'nyong-nyong	Man, monkey?	Africa	Mosquito: *Anopheles* spp.
Zika	Man, monkey	Africa, Asia	Mosquito: *Aedes* spp.
Apeu, curaparu, itaqui, marituba, maratucu, oriboca	Rodents, man, monkey?	South America	Mosquito: *Culex* spp.
Catu	Rodents, monkey?, man?	South America	Mosquito: *Culex* spp., *Mansonia* spp.
Oropouche	Sloth, monkey?, man?	South America	Mosquito: *Mansonia* spp., *Aedes* spp.
Guama	Rodents, monkey?	South America	Mosquito: *Culex* spp., *Limatis* spp., *Aedes* spp.

specific and non-pathogenic to rhesus monkeys. In the production of the first inactivated polio vaccine, the product was contaminated with SV40 virus, and many children were vaccinated with live SV40. Antibody to SV40 is found in these vaccinated children and in people who have contact with rhesus monkeys. Experimentally, the virus is oncogenic in hamsters and some primates. There is apparently no recognized disease caused by this virus in man.

Numerous other simian viruses (SV5, SV20, and others) have been recovered from humans, or their presence has been implicated by sero-logic evidence. This supports the belief that a virus rarely is capable of infecting a non-human primate without infecting man, and vice versa.

SUPPLEMENTAL READING

Andrewes, C.H., and Walton, J.R.: *Animal and Human Health: Viral and Bacterial Zoonoses*. London, Bailliere Tindall, 1977.

Hubbert, W.T., McCulloch, W.P., and Schnurrenberger, P.R. (eds.): *Diseases Transmitted from Animals to Man*, 6th ed. Springfield, Ill., Charles C Thomas, 1975.

Thorn, G.W., et al.: *Harrison's Principles of Internal Medicine*, 8th ed. New York, McGraw-Hill, 1977.

T-W-Fiennes, R.N. (ed.): *Pathology of Simian Primates*. Basel, Switzerland, S. Karger, 1972.

INDIVIDUAL CARE AND TREATMENT OF RABBITS, MICE, RATS, GUINEA PIGS, HAMSTERS, AND GERBILS

STEPHEN M. SCHUCHMAN, D.V.M.

Castro Valley, California

Diagnosis and treatment of diseases of laboratory animals is not unlike those of other, more familiar, species. Their differences and similarities are neither more nor less than those between horses and cows or dogs and cats. Once this mental bridge is spanned from familiar species to laboratory species, cross-application of principles of diagnosis, treatment, and prevention of disease becomes possible.

PHYSICAL EXAMINATION

The physical examination is divided into two parts: (1) general information and (2) systematic examination of the animal.

GENERAL INFORMATION

The questions listed are designed to obtain basic information from the client as to the animal's care, general condition, and micro- and macroenvironment.

CHECK LIST

1. Species
2. Sex
3. Age
4. Weight in grams, pounds, or ounces
5. What kind of diet is fed and by whom?
6. How is water dispensed and by whom?
7. Room and cage temperature
8. Humidity
9. Type of cage
10. Frequency of cage cleaning
11. Number and kind of animals owned
12. What age group is affected?
13. What is the major complaint? How long has it been going on?
14. What does the client think is the problem?
15. Has the animal had a litter or has it been bred?
16. Has the animal been on medication in the past?

SYSTEMATIC EXAMINATION OF THE ANIMAL

Under each system, specific items are listed. These are guides to help identify clinical signs. It should be remembered that a high percentage of clinical illnesses seen in laboratory species are either primary or secondary to nutritionally deficient diets or poor animal husbandry practices.

Table 1. *Useful Information*

	HAMSTER	RABBIT	MOUSE	RAT	GERBIL	GUINEA PIG
Weight at birth	2 gm	100 gm	1.5 gm	5.5 gm	3 gm	100 gm
Puberty	(F) 28–31 days (M) 45 days (best to breed 70 days)	4–9 months	35 days	50–60 days	(F) 3–5 months (M) 10–12 weeks	(F) 20–30 days (M) 70 days
Duration of estrous cycle°	4 days	Ovulation not spontaneous; stimulated by copulation, doe ovulates 10 to 13 hr after	4 days	4 days	4 days	16 days
Gestation (days)	16	28–36	19–21	21–23	24	62–72
Separation of adults during parturition and weaning	Yes	Yes	No	No	No (mates for life)	No
Number per litter	4 to 10	7	10	8–10	1–12	1–4
Eyes open	15 days	10 days	11–14 days	14–17 days	16–20 days	Prior to birth
Wean at	25 days	42–56 days	21 days	21 days	21 days	14–21 days or 160 gm
Postpartum estrus	Within 24 hours	14 days	Within 24–48 hours	Within 24–48 hours	Within 24–72 hours	Within 24 hours
Breeding life	11–18 months	1–3 years (maximum 6 years)	12–18 months	14 months	15–20 months	3–4 years
Adult weight	(F) 120 gm (M) 108 gm	(F) 4 kg (M) 4.3 kg	(F) 30 gm (M) 30 gm	(F) 300 gm (M) 500 gm	(F) 75 gm (M) 85 gm	(F) 850 gm (M) 1000 gm
Life span (years)	2–3	5–7	3–3½	3	4	4–5
Body temperature (°F)	97–101	101–103.2	96.4–100	99.5–100.6	100.8	100.4–102.5
Daily adult water consumption	8–12 ml/day	80 ml/kg body weight	3–3.5 ml/day	20–30 ml/day	4 ml/day	10 ml/100 gm body weight
Daily adult food consumption (varies with age and condition)	7–12 gm/day	100–150 gm/day	2.5–4 gm/day	20–40 gm/day	10–15 gm/day	30–35 gm/day
Diet	Commercial rat, mouse, or hamster chow supplemented with kale†, cabbage†, apples, milk	Commercial rabbit pellets, greens in moderation	Commercial mouse chow	Commercial rat or mouse chow	Commercial mouse or rat chow (lowest fat possible); sunflower seeds	Commercial guinea pig chow, good-quality hay, kale, cabbage, fruits (cannot rely on vitamin C levels of commercial ration)
Room temperature (°F)	65–75	62–68	70–80	76–78	65–80	65–75
Humidity (percent)	50	50	50	50	less than 50	50

°All species listed except rabbits are seasonally polyestrus
†Better source of vitamin C than lettuce

EXAMINATION

1. Integument and hair coat:
   a. General condition
   b. Signs of scratching or fighting
   c. Alopecia; distribution
   d. Pustules
   e. Fluorescence of hair shafts that are not considered normal (Wood's light examination)
   f. Cutaneous swelling (neoplastic/non-neoplastic or infectious)
   g. Skin scraping, cellophane tape test for mites, black paper test for mites.
2. Digits and tail:
   a. Necrosis of digits
   b. Ulcerated or abscessed foot pads
   c. Circumscribed lesions or sores around base of tail
   d. Sores randomly spaced anywhere on tail
   e. Gray-blue coloration of tail of mice (cyanosis)
   f. Fecal soiling of ventral surface of tail near base
   g. Congenital absence of tail or loss of tail
   h. Presence of ingrown toenails
3. Ears:
   a. Examination of ear canal
   b. Scratching around ears
   c. Sores on ears
   d. Drooping ears in rabbits (in which this is not a breed characteristic)
   e. Cyanotic appearance of pinna
   f. Congenital absence of ears or evidence of traumatic loss of part or all of the pinna
4. Locomotion:
   a. Reluctance to move
   b. General weakness of all four limbs
   c. Paraparesis or paraplegia
   d. Palpate appendicular skeleton
   e. Lameness
   f. Favors a particular side when lying down (fractures or soreness on opposite side)
   g. Radiographic examination
5. Musculature:
   a. Relative amount and condition of muscle mass
   b. Pain on palpation.
6. Central nervous system:
   a. Cranial nerve deficit
   b. Spinal reflexes
   c. Postural reflexes
   d. Gross CNS disturbance (head tilt, paraplegia, circling, convulsions, flaccid or spastic paralysis)
   e. Ophthalmoscopic examination (in species in which this is practical)
7. Respiratory system:
   a. Labored breathing
   b. Open-mouth breathing
   c. Sneezing, epistaxis
   d. Evidence of nasal discharge, staining of nares, staining of medial surface of forelegs
   e. Cyanotic coloration of pinna and tail
   f. Auscultation of thorax
   g. Radiographic examination of thorax
8. Circulatory system:
   a. Auscultation of chest
   b. Palpate pulse
   c. Radiographic examination of thorax
   d. Electrocardiogram
   e. CBC and necessary blood chemistries
   f. Color of mucous membranes
9. Gastrointestinal system:
   a. Check incisors and molars
   b. Check cheek pouches for impaction or other abnormalities
   c. Examine tongue and oral mucosa
   d. Palpate abdomen
   e. Examine anus and surrounding area for signs of diarrhea or other abnormalities
   f. Check consistency and number of fecal pellets
   g. Fecal flotation, sedimentation examination, protozoan examination, and fecal culture
   h. Radiographic examination of abdomen
10. Lymphatic system:
    a. Examine for lymphadenopathy
    b. Abscessation of nodes
    c. Neoplasms
11. Mammary glands:
    a. Neoplasm
    b. Mastitis
    c. Enlargement of glands in milk production
12. Urogenital system:
    a. Determine sex
    b. Penis — sores, ulcerations
    c. Vaginal discharge
    d. Palpate for fetus
    e. Urinalysis
    f. Palpate urinary bladder for calculi

Sexing Mature and Immature Laboratory Animals. A standard rule used to determine the sex of any mature laboratory species is that the anogenital distance is longer in the male than in the female. This is easiest to determine when both sexes are present, as is the usual case when a litter is born. To determine the sex of a mature laboratory animal, consult Table 2. To determine the sex of an immature rabbit, see Figure 1. Figure 2 illustrates sex determination in gerbils, rats, guinea pigs, and hamsters.

MANUAL RESTRAINT OF RODENTS AND LAGOMORPHS

Two basic methods are described that allow for secure and safe manual restraint of rodents. The restraining procedure for rabbits differs and is described separately. Familiarity with each species minimizes the necessity of excessive restraint.

Long-tailed rodents may be removed from their cages by gently lifting them near the base of the tail and placing them either in the hand or on a non-slip surface such as a wire cage top. Short-tailed species, if too aggressive to be picked up by the palm or cupped hands, can be removed by grasping the loose skin over the neck with long-nosed forceps.

Most routine examinations are done without any restraint other than gently holding the animal in the hand. If a procedure requires more than this, the following methods are used.

Small jumpy rodents (hamsters, mice, gerbils) should be examined at ground level to prevent injuries resulting from falls from the examining table. It is important to assure that all exits from the examining room are closed.

TOWEL METHOD

This method is used for an aggressive animal or for one that might bite as a result of a required procedure. An opened towel of desired thickness (depending on the size of the animal's teeth) is placed in the hand used to hold the patient. The rodent is allowed to walk on a wired surface while the tail (if present) is held taut. The animal is then gently grasped behind the head, using the toweled hand. Once a secure hold is established, the body can be supported in the palm of the same hand or with the free hand. Routine injections, laboratory collection of specimens, minor surgical procedures, or close examination of the oral cavity can be accomplished using this procedure.

NO-TOWEL METHOD

Small rodents or less aggressive large ones may be securely restrained by placing the animal on a non-slip surface and, while holding the tail or caudal end of the animal, slowly and gently grasping enough loose skin over the neck region so that the animal's head and neck are restricted in movement. The rest of the body is held in the palm or supported with the other hand.

LIFTING, CARRYING, AND MANUALLY RESTRAINING RABBITS

Care should be taken when removing rabbits from their cages. The animal's quick, jerky motions can result in fracture of its back. The animal is removed by grasping the loose skin over the dorsum of the neck and lifting gently while the hind legs are supported with the other hand. The animal can be carried in this manner if held close to the chest.

Text continued on page 749

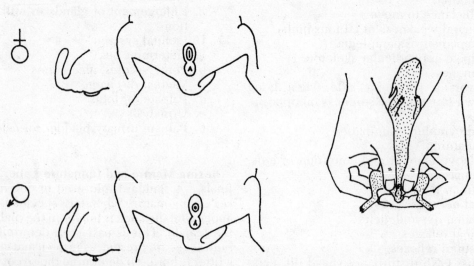

Figure 1. Sexing young rabbits. The penis of the male is a rounded protrusion 1.2 mm dorsal to the anus; a pair of reddish-brown specks occur near the vent. The vulva of the female has a slit-like opening and is less than 1.2 mm from the anus; no specks are apparent. (From Sanford: Reproduction and Breeding of Rabbits. Fur & Feather, Yorkshire, England, 1958.)

Table 2. *Determination of the Sex of Mature and Immature Laboratory Rodents and Lagomorphs*

MALE	FEMALE
Mature Hamsters, Mice, Rats, Guinea Pigs, and Gerbils	
1. Anogenital distance longer in the male.	1. Anogenital distance shorter in the female.
2. Manipulate "genital papilla" (prepuce) to protrude penis.	2. Look for three external openings in the inguinal area:
3. Palpate for testicles either in a scrotal sac (if present) or subcutaneous in inguinal region.	(a) anus (most caudal opening),
4. Males have only two external openings in the inguinal area:	(b) vaginal orifice (middle opening)—look carefully— and
(a) anus,	(c) urethral orifice at tip of urethral papilla (most anterior opening).
(b) urethral orifice at tip of penis.	In these animals the urethral papilla is located outside the vagina (unlike the dog or cat).
In very fat males there may be a depression between the penis and anus. This depression can be obliterated by manipulating the skin in that area.	In very fat females or young females, the vaginal orifice may be either hidden by folds of skin (the former) or sealed (latter). Gentle manipulation of the skin in this area will divulge the orifice.

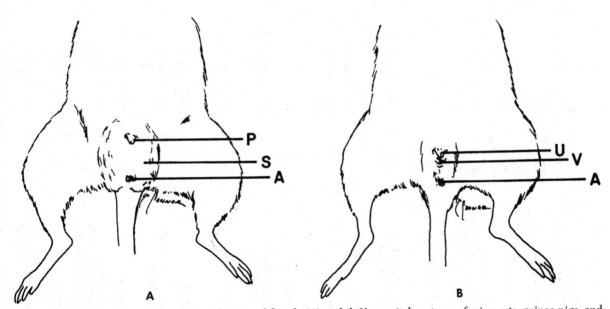

Figure 2. External genitalia of the male (*A*) and female (*B*) gerbil. Urogenital anatomy of mice, rats, guinea pigs, and hamsters is similar to that of gerbils. *P* = tip of prepuce; *S* = scrotal sac; *A* = anus; *U* = urethral orifice; and *V* = vaginal orifice. (From Harkness, J. E., and Wagner, J. E.: *The Biology and Medicine of Rabbits and Rodents.* Philadelphia, Lea & Febiger, 1977.)

Mature Rabbits	
1. Protrude penis by manipulating skin of prepuce.	1. There is a common orifice for both the vagina and urethra (like the dog and cat).
2. Palpate for testicles.	2. No structure like a "penis" can be protruded from the urogenital orifice.
3. Anogenital distance is longer.	3. Anogenital distance is shorter.

Table 3. Techniques for Performing Routine Blood Chemistries on Small Laboratory Animals

| TEST | METHOD | AMOUNT OF SAMPLE (λ)* | | | INSTRUMENT USED | WAVE LENGTH | COMMENTS** |
		Regular Plasma	or	Serum			
Glucose†	Ortho-toluidine (Communicable Dis. Center, U.S. DHEW, PHS, 1965)	20	or	20	Coleman 6/20	630	Plasma or serum must be removed from cells within 40 minutes
Glucose‡	Ortho-toluidine	25	or	25	Coleman Jr. II	595	Use Dow reagent, which uses 100 μl; can use 25 μl by cutting all solutions by 75%
BUN†	Diacetylmonoxime (Crocker, 1967)	10	or	10	Coleman 6/20	520	Use Pfizer BUN-tel, which uses 20 lambda; can use 10 lambda by cutting all solutions by 50%
BUN§	Eskalab	2	or	2	Eskalab		
Calcium or Phosphorus	Harleco	— —		250 100	Eskalab		Standard Harleco procedure requires twice the serum; solutions used are cut by 50%
Calcium§	Harleco calcium	—		500			Titration with EDTA
Calcium‡	O-cresophthalein complexone	—		25	Perkin-Elmer Coleman 55	565	Use Dow reagent, which uses 50 μl; can use 25 μl by cutting all solutions by 50%
SGPT†	Sigma Frankel	100	or	100	Coleman 6/20	505	Sigma Frankel uses 200 lambda; use 100 lambda by cutting all solutions by 50%
SGPT§	Eskalab	50	or	50	Eskalab		
SGPT‡	Henry et al. (1960) (modified)	50	or	50	Chemetrics Analyzer Computer	340	
SGPT§	Eskalab	50	or	50	Eskalab		
SCOT§	Henry (1960) Amador and Wacker (1962) (modified)	50	or	50	Chemetrics Analyzer Computer	340	
Alkaline phosphatase§	Eskalab			25	Eskalab		
Alkaline phosphatase†	Berger and Rudolph (1965) (kinetic PNP)	—		25	Perkin-Elmer Coleman 55	405	Use 1 ml of substrate

Test	Method				Instrument	Wavelength	Remarks
Sodium and potassium†	Coleman flame photometer	50	or	50	Coleman flame photometer		Add 50 lambda plasma or serum to 5 ml of working diluent
Potassium and sodium	IL flame photometer	–		50	IL flame photometer		
Bilirubin, total and direct	Evelyn Malloy (diazo technique)	100 (Add 100 more for direct)	or	100	Coleman 6/20	550	Add 100 lambda to volume of 1 ml water; this is 10% of regular method and must use micro-cuvettes
Bilirubin, total and direct‡	Jendrassik bilirubin; Nosslin (modified)	50 (Add 50 more for direct)	or	50	Coleman Jr. II	600	
Amylase†	DyAmyl-L® (dyed amylopectin)	–		50	Perkin-Elmer Coleman 55	540	For sample, dilute 50 µl with 0.95 ml saline
Amylase†	Caraway	–		50	Coleman 6/20	660	Use dilution of 50 lambda to 0.2 ml saline; use 1–5 dilution in technique
Cholesterol‡	Lieberman direct	200		–	Coleman 6/20	640	
Cholesterol‡	Lieberman direct (modified)	–		25	Coleman Jr. II	625	Use 1.5 ml color reagent with microcuvettes
Cholinesterase‡	S-butyrylthiocholine hydrolysis	–		10	Perkin-Elmer Coleman 55	405	
Chloride‡	Schales and Schales	–		50			Titration with mercuric nitrate (0.01 N)
CO_2‡	Van Slyke (modified)	50 (Heparinized only)	or	50			Titration with NaOH (0.50 N) diluted 1:10 for use
Triglycerides‡	Pinter et al. (1967) Garland and Randle (1962)	–		200	Gilford 3400 E	340	(Worthington Biochemical Corp.)
Uric Acid‡	Urica-Quant	250	or	250	Perkin-Elmer Coleman 55	405	Use BMC, which uses 500 µl; can use 250 µl by cutting reagents by 50%
LDH‡	Amador et al. (1963) Wacker et al. (1956) (modified)	–		25	Chemetrics Analyzer Computer	340	
Phosphorus‡	Hycel	–		100	Coleman Jr. II	650	Use Hycel, which uses 200 µl; can use 100 µl by cutting reagents by 50%

°10 lambda = 0.01 ml
†Techniques of H. Weitzman, Director of Hayward Medical Laboratory, Hayward, Cal.
‡Techniques of J. Alberti and L. Krusee, Veterinary Disease Laboratory, Campbell, Cal.
§Technique of A. Ramans, Valley Veterinary Hospital, Ygnacio Valley Road, Walnut Creek, Cal.
°°10 microliters (µl) = 0.01 ml

Table 4. Hospital Colony Study Using Techniques† from Table 3*

TEST	SPECIES	NO. OF TESTS RUN	MEAN	UNITS	S.D.	CV (%)
BUN	Mouse	3	21.0	mg/dl	2.64	12.50
	Rat	6	15.3	mg/dl	1.21	7.89
	Hamster	6	15.6	mg/dl	1.14	7.30
	Guinea pig	6	22.3	mg/dl	2.94	13.10
	Rabbit	4	15.0	mg/dl	2.58	17.20
SGPT	Mouse	2	26.0	IU/l	1.41	5.43
	Rat	4	16.7	IU/l	2.21	13.20
	Hamster	7	59.1	IU/l	26.20	44.40
	Guinea pig	6	23.0	IU/l	2.09	9.12
	Rabbit	3	39.3	IU/l	10.00	25.40
Alkaline phosphatase	Mouse	3	76.0	IU/l	2.51	3.29
	Rat	7	125.0	IU/l	20.10	16.00
	Hamster	8	54.6	IU/l	9.39	17.10
	Guinea pig	6	23.1	IU/l	4.95	21.30
	Rabbit	4	60.7	IU/l	8.53	14.00
Sodium	Mouse	2	152.0	mEq/l	2.82	1.86
	Rat	6	138.0	mEq/l	2.17	1.56
	Hamster	8	141.0	mEq/l	3.44	2.43
	Guinea pig	6	133.0	mEq/l	0.81	0.61
	Rabbit	3	144.6	mEq/l	6.11	4.22
Potassium	Mouse	2	7.00	mEq/l	0.14	2.02
	Rat	6	5.06	mEq/l	0.51	10.10
	Hamster	8	4.72	mEq/l	0.76	16.20
	Guinea pig	6	4.76	mEq/l	0.27	5.72
	Rabbit	3	4.70	mEq/l	0.45	9.75
Total protein	Mouse	3	5.90	gm/dl	0.23	3.89
	Rat	6	5.88	gm/dl	0.36	6.21
	Hamster	7	5.67	gm/dl	0.31	5.64
	Guinea pig	6	5.01	gm/dl	0.20	4.06
	Rabbit	3	6.10	gm/dl	0.51	5.21
Total bilirubin	Mouse	QNS	—	—	—	—
	Rat	6	0.42	mg/dl	0.14	35.30
	Hamster	6	0.77	mg/dl	0.28	36.50
	Guinea pig	6	0.57	mg/dl	0.08	14.40
	Rabbit	3	0.40	mg/dl	0.10	25.00
Cholesterol	Mouse	2	119.50	mg/dl	4.94	4.14
	Rat	3	40.00	mg/dl	3.46	8.66
	Hamster	3	88.00	mg/dl	14.70	16.70
	Guinea pig	2	60.00	mg/dl	6.36	10.50
	Rabbit	QNS	—	—	—	—
Creatinine	Mouse	QNS	—	—	—	—
	Rat	3	0.43	mg/dl	0.15	35.20
	Hamster	3	0.20	mg/dl	0.10	50.00
	Guinea pig	3	0.57	mg/dl	0.05	10.10
	Rabbit	QNS	—	—	—	—
Lipase	Mouse	2	0.025	Tietz	0.01	28.20
	Rat	6	0.072	Tietz	0.01	24.00
	Hamster	7	0.130	Tietz	0.02	20.30
	Guinea pig	6	0.060	Tietz	0.02	43.90
	Rabbit	3	0.190	Tietz	0.03	19.50

*Boulevard Pet Hospital, Castro Valley, Cal.
†Techniques of J. Alberti and L. Krusee, Veterinary Disease Laboratory, Campbell, Cal.

Table 5.   *Blood Values and Some Values of Chemical Constituents of Serum**

	RATS	MICE	HAMSTERS	GUINEA PIGS	RABBITS	MONGOLIAN GERBIL
SGPT (Sigma-Frankel units)	25–42	32–41	22–36	10–25	14–27	–
Alkaline phosphatase (Bodansky units)	4.1–8.6	2.4–4.0	2–3.5	1.5–8.1	2.1–3.2	–
BUN (mg/dl)	10–20	8–30	10–40	8–20	5–30	18–24
Sodium (mEq/liter)	144	114–154	106–185	120–155	100–145	144–158
Potassium (mEq/liter)	5.9	3.0–9.6	2.3–9.8	6.5–8.2	3.0–7.0	3.8–5.2
Bilirubin total (mg/dl)	0.42	0.18–0.54	0.3–0.4	0.24–0.30	0.15–0.20	–
Blood glucose (mg/dl)	50–115	108–192	32.6–118.4	60–125	50–140	69–119
RBC (10^6/mm^3)	7.2–9.6	9.3–10.5	4–9.3	4.5–7	3.2–7.5	8.3–9.3
Hemoglobin (gm/dl)	14.8	12–14.9	9.7–16.8	11–15	10–15	10–16
Hematocrit (percent)	40–50	35–50	40–52	35–50	35–45	35–45
WBC (10^3/mm^3)	8–14	8–14	7–15	5–12	8–10	9–14
Segmented	30	26	16–28	42	30–50	10–20
Nonsegmented	0	0	8	0	0	0
Lymphocyte	65–77	55–80	64–78	45–81	30–50	70–89
Eosinophil	1	3	1	5	1	1
Monocyte	4	5	2	8	9	0
Basophil	0	0	0	2	0	0

*These are values found in healthy-appearing animals and can be used as guides but should not be interpreted as physiologic normals for the species listed.

When ordinary means of restraint are undesirable, the following method can be used. The rabbit is placed on a non-slip surface of a table and positioned on either its back or sternum. Both fore and hind limbs are tied individually and gently but firmly stretched in their respective directions. The bindings are secured at the ends of the table. An assistant (standing in front of the animal) places each hand on the respective side of the animal's head and applies gentle but firm traction in an anterior direction. Traction is continued until the desired procedure is completed. It is thought that this procedure places the animal in a cataleptic state. Once traction is released and the animal is untied, it immediately becomes active.

BLOOD AND SERUM COLLECTING TECHNIQUES

When first using either of the following techniques, the clinician is asked to recall his or her first experience in collecting blood from a cat and how difficult it was until the technique was perfected. This experience will apply to the collection of blood from laboratory species. (See Tables 3 and 4.) A study was done on our Hospital Colony using the technique from Table 3; the results are reported in Table 5.

Needle-hub venipuncture and orbital bleeding are two methods of blood collecting that are safe, supply adequate amounts of blood, and are cosmetically acceptable. Both procedures are carried out with manual restraint only. Sedation or anesthesia is unnecessary and often contraindicated. Routine research blood collecting techniques such as cardiac puncture and cutting digits or tails have a high risk factor or are otherwise unsuitable for use on a client's animal.

Total blood volume for rodents and lagomorphs averages 5 to 7 ml/100 gm of body weight. This figure is helpful in determining amounts of blood that can safely be collected.

NEEDLE-HUB VENIPUNCTURE TECHNIQUE

The needle-hub venipuncture method can be used on laboratory species that have veins large enough to be cannulated with a 25-gauge needle. It can be used on rabbits, guinea pigs, mature rats, and hamsters. Each species is restrained in an appropriate manner by an assistant. A rubber band tourniquet is placed above the elbow or stifle. Rabbits and guinea pigs can be bled from the cephalic vein, while rats and hamsters are sampled from a large vein on the lateral surface of the thigh. Clipping the hair and extending the limb facilitate visualization of the vein. A 25-gauge, ⅝-inch hypodermic needle (without syringe) is inserted into the occluded vessel. Blood will flow into the hub of the needle. Collection is made (*in situ*) directly from the hub of the needle with a micro-hematocrit tube* or a capillary micro-container† for serum or whole blood. If skin contamination will not affect the sample, lancing of the occluded vessel without cannulation can be done. The blood sample is then collected directly from the surface of the skin.

ORBITAL BLEEDING TECHNIQUE

The orbital bleeding technique (Riley, 1960) is used when venipuncture or lancing a vein is not practical. This is the method of choice for mice but can be used on rats, hamsters, and gerbils. An assistant is not required. The animal is placed on a non-slip surface to facilitate handling.

The thumb and forefinger stabilize the head and neck and tighten the loose skin in this area. The index finger is free to lightly bulge the eye outward. With the clinician's free hand, a micro-hematocrit tube is placed just lateral to the medial canthus and gently but firmly slid posteriorly and medially under the globe to the venous plexus that lines the back of the orbit. A controlled thrust is required when collecting samples from rats or hamsters. In the mouse, the vessels of the plexus rupture easily when the tube contacts them. Slight withdrawal of the tube allows blood to fill the capillary tube.

When collecting is completed, direct pressure over the lid expedites hemostasis. Weekly sampling has been done on the same animals without clinically affecting their health. A 40-gm mouse has a total blood volume of 2 ml. If the animal is healthy, 0.1 to 0.2 ml can be safely collected. The capacity of a micro-hematocrit tube is 0.02 ml.

CBC, PLASMA AND SERUM COLLECTION

White blood cell pipettes‡ can be filled and blood smears made directly from the pooling blood.

Specimens for routine serologic studies are obtained by using plain hematocrit tubes. When plasma is needed, heparinized tubes are substituted. After the tube is filled and spun, the clot or red cell layer can be broken off and discarded, leaving a column of plasma or serum for diagnostic testing.

VIRUS DIAGNOSTIC TESTING†

Table 6 indicates viral infections that can be serologically identified and the species of laboratory animals usually tested. Testing programs such as these are used mainly for commercial colonies but have been modified for clinical application.

URINE COLLECTION

Collection techniques vary depending upon species. Mice and rats will urinate if picked up quickly. Urine may then be collected from the table surface (if clean) with a micro-hematocrit tube. Animals that will not urinate spontaneously can be placed in modified metabolic cages. These can be made by placing a plastic bag or sheet of plastic on the floor of a cage that has been elevated slightly at one end. Usually within one hour, an adequate sample is obtained. It should be remembered that gerbils produce only 2 to 3 drops of concentrated urine a day (appreciably less than other laboratory species). Rabbits' urine may be collected either by manual expression of the bladder or by centesis. Catheterization is only practical in the male. A no. 3½ French urinary catheter is used, although the urethra will accommodate a larger size. Extreme caution should be used when attempting this procedure, since the urethra in this species is easily traumatized and ruptured.

URINALYSIS

Bili-Labstix®‡ are used to check urine for pH, protein, glucose, ketones, bilirubin, and blood. The small volume of urine obtainable in some species necessitates multiple collections to complete an analysis. Specific gravity is measured with a refractometer.§ Centrifuged urine sediment samples can be obtained by filling a micro-hematocrit tube and centrifuging.

Lithuria and basic urine may be found in hamsters, guinea pigs, and rabbits. Amorphous calcium carbonate and triple phosphate crystals are the predominant types found. Rat and mouse urine is acid-reacting and comparatively free of crystals. Proteinuria is a consistent finding in these two species.

---

*Micro-hematocrit tubes (length, 75 mm; OD, 1.47 mm; ID, 0.56 mm; a larger size can be used accordingly), Clay Adams, a division of Becton-Dickinson and Co.

†Microtainer capillary whole blood collector, capillary blood serum separator, Becton-Dickinson, Rutherford, N.J.

‡Unopette®, Becton-Dickinson, Rutherford, N.J.

†Laboratory Animal Virus Testing Service, Microbiological Associates, Inc., 4733 Bethesda Ave., Bethesda, Md. 20014.

‡Ames Co., Elkhart, Ind. 46514.

§Protometer B5991 or Total Solids Meter B5996, Scientific Products, 1430 Waukegan Road, McGaw Park, Ill. 60085.

Table 6. *Serologically Identifiable Viral Infections and Laboratory Animals Used**

VIRAL INFECTION	HAMSTER	GUINEA PIG	RAT	MOUSE
Reovirus, type 3	X	X	X	X
Pneumonia virus of mice (PVM)	X	X	X	
K virus (newborn mouse pneumonitis)				X
Theiler's encephalomyelitis (GD–VIII)	X	X	X	
Polyoma				X
Sendai	X	X	X	X
Minute virus of mice (MVM)			X	X
Mouse adenovirus (MAdV)			X	X
Mouse hepatitis (MHV)			X	X
Lymphocytic choriomeningitis (LCM)	X	X	X	X
Ectromelia				X
Toolan H-1		X	X	
Simian myxovirus (SV5)	X	X	X	X
Kilham rat virus			X	
Rat coronavirus			X	

*Laboratory Animal Virus Testing Service, Microbiological Associates, Inc., 4733 Bethesda Ave., Bethesda, Md. 20014.

ECTOPARASITE MONITORING

Mite and fungal infestations are two of the more common dermatologic problems encountered. Examination of the animal may be expedited by the use of a hand lens or binocular loupe. Scrapings, Wood's light examination and fungal culture are the tests of choice. When mite infestation is suspected but cannot be demonstrated by skin scraping, it may be helpful to place an anesthetized or chemically immobilized animal on black paper. If the test is conducted long enough and infestation is moderate to heavy, the mites will migrate from the skin to the hair shafts where they can be seen. They may also be visible on the black paper.

FECAL ANALYSIS FOR HELMINTHS, PROTOZOA, AND BACTERIA

Analysis of feces is an important part of a laboratory animal's health program, whether the animal is used for research or as a pet. The examination should consist of (1) fecal sedimentation examination, (2) fecal flotation examination, (3) protozoan smear examination, and (4) bacterial culture of feces on selective media. The analysis should specifically check for (1) ova of *Hymenolepis nana*, (2) ova of *Syphacia*, *Aspicularis*, and other nematodes, (3) overgrowth of protozoa, and (4) *Salmonella* and *Pseudomonas*.

Coprophagy, feces-contaminated food or bedding, and contamination of feed during processing all contribute to heavy infestation if the life cycle of the pathogenic organism is direct. Semi-yearly examinations are advised if the animal population remains closed. If new animals enter the household, testing should be more frequent.

CLINICAL SIGNS AND DISEASES MOST COMMONLY SEEN*

The following information is tabulated (Tables 7 to 11) for each species:
1. The systems most commonly affected by diseases
2. Clinical signs most commonly seen when that system is affected
3. Description of disease
4. Brief approach to treatment
5. Differential diagnosis in some cases
The systems and diseases are listed in order of decreasing frequency.*

DIAGNOSTIC RADIOGRAPHY FOR SMALL RODENTS

Diagnostic radiographs can be obtained by using the technique chart (Table 12). Individual calibration of the machine to be used is necessary for best results. Rabbits and large rats require the same technique as that for cats. Kodak Blue Brand® or Sakura® medical x-ray film is used in high-speed cassettes. Kodak no-screen film is also used especially when patient movement is not a problem and greater detail is needed.

To facilitate positioning of a small mammal, 4 strips of adhesive tape, ½ × 12 inches long, are wrapped around the individual extremities. Thus, adequate positioning can be obtained even while wearing lead gloves. Placing small

*Based on the author's experience.

Text continued on page 762

Table 7. Diseases of Rabbits

CLINICAL SIGNS	AGE GROUP	MORBIDITY	MORTALITY	TESTS	ETIOLOGIC AGENT	TREATMENT	COMMENT
Respiratory System							
Unilateral or bilateral purulent nasal discharge; stained hairs around nostrils; sometimes staining of medial aspect of paws; nasal discharge may be present only on exercise; conjunctivitis; some cases may show marked dyspnea	Usually mature	H(±)	±	Culture; radiographs of thorax	*Pasteurella multocida*	A. Antibiotics 1. Penicillin 2. Furazolidone 3. Tetracyclines 4. Sulfonamides 5. Sulfaquinoxaline B. Nebulization, vaporization	Common name: "snuffles"; primarily a respiratory disease, but same organism can cause septicemia, abscess, urogenital disease in males and females
							Other less common diseases that can cause respiratory signs:
					Pasteurella pseudotuberculosis		Pseudotuberculosis
					Vaccinia virus		Rabbitpox: Usually rash, pock-type lesions on skin and ears
					Myxoma virus		Myxomatosis: Very high morbidity and mortality; may see edema of head resulting in drooping of ears; also, in chronic cases, fibrotic nodules on nose and ears
							Non-specific conjunctivitis, (conjunctivitis only sign)
Integument and Ears							
Crusty accumulation in ear canals; shaking head; scratching at ears	Any	±	L	Otoscopic and microscopic examination	*Psoroptes cuniculi; Chorioptes cuniculi*	Rotenone in oil; clean cage	Common name: ear canker
Crusty skin; pruritus; alopecia (patchy or generalized); usually head and ears affected but can be any place on body	Any	±	L	UV light; KOH preparations; fungal culture	*Microsporum* sp.; *Trichophyton* sp.	Griseofulvin	Communicable disease
Alopecia on chest area; animal biting out hair	Mature female	0	0	Rule out other dermatologic diseases	Hair pulling for nesting behavior	Nothing	Other pruritic disease: *Sarcoptes*
Large subcutaneous abscess anywhere on body, usually underside of neck	Any (but more in males)	L	L	Culture	*Pasteurella multocida* (unless proved otherwise)	Open drain; appropriate antibiotics (penicillin)	Usually associated with fighting or from a chronically irritated area; staphylococcus second most common cause

Digestive System

Signs	Age/Sex Affected		Diagnosis	Cause		Treatment	Comments
Slobbering; difficulty eating; may get teeth caught on wire cage	Usually mature	L	Examination of oral cavity	Probable congenital malocclusion	L	Routine cutting of overgrown or ingrown incisors or molars	Continuous-growing incisors must be continually worn down; if not, this condition may result. Lack of gnawing on hard objects is not a major cause; malocclusion is.
Small warts on tongue and oral mucosa	Any over a month old	±	Biopsy	Rabbit oral papillomatosis	±	Remove wart or vaccinate	
Bloat; profuse mucoid diarrhea; anorexia; borborygmus; huddling	Any	+	Fecal analysis to check for other problems	Unknown; may be: 1. Due to deficiency of amylase 2. Nutritional 3. Bacterial 4. Viral 5. Irritant 6. Toxin 7. Stress	± (young)	Increase roughage in diet; prevent secondary septicemia and dehydration; increase fiber in diet to 15–25%; dimetridazole powder 0.025 to 0.1% in drinking water during 3–8 weeks of age	Commonly referred to as mucoid enteritis or mucoid enteropathy. Other less common diarrhea-causing diseases 1. Salmonellosis 2. Coccidiosis

Mammary Gland

Signs	Age/Sex Affected		Diagnosis	Cause		Treatment	Comments
Anorexia; polydipsia; mastitis	Mature female	L	Culture	Streptococcus; Staphylococcus; Pasteurella	±	Antibiotics; drain; hot pack	Usually associated with nursing

Urogenital System

Signs	Age/Sex Affected		Diagnosis	Cause		Treatment	Comments
Lithuresis; pH urine 8–9; urine dries and leaves large amount of white crystals; sometimes urine may be brown or red-brown	Any; usually mature when noticed	0	Urinalysis	Normal rabbit urine	0	None	When urine dries, it has chemical consistency similar to that of boiler scale; use mild acid solution such as vinegar to clean area.
Ulceration; scab-covered lesion about genitals, either sex; can have ulcers in other areas; vesicles may be on skin surrounding genitals	Mature		Look for organism in exudate using dark field microscopy	Treponema cuniculi		Penicillin	Not communicable disease

Miscellaneous

Signs	Age/Sex Affected		Diagnosis	Cause		Treatment	Comments
Hepatomegaly; irregular surface to liver; abdominal enlargement; poor general condition; diarrhea (±); in young, mild hemorrhagic diarrhea (a healthy rabbit usually seen; hepatic lesions may only be seen as an incidental finding)	Any	±	Microscopic examination of feces; both types have oocysts that appear in stool	Eimeria sp.; both intestinal and hepatic types occur in rabbit	±	Wire floors; sulfaquinoxaline; sulfamethazine; sulfaquinoxaline 0.1% solution in drinking water for 2 weeks	Other less common diseases affecting liver 1. Pasteurella tularensis causes small yellow-gray necrotic foci on liver; spleen is covered with miliary necrotic foci 2. Tyzzer's disease; necrotic foci on liver, along with enteritis
Subcutaneous swellings	Any	L	Biopsy	Pox virus	L		Shope fibroma only seen in wild cottontails

Table 8. Diseases of Guinea Pigs

CLINICAL SIGNS	AGE GROUP	MORBIDITY	MORTALITY	TESTS	ETIOLOGIC AGENT	TREATMENT	COMMENT
Lymph System; Respiratory System							
Active, healthy looking animal with enlarged lymph nodes; nodes may discharge pus	Usually mature	±	±	Culture	β-Hemolytic streptococci, Lancefield type C	Antibiotics; drainage; quarantine	Called "lumps"; other diseases (less common) with same signs: pseudotuberculosis, streptobacillosis
Acute death	Any	±	H	Culture; necropsy	β-Hemolytic streptococci		Generalized septicemia; other diseases causing acute death: salmonellosis, pseudotuberculosis
Chronic duration: anorexia, ruffled haircoat, huddling, dyspnea, nasal discharge, crusty dried mucus on medial aspect of forelegs, purulent conjunctivitis, lymphadenitis	Usually mature	±	H	Culture	β-Hemolytic streptococci, Lancefield type C	Antibiotics; supportive care. Oxytetracycline at a rate of 0.1 mg/ml of drinking H_2O for 7 days can be used to control epidemic but does not eliminate condition[*]	*Other diseases with similar signs:*
					Bordetella bronchisepticus		*Bordetella:* usually just confined to respiratory tract
					Salmonella typhimurium or *Salmonella enteriditis*		*Salmonella:* respiratory signs usually lacking; may not have diarrhea
					Pasteurella pseudotuberculosis		Pseudotuberculosis: palpate for enlarged mesenteric lymph nodes; chronic emaciation may be only sign
							Pneumococcal pneumonia
							Virus pneumonia
							Pseudomonas
							Klebsiella
							Corynebacterium
Integument and Hair							
Alopecia (can be generalized or patchy), may be symmetrical in distribution; non-pruritic	Any age	±	L	Rule out other dermatologic diseases	Unknown; in weanlings or females, may be due to stress; in males, a similar-looking disorder is due to grooming between two animals	Feed hay, cabbage, or kale or do nothing	Usually seen only in colony or heavy stress situations
Pruritus, scab-like lesions, owner usually sees small, white elongated insects	Any age	±	L	Examine hair and skin closely	Lice (*Gliricola Gyropus*)	Carbamate powders, dichlorvos strips	Good husbandry necessary for control

Clinical Signs	Age			Diagnosis	Etiology	Treatment	Remarks
Scaly, patchy skin lesions; broken hair shafts, can be generalized; pruritic	Any	±	L	UV light; KOH preparation culture	*Tricophyton Microsporum*	Griseofulvin (use cautiously, since derived from *Penicillium* cultures)	Communicable disease
Sores on hocks or plantar surface of foot; abscesses	Mature	±	L	Culture	*Corynebacterium pyogenes*	Put on softer surface; treat symptomatically (daily medicated dressings)	Problem encountered when animal is usually raised on wire
Diseases of Pregnant Females							
Sow in late pregnancy; lethargy; anorexia; huddling; may die within 24 hours	Mature	±	+		Pregnancy toxemia	Steroids; supportive care; calcium gluconate Cesarean section	Friable yellow liver on necropsy; normal fetus; may be prevented by feeding good-quality diet last part of gestation
Digestive Tract							
Difficulty chewing or moving mouth; slobbering when eating; overgrowth of molars	Mature	±	L	Physical examination; radiography	Probable congenital malocclusion; poor quality hay diet; chronic fluorosis	Correct diet; file or cut molars to proper size	Disease of salivary glands may mimic clinical signs; chemical restraints may be needed to examine molars
Blood-tinged diarrhea; acute death sometimes in young; usually asymptomatic	Young	±	±(L)	Fecal analysis	*Eimeria caviae* or protozoan overgrowth (*Trichomonas*)	Coccidiostats	Coccidiosis usually not a problem; other internal parasites not usually a problem but should check for them; nematode of cecum (*Paraspidodera*) is reported to be most common
Miscellaneous							
Poor weight gain; rough coat; greater incidence of disease; increased huddling; hesitancy to move about; enlarged joints (±); subconjunctival hemorrhage (±)	Any	±	±	Serum ascorbic acid levels of feed and analysis	Ascorbic acid deficiency	Ascorbic acid in water and feed; kale, cabbage, citrus fruits, orange juice instead of water; ascorbic acid supplement 1–3 mg/100 gm/day or 100 mg tablet dissolved in 500 ml of drinking H_2O, change daily	Occurs even on fortified commercial diet 1. Poor quality control of commercial ration 2. Shelf life of guinea pig feed is short. Other diseases causing soreness of limbs or inability to move 1. Fractures 2. Muscular dystrophy (vitamin E deficiency) 3. Myositis (viral?) 4. Guinea pig paralysis (viral?)
Cachexia; generalized loss of condition	Usually mature males	±	±	Possibly radiography and/or electrolyte studies	Thought to be improper Ca:P ratio or its relationship to Mg	Put on balanced diet	Diffuse calcification of internal viscera
Straining to urinate; small amount of urine; blood-tinged urine, arching back, standing higher on hind feet	Mature males mostly	±	±	Palpate bladder for urinary calculi, X-ray abdomen	Unknown	Cystotomy	May cause intermittent or complete obstruction. It is an operable condition

*Harkness, J. E., and Wagner, J. E.: The Biology and Medicine of Rabbits and Rodents. Philadelphia, Lea & Febiger, 1977.

Table 9. Diseases of Hamsters

CLINICAL SIGNS	AGE GROUP	MORBIDITY	MORTALITY	TESTS	ETIOLOGIC AGENT	TREATMENT	COMMENT
Gastrointestinal Tract							
Diarrhea-stained anus; lethargy; anorexia; prolapsed rectum; can die within 48 hours to 1 week after symptoms start	Any	±	H	Culture feces; fecal analysis; direct smear	Proliferative ileitis "Wet tail"; exact etiology unknown; overgrowth of *E. coli* and protozoan organisms (trichomonads); improper caging; overcrowding; lack of fresh water	Supportive care 1. Fluids sq. 2. Antibiotics (Gentocin) 3. Sulfonamides 4. Improve husbandry 5. Fresh food 6. Whole milk or buttermilk 7. Surgery for intussusception	Very common; guarded prognosis; normal bacteria, flora and fauna are gram-negative bacilli resembling *Bacterioides, Lactobacilli* (gram-positive type), *Streptococcus bacillus, Escherichia, Staphylococcus,* spirochetes, large coccus forms, *Giardia* and trichomonads; prolapsed rectum is usually accompanied by an intussusception of the colon
Mild diarrhea; animal relatively healthy in appearance	Mature	L	L	Microscopic examination of stool	Overgrowth of *Trichomonas, Giardia, Chilomastix*	High protein diet fed for 7 days; 45% ground beef liver, 42% lean ground beef, 11% lard, 2% calcium carbonate or carbarsone per os; 15.6 mg/100 gm body weight per day for 21 days	
Constipation; diarrhea may be associated with it	Young	±	±	Palpate abdomen; x-ray abdomen	Inadequate amount of water to drink	Assure adequate water intake; milk of magnesia	

Clinical Signs	Age			Diagnosis	Etiology	Treatment	Comments
Usually no clinical signs other than mild enteritis	Any	±	L	Fecal analysis	*Hymenolepis nana; Syphacia obvelata,* and others	Proper anthelmintic; piperazine, Yomesan	*H. nana*; communicable disease
				Integument			
Alopecia about the face, but can be generalized	Usually mature	±	±	Skin scrapings	*Demodex* sp.; *Notoedres* sp.	Pyrethrum insecticides; Eurax (crotomiton)	Common; although looks like a poor prognosis they respond; pruritus is not a major finding
				Miscellaneous			
Paresis; inactivity; inability to lift head; crawls	Mature	±	±	Physical examination, radiographs	Nutritional deficiency	Vitamin D	Commonly called cage paralysis; other musculoskeletal diseases: 1. Nutritional muscular dystrophy (vitamin E deficiency) 2. Polymyopathy and myocardial necrosis (congenital and genetically controlled gradual onset)
Ocular discharge; chattering; ruffled haircoat; huddling; nasal discharge ±	Young; more susceptible	±	L	Possible viral etiology and/or pneumococcus, streptococcus		Antibiotics: chloramphenicol; tetracyclines	
Change in behavior; lethargy; inactivity; sleeping long periods; slow heart rate; respiratory rate slow; all animals in group may not be in this condition; low body temperature	Usually not in very old animals	±	±	Physical examination	Hibernation: large fluctuation in ambient temperatures; precold exposure in history	Raise environmental temperature	Animal will go into hibernation for a few days, then out; may be repeated; heart rate can be as slow as 4–15 beats/minute

Table 10. Diseases of Mice and Rats

CLINICAL SIGNS	AGE GROUP	MORBIDITY	MORTALITY	TESTS	ETIOLOGIC AGENT	TREATMENT	COMMENT	SPECIES
Integument and Appendages								
Scratching around head and ears; abrasions; scabs; bald spots	Haired animals	±	L	Skin scraping; blue paper test	*Myobia; Myocoptes; Radfordia; Notoedres*	Dichlorovos strips; ectocide; pyrethrum powder	Common in mice	Mice, rats
Sores around ears and on pinna; scabs and wounds randomly positioned on caudal two-thirds of tail	Mature males	L	L	Observation	Fighting	Separate males		Mice
Circumscribed necrotic lesion usually at base of tail	Any	±	L		Humidity too low	Adjust humidity to 50-55 per cent	Ringtail syndrome	Mice
Congenital absence of tail	At birth	O	O	Genetic studies	Hereditary			Mice
Bluish or pale color of pinna or tail	Any	±	H	Any that are necessary	Cyanosis, usually associated with severe respiratory illness or septicemia	Antibiotics; fluids; general supportive care	Poor prognostic sign	Mice
Bald spots; scaliness; pruritus (±)	Haired	+	L	Wood's light examination; KOH slide culture	*Trichophyton; Microsporum*	Griseofulvin; tolnaftate cream 1 per cent	There may be some normal fluorescence of hair shafts	Mice, rats
Sloughing and/or necrosis of digits and tail; papules or pustules (±)	Any	H	H	Serology	Pox virus (ectromelia)	Vaccination; supportive care if requested; euthanasia advised	Often a latent infection; vaccination of healthy stock	Mice
Respiratory System								
Sneezing; chattering; labored breathing; nasal discharge; pawing at nose; epistaxis; cachexia; unkempt coat; arching of back; generalized depression; vestibular disease; conjunctivitis	Usually mature	±	±	Culture if possible; serology	Not a specific disease entity but due to one or more of the following: enzootic bronchiectasis (rats) (probable virus); infectious catarrh (*Mycoplasma pulmonis*); disease syndrome referred to as chronic murine pneumonia	Antibiotics; long-term if necessary 1. Tylosin 2. Sulfonamides 3. Tetracycline, 2-5 mg to each ml H_2O 4. Sulfamerazine 0.02% solution	Other less common diseases with similar signs: *Pasteurella pneumotropica; Bordetella bronchiseptica;* pneumonia virus of mice; adenovirus; K virus; *Diplococcus pneumoniae* (common in rats); streptococcal infections	Mice, rats

Gastrointestinal Disease

Sign	Age			Diagnosis	Cause	Treatment	Remarks	Species
Prolapsed rectum	3 weeks and older	±	L	Fecal analysis; cellophane tape test not reliable	*Aspicularis tetraptera; Syphacia obvelata* or other heavy parasite infestation	Appropriate anthelmintic therapy: 1. Piperazine compounds 2. Yomesan	Pinworms and *Hymenolepis nana* are common (M)	Mice, rats
Mustard-color soiling around tail and caudal part of body; watery stools; acute death; fecal impaction	Suckling age	H	H	Fecal cultures if necessary to rule out other diseases	Epizootic diarrhea of infant mice (EDIM); epizootic diarrhea of suckling rats	Filter caps over top of cage prevent transmission; antibiotic therapy sometimes helpful	Filter caps and sanitation are effective in stopping outbreaks	Mice, rats
Mild diarrhea; usually healthy-looking animal	Any age	±	L		*Giardia* or other protozoan overgrowth	Feed apples, cabbage, ground beef; furazolidone, antibiotics		
Acute death; focal necrosis of liver (white spots); may have enteritis; diarrhea may be present	Any age	±	H	Difficult to culture; histopathology with special staining technique may demonstrate organisms	Tyzzer's disease; *Bacillus piliformes*	Antibiotics	Can be latent; other diseases with similar signs; salmonellosis; *Pseudomonas*, septicemia following stress	Mice, rats

Central Nervous System

Head tilt; circling	Mature	L	L	Radiography; neurologic examination	*Mycoplasma* or bacterial infection of vestibular apparatus associated with upper respiratory infection	Antibiotics; steroids		Mice, rats

Mammary Glands

Neoplasm	Mature female	L	L	Biopsy	Mammary tumor, fibroadenoma, adenocarcinoma (M); fibrosarcoma (R)	Surgical excision	Usually recur after removal; located anywhere on body	Mice, rats

Lymph Nodes

Lymphadenopathy	Mature	L	±	Culture or biopsy	*Pasteurella pseudotuberculosis*	Antibiotic if bacterial		Mice, rats

Table continued on next page

Table 10. Diseases of Mice and Rats (Continued)

CLINICAL SIGNS	AGE GROUP	MORBIDITY	MORTALITY	TESTS	ETIOLOGIC AGENT	TREATMENT	COMMENT	SPECIES
Miscellaneous								
Enlargement of salivary glands causing swelling of neck region	Mature	±	L	Biopsy	Sialodacryadenitis; viral etiology	Steroids; antibiotics	Usually latent	Rats
Marked depression; hunched-up posture; roughened coat; conjunctivitis; anorexia; lethargy; death; stunting in surviving animals	Any; young more commonly affected	±	±	Fecal culture	*Salmonella, Pseudomonas*	Antibiotics; hyperchlorination of water (10 ppm); euthanasia advised (if communicable disease)	These are non-specific signs of septicemia; any latent disease can cause infection if animal is stressed; examples are mouse hepatitis virus, reovirus, heavy parasitism	Mice

*Table 11.   Diseases of Gerbils**

CLINICAL SIGNS	AGE GROUP	MORBID-ITY	MORTAL-ITY	TESTS	ETIOLOGIC AGENT	TREATMENT	COMMENT
				Miscellaneous			
Bare spots on base of tail	Mature	±	L		Fighting due to overcrowding	Correct over-crowding	
Inflammation and ulceration around the nose and jaw	Mature			Rule out other dermatologic problems	Thought to be from mechanical abrasion	Remove source of mechanical abrasion	
Protrusion of nictitating membrane, conjunctiva, and eye itself	Older animals	?	?		Unknown		Evaluate for glaucoma or retrobulbar pressure
Scanty or patchy growth of hair	Young not weaned	?	?		Unknown	None; hair will grow in as animal gets older	Seen in some strains of mice also
Seizures when handled: body stiffens; legs stiffen and tremble	More common in young animals				Thought to be a form of catalepsy	Dilantin has been used but may be unnecessary	Seizures occur with less frequency as the animal gets older
Sneezing; chattering; labored breathing	Any	±	±	Physical; culture; radiography	Virus? Bacterial? Mycoplasm?	Penicillin; tetracyclines	Usually follows stress
Diarrhea, mild	Any	±	±				No one enteric disease is prevalent but should consider enteritis due to: 1. *Salmonella* 2. Unwashed vegetables 3. Parasitism, although very few natural parasites; gerbils are very susceptible to most experimental infestation 4. Protozoan overgrowth (*Entamoeba* may be a normal finding)

*From: Schwentker, V., Tumblebrook Farm, West Brookfield, Mass.: Personal communication.

Table 12. *Radiographic Technique for Small Mammals**

THICKNESS (cm.)	FFD (inches)	KVP	MA	SECONDS	MAS
			Bone†		
0.5	36	40	100 (Fine Focal Spot)	1/30	3.3
1		42			
2		44			
3		46			
4		48			
5		50			
6		52			
7		54			
			Soft Tissue		
1	36	38	100 (Fine Focal Spot)	1/30	3.3
2		40			
3		42			
4		44			
5		46			
6		48			
7		50			
8		52			
9		54			
			Thoracic		
2	36	34	200	1/60	3.3
3		36			
4		38			
5		40			
6		42			
7		44			
8		46			

*Radiographic technique of R. P. Barrett, Castro Valley, Cal.

†If animal is immature, it might be better to use 50 ma.

rodents in a stockinette tube or radiolucent plastic cylinder is also helpful in taking radiographs of non-anesthetized patients.

PARENTERAL ROUTES OF MEDICATION

Intramuscular and subcutaneous injections are the preferred routes of parenteral administration of medications. Accurate dosing is accomplished by using a tuberculin or a microliter syringe* equipped with a 25- to 27-gauge needle. Microliter syringes are used when doses are 0.1 ml or less.

Intravenous injections can be given when necessary. A 25- to 27-gauge needle is chosen according to vein size. The vein of choice for an intravenous injection in each species is listed at the top of the next column.

*Microliter syringe (0.001 to 0.1 ml), The Hamilton Co., Reno, Nevada.

SPECIES	VEIN OF CHOICE
Rabbit	Marginal ear vein or cephalic vein
Guinea pig	Cephalic vein
Rat	Vein on the caudolateral aspect of the thigh or the vein on the dorsal surface of the tail*
Hamster	Vein on the caudolateral aspect of the thigh
Mouse	Tail vein* (very difficult without practice)

*Wrap or immerse the tail in warm water prior to venipuncture.

INTRAGASTRIC INTUBATION AND ARTIFICIAL ALIMENTATION

Oral alimentation by eye dropper or intragastric intubation of a liquid replacement diet can help support an anorectic patient's nutritional needs. Liquid diets* fortified with baby foods (fruits, vegetables, cereals, meats) have been used satisfactorily. Usually, a volume of 2 to 3 ml/100 gm of body weight is infused at one time. Karo syrup, honey, or vegetable oil can be added if caloric requirements necessitate it. The daily caloric requirement for a healthy mature rodent is roughly 15 to 35 kcal/100 gm of body weight. The higher caloric requirement pertains to mice and hamsters, while the lower requirement is for rats, guinea pigs, and rabbits. Growth, lactation, or a febrile condition can double the daily caloric requirement. Table 13 gives several purée recipes. The purées can be given by eye dropper, gastric intubation, or free choice. Anorectic guinea pigs that would not take solid food have been fed these diets as their only source of nutrition for up to two months. Purées should be fed at room temperature. Refrigeration life is short, less than two days.

Intragastric intubation can be accomplished with either a flexible rubber tube† or a rigid metal cannula‡ with a ball-tipped end. Sharp incisors can easily cut a flexible tube unless the jaws are manually held open. Passage of the tube through the interdental space (between incisors and molars) may help avoid this problem. If this is not possible, a tongue depressor or a small flat stick with a hole drilled in its center can be used as a mouth gag. The gag is placed on edge just behind the incisors. A tube can then be passed through the hole in the mouth gag. Specula are not needed when using metal cannulas. These are designed specifically for use in laboratory species. With a little prac-

*Esbilac® (Borden), Initol® (Hill), Neo-Mull-Soy® (Borden) and Pet Kalorie® (Haver-Lockhart) made into a slurry.

†Number 3 to 12 French rubber stomach tube by Davol.

‡Oral Administration Needle, Aloe Scientific, 1831 Olive Street, St. Louis, Mo. 63103; or Biomedical Needles, Animal Feeding Stainless Steel, Popper & Sons, Inc., New York, N.Y. 10010.

*Table 13.   Purée Recipes**

	PELLET	APPLE	ENDIVE	BABY FOOD	ESBILAC	NUTRICAL
Main ingredient	1/2 cup rabbit or guinea pig pellets	1 cut-up apple (Carrots or fresh corn may be substituted)	2 cups chopped endive (Other greens may be substituted)	Feed from jar: Strained creamed spinach Strained pears Strained applesauce	1 tsp Esbilac powder	1/3 tsp Nutrical
Amount of water	3/4 cup	1/8 cup	1/4 cup	none	1 tsp	1/3 tsp
Comments	Soaking pellets before blending gives best results	←————— Mix in blender to desired consistency —————→				May be fed separately or mixed with Esbilac

GENERAL COMMENTS

A blender is suggested for preparing purées.
Amounts of liquids in the above recipes can be adjusted to change mixtures to desired consistency.
It is preferable to prepare puréed foods daily.
Use plastic medicine droppers to feed purées. If opening at tip of dropper is not large enough, it can be made bigger by cutting a little off the tip with a strong pair of scissors.
It is always advisable to present a variety of foods. A sick pet may turn away from the first entrée offered but take another with no hesitation.
Add ascorbic acid—200 mg per 500 ml of purée—for guinea pigs.

*Purée recipes from Manuel Rood, Berkeley, Cal.

Table 14. Drug Dosage*

DRUG	MANUFACTURER'S CONCENTRATION	DOSAGE BY WEIGHT (mg/body weight)	ROUTE	DOSAGE BY VOLUME (ml/body weight)†	COMMENT
Fluothane	U.S.P.	Give to effect	Inhaled	Give to effect	Found to be very safe and well tolerated. I do not use nitrous oxide when anesthetizing rodents or rabbits. Halothane is my drug of choice for immobilization or anesthetization.
Innovar-Vet	Comes in a standard concentration containing a mixture of Fentanyl, 0.4 mg/ml, and Droperidol, 20.0 mg/ml	—	Intramuscular	0.02–0.05 ml/100 gm	Up to 0.15 ml/100 gm may be necessary in hamsters; 0.02–0.05 ml dose works best in rats, guinea pigs, and mice; 0.02 ml for rabbits.
Nalline	5 mg/ml	0.5 mg/100 gm	Subcutaneous; intramuscular; intravenous	0.1 ml/100 gm	Intravenous route for quickest response; 5 mg is the largest dose usually given.
Ketamine HCL	100 mg/ml	4.4 mg/100 gm	Intramuscular	0.05 ml/100 gm	Produces a mild form of sedation; good for minor surgical procedures and oral examination; short duration; less than 20 minutes.
Ketamine HCL	100 mg/ml	11 mg/kg	Intravenous	0.11 ml/kg	Used in rabbits; good for endotracheal intubation and minor surgical procedures; very short duration (less than 10 minutes).
Surital (5 gm) stock bottle	2% solution	—	Intravenous	1.0 ml/2.27 kg (1.0 ml/5 lb)	Used in rabbits for endotracheal intubation; use anesthetic to effect.
Atropine sulfate	1/150 gr/ml or 0.4 mg/ml	0.004–0.01 mg/100 gm	Subcutaneous; intramuscular; intravenous	0.01–0.025 ml/100 gm	More than 30% of domestic rabbits have serum atropenesterase in their bodies. This enzyme hydrolizes atropine.
Dexamethasone	1 mg/ml	0.06 mg/100 gm	Subcutaneous; intramuscular; intravenous; intraperitoneal	0.06 ml/100 gm	
Prednisone	10 mg/ml	0.05–0.22 mg/100 gm	Subcutaneous; intramuscular	0.005–0.022 ml/100 gm	
Yomesan	500 mg tablets (active ingredients)	3–9 mg/100 gm	Oral	Feed medicated ration or a single dose per os	Mix thoroughly one pulverized tablet/1 lb of finely ground feed; small amounts of water are added to ground mixture to facilitate reshaping into a kibble type ration; air dry or feed as mash. We have used it on large numbers of mice (male, female, some pregnant) without problems; have not had opportunity to use on large numbers of other species. Medicated feed is fed for 3 days, off for 3 days, on for 3 days; repeat in 2 weeks if necessary. Procedure described can also be used in hamsters, although its efficacy has not been documented; I have no personal experience using it in guinea pigs, rabbits or gerbils.

Drug	Formulation	Dosage	Route	Amount	Remarks
Piperazine citrate or adipate	500 mg tablets or in bulk	50–100 mg/100 gm	Oral	½–1 tablet/50 ml water	Put in drinking water; use the following regimen for pinworms (in mice and rats): 7 days on medication; 7 days off medication; 7 days on medication. Clean cages thoroughly just before putting animal on medication and when taking it off medication; do all animals in same room at same time. Pinworm eggs may be airborne; filter caps may help. Five percent sucrose solution may increase palatability of medicated water.
Sucrose			Oral	25 gm/487 ml of water	Used to increase palatability of medicated water.
Griseofulvin	50 mg/tablet	2 mg/100 gm	Oral	Consult chart for amount of feed consumed	Mix one (50 mg) tablet/lb of feed; follow mixing instructions for yomesan; use cautiously in guinea pig since griseofulvin is derived from *Penicillium griseofulvin*.
Shell Pest Strips (DDVP)		—	—	—	Place a strip 1 × 2 × 2 inches on top of average-size mouse cage; keep it away from animal so it will not chew on it; use for 3 days; take off for 3 days. Serum cholinesterase levels will fall with long-term use but will go back to normal when strips are removed; production may be lowered. Can be used safely on mature, healthy (not systemically ill) animals.
Methyl carbamate-type flea powder			—	1/16 tsp/100 gm if nursing; 1/64 tsp/adult	Put desired amount of powder into a paper bag (lunch bag size); place animal in bag and shake; this method distributes medication evenly over animal; *only for mature animals* for lice, fleas, and superficial mites.
Crotomiton (Eurax)	10% lotion	—	Topical	—	Apply one to two times a day.
Chloramphenicol palmitate	125 mg/4 ml	2–5 mg/100 gm	Oral	0.07–0.16 ml/100 gm	Give two to three times a day. Add 4 ml of chloramphenicol to 3 oz water.
Chloramphenicol succinate	100 mg/ml	5 mg/100 gm	Intramuscular	0.05 ml/100 mg	Give one to two times a day (dose can be doubled if needed).
Tylosin	50 mg/ml	0.2–0.4 mg/100 gm	Intramuscular	0.004–0.008 ml/100 gm	Give one to two times a day (dose can be doubled if needed).
Gentamicin sulfate (Gentocin)	50 mg/ml	0.44–0.88 mg/100 gm	Intramuscular	0.008–0.016 ml/100 gm	Give one to two times a day; has been used with good results in hamsters with wet tail.
Tetracycline (Panmycin)	100 mg/ml	1.5–2 mg/100 gm	Oral	0.015–0.02 ml/100 gm	Give two to three times a day or add 0.1 ml tetracycline to 3 oz water.
Sulfamerazine		5–8 mg/100 gm	Oral	30–80 mg added to sufficient quantity of water to make 100 ml of solution.	Put in drinking water or administer proper dosage for weight per os.
Sulfaquinoxaline	Concentrate stock solution: 20 gm/100 ml or 20%	—	Oral	0.25–1.0 gm/1000 ml of water (0.025–0.1% solution) or 0.256 gm/500 gm of feed (0.05% ration)	Medicate for 30 days; improve sanitation and animal husbandry methods. Add 5 ml of stock solution to 1000 ml of drinking water, giving a 0.1% solution in drinking water.

Table continued on following page

Table 14.   *Drug Dosages** (Continued)

DRUG	MANUFACTURER'S CONCENTRATION	DOSAGE BY WEIGHT (mg/body weight)	ROUTE	DOSAGE BY VOLUME (ml/body weight)†	COMMENT
Sulfadimethoxine (Albon)	5% oral suspension	2.0–5.0 mg/100 gm 100 gm	Oral	0.016–0.04 ml/100 gm	Give once a day per os or 1 ml of oral suspension to 3 oz drinking water.
	Also available in 12.5% solution	2–5 mg/100 ml	Oral	0.016–0.04 ml/100 gm	0.5 ml stock solution to 3 oz water.
Procaine penicillin G	300,000 units/ml	2000 units/100 gm	Intramuscular	0.0066 ml/100 gm	Has been used in all laboratory species; anaphylaxis can occur in guinea pigs; use other antibiotics if possible.
Furazolidone (Furoxone)	100 mg/ml	0.5 mg/100 gm	Oral	0.005 ml/100 gm	0.55 gm/100 ml of water = 0.055% solution or 5 mg/100 gm of feed for long-term therapy (30 days); used mainly in rabbits.
Nitrofurazone (Furacin)	0.2% solution (0.2 gm/100 ml)	8 mg/kg	Oral	4 ml/kg added to daily water	100 mg/1000 ml of water or 0.01% solution for long-term therapy in rabbits, or add 50 ml of Furacin to 1000 ml of water (2 tblsp per qt H_2O).
Vitamin A, U.S.P.	100,000 units/ml	50–500 units/100 gm	Intramuscular	0.0005–0.005 ml/100 gm	
Vitamin D, U.S.P.	100,000 units/ml (1 ml of stock solution can be diluted with 10 ml of saline)	20–40 units/100 gm	Intramuscular	0.002–0.004 ml of diluted stock solution/100 gm	
Vitamin C, U.S.P.	100 mg/ml	2–20 mg/100 gm	Intramuscular	0.02–0.2 ml/100 gm	100 mg tablet to 500 ml of water.
B complex (Vitaxin) B_1	100 mg/ml	—	Intramuscular	0.002–0.02 ml/100 gm	
B_2	2.0 mg/ml				
B_{12}	100 µg/ml				

* Long-term antibiotic therapy (more than 5 days at therapeutic levels) may result in fatalities due to destruction of symbiotic bacteria in the gastrointestinal tract. This is especially true in guinea pigs and hamsters. Unless otherwise stated, chemotherapeutic agents may be used on any species.

† Except where otherwise noted.

tice, they can be passed quickly and atraumatically. With either method of gastric intubation, two points of resistance are usually encountered. The first is just before the tube reaches the esophagus and the second is just before the tube reaches the cardia. Gentle manipulation of the tube (not pressure) will help it pass atraumatically.

ENDOTRACHEAL INTUBATION IN THE RABBIT

See page 709.

DRUG DOSAGES

The dosages in Table 14 are ones that I have used in my practice. They have a fair degree of safety and efficacy. Serum level studies of the chemotherapeutics have not been carried out by the author and will not be discussed here.

SURGERY AND ANESTHESIA

Surgical and anesthetic procedures are routine with just a few exceptions. Induction is accomplished by masking with halothane. I do not use nitrous oxide on rodents. Intubation is not done routinely. If it is needed, intubation is done only in the rabbit, since this is the species for which it is most practical. Planes of anesthesia can be maintained by observing respiration rate and color of the albinotic iris in those species where it is present.

Routine surgical procedures include excision of neoplasms, débridement of abscesses, ovariohysterectomy, castration, exploratory laparotomy, and cystotomy for the removal of urinary calculi in guinea pigs.

Suturing techniques are routine except for the small size of the material needed. Preplacement of sutures during surgery of visceral organs is a helpful technique. For example, closure of the urinary bladder is easier if 4–0 catgut sutures are preplaced before the initial incision into the bladder is made. Closure of incisions is routine. Catgut is used internally and subcutaneously, and stainless steel is used in the skin. Rabbits present the main problem of chewing at incision sites. An Elizabethan collar will usually control this. Hamsters, guinea pigs, rats, and mice seem to tolerate cutaneous sutures.

Postsurgical care of laboratory animals presents particular problems. Temperature regulation and body heat conservation are paramount problems in very small rodents. Small body size and its relationship to exposed surface area make them more vulnerable to heat loss. Exogenous heat sources, such as hot water bags or a well-covered heating pad on a low setting, are indicated. Full recovery from anesthesia should be accomplished before the animal is returned to its cage.

For specific information and particular surgical procedures of either a clinical or experimental nature, the reader should consult Farris and Griffith, 1967, pp. 168–180, 434–452; and Markowitz, Archibald, and Downie, 1959.

COMMUNICABLE DISEASES

Dermatomycosis, salmonellosis, and hymenolepiasis are relatively common in laboratory animals. If diagnosed, the disease's public health significance should be explained to the client. Consultation with a physician familiar with communicable diseases can be helpful.

Leptospirosis, tularemia, sylvatic plague, lymphocytic choriomeningitis, and rabies can occur as natural diseases in laboratory species. Although extremely uncommon, their existence and significance should not be forgotten.

Vaccination against rabies and leptospirosis is not performed routinely unless the incidence of the disease in a specific area warrants it or an owner specifically requests it. Killed vaccines are used if they must be given.

SUPPLEMENTAL READING

Crocker, C.L.: Rapid determination of urea nitrogen in serum or plasma without deproteinization. Am. J. Med. Techn., *33*:361–365, 1967.

Farris, E.J., and Griffith, J.Q.: *The Rat in Laboratory Investigation.* Rpt. 1963. Philadelphia, J. B. Lippincott Co., 1967.

Green, E.L., et al.: *Biology of the Laboratory Mouse*, 2nd ed. New York, McGraw-Hill Book Co., 1966.

Hafez, E. S. E.: *Reproduction and Breeding Techniques for Laboratory Animals.* Philadelphia, Lea & Febiger, 1970.

Harkness, J.E., and Wagner, J.E.: *The Biology and Medicine of Rabbits and Rodents.* Philadelphia, Lea & Febiger, 1977.

Hoffman, R. A., Robinson, P.F., and Magalhaes, H.: *The Golden Hamster, Its Biology and Use in Medical Research.* Ames, Iowa, The Iowa State University Press, 1968.

Laboratory Animals. J. Lab. Animal Sci. Assoc., Laboratory Animals Ltd., 7 Warwick Court, London, WCIR 5DP.

Laboratory Animal Science. Joliet, Ill., American Association for Laboratory Animal Science.

Markowitz, J., Archibald, J., and Downie, H.G.: *Experimental Surgery*, 4th ed. Baltimore, Williams & Wilkins Co., 1959.

Melby, E.C., Jr., and Altman, N.H.: *Handbook of Laboratory Animal Science*, Vols I and II. Cleveland, Ohio, CRC Press Inc., 1974.

Riley, V.: Adaptation of orbital bleeding technique to rapid serial blood studies. Proc. Soc. Exp. Biol. Med., *104*:751–754, 1960.

Schwentker, V.: *The Gerbil: An Annotated Bibliography.* Presented by Tumblebrook Farm, West Brookfield, Mass.

Wagner, J.E., and Manning, P.J.: *The Biology of the Guinea Pig.* New York, Academic Press, 1976.

Weisbroth, S.H., Flatt, R.E., and Kraus, A.L.: *The Biology of the Laboratory Rabbit.* New York, Academic Press, 1974.

Wescott, R.B.: *An Outline of Diseases of Laboratory Animals.* Columbia, Mo., University of Missouri Press, 1969.

Section
9

NEUROLOGIC AND MUSCULOSKELETAL DISORDERS

ALEXANDER DE LAHUNTA, D.V.M.
Consulting Editor

Cerebrospinal Fluid Analysis.. 769
Botulism, Tick Paralysis, and Acute Polyradiculoneuritis
(Coonhound Paralysis).. 773
Tick Paralysis in Australia... 777
Inflammatory Muscle Disease in the Dog............................. 779
Exertional Rhabdomyolysis (Myoglobinuria) in the Racing
Greyhound.. 783
Myotonia in the Dog... 787
Episodic Weakness 791
Canine Polyarthritis.. 795
Canine Hip Dysplasia.. 802
Osteochondrosis in the Dog.. 807
Intracranial Injury.. 815
Storage Diseases... 821
Canine Hepatic Encephalopathy 822
Treatment of Feline and Canine Seizure Disorders 830
Diagnosis and Treatment of Narcolepsy in Animals............. 837
Clinical Behavioral Problems: Aggression............................. 841
Feline and Canine Behavior Control: Progestin Therapy...... 845

Additional Pertinent Information, Still Current, Found in
Current Veterinary Therapy VI:

Baker, H. J.: Inherited Metabolic Disorders of the Nervous
System in Dogs and Cats, p. 868.
Brasmer, T. H.: Evaluation and Therapy of Spinal Cord
Trauma, p. 837.
Cummings, J. F., and deLahunta, A.: Canine Polyneuritis,
p. 825.
deLahunta, A.: Feline Ischemic Encephalopathy — A Cere-
bral Infarction Syndrome, p. 906.
deLahunta, A.: Fibrocartilaginous Embolic Ischemic Mye-
lopathy, p. 908.
Gambardella, P. C.: Multiple Cartilaginous Exostoses in
Dogs, p. 886.
Griffiths, I. R.: Avulsion of the Brachial Plexus in the Dog,
p. 828.

Hoffer, R. E.: Otitis Externa and Media, p. 848.
Kay, W. J., and Fenner, W. R.: Epilepsy, p. 853.
Lorenz, M. D.: The "Swimming Puppy" Syndrome, p.
905.
Trotter, E. J.: Canine Intervertebral Disk Disease, p. 841.

Additional Pertinent Information, Still Current, Found in
Current Veterinary Therapy V:

deLahunta, A.: Progressive Cervical Spinal Cord Compres-
sion in Great Dane and Doberman Pinscher Dogs (A
Wobbler Syndrome), p. 674.
Fox, M. W.: Normal and Abnormal Behavioral Develop-
ment of the Dog, p. 703.
Knecht, C. D.: Radial-Brachial Paralysis, p. 658.
Reid, J. S.: Osteoarthritis, p. 707.

CEREBROSPINAL FLUID ANALYSIS

JAMES W. WILSON, D.V.M.
Roseville, Minnesota

Cerebrospinal fluid (CSF) is a liquid produced by the central nervous system (CNS). It covers the entire surface of the brain and spinal cord, penetrates the CNS parenchyma, and functions to protect, support, and sustain the CNS. Although classically considered to be produced by the choroid plexuses, other CNS components do contribute in total production. The major flow of CSF is from the lateral ventricles to the third ventricle, then to the fourth ventricle via the mesencephalic aqueduct. From the fourth ventricle it enters the central canal or the subarachnoid space, where it passes dorsally over the cerebrum or caudally over the spinal cord. Recent experimental evidence suggests that some degree of retrograde flow and also some intermixing probably occur within the subarachnoid space. The major site of CSF absorption is at the arachnoid villi located within the cranial venous sinuses. Additional sites of absorption include the lymphatics and veins around spinal nerve roots, the subarachnoid blood vessels, and the CNS parenchyma.

There is evidence to suggest that the CSF found in the subarachnoid space may actually have the same composition as the interstitial fluid surrounding the neurons and glial elements in the CNS. Changes from normal in CSF should therefore, theoretically, reflect changes within the CNS. Sampling and analysis of CSF may thus aid in the diagnosis and prognosis of neurologic disorders and should be considered in all data bases collected from patients with such disorders.

Samples of CSF can be obtained either from the cerebellomedullary cistern or from a lumbar puncture. Both of these sampling sites have their strong advocates and adversaries. In either case, fluid can be obtained easily and with minimal danger to the patient when the procedures are performed correctly. The techniques for obtaining samples from either site are adequately described in the publications listed in the supplemental readings.

ANALYSIS

CHARACTER

CSF is normally a clear, colorless liquid of low viscosity. Any change from this watery character is abnormal. Probably the most common reason for change in character of CSF is the presence of blood. Recent hemorrhage, not caused by sampling, will result in a uniform red tinge to the CSF. The degree of discoloration corresponds to the number of red blood cells (RBCs) present. The CSF normally has a different chemical composition and a higher osmolality than plasma. Because of this, RBCs begin to crenate soon after contact with CSF. Actual hemolysis can begin within 24 hours. Xanthochromia (yellow discoloration), which results from the chemical breakdown of the heme released by hemolysis, may be evident within 12 hours following hemorrhage. Whole blood can also be eliminated from the subarachnoid space quite rapidly. Investigators have found that injected blood cells disappear from the subarachnoid space of dogs within 2 to 24 hours after injection, depending on the type of experiment. Thus, pathologic hemorrhage can be difficult to identify by CSF sampling.

By far the most common reason for the presence of RBCs within the CSF is iatrogenic trauma and contamination with blood at the time of sampling. A swirl of blood within clear CSF is seen during sampling. Repeated changing of the collection chamber will usually aid in obtaining an uncontaminated or minimally contaminated sample. In contaminated samples, centrifugation will produce a clear supernatant with a button of RBCs at the bottom of the tube. In contrast, a xanthochromic supernatant is expected with presampling hemorrhage. In either case, if blood is suspected within the CSF, an anticoagulant should be added to the sample to facilitate microscopic inspection of the cells present.

Other changes in character may be seen. CSF is normally very watery. If it contains more than 500 white blood cells (WBCs)/cu mm it can become turbid. In meningeal infections the fluid may appear frankly purulent. CSF also does not normally coagulate. Coagulation can occur only if coagulation factors have been introduced into the CSF. Fibrinogen must be present. This may occur with bacterial infection or previous internal hemorrhage, but in most cases it is the result of iatrogenic blood contamination. In actuality, coagulation of a CSF sample should hardly ever be seen. Whenever a sample appears to have blood present or is turbid, an anticoagulant should be added to aid cytologic evaluation of the sample.

PRESSURE

Pressure of CSF in the normal anesthetized dog can vary from 0 to 180 mm H_2O. Thus, only elevated pressures are significant. Pressures can be obtained by direct objective measurement during sampling using a manometer or by direct subjective evaluation of the flow of CSF from the sampling needle. Techniques for direct manometer measurement are adequately described in the supplemental readings. Subjective evaluation can be gained through experience and, although not precise, when added to other findings may yield as much useful information as precise measurement.

Abnormally high CSF pressure can be caused by anything that produces an increase in intracranial contents, an increased fluid secretion, or a decreased absorption. Thus, pressure readings alone are not diagnostic. They may, however, supplement other findings and support a specific diagnosis. High pressures are commonly recorded with intracranial neoplasia. Other conditions in which elevated pressures have been documented include CNS abscesses, meningitis, both non-communicating hypertensive and communicating hydrocephalus, cerebral edema, and CNS hemorrhage.

CYTOLOGY

CELL COUNT

The freshly obtained CSF sample should be thoroughly mixed and a sufficient aliquot pipetted to fill a standard hemocytometer. Cells in all nine of the large millimeter squares on one side are counted. This count is multiplied by 1.1 to give the total cell count/cu mm. A WBC diluting pipette is rinsed with glacial acetic acid, filled with CSF, and agitated for five minutes. This causes lysis of the RBCs present in the sample. The hemocytometer is reloaded using this treated CSF, and the cells in all nine large millimeter squares on both sides of the chamber are counted. The WBC count/cu mm is obtained by multiplying the resultant count by 0.55. Subtraction of the WBC count from the total cell count gives the RBC count/cu mm.

Of 71 samples I obtained from clinically normal dogs, only two contained WBCs. Both samples were obtained from two colony dogs from which CSF samples had been taken weekly for the previous month. The normalcy of these two dogs was not verified by necropsy. Thus, WBCs should be considered a rare finding in normal animals.

Iatrogenic blood contamination during sampling is a frequent problem. A formula that utilizes the ratio of venous RBCs to venous total protein, WBCs, or enzyme activities has been used to correct values obtained from CSF contaminated with blood (Table 1). The formula to correct for blood contamination assumes that the amount of a substance in the CSF due to blood contamination is proportional to the number of RBCs in the CSF compared with that in venous blood. The accuracy of correction using this formula was evaluated in 190 CSF samples. Blood contamination was identified in 115 samples by the presence of intact RBCs. Ninety-one of these samples contained no WBCs, although use of the correction formula predicted 1 to 573 WBCs could have been present from blood contamination alone. Of 24 samples containing both RBCs and WBCs, 22 were obtained from animals having neurologic disease that could easily account for all the WBCs. Use of the formula led to misleading WBC counts in several instances. This formula would appear to be an unreliable method to determine corrected or "uncontaminated" values for WBC.

CELL IDENTIFICATION

Identification of the type(s) of WBCs present or the presence of other cell types within the

---

Table 1. *Correction Formula for Contaminated CSF*

$$X_c = X_{CSF} - (X_b \times RBC_{CSF}/RBC_b)$$

where:

X_c = corrected value for WBC, TP, or enzyme in CSF;
X_{CSF} = observed WBC, TP, or enzyme in CSF;
X_b = WBC, TP, or enzyme in venous blood;
RBC_{CSF} = observed RBC in CSF;
RBC_b = RBC in venous blood.

CSF sample can be accomplished by several methods. The simplest of these is to make a representative smear from thoroughly mixed CSF and stain the air-dried preparation. This is not recommended in most cases because cell populations in CSF are usually very low. A more reliable method is to centrifuge the CSF and prepare a smear from the precipitate. Adding several drops of patient serum to the precipitate helps preserve cytologic detail. Routine or special stains can then be utilized. The remaining technique is ultrafiltration. Several systems that trap cells and debris on a porous filter are now commercially available. After filtration, the membrane and deposited cells can be fixed and stained. No matter which technique is used the results depend considerably on the skill of the preparing technician.

The prepared slide should be handled exactly like any other cytologic preparation. It can be stained with methylene blue, hematoxylin and eosin, Gram's stain, India ink, or another stain. In all cases, a differential WBC count should be obtained. Individual cells should be examined closely, checking for toxic changes or the presence of ingested organisms. Samples containing suspicious cells can then be stained differentially to resolve the question.

CHEMISTRY

SPECIFIC GRAVITY

Specific gravity (sp gr) is the ratio of the density of a liquid to that of water under identical testing conditions. This property can be indirectly obtained for CSF through direct measurement of the refractive index using a hand-held, temperature-compensated refractometer.* Values for sp gr can be read directly from the reticle within the eyepiece of the instrument. The normal CSF sp gr range, obtained by measurement from 71 clinically normal dogs, is 1.004 to 1.006. Although wider normal ranges have been stated elsewhere, other methods of assessing sp gr support this narrower range as being more accurate.

A retrospective review of 124 CSF analyses from animals with suspected neurologic disease revealed a range of 1.004 to 1.016. Only 30 (24.2 percent) of the total were greater than 1.006. Few diseases were associated with an abnormal sp gr. In addition, the number of neurologically diseased animals with CSF sp gr values within the normal range was far too great to derive any clinical application. There was no correlation

*American Optical T-S Meter, American Optical Corporation, Buffalo, N.Y.

between sp gr values and etiologic diagnosis, type of disease, prognosis, or survival.

PROTEIN

CSF protein can be evaluated both quantitatively and qualitatively. Total protein content can be determined by several methods. One of the easiest is the trichloroacetic acid (TCA) turbidimetric procedure. For this test, 0.5 ml of the supernatant from centrifuged CSF is combined with 1.5 ml of 5 percent TCA and allowed to react at room temperature for five minutes. The sample is then agitated and the protein content determined by measuring the resultant turbidity at 420 mu. The protein content is expressed as mg/dl. Using this method, the normal CSF total protein range, obtained by sampling 61 clinically normal dogs, is 7 to 24 mg/dl. Other methods yield a wider and higher range; thus, sufficient control values should always be obtained to determine the range for the laboratory method utilized.

Precise separation of CSF protein types is difficult and expensive. A less precise measurement of CSF globulin content can be obtained from two easier methods, Pándy's test and the Nonne-Apelt test. Pándy's test is performed by combining 1 ml of saturated phenol solution with 1 drop of CSF. After agitation, the produced turbidity is reported from 1 to 4 plus (globulin). Normal CSF gives a negative to trace reaction. Thus, normal CSF contains very little protein and that present is almost entirely albumin.

Determination of total protein content and reaction to Pándy's reagent should always be performed as part of the routine analysis of CSF. A retrospective review of 145 analyses from animals with suspected neurologic diseases revealed that 69 (47.5 percent) of the samples had abnormally high values. Abnormal amounts of protein were found in 10 of 14 cases of cranial neoplasia, 5 of 6 cases of congenital abnormalities, 3 of 6 cases of CNS trauma, 10 of 17 cases of degenerative disorders, 16 of 24 cases of inflammatory disease, plus occasional other disorders. Pándy's test was performed on 66 samples. Although only 15 positive reactions were seen, negative test results are equally informative through identification of a protein elevation due solely to increased amounts of albumin.

It would seem logical to assume that the effect of blood contamination on CSF total protein should be remarkable, inasmuch as plasma contains several thousand milligrams of protein/dl, whereas CSF contains less than 24 mg of protein/dl. However, of 35 contaminated CSF samples obtained from clinically normal dogs, the total protein concentration was greater than normal in only one sample. Use of the formula to correct CSF protein values in contaminated samples led to corrected values less than zero in several analyses. The formula would therefore appear to be just as unreliable in determining corrected CSF total protein values as it was with WBC values. It is equally unreliable in determining "uncontaminated" CSF enzyme values.

CREATINE PHOSPHOKINASE

Creatine phosphokinase (CPK) is an enzyme that is abundant in mammalian skeletal muscle, cardiac muscle, and neural tissue. Plasma CPK does not normally cross the blood-brain-CSF barrier, and normal CSF CPK activity appears to be derived from the CNS. The CPK activity can be determined by a commercially available colorimetric method.† The normally low CSF CPK content requires some modification of the methodology. Instead of a ten-fold dilution in water, undiluted CSF is allowed to react with the substrates. The formed product is then coupled to produce a color complex that is measured. Enzyme activity is expressed in sigma units (SU)/ml. The normal CSF CPK activity for the dog, determined for 67 samples from clinically normal dogs utilizing this method, is less than 1 SU/ml. Temporal variability within individuals is minimal. The enzyme is stable for 48 hours when stored at refrigerator temperatures or colder.

Of 126 analyses from animals with suspected neurologic disease, 32 samples had elevated CPK activity ranging from 1.3 to 38 SU/ml. Elevated enzyme activity was identified in all of four cases of feline infectious peritonitis and in both of two cases of feline toxoplasmosis. Elevated CSF CPK was found in many other disorders but not frequently enough to aid in diagnosis. Of the 32 animals with an elevated CSF CPK, 18 (56 percent) died or were euthanized and 4 (13 percent) became progressively worse. A total of 22 (69 percent) failed to recov-

---

†Procedure No. 520, Sigma Chemical Company, St. Louis, MO.

Table 2.　*Normal Canine CSF Composition*

Color, character	Crystal clear
Specific gravity	1.004–1.006
Total protein	7–24 mg/dl
Pandy's reaction	Negative to trace
CPK	<1 SU
Cell count	Occasional WBC

er. None of the animals with CSF CPK higher than 5 SU/ml recovered.

CHANGES WITH DISEASE

Analysis of CSF should be considered for all cases of suspected neurologic disease. After obtaining a sample, the opening pressure, occurrence or lack of iatrogenic blood contamination during sampling, and the resulting sample character should be recorded. The sample should then be mixed thoroughly and appropriate aliquots obtained for cell count and culture. Differentiation of the cells present should be performed by preparation of a direct smear, ultrafiltration, or centrifugation and collection of precipitate. The total protein content, Pándy's reaction, and CPK activity can then be obtained from the supernatant. The remaining supernatant should be frozen for further reference.

Unfortunately, there is no reliable formula to correct for iatrogenic blood contamination of a sample. If RBCs are present and intact, iatrogenic contamination should be suspected. If they are crenated or the supernatant is xanthochromic, previous hemorrhage is likely. Many hydrocephalics have xanthochromic CSF containing crenated RBCs resulting from damage to blood vessels within the white matter lining the enlarged ventricles. Presence of WBCs should be critically evaluated and most probably indicates an active inflammatory process. High counts can be seen with encephalitis, meningitis, and myelitis as a result of generalized inflammation. The presence of WBCs is also seen in neoplasia, degenerative disorders, and congenital abnormalities owing to local inflammation incited by the disease process.

Microscopic examination of the CSF and differential cell count is extremely important for disease state identification. If an increase in WBC is predominately neutrophilic, a bacterial infection is usually present. A lymphocytic or mixed mononuclear reaction is seen in viral or fungal infections, tumors, and degenerative disorders. A WBC elevation due solely to eosinophils was observed in one case seen by the author, thus pointing toward *Dirofilarial* encephalitis in an otherwise confusing case. Occasionally, organisms can be seen within WBCs during a differential count, thereby narrowing the diagnosis. Finding desquamated neoplastic cells would support a diagnosis of a CNS tumor.

In an uncontaminated sample, an increased protein content and a negative Pándy's reaction may indicate CNS edema from a space-occupying lesion or damage to the blood-brain-CSF barrier by systemic or CNS disorders. This can be seen in cases of cranial neoplasia, trauma, poisoning, and seizures. An elevated protein content and a positive Pándy's reaction indicate the presence of increased amounts of globulin and are usually due to active inflammation or the presence of plasma from vascular damage. This is a frequent finding with CNS infectious processes.

Evaluation of CPK enzyme activity aids prognosis. An increase may reflect nerve cell dysfunction or death or a change in blood-brain-CSF permeability. In either case, high values indicate an active, severe process. Poor response to therapy, progression of the disorder, or death can be expected.

A complete analysis should always include a culture. If cell count and differential do not identify the presence of WBCs, clinical judgment can determine if culture is necessary. In all cases where WBCs are present, the likelihood of infection is good, and identification of an organism should be attempted. The presence of organisms within WBCs mandates culture. Identification of the organism and its antibiotic sensitivity greatly aids therapy and resulting prognosis.

SUPPLEMENTAL READING

Coles, E. H.: Cerebrospinal fluid. In Kaneko, J. J., and Cornelius, C. E. (eds.): *Clinical Biochemistry of Domestic Animals*, 2nd ed., Vol. 2. New York, Academic Press, 1971.
deLahunta, A.: *Veterinary Neuroanatomy and Clinical Neurology*. Philadelphia, W. B. Saunders Co., 1977.
Hoerlein, B. F.: *Canine Neurology: Diagnosis and Treatment*, 2nd ed. Philadelphia, W. B. Saunders Co., 1971.
Jenkins, T. W.: *Functional Mammalian Neuroanatomy*. Philadelphia, Lea & Febiger, 1972.
Kay, W. J., Israel, E., and Prata, R. G.: Cerebrospinal fluid. Vet. Clin. North Am., *4*(2):419–435, 1974.
Medway, W., Prier, J. E., and Wilkinson, J. S.: *Textbook of Veterinary Clinical Pathology*. Baltimore, Williams & Wilkins Co., 1969.
Rozel, J. F.: Membrane filtration of canine and feline cerebrospinal fluid for cytologic evaluation. J. Am. Vet. Med. Assoc., *160*:720, 1972.

BOTULISM, TICK PARALYSIS, AND ACUTE POLYRADICULONEURITIS (COONHOUND PARALYSIS)

JEANNE A. BARSANTI, D.V.M.
Athens, Georgia

It is important for treatment and prognosis to differentiate among these diseases in the dog. This can be difficult, since all present clinically with generalized lower motor neuron dysfunction. Functionally, the lower motor neuron is the final common efferent pathway of the nervous system. Anatomically, it includes the motor neuron, nerve root, spinal or cranial nerve, neuromuscular junction, and muscle. Dysfunction of any of these components causes clinical signs varying from paresis to paralysis, with hypotonia and hyporeflexia. Hypotonia can be determined by decreased resistance to passive manipulation of the limbs of a recumbent animal. Hyporeflexia is determined by examination of cranial nerve reflexes, limb reflexes such as patellar and flexor reflexes, and the perineal reflex.

Although botulism, tick paralysis, and polyradiculoneuritis all affect the lower motor neuron system, the pathophysiologic mechanism varies with each. Toxin produced by *Clostridium botulinum* blocks the release of acetylcholine at the neuromuscular junction. The neurotoxin secreted by the salivary glands of feeding female ticks either inhibits depolarization in the terminal portions of motor nerves or blocks release of acetylcholine at the neuromuscular junction. Acute polyradiculoneuritis is theorized to be due to a cell-mediated immunologic disorder in which peripheral nervous tissue and, in particular, myelin are attacked by specifically sensitized lymphocytes. Based on these pathophysiologic differences, the history and some of the clinical signs vary. .

HISTORY

An accurate history is important in differentiating these diseases. Ingestion of carrion within six days of the development of clinical signs is suggestive of botulism. All reported cases in dogs have been due to type C toxin, which is found in carrion, in contrast with human cases, which are primarily due to type A or B toxin, found in improperly prepared food. The onset of clinical signs can be very rapid, within hours of ingestion. The more rapidly severe signs develop, the poorer the prognosis.

Exposure to feeding female ticks of certain species, usually *Dermacentor andersoni* or *D. variabilis* in the United States, is necessary to produce tick paralysis. Clinical signs develop seven to nine days after attachment of the tick and may be transient if the feeding ticks disengage and fall off. One feeding tick is sufficient to cause clinical signs.

Many cases of acute polyradiculoneuritis develop 7 to 14 days after exposure to a raccoon bite (coonhound paralysis). Not all dogs bitten by the same raccoon will be affected, suggesting that the individual susceptibility of the dog is as important as the raccoon bite itself. Not all animals with polyradiculoneuritis have had exposure to raccoons. In these cases, the inciting cause is usually unknown. A similar acute polyradiculoneuritis in man (Landry-Guillain-Barré syndrome) has been associated with many causes, including mild antecedent infections of the respiratory or gastrointestinal tracts and measles and influenza vaccinations.

PHYSICAL EXAMINATION

Physical examination helps differentiate these three diseases if an engorged, feeding female tick is found, suggestive but not definitive of tick paralysis, or if muscle wasting, characteristic of polyradiculoneuritis, is evident. Muscle atrophy in canine polyradiculoneuritis can develop rapidly (within one week). Some dogs with botulism have slow cardiac rates, but this is not a consistent finding. Most abnormal findings on physical examination in all three diseases are secondary to the neurologic dysfunction and include dehydration and respiratory and urinary tract infection.

These diseases are characterized on neuro-logic examination by generalized symmetric paresis or paralysis with hypotonia and hyporeflexia. The degree of lower motor neuron dysfunction varies with each case. In the most severe cases, incipient respiratory failure may be indicated by diaphragmatic respiration secondary to marked paresis of the intercostal muscles. In tick paralysis and polyradiculoneuritis, paresis begins in the pelvic limbs and ascends. In tick paralysis signs generalize within one to two days, while in polyradiculoneuritis signs may increase in severity up to approximately ten days. In botulism both generalized weakness leading directly to quadriplegia and paraparesis ascending to the front limbs and cranial nerves have been noted. This is in contrast to human botulism, which is characterized by descending paralysis beginning with the cranial nerves. Voluntary tail wag and ability to move the head are usually maintained even in severe cases of all three diseases. A weak bark is also characteristic of these diseases.

The degree of cranial nerve involvement in each disease varies. Multiple cranial nerves are involved in botulism in both dogs and man. Mydriasis with sluggish pupillary response to light, decreased jaw tone, dysphagia, and diminished palpebral reflexes have been found in dogs with botulism. Two dogs have developed megaesophagus with regurgitation. Ophthalmoplegia and weakness of the tongue, which are noted in human cases, have not been reported in dogs to date. Cranial nerve abnormalities are less prominent in dogs with tick paralysis or acute polyradiculoneuritis. If present they are usually limited to facial nerve diplegia and mildly depressed gag reflexes. There may be mydriasis and anisocoria. This difference is of degree only and varies with the severity of the individual case, since all these diseases can affect the motor component of cranial as well as peripheral nerves.

Sensory abnormalities are found only in acute polyradiculoneuritis, since the disease process can involve dorsal as well as ventral spinal roots. The usual manifestation is hyperesthesia on palpation of limb musculature. However, this is not a consistent finding in all cases of polyradiculoneuritis. In all three diseases, affected animals remain bright and alert, unless severe dehydration or an overwhelming secondary infection develops.

LABORATORY TESTS

Hematologic tests, blood chemistry, and urinalysis either are normal or reflect only secondary infection in all three diseases. Cerebrospinal fluid analysis is also normal. This is in contrast with the increased protein concentration and normal cell count (albuminocytologic dissociation) found in acute polyradiculoneuritis in man. This difference may reflect a difference in technique, since mainly cisternal taps have been evaluated in dogs and mainly lumbar taps in man.

Since electromyography (EMG) can identify the component of the lower motor neuron system most severely affected by the disease process, it is useful in differentiating these diseases. EMG abnormalities become apparent approximately five days after peripheral weakness develops. In polyradiculoneuritis nerve conduction velocities are slower than normal because of demyelination of peripheral nerves. In severe cases positive sharp waves and fibrillation potentials are present in resting muscles, indicating denervation of muscle fibers from axonal degeneration. The motor unit action potential may be polyphasic and increased in amplitude. An evoked motor response to a supramaximal electrical stimulus is normal, indicating normal function of the neuromuscular junction.

Few, if any, fibrillation potentials or positive sharp waves are found on EMG in botulism or tick paralysis, since denervation does not occur. The main abnormality is marked reduction in amplitude of evoked motor potentials to a single supramaximal electrical stimulus, indicating abnormal transmission at the neuromuscular junction. In both diseases nerve conduction velocity may be slightly slower than normal and terminal conduction times prolonged. The slower conduction velocity (probably due to temperature reduction of the limb) is mild in relation to the marked reduction in amplitude of the muscle action potential. A slower than normal nerve conduction velocity is a consistent finding in people with tick paralysis and occasionally is reported in humans with botulism. This finding leads to the theory that the toxin in tick paralysis prevents depolarization of the terminal part of the motor neuron rather than inhibiting the release of acetylcholine at the neuromuscular junction.

If an affected animal dies, acute polyradiculoneuritis can be differentiated from botulism and tick paralysis because light microscopic abnormalities can be found. In polyradiculoneuritis segmental demyelination occurs primarily in the ventral spinal roots, but changes also occur in the dorsal roots and spinal and peripheral nerves. A perivascular leukocytic infiltration mainly of lymphocytes is found. In severe cases degeneration of axons is also present.

A definitive diagnosis of botulism can be made by finding that serum, feces, vomitus, or the suspect ingested substance produces certain signs when injected into mice and that the development of these signs can be prevented by concomitant injection of botulinal antitoxin of the appropriate type (mouse neutralization test). Approximately 8 to 10 ml of serum or 50 gm of feces, vomitus, or food is necessary to conduct these tests. The Center for Disease Control, Atlanta, Georgia, has been very cooperative in conducting or providing instructions for performing these tests. Poultry disease laboratories also may have diagnostic capabilities, since type C botulism causes poultry losses. Isolation of the organism *Clostridium botulinum* from the GI tract or liver is not sufficient for diagnosis, since it can be isolated from normal animals.

TREATMENT AND PROGNOSIS

The treatment of tick paralysis as found in the USA is simple and provides a diagnostic test (see page 778 for treatment of tick paralysis in Australia). Removal of the tick or ticks results in marked improvement within 24 hours and complete recovery within days. Without tick removal, signs increase in severity and death (from respiratory paralysis) can occur within five days of onset of signs. The fatality rate in humans from lack of recognition of the disease has been about 10 percent. To avoid this fatality rate, all dogs in which tick paralysis is being seriously considered in the differential diagnosis should be thoroughly examined for ticks, including the ear canals and interdigital areas. If a tick is not found but tick paralysis is still highly suspected, the dog should be dipped in an insecticide solution.

There is no proved, specific treatment for cases of botulism. The use of appropriate antitoxin can prevent the development of clinical signs but will not reverse clinical signs already present. If the toxin type is unknown in affected dogs and antitoxin is available, type C antitoxin should be given, since all reported cases in dogs have involved type C toxin. The use of penicillin has been advocated to reduce the intestinal population of clostridial organisms. The efficacy of this treatment has not been documented, since most often the toxin itself is ingested rather than produced in the intestinal tract. The benefits of the use of guanidine hydrochloride (15 to 30 mg/kg/day orally in divided doses) to increase acetylcholine release have been debated. Aminopyridine, 2 to 3 mg/kg intraperitoneally, has reversed paralysis due to experimentally induced botulism in rats. As in other oral intoxications, vomiting should be induced and gastric lavage performed if ingestion is recent, and cathartics and enemas should be given to evacuate any remaining gastrointestinal contents.

Supportive care is the most important treatment for cases of botulism. Patients must be assisted to eat, drink, urinate, and defecate. They should be comfortably bedded and turned often. Respiratory paralysis requires a respirator. Urinary and respiratory tracts should be monitored for signs of infection and treated appropriately. Most dogs that recover have responded within 14 days, although two cases remained mildly paretic after 24 days. Affected dogs recover motor functions in the reverse order in which they were lost. Surviving dogs have recovered completely with no residual effects.

There is also no specific therapy for acute polyradiculoneuritis. Glucocorticoids have been suggested, but there is no conclusive evidence that their use influences the course of the disease, especially since slow spontaneous recovery is the rule with or without treatment. Their use may increase the chance of development and the severity of secondary infections.

Supportive therapy is also most important in the management of cases of acute polyradiculoneuritis. Similar care to that given for botulism is used. An additional problem is that with severe muscle atrophy decubital ulcers and fibrous muscular contraction may occur. A very well-cushioned bed (thick straw or a water bed has been beneficial) and hourly turning if possible will help prevent or decrease the number of decubital ulcers. Warm whirlpool baths for 20 minutes twice a day will stimulate the appendicular musculature and help prevent contracture. Recovery generally occurs in three to four weeks, with the most rapid canine recovery reported to be 16 days. As in botulism, the paralysis regresses in the reverse sequence to which it developed. The prognosis is guarded in the progressive phase of the paralysis, since respiratory failure may occur. The prognosis is usually good after this phase, although occasionally recovery may be slower than four weeks and may be incomplete. Delayed recovery probably relates to axonal degeneration rather than segmental demyelination. If the initiating factor was a raccoon bite, the dog is predisposed to develop the condition again after another exposure to raccoons.

CONCLUSION

Even though their main presenting clinical signs are similar, these three diseases can be differentiated by assessing the history, clinical signs, course of the disease, and laboratory tests. Tick paralysis is diagnosed by the rapid improvement after removal of engorged female ticks. Botulism is suggested by the history of ingestion of carrion, cranial nerve dysfunction, rapidity of development of clinical signs, electromyographic findings of reduced muscle action potentials, and gradual improvement over one to three weeks, depending on the amount of toxin ingested. A definitive diagnosis of botulism can be made by identifying the toxin in serum, feces, vomitus, or ingested material using the mouse neutralization test. Acute polyradiculoneuritis is suggested by a history of exposure to raccoons, severe muscle wasting, hyperesthesia on palpation of limb muscles, onset of paralysis beginning in the rear limbs and progressing cranially over about a five to ten day period, electromyographic evidence of decreased nerve conduction velocity and perhaps denervation, and slow recovery over three to four weeks. If death occurs, the diagnosis can be confirmed histologically.

SUPPLEMENTAL READING

Barsanti, J.A., Walser, M., Hatheway, C.L., Bowen, J.M., and Crowell, W.: Type C botulism in American foxhounds. J. Am. Vet. Med. Assoc., *172*:809–813, 1978.
Center for Disease Control: Botulism in the United States, 1899–1973. Handbook for epidemiologists, clinicians, and laboratory workers. Atlanta, Center for Disease Control, 1974.
Chrisman, C.L.: Differentiation of tick paralysis and acute idiopathic polyradiculoneuritis in the dog using electromyography. J. Am. Anim. Hosp. Assoc., *11*:445–458, 1975.
Cummings, J.F., and Haas, D.C.: Coonhound paralysis: An acute idiopathic polyradiculoneuritis resembling the Landry-Guillain-Barré syndrome. J. Neurol. Sci., *4*:51–81, 1967.
Darke, P.G.G., Roberts, T.A., Smart, J.L., and Bradshaw, P.R.: Suspected botulism in foxhounds. Vet. Rec., *99*:98–99, 1978.
Murnaghan, M.F.: Tick paralysis in the dog: A neurophysiological study. Proceedings of the 10th International Congress of Entomology, 1956, pp. 841–847.

TICK PARALYSIS IN AUSTRALIA

JAN E. ILKIW, B.V.Sc.
Sydney, Australia

Tick paralysis in Australia is a disease produced by *Ixodes holocyclus* (Neumann). Other species, *I. cornuatus* and *I. hirsti*, have been reported associated with cases of tick paralysis.

Ixodes holocyclus is a three-host tick that engorges and then falls off the host between each successive stage of the life cycle. The disease usually follows infestation with adult female ticks but may follow infestation with nymphs or larvae.

Cases of tick paralysis are restricted to the coastal areas of eastern Australia, especially in bush and scrub country.

CLINICAL SIGNS

Severe disease with death is reported in all species: man (principally infants), foals, calves, pigs, sheep, and poultry, but it is most common in the dog and cat. In contrast, death is rarely observed in native fauna. In the dog one tick is sufficient to cause paralysis with progression to death, but not all adult female ticks are capable of causing the disease. Clinical signs are usually observed six to seven days after attachment of the tick, and even with mass infestation signs do not appear before the fourth day.

In the dog the signs are those of a rapidly ascending, flaccid motor paralysis. Altered voice, cough and dysphagia may be early signs, but the first consistent sign is a slight incoordination of the hindquarters. Whether the ticks are removed at this stage or not, the incoordination becomes more marked and soon the dog is unable to stand. Respiration is slow and embarrassed, and violent retching occurs in some animals. The disease progresses to the forelimbs until the dog lies in lateral recumbency; the pupils are usually dilated and unresponsive to light, and the dog makes feeble convulsive movements usually associated with respiration. In contrast with the severity of the motor disturbance, other signs are slight. The afferent sensory pathways are usually not affected; consciousness is not lost, and the animal is aware of activity in its immediate surroundings.

In the cat the signs are similar to those seen in dogs, but vomiting is uncommon.

PATHOGENESIS OF THE DISEASE

Studies by Cooper (1976) indicated that the paralysis is produced by an abnormality in the mechanism that couples nerve terminal depolarization and acetylcholine release. No abnormality in nerve conduction was found, but the release of acetylcholine in response to nerve stimulation was depressed due to a reduction in quantal content rather than quantal size. This effect was found to be markedly temperature-dependent, in that lowering the temperature resulted in a reduction of the effect.

Studies of the cardiovascular and respiratory effects of *Ixodes holocyclus* in the dog (Ilkiw, 1979) have shown that both these systems also are involved. There is a progressive fall in respiratory rate with no change in tidal volume. This contrasts with other diseases that cause neuromuscular paralysis in which respiration is rapid and shallow. In tick paralysis this is probably the result of central respiratory depression. The "grunting" type of respiration characteristic of a dog with tick paralysis is due to closure of the vocal cords during expiration. No abnormalities in blood-gas or acid-base status are found until quite late in the disease. Just prior to death, moderate hypoxemia with acute ventilatory failure and a mild metabolic acidosis are present. Abnormalities in the electrocardiogram (sinus tachycardia, ventricular tachycardia, sinus arrest, and sinus bradycardia) frequently are found. The sinus bradycardia observed terminally is due to increased vagal tone. Within the cardiovascular system there is an increase in peripheral vascular resistance, leading to a significant elevation in mean arterial pressure. The elevation in pulmonary arterial pressure despite a fall in cardiac output indicates an increase in pulmonary vascular resistance. These changes appear to be due to central sympathetic stimulation.

777

IMMUNITY

It is possible to produce immunity to tick paralysis by allowing ticks to engorge for short periods of time. After two to three months the dog can tolerate a number of ticks to full engorgement. The serum from such dogs was found to be beneficial in the treatment of tick paralysis and is now commercially available.

TREATMENT

Treatment of animals with tick paralysis falls into three categories.

REMOVAL OF THE TICK OR TICKS

Once the diagnosis has been made, a thorough search by palpation should be made. In small animals the favorite sites for attachment are on the head and neck, especially in the ears or under the collar; behind the elbows; and between the scapulae. Although one tick may be found, the search should be a complete one, because other ticks will prevent recovery, even with treatment.

Ticks are best removed with tweezers or fingernails, taking care not to squeeze the body of the tick, because further toxin may be expressed into the animal. If the animal is showing signs of the disease, removal of the tick is not enough, as the disease may progress for 48 more hours.

NEUTRALIZATION OF THE TOXIN

Hyperimmune serum should then be injected slowly intravenously. The dose administered depends on the severity of the clinical signs and the size of the animal, but as a guide a dose rate of 0.5 ml/kg body weight may be used. In the cat care should be taken to avoid reactions to the serum. Hyperimmune dog serum may be administered intravenously to cats after an antihistamine, or it may be given intraperitoneally.

It appears that hyperimmune serum is totally effective in those animals with a straightforward ascending paralysis (Allan and Pursell, 1971). However, some deaths can be expected if the animal is showing signs of vomiting, laryngeal paralysis, sialosis, and pulmonary edema.

SUPPORTIVE TREATMENT

Good nursing care is vitally important in animals with tick paralysis. Dogs should be watched carefully for changes in respiratory and heart rates and nursed through crisis periods. After retching or vomiting the pharynx should be swabbed clean, and if the animal is in lateral recumbency it should be turned every four to six hours to prevent the development of hypostatic pneumonia.

Stress of any type, such as excitement, fear, or heat, has an adverse effect on the course of the disease. Quiet cage rest with minimal interference should be provided in a cool environment. All water and food should be withheld until the patient is mobile and has been free from vomiting for 12 to 24 hours. Water can then be given in small amounts, and if no vomiting occurs food can be given.

Antimicrobial therapy by a parenteral route should be administered in advanced cases to prevent the development of pneumonia.

Although symptomatic treatment of tick paralysis with various drugs is common, some of these drugs can have deleterious effects. Atropine sulfate, which is administered to dry up salivary and bronchial secretions, should not be given if the animal is in an advanced stage of the disease or if bradycardia is present. Intravenous fluid replacement is generally not required unless recovery is prolonged. If fluids are administered, they should be given very slowly, with careful monitoring of the patient for signs of pulmonary congestion.

Recent work (Ilkiw, 1979) has demonstrated that phenoxybenzamine hydrochloride (Dibenyline, Smith Kline and French), an α-adrenergic blocking drug, is beneficial when used in conjunction with hyperimmune serum in the treatment of dogs presented in advanced stages of the disease. It should be administered at a dose rate of 1 mg/kg body weight, diluted in at least 20 ml of normal saline, and given slowly intravenously over a period of at least 20 minutes. Care must be taken not to overload the circulation if the drug is administered in a large volume of diluent. To aid removal of fluid from the lungs, a diuretic may be given.

If respiratory arrest is imminent or excessive secretions in the trachea are impairing respiration, tracheostomy may be performed. This allows suction of fluid from the trachea and intermittent positive pressure ventilation (IPPV) to be initiated. Constant cleaning of the tracheotomy tube is important to prevent respiratory obstruction. Postural drainage may also be advantageous.

After recovery, a convalescent period of up to two weeks with restricted exercise and avoidance of high temperatures should be advised to prevent death from cardiac complications.

PREVENTION

Bathing with the organophosphate Asuntol (Bayer Australia Ltd.) according to the manufacturer's instructions has been shown to give complete protection against *Ixodes holocyclus* for one week.

Daily searching of the animal is also a very effective means of protection, because the disease cannot be produced from attachment of the tick in less than four days.

There has been some controversy over the efficiency of drug-impregnated collars in providing complete protection against *Ixodes holocyclus*.

SUPPLEMENTAL READING

Allan, G.S., and Pursell, R.T.: Pulmonary involvement and other sequelae of tick poisoning. Aust. Vet. Pract. *1*:39–40, 1971.
Cooper, B.J.: *Studies on the Pathogenesis of Tick Paralysis*. Ph.D. thesis, University of Sydney, Sydney, Australia, 1976.
Ilkiw, J.E.: *A Study of the Effects in the Dog of* Ixodes holocyclus. Ph.D. Thesis, University of Sydney, Sydney, Australia, 1979.

INFLAMMATORY MUSCLE DISEASE IN THE DOG

I. D. DUNCAN, B.V.M.S.
Montreal, Canada

and I. R. GRIFFITHS, B.V.M.S.
Glasgow, Scotland

Inflammation of skeletal muscle of either infectious or idiopathic origin is a fairly common canine neuromuscular disease. Masticatory muscle myositis, which can present either as an acute or chronic clinical condition, is the best known of these diseases in the dog. The more generalized form of this type of idiopathic disease, or polymyositis, has been less well described in the veterinary literature. Muscle inflammation can also result from local or systemic microbial infection. The clinical signs that result in these conditions depend on the muscles affected and the severity and extent of the lesion. Muscle weakness and stiffness are often two of the most important presenting signs in affected dogs.

IDIOPATHIC MYOSITIS

MASTICATORY MUSCLE MYOSITIS

In the past, the terms *eosinophilic myositis* and *atrophic myositis* have been used to describe the syndromes that have had, respectively, acute or chronic onsets (Harding and Owen; Griffiths, et al.). It has been suggested that atrophic myositis may follow acute attacks of disease (Whitney); however, insidious muscle atrophy can occur without previous history of acute attack, and the acute disease can occur unassociated with eosinophilia (Griffiths, et al.).

CLINICAL SIGNS

Cases presenting with an acute onset, pain, and swelling of the temporal and masseter muscles often result in reticence to open the mouth. All breeds of dogs may be affected, although in the past a higher incidence has been reported in the German shepherd. Exophthalmos may be noted as a result of swollen muscles, and conjunctivitis can occur. Affected dogs are usually dull and unwilling to eat and may be pyrexic. Inspection of the tonsils and submaxillary lymph nodes may reveal some swelling; there may be splenomegaly, and the dog may be anemic. Hematologic studies will confirm the anemia, and leukocytosis is often present, most often associated with neutrophilia. The differential count may show eosinophilia, but without a muscle biopsy this should not be taken as unequivocal evidence of eosinophilic myositis. Blood biochemistry usually shows raised gamma globulin and serum creatine phosphokinase (CPK) levels. The chronic form may occur without report of previous acute attacks or any periods of unexplained malaise. In some instances, however, chronic atrophy apparently follows acute or subacute bouts of muscle inflammation, but in our experience this is rare. The chronic disease is usually first noticed by the owner as an insidious, progressive atrophy of the temporal and masseter muscles that may be accompanied by increasing difficulty in opening the mouth. This may be so severe that it prevents eating, and the dog will lose weight. In some cases masticatory muscle atrophy may be unilateral, but in most instances it is bilateral.

ELECTROMYOGRAPHY

This has limited value in both these conditions, in our experience. In both the acute and chronic diseases, spontaneous activity that consists of fibrillation potentials and positive sharp waves can be seen. These are, however, not as profuse as those seen in denervation. Bizarre high frequency discharges (pseudomyotonia) can also be found. Examination of individual motor unit potentials may be of more use in diagnosing this disease electromyographically.

ETIOLOGY

The cause of masticatory muscle myositis remains an enigma, especially the apparent predilection for this group of muscles. Although there is no directly analogous disease in human medicine, a syndrome of hypertrophy of the muscles of branchial cleft origin (i.e., muscles of mastication) does occur (Lambert and Young). To date, there have been no thorough studies of this area in canine medicine, and only speculative ideas have been advanced. Certainly the pathology that has been found in our cases (Griffiths, et al.) suggests that the disease may have an autoimmune basis. It may be possible that this process is directed predominantly against the masticatory muscles, for they may have different surface antigens as a result of their different embryologic origin (branchial arch) from that of other skeletal muscles. It is also possible that a viral infection such as a coxsackievirus, which has been implicated in human polymyositis, could be responsible or that it could sensitize the muscle. It is also possible that a viral upper respiratory tract infection may result in local spread of the virus, with the masticatory muscles being secondarily

infected. The clinical signs of enlargement of the tonsils, submaxillary lymph nodes, and spleen, which are seen in many acute cases, might suggest a viral infection. In the report of Harding and Owen, local salivary gland inflammation was also noted. Further studies in this area are necessary.

PATHOLOGY

In both the acute and chronic forms of the disease, muscle biopsy can be useful. In the acute form, biopsy can help distinguish the disease from infectious causes of myositis (see later in this article) and can help determine therapy. In the chronic disease a biopsy may help distinguish between chronic inflammatory muscle disease and neurogenic atrophy, which can be confused clinically. In the acute disease massive inflammatory cell invasion of the masticatory muscles takes place, with diffuse necrosis resulting in a severe necrotizing myopathy or myolysis (Fig. 1). The cellular infiltrate is composed of macrophages, lymphocytes, plasma cells and, in certain areas, neutrophils. Degenerating fibers are often surrounded by macrophages that are digesting sarcoplasm, but occasionally lymphocytes are seen to initiate the infiltration of the cell. Although muscle necrosis is often predominant, vigorous regenerative activity also is usually seen. Other reports (Harding and Owen) have stressed the predominance of eosinophils in affected muscles. These may represent up to 70 percent of the total cellular infiltrate. Despite this and other reports, we have found the reverse to be true and that eosinophils were rare, even in cases biopsied within one week of the appearance of clinical signs. In the report of Harding and Owen it was noted that numerous other muscles were found to be infiltrated with inflammatory cells. These included the tongue, esophagus, sternothyroid, biceps, and triceps muscles. While there was only superficial mention of any one of these cases showing clinical evidence of generalized muscle inflammation (polymyositis), the possibility still remains that masticatory myositis and polymyositis are the same disease. The apparent current success of treatment of the acute form prevents full muscle surveys of the acute masticatory disease, but future cases should, if possible, be biopsied in other sites (e.g., biceps and triceps) to check for generalized muscle involvement. In the chronic disease, inflammatory cell infiltrates are seen but often only in a focal pattern compared with the diffuse infiltration in the acute disease. The cells in these areas are similar to those seen in

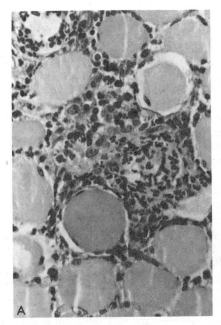
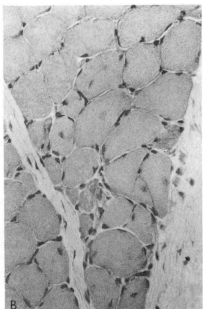

Figure 1. *A.* Mildly affected area from the temporal muscle of a patient with acute masticatory muscle myositis. A necrotic fiber is engulfed by macrophages and lymphocytes. *B.* The contralateral temporal muscle to that seen in *A*, one year after treatment of the acute disease. Note the complete lack of inflammatory cells in this area, although a few may still be present in the perimysium. A few atrophic fibers are present; there are some internal nuclei, and there is an increase in perimysial connective tissue.

the acute disease, but muscle necrosis is not so marked. There is obvious perimysial and endomysial connective tissue proliferation and other evidence of a chronic myopathic process.

TREATMENT

Once a diagnosis of acute masticatory muscle myositis of non-infectious origin has been made, high doses of steroids (betamethasone) in doses of 2 mg per day (small dogs) or 4 mg per day (large dogs) should be prescribed and maintained for two weeks. This dose should then be reduced over the following two weeks. Repeated courses of this drug may be necessary because further bouts of acute inflammation may occur. The indication of further damage may be achieved by monitoring CPK levels at regular intervals (Averill). It is known that this enzyme may start to "leak" from the muscle fiber membrane before structural changes can be noted. The chronic cases of the disease are often more difficult to treat because of the marked restriction in jaw opening that develops as a result of the connective tissue proliferation in the atrophic masticatory muscles. It may be necessary to open the mouth forcibly by applying traction to the mandible and maxilla while the dog is anesthetized. It is possible to hear the tearing of fibrous tissue during this maneuver. Care must be taken not to stretch the jaw too far, or inability to close the mouth may result. Steroid therapy after stretching will help to limit the formation of new connective tissue and will also suppress the putative autoimmune reaction.

POLYMYOSITIS

This is one of the most common muscle diseases in man. Its importance in the dog has only recently been recognized, but to date an adequate series of clinical or pathologic correlations has not been published. Meier described two cases of polymyositis in the dog, one with an acute onset and the other more chronic. In both instances the pathologic changes were severe and similar to those seen in our cases of acute masticatory muscle myositis. In man polymyositis is either seen alone or, more commonly, in association with skin inflammation (dermatomyositis), with one of the connective tissue disorders such as systemic lupus erythematosus (SLE), or with malignancy (carcinomatous myopathy) (Walton). There has been a single canine case report of polymyositis in association with SLE (Krum, et al.), but it is likely that more will be found as the connective tissue disorders become more frequently recognized in the dog. The incidence of canine polymyositis in the UK appears to be lower than that seen in the USA, where German shepherds appear to be most frequently involved.

CLINICAL SIGNS

From the published reports the presenting signs are usually of a dog that weakens on exercise with or without muscle stiffness and pain (Averill). Problems in chewing and swallowing that result in regurgitation can often be present. Some differentiation between muscle weakness as a result of myasthenia gravis (MG) or from lower motor neuron disturbances may be necessary. In the latter case there will be decreased muscle tone, loss of tendon reflexes, and possibly some ataxia. Ancillary aids may be necessary to differentiate polymyositis from MG. Blood biochemistry will show elevated CPK and aldolase levels in polymyositis. Electromyography may reveal the presence of spontaneous activity in many muscles in polymyositis, and the motor unit potentials during voluntary movement should be examined. Repetitive nerve stimulation may be necessary to distinguish between polymyositis and MG, and an anticholinesterase test may have to be carried out. In addition, muscle biochemistry and biopsy will usually be normal in MG. Muscle biopsy should be carried out from muscles that are thought to be clinically affected. This should help distinguish the idiopathic disease from infectious causes of myositis.

ETIOLOGY

As with masticatory muscle myositis, little is known about the etiology, although the pathologic findings would suggest an autoimmune origin.

PATHOLOGY

The focal nature of the inflammatory cell infiltrate often makes diagnosis from a single biopsy difficult, and often multiple biopsies may be necessary. The cellular infiltrate is similar to that seen in masticatory muscle myositis, although one case of eosinophilic polymyositis has been reported (Scott and deLahunta).

TREATMENT

This is the same as described for acute masticatory myositis. The prognosis in these cases in normally good.

INFECTIOUS CAUSES OF MUSCLE INFLAMMATION

Bacterial infection is an uncommon cause of myositis. Acute or chronic muscle inflammation can result from local infection such as infected fractures. Treatment should be aimed at local wound care, systemic administration of the appropriate antibiotic, and surgical intervention if this is indicated. *Leptospira icterohaemorrhagia* can cause a more specific, severe, and generalized hemorrhagic necrotizing myopathy. Affected dogs are usually severely ill as a result of the systemic infection and, although there may be muscle pain and weakness, this can often be missed.

The protozoal organism *Toxoplasma gondii* can cause myositis in two different age groups of dogs. In the old dog, a focal necrotizing myositis can be found in cases with CNS infection of *T. gondii*, although the CNS infection usually masks the muscle changes. In the puppy, *T. gondii* infection can be found as a congenital disease. Affected dogs are noted shortly after birth and are found to be paraplegic or paraparetic. There is marked extensor rigidity of the hind limbs; flexion may be difficult, and slight muscle atrophy may be detected. A pedal reflex cannot be elicited because of the rigidity, but pain sensation is intact. Electromyography may demonstrate the presence of spontaneous activity in affected muscles that is suggestive of denervation. Pathologically, there is a severe necrotizing myopathy, with a marked mononuclear cell infiltrate and occasional *T. gondii* cysts (Griffiths and Duncan, unpublished). In the nervous system myelitis, radiculitis, and ganglionitis are often present, resulting in neurogenic muscle atrophy that is found concurrently with the myositis.

SUPPLEMENTAL READING

Averill, D.R.: Polymyositis in the dog. In Kirk, R.W. (ed.): *Current Veterinary Therapy VI*. Philadelphia, W.B. Saunders, 1977, pp. 822–825.

Griffiths, I.R., Duncan, I.D., McQueen, A., Quirk, C., and Miller, R.: Neuromuscular disease in dogs: Some aspects of its investigation and diagnosis. J. Small Anim. Pract., *14*:533, 1973.

Harding, H.P., and Owen, L.N.: Eosinophilic myositis in the dog. J. Comp. Pathol., *66*:109, 1956.

Krum, S.H., Cardinet, G.H., Anderson, B.C., and Holliday, J.A.: Polymyositis and polyarthritis associated with systemic lupus erythematosus in a dog. J. Am. Vet. Med. Assoc., *61*:1, 1977.

Lambert, C.D., and Young, J.R.B.: Hypertrophy of the branchial muscles. J. Neurol. Neurosurg. Psychiatry, *39*:810, 1976.

Meier, H.: Myopathies in dogs. Cornell Vet., *48*:313, 1958.

Scott, D.W., and deLahunta, A.: Eosinophilic polymyositis in a dog. Cornell Vet., *64*:49, 1974.

Walton, J.N. (ed.): *Disorders of Voluntary Muscle*, 3rd ed. New York, Longman, 1974.

Whitney, J.C.: Atrophic myositis in a dog: The differentiation of this disease from eosinophilic myositis. Vet. Rec., *69*:130, 1957.

EXERTIONAL RHABDOMYOLYSIS (MYOGLOBINURIA) IN THE RACING GREYHOUND

JAMES R. GANNON, B.V.Sc.
Balwyn, Victoria, Australia

INTRODUCTION

Myoglobinuria is not a disease — it is a symptom. To be more specific, it is part of a syndrome seen in racing greyhounds throughout the world. It has been reported in the USA (Keene and Yarborough), where it is known as the "Grueller syndrome" or "running the back off the dog"; in the UK (Prole) it is known as azoturia and myoglobinuria; in Australia (Davis and Paris) it is called metabolic acidosis, azoturia, and exertional rhabdomyolysis. A similar condition is recognized in humans as exertional rhabdomyolsis (Champion, et al.). There seems little doubt, in the face of histopathologic records in the human, canine, and equine fields, that the ultimate cause of exertional rhabdomyolsis is local muscle ischemia resulting in lysis of the muscle cell wall. However, one must endeavor to obtain a fuller understanding of the underlying causes of the ischemia if any rational therapeutic or prophylactic measures are to be instituted.

CLINICAL CATEGORIES

Exertional rhabdomyolysis may be subdivided arbitrarily into the following types, based on severity of symptoms and acuteness of onset:

1. Hyperacute. This occurs during a race or trial. The patient exhibits extreme distress with hyperpnea and generalized muscular pain. Handling is resented, particularly along the back and over the hindquarters. When the dog is walked, the nails of its hind limbs are scuffed along the ground. There is pronounced myoglobinuria. Changing position from standing to lying or vice versa is extremely difficult and achieved only with obvious pain and distress. Death is common within 48 hours from acute renal failure due to massive nephron blockage with myoglobin.

2. Acute. This also occurs during the race or trial. The patient exhibits distress with acute pain on palpation of the longissimus, quadriceps and biceps femoris muscles. Myoglobinuria is observed on one or two occasions only; thereafter, the urine shows no obvious discoloration when voided. Death may occur if the condition is not treated, but the mortality rate is low.

3. Subacute. This form is never fatal, and myoglobinuria is rarely observed macroscopically. The patient is never noticeably distressed because muscle pain is confined to the longissimus thoracis muscle only and may not be apparent on palpation for 24 to 72 hours after the trial or race.

PREDISPOSING FACTORS

Exertional rhabdomyolysis is a metabolic disease affecting healthy adolescent and adult canine athletes. It is neither a deficiency nor an infectious problem. It is predictable in some greyhounds, given certain environmental and managerial circumstances, namely (a) an absolute lack of physical fitness in relation to the exercise load, (b) the tendency of highly strung greyhounds to become very tense and excitable prior to running, (c) hot and humid climatic conditions during traveling or in the kennels before the race, and (d) subjection of a physically fit and regularly run greyhound to an excessive frequency of running in either trials or races.

SEVERITY OF CASES

Although any of the predisposing factors mentioned may produce any one of the clinical categories previously described, given the correct circumstances, observation would suggest that (1) hyperacute cases are more often associated with predisposing factor (a), (2) acute cases are usually associated with predisposing factors (b) and (c), and (3) subacute cases are more often associated with predisposing factor (d). It is apparent that the condition of exertional rhabdomyolysis is multifactorial in origin but that the end result in each case is focal necrosis of the muscle cell wall caused by ischemia and release of myoglobin. One must therefore consider the pathophysiology of each of the predisposing factors before adequate therapy and prophylaxis can be prescribed.

THE UNFIT GREYHOUND SUBJECTED TO EXCESSIVE FAST WORK

PATHOPHYSIOLOGY

The end products of muscular exercise are heat, energy output (work), and hydrogen ions. Heat is dissipated via the circulatory system. Hydrogen ions are eliminated by the body's buffer systems. These buffer systems consist of (in order of activity) the intracellular bicarbonate ions, the intracellular protein buffers, and the active transfer of hydrogen ions by the ion pump of the cell wall to the extracellular fluid bicarbonate buffer system. It will be recalled that the ion pump of the cell wall is an energy-using mechanism requiring glucose and oxygen for the active transport of sodium ions out of the cell and of potassium ions into the cell, thereby maintaining the sodium-potassium differential of the extracellular and intracellular fluids. Although ion levels of sodium and potassium and their shifts markedly affect electrolyte balance, one should remember that calcium ions also have a profound effect on muscle contraction, so attention should be given to proper maintenance of the levels of this ion also.

When the unfit greyhound is subjected to excessive fast work there is an enormous production of hydrogen ions that is beyond the buffering capability of the intracellular buffers. The intracellular buffers of bicarbonate and protein soon fail to cope with the load. The ion pump of the unfit muscle cell also fails. Sodium ions that now enter the muscle cell are not returned to the extracellular fluid because of ion pump failure. Osmotic pressure within the cell increases, and water is drawn into the muscle cell. Hence, the muscle cells swell. The now-enlarged muscle cells restrict local circulation by direct pressure on the arterioles, venules, and capillary bed. The result is a hyperacute form of rhabdomyolysis due to local ischemia together with reduced heat dissipation from the muscles. The mortality rate is high, and therapy must be instituted promptly to be effective.

RELATED CLINICAL SIGNS

The muscles appear swollen and tense ("blown up over the back") and are painful on palpation. They feel hot to the touch as a result of diminished heat dissipation resulting from locally restricted circulation. Myoglobinuria occurs because of lysis of the cell wall, and movement becomes difficult and painful. Urine pH is alkaline (7.5 to 8.5) owing to respiratory alkalosis for the first hour after the run, but it becomes markedly acidotic after four to six hours (pH 5.2 to 5.8) compared with the normal pH range of 6.0 to 6.5 for the resting greyhound.

RECOMMENDED THERAPY

Supply fluids intravenously; 45 ml/kg of any normal extracellular replacement fluid (ECF) will prevent hypovolemic shock and aid renal excretion of myoglobin, both of which are consequent upon extensive muscle trauma. Repeat the administration of ECF daily for the next two to three days.

Supply buffer; 20 ml/kg of 4.2 percent bicarbonate solution should be given intravenously at the same time as or immediately following the administration of ECF. Use 20 ml/kg of 1.4 percent bicarbonate solution daily for the following two to three days. This massive bicarbonate input increases ECF buffer at a time when it is desperately required. It also maintains nephron viability and function, because an alkaline medium is less conducive to precipitation of the myoglobin protein than is an acid medium. In normal greyhounds blood bicarbonate levels average 25 to 28 mEq/liter, while the cases under discussion average 8 to 12 mEq/liter.

Cool the patient during the first few hours to remove excess local heat. Use cold wet towels, ice packs applied locally, and fans until body temperature is normal; then maintain a steady warm environment of 70 to 75° F.

Since the patient will be in a negative nitrogen balance for some time, anabolic steroids are indicated. An initial dose of 1.0 mg/kg intramuscularly should be followed by 0.5 mg/kg every third day for four more doses. Because the patient is acutely stressed, prophylactic antibiotic (Lincomycin or Pen-Strep) should be given for five days to prevent secondary infections. Good nursing consists of three daily meals of high-protein commercial food, fluid *ad lib.*, and soft bedding. Allow voluntary walking exercise as soon as the patient is capable — usually after 36 hours. Keep the urine alkaline with oral sodium bicarbonate, 100 mg/kg, *or* potassium citrate, 5 mg/kg, for the ten days following the onset of the attack to protect nephrons during the period of protein excretion. Restoration of glycogen reserves in regenerating muscle fibers may be aided by adding 8 to 10 grams of glucose to each meal, together with intramuscular administration of vitamin B_{15} (pangamic acid, 1 mg/kg) daily for seven days. Phenylbutazone, 100 mg/25 kg t.i.d. with or after food orally for five days aids in relief of joint pain, and its anti-inflammatory effects secondarily reduce muscular pain and offer symptomatic relief. A convalescence of eight weeks is to be anticipated before most patients can return running trials.

GREYHOUNDS UNDULY EXCITED BEFORE RACING

PATHOPHYSIOLOGY

The prolonged barking, puffing, and deep panting result in a condition of respiratory alkalosis because of loss of CO_2 (H^+ ions). Renal compensation occurs, with excretion of plasma bicarbonate in the urine. The patient now suffers a loss of alkaline reserve when its urinary pH increases from the normal 6.0 to 6.5 to 7.5 to 8.5. The patient enters the race with a reduced capacity to handle the hydrogen ions produced by physical exertion. It is not that the patient lacks physical fitness or that the intracellular buffering and ion transport systems are unsatisfactory. The problem results from an inability to buffer the hydrogen ions at the end of chain of events, i.e., in the ECF. This time the ion pump in the cell wall is overloaded and fails because of a blocking effect at its outlet. The overall effect is as previously summarized and again results in local ischemia and an acute form of exertional rhabdomyolysis. Mortality in these acute cases reaches 25 percent if untreated, but recovery rates of 100 percent are now achieved if therapy is instituted within 12 hours of onset and if a convalescence of eight weeks is given.

RECOMMENDED THERAPY

This is the same as that discussed earlier in the article.

RECOMMENDED PROPHYLAXIS

The induction of a mild metabolic alkalosis prior to traveling and kenneling has been found to minimize the risk of acute exertional rhabdomyolysis in tempermental patients in the predisposing circumstances outlined. Administer 100 mg/kg bicarbonate of soda with 400 mg/kg glucodin in 150 ml water and 50 ml milk (for palatability) about 15 to 30 minutes before traveling or kenneling.

HOT HUMID CONDITIONS

PATHOPHYSIOLOGY

The greyhound is virtually a non-sweating animal. Loss of body heat is dependent to a small degree on conduction (contact with cooler surfaces) and convection (cooling draughts) but mainly depends upon evaporative cooling from the respiratory system. Greyhounds prior to racing are confined in a single kennel, which is then itself confined to a room of similar kennels. The progressive panting and barking of these excited greyhounds results in a considerable moisture loss to the atmosphere of the kennel room. If the weather is already humid the evaporative cooling available to the respiratory system of the confined greyhounds is likely to be almost zero. In such situations one observes marked hyperpnea and considerable salivary drooling (200 to 300 ml saliva) in some patients. The greyhound is then presented for the race with an elevated body temperature (104° F [40° C]) and a lowered alkali reserve as a result of the respiratory alkalosis associated with hyperpnea. Both of these combine to produce an acute exertional rhabdomyolysis.

RECOMMENDED THERAPY

Therapy is as previously discussed. Recovery and mortality rates are the same as those associated with the acute condition.

RECOMMENDED PROPHYLAXIS

Air conditioning in the kennels to reduce environmental humidity and temperatures is a good solution. If this is not available then promotion of air movement should be specified, using forced draught fans or extractor fans. Reduction of body temperature before the race by hosing (if permissible) or fanning will also help. Another technique is administration of oral bicarbonate-glucose solution prior to kenneling to minimize alkali reserve deficit.

EXCESS FREQUENCY OF RUNS FOR FIT GREYHOUNDS

PATHOPHYSIOLOGY

Knochel and Schlein showed that in dogs, when a muscle cell contracts, there is an outflow of potassium ions. These potassium ions act upon the arterioles and the capillary bed, producing vasodilation. In effect, this opens up the ventilation system within the muscle bed, thus dissipating heat, removing waste metabolites (including H^+), and increasing the inflow of glucose, oxygen, and bicarbonate buffer available to the ion pump and muscle cell. If the intracellular level of potassium progressively falls (i.e., reaches a stage of a relative K^+ deficit), there is an insufficient outflow of K^+ ions on muscular contraction to stimulate the local vasodilation. In fact, it was possible to produce all of the histologic changes of exertional rhabdomyolysis in canine muscle cells by inducing an intracellular potassium deficit with chlorothiazide diuretics or desoxycorticosterone acetate (Doca) injections. There is also a considerable body of evidence to show that an increased amount of potassium and hydrogen ions are excreted in the urine after severe muscular exertion. This process is exacerbated by the increased levels of cortisol and aldosterone produced by the greyhound subjected to a stressful training-racing program (sodium retention and potassium excretion). It appears, therefore, that some greyhounds subjected to a stressful racing program (2 races or trials weekly) suffer a relative potassium deficit — relative in the sense that, while the deficit is not sufficient to produce marked changes in the ECF potassium levels, it is sufficient to fail to induce vasodilation on muscular contraction.

When the intracellular levels of potassium fall to a critical level and fail to induce a vasodilation of the arteriole–capillary bed following muscular contraction, the result is local hyperthermia and ischemia leading to a subacute form of exertional rhabdomyolysis. In such cases death does not occur. Myoglobinuria may or may not be observed, depending on the extent of the muscle damage. ECF potassium levels are not likely to reflect the intracellular K^+ status, since this requires major ICF changes of K^+.

Clinically, the trainer reports that the greyhound did not run well and appeared "tied up" or "shortened stride." The patient is usually presented 24 to 72 hours after the run, because the myositis is not severe and escapes attention until then. Observation suggests that the inflammatory changes of myositis associated with the localized lysis of the cell wall do not reach a peak for 24 to 48 hours after the race.

RECOMMENDED THERAPY

Treatment and prophylaxis are based on the understanding that the subacute form of exertional rhabdomyolysis is associated with a relative potassium deficit rather than with a failure of the ion pump and alkali reserve. Therefore, therapy should include (1) alkalinization of the urine to minimize protein precipitation in the nephron, (2) the use of anabolic steroids, as previous mentioned, (3) good nursing that includes provision of warmth, customary walking exercise only for 14 days, and the usual racing diet. Phenylbutazone may be used to relieve muscular discomfort.

RECOMMENDED PROPHYLAXIS

Herein lies the main approach to this form of exertional rhabdomyolysis. The normal urinary pH for maximum performance of racing greyhounds is 6.0 to 6.5. This is based on testing a midstream collection of the first sample of the morning. The sample must be taken at least eight hours after feeding and two days or more after a hard run and be from a patient receiving no medication for two days. Such samples are collected and submitted for testing on an average of two to four times monthly by regular clients.

Some greyhounds, even when physically fit, if subjected to excessive frequency and stress of fast work (2 to 3 races or trials per week) develop more acidotic urine, with a pH range of 5.3 to 5.8. A prolonged acidotic state (three to six weeks' duration) in these greyhounds will induce a relative potassium deficit. This critical stage is reached when the urine pH undergoes a dramatic swing from acidotic (5.3 to 5.8) to alkalotic (7.3 to 8.3), indicating a metabolic alkalosis associated with a relative potassium deficit, as indicated by Hall. If the greyhound is raced at this stage a subacute exertional rhabdomyolysis will result.

Prophylaxis is based on monitoring the urine sample (which must be collected as specified) for a change from acidotic to alkalotic and administering potassium supplements in a slow-release inert wax base orally at the rate of 25 mg/kg b.i.d. In addition, it should be strongly recommended that the owner reduce the frequency of trials and races to a level at which the work load is sufficient to maintain urinary pH at 6.0 to 6.5. For dogs with cooperative trainers it is preferable to alkalinize the urine with potassium citrate or acetate when the pH is first detected to be below 6.0 and to adjust the training program at that stage. However, this ideal is not always readily achievable.

SUPPLEMENTAL READING

Champion, D.S., Arias, J. M., and Carter, N.W.: Rhabdomyolysis and myoglobinuria — association with hypokalemia of renal tubular acidosis. J.A.M.A., *220*:967–969, 1972.

Davis, P.E., and Paris, R.: Azoturia in a greyhound: Clinical pathology aids in diagnosis. In *The Racing Greyhound*, vol. 2. London, World Greyhound Racing Federation, 1977, pp. 119–131.

Hall, L.W.: *Fluid Balance in Canine Surgery*. Baltimore, Williams & Wilkins Co., 1967.

Keene, R.B., and Yarborough, J.H.: Lamenesses of the racing greyhound. Vetscope, *11*:2–9, 1966.

Knochel, J.P., and Schlein, E.M.: On the mechanism of rhabdomyolysis in potassium depletion. J. Clin. Invest., *51*:1750, 1972.

Prole, J.H.B.: A survey of racing injuries in the greyhound. In *The Racing Greyhound*, vol. 2. London, World Greyhound Racing Federation, 1977, pp. 119–131.

MYOTONIA IN THE DOG

I.D. DUNCAN, B.V.M.S.

Montreal, Canada

Myotonia is a disorder of skeletal muscle characterized clinically by active contraction of a muscle that persists after the cessation of voluntary effort or stimulation (Walton). The underlying defect is thought to originate in an abnormal muscle membrane that discharges trains of repetitive action potentials in response to depolarization (Bryant). In man myotonia is found in a number of different muscle diseases, the most important of which are myotonia dystrophica and myotonia congenita. Myotonia has been found in association with several different muscle diseases in the dog, a number of which appear to be breed-specific.

MYOTONIA IN THE CHOW

Myotonia has been reported as occurring in this breed in four countries: the United Kingdom (Griffiths and Duncan), Holland (Wentink, et al.), Australia (Farrow, personal communication), and New Zealand (Jones, et al.). It therefore seems likely that myotonia is more widespread in the chow than in any other breed. To date there is no definite proof that the disease is inherited in the chow, but in the report of Wentink, et al., affected cases were found in two successive litters bred from the same parents. In the report of Jones, et al., three members of the same litter were found to be affected. In our experience of four chows with the disorder (two male, two female), all have come from litters produced by normal parents, and each has been the only member of the litter to be affected. With this evidence it could therefore be postulated that the disease is transmitted as an autosomal recessive trait.

ETIOLOGY

Much of the investigation into the origin of myotonia has been carried out in the myotonic goat and in carboxylic acid–induced myotonia in laboratory animals (Bryant). In both these cases a low membrane chloride conductance is thought to play a key role in the pathophysiology of the disease (Furman and Barchi). This is related to accumulation of potassium in the t-tubular system, which leads to progressive postexcitation depolarization of the muscle membrane. 20,25-Diazacholesterol, a cholesterol-lowering agent, has also been used to induce myotonia in experimental animals following the discovery that chronic administration of the drug to human patients could produce myotonia. The mechanism by which this drug produces myotonia is not known for certain, but it has been suggested it may be due to an alteration of the muscle membrane lipid structure.

CLINICAL SIGNS

In all instances the clinical signs appear as early as two to three months of age, but whether myotonia is present at birth is not known. The signs are first noted when the animal attempts to rise. Marked abduction of the forelimbs often occurs, and after struggling to rise the dog walks with a stiff gait and arched back. There is marked inability to flex the stifle joints, and the dog may move with a 'bunny-hop gait' and find it impossible to climb stairs. In all reported cases this stiffness lessens with exercise but worsens with cold weather. If the dog is suddenly rotated onto its side or back, the resultant hyperextension of the limbs will persist for up to a minute and will prevent the dog from righting itself. On palpation of skeletal muscle (proximal and distal muscles in the fore and hind limbs and the masticatory muscles), marked hypertrophy can be detected. This can perhaps be felt best in the proximal muscles of the fore and hind limbs, where individual muscles can easily be palpated as a result of their hypertrophy.

An additional clinical test can be of signifi-

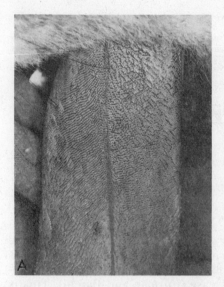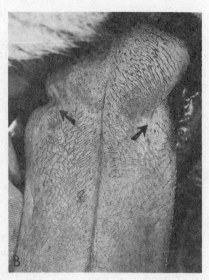

Figure 1. *A.* Tongue of a myotonic chow prior to percussion. *B.* After percussion with a blunt instrument a furrow forms (*arrows*) and persists for 30 to 45 seconds.

cant value in diagnosing the disease. Percussion of a muscle with a blunt instrument will result in a furrow that will persist for up to 30 to 45 seconds (myotonic dimple) (Fig. 1). Either a proximal fore or hind limb muscle can be percussed with the animal lying on its side, although the hair has to be clipped over the muscle in order to visualize the dimple. If the dog is anesthetized, percussion of the tongue will often reveal a very obvious myotonic dimple.

Care should be taken when anesthetizing suspected cases, because stenosis of the laryngeal glottis can result in difficulties in intubation. In one case stenosis of the glottis was thought to be responsible for the moderate dyspnea from which the dog was suffering. (Griffiths and Duncan). Muscle tone as judged by passive flexion of the joints is not increased, and no other neurologic abnormalities other than occasional dysphagia are noted. In some cases of the disease patellar luxation and secondary arthritis may be found, possibly as an initial result of the continued contraction of the hind limb extensor muscles. Abnormalities of other organs apart from the muscular system have not been reported. Measurement of serum creatine phosphokinase (CPK) should be carried out, for in some cases this may be raised and indicate myopathic damage.

ELECTROMYOGRAPHY (EMG)

An unequivocal diagnosis of myotonia in the chow can be made on EMG examination, although the clinical signs, breed, and presence of a myotonic dimple should enable a diagnosis to be made without an EMG. The insertion of a concentric needle electrode into almost any muscle in the resting or anesthetized dog will induce high-frequency discharges that can be heard on the EMG loudspeaker. These sounds, which have been likened to noise produced by a "dive bomber," are the result of waxing and waning of the amplitude and frequency of the discharges. Currently, the analogy between these sounds and a motor bike "revving up" might be more appropriate. Insertion of the needle and needle movement will elicit these discharges, but following this activity spontaneous discharges also will occur (Fig. 2). Percussion of the muscle while the needle is in place also will induce myotonic discharges. In general these discharges have a frequency of 100 to 200 per second and last for ½ to 1 second. They persist both after depolarizing and nondepolarizing muscle relaxants are given, thus proving that the activity arises in the muscle. The reaction to succinyl choline is somewhat unusual in that, instead of the normal fasciculations that occur shortly after the drug is given, opisthotonos, tonic spasm of all the limbs, and apnea as a result of fixation of the thorax are found (Griffiths and Duncan; Jones, et al.) This has also been noted in human patients with myotonia and in the myotonic goat (Bryant). To date there have been insufficient reports of the EMG of voluntary activity, but in one case the interference pattern was normal (Griffiths and Duncan). Nerve conduction velocities are within normal range.

PATHOLOGY

While muscle biopsy is not an essential part of the investigation of this disease, it can provide some useful information. To date there has been some variance (Duncan, Griffiths, and

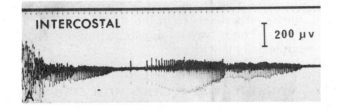
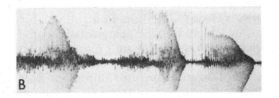
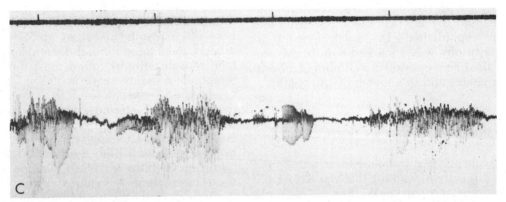

Figure 2. Typical myotonic discharges. A. Intercostal muscle. Note the increase and decrease in both frequency and amplitude of the high-frequency potentials. B. Lateral triceps. C. Biceps femoris. In B and C time marker = 1 second.

McQueen; Wentink, et al.; Jones, et al.) in the description of the pathologic changes found, and in our recent cases there have been differences among individual chows. In two of our cases the only abnormality noted in the proximal muscle biopsies from the fore and hind limbs was pronounced hypertrophy, probably of both type I and II muscle fibers. In the remaining cases there was a marked variation in muscle fiber size in biopsies from the same muscles, with both hypertrophic and atrophic fibers (Duncan, et al.), as was described by Jones, et al. The incidence of other myopathic change in our cases and in those of Jones, et al., is variable. These changes include muscle fiber degeneration and regeneration, hyaline fibers, split fibers, internal nuclei, and increased connective tissue and have led us to suggest that these cases may represent a true muscular dystrophy (Walton); i.e., there is evidence of a primary inherited progressive degenerative myopathy. However, there is no evidence of the changes that are regarded as the hallmark of human myotonia dystrophica, that is, ringed fibers and sarcoplasmic masses. Interestingly, however, it appears probable that some groups of muscle (for example, the ventral neck muscles) may be more severely 'myopathic' than the limb muscles (Duncan, et al.) This may be analogous to many of the human dystrophies in which the predilection for various groups of muscles to be more severely affected has given

rise to many of their appelations, e.g., facioscapulohumeral dystrophy.

TREATMENT

Attempts at treating myotonia are aimed at "stabilizing" the muscle fiber membrane using such compounds as procainamide and phenytoin. The mode of action of these compounds is to block dynamic sodium-conducting channels (Bryant). Despite the success of these drugs in human myotonia congenita they have had little success in the dog, although procainamide therapy has not been thoroughly evaluated (Griffiths and Duncan). Their success is likely to be limited if dystrophic muscle changes predominate, but further attempts at drug therapy should be made in the future in affected chows, since the main muscle pathology seen in that breed is hypertrophy. Once the diagnosis has been established, the owner should be advised that current known treatment is unsuccessful and that, while there may be no progression of signs, improvement is unlikely. Advice should be given to avoid exposure to cold weather. Because of the possible inherited nature of this condition, affected dogs and their parents should not be used for breeding.

In summary, myotonia in the chow has many similarities to human myotonia congenita (Thomsen's disease) on the basis of its very early onset, clinical signs, muscle hypertrophy, and significant lack of involvement of other organs. It is unlike human myotonia dystrophica, in which alopecia, cataracts, gonadal hypoplasia, and endocrine and immunoglobulin abnormalities are found. Unequivocal evidence of a familial nature remains unproved, and, while similarities between it and its human counterparts remain interesting, caution should be exercised in further extrapolation.

Myotonia has been seen in other single cases involving a West Highland terrier (Griffiths and Duncan) and a black Labrador (Griffiths and Duncan, unpublished). In the latter case muscle hypertrophy was a marked feature. Myotonia has also been reported in a number of inherited myopathies and in a metabolic myopathy.

SEX-LINKED MYOPATHY IN IRISH TERRIERS

Five male puppies from one litter were found to have difficulty in walking that was associated with stiffness and weakness, from eight weeks of age onward (Wentink, et al.). Dysphagia was present in all cases and there was lumbar kyphosis and muscle atrophy. A myotonic dimple was not elicitable on percussion. Myopathic changes were prominent in the skeletal muscles examined and consisted of degeneration, regeneration, calcification, and some inflammatory cell infiltration. Prolonged high-frequency discharges that decreased in frequency were found on EMG examination. These are unlike the discharges seen in the myotonic chow, which are short-lasting and increase and decrease both in amplitude and frequency.

AUTOSOMAL RECESSIVE MYOPATHY ASSOCIATED WITH MYOTONIA AND A DEFICIENCY OF TYPE II MUSCLE FIBERS IN LABRADOR RETRIEVERS

This disease was described in five retrievers from three separate litters and was first seen at the age of six months or less (Kramer, et al.). The dogs were stiff, walked with a hopping gait, and had abnormal head and neck posture. Muscle atrophy was noticeable. Unlike that condition seen in the chow and human cases of myotonia congenita, exercise increased the weakness, and cold weather also exacerbated the signs. There was no note of the presence of a myotonic dimple. Serum CPK levels were lower than normal, unlike the values found in the chow (Griffiths and Duncan; Jones, et al.). Discharges were found on EMG examination that were classified as myotonic. Muscle biopsy showed a variation in fiber size and an increase

in connective tissue, and histochemistry demonstrated a decrease in the number of type II fibers. There was no apparent progression of clinical signs with age.

MYOPATHY IN ASSOCIATION WITH CUSHING'S DISEASE

The clinical signs of muscle weakness and atrophy in the majority of dogs with hyperadrenocorticism are well known. Muscle weakness often results in excess abduction of the elbows and a pendulous abdomen, and generalized muscle atrophy, often most noted in the temporal muscles, can be seen. Iatrogenic Cushing's disease can result from the protracted over-dosage of steroids, and such cases can present with a myopathy. In both spontaneous and iatrogenic Cushing's disease a few cases may present with limb rigidity and a stiff gait (Duncan, Griffiths and Nash; Greene, et al.). In these cases there is hyperextension of all four limbs, especially the hind limbs, and flexion of the limb may be impossible even under general anesthesia. A myotonic dimple can be found on percussion of the muscles, which are often hypertrophic. Electromyography of dogs with Cushing's disease either with muscle weakness and atrophy or stiffness revealed the presence of high-frequency discharges, mainly in proximal muscles (Duncan, et al.; Greene, et al.). These discharges were mainly pseudomyotonic (Fig. 3); i.e., they did not wax and wane. They were often stimulated by needle insertion and started and stopped abruptly after periods of up to 30 seconds. After careful searching, however, spontaneous myotonic discharges were also found (Duncan, et al.). Pseudomyotonic discharges can be found in many primary disorders of muscle and can also be found in neurogenic atrophy. Use of the term "pseudomyotonic" should perhaps be discontinued in favor of the more accurate term, "bizarre high-frequency discharge" (Eisen and Karpati). The origin of these high-frequency discharges is not known, but the association between them and the abnormal calcium metabolism that is found in canine Cushing's disease has been suggested. Muscle biopsy from affected cases shows atrophy, some fiber necrosis and regeneration, and an increase in fat and connective tissue. Skeletal muscle calcification can occasionally be seen. Treatment of Cushing's disease using adrenocorticolytic drugs can occasionally result in resolution of the weakness and muscle atrophy (Greene, et al.), but in most instances, although polydipsia and polyuria may be reduced, the weakness remains and myotonic discharges can still be found.

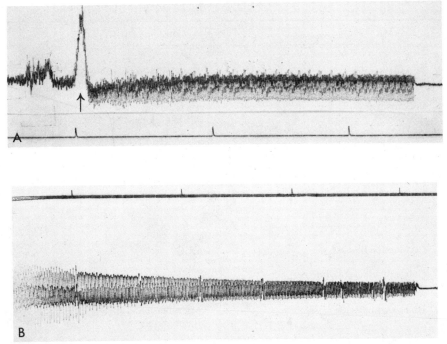

Figure 3. Typical bizarre high-frequency discharge (pseudomyotonia). Needle movement *(arrow)* has triggered this discharge, which does not vary in frequency or amplitude and terminates abruptly. *B.* In this high-frequency discharge (pseudomyotonic) there is a slight variation in frequency and amplitude. In *A* and *B* time marker = 1 second.

SUPPLEMENTAL READING

Bryant, S. H.: The electrophysiology of myotonia, with a review of congenital myotonia in goats. In Desmedt, J. E. (ed.): *New Developments in Electromyography and Clinical Neurophysiology.* Vol. 1. Basel, Karger, 1974, p. 420.

Duncan, I. D., Griffiths, I. R., and McQueen, A.: A myopathy associated with myotonia in the dog. Acta Neuropathol., *31*:297, 1975.

Duncan, I. D., Griffiths, I. R., and Nash, A. S.: Myotonia in canine Cushing's disease. Vet. Rec., *100*:30, 1977.

Eisen, A. A., and Karpati, G.: Spontaneous electrical activity in muscle description of two patients with motor neuron disease. J. Neurol. Sci., *12*:121, 1971.

Furman, R. E., and Barchi, R. L.: The pathophysiology of myotonia produced by aromatic carboxylic acids. Ann. Neurol., *4*:357, 1978.

Greene, C. E., Lorenz, M. D., Munnell, J., Jr., Praase, K. W., White, L. A., and Bowen, J. M.: Myopathy associated with hyperadreno-corticism in the dog. J. Am. Vet. Med. Assoc., *174*:1310–1315, 1979.

Griffiths, I. R., and Duncan, I. D.: Myotonia in the dog: A report of four cases. Vet. Rec., *93*:184, 1973.

Jones, B. R., Anderson, L. J., Barnes, G. R. G., Johnstone, A. C., and Juby, W. D.: Myotonia in related chow chow dogs. N.Z. Vet. J., *25*:217, 1978.

Kramer, J. W., Hegreberg, G. A., Braun, G. M., Meyers, K., and Ott, R. L.: A muscle disorder of Labrador retrievers characterized by deficiency of type II muscle fibers. J. Am. Vet. Med. Assoc., *169*:817, 1976.

Walton, J. N.: *Disorders of Voluntary Muscle,* 3rd ed. New York, Longman, 1974.

Wentink, G. H., van der Linde-Sipman, J. S., Keijer, A. E. F. H., Kamphuisen, H. A. C., van Vorstenbosch, C. J. A. H. V., Hartman, W., and Hendriks, H. J.: Myopathy with a possible recessive x-linked inheritance in a litter of Irish terriers. Vet. Pathol., *9*:328, 1972.

Wentink, G. H., Hartman, D., and Koeman, J. P.: Three cases of myotonia in a family of chows. Tijdschr. Diergeneeskd., *99*:729, 1974.

EPISODIC WEAKNESS

BRIAN R. H. FARROW, B.V.Sc.

Sydney, Australia

Episodic weakness may be a manifestation of a variety of different diseases and presents an interesting diagnostic problem for the clinician. Weakness interspersed with periods of apparent normality can result from neuromuscular, cardiovascular, or metabolic diseases. Diseases that may produce weakness of an episodic nature are indicated in Table 1, together with pertinent diagnostic aids and appropriate therapy.

Table 1. *Episodic Weakness*

DISEASE	DIAGNOSTIC AIDS	TREATMENT
Neuromuscular		
Myasthenia gravis	Anticholinesterase response	Prostigmine
	Electromyographic studies	Pyridostigmine
Polymyopathy	Enzymology: SGOT↑, CPK↑	Specific therapy where indicated
	Muscle biopsy	Glucocorticosteroids
Cardiovascular		
Arrhythmias	ECG	Antiarrhythmic agents (ventricular)
		Lidocaine
		Quinidine
		Procainamide
		Phenytoin
		Cardiac glycosides (supraventricular)
Conduction blocks	ECG	Depends on degree and course (see elsewhere in text)
Congestive heart failure	Radiography	Cardiac glycosides
		Diuretics
Heartworm disease	Microfilariae in blood	Treat CHF if necessary
	Radiography	Caparsolate
Metabolic		
Hypoglycemia	Fasting blood glucose	Surgery (pancreatic neoplasia)
		Diazoxide
		Phenytoin
Adrenal insufficiency	Na↓, K↑	Fludrocortisone acetate
	ECG	Glucocorticosteroids, when
	Plasma cortisol↓	necessary
	ACTH response	
Other disturbances	Electrolyte determinations	Appropriate fluid therapy
		Specific treatment as indicated

NEUROMUSCULAR DISEASES

MYASTHENIA GRAVIS

Myasthenia gravis (MG) is a neuromuscular disorder manifested by weakness and fatigability of muscles. The weakness is alleviated by rest or the administration of anticholinesterase drugs. After variable amounts of exercise, weakness in the appendicular muscles is evident. Affected animals become fatigued and shorten stride before lying down and refusing to move. After a short period of rest they are able to walk again before the weakness returns. Drooping of facial features reflects facial muscle weakness in some cases. Sialosis, regurgitation of food, and megaesophagus in a high percentage of cases are manifestations of pharyngeal and esophageal striated muscle weakness. The response in MG to the administration of anticholinesterase drugs is diagnostic. Edrophonium chloride,* a short-acting anticholinesterase drug, or neostigmine methylsulfate,† a longer-

acting drug, may be used for diagnostic testing.

Following IV administration of edrophonium chloride (total dose 0.5 to 5.0 mg, depending on size), there is obvious clinical improvement within 10 to 30 seconds and then a return of weakness within five minutes. Neostigmine methylsulfate is given by intramuscular injection (0.05 mg/kg), following which there is a clinical improvement in 15 to 30 minutes that lasts for some hours. Undesirable muscarinic effects such as vomiting or defecation should be prevented by prior administration of atropine. Care should be taken with anticholinesterase test-dosing, since the possibility of a cholinergic crisis (i.e., excessive muscle depolarization and weakness) exists from dosage of nonmyasthenic individuals or overdosage. Facilities for resuscitation should be readily accessible should the need arise. The use of electrodiagnostic testing, when available, enables demonstration of characteristic decremental responses to repetitive nerve stimulation. Repetitive supramaximal stimuli are applied to a peripheral nerve (e.g., the ulnar nerve), and the

*Tensilon, Roche Laboratories, Nutley, N. J.
†Prostigmin Injection, Roche Laboratories, Nutley, N. J.

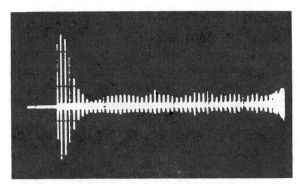

Figure 1. Electromyographic recording of evoked motor unit potentials from a dog with myasthenia gravis. The potentials were recorded from the palmar interosseous muscles during repetitive supramaximal stimulation of the ulnar nerve at a rate of 30 per second. Note the significant and progressive decrease in successive responses in the early phase of stimulation.

Table 2. *Anticholinesterase Therapy in Myasthenia Gravis*

DRUG	DOSAGE*
Neostigmine bromide†	0.5 mg/kg per os
Pyridostigmine bromide‡	2.0 mg/kg per os

* Dosages of both drugs to be administered as required.
† Prostigmin, Roche Laboratories, Nutley, N.J.
‡ Mestinon, Roche Laboratories, Nutley, N.J.

induced action potentials are observed in an appropriate muscle (e.g., the interosseus muscles). In normal animals successive stimuli produce action potentials of the same magnitude, whereas in myasthenic individuals successive stimuli produce action potentials of decreasing magnitude (Fig. 1).

The basic defect in MG is a reduction of available acetylcholine receptors at neuromuscular junctions, which in the majority of adult onset cases is the result of an antibody-mediated autoimmune attack directed against the postsynaptic neuromuscular junction. The decreased number of available receptors reduces the probability of interactions between acetylcholine and receptor molecules.

Therapy in MG is based on symptomatic control by the use of anticholinesterases. Although therapy does nothing to repair the basic deficiency in receptors, it does delay the degradation of acetylcholine released by the nerve and allows it to interact with more receptors, thereby improving neuromuscular transmission and the animal's strength. Neostigmine bromide‡ or pyridostigmine bromide§ are the anticholinesterase drugs generally used for oral administration in MG. Pyridostigmine bromide is also available as a sustained-release tablet**, making less frequent administration possible. There is marked variability in dosage requirements, and it is necessary to individualize the dose for each case. Suggested starting doses are indicated in Table 2. Glucocorticosteroid therapy, directed against the autoimmune mechanisms involved in the pathogenesis of the disease in adults, may also be indicated as an adjunct to

anticholinesterase therapy in certain individuals.

Although the association between thymic disorders and MG is not as well documented in dogs as it is in people, thymoma has been reported in some dogs with MG. For this reason the cranial mediastinum of dogs with MG should be evaluated radiographically. The etiologic connection between thymic abnormalities and MG remains the subject of speculation.

MG in dogs is often of a transitory nature, with spontaneous remissions occurring after some weeks. During this time appropriate anticholinesterase medication is necessary to provide adequate muscular strength and minimize the risk of aspiration pneumonia. In many cases the need for therapy diminishes with time, and treatment may be discontinued after several weeks when strength returns to normal.

MG has also been reported in puppies and, although it is difficult to tell with certainty, it seems that the onset of the disease is some weeks after birth. Slightly different mechanisms may be involved in the pathogenesis of the neuromuscular disorder in these cases, but the approach to therapy is the same. The disease has also been recorded in cats.

POLYMYOPATHY

The weakness that accompanies various myopathies can be difficult to distinguish clinically from MG. The disability in dogs with myopathic weakness tends to be progressive but may vary in intensity and is generally made worse with exercise. Pain may be present on palpation of muscle groups but is frequently absent.

In addition to weakness, muscle trembling may be apparent following minimal exercise. Diagnosis is confirmed by demonstration of elevated levels of serum enzymes of muscle origin, particularly creatinine phosphokinase (CPK), and by the presence of histologic changes in muscle biopsies. Where electromyographic facilities are available, detection of increased insertional activity, trains of high-frequency discharges that start and stop suddenly, and muscle unit action potentials that are

‡ Prostigmin Tablets, Roche Laboratories, N. J.
§ Mestinon Tablets, Roche Laboratories, Nutley, N. J.
** Mestinon Timespan Tablets, Roche Laboratories, Nutley, N. J.

reduced in amplitude and duration are all suggestive of myopathy. Some specific infectious agents, such as *Toxoplasma gondii* and *Leptospira icterohaemorrhagiae*, may produce a polymyositis, but in most cases of polymyositis the etiology is obscure. The nature of the inflammatory infiltrate in many cases suggests that immune mechanisms may be involved. When biopsies fail to implicate an infectious agent, vigorous use of glucocorticosteroid therapy generally produces a favorable response. Other acquired and congenital myopathies of a non-inflammatory nature have also been observed in dogs but have not been well documented to date. However, the diagnosis should be considered in young animals presented because of weakness.

CARDIOVASCULAR DISEASES

The initial physical examination of the animal presented for episodic weakness could reveal the presence of congestive heart failure (CHF) and other cardiovascular abnormalities, if present. Careful auscultation of the chest will detect the presence of valvular abnormalities. Arrhythmias may also be detected at this time, although the arrhythmias may not always be present or detectable at the time of the examination. Electrocardiographic examination is necessary to define the arrhythmias and conduction disturbances more precisely in order to select the appropriate therapy. This aspect of therapy is discussed in detail elsewhere in the text (see Section 4, Cardiovascular Diseases).

Dogs with heartworm disease are occasionally presented with a history of episodic weakness and no other signs of CHF. In these cases physical examination may be unrewarding, and the diagnosis depends on demonstration of microfilariae in the peripheral circulation together with characteristic changes on thoracic radiography. A detailed discussion of diagnosis and treatment of heartworm disease may be found elsewhere in the text.

METABOLIC DISEASES

HYPOGLYCEMIA

Hypoglycemia is probably the most frequently encountered metabolic change that results in weakness of an episodic nature. This may result from increased utilization of glucose, as in hyperinsulinism, or from interference with normal glucose availability, as in the glycogen storage diseases, adrenal insufficiency, hepatic insufficiency, and starvation.

Blood glucose determination should be part of the initial laboratory investigation of animals presented with episodic weakness in which examination fails to implicate neuromuscular or cardiovascular disease. It is important to remember that blood glucose levels may be normal at the time of presentation or at a single sampling in cases in which the weakness is in fact of hypoglycemic origin. It is therefore necessary in some cases to repeat blood glucose determinations after withholding food for 12 to 24 hours before hypoglycemia can be excluded as a possible cause.

The clinical signs of hypoglycemia vary in severity from mild weakness and behavioral changes to grand mal seizure episodes. Which particular clinical picture dominates is not so much a manifestation of the degree of hypoglycemia as of the rapidity with which the blood glucose level is lowered. Some animals can adapt to changes in blood glucose that occur slowly over a long period and so display neurologic signs infrequently. Others, in which hypoglycemia occurs precipitously, manifest severe signs.

Once established, the precise cause of hypoglycemia should be investigated. Young puppies may develop transient hypoglycemia as a result of starvation or gastrointestinal disease that interferes with glucose uptake. A persistent or recurrent hypoglycemia occurs in young puppies, particularly of the toy breeds, that have inherited abnormalities in carbohydrate metabolism. These diseases (glycogen storage diseases) are not well defined in the dog.

Hyperinsulinism. The commonest cause of maturity-onset hypoglycemia is hyperinsulinism from a functional pancreatic beta-cell neoplasm. In cases in which hypoglycemia is established as the cause of neurologic dysfunction in a mature dog that is free of significant liver disease, exploratory laparotomy and a search for a pancreatic tumor is warranted. It should be remembered that these tumors are frequently small and may be difficult to find. It should also be remembered that in dogs these tumors tend to be malignant, metastasizing to portal lymph nodes and the liver early in the course of disease. Where facilities allow, establishment of the diagnosis by demonstration of inappropriately high insulin levels is desirable. This should be performed in conjunction with blood glucose estimations. Provocative testing utilizing intravenous tolbutamide is rarely necessary to establish the diagnosis in the clinical situation.

The treatment of choice is surgical removal of the tumor. However, because of the highly metastatic behavior of this tumor in dogs, surgery may not be successful. In these cases symptomatic relief can frequently be attained by the use of oral diazoxide (10 mg/kg initially, increasing as required up to 40 mg/kg daily), a non-diuretic thiazide with hyperglycemic effects. Streptozotocin, an antibiotic and cytotoxic agent derived from *Streptomyces achromogenes*, is known to have cytotoxic effects against both normal and neoplastic pancreatic beta-cells and has been used for the treatment of metastatic insulinomas in people. The drug has not been adequately evaluated in the dog; however, it is very expensive and has a fairly narrow margin of safety, with toxic effects predominantly on the renal tubules. Therefore, further work is necessary to evaluate the role, if any, of streptozotocin in the management of metastatic pancreatic beta-cell neoplasia in the dog. When owners request further treatment of these cases, it may be preferable to use diazoxide in conjunction with phenytoin, which has anticonvulsant activity and also tends to inhibit insulin secretion.

ADRENOCORTICAL INSUFFICIENCY

The fluctuating and often severe electrolyte disturbances and changes in blood pressure that result from adrenocortical insufficiency are responsible for the episodic weakness associated with this disease. A history of gastrointestinal disturbances is frequently present in these cases. On physical examination bradycardia may be present. Flattened P waves and tall, peaked T waves on the electrocardiogram reflect the hyperkalemia that may be present at the time of examination. Hematologic examination often reveals eosinophilia and lymphocyto-

sis, and plasma electrolyte determinations may show hyperkalemia and hyponatremia. However, the laboratory features traditionally ascribed to hypoadrenocorticism often are absent at the time of examination, particularly in mild cases, and in cases in which the index of suspicion is high, confirmation of the diagnosis should be sought by direct assay of plasma cortisol levels before and after administration of ACTH. Cases of adrenocortical insufficiency should receive specific hormone replacement therapy consisting of 9α-fluorohydrocortisone, together with glucocorticosteroid supplementation at times of stress. The detailed managementof these animals and those that may be presented in a more critical state is dealt with in Section 11, Endocrine and Metabolic Disorders.

OTHER METABOLIC CAUSES

Other electrolyte disturbances secondary to such events as severe vomiting or diarrhea or diabetic ketoacidosis may also produce weakness. These disorders are less likely to be episodic in their manifestations. Therapy should be directed at correction of the electrolyte disturbances and treatment of the fundamental disorder.

SUPPLEMENTAL READING

Capen, C.C., Belshaw, B.E., and Martin, S.C.: Endocrine disorders. In Ettinger, S.J. (ed.): *Textbook of Veterinary Internal Medicine*, Philadelphia, W.B. Saunders Co., 1975, pp. 1351–1452.
Drachman, D.B.: Myasthenia gravis. N. Engl. J. Med., 298:136–142, 186–192, 1978.
Ettinger, S.J., and Suter, P.F.: *Canine Cardiology*. Philadelphia, W.B. Saunders Co., 1970.

CANINE POLYARTHRITIS

RALPH E. BARRETT, D.V.M.
Carmichael, California

INTRODUCTION

Polyarthritis is defined as the simultaneous inflammation of several joints. There are numerous causes of polyarthritis. It may present as a specific disease entity (e.g., rheumatoid arthritis), but more commonly it is a manifestation of, or is present concurrently with, another poly-

systemic disease (e.g., systemic lupus erythematosus, chronic infection, septicemia, neoplasia, or other disease). Table 1 presents the conditions that should be considered in the differential diagnosis of polyarthritis. Included in the table are conditions that may be confused with polyarthritis prior to localization of the lesion to the joints. In addition to the causes of polyarthritis, there are many conditions that may affect single joints. These include synovial neoplasia, neoplastic extension from surrounding soft tissues, and bacterial infection from penetrating trauma or extension from surrounding soft tissues. Also, the causes of polyarthritis may occasionally present as monarthric disease initially or when one joint is disproportionately affected.

Since the etiology, clinical course, prognosis, and therapy vary widely in polyarthritis, a thorough diagnostic workup is emphasized. Clinical pathology, radiography, special serology, joint fluid analysis and synovial biopsy are usually necessary for a definitive diagnosis. Several of the more common causes of polyarthritis, including degenerative joint disease, bacterial polyarthritis, systemic lupus erythematosus (SLE) and other inflammatory non-erosive polyarthritides and rheumatoid arthritis (RA), will be discussed.

NON-INFLAMMATORY POLYARTHRITIS

DEGENERATIVE JOINT DISEASE

DEFINITION

Degenerative joint disease (osteoarthrosis, osteoarthritis) is a non-inflammatory chronic joint disease characterized by degenerative and proliferative joint changes. Degenerative joint disease is not usually classified as a form of polyarthritis because the lesions are not inflammatory and it usually does not involve multiple joints. It is included in this discussion because it is the most common cause of canine joint disease and must be considered in the differential diagnosis. It is classified as primary or secondary. Primary degenerative joint disease, which is common in man, is the result of the wear and tear of cartilage during aging and pathologically is considered a "normal" response to aging. Few clinical cases of possible primary canine degenerative joint disease have been described, but autopsy evidence of primary degenerative joint disease in the dog is not uncommon. Secondary degenerative joint disease occurs when abnormal stresses are placed on the joints that hasten the rate of cartilage loss.

ETIOPATHOGENESIS

The etiopathogenesis is not known. Secondary stress may arise from acquired and congenital postural and orthopedic abnormalities, dysplastic joints, trauma, inflammatory joint

Table 1. *Differential Diagnosis of Polyarthritis*

A. Non-inflammatory
  1. Degenerative joint disease (osteoarthritis)
    a. Primary
    b. Secondary
B. Inflammatory
  1. Infectious
    a. Bacterial
    b. Fungal
    c. *Mycoplasma*
    d. Protozoal (e.g., *Leishmania*)
  2. Non-infectious
    a. Immune-mediated
      (1) Non-erosive
        (a) Systemic lupus erythematosus
        (b) Polyarthritis occurring secondary to primary infectious and neoplastic processes or idiopathically
      (2) Erosive
        (a) Rheumatoid arthritis–like
    b. Non-immunologic
      (1) Crystal-induced arthritis (gout, pseudogout)
      (2) Hemarthrosis
        (a) Hemophilia
        (b) Multiple myeloma with hyperviscosity syndrome
        (c) Many bleeding diatheses
C. Non-articular conditions that may mimic polyarthritis
  1. Hypertrophic osteodystrophy
  2. Pulmonary hypertrophic osteoarthropathy
  3. Eosinophilic panosteitis
  4. Polymyositis
  5. Peripheral neuropathy
  6. Spinal cord dysfunction

diseases, damage to supporting structure of the joints, and obesity. Conditions in the dog that predispose to this instability and premature aging of cartilage include osteochondrosis, ununited anconeal and coronoid processes, hip dysplasia, patellar luxation, achondroplasia, trauma to cartilage and epiphyses, postinflammatory cartilage damage, trauma to structural support of the joint, Legg-Perthes disease, and improper repair of a fracture or other orthopedic problem.

CLINICAL MANIFESTATIONS

Clinical signs may be absent early in the disease. Later signs may include lameness, mild joint pain on palpation, stiffness, limitation of movement, and disuse atrophy of muscles. If only one joint is involved, differentiation from other polyarthritic conditions is not difficult. However, hip dysplasia, osteochondrosis and un-united anconeal process, which precede degenerative joint disease, can be bilateral, or multiple conditions may be present in some dogs.

DIAGNOSIS

Age and breed of dog should be considered for genetic predisposition. Joint swellings are due to bone changes rather than to soft tissue changes such as occur in infectious or immune-mediated non-erosive arthritic diseases.

Degenerative joint disease is characterized radiographically by periarticular new bone proliferation, a decreased joint space (articular degeneration), deformation of subchondral bone, and increased density of subchondral bone. Very rarely, bone cyst formation occurs. There is poor correlation between severity of radiographic changes and clinical signs.

Joint fluid is usually normal (see Table 3). There is a small volume of clear, non-clotting fluid with a normal or slightly elevated total WBC count (< 3000 WBC/cu mm). Mononuclear cells predominate. Viscosity is normal.

THERAPY

There is no specific treatment for degenerative joint disease. The goals of therapy are to relieve pain, to allow continued joint function, and to slow the progression of degeneration.

1. *Restricted exercise.* Abnormal weight-bearing activities and strenuous exercise are harmful, but normal exercise may be helpful.

2. *Analgesics.* Salicylates (buffered aspirin) at a dosage of 30 mg/kg t.i.d. is often beneficial. Arquel® (Parke-Davis), at a dosage of 2 mg/kg per os once daily indefinitely, has been used with success experimentally to control the pain in chronic, severe degenerative joint disease. Toxic gastroenteritis can be observed as an uncommon side effect. Phenylbutazone (Butazolidin®, Geigy) may be used as a short-term analgesic and anti-inflammatory agent. Long-term usage is contraindicated because of potential ulcerogenic effects and hematopoietic toxicities. Dosage is 50 to 200 mg per os every eight hours.

3. *Anti-inflammatory drugs.* Use of systemic and intra-articular corticosteroids is controversial. Their usage may make the animal more comfortable and decrease secondary inflammation and pain; however, this may allow for increased traumatization and may hasten the degenerative process.

4. *Diet.* Reduce body weight.

5. *Surgery.* Several orthopedic techniques may slow or eliminate the degenerative process by restabilizing the joint, re-establishing alignment, or eliminating pain. Examples include cranial cruciate repair, patellar luxation and stifle deformity repair, femoral head excision, curettage of osteochondrosis lesions, un-united anconeal process removal or repair and arthrodesis.

Prognosis for total remission in degenerative joint disease is poor. These animals usually experience a slow, progressive clinical deterioration. However, properly treated cases can be maintained satisfactorily for years.

INFLAMMATORY POLYARTHRITIS — INFECTIOUS

BACTERIAL POLYARTHRITIS

Although viral, *Mycoplasma*, protozoal, and mycotic infections are possible, the most common type of infectious polyarthritis in the dog is bacterial. Monarthric bacterial arthritis due to localized joint damage or extension from surrounding soft tissue infection is more common than polyarthritis associated with septicemia. The polyarthritis of subacute bacterial endocarditis may be caused by hematogenously spread bacteria or by the deposition of antigen-antibody complexes in the synovial membrane (see inflammatory non-erosive joint diseases). Septic polyarthritis will be discussed here.

When true septicemia is present, involvement of other organ systems may also occur. Pneumonia, endocarditis, and pyelonephritis are often present concurrently. Bacterial polyarthritis associated with sepsis is an uncommon disease and accounts for only a small percentage of polyarthritis cases.

ETIOLOGY

The most common organisms involved are *Streptococcus* spp. and *Staphylococcus* spp., but *E. coli*, *Pseudomonas* spp., and other enterics are less commonly involved.

CLINICAL MANIFESTATIONS

Signs of septic arthritis include lethargy, weakness, anorexia, lameness, and reluctance to walk. Pyrexia is present in acute cases, while recurrent fever may be seen in chronic cases. The joints affected by the polyarthritis are inflamed. Pain, swelling, heat, and erythema are often present. A previous systemic disease or infection may be of historical significance. A local infection of the skin, bone, teeth, pharynx, prostate, anal glands, uterus, or umbilicus of neonates may be concurrent. Bacterial endocarditis with a systolic or, rarely, a diastolic (aortic valve) murmur may be present. Mitral valve involvement is most common. Cardiac arrhythmias are uncommon but may be found if myocarditis has occurred. Evidence of pyelonephritis with lumbar pain, hematuria, pyuria, proteinuria, and bacteriuria may also be present. Petechial hemorrhages of mucous membranes due to endotoxemia and vasculitis are rarely seen.

DIAGNOSIS

Diagnosis can be made only after identification of the microorganism. Routine aerobic and anaerobic cultures of joint fluid are employed as well as direct Gram stains of synovial fluid. In addition, two or three serial blood cultures prior to antibiotic therapy are recommended. Bacteriologic studies of other organ systems (e.g., urinary) may be helpful in identifying the source and type of organism.

The joint fluid has a decreased viscosity and will clot on exposure to air. Total synovial fluid WBC counts are typically over 100,000 WBC/cu mm (see Table 3). More than 90 percent are neutrophils, and floccules of mucopurulent material may be present. Phagocytized or free bacteria may be observed in the fluid. An elevated RBC count due to severe inflammation is common.

Radiographic signs are uncommon during the first week. Later radiographic abnormalities include destruction of periarticular bone, articular erosion, and massive bone proliferation around the joint margins.

THERAPY

Identification of the organism and use of the appropriate systemic antibiotics are imperative. Symptomatic therapy should be instituted after cultures have been acquired if the dog is critically ill. Parenteral sodium penicillin in dosages of 40,000 to 100,000 units/kg IV every six hours or procaine penicillin IM b.i.d., with streptomycin at 10 to 20 mg/kg IM b.i.d., is usually effective. In resistant cases, penicillin and kanamycin at 6 mg/kg IM b.i.d. is more effective. *Pseudomonas* infections may only be sensitive to gentamicin at 2 mg/kg IM b.i.d. When possible, the antibiotics should be changed to the oral route and administration continued for four to six weeks. Response to therapy should be monitored, with blood and joint fluid cultures as indicated. Rarely, one or two severely affected joints may require needle aspiration or surgical drainage for decompression and to facilitate response to systemic therapy. Intra-articular therapy is rarely required, owing to the excellent vascular supply of the joint. With vigorous, appropriate antibiotic therapy, the prognosis for complete elimination of the organism is good.

INFLAMMATORY POLYARTHRITIS — NON-INFECTIOUS

IMMUNE-MEDIATED/NON-EROSIVE

SYSTEMIC LUPUS ERYTHEMATOSUS (SLE) POLYARTHRITIS

DEFINITION

SLE is a chronic multisystem inflammatory disease. It is characterized by autoimmune phenomena. Many organ systems can be affected and clinical signs, including autoimmune hemolytic anemia, thrombocytopenia, glomerulonephritis, skin lesions, polymyositis, meningitis, myelopathy, and polyarthritis, have been observed in the dog. The most common clinical sign in the dog is polyarthritis.

ETIOPATHOGENESIS

Many factors have been shown to be associated with exacerbations of SLE. Exposure to sunlight, certain drugs, infectious agents, endocrine factors, and genetic factors have all been incriminated. Virus participation is highly suspected. Cell-free filtrates have been prepared from dog spleens. When injected into normal dogs and mice, antinuclear antibodies are formed. Also, positive LE clot tests and autoimmune hemolytic anemia have been seen in cats infected with feline leukemia virus. SLE in the NZB strain of mice is possibly related to an underlying leukemia virus infection. Present information suggests that an abnormal immune response in genetically predisposed SLE patients may result in the development of cell-mediated immunity and autoantibodies to cellular contents released during chronic viral infection or to new cell antigens that result from the viral infection. Although autoantibodies may affect numerous tissues they have not been shown to be cytotoxic, but they will cause formation of antigen-antibody complexes. Many of the clinical manifestations of SLE are due to deposition of these immune complexes in the tissues. Activation of complement and noncomplement systems has been incriminated as producing the lesions seen, particularly those occurring in the glomerulus of the kidney.

CLINICAL MANIFESTATIONS

The polyarthritis form of the disease often presents with a history of a shifting leg lameness and chronic relapsing pyrexia, which is not responsive to antibiotics. The lameness often undergoes periods of exacerbation and remission. Enlargements of the joints are seen in about half the cases. In acute cases local redness, swelling, and heat or only arthralgia may be seen. Joint enlargements in chronic cases are usually due to fibrosis of the joint capsule. Lymphadenopathy may be seen during periods of exacerbation. Cachexia and generalized muscle atrophy are proportional to the severity and chronicity of the disease.

DIAGNOSIS

Definitive diagnosis of the non-erosive polyarthritis of canine SLE can only be reached by positive serologic tests and elimination of other causes of polyarthritis. Radiographs are usually negative for joint abnormalities other than periarticular soft tissue swelling. The hematologic examination may show a leukocytosis, neutrophilia, and moderate anemia. A mild increase in serum globulins may be seen.

The joint fluid in SLE often has a reduced viscosity and will form a clot on exposure to air. The fluid is turbid and the color is occasionally yellow owing to the presence of hemosiderin. The total WBC count is over 3000 WBC/cu mm and may be as high as 400,000/cu mm. The percentage of neutrophils is increased to 20 to 85 percent of the cells (normally 10 percent) (see Table 3). Bacterial, *Mycoplasma, Chlamydia,* and virus cultures are negative. Rarely, LE cells may be seen in direct smears of joint fluid; however, LE cells may be seen non-specifically in inflamed joints regardless of the cause and are therefore not specific for SLE.

Serologic diagnosis is based on the finding of a positive LE cell test and a positive fluorescent antinuclear antibody (FANA) test. However, at present, available commercial tests may often be inaccurate. The LE clot test is subject to human error and is a more indirect test than the FANA test. The LE cell can rarely be seen in chronic infectious diseases of the dog but is still the most specific for SLE. The FANA test is the most sensitive test for SLE, but false positives can occur. Other evidence of autoimmune disease, including autoimmune hemolytic anemia with a positive Coombs' test, thrombocytopenia, immune complex glomerulonephritis, polymyositis, meningitis, and myelopathy, would add further support to a diagnosis of SLE. Rheumatoid factor test is usually negative but may be positive in SLE.

Histologically, the synovial membrane may be swollen and a primarily neutrophilic infiltrate is present. The largest number of these cells are found within and adjacent to the synovial cell layer. There are usually a few small aggregates of plasma cells near small blood vessels beneath the synovium. Joint destruction, deformity, and narrowing are rare. If these are present, a diagnosis of an overlap syndrome (rheumatoid arthritis–lupus) should be suspected.

THERAPY

The goals of therapy are to control the arthralgia symptomatically and to slow or stop progression of the arthritis. The immune-mediated polyarthritis of SLE is responsive to corticosteroids in over half the cases. Prednisolone is recommended at a dosage of 2 to 4 mg/kg per os divided b.i.d. for two to four weeks; it is then reduced to 1 mg/kg divided b.i.d. for two weeks, reduced again to 0.5 mg/kg divided b.i.d. for two weeks, and then stopped. If exacerbation of clinical signs occurs, maintenance for life at the lowest effective dosage is indicated. Often periods of months may lapse before relapse occurs. Alternate-day prednisolone therapy with the total dosage given every other morning is occasionally satisfactory. This will reduce the side effects of long-term corticosteroid therapy, allow the hypothalamic-pituitary-adrenal axis to recover and prevent prolonged immunosuppression.

In cases resistant to corticosteroid therapy Pedersen et al. (1976*b*) have produced remissions using more potent immunosuppressive drugs. Cyclophosphamide (Cytoxan®, Mead Johnson) is given at a dose of 1.5 to 2.5 mg/kg daily for four consecutive days of each week. Dogs weighing 10 kg or less receive 2.5 mg/kg daily; dogs weighing 10 to 20 kg receive 2.0 mg/kg daily, and dogs weighing more than 20 kg receive 1.5 mg/kg daily for four consecutive days of each week. Azathioprine (Imuran®, Burroughs Wellcome) is given at a dose of 2 mg/kg per os daily.

After two weeks on combination drug therapy the prednisolone dose is reduced to half the initial dose and, after the arthritis is in complete remission, half the initial dose is given every other morning, if possible. Complete blood counts are done weekly for the first month, every two weeks for the second month and monthly thereafter on all dogs receiving cyclophosphamide and azathioprine. If the white blood cell counts remain above 7000/cu mm, the doses of these two drugs are not changed. If the white blood cell count falls to between 5000 and 7000/cu mm, the doses of these two drugs are reduced by one-fourth. If the white blood cell count falls below 5000/cu mm, cyclophosphamide and azathioprine are discontinued until the count increases, and then they are reinstituted at half the initial doses. Remission usually occurs within 2 to 12 weeks. Only a small percentage of dogs fail to respond completely. Dogs with residual joint damage may show pronounced improvement but may retain some minimal lameness.

After the arthritis is in remission for at least two months, the dose of azathioprine is reduced to 2 mg/kg every other morning. When the disease is in complete remission for at least four months, an attempt is made to withdraw all cytotoxic drugs. If this is successful, corticosteroids are eventually discontinued. If the joint disease recurs, the disease is maintained in remission with the lowest possible dose of these drugs.

Side effects from chronic use of these drugs are not a problem in most cases. Delayed hair growth or hair loss may occur as an effect of the cytotoxic drugs. Sterile hemorrhagic cystitis can be a side effect of prolonged cyclophosphamide usage. Bone marrow depression due to cytotoxic drugs is occasionally seen, but the dosages can usually be readjusted before it becomes a problem. Liver disease resulting from chronic use of azathioprine is not a problem at this dosage, although dogs with pre-existing liver problems should not be given this drug.

OTHER CAUSES

A polyarthritis clinically and pathologically similar to canine non-erosive SLE polyarthritis has been observed in dogs with chronic bacterial infections, chronic fungal infections, bacterial endocarditis, dirofilariasis and neoplastic diseases, and some cases have no known cause (idiopathic). In some of these cases, the joint disease may be the main manifestation of the underlying infectious disease process. As in SLE, the pathogenesis of the joint disease in these animals probably involves the deposition of immune complexes in the synovial membrane. The joint disease usually subsides with correction of the primary disease process. However, corticosteroids may be needed to hasten resolution of the lameness if it is severe. Concurrent use of cyclophosphamide, azathioprine, and prednisolone as described before may be necessary.

IMMUNE-MEDIATED/EROSIVE

RHEUMATOID ARTHRITIS

DEFINITION

Rheumatoid arthritis (RA) is a severe, erosive, often progressive polyarthritis associated with immunologic mechanisms. Numerous cases of RA have been reported in the dog but not in the cat. RA is not a common disease, but reported incidence is increasing as diagnostic techniques improve and awareness of the disease increases. RA is a specific disease entity in the dog, and the term RA should not be used unless diagnosis has been confirmed.

ETIOPATHOGENESIS

Exact etiology and pathogenesis of RA are unknown. Most present theories on etiology propose that an unknown infectious organism initiates RA, and this agent directly or indirectly results in immune-complex disease, hypersensitivity, and autoimmunity. Numerous agents, including bacteria, viruses, phages, *Mycoplasma*, protozoa, and physical agents, have been suspected as initiators. Pathogenesis of the joint destruction in RA has been postulated to involve several immune-mediated steps: (1) An altered immunoglobulin G (IgG), possibly as a result of reaction with antigen, is produced. (2) Rheumatoid factor (RF), produced by B-lymphocytes and plasma cells in the synovial membrane, reacts with the altered IgG. (3) RF-IgG complexes are formed near the joint capsule and fix complement (C). (4) Chemotactic factors are released and attract neutrophils to the joint. (5) RF-IgG-C complexes are phagocytized in the joint space by neutrophils. (6) Lysosomal enzymes are released by the neutrophils and cause the tissue damage. Evidence for the presence of T cell–mediated destruction has also been suggested.

CLINICAL MANIFESTATIONS

History of a chronic, relapsing, and progressively worsening lameness involving several limbs or generalized stiffness is common. Initially there is a shifting lameness, with soft tissue swelling around involved joints. There is pain on palpation and movement of the joints. Depression, fatigue, anorexia, and weight loss are often present. Advanced cases may have crepitus or may present with non-functioning joints due to destruction and ankylosis. Pyrexia, lymphadenopathy, and splenomegaly are often present. Joint involvement is most severe in the carpal and tarsal joints, but in some cases elbows and stifles may show severe changes. Other joints usually do not become as severely involved. Small breeds are most commonly affected. RA can occur at any age but usually is seen after the first year of life. Subcutaneous nodules, pleuritis, interstitial pneumonia, ocular lesions, and vasculitis reported in man have not been seen in the dog.

DIAGNOSIS

Nine criteria should be evaluated in the diagnosis of RA in the dog (Table 2). Six of the nine criteria should be satisfied for a diagnosis of

Table 2. *Diagnostic Guidelines in Canine Rheumatoid Arthritis*

1. Morning stiffness.
2. Pain or tenderness in one or more joints.
3. Soft tissue swelling or effusion in one or more joints.
4. Swelling of any other joint.
5. Symmetric onset of joint symptoms and swelling.
6. Roentgenographic evidence of RA.
7. Positive RF test.
8. Poor mucin precipitate of synovial fluid.
9. Characteristic histologic changes in the synovium.

classic canine RA. Diagnostic emphasis should be placed on the radiographic appearance of RA and the presence of characteristic histologic changes in the synovium.

Several non-specific clinical pathologic abnormalities may be present. A normochromic, normocytic anemia not responsive to hematinics is occasionally seen. Mild leukocytosis and neutrophilia may be present. Serum protein determinations and electrophoresis are variable but often reveal hypoalbuminemia, hyperglobulinemia, and elevations of the alpha²- and beta-globulin fractions. Proteinuria associated with renal amyloidosis may be present.

Rheumatoid factors (RF) are autoantibodies to altered IgG (see "Laboratory Diagnosis of Immunologic Disorders," page 392). RF is mainly immunoglobulin M (IgM), and immunoglobulin A (IgA) may be involved as RF in certain cases. IgM is the predominant RF detected by standard agglutination tests. RF titer is determined by the sensitized sheep red blood cell (Rose-Waaler) method or by the latex particle agglutination (LPA) method. Human rheumatoid latex reagent is unsatisfactory in the dog. A specific latex reagent must be prepared for dogs. Positive RF titers in dogs by the Rose-Waaler method range from 1:16 to 1:128. RF may be positive in dogs with other autoimmune (e.g., SLE) or chronic infectious diseases. Also,

serologic abnormalities such as LE cell factor and antinuclear antibodies can be seen in dogs with RA but less frequently than in SLE. Because there is some degree of overlap of these factors, it seems unwise to separate SLE and RA based on serologic tests alone. Separation should be based on the type of joint disease associated with each. RA is usually erosive in nature; SLE and other hypersensitivity arthritides are usually non-erosive.

Characteristic radiographic changes develop within weeks to months as the condition progresses. Signs include soft tissue swelling or joint capsule distention, subchondral bone rarefaction, marginal erosions at the site of attachment of the joint capsule, joint space widening or narrowing, periarticular soft tissue or joint capsule calcification, irregular articular surfaces, disuse atrophy of muscles, and osteoporosis. Severe joint deformity and ankylosis may be present in advanced cases. These changes are symmetric, involving several joints.

An exudative joint fluid similar to SLE is characteristic (Table 3). Total WBC count is usually not as high. Recent studies have shown that a characteristic finding in canine RA is the presence of IgG and the absence of C3 in mononuclear cells in the synovial fluid.

Histologic evaluation of synovial membrane biopsies are characterized by a diffuse, proliferative synovitis, with a dense infiltration of lymphocytes and plasma cells. Increased collagenous connective tissue and hyperplastic synoviocytes are present. Villous hypertrophy occurs and may protrude into the articular space and attach to a fibrous pannus that has replaced an eroded articular cartilage.

THERAPY

The goals of therapy are to control pain and slow the progressive, erosive joint damage. Quinacrine and gold salts have been shown to

Table 3. *Synovial Fluid in Various Types of Canine Arthritis**

| CONDITION | NUCLEATED CELLS/CU MM | DIFFERENTIAL (% TOTAL) | | MICRO-ORGANISMS | IgG AND C3 INCLUSIONS |
		Mononuclear Cells	*Neutrophils*		
Normal†	<3000	90–100	0–12	Absent	Absent
Degenerative† joint disease	<5000	88–100	0–12	Absent	Absent
Rheumatoid-like arthritis (6 cases)	3000–38,000	20–80	20–80	Absent	Present
Non-erosive, non-infectious arthritis (51 cases)	3000–375,000	5–85	15–95	Absent	Absent to rare
Septic arthritis (10 cases)	100,000–450,000	1–10	90–99	Present in 90% of cases	Not tested

*Adapted from Pedersen, N. C.: Proc. AAHA Convention, May 1976.
†Cell count and differential values reconstructed from Sawyer (1963).

be beneficial in human RA but have not been evaluated in the dog. D-Penicillamine has been used with some success in treating human RA, and a few cases of canine RA appear to have benefited from its use. Buffered aspirin will occasionally control symptoms and pain associated with RA, but the disease usually progresses in spite of therapy. A dosage of 30 mg/kg t.i.d. is recommended, but higher dosages may be necessary. Corticosteroids have a temporary beneficial effect on canine RA, but progressively higher dosages become necessary with time, and they do not change the progressive course of the joint destruction. Short-term benefits may be seen with prednisolone at a dosage of 2 mg/kg/day divided b.i.d. Immunosuppressive drug therapy with cyclophosphamide, azathioprine, and prednisolone has arrested the progression of the disease in several cases in which it has been tried (Pedersen et al., 1976a) (regimen described in the SLE discussion). It is important that therapy be instituted before advanced joint destruction occurs. In cases of advanced joint destruction with only a few joints involved, arthrodesis may allow the return of some function.

SUMMARY OF IMPORTANT CLINICAL ASPECTS OF POLYARTHRITIS

1. True polyarthritis involves inflammation of the joints, but multiple joint involvement with degenerative joint disease may present with similar clinical signs.

2. Polyarthritis may occur as the predominant presenting problem, but usually it is associated with another systemic disease.

3. Presenting signs in decreasing frequency include (a) general body stiffness, (b) fever of unknown origin, (c) joint pain, and (d) joint swelling.

4. Causes of true polyarthritis (multiple joint inflammation) include (a) rheumatoid arthritis, (b) systemic lupus erythematosus, (c) secondary infection or neoplasia elsewhere in the body, (d) sepsis (septicemia with hematogenous spread), and (e) idiopathic causes (i.e., none of the previously described causes can be confirmed).

5. Since treatment and prognosis vary greatly, it is imperative that ancillary diagnostic tests be performed completely for a definitive diagnosis.

SUPPLEMENTAL READING

Biery, D. N., and Newton, C. D.: Radiographic appearance of rheumatoid arthritis in the dog. J. Am. Anim. Hosp. Assn., 11:607–612, 1975.
Hardy, R. M., and Wallace, L. J.: Arthrocentesis and synovial membrane biopsy. Vet. Clin. N. Am., 4:449–462, 1974.
Miller, J. B., Perman, U., Osborne, C. A., Hammer, R. F., and Gambardella, P. C.: Synovial fluid analysis in canine arthritis. J. Am. Anim. Hosp. Assn., 10:293–398, 1974.
Pedersen, N. C., Pool, R. C., Castles, J. J., and Weisner, K.: Non-infectious canine arthritis. II. Rheumatoid-like arthritis. J. Am. Vet. Med. Assn., 169:295–303, 1976a.
Pedersen, N. C., Weisner, K., Castles, J. J., Ling, G. V., and Weiser, G.: Non-infectious canine arthritis. I. The inflammatory, non-erosive arthritides. J. Am. Vet. Med. Assn., 169:304–310, 1976b.
Sawyer, D. C.: Synovial fluid analysis of canine joints. J. Am. Vet. Med. Assn., 143:609, 1963.
Schultz, R. D.: Immunologic disorders in the dog and cat. Vet. Clin. N. Am., 4:153–173, 1974.

CANINE HIP DYSPLASIA

STEN-ERIK OLSSON, V.M.D.

Stockholm, Sweden

INTRODUCTION

In the dog hip dysplasia is a developmental condition and not a congenital anomaly (Olsson and Kasström; Riser; Gustafsson et al.). Subluxation of the femoral head leads to abnormal wear, with erosion of its cartilage (Fig. 1), interference with the endochondral ossification of the acetabular rim (Figs. 2 and 3), fibrillation of the round ligament, synovitis,

thickening of the joint capsule and, eventually, formation of osteophytes. The pathologic changes in the cartilage and the soft tissues of the hip joint may start at three to five months of age. They are usually not very severe until the time when osteophytes appear — i.e., in late adolescence or early adulthood.

The radiographic appearance of hip dysplasia in a young dog is a shallower than normal acetabulum and a flattened femoral head that is

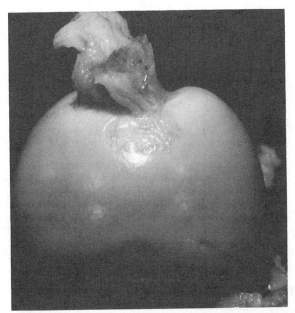

Figure 1. Femoral head from a 37-week-old German shepherd with very slight hip dysplasia. There is an area of cartilage erosion close to the round ligament.

slightly subluxated (Fig. 4). The trigger mechanism in hip dysplasia may be either slight joint laxity or poor support in weight-bearing from a slanting roof of the acetabulum. Either way, a vicious circle of increased luxation, increased remodeling with more flattening, and an even shallower acetabulum is started. Osteoarthrosis, increasing in severity over the years, is always seen.

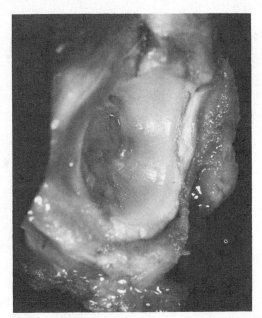

Figure 2. Left acetabulum from an 11-month-old golden retriever with moderate hip dysplasia. Part of the acetabular rim seems to be detached from the joint cartilage. The joint capsule is thickened.

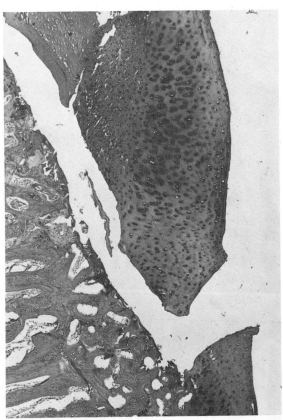

Figure 3. Histologic section from the craniodorsal rim of the acetabulum in a Labrador retriever, 9 months old. The joint cartilage of the rim has been detached in a fashion very similar to that seen in osteochondritis dissecans in other joints. (hematoxylin-eosin stain, × 50.)

ETIOLOGY AND PATHOGENESIS

The etiology of hip dysplasia is multifactorial. Anything that causes abnormal weight-bearing by the hip joint in a growing dog can lead to the morphologic changes characteristic of hip dysplasia. The cause of hip dysplasia can be local — for example, a fracture of the femoral shaft healed in malalignment — or it can be a unilateral sacralization of the seventh lumbar vertebra, giving rise to an asymmetric pelvis (Fig. 5). In these cases hip dysplasia is usually unilateral. Most cases of hip dysplasia are, however, caused by generalized constitutional factors governing the growth and development of the skeleton. The reaction of the hip joints to these generalized stimuli is due to their anatomic shape — the hip joints are unique in that they are the only joints with no horizontal support in weight-bearing.

The pathologic changes found in the cartilage of the acetabular rim are similar to those seen in osteochondrosis in other joints. However, no correlation between the occurrence of hip dysplasia and osteochondrosis has been established.

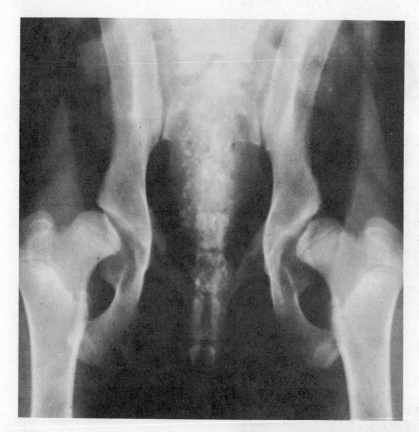

Figure 4. Radiograph of the pelvis and hip joints of a 5-month-old German shepherd with severe hip dysplasia. The acetabula are shallow and the femoral heads are flattened and slightly subluxated.

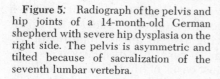

Figure 5. Radiograph of the pelvis and hip joints of a 14-month-old German shepherd with severe hip dysplasia on the right side. The pelvis is asymmetric and tilted because of sacralization of the seventh lumbar vertebra.

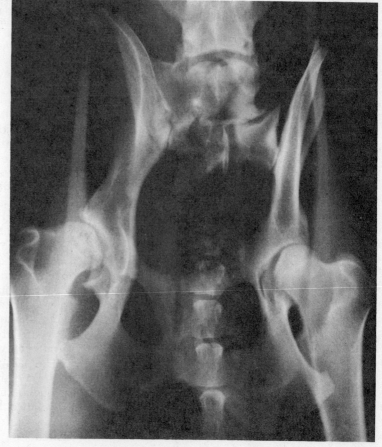

DIAGNOSIS

The diagnosis of hip dysplasia is usually made on the basis of radiographs. It must be understood that in dogs under the age of one year it is sometimes difficult to differentiate between a normal and a slightly abnormal hip joint. In severe cases diagnosis can be made at an age of three to four months, but a dog must be about 18 months old before a definite "diagnosis" of normal hip joints can be made. In dogs older than five to six years it is difficult to decide whether osteoarthrosis of the hip joints is primary or secondary to hip dysplasia.

Palpation at an early age (Bardens and Hardwick) — i.e., estimation of the amount of laxity of the hip joint — has limited prognostic value except in puppies in which the hip joints are very tight. There is a great chance that these hip joints will develop into sound joints (Kasström).

GENETICS AND PREVENTION

Hip dysplasia as it is seen in most breeds of large dogs is an inherited defect with a polygenic mode of inheritance. This means that many genes are responsible for its development. It is also quantitative in nature, because its phenotypic expression can vary from very minor changes to complete luxation with almost no acetabulum. As with any other inherited defect having a polygenic mode of inheritance, the expression of hip dysplasia is subject to modification by a variety of environmental factors. The amount of influence by the environment can be estimated and expressed as a heritability index. (A condition that is completely genetically controlled has a heritability index of 1. If there is no hereditary influence, the heritability index is 0).

The most recent heritability index estimated on the hitherto largest series of unbiased data (2404 German shepherd dogs of 401 litters from one kennel) was found to be from 0.4 to 0.5 (Hedhammar et al.). Such a heritability index means that heritability is moderate, indicating that it is possible to lower the incidence and severity of hip dysplasia considerably by genetic selection. Breeding of phenotypically normal individuals (dogs with radiographically normal hip joints) is usually what is recommended and practically possible. This is, of course, better than no selection at all, but the limitation of the method is obvious when one knows that male dogs with excellent hip joints may have offspring in whom the frequency of hip dysplasia varies from 21 percent to 68 percent (Hedhammar et al.). Such a difference in frequency is what can be expected in offspring of sires that have unknown parental hip joint status. Rather than using individual selection (mass selection), it is recommended that individual performance (progeny testing) and family performance (sibling evaluation and pedigree depth) be used. This was done in the aforementioned kennel once the heritability index had been estimated. The result was striking. Hip dysplasia frequency was lowered from 50 percent to 28 percent (Hedhammar et al.). This kind of selection is difficult to accomplish in privately owned dogs, since most breeding occurs on a small scale.

Breeders must understand that one can expect a significant lowering in frequency of hip dysplasia only if good hip joints are the only factor considered as a criterion for breeding. However, this is very rarely the case. Instead, many other desirable characteristics such as certain conformation, good disposition, and good working ability are also of importance. This makes it difficult to obtain immediate results.

It has been shown that the incidence and severity of hip dysplasia can be influenced by nutrition during growth in the offspring of dogs with hip dysplasia (Kasström). A high-calorie diet increases incidence and makes dysplasia more severe, whereas a low-calorie diet decreases incidence and makes hip dysplasia less severe. This finding and the observation that overfeeding (*ad lib*) of puppies causes many other skeletal problems in fast-growing dogs clearly demonstrate that restrictive feeding of growing dogs is important for normal development. On the other hand, puppies that develop normal hip joints despite overfeeding probably have a better genetic constitution (genotype).

It is imperative for breeders to decide what kind of dog they want. If good function and working ability is high on the priority list, special attention should be paid to good hip joints in breeding. If less practical characteristics such as conformation and color have top priority, hip dysplasia may be of less concern. It should always be remembered that the radiographic diagnosis of hip dysplasia and the clinical recognition of it are two different matters. Many times there is poor correlation between the degree of hip dysplasia as seen on radiographs and the clinical signs. Many dogs with hip dysplasia have no noticeable clinical signs. One must understand that the radiographic diagnosis of hip dysplasia in a clinically healthy dog is nothing but a memo to the owner, saying that the owner must put the status of the dog's hip joints on the negative side of the balance sheet when summing up the factors that make the animal suitable or unsuitable for breeding.

CLINICAL SIGNS AND TREATMENT

The clinical signs of hip dysplasia vary widely from very slight discomfort to severe crippling disease. There are great differences in individual temperament, which will influence the signs of hip dysplasia. Young dogs may walk with a swaying gait and may "bunny hop" on the hind limbs when running. Pain on abduction and extension of the hip joints can usually be elicited. One should not forget that improvement or even disappearance of signs is not uncommon, and adult dogs may not show any evidence of hip dysplasia until old age, when severe osteoarthrosis complicates the picture.

Dogs with clinical signs of hip dysplasia should be allowed to choose their own level of exercise, but if necessary they may be encouraged to a moderate level of activity. Forced sudden activity such as playing ball or jumping should be discouraged. Older dogs can be given the usual medication for pain caused by osteoarthrosis.

At the present time there are four surgical procedures available for cases in which, for various reasons, surgery is indicated. The simplest and most "innocuous" method is pectineomyotomy, for which there is wide indication. Following this type of surgery, improvement has been seen both in young dogs with unstable hips and in old dogs with osteoarthrosis (Wallace). Pectineomyotomy changes the gait pattern of the hind legs somewhat, allowing for more abduction in weight-bearing. This is probably why it seems to alleviate pain. A less enthusiastic report about the effectiveness of pectineomyotomy was reported by Vaughan and co-workers.

Another surgical procedure is pelvic osteotomy (Hohn and Janes). It is aimed at improving the support of the acetabular roof. The acetabulum is rotated over the femoral head, and in this way further subluxation is prevented. This procedure is technically difficult and requires long-term postoperative care. The long-term result is questionable.

Resection arthroplasty (i.e., removal of the femoral head) is a salvage procedure for dogs with severe hip dysplasia. This operation is comparatively easy to perform, but postoperative care and rehabilitation are time-consuming. Intensive physical training and exercise such as swimming and running are imperative during the first four to six months after the operation in order to get good functional nearthrosis. Resection arthroplasty should be reserved for young active dogs and preferably should be done on both sides at the same operation (Olsson et al.).

In recent years the total hip prosthesis has been used successfully in dogs with severe hip dysplasia, but nothing is known about the long-term result. One should remember, however, that manufacturing, fitting, and insertion of a well-functioning total hip prosthesis is a technically difficult and expensive procedure.

SUPPLEMENTAL READING

Bardens, J. W., and Hardwick, H.: New observations on the diagnosis and cause of hip dysplasia. Vet. Med. Small Anim. Clin., 63:238–245, 1968.

Gustafsson, P.-O., Olsson, S.-E., Kasström, H., and Wennman B.: Skeletal development of greyhounds, German shepherd dogs, and their crossbreed offspring. Acta Radiol. 344(Suppl):81–107, 1975.

Hedhammar, Å., Olsson, S.-E., Andersson, S.-Å., Persson, L., Pettersson, L., Olausson, A. and Sundgren, P.-E.: Canine hip dysplasia: Study of heritability in 401 litters of German shepherd dogs. J. Am. Vet. Med. Assoc., 9:1012–1016, 1979.

Hohn, R. B., and Janes, J. M.: Pelvic osteotomy in the treatment of canine hip dysplasia. Clin Orthop., 62:70–78, 1969.

Kasström, H.: Nutrition, weight gain, and development of hip dysplasia. An experimental investigation in growing dogs with special reference to the effect of feeding intensity. Acta Radiol., 344 (Suppl.):135–179, 1975.

Olsson, S.-E., Figarola, F., and Suzuki, K.: Femoral head excision arthroplasty. A salvage operation in severe hip dysplasia in dogs. Clin. Orthop., 62:104–112, 1969.

Olsson, S.-E., and Kasström, H.: Etiology and pathogenesis of canine hip dysplasia. Introduction of a new concept. Proceedings of the Canine Hip Dysplasia Symposium and Workshop, St. Louis, Missouri, October 19–20, 1972. St. Louis, Missouri, Orthopaedic Foundation for Animals, Inc., 1973, pp. 1–52.

Riser, W. H.: Growth and development of the normal canine pelvis, hip joints, and femurs from birth to maturity: A radiographic study. J. Am. Vet. Radiol. Soc., 14:24–34, 1979.

Riser, W. H.: The dysplastic hip joint: Its radiographic and histologic development. J. Am. Vet. Radiol. Soc., 14:35–50, 1973.

Vaughan, L. C., Clayton-Jones, D. G., and Lane, J. G.: Pectineus muscle resection as a treatment for hip dysplasia in dogs. Vet. Rec., 96:145–148, 1975.

Wallace, L. J.: Pectineus tendonectomy or tenotomy for treating clinical canine hip dysplasia. Vet. Clin. North Am., 3:455–465, 1971.

OSTEOCHONDROSIS IN THE DOG

STEN-ERIK OLSSON, V.M.D.

Stockholm, Sweden

It has long been known that there are certain skeletal problems characteristic of growing dogs of large breeds. Several conditions, such as osteochondritis dissecans of the shoulder, un-united anconeal process of the elbow, and retained cartilage of the distal ulna, were described in the 1950's and 1960's. Lesions of similar nature in the hind limbs, such as hip dysplasia and *genu valgum*, have also been known for a long time. More recently, lesions such as osteochondritis dissecans of the medial condyle of the humerus and fragmentation of the coronoid process (un-united coronoid process) of the ulna have been described. In studies of the hind limbs interest is now focused on epiphysiolysis of the femoral head and osteochondritis dissecans of the stifle and hock.

The various lesions have been looked upon as separate entities, and not until lately was there an understanding of the morphologic similarities and the generalized background of these lesions. Similar lesions in horses, cattle, pigs, turkeys, and poultry have been studied, and this has contributed to an even better understanding of the generalized nature of the condition now called osteochondrosis.

Of all the lesions mentioned, hip dysplasia is the only one that does not fit into the classification of osteochondrosis, even though some of the changes in the acetabulum in hip dysplasia are very similar to those seen in osteochondritis dissecans.

ETIOLOGY

The basic mechanism influencing the development of osteochondrosis is a disturbance of endochondral ossification. The various lesions considered to be manifestations of osteochondrosis apparently occur at sites at which cartilage is exposed to pressure or tension. It should be pointed out that all cartilage in the growing skeleton may be affected (i.e., both the growth plates and the joint cartilage). Although it has been recognized that certain lesions in the growth plates, such as retained cartilage of the distal ulna, are the result of overgrowth and a failure of calcification and ossification, the nature of the lesion in the joint cartilage (osteochondritis dissecans) was previously not understood. It has been a common misconception that the defect seen, for example, in osteochondritis dissecans of the shoulder is an aseptic necrosis of bone. Obviously, one has not reckoned with the concept of joint cartilage as a growth cartilage. It should therefore be emphasized that the joint cartilage is in fact the growth cartilage of the epiphysis in the same manner that the cartilage of the growth plates of the long bones is the growth cartilage of the metaphysis.

Normal growth of the epiphysis takes place by proliferation of chondrocytes near the joint surface. As cartilage continues to grow, vesiculation, degeneration, and calcification of the cells take place. The calcified layer of the cartilage is invaded by vessels from the bone marrow. Some of the calcified cartilage is resorbed, but remnants of cartilage are used as a framework for bone, which is laid down by osteoblasts. The process is called endochondral ossification.

In osteochondrosis, the normal differentiation process of the chondrocytes is disturbed — i.e., vesiculation, degeneration, and calcification do not take place in a normal way — and the cartilage gets thicker than normal. At certain sites of pressure or tension, vessels from the bone marrow do not penetrate the cartilage, and bone is not formed. If this process is localized to only a part of the joint cartilage and formation of bone continues in the calcified layer of the surrounding cartilage, the radiographic appearance will be that of an osseous defect. The basal layer of the thickened articular cartilage becomes necrotic and serves as a starting point for fissures in the cartilage. When a fissure reaches the surface of the joint cartilage, the condition is called osteochondritis dissecans (Fig. 1). It should be emphasized that the defect in the bone is there because cartilage did not undergo endochondral ossification. Hence, necrosis of pre-formed bone is not the cause of the defect (Fig. 2).

If changes such as the foregoing take place in a metaphyseal growth plate, epiphysiolysis may

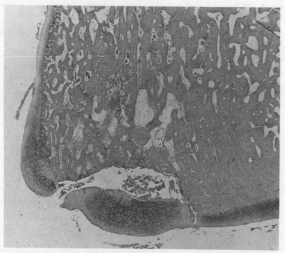

Figure 1. Histologic section of the medial humeral condyle in the elbow joint of a 10-month-old German shepherd. There is a defect in the subchondral bone, partly covered by a thickened joint cartilage. Necrotic debris can be seen between the floor of the defect and the cartilage flap. The trabeculae of the subchondral bone are thickened and there is marrow fibrosis. The picture is typical of advanced osteochondritis dissecans. (hematoxylin-eosin, × 50.)

occur or the normal shape of the bone may be changed because the growth process is interrupted. It should be emphasized, however, that many lesions do not advance that far. Some lesions are seen only on radiographs and heal spontaneously, never causing any clinical problems.

Radiographic and pathologic investigations have demonstrated that osteochondrosis is truly generalized, since pathologic lesions are often found at several sites in the same animal. Osteochondritis dissecans, for example, is often bilateral and symmetric, and it frequently occurs in more than one pair of joints.

In certain breeds of pigs that are bred and fed to grow fast, osteochondrosis occurs with a frequency of more than 80 per cent, and osteochondritis dissecans may be found in almost all joints. If growth is slowed down by nutritional or genetic means, osteochondrosis does not occur in these animals. In the dog osteochondrosis also is obviously related to rapid growth. Retained cartilage of various growth plates and osteochondritis dissecans of different joints are found only in dogs of medium or large size. Male dogs, which usually grow faster than females, are affected twice as often as females.

OSTEOCHONDRITIS DISSECANS OF THE SHOULDER JOINT

For a long time, osteochondritis dissecans was known to exist in the dog only in the shoulder. It was first recognized in the 1950's, and a large number of papers have appeared on the subject. Osteochondritis dissecans of the shoulder joint may be seen in medium and large size dogs, predominantly in males. The first clinical signs are usually noticed between the ages of four and seven months. Lameness of one or both forelimbs that is insidious in onset and gets worse after exercise is the most prominent sign. Stiffness after rest is another important sign. Pain can usually be elicited by palpation, flexion, and extension of the shoulder. The clinical signs may vary in severity over periods of weeks or months.

DIAGNOSIS

Definitive diagnosis is made by means of radiographic examination. A mediolateral radiograph of the extended shoulder usually reveals a defect in the subchondral bone of the humeral head. In mild or early cases, only a flattening of the dorsocaudal contour of the humeral head is seen. It is imperative that radiographs be of good quality. Sedation or anesthesia is necessa-

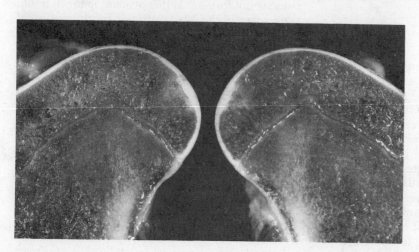

Figure 2. The cut surfaces of the humeral head of a 9-month-old German shepherd with osteochondrosis. In the caudal part of the humeral head the joint cartilage is thickened. Osteochondritis dissecans has not yet developed, as the surface of the cartilage is intact.

ry, as a rule. The dog is placed on the cassette with the side to be radiographed toward the table. The affected limb is pulled in a cranioventral direction, and the opposite limb is pulled caudally out of reach of the well-collimated x-ray beams.

In dogs with advanced lesions there is usually sclerosis of the subchondral bone and sometimes calcification of the cartilage flap that covers the defect. In many cases the defect is located on the caudolateral instead of the caudal side of the humeral head. Hence, a radiograph made in lateral projection does not visualize the lesion as a defect in the contour of the bone but rather as an area of decreased density in the caudal part of the head. It should be remembered that the lesion in most cases is bilateral, and for this reason both shoulders should always be radiographed, even if there is no history or sign of bilateral lameness.

THERAPY

It is usually easier to make the diagnosis of osteochondritis dissecans of the shoulder than to decide what kind of therapy to use, because many cases of osteochondritis dissecans of the shoulder heal spontaneously. The pedicle of the cartilage flap may rupture and the flap may become dislodged. Eventually this flap, now turned into a joint mouse, is resorbed by the joint fluid through enzyme activity. Sometimes the natural course is entirely different; the flap remains intact, and as long as it covers the floor of the defect, no outgrowth of scar tissue takes place. It is not unusual to find that the lesion in the humeral head on one side heals spontaneously, while the one in the humeral head of the other limb continues to cause problems.

Because the animal shows pain and lameness, restriction of exercise has been recommended as part of the treatment by many investigators. In contrast, the author is of the opinion that a dog with osteochondritis dissecans of the shoulder should be allowed to move around as much as possible, because in this way the chance is greater that the flap will be dislodged. If necessary, the dog can be given analgesics. If there is no obvious improvement after four to six weeks, surgery should be seriously contemplated. If one can prove the presence of a calcified flap or a piece of cartilage in the defect, surgery should be performed with no further delay. Even in cases in which the signs are not severe or may have subsided it is safe to repeat the radiographic examination. If the radiographs reveal that bone has not begun to fill the defect, an arthrogram should be made to demonstrate whether or not there is a flap or a loose piece of cartilage in the defect. If the arthrogram is positive, surgery is indicated; however, surgery is not necessary if there is no loose piece of flap in the defect, as in this case healing will take place spontaneously. If there is a joint mouse it is usually lodged in the ventrocaudal pouch of the joint, where in most cases it does not cause any clinical signs. Eventually it will be resorbed, but it can also remain viable and grow in size and cause some discomfort later. If a joint mouse is lodged in the sheath of the biceps tendon, it usually gives rise to pain and lameness and necessitates surgery.

Arthrography of the shoulder is easy to perform. The anesthetized dog is placed on the table with the side to be examined facing upward. A needle is inserted into the shoulder slightly caudally to the tip of the acromion. Depending on the dog's size, 4 to 6 ml of a 20 percent solution of methiodal sodium (Skiodan®, Winthrop) or a similar compound is injected. The dog is turned over on its other side, and the limb is moved passively for about one minute in order to distribute the contrast medium evenly in the joint. Two films are then taken at an interval of about two to three minutes. If it is seen on previous plain films that the defect is located in the caudolateral part of the humeral head, the limb should be held in five to ten degrees of supination during the second exposure to make the central beam hit the floor of the defect as tangentially as possible.

Surgery consists of removing the cartilage flap or piece of cartilage that is lying in the defect and trimming the edges of the defect. Postoperative care includes restricted exercise for about four weeks.

MANIFESTATIONS OF OSTEOCHONDROSIS IN THE ELBOW JOINT

In the very young dog it is sometimes not easy to differentiate between lameness caused by pain in the elbow and that caused by pain in the shoulder. It is therefore recommended that in doubtful cases both the elbow and the shoulder be radiographed. Radiographic examination is of great importance for early diagnosis of lesions in the elbow, provided that proper technique is used. Two projections are necessary, one mediolateral with the elbow fully flexed and one craniocaudal with about 30 to 40 degrees of flexion of the elbow. It is sometimes useful also to have a mediolateral view of the elbow in only a few degrees of flexion.

There are three lesions in the elbow, all of which are manifestations of osteochondrosis:

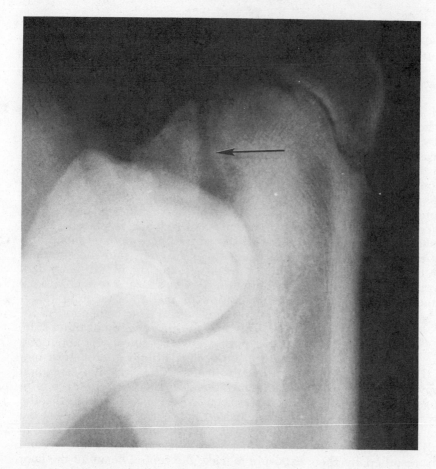

Figure 3. Lateral radiograph of the elbow joint of a 20-week-old giant schnauzer with an un-united anconeal process. The arrow indicates the irregular line (the cartilage) that separates the anconeal process from the olecranon. (For early diagnosis of the lesion it is imperative that the elbow joint be maximally flexed, as in this picture.)

osteochondritis dissecans of the medial condyle of the humerus, fragmentation of the coronoid process (un-united coronoid process), and un-united anconeal process. They are all very important because they lead to severe osteoarthrosis and lameness.

The three lesions have a similar clinical appearance, at least in the early stages. The owner of a dog with any of these elbow lesions usually complains that the animal has a stiff gait during the first few minutes after a period of rest. This sign is usually seen when the dog is about four to five months old. Forelimb lameness is rarely noticed until the dog gets a little older, and the lesions are often bilateral. For this reason the dog becomes lame on both forelimbs, and this is difficult for the owner to observe. The bilateral lameness is usually seen as a slightly stiff, stilted gait of the forelimbs, which are usually held slightly laterally rotated, with elbows close to the chest. Careful clinical examination reveals some pain in the elbows on extension and sometimes on flexion.

Radiographic examination of the elbows at the age of about five months is essential for the diagnosis of one of the three lesions, in fact, one that seems to be the least common — the un-united anconeal process. The other two lesions do not give rise to radiographic signs at this age.

UN-UNITED ANCONEAL PROCESS
(ELBOW DYSPLASIA)

The un-united anconeal process has long been recognized and was recently considered to be the most common cause of osteoarthrosis of the elbow. It is found in many breeds of large dogs but seems to be a problem mainly in the German shepherd. The condition may be a genetic trait, because the lesion is frequently found in littermates. It is therefore not advisable to use a dog with un-united anconeal process for breeding.

In the German shepherd, the anconeal process ossifies at about the age of 10 to 13 weeks and unites with the rest of the ulna about two to four weeks later. In a normal dog the anconeal process should be united with the ulna by age 18 to 20 weeks, at the latest. If not united at that time, there is little question that the anconeal process will remain un-united (Fig. 3). In such a case degeneration, necrosis, and fissures can be seen histologically in the cartilage that separates the ossification center of the anconeal process from the olecranon. In the adult dog the end result is a highly pathologic anconeal process consisting of a large piece of bone that is connected to the ulna only by a bridge of fibrous cartilage or connective tissue.

THERAPY

Treatment of a dog with un-united anconeal process is surgical. The most common procedure is to remove the un-united process via a lateral incision between the lateral epicondyle and the olecranon. It has also been suggested that osteosynthesis be done; i.e., the anconeal process is screwed to the ulna in order to avoid instability, which is said to occur when the anconeal process is loose or removed. More research seems to be needed in order to evaluate the result of this kind of treatment. There is a time factor to consider when one decides to perform surgery. Indications that surgery should not be done until the dog has reached an age of 9 to 12 months exist. If it is performed earlier, during the period of very fast growth (four to eight months), secondary changes (remodeling and osteoarthrosis) seem to develop more easily after surgery than if the un-united anconeal process is left in place until a time when growth is almost completed.

FRAGMENTATION OF THE CORONOID PROCESS OF THE ULNA (UN-UNITED CORONOID PROCESS) AND OSTEOCHONDRITIS DISSECANS OF THE MEDIAL CONDYLE OF THE HUMERUS

These two lesions were recently described as causes of osteoarthrosis of the elbow and were found to be more common than the un-united anconeal process, at least in certain breeds. The author has found the condition to be a particular problem in golden, Labrador, and flat-coated retrievers, but the two lesions may occur, separately or together, in most breeds of large dogs.

DIAGNOSIS

Although the clinical signs of the two lesions are very similar to those of the un-united anconeal process in the early stages, the radiographic picture is entirely different. As a rule, nothing abnormal can be seen on radiographs before the dog is about seven months of age, although clinical signs may have been present since the age of four to five months. It is therefore imperative to advise the owner of a young dog with slight clinical signs of the elbow to return the dog for a repeat radiographic examination four to eight weeks after the first examination. Too many cases have hitherto been missed by veterinarians who have fallen back on the erroneous and diffuse diagnosis of "growing pain." There is no justification for making this diagnosis or, even worse, for injecting corticosteroids intra-articularly, even if the clinical signs are vague and the radiographic picture is normal in a young dog.

The fragments of the coronoid process usually cannot be visualized on radiographs. The first radiographic signs in fragmentation of the coronoid process are small osteophytes on the dorsal aspect of the anconeal process (Fig. 4) and on the medial aspect of the coronoid process. The osteophytes on the anconeal process can be seen only if the radiograph is made with the elbow in full flexion. If there is a lesion on one side only, the diagnosis is usually compara-

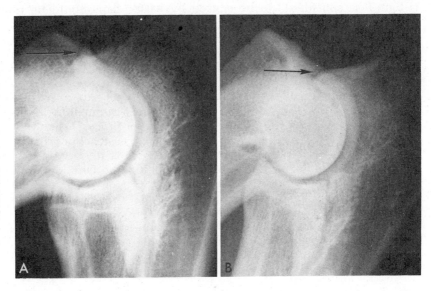

Figure 4. Lateral radiograph of both elbows of an 11-month-old mongrel. It was euthanatized because of severe right forelimb lameness caused by pain in the elbow joint. *A.* The right elbow. There are osteophytes on the proximal part of the anconeal process *(arrow)* as a sign of osteoarthrosis. *B.* The left elbow. The proximal part of the anconeal process is smooth *(arrow)*. At necropsy it was demonstrated that the cause of osteoarthrosis of the right elbow joint was fragmentation of the coronoid process.

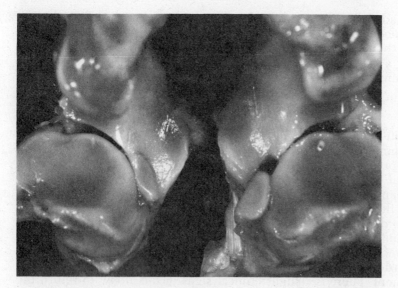

Figure 5. Specimens from the elbow joint of a 10-month-old Labrador retriever. The figure shows the joint surfaces of the radius and ulna. On each side there is an ossicle between the coronoid process of the ulna and the head of the radius. On the left limb (to the right of the picture), the ossicle is large and has "popped out." It is attached to the coronoid process by a fibrous band and to the anular ligament of the radial head. In the right elbow joint the ossicle is more firmly attached to the coronoid process. The ossicle in the left elbow joint had caused severe erosion on the corresponding joint surface of the medial condyle of the humerus.

tively easy to make, since the difference between the normal and diseased side will be obvious, provided that one knows what to look for (Fig. 4). The differential diagnosis between a case of fragmentation of the coronoid process and a case of osteochondritis dissecans of the medial condyle of the humerus is more difficult. In typical cases of the latter lesion a small triangular defect can be seen in the weight-bearing surface of the medial condyle. This defect is often surrounded by a sclerotic zone.

It is obvious that the two lesions have gone unrecognized until recently, mainly because the early radiographic changes have been overlooked. Once the dog is older than one year of age, the radiographic signs are usually obvious, and the diagnosis of osteoarthrosis is made. This often means a negative attitude by the veterinarian toward a search for rational treatment, since osteoarthrosis (if no obvious cause is found) is considered to be caused by wear and tear. It should be mentioned that there are cases in which the radiographic findings are minimal, even at an age of two to three years. These dogs may have slight recurrent lameness, the cause of which can be traced to the elbow. These dogs are excellent candidates for successful surgery.

SURGICAL TREATMENT

In most cases of fragmentation of the coronoid process and osteochondritis dissecans of the medial condyle of the humerus, surgery preferably should be done at the age of 8 to 11 months. Only the medial approach to the elbow can be used. A slightly bowed incision in the skin and underlying fascia is made from over the distal part of the humeral shaft, over the protuberance of the medial condyle, and down over the forearm. The pronator teres muscle and the flexor carpi radialis muscle are then dissected and cut as close as possible to their origins at the medial condyle of the humerus. This gives free access to the joint capsule and allows the median nerve to be seen and the position of the underlying artery and vein to be known. The joint capsule and the medial collateral ligament can thereafter be incised along the joint space without risk of damaging any of these structures. The incision must be long enough to allow some luxation of the joint, which makes possible the inspection of the joint surface of the medial condyle of the humerus and of the coronoid process of the ulna.

In early cases of osteochondritis dissecans of the medial condyle of the humerus, there is a defect in the weight-bearing surface that is covered by a flap of cartilage (see Fig. 1). The flap should be removed and the edges of the defect trimmed. In later cases there usually is no flap. Instead, it may have been turned into a large cartilaginous body that may be found adhering to the joint capsule. It may even have been resorbed. In a joint with only a defect and no flap, only the edges of the defect should be trimmed. Whatever the findings, the coronoid process should be inspected carefully, since osteochondritis dissecans of the medial condyle is frequently combined with fragmentation of the coronoid process. The most common finding in fragmentation of the coronoid process is an elongated ossicle, covered with cartilage, that lies between the coronoid process and the head of the radius (Fig. 5). The fragment contains bone apparently because it is vascularized from the anular ligament of the radial head, allowing for endochondral ossification. Sometimes the coronoid process is fragmented in several small pieces. On the opposing joint surface there is always considerable erosion caused by the loose fragments. All fragments should be removed. The operation is completed by closure of the joint capsule, muscles and skin. The dog is caged for about ten days and allowed only restricted exercise for four to six weeks.

If the only finding at early operation is fragmentation of the coronoid process and if the fragments can be completely removed, prognosis is good. If the procedure is done late and severe osteoarthrosis has developed, prognosis is guarded. The joint will usually become pain-free, but range of motion will remain limited. In cases of osteochondritis dissecans of the humeral condyle or those in which the two lesions are combined, prognosis is always guarded, even if the operation is performed early. However, surgical treatment should always be tried, since an untreated case of either of the two lesions or a case with the two lesions combined usually develops into very severe osteoarthrosis. It should be remembered, however, that in many dogs with fragmentation of the coronoid process the lesion can remain undetected for years. This usually happens in dogs with bilateral lesions and in those whose owners are not very observant. These dogs are often not brought to a veterinarian until there is acute unilateral lameness due to trauma of one of the severely osteoarthrotic elbows.

OSTEOCHONDRITIS DISSECANS OF THE KNEE (STIFLE)

Osteochondritis dissecans of the knee is a much more common lesion in large dogs than was previously assumed. Diagnosis is often difficult, since the clinical signs in most cases are diffuse in the young dog. The hips rather than the stifles are apt to be suspected as the cause of the lameness. There is no obvious lameness but rather a disturbed gait pattern of the hind limbs somewhat similar to the "slinky gait" of hip dysplasia. Radiographs are essential for early diagnosis, but only technically good radiographs made in the right projections will reveal a flattening or defect of the lateral or medial condyle, particularly if the lesion is small. Two craniocaudal views with the stifle in different angulations and one mediolateral view are usually necessary for correct diagnosis.

The most common site of a defect is the lateral femoral condyle, particularly its weight-bearing surface. The lesion can easily be missed if the central beam from the x-ray tube does not hit the lesion tangentially.

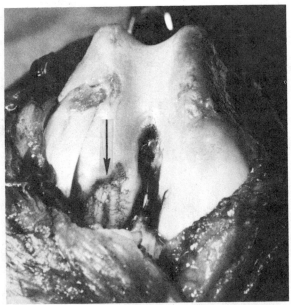

Figure 6. Picture of the stifle taken during surgery on a 4-year-old German shepherd. The clinical signs included severe lameness because of pain in the stifle. The radiographic appearance was that of severe osteoarthrosis. Explorative arthrotomy revealed a large, poorly healed osteochondritis dissecans defect (*arrow*) and large osteophytes. The menisci and the cruciate ligaments were intact.

Many cases of osteochondritis dissecans of the stifle remain undetected and heal by themselves, sometimes leaving only a scar in the condyle. In other cases severe osteoarthrosis develops (Fig. 6). Roughly 10 to 15 per cent of all cases of osteoarthrosis in the stifle seen in the larger breeds are caused by osteochondritis dissecans. Once osteoarthrosis has developed, there seems to be little one can do to improve the situation other than provide the conventional medical and physical therapy. If it is a young dog with acute lameness and a large lesion in either the lateral or medial condyle, an exploratory arthrotomy should be contemplated, and a flap or joint mouse should be removed.

More research must be done before any definite conclusions can be drawn about why some cases of osteochondritis dissecans of the stifle heal without secondary changes, whereas others give rise to very severe osteoarthrosis. There seems to be no straightforward indication for surgery at the present time other than in cases of acute lameness in which a large flap or a joint mouse can be seen.

OSTEOCHONDRITIS DISSECANS OF THE HOCK

Osteochondritis dissecans of the hock is not as common as in the shoulder, elbow, or stifle but is common enough to warrant special atten-

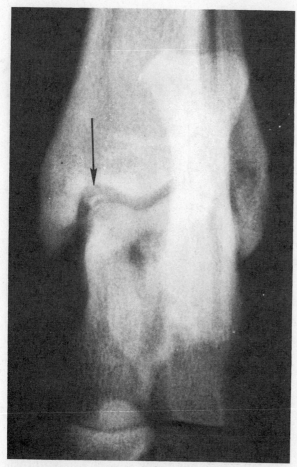

Figure 7. Dorsoplantar radiograph of the left hock joint of a 13-month-old Rottweiler. The dog was limping on the limb and there was swelling of the hock and pain on flexion and extension. The range of flexion was markedly decreased. The radiograph demonstrates an increased joint space between the tibia and the medial ridge of the talus, as well as a calcified joint mouse (*arrow*).

Sometimes a fragment can be seen because it is calcified or ossified (see Fig. 7). In old cases, the fragments can be very large. Sometimes a lateral radiograph with the hock in as much flexion as possible is useful.

A rather high percentage of fragments removed from hocks contain bone, because vessels from the collateral ligament enter the fragment and make it possible for the cartilage to undergo endochondral ossification. The finding of bone in the fragment in osteochondritis dissecans of the hock is in contrast to what is seen in osteochondritis dissecans in other joints of the dog. Here, ossicles are very rare.

Surgery is the treatment of choice in osteochondritis dissecans of the hock. The joint can be reached by a longitudinal incision caudal to the medial malleolus. With the limb in flexion, the fragments can easily be removed. Prognosis is good if surgery is performed early.

OTHER MANIFESTATIONS OF OSTEOCHONDROSIS

In most cases of osteochondrosis, retained cartilage of various growth plates is seen. Clinical signs are not caused by these changes, and they usually heal spontaneously. Only advanced lesions in the growth plates of the distal ulna, the distal femur, or the proximal tibia seem to cause disturbance of growth and subsequent deformation. In cases of ulnar involvement, decrease in growth rate of the ulna leads to asymmetry of the forelimb. The distal part of the radius is bowed around the distal metaphysis and epiphysis of the slower-growing ulna. This leads to lateral deviation of the distal part of the forelimb. When the distal femur and proximal tibia are involved, it usually leads to *genu valgum*. Once there is deformation, surgical correction must be performed, but it is safe to wait until growth is completed. If a dog is seen at an early stage of osteochondrosis with only slight deformation, it should be put on a restricted but well-balanced diet, and exercise should also be restricted.

Slipped femoral capital epiphysis is a common lesion in osteochondrosis of pigs, and there is good reason to suspect that osteochondrosis may be involved in the etiology of slipped epiphysis in dogs also.

PREVENTION OF OSTEOCHONDROSIS

It is obvious that we must know more about the etiology and pathogenesis of osteochondro-

tion in cases of slight lameness in the hind limbs of young dogs. The lesion seems to be particularly common in Labrador and golden retrievers, but it does occur in other breeds. Clinical signs usually begin at four to five months of age and are usually very vague. The lesion is more often unilateral than is osteochondritis dissecans in other joints. The most typical findings are a slightly shorter step than normal for the affected limb and pain on extension and flexion of the hock. Rather early, the range of flexion is decreased considerably. It should be emphasized that this is an almost pathognomonic sign in young dogs. In some dogs there is obvious joint effusion. As in osteochondritis dissecans of other joints, the radiographic examination provides the diagnosis (Fig. 7). The lesion is located at the medial ridge of the talus, and it is best demonstrated as a defect in the ridge on a dorsoplantar film.

sis before we can effectively prevent the condition. However, there are enough indications of a genetic disposition that we should recommend that breeders not use dogs with osteochondrosis or those that have had several cases of osteochondrosis in their offspring.

Owners of dogs belonging to breeds known to develop osteochondrosis should be given the following advice: Don't overfeed your puppy! The "fat, happy puppy" that is growing at maximal genetic capacity because of *ad lib.* feeding runs a considerable risk of developing osteochondrosis.

SUPPLEMENTAL READING

Olssen, S.-E. (ed.): Osteochondrosis in domestic animals. I. Pathogenesis and pathology in pigs, horses, bulls, turkeys, and broilers, with comparative aspects on osteochondritis dissecans in man. Acta Radiol., Suppl. 358, 1978.

INTRACRANIAL INJURY

J. E. OLIVER, JR. D.V.M.
Athens, Georgia

Trauma cases accounted for 12.8 percent of admissions at one metropolitan teaching hospital (Kolata, et al., 1974), the distribution between dogs and cats being about the same as that for the total hospital population. Motor vehicle accidents accounted for over half the injuries in dogs but for only 16.3 percent in cats, and head injuries from these accidents occurred in about 25 per cent of dogs and in almost 40 percent of cats. In a survey of 600 dogs involved in motor vehicle accidents, 30 had skull injuries and 12 had brain injuries (Kolata and Johnston, 1975). Seventy-five dogs died or were euthanatized as a result of their injuries. None of the dogs with brain injuries died, but two were euthanatized. Similar data on human motor vehicle accidents indicate that 50,000 deaths occur each year in the United States and that more than two-thirds of these include head injuries (Javid).

These data suggest that the dog is relatively resistant to intracranial injury as compared with man. Considering the heavy temporal muscle and relatively thick skull of most dogs, this is probably true. However, many injured dogs die and are not accounted for in hospital statistics.

Management of acute intracranial injury must be instituted at the earliest possible moment if brain function is to be preserved. In man, 60 percent of deaths from brain injury occur in the first 24 hours (Javid). Animals with acute intracranial injury frequently are in shock and have incurred injuries to other body systems. Emergency treatment, as outlined later in this article, may be necessary to preserve life before a complete evaluation can be made.

DIAGNOSIS

A rapid but thorough physical examination should be made. Open chest wounds or gross hemorrhage may require immediate attention. A general assessment of the patient's injuries provides a more accurate prognosis and estimates of the therapy required and the probable duration and cost of hospitalization. A neurologic evaluation is then made to determine the location and extent of brain injury.

NEUROLOGIC EXAMINATION

Clinical evaluation of the levels of consciousness, motor function, and neuro-ophthalmologic signs (pupils, eye movements) provides sufficient information to localize the level of the brain injury and to make a reasonably accurate prognosis (Oliver, 1972, Ommaya and Gennarelli; Overgaard, et al.).

Consciousness is maintained by pathways from the rostral reticular formation in the brain stem (reticular activating system) to the cerebral cortex. Decreasing levels of consciousness indicate increasing disconnection of this system. Loss of consciousness indicates complete disconnection.

Consciousness may be graded as awake and alert, lethargic, stuporous, or comatose. The patient that is lethargic will tend to sleep when undisturbed but is easily aroused with mild stimulation. The stuporous patient can only be aroused with strong, usually painful, stimulation. Strong, painful stimulation does not arouse the patient in coma, although some motor activity can be elicited.

Table 1. *Signs Characteristic of Focal Brain Stem Hemorrhage at One Level*[*]

LEVEL	CONSCIOUSNESS	PUPILS	EYE MOVEMENT	MOTOR FUNCTION	AUTONOMIC RESPONSES
Diencephalic	Apathy to stupor	Small but reactive	Normal	Hemiparesis to tetraparesis	Normal to Cheyne-Stokes respiration
Midbrain	Stupor to coma	Bilateral dilated or midposition, unresponsive	Ventrolateral strabismus, bilateral	Decerebrate rigidity	Hyperventilation (variable)
Pons	Coma	Midposition, unresponsive	Oculocephalic reflexes absent	Decerebrate rigidity to flaccid paralysis	Rapid shallow respiration, loss of micturition reflex
Medulla	Coma	Midposition, dilated terminally	Absent	Flaccid paralysis	Irregular to apnea

[*]Assuming a large intramedullary hemorrhage confined primarily to one level. The most frequent is in the caudal midbrain and pons following acute head injury. Asymmetric or smaller lesions will produce less severe signs.

Motor function includes voluntary and involuntary (reflex) activity. An awake animal will usually have intact voluntary motor activity, although some degree of paresis may be present. Severe paresis or paralysis in an awake, alert animal is likely to indicate spinal cord damage. A lethargic animal may have some paresis but usually will still have voluntary motor function. A stuporous animal will often exhibit a hemiparesis or tetraparesis. Some voluntary activity is usually preserved. Myotatic reflexes may be exaggerated. Voluntary motor activity is lost in coma. Coma may be further graded as (1) normal spinal reflex responses; (2) decerebrate rigidity, including extension of all four limbs, "clasp-knife response" and possibly opisthotonos; or (3) hypotonia of the muscles and depression of spinal reflexes.

Pupillary light reflexes and oculocephalic responses are also useful indications of the extent of intracranial injury. Constricted pupils are usually seen with lesions in the diencephalon (hypothalamus). Lesions of the oculomotor nucleus (midbrain) or nerves produce pupillary dilation that is unresponsive to light. Brainstem lesions encompassing the oculomotor nuclei and descending sympathetic pathways will result in a pupil in midposition that is unresponsive to light.

A summary of the clinical findings with lesions at various levels of the brain stem is presented in Table 1. It is important to realize that the level of the lesion indicated by clinical signs is the lowest level of significant injury. Areas rostral to that level may have suffered serious damage also (Ommaya and Gennarelli).

The time course of the clinical signs and the presence of lateralizing signs are also of importance in establishing a diagnosis and prognosis. Brain-stem hemorrhage, the most frequently encountered lesion in severe head injury, is characterized by loss of consciousness immediately after injury. Herniation of the cerebrum under the tentorium cerebelli, compressing the brain stem, occurs more slowly and may be accompanied by unilateral or bilateral clinical signs (see Tables 2 and 3 and Fig. 1).

PROGNOSIS

Clinical evaluation of levels of consciousness, neuroophthalmologic signs, and motor signs provides an accurate prognosis (Oliver, 1972; Ommaya and Gennarelli; Overgaard et al). Animals that are unconscious from the time of injury and remain unconscious for 48 hours rarely recover. Those that do recover usually have severe motor deficits.

Slowly progressive signs of loss of consciousness, decreasing voluntary motor activity, and pupillary dilation indicate increasing intracranial pressure from an expanding hematoma or from brain swelling. These cases can be saved if adequate treatment is instituted early (Table 4).

PATHOLOGY

Because the brain is encased in an inelastic compartment, virtually all the pathologic sequelae to head injury result in increased intracranial pressure. Depressed skull fractures, intracranial hemorrhage, and brain swelling all increase the volume of material within the calvaria. Brain tissue is compressed or displaced, creating focal or generalized dysfunction. Increased pressure causes displacement of the cerebral hemispheres under the tentorium cerebelli caudally, causing compression of the brain stem. Further increases in pressure will produce herniation of the cerebellum through the

Table 2. *Signs Characteristic of Progressive Bilateral Tentorial Herniation**

LEVEL	CONSCIOUSNESS	PUPILS	EYE MOVEMENTS	MOTOR FUNCTION	AUTONOMIC RESPONSES
Early diencephalic	Apathy	Small but reactive	Normal	Hemiparesis	Normal to irregular respirations
Late diencephalic	Stupor	Small but reactive	Normal	Hemiparesis to tetraparesis	Cheyne-Stokes respiration
Midbrain	Coma	Bilateral dilation	Poor oculocephalic response	Decerebrate rigidity	Hyperventilation
Pons	Coma	Midposition, unresponsive	Oculocephalic response absent	Flaccid paralysis	Rapid shallow respirations
Medulla	Coma	Misposition, dilated terminally	Absent	Flaccid paralysis	Irregular to apnea, pulse slowing

*Modified from Plum and Posner: *The Diagnosis of Stupor and Coma*, 1966; and Oliver, J. E., Jr.: Vet. Clin. North Am., 2:341, 1972.

Table 3. *Signs Characteristic of Progressive Unilateral Tentorial Herniation**

LEVEL	CONSCIOUSNESS	PUPILS	EYE MOVEMENTS	MOTOR FUNCTION	AUTONOMIC RESPONSES
III N.	Normal to stupor	Ipsilateral dilation	Normal to slight lateral strabismus	Normal to hemiparesis	Normal
Early midbrain	Stupor	Ipsilateral to bilateral dilation	Ipsilateral ventrolateral strabismus	Hemiparesis ipsi- or contralateral	Normal
Late midbrain to pons	Coma	Dilated bilateral to fixed midposition	Ventrolateral strabismus to fixed midposition	Decerebrate rigidity	Hyperventilation
Pons	Coma	Midposition, unresponsive	Oculocephalic response absent	Flaccid paralysis	Rapid, shallow respirations
Medulla	Coma	Midposition, dilated terminally	Absent	Flaccid paralysis	Irregular to apnea, pulse slowing

*Modified from Plum and Posner: *The Diagnosis of Stupor and Coma*, 1966; and Oliver, J. E., Jr.: Vet. Clin. North Am., 2:341, 1972.

818   INTRACRANIAL INJURY—*Continued*

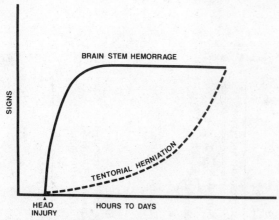

Figure 1. Sign-time graph of head injury. Tentorial herniation and brain stem hemorrhage may be differentiated by the clinical course. (From Oliver: Vet. Clin. North Am., 2:341, 1972.)

foramen magnum, compressing the medulla oblongata. Death from respiratory arrest rapidly ensues.

Brain swelling or cerebral edema is an increase in fluid, primarily extracellular in white matter and intracellular in gray matter. Edema may be a sequela to any insult to nervous tissue, including trauma, hypoxia, hypercarbia, cold, heat, toxins, and others. It is safe to assume that any significant head trauma will produce some degree of cerebral edema.

Hemorrhage may be extradural, subdural, subarachnoid, or intracerebral. Subarachnoid hemorrhage is probably the most frequent, with intracerebral hemorrhage the most severe.

Fractures may be linear or depressed, simple or comminuted, and closed or compound. Fractures may be significant if they are depressed into the brain, if they lacerate a blood vessel, or if they are compound with the possibility of introducing infection into the brain. Basilar fractures may lacerate the cavernous sinus; dorsal calvarial fractures may lacerate the dorsal sagittal sinus, and lateral calvarial fractures may lacerate the middle meningeal artery.

MANAGEMENT

Acute head injury requires treatment as early as possible and careful monitoring for changes in the condition of the animal. Stuporous or comatose animals should be monitored continuously if treatment is to be successful. Figure 2 provides a guide to management based on the clinical signs of the animal.

Unconscious animals may need attention before they reach the veterinary clinic. Owners can be instructed on the telephone to maintain a patent airway by extending the animal's head and neck and pulling the tongue forward. If possible, the animal should be carried on a piece of plywood or some similar rigid support to avoid displacement of the spinal column.

When the animal is presented for treatment, maintenance of a patent airway is still the most important consideration. An endotracheal catheter or tracheostomy tube should be used if any difficulties in respiration are encountered. Hypoxia and hypercarbia are primary causes of brain swelling.

Treatment of shock, gross hemorrhage, and penetrating chest wounds must be instituted to maintain life. (Details of management are described in other articles.)

Glucocorticoids are usually given for shock and probably are beneficial in the treatment of trauma-induced cerebral edema. The effectiveness of glucocorticoids in edema from brain tumors and from several experimental models of edema (cold, psyllium seed) is well established (Fishman), but efficacy in trauma-induced edema is less clear (Tornheim and McLaurin). Until more definitive evidence is presented I still recommend giving dexamethasone at a dose of 2 mg/kg body weight intravenously. Other glucocorticoids may be substituted, but the potential for harmful side effects at this dosage must be considered.

The efficacy of osmotic diuretics has also been questioned (Fishman) but the bulk of the evidence supports the use of mannitol or other

Table 4. *Comparison of Acute Brain-Stem Hemorrhage with Tentorial Herniation Following Head Injury**

	BRAIN-STEM HEMORRHAGE	TENTORIAL HERNIATION
Onset	Early	Delayed
Course	Static to progressive	Progressive
Pupils	Constricted early, dilated late	Unilateral dilation progressing to bilateral dilation
Consciousness	Stuporous to comatose	Alert or apathetic, progressing to coma
Muscle Tone	Decerebrate rigidity or flaccid paralysis	Normal or weak progressing to decerebrate rigidity to flaccid paralysis
Reflexes	Usually symmetrical	Often unilateral asymmetry

*From Oliver, J. E., Jr.: Vet. Clin. North Am., 2:341, 1972.

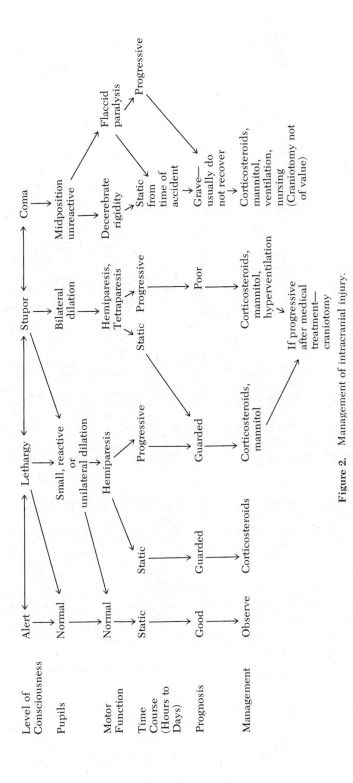

Figure 2. Management of intracranial injury.

osmotic diuretics (James, et al.). I recommend that a stuporous or comatose animal be given mannitol (20 percent solution) at a dose of 2 gm/kg IV, 2 doses six hours apart in a slow drip (approximately 30 drops per minute). A recent report indicates that much lower doses of mannitol (0.25 gm/kg) are almost as effective in the treatment of brain-injured human patients, although the response does not last as long as with higher doses (Marshall, et al.). If the lower dose can be proved effective in dogs, some of the complications of hyperosmolar therapy may be avoided.

Patients receiving osmotic diuretics should be monitored carefully for renal output. An indwelling urethral catheter should be used in comatose patients. Hydration should be monitored by checking the elasticity of the skin, packed cell volume, and total solids of the plasma (see article on fluid therapy). Dehydration is not necessary to reduce cerebral edema, but overhydration must also be avoided. Central venous pressure measurements may be useful for evaluation of fluid therapy. Mannitol may be dangerous in animals with severe blood loss (Parker).

Several experimental studies have suggested that dimethyl sulfoxide (DMSO) is effective in treating cerebral edema. Adequate data are not available to make a final judgment, so use of DMSO should be considered experimental at this time.

Coma starting at the time of injury and persisting for 48 hours in spite of medical treatment is evidence of brain-stem hemorrhage (Tables 1 and 4). Prognosis for recovery is grave, and treatment is limited to nursing care. The animal should be turned frequently to prevent hypostatic congestion; the bladder should be emptied at least three times daily; body temperature should be maintained in the normal range, and fluid balance should be maintained.

Progressive deterioration indicates an expanding mass or uncontrolled cerebral edema. Hematomas will usually produce signs of unilateral compression (see Table 3). Progressive signs constitute an emergency and indicate the need for craniotomy. Bur holes may be placed and the hematoma evacuated or a lateral craniotomy performed for complete decompression (Oliver, 1966, 1968, 1975).

Surgery is warranted in the first 24 to 48 hours in the absence of progressive signs if there is a skull fracture depressed more than the thickness of the calvaria, if the fracture is compound, or if there are bone fragments in the brain.

Postoperative and medical treatment includes good nursing care, as previously described. Antibiotics are usually indicated, especially if shock or open wounds are present.

Post-traumatic epilepsy is a possible sequela to head injury. Prophylactic anticonvulsants have been recommended, but their efficacy is not clearly established. Phenobarbital (2 mg/kg/day) is given to all animals with open head injury or following craniotomy.

SUPPLEMENTAL READING

deLahunta, A: *Veterinary Neuroanatomy and Clinical Neurology.* Philadelphia, W. B. Saunders Co., 1977.

de la Torre, J.C., Kawanaga, H.M., Rowed, D.W., Johnson, C.M., Goode, O.J., Kajihara, K., and Mullan, S.: Dimethyl sulfoxide in central nervous system trauma. Ann. N.Y. Acad. Sci., 243:362, 1975.

Fishman, R.A.: Brain edema. N. Engl. J. Med., 293:706, 1975.

Hoerlein, B.F.: *Canine Neurology,* 3rd ed. Philadelphia, W.B. Saunders Co., 1978.

James, H.E., Langfitt, T.W., and Kumar, V.S.: Analysis of the response to therapeutic measures to reduce intracranial pressure in head-injured patients. J. Trauma, 16:437, 1976.

Javid, M.: Current concepts — Head injuries. N. Engl. J. Med., 291:890, 1974.

Kolata, R.J., and Johnston, O.E.: Motor vehicle accidents in urban dogs: A study of 600 cases. J. Am. Vet. Med. Assoc., 167:938, 1975.

Kolata, R.J., Krant, N.H., and Johnston, O.E.: Patterns of trauma in urban dogs and cats: A study of 1000 cases. J. Am. Vet. Med. Assoc., 164:499, 1974.

Marshall, L.F., Smith, R.W., Rauscher, L.A., and Shapiro, H.M.: Mannitol dose requirements in brain-injured patients. J. Neurosurg., 48:169, 1978.

Oliver, J.E., Jr.: Principles of canine brain surgery. Animal Hosp., 2:73, 1966.

Oliver, J.E., Jr.: Surgical approaches to the canine brain. Am. J. Vet. Res., 29:353, 1968.

Oliver, J.E., Jr.: Management of the patient with acute head injury. Proc. Gaines Veterinary Symposium, Purdue University, Lafayette, Indiana, 1969.

Oliver, J.E., Jr.: Neurologic emergencies in small animals. Vet. Clin. North Am., 2:341, 1972.

Oliver, J.E., Jr.: Craniotomy, craniectomy and skull fractures. *In* Bojrab, M.E. (ed.): *Current Techniques in Small Animal Surgery.* Philadelphia, Lea & Febiger, 1975.

Ommaya, A.K., and Gennarelli, T.A.: Cerebral concussion and traumatic unconsciousness. Brain, 97:633, 1974.

Overgaard, J., Christensen, S., Hvid-Hansen, O., Haase, J., Land, A., Hein, O., Pedersen, K., and Tweed, W.A.: Prognosis after head injury based on early clinical examination. Lancet, 2:631, 1973.

Parker, A.J.: Blood pressure changes and lethality of mannitol infusions in dogs. Am. J. Vet. Res., 34:1523, 1973.

Plum, E., and Posner, J.B.: *The Diagnosis of Stupor and Coma.* Philadelphia, F.A. Davis Co., 1966.

Sabin, T.O.: The differential diagnosis of coma. N. Engl. J. Med. 290:1062, 1974.

Tornheim, P.A., and McLaurin, R.L.: Effect of dexamethasone on cerebral edema from cranial impact in the cat. J. Neurosurg., 48:220, 1978.

STORAGE DISEASES

BRIAN R.H. FARROW, B.V.Sc.
Sydney, Australia

The storage diseases are a relatively rare group of diseases that result from deficiency of specific intracellular enzymes contained within membrane-bound structures in the cell known as lysosomes. These enzymes are responsible for the normal degradation of proteins, polysaccharides, and nucleic acids. When a particular enzyme deficiency exists, that enzyme's substrate accumulates within cells, and this ultimately interferes with function. The tissue distribution of the undegradable substrate determines the organs most affected and the clinical signs.

Certain characteristic features of the storage diseases, summarized here, are adapted from Blakemore (1975).

1. Animals are normal at birth.

2. Affected animals may fail to grow as rapidly as their littermates.

3. There is usually a recessive mode of inheritance, with only certain members of a litter likely to be affected.

4. There often is a history of inbreeding, clinical signs being expressed in the homozygous recessive individual.

5. Specific deficiencies of single enzymes are known to occur in certain breeds.

6. Young animals are presented with signs of multifocal neurologic disease that is progressive in nature and ultimately fatal.

7. Systems other than the nervous system may be involved.

In people, more than 20 of these inborn errors of metabolism are known to occur, and in domestic animals a smaller but increasing number have been described. The diseases are named after the main substance stored, the enzyme that is deficient, or the person who first described the syndrome. Examples of storage diseases in dogs and cats are shown in Table 1. Most of the inherited lysosomal storage diseases are accompanied by severe neurologic disease. In the case of the glycogen storage diseases, although there are neuronal lesions and neurologic disturbances, the main clinical sign is weakness.

Diagnosis in suspected cases can be confirmed by enzymatic analysis of peripheral blood leukocytes or tissues such as skin, which can be biopsied, cell-cultured, and subsequently analyzed. Laboratories with facilities for lysosomal enzyme assay should be consulted regarding particular specimen requirements. Diagnosis can also be confirmed by histologic

Table 1. *Examples of Storage Diseases in the Dog and Cat*

DISEASE	BREEDS AFFECTED	SELECTED REFERENCE
Glycogenoses		
α-Glucosidase deficiency (Pompe's disease)	Dog	Mostafa, 1970
α-Glucosidase deficiency	Cat (DSH)*	Sandstrom et al., 1969
Sphingolipidoses		
β-Galactocerebrosidase deficiency (Krabbe's disease)	Dog (Cairn terrier, WHW,† beagle, miniature poodle) Cat (DSH)	Fletcher et al., 1971
β-Glucocerebrosidase deficiency (Gaucher's disease)	Dog (Australian silkie terrier)	Hartley and Blakemore, 1973
Hexosaminidase deficiency (GM$_2$ gangliosidosis; Tay-Sachs disease)	Dog (German short-haired pointer) Cat (DSH)	Karbe, 1973
β-Galactosidase deficiency (GM$_1$ gangliosidosis, type I)	Cat (DSH)	Blakemore, 1972
Partial β-galactosidase deficiency	Cat (Siamese)	Baker et al., 1971
Sphingomyelinase deficiency (Niemann-Pick disease)	Cat (DSH, Siamese)	Chrisp et al., 1970 Percy and Jortner, 1971

*Domestic short-haired cat.
†West Highland white terrier.

examination of appropriate biopsy or necropsy material in which the stored substrate may cause characteristic ultrastructural changes. Biochemical identification of the stored material enables specific diagnosis.

INHERITANCE

Most of the diseases due to deficiency of a lysosomal enzyme are inherited as autosomal recessive traits. Heterozygotes, having one normal and one defective gene, are clinically normal, although their specific lysosomal enzyme level is intermediate between homozygous recessive and homozygous normal individuals. It is therefore possible, using lysosomal enzyme assays, to detect the heterozygote carrier animals and manage breeding programs accordingly. Peripheral blood leukocyte enzyme assay of puppies may also be used to detect homozygous recessive individuals that will subsequently develop the disease.

TREATMENT

Treatment for the lysosomal storage diseases is not available at present. In veterinary medicine attention should be directed toward detection and elimination from the breeding population of carrier animals. Current emphasis in research on storage diseases is directed toward enzyme replacement therapy. The rationale for this is based on the assumption that exogenously administered enzyme can enter lysosomes through a process of endocytosis and function in the degradation of accumulated substrate. Although this approach is promising, problems with enzyme uptake and inactivation have prevented successful application of it. The use of lipid vesicles (liposomes) to protect and stabilize replacement enzymes and enhance uptake and subcellular distribution holds some promise for the treatment of people with these disorders. The naturally occurring storage diseases of animals provide valuable models in which new approaches to therapy may be studied.

SUPPLEMENTAL READING

Baker, H.J., Lindsey, J.R., McKhann, G.M., and Farrel, D.F.: Neuronal GM₁ gangliosidosis in a Siamese cat with beta-galactosidase deficiency. Science, 174:838, 1971.

Blakemore, W.F.: Lysosomal storage diseases. In Grunsell, C.S.G., and Hill, F.W.G. (eds.) Veterinary Annual, 15th issue. Bristol, England, Wright-Scientechnica, 1974, p. 242.

Blakemore, W.F.: GM₁ gangliosidosis in the cat. J. Comp. Pathol., 82:179, 1972.

Chrisp, C.E., Ringler, D.H., Abrahams, G.D., Radins, N.S., and Brenkert, A.: Lipid storage disease in a Siamese cat. J. Am. Vet. Med. Assoc., 156:616, 1970.

Fletcher, T.F., Lee, D.G., and Hammer, R.F.: Ultrastructural features of globoid-cell leukodystrophy in the dog. Am. J. Vet. Res., 32:177, 1971.

Hartley, W.J., and Blakenmore, W.F.: Neurovisceral glucocerebroside storage (Gaucher's disease) in a dog. Vet. Pathol., 10:191, 1973.

Jolly, R.D., and Hartley, W.J.: Storage diseases of domestic animals. Aust. Vet. J., 53:1, 1977.

Karbe, E.: Animal model of human disease: GM₂-gangliosidoses (amaurotic idiocies) types I, II, and III. Animal model: canine GM₂ gangliosidosis. Am. J. Pathol., 71:151, 1973.

Kolodny, E.H.: Lysosomal storage diseases. N. Engl. J. Med., 294:1217, 1976.

Mostafa, I.R.: A case of glycogenic cardiomegaly in the dog. Acta Vet. Scand., 11:197, 1970.

Percy, D.H., and Jortner, B.S.: Feline lipidosis. Arch. Pathol., 92:136, 1971.

Reynolds, G.D., Baker, H.J., and Reynolds, R.H.: Enzyme replacement using liposome carriers in feline GM₁ gangliosidosis fibroblasts. Nature, 275:754, 1978.

Sandstrom, B., Westman, J., and Ockerman, P.A.: Glycogenesis of the central nervous system in the cat. Acta Neuropathol. (Berl.), 14:194, 1969.

CANINE HEPATIC ENCEPHALOPATHY

RALPH E. BARRETT, D.V.M.
Carmichael, California

INTRODUCTION

Hepatic encephalopathy (HE) is a clinical syndrome that consists of diverse neurologic abnormalities and characteristic but non-diagnostic laboratory findings that develop in the presence of hepatic disease. This condition is being diagnosed with increased frequency in dogs as veterinarians become more aware of the variable clinical syndromes of HE.

Neurologic signs of HE (see Table 3) have been seen in dogs with three types of liver

Table 1. *Differential Diagnosis of Hepatic Encephalopathy in the Dog*

I. Hepatic diseases
    A. Congenital portal vein anomalies
    B. Acquired portal vein anomalies
    C. Urea cycle enzyme deficiencies
    D. Advanced liver failure
        1. Cirrhosis
        2. Neoplastic infiltration
        3. Toxicosis
II. Non-hepatic diseases
    A. Metabolic
        1. Hypoglycemia
        2. Uremia
        3. Barbiturate toxicity
        4. Lead toxicity
        5. Other toxicities
    B. Central nervous system diseases
        1. Neoplasia
        2. Trauma
        3. Abscess
        4. Encephalitis/meningitis
        5. Thrombosis
        6. Idiopathic epilepsy
        7. Hydrocephalus
        8. Degenerative congenital CNS diseases
        9. Systemic lupus erythematosus

diseases: (1) congenital portal vein anomalies, (2) urea cycle enzyme deficiencies, and (3) advanced liver disease (Table 1). Signs of HE are not seen in the common canine liver conditions of fatty infiltration, chronic or acute obstructive jaundice, and chronic passive congestion. Also, HE is extremely uncommon in infectious canine hepatitis.

PATHOGENESIS

There are two requirements for development of HE: (1) shunts around the liver that allow toxins that normally are removed or modified to reach the brain and (2) a degree of hepatic insufficiency. The liver is necessary for the maintenance of normal brain metabolism by producing compounds the brain cannot manufacture or by disposing of other compounds originating in the gut that are toxic to the brain. Ingested proteins and amino acids along with urea are broken down by bacteria in the colon to ammonia. This is absorbed and converted to urea in the liver. Gastrointestinal bleeding, shock, and hypoxia can overwhelm the marginally functioning liver and precipitate HE. In the brain ammonia is converted to glutamine. Whether ammonia has a neurotoxic effect is uncertain, since blood ammonia concentrations correlate poorly with the severity of HE. The exact pathogenesis of hepatic encephalopathy remains unknown, but present theories revolve around the three interrelated factors of increased cerebral sensitivity, metabolic derangements, and cerebral toxins. The last-named factor appears most important.

Increased cerebral sensitivity relates to the fact that the brains of patients with severe liver disease exhibit increased sensitivity to factors that depress the level of consciousness (e.g., sedatives, infection, electrolyte disturbances, hypoxia, and others). Patients without liver disease are more tolerant of these factors. This increased sensitivity suggests that the liver produces substances that are important to brain function.

Several *metabolic derangements* may precipitate hepatic encephalopathy in susceptible patients (Table 2). These factors summate with the effects of cerebral toxins and may precipitate an episode of HE. The most common cause of HE in advanced liver disease is excessive gut protein.

Cerebral toxins produced in the gut and not cleared by the diseased liver may be the most important aspect of the pathogenesis of HE. It is no longer valid to consider the simplistic view that hyperammonemia is the sole cause of HE. Many substances have been incriminated in the induction of HE. Ammonia, methionine (and methanethiol derived from methionine), phenylalanine, tyrosine, tryptophan (and indoles and skatoles from tryptophan), a decrease in the branched-chain amino acids (valine, leucine, and isoleucine), glutamine, alpha-ketoglutaramate, citrulline, short-chain fatty acids, serotonin and false neurotransmitters (octopamine, gamma-aminobenzoic acid, and beta-phenylethanolamines), and a decrease in the normal neurotransmitters have all been suspected.

Although the pathogenesis of HE is a complex phenomenon probably caused by a multiplicity of factors, most researchers believe that ammonia may still be a key cerebral toxin. This is based on the findings that (1) increased blood and cerebrospinal fluid (CSF) ammonia concentrations are usually found in patients with HE, (2) elevated glutamine levels (the end product of cerebral ammonia detoxication) are usually found in the CSF of patients with HE, (3) patients with congenital urea cycle enzyme deficiencies often have hyperammonemia, and (4) ammonia will precipitate HE in experimental animals. Evidence against the sole role of hyperammonemia as a cause of HE includes the observations that (1) some patients with HE have normal or only slightly elevated blood ammonia levels and (2) massive doses of ammonia are necessary to produce HE in experimental animals.

Table 2. *Conditions that May Precipitate Hepatic Encephalopathy*

CONDITION	MECHANISM(S)
Increased protein intake	Increased substrate for production of nitrogenous substances
Gastrointestinal hemorrhage	Increases protein substrate Hypovolemia compromises hepatic, cerebral and renal function Hepatic hypoxia
Alkalosis	Increases intracellular transport of ammonia and amines; shifts $NH_3 + H^+ \leftrightarrows NH_4^+$ to the left; NH_3 is more diffusible across cell membranes and is "trapped" intracellularly
Hypokalemia	Reduced conversion of NH_3 to glutamine by liver mitrochondria Causes extracellular fluid alkalosis Increased production of NH_3 by renal tubular cells
Uremia	Increased enterohepatic circulation of urea nitrogen with increased ammonia production Direct cerebral effect of uremia
Hypovolemia	Compromises hepatic, cerebral, and renal function Compromise of renal function increases enterohepatic urea nitrogen cycle and increases ammonia production
Infections	Increased tissue catabolism leads to increased endogeneous nitrogen load and increased ammonia production Dehydration and decreased renal function Hypoxia and hyperthermia potentiate ammonia toxicity
Constipation	Increased production and absorption of nitrogenous substances
Methionine	Metabolic products (e.g., methanethiol) are neurotoxic
Increased fatty acids in diet	Synergistic toxicity with methanethiol and ammonia
Stored blood for transfusion	Contributes ammonia
Commercial protein hydrolysates	Amino acid imbalances contribute to HE
Diuretics	Induce hypokalemic alkalosis Increase renal vein ammonia output Overvigorous→hypovolemia and prerenal azotemia
Tranquilizers and anesthetics°	Direct depressive effect on brain Hypoxia Prolonged metabolism in liver disease

°Chlordiazepoxide (Librium®, Roche), barbiturates, chlorpromazine, diazepam (Valium®, Roche), morphine, meperidine.

The basic cerebral mechanisms for ammonia toxicity are not known. Suggested causes include (1) interference with brain energy metabolism; (2) an accumulation of an inhibitory neurotransmitter, gamma-aminobutyric acid; (3) a decrease in the neurotransmitter acetylcholine; (4) a direct inhibitory effect on the neuronal membrane; and (5) toxicity of the intermediary metabolite alpha-ketoglutaramate.

PATHOLOGY

Since both acute HE and HE seen in chronic liver injury are potentially clinically reversible, it is assumed that HE is not associated with permanent morphologic abnormalities of the brain. Thus, HE is considered to be a metabolic abnormality in which there is some biochemical alteration of cerebral function.

In spite of the severe clinical signs, neurohistologic findings in HE are few. In acute HE no morphologic abnormalities in the brain are seen, although cerebral edema may be present in rare cases. In dogs with chronic congenital portosystemic shunting a spongy degeneration, called polymicrocavitation, and hyperplasia and nuclear enlargement of astrocytes, which are referred to as Alzheimer type II astrocytes, may be seen. Alzheimer type II astrocytosis may reflect an attempt of the glia to maintain brain homeostasis or may be a toxic pathologic response. The exact nature and pathogenesis of the polymicrocavitation is not understood. Most assume these cavities to be dilated interstitial spaces in myelin sheaths without axonal degeneration and with no cellular response. Recent studies suggest that this vacuolization may be due to disturbances of protein synthesis. In advanced hepatocellular degeneration the brain may show irreversible neural damage, degeneration, and demyelination.

DIAGNOSIS

The clinical features of hepatic encephalopathy in the dog are extremely variable. Thus the clinician must have a high index of suspicion. In addition to the primary liver diseases that cause HE, several metabolic and central nervous system diseases must be considered and eliminated from the differential diagnosis (Table 1). Numerous neurologic signs have been observed in dogs with HE (Table 3). Clinical signs often follow a large meal, especially if it is high in protein.

The syndrome most often associated with canine HE is *congenital portal vein anomaly.* In this syndrome variable amounts of portal venous blood are shunted away from the liver. Seven types of anomalies have been identified: (1) persistent ductus venosus, (2) portal vein atresia, (3) portal vein–to–caudal vena cava shunt caudal to the liver, (4) anomalous connection of the portal vein to the azygos vein, (5) shunting of the portal vein and caudal vena cava into the azygos vein, (6) splenic vein–to–caudal vena cava shunt, and (7) mesenteric veins–to–caudal vena cava shunts.

The history usually consists of a variable combination of neurologic (Table 3), urinary tract, and gastrointestinal signs. Clinical signs other than neurologic signs that may be observed include (1) polyuria and polydipsia, (2)

stunted growth, (3) ascites, (4) anorexia, (5) weight loss, (6) vomiting, (7) diarrhea, (8) cystic calculi (urate or ammonium biurate), (9) hypersalivation, (10) bloating after eating, (11) anesthetic or tranquilizer intolerance, and (12) enlarged kidneys. It must be emphasized that animals with congenital portal vein anomalies may present with any one or several of the neurologic or non-neurologic signs. Thus, this syndrome should be included in the differential diagnosis of polyuria and polydipsia, ascites, cystic calculi, CNS disease, poor growth, and weight loss.

Ancillary diagnostic aids include routine and special clinical pathologic studies and radiography. The two consistent biochemical abnormalities in this syndrome are an increased retention of plasma sulfobromophthalein (BSP) and elevated fasting and postprandial levels of blood ammonia. Postprandial values can be obtained by feeding the dog a high-protein meal (e.g., Prescription Diet p/d, Hill's Packing Co., Topeka, Kansas) and sampling blood ammonia in two hours. Another ammonia tolerance test involves the administration of ammonium chloride. One hundred milligrams per kilogram of body weight, with a maximal dose of 3 gm, is dissolved in 20 to 50 ml of warm water. A presample of venous blood is taken following a 12-hour fast. The ammonium chloride solution is given orally with a syringe, and a second blood sample is taken in 30 minutes. These ammonia challenge tests are used to differentiate normal dogs from dogs with hepatic encephalopathy that have normal fasting blood ammonias. (Myers, et al.) Since techniques for blood ammonia determination vary among laboratories, the normal values for each laboratory should be consulted. The increased BSP retention (>5 percent at 30 minutes) may be moderate (5 to 10 percent) but is usually quite high (15 to 20 percent).

There are variable abnormalities in several other blood biochemistry determinations. There may be hypoproteinemia, hypoalbuminemia, slightly elevated serum glutamic pyruvic transaminase (SGPT), slightly elevated serum alkaline phosphatase (SAP), and a below-normal blood urea nitrogen (BUN) level (Table 4). In a significant number of these cases, urate or ammonium biurate crystals or calculi are found in the urine. Repeated urinalyses may be necessary before these crystals are detected. The pathophysiology of these abnormalities has been described elsewhere (Barrett, et al.; Ewing, et al.). It is important to remember that the results of the hepatic function tests and blood ammonia level determinations do not correlate with the severity of HE.

Table 3. Neurologic Signs Observed in Canine Hepatic Encephalopathy

Listlessness and depression
Compulsive pacing or circling
Head pressing
Ataxia
Grand mal seizures
Sudden viciousness
Disorientation and staring
Blindness
Craving attention
Tremors
Walking along walls
Climbing walls
Hypermetria
Coma or stupor

Table 4. *Clinical Chemistry Values Seen in Canine HE*

VALUE	LEVEL
BSP retention	Prolonged
Fasting blood ammonia	Elevated or normal
Postprandial ammonia	Elevated
Total protein	Decreased or normal
Albumin	Decreased or normal
Globulin	Decreased or normal
SGPT	Elevated or normal
SAP	Elevated or normal
BUN	Decreased or normal

Plain and contrast abdominal radiography are beneficial in diagnosing congenital portal vein anomalies. Plain radiographs often demonstrate a small liver. If ascites is present, fluid drainage and a pneumoperitoneogram may be necessary to evaluate the liver silhouette. Differentiation from other causes of reduced liver size must be made by means of liver biopsy and contrast radiographic techniques.

Selective arteriography of the cranial mesenteric or celiac artery, percutaneous splenoportography, and portal or splenic venography have been utilized to diagnose portal vein anomalies. Fluoroscopic monitoring is necessary for positioning the catheter in selective arteriography. Splenoportography has three disadvantages: (1) it is often difficult to isolate the spleen percutaneously; (2) the contrast agents may damage the spleen; and (3) the density of the contrast agent as it passes through the portal circulation is less than with other techniques. Portal venography performed following laparotomy and placement of a Silastic intravenous catheter into the portal vein via a jejunal vein offers excellent visualization of the shunts following contrast agent injection in the majority of cases and does not have the aforementioned disadvantages (Fig. 1). Sodium isothalamate at a dosage of 1 ml/kg can be used as the contrast medium. Hand pressure injection followed by immediate exposure of the radiographs is usually adequate for diagnosis. A single study using only one of these techniques may occasionally be inadequate for diagnosis. Multiple contrast studies should be considered if there is a high index of suspicion for this syndrome. It must be emphasized that contrast radiography is the most reliable diagnostic aid in this syndrome. Abnormal shunting is often difficult to detect on exploratory laparotomy or gross necropsy.

Hepatic encephalopathy may rarely be seen in end-stage hepatic disease. Dogs with *chronic cirrhosis, diffuse hepatic neoplastic infiltration,* and advanced *hepatic toxicosis* may have hyperammonemia and show signs of ataxia, stupor, coma and seizures shortly before death. HE

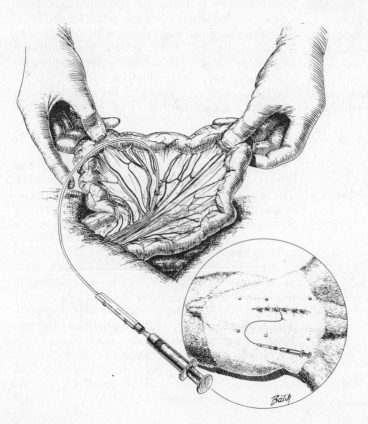

Figure 1. Jejunal catheterization for portography.

is not the dominant clinical syndrome. Signs of chronic, advanced liver failure, such as emaciation, anorexia, vomiting, diarrhea, polyuria and polydipsia, jaundice and ascites, are more prevalent. Hematologic examination, clinical biochemistries, radiography, and liver biopsies will establish the diagnosis of these conditions.

Two cases of *urea cycle enzyme deficiency* in the dog associated with hyperammonemia have been reported (Strombeck, et al., 1975a). One dog showed signs of anorexia, listlessness, depression, vomiting, emaciation, and chronic diarrhea. The other dog had signs of stunted growth, occasional vomiting, and seizures characterized by shaking, muscle stiffness, and disorientation. Routine laboratory tests for liver function, including SGPT, SAP, and BSP retention, were normal. The hyperammonemia was associated with a deficiency of arginosuccinate synthetase, one of the urea cycle enzymes.

Since the diagnosis of HE may be difficult to differentiate from other causes of encephalopathy, other diagnostic tests may be done prior to evaluation of liver function or blood ammonia. The cerebrospinal fluid in HE is clear, normocellular, and under normal pressure, except when cerebral edema is present. The electroencephalogram (EEG) may be of diagnostic value. The lack of focal abnormalities in the EEG is a clue in differentiating metabolic coma from localizing neurologic disorders. The EEG shows bilateral, synchronous, symmetrical high-voltage slow waves. This EEG pattern will help differentiate the causes of metabolic CNS diseases from organic CNS diseases but is not specific for HE. These EEG changes can also be seen in canine hypoglycemia, uremia, and anoxia.

In summary, the diagnosis of HE depends on the presence of hepatic failure and neurologic signs and elimination of other potential causes of encephalopathy. Laboratory tests, including a BSP retention, SGPT, SAP, total protein, albumin, globulin, BUN, urinalysis, fasting, and post-ammonia challenge or postprandial blood ammonia, should be done if HE is suspected. Additional diagnostic aids such as plain and contrast liver radiographs, liver biopsy, urea cycle enzyme analysis, and EEG may be necessary. To eliminate other causes of encephalopathy, electrolytes, fasting blood glucose, blood lead, lupus erythematosus cell test, and CSF tap should be normal.

THERAPY

There are two primary goals in the treatment of hepatic encephalopathy: (1) reversal of the presenting HE crisis and (2) long-term prophy-

lactic and supportive management of the precipitating factors of HE (Table 5).

Treatment of the HE Crisis. Severe encephalopathy can be precipitated by numerous factors (Table 2). It must be considered to be a life-threatening metabolic emergency that requires immediate correction. Total *withdrawal of dietary protein* is mandatory. This removes the substrate for production of further nitrogenous toxins. *Cessation of drugs* such as diuretics, tranquilizers, and methionine that may have precipitated HE is necessary. Barbiturates can be removed by peritoneal dialysis. *Gastrointestinal bleeding* that increases protein substrate and worsens hypovolemia should be corrected. *Blood transfusions* or *parenteral hyperalimentation* that may have initiated the HE crisis should be stopped. *Intravenous fluid therapy* for correction of dehydration, alkalosis, and hypokalemia is beneficial in several ways. Correction of hypovolemia enhances renal elimination of NH_3, corrects prerenal azotemia, and decreases enterohepatic urea nitrogen cycling. Correction of alkalosis and hypokalemia will reduce the intracellular transfer of ammonia and amines. *Cleansing enemas* with warm water will help reduce the colonic content of bacteria and nitrogenous products. Instillation of neomycin in the colon after the enemas may help reduce bacterial production of NH_3. *Intravenous antibiotic therapy* is indicated if concurrent infection is thought to be a precipitating

Table 5. *Current Established Therapeutic Measures for Hepatic Encephalopathy*

I. General supportive care
  A. Correct fluid and electrolyte imbalances
  B. Reverse precipitating causes (see Table 2)
II. Prevention of ammonia and other nitrogenous substances from entering circulation from gastrointestinal tract
  A. Protein restriction
    1. Homemade low-protein diets °
    2. Commercial low-protein diets (k/d,† u/d,† Nephro Diet,‡ Diet N,§ Clinicare N‖)
  B. Sterilization of intestinal tract
    1. Neomycin (and other antibiotics)
  C. Gastrointestinal cleansing
    1. Cathartics
    2. Enemas
  D. Altered gastrointestinal environment
    1. Lactulose therapy
III. Correction of portal vein anomaly by partial ligation of shunt.

°Bovee, K. C.: What constitutes a low-protein diet for dogs with chronic renal failure? J. Am. Anim. Hosp. Assoc., 8:246–253, 1972
†Hill Packing Company, Topeka, Kansas
‡Atlas Canine Products, Inc., Glendale, L.I., New York
§C. P. Bernard Packing Company, Camden, New Jersey
‖Chas. Pfizer & Company, New York, New York

factor. Chloramphenicol at a dosage of 40 mg/kg IV t.i.d. and high dosages of sodium penicillin (100,000 U/kg) IV q.i.d. with kanamycin at 6 mg/kg IM b.i.d. are often beneficial in treating septicemias. *Oxygen therapy* may be helpful in correcting renal and hepatic hypoxia. Resultant increased renal and hepatic function will decrease the enterohepatic circulation of urea nitrogen. There is no evidence that corticosteroid therapy is beneficial in HE. Corticosteroids have been shown to be of value only in chronic active hepatitis in man and the dog.

Long-term Prophylactic Therapy. Therapy in chronic HE is aimed at preventing entrance of ammonia and other nitrogenous toxins from the gastrointestinal tract into the circulation. Three techniques are utilized to manage HE in patients with no precipitating cause: (1) protein restriction, (2) "sterilization" of the intestinal tract, and (3) alteration of the colonic environment to reduce ammonia absorption.

Dietary protein restriction reduces intraluminal nitrogenous substances responsible for ammonia formation and may reduce the total-body urea pool. Urea plays an important role in the control of ammonia production. Enterohepatic circulation of urea is present in animals. Circulating urea diffuses into the small intestine and is hydrolyzed to ammonia by urea-splitting bacteria and mucosal urease in the colon. The ammonia is absorbed back into the circulation and reconverted to urea by the liver. Whenever hepatocellular disease or portosystemic shunting is present, the ammonia is not converted to urea and enters the circulation.

Dietary protein restriction can be accomplished by feeding commercially prepared low-protein diets or, more efficient, homemade low-protein diets. Dogs with congenital and experimentally produced portacaval shunts have been maintained for years with minimal clinical signs of HE using protein restriction as the only means of therapy. The recommended diet for chronic HE is a high-carbohydrate, low-fat, low-quantity, and high-biologic-value-protein diet. Certain short-chain fatty acids have been shown experimentally to potentiate the signs of HE. Thus, high-fat diets should be avoided.

Oral broad-spectrum antibiotics have also been used to decrease urease-producing bowel flora, thereby decreasing the production of ammonia. Controlled therapeutic trials have not been conducted in the dog. However, oral antibiotics have been of little value in dogs with severe portosystemic shunting, and protein restriction alone has been sufficient in some dogs with less severe shunting.

Neomycin is the most commonly used antibiotic in the dog. An initial dosage of 20 mg/kg b.i.d. of neomycin is recommended. The dosage is gradually reduced until the drug is stopped or until the minimal dosage that prevents the signs of HE is found. Other antibiotics (e.g., tetracycline, kanamycin, paromomycin, and sulfonamides) may also be effective. Animals with renal disease should be monitored closely while receiving neomycin, since a small amount of neomycin is absorbed from the gastrointestinal tract, and it is potentially ototoxic and nephrotoxic.

If ascites is present it should be controlled symptomatically. A low-sodium diet (Prescription Diet h/d, Hill's Division, Riviana Foods, Topeka, Kansas) and diuretics are recommended. Since diuretics (e.g., thiazides and furosemide) may cause potassium depletion, they should be used cautiously or with oral potassium supplementation.

Lactulose is a non-absorbable synthetic disaccharide (beta-1, 4-galactoside fructose). Several studies in man have shown it to be as effective as neomycin therapy in treating and preventing recurrent HE. Recent use by this author in dogs with advanced portal-systemic shunting in which protein restriction and neomycin have failed to produce a remission has met with minimal success. The mechanism of action of lactulose is probably due to colonic acidification with decreased ammonia flux ($NH_3 \rightarrow NH_4^+$, which is less diffusible). The catharsis produced may also be beneficial. Lactulose is not hydrolyzed in the small intestine owing to a lack of appropriate intestinal disaccharidases. It is hydrolyzed by colonic bacteria to acetic, lactic and formic acids. The acid environment in the colon also favors growth of *Lactobacillus* organisms, which have no urease and, in contrast with the usual colonic bacteria, cannot convert urea to ammonia. The dosage of lactulose is adjusted until two to three semiformed stools are produced daily or stool pH decreases to 5.5 or less. The human dosage is approximately 60 to 160 gm/day divided t.i.d. Lactose rectal enemas may be of benefit in the reversal of severe coma; 300 ml of lactulose syrup is diluted with 700 ml of water and is administered through a rectal tube with an occluding balloon and drained in 20 to 30 minutes. This is repeated every two hours for three administrations. Lactulose therapy would be indicated in patients with HE that are nonresponsive to protein restriction and neomycin therapy. In man it appears equal in efficacy to neomycin therapy. Recent studies suggest neomycin and lactulose given together may be synergistic. Side effects of lactulose therapy include abdominal pain, flatulence, anorexia, vomiting, and diarrhea. Lactulose (Cephulac®)

is available from Merrell-National Laboratories. It would cost around $100/month to treat a 30-pound dog with lactulose.

EXPERIMENTAL AND THEORETICAL THERAPEUTIC MEASURES

Many methods of therapy for human HE are currently under investigation. Some are expensive and require elaborate technical facilities. Several of these procedures have not been particularly successful. Administration of *Lactobacillus acidophilus* will replace the normal colonic flora with these non-urease–producing organisms, but very large amounts of bacterial culture are needed and clinical effects are variable. *Antibodies to urease* can be induced by parenteral administration of jack bean urease. In clinical trials severe reactions to the jack bean extract occurred, and clinical benefits in patients with HE were not apparent. Administration of *acetohydroxamic acid*, an inhibitor of urease, will lower blood ammonia levels, but little clinical improvement occurred in a small number of human cases. *Colonic bypass* surgery is a radical technique that appears to have little justification in veterinary patients. *Perfusion techniques* including exchange transfusions, plasmapheresis, cross-circulation, hemodialysis, activated charcoal hemoperfusion, and perfusion of isolated animal livers have resulted in some reports of reversal of acute HE, but long-term survival has not been increased.

Administration of L-dopa to human patients with unresponsive HE has recently received much attention. Its use is based in part on the false neurotransmitter hypothesis. This theory states that in HE the toxic amines or their precursors accumulate in the CNS in adrenergic neurons and displace the putative transmitters norepinephrine and dopamine. L-Dopa may replace false neurotransmitters. However, the effects of L-dopa in HE may be secondary to a variety of actions. In experimental animals with HE secondary to end-to-side portacaval shunt L-dopa administration may lower blood ammonia levels and protect against HE.

Dogs with chronic portacaval shunts possess a severe imbalance in amino acid composition. Plasma levels of phenylalanine, methionine, and tyrosine are high, and levels of the branched-chain amino acids valine, leucine, and isoleucine are reduced. Experimental systemic administration of amino acids in proportions that normalize the amino acid pattern has been shown to reverse the signs of HE, even though ammonia concentrations remain high (Fischer, et al., 1975). Further evaluation of this therapy is awaited eagerly by clinicians.

Partial ligation of portal-systemic shunts in dogs has recently received much attention. Results have been variable. Some case studies indicate that surgery may be an alternative to medical therapy in selected cases.

SUPPLEMENTAL READING

Barrett, R.E., deLahunta, A., Roenigk, W.J., Hoffer, R.E., and Coons, F.H.: Four cases of congenital portacaval shunt in the dog. J. Small Anim. Pract., *17*:71–85, 1976.

Ewing, G.O., Suter, P.F., and Bailey, C.S.: Hepatic insufficiency associated with congenital anomalies of the portal vein in dogs. J. Am. Anim. Hosp. Assoc., *10*:463–475, 1974.

Fischer, J.E., et al.: Pathogenesis and treatment of hepatic coma. Prog. Liver Dis., *5*:363–397, 1976.

Fischer, J.E., et al.: The role of plasma amino acids in hepatic encephalopathy. Surgery, *78*:226–290, 1975.

Myers, D.J., Strombeck, D.R., Stone, E.A., Zenoble, R.D., and Buss, D.D.: Ammonia tolerance test in clinically normal dogs and in dogs with portosystemic shunts. J. Am. Vet. Med. Assoc., *173*:377–379, 1978.

Schenker, S., Breen, K.J., and Hoyumpa, A.M.: Hepatic encephalopathy: Current status. Gastroenterology, *66*:121–151, 1974.

Strombeck, D.R., Meyer, D.J., and Freedland, R.A.: Hyperammonemia due to a urea cycle enzyme deficiency in two dogs. J. Am. Vet. Med. Assoc., *166*:1109–1111, 1975*a*.

Strombeck, D.R., Weiser, M.G., and Kaneko, J.J.: Hyperammonemia and hepatic encephalopathy in the dog. J. Am. Vet. Med. Assoc., *166*:1105–1108, 1975*b*.

TREATMENT OF FELINE AND CANINE SEIZURE DISORDERS

ALAN J. PARKER, M.R.C.V.S.
Urbana, Illinois

To treat seizure disorders effectively one must first understand the seizure phenomenon and be able to transmit a good deal of this knowledge to the client; 90 percent of the treatment of seizure cases is client education. Hence, the major objective of this article is briefly to explain the signs, causes, types, and differential diagnoses of and client education for seizures in the cat and dog, as well as the treatment.

The four major mistakes made by clinicians handling seizure cases are (1) failure to recognize a seizure, (2) failure to use adequate diagnostic tests, (3) failure to explain the disorder to the client, and (4) failure to use drugs correctly. This discussion will concentrate on information to help clinicians avoid these mistakes.

DEFINITIONS

A *seizure* or *convulsion* (also referred to as an *ictus* or *fit*) is best defined as the presence of all, any one, or any combination of the following signs:

1. Loss or derangement of consciousness (unconscious, dull, glassy-eyed, excited).
2. Loss of or excess muscle tone or movement (constant rigidity [tonus] or intermittent rigidity [clonus, paddling, flaccidity]).
3. Alteration of sensation (pain, pruritus, self-mutilation), including hallucinations of special senses (sound, vision, taste).
4. Changes in the autonomic nervous system (urination, salivation, defecation, vagal bradycardia, rapid peristalsis with diarrhea, vomiting).
5. Behavioral signs (non-recognition of owner, barking, howling, viciousness, pacing, running in circles, "snapping at flies").

These five general types of signs are caused by intermittent (paroxysmal) intracranial dysrhythmias (abnormal electrical activity), which may not produce the signs every time the dysrhythmias occur. The primary molecular disturbance that triggers the dysrhythmias is as poorly understood as the mechanism that permits the dysrhythmia to cause signs at some times but not at others. However, a number of agents and events are known to influence this process (e.g., anticonvulsant drugs, estrogens, pruritus, otitis externa, and emotions).

There are many causes of seizures but one cause that requires careful definition is epilepsy. *Epilepsy* is simply defined as a state of repetitive seizures. Hence epilepsy is not a true disease; it is a state or syndrome. It is customary not to refer to animals that have seizures from brain tumors, acute encephalitis, or hydrocephalus as epileptics. There is also no sharp time line separating the acute encephalitic having seizures from the post-encephalitic epilepsy case, except that when the acute problem persists longer than a few weeks it becomes "epilepsy."

RECOGNIZING A SEIZURE

The clinician must pay careful attention to all possibilities that the definition of seizures presents. The most frequent signs seen in a convulsion are a loss of consciousness, complete rigidity (tonus) followed by intermittent rigidity/relaxation (clonus), salivation, urination, paddling, and a few minutes' disorientation after recovery. The whole episode takes one to five minutes. Prior to a full generalized seizure one limb may become stiff and be raised, or the head may turn. These are *localizing signs* and tend to indicate which area of the brain is affected first. Such signs are not "jacksonian seizures." The animal may act unusual (quiet, hyperactive, anxious) for minutes or days before a seizure; this is called an *aura*. After the seizure the animal may not recognize the owner, may be blind or ataxic, or may wander and pace aimlessly for hours or several days; these are called *postictal* signs. Some animals may eat and drink excessively after a seizure. This is interpreted as a hypothalamic effect of the seizure.

Most recognition problems arise when only a few signs are seen or with psychomotor seizures. Some animals may show diarrhea or vomiting as the only evidence of a seizure. Others may awaken from a normal sleep disorientated and glassy-eyed. Others may attack something for no apparent reason. Some dogs (especially spaniels) may snap at the air as if a fly were there. Some may do nothing more than collapse and then get up, although such a sign is more typical of narcolepsy or cardiac syncope. One of the rarest types in man involves unusual hypothalamic signs such as pyrexia; this is, however, not a diagnosis to be used for every case with paroxysmal fever of unknown origin.

Minor episodes of jaw chomping or twitching of one limb are called *"focal" seizures* and are not considered petit mal. Some dogs (especially Dobermans) may also snap their jaws when nervous; this is not a seizure.

When considering that an episode may be a seizure, one must look for evidence of intermittent occurrence and some of the signs listed in the definition of convulsions.

DIFFERENTIAL DIAGNOSIS OF SEIZURES

Table 1 lists the causes of seizures in the dog and cat as well as the methods of diagnosing the cause. The clinician must consider all causes, but after a careful history, physical and neurologic examination, the average diagnostic workup is (1) a complete blood count, (2) a chemistry profile including glucose, calcium, blood urea nitrogen, creatinine, SGPT, alkaline phosphatase, and blood protein determinations, (3) a blood lead evaluation run on heparinized blood, (4) a cerebrospinal fluid sample (if indicated), and (5) an electroencephalogram (EEG), if indicated. Other tests may also be indicated, such as electrolytes, BSP, glucagon or ammonia tolerance test, radiographs, ECG, serologic studies, microbiologic tests, and biopsy. We suggest the first three tests be done routinely, followed by a CSF sample and analysis only if brain tumor or recent encephalitis is suspected. An EEG is a helpful tool if available but is not essential.

The clinician must be satisfied with a diagnosis of elimination in most seizure cases, because without the EEG over 80 percent of seizure cases are labeled idiopathic epilepsy. There is no positive blood test for epilepsy. Only the EEG will show abnormal brain electrical activi-

ty and will not do so in every case. The EEG permits reduction of the idiopathic group by identifying some of the subgroups of epilepsy, but it does not really change the therapeutic approach.

It is not wise to regard any type, pattern, or age of onset of seizures as diagnostic for any cause of seizures; one can only suspect a diagnosis with such information. For example, sudden onset of many seizures suggests toxicity or infection, as does onset in animals less than one year of age, and fits of focal chomping without loss of consciousness suggest canine distemper.

The clinician must learn self-confidence and be satisfied with (1) diagnostic elimination of conditions treated by means other than anticonvulsants and (2) effective test therapy using each anticonvulsant drug or a combination. One in three animals will remain uncontrolled — that is a fact of life. Spending a fortune on tests and "witch doctors" will not change the odds unless some unforeseen breakthrough in our knowledge appears.

TYPES OF EPILEPSY

Once all other causes of seizures have been eliminated from the differential diagnosis, one is left with a group of cases called "epilepsy." Not all cases of epilepsy have a common cause. Many are acquired (Table 1), but some are idiopathic and may be genetic in origin. In man the types of epilepsy are classified largely on the basis of the EEG. Terms such as petit mal and grand mal have very specific meanings. Three common veterinary mistakes are to refer to minor focal seizures (e.g., chomping) as "petit mal," to localizing signs as "jacksonian seizures," and to any generalized seizure as "grand mal." It is best to forget the human terms in veterinary medicine. Petit mal seizures in man involve short muscle jerks or absences characterized by specific EEG changes that are very rarely found in animals. Jacksonian seizures are caused by specific motor cortex lesions, and the human motor cortex is much larger and physiologically very different from that of the cat or dog. In man grand mal seizures are primary generalized seizures of a frequently inherited type caused by deep lesions in the brain.

The cat and dog usually suffer from acquired epilepsy with focal lesions of known or unknown cause that produce secondary generalized seizures. Such acquired lesions can frequently be seen to start the electrical discharge in one part of the brain. Hence animals with

Table 1. Differential Diagnosis of Seizures

CAUSES	MEANS OF DIAGNOSIS*
Acquired epilepsy (also called secondary or partial epilepsy)	Elimination of other causes; H, P, N, CP, EEG, CSF
Postencephalitis	
Birth injury or anoxia	
Head trauma	
Postanoxia (e.g., anesthesia or cardiac arrest)	
Post–cerebrovascular accident (CVA)	
Idiopathic epilepsy (causes hard to document by history or EEG. Conditions such as migrating larvae or microemboli; genetic reasons?)	Same
Primary epilepsy (as demonstrated by the EEG and thus assumed to be inherited)	Same
Acute encephalitis	H, P, N, CSF, EEG, CP, S, B
Canine distemper	
Feline infectious peritonitis	
Toxoplasmosis	
Feline leukemia viremia?	
Rabies	
Other viruses or bacteria	
Toxicity (exogenous)	H, P, N, CP, T, EEG
Lead	
Chlorinated hydrocarbon derivatives	
Strychnine	
Others	
Toxicity (endogenous)	
Hepatic encephalopathy	
Portacaval shunt	H, P, N, CP (especially protein BUN, BSP,
Chronic liver insufficiency (cirrhosis and other problems, natural or drug-induced)	glucagon or ammonia tolerance), liver radiography (gross and angiographic), EEG, B
Azotemia (usually terminal)	H, P, N, CP
Hydrocephalus	H, P, N, EEG, radiography (mainly pneumoventriculogram)
Juvenile	
Occult	
Decompensating	
Brain tumor	H, P, N, CSF, EEG, radiography of skull (very rare) and chest (primary focus)
Primary	
Metastatic	
Multifocal	
Hypoglycemia (pancreatic beta-cell tumor, juvenile enzyme immaturity, and hunting dog types)	H, P, N, blood glucose
Hypocalcemia	H, P, N, blood calcium, protein,
Eclampsia, and others	ionized calcium
Acute meningitis	H, P, N, CSF, EEG, M, S
Bacterial	
Fungal	
Viral (see Acute encephalitis)	
Acute cranial trauma	H, P, N, CSF, EEG, radiography (rarely diagnostic)
Acute cerebrovascular accident (CVA)	H, P, N, CSF, EEG
Acute anoxias	H, P, N, EEG, ECG, radiography of chest
Cardiac	
Pulmonic	
Vascular	
Thiamin deficiency (thiaminase toxicity) in cats	H, P, N, therapy
"Worm fits" of young animals	?
Hyperthermia (105°+)	Usually caused by the seizure, and not the reverse
"Flashing lights"	H
Neuronal glycoproteinosis (Lafora's disease)	B or necropsy
Other inherited lysosomal enzyme deficiency or CNS degenerative diseases	H, P, N, CSF, EEG, S, B
Narcolepsy (not a true seizure but a collapse)	H, P, N, EEG

*Key: H = history and signalment, P = physical examination (including ophthalmic), N = neurologic examination, CP = clinical pathologic tests, CSF = cerebrospinal fluid pressure and analysis, EEG = electroencephalography, ECG = electrocardiography, S = serologic studies, B = biopsy, M = microbiologic tests, T = toxicologic testing.

such lesions are also called "partial" epileptics (an inaccurate description). Epileptic animals with seizures that seem to be of a focal origin but of which the cause is not understood are called idiopathic epileptics. In the dog some of these cases are apparently genetic in origin. A few animals can be shown to be primary generalized epileptics with true grand mal seizures on the EEG. Their seizures start electrically in all areas of the brain at once. These are assumed to be genetic. Focal lesions are said to cause secondary generalized seizures because the electrical disturbance starts in one area and then spreads. Classifications of epilepsy are cumbersome and of little clinical significance in veterinary medicine. It is best to recognize (1) focal (limited to one area of the body) or generalized seizures, (2) localizing signs, aura, and postictal signs, and (3) a known cause of the epilepsy or an idiopathic state, some of which are genetic. Further classification is not fruitful to the generalist at the moment.

The term *psychomotor seizure* is used in cats and dogs to indicate the presence of considerable personality or behavioral changes ("fly snapping," abnormal but coordinated movements, viciousness, and others) during or just after the seizure. It is assumed in such cases that behavioral areas of the brain have been affected. The main clinical significance of this classification is that phenobarbital, primidone, and progesterones work better on such cases. Regular seizures are called *motor seizures*. Both motor and psychomotor types are seen with acquired or idiopathic epilepsy (Table 1).

AGE OF ONSET OF SEIZURES

Pancreatic beta-cell tumors and other tumors tend to occur in middle-aged or older animals, and hence a late onset of seizures suggests such a cause. However, several other causes of acquired epilepsy or seizures (trauma, CVA, encephalitis, meningitis) can affect older animals as well. The animal less than one year of age is a prime candidate for toxicity or encephalitis. Cases with genetic, birth, and neonatal causes of epilepsy usually have their first seizure between one and four years of age.

SEIZURE PATTERNS

Seizure patterns often surprise owners and veterinarians. An accurate generalization is that *seizure patterns are completely unpredictable.* Some epileptics start with irregular short seizures that become more frequent and longer over the first year. Others start with status epilepticus. Initial status epilepticus does

suggest some cause other than epilepsy. Some animals have fewer seizures as they grow older, and other have more. Some may have seizures irregularly, or exactly at the same time of day, or always on Sunday, or at exact intervals of a few days or weeks. Some are even associated with the full moon. Gastrointestinal irritation, pruritic conditions, estrus, pseudocyesis, pregnancy, diethylstilbestrol, excitement, and boredom can all be associated in some cases with an increased number of seizures.

There are explanations for all of these patterns but little proof. Seizures will occur most frequently as epileptics sleep or doze, particularly after excitement. This accounts for night seizures and weekend seizures (after visitors, visits, or family play). The brain receives vast amounts of information that never reaches consciousness but does affect areas of the brain that can raise or lower seizure activity. Hence the exacerbation of seizure patterns by disease states, some drugs, and emotions. The full moon is a little more difficult to explain within the constraints of Western medicine, but humans are well known to be affected by the full moon. Dogs key their emotions from their owners; hence, a worried dog and thus a seizure may occur at the time of a full moon. The regular seizure cycles are hard to explain, but most clients respond well to the idea that the brain "winds up" to a seizure.

One must beware of a seizure pattern that suddenly worsens after a long period of control with drugs (especially primidone), because the drug may be damaging the liver, which in turn can cause hepatic encephalopathy.

Seizures caused by hypoglycemia will be associated with postprandial insulin overdose (in pancreatic beta-cell tumors only), long periods without food, or strenuous prolonged exercise. Hydrocephalics often will have seizures after mild head trauma. Hepatic encephalopathy cases frequently show cycles with a few days of good appetite followed by a few days of depression and seizures. They may also show seizures one to three hours after eating, especially if stressed. Toxic agents may cause immediate seizures, or the onset may be delayed hours or days.

CLIENT EDUCATION

The education of the client about epilepsy is critical in patient management. It is possible to get client education materials dealing with human epilepsy from the Epilepsy Foundation of America in Washington, D. C. Their materials explain epilepsy and its control in man, thus permitting comparison of the problems encountered in controlling human epileptics with those of the dog or cat.

It is necessary to explain to the client what a seizure is, what epilepsy is, how epilepsy is diagnosed by elimination, what is meant by "idiopathic," the fact that epilepsy is controlled but not cured, the fact that only two-thirds of cases of animal epilepsy can be controlled, and the fact that there are various causes of epilepsy, including genetic ones. I always advise clients not to breed epileptic dogs of any type and suggest neutering to make control easier. One must mention breed incidences (epilepsy is common in several breeds including German shepherds, Saint Bernards, schnauzers, poodles, Irish setters, and Labradors) but emphasize that an individual of any breed can be affected. Individuals of certain breeds, such as German shepherds, are much harder to control than others (e.g., less than one third of German shepherds with epilepsy are controlled well). Explanations of the varied seizure patterns, the aura, postictal signs, and the absence of pain during a seizure are also necessary. Clients must be particularly advised to keep their hands out of the animal's mouth during a seizure; animals do not swallow their tongues. Carefully advise the client when to call the veterinarian after a seizure but specify that they should call at once if the seizure lasts longer than ten minutes. Explain all the side effects of anticonvulsant drugs, the need to split doses daily, and the need not to miss doses.

CASE HANDLING

CONVULSION IN PROGRESS LESS THAN FIVE MINUTES

Wait for recovery but ensure that the animal is breathing effectively. If not, then treat as status epilepticus. Obtain necessary blood samples at once and perhaps give a heavy sedative dose of phenobarbital (5 to 10 mg/kg); do not use phenothiazine-derivative tranquilizers, which can cause seizures in epileptics. Do not treat chronically unless diagnostic efforts have been made or the animal's seizure pattern is known and control is needed. Do not treat chronically after the first seizure unless the client demands it. If physical, neurologic, and blood examinations are normal, wait to see the pattern develop.

STATUS EPILEPTICUS

Status epilepticus is loosely defined as seizures lasting longer than 15 to 30 minutes. This is an inaccurate description because not all "status" cases are epileptics. Use IV diazepam (5 to 50 mg total dose) to abolish the seizure. If this is not effective, use IV phenobarbital, 30 to 60 mg, in a small dog or a cat. In actuality the drug is given slowly to effect, because there are wide dose variations (up to 30 mg/kg) in my experience. The major problem encountered using phenobarbital is an unwillingness to give enough. The drug is usually sold in 120-mg (2-grain) vials, and the use of several vials seems to be a large dose. The diazepam dose may have to be repeated hourly if the abnormal electrical activity persists. The phenobarbital dose may need repeating every four to six hours in the same situation. Pentobarbital, thiopentone, or thiamylal are used only if phenobarbital is not available, because these drugs have no anticonvulsant effect except via anesthesia. An animal may start seizures as soon as the effect of these three anesthetic agents wears off. Phenobarbital permits a lighter plane of sedation/anesthesia to be reached with control of seizures, and hence it is easier to change such an animal to oral medication. Any animal with status epilepticus should be switched to oral phenobarbital at a dose of 2 to 10 mg/kg (split b.i.d. or t.i.d.) by force-feeding as soon as possible. "Topping up" with IV phenobarbital may be necessary until the correct dose is achieved. It is better to err on the side of oversedation at first. "Status" is a life-threatening condition and is an indication for immediate chronic therapy even after the first seizure — at least until a diagnosis is made.

Once status epilepticus is controlled and the animal is breathing well, blood samples should be taken. Glucose (20 to 50 ml of 10 percent solution) and calcium gluconate (2 to 5 ml of 5 percent solution) should be given slowly IV once blood samples have been taken. Conditions suggestive of hypoglycemia can be treated with glucose before the anticonvulsant but preferably not before a blood sample has been obtained to prove the diagnosis. It is apparently helpful to give IV dexamethasone (2 to 4 mg/kg) after long seizures to reduce hypoxic brain swelling. Hyperosmotic agents are not indicated. Lower doses of dexamethasone (0.1 to 1 mg/kg) can be repeated b.i.d. or t.i.d. for several days as needed. The possibility of exposure to toxic materials must be considered and appropriate specific treatments provided in all "status" cases.

REPEATED SEIZURES OF KNOWN FREQUENCY

Animals that have such repeated seizures should be treated if the client requests it. Most clients will not tolerate more than two or three seizures a year, but others do not want the bother of treatment until the seizures are more frequent. It is a personal decision because occasional short seizures are not life-threatening. We advise treatment if the seizures occur four times per year or more, are getting longer or more frequent, or if status epilepticus has occurred. If laboratory tests show no evidence of abnormality and the history, physical, and neurologic examinations are normal, such animals should be treated as epileptics.

TREATMENT OF CAUSES OTHER THAN EPILEPSY

Seizures due to acute encephalitis or meningitis should be treated with phenobarbital (2 to 5 mg/kg/day) split t.i.d. as a baseline dose, but the actual dose given depends on the amount needed to control seizures and the dose tolerated before ataxia or sedation develops. Doses up to 12 mg/kg/day are not uncommon. Many animals are ataxic during the first few days on phenobarbital, so do not reduce doses too hastily. Be prepared to raise doses slowly because tolerance will develop. After six months of control, withhold the drug slowly over a two-month period to see if the animal has become a postmeningitic or postencephalitic epileptic and hence needs the drug permanently. We find that prophylactic phenobarbital even before seizures appear in encephalitics seems to reduce the future incidence of seizures.

Seizures due to exogenous toxicity are handled as "status," but emesis, lavage, purgation, shampoos, and specific antidotes may also be needed.

Endogenous toxicity cases require careful management of the failing organ system, and the dose of any anticonvulsant drug is usually lower. Phenobarbital is best to use because its effects are easily titrated.

Convulsing hydrocephalics of the juvenile type should receive euthanasia. The occult types (seizures only) are handled as regular epilepticus. The decompensating types are treated for acute decompensation with steroids, furosemide, and perhaps emergency ventriculotomy (temporary or permanent), as well as with phenobarbital. Beware of respiratory depression and be prepared to use an oxygen cage or respiratory assistance.

Hypoglycemia and hypocalcemia cases should have the primary disease treated. They do not need anticonvulsants. Juvenile cases usually mature to normal by six to nine months. The hunting dog types do well on a "cookie-a-mile" basis, but are best handled by also providing a light, fat-free meal one hour before exercise. A high percentage of pancreatic beta-cell tumors are malignant.

Acute intracranial trauma and CVA (stroke) cases rarely show seizures acutely and even then only need small (1 to 2 mg/kg) IV doses of phenobarbital for control. It is not customary to use prophylactic phenobarbital in such cases after recovery.

Acute anoxias require attention to the primary cause but phenytoin (10 to 100 mg/kg/day) is the first-choice anticonvulsant to help stabilize CNS membranes against anoxia. Digitalis-like drugs may aid cardiac cases. A significant group of anoxic cases are also obese, often because of hypothyroidism. Hence a combination of cardiac glycoside and thyroid replacement drugs will help some cases without the use of anticonvulsants. Perhaps this accounts for the illogical use of these drugs in treatment of all epileptics — with some success.

Thiamin deficiency can occur even in cats fed good commercial diets. A dose of subcutaneous thiamin may be indicated as a routine part of therapy for any acute CNS sign in the cat.

If "worm fits" really occur, the treatment is obvious. Hyperthermia in the dog or cat is not critical until 106°F has been passed, although simple cooling measures should be taken before this. Seizures themselves frequently raise the body temperature to 105 to 106°F, and most heat stroke cases do not have convulsions. We think true febrile convulsions are rare in companion animals. If they occur, diazepam or phenobarbital or both should be given as the animal is rapidly cooled.

Lafora's disease is untreatable and rare. The lysosomal enzyme and other CNS metabolic diseases rarely cause seizures, except terminally. They are all unresponsive to therapy.

TREATMENT OF EPILEPSY

The aim of treatment is control. Control is defined as an absence of seizures or a greatly reduced incidence limited only to short single seizures, with minimal postictal signs and no tendency to status epilepticus. About two-thirds of all epileptics will be controlled eventually, but this figure drops to one-third in some breeds, e.g., German shepherds. Some owners may be satisfied with less than total control, but others demand perfection. The owner's criteria are thus significant factors. Once the seizures are controlled the animal may appear to improve in general attitude and often becomes more playful.

When using anticonvulsants the clinician must be aware of the frequent dose differences among dogs, cats, and man. The dog often requires up to ten times the human dose/kg, while cats can require only one-tenth the human dose. Switching medications must be done gradually over a period of one to two weeks. No phenothiazine derivatives (antihistamines, antiemetics, or tranquilizers) should be given to epileptics, because these drugs may cause seizures. Doses must always be divided into b.i.d, t.i.d., or even q.i.d. doses, but higher fractions of the dose can be given at night, when most seizures occur. This method is best reserved for cases needing high sedative doses of the drugs. Human petit mal drugs are sometimes used successfully in veterinary medicine, but one should not assume that animals that respond to these drugs have petit mal seizures.

Dogs

There are four classic anticonvulsant drugs used in the dog. They are in suggested order of use:

1. Phenytoin (30 to 100 mg/kg/day divided t.i.d.). Only Parke-Davis' product, Dilantin, should be used because of its better absorption properties.

2. Phenobarbital (2 to 5 mg/kg/day as a baseline, but up to 12 mg/kg/day divided b.i.d. or t.i.d. to effect; rarely, up to 20 mg/kg/day).

3. Primidone (20 to 40 mg/kg/day divided b.i.d. or t.i.d.).

4. Diazepam (1 to 4 mg/kg/day divided q.i.d.).

The blood levels of these drugs can be monitored, but the clinical effects (control vs. side effects) are adequate guides in practice. Before changing a drug be sure to give it a chance at the maximum tolerated dose and divide the dose at least t.i.d. or q.i.d., because this gives optimal blood levels. Dogs with unusual seizures that have pure visceral or psychomotor signs and those known to be postencephalitics rarely do well on phenytoin. Diazepam is often inconvenient to use in dogs because of prescription regulations, dose size, expense, and frequency of dose. Dogs that have had status epilepticus or multiple seizures in one day should be started on phenytoin and phenobarbital; phenytoin should never be used alone. Cocktails of combinations of drugs should be tried if each drug alone fails. The usual cocktails are phenytoin-phenobarbital or phenobarbital-primidone, but any combination in maximum tolerated doses can be tried. One should be aware of microsomal enzyme induction and the appearance of tolerance to a drug.

This will be observed either as initial sedation/ataxia that resolves in three to four days without a lowering of the dose or as a long-term need to raise the dose. This is especially true of phenobarbital and primidone.

There are side effects with all anticonvulsants. Phenytoin seems the least toxic to the dog but is the least effective drug. It will cause polyphagia, polydipsia, and polyuria. Phenobarbital and primidone are more potent causes of these signs and may lead to obesity. They also cause marked sedation and ataxia in overdose; phenytoin is much less of a problem. Any of these drugs, but especially phenobarbital and primidone, may have a hyperkinetic effect in some individuals (especially "high-strung" animals) that may be manifested by constant pacing and crying. Primidone causes marked elevation in alkaline phosphatase and moderate elevation in SGPT. Phenobarbital and phenytoin have a lesser effect. These changes can mimic liver failure and hide true liver failure if ignored. A few dogs receiving primidone may show partial or severe liver failure and may have seizures because of induced hepatic encephalopathy. Reduction of medication, a switch to phenobarbital, or both, seems to help.

If the four classic drugs are not satisfactory alone or in combination there are others to try, but sudden withdrawal of all drugs should be avoided. It is wise to try the following drugs at first in combination with phenobarbital, at the maximum tolerated doses of each drug. Reduction of phenobarbital should be started only after a few months of control.

1. Valproate (Depakene), 15 to 100 mg/kg/day divided t.i.d.

2. Paramethadione (Paradione) 30 to 50 mg/kg/day divided t.i.d.

3. Carbamazepine (Tegretol), 4 to 10 mg/kg/day divided t.i.d. is of little value in our experience.

4. Carbonic anhydrase inhibitors (Diamox) are useless in long therapy for the dog.

5. Progesterones such as Depo-provera and megestrol acetate. Ovaban can be used at 5 to 20 mg/kg given once every four to six weeks or in smaller doses daily. In either case a week-long "loading period" is required for large daily doses.

Acupuncture is not an inconceivable treatment for epilepsy, but we have no knowledge of its effective use under controlled conditions in a large number of dogs.

"Last resort" ideas for treating epileptics are desperate measures to avoid euthanasia but are worth consideration:

1. Is the dog really getting the drug regularly and in the correct dose?

2. Are the doses high enough?

3. Have combinations been tried?

4. Have all possible drugs been tried?

5. Is the diagnosis accurate? For example, is there liver disease or a brain tumor?

The best last-resort idea is to put the dog on the maximum tolerated maintenance dose of phenobarbital and have the owner give large sedative doses when an aura is seen, after the dog gets excited, or after any seizure (which will at least stop status epilepticus). The drug can be given orally or by injection (IM and occasionally IV).

CATS

Epilepsy in the cat is uncommon. Cats do not suffer from canine distemper, an epileptogenic disease, and we have not yet encountered evidence of genetic epilepsy in cats.

Cats require lower doses of anticonvulsants than man or dogs and are almost intolerant of some drugs. Phenobarbital is the drug of choice, at 2 to 3 mg/kg/day split b.i.d. or t.i.d., but doses of up to 10 mg/kg may be needed on rare occasions. Diazepam is the second-choice drug (1 to 4 mg/kg/day divided t.i.d.). Phenytoin is poorly metabolized by the cat's liver and should not be used unless blood levels are assayed as in man. Cats can sometimes tolerate 0.5 to 1 mg/kg/day. I have seen many phenytoin-poisoned cats because of their intolerance to the drug and the fact that Dilantin, being a human drug, carries no veterinary warnings. Primidone can be given to some cats (2 to 5 mg/kg/day) but many develop liver toxicities. If phenobarbital or diazepam do not help it is likely that the diagnosis is wrong (FIP?). Thiamin should be given to any cat that has acute-onset seizures or any severe CNS signs.

SUPPLEMENTAL READING

Bielfelt, S.W., et al.: Sire and sex related differences in rates of epileptiform seizures in a pure-bred beagle dog colony. Am. J. Vet. Res., 32:2039–2048, 1970.

Clinical and EEG classification of epileptic seizures. Epilepsia, 10 (Suppl.):52–13, 1969.

Cunningham, J.G.: Canine seizure disorders. J. Am. Vet. Med. Assoc., 158:589–597, 1971.

deLahunta, A.: Veterinary Neuroanatomy and Clinical Neurology. Philadelphia, W. B. Saunders Co., 1977, pp. 303–317.

Falco, M.J., et al.: The genetics of epilepsy in the British Alsatian (German shepherd). J. Small Anim. Pract., 15:685–692, 1974.

Lennox, W.G.: Epilepsy and Related Disorders, vols. 1 and 2. Boston, Little, Brown and Co., 1960.

Redding, R.W.: Canine electroencephalography. In Hoerlein, B.F. (ed.): Canine Neurology. Philadelphia, W. B. Saunders Co., 1978, pp. 150–206.

Roye, D.B., et al.: Plasma kinetics of diphenylhydantoin in dogs and cats. Am. J. Vet. Res., 34:947–950, 1973.

DIAGNOSIS AND TREATMENT OF NARCOLEPSY IN ANIMALS*

MERRILL M. MITLER, Ph.D.,
Stony Brook, New York

and ARTHUR S. FOUTZ, Ph.D.
Stanford, California

INTRODUCTION

The First International Symposium on Narcolepsy (La Grande Motte, France, 1975) made this conclusion:

Narcolepsy refers to a syndrome of unknown origin that is characterized by abnormal sleep tendencies including excessive daytime sleepiness and often disturbed nocturnal sleep and pathological manifestations of REM sleep. The REM sleep abnormalities include sleep onset REM periods and the dissociated REM sleep inhibitory processes; ca-

*The authors wish to thank Dr. William C. Dement. Without his scientific leadership and administrative skills, this and all other work with the Narcoleptic Dog Colony would not be possible.

taplexy and sleep paralysis and hypnagogic hallucinations are the major symptoms of the disease.

Thus, narcolepsy is a clear-cut neurologic condition that can be evaluated by polysomnographic techniques in terms of excessive somnolence and abnormalities in the tendency to develop REM sleep. Current estimates suggest that as many as 250,000 Americans suffer from narcolepsy. Disability ranges from minor to complete in terms of ability to function during desired waking hours. Treatment in humans is tailored to individuals and involves stimulants such as amphetamine-like compounds to control somnolence and tricyclic antidepressants such as imipramine and protriptyline to control REM sleep–related symptoms such as cataplexy.

In 1973 Knecht and his colleagues and in 1974 Mitler and his colleagues independently reported a syndrome in the dog that resembles human narcolepsy. Later in 1974 Mitler and Dement began acquisition of narcoleptic dogs to establish a colony for the purposes of studying ontogenetic, pharmacologic, physiologic, electrographic, and hereditary issues associated with this canine disorder.

In December 1978 the colony at Stanford consisted of some 65 dogs, of which 38 animals (16 females) were affected with narcolepsy. More than 15 pure- and mixed-breed dogs had been diagnosed as having the disease, including the poodle, Doberman pinscher, dachshund, beagle, wirehaired griffon, Saint Bernard, cocker spaniel, Welsh corgi, and Labrador. The Stanford group also keeps records of clinical encounters from veterinarians throughout the country with respect to dogs having probable narcolepsy. Additionally, the Stanford group in collaboration with colleagues at the University of California at Davis School of Veterinary Medicine are evaluating several ponies and a miniature horse with a syndrome clinically identical to that affecting dogs. Collectively these data suggest that narcolepsy in animals is far more prevalent than could have been predicted from a review of the veterinary literature. Furthermore, the data suggest that animals affected with narcolepsy are frequently misdiagnosed.

CLINICAL SIGNS

Narcoleptic canines and equines present with paralytic episodes that are flaccid in nature and of rapid onset and termination (cataplexy). Cataplexy is first noted by the client during the adolescent or pre-adolescent period in the patient's life. Of 54 known cases, to date, 46 developed the disease between one and six months of age. In every instance in which precise observations were possible it was noted that the disease developed quite abruptly, usually within a week. Afterward, little change is observed throughout the patient's life. Cataplectic episodes frequently are precipitated by play or the pursuit of desired goals such as food and water. Cataplexy can also occur in what appears to be a spontaneous fashion.

It is important to determine whether any ancillary epileptiform behavior is present during suspected paralytic episodes. During cataplexy there is no fecal or urinary incontinence; there is no excessive salivation; and there is no tonic rigidity of any musculature. Cataplectic attacks can last from several sec-

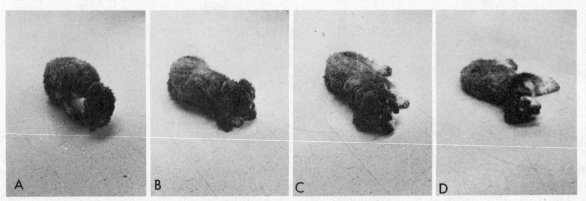

Figure 1. Cataplectic attack. These selected time-lapse photographs (from a series, shot during an interval of approximately 2500 milliseconds) show the development of a cataplectic episode in an adult female miniature poodle. The attack begins with hind limb flaccidity *(A)* that spreads to the forelimbs *(B)* and neck *(C)*. In *D* the dog has regained some head and neck control and has managed to look at the photographer.

onds to more than 20 minutes. Some attacks involve all skeletal musculature; others are isolated to the front or the hind quarters (Figure 1). Vegetative function is not impaired during cataplexy. During long attacks the client may notice the patient struggling slightly, showing brief twitches of the distal musculature, weakly vocalizing, and perhaps making facial grimaces in association with rapid eye movements.

Cataplectic episodes are quite reversible in nature. Petting the patient or making loud, startling noises can completely reverse an attack and reinstitute normal locomotor behavior. In some cases attack frequency is as low as one to two per day, but other animals may seem totally incapacitated by hundreds of paralytic episodes per day. Frequently the client may report that the patient has "bad days and good days." Questioning further, the clinician frequently will notice that the good days are associated with some change in the daily pattern of the animal such as a bath, an automobile ride, or other activity.

FAMILY HISTORY

The client may disclose evidence that the patient's littermates or other less closely related relatives had been observed to show similar cataplectic behavior. The evidence for a hereditary component to canine narcolepsy is quite strong for Doberman pinschers and Labradors. The Stanford colony has successfully produced affected offspring by breeding affected male Doberman pinschers to affected female Doberman pinschers. These direct observations, coupled with several extremely positive family histories, suggest a transmission in Dobermans by an autosomal recessive gene. However, crosses between affected male and affected female poodles and beagles have failed to yield affected offspring. These findings are consistent with at least two hypotheses: (1) different single-allele, recessive genotypes for narcolepsy subtend one phenotype and (2) narcolepsy derives from one or more developmental accidents.

CLINICAL TESTING

The clinician may elect to do clinical tests to confirm the presumptive diagnosis of narcolepsy. Such tests should be aimed at distinguishing cataplexy from epileptic phenomena and from other flaccid reversible paralytic disorders such as myasthenia and hypokalemia. In such diagnostic tests the clinician must be certain that any changes in the frequency or duration of paralytic episodes are due to experimental factors that he or she controls and not due to changes in environment or the stress of drug administration. Thus, baseline and recovery placebo measures of the frequency and duration of the episodes in question should be gathered for comparison with those taken during experimental manipulations.

To rule out epilepsy, suspect animals should not show significant improvement with anticonvulsants such as phenytoin or phenobarbitol. To rule out myasthenia, suspect animals should not worsen with repetitive electric stimulation of the limb or improve with anticholinesterases given in sufficient doses to produce peripheral effects. Anticholinesterase drugs that penetrate the blood-brain barrier, such as physostigmine, aggravate cataplexy. Short-term improvements with stimulant medication, such as amphetamine-like compounds, can be documented. Finally, short-term clinical improvement can be documented for antidepressant medication such as imipramine.

The actual protocol for behavioral testing can vary, depending on the pattern of clinical signs presented by the patient. Several minutes of controlled observation during play with other animals might suffice for certain patients. For others, quantifying attacks during the eating of a specified amount of food may be useful.

TREATMENT

Few data are available on long-term treatment regimens for narcolepsy in animals. In narcoleptic humans pharmacologic interventions are divided into two groups: therapy to control excessive somnolence and therapy to control cataplexy. Electroencephalographic evidence in dogs suggests that canine narcolepsy does have both an excessive somnolence component and a paralytic component. Narcoleptic dogs, when given multiple opportunities to sleep interspersed with longer periods of wakefulness—such as 30 minutes of enforced wakefulness alternated with 30 minutes of *ad libitum* sleep — differ from control dogs with respect to the rapidity with which they fall asleep. Furthermore, once sleep begins narcoleptic animals show an increased tendency to have REM sleep shortly after sleep onset. This observation is consistent with analogous observations on human narcoleptics.

In treating animals, however, the control of excessive somnolence may not be a high clinical priority. Of greater concern to the client may be cataplectic episodes. In some cases it may be possible to satisfy the client by explaining that cataplexy is not, in and of itself, a life-threatening problem to the patient and by instructing the client to avoid placing the patient in situations (e.g., hunting and roaming in dangerous terrain) in which cataplexy could become a dangerous liability. This education may also be supplemented with therapeutic trials of anticataplectic agents such as imipramine or a general stimulant such as methylphenidate. Available data on these drugs in dogs can only confirm short-term efficacy. The use of methylphenidate to control cataplexy in humans is not thought to be of permanent effectiveness. There are no long-term data available for either antidepressant compounds or stimulating compounds in the treatment of narcolepsy in animals.

Another treatment possibility is the use of inhibitors of the enzyme monoamine oxidase (MAOI); however, MAOI drugs such as pargyline and phenelzine have been discontinued in humans, in spite of their high anticataplectic potency, because they have dangerous cardiovascular side effects when the diet contains tyramine.

SELECTING PROPER DOSE LEVELS

The optimum dose levels for drugs that control cataplexy are not readily definable. For humans the physician titrates anticataplectic and stimulant drugs to individual needs. The veterinary practitioner who chooses to treat narcolepsy must use an analogous titration procedure.

A reasonable beginning range for imipramine is 0.5 to 1 mg/kg three times a day. The only route of administration tested to date has been IV, but forms suitable for oral administration are available in various milligram levels. The practitioner should be aware of an important side effect in human males: impotency, which is thought to be related to imipramine's anticholinergic properties.

A reasonable beginning range for methylphenidate is 0.25 mg/kg IV. For oral administration, appropriate divisions and multiples of 5-mg tablets may be tried.

As a final point about dose level, the practitioner should not hope to block cataplexy completely, because the required dose levels may run dangerously high. Rather, some acceptable reduction in frequency and duration of cataplexy should be sought.

TREATMENT RATIONALE

The efficacy of imipramine in controlling cataplexy probably derives from its blockade of serotonin uptake, thus potentiating serotonergic mechanisms, thought by some theorists to control the REM sleep mechanisms and to sequester REM sleep episodes within relatively long periods of sleep.

The hypothesis that narcolepsy stems from the impaired serotonergic mechanisms' ability to control REM sleep mechanisms has received some support recently from studies of monoamine metabolites in cerebrospinal fluid samples from control and narcoleptic dogs. Using gas chromatography–mass spectrometry, Faull and his colleagues at Stanford developed data suggesting that narcoleptic dogs have a decreased concentration and a decreased turnover of serotonin. Additionally, they show a decreased turnover of norepinephrine and a decreased concentration of dopamine. These data are consistent with clinical findings that serotonin-uptake blocking agents have therapeutic efficacy in controlling cataplexy and further suggest that norepinephrine agonists may also be of some therapeutic value in canine narcolepsy. Most drugs suppressing REM sleep are thought to effectively reduce cataplexy.

There are, however, other data suggesting that potent anticataplectic drugs such as imipramine derive their efficacy not from serotonin uptake blockade but from their anticholinergic properties. The Stanford group has data indicating, for example, that other anticholinergics like atropine and scopolamine have marked anticataplectic properties.

Finally, it should be noted that narcolepsy in all animals studied to date is an incurable neurologic disorder. In humans chemotherapies are useful in controlling symptoms but are eventually only palliative. Thus, in animal patients that present clinical management problems it may be better to discuss the possibility of donating the animal for research purposes† rather than have the client administer the various drug regimes and manage the necessary periodic drug withdrawal programs when tolerance develops to therapeutic agents.

---

†Further information may be obtained from the Director, Narcoleptic Dog Colony, Stanford University, (415) 497-6601.

SUPPLEMENTAL READING

Babcock, D., Narver, E., Dement, W., and Mitler, M.: The effects of imipramine, chlorimipramine, and fluoxetine on cataplexy in dogs. Pharmacol. Biochem. Behav., 5:599–602, 1976.

Knecht, C., Oliver, J., Redding, R., Selcer, R., and Johnson, G.: Narcolepsy in a dog and a cat. J. Am. Vet. Med. Assoc., 162:1052–1053, 1973.

Mitler, M.: Toward an animal model of canine narcolepsy cataplexy. In Guilleminault, C., Dement, W., and Passouant P. (eds.): Narcolepsy. Vol. 3 of Advances In Sleep Research. New York, Spectrum Publications, 1976, pp. 387–410.

Mitler, M., and Dement, W.: Sleep studies on canine narcolepsy: Pattern any cycle comparisons between affected and normal dogs. Electroencephalogr. Clin. Neurophysiol., 43:691–699, 1977.

Mitler, M., and Dement, W.: Canine narcolepsy. In Andrews, E., Ward, B., and Altman, N. (eds.): Spontaneous Animal Models of Human Disease. vol. 2. New York, Academic Press, 1979, pp. 165–170.

Mitler, M., Boysen, B., Campbell, L., and Dement, W.: Narcolepsy-cataplexy in a female dog. Exp. Neurol., 45:332–340, 1974.

Mitler, M., Soave, O., and Dement, W.: Narcolepsy in seven dogs. J. Am. Vet. Med. Assoc., 168:1036–1038, 1976.

CLINICAL BEHAVIORAL PROBLEMS: AGGRESSION

KATHERINE A. HOUPT, V.M.D.

Ithaca, New York

The three most common behavioral problems presented to small animal practitioners are (1) house-soiling with urine or feces due to a failure to learn or to retain bladder or bowel control, (2) destructiveness in the owner's absence, and (3) aggression. House-soiling may be primarily a medical problem if due to enteritis, cystitis, or diabetes, but more commonly it is entirely a behavioral problem that must be dealt with psychologically. Destructiveness in the home has a simple but often impractical solution: Do not leave a dog alone in the house for long periods of time. Fortunately, there are also behavioral means to cope with this problem when a dog must be left alone. Aggression is the most serious of these common behavioral problems and can be treated medically, surgically, or behaviorally.

Aggression can take several forms, and it is important to determine the type of aggression because the treatments differ. Aggression can be intraspecific or interspecific. If interspecific, it may be directed at other animals or at people. A good behavioral history will reveal whether the major behavioral problem is interspecific or intraspecific aggression. The character of the onset of the aggressiveness is also worth noting. Aggression of sudden onset is more likely to be the result of organic disease or a drastic change in the animal's environment. Such changes in the environment need not be limited to physical or geographic changes. An alteration of the social environment by the addition or subtraction of an animal or person may influence ag-gressive behavior. Dogs often show aggression toward a new pet and, not uncommonly, toward a new infant or new spouse.

INTRASPECIES AGGRESSION

Intraspecific aggression occurs among strange dogs. A group of dogs will normally form a dominance hierarchy, that is, a social order that determines which animal has first access to food, shelter, and sexual partners. Overt violence is often evident at first, but as the hierarchy is established, subtle threats replace such violence. Nearly all social species form hierarchies in order to reduce aggression and to ensure that the fittest will survive when supplies of food are limited. Cats are not a social species and form dominance hierarchies with difficulty. As a result, aggression may persist for prolonged periods, especially when adult cats are mixed.

There are several factors that may contribute to the development of intraspecies aggression. Scarcity of any necessity, food in particular, increases aggression. Crowding also increases the incidence of aggressive behavior. If possible, animals should be fed individually or, if that is not possible, individual dishes and an abundant amount of food should be provided. A less palatable, bulkier diet, such as meal, rather than a highly palatable diet of meat, should be used in group feeding situations. Crowded conditions not only increase the level of aggression but also prevent the loser of a battle from fleeing to a safe distance.

Intraspecies aggression can usually be avoided by housing dogs individually and by using proper restraint. The most serious problems arise in dogs that must work together as a team. Prefrontal lobotomy, although still in the experimental stage in veterinary medicine, has been shown successfully to attenuate intraspecific aggression in malamutes and to permit formerly aggressive dogs to work together in harness with other dogs (Allen, et al.).

INTERSPECIES AGGRESSION

Interspecies aggression can be directed at other animals (predatory behavior) or toward humans. Predatory behavior or hunting is probably not innate but rather is learned behavior. Cats may chase small, fast-moving objects like mice but usually will not kill them unless they have seen an adult cat, usually their mother, do so. Kittens raised in an environment in which they did not observe adult cats killing rats seldom kill rodents, and kittens raised with rats never kill rats. In general, of course, predatory behavior in cats is not considered misbehavior unless it is directed against songbirds, but predatory behavior by dogs is often a clinical problem. Dogs that kill chickens, deer, lambs, or cats are frequently presented for treatment. The easiest approach is proper restraint of the dog. A dog on a leash or in a pen not only is prevented from killing other animals but also is no longer at risk of automobile-induced trauma. A more drastic treatment may also be used. Many mammals, including canids, are able to learn to avoid a food that they associate with illness. If the dog not only kills but also eats its prey, this phenomenon of taste aversion can be used to eliminate predatory behavior. For example, if the dog kills and eats chickens, it can be allowed to do so and shortly afterward can be given a tablet of apomorphine hydrochloride, 3 mg/dog orally, or the apomorphine can be placed in a dead chicken. Two or three exposures to the nausea and vomiting associated with apomorphine should suffice to teach the dog to avoid attacking chickens. Similar treatment taught coyotes that formerly killed lambs to avoid both live and dead lambs (Gustafson *et al.*).

AGGRESSION TOWARD HUMANS

The most common type of aggression presented to veterinarians is aggression directed toward humans. The practitioner is particularly concerned with aggression toward the veterinarian and soon learns to recognize the two potentially difficult types of aggressive dogs: the dominant and threatening dog, with erect ears and slowly wagging tail but whose teeth are bared; and the fear-biter, the submissive dog with ears flattened against its head and its tail between its legs but which also bares its teeth. The fear-biter will bite when its "critical distance" is invaded by the veterinarian in order to examine it and it cannot escape. Small dogs can be restrained manually and larger dogs can be restrained chemically. The introduction of tranquilizers and sedatives that can be administered intramuscularly or orally has greatly facilitated handling of large intractable dogs. Xylazine (Rompun®, Chemagro), 2 ml/kg IM, and piperacetazine (Psymod®, Pitman-Moore), 0.5 mg/4.5 kg orally, have proved particularly useful. One drawback is the masking of clinical signs by tranquilization. Another is that powerful sedative drugs should not be used on dogs with serious liver or kidney disease because the drugs will not be excreted or metabolized at the normal rate.

Aggression toward humans is by far the most serious veterinary behavior problem. One million dog bites are reported in the United States per year, and many biting episodes that occur within the dog's home probably go unreported. Since most of the victims of dog bites are children, the problem can not be dismissed as affecting only the dog and its owner. The clinician should develop a therapeutic approach to aggression that first uses a purely behavioral approach and then escalates to medical and finally to surgical treatments (Fig. 1). Of course, if the patient is a large dog that has already

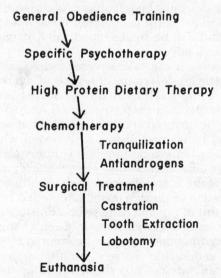

Figure 1. Progressive therapies for aggression.

inflicted serious wounds and there are small children in the household, the most efficacious treatments should be used.

THERAPY

BEHAVIORAL APPROACH

The behavioral approach to therapy involves counseling owners of dogs that are genetically predisposed to aggressive problems, e.g., German shepherds and malamutes. When large-breed dogs are puppies, the owner should make every effort to establish dominance over the animal, because many behavioral problems develop when there is a question of dominance or when a dog is dominant over the owner. Picking up a dog is a good and non-painful way to establish dominance. Play-fighting should be discouraged as well as the slightest indication of threats toward strangers.

If aggression has not been prevented in the developing animal and an aggressive adult dog is presented for treatment, the following should be recommended: (1) adequate restraint, (2) good obedience training, and (3) specific psychotherapy or behavior modification.

Restraint of the aggressive dog is essential to protect both the general public and the owner from attack. No dog should run free, but the aggressive dog in particular should be confined behind a fence or on a leash. A very useful means of further restraint is a muzzle. In order to control the aggression of a dog, the owner must exert dominance over it. If the dog is vicious, the owner may be frightened of it. If the dog is muzzled and therefore cannot bite, the owner will be at ease and able to dominate the dog. Once the dog is adequately restrained it should be enrolled in a good obedience training course. Well-trained dogs are seldom aggressive, both because they are under voice control and because the training can usually proceed only when the dog is submissive to the owner. If possible, the owner rather than a professional trainer should do the actual training, because it is the owner who must control the dog.

The next step in the treatment of the aggressive dog is training directed specifically toward making the dog more submissive. Once the dog has learned to lie down and to stay in an obedience class, use can be made of these commands to reduce aggressive behavior. It may be necessary for the member of the family who is most dominant over the dog to make it lie down at first, but once the dog obeys and stays down for a minute or so for a food reward, then other family members and, eventually, non-family members should give the command.

The dog should be made to lie down before it is fed, before it is taken outside, and so on, until the dog learns that only by assuming a submissive posture, i.e., lying down, will it obtain its needs and desires. This and similar methods have been successful in reducing aggression (Tortora; Campbell).

MEDICAL APPROACH

High-protein diets (24 percent) have been recommended to reduce aggression and hyperactivity in dogs. High-protein diets may alter behavior by increasing the level of the brain neurotransmitter serotonin, which would tend to sedate the animal.

Tranquilization is the next level of treatment. The major tranquilizers like promazine are commonly used in veterinary practice for this purpose, but some clinicians have seen increases rather than decreases of aggression after such tranquilizers have been given. When this occurs, the dog is probably a fundamentally dominant and aggressive animal that has developed inhibitions against attacking. These inhibitions are removed by the central nervous system depressant effect of the tranquilizers. Tranquilizers will be most effective in dogs that are fundamentally fear-biters. Diazepam (Valium®, Roche) 0.5 mg/kg, is particularly effective in reducing anxiety in humans and animals. It may be more useful than the major tranquilizers in reducing aggressive behavior.

SURGICAL APPROACH

Testosterone not only organizes those cells in the fetal brain that are involved in emotional behavior so that the male has a lower threshold for aggression but also stimulates aggression in the adult. The effect of castration on aggressive behavior has been known for centuries, although many dog owners are unwilling to consider it. Castration is particularly effective in young dogs and in middle-aged terrier-type dogs (six to seven years old) that are becoming increasingly aggressive with age. Removing the source of testosterone will probably not be effective in a mature dog that either has been aggressive for much of its life or has shown a sudden onset of marked aggression rather than a gradual increase in grouchiness. Owners should be convinced that it is not cruel to castrate male dogs and that it is as irresponsible to allow a dog with aggressive traits to breed as it is to allow a dog with any other inheritable physical defect to do so. If owners still object to surgical castration, temporary chemical castration may be achieved with 2.2 mg/kg megestrol acetate

(Ovaban®, Schering) orally per day. Castration is of particular value in reducing intraspecies aggression. The American public has long accepted castration as a means of preventing fighting among male cats but seems unwilling to recognize its value in dogs. The female hormones do not, as a rule, stimulate aggression, so that ovariectomy seldom attenuates aggression in female dogs or cats. The exception is bitches that are prone to pseudopregnancy with accompanying aggression. Ovariohysterectomy will usually eliminate the aggression.

In particularly vicious dogs castration followed by treatment with megestrol acetate has been effective in reducing aggression. Specific psychotherapy in the form of submissiveness training as described previously should accompany medical and surgical treatment, or else a re-emergence of aggression may occur.

Aggression of sudden onset may be caused by tumors or abscesses in the brain. Lesions of the hypothalamus or other limbic system structures that inhibit aggression may cause aggression. Conversely, removing those areas of the brain that facilitate aggressive behavior has been advocated in both human and veterinary medicine. As discussed before, prefrontal lobotomy does appear useful for eliminating intraspecific aggression but does not appear to reduce interspecific aggression. Those dogs and cats that were returned to their home environment gradually increased in aggressiveness postoperatively. Obviously, further studies should be undertaken to refine the surgical techniques and to determine which areas should be abolished in order to reduce aggression most effectively. The ethical problems troubling the human psychosurgeon need not be a concern as long as the animal can function as a healthy pet.

If the more moderate forms of therapy for aggression do not attenuate the problem, or if the dog has already inflicted serious injury, a more drastic surgical approach can be used. The incisor and canine teeth can be extracted, thus rendering the dog relatively harmless. Interestingly, dogs so treated appear to decrease in aggressive behavior, as if aggressiveness without the pleasure of an ounce of human flesh, or at least a marked human fear reaction, is not rewarding. Dogs can still prehend and masticate commercial foods, so there is no nutritional disadvantage to the procedure. However, there is eventually an unfortunate cosmetic result, because the muzzle conformation will change as the gums atrophy. Nevertheless, tooth extraction is the most certain way to prevent further harm to the dog's victims. The only other alternative with a more certain outcome is euthanasia. In a situation in which the owners are reluctant to consent to the death of a beloved pet but are concerned about the safety of their children, their friends, and themselves, dental extraction has much to recommend it.

None of the suggested treatments for aggression — behavioral, medical or surgical — is guaranteed to eliminate aggression, although all may attenuate it. The owner of an aggressive dog must be made aware that aggression is of a complicated genetic and environmental etiology and is no more easily eliminated than is any chronic disease, such as arthritis or valvular heart disease. In particular, the client should be made to feel that euthanasia of a large aggressive dog is often wise. If the household consists of adults who are willing to take the risks of serious bites, behavioral techniques, tranquilization, and castration should be utilized. If there are small children in the household, no risks should be taken.

SUPPLEMENTAL READING

Allen, B. D., Cummings, J. F., and de Lahunta, A.: The effects of prefrontal lobotomy on aggressive behavior in dogs. Cornell Vet., 64:201, 1974.

Campbell, W. E.: *Behavior Problems in Dogs.* Santa Barbara, California, American Veterinary Publications, 1975.

Fox, M. W.: *Abnormal Behavior in Animals.* Philadelphia, W. B. Saunders Co., 1968.

Gustafson, C. R., Garcia, J., Hankins, W. G., and Rusiniak, K. W.: Coyote predation control by aversive conditioning. Science, 184:581, 1974.

Hart, B.: Drug choice in feline psychopharmacology. Feline Practice, 3:8, 1974.

Tortora, D. F.: *Help! This Animal Is Driving Me Crazy.* Chicago, Playboy Press, 1977.

FELINE AND CANINE BEHAVIOR CONTROL: PROGESTIN THERAPY

PAUL L. PEMBERTON, B.V.Sc.

Avalon, N.S.W., Australia

INTRODUCTION

Dogs and cats are not as inclined to exercise social self-control as humans are. We can crowd ourselves into cities because our inhibitions are strong enough to avoid territorial brawls. Unfortunately, our companion animals are not able to adapt so well to a crowded life, and veterinarians are now being asked to cure behavior in their patients that is annoying to humans and has a purely psychologic basis. The standard cures in the past have been castration and euthanasia. Progestin therapy often will remove excess aggression from and soothe the troubled minds of pet animals.

NORMAL DEVELOPMENT OF AGGRESSION

Pups of age six weeks and older will wag their tails at every human they meet. They will lick anyone's face, given a chance. As they grow older they become more selective in their displays of affection, until by the end of puberty most dogs are only really affectionate to the members of their human family and to other people they know well. Soon after this they begin protecting their human friends and what they consider to be their territory, which usually includes portions of the street. This protectiveness increases in intensity until about three years of age, when it often becomes a social nuisance. Three-year-old male dogs are the most likely to show excess territorial aggression toward tradespeople, other dogs, wildlife, and vehicles.

Male dogs are more interested in what is happening outside than inside the home. They are more exploratory and like to travel far from home. Female dogs rarely wander far from home and are much more interested in events inside the house.

PHYSIOLOGY OF BEHAVIOR

There are many classic experiments to show that certain specific areas of the brain control behavior. The hypothalamus and related structures — older areas of the cerebrum that are located on the medial and ventral portions of the cerebral cortex — are grouped together and called the limbic system. Different areas of the system have specific and separate functions. These include the control and regulation of (1) visceral and somatic reactions associated with defense and attack; (2) emotions, especially fear, anger, pleasure, and love; (3) fat, carbohydrate, and water metabolism; (4) body temperature; (5) gastric movements; (6) genital functions; (7) hunger, thirst, satiety; (8) sleep rhythm; and (9) aggression.

The limbic system also has to do with the interpretation of sensations, whether pleasant or painful, and with feelings of reward and punishment. Electric stimulation of certain areas soothes the animal, and in other areas it causes extreme pain, fear and defense and escape reactions. The main reward centers are in the ventromedial nuclei of the hypothalamus. The principal centers for pain, punishment, and escape are in the midbrain and the periventricular area of the dorsomedial tegmentum, extending upward into the periventricular structures of the hypothalamus and thalamus.

Tranquillizers like acetylpromazine inhibit both the reward and punishment centers, greatly decreasing the effective reactivity of the animal. The progestins, medroxyprogesterone acetate and megestrol, appear to suppress only the pain and punishment centers, leaving the animal "happy" and still reactive to pleasant sensations.

Stimulation of the perifornical nuclei of the hypothalamus, which are the hypothalamic regions that give the most intense sensation of punishment, causes the animal (e.g., the cat) to develop defensive posture, extend its claws, lift its tail, hiss, spit, growl, develop piloerection, open its eyes wide, and dilate the pupils. The slightest provocation causes a savage attack. Stimulation of the more rostral area of the punishment center, that is, the midline preoptic and septal areas, mainly causes fear and anxiety.

Exactly the opposite emotions and behavior — docility and tameness — occur when the reward centers are stimulated.

Destructive lesions deliberately placed in the caudal hypothalamic nuclei cause hyperglycemia, glycosuria, drowsiness, and docility.

EFFECT OF PROGESTINS ON THE LIMBIC SYSTEM AND MIDBRAIN

CHEMICAL NATURE OF PROGESTINS

Natural progesterone is not active orally and when given by injection is fully metabolized in less than 24 hours. These properties have hampered experimental work and therapeutic application.

In the 1950's a new class of progesterone-like steroid chemicals were synthesized that have prolonged activity and enhanced oral effectiveness. The increased availability of the progestins and our detailed knowledge of them result from their commercial value as human and animal contraceptives.

All progestins have the same basic steroid structure. Some have estrogenic and some androgenic effects; some have mixtures of the two, and some resemble progesterone very closely.

MEGESTROL ACETATE

This is a purely progestational progestin of high potency. In the dog it is metabolized mainly in the liver; 10 percent is excreted by the kidneys. Its half-life is eight days. It inhibits gonadotrophin release and the release of leuteotrophic factors, and has a direct effect on the prostate and mammary glands. Small doses stimulate and large doses inhibit lactation, and very large doses cause male genital atrophy. Megestrol acetate is absorbed into receptor cells in the limbic system, altering their function to produce changes in the sex behavior of dogs. The drug also produces physical signs associated with altered hypothalamic function (appetite, thirst, sleep, carbohydrate metabolism) and changes in behavior brought about by its effect on receptor cells in the midbrain and limbic system. The lethal dose in rats is 200 mg/kg.

MEDROXYPROGESTERONE ACETATE (MPA)

MPA has the same actions as megestrol but is "long-acting." After subcutaneous injection of an aqueous suspension of MPA the water is absorbed quickly, leaving a plaque of MPA that is poorly soluble in body fluids. Studies using labeled MPA showed 75 percent excretion after 7½ months. MPA is less potent than megestrol in producing behavior changes and less likely to produce side effects. It is also slower to take effect than megestrol.

BINDING, METABOLISM, AND ACTION OF STEROID HORMONES ON THE CENTRAL NERVOUS SYSTEM

During the past sixteen years a great deal of biochemical and histochemical work has been devoted to studying the interaction of steroid hormones with the nervous system.

Evidence that steroid hormones can act directly on the central nervous system comes mainly from implantation studies. Many of the effects on behavior produced by peripheral injections of the steroid hormones can also be produced by implantation of these substances in certain areas of the brain. Effective sites are clustered in the preoptic area and the hypothalamus. Implants in many other regions of the brain had no effect.

Scintillation counting of peripherally injected isotope-labeled steroids indicates that certain cells in the limbic system are able to concentrate these hormones. Each hormone differs in the anatomic distribution and chemical specificity of its "binding macromolecules." It is not yet clear whether these binding macromolecules are actually receptors that mediate the hormones' effects on the nervous system.

Testosterone is now regarded as a "prehormone" that must be converted to dihydrotestosterone by 5α-steroid reductase to be active. Progestins are metabolized by the same enzyme and so reduce testosterone activity by competitive inhibition. There is no evidence for a direct effect of Leydig cells, but progestins do act directly on the hypothalamus to regulate the synthesis and secretion of gonadotrophin releasing factors, thus further reducing plasma testosterone. These effects of progestins explain their well-known "antiandrogen" action.

Progesterone itself is the most potent steroid in producing lordosis behavior in estrogen-primed rats, but some of its metabolites (e.g., pregnanedione) and the synthetic progestins, while having weaker sexual effects, are more potent in producing other behavior changes. Progestins are useful in studying the biochemical and physiologic effects of progesterone both because of their potency and because of the possibility of distinguishing different aspects of progesterone function using different steroids. High doses of MPA, for instance, produce anesthesia, whereas megestrol does not. MPA "cures" neurotic cats better than megestrol, but megestrol stops aggression in male dogs better than MPA.

These and many other differences in progestin action are due (at least in part) to the varying areas of the midbrain and limbic system affected by them. Some effort has been made to understand the uneven distribution of progestins in the brain. Corticosterone, estradiol, and progesterone have the same regional distribution: midbrain > hypothalamus > cortex. The extent of retention of these compounds in all brain areas is inversely related to their polarity; i.e., progesterone > 20α-hydroxy-4-pregnan-3-one > estradiol > corticosterone. These results suggest that the high midbrain concentration of progesterone may not be due to the presence of specific binding sites but to the ability of this brain region to retain non-polar steroids.

The progesterone binding ability demonstrable in target tissues is increased by pretreatment of animals with estrogen. Estrogen priming should never be undertaken in the unspayed bitch as it will almost certainly lead to pyometra.

Following the binding to a cytoplasmic receptor protein the steroid is transported to the nucleus, where it takes place in reactions that increase chromating template activity and produce new species of RNA.

This combination of the antiandrogen and hypothalamic-modifying effects of progestins explains why they are so much better than castration for improving behavior. Castration only reduces plasma testosterone, but adrenal-origin steroids and gonadotropins both have a direct effect on behavior.

EXPECTATION OF SUCCESS

The clinician must beware of being talked into treating uncontrolled neurotic dogs presented by neurotic clients who are not suitable pet owners. With cats, too, care should be taken not to choose animals for progestin therapy in cases in which the owner or the other animals in the house are the sole cause of the abnormal behavior. Even in cases in which the limbic system is largely responsible, progestin therapy is surprisingly variable, and prognostication is always cautious. In biting dogs, for instance, results will vary from astounding success to complete failure. If progestins work in canine neurotics they induce, among other things, increased obedience and trainability. Owners should take advantage of this and retrain their pets.

Because progestins may cause cystic endometrial hyperplasia, mucometra, or pyometra, depending on the dose rate and duration of administration, they should only be used for behavior control in entire bitches for up to eight days. This means that, for a nervous young greyhound bitch, eight days on megestrol is safe. The prolonged effect of medroxyprogesterone acetate (MPA) (Depo-Provera, Upjohn; Perlutex, Leo; Promone E, Upjohn [UK, Australia]; Ovaban, Schering; Ovarid, Glaxo [UK, Australia]) at the high dose necessary to cause behavior change probably would not be safe for the uterus. It is wise to avoid progestin therapy is unspayed bitches and surprising how rarely they require it.

Because of its very low solubility in tissue fluids, MPA is not fully absorbed, sometimes for a year or more. Clients should be informed that quite often, especially in large dogs, the beneficial effects of MPA therapy may not be seen at all for two or three months after the injection. Megestrol, being much quicker-acting, may be used during the waiting period. Diazepam (Valium, Roche) and nitrazepam (Mogadon, Roche) are sometimes useful in preventing forced euthanasia of the patient while the progestin has time to take effect. Dose rates are mentioned in Tables 1 and 2, but these vary enormously and can be given to effect without risk. Nitrazepam is particularly useful when sexual desire lies at the heart of the problem.

PROGESTIN THERAPY

INDICATIONS IN DOGS

EXCESSIVE TERRITORIAL AGGRESSION

Overcrowding makes a nuisance of the normally important territorial instinct. Dogs that are reaching their physical prime (usually about 1½ to 2 years old) begin by attacking other dogs that enter their territory. This has to be considered normal, especially in large male dogs. They then graduate to biting mail carriers and then other people of all types, especially children. Note, however, that these are *unpremeditated* attacks provoked by impingement onto

Table 1. Progestin Therapy for Dogs

CONDITION	DRUG OF CHOICE	DOSE RATE	SUPPLEMENTARY THERAPY	PROBABLE SUCCESS
Excess territorial aggressiveness (male-to-male aggression)	Miniature dogs: MPA Medium to large dogs: megestrol	10 mg/kg SC; repeat in 4–6 months 15 mg/kg daily until result obtained, then reduce by 50% weekly until minimum effective dose is found	Diazepam, 1 mg/10–30 kg Nitrazepam, 1 mg/kg Prime with 1–5 mg diethylstilbestrol 48 hours before progestin Retrain dog	Good in small dogs, decreasing to about 50% in large breeds
Hyperkinesis; excess barking	MPA and megestrol combined	MPA, 10 mg/kg SC Megestrol, 5.0 mg/kg	Instruct owner not to excite dog 10–25 mg acetylpromazine	High
Unacceptable sexual activity	MPA	10 mg/kg SC	Castration	High
Hereditary biting	Megestrol	15 mg/kg daily to effect, then reduce	Owner education about discipline	Fair
Destructiveness	Megestrol and MPA combined	MPA, 10 mg/kg SC Megestrol, 5.0 mg/kg	Diazepam, 1 mg/10–30 kg	Good
Night howling in newly purchased pups	Megestrol	15 mg/kg daily for 3 or 4 days	Owner not to respond to howling in any way	Good
Timidity	Megestrol	15 mg/kg daily	Retrain dog; ovaro-hysterectomy if unspayed female	Good
Jealousy and possessiveness	Megestrol and MPA combined	MPA, 10 mg/kg SC Megestrol, 15 mg/kg	Diazepam, 1 mg/10–30 kg	Low
Anorexia nervosa	Megestrol	15 mg/kg for 2–3 weeks	Soft, moist dog food and nothing else	High
Wandering or roaming	MPA	10 mg/kg SC	Castration	Low
Tail chasing	Megestrol	10 mg/kg	Carbamazepine, 50–400 mg every 12 hours Phenytoin, 8 mg/kg	Low when habit is well established; fair if caught early

Table 2. Progestin Therapy for Cats

CONDITION	DRUG OF CHOICE	DOSE RATE	SUPPLEMENTARY THERAPY	PROBABLE SUCCESS
Overgrooming	Megestrol	5 mg/day, reduced quickly to 2.5 mg/week	PERFECT FLEA CONTROL; remove cause of neurosis	High
Inappropriate urination and defecation	MPA plus diazepam	10 mg/kg SC 2 mg daily	Alter social structure causing jealousy or territorial frustration	Low
Spraying	MPA	10 mg/kg SC	Castration	Fair
Bizarre behaviour and sucking	MPA	10 mg/kg every 6 months		High
Viciousness	MPA	10 mg/kg every 6 months		Fair
Fighting	MPA	10 mg/kg every 6 months	Castration	High, but other cats initiate fights
Miliary eczema	Megestrol	5 mg/day, quickly reduced to 2.5–5 mg once or twice a week	PERFECT FLEA CONTROL; while progestins have an antiallergic action in some test systems and are useful for itchiness in dogs and cats, miliary eczema has a strong neurotic component	High

the territory already established by the attacker. They are not the premeditated cortical acts of an undisciplined dog that may have some other motivation, such as attention-getting or jealousy. Progestins are not a substitute for training, discipline, or fences.

HYPERKINESIS

Some dogs cannot keep still or quiet no matter how much training they receive. They jump on and off the examination table several times before they can be restrained, or they run around their owners' legs until restrained by being bound with the lead. At home they are constantly on the move, destroying furniture, digging holes, or barking at things far out of their reach. If they are allowed to join in games they will often bite someone in their excitement. Excessive pointless barking, whatever the cause, is included here under hyperkinesis.

Hyperkinetic dogs chase things like falling leaves and bird shadows. Such animals are usually referred to by their owners as being "high-strung." Most hyperkinetic dogs are female and underweight. Select for therapy only those who have reasonably calm owners.

TIMIDITY

Dogs that exhibit excessive negative avoidance behavior such as cringing, hiding, trembling, involuntary urination and defecation, and biting when cornered (fear biting) can be classed as timid. This behavior may be hereditary or may result from lack of socialization with humans at the critical age of 7 to 12 weeks. It is seen often in dogs purchased from shelters after they have reached adulthood. With great patience they may become confident of one human, but they will remain timid of all other people and of unexpected noises or movements. They overreact to painful stimuli like injections and sometimes have to be dragged or carried into the clinic screaming and urinating.

UNACCEPTABLE SEXUAL ACTIVITY

While libido is basically a product of instinctive limbic-system function, sexual activity is also greatly influenced by the gonadotropins, the sex hormones, and parts of the cerebral cortex. The sense of smell is important in dog sex behavior, and it is interesting to note that the afferent olfactory tract has two branches, one to the cerebral cortex and one directly to the limbic system, the latter being unique among peripheral nerves.

Nearly all complaints about dog sex behavior concern male dogs, but by no means only uncastrated male dogs, thus indicating that not all sexual behavior objectionable to humans is androgen-dependent. There seems no doubt that most of the so-called "hypersexuality" of male dogs is normal libido confused and frustrated by urban situations and the lack of unspayed females. Much of it, too, is due to a lack of owner control. A dog, for instance, that persists in mounting little boys has enough cortical control over its behavior to stop when told to do so, provided the command is firm enough.

Mounting behavior upsets human onlookers more than any other sex-related phenomenon. In one study of male dogs in Sydney, Australia, 4 percent of the 416 dogs presented for euthanasia on the grounds of social misbehavior preferred to mount other male dogs, 8 percent preferred to mount children or adults, and a further 20 percent had mounting as one of their faults but were not particular about what they mounted.

Excess territory-marking by urination in the house is usually ascribed to sexual overactivity. Aggression is also frequently put into the same category, but it is very hard to say whether either urinating in the house or superaggressiveness is due to sexual frustration, territory-marking, jealousy, learned behavior, or lack of discipline, in any one case. The clinician should therefore beware of anticipating an improvement in house-training problems by the use of progestins on the assumption that these problems are based entirely on sex.

Masturbation is a rare complaint, except in male dogs that are kept kenneled nearly all the time, for instance, racing greyhounds. It is usually performed by swinging the extruded penis from side to side, slapping the abdominal skin. Semen is found inside the dog's thighs and on the kennel walls. Dogs are secretive about masturbating but may be discovered because they develop balanoposthitis and cystitis. While masturbation responds well to progestin therapy, for greyhounds in training it is better to increase the work load because progestins may cause loss of keenness to race.

Roaming and excessive barking may sometimes have a sexual basis, but they do not respond well to progestin therapy.

HEREDITARY BITERS

Some pups show very early in their lives that they will bite without warning or provocation. A pup as young as ten weeks of age may bite people on the hand and arm when they attempt to feed, groom, or even touch it. This behavior usually continues for life and does not respond to punishment.

DESTRUCTIVENESS

Dogs left alone in the house frequently destroy furniture, draperies, and rugs. This activity has been observed also in dogs that act terrified of approaching storms. The cost of the damage done is usually far more than the cost of progestin therapy.

NIGHT HOWLING

Newly purchased pups are often presented to the clinician because they have howled all night for several successive nights. Dispensing phenothiazine-derivative tranquilizers to young pups distresses owners because of the degree of stupefaction produced. Frequently owners will call late at night, afraid that the pup is dying. Megestrol is quick-acting enough to solve this problem, and only three or four days' treatment is necessary.

JEALOUSY AND POSSESSIVENESS

These emotions usually involve humans; for example, a dog may refuse to let a husband touch his wife, or a bitch may bite any stranger who approaches a member of her family, whether in her territory or not. A dog that once enjoyed the position of child-substitute will sometimes bite a new human infant entering its territory. Such a dog may also continue to regard all children as competitors for the available attention and comfort. Progestins will only be successful in deterring this kind of behavior if it originates in the limbic system.

ANOREXIA NERVOSA

This responds well to progestin therapy, but animals tend to lose their appetites again when the progestin is withdrawn.

TAIL CHASING

Some severely affected dogs snarl at their own tails and attack them as if they were a threat. Most tail chasers just go around and around, particularly when they become excited. This is regarded by some as subepileptic episodic behavior. Phenytoin sodium (Dilantin, Parke-Davis) has been used with very mixed success at a dose of 4 mg/kg. It should be remembered that this drug takes at least a week to reach therapeutic blood levels. Another an-

tiepileptic drug, carbamazepine (Tegretol, Geigy) has also been tried at between 100 mg and 400 mg per dog every twelve hours with some success. Progestins are not highly effective either, but it helps if the behavior is treated as soon as it is noticed. Many owners think it funny or part of the animal's normal play and so leave the habit until it is too well established to be stopped.

SPECIAL PROBLEMS OF GREYHOUNDS

Greyhounds occasionally try to bite other competitors during a race. Overuse of testosterone or anabolic steroids should be excluded as a cause before the dog is branded a "fighter." Trainers usually blame a real or imaginary painful physical condition, but this rarely is the case. Megestrol is the drug of choice because the dose rate is adjustable and can be withdrawn quickly in case of weight gain or a loss of interest in chasing.

Some greyhounds, usually female, are too timid or spoiled to be broken in. Megestrol therapy for a week is effective, and such short-term therapy does not have any reproductive consequences.

INDICATIONS IN CATS

OVERGROOMING

Cats whose territorial requirements cannot be met because of overcrowding turn to neurotic activities. The commonest of these is overgrooming. Two types of damage can occur: All the cat's body hair, except that of the head and neck, become stained reddish-brown from constant wetting with saliva. Alternatively, eosinophilic plaques and linear dermatitis of the trunk and limbs and eosinophilic ulceration of the lips and nose may develop. Disturbance of territorial instinct can be brought about by such things as (1) a cat and its owners moving to a new house where the cat must try to establish a new territory in an already overcrowded set of backyards; (2) a new cat moving in next door; or (3) the owners' taking in a new cat or dog. *Great care must be taken to see that overgrooming cats do not have fleas.*

INAPPROPRIATE URINATION AND DEFECATION

This common complaint probably has many etiologic factors. Three of them are territorial disturbances, such as those mentioned under overgrooming; the loss of a close companion, whether human or animal; and senility. Progestin therapy does not alter inappropriate excretory patterns in senile cats. Cats suffering from this neurosis will urinate or defecate in places designed to attract the maximum attention — for instance, in the sink, in the middle of the carpet, or on the bed cover. The urine is found in pools on the floor, not sprayed on the walls.

URINE SPRAYING

Inside and outside walls and trees may be sprayed with urine at the same height as the cat's urethra. This occurs mostly for sexual reasons. It may be observed in castrates as well as uncastrated males. It is commonest in the mating season and responds better to progestin therapy than inappropriate urination.

SUCKING

This is a neurotic habit seen most often in inbred "fancy" cats. Animals with mild cases suck the tips of their tails. Those with severe cases suck their tails, dewclaws, toes, and footpads. Skin lesions typical of self-mutilation appear. Some badly affected animals will suckle inanimate objects like a baby pacifier or "dummy." While the foregoing cats respond well to six monthly injections of medroxyprogesterone acetate, those that suck on or eat blankets do not. The condition is seen in the Siamese more often than in other breeds, and woolen blankets are usually preferred.

VICIOUSNESS

The senseless desire to bite and scratch humans is seen frequently in long-haired cats. It responds well to six monthly injections of medroxyprogesterone acetate.

FIGHTING

If a cat has been proved to be the aggressor in fights over territory, sex, or food, it will fight much less after progestin therapy. However, other cats will still attack the treated animal. The end result is a reduction in the number of abscessed wounds and a shift in their position from the front of the body, where they were when the cat was the aggressor, to the rear of the body, where the aggressor-turned victim was bitten while running away.

CONTRAINDICATIONS

1. Diabetes mellitus. Progestins also may occasionally precipitate incipient diabetes mellitus.

2. Pregnancy. Megestrol is claimed not to be teratogenic and not to prolong pregnancy, but the same cannot be said for MPA. Depot injections of MPA can safely be given only to unspayed bitches during anestrus and even then may cause a very long interestrus delay.

3. Estrus. The possibility of causing uterine disease must be considered.

4. Stud dogs. Progestins reduce libido but do not inhibit spermatogenesis completely. The time needed to return to normal is approximately the same as the period of treatment.

SIDE EFFECTS

The side effects of prolonged progestin therapy resemble those of prolonged corticosteroid use. They are fairly obvious, and unless the client is warned he or she may cease therapy because of the side effects without first checking with the veterinarian. *Owners must be thoroughly appraised of side effects before prescribing progestins.* The side effects include:

1. Obesity. This may be due to (a) the drugs' direct effect on the hunger and satiety areas of the hypothalamus; (b) decreased excretion of sodium by the kidney, leading to sodium and thus water retention; (c) altered carbohydrate metabolism, because, while the exact mechanism by which progestins alter carbohydrate metabolism is not known, they do have a glucocorticoid-like effect that, in the case of MPA, is prolonged and may be irreversible, and (d) decreased mental and physical activity. Obesity can be controlled by diet and exercise and by quickly establishing the minimum effective dose. The subject of obesity is well covered in *Current Veterinary Therapy VI* and elsewhere in this volume.

2. Polydypsia. Patients will sometimes drink so much that they begin to urinate in the house. This problem usually only lasts a few days. If it persists, dose reduction is indicated.

3. Stump pyometra. Bitches and queens who have had ovariectomy or ovariectomy and partial hysterectomy are quite likely to develop pyometra in what is left of the uterus after prolonged high-dosage treatment.

4. Eosinopenia. In all 12 dogs on which hematologic studies were made before and after eight days of megestrol treatment at 15 mg/kg, eosinophils were reduced from an average of 7 percent to nil. All these dogs were itchy at the commencement of therapy but much less so at the end.

5. Local alopecia. It is important to inject MPA into curly-haired breeds on a part of the body where it will not show, because the hair over the injection site will sometimes fall out. It takes at least a year to grow back, and when it does it may be white and coarse.

6. Rebound effect. For about two weeks after the effect of progestin wears off, a small percentage of dogs and cats become much worse than they were before. This can be used as a guide to determine when the next injection is due.

SUPPLEMENTAL READING

Anderson, G., and Lewis, L.: Obesity. In Kirk, R.W. (ed.): *Current Veterinary Therapy VII* (this volume). Philadelphia, W.B. Saunders Co., 1980.

Evans, J.M.: Sexual behaviour patterns in dogs. In Post-graduate Committee in Veterinary Science Proceedings, No. 37: *Canine Medicine.* Sydney, Australia. Post-graduate Committee, 280 Pitt Street, 1978.

Garben, H.A., Jockle, W., and Sulman, F.G.: Control of reproduction and undesirable social and sexual behavior in dogs and cats. J. Small Anim. Pract., 14:151–158, 1973.

Iversen, L., et al. (eds.): *Handbook of Psychopharmacology,* vol. 5. New York, Plenum Press, 1975.

Pemberton, P.L.: The use of progestogens in certain behavioural abnormalities of dogs and cats. In Post-graduate Committee in Veterinary Science Proceedings. No. 30: *Neurology.* Sydney, Australia, Post-graduate Committee, 280 Pitt Street, 1976.

Section

10

GASTROINTESTINAL DISORDERS

DONALD R. STROMBECK, D.V.M.
Consulting Editor

The Oral Cavity 855
Clinical Pathology of the Liver 875
Management of Canine Chronic Active Hepatitis 885
Feline Liver Disease 891
Acute Gastric Dilation–Volvulus 896
Microbiology of the Gastrointestinal Tract: Microflora
    and Immunology 901
The Use of Antimicrobial Drugs in the Treatment of
    Gastrointestinal Disorders 913
Management of Diarrhea: Motility Modifiers and Adjunct
    Therapy 914
Diet and Nutrition in the Management of Gastrointestinal
    Problems 919
Malassimilation Syndrome: Maldigestion/Malabsorption 930
Gastrointestinal Parasitism 935
The Management of Colitis 948
Perianal Fistulas 952
Gastrointestinal Fiberoptic Endoscopy 954
Gastrointestinal Biopsy Techniques 962
Laparoscopy in Small Animal Medicine 969

Additional Pertinent Information, Still Current, Found in
Current Veterinary Therapy VI:

Hardy, R.M., and Stevens, J.B.: Chronic progressive hepatitis in Bedlington terriers (Bedlington liver disease), pp. 995–998.

Hoffer, R.E.: Diseases of the esophagus, pp. 931–935.
Hornbuckle, W.E., and Kleine, L.J.: Obstruction of the small intestine, pp. 952–958.
Lorenz, M.D.: A diagnostic approach to chronic diarrhea, pp. 971–973.
Parks, J.L.: Acute pancreatitis, pp. 973–977.

THE ORAL CAVITY

RAY DILLON, D.V.M.
Auburn, Alabama

INTRODUCTION

The oral cavity is a routinely examined area in small animal practice. The amount of disease found is directly related to the clinician's attention to detail and knowledge of normal anatomy. Subtle oral disease is often overlooked during a routine physical examination when the mouth is opened "to catch a passing glance at the tonsils." The oral cavity is unique in that diagnosis of disease there can often be made based on physical examination alone.

The simple task of counting the teeth will often reveal anomalies. Other congenital anomalies such as cleft palate should be identified on the initial examination of the neonate. The deciduous teeth of puppies and kittens as well as the teeth of adult animals should be counted. Early detection of retained deciduous teeth and impacted teeth is paramount to the development of a normal occlusal pattern. In older animals loose teeth may later be lost, and caries may develop, resulting in fractured teeth predisposing to osteomyelitis.

The occlusal pattern should always be examined regardless of the age of the animal. Abnormal wearing of the teeth may be a clue to problems that are not obvious on physical examination. The problems associated with malocclusion and possible pulp necrosis in excessive wearing should be outlined for the owner.

The gingivae should be examined, with particular attention paid to the gingival margins. Hyperemic and edematous areas should be investigated. The use of a dental probe is indicated to isolate subgingival calculus. Supragingival and subgingival calculus should be pointed out.

The problem of halitosis can usually be resolved in the diagnosis of periodontal disease and calculus. However, stomatitis, oral neoplasia, respiratory disease, or cheilitis can often be the origin of the odor. A careful search for the cause usually necessitates anesthesia in patients with stomatitis. Exfoliative cytologic studies, culture, and biopsy are often required for a definitive diagnosis. On physical examination, careful attention should be paid to identifying the exact areas of the mouth affected and speculating about whether some of the condition was self-induced.

Masses within the mouth should be considered malignant until proven otherwise. Therefore, suspicious lesions should be carefully examined to determine size, consistency, location, and depth of involvement. Radiologic studies will often help to define the problem further.

DECIDUOUS TEETH — DEVELOPMENT AND RETENTION

The first indication of a tooth in the fetus is an invagination of the oral ectoderm known as the dental lamina. From this, the tooth bud forms and develops into a cap-shaped dome over an area of mesoderm (the dental papillae) that becomes the dentin and pulp tissue. The enamel covering is formed from the ectoderm and determines the shape and size of the root and crown portions. Cementum and periodontal fibers that attach the tooth to the alveolar bone are formed from the dental sac (mesodermal origin). The chemical contents of teeth are shown in Table 1.

Table 1. *Chemical Composition of Teeth*

CONSTITUENT	ENAMEL	DENTIN	CEMENTUM AND COMPACT BONE
Water (%)	2.3	13.2	32
Organic matter (%)	1.7	17.5	22
Ash (%)	96	69.3	46

One hundred grams of ash contains 35 grams calcium, 17 grams phosphorus, 3 grams CO_2, and small amounts of almost all of the elements.

SECTION CANINE TOOTH

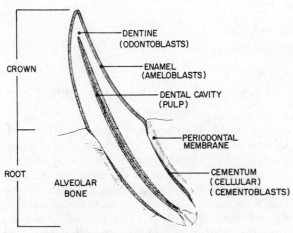

Figure 1. Normal tooth and periodontium.

The dental pulp contains blood vessels and nerves, furnishes nourishment to the tooth, produces dentin through the odontoblastic process, and registers pain from heat, cold, and chemical or traumatic stimuli (Fig. 1).

Dentin makes up the bulk of the tooth. It is a lining tissue that is slightly compressible and highly elastic. Collagen and water compose the 30 percent organic matter content, and apatite (mineral matrix) makes up the remaining 70 percent inorganic portion. The high sensitivity of dentin to pain may possibly be a result of changes in surface tension and electrical charges. Caries spread rapidly through dentin when penetration of the enamel occurs. Dogs are born edentulous; eruption of deciduous teeth begins at two to four weeks. The eruption time varies with the individual. Generally the following pattern is observed: Central and intermediate incisors and canines appear at about 1 month of age, corner incisors at five to six weeks, and molars at four to eight weeks. The eruption process can take as short a time as ten days. Eruption of teeth in larger breeds usually occurs a few days before that in smaller breeds. On the average, the latest emergence is at day 35, with variation according to breed (Ross). By eight weeks the eruption process should be complete. The dental formula at this time is

$$2(I\frac{3}{3}, C\frac{1}{1}, P\frac{3}{3}) = 28.$$

Almost all deciduous teeth resemble their permanent functional successors except in their smaller size and pointed cusps. The second deciduous molar is very similar to the permanent upper carnassial tooth, and the third deciduous molar is similar to the permanent first upper molar. Lower incisors should occlude caudal to the upper incisors. Centric occlusion of the deciduous molars does not occur because the lower second and third lie completely inside the upper teeth.

Resorptive processes start almost as soon as the deciduous tooth has erupted. Eventually most of the dentin and crown is removed, leaving only an enamel cap. This process is complete by the time permanent teeth begin eruption. As before, the larger breeds of dogs begin the process before the smaller breeds. Incisors are first to erupt, followed by premolars and canines. Molars are last to erupt. Table 2 gives the approximate timetable. At this time the permanent dental formula (Fig. 2) is

$$2(I\frac{3}{3}, C\frac{1}{1}, P\frac{4}{4}, M\frac{2}{3}) = 42.$$

The pathologic process involved in retention of deciduous teeth is not totally understood. Failure of the periodontal membrane to detach from the tooth is a possible cause. Osteoclasts that progressively resorb the cementum and dentin of the deciduous root exert their effort in response to the pressure exerted by the erupting permanent tooth. If the deciduous roots are not in the direct path of the erupting permanent tooth, the roots may escape resorption. This is primarily a mechanical failure, since the normal position of the permanent incisors is not directly beneath the deciduous incisors and the permanent canines generally are rostral (anterior) to the deciduous canines.

The sequelae to retention of deciduous teeth are varied. Malocclusion of the permanent teeth is of primary concern. The maintenance of deciduous teeth even for two to three weeks can cause permanent displacement. The displacement of one tooth may cause overcrowding on the entire arcade. Each tooth has a characteristic path of eruption. The maxillary canine tends to erupt rostral to the deciduous canine. Retention of a lower deciduous canine forces the lower permanent canine forward, and the lower in-

Table 2. *Eruption of Permanent Teeth*

TOOTH	TIME OF ERUPTION
Incisors	2–5 months
Canines	5–6 months
Premolars	
1st	5–6 months
2nd	6 months
3rd	6 months
4th	4–5 months
Molars	
1st	5–6 months
2nd	6–7 months
3rd	6–7 months

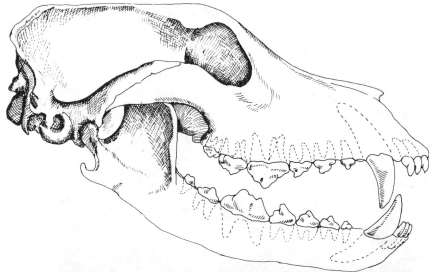

Figure 2. Relation of permanent teeth, shown schematically (A) and radiographically (B). Note the position of the upper and lower arcades.

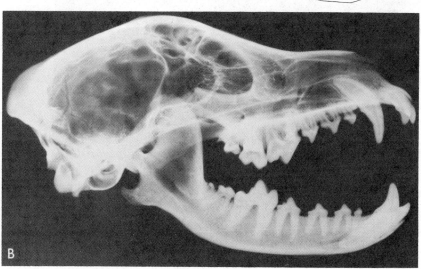

cisors either crowd and rotate or move forward to form an abnormal scissors bite. The maxillary incisors tend to erupt lingual to the deciduous incisors, and a rostral crossbite with ventral deviation of the incisive bone usually follows if a sufficient deviation of eruption position has occurred. Trauma to the roof of the mouth occurs when the lower canine is retained owing to eruption of the permanent canine lingual to it. The lower incisors erupt lingual to the deciduous ones and retention causes overcrowding, with rotation or staggering of teeth, or both. Food entrapment is common in overcrowded teeth and leads to periodontal damage, gingivitis, and reduction of tooth life.

TREATMENT

There should be no waiting period to see if these teeth will "fall out" naturally. A good rule of thumb is that two teeth of the same type should never be in the same part of the mouth at the same time. To prevent abnormal positioning of permanent teeth, extraction of retained deciduous teeth should be performed at the time the permanent canine breaks through the gingival tissue, or at six to seven months of age. Care should always be taken to avoid damage to the underlying permanent tooth bud. Using a dental elevator, the gum is loosened around the neck, and with further manipulation the root is separated from its alveolar attachment. Forceps may be used to lift the tooth out. Good drainage aids healing, and if considerable tissue damage has occurred, administration of a systemic antibiotic for 48 hours is indicated. Removal of the entire root is desirable but, if not possible, the remaining deciduous root seldom causes trouble and is usually resorbed or sloughed as a sequestrum. Problems with de-

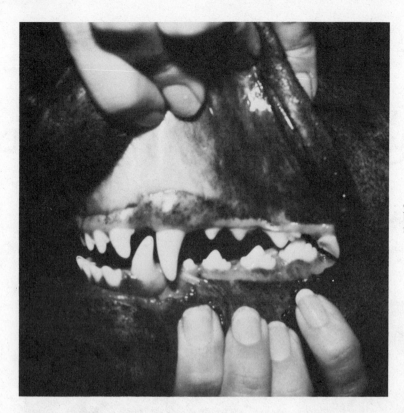

Figure 3. Normal alignment of the canine and premolar teeth. Rostral crossbite causes contact of the maxillary and mandibular incisors.

ciduous teeth are rare when compared with those of permanent teeth. Fractured deciduous teeth should be extracted if more than seven to ten days will elapse before natural loss would normally occur.

DEVELOPMENTAL PROBLEMS

Sequential dental examination is extremely important, especially in the pure-bred pet. The previously discussed initial dental examination includes a careful examination for difficult eruption of any deciduous teeth. A small longitudinal incision of the gum over the unerupted tooth generally eases the eruption. Malocclusion problems should be examined throughout the animal's development. Although the uncoordinated growth pattern of the oral bone structures generally is of genetic origin, developmental factors may be synergistic or antagonistic with the phenotypic expression of the traits. The deciduous teeth and the role they may play in interdigitation may regulate growth of the jaw. The removal of deciduous incisors or canines that seem to be inhibiting the forward growth of the shorter jaw is recommended at 10 to 12 weeks of age. The occlusal position of the lower canine and the lower fourth premolar should be used to evaluate occlusion. It should be remembered that in the normal bite of the dog and cat the maxillary incisors overlap the

mandibular incisors; the mandibular canines articulate rostral to the maxillary canines, and the mandibular premolars close into the interproximal space rostral to their maxillary counterparts (see Fig. 2). However, due to repeated selective breeding over the years, dictated by the esthetic considerations of owners, distortion of this normal pattern has occurred. In the small breeds, especially, alterations in the size and shape of the mouth occur faster and more easily than changes in the size and shape of the teeth.

Many abnormalities may occur in the dental arcade, and close inspection of the mouth at 9 to 12 months of age is essential to prevent future problems of permanent teeth.

Rostral crossbite is generally considered to be a developmental problem, although the genetic influence is difficult to determine. The defect is commonly misdiagnosed as prognathism. Anterior crossbite may be differentiated on the basis that the lower canines and premolars are in proper occlusion and only the incisors are out of proper alignment (Fig. 3). The maxillary incisors generally receive most of the trauma, and flatness and blunting usually result. Orthodontic treatment may correct this anomaly if diagnosed early in its course.

If the canine teeth interdigitate correctly, the condition of anterior crossbite is traumatic in origin. If the mandibular canine teeth strongly contact the maxillary lateral incisor or displace the lateral incisor rostrally, then a degree of prognathism exists. If the mandibular third premolar is displaced from the normal position, pointing between the maxillary third and fourth premolars, it strongly indicates that the problem is of genetic origin rather than being traumatic or developmental in nature.

A unique form of prognathism is generally not expressed until the permanent dentition is in place and the animal is seven to ten months of age. During this particular growth phase, the mandible lengthens more than the maxilla and the occlusal pattern may rapidly be altered.

Rotation of the corner incisors is common. They are positioned rostral to the canine teeth and behind the intermediate incisors. The intermediate incisors may also be lingual to the other incisors. The corner incisors should be extracted to give proper room for the main incisors and to prevent impaction and abscessation.

If the cartilaginous attachment at the mandibular symphysis fails to mature, the central incisors are deprived of supporting alveolar bone. Possible sequelae to this condition include periodontal disease and drifting of the incisors, and occasionally separation of the mandible may occur. If periodontal disease develops, removal of affected teeth may be necessary to prevent osteomyelitis or loss of the mandibular symphysis.

In brachiocephalic breeds, the second and third premolars may be rotated and impacted, and the roots may be exposed on the buccal surface. The premolar with the greater impactions should be extracted to prevent future problems.

Anodontia is a condition in which one or more teeth are absent. This condition is generally considered to be inheritable, especially if several teeth are absent in one area or the same tooth is absent on both sides of the dental arcade. A deciduous tooth may be present and a permanent replacement tooth missing, but the reverse is very rare.

Improper germination may result in splitting of the tooth bud to form two teeth, resulting in rotation or crowding. A unique condition called *dens in dente* results from an enfolding of the enamel, dentin, and pulp within the tooth bud. This generally results in exposure of the dentin at the time of the tooth eruption. Endodontic procedures generally will save the normal portion of the tooth.

MICROBIOLOGY

The mouth supports one of the most concentrated and varied microbiotic systems found in the body, quite distinct from those found in nearby tissues of the nares, nasopharynx, and oropharynx. In early life the main focus seems to be the dorsum of the tongue. With the eruption of teeth, distinctive groups of microorganisms begin to colonize on tooth surfaces, first about the gingival sulcus and then on crowns, to form dental plaque. Dental plaque averages 2×10^{12} bacteria per gram, similar to the number in a bacterial colony on solid medium (Schluger). Within the first days of life, a predominantly (90 percent) streptococcal flora has been established. Other bacteria develop with maturation. Some microorganisms such as spirochetes and *Bacteroides,* whose habitat is the gingival sulcus, await eruption of teeth. Although bacteria regularly find their way into the oral soft tissue, because of local resistance infection is rarely established. This flora has potentially great virulence when introduced into other tissues, such as in bite wounds. Some gram-positive organisms may precipitate dental caries. Accumulation and mineralization of gingival plaque form dental calculus.

The indigenous microbial population of the mouth tends to maintain its balance and resist invasion of its territories by exogenous organisms. Exogenous mouth infections are rare; clinical infections of endogenous organisms occur when one group becomes dominant.

Table 3 lists normal canine oral flora (Sapher and Carter).

DISEASE OF THE PULP

The pulp can be classified as soft tissue composed of blood vessels, nerves, and connective tissue. The pulp supplies nutritive and sensory functions to the dentin and has *no* role in the stability of the tooth in the alveolar socket. Be-

Table 3. Normal Canine Oral Flora*

AEROBIC BACTERIA	INCIDENCE (%)
Streptococcus	82
Staphylococcus	60
Actinomyces	14
E. coli	22
Corynebacterium	26
Pasteurella	22
Caryophanon	20
Mycoplasma	83
Actinobacter	10
Moraxella	40
Neisseria	20
Enterobacter	2
Bacillus	12

*From: Sapher, D. A., and Carter, G. R.: Gingival flora of the dog, with special reference to bacteria associated with bites. J. Clin. Microbiol., 3:344–349, 1976.

cause of the route of entry (through the apex) and the "walled-off" nature of the pulp in the mineral shell, infection and trauma are poorly tolerated by the pulp. Damage may occur through direct exposure of the pulp to the oral cavity, extension of periodontal disease to the apex of the tooth, or trauma.

Fractures and caries may result in exposure of the pulp to the oral flora. Necrosis of the pulp in a chronic condition is evidenced by a dark discoloration. Exposure of the pulp for 12 hours is an indication for endodontic therapy. Brown or tan dentin around the pulp indicates repair of the tooth by secondary dentin over the pulp as it recedes. This condition is most commonly noted in the canines and incisors of older dogs or in dogs with a history of constant wear of the teeth by chewing on foreign objects. These worn-down teeth should remain viable, but the animal's owner should be alerted to watch for color changes or painful prehensive habits. A red or pink color can be interpreted as recent pulp exposure; pulp death can be anticipated in 6 to 12 months.

Trauma may result in pulpal hemorrhage, as indicated by a pink translucent color of the crown. This will usually result in pulpal necrosis, and endodontic therapy is indicated to prevent periapical abscesses. Fracture lines in the rostral teeth may be seen coursing in any direction in the enamel. Fractures usually run rostral to caudal on either the labial or lingual surfaces. The lines may be difficult to see unless observed carefully with reflected light or transillumination. Crown fractures may be simply transverse or oblique with no pathologic damage to the alveolus or pulp cavity. In this case, the tooth should be left *in situ*. Longitudinal fractures with damage to or exposure of the pulp cavity require either repair or extraction. Fractures below the gum line are uncommon except those produced iatrogenically during extraction. Radiography may be indicated to determine whether a fracture is present below the gum line or whether excessive mobility is due to loosening of the periodontal ligaments.

Invasion of apical tissue from periodontal disease is uncommon in the dog and cat but may induce pulpal necrosis. Generally, periapical abscesses are secondary to pulp disease rather than being the inciting pathologic process. If endodontic therapy is not performed, extraction of the affected tooth is recommended when periodontal disease has induced an apical abscess and pulpal necrosis (Ridgway and Zielke).

When necrosis of pulp material occurs, bacteria invade the root canal and rapidly spread through the pulp, eventually causing a periapical abscess. Root resorption due to necrosis of the periodontal ligaments and alveolar bone may eventually result in loss of the tooth. Pain may be evidenced intermittently. As the condition progresses, the dog may hold its head to one side, alter its eating habits, lose weight, and paw at the mouth. Sensitivity is particularly noticeable following eating or drinking. Radiographic signs of a periapical abscess include distention of the periodontal membrane, sclerosis of apical bone, cyst formation or radiolucency at the apex, or osteomyelitis. Fistulas associated with apical abscesses are rare except when associated with the upper fourth premolar.

CAVITIES

Microbial activity is responsible for the initiation of enamel caries. The cariogenic bacteria of plaque induce acidogenic demineralization of enamel. Thus, caries are initiated on enamel surface areas where plaque stagnates, and oral microbial flora finds an environment for colonization and metabolism of carbohydrates to form organic acids. These acids demineralize enamel and alter the permeability of deeper structures. Remineralization is the only natural route of defense.

Dentin caries are common in the dog and cat. Twenty percent of all teeth lost in the cat can be traced to dentin decay, compared with 10 percent or less in the dog (Ross). Like enamel caries, dentin caries are a plaque-dependent infectious disease. Plaque-generated acids penetrate and demineralize the dentin, and proteolytic degeneration of the matrix follows. The progress of caries through dentin is faster than through enamel, and therefore an increased susceptibility in the dog and cat can be expected on any exposed root surface. Lesions often start at the enamel-cementum junction in the gingival sulcus. The cementum will not tolerate exposure to the oral environment and recedes, leaving dentin exposed. The dentin has a tubular structure that permits rapid passage of material; has a higher organic content than enamel, permitting more rapid diffusion of acids; and has smaller apatite crystals, allowing easier acid demineralization. A combination of dentinal resorption, lysis, and infection of pulp tissues results in a weak tooth that is susceptible to periapical abscesses, trauma, and fractures at or below the gum line (Fig. 4). Rarely can such teeth be extracted in one piece, and broken roots can remain as nidi for continued osteomyelitis.

Early detection may prevent loss of teeth

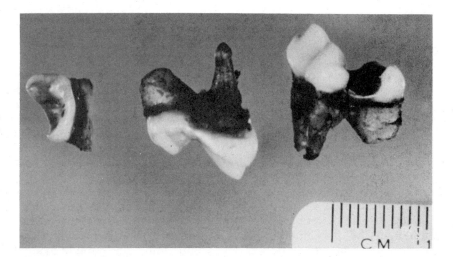

Figure 4. Tooth loss due to caries. Note resorption of the roots.

through restoration. Avoiding introduction of bacteria during restoration at the gingival margin is especially important. A gingivectomy may be needed to identify the caries for drilling and filling. If these cavities are located in interproximal areas, the amount of gingival tissue that must be removed makes restoration impractical. Careful extractions are then indicated. Involvement of more than one tooth is common, and the client should be advised of this predisposition. Because of the location of the caries, the patient may present with what appears clinically to be periodontal disease. In the susceptible animal it is not uncommon to see three to ten teeth affected at the same time. A diagnosis of gingivitis with involvement of the periodontal ligaments resulting in loss of teeth is often made erroneously.

Prophylaxis in susceptible animals includes decreasing gingival plaque formation and bacterial concentrations through daily oral hygiene at home, i.e., diet, chewing exercises, and cleaning the teeth.

THE NORMAL PERIODONTIUM

Because of the importance of the periodontium in oral problems in the dog and cat, understanding the anatomy of this supporting structure of the teeth is important (Fig. 5). The periodontium is essentially composed of four structures: (1) the gingivae, (2) the periodontal ligament, (3) the cementum, and (4) the alveolar process.

The gingivae are the oral mucous membranes and essentially consist of two layers: surface epithelium and lamina propria. The surface epithelium is of stratified squamous type. Only the masticatory mucosa and specialized mucosa of the tongue are keratinized; the sulcar epithe-

lium and epithelial attachment are never keratinized. The lamina propria of the gingivae represents several fiber groups. The basic function of the gingival fiber apparatus is to maintain the free gingiva in close approximation to the tooth. The blood supply to the gingivae is derived mainly from the supraperiosteal branches of the lingual and buccinator arteries. The gingival sulcus (approximately 1 to 3 mm) is the area from the epithelial attachment of the gingiva on

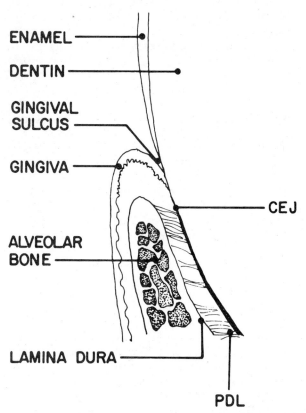

Figure 5. Normal sulcus. PDL = periodontal ligament; CEJ = cementum-enamel junction.

the root surface to the top of the gingival margin. This attachment is generally at the cementum-enamel junction. The thin edge of the gingiva that lies against the enamel is the important sulcus area where most periodontal disease originates.

The periodontal ligament is the connective tissue that surrounds the root of the tooth, attaches it to alveolar bone, and serves as a shock absorber. The ligament is continuous with the connective tissue of the gingiva and communicates with the marrow space of the alveolar bone through the lamina dura. This communication is an important aspect of periodontal disease. There are essentially no elastic fibers in the periodontal ligament; however, part of these fibers are imbedded in bone and cementum via Sharpey's fibers. The metabolic activity of these bundles is greater on the alveolar bone side than on the cementum bone side, with a greater number of individual fibers and a greater collagen turnover rate being noted on the alveolar bone side. The normal periodontal ligament is eyeglass-shaped and is wider at the cementum-enamel junction and apical areas than at the midroot area. These factors allow subgingival pockets to be a common and detrimental syndrome (Socransky). Innervation of the periodontal ligament is through unmyelinated sensory fibers whose proprioceptive functions are a very important neural mechanism for normal masticatory function. Tension on the periodontal ligament, such as occurs in orthodontic movement, will eventually result in bone apposition, whereas prolonged compression of the periodontal ligament will result in bone resorption. Changes in the length of the periodontal ligaments occur before osseous changes develop.

The cementum is a modified osseous tissue serving to attach the periodontal ligament to the dentin of the tooth root. As is true of most osseous structures, cementum has the vital capacity to repair and regenerate. The functions of the cementum can be summarized as (1) attachment of the periodontal ligament fibers to the tooth, (2) compensation by apposition for loss of tooth length in the continuous eruption noted in some animals, (3) repair of horizontal root fractures, and (4) regulation of the width of the periodontal ligaments relative to alveolar bone. The cementum-enamel junction has not been thoroughly investigated in canine and feline patients; however, as is noted in other animals, the cementum and enamel may fail to meet or may overlap in various combinations in some individuals. If the cementum and enamel fail to meet, the dentin is exposed to the oral environment at the epithelial attachment of the gingiva.

Although the cementum has the ability to repair, exposure of the cementum to the oral environment, as occurs in severe periodontal disease, will induce recession of the cementum and exposure of the dentin.

The alveolar process is the portion of the maxilla and mandible that forms and supports the sockets that contain the teeth. The alveolar process is dependent upon the tooth for its formation and existence and does not become evidenced until eruption of teeth has occurred. The portion of the alveolar bone that appears radiographically as an opaque line paralleling the tooth is called the lamina dura (see Fig. 2). Other parts of the alveolar process include the area in which the periodontal ligament fibers are imbedded and the supporting alveolar bone, which gives strength to the socket in the form of cortical compact bone and cancellous bone. Bone is perhaps the least stable of all the periodontal tissues. When bone resorption occurs, it is seldom replaced by osseous tissues. Where bone is covered by vascularized connective tissue, it is extremely sensitive to pressure and tension. As stated previously, because bone is much more active metabolically than cementum, pressure results in bone resorption, and tension placed on periodontal ligaments results in bony apposition.

LOOSE TEETH

The problem of loose teeth is one that confronts all practitioners and can be classified in two etiologic categories: (1) traumatic and (2) chronic pathologic. The fate of a tooth is not totally dependent on its degree of mobility. Initially, movement can be due to intra-alveolar changes confined to the socket and is associated with redistribution of the fluids, interstitial contents, and fibers. A secondary stage occurs that involves progressive deformation of the alveolar bone. Therefore, bone loss is not the sole cause of tooth mobility, and the severity of mobility does not necessarily correspond with the amount of bone loss. In the absence of severe weakening or loss of apical periodontal attachments, a correlation can be found between the loss of bone and tooth mobility but only after more than half of the bone surrounding the tooth has been lost. Therefore, recurrent gingivitis resulting in absorption of the gingival margin and exposure of the root is not necessarily an indication for the extraction of the tooth. Based on the information just discussed, proper dental hygiene, prevention of occlusal forces, and prevention of excessive mobility would facilitate reattachment of periodontal ligaments.

Local etiologic factors concerning pocket formation and periodontitis are covered elsewhere in this article. A careful examination of malpositioned mobile teeth is extremely important, and extraction of an improperly aligned tooth may result in decreased mobility and correction of any pathologic condition in the occlusal tooth. Clinically, tooth mobility is most often due to loss of the attachment apparatus as a result of periodontal disease.

TREATMENT

Splinting is based on the concept that teeth bound together create a multiple-rooted unit that increases the total area of root resistance. In altering the center of rotation greater resistance is created, especially to rostral-caudal forces. In the acute trauma case in which extreme mobility of several teeth is noted, temporary measures may be performed. External splints are easy to apply, and a measure as simple as placing stainless steel wire around the affected teeth or across the arcade may be advantageous. Wire-extending techniques have included acrylic resins, metal bands attached through brackets or buttons, and permanent procedures involving wire passed through amalgam-filled holes in the teeth. The length of time necessary for reattachment is highly variable, but it has been demonstrated that, after gingival flap surgery in man, 10 to 14 days are needed before initial reattachment occurs (Schluger, et al.). Full maturation of collagen and complete renewal of the gingival reattachment may take a minimum of five to six weeks. Devices applied too tightly or malaligned may cause excessive mobility after splints are removed. In trauma cases, when wire banding techniques of the canine or incisor teeth are being used, a period of three weeks before removal is often workable.

In the trauma case in which a tooth has been totally dislodged, replacement of the tooth in the socket within 30 minutes has been used as a rule of thumb in man. Adequate splinting of the tooth is essential for attachment.

PERIODONTAL DISEASE

Periodontal disease is the most common oral problem encountered in the average small animal practice, and the periodontium should never be excluded from a dental examination. The signs most highly predictive of periodontal disease include (1) color changes; (2) swelling, enlargement, or cratering of the marginal and papillary gingivae; (3) bleeding on gentle probing; and (4) periodontal pockets. Less predictive signs include recession of gingival margins, tooth mobility, and bone loss. Signs may be related to current periodontal disease but may also be related to other disease or have resulted from periodontal disease that is no longer actively present.

The first two of the more predictive signs can be detected visually. If they are absent, a probe can be used to check for the latter two signs. Probing of the rostral surface of the teeth usually reveals the most severe disease.

Dental deposits can be classified as (1) plaque, (2) supragingival calculus, or (3) subgingival calculus.

Plaque is a concentrated bacterial aggregation that is lightly adherent and constantly growing. Composed mostly of bacteria, plaque induces gingival changes that are initially reversible. As new colonies of bacteria grow, gram-positive cocci are overgrown by gram-negative cocci. Calculus is mineralized plaque. Supragingival calculus is usually creamy white or yellow but can be stained. Subgingival calculus is harder and is formed in the gingival sulcus. Because the pathogenic potential of plaque is the organism itself and not the mechanical irritation, the beneficial effects of simple mechanical cleaning away of calculus are short lived (Fig. 6).

The mechanisms that initiate periodontal disease may be considered as follows (Mergenhagen, et al.) (Fig. 7):

1. Bacterial enzymes disrupt the integrity of the intercellular matrix of the gingival epithelium.

2. Toxic metabolites from plaque bacteria affect the cellular capacity to maintain the integrity of the periodontium.

3. With loss of epithelial integrity, bacterial endotoxins and chemotoxic fibers gain access to the lamina propria, initiating the complement fixation process.

4. The resultant inflammation eventually leads to destruction of the periodontal tissue via lysosomal hydrolytic enzymes.

Subclinical or minor clinical involvement occurs over a three to five year period before the onset of obvious signs. Often by this time irreparable damage has occurred. A change in eating habits and halitosis may be the first signs noted by the owner. Inflammation of the gingival margins, calculus, increased area of food entrapment, and minor changes in gingival contour precede stages of purulent infection, gingivitis, gum recession, pyorrhea, loose teeth, pain with chewing, depression, and weight loss. In the final stages, tooth roots are destroyed, and depression may be severe. The progression of the disease at this point is very slow, and the owner may associate the changes with old age and natural loss of spirit. In the rarely affected young dog, periodontal disease is primarily characterized by gingivitis, whereas in older dogs bone loss is the common sequela (Fig. 8). Bone loss primarily occurs on the buccal surface of the arcade rather than interdentally, as in man. This loss on the buccal surface results in the early involvement of the bifurcation and trifurcation areas of multiple-rooted teeth. Histologically the changes in the epithelium and connective tissue are similar to those described in man (Hull, et al.). Normally, a few scattered cells — primarily of the plasma cell and polymorphonuclear neutrophil (PMN) leukocyte types — are observed beneath the sulcular and junctional epithelium. When periodontal disease is present, the population of inflammatory cells greatly increases. Plasma cells, a few small lymphocytes, and large numbers of leukocytes are found within the sulcular epithelium, the coronal part of the junctional epithelium, and the gingival crevice. Proliferative response by the junctional epithelium causes the formation of rete ridges into the underlying connective tissue. The migration and accumulation of PMN leukocytes into the crevice is the result of chemotactic factors released from bacterial deposits on the tooth surface. Because plasma cells are the site of antibody synthesis, their presence has been interpreted to indicate the immunologic nature of gingivitis and periodontal disease (Mergenhagen, et al.).

There are six gross stages of gingivitis: (1) insult caused by plaque, (2) hyperemia of capillaries, (3) inflammatory response (exudation),

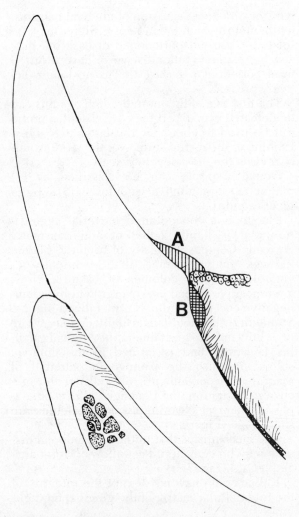

Figure 6.   Calculus. *A.* Supragingival. *B.* Subgingival.

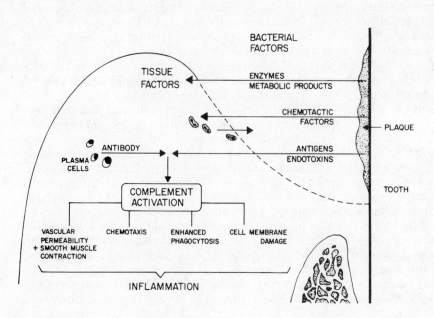

Figure 7. Schematic illustration of the role of complement in gingival inflammation initiated by bacteria.

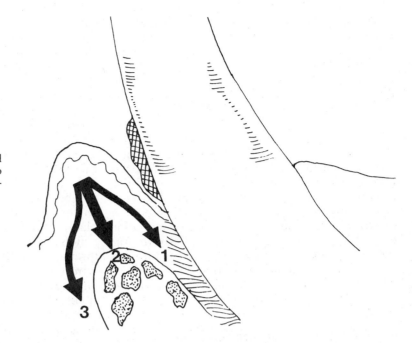

Figure 8. Inflammation may spread into the periodontal ligament (*1*), into the alveolar bone (*2*), or along the attached gingiva (*3*).

(4) destruction of irritant, (5) limitation of inflammation and proliferation of fibrous connective tissue, and (6) repair.

The resultant enlargement of the gingivae can be edematous, as a result of hypertrophy in the acute stages, or fibrotic, owing to hyperplasia in the chronic stages. In judging color changes, the area most likely to be inflamed — the margins and papillae — should be compared with the rest of the attached gingiva. Hyperplasia, interproximal cratering, and retraction of gingival margins are chronic morphologic changes.

In the "breakdown" phase of inflammation the tissues are engorged with fluid, soft, edematous, and lacking in resiliency. An instrument such as a probe, pressed slightly against the tissue and then removed, will leave a momentary indentation or pit. In fibrosis the gingivae are firm and leathery in consistency.

In the careful examination of the chronic gingivitis patient the single most reliable method of determining the presence or absence of periodontal pockets is the probe. If inflammation persists at the gingival margin, it leads to a deepening of the sulcus, producing a periodontal pocket. This environment perpetuates the inflammatory process and "protects" the bacteria. The pocket deepens, and supporting structures are lost. The pocket is therefore the *sine qua non* of periodontal disease. Identification and elimination of the periodontal pocket will help preclude tooth mobility and premature loss of teeth.

Even though pocket depth is recorded as the distance from the marginal gingiva to the base of the pocket, the veterinarian should constantly be aware that the most important consideration is gingival recession plus pocket depth, i.e., the distance from the cementum-enamel junction to the bottom of the sulcus.

A periodontal probe should be of small diameter so that it can penetrate the depth of the pocket. Only mild sedation may be necessary for examination. Probes are available in a double-ended combination with the curved explorer. The probe should be calibrated for measurement for future reference. Usually the probe can be inserted into the pocket. At other times calculus may block the probe and feel hard. The pocket bottom is soft tissue, not bone. The force used in probing should be approximately that which would produce blanching when pressing the end of the probe against the back of a finger. Interproximal areas are important locations to probe. Sulcular bleeding in response to gentle probing is one of the most reliable indications of periodontal inflammation. If neither pockets nor bleeding is found, even in the presence of calculus, there is a high probability that no significant inflammation is present.

Because bacteria are the primary cause of periodontal disease, scaling and polishing are the initial steps in the treatment of simple gingivitis. The readily visible supragingival calculus can be removed either by hand scaling or by ultrasonic instruments. Improper cleaning can induce more damage than the disease itself. The use of ultrasonic instruments to remove subgingival calculus is not recommended, owing to the vibration, the heat of the instrument, and the size of the cleaning tip. Although the supragingival calculus is more noticeable, the subgingival calculus is more important to the health of the patient. Subgingival calculus can be located in three ways: (1) By passing an explorer or the working end of a scaler vertically and subgingivally along the root surface, the examiner can feel the irregular calculus. (2) By examining the marginal surface of the gingivae, the practitioner will often see localized edematous areas or a darkened color caused by subgingival calculus. (3) By drying the tissue and directing a stream of air into the sulcus, the examiner can retract the gingival tissue away from the tooth and have a direct view of the subgingival tissues.

CLINICAL TECHNIQUE FOR SCALING

The scaler is effective in removing subgingival calculus, but a curet is often more efficient. This sharp instrument can remove calculus and is used to plane exposed root surfaces.

There are different methods of scaling, but the removal of subgingival calculus depends largely on the sense of touch. Scalers and curets *must be sharpened frequently.* Dull instruments discourage good dental hygiene.

Ultrasonic cleaning instruments vibrate at as much as 29,000 cycles per second. These vibrations disrupt the attachment of calculus to the tooth. Ultrasonic cleaning will produce a shower of bacteria, and therefore the operator should always wear a surgical mask to prevent inhalation of bacteria. Ultrasonic scaling has become widely accepted and is very beneficial. Because of the possibility of burning gingival tissue, etching the enamel, and causing thermal irritation of pulp tissue, extra care must be taken when using ultrasound. The ultrasonic Cavitron* vibrates at 25,000 to 28,000 cycles per second, and a lack of water for one or two seconds produces damaging heat. Less than one gram of force should be applied to the tooth, because the vibration and not the amount of force causes the loosening of tartar. Ultrasound is not effective in removing stain and also leaves a rough surface that will encourage new plaque formation within 24 hours (Dietrich).

Removal of subgingival calculus must be performed carefully but thoroughly. The use of the ultrasonic unit is not recommended below the gingival margin unless extreme care and respect for tissues are maintained. Instrument vibration makes tactile sensation extremely limited, and therefore injury from overzealous pressure applied to sensitive tissue is a common sequela. Although supragingival calculus is often the owner's primary complaint, the most important step in the cleaning operation is removal of the subgingival calculus. The normal depth of the gingival sulcus is approximately 1 to 3 mm. It is important to use the dental probe to explore the depth of subgingival pockets. Inflammation and edema of the gingival crest may swell the gingival tissues and cause the appearance of gingival pockets without actual recession of the underlying periodontal ligaments and subgingival tissues. Careful probing

---

*Cavitron, Model 1010 or 30, produced by the Dentsply Corporation, 500 W. College Avenue, York, PA 17407. The approximate cost is $1010.

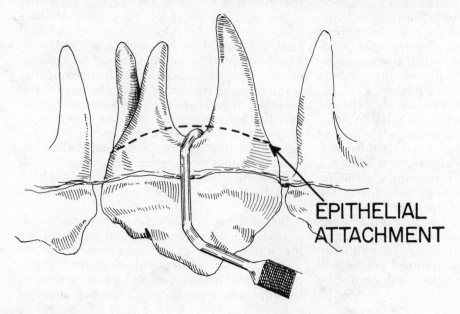

EPITHELIAL ATTACHMENT

Figure 9. Exploring the furca of a multiple-rooted tooth.

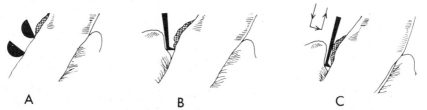

Figure 10. *A.* Curet applied correctly (*bottom*) and inefficiently (*top*). *B.* Incorrect angle for scaler. *C.* Periodontal hoe is inserted gently into the sulcus and, upon reaching the apical limit of calculus, is moved coronally.

is necessary to investigate the bifurcation of the tooth roots (Fig. 9). Although bacterial plaque may extend to the bottom of the subgingival sulcus, it is unusual for calculus to develop at the very bottom of the sulcus. Therefore, once the probe or scaler has found the depth of the sulcus, most of the movements with the instruments should be in a gingival direction from the bottom of the sulcus (Fig. 10). The scaler is the instrument of choice for subgingival calculus of the canines and larger incisors. The number u-15 scaler is best to use in the area of the molar and premolar arcade. The area of the cementum-enamel junction normally has a roughened texture, and a slight bulge may be felt even when the area is free of calculus. When the depth of the gingival pocket has been reached, use a pulling motion with the instrument held at a 40- to 25-degree angle to the tooth. Repeated pulling strokes will pull the calculus out of the gingival sulcus without difficulty. Pushing strokes are not recommended because of the ease with which such sharp instruments can damage the gingival epithelium lining the depth of the sulcus. Sharp instruments are essential to this procedure; dull instruments are a waste of time and excessively traumatic. When a deep periodontal pocket has been identified and the calculus has been removed, the tooth root must be smoothed. Small curets are the most desirable instruments for root planing and débridement of soft tissue (Fig. 11). By moving the instrument in various directions, up and down and back and forth, the root cementum is smoothed and small indentations made by the scaling procedure are eliminated. Directing the cutting edges of the curet toward the soft tissue removes the damaged epithelial lining of the pocket and produces a suitable site for re-epithelialization (see Fig. 10). If the pocket appears to be supraosseous or intraosseous in nature, more extensive curettage is necessary before re-epithelialization can be successful (see Fig. 8).

Careful scaling and curettage is essential to eliminate subgingival disease. Simple scaling of supragingival calculus is not adequate treatment. If the gingival tissue does not return to normal following careful scaling and polishing, surgical removal of periodontal pockets (gingivectomy) is indicated. Removal of this soft tissue wall reduces the amount of food and bacteria that can be held in contact with the periodontium. Periodontal probing to detect pocket depth is done before gingivectomy. It should be emphasized that there is a normal increase in the depth of the sulcus with age. The boxer breed is particularly predisposed to loss of tissue attachments.

GINGIVECTOMY

For gingivectomy the gingival incision should be at a 45-degree angle away from the crown of the tooth. The main point of interest is

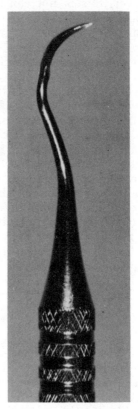

Figure 11. Curet used for debriding and scaling.

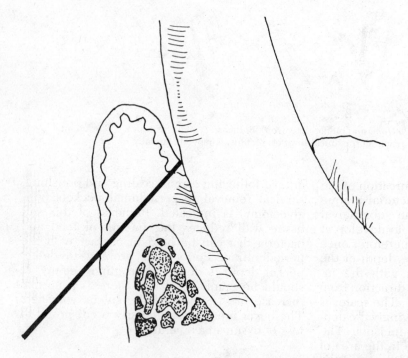

Figure 12. Correct angle of a gingivoplasty incision.

the bottom of the pocket (Fig. 12). All exposed root is planed smooth, and four to five coats of tincture of benzoin and myrrh are applied for protection of the cut surface. The use of electrocautery reduces hemorrhage during gingivectomy; however, this is not considered to be necessary, and improper use of the unit may damage adjacent tissues. Following this procedure the dog will return to normal eating habits within a few days, with total healing generally complete in two to four weeks. It should be emphasized that this procedure will produce an unattractive appearance but is essential to the animal's health and necessary to prevent future loss of teeth. Owing to the nature of periodontal disease, more than one tooth is generally involved, and therefore large areas of the gingivae are often removed at one time.

A mandibular frenectomy may be performed when the frenulum enhances the development of periodontal disease around the mandibular canines. A flaccid frenulum may become included in gingival pockets, causing increased food retention and making cleaning of the area more difficult. The procedure involves removal of the frenulum on the buccal surface of the mandible.

POLISHING AND AFTERCARE

After all teeth have been scaled, polishing is performed to remove all plaque. Rubber cups or brushes can be used with a dental handpiece or a small, variable-speed hand drill. Medium-grit pumice should be mixed into a fine consistency with water. The rubber cups will flatten out as they are placed against the tooth. By operating the drill at a slow rate and carefully directing the rubber cup, the surface of the tooth beneath the gingival margin as well as the crown can be polished.

Following proper scaling, tissue repair occurs in the following sequence (Schluger, et al.): (1) epithelial migration, 1 to 2 days; (2) epithelial coverage, 4 days; (3) complete epithelial coverage, 6 to 10 days; (4) clinically normal gingivae, 10 days; and (5) complete repair, 14 to 21 days. However, if substantial bony defects are present, epithelial regeneration outgrows bone repair, and bony defects are replaced with epithelial tissue.

Oral bacteria can be cultured from the peripheral blood of dogs with periodontal disease 15 to 20 minutes following eating, scaling, or extraction. Obviously, oral pathogens and toxic products have access to the body tissues. Correlation has been found between periodontal disease and bacterial endocarditis in humans and some laboratory animals (Schluger, et al.). Digestive and urinary complications have also been incriminated, but controlled studies have failed to show a true statistical correlation between periodontal disease and malfunction of these organ systems.

The use of antibiotics in periodontal therapy is a well-established clinical practice. Because of the vascularity and suppuration commonly encountered, bactericidal antibiotics are indicated. Topical antibiotics for periodontal disease are of questionable efficacy. Cautery agents and teeth whiteners, usually acidic compounds, can do more harm than good.

OTHER PREDISPOSING FACTORS

In addition to bacteria, several other factors predispose to periodontal disease. Incorrect and abusive oral hygiene procedures, including careless technique in hand scaling, ultrasonic scaling, and home oral hygiene, may lead to early separation of the periodontal ligament. Temporary improvement following improper procedures is often observed, but the condition soon worsens even more quickly. Heredity may be a factor, inasmuch as it influences gingival morphology, tooth formation, tooth placement, and individual resistance to bacteria. In a study of a colony of beagles the severity of the periodontal condition varied considerably even when the dogs were maintained under identical conditions and diets (Hull, et al.). Confinement and soft foods add to the problem. Dogs with food available constantly are more likely to have problems. Because they greatly increase the time necessary for periodontal repair, stress and malnutrition also play a role.

ORAL HYGIENE

Almost 90 percent of successful therapy depends on regular and thorough home care; without it, relief is brief despite the efforts of the veterinarian. Although many owners and practitioners scoff at the idea, daily brushing of the affected dog's teeth is extremely important. A small, soft toothbrush is most effective; an adult's or child's toothbrush with the bristles shortened to a length of approximately ⅜ inch works well. All plaque should be removed from the teeth and the surrounding tissues without disturbing other areas of the mouth. Areas of special interest are the interproximal areas of the teeth, exposed roots in the area of the bifurcation in molars, and the deep gingival sulcus of the canine teeth. This procedure, in addition to removing debris, stimulates circulation that will in turn stimulate gingival attachments to the teeth. A digestible, meat-flavored toothpaste such as Doggy Dent or a *nondetergent* toothpaste for humans may be used as dentifrice. Most toothpastes are detergent-based and are not recommended. The use of chemicals such as hydrogen peroxide and baking soda is of questionable efficacy and may be detrimental to the animal when the substances are used and subsequently swallowed on a regular basis. Experiments have demonstrated

that bacterial plaque should be removed once every 48 hours to prevent calcification of plaque into hard deposits that are not removable by brushing (Schluger, et al.). Most dogs will tolerate brushing after a period of familiarization (two weeks), but if they will not, simply wiping debris from the tooth surface with a soft cloth is of some help. Emphasis should be placed on the gingival margins in this procedure.

Demonstration of proper technique is necessary if the veterinarian expects the client to utilize this procedure. Simply stating that the animal's teeth should be brushed is inadequate motivation. The brushing technique is essentially the same as the proper technique for people. The easiest way to reach the molar area is to hold the brush at a 75° angle, cleaning the inside and outside surfaces of these teeth. The anterior arcade is best cleaned by using circular brush strokes, with emphasis placed at the gingival margin. Dog biscuits (such as Milk Bones), vinyl chew toys, and dry dog foods, which exercise the teeth and gums, have been advocated as aids in reducing plaque formation. Although these can decrease calculus formation supragingivally on the exposed tooth surfaces, it is unlikely that they will prevent the formation of bacterial plaque and resulting calculus in the gingival sulcus, where the true disease process occurs. Chewing exercises stimulate the flow of alkaline saliva, which may neutralize some of the acid-producing capacity of the bacteria. Because the carbohydrate content of the diet is considered to be the rate-limiting factor influencing the number and distribution of oral bacteria, most carbohydrates, and especially sweet snacks, should be avoided. Mouthwashes and breath cleaners are of questionable effectiveness in the mouth. Most dogs will not tolerate the foaming sensation, and swallowing these mixtures may produce untoward effects. For the extremely conscientious client, additional procedures in the form of oral irrigation can be advocated. This procedure can be accomplished using a variety of equipment, from an electric Water-Pic to a water pistol or syringe. Irrigation will help dislodge plaque from subgingival areas and promote better oral hygiene.

PERIAPICAL DISEASE

Periapical disease is a common condition in dogs. Often it is unnoticed by the owner until irreparable damage has occurred. This characteristically slow and insidious process can be present in any tooth but is most common in the canine and carnassial teeth, where destruction and eventual loss may take up to five years.

Most periapical disease originates as an extension of inflammation and necrosis of the pulp cavity. Bacteria may gain access to the pulp cavity as a result of periodontal disease or of tooth fracture caused by trauma. Cysts and tumors can also cause periapical disease. The rich vascular supply at the tooth root apex may help a septicemia to localize and manifest itself as a periapical disease. Variation of root involvement determines which external signs are manifested (see Fig. 2): Upper teeth — incisor and canine, one root; first cheek tooth, one root; second and third cheek teeth, two roots; and fourth, fifth, and sixth cheek teeth, three roots. Lower teeth — incisor and canine, one root; first cheek tooth, one root; second, third, fourth, and fifth cheek teeth, two roots; and the sixth cheek tooth, one root.

ABSCESSES

Carnassial tooth abscesses are the most widely recognized form of periapical disease. The external draining fistula ventral to the eye is the classic sign; however, external signs are variable. The lesion may be a small, hard swelling with subcutaneous cellulitis or a persistent or recurring fistula below the nasal canthus of the eyelid. When pus collects between the skin and bone, osteolysis of the maxilla is often the cause. A controversy exists about whether the single large caudal root or the rostral buccal root is most often involved. Both can cause the characteristic bulging and fistulous tract ventral to the eye. Draining may also occur into the conjunctival sac and out of the eye. If the lingual root is involved, unilateral chronic epistaxis often occurs. One case was reported in which a draining fistula appeared dorsal to the eye and caused blepharitis, conjunctivitis, and mucopurulent discharge. Fistulous tracts from mandibular tooth abscesses that drain through the skin are not as common. Radiologic evaluation may be required to detect nondraining periapical abscesses.

Extraction of the infected tooth is the primary treatment for periapical disease. However, if chronic infection and fistula formation do not exist, removal of the tooth is not necessary. As long as the root is firmly in the alveolus and the periodontal membrane is intact, an apicoectomy can be performed to save the tooth. A resolved chronic case will actually form new cementum and bone to anchor the tooth even more firmly than before. Extraction of the carnassial tooth may be performed using any one of several methods:

1. Splitting the tooth is usually not required. After elevating the gingiva away from all surfaces of the tooth, the tooth is lifted from the socket. Dental forceps are then used to lift and rotate the tooth from its deeper attachment.

2. The single caudal root is separated from the rostral pair by using a hacksaw blade to split the tooth to the gum line. The final splitting is performed with a tooth splitter, and the separate roots are elevated and removed.

3. In alveolar resection, the gum is incised vertically between the rostral and caudal roots and reflected from the tooth. The lateral aspect of the alveolus is then removed. Using a mallet and chisel, a ¼-inch chisel or root elevator is driven between the roots and rocked up and down to loosen them from the periodontal membrane. The tooth is removed using non-crushing molar forceps, and the cut edges of the gum line are apposed with catgut sutures.

4. A high-speed drill is used to cut a hole between the roots, then a needle containing a cutting wire is passed through the hole. The tooth is then sawed in two from the gingival surface.

5. A dental drill with a diamond disk in the handpiece is used to split the tooth roots to the gum line.

Before closure in any of these techniques, good ventral drainage should be established. The entire abscessed alveolus should be curetted by hand or with a high-speed drill. If a lingual root abscess has involved the sinus, it may be necessary to drive a Steinmann pin into the medial alveolus to penetrate the sinus and establish drainage. If a fistula is present, a seton soaked in a suitable antibiotic ointment or mild tincture of iodine may be passed through it to aid in drainage. With good drainage through the alveolus, the fistula may be closed using routine surgical procedure.

Osteomyelitis, endocarditis, and suppurative arthritis may occur following oral surgery. When possible, the patient should begin receiving bactericidal antibiotics 24 hours preoperatively, and they should be continued for three days postoperatively. Penicillin is usually effective.

A commonly encountered condition in the older patient with chronic periodontal disease is osteomyelitis. This generally occurs in the patient who has lost teeth either naturally or through extraction. Sequestered roots of lost teeth will often be noted radiographically. When this is noted concomitant with osteomyelitis and substantial loss of bone, extraction of the roots and curettage are inadvisable until the osteomyelitis is brought under control. Evaluation of individual cases as to the danger of a fractured mandible versus osteomyelitis must be weighed carefully.

Firm, non-painful swelling of gingival tissue unilaterally has been a primary complaint in cases of actinomycosis. The gingival margin may be normal. Filamentous organisms can be obtained by fine-needle aspiration of the gingiva. Anaerobic incubation of the aspirate is required for the culture of *Actinomyces* spp. Long-term ampicillin therapy is usually effective.

STOMATITIS

Endogenous mouth infections are rare. Clinical infections of endogenous organisms occur when one group becomes dominant or when host defense mechanisms are depressed. Attention must be paid particularly to culture and antibiotic sensitivity tests in recurring stomatitis. Cultures should be taken from deep lesions after necrotic tissue has been carefully debrided. Cytologic studies are an important adjunct procedure and can be revealing in selected cases.

Spirochete and fusiform bacilli are normal inhabitants of the oral cavity (Sapher, et al.). Because the clinical signs have an acute onset, it has been generally assumed that another agent or factor is responsible for initiation of Vincent's stomatitis. Severe necrosis of mucous membranes, with periodontal invasion resulting in apical abscesses, has been observed. Halitosis in these cases is severe, and pain, anorexia, and viscous salivation are commonly encountered. The mucous membranes denude readily, and gingival bleeding is common. Exfoliative cytology will demonstrate an abundance of the organisms. Isolation of spirochetes is difficult and must depend upon the ability of motile spirochetes to penetrate the culture medium and migrate away from the remainder of the oral microorganisms.

Therapy is aimed at long-term systemic and local penicillin therapy. Two to three weeks may be necessary for recovery. The condition may recur if therapy is not administered properly. Topical penicillin should be applied orally in solution or spray three to four times daily. Oxygenating mouth rinses (3 percent hydrogen peroxide in equal volume with water) are helpful. If severe necrosis is present, débridement by mechanical and chemical (2 to 5 percent silver nitrate) cautery is necessary. The nutritional status of the patient should be assessed and soft food should be provided to prevent further trauma and ensure adequate caloric intake. The degree to which this condition is communicable has not been determined in dogs and cats and probably depends on individual susceptibility and the inciting pathologic process.

Thrush is due to an overgrowth of *Candida albicans* and is characterized by creamy white patches anywhere in the mouth. The adjacent mucosa is usually erythematous, and scraping of the lesions produces a raw, bleeding surface. The tongue and palate are preferentially affected. Pain, ropy salivation, and anorexia are often present. Although this fungus occurs in about one third of normal mouths, overgrowth does not occur unless the balance of the oral flora is disturbed by debilitating illness or antibiotic therapy. Concomitant candidiasis of the gastrointestinal tract rarely occurs. The diagnosis is based on clinical signs, exfoliative cytology, culture, and a biopsy revealing the hyphae of *Candida* invading epithelium (PAS stain). Treatment is not uniformly successful. Specific antifungal therapy consists of nystatin, 500,000 units three times daily (100,000 units/ml in a flavored vehicle). Nystatin powder or Mystectin-F suspensions have been used with success for painting the mucous membranes. One percent aqueous gentian violet solution has been advocated, but staining makes it unattractive to clients. A 2 percent solution of potassium permanganate mouthwash is an effective alternative.

FELINE STOMATITIS

Although the vesiculation and ulceration of feline calcivirus infections typically involve the rostral and lateral margins of the tongue, the hard palate, lips, external nares, and foot pads can also be affected. Excessive salivation, discomfort, and changes in eating habits may not be evident even when lesions are extensive. The oral lesions can be present in the absence of respiratory signs.

FELINE GLOSSOPHARYNGITIS

Glossopharyngitis (bilateral ulcers of the caudal oral cavity) is often observed in the cat. The ulcers usually are observed just caudal to the last molars at the angle of the junction of the upper and lower arcade. The clinical appearance and size are variable, but usually they are ¼ to 1 cm in diameter with a granulomatous appearance. Culture of the area does not reveal any significant pathogens. Chronic inflammation with invasion of eosinophils and plasma cells is usually noted histopathologically. The cat may present with anorexia and weight loss as the only signs. Although these oropharyngeal lesions can occur in cats without underlying disease, they have been associated with chronic calicivirus infections and feline leukemia virus infections. A lowered resistance to oral infection has been noted in feline leukemia virus–positive cats.

Treatment of the condition involves a long-term series of recoveries and relapses. Supportive care is of paramount importance. Initial therapy with topical and systemic antibiotics is usually ineffective. Vigorous cautery, both mechanical and chemical, combined with steroid therapy seems to be the treatment of choice, but total control of the problem is uncommon. Mechanical débridement can be followed by cautery with silver nitrate. Systemic antibiotics, topical penicillin, and hydrogen peroxide mouthwash are used for one week. Prednisolone (0.5 mg/kg) is instituted on the fifth day and administered on an alternate-day basis for two weeks. The lesions may decrease in size and the cat may become clinically normal for four to six months before the condition recurs. Rarely, the lesion will totally disappear without exacerbation.*

Oral lesions are less common with feline rhinotracheitis. The small, elongated ulcers and vesicles of the tongue and pharyngeal area are rarely extensive. Stomatitis is not observed with other feline respiratory infections but can occur with panleukopenia, uremia, vitamin A deficiency, and the ingestion of irritant plants and chemicals.

The eosinophilic granuloma of cats is seen in the area where the maxillary canine teeth normally contact the upper arcade. Continuous self-inflicted trauma by licking may cause the lesion to appear raw and has been incriminated as a mechanism for spreading the lesions to other areas of the body. The use of local and systemic steroids has met with varying degrees of success. Megestrol acetate, at a dose of 5 mg every other day for 10 to 14 doses, in combination with Depo-Medrol, has been reported to be successful. Because of resultant scarring, infection, and recurrence, surgical removal of the lesions should not be attempted. Beta-radiation has also been used successfully.

SYMPTOMATIC APPROACH

In many patients no specific etiology can be determined for focal or diffuse stomatitis. Foreign bodies may incite the initial damage. Affected animals will be presented in various phases of recovery. Secondary bacterial infection and scar tissue may camouflage the foreign body, so careful inspection under sedation is

*Editor's note: These may be manifestations of the feline eosinophilic complex.

often necessary. Removal of bones, wood splinters, hooks, and needles usually can be performed without incident. Intermittent problems caused by migrating grass awns and porcupine quills may be eliminated only by careful dissection of scar tissue.

Systemic conditions may also produce stomatitis. Resolution of the oral lesions is generally rapid once the underlying cause is corrected. Uremia, vitamin deficiency, caustic chemicals, heavy-metal poisoning, diabetes, and immune-mediated diseases such as pemphigus and lupus erythematosus can produce oral lesions that appear grossly as stomatitis.

Many ulcerative and inflammatory lesions of the mouth are *early signs of malignancy or autoimmune diseases*. After underlying systemic causes have been ruled out, a biopsy of the edge of newly developing lesions is indicated in cases that do not respond to conventional therapy. Owing to the presence of secondary bacterial infections, the neoplastic and autoimmune diseases may appear to respond transiently to antibiotic therapy. The importance of early diagnosis and treatment of pemphigus-like diseases and neoplastic conditions cannot be overstated.

A specific etiology of simple stomatitis cannot be determined in many cases. Culture often reveals the normal mixed flora of the mouth; therefore, antibiotic sensitivity testing is unreliable. Symptomatic therapy is often effective. A gauze sponge can be used for mechanical débridement of mucosal surfaces. Hydrogen peroxide (3 percent) will help clean affected areas. Chemical cautery with 5 to 10 percent silver nitrate is useful in cases in which the underlying mucosa is ulcerated and necrotic. Avoid collection of silver nitrate in the pharyngeal area, or edema of the larynx may result. Cautery may have to be repeated in five days. Penicillin should be instilled into the mouth three times daily. Systemic penicillin therapy is indicated for ten days. Soft food and analgesics may be needed for several days following vigorous cautery.

TONSILS

The paired tonsils lie in the tonsillar fossa in the lateral wall of the oropharynx. They can be located caudal to the palatoglossal arch and ventral to the soft palate. Although the tonsils are elongated, they can be divided into a small submucosal portion and a larger protruding portion.

The true physiologic function of the tonsils is questionable. However, since the palatine tonsils consist mostly of lymphoreticular tissue, they are presumed to be part of the body's defense system. The lack of a well-defined afferent lymphatic system poses questions as to their functional role. The medial retropharyngeal lymph nodes receive the efferent lymphatics from the tonsils. In addition to the palatine tonsils, other lymphatic tissue is scattered in the mucous membranes of the pharynx and on close inspection can be observed as elevated plaques.

Examination of the tonsils is performed routinely in clinical practice. If a pathologic condition of the tonsils is suspected, close examination is required. Mere observation of phlegm in the pharyngeal area should not be used to diagnose tonsillitis. With the tongue pulled forward, the palatine tonsils are usually observed as pink, elongated structures in the pharynx. A fold of mucous membrane that forms a pocket at the base of the tonsil can be grasped gently, then the minor portion is drawn forward and appears caudally as a bulge in the mucosa. Ventral pressure on the base of the tongue may induce prolapsing of tonsils from the crypt.

Depending on the animal's age and breed, the tonsils differ greatly in size, shape, and percentage of tonsil within the crypt. The physical size and shape of the tonsils often have no correlation with the pathologic condition. Observation of the tonsils protruding from the crypts is not sufficient to support a diagnosis of tonsillitis. Color is considered to be the best criterion of the inflammatory status of the tonsils. Acutely inflamed tonsils appear red and edematous. The surrounding mucosa and other oral lymphatics may appear inflamed, and the tonsils may not protrude from the crypt. Under close observation, petechial hemorrhage may be seen on the surface. In subacute inflammation a mottled appearance of the tonsils may represent necrotic foci, small abscesses, or areas of resolution. The inflamed tonsils are soft and friable and bleed easily when manipulated.

Most pathologic conditions of the tonsils are bilateral. Unilateral involvement dictates close observation for a neoplastic condition, tonsillar cysts, foreign bodies, or localized pharyngeal abscessation.

Primary tonsillitis denotes a lack of any predisposing factors for the inflammation. Small-breed dogs are the most frequently affected. Primary tonsillitis in dogs older than one year is uncommon. Anorexia, lethargy, dysphagia, coughing, excessive phlegm, retching, and pyrexia may be present as clinical complaints. Clinical improvement is generally noted after systemic antibiotic therapy. Based on physical examination of the tonsils, clinical improvement generally precedes resolution of the inflammatory process. Recurrence can be anticipated in selected cases, with exacerbations lasting several days. Tonsillectomy is rarely required in chronic primary tonsillitis cases unless tonsillar enlargement significantly obstructs the pharynx or the dog demonstrates poor health between acute exacerbations. Most dogs can be managed medically and appear to "outgrow" this problem. In chronic cases a careful physical examination is required to rule out undetected predisposing factors.

In secondary tonsillitis the inflammatory process of the tonsils can be attributed to concomitant systemic or local predisposing factors. The presence of obvious tonsillitis does not indicate the site of primary disease and should not be used as a "catch-all" diagnosis. Because of the lymphoreticular nature of the tonsils, any chronic irritation or inflammatory process of the oral cavity or pharynx, e.g., abscessation, gingivitis, chronic oral foreign body, chronic vomiting, or regurgitation, may induce a tonsillar reaction. The gagging and spitting up of foam described in cases of tonsillitis necessitate the differentiation of megaesophagus, pylorospasm, cricopharyngeal achalasia, chronic productive coughs, retropharyngeal abscesses, foreign bodies, and other conditions from primary tonsillitis.

Medical treatment of tonsillitis through the use of systemic broad-spectrum antibiotics, supportive care, and analgesics is generally rewarding. Culture of inflamed tonsils produces *Streptococcus* (beta-hemolytic), coliform organisms, and normal oral flora. Tonsillectomy is usually not needed in the acute inflammatory stage.

Gross tonsillar enlargement may cause dysphagia and dyspnea in breeds with a narrow oropharynx, such as cocker spaniels and brachycephalic breeds with a predisposition to upper airway disease. Primary or secondary metastatic neoplasia should always be suspected in cases of chronic tonsillitis. The predilection for squamous cell carcinomas to metastasize to regional lymph nodes and to be locally invasive dictates early diagnosis if extirpation is to be successful. Unlike squamous cell carcinomas, which are most commonly unilateral, lymphosarcoma usually occurs bilaterally, with enlargement of the retropharyngeal lymph nodes.

PREHENSILE DYSFUNCTION

The common clinical complaint of anorexia may often be related to an animal's inability to open its mouth or pain on opening the mouth. Differential diagnosis of such a condition should include retrobulbar abscess, abscess of the zygomatic gland, oral foreign bodies, inflammatory myositis, myofascitis, fractures of the mandibular joint, cranial mandibular osteoarthropathy, and trauma to soft tissues or periosteum. Pain on opening the jaws concomitant with pyrexia and exophthalmos should be an indication for careful examination for a retrobulbar abscess, either secondary to a penetrating foreign body or due to sialadenitis of the zygomatic gland. Careful examination under sedation may demonstrate inflammation of the oral tissues caudal to the last upper molar, with a focal area of inflammation or edema. Draining of the abscess through an incision in this area, combined with 14 days of systemic antibiotic therapy, is generally effective treatment. Both of these steps are indicated and adequate drainage is an important step.

Other conditions may present with pyrexia that is due to pain or inflammation. Myositis can be attributed to several causes. Eosinophilic myositis has been described in larger breeds of dogs such as the German shepherd. There is bilaterally symmetric swelling of the masseter, temporalis, and pterygoid muscles, and other skeletal musculature may be involved. Exophthalmos may lead to exposure keratitis. Extreme pain is a classic sign in the acute syndrome; however, pain may be absent if fibrosis has become a sequela to repeated attacks. The hemogram may reveal a marked absolute eosinophilia; however, this varies with the stage of the disease. Electromyographic studies have demonstrated positive spike waves with fibrillation potentials. Muscle biopsy is necessary for definitive diagnosis. Histologically, mononuclear cells, hemorrhage, and muscle fiber necrosis are noted. Treatment generally involves supportive therapy and corticosteroids in an effort to allow the animal to maintain adequate body functions until mastication becomes normal. However, inability to open the mouth may be noted in recurrent cases when atrophy and fibrosis are evident. This condition may appear unilaterally and must be differentiated from acute trauma. In severe trauma to the masseter muscle area, periostitis may be demonstrated radiographically. Electromyographic studies of acute trauma conditions are generally normal. However, if disuse atrophy is severe, fibrosis may be noted. Included in the differential diagnosis should be deinnervation atrophy. An electromyographic examination seven to ten days after the insult may demonstrate deinnervation changes. In the acute trauma case corticosteroid therapy and rest, in addition to tube feeding or feeding through an esophagostomy tube, are indicated.

Myofascitis has been noted in several young dogs that showed extreme pain. As in any myositis condition, fibrosis at the time of presentation may be noted as an inability to open the mouth. Generally, a mild or moderate attack of myofascitis is noted at 8 to 12 months of age and may last from several days to two weeks. The attacks occur with regular frequency until the animal is 1½ to 2 years old. The symptoms seem to be responsive to corticosteroid therapy. As the dog matures, the attacks decrease in intensity and duration until the animal becomes asymptomatic. However, repeated attacks, if they are not treated, may result in permanent fibrosis.

Regardless of the etiology, atrophic myositis may be diagnosed clinically when the animal is presented with atrophy of the head musculature and the masseter muscles. Common presenting signs include the observation that the dog chews bones with its front teeth only or is unable to open its mouth wide enough to catch a ball or stick. It may affect any breed of dog, and the presentation with inability to open the mouth even under general anesthesia is diagnostic. This condition may be unilateral or bilateral.

Inflammation and fibrosis on one side may lead to disuse atrophy on the opposite side. Electromyographically, the abnormal side demonstrates increased insertional activity, positive sharp waves, fibrillation potentials, and myopathic potentials. Large muscle areas may have complete electrical silence, which is indicative of complete fibrosis. Several muscle biopsies are needed to demonstrate the pathologic state, which is a mixture of fibrosis, lymphocytic infiltration, and adipose tissue deposition. In these cases the prognosis is poor. Mechanical methods for opening the mouth and breaking down fibrotic tissue are not recommended. The resulting trauma and muscle tearing may only aggravate the course of the condition. Corticosteroids (1.0 mg/kg prednisolone, every other day) and emphasis on jaw exercises for the dog are important in the clinical management. The client should be encouraged to make the dog chew in an effort to decrease the changes of disuse atrophy and keep fibrosis at a minimum. Inability to open the mouth as a sequela always dictates a poor prognosis. It is not uncommon for a patient with an inability to open the mouth and a tentative diagnosis of myositis to be diagnosed ultimately as having masseter muscle atrophy secondary to arthritis of the temporomandibular joint.

Fractures of the mandible or temporomandibular joint and dislocation of the temporomandibular joint often present with pain on manipulation of the jaws. If crepitation is noted on opening the jaw and is localized to the temporomandibular joint, luxation in this joint should not be presumed automatically. Radiographs are necessary to rule out fractures in this area. If luxation is noted in the absence of any fractures, a ½-inch piece of wood can be placed between the last molars on the affected side. Utilizing the wood as a fulcrum, the mandibular symphysis and nose are pulled together, as if to close the jaws. This maneuver elevates the temporomandibular joint into proper apposition. It should be emphasized that this should be performed only in the confirmed absence of any fractures of the oral structures. When luxation of the mandible, including locking of the coronoid process with the zygomatic arch, is present, the dog is unable to close its mouth. The structures can be disarticulated under general anesthesia.

Cranial mandibular osteoarthropathy may also present as the inability to open the mouth. This periosteal exostosis is classically observed in young West Highland white and Scottish terriers. Although other breeds can be affected, age, breed, and clinical presentation make the diagnosis obvious. It is generally considered to be a self-limiting disease; however, supportive therapy is often needed to maintain these animals in a proper state of nutrition until recovery. An esophagostomy tube is rarely needed in this condition.

Other conditions that may present with pain on opening the jaws include oral foreign bodies, acute stomatitis, and insect bites involving the oral mucous membranes. Differential diagnosis is usually based on physical examination. As in any condition involving the oral structures, in which adequate examination cannot be performed on the examination table, general anesthesia or sedation is indicated. This will facilitate a proper, adequate, and thorough oral examination.

SUPPLEMENTAL READING

Brody, R.S.: Canine and feline neoplasma. Adv. Vet. Sci. Comp. Med., *14*:309–354, 1970.
Dietrich, U.B.: Dental care: Prophylaxis and therapy. Canine Practice, *3*:44–53, April 1976.
Harvey, C.E., and O'Brien, J.A.: Disorders of oropharynx and salivary glands. In Ettinger, S.J.: *Veterinary Internal Medicine.* Philadelphia, W.B. Saunders Co., 1975.
Hess, P.W., and Meierhenry, E.F.: Management of canine and feline oral and pharyngeal tumors. Proceedings of 41st Annual Meeting, AAHA, 1974, pp. 122–125.
Hull, P.S., Soames, J.V., and Davies, R.M.: Periodontal disease in a beagle colony. J. Comp. Pathol., *84*:143, 1974.
Mergenhagen, S.E., Tempel, T.R., and Snyderman, R.: Immunologic reactions and periodontal inflammation. J. Dent. Res., *49*:256, 1970.
Ridgway, R.L., and Zielke, D.R.: Non-surgical endodontic technique for dogs. J. Am. Vet. Med. Assoc., *174*:82, 1979.
Ross, D.L.: The oral cavity. In Kirk, R.W. (ed.): *Current Veterinary Therapy VII.* Philadelphia, W.B. Saunders Co., 1977.
Saphir, D.A., and Carter, G.R.: Gingival flora of the dog, with special reference to bacteria associated with bites. J. Clin. Microbiol., *3*:344–349, 1976.
Schluger, S., Yuodelis, R.A., and Page, R.C., *Periodontal Disease.* Philadelphia, Lea & Febiger, 1977.
Socransky, S.S.: Relationship of bacteria to the etiology of periodontal disease. J. Dent. Res., *49*:203, 1970.

CLINICAL PATHOLOGY OF THE LIVER

BERNARD F. FELDMAN, D.V.M.

Davis, California

The liver is the factory of the body. It manufactures plasma proteins, including albumin and the alpha and beta globulins, as well as most of the coagulation proteins. It manufactures lipids and esterifies cholesterol. It synthesizes glycogen for energy storage and stores vitamins D and B_{12} and iron. It detoxifies or inactivates many drugs and other substances, including ammonia and the steroid hormones. It secretes cholesterol, bile pigments, and bile salts; bile salts aid in the emulsification of dietary fats prior to digestion. Liver function tests are based on these activities. Other tests indicate liver cell damage or death by demonstrating the activity of enzymes released in these processes.

No single test can be used alone to evaluate liver function fully in health or disease. Hence, examination of the liver begins with the history and physical examination and progresses

Table 1. *Hemogram Parameters Affected by Liver Disease*

Hematocrit, hemoglobin, red blood cell count: May be decreased

Red cell indices: In advanced liver disease may be macrocytic and normochromic

Icterus index: Elevated

Total protein: Decreases because of decrease in albumin with advanced disease; increases in globulin may offset the albumin decrease

Fibrinogen: Variable, but may decrease with advanced disease

Red cell morphology: Elevation in serum lipid levels may cause spiculation (acanthocytes)

Neutrophils: May be toxic (Döhle bodies, toxic granulation, vacuolization)

Table 3. *Biochemical Parameters Affected by Liver Disease*

Alanine aminotransferase (GPT): Elevated in liver cell damage; hepatospecific in dog, cat, man and non-human primates

Alkaline phosphatase: Obstruction of biliary tree causes enzyme induction (occurs on the hepatocyte membrane)

Asparate aminotransferase (GOT): Elevations exhibited in liver cell damage as well as in muscle damage

Bilirubin (direct, indirect, and total): Variable, depending on the problem

Calcium: May be a physiologic decrease caused by decrease in albumin

Cholesterol: Variable, depending on problems; elevated in obstructive disease, decreased in severe diffuse liver disease

Glucose: Severe diffuse liver disease as well as glycogen storage diseases may cause decreases

Lactate dehydrogenase: Slow-moving fraction elevated with liver cell damage

Sorbitol dehydrogenase: Hepatocellular damage causes increases in common domestic animals

Urea nitrogen: May be lower than normal in diffuse liver disease; in any case, is no longer reflective of glomerular filtration rate

through hematologic studies, urinalyses, clinical biochemistries (Tables 1 to 3), radiology and histopathologic tests. Most laboratory parameters are innocuous and non-specific in determining hepatic involvement. No single liver test is always reliable, and a single test may be normal despite abnormal results in other liver tests. Because of the unreliability of any single test for diagnosing liver disease, a large number of liver tests have been developed and new ones are being developed every year. The purpose of this article is to review the currently most widely used liver tests and the basis for their use in terms of the physiologic function of the liver. Liver tests will be discussed in the following functional categories: (1) cholestasis, (2) hepatocellular disease and leakage, (3) acquired blood coagulation defects, (4) reduction of functional hepatic mass, (5) lipid metabolism in liver disease, (6) tests of synthesizing and detoxifying ability as liver tests, and (7) liver biopsy. A discussion based on the diagnostic parameters of specific disease processes follows these discussions.

CHOLESTASIS

In general, serum bilirubin measurements are not sensitive indicators of hepatic damage

Table 2. *Urine Parameters Affected by Liver Disease*

Bilirubin: Presence is compared with serum levels

Urobilinogen: Increased in hemolytic disease; decreased in obstructive hepatic lesions (see text)

Crystals:
1. Ammonium biurate: Elevated in portosystemic shunting (*normal* in the Dalmatian)
2. Aminoaciduria: Leucine or tyrosine crystals in the urinary sediment (an overflow effect)
3. Bilirubin crystals: May reflect hyperbilirubinuria

but, in spite of their insensitivity, various tests of bilirubin and its metabolic products can yield useful information in evaluating liver disease. Bilirubin is a yellow pigment composed of four pyrrole rings. It is derived largely (80 to 90 percent) from hemoglobin released in the destruction of red blood cells by cells of the reticuloendothelial system — especially those of the spleen. Some additional bilirubin comes from catabolism of related substances, including myoglobin and the cytochromes. Bilirubin is insoluble in water at normal blood pH but is carried in the plasma bound to albumin. In the liver it crosses the parenchymal cell membranes, is conjugated in the presence of glucuronyl transferase to bilirubin diglucuronide (which is water-soluble), and is then secreted into the bile. Conjugated (but *not* unconjugated) bilirubin is excreted into the urine.* The canine kidney has a low threshold for conjugated bilirubin. However, most of it passes into the bile and is converted to fecal urobilinogen in the small and large bowels by bacterial enzymes. Some urobilinogen is reabsorbed into the blood stream and subsequently excreted into the urine or back into the bile. Most is oxidized to stercobilin, a brown pigment excreted in the feces. When there is excessive production of bilirubin, as occurs in the hemolytic anemias, the concentration of unconjugated bilirubin in the serum is elevated. This may also

---

*Synonyms for bilirubin: *Unconjugated* bilirubin: protein-bound, water-insoluble, fat-soluble, free or *indirect* reacting. *Conjugated* bilirubin: water-soluble, fat-insoluble, *direct* reacting.

occur as the result of decreased liver uptake of bilirubin (Gilbert's syndrome in man) and reduced conjugation in the liver (Crigler-Najjar syndrome in man). In diseases causing liver cell damage the unconjugated bilirubin level is also evaluated.

The term "direct reacting bilirubin" refers to bilirubin diglucuronide, which, because it is water-soluble, reacts directly with Ehrlich's color reagent (diazotized sulfanilic acid). Unconjugated bilirubin has been called "indirect reacting" because, being water-soluble, it requires the addition of alcohol or some other similar reagent to enable it to react with the color reagent. Obstruction of the flow of bile causes elevated serum levels of conjugated bilirubin. This fraction is also elevated in diseases causing liver cell damage. Jaundice (icterus) can occur as a result of excessive production of bilirubin, impaired conjugation or excretion of bilirubin by liver cells, or obstruction of bile flow. Jaundice becomes clinically apparent when the total serum bilirubin level reaches about double the upper limit of normal.

The numerical difference between the total bilirubin and conjugated bilirubin values equals the unconjugated bilirubin value. This test has no value unless the total bilirubin level is elevated. At low concentrations the test is not sensitive enough to differentiate conjugated from unconjugated bilirubin. This simple test, however, often suffices to identify the cause of jaundice. When jaundice results from excessive hemolysis, 85 percent or more of serum bilirubin is unconjugated and, while there is no increase in urine bilirubin levels, urine and stool urobilinogen concentrations are increased. When jaundice results from defective liver cell function, as occurs in hepatitis, or

when it results from obstruction of the flow of bile, usually less than 50 percent of serum bilirubin is unconjugated; urine bilirubin levels are increased, urine urobilinogen and stool urobilinogen levels are decreased. When there is complete obstruction, as may result from carcinoma of the head of the pancreas, urine and stool urobilinogen values may be totally absent. Patients with cirrhosis have 50 to 70 percent unconjugated serum bilirubin. Bilirubinuria caused by cholestasis often precedes the onset of or occurs in the absence of hyperbilirubinemia. It should accompany a high serum alkaline phosphatase level. Bilirubinuria is occasionally observed in animals with hemolytic disease. There is some indication that the canine kidney can degrade increased levels of hemoglobin to bilirubin.

Urinary urobilinogen determination may be useful to differentiate partial or complete biliary obstruction. A positive urine urobilinogen test indicates that the bile duct is at least partially patent. A negative urobilinogen test, while it can occur with complete bile duct obstruction, occurs more commonly as the result of improper urine handling (excessive time from sampling to test), oral antibiotic therapy, or diarrhea. Laboratory findings in cholestatic and hemolytic hyperbilirubinemic disorders are summarized in Table 4.

Of course, it is important to distinguish liver cell damage from extrahepatic obstruction, because the latter is an indication for exploratory surgery, whereas the prognosis may be worsened if laparotomy is performed in patients with hepatitis. One useful laboratory test for this purpose is a measurement of serum alkaline phosphatase. This serum enzyme may come from liver, bone, and intestine. The liver frac-

Table 4. *Use of Bilirubin in the Differential Diagnosis of Jaundice*

TEST	SAMPLE	NORMAL RANGE (Dog)	HEMOLYTIC	OBSTRUCTIVE	HEPATOCELLULAR
BLOOD					
Bilirubin (mg/dl)	Serum				
Total		0–0.6	Greatly increased	Increased	Increased
Direct		0–0.3	Normal or increased	Increased	Increased
Indirect		0–0.3	Increased	Increased	Increased
Alkaline phosphatase (IU/liter)	Serum	42.6–201	Normal	3- to 8-fold increase	1- to 3-fold increase
URINE					
Bilirubin	Fresh urine	0	0	Positive	Positive
Urobilirubin	Fresh urine	1–2+	Normal or increased	Normal or decreased	Increased

tion is normally excreted in the bile. Elevation of serum alkaline phosphatase to levels three times the upper level of normal or more occurs in obstructive jaundice, whereas the majority of patients with liver cell damage have values lower than that. Serum alkaline phosphatase activity also increases through induction by corticosteroids, either iatrogenic or in hyperadrenocorticism. Increased osteoblastic activity in hyperparathyroidism and canine panosteitis also increases serum alkaline phosphatase. Many forms of neoplasia, e.g., sarcomas, carcinomas, and mixed mammary tumors, cause increases in serum alkaline phosphatase, although the source is unknown. With liver cell damage the elevation of alkaline phosphatase results from some degree of intrahepatic cholestasis. Patients with liver cell damage also tend to have elevations in alanine aminotransferase (ALT,GPT), aspartate aminotransferase (AST,GOT) and gamma glutamyl transpeptidase (GGT), the most sensitive indicator of liver damage.

When a diagnosis of hepatic obstruction is suspected, increased activity of 5'-nucleotidase is further evidence for this diagnosis. Patients with hepatic obstruction need to be further differentiated into those with intrahepatic obstruction and those with extrahepatic obstruction, but this is often impossible by means of laboratory tests. True negative urine urobilinogen (the test is very insensitive to small amounts) implies extrahepatic obstruction.

Cholesterol increases in serum as the result of cholestasis or extrahepatic obstruction. Cholesterol levels are normal or decreased in hepatitis and cirrhosis. In dogs with hepatic disease causing increased serum cholesterol levels, a spur cell anemia has been described. Although the exact cause of the spur cell formation is not known, abnormalities of serum lipids and red cell membrane lipids are likely to be involved. In man deficiency of lecithin-cholesterol acyl transferase (LCAT), a red cell membrane enzyme, has been implicated in red cell spiculation seen in hepatocellular disease. Examination of serum lipoproteins may offer some revealing clues in this disorder.

HEPATOCELLULAR DISEASE: LEAKAGE

Hepatocellular disease may be detected by measuring substances in serum that originate in hepatocyte cytoplasm and that, during disease, leak into extracellular fluid. Increased activity of alanine aminotransferase (ALT,GPT) and aspartate aminotransferase (AST,GOT) is seen in liver cell damage. AST is not specific for the liver, since it may also originate in muscle. AST and arginase are normally located within mitochondria. As a result, elevations in these enzymes are less likely to occur as the result of plasma membrane leakage. Sorbitol dehydrogenase (SDH) is hepatospecific in all the common domestic animals, and its activity parallels that of ALT. Lactate dehydrogenase (LDH) is rarely used in the diagnosis of liver disease because it is too non-specific and too insensitive to liver disease. LDH isoenzymes are used to differentiate liver, muscle, and cardiac disease. They are not frequently needed for this purpose. Other enzymes less commonly used include ornithine carbamyl transferase (OCT), glutamate dehydrogenase (GDH), and isocitrate dehydrogenase (ICD). These enzymes are used to detect liver cell damage and largely parallel the activity of ALT.

The magnitude of the enzyme increase is directly proportional to the number of hepatocytes affected. Enzyme elevations cannot be viewed as significant unless the upper limit of normal is at least doubled. The magnitude of the increase is not related to the reversibility of the condition. Reversible biochemical conditions or hepatocellular degeneration cannot be differentiated from irreversible hepatocellular degeneration or necrosis on the basis of the serum enzyme values. Diffuse hepatocellular hypoxia due to shock may cause a marked increase in enzyme activities, whereas focal necrosis may be reflected by modest increases. The duration of increased serum enzyme values is dependent on the persistence of leakage from hepatocytes and the rate of disappearance from plasma. ALT, AST, and SDH are not excreted from plasma, because their molecular weight precludes glomerular filtration. These enzymes become stereochemically denatured, lose their catalytic ability, and can no longer be detected as measured. The plasma half-life of these enzymes is approximately two to five hours. This is significant when considering the progress of hepatic disease marked by enzyme leakage. If values diminish by 50 percent every one to two days, prognosis is good, whereas continuing elevations suggest the probability of persistent hepatocellular disease.

Severe or chronic damage to liver cells is also reflected by other laboratory abnormalities (see later in this article), including decreased albumin concentration and increased prothrombin time. When the pathologic process in the liver fails to resolve and progresses to cirrhosis these laboratory changes are often marked, and the beta and gamma globulin fractions of serum protein are typically elevated, with beta-gamma "bridging" on electrophoresis, especially when the disease is active. When it is not active, or when damage is not severe, the only changes detected may be borderline elevations of ALT and abnormal retention in the serum (over 5 percent) of sulfobromophthalein (BSP). In advanced chronic cirrhotic liver disease the hepatospecific "leakage" enzymes are often normal, suggesting that few viable hepatic cells remain. Sometimes the only change is elevated gamma glutamyl transpeptidase (GGT).

There is an indication that, in active liver cell damage, polymorphonuclear leukocyte microbicidal function may be impaired, contributing to the increased susceptibility of these patients to infection. In addition, serum complement levels have been shown to be decreased in active liver cell damage, further aggravating an already compromised situation.

ACQUIRED BLOOD COAGULATION DEFECTS

Hemostatic problems in liver disease frequently are multifactorial, for numerous reasons. All clotting factors, with the exception of Factor VIII and calcium, are synthesized in the liver. Therefore, depending on the severity of the liver disease, there may be variable depression of all clotting factors except Factor VIII and calcium. This would cause prolongation of the activated clotting time (ACT), which is a general screen of clotting factor deficiencies. Prolongation of the prothrombin time (PT), which screens the extrinsic system and the common coagulation pathway, and prolongation of the partial thromboplastin time (PTT), which screens the intrinsic system and the common coagulation pathway, is known to occur in severe diffuse liver disease.

Patients with portal hypertension and congestive splenomegaly secondary to right heart failure will have a redistribution of platelets to the red pulp of the spleen and moderate depressions in platelet counts. Occasional patients with chronic liver disease have been reported to have ill-defined qualitative platelet defects.

Bile duct obstruction may be the cause of vitamin K deficiency, since bile is necessary for absorption of this vitamin. Vitamin K is necessary for the carboxylation of glutamic acid residues in Factors II, VII, IX, and X. When these factors are synthesized in the absence of vitamin K, they are functionally inactive, causing a prolongation of PT and PTT. (See later discussion of tests of hepatic synthesizing and detoxifying ability as liver tests.)

Chronic liver disease may cause primary fi-

Table 5. *Laboratory Abnormalities That May Occur in Primary Fibrinogenolysis Associated with Chronic Liver Disease*

Low fibrinogen
Fibrinogen degradation products in serum
Evidence of clot lysis *in vitro*
Short euglobulin lysis time
Protamine test negative
Platelets: normal in number but may have a qualitative defect
Screening tests: PTT, PT may be normal

brinogenolysis (Table 5). Primary fibrinogenolysis results from the release of plasminogen activators into the circulation. Plasminogen is converted into plasmin within the circulation, and the end products are fibrinogen degradation products.

Occasionally patients with chronic liver disease will develop bacteremia and therefore may develop disseminated intravascular coagulation (DIC) secondary to endotoxemia or exotoxemia (Table 6). Patients with acute hepatic necrosis due to any cause may develop DIC. DIC is a disorder characterized by activation of the blood coagulation system, which in most instances results in the generation of excess thrombin in the systemic circulation.

REDUCED FUNCTIONAL HEPATIC MASS

This is usually a late occurrence in chronic or end-stage liver disease. The laboratory tests that detect reduced hepatic mass are sulfobromophthalein (BSP) excretion, blood ammon-

Table 6. *Laboratory Diagnosis of Disseminated Intravascular Coagulation Resulting from Chronic Liver Disease*

PT, PTT: Prolonged, owing to depression of Factors I (fibrinogen), V, and VIII
Thrombin time: Prolonged, owing to circulating fibrin degradation products (FDPs), which inhibit fibrin polymerization
Fibrinogen concentration: Frequently low, owing to action of thrombin (stress increases fibrinogen and Factor VIII levels)
Protamine sulfate test: Positive, owing to circulating fibrin monomer and/or FDPs
Fibrin degradation products: Elevated, owing to lysis of fibrin in microcirculation
Euglobulin lysis time: Normal; no circulating lytic enzymes
Platelet count: Reduced, owing to action of thrombin
Peripheral blood smear: Fragmented red cells (schistocytes) may be present

ium concentration and tolerance, and serum protein concentration.

In the dog and cat the amount of BSP retention in blood is determined 30 minutes after a single intravenous injection of 5 mg BSP/kg body weight. The dye is rapidly removed from blood, conjugated by hepatocytes, and excreted in bile. The rate of excretion may be used as an index of the functional hepatic mass but in reality is an index of hepatic blood flow, hepatic uptake of dye, and hepatic conjugation of the dye. Approximately 55 percent of the functional mass of the liver is lost before BSP retention or reduced clearance occurs. The principal causative lesions are atrophy and fibrosis. It has been reported that in hyperbilirubinemic conditions BSP clearance values are misleading, because both bilirubin and BSP are carried by albumin, and competition for albumin binding occurs between bilirubin and BSP. However, BSP is highly competitive for the albumin binding site and will actually dislodge bilirubin. Since binding and hepatocyte uptake are competitive, BSP may be falsely elevated in excessive (greater than 5 mg/dl) hyperbilirubinemia. Values of bilirubin lower than this do not preclude use of the BSP test.

Hypoalbuminemia occurs late in chronic liver disease. Lack of BSP binding caused by hypoalbuminemic conditions allows increased clearance of the dye. Therefore, the BSP value in this state may cause underestimation of the severity of the hepatic lesion. Since the BSP molecule bound to albumin is small, it will be lost in ascitic fluid or in albumin-loss states. Thus, with ascites or with increased albumin-loss states (in urine or in protein-losing gastroenteropathies), BSP values may cause underestimation of hepatic disease. Some drugs are also competitive for hepatocyte binding sites, falsely increasing BSP values. Conversely, phenobarbital stimulates increased hepatic uptake and excretion, falsely lowering BSP values. The BSP test is probably the most sensitive routine test of hepatocellular function available at present. Its principal value lies in the detection of improved function of the liver and in the subsequent followup of patients whose other liver tests are either normal or only slightly abnormal, as most commonly occurs with cirrhosis.

One function of the liver is synthesis of urea from various sources of ammonium, most of which come from protein-splitting bacteria in the gastrointestinal tract. In cirrhosis there is extensive liver cell destruction and fibrous tissue replacement in areas between nodules or irregularly regenerating liver cells. This architectural distortion also distorts the hepatic blood supply and leads to shunting into the systemic venous system. Thus, two conditions should exist for normal liver breakdown of ammonium: (1) enough functioning liver cells must be present and (2) enough ammonia must reach these liver cells. With normal hepatic blood flow, blood ammonium elevation occurs only in extremely severe liver decompensation. With altered blood flow in cirrhosis or, more commonly, in portosystemic shunting, less severe decompensation is needed to produce elevated blood ammonium levels. Hepatic failure produces a syndrome known as prehepatic coma (hepatic encephalopathy). This syndrome may be simulated by hyponatremia or hypokalemia, which cirrhotic patients often manifest. Blood ammonium shows the best correlation with hepatic encephalopathy or coma of any current laboratory test, although it is not wholly dependable. However, blood ammonium is not elevated in all of these patients, so a normal test value does not rule out the diagnosis. An ammonium tolerance test in the dog may be accomplished by administering 0.1 gram of ammonium chloride per kilogram of body weight per os to a fasting patient; serum samples are collected at 30 minutes after administration. Prolonged ammonium level elevation caused by this provocative test suggests portosystemic shunting or cirrhosis, and prognosis must be guarded. Blood ammonium levels are pathologically increased in congenital urea cycle enzyme deficiency and acute hepatic necrosis. Levels are also increased after a high-protein meal. Samples for ammonium assay require special handling and consultation with the testing laboratory.

Concomitant low blood urea nitrogen levels are anticipated with elevated ammonium values. Significant decreases in urea occur late in hepatic disease. The urea value may be lowered but may not drop below the low end of normal range. In our hospital most low urea nitrogen values are associated with prolonged inanition rather than with hepatic disease. The importance of impaired urea formation in hepatic disease is that blood urea nitrogen measurements lose much of their value as an index of renal function in these patients. Creatinine levels should be used as an index of renal function in patients with hepatic disease.

The liver synthesizes almost all plasma protein except the immunoglobulins, which are synthesized by lymphoid tissues. Total serum protein concentration ranges from 6.0 to 8.0 gm/dl. Hemoconcentration resulting from dehydration increases these values. There is no known disease otherwise associated with an elevation of serum albumin concentration. The globulin fractions (and so the total protein concentration) may be elevated in a variety of chronic disorders, such as chronic inflammatory disease, liver disease, and malignant disease. Decreased serum protein concentration may result from decreased protein intake (starvation), poor absorption, decreased protein synthesis (liver disease), increased rate of destruction, or excessive losses from the genitourinary or gastrointestinal tract. Discovery of abnormal serum protein concentration is one indication for serum protein electrophoresis (Table 7). By this technique five bands can readily be distinguished. Of these the fastest and most dense is albumin, followed by α_1-, α_2-, β-, and γ- globulins, the last appearing on both sides of the application point. Hyperproteinemic conditions are generally reflective of increased levels of globulins, whereas hypoproteinemic conditions are generally reflective of hypoalbuminemic conditions. Hypoalbuminemia associated with liver disease is evidence of end-stage liver disease. This is a late finding because of the long half-life of serum albumin (in excess of 24 days). About 80 percent reduction in functional mass occurs before hypoalbuminemia is detectable. Since albumin is normally catabolized by the liver, liver disease decreases albumin catabolism, functionally lengthening the serum half-life, which further delays the onset of hypoalbuminemia. Compensatory increases in globulin concentrations may occur during hypoalbuminemic states and will obscure hypoalbuminemia if only total proteins are measured. As stated before, concomitant dehydration can also obscure the extent of hypoproteinemia.

About half of serum calcium is bound to albumin. Albumin also binds bilirubin, fatty acids, small fractions of thyroxine and cortisol, and numerous drugs, such as BSP. The clinical significance of low serum calcium concentration depends on albumin concentration. For each decrease of 1 gm/dl in serum albumin, there is a decrease of about 1 mg/dl in serum calcium concentration, without evidence of altered physiology. This is because the biologically active fraction of serum calcium is free ionized calcium.

The α_1-globulins include α_1-antitrypsin (an antithrombin), α_1-glycoprotein, α_1-lipoprotein, thyroxine binding globulin, and transcortin. Low values of α_1-globulin are rare in diseases not characterized by total protein losses. Elevation of α_1-globulin levels is common in patients with malignant neoplasms but may also occur in acute inflammation or with obstructive or inflammatory conditions of the biliary tract.

The α_2-globulins include macroglobulin (another antithrombin), haptoglobin, glycoprotein, ceruloplasmin, and numerous enzymes. Increases in α_2-globulin concentrations are usually associated with tissue destruction or proliferation, including infection, inflammation, collagen diseases, neoplastic diseases, and trauma.

Table 7. *Serum Protein Electrophoretic Patterns in Diseases Affecting the Liver*

CONDITION	CHANGES IN CONCENTRATION				
	Albumin	*α_1-Globulin*	*α_2-Globulin*	*β-Globulin*	*γ-Globulin*
Active inflammation and infection	N°	I	NI	N	N
Inflammatory, obstructive lesions of biliary tract	N	I	N	I	N
Malignancy	D	I	I	N	N
Chronic infection	D	NI	I	N	I
Collagen disease (lupoid hepatitis)	N	N	I	N	I
Hemolytic syndrome	N	N	D	N	N
Cirrhosis	D	N	D	I bridging	I
Malabsorption/ malnutrition	D	N	D	N	D
Protein-losing enteropathy	D	D	D	D	D

°Key: N = normal; I = increased; D = decreased

Decreased levels are seen in hepatocellular disease, malabsorption, and hemolytic anemias.

Thrombin inhibitors (plasma α_2-macroglobulin, plasma α_1-antitrypsin, and antithrombin III) localize the conversion of fibrinogen to fibrin when thrombin is generated. This is part of the coagulation check-and-balance system; otherwise, any trivial injury could lead to progressive thrombosis throughout the vascular circulation. Decreases in this antithrombin activity are associated with severe liver disease and, hence, with coagulopathies (see preceding discussion). Increased plasma antithrombin activity is associated with obstructive liver disease. There may be increased antithrombin titers as well as hypothrombinemia, low Factor VII levels, increased capillary fragility and, thus, coagulopathies.

The β-globulins may separate into two bands: β-1, which includes transferrin and hemopexin, and β-2, which includes the lipoproteins as well as complement fractions and enzymes. The usual cause of an overall β-globulin increase is an elevation of β-lipoproteins.

The γ-globulins include the immunoglobulins (IgG, IgA, IgM), although these globulins are also detectable in the α and β regions. The other immunoglobulins (IgD and IgE) are usually detectable only by immunologic methods. IgA constitutes approximately 12 percent of the γ-globulins. It is the fastest migrating of the three, and elevations of its concentration cause "bridging" of electrophoretic patterns between the β and γ fractions. Increases are seen in patients with cirrhosis and chronic infections.

LIPID METABOLISM IN LIVER DISEASE

Because of its importance in cholesterol metabolism, especially esterification and excretion, the total serum cholesterol level and cholesterol fractionation into free and esterified cholesterol were previously used as a measure of hepatic damage. Currently, the serum cholesterol esters and free cholesterol levels are thought to have very limited value as practical clinical tests of hepatic function in man. In the dog and the cat, as more is learned about liver disease, these determinations may have some clinical application. Table 8 considers the fractionation of cholesterol as it occurs in human liver disease.

TESTS OF SYNTHESIZING AND DETOXIFYING ABILITY AS LIVER TESTS

PROTHROMBIN TIME

The response of prothrombin time (PT) to vitamin K, which is dependent upon the synthesis of several coagulation factors made in the liver (Factors II, VII, IX, X), is an ideal test that can be used clinically to measure liver synthesizing and detoxifying ability. The PT response to vitamin K injection cannot be used when the PT is normal. The PT is not a sensitive index of liver disease, since the liver has a large reserve capacity for PT factor synthesis. The PT response to intramuscular versus oral vitamin K may differentiate between intrahepatic and obstructive liver disease. A significant response (shortening of the PT) to intramuscular vitamin K suggests obstructive, not intrahepatic, disease. PT prolongation may have diagnostic value. A PT that is less than 40 percent of control with parenteral vitamin K suggests active hepatitis. With intramuscular injection of vitamin K, a PT more than four seconds longer than the control denotes advanced cirrhosis and a guarded prognosis.

Table 8.   *Cholesterol Fractionation in Liver Disease in Man*

CONDITION	TOTAL CHOLESTEROL	ESTERIFIED CHOLESTEROL	FREE CHOLESTEROL
Normal	150–259 mg/dl	66%	33%
Hepatitis	Normal or low	Normal or low, 50%	Normal or low, 50%
Cirrhosis	Marked elevation	66%, elevated	33%, elevated
Extrabiliary obstruction	Moderate elevation	66%, elevated	33%, elevated

Note 1: In general, the esterified:total cholesterol ratio of 2:3 is maintained in obstructive hepatic disease, and the relative amount of esterified cholesterol is decreased in liver cell damage.

Note 2: Of 266 dogs with morphologically determined hepatopathy, 90 were found to have lowered esterified cholesterol levels. The decrease in serum esterified cholesterol occurred in acute hepatopathy, obstructive jaundice, hepatic cirrhosis, and hepatic tumors. Those dogs, for the most part, exhibited hyperbilirubinemia. The decrease in serum esterified cholesterol is not a reliable indicator for the degree of severity in hepatic disease.

MEASUREMENTS OF CARBOHYDRATE METABOLISM

Except as screening tests for suspected glycogen storage disease, tests of carbohydrate metabolism are not clinically useful as liver tests. Glucagon or epinephrine causes mobilization of hepatic glycogen in normally fed patients. An anticipated normal response to an appropriate dose of epinephrine or glucagon would be a 40 to 60 percent increase in blood sugar over preinjection values. The mobilization of liver glycogen by glucagon or epinephrine is markedly decreased in diffuse liver cell damage and in types I, II, and III glycogen storage diseases. Glycogen storage diseases types IV, V, and VI in man are poorly responsive to epinephrine or glucagon.

LIVER BIOPSY

This procedure has been greatly simplified and its morbidity and mortality markedly reduced by the introduction of the small-caliber biopsy needle. Contraindications to biopsy include prolongation of the prothrombin time and a platelet count of less than $50,000/\mu l$. Liver biopsy is especially useful to differentiate among cirrhosis, hepatitis, and extrahepatic obstruction and as an additional diagnostic aid when the clinical picture or laboratory values are confusing or atypical. Liver biopsy is of particular value in proving the diagnosis of metastatic or primary hepatic malignancy, in determining the cause of hepatomegaly of unknown origin, and in the few patients that have systemic diseases affecting the liver.

A discussion of liver biopsy should include a few words of caution. Two disadvantages are soon recognized by anyone dealing with a large number of liver specimens. First, the procedure is a needle biopsy, which means that a very small fragment of tissue, often partially destroyed, is taken in a random-sample manner from a large organ. Localized disease is easily missed. Second, many diseases produce nonspecific changes that may be spotty, healing, or minimal. Even with an autopsy specimen it may be difficult to make a definite diagnosis or to determine the etiology of many cases. The pathologist should be furnished with the pertinent history, physical findings, and laboratory data; sometimes these have as much value for interpretation of the microscopic findings as the histologic changes themselves. Prior to storing the specimens in formalin, touch impressions submitted to a clinical pathologist for exfoliative cytologic examination may be rewarding. In summary, liver biopsy is often indicated in

Table 9. Laboratory Findings in Dogs with Chronic Active Hepatitis

ABNORMALITY	INCIDENCE (%)
ALT (GPT)	91
Alkaline phosphatase	100
Bilirubin, total	82
BSP retention in 30 minutes	100
Serum albumin (decreases)	27
Serum globulins (increases)	27

difficult cases, but it should not be expected to be infallible or even invariably helpful.

LABORATORY FINDINGS IN SOME LIVER DISEASES

CHRONIC ACTIVE HEPATITIS

Chronic hepatic disease can be classified into a number of types based on histologic changes. A common form of hepatic disease seen in dogs at the University of California Veterinary Medical Teaching Hospital is chronic active hepatitis. Table 9 outlines the most significant biochemical alterations. Hemograms were unremarkable and, in the dogs examined, decreases in plasma concentrations of the branched-chain amino acids (valine, isoleucine, and leucine) and the aromatic amino acids (tyrosine and phenylalanine) were noted.

PRIMARY AND METASTATIC NEOPLASTIC DISEASE OF THE LIVER

The liver can be the site of primary and metastatic neoplastic disease. Primary malignant neoplasms include hepatocellular carcinomas, cholangiosarcomas, fibrosarcomas, and hemangiosarcomas. Benign primary neoplasms include adenomas, fibromas, and hemangiomas. Metastatic disease of the liver appears following spread from primary sites, including the spleen, lymph nodes, adrenal glands, pancreas, bone, lungs, mammary glands, and the gastrointestinal tract. Tables 10 and 11 outline the

Table 10. Laboratory Findings in Dogs with Primary Hepatocellular Carcinoma

ABNORMALITY	INCIDENCE (%)
ALT (GPT)	100
Alkaline phosphatase	100
Serum albumin (decreases)	83
Serum globulins (increases)	83
Blood glucose (decreases)	38
Bilirubin, total	25
BSP retention in 30 minutes	33

Table 11. *Laboratory Findings in Dogs with Metastatic Neoplastic Disease of the Liver*

ABNORMALITY	INCIDENCE (%)
ALT (GPT)	46
Alkaline phosphatase	50
Bilirubin, total	46

laboratory findings in hepatic neoplastic disease.

GLUCOCORTICOID-INDUCED HEPATOPATHY

Hepatopathy associated with glucocorticoid therapy or with naturally occurring hyperadrenocorticism has been reported. On histologic review, the hepatopathy was characterized by centrilobular vacuolization, perivascular glycogen accumulation within hepatocytes, and focal centrilobular necrosis. The predominant clinical findings (Table 12) were hepatomegaly, increased levels of serum enzymes associated with hepatic disease, and increased BSP retention. The hepatopathy appeared to be reversible.

PORTOSYSTEMIC DISEASE

Portosystemic shunting causes a wide variety of clinical signs that are attributable to hepatic encephalopathy, which is more specifically caused by a combination of hyperammonemia, increased blood concentrations of mercaptans and short-chain fatty acids, altered ratios of blood concentrations of amino acids, and increased blood concentrations of false neurotransmitters.

Portal vein hypertension can result from lesions that cause increased portal blood flow (e.g., arteriovenous fistula) or, more commonly, increased resistance to portal blood flow. Based on the location of the obstructing lesion, three types of portal hypertension are recognized: (1)

blockage in the prehepatic section of the portal vein, i.e., extrahepatic presinusoidal block; (2) blockage within the hepatic parenchyma, i.e., intrahepatic presinusoidal, sinusoidal, or postsinusoidal block; and (3) impairment of the hepatic vein outflow, i.e., extrahepatic postsinusoidal block. Table 13 summarizes significant diagnostic laboratory parameters.

FATTY LIVER

Fatty liver is a common cause for hepatomegaly. The etiology may be unknown or referable to diabetes mellitus or hyperadrenocorticism. The majority of patients with this condition (75 percent) have abnormal BSP values, the degree of abnormality being variable. Alkaline phosphatase may be elevated in 48 percent of patients, less than five times the top level of normal, and more often with severe degrees of fatty metamorphosis. Serum bilirubin may be raised in 35 percent of patients but most have minimal abnormality, usually less than twice normal and without jaundice. Severe cases of fatty liver may present with jaundice, but this is very uncommon.

CIRRHOSIS

A wide spectrum of test results is exhibited by cirrhosis, depending on whether the disease is active or inactive and the degree of liver cell damage. With inactive cirrhosis, the most frequent abnormality (if found) is the BSP value. Early cases may not show any abnormal test results or may have an elevated BSP. In more advanced cases the BSP is abnormal to a varying degree. In moderate degrees of cirrhosis there may be minimal or mild abnormalities in ALT (GPT), alkaline phosphatase, and serum bilirubin, though with no definite patterns. In advanced cases other liver tests may show abnormalities.

Table 12. *Clinical and Laboratory Findings in Dogs with Probable Glucocorticoid-Induced Hepatopathy*

ABNORMALITY	INCIDENCE (%)
ALT (GPT)	72
Alkaline phosphatase	94
Gamma glutamyl transpeptidase	75
BSP retention in 30 minutes	73
Resting blood ammonium (increase)	0
Hepatomegaly	55
Polydipsia and polyuria	64

Table 13. *Significant Laboratory Parameters Altered in Portosystemic Disease*

TEST	ABNORMALITY
Blood ammonium	
Fasting level	Elevated
After 0.1 gm NH_4Cl/kg body weight, orally	Markedly elevated
BSP retention in 30 minutes	Elevated
ALT (GPT)	Slight increase
Alkaline phosphatase	Slight increase
Total protein	Slight decrease
Biopsy	Contributory
Prothrombin time	Normal to slight prolongation

BEDLINGTON LIVER DISEASE

Chronic progressive hepatitis ("Wilson's-like" disease) has been described in the Bedlington terrier. The disease is characterized by (1) being discovered after some stressful event, (2) a chronic form, and (3) a clinically asymptomatic group with persistent elevations of ALT. Normal serum levels of copper and ceruloplasmin, which is different from the manifestations of Wilson's disease in man, have been noted. Elevations of hepatic copper levels have been striking.

SUPPLEMENTAL READING

Cutler, R. W. P.: Wilson's disease. In Rubenstein, E., and Federman, D. D. (eds.) *Scientific American Medicine: Neurology.* New York, Scientific American, 1978.

Duncan, J. R., and Prasse, K. W.: *Veterinary Laboratory Medicine.* Ames, Iowa, Iowa State University Press, 1977.

Edwards, D. F., et al.: Portal hypertension secondary to a right atrial tumor in a dog. J. Am. Vet. Med. Assoc., 173:6, 1978.

Meyer, D. J., et al.: Ammonia tolerance test in clinically normal dogs and in dogs with portosystemic shunts. J. Am. Vet. Med. Assoc., 173:4, 1978.

Rogers, W. A., and Ruebner, B. H.: A retrospective study of probable glucocorticoid-induced hepatopathy in dogs. J. Am. Vet. Med. Assoc., 170:6, 1977.

Shull, R. M., et al.: Spur cell anemia in the dog. J. Am. Vet. Med. Assoc., 173:8, 1978.

Strombeck, D. R.: Clinicopathologic features of primary and metastatic neoplastic disease of the liver in dogs. J. Am. Vet. Med. Assoc., 173:3, 1978.

Strombeck, D. R., and Gribble, D.: Chronic active hepatitis in the dog. J. Am. Vet. Med. Assoc., 173:4, 1978.

Strombeck, D. R., and Qualls, C.: Hepatic sulfobromophthalein uptake and defect in a dog. J. Am. Vet. Med. Assoc., 172:12, 1978.

Strombeck, D. R., Breznock, E. M., and McNeel, S.: Surgical treatment of portosystemic shunts in two dogs. J. Am. Vet. Med. Assoc., 170:11, 1977.

MANAGEMENT OF CANINE CHRONIC ACTIVE HEPATITIS

DONALD R. STROMBECK, D.V.M.

Davis, California

Hepatic disease constitutes a wide variety of different acute and chronic pathologic processes that can affect animals of any age. Chronic hepatic disease can be classified into a number of types on the basis of histologic changes. The cause and pathogenesis of chronic hepatic disease are usually unknown. This lack of understanding extends to treatment, which is usually non-specific, and to prognosis, which is usually thought to be poor.

Treatment of chronic hepatitis is directed at arresting inflammation, correcting nutritional derangements, resolving fibrosis, and managing complications. No therapy for chronic hepatitis has been evaluated for effectiveness in a controlled study. Therapy is often empirical and based on old concepts of hepatic disease. Other therapy may have a more scientific basis but is predicated on pathology being similar in most hepatic diseases. The most important specific therapy involves the use of immunosuppressive or anti-inflammatory drugs and diets designed to correct abnormal nitrogen metabolism.

CORTICOSTEROIDS

The anti-inflammatory drugs used most widely for treating chronic active hepatitis are the corticosteroids. Prednisolone is preferred, since it is already biologically active. Since its precursor, prednisone, must be metabolized by the liver to produce the active form, achieving desired blood levels is less predictable when prednisone is used. Signs of hypercorticism can appear with chronic hepatic disease because steroids are not adequately metabolized and prepared for renal excretion, and continued stress stimulates secretion of excess adrenal corticosteroids. When a steroid is used for treatment, its half-life is predictably longer than normal, making an overdose possible. To minimize that problem, the initial dose used is 1.0 to 2.0 mg/kg body weight. The dose is subsequently reduced on remission to 0.4 mg/kg or less.

The indication for corticosteroid therapy is a diagnosis of chronic active hepatitis, in which the morphologic lesion is destruction of hepato-

Table 1. *Results of Treatment* of 16 Dogs with Chronic Active Hepatitis*

RESULT	PERCENTAGE
Long-term improvement†, 6–20 months	56
Short-term improvement, then euthanasia	25
Died within 4 days of onset of therapy	19‡

*Treatment consisted primarily of corticosteroids and controlled diet.

†Improvement based on blood chemistries, clinical signs, and results of rebiopsy of the liver.

‡One dog died within 18 hours after beginning of treatment.

cytes by lymphocytes and plasma cells. Whether these cells are directly cytotoxic or are destructive because of the antibodies they produce, corticosteroids cause their disappearance.

Corticosteroids should not be used in acute hepatitis with an etiology that is unknown but suspected of being viral. Mortality and morbidity rates increase when corticosteroids are used in animals with viral hepatitis or in humans with some forms of acute hepatitis. Viruses may be able to replicate more rapidly when steroids are used in clinical cases, as happens in experimental animals. Corticosteroids have important catabolic effects that stimulate a breakdown of body proteins at a time when protein synthesis must be promoted in order to restore many hepatic functions. Corticosteroids increase urea cycle activity by stimulating hepatic enzyme synthesis. The diseased liver is handicapped in its ability to synthesize protein, however, and the increase in ammonia produced by corticosteroid-directed protein catabolism may cause clinical signs to worsen.

More than three-fourths of animals recognized as having chronic active hepatitis at the Veterinary Medical Teaching Hospital at Davis are treated with corticosteroids (Table 1). The remainder are given euthanasia or are discharged without treatment, with no followup possible. A few treated cases improved but later died of complications or were given euthanasia. Less than 19 percent of the cases treated with steroids died from hepatitis, with death occurring within four days of initiation of treatment. In one case (death in less than 18 hours), steroid therapy was judged to have been initiated too late to affect the course of the disease. About half of treated cases showed long-term improvement. The longest successful treatment has lasted more than 24 months. Rebiopsies of the liver showed marked improvement in all parameters used to identify chronic active hepatitis. Long-term therapy appears to

be important, since acute relapse after discontinuation of steroid therapy results in more severe hepatic disease. There is no evidence that animals with chronic active hepatitis can recover spontaneously without the help of immunosuppressive drugs. The results of corticosteroid therapy should be evaluated by blood biochemical testing and by rebiopsy of the liver.

DIET

Dietary management is required to minimize the abnormalities in nitrogen metabolism, which consist of hyperammonemia and alterations in plasma levels of amino acids. Hyperammonemia can be managed in part by feeding a low-protein diet, an acceptable procedure as long as synthesis of body proteins is not severely reduced. Overall protein synthetic functions are evaluated by measurement of plasma proteins. The levels of these proteins are not low in dogs with chronic active hepatitis, so such patients should not suffer major nitrogen deficiencies if fed a low-protein diet. When hypoproteinemia is a major problem, however, restriction of dietary protein will worsen the condition. In general, the patient should be fed as much protein as can be tolerated; an insufficient amount will result in hypoproteinemia, and an excessive amount will produce signs of hepatic encephalopathy. The restoration of hepatic function requires synthesis of both hepatocyte structures and enzymes. Reduction of dietary protein prevents synthesis from taking place.

Even more important than restricting the total protein content of the diet is restriction of the amount introduced into the intestinal tract at any one time. Feeding small amounts of readily digested protein frequently allows assimilation to be completed in the small intestine. Little is left to enter the large intestine, where there are large numbers of bacteria responsible for ammonia production. Thus, multiple feedings of smaller quantities of food are recommended.

The minimum amount of protein to feed daily is 1.0 gm/20 kcal. If greater amounts can be tolerated, they will be beneficial. If early clinical signs of hepatic encephalopathy (depression, anorexia) appear, the amount of protein should be reduced. Caloric requirements must be met with carbohydrate; otherwise, energy needs will be met by metabolizing proteins in the diet, with ammonia produced as the byproduct. In addition, adequate carbohydrates diminish the catabolism of body protein for energy and reduce the ammonia produced.

The diet can indirectly reduce intestinal ammonia production and absorption. Ammonia is produced from plasma proteins escaping into the colon and from desquamated villous epithelial cells. Events that accelerate this loss, such as intestinal inflammation and circulatory problems, increase the amount of protein entering the colon. When diets improve any existing protein-losing enteropathy, ammonia production is reduced. In general, complete restriction of food intake reduces the turnover rate of intestinal epithelial cells. Low-residue diets have a similar effect and reduce the amount of protein entering the colon.

Dietary measures may partially correct plasma amino acid imbalances. Correction of amino acid imbalances in experimental dogs allows them to survive with hepatic insufficiency when they normally would not. More normal concentrations of plasma amino acids can be attained by feeding a protein composed of many branched-chain amino acids and few aromatic amino acids. Milk proteins are beneficial to humans with hepatic disease. The benefits may be due to the composition of the protein's amino acids. The ratio between these types of amino acids, however, is essentially the same for proteins in cottage cheese, meat, and fish, so the benefits of cottage cheese must be due to properties other than amino acid composition. Cottage cheese is a valuable adjunct in treating chronic hepatitis in humans. It has optimal digestibility and biologic value and is utilized completely without forming large amounts of ammonia. Protein requirements are much lower when the source is used completely than when it is not. Cottage cheese may also reduce the formation and absorption of toxins and antigens in the colon. It affects the numbers of colonic bacteria because it is free of residue and is completely digested and absorbed. With fewer bacteria, fewer toxins are produced. Diet also influences the type of bacteria flourishing in the intestine and may be a factor in improving chronic hepatitis. Control of diet allows additives to be eliminated. Commercial pet foods contain additives that can be metabolized by intestinal bacteria to produce potent hepatotoxins. A disadvantage of cottage cheese is its poor palatability. Clients may fail to adhere to such a diet, especially if it does not yield dramatic results. A cottage cheese–based diet may have to be continued indefinitely, and the distribution of plasma amino acids may continue to be abnormal despite improvement in clinical signs and liver histology. Little is known about the value of other proteins in managing hepatic encephalopathy, but vegetable proteins are thought to be more beneficial than animal proteins.

Dietary therapy cannot correct plasma amino acid abnormalities when conventional foods are fed. They can be corrected by intravenous infusion of the proper amounts of individual amino acids or by supplementation of conventional foods with branched-chain amino acids given orally.

Although the amount and quality of protein in the diet is important, the manner in which it is used is determined by other dietary constituents. The carbohydrate should be readily digested and absorbed so that little is available for fermentation to volatile free fatty acids in the colon. Boiled white rice is an example. Include lipids primarily to satisfy the requirements for unsaturated fatty acids. Minimize fat to prevent the large increases in plasma free fatty acid concentrations that can follow a meal. Multiple feedings are important to minimize the increases in plasma fatty acid concentrations found during fasting. Palmitic acid, a long-chain fatty acid, is oxidized only partially by the diseased liver, resulting in large amounts of octanoic acid. Any fatty acid interferes with the conversion of ammonia to urea, and octanoic acid contributes to hepatic encephalopathy. Balance the diet with vitamins and mineral supplementation if needed. Since the dog's requirements for vitamins are determined by its caloric intake, the patient that is not eating does not require vitamin supplementation.

RESOLUTION OF FIBROSIS

Treatment may help correct advanced fibrosis and cirrhosis. A moderate amount of fibrosis will disappear with corticosteroid therapy and dietary management, so no specific drug therapy for fibrosis is necessary. Fibrosis that remains despite this form of management can be resolved by other means. Experimental fibrosis in dogs can be treated successfully with colchicine. Controlled studies have shown that the drug resolves cirrhosis in humans. Long-term colchicine treatment dramatically improves hyperbilirubinemia, ascites, acute bouts of hepatic encephalopathy, and survival rate. Colchicine disrupts microtubule formation, interrupting intracellular transport, and increases collagenase activity. By inhibiting microtubule assembly, colchicine interferes with transcellular movement of collagen, so that it is not deposited in the liver. Stimulation of collagenase activity removes collagen that is already deposited. Colchicine is more effective in resolving fibrosis than are proline analogs, which have only a single mechanism to interfere with collagen synthesis. The side effects of colchicine (vomiting, diarrhea, depression, and anorexia) are caused by interference with the function of gastrointestinal epithelial cells. Less common complications of the drug include fever, loss of hair, hypocalcemia, blood dyscrasias, and possible liver damage. Corticosteroids and estrogens have non-specific effects in treating fibrosis. Penicillamine interferes with collagen deposition by inhibiting its cross-linking and maturation.

ANTIBIOTICS

Antibiotics are used with signs of acute hepatitis, though not with the goal of sterilizing the gut. Antibiotics are directed primarily against bacteria absorbed from the intestine and not removed by the liver. Hepatic reticuloendothelial function is reduced with hepatitis, so bacteria are not removed from the portal circulation. Antibiotics are directed against intestinal anaerobes and aerobes, with penicillin the choice against the former and kanamycin or gentamicin against the latter. Chloromycetin is useful against both types of bacteria, but many bacteria have become resistant to its effects. Septicemia severely aggravates hyperammonemia and hepatic encephalopathy, and this complication is minimized by antibiotics. Parenteral antibiotics are more effective for this purpose than unabsorbed antibiotics.

HEPATIC ENCEPHALOPATHY

Severe hepatic encephalopathy is a major complication occurring if protein intake is restricted insufficiently or if there is massive loss of blood or plasma proteins into the alimentary tract. The signs of hepatic encephalopathy are precipitated by absorption of ammonia, mercaptans, and volatile short-chain fatty acids from the intestine. This is treated by colonic irrigation to remove all the contents. Enemas and cathartics reduce bacterial numbers and the substrates and agents for ammonia production. Ammonia absorption is reduced by using saline cathartics and mildly acidic enemas. At lower pHs, ammonia exists primarily in ionized form and, being a charged ion, is not absorbed. A cathartic and pH-reducing effect is also produced by lactulose, a disaccharide used to treat hepatic encephalopathy in humans. This sugar is not digested in the small intestine but fermented in the colon, forming metabolites that cause an osmotic diarrhea.

Ammonia is also produced by colonic urease-producing bacteria, in amounts proportional to blood urea nitrogen levels. Reducing blood urea nitrogen levels is important in treating hyperammonemia. Ammonia production can be decreased by reducing the numbers of colonic bacteria. However, it is difficult to maintain for more than a few days even when effective antibiotics are used. Bacteria, especially aerobes, rapidly develop drug resistance, and the drug's effectiveness is terminated. Penicillin does not affect numbers of colonic bacteria. Non-absorbed antibiotics must be used against anaerobes, with vancomycin one of the few that are effective. Gentamicin or kanamycin, given orally, is effective against aerobes. Neomycin, an aminoglycoside similar to kanamycin, is used to reduce colonic bacterial numbers in humans with hepatic encephalopathy, but many bacteria are now resistant to its effects. Clinical studies in humans with hyperammonemia and hepatic encephalopathy show that neomycin does not significantly lower blood ammonia levels. A combination of sorbitol and neomycin gives an improvement in clinical signs that is related to an increase in stool frequency. The beneficial effects of neomycin may be due to its ability to produce diarrhea and empty the colon. Diarrhea due to any cause, even laxatives, reduces colonic bacterial numbers.

Colonic bacterial activity is thought to be altered by introducing non-urease–producing bacteria with the idea that they will displace those producing urease. *Lactobacillus* cultures have been advocated to repopulate the colonic microflora. Such therapy is ineffective in humans. Both animal and human studies show that it is difficult to alter bacterial populations in the colon. Bacteria given orally do not remain and multiply in the intestine but pass out in the feces. Transient bacteria entering through the oral cavity are able to populate the colon only when the bacterial flora is disrupted. An alternate approach of management is to inhibit bacterial urease activity. Some immunity can be produced following immunization of animals with urease or urease-producing bacteria. This results in some reduction of colonic urease activity.

Hyperammonemia has been treated with substances that augment the fixation of ammonia into non-toxic products. Ammonia is mostly converted to urea, and any substance supporting urea cycle activity increases the conversion. Krebs cycle intermediates providing aspartate are required to maintain urea cycle activity. Thus blood glucose levels are maintained, which is obviously important when hepatic disease produces hypoglycemia. Acute hyperammonemia during fasting reduces plasma alanine concentrations, which reflects its deamination and conversion to glucose. Increased urea cycle activity requires arginine, and acute ammonia toxicity reduces plasma arginine levels. Arginine infusions have been used to treat hyperammonemia in animals and humans, although with uncertain effectiveness. Arginine infusion decreases high blood ammonia levels but is not accompanied by clinical improvement. Ammonia is also fixed and detoxified by forming glutamine from glutamic acid and by providing alpha keto acids for amination by ammonia to form amino acids.

The effects of hyperammonemia in inducing hepatic encephalopathy are reduced by decreasing ammonia diffusion into the brain. Ammonia enters the brain more rapidly during alkalosis, when larger amounts of ammonia are un-ionized, lipid-soluble, and more readily diffusible. Thus, any existing alkalosis is corrected. (In most cases the alkalosis is a metabolic type, owing to loss of gastrointestinal secretions from vomiting.) Alkalosis is treated by replacing fluid deficits and by continuing fluid therapy to initiate diuresis. Since animals become potassium-depleted from vomiting, potassium must be replaced in managing hyperammonemia and alkalosis. Electrolyte solutions containing glucose will worsen hypokalemia by promoting potassium movement into cells. Potassium deficiency in itself can cause hyperammonemia.

It has been suggested that the major effects of hepatic encephalopathy are due to an unknown toxic effect of ammonia and an alteration of the level of neural transmitters. The increased levels of inhibitory transmitters and reduced levels of excitatory transmitters have been treated by increasing brain levels of the neurotransmitter dopamine, using its precursor L-dopa. This treatment has given variable results in humans with severe hepatic encephalopathy, although a general effect is to cause arousal from coma.

RENAL INSUFFICIENCY

Successful management of complicating renal failure is dependent on early recognition. Early recognition of oliguria is followed by measures to improve renal circulation and initiate diuresis. Therapy is directed at improving effective circulating plasma volume. Fluids, fortified with potassium as necessary, are administered to replace deficits and restore renal circulation. Fluid replacement is monitored by central venous pressure. Replacement of fluid to correct renal insufficiency can increase amounts of ascitic fluid. Mannitol can be used to improve renal circulation and initiate diuresis. Diuretics such as furosemide are not used, because they are metabolized in the liver and are a potential cause of drug-induced hepatopathy. Since hepatic circulation is reduced along with the effective circulating plasma volume, treatment of the hepatorenal syndrome also improves splanchnic circulation. Unfortunately, treatment for the hepatorenal syndrome is nonspecific, since no specific measures are very effective in restoring normal renal function in patients with chronic hepatitis. The prognosis is poor when oliguria, uremia, and ascites develop. Uremia increases the amount of substrate for bacterial ureases to produce ammonia, which causes signs of hepatitis to worsen. The hepatorenal syndrome in humans has been treated successfully by surgically created portacaval shunts.

ASCITES AND FLUID AND ELECTROLYTE IMBALANCES

Diuretics are the only means used to manage most cases of ascites in small animals. A number of potent diuretics are used in long-term treatment when the cause of portal hypertension and hypoproteinemia cannot be removed. Diuretics can readily induce severe electrolyte disturbances in patients with ascites and liver disease. Total-body exchangeable potassium is low in patients with chronic hepatic fibrosis. Thus, in treating ascites, potassium chloride should be supplemented, potassium-sparing diuretics should be used, or the two methods can be combined. The diuretics, in order of increasing potency, are the thiazides, ethacrynic acid, and furosemide, with the latter not used for reasons stated earlier. They all inhibit proximal sodium reabsorption, thereby increasing the amounts of sodium delivered to the distal nephron. The high levels of sodium in the distal nephron stimulate the sodium-potassium exchange mechanism for secreting potassium. Acetazolamide, a carbonic anhydrase inhibitor, is a diuretic that is a more potent potassium waster. Two diuretics with potassium-retaining properties are spironolactone and triamterene. The former drug competitively inhibits the action of aldosterone on the distal tubule, enhancing sodium excretion while potassium excretion decreases. Triamterene interferes with sodium reabsorption in the distal tubule, enhancing sodium excretion while potassium excretion is reduced. Triamterene and spironolactone differ in the manner in which they interfere with sodium reabsorption in the distal tubule. Both drugs can cause abnormal potassium retention, producing hyperkalemia. For this reason, potassium-retaining diuretics are combined with potassium-wasting ones to achieve the desired goal.

It is unrealistic to expect diuretics to mobilize and excrete the excess fluid in patients with ascites. A more realistic goal is to use them to prevent further sodium retention. Restriction of dietary sodium is an important adjunct to the use of diuretics.

Marked diuresis removes ascitic fluid, so a cardiac output that is below normal is reduced further. Other complications of diuretics include water retention, hyponatremia, and increased plasma urea and creatinine. Hyponatremia, frequently a problem before treatment, is aggravated by diuretics. A number of vasoactive drugs have been tried to improve renal blood flow, but they are generally less effective than diuretics in increasing sodium excretion.

Another means of stimulating diuresis and natriuresis is through expansion of the plasma compartment to increase the effective plasma volume. Volume expansion involves Third factor to excrete sodium. The plasma volume is expanded with albumin, ascitic fluid, or dextran, but these agents should not be used if central venous pressure is abnormally high and contributing to the portal hypertension. Measurement of central venous pressure aids in determining the amount of fluid to give.

Ascites is commonly treated by removal of ascitic fluid via paracentesis. However, it may re-form within hours. The fluid removed contains plasma proteins that are lost from the body. The removal of ascitic fluid from hypoproteinemic patients results in a further decrease in plasma proteins as ascites fluid reforms. Serum albumin synthesis usually is too slow to replace losses from repeated paracentesis. There are advantages in removing ascitic fluid, in that its removal from some patients results in increased cardiac output and plasma volume. These effects may result from relieving compression on the caudal vena cava, portal vein, or renal veins. Paracentesis limited to removal of small volumes two or three times a day is recommended.

Paracentesis can be combined with plasma volume expansion so that fluid removed from the abdominal cavity is infused intravenously. Central venous pressure is monitored to determine the rate of infusion. Vigorous treatment with diuretics can be combined with the infusion to maximize the benefits of albumin reinfusion. This procedure speeds the return to normal plasma protein levels. Another means of chronically reinfusing ascitic fluid into the vascular compartment involves permanent placement of Silastic tubing (containing a valve) to connect the peritoneal cavity with the central venous system.

An effective means of reducing portal hypertension and effecting a reasonable cure for ascites is to create a portosystemic shunt. It can be effective only if the cause of the hypertension is either prehepatic or hepatic and not if the cause is in the heart or vena cava. There are many examples of the naturally occurring model of portosystemic shunts in dogs to illustrate the problems that can occur. A portosystemic shunt to treat ascites is a choice of treatment that is likely to create more problems than the original one. Proceeding one step further, however, may eliminate many of those complications. Portosystemic shunts have been created experimentally in dogs to produce a situation that terminates in death within two to three months. If, in addition, the portal venous system is arterialized by anastomosing a small artery with one of the portal vessels, the dogs survive with surprisingly few problems. It remains to be seen whether this two-step procedure can be used to achieve improvement in clinical cases of portal hypertension and ascites in small animals. Some animals have hydrothorax complicating ascites with hepatic disease. This has been managed in humans with tetracycline-induced pleural symphysis.

Alkalosis, which often accompanies chronic hepatitis, is corrected by fluid therapy. Potassium deficits may require oral supplementation or balanced electrolyte solutions fortified with additional potassium. Correction of a total-body potassium deficit may take weeks. Magnesium is usually depleted along with potassium during hepatic disease. Occasionally the potassium deficit cannot be repaired unless magnesium is given first. Magnesium is not a constituent of Ringer's solution.

COAGULOPATHIES

The treatment of coagulopathy associated with chronic active hepatitis is based on the premise that disseminated intravascular coagulation (DIC) and clotting-factor deficiencies coexist. Fibrinolysis is a likely problem, and treatment for DIC and clotting-factor deficiencies can improve fibrinolysis. Heparin (100 units/kg, three times a day) given to treat DIC results in decreased plasmin activity and blocks the clotting mechanism. The clotting factors are replaced by transfusions of fresh blood. Using heparin without replacing clotting factors causes a high incidence of uncontrolled fatal hemorrhage in humans with hepatitis. Thus, heparin should not be given alone. Whole blood also provides antiplasmin activity, which inhibits fibrinolysis. Results from experimental dogs indicate that resistance to heparin therapy develops after four to five days, and the prognosis is poor when the coagulopathy does not respond within 24 to 48 hours.

Treatment specifically for fibrinolysis must be considered experimental at present. The treatment has consisted of administration of epsilon-aminocaproic acid in conjunction with the use of heparin and blood clotting factor replacement.

There is little hope for successful treatment of an animal with hepatic disease that is hemorrhaging into the intestine. Gastrointestinal hemorrhage is difficult enough to manage in patients that do not have associated hepatic disease.

SUPPLEMENTAL READING

Fischer, J. E., and Baldessarini, R. J.: Pathogenesis and therapy of hepatic coma. In Popper, H., and Schaffner, F. (eds.): *Progress of Liver Diseases*, vol. 5. New York, Grune & Stratton, 1976, pp. 363–397.
Strombeck, D. R.: *Small Animal Gastroenterology.* Davis, Calif., Stonegate Publishing Co. 1979.
Strombeck, D. R., and Gribble, D.: Chronic active hepatitis in the dog. J. Am. Vet. Med. Assoc., *173*:380–386, 1978.

FELINE LIVER DISEASE

WILLIAM E. HORNBUCKLE, D.V.M.
Ithaca, New York,

and GRAEME S. ALLAN, M.V.Sc.
Sydney, Australia

The clinical diagnosis of liver disease in the domestic cat can be elusive. Affected cats can remain asymptomatic for long periods of time, and signs of illness, if present, may be vague or non-specific. Morphologic liver disease, abnormal liver function tests, or both, can have a variety of primary and secondary causes. The types of liver disease, diagnostic features of clinical examinations, and supportive medication will be discussed.

OVERVIEW

Acute cholestatic liver disease is one of the most frequent diagnoses in cats examined at the New York State College of Veterinary Medicine (NYSCVM). Many cats respond to supportive medication and recover, so histopathologic examination of the liver is not done. Liver disease associated with fever is suspicious of viral or bacterial infection. Drugs and certain toxins also may cause liver disease.

Chronic hepatobiliary disease includes the histopathologic complex of pericholangeal inflammation, cholangitis, cholangiohepatitis, and biliary cirrhosis. The syndrome may occur with or without coincident pancreatitis. The cause cannot be determined in most cases. However, environmental toxins or viral antigens should be suspected if bacterial infection and liver flukes have been ruled out. Persistent cholangiohepatitis can remain subclinical for indefinite periods of time. Clinical signs (e.g., inappetence, vomiting, and weight loss) can be intermittent or progressive. Tissue or serum jaundice, or both, may or may not be observed, and definitive diagnosis requires histopathologic examination of biopsied liver tissue.

Hepatic lipidosis (fatty degeneration) is common and can be complicated by cholestasis and necrosis. The cause is often unknown, although nutritional imbalances, prolonged anorexia (Barsanti, et al.), metabolic diseases (e.g., diabetes mellitus), certain toxins and drugs, and conditions causing hypoxemia may be implicated.

Cholelithiasis is rare in the domestic cat, but inspissated bile can present a clinical picture of obstructive jaundice. Rarely, congenital anomalies (e.g., bile duct agenesis, cysts, or accessory gallbladders) will cause clinical disease. Large liver abscesses with or without foreign bodies are also rare.

Clinical and biochemical evidence of liver disease can result from diseases occurring in the pancreas or small intestine and has also been observed in some cats with diaphragmatic hernia. Chronic or subacute pancreatitis, pancreatic neoplasms and, rarely, acute pancreatitis can cause extrahepatic or intrahepatic cholestasis, or both, as can metastatic infection or neoplasia of the liver. Icterus is common in cats with diabetes mellitus. Severe enteritis, intestinal foreign bodies, and neoplasia can cause ascending infection, injury, or obstruction of pancreatic and biliary ducts. Injury to the liver can result in fatal hemoperitoneum or bile peritonitis.

The liver is commonly involved in feline infectious peritonitis (FIP). This disease is caused by a coronavirus that, under experimental conditions, can cause acute multifocal hepatitis. Feline leukemia virus (FeLV) should be ruled out when immunosuppression or neoplasia is suspected. Toxoplasmosis is an infrequent cause of primary liver disease. Increased liver enzyme activity and hepatomegaly occur in hemobartonellosis, and cats with infectious enteritis (parvovirus) occasionally become icteric. Systemic fungus infections, hepatozoonosis (Ewing), cytauxzoonosis (Wagner), and Tyzzer's disease (Kovatch and Zebarth) are rare.

Neoplastic liver disease can be primary, secondary, or part of a multicentric distribution (e.g. lymphosarcoma or myeloproliferative disease). Vascular anomalies of the liver are rare. An intrahepatic arteriovenous fistula has been reported in a cat with ascites (Legendre, et al.). A four-month-old kitten with a portosystemic shunt was recently examined at NYSCVM because of neurologic signs. Centrolobular congestion is common and can have a variety of causes, including congestive heart failure.

HISTORY

The animal's vaccination coverage, outdoor activity, hunting prowess and daily nutrition, and the number of healthy and sick cats in the same environment should be determined. Previous illness, medication, and injury should be documented. Diagnostic suspicion increases in areas in which there is known incidence of systemic fungus, liver flukes, cytauxzoonosis, or toxic plants or chemicals. FeLV and FIP should be considered in environments that have many cats. Toxoplasmosis is a consideration in hunting cats and in situations in which raw meat is fed. A cat's habit of playing with string, cellophane, or other forms of foreign material should be determined.

The most common signs observed in cats with liver disease are inappetence, lethargy, diarrhea or vomiting (or both), and weight loss. Weakness, abdominal distention, polyuria or polydipsia (or both), and jaundice are some-

times seen. Jaundice can be a primary complaint that is detected by an observant owner who is aware of color change in the cat's ears, skin, or eyes. Icteric cats with blue eyes have been presented with the complaint that their eyes (irises) had turned green. Hemorrhage is rarely reported. Neurologic signs can result from the polysystemic effects of toxins or diseases such as FIP, lymphosarcoma, toxoplasmosis, or cryptococcosis. The previously mentioned kitten that had a portosystemic shunt presented with alternating periods of aggressiveness and somnolence.

PHYSICAL EXAMINATION

The primary physical findings that focus on liver diseases are hepatomegaly, jaundice, or both. Abdominal distention can result from hepatomegaly, peritoneal effusion, or extrahepatic soft tissue masses (e.g., pancreatitis or neoplasia). Rarely, gallbladder distention resulting from common bile duct obstruction or large liver cysts will cause abdominal distention. Peritoneal effusions can result from neoplasia, transudation (e.g., cirrhosis or arteriovenous fistulas), FIP, or other exudates.

Tissue jaundice is detected at serum bilirubin levels of 2 to 5 mg/dl. Faint degrees of jaundice are best detected in the caudal palate. Depression anemia is common in sick cats, and careful examination is necessary to differentiate it from hemolytic anemia. The majority of icteric cats examined by NYSCVM have intrahepatic cholestasis (Table 1). Not all icteric cats have liver disease. Extrahepatic cholestasis (obstructive jaundice) and hemolytic jaundice are less common.

Hemorrhage is not a common physical finding in cats with liver disease. Disseminated intravascular coagulopathy (DIC) has been observed in experimental cats infected with FIP-coronavirus at NYSCVM. Other coincidental physical findings that may influence diagnosis or treatment include fever, dehydration, splenomegaly, and respiratory signs. Because FIP, toxoplasmosis, systemic fungi, and lymphosarcoma cause suggestive ocular lesions, routine ophthalmoscopic examination is advised.

RADIOLOGY

The patient is positioned so that ventrodorsal and right lateral recumbent radiographs of the abdomen are obtained. The primary beam is centered over the last rib; the film should be of sufficient size to include the diaphragm and

Table 1. *Fifty-Six Cats with Tissue and/or Serum Jaundice**

CONDITION	NUMBER
Neoplasia (secondary, multicentric, or primary)	13
Lymphosarcoma (8)	
Myeloproliferative disease (2)	
Lymphoproliferative disease (1)	
Biliary adenocarcinoma (1)	
Pancreatic adenocarcinoma (1)	
Feline infectious peritonitis	9
Acute cholestatic liver disease	
(laboratory diagnosis)	9
Hepatic lipidosis	5
Cholangiohepatitis	4
Hemobartonellosis	3
Pancreatitis	3
Diabetes mellitus†	2
Panleukopenia (parvovirus)	2
Panleukopenia (FeLV)	2
Toxoplasmosis	1
Cholangiohepatitis (liver flukes)	1
Inspissated bile (accessory gallbladders)	1
Cholecystitis (accessory gallbladders)	1

*New York State College of Veterinary Medicine, 1975–1978.

†One cat also had cholangiohepatitis and the other had hepatic lipidosis.

kidneys. The liver is mainly contained within the costal arch, but its ventrocaudal surface lies slightly caudal to the arch and is readily recognized silhouetted against the fat of the falciform ligament. It may be displaced caudally during deep inspiration, in obese patients, and in patients with pleural effusion, emphysema, and hepatomegaly. When interpreting abdominal radiographs, note the axis of the stomach, which usually lies in the same plane as the tenth intercostal space. Dorsal and caudal displacement is seen in hepatomegaly, and cranial displacement in a vertical plane is seen with decreased hepatic mass (Root). Where there is inadequate intrinsic gastric contrast to allow appreciation of suspected hepatomegaly, air or barium should be placed in the stomach before the patient is radiographed again.

Radiographic criteria for diagnosing hepatomegaly are (1) rounding of the margins of the left lateral and right middle lobes where they are silhouetted against the falciform ligament and (2) caudal displacement of contiguous viscera (stomach, proximal duodenum, right kidney, and transverse colon). Generalized hepatomegaly occurs in hepatic venous stasis, extrahepatic biliary duct obstruction, neoplasia, diffuse inflammation, nodular hyperplasia, cirrhosis, and metabolic disorders such as amyloidosis and lipidosis. The liver silhouette may be reduced in chronic cirrhosis, hepatic necrosis, diaphragmatic tears with herniation of part of the liver, and portal vein shunting disorders that result in hepatic hypoperfusion. Localized hepatomegaly may be seen where there are abscesses, biliary cysts, intrahepatic bile duct obstruction, and neoplasia. Hepatosplenomegaly may be seen with right-sided cardiac failure, and hepatonephromegaly may be seen with FIP and diabetes mellitus. Hepatonephrosplenomegaly may occur with hepatitis, metabolic infiltrative diseases (amyloidosis, lipidosis) and infiltrative neoplasms (e.g., lymphoma) (O'Brien).

Focal increases in tissue density may result from mineralization of foci of necrotic hepatic tissue and where radiodense choleliths are present. Areas of decreased density may occur with gas-producing hepatic disease, septic cholecystitis, and disorders in which gas may enter the liver via the portal circulation.

Radiographically identifiable extrahepatic signs of liver disease include ascites and focal loss of radiographic detail adjacent to the liver. These latter changes may accompany focal bile peritonitis or hemorrhage following biliary and hepatic trauma, respectively.

Additional special studies may be performed for more complete hepatic examination. Pneumoperitoneography or capnoperitoneography is useful to define the liver size and contour when used with appropriate projections (e.g., the erect dorsoventral and lateral views). Angiography is useful for defining patterns of liver perfusion and vascular "shunts." Cholecystography has been useful in cats with diaphragmatic hernias in which the liver was the only viscus displaced into the thorax, and it should also be employed when radiolucent (cholesterol and bile salt) choleliths or choledocholiths are suspected. In interpreting cholecystograms, the reader should be aware that cholecystic duplication and triplication are common in the domestic cat (Boyden; Carlisle).

Liver scintigraphy is a nuclear medical procedure in which a gamma ray–emitting radioisotope is administered to the patient. After administration of a suitable isotope, the area of interest is examined using either a gamma ray camera or a rectilinear scanner, and areas of increased or decreased gamma ray emission are identified. This technique may be useful to identify focal space-occupying lesions of the liver, such as tumors, cysts, or abscesses.

LABORATORY EXAMINATION

The hemogram, bone marrow examination, or both, can shorten the diagnostic process in some cats with primary or secondary liver disease. Leukemia, myeloproliferative disease, myeloma, and hemobartonellosis are examples of diseases that can be diagnosed by these tests. Hematologic examinations can also aid in the characterization of anemia and in monitoring the course and treatment of disease.

Bilirubinuria is a reliable indicator of cholestasis in the cat. Ictotest® reagent tablets should be used if discoloration of urine causes difficulty in the interpretation of reagent sticks. Excessive urobilinogen can occur with hemolytic or hepatocellular disease. The absence of urobilinogen on several examinations is equivocal evidence of obstructive cholestasis in icteric cats. Bilirubin, tyrosine, and leucine crystals have been observed in the urine of cats with liver disease.

Both alanine aminotransferase (formerly SGPT) and aspartate aminotransferase (formerly SGOT) activity should be evaluated. When both enzymes were examined in a group of clinical and experimental cats with liver disease at NYSCVM, SGOT was often the predominant enzyme activity. There were case examples in which only SGPT or only SGOT activity was increased.

Increased serum alkaline phosphatase activity is usually indicative of liver disease in the cat. Alkaline phosphatase is metabolically degraded in plasma and has a half-life of six hours. This is why the degree of alkaline phosphatase activity in cats with obstructive jaundice is less than that in the dog. The plasma half-life of alkaline phosphatase in the dog is 72 hours. Glucocorticoids and phenobarbital do not induce alkaline phosphatase activity in the cat as they do in the dog (Hoffman and Dorner).

The van den Bergh test (total serum bilirubin, conjugated and unconjugated) often contributes no more information about the pathogenesis of jaundice than the physical, hematocrit, and urine bilirubin examinations. Unconjugated hyperbilirubinemia can occur in hemolytic anemia and liver disease characterized by insufficient numbers or function of hepatocytes (e.g., cirrhosis and kernicterus) (Tryphona and Rozdilsky). Predominately conjugated hyperbilirubinemia is expected with extrahepatic and intrahepatic cholestasis.

Bromsulphalein (BSP) dye retention, blood ammonia, and serum protein levels are of diagnostic value in select cases. The first two tests assess alterations in functional hepatocyte mass (e.g., diffuse fibrosis or lipidosis, cirrhosis, neoplasia) and the blood supply of the liver (e.g., cirrhosis and portosystemic shunts). Factors such as jaundice and cardiovascular disease can increase dye retention, and hypoproteinemia can "normalize" BSP test results. Blood ammonia requires special collection techniques and can be an expensive test. It is indicated in cases in which significant liver disease is suspected and BSP test results are normal or equivocal. Hyperammonemia was determined in the previously mentioned kitten with a portosystemic shunt. Hyperglobulinemia can result from chronic inflammation or neoplasia. Hypoalbuminemia can result from decreased liver synthesis but also results from gastrointestinal or renal loss, hemorrhage, or sequestration of body fluids.

Blood and urine should be examined for glucose. Hyperglycemia commonly occurs in stressed or sick cats. One quarter of the cats in Table 1 had increased blood glucose levels, but only two actually had diabetes mellitus. Hypoglycemia has also been documented in some cats with liver disease.

Coagulation studies are advised for cats with jaundice or obvious hemorrhage and should be made prior to surgical procedures. Analysis or cultures of thoracic and abdominal fluid may be diagnostically rewarding (e.g., in FIP and neoplasia). Testing for FeLV, FIP, toxoplasmosis, system fungus, and other conditions requires the use of accredited laboratories to minimize equivocal or erroneous interpretation. Routine fecal examinations are necessary for the detection of trematodes.

LIVER BIOPSY

Biochemical evidence of liver disease does not discriminate among the varied forms of morphologic disease. Histopathologic examination provides this information and in many cases results in definitive diagnosis. The condition of the cat and individual preference determine whether liver tissue is obtained by percutaneous, key-hole, laparoscopic, or laparotomy techniques (Osborne, et al.). The last two techniques allow more selective tissue collection, and laparotomy offers the opportunity for corrective surgery.

TREATMENT

Medical treatment is generally supportive and is determined by clinical signs and laboratory data compatible with liver disease. Surgery is necessary to treat diaphragmatic hernias (liver entrapment), local parenchymal lesions (cysts, neoplasia, and abscesses), vascular anomalies, and conditions causing extrahepatic cholestasis.

If there are no contraindications for oral alimentation, small amounts of palatable food are given two to three times per day. Periodic checks of body weight are made to evaluate the adequacy of total daily nutrition. A balanced commercial ration approved for cats by the NRC is usually adequate. Additional protein should be of high biologic value (e.g., cottage cheese). Nutritional adjustments for salt retention (ascites) and, rarely, for protein or fat intolerance (encephalopathy, steatorrhea) are discussed elsewhere. If a cat does not eat satisfactory amounts within 36 to 48 hours, forced feeding is needed (by hand or nasogastric or orogastric intubation).

Vitamins, anabolic steroids, and lipotrophic agents (methionine, choline, inositol) are often administered for empirical or theoretical reasons. Only two vitamins will be mentioned. Vitamin B–complex administration is recommended. Vitamin K (aquamephyton) is administered to cats with significant cholestasis or coagulopathies. The therapeutic benefits of anabolic steroids (stanozolol) are difficult to measure, but occasionally cats show a dramatic improvement in general demeanor. Adequate calories and protein of high biologic value are needed to enhance the effects of anabolic steroids. There may be some indication for lipotrophic agents in inappetent or malnourished cats. However, there is no convincing evidence that methionine and choline are useful in hepatic lipidosis that is not caused by choline deficiency. Methionine is contraindicated in suspected cases of hepatic encephalopathy.

Balanced electrolyte solutions are used to correct and maintain hydration. Intravenous dextrose solutions correct signs of hypoglycemia, provide a source of calories, and have a protective influence on toxic hepatocytes. Hyperglycemia occasionally occurs in sick cats, and rapid screening tests for blood glucose should be done prior to dextrose infusions. If increased blood glucose levels do not return to normal levels after rehydration, diabetes mellitus is suspected.

Various sources indicate that the following antimicrobial agents are potentially toxic in the presence of liver disease: chloramphenicol, chlortetracycline, erythromycin, oxytetracycline, neomycin, streptomycin, and the sulfonamides (Aronson; Wilkinson). Tetracycline can cause increased fat deposition in the liver through the inhibition of the release of lipoproteins (Barsanti, et al.). However, tetracycline is useful in some cases of liver disease because it is concentrated there. Penicillin, ampicillin, cephalosporins, and gentamycin have been used safely in cats with liver disease.

Histopathologic examination of the liver and/or hematologic examinations are preferred prior to the administration of glucocorticoids. Prednisolone is preferred instead of prednisone because it does not require metabolic activation by the liver; single daily doses should be administered in the evening to cats. Indications for the use of glucocorticoids are often vague and require prudent clinical judgments. States of inappetence, listlessness, and weight loss that have been refractory to other treatments are common indications for their use. Certain neoplasms and some forms of chronic inflammation may be more specific indications.

Ascites with or without peripheral edema is treated with diuretics, paracentesis, and low-salt diets. To avoid complete inappetence and loss in body weight, rations are often not changed, and therapy is limited to the use of diuretics. Hepatic encephalopathy is rare in the cat and is discussed elsewhere.

Many cats infected with liver flukes are asymptomatic. Additional factors such as environmental stress, malnutrition, or intestinal parasitism are usually necessary to precipitate clinical signs of the disease. The administration of hexachloroparaxylol has been suggested as a possible treatment (Chung, et al.).

SUPPLEMENTAL READING

Aronson, A.L.: Diseases caused by chemical and physical agents. In Catcott, E.J., (ed.): *Feline Medicine and Surgery.* Santa Barbara, American Veterinary Publications, 1975, pp. 113–130.

Barsanti, J.A., Jones, B.D., Spano, J.S., and Taylor, H.W.: Prolonged anorexia associated with hepatic lipidosis in three cats. Feline Pract., 7:52–57, 1977.

Boyden, E.A.: The accessory gallbladder: An embryological and comparative study of aberrant biliary vesicles in man and his domestic animals. Am. J. Anat., 38:177–222, 1926.

Carlisle, C.H.: A comparison of techniques for cholecystography in the cat. J. Am. Vet. Radiol. Soc., 18:173–176, 1977.

Chung, N.Y., Miyahara, A.Y., and Chung, G.: The prevalence of feline liver flukes in the city and county of Honolulu. J. Anim. Hospital Assoc., 13:258–262, 1977.

Hoffmann, W.E., and Dorner, J.L.: Feline practitioners' seminar. American Animal Hospital Association Meeting, Boston, 1977.

Ewing, G.O.: Granulomatous cholangiohepatitis in a cat due to a protozoan parasite resembling *Hepatozoon canis.* Feline Pract., 7:37, 1977.

Kovatch, R.M., and Zebarth, G.: Naturally occurring Tyzzer's disease in a cat. J. Am. Vet. Med. Assoc., 162:136–137, 1973.

Legendre, A.M., Krahwinkel, D.J., Carrig, C.B., and Michel, R.L.: Ascites associated with intrahepatic arteriovenous fistula in a cat. J. Am. Vet. Med. Assoc., 168:589–591, 1976.

O'Brien, T.R.: *Radiographic Diagnosis of Abdominal Disorders in the Dog and Cat.* Philadelphia, W. B. Saunders Co., 1978.

Osborne, C.A., Hardy, R.M., Stevens, J.B., and Perman, V.: Liver biopsy. Vet. Clin. North Am., 4:333–348, 1974.

Root, C.R.: Interpretation of abdominal survey radiographs. Vet. Clin. North Am., 4:763–803, 1977.

Tryphona, L., and Rozdilsky, B.: Nuclear jaundice (kernicterus) in a newborn kitten. J. Am. Vet. Med. Assoc., 157:1084–1087, 1970.

Wagner, J.E.: A fatal cytauxzoonosis-like disease in cats. J. Am. Vet. Med. Assoc., 168:585–588, 1976.

Wilkinson, G.T.: A review of drug toxicity in the cat. J. Small Anim. Pract., 9:21–32, 1968.

ACUTE GASTRIC DILATION–VOLVULUS

DONALD R. STROMBECK, D.V.M.
Davis, California

INTRODUCTION

The cause of acute gastric dilation is unknown. It occurs almost invariably in large breeds of dogs of any age, with males outnumbering females 2 to 1. It is a disease of domestication, since the incidence is greater with diets of commercial dog foods than with natural diets. The incidence of acute gastric dilation may be related to the cereal content of commercial dog foods. Single rather than multiple daily feeding is associated with the problem. At present, comprehensive data are lacking on breed incidence, heritability pattern, and relationship to diet, frequency of feeding, and postprandial activity. Acute gastric dilation develops because the stomach cannot be emptied and so intragastric pressure increases. Such pressure is normally relieved by eructation and vomiting. In this condition, however, the gas, liquid, and solid gastric contents accumulate and are all retained.

Dilation of the stomach causes it to rotate on its long axis, producing a torsion of the gastroesophageal junction in a clockwise direction when the dog is in dorsal recumbency and is viewed cranially. Distention causes the greater curvature to move ventrally and the pylorus to move dorsally and to the left, becoming adjacent to the esophagus on the right. The spleen, following gastric movement, can be drawn in a complete circle and can also undergo torsion by rotating on its own attachments.

The pathogenesis of acute gastric dilation may involve the generation of normal amounts of gastric gas and fluid that are unable to escape. It may also involve the generation of more gas and fluid than can be disposed of.

ABNORMAL GASTROESOPHAGEAL JUNCTION

The correlation of acute gastric dilation with the animal's size and conformation suggests that an anatomic factor may contribute to the problem. Many dogs of the larger breeds have relatively deep chests, which alters the anatomic relationships of the stomach, esophagus, gastroesophageal junction, and diaphragm. Eructation

is not possible in dogs with acute gastric dilation, most likely because the gastroesophageal junction and sphincter fail to open. Alteration of the anatomic relationships may be the most important reason for this failure. The anatomic arrangements of this area are designed to prevent gastroesophageal reflux; therefore, any exaggeration of the normal antireflux mechanisms could prevent normal eructation. The angle at which the esophagus enters the stomach determines whether the junction opens in response to increased intragastric pressure. With gastric filling the angle between the esophagus and stomach becomes acute, and increased intragastric pressure closes the valve of His. The diaphragm contributes to the antireflux mechanism by maintaining the oblique angle at which the esophagus enters the stomach. The angle is maintained by the crura of the diaphragm, sectioning of which results in gastroesophageal reflux. Thus, the length of the intra-abdominal esophagus, the angle between esophagus and stomach, and intragastric pressure all contribute to the prevention of reflux and may be abnormal in large, deep-chested breeds of dogs.

The intra-abdominal segment of esophagus is retracted into the thoracic cavity as part of the vomiting reflex. This is mediated by vagal nerves that cause contraction of esophageal longitudinal muscles. Selective vagotomy of the caudal canine esophagus abolishes the ability to retract its intra-abdominal segment. This surgery has been proposed as a means of treating reflux in humans. These features of normal esophageal function suggest that failure of the animal to vomit or eructate may be due in part to a loss of normal vagal innervation to the caudal esophagus.

ABNORMAL GASTROESOPHAGEAL SPHINCTER

Alteration of gastroesophageal sphincter function cannot by itself result in its failure to open. Its function is controlled by both neural and humoral factors, the losses of which contribute to incompetence and reflux. No known control, even by exerting its maximal influence, can prevent the sphincter from opening when

896

intragastric pressure increases. The role of the sphincter in controlling movement of gastric contents into the esophagus is questionable, since replacement of the sphincter with an inert tube does not result in reflux. Thus, there is little reason to believe that malfunction of the sphincter itself produces acute gastric dilation.

ABNORMAL GAS AND FLUID PRODUCTION

Acute gastric dilation is associated with retention of gas in both the postprandial and fasting stomach. It has been suggested that the gas is swallowed air or that it is produced by bacterial activity on gastric contents or by the reaction of gastric acid with secretions containing bicarbonate. One study reports that the gas that produces acute gastric dilation is similar in composition to atmospheric gas, which supports the idea that most of it is swallowed air. In some dogs the concentration of carbon dioxide was 10 percent, indicating that production of this gas contributes to gastric dilation. Another study reports the gas to be primarily carbon dioxide, supporting the theory that gas-producing bacteria are involved. Air is swallowed during drinking and eating; rapid eating and gulping of liquids increase the amounts. This air escapes by eructation in normal dogs.

Gas is not produced by fermentation in the normal empty stomach, because bacteria are virtually non-existent. During feeding, bacterial numbers increase to 10^5 per gm of contents, the sources being the oral cavity and the diet. Numerous species are found, including almost every organism found in the fecal flora. Increased numbers of gas-producing bacteria in the stomach could predispose to acute gastric dilation. Cultures of gas-producing clostridia were found in one study but not in another. Increased bacterial numbers in the residual secretions of the empty stomach reflect a reduced secretion of hydrochloric acid. Gastric bacterial numbers are kept low by the normal pH of 3.0 or less. It has not been determined whether large dogs that are predisposed to acute gastric dilation have a reduced capacity to secrete hydrochloric acid. Morphologic findings indicate that these dogs have normal numbers of oxyntic cells. Severe gastric dilation may damage the stomach enough that normal gastric acid secretion is lost, predisposing to subsequent dilation.

Gas can be formed by the interaction of gastric hydrochloric acid and bicarbonate-containing secretions. The bicarbonate content of saliva is high, making swallowed saliva a source for the carbon dioxide produced. Gastric secretion of plasmalike fluid is normally mini-

mal. With acute gastric dilation, however, extracellular fluid moves into the gastrointestinal tract. The influx of fluid is secondary to altered circulation throughout the abdomen, but especially in the portal system. Gastric mucosal permeability increases, contributing to the influx of fluid. The addition of bicarbonate-containing extracellular fluid to the large amounts of acid secreted following feeding will generate substantial amounts of carbon dioxide.

Acute gastric dilation can appear after trauma, spinal surgery, and major abdominal surgery, in which a stimulation of the sympathetic nerves produces acute loss of gastrointestinal motility. Acute gastric atony and paralytic ileus describe the loss of motor function. Gas and fluid accumulate throughout the gastrointestinal tract. General anesthesia can cause gastric dilation, which may also be mediated by effects on the nervous system. The stomach can also dilate and become atonic secondary to gastric outlet obstruction.

PATHOPHYSIOLOGY

The pathophysiology of acute gastric dilation includes impairment of gastric mucosal circulation with resulting mucosal degeneration. As dilation progresses, the increased pressure occludes circulation through the portal vein and caudal vena cava. The consequence is reduced effective circulating blood volume, which contributes to shock.

Experimental obstruction of a dog's portal vein for as short a time as 30 minutes results in death within 24 hours. The cause of death is unknown but is suggested to be endotoxin absorbed from the gut and not removed by the liver during portal occlusion. Shock becomes irreversible when tissue hypoperfusion persists for several hours in hemorrhagic shock models. Irreversibility is signaled by the failure of any treatment to restore blood pressure and cardiac output.

Shock is probably also produced by peptides with vasoactive properties and myocardial depressant effects. These peptides are produced by pancreatic lysosomal enzymes acting on plasma proteins, the enzymes being released when pancreatic circulation is reduced, producing ischemia and hypoxia.

Reduced cardiac output, hypoxemia, and the effects of toxic peptides contribute to myocardial ischemia and hypoxia-producing cardiac dysrhythmias that can be fatal. These dysrhythmias are similar to clinicopathologic features of arrhythmias found in dogs with experimental occlusion of coronary arteries. They include ventricular premature depolarizations, slow ventricular rhythms, paroxysmal ventricular tachycardia, ventricular tachycardia, and multifocal ventricular tachycardia.

Disseminated intravascular coagulation (DIC) can complicate acute gastric dilation.

Acute gastric dilation results in hemoconcentration from loss of fluid into the gut. These changes are reflected in increases in hematocrit value and plasma protein concentration. No consistent changes are seen in plasma sodium, potassium, and chloride concentrations in the natural disease. Plasma potassium can increase following decompression, the concentration reaching almost twice normal within two hours. Acidosis is caused by a great increase in plasma organic acids such as lactic acid, which is elevated with acute gastric dilation.

Hepatic and renal function are usually affected by acute gastric dilation. Hepatic necrosis is identified by slight to moderate increases in serum glutamic-pyruvic transaminase (GPT) activity. The activity of this enzyme does not increase for the first two hours of acute gastric dilation but increases up to 50 times normal by two hours after decompression. Renal function is reduced, as shown by slight increases in blood urea nitrogen and creatinine levels.

Acute gastric distention applies pressure on the diaphragm and thorax, restricting pulmonary function and reducing tidal volume. Compensation is made by increased respiratory rate but, as dilation worsens, normal minute volumes cannot be maintained. The result of respiratory impairment is decreased blood oxygen tension, with the fall greatest in the caudal vena cava. The hypoxemia associated with the circulatory changes accelerates tissue death from hypoxia.

RADIOGRAPHIC FINDINGS

Gastric dilation is readily identified radiographically by finding a large gas- and fluid-filled stomach. Radiographs are taken primarily to determine whether volvulus has developed and only after decompression has been attempted or accomplished. Volvulus or splenic torsion can remain after successful decompression, which makes it essential to evaluate all dogs radiographically following a decompression that did not require celiotomy. Some dogs will eat and bloat only intermittently, despite having persistent volvulus.

MANAGEMENT

The immediate measures deal with life-threatening problems. They consist of decompression of the acute dilation and management of cardiovascular failure. Any complications found, such as cardiac dysrhythmias and DIC, are treated.

GASTRIC DECOMPRESSION AND SURGERY

Decompression of acute gastric dilation is achieved most quickly by passing a stomach tube or by trocarization. When a colt-size tube (¼-inch inside diameter) can be passed, the contents of the stomach can be removed by lavage assisted by vacuum. This tube is too large to pass in some dogs without rupturing the gastroesophageal junction or stomach. In many dogs a relatively inflexible tube of smaller diameter can be passed and directed through the gastroesophageal junction under fluoroscopic control. Inability to pass a stomach tube is not diagnostic for volvulus. Furthermore, a stomach tube can be passed in some dogs that have volvulus. When time does not permit attempting to pass a stomach tube or when a tube cannot be passed, decompression is achieved by trocarization of the stomach with 14 to 18 gauge needles. Following partial decompression, attempts are made to pass a large-bore stomach tube. Decompression is attempted by whatever means is necessary to relieve the critical condition. Trocarization can save the patient's life, and if peritonitis develops as a complication, it can be managed later. The mortality rate of treated acute gastric dilation continues to be high. The most important treatment must be directed at the causes of high mortality (not peritonitis). When acute dilation does not recur, time is available for proper radiographic evaluation of the patient and for surgery to correct volvulus when the patient's condition improves.

Decompression can be achieved by gastrotomy, which is performed under local anesthesia. The introduction of decompression via gastrotomy as part of the management has reduced mortality at one institution from 68 to 33 percent. Gastrotomy also fixes the stomach to the abdominal wall and, if the stomach is rotated to cause volvulus, this procedure prevents it from returning to its normal position after decompression. Decompression can be maintained by gastrotomy or by a pharyngostomy tube until the patient's condition stabilizes and normal gastric motility returns.

Surgical intervention to decompress acute gastric dilation is associated with a high mortality rate, exceeding 33 percent even in cases in which care is optimal. Surgeons believe that rapid surgical intervention offers the best chance for survival in dogs with acute gastric dilation involving volvulus. Surgery is performed to return the stomach to its normal position and facilitate passage of a stomach tube for gastric larvage or to remove the gastric contents via gastrotomy. Surgery may include splenectomy to remove a twisted or severely damaged spleen, pyloromyotomy to accelerate gastric emptying, and fixation of the stomach to the abdominal wall or colon. Splenectomy does not prevent recurrence of acute gastric dilation, nor does gastropexy (surgical fixation of the greater curvature of the stomach to the left abdominal wall), since the adhesions formed eventually break down. A more permanent type of gastropexy involves incorporation of part of the stomach into the left lateral abdominal wall. Gastric muscles are sutured to muscles of the abdominal wall with the anticipation that the adhesions will remain. There is no evidence that this surgery hampers normal gastric function. Another procedure for incorporation of the stomach wall into the wall of the abdomen involves creation of a gastrotomy using a Foley catheter. This binds the stomach wall to the abdominal wall and, after adhesions are formed, a gastropexy is created. Until the Foley catheter is removed (five to seven days), decompression is maintained. Gastrocolopexy, the fixation of the greater curvature of the stomach to the transverse colon, has been used successfully to prevent recurrence of acute gastric dilation. Partial gastric resection is indicated in cases in which irreversible changes are apparent in parts of the stomach. A recurrence of acute gastric dilation may be prevented by eliminating factors that contribute to the competence of the gastroesophageal junction to prevent reflux. Possibilities include elimination of the intra-abdominal esophagus and fundusectomy to eliminate the valve of His. Gastroesophageal reflux, an undesirable complication, would develop with the first-mentioned procedure. Gastric retention is associated with a loss of motility in the fundus, in which case fundusectomy would accelerate gastric emptying and could help prevent recurrence.

FLUIDS

An immediate goal of initial treatment for acute gastric dilation is to improve cardiovascular function. Short-term improvement can be achieved by rapid administration of fluids. Rate of administration and response to therapy are evaluated by measuring central venous and arterial blood pressures. Balanced electrolyte solutions such as Ringer's are used, to which bicarbonate can be added. Plasma potassium concentrations are not often increased in clinical cases. Moreover, hypokalemia can develop, which is not surprising since fluid secreted into the gut has a higher potassium concentration than extracellular fluid. With the loss of large amounts of fluid into the stomach, total body potassium is reduced. Hypokalemia develops despite acidosis, which promotes the movement of intracellular potassium into extracellular fluid. The potassium is then lost from the extracellular fluid, producing hypokalemia. If mild hyperkalemia is a problem in clinical cases, as it is in experimental models, it will be resolved by the bicarbonate used to treat acidosis. In potassium depletion the use of a solution containing no potassium could produce signs of hypokalemia. Shock therapy should include the use of solutions containing glucose. Glucose can be added to a level of 5 percent in one of the balanced electrolyte solutions. Acidosis is treated by adding bicarbonate to the balanced solution or by giving it slowly as a separate injection. Plasma bicarbonate deficits of 5 to 15 mEq/liter are predictable, and bicarbonate is given to replace the extracellular fluid deficit. Intracellular bicarbonate deficits are corrected more slowly.

Large dogs are often undertreated with fluids. When fluid therapy is delayed, a patient becomes less responsive to subsequent fluid administration. Fluids are given as rapidly as possible and in amounts required to improve cardiac output. At least two venous catheters should be placed, with one to measure central venous pressure. Fluids are given to return central venous pressure to upper normal values (4 to 5 mm Hg). When central venous pressure is normal or elevated in an animal that is hypovolemic and in shock, fluid is given until the central venous pressure increases. Humans with an elevated central venous pressure are often hypovolemic and respond favorably to large amounts of fluid, with no increase in central venous pressure.

Plasma protein concentration increases during acute gastric dilation and decreases with decompression and fluid therapy. Plasma proteins are lost into the gut with congestion produced by portal hypertension. Whole plasma may be needed to improve cardiac output if fluids are effective for only a short period. A lack of response to colloids suggests that shock is irreversible. Dextrans can be used to restore the circulating blood volume to effective levels. They are excreted in a short time. Excessive amounts increase bleeding time.

DRUGS

Corticosteroids are used routinely in managing shock. No controlled studies have shown that steroids increase survival rate in animals in shock, but beneficial effects are attributed to the ability of steroids to improve cardiac performance, stabilize membranes, and improve cell metabolism. The high doses of steroids recommended would create no problems if they were without side effects. High doses can cause acute pancreatitis and immunosuppression, permitting and potentiating bacteremia. The ability of the reticuloendothelial system to remove circulating bacteria is reduced in shock, and pharmacologic immunosuppression further handicaps the ability to respond to infection.

Cardiovascular function would be improved in shock cases by drugs that increase cardiac output and systemic arterial blood pressure and reduce peripheral vasoconstriction. Most agents (e.g., the catecholamines) that increase cardiac output and blood pressure, however, constrict microcirculation in the splanchnic viscera, contraindicating their use. Other agents (e.g., isoproterenol) reduce peripheral resistance but are likely to make shock patients more hypotensive. Newer agents appear to be quite effective in reducing mortality in dogs with endotoxin shock.

Antibiotics. The use of antibiotics is directed against microorganisms absorbed from the gastrointestinal tract and ineffectively removed by the reticuloendothelial system. Both anaerobic and aerobic bacteria are absorbed, and no single antibiotic is usually effective against both. Penicillin is an effective antibiotic against anaerobes entering the stomach, and it does not disrupt the normal intestinal microflora. Such anaerobic bacteria develop resistance to antibiotics with speed and ease, so effective antibiotics may differ from one patient to another. Kanamycin is usually effective against aerobes. Chloromycetin is less effective against aerobes but is also effective against anaerobes. Resistance to gentamicin is less likely to develop than resistance to other antibiotics. Aerobic bacteria and their endotoxins are responsible for the high mortality rates associated with abdominal contamination by the gut microflora. Abdominal infection by anaerobic contamination results in abscess formation.

Increased numbers of gas-producing bacteria are thought to contribute to excess gas formation and acute gastric dilation. This would have to be associated with a loss of the normal mechanisms for maintaining relatively sterile conditions in the empty stomach. Colonization of the stomach by gas-producing bacteria would depend on a reduction in normal acid secretion. Antibiotics are not likely to control abnormal numbers of stomach bacteria. Antibiotics given orally are not absorbed in the stomach, but neither are they retained. Furthermore, bacteria continually enter the stomach from the oral cavity.

Other Agents. Cardiac dysrhythmias are treated with lidocaine hydrochloride (4 mg/kg IV as initial bolus, 2 mg/kg as repeated bolus, and 25 to 50 mg/kg/min to continue treatment) or procainamide hydrochloride (2 mg/kg IV as initial bolus, 1 mg/kg as repeated bolus, and 20 to 40 mg/kg/min to continue treatment). DIC is treated with heparin (50 to 150 units/kg body weight at four- to six-hour intervals).

Management to prevent recurrence consists of feeding three to four times a day instead of once. Many clinicians believe that diets formulated by the owner should replace commercial dry dog foods. If feeding practices growing out of domestication predispose to acute gastric dilation, diets that are natural for carnivores should help prevent recurrence. However, no relationship has been proved between diet and acute gastric dilation. Management also includes restriction of water consumption and activity immediately after eating.

Antifoaming agents would be of value in preventing frothy bloat, but dogs with acute gastric dilation retain free air, and such chemicals would have no value in preventing recurrence.

PROGNOSIS

The mortality rate is at least 30 percent and will be higher if surgery is required. After decompression by non-surgical techniques, radiographic studies are conducted to identify any volvulus, which is surgically corrected 24 to 72 hours later or when the patient's condition improves.

The recurrence of acute gastric dilation is usually unpredictable but is greater if there is a radiographically identifiable loss of gastric motility. Normal fundic and antral motility are required for normal gastric emptying, the loss of which predisposes to acute dilation. The prognosis is less optimistic when surgery is indicated to resect atonic parts of the stomach.

SUPPLEMENTAL READING

Betts, C. W., Wingfield, W. E., and Greene, R. W.: A retrospective study of gastric dilation—torsion in the dog. J. Small Anim. Pract., 15:727–734, 1974.

Betts, C. W., Wingfield, W. E., and Rosin, E.: "Permanent" gastropexy as a prophylactic measure against gastric volvulus. J. Anim. Hospital Assoc., *12*:177–181, 1976.

Caywood, D., Teaque, H. D., Jackson, D. A., Levitt, M.D., and Bond, J. H.: Gastric gas analysis in the canine gastric dilation–volvulus syndrome. J. Anim. Hospital Assoc., *13*:459–462, 1977.

Christie, T. R., and Smith, C. W.: Gastrocolopexy for prevention of recurrent gastric volvulus. J. Anim. Hospital Assoc., *12*:173–176, 1976.

DeHoff, W. D., and Greene, R. E.: Gastric dilatation and the gastric torsion complex. Vet. Clin. North Am., *1*:141–153, 1972.

Muir, W. W., and Lipowitz, A. J.: Cardiac dysrhythmias associated with gastric dilatation–volvulus in the dog. J. Am. Vet. Med. Assoc., *172*:683–689, 1978.

Parks, J. L., and Greene, R. W.: Tube gastrostomy for the treatment of gastric volvulus. J. Anim. Hospital Assoc., *12*:168–172, 1976.

Strombeck, D. R.: *Small Animal Gastroenterology.* Davis, Calif. Stonegate Publishing Co., 1979.

Van Kruiningen, H. J., Gregoire, K., and Meuten, D. J.: Acute gastric dilatation: A review of comparative aspects by species and a study in dogs and monkeys. J. Anim. Hospital Assoc., *10*:294–324, 1974.

Walshaw, R., and Johnston, D. E.: Treatment of gastric dilatation–volvulus by gastric decompression and patient stabilization before major surgery. J. Anim. Hospital Assoc., *12*:162–167, 1976.

Wilson, R. F., and Sibbald, W. J.: (Editorial) A new look at an old approach to resuscitation: Early aggressive fluid administration. Circulatory Shock, 2:1–3, 1975.

Wingfield, W. E., Betts, C. W., and Greene, R. W.: Operative techniques and recurrence rates associated with gastric volvulus in the dog. J. Small Anim. Pract., 16:427–432, 1975.

Wingfield, W. E., Cornelius, L. M., and DeYoung, D. W.: Pathophysiology of the gastric dilation–torsion complex in the dog. J. Small Anim. Pract., *15*:735–739, 1974.

MICROBIOLOGY OF THE GASTROINTESTINAL TRACT:

Microflora and Immunology

DWIGHT C. HIRSH, D.V.M.

Davis, California

MICROFLORA OF THE GASTROINTESTINAL TRACT

INTRODUCTION

The gastrointestinal tract is a complex ecosystem made up of bacteria, fungi, and protozoa living in close association with the host. For example, in the colon there are 10^{11} organisms per gram of feces. Some have estimated that there may be 400 to 500 different species represented, many of which have not been cultured. All of these microbes live in a special relationship with the host. They are not arranged in a random, haphazard manner, but rather each species inhabits its special place, or niche, throughout the tract. The relationship is in a delicate balance that is easily upset. Such imbalances result in increased susceptibility to disease.

The normal flora of the gastrointestinal tract has been shown to serve at least three different purposes. First, and most important, it serves as a barrier between disease-producing organisms and the host; second, it may provide a source of energy; and third, it conditions the immunologic components of the gastrointestinal tract to respond in a highly efficient manner to antigenic materials introduced along the tract.

NORMAL FLORA

At birth the gastrointestinal tract is sterile. Within minutes of birth, however, the canal is flooded with microorganisms acquired from the immediate environment. The most important contributor to this microbial environment is the animal's dam.

As the diet changes from milk to solid food, the flora of the gastrointestinal tract also changes. This change in flora may be dramatically different, depending upon the character and nature of the food ingested, and takes place in a sequential manner.

Tables 1 to 4 show the composition of the bacterial flora of newborn puppies and kittens and of adult animals. From the moment of birth onward, the microbial flora is in a constant state of flux. Changes occur until the so-called normal flora is established. Once established, it is very stable.

Table 1. *Microbial Flora of the Gastrointestinal Tract of a Normal 14-day-old Puppy*[*]

| ORGANISM | Stomach | NUMBER/GRAM OF CONTENTS (log_{10}) Small Intestine | | Cecum | Feces |
		Anterior	Posterior		
Total	5–6	5	7	8–9	10
Anaerobes (Bacteroidaceae) (excluding *Lactobacillus*)	–[†]	–	–	8–9	9–10
Enterobacteriaceae	2–4	3	2–7	4–8	7–8
Streptococci (including enterococci)	3–6	2–5	2–7	4–8	9
Staphylococcus aureus	2–5	3–5	2–4	3	4
Lactobacillus spp.	2–5	2–4	5–6	4–7	9

[*]Data from: Smith, H. W.: J. Pathol. Bacteriol. *90*:495–513, 1965; and from Mitsuoka, T., and Kaneuchi, C.: Am. J. Clin. Nutr., *30*:1799–1810, 1977
[†]None detected

RELATION OF NORMAL FLORA TO STRUCTURE AND FUNCTION OF THE GASTROINTESTINAL TRACT

The microbial flora has been shown to influence the anatomic structures that line the gastrointestinal tract. Epithelial cell renewal has been shown to be faster in animals that have acquired a microbial flora. Likewise, the crypts are longer and there is more surface area, compared with the germ-free state. In addition to structural changes or differences, there are also changes that occur in the cellular content and reactions of cells that are not part of the gastrointestinal tract per se. The microbial flora aids or stimulates the formation of lymphatic tissue that lies beneath the tract.

In addition to the changes in the lymphoid system that take place following the acquisition of the microbial flora, changes occur in the activity of macrophage-type cells. Macrophages from conventional animals have been shown to digest phagocytosed material better, compared with macrophages taken from germ-free animals. Macrophage mobilization and subsequent participation in immune-related phenomena have been shown to be increased in animals possessing a microbial flora.

In addition to anatomic changes in the tract, functional activity has also been shown to be related to the microbial flora. If germ-free and conventional animals are compared with respect to the transit time of non-absorbable substances, it will be seen that these substances

Table 2. *Microbial Flora of the Gastrointestinal Tract of a Normal 14-day-old Kitten*[*]

| ORGANISM | Stomach | NUMBER/GRAM OF CONTENTS (log_{10}) Small Intestine | | Cecum | Feces |
		Anterior	Posterior		
Total	>6	3–6	4–8	8–9	10
Anaerobes (Bacteroidaceae) (excluding *Lactobacillus*)	–[†]	–	–	8–9	9
Enterobacteriaceae	–	3	3–4	8–9	7–8
Streptococci (including enterococci)	–	–	–	4–8	8
Lactobacillus spp.	>6	6	4–8	7–8	5–6

[*]Data from: Smith, H. W.: J. Pathol. Bacteriol. *90*:495–513, 1965; and from Mitsuoka, T., and Kaneuchi, C.: Am. J. Clin. Nutr., *30*:1799–1810, 1977
[†]None detected

Table 3. *Microbial Flora of the Gastrointestinal Tract of a Normal Adult Canine**

| | NUMBER/GRAM OF CONTENTS (log_{10}) | | | | |
| | | Small Intestine | | | |
ORGANISM	Stomach	Anterior	Posterior	Cecum	Feces
Total	6	6	7	8–9	10–11
Anaerobes (Bacteroidaceae) (excluding *Lactobacillus*)	1–2	5–6	4–5	8–9	10–11
Enterobacteriaceae	1–5	2–4	4–6	7–8	7–8
Streptococci (including enterococci)	1–6	5–6	5–7	8–9	9–10
Staphylococcus aureus	1	NA†	1–2	NA	4–5
Lactobacillus spp.	4–5	3–5	4–6	8–9	9
Spirochetes (relative amounts)	1+	1+	1+	2+‡	–§
Spirillaceae	NA	NA	NA	NA	–

*Data from: Smith, H. W.: J. Pathol. Bacteriol., *90*:495–513, 1965; and from Mitsuoka, T., and Kaneuchi, C.: Am. J. Clin. Nutr., *30*:1799–1810, 1977
  †Not available
  ‡4+ in the colon
  §None detected

move through the tract at a significantly higher rate when a microbial flora is present. This increase in peristaltic activity may appear to be a detriment. But, more important, the peristaltic activity of the small bowel is a host defense mechanism that sweeps microorganisms that do not belong there (i.e., pathogens) distally into an environment more noxious to them.

NORMAL FLORA AS AN ECOSYSTEM

Studies have shown that the flora is remarkably stable. Fluctuations that occur as the result of various stimuli are transient and, following the removal of such disruptive influences, the flora returns to the state that existed prior to the change. Because of this stability, it has been

Table 4. *Microbial Flora of the Gastrointestinal Tract of a Normal Adult Feline**

| | NUMBER/GRAM CONTENTS (log_{10}) | | | | |
| | | Small Intestine | | | |
ORGANISM	Stomach	Anterior	Posterior	Cecum	Feces
Total	4–6	3–4	7–8	8–9	9–10
Anaerobes (Bacteroidaceae) (excluding *Lactobacillus*)	–†	–	–	8–9	9–10
Enterobacteriaceae	4–5	3–4	4–5	5–6	6–9
Streptococci (including enterococci)	6	4	5–6	8–9	8–9
Lactobacillus spp.	–	–	7	8–9	5–9
Spirochetes	NA‡	NA	NA	NA	7–8
Spirillaceae	NA	NA	NA	NA	9

*Data from: Smith, H. W.: J. Pathol. Bacteriol., *90*:495–513, 1965; and from Mitsuoka, T., and Kaneuchi, C.: Am. J. Clin. Nutr., *30*:1799–1810, 1977
  †None detected
  ‡Not available

postulated that the relationship between the normal host and its flora is optimal. In other words, each location or site along the gastrointestinal tract is especially suited for a particular species of microorganism. Each particular strain of microbe occupies a particular site, or niche, and all others are excluded. In most instances, bacteria fed to a normal animal will be eliminated from that animal within 24 to 48 hours. If microorganisms with pathogenic potential are excluded in a similar manner, then the relationship between the host and its flora results in a defense barrier against bacterial species with pathogenic potential. This barrier and how it is formed will be discussed here.

In order to better understand how the stabilized, normal microbial flora acts as a barrier to bacterial species with pathogenic potential, it is first necessary to describe in general terms the events leading up to a disease process caused by a pathogenic agent.

Bacterial pathogens go through a two-step process in the initiation of a disease state. The first step is attachment of the pathogen to the epithelial cells of the gastrointestinal tract; the second is an activity that results in the production of the disease state.

Most if not all bacterial pathogens, as a first step in producing disease, must attach to a so-called "target cell." The concept of a target cell was formulated because disease produced by various pathogenic species of bacteria almost always occurs at a particular site along the gastrointestinal tract. Following attachment to the target cell, the bacterial pathogen multiplies on the epithelial cell, with resultant disease.

The normal microbial flora acts as a defense barrier either by making the target cell unavailable to the pathogen or by creating an environment that is detrimental to the pathogen. In other words, if the normal inhabitants of the gastrointestinal tract are secure in their niches, then species of bacteria with pathogenic potential may not be able to compete successfully with them for a site of attachment. Without a site of attachment, the pathogen would be swept distally by peristalsis, away from the susceptible target cell. Thus, anything that upsets the balance between host and normal flora may give a pathogen easy access to its target cell or allow it to multiply to high enough numbers so that competition for the target cell is easier.

The mechanisms whereby members of the normal flora establish their particular niches and exclude other species of bacteria as well as potential pathogens can be divided into bacterial properties and host properties.

BACTERIAL PROPERTIES

Surface Structures. Structures on the surface of microorganisms living in the gastrointestinal tract are probably one of the most important of all the properties a bacterium may possess that are involved in the establishment of the ecosystem. These structures are important because it is through them that the microorganism comes in intimate contact with the host.

Adhesin is a term used by some to describe surface structures that account for the "stickiness" certain bacteria have for certain epithelial cells. Adhesins may be classified in three general categories: fimbria, agglutinins, and capsular structures.

FIMBRIA. Fimbria are whisker-like protrusions on the surface of a microorganism. Chemically, they are proteins. The best-studied fimbrial structure relative to the gastrointestinal tract is the K-88 antigen. Though this antigen is used by enterotoxigenic *E. coli* to stick to toxin-sensitive cells of the small intestine of the newborn pig, it can be hypothesized that similar structures may be present on the surface of microorganisms that constitute the normal flora. K-88 antigens have an affinity for certain substrates found on or as part of the epithelial cells of the distal small intestine. Similar structures with different site specificity may account for the locational stability of the normal flora.

AGGLUTININS. Agglutinins, so named because they will agglutinate red blood cells, are a group of substances found on the surface of various microorganisms occupying the gastrointestinal tract. These substances have not been defined chemically. Experimentally, bacteria possessing these substances have been shown also to adhere to the brush border of rabbit intestinal cells. It can be theorized tht certain agglutinins have affinity for various substrates throughout the GI tract.

CAPSULAR STRUCTURES. Capsules, chemically polysaccharides in nature, are sticky, especially in relation to the surfaces of epithelial cells. Though proof of specificity is lacking, it is hypothesized that some capsular types will stick to certain cell surfaces. An example of the possible specificity of capsular antigens is seen in the specific adherence of certain capsular types of *E. coli* to urinary bladder epithelial cells. Again, it is tempting to speculate that the same sort of specificity occurs in the gastrointestinal tract.

Metabolic By-products. The secretion of certain substances into the immediate environment of a niche may be important in keeping the population size in check in addition to making conditions undesirable for other competing species of microorganisms. There are two classes of metabolic by-products that will be discussed: (1) fatty acids and (2) deconjugated bile salts.

FATTY ACIDS. The fatty acids, especially acetic and butyric acids, are powerful stabilizing influences in the gastrointestinal tract. These substances are secreted as metabolic by-products by the species of obligate anaerobes that live in the GI tract. These substances do not act alone, however. To be most effective, the fatty acids work in concert with the pH and oxidation-reduction potential (Eh) of the bowel. When the pH is between 5 and 6 (the normal pH of the large intestine) and the Eh is approximately -200 mV or less (the normal Eh of the large intestine is approximately -500 mV), the fatty acids present are extremely toxic to members of the family Enterobacteriaceae. It is probably the fatty acids in cooperation with the pH and Eh that are responsible for the precipitous drop that occurs in the numbers of enteric bacteria following the colonization of the large bowel with anaerobes. Even more spectacular than that are the effects of these particular by-products upon members of the family Enterobacteriaceae that possess pathogenic potential.

DECONJUGATED BILE SALTS. Free bile acids (e.g., deoxycholic and cholic acid are inhibitory to the flora of the large bowel. This flora will deconjugate the conjugated bile acids (e.g., taurocholic acid) traveling down the small intestine. The resulting deconjugated acid is toxic at concentrations of 1 to 2 millimoles/liter and at pH 5.8, the conditions of the terminal ileum. Though this phenomenon probably does not play a role at the niche level, it has been postulated to be a mechanism that prevents retrograde bacterial colonization by large bowel organisms in the upper small gut.

Nutritional. Nutritional substrate availability is probably a mixture of host and bacterial properties. In its simplest terms, nutritional substrate availability means that some strains of bacteria eat what others need. It has been shown that competition occurs for fermentable carbon sources under highly anaerobic conditions. If an invader can out-compete an inhabitant of a particular niche for a carbon source, than the invader will probably take over the niche.

HOST PROPERTIES

Very little is known concerning the host's contribution to the host-parasite relationship.

Epithelial surfaces and the substances bathing them are the structures in most intimate contact with the microorganisms living in the gastrointestinal tract. The nature of the substances within the cell membrane or within the substances secreted by the epithelial cells is just now being studied. The most probable sites for bacterial adhesion appear to be the brush borders and the overlying mucous gel.

Peristalsis. Peristalsis has been used throughout this discussion to describe the mechanism whereby microorganisms that are not anchored are swept distally. In the small bowel, peristaltic activity plays a major role in host defense of the intestinal tract. The most important regulator of the size of the population of pathogenic bacteria in the small intestine is peristaltic activity. The normal flora contributes to the defense of the small bowel by stimulating peristalsis.

Immune System. It is known that the local immune response at an epithelial cell surface will prevent the binding of pathogenic microorganisms. Presumably this is due to antibody made against antigenic determinants on the surface of the pathogen. Since the pathogen can no longer stick to the epithelial cell, it will be swept distally away from the target cell. This immunologic phenomenon is easily understood in terms of host response to a pathogen. But what about the response to normal flora?

Experimental evidence suggests that animals do not form much of an immune response to antigenic determinants possessed by members of their own flora. There is a great deal of similarity between the antigen determinants on the surface of epithelial cells that line the intestinal tract and the microorganisms that live there. If this is so, then it is unlikely that an immune response will be made against the normal flora. But even if an immune response were made against the members of the normal flora, only those organisms that must adhere to an epithelial surface will be affected, and these can only be influenced if their numbers are small.

On the other hand, the microorganisms can change under the influence of an immune response. It has been shown that certain species of epithelial cell dwellers constantly change surface antigenic determinants, presumably under antibody pressure. Conceivably these sorts of changes would occur until antibodies were no longer made, i.e., when the determinants on the surface of the microbe were similar to the determinants on the surface of the epithelial cells.

One might ask why this could not occur with

the pathogenic species of microorganisms. It is possible, except that it has been shown that antibody and bacterial antagonism work in a synergistic manner. Pathogenic microorganisms (in small numbers) would have to contend with both an immune response and bacterial antagonism to be able to adhere to target cells.

All of these factors have been hypothesized to account for the stability of the normal flora — normal flora that acts as a primary protective barrier to block selective adsorption of pathogenic species of bacteria to their target tissue. One might then ask how the ecosystem can be changed to favor microorganisms with pathogenic potential?

Obviously, the newborn animal would be the most susceptible to disease, since there are no established niches. This is exactly what happens when the newborn animal does not receive colostrum. Colostrum contains the antibodies that are specific for surface structures on potential pathogens. Combination of these antibodies with these surface structures blocks attachment of the pathogen to its target cell.

Antimicrobic agents can interfere with the normal defense barrier of the gastrointestinal tract to such a degree that serious illness can result secondary to antimicrobic treatment. This is because the bulk of the normal microbial flora (prokaryotic) is inhibited or killed by the commonly used antibacterial agents. However, there are two segments of the normal flora that may not be affected as seriously as the rest. These are fungi and members of the family Enterobacteriaceae.

Members of the family Enterobacteriaceae may acquire the genes necessary to either inactivate an antimicrobic agent or become resistant directly. The pieces of DNA upon which the resistance genes reside belong to a family of genetic elements called *plasmids*. Plasmids exist inside the bacterial cell membrane in the cytoplasm and are unassociated with the chromosomal DNA. In fact, plasmid DNA replicates autonomously and for the most part is not controlled by chromosomal DNA. Most plasmid DNA molecules that carry genes for antimicrobic resistance (R plasmids) are transmissible. This means that R plasmids and their antimicrobial resistances can be passed, by conjugation, from one bacterium to another. This can be done at any time but is very efficient during log phase growth. Thus, a resistant bacterium can pass antimicrobic resistance to any member of the family Enterobacteriaceae and, provided the particular plasmid that is passed is compatible in the new host cell, the recipient will also be resistant. R plasmids may carry any number or combination of resistance genes. Bacteria possessing R plasmids are resistant to two or more antimicrobic agents. In our experience, the median number of resistance genes is three to four. Thus, selection of a resistant bacterium through the use of antimicrobic agents (either prophylactically or therapeutically) results in the selection of a bacterium resistant to other antimicrobics as well. Over the years, the environmental pool of the plasmids has grown tremendously. The reason for this is beyond the scope of this discussion, but the fact remains that most of the members of the family Enterobacteriaceae (pathogen and non-pathogen alike) possess R plasmids. And since most of the enteric pathogens belong to the family Enterobacteriaceae, antimicrobics will select for these bacteria at the expense of other non-Enterobacteriaceae, especially the obligate anaerobes. If this later group of microorganisms is removed, so also is a powerful regulatory substance — fatty acids.

Fungi can also be affected by antimicrobic agents, albeit indirectly. These microorganisms are kept in check, as are members of the family Enterobacteriaceae, by low pH, low Eh, and volatile fatty acids. Antimicrobic agents, by removing the producers of the volatile fatty acids, also remove an important restraint on the fungi. In addition, there is some evidence to suggest that yeasts (especially of the genus *Candida*) are affected directly by antimicrobics in such a manner as to make them more invasive.

Stress. Stress, whether nutritional or emotional, appears to increase the likelihood of disease of any kind, especially intestinal disease. Experimentally, stress will result in a change in the normal intestinal flora. These changes, at least in experimental animals, stem from a drop in the anaerobic component of the normal flora. Subsequently, the numbers of coliform bacteria rise to very high levels. What appears to be occurring is a change in the major regulatory mechanism of the intestinal tract, the fatty acid production. Most, if not all, enteric pathogens belong to the family Enterobacteriaceae. Without fatty acid control these pathogens would be able to grow to numbers that would allow for successful competition for attachment to a target cell site. The key question appears to be, why did the population of anaerobic bacteria drop? The answer is not known. One possibility may be substrate availability for the anaerobic species. It is known that the amount of mucin secreted into the gastrointestinal tract can be influenced by corticosteroids. If the stress were of sufficient magnitude and chronicity to result in a level of corticosteroids that would be sufficient to decrease mucin production, then conceivably the numbers of anaerobic bacteria that utilize the mucin as an energy source would also be reduced.

IMMUNITY OF THE GASTROINTESTINAL TRACT

PASSIVE IMMUNITY

At birth most, if not all, species of animals have a lowered ability to respond immunologically to externally introduced antigens, but not because they are unable to do so. On the contrary, in those species studied a specific immune response *in utero* can be generated toward antigenic determinants carried by certain antigens. The maturation of the propensity of an animal to respond to certain antigenic determinants progresses in a sequential fashion, starting *in utero*. The sequence depends upon the species of animal. It has been found that the response of the fetus is not of the same magnitude, by any means, as that seen after birth, but it is sufficient to abort disease following infection by certain agents.

The lowered ability to respond to antigenic determinants presented neonatally may in part be due to increased levels of corticosteroids found in the fetal and neonatal circulations and in part to the relative immaturity of certain elements of the immune system. Whatever the reason, the neonate is at risk. the antigenic determinants that place the animal at risk for the most part are carried by species of bacteria with pathogenic potential whose target cell resides in the intestinal tract.

Protection of the neonate from such insults is acquired from the dam by way of antibodies. It must be stressed that this is not just any antibody, but antibody with specificity for antigenic determinants possessed by the pathogen; i.e., the dam has to have been exposed to the antigenic determinants. This protection is passed to the offspring prenatally, postnatally, or both, depending on the species of animal. Horses, pigs, and ruminants acquire no immunoglobulins from the dam prenatally, whereas 5 percent of the passively acquired immunoglobulins are passed prenatally in the dog and 95 percent postnatally. In man and rabbits the process is entirely prenatal.

Passage of antibody across the placenta depends upon the placentation and the possession of appropriate receptors for the Fc portion of IgG. The placentation and receptors of human, dog, cat, and rabbit are sufficient for passage of all (human and rabbit) or part (dog and cat) of passively acquired immunity. All acquired immunity with placental passage comes from IgG.

Acquisition of antibody after birth is a process that starts with the ingestion of colostrum and continues with the ingestion of milk until weaning. The most abundant immunoglobulin in colostrum is IgG, followed by IgA and IgM. In milk, IgA is the predominant immunoglobulin.

Immunoglobulins acquired neonatally protect the newborn in two ways: (1) they provide circulating antibody to help prevent systemic disease and (2) they provide antibody at the level of the intestinal epithelial cell to block subsequent attachment of potential pathogenic microorganisms to target cells. In order to provide protection in the systemic circulation of the newborn, colostral antibodies must be able to cross the epithelial boundary of the intestinal tract and gain entrance, intact, into the lymphatic and vascular systems. During the first 24 to 48 hours, depending on species, the epithelial cells of the small intestine will absorb Ig from the lumen of the bowel. This absorption is relatively non-selective as far as isotype of immunoglobulin is concerned. Diet or feeding practices may influence absorption time. The mechanism behind the phenomenon appears to be the following: Ig adsorbs to receptors (for Fc) at the base of the microvilli of the small intestine. A pinocytic vesicle then forms, with the Ig attached to the pinocytic vacuole wall. The Ig as such passes through the epithelial cell to the lamina propria. It is only during the time of absorption of Ig that the receptors are present. The result of pinocytic events that take place after the receptor is gone, and the result when intestinal absorption of Ig does not occur (as is the case with humans and rabbits), is the fusion of the pinocytic vesicle (containing the Ig) with a lysosome and the ultimate enzymatic degradation of the immunoglobulin protein.

Immunoglobulins acquired in colostrum are exposed to enzymatic processes in the oral cavity and gastrointestinal tract of the newborn. The most labile, in terms of enzymatic degradation in the gastrointestinal tract, is IgG, whereas IgA and IgM, because of their association with secretory component (SC), are less so. (This topic will be discussed in greater detail later.) However, colostral secretions have been shown to contain a trypsin-inhibitory factor. This factor, and others like it, has been postulated to account for the survival of IgG (and IgM not associated with SC) during the first day or two after birth. In addition, the levels of enzymatic activity of the secretions of the neonate are only a fraction of what they will be later. This, in conjunction with enzyme inhibitors in colostrum, serves to protect enzymatically labile immunoglobulins. After the first days of lactation, the levels of IgG and IgM fall drastically, whereas the concentration of IgA falls relatively little. As a result, the major immunoglobulin in the milk of all species except the ruminant is IgA. This change in emphasis suits the situation beautifully. IgG is no longer able to cross the epithelial surface of the intestinal tract, and the enzyme-inhibitors are no longer being secreted. Yet the intestinal tract is vulnerable to attack by pathogenic species of micoorganisms. There are two reasons for this: (1) the normal microflora of the gastrointestinal tract has not yet been established, and competition for ecologic niches is still going on at a great pace; and (2) the immune system may not be competent enough to respond to the antigenic determinants of a potential pathogen (this depends on the determinant and the species of animal). If able to respond, it will take time for enough specific antibody to be made in order to block adsorption of the pathogen to a target cell. Thus, the change in the immunoglobulin isotype is fortuitous, because IgA is aptly suited for survival in the milieu of the gastrointestinal tract.

ACTIVE IMMUNITY — GENERAL

The immune response to antigens presented to the animal by way of the gastrointestinal tract is in many ways similar to and in some ways different from the response to antigens presented parenterally. The similarities of the responses encompass the cells involved and the end products (antibody and cell-mediated immunity). The dissimilarities are seen in the traffic patterns that stimulated cells take after contact with antigen and in the major type of antibody that is made (IgA).

There are three cell types involved with the initiation and elicitation of the immune response: macrophages, T cells, and B cells.

MACROPHAGES

Macrophages are large phagocytic cells that arise in the bone marrow, traverse the peripheral circulation as monocytes, and reside in the tissues as wandering phagocytic cells. Aside from their phagocytic activities, these cells appear to play an important role in the initiation of the immune response. In particular, macrophages have been shown to somehow enable the response to proceed in the most efficient fashion, i.e., a maximal immune response per unit of antigen. Macrophages "process" antigen in such a way as to make the antigen more presentable to the other cells of the immune response (the T and B cells). Without the participation of the macrophage, most immune responses to antigens are weak and meager, and with some antigenic systems immunologic tolerance may result.

Included in the macrophage pool are the dendritic macrophages, which sit on the reticular fibers of lymph nodes, and the phagocytic cells of the spleen. The Kupffer cells of the liver, on the other hand, do not appear to act beyond the function of phagocytic cells.

T CELLS

The second cell of the immune response, the T cell, arises in the bone marrow. In order to function to its fullest capacity, it must first travel to the thymus. After leaving the thymus, T cells travel to peripheral lymphoid tissue and accumulate in T cell–dependent areas of the spleen (periarteriolar cuff of the white pulp) and lymph nodes (diffuse cortex and corticomedullary junction). There are at least three subpopulations of T cells: (1) T-helper cells, (2) T-suppressor cells, and (3) the T cell subpopulation that is involved in cell-mediated immunity (CMI).

T-helper cells are those T cells that cooperate with the macrophage (containing the "processed" antigenic determinants) and the B cell, the end result being the formation of antibody specific for the antigenic determinants (in or on the macrophage) by cells of the B cell line. How the T cell does this is not known. A T cell specific for the antigen will recognize a portion of the antigen (an antigenic determinant) via a receptor on the surface of the T cell in a fashion somewhat analogous to a lock and key. The antigenic determinant–recognizing receptor has not yet been defined, but its existence is well documented. Once the correct contact is made, the helper T cell stimulates the B cell (also associated with other antigenic determinants via a receptor) to undergo blastogenesis and division and finally to make antibody specific for the antigenic determinant recognized by the B cell. At the same time that the B cell is dividing (cloning), the T-helper cells are doing the same. This enlarging population, in addition to aiding the B cell to clone, also regulates the size of the B cell clone. The expanded clone of T cells, after antigens have left the system, remains as a "memory" compartment waiting for contact with the same antigenic determinant again. When this contact occurs, a response characteristic of a secondary response will arise; i.e., more antibody will be made in a shorter length of time.

The T cells involved with cell-mediated responses (tumor and graft rejection, macrophage activation) are different from the T-helper cell population. Tumor immunity is the result of specific T cells that recognize specific non-self antigenic determinants on the surface of tumor cells. T cells then respond by the liberation of substances called *lymphokines* that have detrimental effects on the tumor (or non-self cell in the case of an allograft). An analogous T cell response may occur in viral infections. Here virus-determined antigenic determinants (non-self) are exhibited by the infected cell.

T cell–mediated immunity is also important in diseases caused by certain infectious agents. The classic agents are *Brucella, Listeria, Mycobacterium, Salmonella,* and *Toxoplasma.* These agents reside quite happily inside macrophage cells. Antibody, though specifically made against antigenic determinants on their cell surfaces, cannot bind with them because of their intracellular location. The T cell, however, following contact with antigenic determinants on their surfaces, liberates lymphokines that will activate the macrophages to kill very efficiently the bacteria living in their cytoplasm.

The third subpopulation of T cell is the T-suppressor cell. This subpopulation, recognized relatively recently, has been called by some the regulatory cell type. Instead of aiding the immune response, this subpopulation turns it off. T-suppressor cells, like T cells in general, take part in the immune response in a specific fashion; i.e., they recognize specific antigen determinants. Thus, it can be said that the magnitude of an immune response is dependent upon the relative proportions of T-suppressor cells and T-helper cells.

B Cells

B cells, like macrophages and T cells, are a population of lymphocytes that arise in the bone marrow. But unlike macrophages and T cells, they travel to a site in the body that has yet to be identified (possibilities are the fetal liver, lymphoid follicles, or bone marrow itself). This site is analogous to the bursa of Fabricius in birds and mammals and is called the bursal equivalent (thus the epithet *B cell*). Before they can realize their full potential, B cells must go to the bursal equivalent. Following induction to further differentiation in the bursal equivalent, they are full-fledged B cells with certain characteristics that enable the observer to tell them from T cells, i.e., receptors for complement, immunoglobulins on their surfaces and, most important, the ability, following exposure to antigen, to make antibody. After leaving the bursal equivalent, B cells travel to B cell–dependent areas of the spleen (germinal centers in the white pulp) and lymph nodes (germinal centers). The B cell possesses antigenic determinant–recognizing receptors on its surface that have been defined in considerable detail. These receptors are immunoglobulins in nature and in fact contain the combining site of the same specificity of the antibody the cell will ultimately make.

The B cell cooperates with the helper T cell together with the antigenic determinants on the surface of the macrophage. The B cell, after receiving a signal from the T-helper cell along with a signal from its own surface via the combination of receptor and antigenic determinant, undergoes blastogenesis, division, and production of antibody. As mentioned before, the helper T cell continuously controls the B cell clone size. In addition, the helper T cell will signal the B cell to stop making IgM, the immunoglobulin that the B cell will make first, and to make another isotype. (Depending upon the location of the cell, this might be IgG, IgA, or IgE.) Some of the B cell clones will stop their cloning process and, like the T-helper cells, remain as memory cells. It is doubtful that memory cells per se are evolved. Rather, the cloning process is interrupted because of the lack of antigen and T-helper cell signals. Other B cells, probably those that were first stimulated by the newly arrived antigen, will differentiate all the way to plasma cells. The prime function of these cells is to produce antibody, and by this time almost all the antibody that they will make will be IgG, IgA, or IgE.

The immune response against antigens introduced parenterally takes place in organized lymphoid tissues (lymph nodes and spleen). Antigens finding their way into the systemic circulation will be phagocytosed by macrophages of the spleen and presented to appropriate T and B cells in the white pulp. Here antibodies to specific antigenic determinants are made along with memory B cells, memory T cells, and T cells that will respond in the CMI response.

The same sort of activity will be found when antigen is introduced into the tissue spaces. Depending upon their physical state (particulate vs. soluble), either the antigen will come in contact with and be phagocytosed by macrophages at the site of antigen deposition and then taken to the draining lymph node or, as is the case of most soluble antigens, the antigen will go directly through the afferent lymphatic system and be filtered out by the dendritic macrophages of the lymph node. It is in the cortex of the lymph node that specific T and B cells come in contact with the antigenic determinants and there that triggering of the immune response takes place.

Shortly after the primary immune response occurs, some memory B and memory T cells leave the lymph node (via the efferent lymphatics) or spleen (via the splenic vein or efferent splenic lymphatic) and become distributed through the body. Those cells in lymphatic channels get back into the blood via the thoracic duct by way of the posterior vena cava near the thoracic inlet. Once in the blood stream, these cells can go to any lymphoid tissue in the body via the various postcapillary venules of lymph nodes that possess a special type of endothelial lining (high endothelial cells). Lymphoid cells wishing to gain entrance into the lymph node do so by passing between the high endothelial cells and thereby find themselves in the cortex of the lymph node.

The end result is that, after a primary immune response, every lymphatic structure in the body becomes seeded with T cells and B cells specific for the antigenic determinant on the antigen that first elicited the primary response. Thus, the same antigen introduced a second time will come in contact with an expanded population (relative to the first exposure) of lymphocytes specific for the determinant on the antigen. The response is therefore quicker (recruitment of virgin B and T cells is not necessary) and more vigorous (more cells are responding).

ACTIVE IMMUNITY — INTESTINAL

Antigens that contact the animal by way of the gastrointestinal tract elicit the production of antibody (mainly IgA but other isotypes as well) and the formation of cell-mediated immunity. The manner in which the immune system accomplishes this is somewhat different from that seen with parenterally introduced antigen. This is because the gastrointestinal tract is unique in regard to exposure to antigenic materials. Being a long tube, it possesses an enormous surface area that is in contact with a variety of antigens, yet the initial antigenic stimulus is localized at a particular site. To be effective the immune response must be triggered locally, but at the same time it must be able to "protect" a relatively large surface area.

In addition to these considerations, the products of the immune response must be able to function along the entire length of the tract. Thus, antibodies that find their way into the lumen must be able to withstand the enzymatic assaults of proteolytic enzymes that exist there. Too, the antibodies must be able to do their jobs at a site that possesses no phagocytic cells and in a milieu that is anticomplementary.

Before discussing how this occurs, it would be best to review the microanatomy of the gastrointestinal tract with emphasis on cells and cell types involved in the immune response. Macrophages, lymphocytes, and plasma cells are found in great numbers throughout the length of the gastrointestinal tract. These cells are found in the lamina propria as diffuse collections of cells, as nodules with germinal centers, or as a collection of nodules with a unique association with the epithelial surface (Peyer's patches).

The diffuse collections of these cell types can be found in the lamina propria running from stomach to rectum. Some lymphocytes can be seen between the columnar epithelial cells and the epithelium (interepithelial cell lymphocytes). The lymphoid cell types are both B and T cells. At one time it was thought that the interepithelial cells represented old and retired lymphocytes being excreted into the intestinal lumen. This is not the case. They are B and T cells, and their presence seems to be dependent upon antigen in the gut.

The lymphoid nodule, the surrounding cells, and the relation of the nodule to the epithelial surface deserve special note. The nodules are found scattered throughout the length of the tract. Groups of nodules occur as Peyer's patches near the terminal end of the small intestine. These nodules arise in the lamina propria and extend down through the muscularis mucosa into the submucosa. The epithelial cells lining the mucosal surface over the lymphoid nodule change from columnar to cuboidal. The cell type overlying the lymphoid nodules requires special mention. These cells, recently termed *M cells* (membranous epithelial), lack microvilli and glycocalyx and possess no terminal webs. M cells, unlike adjacent columnar cells with interlocking tight junctions and terminal webs, permit the passage of substances from the luminal surface through the cytoplasm into the lamina propria.

The nodule itself is divided into three areas: dome, T-dependent area, and follicle. The dome-follicle complex contains B cells almost exclusively, whereas the interfollicle area contains T cells. There are macrophage-type cells present in the nodule, although there is debate on this subject.

Antigenic materials can be absorbed intact from the gastrointestinal tract. Some antigens not only are absorbed but also will stimulate lymphoid cells located in tissues peripheral to the intestinal tract. This has been shown to be a size-related phenomenon. A great deal of research has been done about where these materials are absorbed. Apparently there are two ways that antigenic material can be absorbed from the gastrointestinal tract. The major way is through pinocytic vacuoles of the M cell. Another, though minor, way is through the columnar epithelium. In the latter instance there is a balance between what is digested within the pinocytic vacuole and what is not. After an animal reaches a certain age, most of the macromolecules that enter the columnar cells are digested before they reach the lamina propria.

Whichever way the antigenic material gains entrance to the lamina propria, macrophage cells phagocytose (pinocytose) the antigen and initiate the immune response. The M cell itself may act directly in this capacity. Very close associations between lymphocytes in nodules with M cells have been observed.

If the antigen is invasive (e.g., *Salmonella*), macrophages may phagocytose, process, and present antigenic determinants to appropriate B and T cells in the nodule or mesenteric lymph node.

What happens next is poorly understood. Macrophages probably initiate the response. The T and B cells that form the "triplex" are specific, in that they have receptors that "fit" an antigenic determinant. The triplex probably forms in the nodule, but there is little evidence to say that it cannot form in the mesenteric lymph node. It is at this stage that similarities between the immune responses to parenterally introduced antigens and antigens absorbed via the gastrointestinal tract end. The majority of the B cells that are stimulated in Peyer's patches will ultimately differentiate into plasma cells that will secrete IgA.

T and B cells, following stimulation by antigen, undergo blastogenesis and division. Most of the division is observed with the T cell population. After stimulation, the T and B cells leave the nodule and travel via efferent lymphatics to the mesenteric lymph nodes and then through these nodes to the thoracic duct. After a brief stay in the spleen, these cells will "home" to the lamina propria of the intestinal tract (though not exclusively), but for every cell that goes elsewhere, four to five go to the intestinal tract. In the lamina propria they finish differentiation to plasma cells and secrete IgA. Smaller numbers of IgM- and IgG-secreting lymphocytes find their way to the intestinal tract. Stimulated precursors of IgA production taken from peripheral lymphoid tissue or spleen do not "home" to the lamina propria of the gastrointestinal tract.

The homing phenomenon is poorly understood. It does not seem to be dependent upon antigen or related to IgA on the surface, to secretory component (see following discussion) on the basal side of the epithelial cell surface, or to B or T cells. Whatever the nature of this attraction, it is efficient indeed, for what started at a single locus (a lymphoid nodule) ends up as a generalized deposition of antibody-forming cells along the entire length of the gastrointestinal tract.

In all of the domestic species, except the ruminants, IgA is the major immunoglobulin in intestinal secretions, followed by IgM and then by IgG. Very little if any IgE is found. This is reflected in the relative numbers of IgA-, IgM, and IgG-secreting plasma cells in the lamina propria. All of the IgA found in intestinal secretions comes from local production, whereas IgM and IgG come from both local production and passive diffusion from serum.

The plasma cells that "home" to the lamina propria of the gastrointestinal tract secrete antibody (IgA, IgM, IgG) into the tissue space beneath the epithelial cells lining the tract. IgA is unique among these isotypes, for it is not only the most concentrated (ruminants excluded) but is also aptly suited to function in the biochemically hostile environment of the intestinal tract. IgA is made as a 7S monomer inside a plasma cell. Two 7S monomers are hooked together to form an 11S dimer. (The sedimentation coefficient of the dimer is slightly different, depending upon the species of animal.) The cell hooks the two monomers together with a protein called J-piece. The immunoglobulin is then secreted from the cell and enters the lamina propria. From here it can enter the lymphatics, and in all domestic species studied (dog, ruminant, pig) this dimer constitutes almost all of the IgA found in the serum. However, the major function of the IgA that is secreted is to impart immunity to the mucosal surface of the gastrointestinal tract. It must get to the luminal side of the epithelium and, in addition, must be able to withstand the rather harsh environment of the intestinal lumen. The IgA dimer gets to the lumen by attaching to a glycoprotein (molecular weight of 48,000 to 80,000 daltons, depending on species) that lies on the basal surface of the epithelial cells. This glycoprotein is called secretory component (SC). SC is found on the basal surface of epithelial cells in the villi of the large intestine and in the gland openings and crypt cells of the small intestine. The attachment of dimeric IgA to SC is made via the J-piece. Following attachment, the IgA-SC complex is interiorized, transported to the luminal side of the epithelial cell, and then exteriorized. In this case SC stays attached to the

J-piece of the dimer. This complex is now called secretory IgA (sIgA). The SC of sIgA imparts relative resistance to proteolytic cleavage by the enzymes in the intestinal tract. How this works is not understood.

IgM molecules are made as they are anywhere else in the body; i.e., five 7S monomers are joined together with J-piece. IgM that is secreted into the lamina propria of the gastrointestinal tract will also come in contact with SC, via J-piece, on the basal side of the epithelial cell. Approximately 60 to 75 percent of the IgM in the lamina propria will form a stable enough complex with SC to be transported to the luminal surface of the tract. The rest is secreted with SC in a rather loose association. The attachment of SC to IgM apparently is not the same as with IgA, but the end result, i.e., a relative resistance to proteolytic attack, is the same.

The mucosal surface of the gastrointestinal tract is anticomplementary and does not possess phagocytic cells. IgA, when bound to an antigenic determinant, does not fix complement (at least not by the classic pathway) and has been shown to be a very poor opsonizing antibody (probably because of the lack of receptors on phagocytic cells for the Fc portion of IgA). How then does IgA or any other immunoglobulin impart with immunity on this site? Protection elicited by immunoglobulin in the intestinal tract seems to involve the interaction between the antigen (microorganism) and the epithelial cell. In order to produce disease, most if not all pathogens must first attach to a target cell; interruption of this attachment aborts disease. It is not clear how this blockage occurs. It may be as simple as a steric interference. On the other hand, it may also involve the epithelial cell (the target cell) itself, since metabolic inhibitors will abrogate the blocking mechanism.

The role of the stimulated T cell, aside from acting as a T-helper or T-suppressor, is hard to quantitate. Though most of the lymphocytes in the lamina propria are B cells, there are significant numbers of T cells. Cell-mediated immune responses in the gastrointestinal tract would be involved with tumor rejection and immunity against certain pathogens, such as *Salmonella*, that gain entry into the lamina propria.

Another function of immunoglobulin is to prevent the absorption of food antigens. Food antigens, when bound to specific immunoglobulins, are not absorbed into the body. It is thought by some that this plays an important role in preventing food antigens from stimulating peripheral lymphoid tissue, which would result in a rise in the level of circulating antibody with the concomitant risk of immune complex–mediated disease.

The operation of immunologic memory at the level of the gastrointestinal tract has not been studied to any great degree. Antigens absorbed for the second (or more) time would come in contact with memory B and T cells still in the originally stimulated nodule. However, to be effective the antigen would also have to come in contact with memory B and T cells that arose from the originally stimulated nodule and that are now spread throughout the gastrointestinal tract in the lamina propria. Presumably, the small amount of intact antigen that makes its way through the columnar epithelium would be enough to trigger the cells to finish differentiation to plasma cells, with the resultant production of antibody.

THE USE OF ANTIMICROBIAL DRUGS IN THE TREATMENT OF GASTROINTESTINAL DISORDERS

DWIGHT C. HIRSH, D.V.M.,
and L. REED ENOS, Pharm. D.
Davis, California

Many diarrheal diseases are treated with antimicrobial agents, and this treatment falls into two categories. The first and most common includes those conditions in which the cause is unknown. Antimicrobial therapy in such conditions is irrational. The second category encompasses diarrhea in which a specific microbial etiology is suspected or known. There is no evidence that antimicrobial therapy is of any value in treating these diseases as long as the infectious agent is confined to the gastrointestinal tract. The efficacy of antimicrobial agents in the treatment of these diseases is marginal at best. The deleterious effects of such therapy on the patient and the environment have gone unrecognized. In addition to the intrinsic toxicity of antimicrobial agents, it is now apparent that the effects of these drugs on microbial populations are more far-reaching and potentially more dangerous than were known at first.

Rational or irrational use of an antimicrobial agent results in changes in the normal flora throughout the body. The changes in the normal flora can have such deleterious effects that it is imperative to give serious thought prior to prescribing them.

The normal flora acts as a primary host defense barrier. As such it is vital to the host that the barrier remain intact. This barrier results from the optimal relationship among microbes in the host. This relationship is part of complex ecosystems that exist anywhere in or on the body. Microbes do not distribute themselves in a random, haphazard manner throughout the ecosystem, but rather each microbe exists in a niche especially suited for it. Put another way, the normal flora "niche dweller" lives in a particular site because it is uniquely suited to live there. If another microbe can out-compete the niche dweller, then the newcomer will occupy the niche.

In order to produce disease most bacterial pathogens must first attach to or interact with a target cell. Following this interaction, the microbe will produce disease by a variety of means, e.g., toxin production or invasion. However, if the target cell occurs in a niche occupied by another group of microbes, then the pathogen must out-compete these niche dwellers in order to gain access to the target cell. Most bacterial pathogens cannot do this without help.

A major way to disrupt the ecosystem and thereby help the pathogen successfully compete with the niche dweller is through the use of antimicrobial agents. There is no more efficient method of producing such an effect. For example, it takes one million times more *Salmonella* organisms to produce disease in an untreated animal than in an animal pretreated with an antimicrobial agent. The only difference between these animals is the presence or absence of an intact normal flora. In our opinion, the risk is unwarranted in view of the limited efficacy of antimicrobial agents in treating disease of the gastrointestinal tract.

In addition to allowing a potential pathogen access to target cells, antimicrobial agents will shift the microbial flora from a normal, well-studied, and well-characterized condition to one that is largely unknown. If the aim of therapy is to cover or protect a compromised site near a microbial ecosystem then, when infection does occur, identification of the infecting microorganism will become impossible.

In addition to immediate changes in the microenvironment of the animal, more far-reaching changes occur in the environment directly related to antimicrobial usage. The changes are so serious that antimicrobial agents must be used only in a rational and responsible fashion. The environmental changes include the creation of a vast pool of resistance genes. It now seems certain that the resistance genes found in previously sensitive strains of *Hemophilus influenzae* (the leading cause of meningitis in children), *Neisseria gonorrhoeae*, *Pasteurella multocida* (in poultry and cattle), and *P. haemolytica* (in cattle) arose from this environmental pool. Each time an antimicrobial agent is used, the environmental pool grows larger. As the pool of resistance genes becomes larger, more and more previously sensitive strains become resistant, and bacterial infections thus become refractory to treatment.

MANAGEMENT OF DIARRHEA: MOTILITY MODIFIERS AND ADJUNCT THERAPY

DONALD R. STROMBECK, D.V.M.
Davis, California

PATHOPHYSIOLOGY OF INTESTINAL MOTILITY IN DIARRHEA

The small intestine contains smooth muscle that performs two basic functions. It retards the passage of intestinal contents, thereby ensuring the completeness of digestion and absorption, and it moves contents continuously in the aboral direction. The type of motility that slows transit is rhythmic segmentation, which acts by increasing resistance to flow in the intestinal conduit. Peristalsis is the type of motility that moves intestinal contents in the aboral direction. The movement of material through the small intestine is thus the net effect of the braking action of segmentation and the accelerating effect of peristalsis.

RHYTHMIC SEGMENTATION

Rhythmic segmentation acts by random contractions of the circular intestinal muscles. These contractions are minimal in the fasting intestine and increase in strength with the entry of food. Distention by food increases the muscle activity by reflexes that have pathways through the intrinsic plexuses (Fig. 1). Rhythmic segmentation mixes the intestinal contents with digestive enzymes, brings nutrients into contact with absorptive surfaces, and increases resistance to the passage of nutrients through the intestine. The unstimulated intestine is a flaccid tube that offers little resistance to the flow of liquid material through its lumen. Resistance to flow is increased by reducing the lumen of the tube, as illustrated in Figure 2. Thus, an intestine that has strong rhythmic segmentation contractions is one with considerable motility (hypermotile), whereas the flaccid bowel has little motility (hypomotile).

In general, the strength of normal segmentation in animals with diarrhea is decreased, so the bowel is in a flaccid (hypomotile) state, offering little resistance to the flow of material through it. The rate of contractions is not markedly affected. The goal in treating diarrhea is to restore resistance in the tube by stimulating the strength of rhythmic segmentation.

PERISTALSIS

Peristalsis is defined as waves or rings of constriction moving aborally over the intestine. In each very short section of intestine, peristaltic waves develop at the same frequency as rhythmic segmentation contractions, both rates being determined by electrical properties of the muscle. The rate of peristaltic waves is different in each level of the intestine. The highest rate is found in the duodenum and the lowest in the colon.

The strength of peristaltic contractions is

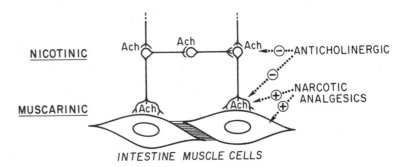

Figure 1. Schematic illustration of control of intestinal smooth muscle activity by the intrinsic nervous system. Two types of receptors are found that are inhibited (−) by anticholinergics. Narcotic analgesics stimulate (+) muscle contraction at the nerve muscle junction and by an effect directly on the muscle. (Ach = acetylcholine.)

minimal during fasting and increases with the entry of food as a result of stimulation of a local reflex and vagal nerve activity. When segmentation and resistance to flow are reduced in the flaccid intestine, very little peristaltic activity is needed to propel liquid contents a long distance with relative ease. In animals with diarrhea the rate of peristaltic activity need not be increased to contribute to the problem.

In any one section of intestine the rate of muscular contraction normally is constant and predetermined, whereas the strength of contractions in rhythmic segmentation and peristalsis is variable and modulated by neural and humoral controls.

Intestinal smooth muscle contraction is mediated by activity in the intrinsic nervous system, which is achieved by the release of acetylcholine at ganglionic synapses and motor end plates (see Fig. 1). Muscle contraction is blocked by atropine and other anticholinergic drugs.

The presence of receptors for serotonin on intestinal smooth muscle cells and on the intrinsic nerves suggests that this biogenic amine is an important neurotransmitter for peristalsis. There is no evidence, however, that antiserotonin drugs reduce peristalsis or that they would be effective in treating diarrhea.

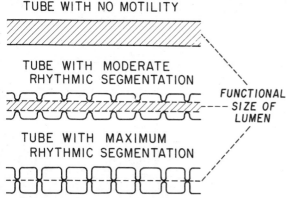

Figure 2. Schematic illustration of the intestinal conduit showing how stimulation of rhythmic segmentation reduces the diameter of the lumen and increases the resistance to flow of the intestinal contents.

COLONIC MOTILITY

An old concept holds that diarrhea reflects a hypermotile state and that constipation results from a hypomotile state. Intraluminal pressure measurements of the colon show that just the opposite is true. The colon that possesses no rhythmic segmentation motility is a flaccid tube in which intraluminal pressure is low. As a consequence there is no resistance to rapid flow through its lumen. This flow is for the most part due to gravity, which is determined by body position. The effects of gravity are reduced when an animal is confined to a hospital cage. The clinician is presented with many chronic cases of diarrhea that are not severe but are frustrating, since these patients respond to cage rest but relapse upon discharge from the hospital. Normal bowel movements are produced in the hospital but become abnormal as soon as regular activity is resumed. Part of the favorable response to cage rest is undoubtedly a reduction in the effects of gravity. With a mild food intolerance, cage rest may be the single change in management necessary to produce normal feces. With strong segmentation contractions, manometric pressure within the colonic lumen is high and colonic transit time is delayed, producing constipation.

The pattern of rates of muscle contractions differs in the colon, producing a reversed gradient of motor activity from the ileocecal valve to the mid-colon that causes intestinal contents to be moved in the oral direction. This results in a bowel segment with a functional obstruction, one in which the transit time of contents is slowed through the cranial half of the colon. When diarrhea due to disease or drugs develops in dogs and cats, multiple pacemakers appear in the cranial part of the colon and the reversed gradient is lost. Thus, segmentation and retrograde peristalsis contribute to the resistance to rapid passage of liquid contents entering the colon.

Distention of the colon stimulates both segmentation and peristalsis, and the amount of residue entering the colon determines the degree of distention in normal animals. The amount of residue in most diets is optimum, so that the colonic contents are adequately processed before they are defecated. Excessive residue in some commercial foods results in more frequent bowel movements. Constipation can be a problem with a normal-residue diet when propulsive activity is insufficient to move the colonic contents aboral at the proper rate. Addition of fiber to the diet frequently corrects the problem, allowing bowel movement frequency to return to normal.

The effects of drugs on colonic function are not well understood. Cholinergic agents actually stimulate contraction of the cranial colon and inhibit motility in the distal colon. Together, these effects evacuate the colon. Anticholinergic drugs have less predictable effects on colonic motility. Any depression of motility is slight and brief.

Diarrhea is associated with an alteration in motility of intestinal smooth muscle. The altered motility either causes intestinal contents to pass through too rapidly for normal assimilation or causes more frequent defecation of completely processed material. The former is associated with reduced resistance to the flow of liquid contents through the lumen. In the latter case colonic inflammation abnormally stimulates the defecation reflex. More extensive inflammation causes a loss of the motility designed to delay transit, resulting in watery feces.

When resistance to flow is minimal in the flaccid intestine, very little peristaltic activity is needed to propel liquid contents over a long distance with relative ease. Peristaltic activity is not increased in diarrhea, and it need not be to contribute to the problem.

MOTILITY MODIFIERS

The theoretical goals of treating diarrhea are to decrease the driving force that moves intestinal contents aborally and to increase the resistance to their flow. Attempts are made to decrease the driving force by inhibiting peristalsis and to increase the resistance to flow by stimulating rhythmic segmentation. However, peristalsis cannot usually be abolished completely with pharmaceutical agents. As long as some peristaltic activity is present, however weak, it can propel liquid contents through a flaccid tube. In some situations peristalsis can be inhibited completely, but when that happens there is also a complete loss of rhythmic segmentation. The result is ileus. The paralyzed section of intestine is unable to move any material, and a functional obstruction results. Drugs used to decrease propulsive activity in the intestine do not abolish peristalsis, and they always reduce segmentation. Thus, the first goal — decreasing the driving force — is difficult to attain with drugs. The second goal — increasing the resistance to flow — is achieved with drugs that stimulate rhythmic segmentation.

NARCOTIC ANALGESICS

Narcotic analgesics are the only drugs that effectively increase resistance to flow by stimulating rhythmic segmentation. They include morphine, meperidine, paregoric, diphenoxylate, and loperamide. Narcotic analgesics increase the amplitude of rhythmic segmentation and decrease propulsive contractions (Table 1). Additional effects are delayed emptying of the stomach and increased tone in the ileocecal valve and anal sphincter. The narcotic analgesics act centrally and on synapses to augment segmentation, but their major action is a direct effect on intestinal smooth muscle (see Fig. 1), producing both tonic and phasic contractions of the circular muscle. Narcotic analgesics either have no effect or cause relaxation of longitudinal intestinal muscle in the dog. The net effect of narcotic analgesics is to inhibit the flow of intestinal contents. The major disadvantage to the use of these drugs is that they are narcotics and can produce central nervous system depression. Because they are narcotics they are controlled by the FDA.

Atropine is added to narcotic analgesics (Table 2) to minimize their abuse by humans, since the effects of atropine toxicity appear before those of narcotic analgesic toxicity. However, the levels of atropine added to narcotic analgesics are 20 to 30 times lower than the usual doses for small animals, so narcotic analgesic toxicity appears before atropine toxicity in those species. Since an anticholinergic drug such as atropine has an effect opposite to that of

Table 1. *Pharmacologic Actions of Narcotic Analgesics*

STOMACH
    Contract antrum
    Decrease antral propulsion
Net effect: delay gastric emptying
General effect: decrease pain

SMALL AND LARGE INTESTINE
    Increase tone and segmentation
    Decrease propulsion
    Contract ileocecal and anal sphincters
Net effect: increase transit time

Table 2. FDA Classification of Drugs Used as Adjunctive Therapy in Treatment of Acute Enterocolitis, Functional Gastrointestinal Disorders, and Diarrhea[*]

EFFECTIVE

Diban[a] (powdered opium, atropine)
Donnagel-PG[a] (powdered opium, atropine, hyoscyamine, kaolin, pectin)
Lomotil[b] (diphenoxylate, atropine)
Parapectolin[c] (paregoric, pectin, kaolin)
Imodium[d] (loperamide)

PROBABLY EFFECTIVE

Pathilon[e] (tridihexethyl chloride)
Pro-Banthine[f] (propantheline bromide)

POSSIBLY EFFECTIVE

Darbazine (Combid)[f] (prochlorperazine maleate, isopropamide iodide)
Bentyl[g] (dicyclomine hydrochloride)
Cantil[g] (mepenzolate bromide)
Librax[h] (chlordiazepoxide hydrochloride, clidinium bromide)
Quarzan[h] (clidinium bromide)

[*]From literature in advertisements, drug inserts, and the *Physician's Desk Reference*, published annually by Medical Economics Co., Oradell, NJ.
[a]A. H. Robins Co., Richmond, VA
[b]Searle & Co., Chicago, IL
[c]W. H. Rorer, Fort Washington, PA
[d]Ortho Pharmaceutical Corp., Raritan, NJ
[e]Lederle Laboratories, Pearl River, NY
[f]Smith Kline and French, Philadelphia, PA
[g]Merrell-National Laboratories, Cincinnati, OH
[h]Roche Laboratories, Nutley, NJ

the narcotic analgesics, the question arises as to which drug's action will prevail. Anticholinergics act at synapses to block transmission, so the muscle is not stimulated to contraction. Since narcotic analgesics stimulate muscle activity by a direct effect, their action will prevail when they are used with an anticholinergic drug that acts at the synaptic level. Thus the paradox of combining two drugs that have opposing activity is resolved.

The ideal motility modifier for treating diarrhea would possess all of the narcotic analgesic's properties that stimulate rhythmic segmentation but none of the effects that depress the central nervous system. Some new drugs such as loperamide approach that ideal.

Intestinal motility sometimes fails to return to normal after correct pharmacologic treatment. Frequently, potassium deficits must be corrected before normal motor function returns. Diarrhea causes an accelerated loss of potassium from the body. If anorexia is associated with diarrhea, the potassium is not replaced until it becomes part of therapy. Potassium-replacement therapy is often required for diarrhea. The amount to be replaced can only be estimated, since the concentration of plasma potassium is often a poor reflection of total-body potassium levels. Potassium deficits may contribute more to the loss of motility than disease-induced stimulation of the sympathetic nervous system does.

ANTICHOLINERGIC DRUGS

Anticholinergics constitute the group of drugs most commonly used in treating diarrhea in small animals. These drugs block the effects of acetylcholine, which is the most important neurotransmitter released during the normal motor functions of intestinal smooth muscle (see Fig. 1). Acetylcholine is the transmitter for contraction of both circular and longitudinal smooth muscle of the intestine, and hence it plays a role in peristalsis as well as in rhythmic segmentation. Large doses of cholinergic drugs, which simulate the effects of acetylcholine, contract smooth muscle in the entire intestine, and the contents are propelled from one end or the other. In only a few clinical situations does this cause diarrhea. Toxicity from cholinesterase inhibitors and cholinergic drugs used as taeniacides produces this effect. A cholinergic effect probably causes sudden diarrhea in some animals during acute stress. There is no evidence that persistent diarrhea is due to stimulation of a cholinergic pathway.

Anticholinergic drugs reduce the physiologic effects of acetycholine, and motility is reduced in both circular and longitudinal smooth muscle. Thus, while peristalsis may be reduced, there is also a major adverse reduction of resistance to flow in the tube (Table 3). Pharmacologists recognize that anticholinergic drugs are contrary to the mode of action of useful antidiarrhea agents. Furthermore, they have been found to be disappointing when used for that purpose. The Food and Drug Administration (FDA) has recently restricted the claims that can be made for them and has questioned their effectiveness (see Table 2).

Most small animal patients with diarrhea recover normal function regardless of therapy. The value of anticholinergic drugs in treating

Table 3. Pharmacologic Actions of Anticholinergic Drugs

Decrease intestinal muscle tone and propulsion
Decrease intestinal motility caused by opiates and serotonin
High doses decrease intestinal motility due to emotional stimuli
Some muscle tone and movement are resistant to anticholinergic drugs

diarrhea should be determined in controlled studies in which alternate unselected cases of diarrhea are treated with and without the drug, with careful evaluation of the results. Anticholinergics are not innocuous drugs. Their use can precipitate ileus by further reducing the decreased motility found in diarrhea.

DRUGS OF CHOICE

Narcotic analgesics remain the preferred drugs for treating diarrhea and dysentery. This preference is based on pharmacologic studies showing that narcotic analgesics comprise the motility-modifying drugs that are effective in treating diarrhea. Evaluation of all motility modifiers has led to the FDA classification shown in Table 2, which is based on a review by the National Academy of Sciences–National Research Council and on other information. The FDA allows literature on narcotic analgesics to state that they are effective as adjunctive therapy in the management of diarrhea. The claims for effectiveness of any of the anticholinergic drugs must be qualified. Despite all the evidence in favor of the use of narcotic analgesics, some studies report that these drugs are no more effective than placebos in treating acute diarrhea in children. It should be understood, of course, that narcotic analgesics are only effective as adjunctive therapy and should not be expected to cure primary problems caused by an infectious agent. Cure in such cases will require additional therapy.

LOCALLY ACTING DRUGS

Long before either antibiotics or motility modifiers were available for treating diarrhea, a wide variety of intestinal protective and absorbent agents were used. As is the case with many other pharmaceuticals that have been used empirically for centuries, no controlled studies have been conducted to prove the effectiveness of these protective and absorbent drugs.

A number of these substances are classified as protective because of their adsorbent properties. Bismuth subcarbonate and magnesium trisilicate adsorb gasses, toxins, and bacteria. As an additional property they supposedly coat and protect the ulcerated mucosal surface, although there is no evidence that either of these compounds has any such ability. Aluminum hydroxide, used as an antacid, also has adsorptive properties.

Activated charcoal, used for many years to adsorb toxic substances, is still incorporated into universal antidotes for treating the ingestion of toxic substances. It has also been used to bind gas in the intestine in managing excessive flatus, though it is questionable whether activated charcoal significantly reduces the amount of intestinal gas. There have been no controlled studies to evaluate its efficacy.

Kaolin (hydrated aluminum silicate) is often used to treat diarrhea and acts by binding toxins and bacteria. When used to treat colitis, it is doubtful whether any appreciable binding activity remains by the time it reaches the colon. Kaolin is indicated for the treatment of intestinal fermentation, but again there is no documentation of its usefulness.

Pectin is a common part of diarrhea medications. It is a carbohydrate (polygalacturonic acid) found in apples and the rinds of citrus fruits. The action of pectin is unknown, but it is suspected to be an adsorbent with protective properties.

Astringents have been used in treating diarrhea. Tannic acid, the best example, acts by precipitating proteins on the mucosal surface, forming a protective coating presumably without entering and damaging the cell. This decreases cell permeability and has a constipating effect. Tannic acid also forms insoluble complexes with heavy-metal ions, alkaloids, and glycosides that otherwise could contribute to diarrhea. Tannic acid is now known to be hepatotoxic, causing severe centrolobular necrosis when appreciable amounts are absorbed.

Antacids have also been used to treat diarrhea. All aluminum-based antacid compounds cause constipation. In the case of aluminum hydroxide this is not due to its astringent effects, since the concentrations used are too low. Aluminum hydroxide inhibits motility in the stomach, delaying gastric emptying. Part of its constipating effects may be due to a very slow delivery of solutes to the small intestine, permitting more complete absorption. Aluminum-based antacids also adsorb many substances, including tetracycline and atropine given orally. These antacids bind phosphates and have been used to treat hyperphosphatemia. Part of the aluminum-based antacids' constipating effects are due to the precipitation of poorly absorbed soluble anions that otherwise can cause an osmotic diarrhea.

Calcium antacids are also constipating and occasionally have been used to treat chronic diarrhea. They may have absorptive properties, and they form insoluble salts with anions such as phosphate. It is not known whether high concentrations of calcium have any effect on intestinal motility. Excessive administration of calcium to treat chronic diarrhea can produce hypercalcemia and renal hypercalciuria, which can progress to nephrocalcinosis and renal failure. In contrast with calcium, magnesium salts are cathartic, since they are soluble and poorly absorbed. Magnesium may also be cathartic by direct effects on smooth-muscle function.

Barium sulfate has been used empirically to treat chronic diarrhea. The use is based on observations that diarrhea sometimes improves after barium sulfate is given to conduct gastrointestinal radiographic studies. There have been no controlled studies to evaluate the usefulness of barium sulfate for treating diarrhea. Barium ions stimulate the release of acetylcholine from nerve synapses in intrinsic ganglia, and when a soluble barium salt is given orally it intensely stimulates all types of muscles in the body. Soluble barium salts cause vomiting, severe diarrhea, and colic. If barium sulfate is effective in treating diarrhea and if it acts by those neurogenic actions, it is possible that very minute amounts of barium ions are absorbed and stimulate acetylcholine release. This would have to be in amounts that augment segmentation but do not stimulate simultaneous contraction of the entire length of the intestine, causing diarrhea.

SUPPLEMENTAL READING

Burks, T.F.: Vascularly perfused isolated intestine. *In,* Proc. 4th Int. Symp.: Gastrointestinal motility, Mitchell, Vancouver, 1974:305–312.

Burks, T.F.: Gastrointestinal pharmacology. Ann. Rev. Pharmacol. Toxicol., *16*:15–31, 1976.

Connell, A.M.: The motility of the pelvic colon. Part II. Paradoxical motility in diarrhea and constipation. Gut, *3*:342–348, 1962.

Christensen, J.: Myoelectric control of the colon. Gastroenterology, *58*:601–609, 1975.

Daniel, E.E.: Pharmacology of the gastrointestinal tract. *In,* Handbook of Physiology, Sect. 6, Alimentary Canal, Edited by C.F. Code, Washington, D.C. Am. Physiol. Soc., Vol. 4, 1968:2267–2324.

Goodman, L.A., and Gilman, A.: The Pharmacological Basis of Therapeutics. New York, Macmillan Co., 1975.

Hightower, N.W.: Motor action of the small bowel. *In,* Handbook of Physiology, Sect. 6, Alimentary Canal, Edited by C.F. Code, Am. Physiol. Soc., Washington, D.C., Vol. 4, 1968:2001–2024.

Ludwick, J.R., Wiley, J.N., and Bass, P.: Extraluminal contractile force and electrical activity of reversed canine duodenum. Gastroenterology, *54*:41–51, 1968.

Mishra, N.K., Appert, H.E., and Howard, J. M.: Studies of paralytic ileus. Effects of intraperitoneal injury on motility of the canine small intestine. Am. J. Surg., *129*:559–563, 1975.

Plant, O.H., and Miller, G.H.: Effects of morphine and some other opium alkaloids on the muscular activity of the alimentary canal. I. Action on the small intestine in unanesthetized dogs and man. J. Pharmacol. Exp. Ther., *27*:361–383, 1926.

Strombeck, D.R.: Small Animal Gastroenterology, Davis, Calif., Stonegate Publ. Co., 1979.

Templeton, R.D., and Alder, H.F.: The influence of morphine on transportation in the colon of the dog. Am. J. Physiol. *131*:428–431, 1940.

Vaughan Williams, E.M., and Streeten, D.H.P.: The action of morphine, pethidine, and amidone upon the intestinal motility of conscious dogs. Br. J. Pharmacol. Chem. Ther., *5*:584–603, 1950.

DIET AND NUTRITION IN THE MANAGEMENT OF GASTROINTESTINAL PROBLEMS

DONALD R. STROMBECK, D.V.M.
Davis, California

An important consequence of gastrointestinal, pancreatic, and hepatic problems is loss of nutritional homeostasis. Since the client's major concern is often the maintenance of adequate nutrition, he or she may continue feeding when gastrointestinal function is not normal. In reality, loss of nutritional homeostasis seldom develops into a life-threatening problem; small animals can manage quite well without any food for two to three weeks. Restoration of nutritional homeostasis in animals with either chronic or acute gastrointestinal problems is usually achieved with dietary management rather than with drugs and conventional diets. The primary reason for treating a gastrointestinal problem is often the nuisance of uncontrolled bowel behavior. In such cases medication often fails, and dietary management is the only solution.

Most small animals with signs of vomiting and diarrhea recover normal gastrointestinal tract function without any therapy. In fact, most recover despite incorrect therapy. For both clinician and owner the ideal goal of management is rapid, complete, and lasting remission. Pharmaceutical agents are usually used to achieve that goal. Since treated animals usually recover within 24 hours, drugs are given credit for the cure, reinforcing the idea that the goal is best achieved with medication. In fact, many chronic gastrointestinal problems are neither cured nor successfully managed with drugs. Often, one drug after another is prescribed in the hope that the correct one will be found and will effect a cure. Numerous formulas are available that contain antibiotics, intestinal sedatives, and intestinal protectives that are ineffective for many chronic gastrointestinal problems. The ideal is seldom attained in treating chronic gastrointestinal problems. A more realistic goal is to find a successful management program in which medication is not needed or is used only intermittently.

Management of gastrointestinal, esophageal, hepatic, and pancreatic problems employs controlled diets, antimicrobial agents, intestinal motility modifiers, bulk producers (fiber), antacids, and gastrointestinal protectives. Chronic problems frequently are managed with nothing but controlled diets. Systemic antibiotics are indicated in acute problems, and unabsorbed antibiotics are rarely indicated for any problem. Motility modifiers are prescribed for only a few days for the control of acute signs. Bulk producers can be important adjunctive therapy, whereas gastrointestinal protectives are completely ineffective. The realistic goal is to produce remission using a controlled diet, which is aided (as necessary) by short-term use of motility modifiers and long-term use of bulking agents. Chronic colitis is the only indication for long-term use of a locally acting antibiotic—sulfasalazine. In one other problem, eosinophilic gastroenteritis, the therapy is also specific — corticosteroids.

The most important treatment for gastrointestinal problems is rest for the tract. In acute problems this is accomplished by complete restriction of food. When complete restriction is required for long periods, nutritional homeostasis can be maintained by total parenteral nutrition. The gastrointestinal function of animals with chronic problems is rested to some degree by feeding controlled diets.

PRINCIPLES IN FORMULATING DIETS

Controlled diets are formulated as a compromise between the ideal and the realistic. Criteria for an ideal diet are followed, whenev-

Table 1. *Criteria for an Ideal Diet and Dietary Management Program*

Requires little or no digestion
Contains minimal amount of fat
Lactose-free
Non-allergenic
Low-residue
Isosmotic
Frequent feeding if possible
Good acceptability
Results in optimal intestinal ecology

er possible, in formulating diets for gastrointestinal problems (Table 1).

Nutrients in these diets should require minimum digestion or, ideally, none at all. This allows absorption to be completed in the cranial small intestine, permitting the remainder of the bowel to rest. Elemental diets are predigested, contain amino acids and simple carbohydrates, and are useful in treating chronic inflammatory bowel disease. Complete rest of the alimentary tract is achieved only by total parenteral alimentation.

The ideal diet is virtually free of fat, which makes the absorption of carbohydrates and proteins optimal. Triglycerides synthesized from medium-chain and short-chain fatty acids are sometimes used, since they are more water-soluble, a property facilitating their digestion and absorption. Fat in chyme delays the absorption of nutrients and fluid. When the absorptive capacity of the intestinal tract is reduced, lipids are the first nutrients to escape complete absorption. Normal animals have a large reserve capacity for digesting and absorbing large amounts of fat, but dogs with chronic bowel problems often are unable to assimilate normal amounts. Excessive fat reaching the colon stimulates the secretion of fluid and electrolytes, which occurs before steatorrhea becomes evident.

The ideal diet also contains no lactose, since the intestinal brush-border enzyme lactase is deficient during diarrhea from any cause. Lactase must split milk sugar into the monosaccharides glucose and galactose before absorption is possible. With a deficiency of lactase, dietary lactose causes osmotic diarrhea as a result of bacterial degradation of undigested lactose in the colon (Table 2). Some of the products of lactose fermentation are not absorbed. This increases the number of osmotically active particles and holds water and electrolytes in the colon. Brush-border lactase levels vary in small animals but are normally low and are reduced further when lactose is not being fed. The levels of sucrase and maltase,

Table 2. *Amount of Lactose in Various Foods*

FOOD	AMOUNT	LACTOSE *(gm)*	PROTEIN *(gm)*
Whole milk	8 oz	11.8	8.0
Buttermilk	8 oz	12.0	8.0
Yogurt	8 oz	9.0	8.0
Cottage cheese	¼ cup	1.5	7.5
Cheddar cheese	1 oz	0.6	7.0

two other brush-border disaccharidases, decrease in enteritis.

The ideal diet is non-allergenic and is formulated by selecting the proteins least likely to be allergenic. In some individuals any protein can be absorbed intact, causing reacting antibodies to be synthesized. After the development of hypersensitivity, reactions will be evoked by subsequent feeding of the protein. Why sensitization occurs in some animals and not in others is unknown. Since any protein can be antigenic, the ideal source of nitrogen is a balanced mixture of amino acids, which can be provided with an enzymatically produced protein hydrolysate. These products are not completely non-allergenic, however, since they contain some incompletely hydrolyzed peptides. Ideally, nitrogen requirements can be met with a mixture of pure amino acids.

The ideal non-allergenic diet is seldom required to manage a chronic gastrointestinal problem. Milk protein is one of the proteins least likely to be allergenic. In contrast with humans, in whom allergies to milk protein are relatively common, small animals are rarely found to be sensitive. Allergies to egg protein and meat proteins are more common. The meat proteins most likely to cause allergic reactions are those that are given most frequently. Since lamb or mutton is seldom fed, the likelihood of allergy to these meats is small. Consequently, mutton is the meat protein contained in one commercially available hypoallergenic diet (D/D Prescription diet, Hill Packing Co.). Vegetable proteins, such as those obtained from soybeans, are used to formulate non-allergenic diets for humans with allergies. Little is known about their use in the formulation of hypoallergenic diets for small animals.

The ideal diet is low in residue, thus decreasing the bulk of intestinal contents and allowing an inflamed bowel to rest. Complete diversion of ileal contents from the colon allows a severely inflamed colon to recover. Diets with no residue, such as elemental diets, are used in a similar manner in successful management of acute and chronic inflammatory bowel disease. On the other hand, some chronic problems are managed by increasing the residue in the diet by adding bran or commercially prepared products of cellulose or seed fiber. Additional residue improves gastrointestinal function for several reasons. Some residue is necessary to stimulate normal colonic segmentation so that transit rates are normal. Dietary fiber is also of benefit because of its ability to bind bile acids and bacteria, both of which may contribute to chronic problems. Paradoxically, the same residue is used to treat both diarrhea and constipation.

The ideal diet is not hypertonic enough to cause extracellular fluids to move into the intestine. The osmolarity of regular diets is 500 to 600 mOsm, twice that of extracellular fluid. Hyperosmolarity seldom exists unless liquid diets that contain a high concentration of monosaccharides or disaccharides and electrolytes are used. Some commercially prepared liquid diets given by stomach tube to anorectic patients and some elemental diets are hyperosmolar. They must be administered continuously over 24 hours at a slow rate. This can be done using a constant-rate infusion pump and a pharyngostomy tube. Hyperosmolar diets cause vomiting when fed as a bolus three to four times a day.

The ideal diet is designed to be fed frequently, thus preventing dietary overload and malabsorption. With frequent feedings, dietary nutrients are used to maintain normal blood glucose levels while minimizing gluconeogenesis at the expense of body proteins.

The physical qualities of the diet are important in managing some problems of the alimentary tract. Abnormal motility of the pharynx and/or esophagus sometimes causes great difficulty in swallowing solid boluses of food, although the swallowing of liquids is little affected. Occasionally the opposite is true. Megaesophagus is usually managed better with liquid diets that are fed with the animal in a vertical position (elevated front quarters). Occasionally, food is not regurgitated, whereas liquid is. Thus, management must be directed by observations of trial and error. With gastric-outlet obstruction, gastric emptying is facilitated by liquid or puréed diets.

Ideally, the nutrients will be totally accepted by the patient and the owner. Controlled diets are generally less palatable than regular diets. Lipids make an important contribution to palatability, and palatability is compromised when the diet is virtually fat-free. Since meat also contributes to palatability, acceptance suffers when non-meat protein is used. Diets in which the greatest percentage of calories comes from carbohydrates are low in palatability, even those containing sucrose or glucose. Controlled diets initiated after complete restriction of feeding are usually accepted readily at first, but later they are rejected because the patient wants a change. Poor acceptability is a problem when long-term dietary control is necessary. The greatest single reason for failure of dietary management of a chronic problem is covert modification of the diet by the client to please the patient. The clinician is often totally unaware of the indiscretion. Strict adherence to a controlled diet depends on effective client education. Owners seldom believe that minor dietary alteration is of any consequence.

The ideal diet should help maintain the optimum intestinal bacterial flora necessary for normal function. Little is known about the ecology of the bowel microflora. In the normal gut every species of bacteria has its own niche or preferred site. At each point in the intestinal tract, one species will be able to thrive much better than any other. It maintains this site as a relatively exclusive niche, aided by the fact that oxygen is or is not abundant or by the organism's ability to elaborate substances that suppress the growth of other bacteria attempting to grow there. When diarrhea develops, the normal pattern of bacterial niches is changed, so that normal bacteria can colonize and thrive in regions that normally they do not populate readily. Although this is generally regarded to be the cause of the diarrhea, it may also be an effect of the diarrhea and subsequently contribute to its chronicity. Normally, if bacteria foreign to an animal are given orally, they will pass out in the feces and are unable to colonize the bowel. If for any reason they displace the normal flora, they are considered pathogenic and can cause diarrhea. Thus, either redistribution of the normal flora or colonization by a foreign "transient" organism can cause diarrhea. What factors can cause these changes? Diet is the important one for this discussion. Other causes are stress, antibiotics, and changes in environment.

Diet has an important effect on the population of the microflora. The rate of bacterial growth is related directly to nutrient availability. When a synthetic diet that contains all the nutrients, such as amino acids and glucose, in digested form is fed, total bacterial counts in the intestines decline. These nutrients are completely absorbed in the proximal small intestine. In addition, since the diet contains no residue, mucus secretion and cell desquamation are at a minimum in the small intestine, and fewer nutrients are delivered to the colon. This reduces the availability of nutrients to colon bacteria. Thus the bacterial flora is "starved," and its total population is reduced.

Ideal diets (the so-called elemental diets that are predigested and given orally) thus give rest to the bowel in another manner, by reducing the total number of bacteria that are either potential invaders or producers of enterotoxins. This reduction in microflora population is important primarily in the small intestine.

Bacterial numbers increase with some diets. When nutrients are not digested and absorbed, bacterial numbers increase by 10^3 to 10^5 per gram of contents above normal. Any type of maldigestion, malabsorption, or dietary overload is a potential cause of this increase.

The relative distribution of different enteric organisms is also determined by the diet. Numbers of colonic aerobes increase with low-protein diets, whereas colonic anaerobes increase with high-protein diets. A reduction in numbers of one member of the normal flora increases susceptibility to colonization by pathogens or by foreign transients that become pathogenic when their numbers increase. A diet-induced redistribution of the normal flora can increase the colonic numbers of *Klebsiella, Aerobacter, Proteus,* and *Pseudomonas,* which can become pathologic and cause clinical signs.

In summary, the ideal diet to prescribe is one that results in a bacterial microflora of the gut that is normal with respect to both total numbers and distribution of the population.

FORMULATION OF DIETS

Chronic diarrhea due to unknown causes is seldom managed with pharmaceuticals alone. Controlled diets offer the best chance for successful management. The diet can usually be formulated from foods readily available, or a commercially prepared prescription diet can be used. Seldom are elemental diets required, and rarer yet is parenteral hyperalimentation needed.

The value of client education in the establishment of the rationale and goals of dietary management can never be underestimated. Unless client education is convincing, unknown variables will often be introduced. For example, an owner may feed the animal a few treats, thinking that such an addition to the diet is inconsequential. The value of a controlled diet cannot be determined unless no other foods are given.

A controlled diet is formulated by using the least possible number of ingredients. It is very difficult to determine the effect of any single constituent of a diet that contains 10 to 12 different ingredients, and the combination does not help the patient. Random selection of such prepared foods seldom allows one to identify intolerance to a specific nutrient.

The goal of the initial diet is to maintain reasonable nutritional homeostasis without attempting to balance the diet. The initial diet contains no glutens, to help screen out gluten-induced enteropathy, and no disaccharides, especially no lactose, since the disaccharidases (lactase, maltase, isomaltase, and sucrase) are lost for a week or more in a diarrhea due to any cause. The diet is virtually fat-free. The amount of protein is not excessive and is from a single source.

CARBOHYDRATES

The initial diet contains boiled rice, potatoes, or tapioca as the source of carbohydrates, all of which are gluten-free. Carbohydrates can be used to provide 80 percent of the total diet. Since this amount of carbohydrates is often greater than normally eaten, initially it may be inadequately digested and absorbed. Pancreatic enzyme secretion is determined by levels of carbohydrates, lipids, and proteins in the diet. When the ratio of dietary nutrients is changed, several days are required before pancreatic enzyme levels increase to meet the changed digestive requirements. Digestion of starch is not completed by pancreatic enzymes; it requires brush-border enzymes for final hydrolysis to glucose. Brush-border enzyme levels are also determined by the amounts of each nutrient in the diet. Thus, a change to a high-carbohydrate diet may not result in rapid remission of diarrhea if the levels of carbohydrate-digesting enzymes are low. Diarrhea further contributes to the problem by reducing brush-border disaccharide activity even more. Digestion and absorption of carbohydrates is incomplete and results in osmotic diarrhea. This problem can be minimized by feeding small meals frequently. Overfeeding delays the recovery of mucosal function.

Incomplete digestion and absorption of starches results in increased numbers of intestinal bacteria, which interfere with the production of normal bowel movements. Starchy diets also change the composition of the normal bacterial flora, which may or may not be beneficial.

PROTEIN

Protein incorporated into the diet can be of either animal or vegetable origin. Vegetable proteins are gluten-free. A single protein of animal origin, especially one with a high biologic value — eggs, cottage cheese, or lean meat — is often used. Cottage cheese is often preferred since it contains a smaller amount of lipid than eggs and meat do (Table 3). The

Table 3. *Composition of Various Foods*
(PER 100 GRAMS)

FOOD	ENERGY (Kcal)	WATER (gm)	PROTEIN (gm)	FAT (gm)	CHO (gm)
Barley, pearl	353	11	8	1	78
Bread, white	270	35	8	3	52
whole wheat	260	37	9	3	49
Brewer's yeast	330	13	42	2	34
Cottage cheese, dehydrated	93	77	20	0.5	2
Eggs, whole	163	74	13	12	0.7
Farina	357	11	11	1	76
Heart	105	78	17	4	1
Kidney, beef	141	75	15	8	1
Liver, beef	136	70	20	3	6
calf	141	71	19	5	4
chicken	141	70	22	4	3
pork	134	72	20	5	2
Meat, fatty	350	50	20	30	—
medium	275	56	20	30	—
lean	200	63	27	10	—
Milk, whole	67	87	3.5	3.8	4.7
skim	35	90	3.5	0.1	5.1
Oatmeal	360	13	16	8	56
Rice, brown	355	12	7	1.7	78
white	350	12	7	0.3	80
Soybean meal	330	13	44	1	36
Tapioca	350	12	1	0.2	86

amounts used in the initial diet should meet protein requirements. One gram of protein can be given for each 20 kcal fed, a level that represents 6 to 8 percent of the diet. When food allergy or sensitivity is the cause, the offending antigen is most likely a protein. Since proteins can be absorbed intact, which stimulates the formation of antibody, minimum levels of protein are fed. Intact-protein absorption increases with mucosal damage. After acute enteritis, problems often continue when the regular diet is resumed. Often a controlled diet must be fed for extended or indefinite periods to maintain normal feces. Antigenic components of the diet may be absorbed long after recovery should have occurred. A number of chronic problems may result in animals sensitized during an acute episode of diarrhea.

Many dogs with chronic bowel disease tolerate little or no meat protein. The pathogenesis of colitis involves colonic bacteria that generate ammonia, and remission is possible when the production of colonic ammonia is reduced. Protein that is not completely digested and absorbed delivers nitrogen to the colon, providing the substrate for ammonia production. Thus, dietary protein should be close to 100 percent digestible and low in amount.

A 25-pound (12-kg) dog can be provided 820 kcal using a diet of cottage cheese and rice made up as follows: An 8 fluid ounce cup is used to measure 7 ounces (190 to 200 gm) of dry rice, which is cooked with two volumes of water. Add 3½ to 4 ounces of cottage cheese to the cooked rice. This diet contains 22 to 25 percent cottage cheese and 18 to 20 percent protein on a dry-matter basis.

RESIDUE

The cottage cheese and rice diet leaves little residue after digestion and absorption, so fecal volume is small. Sometimes the small volume of maximally dehydrated feces causes signs of constipation. Liquid material entering the colon in small amounts sometimes has insufficient bulk to stimulate rhythmic segmentation, the motility necessary to delay the passage of colonic contents long enough for optimum absorption of salts and water. Thus, small volumes of ileal contents entering the colon can result in either constipation or soft bowel movements. Both problems can be managed with bulk producers (e.g., Siblin). Such products may be of benefit both by providing residue and by binding bile acids and toxins produced in the intestine. Paradoxically, these products are used to treat both diarrhea and constipation. The amount of bulking agent used is determined by the amount of fiber in a controlled diet. When the diet contains little fiber, Siblin can be added at a level of 1 teaspoon for a dog of 25 to 30 lb (12 to 14 kg). The dose is adjusted to produce the desired fecal volume.

EVALUATION OF DIET

The effect of a controlled diet is evidenced by changes in the character of the feces and in the incidence of vomiting; however, improvement in other signs associated with chronic problems is of value too. These include intermittent halitosis, bloating, belching, borborygmus, flatulence, anal pruritus, assumption of a praying position, shivering, drooling, depression, restlessness, and polydipsia. The owner is instructed to observe changes in these signs in order to evaluate the effectiveness of the dietary recommendations. Careful observation and recording of the character of the bowel movements is especially important.

Severe gastrointestinal problems usually continue to produce clinical signs during hospitalization. Other patients will have normal bowel movements when fed regular diets in the hospital, making it impossible to evaluate a test diet. Unfortunately, these animals often have recurrent diarrhea promptly after being discharged. Hospitalization almost always improves diarrhea as a result of the physical inactivity. That is due in part to the removal of the effects of gravity, since physical movement facilitates the movement of liquid through a flaccid bowel. Thus, most patients must be managed at home before a controlled diet can be evaluated. The environment also must be controlled so that other variables are not introduced.

The client should return in a week or ten days with fecal samples and progress records. Even then, a significant number of animals will not have normal bowel movements, especially following severe attacks of acute gastroenteritis. The controlled diet is continued until remission is complete; then it can be modified by introducing new foods. One new food is gradually introduced over five to seven days. Observations are continued to evaluate the effects. Eventually, a number of foods will be identified as being tolerated or not tolerated. Finally, a sufficient number of foods will be tolerated to allow formulation of a balanced diet. The long-range goal is to develop a diet suitable for the patient and acceptable to the owner. Some patients can eventually be fed commercial dog foods, whereas others must be fed the controlled diet indefinitely. When these controlled diets are fed for extended periods they are supplemented with vitamins and minerals.

COMMERCIAL CONTROLLED DIETS

A number of different commercial controlled diets are available to manage small animals with chronic gastrointestinal problems. The prescription diet d/d is formulated from mutton and rice, and the new formula for i/d contains cottage cheese, whole egg, brewer's rice, liver, corn grits, corn starch, animal fat, soy grits, and sugar (ground wheat has been removed, making it a gluten-free diet). Any formula containing as many ingredients as i/d is less well controlled, since intolerance to any one ingredient will produce signs of disease. Owners of large dogs often prefer to use a commercial food rather than preparing one themselves. Commercial foods that are most likely to produce remission include Science Maximum-Stress Diet (animal fat, soy flour, animal liver meal, dextrose, whole egg, dried skimmed milk, casein, soy oil, and brewer's dried yeast), Science Dry Canine Growth Diet (brewer's rice, ground corn, soy grits, meat and bone meal, animal fat, dried skimmed milk, dried whole egg, soy oil, and brewer's dried yeast), IAMS chunks or IAMS plus (meat meal, ground yellow corn, animal fat, beet pulp, and brewer's dried yeast), and IAMS Eukanuba (poultry by-products meal, ground yellow corn, meat meal, animal fat, dried beet pulp, brewer's dried yeast, cane molasses, dried whole eggs, and dried fish meal). The fat content of Science Maximum Stress is 25 percent and of IAMS Eukanuba, 20 percent. This makes them less than ideal for treating diarrhea. They also are more expensive than the other diets mentioned. All these diets are gluten-free and are often useful in managing chronic diarrhea. Each is partially controlled, in that they contain fewer ingredients than other commercial pet foods.

The prescription diets c/d and p/d are useful as controlled diets for treating diarrhea in cats. Some cats develop diarrhea when fed dry cat foods and fail to respond to any form of management other than the use of canned food.

COMMERCIAL DEFINED DIETS

When regular or controlled diets cannot be given, modified diets given orally or parenteral hyperalimentation can be used.

Oral nutrients can be formulated into a diet that approaches the ideal more closely than a diet of conventional foods. Some commercial preparations that are bland, low in residue, fat, and lactose, and gluten-free can be given by stomach tube (Ensure, Ross-Abbott; Sustacal, Isocal, Portagen, and Sustagen, Mead Johnson;

Meritene and Precision LR Diet, Doyle). These formulations are defined as to osmolarity, calories, and vitamin and mineral content. Some, such as Sustacal, are high in protein, and they produce a large amount of solutes for renal excretion. Ensure contains less protein (14 percent of the total calories). A lower-protein diet is preferred when hyperosmolar dehydration is a potential problem in patients not easily given water.

A more completely restricted and defined diet can be used to meet the ideal criteria. Isocal is an example of a liquid diet that is virtually isosmotic and lactose-free, contains fats in the form of medium-chain triglycerides, is nutritionally balanced, and contains proper amounts of vitamins and minerals. This diet also provides only 13 percent of its calories from proteins and reduces the amount of solute for renal excretion, so additional water must be given. Another balanced diet, Portagen, contains mostly medium-chain triglycerides as the lipid source. Medium-chain triglycerides are available commercially for use in owner-formulated diets (MCT oil, Mead Johnson). Medium-chain triglycerides are digested and absorbed more efficiently than fats containing long-chain fatty acids. They can be absorbed by way of the portal circulation and are used effectively in treating lymphangiectasia.

Diets can be formulated to modify and control all the parameters of nutrient type and concentration. Carbohydrates in corn-syrup solids are modified to produce oligosaccharides of glucose for oral administration in elemental diets. Oligosaccharides do not have the disadvantage of starch (requiring digestion) or that of glucose (producing a hyperosmolar solution) when given in amounts to meet caloric needs. Commercial hydrolysates of starch (e.g., Polycose, Ross-Abbott) contain small oligosaccharides, half of which range in size from five to nine molecules of glucose. This form of carbohydrate minimizes the disadvantages of starch on the one hand and of glucose on the other.

Dietary protein can be modified further by using protein from a non-animal source. CHO-Free liquid (Syntex) is an example of a soy-protein isolate, free of carbohydrates but otherwise essentially complete. This product is combined with carbohydrate to formulate a controlled diet for evaluations of sensitivity or allergy to animal protein.

ELEMENTAL DIETS

An elemental diet is a balance of nutrients, consisting of carbohydrates and lipids in forms requiring little digestion and nitrogen in the form of amino acids. Nitrogen can be provided by a protein hydrolysate or by pure amino acids, in which case it is described as a chemically defined diet. The elemental diet was originally designed to determine whether its use would minimize the intestinal lesion produced by hemorrhagic shock in dogs. This diet consisted of a fibrin hydrolysate, sucrose, and Lipomul. In less than ten years elemental diets have become important in the treatment of severe gastrointestinal disease, in which the goal is to maintain nutritional homeostasis for short periods.

Flexical (Mead Johnson) is an example of a commercially available elemental diet that is not chemically defined. This diet's nitrogen is provided by an enzymatic hydrolysate of casein, to which are added methionine, tryptophan, and tyrosine. About 70 percent of the nitrogen is in the form of free amino acids. The carbohydrate consists of sucrose and glucoseoligosaccharides (dextrin). Its lipids are 20 percent medium-chain triglycerides and 80 percent long-chain unhydrogenated soy oil. Vivonex (Eaton Labs) is an example of a chemically defined elemental diet containing pure amino acids as the only nitrogen source. Being free of peptides, the chemically defined diet is an ideal hypoallergenic diet. The carbohydrate source is glucose and glucose oligosaccharides, with no sucrose or lactose. The diet is very low in fat, supplying less than 1 percent of the total calories. The fats used consist mostly of triglycerides of linoleic acid.

Several problems or disadvantages are associated with the use of elemental diets. In general, such diets are unpalatable and may have to be given by tube feeding. Most of the diets are hyperosmotic solutions, and problems may develop because their liquid property enables them to leave the stomach more rapidly than a meal of solid food. Hyperosmolar solutions rapidly entering the duodenum cause vomiting, diarrhea, and abdominal distress by intense stimulation of the neural and endocrine mechanisms that control normal gastrointestinal function. Both undigested and digested nutrients should enter the small bowel slowly enough so as not to overwhelm its absorptive capacity, which leads to diarrhea. This limitation applies to isosmotic as well as to hyperosmotic solutions. Elemental diets create fluid and electrolyte imbalances. High-carbohydrate diets result in the production of large amounts of metabolic water, which is retained and produces hyponatremia. On the other hand, when water is not provided with high-protein or hyperosmolar solutions, the large amount of solute causes osmotic diuresis and subsequent dehydration. Diets rich in glucose, which is readily absorbed, can cause hyperglycemia and contribute to osmotic diuresis and dehydration.

The side effects of elemental diets are minimized by initially feeding one-third of the animal's needs distributed over six feedings a day, then gradually increasing the daily intake until total needs are met. A second means of administering the diet is via stomach tube. Tube feeding is as frequent as free-choice acceptance. A pharyngostomy tube can be used to feed small amounts frequently or continuously. A pump can be used to deliver a constantly infused diet, a procedure that minimizes the effects of hyperosmolar solutions entering the duodenum. Feeding by gravity drip is acceptable when the rate is controlled. With tube feeding, additional water must be given. Elemental diet formulation and rates of administration for enteral tube feeding are listed in Table 4.

Table 4. *Enteral Feeding Using an Elemental Diet*

VIVONEX HIGH NITROGEN *(25% solution)°*
Composition

Calories per ml	1.0
Grams nitrogen per 20 kcalories	1.5
Calories from fat	0.78%
Calories from carbohydrates	81%
Milliosmoles/liter	844†

Maximum rate of administration

Day 1	7 ml/kg body wt/hour
Day 2	10 ml/kg body wt/hour
Day 3	13 ml/kg body wt/hour

°Solution is made up by dilution of 80 grams in water to make a total volume of 300 ml (add 8.5 ounces of water).

†Osmolality of solution also contributed to by electrolytes in final solution: sodium, 33.4 mEq/liter; potassium, 17.9 mEq/liter; calcium, 13.3 mEq/liter; and magnesium, 9.6 mEq/liter.

PARENTERAL HYPERALIMENTATION

Nutrient and caloric requirements are not met by conventional parenteral solutions containing glucose or lactate (Table 5). Commercial solu-

Table 5. *Caloric Composition of Commonly Used Parenteral Fluids*

SOLUTION	KCAL/LITER
5% glucose	205
5% protein hydrolysate	<205
28 mEq lactate in Ringer's solution	10
16 mEq acetate in maintenance solution	4

tions of amino acids also do not meet the patient's nitrogen needs, since the nutrients are used for energy unless there is an adequate source of calories. Small amounts of glucose given intravenously reduce nitrogen losses by as much as one half. When nutritional homeostasis is desired, the first consideration is to meet the caloric needs, since all nutrients given are used to provide calories until that requirement is met. When the caloric intake is sufficient, dietary proteins or amino acids are used to build and replace body protein. Dogs require 425 non-protein calories for complete utilization of one gram of dietary protein in the synthesis of body proteins.

Some patients with gastrointestinal problems cannot be given anything orally, and it is necessary to maintain partial or complete nutritional homeostasis using parenteral hyperalimentation. This procedure involves intravenous infusion of nutrient solutions at a constant rate (often continuously) throughout each 24-hour period.

A realistic goal is to use total parenteral nutrition only for short periods. The disadvantages of this treatment are usually not prohibitive for periods of less than a week. The primary disadvantages are expense and the chance of introducing infection. Complete formulation to include vitamins and minerals is not critical for a week or less.

NITROGEN COMPOSITION

Originally, total parenteral nutrition solutions were formulated using nitrogen from protein hydrolysates. However, protein hydrolysates prepared by partial acid hydrolysis of fibrin or partial enzymatic hydrolysis of casein are no longer available. Since peptides are poorly utilized, the protein hydrolysates were classified by the Food and Drug Administration only as "probably effective" in partially reversing the negative nitrogen balance of patients in whom oral feeding is either not possible or ineffective. Concentrations of individual amino acids in hydrolysates varied according to the pattern of protein hydrolysis and were unbalanced with respect to normal plasma amino acid levels. Protein hydrolysates also contained high concentrations of ammonia, which could cause signs of hepatic encephalopathy in patients with liver disease. Antigenic peptides in protein hydrolysates were capable of causing hypersensitivity reactions.

Nitrogen is now provided by pure amino acids (Freeamine, McGaw; Travasol, Travenol; and Veinamine, Cutter). Solutions formulated with pure amino acids do not have the undesir-able effects of protein hydrolysates. They are fully effective in reversing negative nitrogen balance and preventing nitrogen loss. They also can be formulated to meet the animal's amino acid requirements precisely.

CALORIC COMPOSITION

During complete anorexia, body protein and lipids provide energy until their depletion results in death. The purpose of parenteral alimentation is to preserve body protein. This is accomplished by providing adequate amounts of calories in the form of carbohydrates and lipids. These calories cannot be provided by amino acids. Administration of 4 grams protein per kg body weight, representing 16 kcal per kg, is highly toxic and meets only about a third of the animal's caloric needs. Fats are an excellent source of calories and contribute very little to the osmolality of hypertonic parenteral alimentation solutions. Glucose is the primary source of energy in the body; it is metabolized to lactic acid and intermediate substances in the citric acid cycle. The major disadvantage of using glucose is that, in order to supply the number of calories required to meet energy requirements, the solution used must be hyperosmotic.

Ethanol is used as a source of calories in parenteral hyperalimentation solutions. The disadvantages of ethanol's use include its CNS-depressant effects and hyperosmolarity.

A commercial lipid formulation for parenteral hyperalimentation, Intralipid (Cutter), contains 100 to 200 grams soybean oil, 12 grams egg-yolk phospholipids, and 25 grams glycerol in 1000 ml solution. It has been administered to dogs at a rate as high as 9 gm of fat/kg body weight/day for a month with no undesirable effects. Other lipid preparations have been formulated that cause dogs to die. The 10 percent and 20 percent lipid solutions of Intralipid have osmolalities of 280 and 330 mOsmoles/liter, essentially the same as that of plasma. These lipid solutions have been used to provide 75 percent of a dog's daily caloric requirements (6 gm/kg body weight/day) and, when they are administered with glucose and amino acids, a positive nitrogen balance is achieved. Whereas hypertonic glucose solutions can be infused slowly only into large central veins, fat emulsions can be given in peripheral veins without causing phlebitis and thrombosis. This difference in administration also reduces the possibility of infection that accompanies catheterization of central veins. Hyperglycemia caused by glucose solutions, with its attendant hormonal and acid-base disturbances, is avoided when solutions based primarily on fat emulsions are used. The diet

Table 6. *Composition of Total Parenteral Nutrition Formula for a 10-Kg Dog*

NUTRIENT	SOURCE	VOLUME *(ml)*	GRAMS	KCAL
Fat	Intralipid 10%	350	35	325
Carbohydrate	Dextrose 10%	100	10	41
Protein	Travasol* 8.5%	100	8.5	35
	TOTAL	550		401

Potassium and Phosphate: Add 7 ml of potassium acid phosphate solution containing 2 mEq/ml. The total potassium administered is 20 mEq and of phosphate is 20 mEq. Additional potassium in the form of potassium acetate or lactate is added to meet greater needs.
Vitamins: Add multiple vitamins (M.V.I., USV Laboratories U.S. Pharm. Corp.).

*Travasol with electrolytes contains per 100 ml: 7 mEq sodium, 6 mEq potassium, 1 mEq magnesium, 13.5 mEq acetate, 7 mEq chloride, and 6 mEq phosphate. Freeamine can be substituted. Greater amounts of electrolytes are required when the source of nitrogen is not in an electrolyte solution.

formulated in Table 6 contains glucose, amino acids, and fats and has an osmolarity of slightly less than 500 mOsmoles/liter.

WATER AND ELECTROLYTE COMPOSITION

Small animals require about 40 ml water/kg body weight in order to excrete the solutes that must be eliminated through the kidneys. Parenteral hyperalimentation solutions used to provide all the calories also normally supply all the water an animal needs. Inadequate water intake is more likely a problem when therapy causes diuresis, such as in the therapy for hyperglycemia and hyperlactatesemia. A more common problem is the administration of too much water. It is one reason why a hypertonic solution to provide all the calories is needed. The volume of fluid needed to infuse the required number of calories in an isosmotic solution would be more than the animal could excrete.

Plasma levels of potassium, phosphorus, and magnesium are monitored during total parenteral nutrition. Bicarbonate levels are determined to evaluate acid-base homeostasis.

Cells contain high concentrations of potassium — 150 mEq/liter of cell water. One kg of lean body mass contains 100 gm of protein, which is used to provide 400 kcal of energy during starvation. The cellular contents —water (75 percent of mass), potassium (112 mEq), magnesium (16 mEq), and phosphate (80 mEq) — are released into the extracellular fluid. The amount of water released is insufficient for renal excretion of the solutes released; additional water, amounting to 2 liters/kg of lean weight lost, is required. These electrolytes must be replaced during reconstruction of the lean body mass by parenteral hyperalimentation.

Potassium requirements double when parenteral hyperalimentation solutions are infused. A minimum of 3 mEq potassium is required for each gram of body nitrogen replaced. Daily potassium requirements in a 10-kg dog can increase from 15 to more than 30 mEq when the animal is receiving total parenteral nutrition. Urinary excretion of potassium continues at 15 mEq/day in a 10-kg dog, regardless of the amount in the body. The potassium is required because of the high intracellular concentrations that are needed when lean body mass is replaced. Potassium also moves rapidly into cells when glucose is given, and this process is accelerated by insulin. Forty mEq of potassium must be added to each liter of hypertonic glucose solution to maintain normal plasma levels. Potassium depletions can amount to 30 to 40 mEq in a 10-kg animal. These losses should be replaced during the first 24 hours of therapy, after which potassium requirements are lower.

Phosphate-free parenteral hyperalimentation solutions reduce serum phosphorus levels. The complications thus produced include weakness, seizures, reversible hemolytic anemia and, unless corrected, death. Total parenteral nutrition in dogs receiving solutions that lack phosphorus results in death within five to six days. It is essential to maintain normal intracellular stores of phosphorus. During parenteral hyperalimentation, lean body mass is restored, and 80 mEq phosphorus move into the cells for each gain of 1 kg. This phosphate is obtained from extracellular fluid, and when it is not replenished by the diet it is mobilized from bone rapidly enough to prevent hypophosphatemia. Phosphate is added to hyperalimentation solutions to maximum concentrations of 40 mEq/liter.

Magnesium is lost during the catabolic state, but its rate of loss is relatively small, being only 20 percent of the phosphorus loss. Since the body conserves magnesium more efficiently than many other ions, hypomagnesemia is not a problem unless losses have been sustained in prolonged starvation, accompanied by severe losses through the gastrointestinal tract or kidneys. Prolonged total parenteral nutrition with magnesium-free solutions can eventually cause hypomagnesemia. Hyperalimentation solutions should contain 4 to 8 mEq magnesium per liter.

Acid-base homeostasis must be maintained and is achieved by adding the acetate, lactate, and phosphate salts of sodium, potassium, calcium, and magnesium. Bicarbonate can be used, but it precipitates calcium and magnesium.

Sodium and calcium balances are not difficult to maintain during parenteral hyperalimentation. Sodium conservation usually is efficient, and depletion seldom occurs unless hyperglycemia and glycosuria are causing diuresis.

VITAMIN COMPOSITION

A deficiency of water-soluble vitamins appears after two to three weeks of total parenteral nutrition. The vitamin requirement of patients receiving this therapy is unknown, and supplementation at present is based on known oral requirements. There are many incompatibilities between constituents of parenteral hyperalimentation solutions and vitamins.

FORMULATION

Table 7 lists the most important nutritional requirements that are met by parenteral hyperalimentation solutions. The amount of water given should not greatly exceed the requirements. All the nutrients and electrolytes should be administered in a maximum volume of 40 ml/kg body weight/day.

Table 7. Daily Nutritional Requirements of a 10-Kg Dog

NUTRIENT	REQUIREMENT
Protein	10 gm
Calories	400 Kcal
Potassium	20 mEq
Phosphate	15–25 mEq
Water	400 ml

Table 8. Complications of Total Parenteral Nutrition

GLUCOSE-BASED SOLUTIONS	ALL TYPES OF SOLUTIONS
Hyperosmolality	Peptide hypersensitivity
Osmotic dehydration	Potassium depletion
Glycosuria	Phosphate depletion
Metabolic acidosis	Hyperammonemia
Fluid overload	Fluid overload
Phlebitis	Infection

ADMINISTRATION

The lipid solution in the formula in Table 6 is infused into a peripheral vein. The amino acid, glucose, and electrolyte solution is delivered from a separate bottle into the catheter that carries the liquid emulsion. After mixing, the osmolality of the solution entering the peripheral vein is less than 500 milliOsmoles per liter. In a 10-kg dog, this solution is infused over a 10- to 12-hour period, amounting to 45 to 50 ml per hour. The infusion can be given by semicontrolled flow using a gravity drip or can be well regulated by roller pumps. Infusion is repeated 12 hours after completion of the previous day's infusion if the plasma has been cleared of the postinfusion lipemia. The usual precautions are taken to follow aseptic technique in the placement and care of catheters and in the handling of solutions of nutrients. Complications associated with glucose solutions have largely been avoided by the formulation of solutions based on lipids as the primary source of calories (Table 8).

SUPPLEMENTAL READING

Andersson, H., Isaksson, B., and Sjögren, B.: Fat-reduced diet in the symptomatic treatment of small bowel disease. Gut, 15:351–359, 1974.

Bessman, S.P.: Interrelations of various food materials. In Ghadimi, H. (ed.): *Total Parenteral Nutrition*. New York, John Wiley & Sons, 1975, pp. 335–342.

Bounous, G., Sutherland, N.G., McArdle, A.H., and Gurd, F.N.: The prophylactic use of an "elemental" diet in experimental hemorrhagic shock and intestinal ischemia. Ann. Surg., 166:312–343, 1975.

Bury, K.D.: Elemental diets. In Fischer, J.E. (ed.): *Total Parenteral Nutrition*. Boston, Little, Brown and Co., 1976, pp. 395–422.

Grotte, G., Jacobson, S., and Wretlind, A.: Lipid emulsions and technique of peripheral administration in parenteral nutrition. In Fischer, J.E. (ed.): *Total Parenteral Nutrition*. Boston, Little, Brown and Co., 1976, pp. 335–362.

Kronfeld, D.S.: Home cooking for dogs, with emphasis on therapeutic regimens. Presented at third symposium on Diet and Disease in Dogs, University of California at Irvine, Nov. 17, 1976.

Williams, R.E.O., and Grasar, B.S.: Alterations in gut bacterial flora in disease. In Badenoch, J., and Brooke, B.N. (eds.): *Recent Advances in Gastroenterology*. London, Churchill Livingstone, 1972, pp. 31–53.

MALASSIMILATION SYNDROME: MALDIGESTION/MALABSORPTION

GUY PIDGEON, D.V.M.
Auburn, Alabama

CLINICAL SIGNS AND DEFINITIONS

Chronic diarrhea, progressive weight loss, steatorrhea, and failure to respond to symptomatic therapy are the major clinical signs and historical complaints anticipated in the malassimilation syndrome. Typically, fecal volume is markedly increased, whereas defecation frequency is only modestly elevated; fecal consistency varies with the underlying disorder. Other problems encountered are ravenous appetite, pica, flatulence, excessive borborygmus, coprophagia, and poor haircoat. In advanced cases, edema related to hypoalbuminemia and signs associated with a deficiency of fat-soluble vitamins may be observed.

Malassimilation is a collective term implying a disorder at any step in the sequence of digestion and absorption. These conditions are uncommon when compared with other diarrheal diseases of the dog. For the purposes of this discussion, derangements of digestion will be equated with pancreatic exocrine insufficiency (the most common cause of malassimilation) and given primary attention here. Disorders of mastication, salivation, gastric secretion and motility, and bile salt metabolism are rarely encountered as primary clinical entities and will not be considered. Malabsorption is the end result of any diffuse disease affecting the small intestine or its lymphatic drainage that interferes with the passage of digested nutrients into the appropriate circulatory system. Compared with maldigestion, malabsorption is uncommon and will be reviewed only in capsule form.

Malassimilation syndrome has been documented only rarely in felines. This discussion is specifically directed toward canine patients; however, general physiologic principles also apply to cats.

DIAGNOSIS

Perhaps the most important phase of diagnostics involves the exclusion of other conditions either as the primary cause of clinical signs or as contributing factors. Repeated fecal examinations for evidence of intestinal parasitism, especially giardiasis, are mandatory in animals suspected of malassimilation, regardless of the dog's age at presentation. If found, parasites are treated accordingly, and two to three weeks are allowed for clinical improvement before further diagnostic tests are performed. The animal's diet should be assessed for caloric adequacy and the client should be questioned regarding unusual food additives or supplements. If milk or other dairy products are given, these should be excluded from the diet for 10 to 14 days; improvement is indicative of lactase deficiency. Careful history-taking, meticulous physical examination, and appropriate laboratory testing should rule out such diseases as intussusception, Addison's disease, diabetes mellitus, chronic active hepatitis, cardiac cachexia, and wasting associated with neoplastic processes.

This author has little desire to argue against "response to therapy" as an important diagnostic tool in chronic diarrheal diseases; however, two comments seem appropriate. First, if knowledge is to be gained, treatment must be altered systematically. Changes should be made one at a time, and a particular mode of therapy should be adhered to for a minimum of two weeks before it is considered inadequate. Sufficient time for response is particularly important in dietary therapy. Second, it is this author's opinion that pancreatic enzyme supplements are commonly misused by veterinarians. These products are expensive and required by the affected animal for the rest of its life; therefore, empirical therapy must be administered with an open mind in appropriate clinical situations and be accompanied by good client education.

A variety of laboratory procedures have been developed to test for malassimilation and to differentiate between maldigestion and malabsorption. A number of these will be discussed. None of the available, easily performed tests are consistently accurate. A promising new test for maldigestion has been evaluated (Strombeck,

1979) and will be available if FDA approval is forthcoming. In this procedure a synthetic peptide containing para-aminobenzoic acid (PABA) as a tracer is given orally. The bond between the PABA and the remainder of the peptide is specifically cleaved by chymotrypsin in the duodenum; PABA is readily absorbed and is 95 percent excreted in the urine within six hours. Assay of urine for total aromatic amines provides an excellent index of duodenal chymotrypsin activity. The product is under development by Adria Laboratories, Columbus, Ohio, and is tentatively scheduled for release in 1981.

MICROSCOPIC EXAMINATION

A crude assessment of the status of digestion and absorption can be obtained by careful study of appropriately stained fecal material under the microscope. Neutral fat in the feces appears as orange-red droplets when a fecal smear is stained with 3 or 4 drops of Sudan III. More than 3 to 5 droplets per high-power field is considered evidence of maldigestion. Grossly fatty stools from a malabsorptive animal in which digestion is normal should be negative for sudanophilic droplets, and needle-like fatty acid crystals may be observed. Protein maldigestion may lead to the presence of meat fibers in stool from a meat-fed animal. Visualization of muscle striations is improved by staining with iodine or eosin. Excessive starch, demonstrated by iodine stain, is also suggestive of maldigestion; however, there is marked variation in the fecal starch content of normal animals. Because all tests performed on feces are to some extent diet-dependent, control studies should be performed on stools from normal animals fed the same diet. It may be instructive to stain and examine smears made from the animal's food source.

FECAL TRYPSIN ACTIVITY

Enough fresh feces is added to 9 ml of 5 percent sodium bicarbonate solution to make a total volume of 10 ml. A thin strip of x-ray film (undeveloped, or a dark portion of developed film) is immersed in the mixture for two and one-half hours at room temperature or for one hour at 37°C. Clearing of the film after gentle washing in water is a positive test and indicates the presence of fecal trypsin from normal pancreatic secretion. The accuracy of the test can be improved by mixing 1 ml of diluted feces with 2 ml of 7.5 percent gelatin warmed to 37° C. Incubate the mixture as in the film test, then refrigerate for 20 minutes. Failure to gel is

a positive test and again indicates fecal protease activity. Unfortunately, these simple tests are subject to both false negative and false positive results; therefore, obtaining multiple negative results on separate days is recommended prior to basing a diagnosis of maldigestion on this procedure. Malabsorptive animals should have consistently positive test results.

FAT ABSORPTION TEST

Grossly turbid plasma two to three hours following a fatty meal indicates adequate pancreatic lipase secretion and normal absorptive processes. Absence of postprandial lipemia is indicative only of an abnormality at some step in the assimilation scheme. Anticoagulated blood samples are collected prior to and at one-, two-, and three-hour intervals after oral administration of vegetable oil or Lipomul (Upjohn) at a rate of 3 ml/kg. Following centrifugation or adequate settling, plasma is examined for turbidity. If all samples are clear, maldigestion can be confirmed by repeating the study after preincubating the oil with two teaspoons of Viokase powder (A.H. Robins Co.) for 30 to 60 minutes. The post-administration samples should demonstrate lipemia if pancreatic lipase deficiency is the sole cause of the initial negative test. Persistent lack of turbidity implies an absorptive disorder; however, problems with gastric emptying, micelle formation, and the crude visual evaluation of turbidity may affect the reliability of the test.

FAT BALANCE STUDIES

The 72-hour quantitative fecal fat analysis has long been a "data base" test for people with suspected malassimilation disorders. A recent study stresses the usefulness of fecal fat analysis in distinguishing dogs with malassimilation from those with other chronic diarrheal diseases (Burrows et al., 1979). Data presented indicated that normal dogs, fed widely varying diets, excreted a constant small amount of fat (0.2 gm/kg/24 hr). Dogs documented as suffering from malassimilation had a fecal fat content of 1.0 gm/kg/24 hr or higher. Animals with other chronic diarrheal diseases were not different from normal dogs in regard to fecal fat excretion. The authors stress the need to express fecal fat as a function of body weight. Significant steatorrhea will be overlooked in animals of small stature when the accepted criterion for steatorrhea — more than 7 grams of fecal fat per 24-hour period — is utilized. If the animal receives a consistent diet of commercial dog food then carefully collected, commercially analyzed

24-hour fecal samples should yield adequate data.

D-XYLOSE ABSORPTION

D-Xylose is a non-digestable pentose sugar that is readily absorbed from the normal small intestinal tract. Adequate serum levels after oral administration of D-xylose indicate a normal absorptive surface. Impaired digestive function does not affect the test. Unfortunately, the assay for D-xylose is difficult and not available at many laboratories. The test is performed by administering 10 ml/kg of 5 percent D-xylose solution (0.5 gm/kg) by gavage. Blood samples are collected at 0, 30, 60, 120, and 180 minutes. Normal animals have peak concentrations higher than 45 mg/dl during the sampling period, usually within 90 minutes. False negative results may be obtained in conditions associated with bacterial overgrowth of the small bowel or in delayed gastric emptying.

ORAL GLUCOSE TOLERANCE

This test provides a useful index of intestinal absorptive function, although it is less reliable than the D-xylose test. Glucose (2.0 gm/kg) is given in 20 percent solution by stomach tube to a fasting animal. Blood samples are collected as in the D-xylose test and are analyzed for glucose content. Care must be exercised to avoid exciting the animal during the test, and serum should be separated from the cells soon after collection. In normal animals peak glucose levels are obtained after 30 to 60 minutes, and they are approximately 160 mg/dl. Return to the fasting glucose level should occur prior to 180 minutes. Animals with intestinal malabsorption have lowered peak concentrations and rapidly return to fasting levels. Assessment of this test is subjective, and plotting results on graph paper for comparison with normal results may be useful. Non-diabetic maldigestive dogs generally have normal oral glucose tolerance curves; however, prolonged hyperglycemia may indicate a prediabetic state.

SERUM PROTEIN LEVELS

Symmetric reduction in serum gamma globulins and albumin should lead to consideration of the bowel as a route of loss. Protein-losing enteropathy can be documented by radioisotope studies. In practice, the diagnosis is made by excluding other routes of loss (proteinuria or severe skin disease) and by demonstrating normal liver function (BSP retention, ammonia tolerance test, or biopsy is required to assess the liver with certainty).

MELENA

In the absence of coagulation defects, the passage of digested blood in the stool of an animal with other clinical signs of malassimilation is convincing evidence of gastric or primary small bowel disease.

RADIOGRAPHY

Standard x-ray studies, including contrast procedures, rarely are useful in the diagnosis of problems that cause either digestive or absorptive disturbances.

INTESTINAL BIOPSY

Histopathologic study is essentially the only means of definitive diagnosis in malabsorptive diseases. A skilled operator using appropriate instrumentation can obtain duodenal mucosal biopsies via endoscopy. In practice, most biopsies are obtained during exploratory laparotomy. Full-thickness biopsies are recommended; palpable abnormalites of the intestine guide site selection. In the absence of gross disease or in diffuse disorders duodenal, mid-jejunal, and proximal ileal biopsy are suggested. At least one regional lymph node should be sampled or removed in its entirety. All abdominal viscera must be examined, and abnormal structures should be biopsied. Specimens require careful handling to avoid trauma artifact, and intestinal tissue should be pinned to a cardboard backing before fixing so as to maintain anatomic continuity for the pathologist. Animals with suspected malabsorptive disease rarely are good candidates for surgery. Hypoalbuminemia and bowel disease retard healing. Excellent surgical technique, the use of non absorbable sutures, and careful analysis of risk:benefit ratio are recommended.

MALDIGESTION

SIGNALMENT

The clinical signs, previously discussed, of malassimilation due to pancreatic exocrine insufficiency are anticipated in two distinct groups of dogs: those suffering from juvenile pancreatic atrophy (Anderson and Low, 1965) and those presenting with end-stage recurrent inflammatory disease of the pancreas. The German shepherd breed is over-represented in the first group, and clinical signs are expected prior to two years of age. The specific cause of juvenile pancreatic atrophy is unknown; its breed predisposition suggests hereditary factors. This condition is usually uncomplicated, although prediabetic glucose tolerance curves have been demonstrated. Response to therapy is generally adequate.

It is simplistic to list recurrent pancreatitis as the etiologic agent of maldigestion in the second group, since the pathogenesis of that disorder is not well known; however, such considerations are beyond the scope of this discussion. Animals of any breed presenting in middle to old age with appropriate clinical signs should be suspected. Historically recurrent gastrointestinal upset and antecedent obesity are supportive findings. It has been shown that 90 percent of exocrine function must be lost before clinical signs of maldigestion become evident; concurrent endocrine dysfunction is quite possible and should be assessed. Intercurrent geriatric disorders complicate the clinical situation; response to therapy is not as good in this group. The author's limited experience with combination diabetic/exocrine-deficient dogs has been uniformly unpleasant. Rarely, pancreatic maldigestion can be observed in the terminal stage of pancreatic neoplasia, abscessation, amyloidosis, and other diseases. Pathologic changes encountered in pancreatic disease have been described (Thordal-Christensen and Coffin, 1956).

THERAPY

Pancreatic maldigestion is an "end-point" condition. Like other organs with large functional reserves, clinical signs are not appreciated until pathologic processes are advanced and irreversible. Therefore, all therapy is supportive and required for the rest of the animal's life.

Oral pancreatic enzyme replacement is expensive and inefficient; unfortunately the alternatives are even less practical. A number of commercial enzyme preparations are available. Most veterinary experience has been with powdered pancreatin (e.g., Viokase-V, A.H. Robins Co.). It has been demonstrated that 60 to 90 percent of unprotected orally ingested pancreatic enzymes are destroyed by gastric acid. Enteric-coated products have seemed a logical choice; however, none of the previously available products has been satisfactory. At this writing, the human literature contains information regarding a new enteric-coated preparation. The product is pancrealipase in microspheres, individually enteric-coated, and administered in capsule form (Pancrease, Johnson & Johnson). Clinical trials in people demonstrate superiority over other enzyme formulations. To the author's knowledge results of clinical experience with this product in the dog are not yet available.

To improve the viability of orally administered non–enteric-coated enzymes, additional additives and timing maneuvers have been recommended, e.g., sodium bicarbonate, bile salts, antibiotics, and the pre-incubation of enzymes with food. Recent reports in the human literature demonstate the usefulness of cimetidine (Tagamet, Smith Kline & French) as an adjunct to enzyme therapy (Regan et al., 1977; Saunders et al., 1977). Cimetidine, developed for peptic ulcer disease, is a competitive antagonist at histamine type 2 receptor sites, thus blocking the stomach's normal acid secretory response. Cimetidine and traditional therapy for pancreatic maldigestion were recently evaluated in experimental dogs (Pidgeon and Strombeck). Some important findings were as follows: (1) Powdered pancreatin alone significantly reduced steatorrhea and fecal mass. Interestingly, no difference was found between 1- , 2- , and 4-teaspoon doses in 20-kg dogs. (2) Sodium bicarbonate, other antacids, bile salts, and pre-incubation of the enzymes with food did nothing to improve pancreatin function. (3) Neomycin, in addition to oral enzymes, did prove useful. Supporting subjective evidence indicates that bacterial overgrowth of the small bowel may play a role in maldigestive states. (4) Cimetidine in addition to pancreatin significantly improved enzyme availability in the duodenum, as reflected by reduced steatorrhea.

Recommendations for initial therapy in the maldigestive dog include feeding a mixture of commercial dry and canned food that is calorically adequate for the animal's ideal weight plus 10 percent, divided into two or three feedings. Low-fat, low-bulk diets have been recommended but are not generally necessary. For 20-kg dogs, add 1 level teaspoonful of pancreatin powder to each meal. If initial response is inadequate, adjust the dosage upward to a maximum of 2 teaspoonfuls. During the early phase of treatment vitamin supplementation, especially with vitamins A, D, E, and K, and intestinal antibiotics may be indicated. Neomycin or other non-absorbed antibacterial drugs are recommended but should not be given for more than five successive days. Long-term antibiotic therapy in the bowel succeeds only in inducing resistant strains of bacteria and potential "super" infection.

If some response to enzyme therapy is obtained, lending credence to the diagnosis, but objectionable clinical signs persist, cimetidine may be added to the therapeutic scheme. The drug is not currently approved for dogs, nor is dosage information available; therefore, good client education is important. The LD_{50} of cimetidine in dogs is approximately 2.6 gm/kg; death is preceded by tonic or clonic convulsions.

Ninety-day studies in dogs at doses approximately 25 times the normal therapeutic level produced no adverse clinical signs or significant clinical pathologic change (Brimblecombe et al., 1975). In 20-kg dogs 300 mg of cimetidine (15.0 mg/kg) given at the time of the animal's meal in conjunction with powdered pancreatin proved useful, and no drug-associated problems were encountered. The normal adult human dosage is 300 mg of cimetidine three to four times a day.

MALABSORPTION

Malabsorption is tentatively diagnosed in an animal that has typical clinical signs after exocrine pancreatic function is found to be normal. Definitive diagnosis requires the demonstration of a functional abnormality related to small intestinal absorptive activity (see "Diagnosis") and histopathologic examination of small intestinal tissue.

Veterinary literature contains minimal information regarding the etiology and therapy of malabsorptive disorders. Fortunately these conditions are rare. Unfortunately, they are usually documented late, long after etiologic clues have been obliterated. Non-specific therapy is usually unsatisfactory.

It is this author's opinion that little service is provided the veterinary community by comparing the morphologic pathology of canine enteropathies with human disorders. Etiologic and therapeutic implications generated by such discussions have not been useful. Rather, our collective efforts should identify functional changes, carefully describe the nature and location of lesions, and discuss response to specific therapy. Perhaps, as diagnostic efforts become more aggressive, information of use to the practicing clinician will be more readily available.

PRIMARY INTESTINAL MALABSORPTION

Rare conditions are encountered in which small intestinal villi are shortened, thickened, and reduced in number. The lamina propria is infiltrated with lymphocytes and plasma cells. Cases of malabsorption have been described wherein villus morphology is considered normal; however, a dense plasmocytic and lymphocytic infiltrate of the lamina propria is present. Another condition, perhaps more common in German shepherds, involves the infiltration of the bowel wall by eosinophils. Eosinophilic enteritis rarely is severe enough to cause true malabsorption. It is convenient to think that all these conditions represent an inappropriate immune response to either ingested or locally produced antigens. Unfortunately, allergy testing has not proved to be diagnostic, nor has response to controlled diets been satisfactory. Eosinophilic enteritis is thought to be secondary to visceral larval migrans in some dogs (Hayden and Van Kruiningen, 1973). Occasional response to thiabendazole (50 mg/kg once a day for five days) has been obtained. Alternatively, eosinophilic enteritis can be controlled with corticosteroids; however, high doses and long-term use may be necessary. The other primary bowel wall diseases present difficult management problems. Good supportive care and low-fat, high-protein diets are helpful. Some response to corticosteroids and other immunosuppressive drugs may be obtained in plasmocytic enteritis. Intestinal antibiotics and vitamin supplementation have been utilized with variable results.

INTESTINAL LYMPHANGIECTASIA

Dilatation of intestinal lacteals may be encountered as a primary idiopathic process or secondary to other lymphatic disease and leads to a loss of protein into the bowel and interference with fat absorption (Finco et al., 1973). Therapy is aimed at resolution of primary disorders. In idiopathic disease sporadic improvement is found with the institution of low-fat diets supplemented with medium-chain triglycerides (MCT Oil, Mead Johnson). These lipids are directly absorbed into the venous system, significantly reducing lymphatic flow.

SECONDARY INTESTINAL MALABSORPTION

Malabsorption can develop secondary to any advanced, diffuse disease affecting the small intestine. Therefore, neoplastic diseases such as lymphosarcoma and infectious processes like histoplasmosis must be considered in the differential diagnosis. Diagnosis and treatment of these conditions are discussed elsewhere in this text.

Bacterial overgrowth of the small bowel as a primary chronic disease is rare; however, its significance as a complicating factor in other gastrointestinal disturbances should not be overlooked. Abrupt changes in diet are associated with marked changes in intestinal flora and may provide more satisfactory therapy than intestinal antibiotics, which rapidly induce resistant bacterial strains.

Iatrogenic malabsorptive states can theoretically be induced by massive bowel resection, although reported cases are rare. In humans removal of the ileum, especially the distal segment, is associated with deficient bile salt resorption and the development of steatorrhea. To the author's knowledge, this sequela has not been documented in the dog.

SUPPLEMENTAL READING

Anderson, N.V., and Low, D.G.: Juvenile atrophy of the canine pancreas. An Hosp *1*:101–109, 1965.

Brimblecombe, R.W., Duncan, W.A.M., Durant, G.J., et al.: Cimetidine — A non-thiourea H_2-receptor antagonist. J. Int. Med. Res., 3:86–91, 1975.

Burrows, C.F., Merritt, A.M., Chiapella, A.M.: Determination of fecal fat and trypsin output in the evaluation of chronic canine diarrhea. J. Am. Vet. Med. Assoc., *174*:62–66, 1979.

Finco, D.R., Duncan, J.R., Schall, W.D., et al.: Chronic enteric disease and hypoproteinemia in 9 dogs. J. Am. Vet. Med. Assoc., *163*:262–271, 1973.

Hayden, D.W., and Van Kruiningen, H.J.: Eosinophilic gastroenteritis in German shepherd dogs and its relationship to visceral larval migrans. J. Am. Vet. Med. Assoc., *162*:379–384. 1973.

Hill, F.W.G., Osborne, A.D., and Kidder, D.E.: Pancreatic degenerative atrophy in dogs. J. Comp. Path., *81*:321–330, 1971.

Holroyd, J.B.: Canine exocrine pancreatic disease. J. Small Anim. Pract., 9:269–281, 1968.

Pidgeon, G.L., and Strombeck, D.R.: Assessment of therapy in experimental canine exocrine pancreatic insufficiency. (Manuscript in preparation.)

Regan, P.T., Malagelada, J.R., Dimagno, E.P., et al.: Comparative effects of antacids, cimetidine and enteric coating on the therapeutic response to oral enzymes in severe pancreatic insufficiency. N. Engl. J. Med., 297:854–858, 1977.

Saunders, J.H.B., Drummond, S., and Wormsley, K.G.: Inhibition of gastric secretion in treatment of pancreatic insufficiency. Br. Med. J., *1*:418–419, 1977.

Strombeck, D.R.: New method for evaluation of chymotrypsin deficiency in dogs. J. Am. Vet. Med. Assoc., *173*:1319–1323, 1979.

Thordal-Christensen, A., and Coffin, D.L.: Pancreatic diseases in the dog. Nord. Vet. Med., 8:89–114, 1956.

Van Kruiningen, H.J., and Hayden, D.W.: Interpreting problem diarrheas of dogs. Vet. Clin. North Am., 2:29–67, 1972.

GASTROINTESTINAL PARASITISM

EDWARD L. ROBERSON, D.V.M.,
and LARRY M. CORNELIUS, D.V.M.
Athens, Georgia

PREVALENCE OF HELMINTH INFECTIONS IN DOGS

Despite many years of attention to parasitic infections of small animals, the prevalence of ascarids, hookworms, whipworms, and tapeworms is still quite high and widespread. Table 1 presents prevalences of these parasites in pound dogs (all ages) from five different locations in the U.S. Overall, more than 50 percent of these dogs were infected with ascarids, hookworms, or whipworms or a combination of these.

A further study in Georgia (Table 2) compares the prevalences of canine helminths in pups (less than six months old) and adult dogs obtained from pounds. Ascarids (*Toxocara canis*) were very much more prevalent among pups (74 percent) than among dogs more than six months old (13 percent); whipworms (*Trichuris vulpis*) were more prevalent among older dogs (62 percent as compared with 15 percent in pups); and hookworms (*Ancylostoma caninum*) were equally prevalent in both age groups (82 to 85 percent).

The Georgia study also surveyed owned dogs seen as patients at the University of Georgia Veterinary Teaching Hospital. Table 2 suggests that routine and therapeutic deworming of owned animals (and perhaps an increased level of nutrition and improved living conditions) substantially reduces the overall prevalence of ascarids, hookworms, and whipworms.

HOOKWORMS

MEANS OF INFECTION AND CLINICAL SIGNS

Infections of the more common hookworms of dogs (*Ancylostoma caninum* and *Uncinaria stenocephala*) and cats (*Ancylostoma tubaeforme*) may be obtained by the ingestion of food and water contaminated with infective L_3 larvae or by penetration of the skin by these larvae. Another evidently important means of infection documented for *A. caninum* is the passage of L_3 larvae to pups via the bitch's milk. In this transmammary route infective larvae that the

Table 1. *Incidence of Parasitic Infections at Necropsy of Dogs from Five States*

INFECTION[*]	GEORGIA	OHIO	NORTH CAROLINA	TEXAS	CALIF.	OVERALL
No. Dogs Sampled	177	1128	868	737	188	3098
Ascarids % Infected	51	51	40	58	93	52
Hookworms % Infected	81	51	87	82	46	70
Whipworms % Infected	55	72	62	10	27	51
Tapeworms % Infected	NR[†]	19	44	17	9	26[‡]

(Modified from: Hass, D. K., Collins, J. A., and Flick, S. C.: Canine parasitism. Canine Practice, 2(6):42–47, 1975. Used with permission.)

[*]Ascarids: *Toxocara* and *Toxascaris*
　Hookworms: *Ancylostoma* and *Uncinaria*
　Whipworms: *Trichuris*
　Tapeworms: *Taenia* and *Dipylidium*
[†]NR = not recorded by investigator
[‡]Based upon 2921 dogs; the prevalence of tapeworms was not recorded by the Georgia investigators.

pregnant bitch has picked up orally or by skin penetration accumulate in her mammary glands and subsequently pass via the milk to her nursing pups, especially during the first weeks of nursing.

Hookworm larvae obtained orally (via the bitch's milk or contaminated water or food) are confined to development in the digestive tract, especially in young animals. Larvae of *A. caninum*, when ingested orally, enter the gastric glands of the stomach or glands of Lieberkühn in the small intestine, where they develop for a few days and subsequently return to the gut lumen to molt to the fourth stage, then to the fifth stage, after which they mature to adult stage. Hookworm eggs may be seen in the host's feces as early as 15 to 18 days after the initial oral infection.

The blood-letting by hookworms will have begun with the fourth stage larvae (i.e., about eight days following the initial infection, several days before eggs are passed). The fourth-stage larvae, young immature adults (fifth stage), and adult worms feed by pulling a plug of mucosa into the large buccal cavity. The digestion of this plug occurs within approximately 30 minutes, resulting in disruption of the vasculature and loss of blood into the surrounding tissue. After ingesting as many as two or three mucosal plugs, the worms move to another site, leaving the first site bleeding. This graze-type feeding results in numerous punctiform hemorrhages of the small intestinal mucosa.

A. caninum is the most pathogenic hookworm for dogs, and *A. tubaeforme* is most pathogenic

Table 2. *Prevalence of Nematodes in Pound vs. Owned Dogs in North Georgia*

	PERCENT OF DOGS INFECTED			
	POUND DOGS		OWNED DOGS	
ORGANISM	*Pups*	*Adults*	*Pups*	*Adults*
Toxocara canis	74	13	39	6
Ancylostoma caninum	85	82	37	37
Uncinaria stenocephala	12	28	1	1
Trichuris vulpis	15	62	10	23
Toxascaris leonina	0	0	1	<1
Capillaria spp.	0	<1	0	<1
Physaloptera spp.	<1	0	0	0
Spirocera lupi	0	<1	0	0
No parasites	6	6	43	50

(Data obtained by D. E. Burgess and T. M. Burke, Athens, Ga.)

for cats. The pathogenicity of *A. braziliense* and *Uncinaria* is 50 to 100 times less than that of *A. caninum*. Maximum blood loss is seen 10 to 25 days after infection. Pups with 66 to 132 worms (*A. caninum*)/kg of body weight will show approximately a 45 percent decrease in hematocrit value; 165 worms/kg is considered the LD_{50} in young pups.

The loss of blood into the lumen of the canine digestive tract gives a tarry appearance to the feces, which may become foul-smelling and completely fluid. Such pups quickly develop pale mucous membranes and demonstrate signs of weakness and emaciation. Older dogs may develop regenerative microcytic hypochromic anemia as a result of iron deficiency caused by chronic blood loss.

TREATMENT

In young pups and kittens and in older animals that are clinically anemic and listless from hookworm infection it is necessary to eliminate the parasites as quickly as possible. Anthelmintics requiring a single dose (rather than five daily doses) are most satisfactory for these cases. These include dichlorvos (Task® or Task Tabs®), pyrantel pamoate (Nemex®) or disophenol (D.N.P.®) (Table 3). Dichlorvos seems to bring about the most immediate expulsion of worms (within eight hours or so), whereas disophenol given subcutaneously requires 24 hours or more to effect expulsion. Dichlorvos is contraindicated if severe diarrhea accompanies the clinical anemia and listlessness; in these cases pyrantel pamoate or disophenol are preferred. Larval stages in the lungs at the time of treatment are not affected by any of these drugs. Many of these larvae will cycle to the intestine and mature within two weeks. Thus, retreatment should be given two weeks after the initial treatment. To determine if subsequent treatments are needed, feces should be rechecked for eggs at two-week intervals until previously ill young animals are about four months of age.

Necessary supportive therapy will depend upon the severity of the anemia. When the packed cell volume is 15 percent or lower, whole blood probably should be administered, at a rate of about 10 to 15 ml/lb (4.5 to 6.8 ml/kg). This is especially important if the animal's clinical condition seems to be deteriorating. The intravenous route is preferred, but injection into the femoral bone marrow cavity through the trocanteric fossa is simple in pups and kittens and should be used whenever intravenous injection is too difficult. Intraperitoneal transfusion can be done, but results are less

satisfactory. Other supportive measures include keeping the animal warm and quiet, with no undue stress. It is critical that handling of severely anemic animals be gentle during blood transfusion. Excessive struggling can result in the patient's death. Hematinic drugs are generally unnecessary in animals consuming a proper diet; however, nursing pups or kittens probably should receive iron supplementation.

In less critical hookworm infections, in which immediate expulsion of worms is not essential, or in routine dewormings a single treatment with dichlorvos, toluene (Vermiplex®), or thenium closylate (Canopar®) or a five-day treatment with mebendazole (Telmintic®) gives relatively equal and satisfactory results.

Experimentally, fenbendazole at 50 mg/kg body weight for three days has expulsed hookworms satisfactorily (see Table 3). The feces of pups so treated were normal and formed following a three-day treatment with fenbendazole, as compared with the dysenteric stools of untreated infected littermates.

Two older compounds that have little merit in treating hookworms today are *n*-butyl chloride and tetrachloroethylene. The former is only 60 percent effective for hookworms and the latter, although 90 percent effective, has numerous disadvantages (hepatotoxicity and contraindication in debilitated or tapeworm-positive animals) that newer synthetic anthelmintics have overcome.

ASCARIDS

MEANS OF INFECTION AND CLINICAL SIGNS

Two species of ascarids, *Toxocara canis* and *Toxascaris leonina*, infect dogs. Cats are infected by a feline strain of *Toxascaris leonina* and their own species of *Toxocara*, *T. cati*. These three ascarids differ in the extent of larval migration in the host and, thus, in the degree of larval pathogenicity. Larvae of *Toxocara canis* migrate most extensively, i.e., liver-lung migration or somatic tissue migration. Larvae of *Toxocara cati* are confined predominately to a liver-lung migration; somatic migration of this ascarid is fairly insignificant. Larvae of *Toxascaris leonina* are confined to gut mucosal invasion and do not migrate through hepatic, pulmonary, or somatic tissues. Thus the pathogenesis of *Toxascaris* is considerably less than that of either species of *Toxocara*, and treatment for the gut-dwelling *Toxascaris* is less complicated than for *Toxocara*, since none of the currently available anthelmintics significantly reduce the numbers of extraintestinal larvae of *Toxocara*.

Table 3.   Anthelmintics for Dogs and Cats

DRUGS	EFFICACY*					DOSAGE	COMMENTS
	Hook-worms	Ascarids	Whip-worms	Tape-worms	Strongy-loides		
D.N.P.® (disophenol) (American Cyanamid)	95%	—	—	—	—	10 mg/kg SQ	36 mg/kg is fatal. Do not administer to overheated animals or those with respiratory problems. Can be used on nursing young.
Tetrachlorethylene (Several manufacturers)	90%	—	—	—	—	0.22 ml/kg after 12-hr fast	Hepatotoxic. Contraindicated in sick, debilitated, or tapeworm-positive animals.
Canopar® (thenium closylate) (Burroughs Wellcome)	89%	±	—	—	—	1 tablet (500 mg) for dogs over 10 lb (5 kg), regardless of weight; ¼ tablet (125 mg) (q 12 hr) b.i.d. for 5- to 10-lb (2.5- to 5-kg) dogs	Not absorbed from digestive tract. Some emesis. Cannot use in nursing pups or those less than 5 lb (2.5 kg).
Piperazine (Many manufacturers)	—	85%	—	—	—	110 mg/kg orally; maximum of 250 mg for pups under 2.5 kg and for cats and kittens	No contraindications except long-standing renal or liver disease.
Caricide® (diethylcarbamazine) (American Cyanamid)	—	80%	—	—	—	6.6 mg/kg/day orally as a preventive	Most effective prevention against heartworm is within 2 weeks after 3rd-stage larvae infect the host. Contraindicated if microfilariae present.
Whipcide® (phthalofyne) (Pitman-Moore)	—	—	90%	—	—	200 mg/kg orally after 24-hr fast; 250 mg/kg IV, no fasting	Side effects. Foul odor of by-products.
Milibis-V® (glycobiarsol) (Winthrop)	—	—	90%	—	—	220 mg/kg daily × 5 days	Developed for treatment of amebiasis. ½ dose × 10 days recommended for debilitated dogs.

Thiabendazole (Merck Sharp & Dohme)	±	±	—	95%	55 mg/kg daily × 3 days orally	Some emesis. Repeat treatment monthly if needed.
Nemex® (pyrantel pamoate) (Pfizer)	95%	95%	—	—	1 ml suspension per lb (5 mg/kg) orally	Used in dogs of all ages, including nursing pups. No contraindications.
n-Butyl chloride (Several manufacturers)	60%	90%	—	—	1 mg/kg after 12-hr fast	Cathartic recommended.
Task® (dichlorvos) (Shell)	95%	95%	90%	—	Dog: 27–33 mg/kg. Puppy & cat: 11 mg/kg	Contraindications include heartworm disease and liver or kidney damage. Do not use in conjunction with other cholinesterase inhibitors. Split dosage b.i.d. for debilitated animals.
Styquin® (butamisole HCl) (American Cyanimide)	92%	—	99%	—	2.4 mg/kg SQ	A four-fold overdose is lethal; do not use simultaneously with Scolaban
Dizan® (dithiazanine iodide) (Elanco)	80%	80%	80%	85%	11 mg/kg b.i.d. × 5–10 days orally	Requires multiple dosage. Absorbed products may be nephrotoxic. Effective microfilaricide.
Telmintic® (mebendazole) (Pitman-Moore)	95%	95%	95%	85% T† 0% D	22 mg/kg in food daily × 5 days	No contraindications. Approved for dogs; experimental in cats.
Vermiplex® (toluene and dichlorophene) (Pitman-Moore)	95%	90%	—	72% T 85% D	Size capsule as directed by manufacturer	Incoordination, emesis, toxicity in excess.

Table continued on following page

Table 3. *Anthelmintics for Dogs and Cats (Continued)*

DRUGS	EFFICACY					DOSAGE	COMMENTS
	Hook-worms	Ascarids	Whip-worms	Tape-worms	Strongy-loides		
Scolaban® (bunamidine HCl) (Burroughs Wellcome)	—	—	—	100% T 56–90% D	—	25 mg/kg on empty stomach; feed lightly in 3 hr	Occasional idiosyncratic reaction. Do not use simultaneously with Styquin.
Yomesan® (niclosamide) (Chemagro)	—	—	—	80% T 18–56% D	—	100–157 mg/kg orally	Heavy mucus interferes with elimination of scolex.
Nemural® (arecoline-acetarsol) (Winthrop)	—	—	—	50%	—	4–6 mg/kg orally after light feeding	Severe vomiting and diarrhea may occur and may be difficult to control.
Fenbendazole (experimental) (American Hoechst)	98%	99%	100%	100% T 0% D		50 mg/kg/day × 3 days	Granules added to moist food.

°Percentages in "Tapeworms" column refer to % of dogs cleared of infection; all others refer to % of nematodes expelled.

†T = *Taenia* sp.; D = *Dipylidium caninum*

The greatest larval damage occurs to the liver and lungs. Following ingestion of infective eggs of *Toxocara canis* and release of the larvae in the stomach and small intestine of pups (especially pups less than five weeks old), the larvae enter the hepatic portal system, migrate through the liver for several days, are carried in the blood via the heart to the lungs, where additional migration and disruption of tissue occur until they enter the respiratory tree, from which they are coughed up, swallowed, and returned to the gut. Almost all *Toxocara* larvae take this route in very young pups (less than five weeks old) and eventually mature as adult worms in the gut. Assuming that there is a continuous source of infective eggs, as the pup grows older fewer larvae will enter the respiratory passage that returns them to the gut; instead, more and more larvae in the lung will burrow through the pulmonary vein and will be distributed with oxygenated blood to somatic tissues, where they will remain without further development, perhaps for the life of the animal. Practically all larvae infecting three-month-old pups will become somatically located.

For male dogs there is no release from the continually growing burden of somatic ascarid larvae. In females, however, pregnancy and subsequent lactation afford a chance for the bitch to reduce her somatic numbers — at the expense of the pups. Transplacental (prenatal) migration of the bitch's larvae begins following day 35 of pregnancy. These larvae will enter the liver and lung of the fetus and await the birth of the pup before passing to the gut. Extremely heavy prenatal infections may cause stillbirths. Further depletion of the bitch's stored larvae occurs during nursing, when larvae pass via the milk to the pups. A bitch with a moderate somatic infection of ascarids, if prevented from further ingestion of eggs, will require three or four pregnancies to pass all of her larval burden to her pups.

In heavy prenatal and transmammary infections the pulmonary phase may be lethal for pups within a few days of birth. Generally, however, pups do not succumb immediately but clinically become unthrifty, demonstrate evidence of respiratory distress and a dull haircoat, develop a distended abdomen primarily as a result of the physical presence of numerous large worms (potbellied appearance), and experience varying degrees of digestive disturbance (colic, vomiting, diarrhea, or alternating diarrhea and constipation). Only very rarely do adult worms wander into and block the bile or pancreatic ducts. Somewhat more frequently, however, wandering larval stages enter the central nervous system, resulting in meningitis-like signs.

Treatment of young pups or kittens for heavy ascarid burdens (especially *Toxocara*) involves repeated dosing (perhaps three or four treatments at two-week intervals beginning at two weeks of age). Repeated treatments are necessary because none of the currently available drugs have any significant effect against larval stages (L_2 and L_3) that may occur in the liver or lungs at the time medication is administered. Following treatment, some of these larvae will complete their migration, returning to the digestive tract and continuing development through a fourth larval stage and immature adulthood to become adult worms. Another treatment will be necessary to expel these intestinal stages. Meanwhile, as long as the pup is nursing, transmammary infections are continuously occurring and add to the necessity for repeated treatments. Multiple treatment generally is not needed for older animals infected with *Toxocara*.

A wide variety of anthelmintics are available for treating ascarid infections—piperazine, *n*-butyl chloride, dichlorvos, methylbenzene (toluene), mebendazole, and pyrantel pamoate (see Table 3). All are substantially effective, and the selection of one drug over another is not necessary when routinely treating healthy pups, eight weeks of age or older, that are taking solid food (mebendazole is administered in the food). Nursing pups, however, especially those clinically ill from heavy ascarid infections, seem to tolerate the relatively new pyrantel pamoate (Nemex®) best. This compound is supplied in suspension form, is caramel-flavored, and is often easier to administer orally by syringe to nursing pups of small breeds than are tablet and capsule formulations of the other anthelmintics. Nemex® also has excellent activity against hookworms.

Supportive treatment for toxocariasis consists primarily of good nursing care. For nursing pups or kittens, it is beneficial to provide warm, dry housing and to be certain that the bitch or queen is lactating properly. Older animals should be provided a palatable, balanced diet.

In light of the ubiquity of prenatal and transmammary infections of ascarids and hookworms, an anthelmintic that is effective against somatic stages in the bitch, thus preventing infection of her pups, clearly is needed. Such a drug most likely would require daily long-term administration. Preliminary success along these lines has been obtained in Germany with fenbendazole, an anthelmintic that currently is approved in the United States only for use in horses (Panacur®). Studies in this country are underway at this time to assess the potential of fenbendazole against somatic ascarid and hookworm larvae in pregnant bitches.

WHIPWORMS

MEANS OF INFECTION AND CLINICAL SIGNS

Whipworm (*Trichuris vulpis*) infections of dogs occur by direct ingestion of eggs containing the infective stage. The hatched larva burrows into the upper small intestine for approximately one week (without consequent pathology), emerges, and subsequently moves to the cecum to establish a lifelong residency.

Although the morbidity associated with whipworm infection has been suggested in the past to be relatively low, more recent clinical observation has indicated that the opposite is true. At the University of Georgia Veterinary Teaching Hospital whipworms are one of the most common causes of chronic mucoid bloody diarrhea (large bowel diarrhea). Whipworm ova are frequently absent in the feces in such cases, making diagnosis difficult. By using a flexible fiberoptic endoscope we have been able to visualize whipworms in the cecum of dogs with large bowel diarrhea when fecal flotation tests were repeatedly negative. It is suggested that, whenever a cause for chronic large bowel diarrhea cannot be established by routine diagnostic methods, whipworm treatment should be given before resorting to more elaborate diagnostic procedures.

Cats are not infected by the canine species of whipworm. A few reports of feline infection with *Trichuris campanula* have been made in the U.S., South America, Cuba, and the Bahamas.

TREATMENT

Five anthelmintics that give satisfactory activity against canine whipworms are now available. The activity of two of these—phthalofyne (Whipcide®) and glycobiarsol (Milibis V®)—is strictly against whipworms, while the others—butamisole HCl (Styquine®), dichlorvos (Task®) and mebendazole (Telmintic®)—also are effective against ascarids and/or hookworms (see Table 3). The latter three have the advantage of requiring only a single dose; glycobiarsol and mebendazole each require five daily doses. However, dichlorvos is contraindicated in heartworm-positive dogs, and both dichlorvos and phthalofyne are contraindicated in dogs that have chronic nephritis, hepatitis, pancreatitis, or cardiac insufficiencies. Intravenous phthalofyne is seldom used now because of the occurrence of vomiting, ataxia, and drowsiness in approximately 40 percent of dogs treated in this manner. Another disadvantage of intravenous phthalofyne is accidental perivascular leakage, which causes cellulitis and subsequent necrosis. Side effects occur less frequently in dogs given phthalofyne orally; ataxia and drowsiness seldom occur but vomition is fairly common. These disadvantages of phthalofyne favor the routine use of dichlorvos for treating whipworm infections in areas in which heartworms are not endemic.

The degree of success of dichlorvos (and perhaps of the other drugs) seems to be inversely proportional to the whipworm burden. In dogs harboring fewer than 100 worms, greater than 90 percent expulsion can be expected. When the burden exceeds 100 worms, the efficacy of dichlorvos is reduced, and retreatment within one to two weeks is necessary.

In general, the expulsion of whipworms from a treated dog requires a longer period of time (usually 72 hours) than the expulsion of ascarids or hookworms (less than 48 hours). Thus, collection of feces for a post-treatment evaluation of whipworm eggs should not be made within 72 hours of treatment. Submission of a fecal sample one week after treatment is the routine policy of practitioners and is preferred. In obstinate cases, a second regimen of medication can be given in one to two weeks. Such animals should be checked routinely at three-month intervals for the establishment of additional patent infections.

In cases in which clients are adept and conscientious about treating their dogs, the five-day regimen either of glycobiarsol or mebendazole may be handled by the client. No fasting is required with either drug. If there is difficulty in administering the rather large glycobiarsol tablets they can be crushed and added to the food. Mebendazole is prepared as a powder for addition to the food. It is advantageous to use moist food when either drug is added; this allows the drug to stick to it and results in consumption of the entire dose. Again, mebendazole is preferred over glycobiarsol because of its slightly greater activity against whipworms and its broader anthelmintic range (ascarids, hookworms, and *Taenia* but not *Dipylidium* tapeworms).

Supportive therapy generally is unnecessary in whipworm-infected dogs.

TAPEWORMS

MEANS OF INFECTION AND DIAGNOSIS

Tapeworms that commonly infect dogs include *Dipylidium caninum* and *Taenia pisiformis*. Those commonly infecting cats are *D.*

caninum and *T. taeniaformis*. Cats and dogs acquire *Dipylidium* infections by ingesting fleas or biting lice that carry the infective cysticercoid. Dogs become infected with *T. pisiformis* and cats with *T. taeniaformis* by ingestion of infective cysticerci from rabbit and rat or mouse tissues, respectively.

Gravid (egg-filled) proglottids detach from these tapeworms and pass with the feces. The proglottid may be seen crawling on or near freshly passed feces or on the perineum of the dog. In dry weather they desiccate and shrink quickly and thus may go undetected. The proglottid may be identified by teasing it open with forceps in a couple of drops of water on a glass slide, placing a coverslip over it, and examining it under a compound microscope for packets containing several to 20 eggs (*Dipylidium*) or for single eggs with a dark, thick striated wall (*Taenia*). A dried proglottid should be allowed to rehydrate for 15 minutes or more before attempting to tease it open. Identification of the tapeworm is needed in order to advise clients on appropriate preventive measures and to treat the infection effectively. (*Dipylidium* is not eliminated by some drugs that expel *Taenia*.)

Although still uncommon, infections of *Spirometra mansonoides* are being seen with increasing frequency in the southeastern U.S. These tapeworms do not shed proglottids. Fluke-like operculated eggs (slightly larger than those of *A. caninum*) are passed in the feces and are recovered easily by salt flotation procedures that are used routinely to detect nematode eggs. The intermediate hosts of this tapeworm include water copepods (first host) and amphibians or reptiles (second host), on which dogs or cats occasionally feed.

Each of these tapeworm infections is of negligible pathologic importance. In our laboratory T. M. Burke has recovered over 8000 *Dipylidium* scolices from a single three-month-old pup that had normal stool consistency and appetite. However, clients are aesthetically offended by seeing crawling proglottids issuing from their pets and demand that something be done to stop it.

TREATMENT

Bunamidine hydrochloride (Scolaban®) is the only anticestodal drug currently available in the U.S. that has particularly good activity against *Dipylidium caninum* (see Table 3). At the recommended dosage of 25–50 mg/kg of body weight in dogs or cats, 56–90 percent of *Dipylidium*-infected animals and 100 percent of *Taenia*-infected animals can be expected to be cleared. *Echinococcus* also is expelled by this drug. Fewer than one of every ten animals will vomit following dosing with tablets. The enteric-coated tablets should not be crushed for administration in suspension, since the drug is irritating to the oral mucosa, and oral absorption is more liable to result in toxic manifestations (emesis and diarrhea).

Bunamidine hydrochloride can be administered to females during all stages of pregnancy and during lactation without ill effects to the bitch or her pups. Reduced spermatogenesis has been found in male dogs but not in male cats 4 to 28 days following administration of twice the current recommended dosage, i.e., 2 × 25–50 mg/kg.

One rare complication of the use of bunamidine hydrochloride is the occasional sudden death of an apparently healthy dog. This idiosyncratic reaction occurs most often in large, heavily exercised, working-type dogs that have developed ventricular fibrillation and died upon sudden exertion within a 24-hour period following treatment. There is evidence that in these cases the drug had sensitized the heart musculature to epinephrine, the level of which at the time of sudden exercise increased in the blood and may have triggered fibrillation of the cardiac muscle. The occurrence of sudden death appears to be dose-related in view of the greater frequency of deaths in Australia (1 of 3000 dogs treated at a dose of 44 mg/kg) than in the U.S. (1 of an estimated 600,000 dogs treated at a dose of 25 mg/kg). In Canada and the United Kingdom, where even lower doses are used, no drug-related deaths have been reported.

Niclosamide (Yomesan®) has been used widely by veterinary practitioners for tapeworm infections. Whereas this compound clears approximately 80 percent of dogs harboring *Taenia* infections, less than 50 percent of dogs with *Dipylidium* infections will be cleared. The drug does destrobilate (remove the body of) the tapeworm, but the remaining intact scolex will regenerate another body and shed gravid proglottids three to four weeks after treatment. Thus, the client returns again complaining about the "crawly things" on his or her pet. Similarly, mebendazole in five daily treatments is about 85 percent effective for taeniad tapeworms but has no activity against *Dipylidium*.

Vermiplex® and Anaplex® (commercial combinations of toluene and dichlorophene) are frequently used to treat ascarids and hookworms simultaneously (toluene) and to "aid in the control of" tapeworms (dichlorophene) (Table 3). These drugs are used primarily in young dogs and cats during the ascarid-positive months. Studies suggest that the efficacy of these drugs for *Taenia* is 72 percent and for *Dipylidium*, 85 percent but these figures may be high, since no reported search was made following treatment for destrobilated scoleces that may have remained attached to the intestinal mucosa.

Arecoline-acetarsol (Nemural®), an old purging compound used in both dogs and cats, is still used by some practitioners to treat *Taenia* and *Dipylidium* infections. This drug narcotizes the tapeworm for two to three hours, during which it must be expelled; otherwise, reattachment occurs. The purgative action of arecoline, however, usually brings about catharsis within the desired three hours.

It is difficult to assess the efficacy of Nemural® for tapeworms in the absence of any recent experimental investigations. This fact, plus occasional adverse reactions (vomition, salivation, discomfort, restlessness, ataxia, and labored breathing), restrictions against its use in pups less than three months old and cats less than one year old, and contraindications in animals having febrile conditions, intestinal disturbances, or severe cardiac or circulatory disturbances, has greatly limited use of the drug today.

The currently used synthetic anticestodals (Scolaban®, Yomesan®, Telmintic®, and Vermiplex®) kill the tapeworm so that it becomes completely or partially digested before being voided in feces. Detection of voided worms by examination of the feces is therefore not possible. Arecoline-acetarsol, on the other hand, simply narcotizes worms so that they remain alive and can be detected in the feces. The occurrence of some worms in the feces, however, gives no indication of how many tapeworms still remain attached in the gut.

PROTOZOAN INFECTIONS

FLAGELLATES

Giardia sp. and *Pentatrichomonas* sp. are found in approximately 10 percent of dogs and only occasionally in cats. The clinical significance of either of these protozoans is disputed. They may be seen in perfectly normal feces (saline smear), yet they are far more likely to be detected in soft or loose feces, especially in young dogs. It has been suggested that they may be non-pathogenic opportunists, frequently present in the small intestine in low numbers but multiplying to large populations when the gut environment is favorable (for example, in mucoid enteritis). The fact that direct treatment of these organisms favors re-establishment of normal bowel function suggests that these flagellates are primary pathogens. In man *Giardia*-induced diarrhea may occur without evidence of either cysts or trophozoites in the feces. In these cases duodenal aspirates are needed to demonstrate the parasite. The incidence of similar findings in dogs and cats is unknown, but if giardiasis is strongly suspected in a patient with negative fecal findings, it may be prudent to treat for *Giardia*.

Details of diagnostic morphology and procedures other than the direct saline smear can be obtained from the sixth edition of *Current Veterinary Therapy*.

Infections of either *Giardia* or *Pentatrichomonas* respond rather dramatically to treatment with a human trichomonad drug, metronidazole (Flagyl®). The drug is given orally at the rate of 25 mg/kg every 12 hours for five days for *Giardia* and at the rate of 66 mg/kg/day for five days for *Pentatrichomonas*. Treatment with glycobiarsol (Milibis®), using the whipworm regimen, is also suggested to be effective for trichomonads, but its use is not well documented. *Giardia* infections alternately can be treated with quinacrine (Atabrine®) orally at 50 to 100 mg every 12 hours for three days, with rest for three days; then the regimen is repeated.

COCCIDIA

Traditionally, the coccidia of dogs and cats have been viewed as consisting of but a few species of *Isospora*. Closely controlled experimental work in the past five years, however, has uncovered several other genera — a total of 13 feline species and 12 canine species of coccidia (Table 4). Future investigations very likely will discover more. Furthermore, it is now known that, unlike the monoxenous (single-host) infections of *Eimeria* in ruminants and birds, feline and canine coccidian infections can involve an intermediate host. Cat-to-cat or dog-to-dog infections of the species of coccidia listed in Table 4 can occur by direct ingestion of sporulated oocysts. Additionally, certain other animals (listed as intermediate hosts in the table) may become infected by ingesting oocysts from the cat or dog. The coccidian stages in intermediate hosts become located as asexually multiplying cystic forms in extraintestinal tissues (muscles, endothelium, brain, connective tissues, and others) that are infective for felids or canids that prey upon animal tissues. The intermediate hosts do not produce oocysts.

Relative to pathogenicity, it is usually the intermediate hosts rather than the dog or cat (definitive host) that are adversely affected.

Table 4. *Coccidia of Cats and Dogs*

ORGANISM	AVERAGE OOCYST SIZE (μm)	INTERMEDIATE HOST
Coccidia of Cats		
Isospora felis	40 × 30	Mouse
Isospora rivolta	25 × 20	Mouse
Besnoitia besnoiti	15 × 13	Cattle
Besnoitia wallacei	17 × 12	Mouse
Besnoitia darlingi	12 × 12	Opossum
Toxoplasma gondii	12 × 10	Mammals, birds
Hammondia hammondi	12 × 11	Mouse
Sarcocystis hirsuta	12 × 8	Ox
Sarcocystis tenella	12 × 8	Sheep
Sarcocystis porcifelis	13 × 8	Pig
Sarcocystis muris	10 × 8	Mouse
Sarcocystis leporum	10 × 13	Cottontail
Sarcocystis sp.	11 × 8	White-tailed deer
Coccidia of Dogs		
Isospora canis	38 × 30	Mouse
Isopora ohioensis	23 × 19	Mouse
Isospora neorivolta	11 × 13	Mouse
Isospora burrowsi	20 × 17	—
Hammondia heydorni	11 × 12	Ox
Sarcocystis cruzi	16 × 11	Ox
Sarcocystis ovicanis	15 × 10	Sheep
Sarcocystis miescheriana	13 × 10	Pig
Sarcocystis bertrami	15 × 10	Horse
Sarcocystis fayeri	12 × 8	Horse
Sarcocystis hemionilatrantis	14 × 9	Mule deer
Sarcocystis sp.	11 × 15	White-tailed deer

(Prepared by A. K. Prestwood, Athens, Ga.)

Dalmaney disease of cattle, for example, represents the clinical manifestations of damage to bovine vascular endothelium caused by multiplying coccidial stages, the infection having been obtained by cattle ingesting infective oocysts that were shed in the feces of dogs. More information about the effect of these coccidia on cattle and other intermediate hosts can be obtained from references listed in the supplemental reading.

Clinical coccidiosis in dogs or cats apparently is caused only by certain species of *Isospora* and by *Toxoplasma gondii* (toxoplasmosis). The cat is the only definitive host for *T. gondii*, i.e., the only host in which oocysts are produced in the intestine and shed in the feces. Following accidental ingestion of *T. gondii* oocysts, pathogenic extraintestinal infections can develop in virtually all mammals, including dogs and the cat itself. Most of these are subclinical infections, but occasionally a severely pathogenic case is seen, especially in immunologically naive pups and kittens or in immunologically deprived older animals. A detailed discussion of toxoplasmosis may be found elsewhere in this text.

Little is known about clinical coccidiosis due to infections of *Isospora* in dogs and cats. The pathogenicity of the intestinal stages of this coccidium is only now beginning to be evaluated experimentally. For example, recent work by J. P. Dubey (1978) gives evidence that *I. ohioensis* can cause clinical disease in newborn pups — diarrhea resulting from inflammation of the intestinal crypts, with necrosis and massive desquamation of the tips of villi and contents of the lamina propria, especially in the lower part of the small intestine. Only five of 21 newborn pups given large numbers of oocysts, however, developed clinical illness, and none of 26 weaned pups, similarly infected, became ill despite apparent infections as judged by the shedding of oocysts from four days to two weeks after initial exposure. Subsequent re-exposure did not produce apparent reinfection.

Until experimental studies are performed with other species of *Isospora* in dogs and cats, it seems safe to assume that intestinal coccidiosis in general is a self-limiting disease. Apparently most pups and kittens acquire low-level infections soon after birth and rapidly become immune to clinical disease. Clinical disease may result if massive numbers of oocysts are ingested by non-immune animals. Overcrowding, poor sanitation, and inadequate disease control are conditions that may favor clinical coccidiosis. In clinical cases peak numbers of oocysts are shed within the first week following exposure. Shedding of oocysts continues only for about two weeks in weaned pups but may last as long as five weeks in nursing pups, suggesting a delay in acquisition of immunity in younger pups.

DIAGNOSTIC PROCEDURES

Although a saturated solution of $NaNO_3$ used for routine fecal flotations will recover the larger size oocyst of *Isospora*, all coccidian oocysts (especially *Toxoplasma* and *Sarcocystis*) are best recovered by using Sheather's sugar centrifugal flotation technique. Sheather's sugar solution is prepared by mixing 500 gm of regular table sugar with 320 ml of distilled water; add to this 6.5 gm of phenol crystals that have been melted in a hot-water bath (avoid excessive inhalation of fumes).

The procedure for using the Sheather's technique is as follows:

1. Soften feces with tap water to a fluid consistency.

2. Pass the aqueous fecal suspension through a tea strainer or two layers of gauze (to remove excessive debris).

3. Thoroughly mix one part of the strained fecal suspension with two parts of Sheather's sugar solution. Pour into a 15-ml centrifuge tube and add sufficient sugar solution to form a meniscus at the top of the tube. Place a circular coverslip on top. (If an air bubble appears under the coverslip, add more sugar solution to the tube and put the coverslip on again). Balance with a tube of exactly equal weight on the opposite side. Centrifuge at 1500 rpm for 10 minutes.

4. Remove coverslip (twist slightly and lift straight up) and place on a microscope slide. Examine with a $20\times$ or $42\times$ objective (since the eyepiece is $10\times$, the total magnification will be 200 to 420 times actual size).

This technique is especially beneficial in recovering oocysts of *Toxoplasma* and sporocysts of *Sarcocystis*. It also reveals most nematode eggs and protozoan cysts as *Giardia*. Fluke eggs are not demonstrated well nor are tapeworm eggs or nematode larvae.

Differential diagnosis of coccidian infections (whether clinical or subclinical) deserves some attention in light of the specific need to identify oocysts of *T. gondii* in cats and the need to separate the potentially pathogenic *Isospora* from other non-pathogenic coccidia of dogs or cats. Such a separation is fairly easily accomplished on the basis of differences in sizes of oocysts (Table 4), provided that the compound microscope is equipped with a calibrated ocular micrometer. The largest oocysts (more than $20 \times 17\mu$) shed by either dogs or cats are all species of *Isospora*. The other genera of coccidia have smaller oocysts that are relatively similar in size. Morphologic features can be used to separate *Sarcocystis* from the other genera. The oocysts of all of the species of *Sarcocystis* undergo sporulation and rupture before being shed in the feces; thus, small "sporocysts" each containing four minute sporozoites are recovered by flotation of fresh feces. The small, similar-appearing oocysts of *Besnoitia*, *Hammondia*, and *Toxoplasma* are passed unsporulated (as are *Isospora*) and require two days or more for the protoplasmic mass to develop into two sporocysts each containing four sporozoites (all within a single oocyst). Isolation of these three types of oocysts from feces, inoculation of the oocyst into mice, and histosectioning of the mouse brain to check for *Toxoplasma* cysts are procedures that are handled more readily by a diagnostic laboratory. Feces containing unknown oocysts should be fixed in 2 percent potassium dichromate for shipping to a laboratory.

TREATMENT

Several drugs are used as coccidiostatic agents, including intestinal sulfas, sulfadimethoxine, and nitrofurazone. These drugs are probably indicated only in animals showing clinical signs of coccidiosis (see previous discussion). Dosage is according to manufacturers' recommendations for 14 to 21 days. Spiramycin® (Rhone-Pulene, France) and amprolium (Corid®, Merck) are drugs reported to be coccidiocidal. We have not used these drugs in dogs or cats with coccidiosis.

Supportive care is important, especially in puppies and kittens. Parenteral fluid therapy with lactated Ringer's solution should be given according to estimations of percent dehydration. Intestinal protectants such as Kaopectate are helpful when administered in adequate amounts (3 to 5 ml/kg every six to eight hours). Other measures, such as whole blood transfusion (4.5 to 6.8 ml/kg) and the use of blankets or heating pads, may be required in anemic, hypothermic animals. Prolonged use of enteric antibiotics or potent parasympatholytic agents should be avoided because they alter the normal intestinal microflora and cause ileus, thereby favoring multiplication of enteric pathogens and the subsequent production and absorption of their toxins.

PREVENTIVE AND CONTROL MEASURES FOR HELMINTH AND PROTOZOAN PARASITES

All gastrointestinal parasites shed some stage (egg, oocyst or other stage) in feces, which after an appropriate incubation period can directly reinfect dogs or cats or, with certain parasites, intermediate hosts. It is at this point that attempts to break the organism's life cycle can be particularly beneficial. There is no better preventive measure than simple removal of the feces on a regular basis, preferably daily. Parasite eggs are trapped in the fecal mass until it becomes disseminated by rain or tracking. Dogs isolated individually on concrete-floored runs that are hosed down with water daily usually do not track their feces and seldom increase their existing parasite burden. Over a period of one year, even in the absence of anthelmintic treatment, dogs under these ideal conditions probably will lose more GI parasites by natural expulsion of aged worms than they will gain. Housing several dogs in the same run makes thorough removal of feces more difficult but all the more important. Dissemination of the feces (and thus of parasite eggs) by tracking is much more likely to occur. Even so, approximately six days are required for freshly passed hookworm eggs to develop, hatch, and reach the infective larval stage; almost two weeks are needed for ascarid eggs to become infective; and only two days are required for coccidian oocysts to sporulate to the infective stage. Tapeworm eggs are immediately infective for their respective intermediate hosts. Once these stages are spread in cracks and corners of the run, they are not so easily flushed away by water spray. Ascarid eggs have a sticky coat that allows them to adhere easily even to smooth surfaces like glass and especially to rough surfaces like concrete or soil. Thus, every effort should be made to remove the fecal mass while it is intact.

Most clinical cases of whipworm infection seem to occur in dogs confined to a small-yard pen, where defecation continuously seeds the ground with eggs and allows for reinfection of the dog, especially if food is eaten from the ground. This often occurs with hunting-type dogs and is much more likely to occur in clay soil than in sandy soil. Perhaps the physical rain-washing of whipworm eggs deep into the less compact sand prevents access to the eggs, whereas eggs in clay soil remain nearer the surface. The reverse is true of hookworm infective larvae, which seem to infect dogs more readily from sandy soil. It must be remembered, however, that whipworm eggs are not motile, whereas hatched hookworm larvae can migrate deeper in sandy soil when the surface is dry and return to the surface when moisture is favorable.

Direct sunlight is an excellent all-round means of reducing the level of infective stages of parasites on premises (concrete or ground). Hatched hookworm larvae are more susceptible to desiccation than are the intact eggs of ascarids and whipworms; nevertheless, burdens of ascarids or whipworms are generally lower in dogs housed in bright sunlight than in dogs housed in shaded areas. Of course, in geographic areas of uncomfortably high temperatures, some shading may be a necessity.

If heavy hookworm infections are not being controlled by anthelmintics in dogs confined to yard plots where daily removal of feces may not be practical, reduction of the numbers of larvae contaminating the premises can be accomplished chemically. Sodium borate, sold in grocery stores for use in washing clothes, can be sprinkled dry over concrete or dirt areas (10 lb/100 sq ft) and wet by sprinkler. Hookworm larvae are effectively killed by this method. The effect on unhatched hookworm eggs or eggs of ascarids or whipworms is questionable. Repeated application at one- to two-month intervals is recommended during the spring and summer months. Grass is killed but no adverse effects to dogs' feet have been reported. A commercial spray (VIP Hookworm Spray Concentrate®, Florida Veterinary Laboratories) is available for use in a power sprayer for yards and kennels. It can be used at two-week intervals and does not kill grass as sodium borate does. Tests indicate a good level of reduction in infective hookworm larvae. However, the residual activity evidently lasts but a few days, and intact fecal material is not penetrated by the compounds.

Low-level use of diethylcarbamazine (Caricide®, Dirocide®, Cypip®, Filarabits®) has tremendous preventive benefit not only for heartworm but also for ascarid infections. Tablet or syrup formulations are available for daily oral administration, either directly in the mouth or in the food (6.6 mg/kg BW/day). A powdered formulation (Cypip®) for administration in the food requires a daily dosage of 2.75 mg of base/kg BW.

While it is known that diethylcarbamazine prevents heartworm infection by destroying the infective third-stage larvae, which is transmitted from mosquitoes, it is not known with certainty which stages of ascarids are adversely affected by the drug. We do know that patent ascarid infections in the gut are usually prevented. Apparently, there is no effect against somatic stages of ascarid larvae in the extraintestinal tissues.

The addition of styrylpyridinium chloride to diethylcarbamazine (Styrid-Caricide®, American Cyanamid) provides a compound that is effective in "preventing the establishment of patent hookworm infections." Again, somatic hookworm larvae seem to be unaffected. Daily use of Styrid-Caricide® is recommended in pups from the time of weaning until approximately six months of age, when the most critical hookworm period is past. Thereafter, diethylcarbamazine alone may be used for the continued prevention of heartworms. Use of these compounds has the effect of lowering the overall environmental contamination with parasite eggs and, therefore, of reducing the chance of overwhelming infections being obtained by other dogs.

Control of tapeworms depends not only on the effectiveness of the anthelmintic used but also on the availability of reinfections from appropriate intermediate hosts. To control *Dipylidium* in either dogs or cats, fleas and, less frequently, chewing lice must be controlled. The consistent use of flea collars, while not completely effective in eliminating fleas, does much to reduce the total population and thus restricts the opportunity of reinfection with *Dipylidium*. Similarly, *Taenia* infections do not occur if dogs do not eat wild cottontail rabbits and cats do not eat wild rodents. Prevention of these carnivorous habits of outdoor animals is hardly feasible, but clients should at least be told how their animals continue to obtain reinfections of taenid tapeworms.

SUPPLEMENTAL READING

Dubey, J.P.: A review of *Sarcocystis* of domestic animals and of other coccidia of cats and dogs. J. Am. Vet. Med. Assoc., *169*:1061–1080, 1976.
Dubey, J.P.: Pathogenicity of *Isospora ohioensis* infection in dogs. J. Am. Vet. Med. Assoc., *173*:192–197, 1978.
Hass, D.K., Collins, J.A., and Flick, S.C.: Canine parasitism. Canine Practice, *2*(6):42–47, 1975.
Roberson, E.L.: Antinematodal drugs; anticestodal and antitrematodal drugs. In Jones, L.M., Booth, N.H., and McDonald, L.E. (eds.): *Veterinary Pharmacology and Therapeutics*. Ames, Iowa, Iowa State University Press, 1977, pp. 994–1064.

THE MANAGEMENT OF COLITIS

MICHAEL D. LORENZ, D.V.M.
Athens, Georgia

Inflammation of the colon is an important cause of diarrhea in the dog; however, it is relatively rare in the cat. Several diverse causes of colitis exist, and appropriate therapy and prognosis are dictated by establishing the underlying cause of the colonic inflammation. The initial step in the diagnosis of chronic diarrhea is to localize the clinical signs to either the small or large intestine. Several good algorithms have been proposed for the diagnosis of chronic diarrhea, and the reader is referred to them for a logical approach to the diagnosis of diarrhea (Anderson; Lorenz). One should recognize that the term *colitis* implies inflammation of the colon and does not necessarily afford the clinician an etiologic diagnosis. In addition, inflammation of the colon is often associated with inflammation of the small intestine, and the term *enterocolitis* may be more appropriate in this case.

To achieve accurate diagnosis proctoscopic examination, mucosal biopsy, stool culture, and perhaps barium enema are necessary diagnostic procedures. The goal of this article is to describe the management of acute ulcerative colitis, chronic ulcerative colitis, and the spastic (irritable) colon syndrome.

ACUTE COLITIS

The most common causes of acute colitis include trichuriasis, mechanical irritation from foreign bodies with or without bacterial complications, and bacterial infections usually associated with small intestinal disease (bacterial enterocolitis). Although several agents are likely to be responsible for the latter disease, *Salmonella* infections appear to be more frequent than previously reported. The incidence of

Salmonella-associated enterocolitis has increased dramatically in our hospital during the past 10 years and, most alarmingly, the organisms have developed increasing resistance to antibiotic therapy.

Treatment of acute colitis should be directed at the primary cause if it can be established. In many cases the underlying cause is not apparent, and symptomatic therapy is indicated to correct dehydration and electrolyte imbalances and prevent further fluid losses by control of the diarrhea.

In the initial management of acute colitis, multiple fecal samples should be evaluated for parasites (fecal flotation, direct fecal smears, phenol-formalin fixed feces). In *Salmonella*-endemic areas, 1-gram stool samples or rectal swabs should be submitted for bacterial culture and antibiotic sensitivity tests. Food should be withheld for 24 hours and oral glucose-electrolyte solutions given to maintain hydration. Dehydration may be present, so parenteral administration of Ringer's lactate solution may be necessary for 24 to 48 hours. After 24 hours, food is slowly returned to the patient. A bland, low-residue diet such as boiled lean hamburger or chicken with cooked white rice may be beneficial, particularly if the colonic mucosa has been severely ulcerated.

Intestinal protectants and binding agents, such as kaolin-pectin, aluminum hydroxide gel, or bismuth subsalicylate, if given in large volumes every four hours may be beneficial, particularly if colonic hypersecretion is involved in the pathogenesis of the diarrhea. At the dosages routinely used these agents are probably ineffective. A dosage of 4 to 6 ml/kg q four hours is recommended.

If bacterial infection other than *Salmonella* is suspected, tetracycline (15 mg/kg t.i.d.) or chloramphenicol (30 mg/kg t.i.d.) may be given for 7 to 10 days. Antibiotic therapy for the treatment of enteric *Salmonella* infections may actually prolong the clinical course and carrier state. Antibiotic therapy is definitely indicated when systemic signs of salmonellosis accompany the enteric signs. Specific antibiotics are administered, based on sensitivity results; however, prior to receiving this information, gentamycin (2 mg/kg t.i.d. SC or IM) or trimethoprim-sulfadiazine (Tribressin) therapy will likely be effective. Ampicillin and chloramphenicol may be effective; however, isolates of *Salmonella* organisms in our hospital during the past two years have been resistant to these antimicrobial agents. At present, we treat pure *Salmonella* enteric infections with isolation of the patient, oral glucose-electrolyte solutions (Gatorade, Pedilyte), parenteral fluids, and

motility-altering drugs such as diphenoxylate hydrochloride (Lomotil), 1.0 to 2.5 mg q 6 hours, or paregoric. Antibiotics are used for patients with systemic illness. Enteric antibiotics (poorly absorbed sulfonamides, oral aminoglycosides) are not effective, and their use for enteric infections should be condemned.

Opiates prolong fecal transit time by stimulating segmental peristalsis of the gut and may help correct the diarrhea and prevent further fluid loss. In addition, these drugs may decrease colonic distention, abdominal cramping, and tenesmus. Diphenoxylate hydrochloride, 1.0 to 2.5 mg q 6 hours, is the most effective of the drugs available and is usually given for two or three days. Anticholinergic antispasmodics, although often used to decrease intestinal motility, may not be indicated, since hypermotility may not be a contributing factor in the pathogenesis of large-bowel diarrhea. In fact, these drugs may actually hasten fecal transit time by inhibiting segmental peristaltic contractions (contractions that effectively retard movement of luminal contents). Atropine-like antispasmodic agents are indicated if severe tenesmus has produced a rectal prolapse. Even in this situation these drugs should be given in moderation and for short periods of time. Propantheline bromide (Pro-Banthine) has antiparasympathetic activity and decreases intestinal secretion and spasm. Although primarily indicated to decrease gastrointestinal secretions, this drug may also be beneficial in the treatment of acute colitis because of its effect in relieving colonic spasm. A dosage of 7.5 to 15 mg q 6 hours is recommended.

ULCERATIVE COLITIS

Chronic inflammation of the colon is well documented in the dog but is rare in the cat. Chronic ulcerative colitis of dogs can be separated by histologic changes into three categories: histocytic ulcerative colitis (granulomatous colitis, boxer colitis), eosinophilic ulcerative colitis, and idiopathic ulcerative colitis. Treatment and prognosis of these disorders vary; therefore, it is very important to obtain histologic confirmation of the pathologic lesion.

Proctoscopic examination with mucosal biopsy is indicated for every case of chronic colitis. In addition, fecal cultures are indicated, particularly in areas where *Salmonella* is known to be a problem. Barium enema, although sometimes helpful in establishing the presence of disease in the ascending and transverse colon, does not provide morphologic evidence as to the type of colitis present and therefore has limited diagnostic value in most cases.

Although the histopathologic lesions of histo-cytic and idiopathic ulcerative colitis are different, both conditions are usually treated by similar methods. The etiology of both conditions is unknown, and treatment regimens have been based primarily upon those utilized for the management of human ulcerative and granulomatous (Crohn's) colitis. The prognosis for total remission of signs is guarded, and the owner should be warned to expect several relapses during therapy. Remissions can be achieved in less advanced cases, but once the disease becomes severe and scar tissue is present, the chances for successful therapy are poor.

IMMEDIATE MANAGEMENT

The immediate objectives of medical therapy for severe ulcerative colitis or acute fulminating exacerbations include colonic rest with attempts to restore normal intestinal function, maintenance of nutrition, correction of electrolyte and fluid imbalances, and correction of anemia that may accompany prolonged colonic hemorrhage.

Affected dogs should be placed in a quiet environment where they are not likely to be disturbed by daily hospital activities. If at all possible, therapy should be achieved at home. Sedatives such as phenobarbital or tranquilizers such as chlorpromazine (Thorazine) allow the patient to rest. Chlorpromazine and prochlorperazine (Compazine) help to control signs of anxiety and vomiting, which may occur in highly nervous dogs. Anticholinergic antispasmodic agents have variable, often disappointing, effects in controlling diarrhea or tenesmus. These agents may be most effective if administered 30 minutes to one hour prior to feeding because they tend to abolish the gastrocolic reflex. Propantheline bromide (Pro-Banthine L.A.), 15 to 30 mg q 12 hours, may be quite helpful. Excessive use of potent antispasmodic drugs should be avoided because they may totally suppress intestinal motility and produce ileus. This author prefers to administer propantheline bromide tablets before each meal and to use the long-acting tablets at night to prolong nocturnal effects. Diphenoxylate (Lomotil) therapy may also be beneficial; however, it should be used for brief periods of time or discontinued if colonic perforation appears likely. Hydrophilic agents such as Metamucil or binding agents such as aluminum hydroxide gel may thicken the stools and reduce the frequency of diarrheal movements. These agents should be given four times a day, usually after meals and at night.

In fulminant ulcerative colitis or in prolonged cases accompanied by profuse diarrhea, parenteral fluid and electrolyte replacement therapy may be necessary to correct dehydration and electrolyte imbalances. To evaluate the patient fully a complete blood count and biochemical profile should be performed. If bleeding has been prolonged or severe, whole blood transfusions may be indicated. In most cases, the patient is rehydrated over three to four days using Ringer's lactate solution supplemented with potassium chloride if needed. For the first 48 hours it may be desirable to permit nothing by mouth to avoid gastrocolic stimulation and thus reduce tenesmus. In the dog it is usually not possible to achieve total parenteral hyperalimentation for several weeks, as is commonly done for human patients (Driscoll and Rosenberg). Therefore, to assure adequate caloric intake, affected dogs are placed on bland, low-residue diets on the third day of treatment. Dietary substances that are allowed include corn oil, cooked refined corn or rice, rice and wheat cereals, oatmeal, white bread, lean meat, poultry, potatoes, macaroni, and spaghetti. Commercial low-residue diets (I/D) may be substituted for part or all of the diet. The total ration should be divided into three equal meals. B-complex and fat-soluble vitamins should be given by intramuscular injection for three days, followed by oral vitamin supplementation with each meal. Evidence of iron deficiency anemia secondary to chronic blood loss is an indication for daily hematinic therapy.

ANTIBIOTIC THERAPY

Dogs severely affected with histiocytic or idiopathic ulcerative colitis should immediately begin receiving salicylazosulfapyridine (Azulfidine) therapy. This drug is seldom necessary in cases of eosinophilic ulcerative colitis. Its value in the management of ulcerative colitis is debatable, since no controlled studies in the dog are available. Yet on a clinical basis this drug appears to benefit many dogs (Ewing and Gomez), particularly in cases in which client cooperation allows a long-term trial. Studies indicate that intestinal bacteria split the compound into 5-aminosalicylate and sulfapyridine (Goldman). The anti-inflammatory action of 5-aminosalicylate may be responsible for the beneficial effects, since this compound apparently is concentrated in the colonic wall. If the proposed mechanism of Azulfidine is correct, one should avoid concomitant antibiotic therapy. The dose of Azulfidine is 60 mg/kg every eight hours; however, in most cases a maximum dose of 1 gm every eight hours is effective. A total daily dose of 4 to 5 gm should not be exceeded.

In humans, 15 to 20 percent of patients taking Azulfidine experience side effects, but complications in the dog are not common. Vomiting, depression, hemolytic anemia, dermatitis, and cholestatic jaundice have been reported. Response to the drug may be delayed, so therapy should be continued several weeks before one decides that the treatment is not effective.

In early cases, chloramphenicol or tetracycline may be beneficial and should be given for three to four weeks. During this time the patient must be monitored closely for signs of improvement. Worsening of signs during this time is an indication to stop the antibiotics and begin treatment with Azulfidine, as previously described.

CORTICOSTEROID THERAPY

Systemic corticosteroid therapy produces rapid and dramatic improvement in dogs with eosinophilic ulcerative colitis. However, in the other forms of ulcerative colitis systemic corticosteroids should be prescribed with great caution and probably not until all other measures have been given a fair trial. For eosinophilic ulcerative colitis, prednisolone, 1 mg/kg every 12 hours is given five to seven days or until signs of tenesmus, diarrhea, and colonic hemorrhage have greatly improved. Thereafter, the dose is gradually reduced every three days until the medication is discontinued. Many cases do not require constant therapy; however, periodic therapy may be necessary because relapses are occasionally encountered. During initial steroid therapy when the colon is severely ulcerated, broad-spectrum antibiotics such as tetracycline or chloramphenicol are administered.

Systemic corticosteroids should not be given routinely to dogs with idiopathic or histocytic ulcerative colitis until Azulfidine therapy has been thoroughly evaluated. Azulfidine therapy should be continued during corticosteroid administration. Prednisolone, 0.5 to 1.0 mg/kg, should be given every 12 hours for two weeks. Failure to achieve improvement with corticosteroids during this period of time is an indication to stop these agents. If improvement occurs, alternate-day steroid therapy for several months is maintained. Any indication that the dog's condition is worsening necessitates withdrawal of steroid therapy. Some dogs may respond to corticotropin (ACTH) gel, 1.0 unit/kg, given daily by intramuscular injection. Critical evaluations of ACTH therapy in the dog have not been reported, although this therapy is known to be beneficial in many human patients.

Corticosteroid retention enemas may be quite beneficial (although somewhat expensive) in the initial therapy of chronic ulcerative colitis. Hydrocortisone retention enemas (Cortifoam, Cortenema) should be given three times a day for three to five days and then decreased to once a day, usually at night. Hydrocortisone suppositories (Cort-Dome Suppositories) inserted intrarectally three times a day may be beneficial in those cases with severe rectal involvement. Variable systemic absorption may occur following local therapy, and the dosage of systemic corticosteroids should be lowered if steroid side effects become severe.

IMMUNOSUPPRESSIVE THERAPY

For dogs that do not respond to Azulfidine or corticosteroid therapy, immunosuppressive therapy should be considered. Although numerous studies have been reported in humans, studies related to the effects of immunosuppressive agents in the treatment of canine ulcerative colitis are lacking. Recently, immunotherapy in human inflammatory bowel disease was thoroughly reviewed (Sachar and Present). These authors conclude that immunosuppressive drugs are potentially dangerous and that their routine use in ulcerative colitis is not advisable except as short-term measures in patients unresponsive to or intolerant of Azulfidine or corticosteroid therapy. In the treatment of Crohn's colitis (granulomatous colitis) these agents appear to have a steroid-sparing effect and are as beneficial as Azulfidine. The interested reader should consult this article for the various regimens that are reviewed.

Metronidazole (Flagyl) may have immunosuppressive and granuloma-inhibiting properties (Grove, et al.). In one study of Crohn's disease in humans, 13 of 17 patients treated with metronidazole, 20 to 40 mg/kg/day, experienced marked clinical improvement (Ursing and Kamme). Long-term followup studies were not reported. One must wonder whether this drug has any role in the treatment of canine ulcerative colitis, because it is apparently safe for chronic administration in this species.

OTHER POTENTIALLY BENEFICIAL TREATMENTS

Various clinicians have reported favorable results with oral tylosin therapy given for several months. This drug can be given as tablets or as a powder placed in the dog's drinking water. This author has no experience with this therapy, and controlled studies have not been reported.

Hypoallergenic diets are thought to benefit

some dogs with ulcerative colitis because food allergy has been suggested as a cause of this disease. These diets have not benefited patients treated by the author. In the long-term management of ulcerative colitis bulky diets may help some patients (they should be used only after the colon has healed). The addition of wheat bran or hydrophilic agents such as Metamucil to the diet may be of benefit. Recent studies indicate a correlation between low-fiber, highly refined diets and the occurrence of intestinal disease in human beings (Trowell). It is premature to speculate that a similar correlation exists in dogs.

SPASTIC COLON SYNDROME

Although well-documented in humans, the existence of this disease in dogs is based only on clinical observations and the elimination of organic bowel disease by various diagnostic tests. Treatment of this disorder is based on the assumption that the underlying cause is functional rather than organic. Initially, specific food intolerance should be investigated through the use of elimination diets. Bulky diets appear to benefit some dogs, whereas low-bulk diets are beneficial to others. Following these trials, symptomatic therapy is undertaken if the signs cannot be controlled with diet manipulation. Mild sedation with phenobarbital or chlorpromazine is of great benefit in some patients. Antianxiety drugs such as hydroxyzine hydrochloride (Atarax), 10 to 25 mg t.i.d., or diazepam sodium (Valium), 10 mg t.i.d. orally, may be beneficial in nervous, excitable dogs. Diphenoxylate, 1.0 to 2.5 mg q 6 hours, is the antidiarrheal agent of choice for the relief of intractable diarrhea. Clients should be reassured that the cause of the dog's problem is "functional" (perhaps even psychogenic) and that a stable daily routine may be the most beneficial therapy.

SUMMARY

Successful therapy of chronic ulcerative colitis requires both the client and clinician to be diligent. There are no magic cures, and a firm commitment to long-term symptomatic therapy is the basis of management. Absolute adherence to sound diagnostic procedures is mandatory in order to rule out potentially curable disease. Although chronic ulcerative colitis is frustrating to treat because of its unpredictable course, many patients can definitely be benefited and returned to a normal existence.

SUPPLEMENTAL READING

Anderson, N.V.: The malabsorption syndromes. In Kirk, R.W. (ed.): *Current Veterinary Therapy VI*. Philadelphia, W.B. Saunders Co., 1977.
Driscoll, R.H., and Rosenberg, I.H.: Total parenteral nutrition in inflammatory bowel disease. Med. Clin. North Am., 62:185–201, 1978.
Ewing, G.O., and Gomez, J.A.: Canine ulcerative colitis. J. Anim. Hospital Assoc., 9:395, 1973.
Galdman, P.: Therapeutic implications of the intestinal microflora. N. Engl. J. Med., 289:623, 1973.
Grove, D.I., Mahmoud, A.A.F., and Warren, K.S.: Suppression of cell-mediated immunity by metronidazole (abstract). Clin. Res., 24:286A, 1976.
Lorenz, M.D.: A diagnostic approach to chronic diarrhea. In Kirk, R. W. (ed.): *Current Veterinary Therapy VI*. Philadelphia, W.B. Saunders Co., 1977.
Sachar, D.B., and Present, D.H.: Immunotherapy in inflammatory bowel disease. Med. Clin. North Am., 62:173–183, 1978.
Trowell, H.: Definition of dietary fiber and hypothesis that it is a protective factor in certain diseases. Am. J. Clin. Nutr., 29:417–427, 1976.
Ursing, B., and Kamme, C.: Metronidazole for Crohn's disease. Lancet, 1:775–777, 1975.

PERIANAL FISTULAS

RICHARD E. HOFFER, D.V.M.
Park City, Utah

Perianal fistula is a clinical condition characterized by sinus tract and fistulous tract formation in the perianal region. The condition is seen most commonly in German shepherds but has been reported in the Irish setter, Labrador retriever, and cocker spaniel. I have seen it in our practice in a Komondor and a coonhound.

Many different methods of therapy, both medical and surgical, have been utilized to treat perianal fistula. Two methods of therapy that we have utilized will be discussed.

ANATOMY OF THE ANAL AREA

The rectum and anal canal form an epithelial tube that is continuous with the skin at the anus. The transition from rectal mucosa to external skin can be divided into three zones. The cutaneous zone may be divided into an outer hairbearing zone and an inner hairless zone, which contains the anus. This zone contains circumanal glands, which are sebaceous, and tubular glands as well as the hair follicles. The intermediate zone separates the cutaneous zone from the columnar zone, which contains the anal columns, anal sinuses, and the anal glands, which are tubuloalveolar glands. The anal area is surrounded by the external anal sphincter, which contains the anal sacs, diverticula of the cutaneous zone. Glandular masses (para-anal glands) on the surface of the sac secrete into it. The internal anal sphincter is located at the junction of the rectum and anus and is responsible for the anal pucker, which acts to terminate the bowel movement cleanly.

ETIOLOGY

The etiology of perianal fistula is unknown. Three mechanisms have been suggested. The first but least accepted is that it results from chronic infection of the anal sacs. Most investigators feel that anal sac involvement with perianal fistula is secondary rather than primary. The second theory suggests that there are minute fecaliths formed in the anal sinuses. These supposedly erode through the mucosal lining of the sinuses, resulting in the formation of microabscesses that subsequently form fistulas to the outside. The third and probably most widely accepted theory of the etiology suggests that the fistulas and sinuses are from the infected circumanal glands. A dog with a broad tail base or a low tail carriage, or both, may cause a fecal film to develop over the perianal region that can result in circumanal gland infection. The low tail carriage results in poor perianal ventilation that adds to the possibility of anal infection.

SYMPTOMS

The condition is seen most commonly in dogs more than two years of age and affects either sex. German shepherds are most commonly affected. The most common presenting complaints are tenesmus, constipation and, often, anal bleeding.

Many clients report that the dog has undergone a personality change and has become very sensitive around the tail head. The dog will often lick at the anus and show pain on defecation. As the condition persists, the appetite will fall off, with subsequent weight loss. Occasionally, the dog may have anal hemorrhage due to erosion of a blood vessel by the inflammatory process. The longer the condition has been present, the greater the amount of tissue damage.

DIAGNOSIS

The ease of diagnosis depends upon the severity of the condition. Often it is necessary to anesthetize the dog before being able to perform a thorough perianal examination. It is a good idea to examine the perianal region of German shepherds or other breeds that are predisposed to the disease as part of routine physical examinations.

If there is only one tract present, the condition must be differentiated from a rectal abscess. This is done by passing a probe into the tract and seeing if it exits in the rectum or the columnar zone of the anus. A draining tract from an anal sac abscess may be differentiated by palpation of the infected sac. Infusion of the anal sac will also confirm any communication. Trauma can best be differentiated by careful history-taking and by using as a guideline the fact that such lesions are usually acute with trauma, whereas they are chronic with perianal fistula.

Advanced perianal gland adenocarcinomas may resemble old, extensive perianal fistula disease. The only way to distinguish between them is by histopathologic studies.

TREATMENT

Most people agree that some form of surgical therapy is necessary to treat perianal fistulas successfully. The first step in treating perianal fistulas is to remove the anal sacs, since the anal sacs are usually secondarily involved, and most methods of therapy will damage them. One method of surgical therapy involves débridement of the fistulas and medical therapy or cautery. Complete excision of all diseased tissue, including the cutaneous and columnar areas of the anus, has been recommended. This excision includes any diseased muscular tissue. A modification of this technique is to excise the diseased cutaneous tissue and perform an anal pull-through, leaving the subcutaneous tissue and external sphincter intact. This procedure will remove the internal anal sphincter. The main complication of complete excisional therapy is fecal incontinence, which occurred in 28 percent of the patients in one study. Anal stenosis may develop if primary healing does not occur. Flatulence has been reported as a problem, too. Recurrence of fistulas is generally not a problem if the entire 360° area is resected. Cutaneous skin excision with an anal pull-through procedure has a lesser incidence of fecal incontinence. However, the other complications remain. It should be remembered that any procedure that eliminates the internal anal sphincter will result in the dog's inability to terminate a bowel movement cleanly. The owner will have to wipe the dog's anus to prevent staining.

The most recent method of treatment of perianal fistulas utilizes cryosurgery. This procedure rarely produces fecal incontinence or loss of the internal anal sphincter. As discussed elsewhere in this text, cryosurgery destroys the diseased tissue, which subsequently sloughs, granulates, and epithelializes. There are various cryosurgical units available, and the technique used depends upon the unit. The lesions may be opened and frozen individually with a cryoprobe or may be frozen using a very fine spray of liquid nitrogen. This method produces the least amount of tissue destruction and postoperative complications. However, with very extensive lesions it is time-consuming.

Another cryosurgical method is to spray-freeze the entire diseased cutaneous zone with liquid nitrogen. Care is taken not to freeze the columnar zone and to preserve the internal anal sphincter. The area is sprayed to a depth of 0.5 cm, leaving the anus unfrozen. Temperature probes may be utilized to regulate the depth of freezing. The technique produces severe sloughing of the perianal area. One advantage of cryotherapy is the absolute resolution of pain. Most patients show a marked improvement shortly after the final thaw. Freezing kills the superficial nerve endings in the lesion and thus eliminates most of the pain. The area will generally slough in seven to ten days and then gradually contract and epithelialize. An extensive lesion usually requires two separate treatments about four to six weeks apart.

The major complication of cryosurgery is the formation of an anal stricture requiring a stricture revision procedure. The degree of stricture is a direct function of the amount of tissue originally frozen. The incidence of fecal incontinence is very low when the perianal area is properly frozen. The incidence of recurrence is 10 to 15 percent in our practice after the second cryotreatment. Dogs that have recurrences following two treatments tend to continue to have them. These cases can be palliated but usually not cured.

It requires experience and practice to use cryotherapy properly. If the fistulous area is not adequately frozen, a cure cannot be obtained. Conversely, overfreezing can damage the area so much that fecal incontinence or severe anal stricture results.

SUPPLEMENTAL READING

Borthwick, R.B.: The treatment of multiple perianal sinuses in the dog by cryosurgery. J. Anim. Hosp. Assoc., 7:45–51, 1971.

Greiner, T.P., Lisha, W.D., and Withraw, S.J.: Cryosurgery. Vet. Clin. North Am., 5:565–581, 1975.

Harvey, C.E.: Perianal fistula in the dog. Vet. Rec., 91:25–32, 1972.

Lowe, J.G., and Bunch, G.S.: The cryosurgical treatment of canine anal furunculosis. J. Small Anim. Pract., 16:387–392, 1975.

Lowry, C.: The perianal and anovaginal regions. In Bojrab, M.J. (ed.): Current Techniques in Small Animal Surgery I. Philadelphia, Lea & Febiger, 1975, pp. 154–165.

Robins, G.M., and Lowe, J.G.: The management of anal furunculosis. J. Small Anim. Pract., 11:333–341, 1973.

GASTROINTESTINAL FIBEROPTIC ENDOSCOPY

JAMES F. ZIMMER, D.V.M.
Ithaca, New York

Gastrointestinal endoscopy consists of examination of the mucosal aspect of the alimentary canal *in vivo* using any one of a variety of instruments. Although endoscopic examination of the alimentary canal with associated diagnostic procedures represents a major advance in the field of gastroenterology, it must be regarded as only a supplementary procedure in the diagnostic evaluation of cases of gastrointestinal disease. Endoscopy does not reduce the need for a complete history, a thorough physical examination, or laboratory and radiographic evaluations.

INSTRUMENTATION

Gastrointestinal endoscopy cannot be considered a recent development. The history of gastric endoscopy dates back to 1868, when Kussmaul successfully inserted a straight metal-tube gastroscope into the stomach of a professional sword-swallower. It is reported that a seventeenth-century veterinarian devised a hollow tube for the diagnosis and treatment of a bovine fecalith, thus predating the recorded use of endoscopy in man. During the past few decades, technical advancements and enthusiasm for clinical application have resulted in the development of sophisticated endoscopic instruments.

The principle of fiberoptic endoscopy is based on the total internal reflection of light in tiny flexible glass fibers. A spot of light entering one end of a fiber is transmitted by "bouncing" along the walls of that fiber until it emerges at the opposite end. The spot of light that emerges is about 95 percent as bright as that entering the fiber. To minimize the light loss and to prevent light in one fiber from scattering into adjacent fibers, each fiber is wrapped with insulation, usually a glass coating of a different refractive index. Approximately 200,000 of these insulated fibers are combined to form a bundle approximately 1/4 inch in diameter. The fibers of each bundle are joined together only at the proximal and distal ends, allowing greater flexibility of the fiber bundles.

In those endoscopes designed for clinical use there are two separate fiber bundles, one for viewing and one for light transmission. The fibers in the visual bundle are spatially oriented, so that the top of the object viewed at one end is in the same spatial orientation at the other end. A lens system at the distal or mucosal end focuses the image on that end of the bundle, and a lens system at the proximal or observer's end magnifies the image emerging from the bundle. The direct internal transmission of light through this flexible glass bundle enables the projection of a visual image from one end of the bundle to the other through curves, coils, and even knots in the bundle. Light for illumination at the mucosal end of the endoscope is carried from an external light source through a non-spatially oriented bundle. The intensity of this light is sufficient for visualization and photography; however, there is no danger of heat-induced damage to the patient because the light source is outside the patient. Still photography is easily accomplished by the addition of a standard 35 mm camera with an appropriate adapter.

In addition to the fiberoptic light bundle and the fiberoptic viewing bundle, most endoscopes contain a suction channel that can be used to evacuate mucus, fluid, and blood from the viscus being examined. Suction is controlled by a button or valve at the head of the instrument. A similar mechanism allows control of the flow of air from an external air pump into the viscus. This insufflation of air distends the viscus and enables visualization of its mucosa and lumen. Without this distention the walls of the viscus would collapse around the tip of the endoscope and obstruct the examination. Another proximally located mechanism provides control of a fine spray of water over the distal objective lens to rinse away mucus, blood, or other material coating the lens.

Most modern endoscopes also have a channel for the passage of biopsy forceps, cytology brushes, and catheters for the irrigation of lesions and collection of cytologic specimens. This channel usually is the same as that used for suction. The standard biopsy instruments consist of two small opposing cups mounted on the end of a long flexible shaft. The biopsy forceps are passed through the biopsy-suction channel, and mucosal biopsy specimens are taken under direct visualization. The biopsy specimens are small, often only 2 mm² in area and 1 to 2 mm thick, and must be oriented properly for accurate histologic interpretation. The brush cytology technique consists of the introduction of a small brush through the biopsy-suction channel, rubbing or brushing the area under direct visualization, and then spreading the resulting material on slides for staining and examination. The spray cytology technique involves the introduction of a plastic tube with a narrow nozzle through the biopsy-suction channel. Irrigation of the selected lesion is carried out under pressure. The washings are then aspirated, centrifuged, and examined. These latter two procedures require the cooperation of a pathologist experienced in exfoliative cytology.

Perhaps the most significant technologic achievement in the field of endoscopy has been the development of a mechanical system by which the distal (mucosal) end of the endoscope can be moved and controlled by manipulation of a deflection control knob or arm on the observer's end of the endoscope. The tip control systems of the more sophisticated (i.e., more expensive) endoscopes enable movement of the distal tip in two planes and various combinations thereof. The relative limitation of movement in one plane is easily overcome by rotation of the entire endoscope on its long axis. This controlled deflection of the distal end of the endoscope allows thorough examination of the mucosal aspect of the alimentary canal and reduces the danger to the patient. The area of mucosa for biopsy, cytology, or photography can therefore be selected on the basis of appearance rather than accessibility. Controlled selective visualization and "target biopsy" increase the accuracy and effectiveness of gastrointestinal endoscopy.

PROCEDURES

To minimize the risk of injury to the animal and to reduce the possibility of damage to the instrument, veterinary patients undergoing fiberoptic endoscopy are placed under general anesthesia following routine preanesthetic preparation. A fast of 12 to 24 hours is recommended for most patients undergoing upper gastrointestinal endoscopy. However, for those cases with indications of delayed gastric emptying, a longer fast (24 to 48 hours) may be necessary to evacuate the stomach completely. In preparation for colonoscopy, a 24- to 48-hour fast is recommended, and a high warm-water enema is given the evening before and again two to four hours before the procedure. Such an enema should be administered until the return is completely clear.

One basic principle of endoscopy that cannot be overemphasized is that one should never attempt to advance an endoscope by force. If resistance is met, one must withdraw the instrument and attempt to determine the source of the resistance and how it can best be circumvented. The procedures described are those that the author has found to be successful with the instruments available to him.

ESOPHAGOSCOPY

Indications and Technique. Signs indicating esophageal disease include repeated "regurgitation"* of undigested food and/or saliva,

---

*In the veterinary literature, the term *regurgitation* has been equated with esophageal disease. Specifically, the relatively passive act of emptying the dilated esophagus by animals with megaesophagus has been dubbed regurgitation. Thus, it has been stated that regurgitated material does not contain gastric juice and has a basic pH. By strict definition, however, regurgitation is the expulsion of the contents of the stomach in small amounts without the abdominal retching usually associated with vomiting. To be consistent with the other veterinary literature, the term is used here with the former connotation, but this difference in meaning is denoted by the addition of the quotation marks.

ballooning of the cervical esophagus, excessive drooling, anorexia or dysphagia, and recurrent pneumonia (due to aspiration). In addition to a thorough history and a complete physical examination, it is important to evaluate the esophagus radiographically before endoscopic examination is performed. Interpretation of plain radiographs in conjunction with the clinical findings will indicate whether further plain radiographs or contrast studies are needed. Esophagograms are usually performed using a suspension of barium sulfate as the contrast material. However, if there is a possibility of esophageal perforation, a sterile, readily absorbed contrast medium (Hypaque® [Winthrop]) should be used in place of the barium suspension. This radiographic evaluation will help locate radiopaque and radiolucent foreign bodies or suggest the nature of other abnormalities.

Esophagoscopy allows visualization of the mucosal lining of the esophagus, making it possible to detect inflammation, ulcerations, dilations, diverticula, strictures, foreign bodies, tumors and parasitic infestations. The animal is placed under general anesthesia, intubated with a cuffed endotracheal tube, and placed in lateral recumbency. An oral speculum is placed in the mouth. The animal's head and neck are extended and the tongue is pulled forward. The lubricated endoscope is passed dorsal to the larynx and into the esophagus. The esophagus offers little resistance to passage of the endoscope. Insufflation of the esophagus facilitates passage of the endoscope and improves visualization of the mucosa and any pathologic changes. Accumulations of saliva are easily aspirated through the suction channel. Once the instrument is in the lumen of the esophagus, it is advanced slowly to observe the walls of the esophagus. The esophagus extends from the cricopharyngeal sphincter to the cardia of the stomach and is about 30 cm long in medium-sized dogs. The normal esophageal mucosa is pale pink to pink-gray in color, smooth, and glistening. Pulsations of the heart and aorta are transmitted through the wall of the esophagus and are visible at the base of the heart. At this same area, there is a normal slight narrowing of the dilated esophageal lumen. At the gastroesophageal junction, the esophagus normally forms a small closed rosette.

Abnormal Endoscopic Findings. In acute esophagitis, the mucosa is hyperemic and unusually friable, as manifested by bleeding and denudation of the epithelium upon contact with the endoscope. Secretions are increased and may be profuse and blood-tinged. Cases of acute esophagitis in dogs have been reported.

The esophagitis apparently was induced by reflux of gastric fluid into the esophagus as a result of improper positioning during abdominal surgery. Regurgitation of a small amount of grayish fluid during surgery was associated with postoperative anorexia or dysphagia. Spontaneous reflux peptic esophagitis in the dog has also been reported. It was postulated that reflux of gastric contents into the esophagus was related to a defect in the lower esophageal sphincter.

With chronic obstructions of the esophagus, there is usually dilation of the esophagus cranial to the obstruction, with loss of tone of that section. Dilation will be limited to the esophagus cranial to the base of the heart in animals with vascular ring anomalies. Mucosal changes at these sites may be minimal. This is in marked contrast to acquired strictures, in which the normal mucosa is replaced by scar tissue that appears as white ringlike structures or webs.

Endoscopic examination of the esophagus in cases of suspected or diagnosed esophageal foreign bodies is of value in locating the object, identifying any exposed sharp edges, and evaluating the degree of damage to the esophageal wall. In those cases in which there is no evidence of pressure necrosis of the esophageal wall and when the object has no apparent sharp edges, removal of the foreign body can be directed by endoscopic visualization. Long alligator grasping forceps or a probang is carefully guided along the endoscope to the foreign body and used to grasp and extract the object under constant visualization. After removal of the foreign body, endoscopic re-examination of the esophagus is performed to evaluate the severity of damage to the esophageal wall and to determine whether further treatment is necessary.

Generalized megaesophagus is a neuromuscular disease of the esophagus occurring in less than 1 percent of the canine population but producing a high death rate. The condition occurs most frequently in young dogs, particularly German shepherds and great Danes. It is characterized by persistent "regurgitation," dilation of all or part of the body of the esophagus, and respiratory tract disease. Radiography is the most practical method of establishing a definitive diagnosis of this condition. The radiographic hallmark of the disease is a greatly dilated esophagus with narrowing of the lumen at the diaphragm. The entire thoracic and, often, the cervical esophagus is dilated. Since the condition results in a functional abnormality, endoscopic examination of the esophagus is generally unrewarding. With the animal under general anesthesia and with insufflation of the esophagus, the judgment that the esophagus is dilated may be difficult unless there is marked dilation.

Occasionally, a mild esophagitis will be present as a result of retention of ingesta in the esophagus. A rare condition usually associated with pre-existing megaesophagus is gastroesophageal intussusception, also referred to as eversion of the stomach. The clinical signs change from persistent "regurgitation" and vomiting to abrupt depression and the appearance of dark blood in the vomitus. Radiographically, an area of increased density within the thoracic esophagus is evident, and the gas pattern of the fundic portion of the stomach is distorted or absent. Endoscopically, one finds the rugose gastric mucosa filling the lumen of the thoracic esophagus. Immediate surgical intervention is the necessary treatment.

GASTROSCOPY

Indications and Technique. Endoscopic examination of the mucosal aspect of the stomach is indicated when the clinical signs or physical findings suggest the presence of gastric disease and/or when there is a need for confirmation or clarification of radiographic findings. In most cases of gastric disease or dysfunction, persistent vomiting is the chief complaint. To establish clearly what actually is occurring, a detailed description of the act of vomiting should be obtained from the client. The clinician should observe the vomiting act if at all possible. An accurate description of the vomitus itself often provides additional valuable information. Its color and consistency and any changes in these characteristics during the course of the disease should be described. These and other specific details may indicate the seriousness of the disorder and whether symptomatic treatment or an extensive diagnostic evaluation is warranted. Other clinical signs suggestive of potentially serious gastric disease include hematemesis (vomition of blood), melena, weight loss, anemia, and abdominal pain.

Radiographic examination of the abdomen and upper gastrointestinal tract is an important aid in evaluating patients suspected of having gastric dysfunction or disease. Following adequate preparation of the patient, survey radiographs should be taken before other diagnostic procedures are performed, since some radiopaque foreign bodies will be obscured by contrast media. These plain films may reveal the size, shape, position, and contents of the stomach. Upper gastrointestinal contrast studies using either negative or positive contrast media (air or barium sulfate suspensions, respectively) provide some assessment of the function and structure of the stomach. All oral medications and any drugs affecting gastrointestinal motility should be discontinued for an appropriate period prior to such studies.

Gastroscopy allows visualization of the mucosal lining of the stomach, making it possible to detect inflammation, foreign bodies, tumors, and ulcerations. The preparation of the animal and passage of the endoscope are the same as for esophagoscopy. Careful examination of the esophageal mucosa and lumen should be conducted as the endoscope is passed through the esophagus. The stomach lies mainly in a transverse position, more to the left of the median plane than to the right of it. There are four major divisions of the stomach: the cardiac portion, fundus, body and pyloric portion. The cardiac portion blends with the esophagus and includes the functional gastroesophageal sphincter. The fundus of the stomach is a rather large, blind outpocketing located to the left of and dorsal to the cardia. The body is the large middle portion of the stomach that extends from the fundus on the left to the pyloric portion on the right. The pyloric portion makes up approximately the distal third of the stomach and is irregularly funnel-shaped. The thin-walled, conical part is referred to as the pyloric antrum and funnels down to the pyloric canal, which is directed cranially. Since the stomach is an asymmetric organ, positioning of the animal for gastroscopy will influence which portion of the stomach is best visualized. With the patient in right lateral recumbency, any material in the stomach gravitates into the pyloric portion. The lumen of the pyloric antrum is occluded, and the antrum is at least partially collapsed. With the patient in left lateral recumbency, the material settles in the fundus and body, and the lumen of the pyloric antrum distends with trapped gas.

Gastroscopy is usually begun with the patient in left lateral recumbency. After the mucosal end of the endoscope passes through the cardia, the stomach is partially inflated. The mucosa of the stomach is normally thrown into folds, the gastric rugae, which persist even in a moderately distended organ. These folds are mainly longitudinal in direction and are very tortuous. They are most prominent on the greater curvature and persist there longest with increasing distention. The normal color of the mucosa in the body and fundus is pink to grayish-red. In the pyloric region it is lighter in color. Following insufflation, the body of the stomach is carefully examined. The linear rugae on the greater curvature are followed upward into the pyloric antrum. Because of the sharp angulation of the lesser curvature in the dog, it may be necessary to flex the endoscope maximally up-

ward toward the pyloric antrum and to push the endoscope gently into the stomach. This causes the flexed end of the endoscope to "slide by" into the pyloric antrum. From this position, the peristaltic activity in the antrum and the function and conformation of the pylorus can be visualized. Normally there should be active peristalsis, with the waves moving down the antrum to the pylorus. Alternatively, the antrum may be static, with the pylorus closed. Further retroflexion in this position enables one to examine the shelflike structure representing the mucosal aspect of the lesser curvature, commonly referred to as the gastric angle. Even greater retroflexion brings into view the body, cardia, and fundus of the stomach as viewed from the pyloric antrum. With the animal in left lateral recumbency, any saliva or ingesta present will gravitate to the dependent fundus, forming a "mucus lake." In order to examine the fundus and cardia adequately, it may be necessary to place the animal in right lateral recumbency. Then, with the tip of the endoscope just inside the cardia, the stomach is moderately distended. The tip is then flexed upward toward the fundus along the greater curvature. The endoscope is slowly advanced into the stomach as the flexed tip slides along the greater curvature into the gastric fundus. One can usually see the cardia with the body of the endoscope emerging from it. The combination of these procedures enables the examination of all mucosal aspects of the stomach.

Abnormal Endoscopic Findings. Endoscopic examination of the stomach in cases of suspected or diagnosed gastric foreign bodies provides the same advantages and uses as described for esophagoscopy. By definition, acute gastritis is an acute inflammation of the gastric wall, usually limited to the mucosa. Since this condition is commonly characterized by an abrupt onset and a relatively brief course, gastroscopy would be of limited value unless there were indications of more severe involvement, i.e., persistent hematemesis or marked abdominal pain. Chronic gastritis is generally characterized by vague signs, including sporadic vomition unrelated to the time of eating, poor growth rate, dull haircoat, and others. It has been postulated that the causes of chronic gastritis are the same as, but of greater duration than, those of acute gastritis. Pathologically, chronic gastritis is virtually always of the hypertrophic type, characterized by thickening of the mucosa. Therefore, endoscopically one would expect to find the gastric mucosa thickened, velvety, and covered with a tenacious glassy mucus; the gastric rugae may be exaggerated.

Careful endoscopic examination, thorough radiographic evaluation, and a clinical laboratory data base are warranted in such cases.

When an older dog is presented with a history of persistent vomition, anorexia, and weight loss, one must strongly consider the possibility of gastric neoplasia. Other clinical signs include hematemesis, melena, diarrhea, and anemia. Radiographic features supporting a diagnosis of gastric neoplasia include distortion of the lumen, thickening of the gastric wall, filling defects, derangement of the rugal pattern, delayed gastric emptying, and rigidity of the gastric wall as seen on multiple radiographs. Endoscopic findings in cases of gastric neoplasia are quite variable. Based on gross pathologic findings and the author's endoscopic experience, approximately half the gastric neoplasms diagnosed have mucosal ulcerations. Other endoscopic findings correlate well with the radiographic features. These include adenomatous polyps or masses producing filling defects, diffusely infiltrating non-ulcerating tumors that alter the rugal pattern and affect motility, and raised, thickened plaquelike tumors (with or without central ulceration), resulting in a thickened gastric wall. It must be recognized that some gastric tumors will produce no endoscopic abnormalities. Gastric biopsy is necessary to establish the diagnosis of gastric neoplasia. Endoscopic biopsy samples should be taken from the edge of the lesion, rather than from the center, since the center may contain chiefly necrotic tissue and debris. It is important to take as many samples as possible, since some tumors are difficult to document, and one must try to obtain as deep a bite as possible. In some cases it is necessary to perform an exploratory laparotomy and full-thickness biopsy or excision of the gastric lesion in order to substantiate the diagnosis.

Gastric peptic ulcers are erosive lesions of the gastric mucosa caused by the action of the acid gastric juice. Documented cases in the dog and cat are rare. Clinical signs vary but include chronic vomiting, abdominal pain, anemia, variable appetite, weight loss, and sudden collapse and death due to perforation. Vomiting may be associated with eating. Melena and hematemesis may also be observed and may produce anemia. Survey radiographs and contrast studies may be of little value in outlining an ulcer. Based on reported cases and limited endoscopic experience, gastroscopy should reveal round or oval lesions, 1 to 2 cm in diameter, with a sharply punched-out appearance. The walls of the ulcer should be relatively straight, either perpendicular to or slightly overhanging the ulcer base. The principal sites affected are the non-acid–producing areas of the stomach, i.e., the pyloric antrum and the lesser curvature. Peptic ulceration in the dog has usually been associated with other disorders such as liver disease, malignant mastocytosis, and chronic uremia. Some cases of benign gastric ulcers have been drug-induced, aspirin and indomethacin being particularly damaging.

Giant (or chronic) hypertrophic gastritis is a recently recognized disease affecting a variety of breeds of dogs. This gastritis resembles Menetrier's disease in man, which is also known as hypertrophic gastropathy or protein-losing gastropathy. In the dog it is characterized by a history of variable duration of vomiting, diarrhea, weight loss, lethargy, and variable appetite. Abdominal palpation may elicit pain in the region of the stomach or may reveal a mass in this area. Fluid- and gas-filled loops of intestine may also be palpated. Laboratory findings may include hypoproteinemia (due to excessive non-selective loss of serum proteins into the gastric lumen) and anemia (possibly due to defective erythropoiesis resulting from iron deficiency). Plain abdominal radiographs may reveal a distended, fluid- and gas-filled stomach and a thickened gastric wall. Positive contrast studies may outline an irregularly shaped gastric lumen with mucosal filling defects that produce a broadly scalloped margin of the contrast medium. Gastroscopic examination reveals areas of convoluted mucosa in which the rugae are markedly thicker and taller than normal. The convoluted pattern of affected mucosa is reminiscent of cerebral gyri and sulci. There may also be large amounts of thick, tenacious mucus covering the involved mucosa. Insufflation of the stomach does not obliterate the presence of these tortuous giant rugal folds. Affected mucosa may be distributed either generally or in localized patches. Although the distribution of the lesions is quite variable, the body of the stomach, particularly along the greater curvature, is frequently affected. Mucosal biopsy through the endoscope will usually not be deep enough to substantiate a diagnosis. Exploratory laparotomy for resection of the lesion(s), if possible, or for full-thickness biopsy is indicated. Histologic examination of such a biopsy specimen will permit differentiation from lymphoma and carcinoma. Although surgical resection historically has been the only consistently successful treatment, recent reports in the literature indicate that medical management may be helpful in reducing the excessive protein loss and controlling the signs of the disease. Preliminary reports suggest that atropine or cimetidine or both may be beneficial in treatment.

COLONOSCOPY

Indications and Technique. The primary indication for colonoscopy is the presence of any colonic symptom, sign, or abnormality that is unexplained or needs further clarification. The classic sign of colonic disease is tenesmus. The animal strains and makes frequent attempts to defecate but passes only small amounts of feces. The feces are usually liquid or semisolid and often contain visible amounts of fresh blood and excess mucus. Vomiting may occur occasionally with colonic disease. Weight loss is usually not a problem in animals with colonic disease unless it is chronic and severe. A thorough physical examination may reveal other indications of colonic abnormalities. A careful visual examination of the perineum and circumanal area is recommended. Since many diseases involving the colon also produce lesions in the rectum, a digital rectal examination should be done on every patient with signs of colonic disease, unless it would endanger the animal or cause severe discomfort. Following a low warm-water enema, visual examination of the anal canal and rectum can usually be performed on a conscious animal in the standing position. Simple, inexpensive equipment is available for this purpose. Routine laboratory examination of the feces should be done to determine the presence of parasites, protozoa, and abnormal cells. In addition, fecal cultures for pathogenic bacteria, fungi, and algae should be performed. When combined with mucosal biopsy, colonoscopy is a very effective aid in evaluating animals with signs of colonic disease.

The large intestine of the dog and cat is short and relatively unspecialized. In general, it is a simple tube that extends from the ileocolic sphincter to the anus. The large intestine is anatomically divided into cecum, colon, rectum, and anal canal. The colon begins at the ileocolic orifice and ends at the rectum. The colon has three divisions: the ascending colon, the transverse colon, and the descending colon. The short ascending colon courses in a cranial direction from its origin at the ileocolic orifice in the right side of the abdomen. The transverse colon begins at the right colic flexure and forms an arc, which runs from right to left across the abdomen. The descending colon is the longest segment of the colon. It extends from the left colic flexure to the pelvic inlet, where it becomes the rectum without demarcation. The rectum then extends from the pelvic inlet to the anal canal.

Colonoscopy is begun with the animal in right lateral recumbency in order to pool any liquid contents in the transverse and ascending colon. The well-lubricated distal end of the endoscope is inserted into the anal canal and gently advanced into the colon. Insufflation of air dilates the lumen and facilitates insertion. The colonic mucosa is visualized during both insertion and withdrawal of the endoscope. The normal canine colonic mucosa is pale pink, smooth, and glistening and distends evenly with insufflation. The lumen of the colon should always be visible. Passage through the left and right colic flexures is accomplished by the "slide by" technique, as described for gastroscopy. The instrument is cautiously advanced as long as the mucosa can be seen to slide smoothly and easily past the tip. In most dogs, it is possible to reach the ileocolic and cecocolic junctions. Care must be taken to avoid calling the ileocolic junction a sessile polyp. To identify the junction, one should recognize a depression or dimple on the top of the "polyp" and see the cecocolic orifice in the background.

Abnormal Endoscopic Findings. Colonic mucosal diseases produce superficial ulceration and a granularity of the mucosa. The mucosa becomes friable and bleeds easily upon contact with the endoscope, but the colon distends evenly with insufflation, and no strictures are apparent. The colon maintains its normal length and configuration. On the other hand, transmural diseases of the colon produce deep ulcers with rough, irregular edges. The mucosa is firm, friable, and grossly corrugated. The colon tends to distend poorly, and strictures may be apparent. In severe cases, the colon is shortened and contorted.

Colonic polyps may appear as grapelike clusters with pedunculated bases. They are reddish-purple, and the surface may bleed easily. The adjacent colonic mucosa is usually normal. Malignant colonic tumors may appear as grossly ulcerated areas of mucosa. They may bleed easily if traumatized. In other cases of colonic neoplasia, the lumen may be stenotic, with the mucosa intact and appearing normal.

To confirm the diagnosis of colonic disease, biopsy of lesions may be accomplished with endoscopic biopsy forceps, a suction biopsy instrument, or standard human uterine biopsy forceps.

CONCLUSIONS

Following recent advances in the design and manufacture of low-cost, simple endoscopes, flexible fiberoptic endoscopy will soon be within the financial reach of many practicing veterinarians. These technical advances combined with increasingly strict regulation of the use of radiography in veterinary medicine have set the stage for the rapid adoption and utilization of fiberoptic endoscopy by the practitioner. Understanding the basic principles of these instruments and recognizing the indications for and limitations of various basic procedures provide a starting point from which further experience can be gained. With such experience, one can then apply endoscopy to a wider variety of cases, conditions, and species.

Although flexible fiberoptic gastrointestinal endoscopy has been cited as the single most important advance in the diagnosis of diseases of the gastrointestinal tract, it must be regarded as only an adjunctive diagnostic procedure of value in many, but not all, patients with manifestations of gastrointestinal disease.

SUPPLEMENTAL READING

General

Antelyes, J.: Endoscopy and endopalpation. Vet. Med. Small Anim. Clin., *60*:391–397, 1965.

Bockus, H.L. (ed.): *Gastroenterology.* Vol. 1. 3rd ed. Philadelphia, W.B. Saunders Co., 1974.

Bonneau, N.H., and Reed, J.H.: Use of the gastrocamera in the dog. J. Am. Vet. Med. Assoc., *161*:185–189, 1972.

Johnson, G.F., and Twedt, D.C.: Endoscopy and laparoscopy in the diagnosis and management of neoplasia in small animals. Vet. Clin. North Am., 7:77–92, 1977.

Jones, B.D.: The use of fiberoptic endoscopy in veterinary medicine. Scientific Proceedings, American Animal Hospital Association. 1978, pp. 241–244.

Waye, J.D.: Colonoscopy. Surg. Clin. N. Am., 52:1013–1024, 1972.

Esophagoscopy

Grier, R.L.: Esophageal disease as a result of improper patient positioning. Arch. Coll. Vet. Surg., *IV*:4–6, Spring 1975.

Guffy, M.M.: Esophageal disorders. In Ettinger, S.J. (ed.): *Textbook of Veterinary Internal Medicine.* Philadelphia, W.B. Saunders Co., 1975, pp. 1098–1124.

Kleine, L.J.: Radiologic examination of the esophagus in dogs and cats. Vet. Clin. North Am., *4*:663–686, 1974.

O'Brien, J.A.: Esophagoscopy. Vet. Clin. North Am., 2:99–103, 1972.

Rogers, W.A., and Donovan, E.F.: Peptic esophagitis in a dog. J. Am. Vet. Med. Assoc., *163*:462–464, 1973.

Ryan, W.W., and Greene, R.W.: The conservative management of esophageal foreign bodies and their complications: A review of 66 cases in dogs and cats. J. Am. Anim. Hosp. Assoc., *11*:243–249, 1975.

Wilson, G.P.: Ulcerative esophagitis and esophageal stricture. J. Anim. Hospital Assoc., *13*:180–185, 1977.

Gastroscopy

Bonneau, N.H., Reed, J.H., Pennock, P.W., and Little, P.B.: Comparison of gastrophotography and contrast radiography for diagnosis of aspirin-induced gastritis in the dog. J. Am. Vet. Med. Assoc., *161*:190–198, 1972.

Cornelius, L.M., and Wingfield, W.E.: Diseases of the stomach. In Ettinger, S.J. (ed.): *Textbook of Veterinary Internal Medicine.* Philadelphia, W.B. Saunders Co., 1975, pp. 1125–1149.

Demling, L., Ottenjann, R., and Elster, K.: *Endoscopy and Biopsy of the Esophagus and Stomach.* (Translated by K. H. Soergel.) Philadelphia, W.B. Saunders Co., 1972.

Ewing, G.O.: Indomethacin-associated gastrointestinal hemorrhage in a dog. J. Am. Vet. Med. Assoc., *161*:1665–1668, 1972.

Kipnis, R. M.: Focal cystic hypertrophic gastropathy in a dog. J. Am. Vet. Med. Assoc., *173*:182–184, 1978.

Murray, M., McKeating, F. J., and Lauder, I. M.: Peptic ulceration in the dog: A clinicopathological study. Vet. Rec., *91*:441–447, 1972.

Murray, M., McKeating, F.J., and Lauder, I.M.: Primary gastric neoplasia in the dog: A clinicopathological study. Vet. Rec., *91*:474–479, 1972.

Sautter, J.H., and Hanlon, G.F.: Gastric neoplasms in the dog: A report of 20 cases. J. Am. Vet. Med. Assoc., *166*:691–696, 1975.

van der Gaag, I., Happe, R.P., and Wolvekamp, W.T.C.: A boxer dog with chronic hypertrophic gastritis resembling Menetrier's disease in man. Vet. Pathol., *13*:172–185, 1976.

Van Kruiningen, H.J.: Giant hypertrophic gastritis of Basenji dogs. Vet. Pathol., *14*:19–28, 1977.

Colonoscopy

Amand, W.B.: Non-neurogenic disorders of the anus and rectum. Vet. Clin. North Am., *4*:535–550, 1974.

Ewing, G.O., and Gomez, J.A.: Canine ulcerative colitis. J. Anim. Hospital Assoc., 9:395–406, 1973.

Lorenz, M. D.: Disorders of the large bowel. In Ettinger, S.J. (ed.): *Textbook of Veterinary Internal Medicine.* Philadelphia, W.B. Saunders Co., 1975, pp. 1192–1218.

Overholt, B.F.: Colonoscopy. Gastroenterology, *68*:1308–1320, 1975.

Van Kruiningen, H. J.: Granulomatous colitis of boxer dogs: Comparative aspects. Gastroenterology, 53:114–122, 1967.

GASTROINTESTINAL BIOPSY TECHNIQUES

JANINE B. KASPER, D.V.M.

Davis, California,

and ANN M. CHIAPELLA, D.V.M.

Philadelphia, Pennsylvania

INTRODUCTION

Significant advances have been made in the development of gastrointestinal biopsy techniques in the past two decades. Prior to the 1950's, the only methods of access to the gastrointestinal tract were through exploratory laparotomy and rigid endoscopy. With the advent of suction biopsy instruments for blind biopsy and the increased use of flexible fiberoptic endoscopy, surgical intervention has not been necessary for diagnostic tissue sampling in many cases.

Biopsy provides information for histologic diagnosis when radiologic and biochemical results are insufficient. Institution of a specific therapeutic regimen and a more accurate determination of prognosis are possible when biopsy is employed as an adjunct in the management of gastrointestinal disease.

The etiology and development of small intestinal malabsorptive disease and of inflammatory large bowel disease are areas of small animal medicine that need more investigation and research. The increasing use of intestinal biopsy will help to advance this knowledge.

EQUIPMENT

Instruments available for gastrointestinal biopsy are of two general types, forceps and suction. Alligator-jaw forceps (Fig. 1) are used in conjunction with rigid endoscopy equipment (Fig. 2). The forceps are passed through the endoscope and directed toward a visible lesion for biopsy. Most of the flexible endoscopes are equipped with small forceps that pass through a biopsy channel.

Suction biopsy instruments utilize applied suction to draw a knuckle of mucosa into a capsule. The segment of mucosa is cut off by a cylindrical knife blade activated by a pull-wire. The suction biopsy instrument (Quinton) (Fig.

3) can be used in either directed or blind biopsy techniques. It can be passed through a rigid endoscope and visually guided to the biopsy site. Blindly, the instrument can be passed perorally or rectally for biopsy of the esophagus, stomach, colon, and rectum. Fluoroscopic control has permitted intubation and biopsy of the duodenum and proximal jejunum; however, this procedure is tedious and time-consuming owing to difficulty in passing the instrument through the pylorus.

The Crosby-Kugler capsule (a small capsule with a rotating, spring-activated knife that is triggered by suction) is designed for peroral passage and small intestinal biopsy. This instrument has been demonstrated to be of use in the dog (Batt); however, its routine use in veterinary medicine is not reported.

BLIND VS. GUIDED BIOPSY TECHNIQUES

GUIDED BIOPSY

Focal lesions of the gastrointestinal tract — demonstrated radiographically, surgically, or endoscopically — should be biopsied under direct vision. Ideally, the biopsy site should include the junction of normal and abnormal tissues so that the extent of the disease process can be assessed. It is inadvisable to take biopsy specimens only from the central portion of a lesion, since this area may consist solely of necrotic tissue. When surgical excision biopsy is performed, a full-thickness section of the involved area plus an adjacent lymph node should be removed.

BLIND BIOPSY

Blind biopsy techniques do not involve visualization of a biopsy site. The suction biopsy instrument is passed via the mouth or rectum to

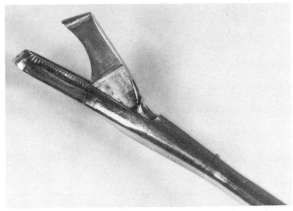

Figure 1. Alligator forceps, 30 cm in length, may be used for mucosal biopsy of the colon.

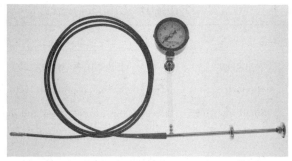

Figure 3. The Quinton° Multipurpose Suction Biopsy Instrument, 4.7 mm × 120 cm, can be used for mucosal biopsy of the esophagus, stomach, small bowel, colon, and rectum. (°Quinton Instrument Company, 2121 Terry Avenue, Seattle, Washington 98121.)

an estimated distance in order to sample areas of the intestinal tract. Since this technique is performed without viewing the biopsy site, its primary application lies in the detection of diffuse mucosal lesions.

Indications for blind biopsy include (1) radiographic, endoscopic, and/or clinical findings suggestive of a diffuse rather than a focal disease process; (2) biopsy of patients at anesthetic risk, since minimal restraint is required for the procedure; and (3) follow-up of a previously diagnosed diffuse lesion with minimal time and effort.

PREBIOPSY CONSIDERATIONS

Several important factors should be considered prior to gastrointestinal biopsy. A selective use of clinical and laboratory data can aid in the choice of a biopsy method.

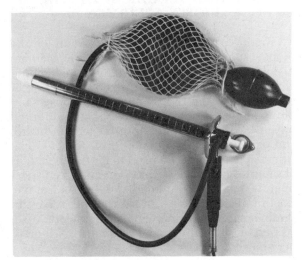

Figure 2. Sigmoidoscope, 1.5 cm × 25 cm, may be used for rigid colonscopy. (Welch Allen Sigmoidoscope set, Model 35103, Skaneateles Falls, N.Y. 13153.)

·Radiographs may indicate the location of a lesion and the extent of its involvement. A localized lesion, for example, would necessitate a guided biopsy technique or total surgical excision. Perforation from forceps or suction biopsy could be avoided by radiographic demonstration of esophageal diverticula or stenosis; in these cases surgical excision biopsy is a better method. Endoscopic examination before biopsy can provide a visual evaluation of the mucosal surface involved and allow selection of focal lesions for biopsy.

Biochemical profiles before biopsy can help to differentiate metabolic disease with secondary GI signs (e.g., vomiting or diarrhea associated with renal, hepatic, or Addison's disease) from primary gastrointestinal disease. Fecal examination, both direct smear and flotation, and careful attention to recent dietary changes can identify the cause of many gastrointestinal signs. Appropriate therapy is then instituted, removing the need for gastrointestinal biopsy. Specific gastrointestinal function tests will help localize the area of the intestine involved and the severity of the disease process. In many instances the cause, e.g., pancreatic insufficiency, becomes evident without biopsy procedures.

A summary of prebiopsy considerations is shown in Table 1.

CONTRAINDICATIONS

Gastrointestinal biopsy is contraindicated in patients with bleeding tendencies. In patients at risk prebiopsy evaluation of clotting capability should include prothrombin time, partial thromboplastin time, and platelet count. This category includes patients with concurrent renal, hepatic, or autoimmune disease. In addition, any past history of clotting abnormalities warrants re-evaluation prior to biopsy. A routine

Table 1. *Clinical and Laboratory Evaluations Prior to Biopsy*

SITE	TESTS
Esophagus	Survey and contrast radiographs, esophagoscopy
Stomach	CBC, biochemical profile, electrolytes, radiography, gastroscopy
Small intestine	Fecal exams (direct smear and flotation), CBC, biochemical profile, electrolytes, fecal digestion tests, fecal fat determination, PABA test, D-xylose absorption test, radiography, endoscopy
Colon	Multiple fecal exams, CBC, electrolytes, colonoscopy, barium enema
Rectum	Multiple fecal exams, digital rectal exam, proctoscopy

screening test, such as the activated clotting time (ACT), ideally should be performed on all biopsy candidates.

Severe ulceration, necrosis, and devitalization of tissue present a potential hazard of perforation in punch or suction biopsy techniques. When these changes are visible endoscopically, surgical excision biopsy is advisable. Risk of perforation is also increased in cases of esophageal diverticula, stenosis, and dilation of the esophageal wall. Surgical intervention should be considered in these cases when biopsy is needed.

Healing of a full-thickness excision biopsy is compromised in the hypoproteinemic patient; punch or suction biopsy alternatively may minimize the risk of dehiscense. If full-thickness biopsy is essential for diagnosis, a plasma transfusion prior to surgery may increase circulating albumin levels. Prompt postoperative therapy based on the histologic diagnosis, e.g., medium-chain triglycerides for lymphangiectasia, may facilitate resolution of the hypoalbuminemia and poor wound healing.

The relative risks of general anesthesia versus sedation must be considered in view of the animal's condition. The risk of general anesthesia in a debilitated patient can be avoided by using a punch or suction biopsy technique that requires minimal restraint.

RESTRAINT

The type of restraint necessary for gastrointestinal biopsy is determined by the biopsy method to be used, the physical condition of the patient, and the cooperative nature of the patient. General anesthesia is used for exploratory laparotomy and for biopsy in conjunction with flexible endoscopic examination. Esophagoscopy and biopsy with rigid instrumentation also require complete anesthesia. Proctoscopic examination with a rigid endoscope can be per-

formed in cooperative patients with minimal or no sedation. Sedation or tranquilization, or both, is recommended when colonic biopsies are performed with alligator forceps, because of the variation of depth of the mucosal biopsy with this procedure. Sedation is accomplished with atropine and Xylazine.*

In most cases the blind biopsy technique with a suction instrument for esophageal, gastric, colonic, and rectal biopsy requires no chemical restraint. For the majority of patients, objections to the passage of the instrument can be overcome with calm verbal assurances and manual restraint.

The decision to perform a biopsy of the gastrointestinal tract in a debilitated, compromised patient must be based on the benefit of a diagnosis versus the risk to the patient. General anesthesia may be avoided if a blind biopsy technique is used initially with the hope of achieving a diagnosis with minimal risk.

CARE AND HANDLING OF THE BIOPSY SPECIMEN

Proper tissue handling and fixation of the biopsy specimen are essential to an accurate histologic evaluation. Tissue should be handled gently and with minimal instrumentation after removal from the biopsy site. The biopsy sample is mounted with the mucosal side oriented upward. Monofilament Saran mesh, cardboard, and paper are common mounting surfaces. The side of a needle can be used to flatten the edges of samples that have curled. The mounted specimen is then placed immediately into a fixative. Gastrointestinal biopsies are routinely fixed in Bouin's solution (5 percent glacial acetic acid, 20 percent formalin, and 75 percent acid) or 10 percent formalin.

---

*Rompun, Haver-Lockhart Co., Cutter Lab, Shawhee, Kansas 66201

INDICATIONS AND METHODS FOR BIOPSY

Palpable masses, endoscopically visualized lesions, and radiographic abnormalities (filling defects, space-occupying masses, abnormal mucosal patterns) are obvious indications for gastrointestinal biopsy. Pain on intestinal palpation, weight loss, vomiting, and diarrhea unresponsive to conventional therapy may also necessitate biopsy after clinical evaluation. In many instances palpable or radiographic signs may not be present. History and clinical laboratory findings suggestive of gastrointestinal tract disease should be followed by biopsy when a histologic diagnosis is essential for therapy, prognosis, and proper patient management.

ESOPHAGUS

Signs of esophageal disease are primarily regurgitation and dysphagia. Weight loss and dehydration may result when the disease process restricts food and water intake. Coughing and fever usually accompany secondary aspiration pneumonia.

Radiographic studies, including survey radiographs and contrast esophagram, should be performed prior to endoscopy or biopsy in all patients with a history suggestive of esophageal disease. Accompanying lateral and dorsoventral thoracic radiographs are recommended to help rule out aspiration pneumonia.

Biopsy of the esophagus is done in conjunction with esophagoscopy in most cases. Blind biopsy is rarely indicated in the esophagus, since diffuse mucosal lesions are uncommon. The majority of esophageal lesions with mucosal involvement are focal and necessitate visual examination (e.g., *Spirocera lupi* granuloma, neoplasia, reflux esophagus). Esophagoscopy and biopsy should be done after radiographic examination is completed. Potential contraindications to esophagoscopy and biopsy can be identified radiographically. Perforation of the esophagus by an endoscope or biopsy instrument can occur when there is a dilated esophageal wall or diverticulum. Surgical excision biopsy is recommended in these instances.

General anesthesia is required for endoscopic examination of the esophagus. Lesions seen endoscopically can be biopsied either with forceps or by directed use of a suction biopsy instrument. When blind esophageal biopsy is performed, no prebiopsy preparation is necessary unless anesthesia is required. Most patients will allow peroral passage of a suction biopsy instrument without sedation. The tube is passed orally (use of a mouth speculum is advisable) to the desired length. Suction is applied by an assistant and a biopsy sample taken by the operator of the instrument. Perforation risk with the suction biopsy instrument is minimal if contraindications are avoided.

STOMACH

Clinical signs of gastric disease include vomiting (after eating or on an empty stomach), anorexia, weight loss, and/or anterior abdominal pain. Many cases of suspected gastritis will respond to symptomatic therapy. In many cases gastric signs may be found to occur secondary to another concurrent disease (renal failure, pancreatitis). However, the possibility of gastric disease should be investigated in the patient with a persistent history of vomiting, anorexia, and weight loss when secondary metabolic or organic diseases have been ruled out.

Survey abdominal radiographs and a barium contrast study should be performed in the patient suspected of gastric disease. Radiographic abnormalities such as increased thickening of rugal folds or stomach wall, filling defects in the mucosa, and space-occupying lesions are indications for gastric biopsy of the stomach.

Gastric biopsy can be accomplished using any of three methods: (1) combined biopsy and endoscopic examination, (2) exploratory laparotomy and full-thickness biopsy, and (3) blind biopsy with a peroral suction instrument.

The technique selected for biopsy should be based on the type of gastric disease suspected. Focal lesions visible radiographically are usually examined endoscopically. If the mucosal surface is abnormal, a directed biopsy through the gastroscope is taken. A non-diagnostic directed mucosal biopsy and a lesion seen radiographically but with no endoscopic mucosal involvement are indications for full-thickness gastric biopsy. Full-thickness biopsy of the stomach is often necessary for the diagnosis of gastric neoplasia. Many gastric tumors (carcinoma, lymphosarcoma, leiomyoma, leiomyosarcoma) are not identified on muscosal biopsy alone. Mucosal biopsy may be sufficient in cases of hypertrophic gastritis, atrophic gastritis, peptic ulceration, and eosinophilic gastritis, in which the disease process extends to the mucosa.

General anesthesia is required for biopsy with gastroscopic examination and for surgical excision biopsy. A 12-hour fast prior to biopsy is recommended; a longer fasting period may be required in cases with delayed gastric emptying. Directed biopsy can be performed with a flexible gastroscope. A lesion should be biopsied at the junction of normal and abnormal tissue. Full-thickness biopsy at exploratory laparotomy should include a section of abnormal tissue and adjacent normal tissue. In some cases, a lesion may be resected. It is advisable to remove an adjacent lymph node in cases of suspected neoplastic disease.

In veterinary medicine blind gastric biopsy techniques can be useful in the detection of diffuse mucosal lesions, e.g., hypertrophic gastritis, atrophic gastritis, and eosinophilic gastritis. A 12-hour fast is also recommended prior to blind biopsy. Delayed gastric emptying may necessitate withholding of food for a longer time period. No chemical restraint is required for passage of the biopsy tube in most patients. A mouth speculum is held in place to prevent the animal from biting the tube. The position of the stomach is estimated by measuring the length from the tip of the nose to the eleventh rib. Since the position of the suction instrument in a blind technique is not standardized, it is advisable to submit at least two tissue samples. The instrument can be rotated 180° to ensure a different biopsy site. The majority of blind gastric biopsies are from the body of the stomach.

In summary, blind gastric biopsy (1) can identify a diffuse gastric mucosal disease, (2) may provide histologic evidence of a gastric disease in patients at anesthetic risk prior to gastroscopy or exploratory laparotomy, and (3) can be used in followup examinations of a previously diagnosed diffuse gastric lesion.

SMALL INTESTINE

Cardinal signs of small intestinal disease include vomiting, weight loss, and large-volume, low-frequency diarrhea. Many cases of suspected small intestinal disease respond to symptomatic therapy. The possibility of small intestinal disease should be investigated further in patients with persistent diarrhea and weight loss. Specific gastrointestinal function tests (see Table 1) are needed to differentiate malabsorption syndromes from maldigestion. Abdominal radiographs and upper gastrointestinal studies are used to evaluate the abdomen for intestinal obstructions and focal intestinal masses. Information regarding bowel wall thickness, mucosal pattern, and intestinal motility may also be obtained from radiographic studies.

Biopsies are necessary to differentiate various malabsorption syndromes, e.g., lymphangiectasia, diffuse infiltrative neoplasia, and chronic enteropathies, and to provide appropriate therapy. Some small intestinal diseases, e.g., eosinophilic enteritis and chronic endoparasitism (*Giardia*), give normal gastrointestinal function test results, but biopsies are needed for diagno-

sis. Focal intestinal lesions palpated during physical examination or seen on radiographic studies are indications for excisional biopsy.

Small intestinal biopsies are obtained routinely by means of an exploratory laparotomy. A 12- to 24-hour fast is usually sufficient preparation. Full-thickness incisional biopsy or total excision of the lesion is performed, depending on the appearance of the intestine.

Many small intestinal diseases are diffuse and do not have obvious visual or palpable abnormalities, in which case multiple bowel biopsies from several levels of the intestine are recommended. Biopsies of the duodenum, jejunum, and ileum, as well as of mesenteric lymph nodes, are routinely performed. Transverse incisional biopsies are taken from the antimesenteric border of the small intestine. The elliptical incision is closed transversely with either an inverted Cushing or simple interrupted pattern, using 000-chromic gut. The biopsy should be of less than 20 percent of the circumference of the intestine to avoid stricture formation.

Other diagnostic procedures performed at the time of small intestinal biopsy are (1) smears of intestinal contents to be examined for *Giardia* and (2) bacterial cultures of small intestinal contents. Significant numbers of *Staphylococcus aureus* and coliforms are abnormal, indicating bacterial overgrowth in the small intestine, which normally contains anaerobes.

In conclusion, an exploratory laparotomy and multiple bowel biopsies are valid diagnostic procedures to document small intestinal disease. Since the surgeon's visual and tactile impressions commonly indicate a normal small intestine, even in diffuse intestinal disease, biopsies are necessary to make a histologic diagnosis.

COLON

The cardinal signs of colonic disease are tenesmus; high-frequency, low-volume defecation; and the presence of frank blood and mucus in the stool. One or several of these clinical signs may be present in inflammatory large bowel disease. Examination of patients with a history of colonic disease should include multiple fecal examinations (both direct smear and flotation). Parasitic causes for colitis in the dog include whipworms (*Trichuris vulpis*), hookworms, Coccidia sp., and *Entamaeba histolitica*. A digital rectal examination associated with transabdominal palpation prior to endoscopy may identify rectal polyps or masses that may cause signs of colonic disease.

Because of the relative ease of colonic biopsy, it is performed in many cases at the initial onset of signs of large bowel disease. Control diets, corticosteroids, and Azulfidine† (sulfasalazine) — alone or in combination — are often used empirically in the treatment of suspected inflammatory disease of the colon. Biopsy of the colon prior to institution of a therapeutic regimen has several advantages:

1. Differentiation of inflammatory vs. non-inflammatory disease is possible.

2. The specific type and extent of the inflammatory process can be identified (e.g., ulcerative colitis, eosinophilic colitis).

3. A rational approach to therapy and prognosis is provided. For example, a case of mild eosinophilic colitis may respond to a control diet and/or corticosteroids, whereas a severe case of histiocytic ulcerative colitis in a boxer carries a poor prognosis even with therapy.

Endoscopic examination of the colon is often performed in conjunction with biopsy. The methods used in veterinary medicine for colonoscopy are rigid and flexible endoscopy. Flexible colonoscopy permits complete examination of the ascending, transverse, and descending colon. While this method allows extensive examination of the large bowel and directed biopsy, it has several disadvantages: (1) general anesthesia is required, (2) equipment is costly and special training is recommended, and (3) patient preparation prior to examination may be time-consuming. Rigid colonoscopes (human sigmoidoscopes) permit examination only of the descending colon and rectum, which is frequently representative of the entire large bowel in a majority of cases. Minimal or no sedation is required for the procedure.

Patient preparation prior to colonic examination with a rigid colonoscope includes a 12- to 24-hour fast and several warm-water enemas. One enema is given the evening before examination, and one or two enemas are given the day of the procedure. The last enema should not be given within one or two hours of biopsy to minimize the artifactual changes of congestion and hyperemia. Irritant enemas, e.g., sodium phosphate or soapy-water enemas, should be avoided since they induce transient histologic changes in the colonic wall that resemble colitis.

Colonic biopsy with rigid endoscopy can be accomplished in several ways. With the animal in right lateral recumbency, the rigid colonoscope is advanced slowly into the colon with the aid of air insufflation. This must be performed slowly to avoid traumatic perforations with the colonoscope. Once the colonoscope is

in place, the obturator (stylus) is removed. The mucosa is examined for texture, color, and friability, as well as for the presence of parasites, erosions, or ulcerations. The normal mucosa is glistening, smooth, and easily distensible. Lymphoid follicles (small, glistening plaques) are normally seen in the mucosa. The position of mucosal disease should be noted as the colonoscope is withdrawn. Biopsies are taken from any visible mucosal lesion or from multiple areas of the colonic mucosa, if diffuse disease is suspected. Alligator-jaw forceps can be passed through the colonoscope and guided to the biopsy site. The jaws of the forceps are opened approximately 2 to 3 mm, and a fold of mucosa is secured. Slight retraction of the mucosa toward the lumen of the colon before closing the jaws helps to separate the mucosa from the submucosal layers, thereby reducing the risk of perforation. A distinct "crunch" is perceived when the biopsy is completed. The most common error of inexperienced operators is to take very shallow, non-diagnostic biopsies or to shred the mucosa in the retraction phase. After each biopsy, the site is observed briefly for hemorrhage. The colonoscope is not reinserted past a biopsy site, since this area is now susceptible to perforation.

Another method of biopsy involves guiding a suction biopsy instrument through the endoscope to the desired biopsy area. After endoscopic examination is completed, the suction instrument alone can be introduced rectally to a desired length and biopsy specimens obtained. This blind method of colon biopsy can be performed in cases in which no focal lesions are present and the disease process is felt to be diffuse. It is advisable to take multiple biopsy samples at various sites in cases of suspected diffuse disease. At least two biopsy specimens should be obtained to rule out inflammatory disease even when endoscopic examination reveals no lesions.

Palpable colonic masses are often intramural. Mucosal biopsy may not provide a diagnostic specimen, since some neoplasms (adenocarcinoma, leiomyoma, leiomyosarcoma, lymphosarcoma) involve only the deeper layers of the colon. In these cases a full-thickness surgical biopsy is necessary for accurate histologic evaluation of the disease process.

RECTUM

The rectum in the dog and cat extends caudally from the brim of the pelvis to the anal sphincter. Many rectal diseases are extensions of disease processes affecting the descending colon. Therefore, signs of rectal involvement

†Azulfidine, Pharmacia Laboratories, Piscataway, New Jersey 08854

are similar to those of colonic disease: tenesmus, increased frequency of defecation, and overt blood and mucus in the stool.

Digital rectal examination should be performed prior to proctoscopy and biopsy, since polyps, strictures, and intraluminal masses often can be palpated. One warm-water enema given one hour prior to endoscopy is often sufficient preparation for proctoscopic examination. Most patients will accept rigid proctoscopic examination with no sedation, but mild sedation may be necessary in apprehensive patients.

Biopsy of the rectum is usually accomplished with a guided biopsy technique. Most rectal conditions are focal in origin (e.g., polyps, pedunculated adenocarcinoma) and require a directed biopsy. In many cases biopsy of these lesions can be performed with forceps, or they can be ligated and excised in their entirety. General anesthesia or sedation is required if lesions are excised rather than simply biopsied. Blind biopsy of the rectum alone is not often performed in veterinary medicine. Biopsy of the rectal mucosa may be obtained in conjunction with biopsy of the colon to ascertain the extent of an inflammatory process.

Large intramural masses in the rectum may require surgical excision biopsy. In some neoplasms (lymphosarcoma, adenocarcinoma, leiomyoma) a mucosal biopsy may not be diagnostic and a full-thickness biopsy will be necessary.

POSTBIOPSY CONSIDERATIONS

SURGICAL BIOPSY

Postoperatively the patient is fasted for 24 hours when surgical excision biopsy is performed. Water is provided *ad libitum*. Fluid balance may be maintained subcutaneously or intravenously, if necessary. Soft food is offered over the next two to three days, with a gradual return to the normal diet. When full-thickness colonic or rectal biopsy is performed, a highly digestible, low-residue diet is advisable to minimize fecal distention of the colon and rectum.

The prophylactic use of antibiotics following surgery of the gastrointestinal tract is controversial. The decision about postoperative antibiotic administration should be based on surgical assessment of aseptic technique on an individual basis.

FORCEPS AND SUCTION BIOPSY

Aftercare is minimal following biopsy with forceps or suction instruments. No dietary restrictions are necessary, but observation for signs of hemorrhage or perforation is advisable.

COMPLICATIONS OF GASTROINTESTINAL BIOPSY

Hemorrhage and perforation (dehiscence) are the two major potenital complications of gastrointestinal biopsy. A clotting profile should be performed prior to necessary biopsy on any patient suspected of bleeding tendencies. Colonic bleeding associated with alligator forceps biopsy should be minimal, i.e., less than 5 ml. Severe hemorrhage is secondary to coagulopathies or laceration of a vessel. In these cases, the animal should be monitored for shock and treated accordingly. A clotting profile and fresh blood transfusions may be necessary to identify and treat a coagulopathy. If laceration of a vessel is suspected, a dilute epinephrine solution (1:10,000 with saline) is sprayed directly on the biopsy site; if possible, cotton pledgets soaked in this solution can also be placed into the colon to control the hemorrhage.

Perforation can be avoided if potential areas of hazard are identified prior to biopsy. A dilated esophageal wall or an esophageal diverticulum could easily be perforated with a punch biopsy forceps or suction instrument. Biopsy of lesions in these circumstances is best performed via surgical excision. There is a slight risk of perforation of the colonic wall with the alligator forceps because the depth of the biopsy is variable. Several steps that minimize the risk of perforation include (1) securing a fold of mucosa with the jaws of the forceps only partially open, (2) gently retracting the mucosa toward the operator until some resistance is felt, and (3) taking the biopsy with the forceps.

Dehiscence may occur following the excision biopsy. Biopsy of patients with potential wound healing problems as a result of hypoproteinemia are best performed with a forceps or suction instrument.

Perforation and dehiscence are manifest in several ways, largely dependent on the site of involvement. Clinical signs of esophageal perforation include regurgitation, dysphagia, anorexia, and fever. A CBC may reveal leukocytosis. Radiographic evidence of mediastinitis may be present, and thoracocentesis may reveal a cloudy, cellular exudate. When perforation occurs in the abdominal cavity (as a result of gastric, small intestinal, colonic, or rectal biopsy), clinical signs indicate peritonitis and may consist of vomiting, anorexia, and abdominal pain. Leukocytosis and fever are usually present. Radiographic findings of increased fluid density in the abdomen and paracentesis of a cloudy, flocculent material confirm the diagnosis. Surgical intervention is necessary when the condition of the patient is critical and deteriorating.

SUPPLEMENTAL READING

Anderson, N.V.: Biopsy of the gastrointestinal system. Vet. Clin. North Am., 4:317, 1974.

Anderson, N.V.: Disorders of the small intestine. In Ettinger, S.J. (ed.): *Textbook of Veterinary Internal Medicine*. Philadelphia, W.B. Saunders Co., 1975, pp. 1150–1191.

Batt, R.M., Jones, P.E., and Peters, T.J.: Peroral jejunal biopsy in the dog. Vet. Record, 99:337, 1976.

Beck, K., Dischler, W., Helms, M., and Oehlert, W.: *Color Atlas of Endoscopy and Biopsy of the Intestine*. (Translated by G.F. Meissner.) Philadelphia, W.B. Saunders Co., 1975.

Brandborg, L.L., Rubin, G.E., and Quinton, B.S.: A multipurpose instrument for suction biopsy of the esophagus, stomach, small bowel, and colon. Gastroenterology, 37:1–16, 1959.

Cornelius, L.M., and Wingfield, W.E.: Diseases of the stomach. In Ettinger, S.J. (ed.): *Textbook of Veterinary Internal Medicine*. Philadelphia, W.B. Saunders Co., 1975, pp. 1125–1149.

Demling, L., Ottenjann, R., and Elster, K.: *Endoscopy and Biopsy of the Esophagus and Stomach*. (Translated by K.H. Soergel.) Philadelphia, W.B. Saunders Co., 1972.

Greiner, T.P., and Betts, C.W.: Diseases of the rectum and anus. In Ettinger, S.J. (ed.): *Textbook of Veterinary Internal Medicine*. Philadelphia, W.B. Saunders Co., 1975, pp. 1307–1333.

Guffy, M.M.: Esophageal disorders. In Ettinger, S.J. (ed.): *Textbook of Veterinary Internal Medicine*. Philadelphia. W.B. Saunders, Co., 1975, pp. 1098–1124.

Lorenz, M.D.: Disorders of the large bowel. In Ettinger, S.J. (ed.): *Textbook of Veterinary Internal Medicine*. Philadelphia, W.B. Saunders Co., 1975. pp. 1192–1218.

LAPAROSCOPY IN SMALL ANIMAL MEDICINE

J. M. PATTERSON, D.V.M.

Guelph, Ontario

INTRODUCTION

Endoscopy, by definition, is the inspection of any body cavity by means of an endoscope. Laparoscopy is an example of an endoscopic procedure for the visual examination of the peritoneal cavity and its contents, following the establishment of a pneumoperitoneum.

Since the turn of the century, great strides have been made in the improvement of both equipment and technique used for laparoscopy in human and veterinary medicine. Most important has been the introduction of fiberoptics, a system whereby both light and images are transmitted through glass fibers. The light source employed in fiberoptics is remote, the light being transmitted from the light source to the laparoscope via a fiberoptic illumination bundle. Because the light source is remote, heat is not transmitted to the patient, a distinct advantage over previous methods, in which small light bulbs were attached directly to the operating end of the scope. These light bulbs offered a minimal amount of light and quickly became hot enough to damage tissue on contact. The light source used by the author is a dual purpose device with a 150 watt incandescent lamp for routine use and a 300 watt arc lamp for generation of high-intensity light for photography (Fig. 1).

Laparoscopes are rigid in design and vary from 2.2 to 10 mm in diameter. The larger laparoscopes contain more glass fibers and can carry more light than the smaller scopes. The optical system employs glass optics, and focusing of the laparoscope is not necessary. In the 180° laparoscope, the objective lens is at the tip of the scope and is surrounded by fiberoptic light fibers. This is a popular instrument, although the optical system is more apt to become clouded when the tip of the scope touches intraperitoneal organs. Frequently the scope may have to be removed from the peritoneal cavity, the optics cleaned, and the instrument reinserted.

Recently, a smaller fiberoptic laparoscope has become available. The Needlescope* measures 1.7 mm or 2.2 mm in diameter and is available from Dyonics, Inc. Because of its size, it is readily inserted into the abdomen without a prior skin incision. This scope has fewer light-

---

*Needlescope, Dyonics Inc., 71 Pine Street, Woburn, Massachusetts

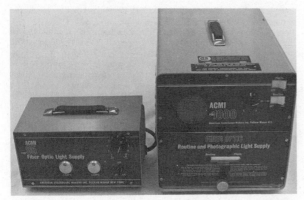

Figure 1. Two fiberoptic light sources from American Cystoscope Makers, Inc.

carrying fibers and requires a bright light source.

EQUIPMENT

Equipment required for laparoscopy includes (Fig. 2)

1. A laparoscope with its trocar and cannula assembly.
2. A light source and fiberoptic cable.
3. A Verres needle and insufflating device to create the pneumoperitoneum.
4. A small surgery pack and two sterile trays 3 inches deep and large enough to hold the laparoscope and accessories. The equipment is placed in a cold sterilization solution in one tray and rinsed and warmed in sterile distilled water in the other.

Useful ancillary equipment includes

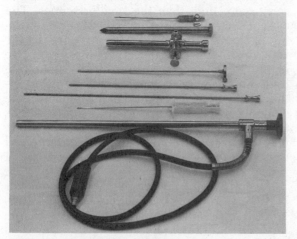

Figure 2. Instruments used for laparoscopy. From top to bottom: Verres needle, primary trocar, primary cannula, tactile cannula, tactile trocar, tactile probe, Tru-Cut disposable biopsy needle, direct vision telescope with fiberoptic illumination bundle.

1. A biopsy needle and supply of 10 percent formalin fixative.
2. A blunt tactile probe with its corresponding trocar and cannula assembly.
3. Photographic equipment that will adapt to the laparoscope.

STERILIZATION OF INSTRUMENTS

The fiberoptic equipment used at present must not be autoclaved. All instruments can be disinfected in standard cold germicidal solutions in accordance with the manufacturer's recommendations. When using any solution with a formaldehyde base, rinsing with sterile water is mandatory. All instruments may also be sterilized with ethylene oxide, but these must be thoroughly aerated prior to use.

The instruments are then carefully rinsed in warm sterile distilled water. When the valved cannula is placed in the cold sterilizing solution, it is necessary to activate the valve so that the solution will enter the cannula. Likewise, when the cannula is rinsed in sterile water, the valve again must be activated to release the antiseptic solution.

Preferably following each use, the cannula should be disassembled and cleaned. The scope should be wiped dry using a soft cloth to avoid damaging the optics.

To prevent the optics from fogging in the warm peritoneal cavity, it is necessary to warm the instrument to 38° C in warm sterile distilled water and then to dry it carefully. The lens is then remoistened with an antifogging detergent such as hexachlorophene, wiped dry, and immediately inserted through the valved cannula into the peritoneal cavity. The lens must be crystal clear for accurate visualization.

PHOTOGRAPHY

Photography for teaching and documentation of laparoscopic findings can be accomplished with the larger scopes. Good laparoscopic photographs can be obtained with the 300 watt arc lamp used in both the American Cystoscope† and the Eder‡ fiberoptic power sources. A single-lens reflex camera is used with an adapter designed to fit the end of the laparoscope. Ektachrome daylight film, ASA rating 160–400, is used with the camera lens focused to infinity at f 2.8 and a shutter speed of from 1/15 to 1/60 of a second.

---

†American Cystoscope Makers Inc., 30 Stillwater Ave., Stamford, Conn. 06902

‡Eder Instrument Co., Inc., 5115 North Ravenswood Ave., Chicago, Illinois 60640

PROCEDURE

Laparoscopy can be performed using general anesthesia, or a local anesthetic may be employed in conjunction with tranquilization and narcotic analgesics. The author prefers the patient to be under general anesthesia, but recent reports have claimed good success using oxymorphone hydrochloride given intravenously in conjunction with local anesthesia (Jones). In the severely depressed patient requiring laparoscopy, a local anesthetic alone may be adequate.

If biopsy is contemplated or bleeding tendencies could be encountered, coagulation tests are advisable.

With the patient adequately restrained, a site for entry of the laparoscope is chosen. Abdominal radiography, palpation, and the anatomic location of the organ system under examination will all aid in determining whether a right, midline, or left lateral abdominal approach would be most useful.

A useful site of entry is approximately 3 to 4 cm caudal to the last rib and midway between the ventral midline and transverse processes of the lumbar vertebrae.

INTRODUCTION OF A PNEUMOPERITONEUM

A pneumoperitoneum is required to produce a gas layer that separates the abdominal wall from the abdominal viscera. The safe introduction of gas into the peritoneal cavity requires a proper needle and a source of gas. By paying particular attention to detail and by acquiring experience one can markedly reduce the incidence of complications during the introduction of the pneumoperitoneum.

The Verres pneumoperitoneum needle is specially designed for the safe initial puncture of the peritoneal cavity. It is an automatic action needle that combines an outer sharp needle with an inner blunt stylet. The blunted stylet is spring-loaded in position so as to obturate and extend beyond the point of the overlying needle. As the device is pressed against the skin, the blunted stylet is forced back, leaving the sharp point free to penetrate the tissue. As the point emerges free into the abdominal cavity the blunt stylet can be felt to spring forward.

After the needle is inserted into the peritoneal cavity, the following safety checks should be made:

1. Move the needle back and forth to be sure that it is in a free space.

2. Attach a syringe, partially filled with saline, for aspiration. If the needle has entered a loop of bowel, intestinal content with or without gas will be obtained. If a blood vessel or spleen has been penetrated, blood will be withdrawn. If nothing can be aspirated, the saline solution is injected; it should flow freely into the peritoneal cavity. Only then should the operator proceed with the injection of gas.

Room air, nitrous oxide, and carbon dioxide are gases that have been used to create a pneumoperitoneum. Reports of air emboli with the use of room air make it a poor choice. Carbon dioxide is both rapidly absorbed and rapidly excreted from the body. Its disadvantage is that it does cause some peritoneal irritation.

Mechanized insufflators are available. These devices inject the gas, record the amount insufflated, and measure the intra-abdominal pressure. Jones describes the use of a gas anesthesia machine that can be used with nitrous oxide as a convenient and safe insufflator for the practitioner.

Once the Verres needle is safely in the peritoneal cavity it is coupled to the anesthetic machine through its flow valve. The flow valve is set at approximately 1 liter per minute. The operator should percuss the abdominal wall as the gas is being introduced. It is important to ascertain that gas is present in the upper as well as the lower abdomen. The abdomen is insufflated until the wall is moderately tense.

LAPAROSCOPIC EXAMINATION

Following surgical preparation and sterile draping, a 1-cm incision is made through the skin at the entry site. The trocar and cannula assembly are then advanced, using a twisting motion, through the skin incision and into the abdomen in a ventrocaudal direction. Prior emptying of the bladder and colon will minimize the chance of these organs being punctured during insertion of the trocar.

The trocar is then removed from the cannula and replaced by the warmed dry laparoscope (Fig. 3). A trumpet valve located on the cannula prevents the loss of gas during this exchange.

The operator is now ready to visualize the abdominal organs. The diaphragm, lobes of the liver, gallbladder, stomach wall, kidneys, adrenal glands, pancreas, spleen, portions of the small and large intestines, peritoneal wall, portions of the male and female reproductive tracts, and the urinary bladder can be clearly visualized. The organs seen are determined to a degree by the location of the entry site.

To manipulate organs, a second 2.5 mm diameter trocar and cannula can be introduced into the peritoneal cavity through a second small skin incision. This trocar is replaced with a

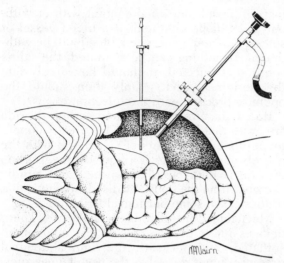

Figure 3. The laparoscope and tactile probe in place in the peritoneal cavity. The peritoneal wall is displaced from the peritoneal contents by a pneumoperitoneum.

blunt probe, which can then be used to shift organs, fat, or mesentery gently out of the way (see Fig. 3). A second helpful technique involves the use of a tilting table to cause the abdominal organs to shift one way or the other to improve the operator's view of selected organs.

The cannula is held firmly in place in the abdominal wall. To allow movement of the scope back and forth within the cannula, the trumpet valve is depressed with the index finger. It is important not to allow the cannula itself to come out of the abdominal wall, because the pneumoperitoneum would be quickly lost and the procedure aborted.

The entire contents of the abdomen on the side being viewed should be examined in a systematic manner and the findings recorded.

Biopsies may be taken at this time. Several biopsy needles and biopsy forceps are available for use with the laparoscope. The Tru-Cut* disposable biopsy needle is 11.4 cm long and yields a core biopsy 20 mm in length. The needle is introduced into the abdomen through a short skin incision proximal to the biopsy site. The distinct advantage is the operator's ability to direct the biopsy needle to an exact location. Biopsies obtained via laparoscopy can be extremely useful in making definitive diagnoses on which to formulate rational treatment and to determine prognosis. Several articles that give detailed instructions regarding liver and kidney biopsies have appeared in recent literature.

After the biopsy is taken the area is checked for bleeding, which is usually minimal. If the

*Tru-Cut Disposable Biopsy Needle, Travenol Laboratories, Inc., Deerfield, Illinois.

biopsy site bleeds more profoundly than expected, the operator should apply internal or external pressure over the bleeding area. A whole blood transfusion may be required. Serious postbiopsy bleeding requires surgical exploration for control.

With the laparoscope removed from the cannula, the gas is slowly released from the abdomen by manipulation of the trumpet valve. The cannula is then removed from the abdomen and a single suture is placed in the peritoneal layer and another in the skin.

DISCUSSION

In order to interpret laparoscopic findings the operator must have a thorough knowledge of gross anatomy and be familiar with the appearance of gross pathologic change. The technique is not meant to replace surgical exploratory laparotomy. Indeed, there are obvious limitations to laparoscopy, including the limited ability to shift readily and simultaneously palpate the abdominal organs.

Laparoscopy and its usefulness in directing liver, kidney, and splenic biopsies has been documented by several investigators. The advantages of being able to visualize the lesion accurately as well as to direct the biopsy needle make the technique safer and ensure a more useful biopsy specimen than those obtained by blind percutaneous biopsy techniques.

For the oncologist, laparoscopy is a valuable tool for diagnosis and documentation of neoplastic change in cancer patients. Followup examination following cancer therapy is made possible with minimal risk to the patient.

In reproductive research the laparoscope has proved its worth in several species, including the cow, pig, sheep, mare, and non-human primates.

In a large series of laparoscopic examinations done on both dogs and cats ranging from 2.0 to 32 kg body weight, it was demonstrated that size of the animal is not a limiting factor (Wildt, et al.). The smaller Needlescope was used in the smaller animals.

There are, however, a number of contraindications for laparoscopy. They include

1. Peritonitis — past or present.
2. Suspicion of extensive abdominal adhesions because of prior abdominal surgery. In such cases puncture of an organ or piece of bowel is more likely.
3. Hernias, including diaphragmatic and inguinal.
4. Coagulation defects.
5. Obesity, because of the difficulty in visualizing the abdomen in a fat patient.

6. Apparent risks that outweigh the benefits that may be derived.

7. Inexperience and improper preparation by the operator.

Complications that have been encountered with laparoscopy include air emboli, cardiac arrest, pneumothorax, damage to internal organs with the Verres needle or trocar, subcutaneous emphysema, and introduction of gas into a hollow viscus. Experience and attention to detail on the part of the operator are essential in avoiding such complications. The procedure is not difficult and, once mastered, is a real aid to diagnosis. With an understanding of its usefulness and limitations, fewer complications will occur.

There are many new and innovative techniques being developed for use with laparoscopy. Johnson has performed gallbladder puncture and subsequent cholecystocholangiography for evaluation of the gallbladder and bile ducts. Many more such procedures are under investigation at this time.

SUGGESTED READING

Cohen, M. R.: *Laparoscopy, Culdoscopy, and Gynecography*, vol. 1. Philadelphia, W. B. Saunders Co., 1970.

Johnson, G. F., and Twedt, D. C.: Endoscopy and laparoscopy in the diagnosis and management of neoplasia in small animals. Vet. Clin. North Am., 7:77–92, 1977.

Jones, B.: The use of endoscopy and laparoscopy as a diagnostic tool in veterinary medicine. Proceedings of the 44th Annual Meeting of the AAHA, 1977.

Wildt, D. E., Kunney, G. M., and Seager, S. W. J.: Laparoscopy for direct observation of internal organs of the domestic cat and dog. Am. J. Vet. Res., 38:1429–1432, 1977.

Section

11

ENDOCRINE AND METABOLIC DISORDERS

JOHN A. MULNIX, D.V.M.
Consulting Editor

Canine Hyperadrenocorticism.. 975
Therapy for Spontaneous Hyperadrenocorticism 979
Hypoadrenocorticism 983
Systemic Glucocorticoid Therapy 988
Hypothyroidism 994
Feline Hyperthyroidism... 998
Primary Hypoparathyroidism 1000
Primary Hyperparathyroidism 1003
Diabetes Insipidus... 1005
Diabetes Mellitus.. 1011
Diabetic Ketoacidosis... 1016
Functional Pancreatic Islet Cell Adenocarcinoma in the Dog 1020
Non-neoplastic Causes of Canine Hypoglycemia....................... 1023
Puerperal Tetany... 1027
The Ovary, Ovarian Hormones, and Contraceptives 1030
Obesity 1034

Additional Pertinent Information, Still Current, Found in
Current Veterinary Therapy VI:

Capen, C. C., and Martin, S. L.: Parathyroid Glands and Calcium Metabolism, p. 1038.
Krook, L.: Nutritional Hypercalcitoninism, p. 1048.
Mattheeuws, D. R. G., and Comhaire, F. H.: Tumors of the Testes, p. 1054.
Osborne, C. A., and Johnston, S. D.: Ectopic Hormone Production by Nonendocrine Neoplasms, p. 1061.
Rijnberk, A., and Leav, I.: Thyroid Tumors, p. 1020.

Additional Pertinent Information, Still Current, Found in
Current Veterinary Therapy V:

Cotton, R. B., and Theran, P.: Diabetic Ketoacidosis, p. 822.
Richards, M. A.: The Diabetes Insipidus Syndrome in Dogs, p. 805.

CANINE HYPERADRENOCORTICISM

JAN C. MEIJER, D.V.M.
Utrecht, The Netherlands

Hyperadrenocorticism is a generalized metabolic disease resulting from glucocorticosteroid excess. The clinical syndrome produced either by excessive and prolonged administration of corticosteroids or adrenocorticotropic hormone (ACTH) is called iatrogenic hyperadrenocorticism. Hyperadrenocorticism may occur spontaneously and principally involves three different entities:

1. Pituitary-dependent hyperadrenocorticism (PDH) is the result of an excessive secretion of ACTH by the pituitary gland and is associated with bilateral adrenocortical hyperplasia. We have found pituitary tumors in about 20 percent of cases of PDH, and this disease entity constitutes 80 percent of cases of spontaneous hyperadrenocorticism.

2. Autonomous secretion of ACTH by a non-pituitary tumor (ectopic ACTH syndrome) potentially may occur but has not been documented in the dog.

3. In approximately 20 percent of cases hyperadrenocorticism is caused by an adrenocortical tumor. These tumors usually occur unilaterally and may be malignant or benign. Their autonomous character is shown by the atrophy of the non-tumorous adrenocortical tissue.

PITUITARY-DEPENDENT HYPERADRENOCORTICISM

CLINICAL DATA

This disease is most often seen in toy poodles, dachshunds and boxers, but all breeds may be affected. It is a disease of middle-aged and older dogs, the median age at diagnosis being seven to eight years. Females tend to be affected more frequently than males.

The clinical signs (Table 1) commonly observed in PDH are the result of the metabolic effects of long-standing hypercortisolism. The number and severity of the signs vary with the duration of the disease and are subject to considerable individual variation. In most cases the owner seeks veterinary help because the dog

Table 1. Clinical and Laboratory Findings in Canine Hyperadrenocorticism

CLINICAL SIGNS	APPROXIMATE % OF CASES
Abdominal enlargement	95
Hepatomegaly	90
Skin atrophy	90
Polydipsia/polyuria/polyphagia	85
Decreased exercise tolerance	80
Muscle atrophy	70
Increased panting	70
Lethargy	65
Obesity	55
Intolerance to hot environment	40
Exophthalmus	30
Anestrus (females)	85
Testicle atrophy (males)	60

LABORATORY ABNORMALITIES	APPROXIMATE % OF CASES
Elevated alkaline phosphatase	90
Eosinopenia	90
Lymphopenia	75
Neutrophilia	60
Elevated SGPT	50
Elevated SGOT	30
Hyperglycemia	30
Hyperglycemia/glucosuria	10
Hypokalemia ($\leq$ 3.5 mmol/liter)	5*, 45†
Hypernatremia ($\geq$ 151 mmol/liter)	30
Subnormal T_4 ($\leq$ 1.5 μg/100 ml)	50

*In dogs with PDH

†In dogs with hyperadrenocorticism due to adrenocortical tumors

has polydipsia and polyuria, frequently accompanied by an increased appetite, weight gain, and the development of a pendulous abdomen. Often there is a non-pruritic bilateral symmetric alopecia. In some cases, especially in toy poodles, this alopecia — which is usually accompanied by increased pigmentation of the skin — is the only sign of the disease. Subtle changes in hair color and texture, retardation of hair growth, and gradually increasing loss of hair — especially on the flanks, the rear side of the hind legs, the base of the auricles, and the ventral abdomen — may develop into generalized alopecia of the trunk, whereas the head and the extremities are spared. Other signs of skin atrophy involve a thin, easily wrinkled skin and cutaneous striae. Keratin-plugged follicles are often found around the nipples and on the ventral abdomen. Calcinosis cutis is an infrequent condition usually found on the dorsal midline. Fatigability, muscle weakness, and decreased exercise tolerance are often mentioned in the history.

Palpation of the abdomen often reveals the presence of an enlarged liver. Hepatomegaly, increased radiodensity of the liver, osteoporosis, and calcification of various tissues, especially bronchial walls and the skin, can be detected radiographically.

LABORATORY DATA

Blood analysis (see Table 1) usually reveals the presence of lymphopenia and eosinopenia. Plasma alkaline phosphatase activity is consistently elevated as a result of the cortisol-induced production of an isoenzyme by the liver. Moderately elevated levels of serum glutamic-oxaloacetic transaminase (SGOT) and serum glutamic-pyruvic transaminase (SGPT) can be found. Plasma glucose levels are usually within normal limits but may be slightly elevated; diabetes mellitus occurs in about 10 percent of dogs with hyperadrenocorticism. Blood urea nitrogen and creatinine concentrations, determined to evaluate renal function, are usually low. Hypokalemia is a rare finding in PDH. If the dog has been deprived of water prior to admission, mild hypernatremia may be found.

Interestingly, plasma thyroxine levels are often subnormal, but this is not associated with hypothyroidism. These low thyroxine levels in dogs with hyperadrenocorticism are probably caused by interference of cortisol with the binding of thyroxine by plasma proteins.

In keeping with the polyuria, the specific gravity of the urine is usually very low. Forty percent of random urine samples had specific gravities ranging from 1.001 to 1.006, and another 40 percent ranged from 1.007 to 1.012. As mentioned previously, glucosuria may be found.

The polyuria that occurs in canine hyperadrenocorticism is most probably due to interference of cortisol with the action of antidiuretic hormone at the level of the collecting tubules. Therefore, the response to the administration of vasopressin is absent or only very moderate.

HYPERADRENOCORTICISM DUE TO ADRENOCORTICAL TUMOR

This disease may affect dogs of any breed; there is no special breed preference. Typically, it is a disease of old dogs, the median age at initial diagnosis being 10 to 11 years. Females are three times more frequently involved than males.

The clinical signs in this disease are identical to those found in PDH and are usually dominated by polydipsia and polyuria. Palpation of the abdomen very seldom reveals the presence of an abnormal, tumorous mass. In addition to the abnormalities that are summarized in Table 1, blood analysis often reveals hypokalemia. Together with the mild hypernatremia that also is frequently found, these mineral disturbances can be attributed to the mineralocorticoid properties of cortisol and possibly to other corticosteroids, secreted by the adrenocortical tumor.

Radiographs of the thorax and abdomen usually fail to indicate the presence and localization of an adrenocortical tumor and its eventual metastases. Urinalysis and blood examination yield the same results as mentioned for PDH.

EVALUATION OF PITUITARY-ADRENOCORTICAL FUNCTION

The clinical signs leading to consideration of hyperadrenocorticism in differential diagnosis are never conclusive evidence of the disease. An objective diagnosis of hyperadrenocorticism can only be reached through evaluation of pituitary-adrenocortical function.

Basically, adrenocortical function is regulated by the pituitary gland through secretion of ACTH, which is modulated by three different mechanisms involving diurnal variation, stress, and the negative feedback control of cortisol.

Since the secretion of cortisol, the major glucocorticosteroid secreted by the dog's adrenal glands, parallels the secretion of ACTH by the pituitary gland, pituitary-adrenocortical function can be evaluated either by measuring plasma ACTH levels or plasma cortisol levels or by measuring cortisol metabolites (17-hydroxycorticosteroids) excreted in the urine.

Single baseline values for these parameters usually have no diagnostic significance because of the considerable overlap between the range of values found in normal dogs and dogs with hyperadrenocorticism. Therefore, evaluation of pituitary-adrenocortical function is based upon the main characteristic of PDH — the decreased sensitivity of the feedback system to dexamethasone. The main characteristic of adrenocortical tumors lies in their autonomous cortisol secretion, which is not suppressed after the administration of high doses of dexamethasone. Pituitary-adrenocortical function is evaluated by judging the decrease in cortisol secretion following the administration of low and high doses of dexamethasone. Decreased but existent suppressibility of cortisol secretion is diagnostic for PDH. Non-suppressibility of cortisol secretion is the hallmark of adrenocortical tumors.

As a parameter for cortisol secretion we measure the concentration of cortisol in the plasma. Since plasma cortisol levels in the dog are low compared with those of man and because extremely low values can be found after dexamethasone administration, special attention should be given to the sensitivity and accuracy of the method used for determination of cortisol levels. We have had experience with both fluorometric and radioimmunoassay techniques, and we strongly prefer the latter method.

DIAGNOSIS

Both diagnosis and differential diagnosis are achieved by dexamethasone (DXM) tests. A low-dose DXM test is used for screening, e.g., to distinguish dogs with hyperadrenocorticism from normal dogs. A high-dose DXM test is used for differential diagnosis and separates dogs with PDH from dogs with autonomous cortisol secretion. The latter group involves all dogs with adrenocortical tumors but also some dogs with PDH, in which incomplete suppressibility after a high dose of DXM is usually associated with a pituitary tumor. In these cases high-dose DXM administration of longer duration usually results in a decline of the plasma cortisol levels, thereby excluding the presence of an autonomously functioning adrenocortical tumor. Ultimately, measurements of plasma ACTH levels, adrenal gland imaging by radiopharmaceuticals, or exploratory laparotomy may assist in the differential diagnosis of hyperadrenocorticism.

The DXM tests and other procedures as well as their interpretation are outlined in the following section and also in Table 2. During the intravenous DXM tests and during the previous

Table 2. *Dexamethasone Tests for Diagnosis of Canine Hyperadrenocorticism*

DXM SCREENING TEST		INTERPRETATION	
8:50 AM Baseline plasma cortisol		100%	
9:00 AM DXM 0.01 mg/kg IV			
12:00 NOON 3-hr plasma cortisol	<50%	<50%	>50%
5:00 PM 8-hr plasma cortisol	<15 ng/ml or	>15 ng/ml or	>15 ng/ml or
	<0.04 µmol/liter	>0.04 µmol/liter	>0.04 µmol/liter
	↓	↓	↓
	normal	PDH	PDH or adrenal tumor

DXM SUPPRESSION TEST		INTERPRETATION		
8:50 AM Baseline plasma cortisol			100%	
9:00 AM DXM 0.1 mg/kg IV				
12:00 NOON 3-hr plasma cortisol	≤50%	≤50%	>50%	>50%
5:00 PM 8-hr plasma cortisol	≤50%	>50%	≤50%	>50%
		PDH		↓
				Adrenal tumor or lesser-suppression PDH

ORAL DXM SUPPRESSION TEST	INTERPRETATION
Day 1 9:00 AM Baseline plasma cortisol: Start DXM 3 dd (1–2 mg) orally	
Day 2 9:00 AM Plasma cortisol: DXM 3 dd (1–2 mg) orally	
Day 3 9:00 AM Plasma cortisol: DXM 3 dd (1–2 mg) orally	
Day 4 9:00 AM Plasma cortisol: ≤50% of baseline value ⟶ PDH or pituitary tumor	
>50% of baseline value ⟶ Adrenal tumor	

night food is withheld, but the dog is allowed to drink. Consecutive tests in the same dog are separated from each other by at least 48 hours.

DXM SCREENING TEST

Indication. The test is used in the diagnosis of hyperadrenocorticism.

Performance. Blood samples are collected immediately before and at three and eight hours after intravenous injection at 9:00 AM of DXM (Oradexon®, Organon) in a dose of 0.01 mg/kg body weight. For each sample, collect 2 ml of blood in tubes with EDTA or heparin as the anticoagulant, centrifuge promptly, and freeze the plasma until it is sent to the laboratory for measurement of cortisol.

Interpretation. In normal dogs plasma cortisol is reduced to essentially 0 ng/ml within three hours and remains suppressed for eight hours or more. Some normal dogs eventually are less suppressed after eight hours, but plasma cortisol then is always below 1.5 μg/100 ml or 15 ng/ml (0.04 μmol/liter).* Dogs with plasma cortisol levels exceeding 15 ng/ml eight hours after the injection of 0.01 mg DXM/kg have hyperadrenocorticism.

In PDH there may be a distinct decrease occurring at three hours or eight hours, to values below 50 percent of the baseline value, but by eight hours the plasma cortisol concentration exceeds 15 ng/ml. A lesser degree of suppression or even absence of suppression in this DXM screening test does not exclude PDH. One must bear in mind that, especially in the early course of PDH, sometimes periods of remission may occur, during which DXM screening may give results as in normal dogs. In these (usually mild) cases, repeated DXM screening tests then are necessary after a few weeks or months. In dogs with adrenocortical tumors, plasma cortisol is not decreased in this test.

DXM SUPPRESSION TEST

Indication. Differentiation between PDH and hyperadrenocorticism due to adrenocortical tumor may be made with this test.

Performance. This test is administered in the same way as the DXM screening test with the exception of the dose of DXM; for the suppression test, inject 0.1 mg/kg body weight intravenously.

Interpretation. In dogs with PDH, plasma cortisol is suppressed to below 50 percent of the baseline value, either at three hours or at eight hours, or both, after the injection of DXM. Most dogs with PDH not associated with pituitary tumor have very low plasma cortisol levels (1.0 to 5.0 ng/ml or 0.003 to 0.014 μmol/liter) three hours after DXM but are beginning to escape suppression at eight hours. Dogs with PDH, which are less suppressible and usually are found to have a pituitary tumor, either show distinct suppression followed by rapid escape from suppression (as evidenced by a low three-hour level and a near-baseline eight-hour level of plasma cortisol) or show a sustained low-grade suppression. There is no suppression of plasma cortisol in very few cases of PDH associated with pituitary tumor. Dogs with adrenocortical tumors have plasma cortisol levels that are essentially not suppressed but that may fluctuate by as much as 30 percent of the baseline value.

ORAL DXM SUPPRESSION TEST

Indication. Inconclusive IV DXM suppression test is an indication for this test.

Performance. After collecting blood at about 9:00 AM for measurement of the baseline plasma cortisol level, DXM (Oradexon®, Organon) tablets are given orally in a dose of 1, 1.5, or 2 mg, according to the size of the dog, three times daily at intervals of eight hours, for three consecutive days. Every 24 hours a blood sample is collected for plasma cortisol determination.

Interpretation. Distinct suppression, evidenced by a final plasma cortisol level below 50 percent of the baseline value, is diagnostic of the non-autonomous nature of the hyperadrenocorticism that may be associated with a pituitary tumor. Non-suppressibility of plasma cortisol in this test, evidenced by a final plasma cortisol concentration higher than 50 percent of the baseline value, is diagnostic for adrenocortical tumor.

We are aware of the fact that these tests do not always result in the correct diagnosis, simply because the secretion rate of cortisol in dogs with adrenocortical tumors may fluctuate spontaneously and so can mimic suppression. In addition, the secretory activity of some pituitary tumors is very hard to suppress with doses of dexamethasone described here. In cases in which the differentiation between apparent autonomous pituitary tumors and adrenocortical tumors proves difficult, the following approaches can be helpful.

---

*To convert μg/100 ml to ng/ml, move the decimal point one position to the right. To convert μg/100 ml to μmol/liter, multiply the value in μg/100 ml by a factor of 0.0276. For example, 1.5 μg/100 ml = 0.04 μmol/liter.

ADRENAL GLAND IMAGING

The intravenous injection of radiolabeled cholesterol (^{131}I-19-iodocholesterol) has permitted diagnostic imaging of normal and hyperfunctioning adrenal glands and adrenocortical tumors. The clinical value of this technique lies in the visualization of functional adrenocortical tumors (with suppressed contralateral gland) and their preoperative localization. The practical application of this technique is limited by the availability of a gamma-ray camera and by the cost of the radiopharmaceutical.

EXPLORATORY LAPAROTOMY

Ultimately, in cases of non-suppressible cortisol production exploratory laparotomy will give the final diagnosis.

ACTH

When measurement of ACTH in canine plasma becomes available for the veterinary profession, it will allow differentiation between cases of less suppressible PDH and adrenocortical tumor. ACTH-secreting pituitary tumors give rise to elevated or high normal plasma ACTH levels, whereas in the case of cortisol-secreting adrenocortical tumors absent or low normal plasma ACTH levels can be expected. Preliminary results confirm this expectation.

SUPPLEMENTAL READING

Lubberink, A. A. M. E.: Diagnosis and Treatment of Canine Cushing's Syndrome. (Thesis) Drukkerij Elinkwijk, Utrecht, University of Utrecht, 1977.

Meijer, J. C., de Bruijne, J. J., Rijnberk, A., and Croughs, R. J. M.: Biochemical characterization of pituitary-dependent hyperadrenocorticism in the dog. J. Endocrinol., 77:111–118, 1978.

Meijer, J. C., Lubberink, A. A. M. E., Rijnberk, A., and Croughs, R. J. M.: Adrenocortical function tests in dogs with hyperfunctioning adrenocortical tumors. J. Endocrinol., 80:315–319, 1979.

Mulnix, J. A., van den Brom, E. W., Lubberink, A. A. M. E., de Bruijne, J. J., and Rijnberk, A.: Gamma camera imaging on bilateral adrenocortical hyperplasia and adrenal tumors in the dog. Am. J. Vet. Res., 37:1467–1471, 1976.

Owens, J. M., and Drucker, W. D.: Hyperadrenocorticism in the dog: Canine Cushing's syndrome. Vet. Clin. North Am. 7:583, 1977.

Scott, D. W.: Hyperadrenocorticism. Vet. Clin. North Am., 9:3–28, 1979.

THERAPY FOR SPONTANEOUS HYPERADRENOCORTICISM

ALEID A. M. E. LUBBERINK, D.V.M.

Utrecht, The Netherlands

PITUITARY-DEPENDENT HYPERADRENOCORTICISM

Treatment of pituitary-dependent hyperadrenocorticism can be accomplished by hypophysectomy, bilateral adrenalectomy, or chemotherapy. The choice of treatment and its success depend upon (1) the surgeon's experience; (2) the breed of the animal — until recently, hypophysectomy proved to be rather difficult in brachycephalic dogs; and (3) an understanding of the possible complications that can be expected in each of the methods of treatment.

HYPOPHYSECTOMY

Hypophysectomy is performed using the technique of Markowitz and associates (1964). After instillation of inhalation anesthesia, accomplished by artificial ventilation and ECG monitoring (plus capnography if possible), the animal is placed in dorsal recumbency at one end of the operating table. During the procedure, lactated Ringer's solution is infused.

The front legs are loosely fixed in the caudal direction. The upper jaw is fixed parallel to the table. Careful attention should be given to the correct horizontal position of the maxilla. The

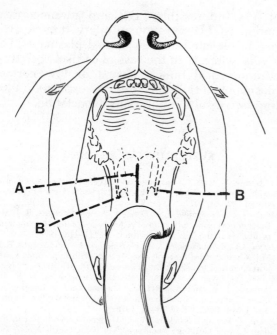

Figure 1. *A.* Incision in soft palate for hypophysectomy. *B.* Hamular process, which can be palpated underneath the soft palate.

mouth is maximally opened by fixing the lower jaw to a metal bar attached to the side of the table and forming an arch over the dog. The mouth and nasopharynx are disinfected with 70 percent alcohol. A midline incision of 3 to 4 cm is made in the soft palate, directly posterior to the hard palate (Fig. 1). When the soft palate is incised, care should be taken not to extend the incision to the hard palate, because this may result in severe hemorrhage from the major palatine artery. The incision is kept open with a small retractor. This allows a view of the sphenoid bone covered with mucoperiosteum. The rather thick mucoperiosteum is incised for 3 cm on the midline between the hamular processes and is stripped to each side. To expose the pituitary gland, a groove is burred in the sphen-

oid bone. The groove is made with a 4 mm diameter dental drill on the midline directly beneath the posterior ends of the hamular processes (Fig. 2). Bleeding from the sphenoid bone can easily be controlled by putting Bonewax* in the grooves of the drill. The groove is very carefully deepened until the pituitary gland becomes visible as a small yellow-pink spot on the midline. Carelessness will result in severe hemorrhage from the horseshoe-shaped venous sinus enclosing the pituitary. If sinus bleeding does occur, the area is packed with gauze soaked in thrombin solution.† Although the bleeding may be controlled within a few minutes, recurrence can be expected when burring is continued. The groove is enlarged until the pituitary can be seen through the dural membrane as a yellowish-pink area bulging slightly (Fig. 3). The dural membrane is then incised crosswise with a small dura knife, allowing the pituitary to bulge out.

The gland is brought further into the bur hole by gentle suction and is removed using fine forceps. Usually the gland is removed in pieces. In most cases the removal does not cause severe bleeding. After removal of the pituitary gland the fossa is inspected carefully for remnants of pituitary tissue. After complete removal there is usually a good view into the pituitary fossa, where arterial pulsations can be seen. The bur hole is closed with Bonewax. The mucoperiosteum is not closed. The soft palate is sutured in one layer using interrupted stitches of nonabsorbable material.

POSTOPERATIVE MEDICATION

On the first postoperative day, the following medication should be given: (1) 2 mg cortisol

---

*Bonewax, Ethicon Ltd., Edinburgh, Scotland (UK)
†Thrombin-Topical®, Parke-Davis Co., Detroit, Michigan.

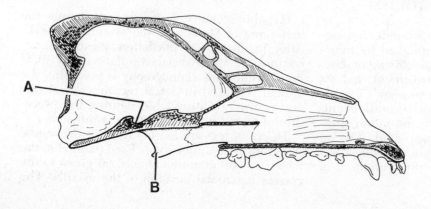

Figure 2. Sagittal section through a dolichocephalic skull, showing the pituitary fossa (*A*) in relation to the main landmark, the hamular process (*B*).

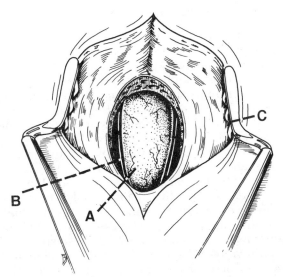

Figure 3. *A.* Pituitary gland covered by dura mater. *B.* Venous sinus. *C.* Wound retractor at the incised soft palate.

acetate*/kg body weight SC every six hours. (2) a broad-spectrum antibiotic, and (3) 3 to 5 IU Pitressin tannate† in oil SC immediately after surgery to control postoperative diabetes insipidus.

On the following days, (1) oral administration of cortisone‡ is started on the second day at a dose of 1 mg/kg every 12 hours if the animal will take it with food; otherwise, the SC administration of cortisol acetate every six hours must be continued; (2) the administration of antibiotics is continued for five days; (3) 48 hours after surgery the injection of Pitressin tannate is repeated, if necessary; and (4) thyroid replacement therapy is started by oral administration of 15 to 20 mg/kg desiccated thyroid§ or 15 to 20 μg/kg of L-thyroxin‖ once daily in the morning.

POSTOPERATIVE COURSE

The following problems may be encountered during the postoperative course: (1) The animals can develop upper respiratory dyspnea, apparently caused by swelling of the soft palate and the mucosa of the nasopharynx. In some cases tracheotomy is necessary. (2) Some dogs may have difficulty in swallowing, which can

delay the oral administration of medications for a few days.

MAINTENANCE THERAPY

At the time of discharge the following maintenance therapy is prescribed: 1 mg cortisone/kg, divided in two equal doses each day, and 15 to 20 mg desiccated thyroid/kg or 15 to 20 μg of L-thyroxin/kg daily.

The usual course of recovery includes a period of excessive skin scaling that occurs from three to eight weeks after the operation. The regrowth of the coat generally is darker than before. At the same time, an improvement in general condition becomes apparent, accompanied by the disappearance of polyphagia, polyuria, pendulous abdomen, and muscle weakness. The animal becomes livelier and, after a period of three months, becomes as normal as possible, relative to its age.

ADRENALECTOMY

With the dog in lateral recumbency and under the same anesthetic conditions as described for hypophysectomy, a paracostal skin incision 8 to 12 cm long is made parallel to and 1 cm caudal to the costal arch, starting just below the muscles of the back. The external and internal oblique abdominal muscles and the transverse abdominal muscle are incised in the same direction as the skin incision. This is followed by incision through the transverse fascia and the peritoneum.

The paracostal approach is preferred to the midline incision because it gives better access to the adrenal gland and prevents possible circulatory collapse, pancreatitis, and peritonitis that may result from unavoidable manipulation of the intestines. The disadvantage of this bilateral approach is that it is impossible to inspect both adrenals from one side, and both adrenals must be removed.

When the abdomen is opened the kidney becomes visible. On the *right* the kidney is displaced caudally only after incision of the hepatorenal ligament. The liver is gently pushed forward by the assistant, thereby exposing the right adrenal gland. The intestines are very carefully displaced in a caudal direction. The phrenicoabdominal vein is ligated at the medial and lateral sides of the gland with artery clamps,* and the adrenal is freed carefully from the surrounding tissues. Usually no special at-

*Hydro-adreson®, N. V. Organon, Oss, The Netherlands
†Pitressin tannate, Parke-Davis Company, Pontypool (UK)
‡Adreson®, N. V. Organon, Oss, the Netherlands
§Thyranon®, N. V. Organon, Oss, The Netherlands
‖Synthroid®, Flint Laboratories, Morton Grove, Illinois

*Ligaclips, Ethicon, Norderstedt, W. Germany

tention needs to be given to the blood supply. After removal of the adrenal it is sometimes necessary to control hemorrhage from one or two small vessels using an artery clamp.

Peritoneum, fascia, and muscles are closed with single sutures of non-absorbable material. The subcutaneous tissues are brought together with absorbable sutures. The skin wound is closed with single sutures of non-absorbable material.

The approach and surgical technique are almost identical for both adrenals. An important difference is that, on the left side, special attention must be given to careful displacement of the stomach and pancreas.

PRE- AND POSTOPERATIVE MEDICATION

The infusion system, which is also used for the measurement of central venous pressure, contains lactated Ringer's solution and 50 to 100 mg of cortisol.* This infusion runs for a period of approximately six hours. Following the removal of the first adrenal, 2 mg of cortisol acetate/kg is given SC. After removal of the second adrenal, a long-acting mineralocorticoid is given as a trimethyl acetate† depot of 25 mg SC. Finally, a broad-spectrum antibiotic is given. During the first 24 postoperative hours the IV infusions are continued and the same parameters are monitored as during the operation. Thereafter, monitoring of the patient is confined to the regular clinical and laboratory observations, including measurements of serum sodium and potassium. The cortisol administration is repeated every six hours.

During the first postoperative week, NaCl (2 to 8 grams per day) is administered orally in capsules. As soon as the animal takes food the glucocorticoid substitution is given orally at a rate of 2 mg/kg, divided in two daily doses.

MAINTENANCE THERAPY

One week after surgery the following maintenance therapy can be started: 1 mg/kg cortisone orally, divided in two daily doses,‡ 2 to 8 grams NaCl with food, and fluorohydrocortisone acetate,§ $1/16$ mg twice daily.

---

*Hydro-adreson Solutio Spirituosa Concentrata, N. V. Organon, Oss, The Netherlands

†Percorten M®, Ciba Ltd., Basel, Switzerland

‡*Editor's Note:* Some clinicians give short acting oral corticosteroids once daily in the morning to dogs and once daily in the evening to cats to mimic the patient's normal diurnal rhythm.

§Fluorhydrocortison®, Nogepha, Alkmaar, The Netherlands

CHEMOTHERAPY WITH o,p'-DDD

o,p'-DDD* is an adrenal cytotoxic agent that particularly affects the zona fasciculata and the zona reticularis, making it an effective agent for the treatment of glucocorticoid overproduction. However, impairment of mineralocorticoid production can also occur, resulting in an addisonion crisis. The schedule of treatment is as follows: 50 mg/kg is given for 10 to 14 consecutive days. To avoid corticosteroid withdrawal symptoms (anorexia and malaise), cortisone acetate is given simultaneously in a dosage of 1 mg/kg twice daily. With this regimen only occasional adverse effects, such as anorexia, nausea, vomiting, and diarrhea, make it necessary to stop the administration of o,p'-DDD. In these situations continuation of cortisone acetate supplementation is, of course, mandatory. Following this period of treatment, a maintenance dose of 50 mg/kg o,p'-DDD is given once every 7 to 14 days and is required indefinitely. The efficacy of this maintenance therapy can be judged by the water intake, other clinical signs, and laboratory parameters (e.g., alkaline phosphatase level). As with hypophysectomy and adrenalectomy, recovery is associated with excessive skin scaling and subsequent regrowth of hair (often darker). Complete recovery may also be obtained with this treatment.

COMMENT

Now that experience has been gained with all three treatments it is possible to indicate the treatment of choice, based upon the advantages and disadvantages of each:

1. During maintenance therapy with o,p'-DDD an animal may quite unexpectedly develop and possibly die from an addisonian crisis.

2. Some animals appear to be quite resistant to o,p'-DDD, and therefore the dosage frequently must be increased.

3. In adrenalectomized animals an occasional addisonian crisis may occur. This can be expected when the animal starts to refuse food and therefore also fails to receive the salt and corticosteroid substitute medication.

4. After one or more years both o,p'-DDD–treated animals and those that have had adrenalectomy may develop a pituitary tumor that grows to such an extent that neurologic signs develop.

5. Hypophysectomy has the advantages of preventing pituitary tumor growth and involv-

---

*Lysodren®, Calbio Pharmaceuticals. Div. of Calbiochem, La Jolla, California

ing simple substitution therapy almost without adjustments. The only disadvantage is that, in a minority of hypophysectomized animals, recovery from surgical damage to the pituitary stalk may take several weeks before the release of antidiuretic hormone is sufficient to allow normal urine output.

We feel that when the surgeon has developed sufficient experience with the technique, hypophysectomy is preferred.

ADRENOCORTICAL TUMOR

Once an autonomous hyperfunctioning adrenocortical tumor is suspected, the patient ideally should be investigated using scintigraphy with labeled cholesterol to locate the tumor. When the clinician does not have access to this technique, a laparotomy must be performed. The ventral midline approach will allow the inspection of both adrenals. However, the associated manipulation of the intestines may result in shock. Therefore, even in this case the paracostal approach is preferred. There is a risk that the wrong side may be opened first and an atrophic adrenal observed. In the majority of cases a tumor of approximately 3 to 5 cm in diameter is found. By meticulous preparation these neoplasms can usually be removed intact together with the atrophied remnant of the gland. The vessels are ligated with artery clamps, as in bilateral adrenalectomy.

In a minority of cases a large tumor that may have metastasized to the liver is observed. In these cases immediate euthanasia is recommended.

Medication during and immediately after the operation is the same as described for bilateral adrenalectomy, except that for obvious reasons there is no need to administer mineralocorticoids and sodium chloride. During the first week after surgery cortisone is administered orally at a rate of 1 mg/kg twice daily. Thereafter, the dosage is lowered to 1 mg/kg once daily for two weeks. After this period medication is continued for two more weeks at a rate of 1 mg/kg every other day. Thereafter medication is discontinued. This regimen is used to allow the hypothalamus-pituitary-adrenal system to recover from long-standing endogenous suppression by the hyperfunctioning adrenocortical tumor and to prevent the animal from a cortisol withdrawal syndrome (anorexia and malaise) immediately after surgery. It takes at least several weeks before the atrophied contralateral adrenal cortex can maintain eucorticism.

SUPPLEMENTAL READING

Johnston, D. E.: Adrenalectomy via retroperitoneal approach in dogs. J. Am. Vet. Med. Assoc., 170:1092, 1977.
Lubberink, A. A. M. E.: Diagnosis and Treatment of Canine Cushing's Syndrome. (Thesis). Drukkerij Elinkwijk, Utrecht, University of Utrecht, 1977.
Markowitz, J., Archibald, J., and Downie, H. G.: Hypophysectomy in dogs. In Experimental Surgery, 5th ed. Baltimore, Williams & Wilkins, 1964.
Schechter, R. D., Stabenfeldt, G. H., Gribbe, D. H., and Ling, G. V.: Treatment of Cushing's syndrome in the dog with an adrenocorticolytic agent (o,p'-DDD). J. Am. Vet. Med. Assoc., 162:629, 1973.
Siegel, E. T., Kelly, D. F., and Berg, P.: Cushing's syndrome in the dog. J. Am. Vet. Med. Assoc., 157:2081, 1970.

HYPOADRENOCORTICISM

MICHAEL SCHAER, D.V.M.
Gainesville, Florida

ETIOLOGY AND INCIDENCE

Primary hypoadrenocorticism, or Addison's disease, in the dog is a well-recognized clinical disorder. The principal gross pathologic finding is bilateral adrenal cortical atrophy, and the usual cause is listed as idiopathic. Although most dogs are found to have idiopathic hypo-adrenocorticism, adrenal insufficiency can also be a sequela of other conditions (Table 1).

There is no breed predilection for hypoadrenocorticism, but most cases reported in the veterinary literature involved female dogs five years old or younger. Adrenal insufficiency has occurred in dogs older than five.

Table 1. *Causes of Adrenal Insufficiency*

Anterior pituitary insufficiency (secondary Addison's disease)
Bilateral adrenalectomy
Mycotic or neoplastic adrenal infiltration
Adrenal thrombosis or hemorrhage
Acute withdrawal following prolonged glucocorticoid therapy
Treatment of Cushing's syndrome with *o,p'*-DDD

PATHOPHYSIOLOGY

The pathophysiologic effects result from decreased production of aldosterone, cortisol, and corticosterone from the adrenal cortex. Aldosterone is produced in the zona glomerulosa, and most of the glucocorticoids are synthesized in the zona fasciculata.

Aldosterone is a mineralocorticoid that is necessary for sodium and potassium homeostasis. Hypoaldosteronism results mainly in renal sodium wasting and potassium retention, causing hyponatremia and hyperkalemia. Other electrolyte imbalances occur, namely, hydrogen ion retention and chloride depletion. The consequences of hyponatremia and hyperkalemia are outlined in Table 2.

Among the numerous effects of glucocorticoid (cortisol and corticosterone) depletion are impaired gluconeogenesis and glycogenolysis, decreased sensitization of blood vessels to catecholamines, impaired excretion of water through the kidneys, decreased appetite, diminished stress tolerance, and decreased mentation characterized by depression.

CLINICAL SIGNS

The histories of dogs with adrenal insufficiency include acute onset of vomiting with or without diarrhea. Hematochezia is sometimes present. The appetite is markedly diminished or lost. Generalized weakness and severe mental depression soon accompany the gastrointestinal dysfunction.

In the acute form of Addison's disease these clinical signs are usually present for one to three days prior to presentation and are sometimes immediately preceded by stressful situations such as trauma. The physical findings of the acute addisonian crisis will vary with the severity of the condition (Table 3).

The historical findings of chronic adrenal insufficiency include gradual weight loss, diminished exercise tolerance, decreased appetite, muscle weakness, and occaisonal episodes of vomiting or diarrhea or both. These signs are usually present for weeks to months prior to examination (Table 3).

DIAGNOSIS

The clinical signs of depression, weakness, decreased appetite, and gastrointestinal dysfunction are compatible with other clinical disorders such as renal failure, exogenous intoxications, acute pancreatitis, and primary gastrointestinal disorders. Therefore, laboratory tests must be made to confirm a tentative clinical diagnosis of Addison's disease (Table 4). The most practical available laboratory findings include hyponatremia, hyperkalemia, and sodium:potassium ratio less than 25:1, and azotemia. The demonstration of these laboratory findings concomitant with appropriate historical and physical findings justifies immediate treatment for hypoadrenocorticism.

The electrocardiogram is of value in diagnosing Addison's disease (Fig. 1). When the serum potassium concentration exceeds 7.0 mEq/liter, certain electrocardiographic changes become apparent. These changes include PQRST wave alterations and arrhythmias. The electrocardiographic changes accompanying hyperkalemia include T wave elevation or depression, shortening and flattening of the P wave with an increased P–R interval, decreased R wave amplitude, diminished or absent P waves with bradycardia, and widening of the QRS complexes, resulting in a sine wave pattern. These myocardiotoxic effects can lead to ventricular fibrillation and cardiac arrest. Lead II is the usual reference lead. It should be noted that the toxic effects of hyperkalemia on the myocardium are more dramatic with concomitant severe hyponatremia (<132 mEq/liter).

The electrocardiogram is especially useful to the practitioner who is confronted with an animal in crisis when laboratory assistance is unavailable. When the history, physical findings, and electrocardiographic abnormalities are compatible with those of Addison's disease,

Table 2. *Effects of Hyponatremia and Hyperkalemia*

HYPONATREMIA	HYPERKALEMIA
Lethargy	Muscle weakness
Mental depression	Hyporeflexia
Nausea	Impaired cardiac conduction
Decreased blood pressure	
Impaired cardiac output	
Decreased renal perfusion	
Hypovolemic shock	

Table 3. *Physical Findings in Acute and Chronic Adrenal Insufficiency*

	ACUTE	CHRONIC
Temperature	Normal, decreased, or increased	Normal
Hydration	Dehydrated or normal	Usually normal
Attitude	Very depressed	Dull
Muscle strength	Profound weakness	Normal or slight weakness
Heart rate	Normal or arrhythmias	Normal or bradycardia
Respiration	Slow, rapid, or normal	Normal
Mucous membranes		
Color	Pink or hyperemic	Normal or slight pallor
Perfusion	Decreased	Normal

it is absolutely appropriate to commence therapy while awaiting the serum biochemical test results.

Radiography frequently demonstrates microcardia in addisonian dogs. This results from the severe hypotension associated with hyponatremia and plasma volume depletion.

TREATMENT OF THE ACUTE ADDISONIAN CRISIS

The acute addisonian crisis is a medical emergency requiring immediate therapy. The therapeutic objectives are (1) to increase plasma volume, (2) to correct hyponatremia and hyperkalemia, (3) to provide glucocorticoid, (4) to correct hypoglycemia, if present, and (5) to recognize and reverse severe cardiac arrhythmias.

An indwelling catheter should be inserted immediately into the jugular vein, using aseptic technique. The initial intravenous fluid of choice is isotonic 0.9 percent saline, which contains 154 mEq/liter of sodium and 154 mEq/liter of chloride. Five percent dextrose in 0.9 percent saline is a hypertonic solution and should not be used initially if the patient is dehydrated, for the solution will enhance volume depletion via osmotic diuresis. If hypoglycemia is present in a dehydrated dog at the time of admission, 50 percent dextrose solution can be given at a volume of 1 ml/kg over a five- to ten-minute period. If the dog is not dehydrated, 5 percent dextrose in 0.9 percent saline solution can also be used initially. The volume and rate of intravenous fluid administration necessary at the start of therapy depends on the degree of dehydration and hypotension. The clinically dehydrated and hypotensive dog should receive the fluids just described at a rate of 20 to 40 ml/kg body weight/hour during the first one to two hours of treatment. Because of the intolerance of the addisonian patient to acute water loading, care should be taken to avoid

Table 4. *Common Laboratory Findings in Canine Addison's Disease*

VALUE	FINDING
Serum potassium	Elevated (greater than 5.5 mEq/l)
Serum sodium	Decreased (less than 137 mEq/l)
Sodium:potassium ratio	Less than 25:1 (normal is 30:1)
Serum chloride	Usually less than 100 mEq/l
BUN	Elevated (can exceed 100 mg/dl)
Creatinine	Frequently elevated (can exceed 8 mg/dl)
Blood glucose	Normal or low
Blood lymphocyte count	Normal or elevated
Blood eosinophil count	Normal or elevated
Packed cell volume	Normal, increased, or decreased
Urine 17-ketogenic steroids	Usually less than 1.0 mg/24 hr in both primary and secondary adrenal insufficiency (normal is 1–4 mg/24 hr)
Urine 17-ketogenic steroids 24 hours after ACTH administration	No increase in primary adrenal insufficiency Slight increase in pituitary insufficiency
Resting plasma 11β-hydroxycorticosteroids	0.1–1.5 μg/dl in adrenal insufficiency
Plasma 11β-hydroxycorticosteroids 2 hours after ACTH gel intramuscularly	Minimal to no rise in primary adrenal insufficiency Greater than 2 μg/dl in secondary adrenal insufficiency

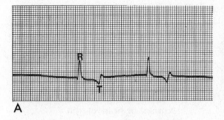 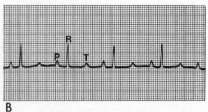

Figure 1. *A.* This electrocardiographic tracing is a lead II rhythm strip from a three-year-old male poodle in addisonian crisis (serum Na=110 mEq/liter; serum K=8.2 mEq/liter). Depicted is atrial standstill (bradycardia with no P waves) with a sinoventricular rhythm. The T waves are biphasic and large in amplitude and the R wave amplitude is small. *B.* Lead II electrocardiogram from the same dog two hours after treatment, illustrating restored sinus rhythm, decreased QT interval, decreased T wave amplitude, and normal R wave.

faster rates of fluid infusion. For the remaining 24-hour period, the isotonic saline is evenly administered at a rate of 50 to 60 ml/kg body weight. By the second treatment day, either 0.9 percent saline or 5 percent dextrose in 0.9 percent saline should be given intravenously at a volume of 50 to 60 ml/kg body weight distributed over a 24-hour period. The intravenous fluids are discontinued when hydration, urine output, serum sodium and potassium levels, and BUN levels are all restored to normal. These therapeutic goals are usually reached after 48 to 72 hours of treatment.

In addition to intravenous fluids, desoxycorticosterone acetate (Doca) should be given intramuscularly at admission. The mineralocorticoid action of this drug enhances renal sodium absorption and potassium excretion. The initial dose ranges from 1 mg for a very small dog to 5 mg for the giant breeds. This drug is given once intramuscularly every 24 hours. Daily in-hospital monitoring of serum electrolyte concentrations is important to avoid iatrogenic hypokalemia due to administration of excess mineralocorticoid.

The rapid intravenous injection of a soluble glucocorticoid is important initially. Prednisolone sodium succinate* is the drug of choice, administered at a dose of 50 to 300 mg, proportional to the size of the dog, during the first hour of therapy. Subsequent glucocorticoid therapy should entail the intramuscular injection of prednisone or prednisolone at a dose of 1 mg/kg body weight every 12 hours. By the third or fourth hospital day the glucocorticoid dose should be reduced to 0.25 to 0.5 mg/kg body weight every 12 hours.

TREATMENT OF HYPERKALEMIC MYOCARDIAL TOXICITY

At serum concentrations higher than 7 mEq/liter, potassium causes progressive depression of excitability and conduction velocity of the myocardium. This occurs because of lowering of the myocardial cell resting membrane potential, which results in a depolarization block.

The early electrocardiographic changes caused by mild to moderate degrees of hyperkalemia (6.5 to 7.5 mEq/liter) include peaking of the T wave and shortening and widening of the P wave. These changes will resolve spontaneously from the combined effects of intravenous saline and intramuscular Doca. However, the electrocardiogram should be repeated in two to four hours to confirm resolution of the abnormal complexes.

The electrocardiographic changes caused by severe hyperkalemia (>7.5 mEq/liter) include disappearance of the P wave, widening of the QRS complex with irregular R–R intervals, and sine wave–type QRS complexes. These changes denote severe myocardial toxicity and frequently require additional measures combined with intravenous saline and intramuscular Doca. These measures include (1) intravenous 10 percent calcium gluconate at a rate of 0.5 to 1.0 ml/kg body weight; it should be administered slowly over a 10- to 20-minute period, accompanied by careful electrocardiographic monitoring; or (2) intravenous sodium bicarbonate administered at a dosage of 1 to 2 mEq/kg over a 15-minute period; or (3) intravenous regular crystalline insulin administered at a dosage of 0.5 unit/kg body weight along with 2 to 3 grams dextrose/unit of insulin. Care should be taken to avoid hypoglycemia because patients with adrenal insufficiency are known to be sensitive to insulin.

These emergency treatments can be given either singly or in combination. (Calcium gluconate should not be mixed in a syringe or infusion bottle with sodium bicarbonate because a precipitate forms.) Frequent electrocardiographic monitoring should be performed until the electrocardiogram rhythm and complexes return to normal. These emergency measures usually are required only once and need not be repeated (Fig. 2).

---

*Solu-delta-Cortef, Upjohn Co., Kalamazoo, Michigan 49001

Figure 2. *A.* This electro-cardiographic tracing is a lead II rhythm strip from an eight-year-old female mixed-breed dog in addisonian crisis (serum Na = 122 mEq/liter; serum K = 8.5 mEq/liter). Depicted is complete heart block (more P waves than QRS complexes with no association). *B.* Lead II electro-

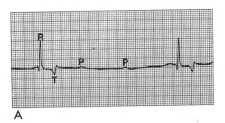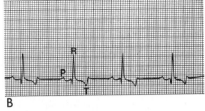

cardiogram from the same dog three hours after treatment with Doca, intravenous saline, calcium gluconate, bicarbonate, and insulin-dextrose, illustrating return of normal sinus rhythm.

TREATMENT OF CHRONIC ADDISON'S DISEASE

Unless a chronic situation characterized by collapse, hypotension, severe azotemia, and cardiac arrhythmias prevails, the therapeutic approach for the patient with chronic adrenal insufficiency is less intense than those methods just described. Saline solution should be administered intravenously if the serum sodium concentration is less than 135 mEq/liter or the BUN level is greater than 60 to 70 mg/dl. If the serum sodium and potassium and BUN levels are not seriously abnormal, Doca is given intramuscularly at a dose of 1.0 to 5.0 mg once daily, and prednisolone (or prednisone) is administered in a divided dose of 2 mg/kg/day, orally or intramuscularly. In addition, the diet should be supplemented with oral sodium chloride at a dose of 1 to 5 grams daily, proportional to the size of the patient. The dog is usually ready to be discharged after 48 hours of in-hospital treatment.

HOME THERAPY FOR ADDISON'S DISEASE

Sodium chloride tablets should be given orally every day at a dose of 1 to 5 grams. These tablets are usually available in a 0.5 gram size.

Daily mineralocorticoid treatment is necessary for dogs. Fluorocortisone acetate† is available in 0.1 mg tablets. The small dog (5 to 10 kg or less) should initially receive 1 tablet daily; the medium-sized dog (10 to 25 kg) should initially receive 1.5 to 3 tablets daily, and the large breeds (over 25 kg) should receive 3 to 5 tablets daily. The dog should have serum sodium and potassium determinations every one to two weeks in order to make the proper dosage adjustments. Once normal serum electrolyte levels are achieved, periodic outpatient check-ups should be scheduled every four to six months. Some patients acquire decreased sensitivity to fludrocortisone acetate, necessitating dosage adjustments.

If the owner is unable to administer the daily mineralocorticoid tablet faithfully, desoxycorticosterone pivilate‡ can be administered intramuscularly every three to four weeks. The average dose is 25 to 75 mg intramuscularly, proportional to the patient's size, every four weeks. The initial dose is 25 mg of desoxycorticosterone pivilate intramuscularly for every 1 mg of desoxycorticosterone acetate required daily for in-hospital correction of the initial electrolyte imbalance. When desoxycorticosterone pivilate is substituted for fludrocortisone acetate tablets, the animal requires 25 mg intramuscularly for every 0.1 mg tablet of fludrocortisone acetate.

In addition to the mineralocorticoid preparations, desoxycorticosterone acetate pellets (125 mg)§ have been used successfully for dogs with adrenal insufficiency. The pellets should be inserted subcutaneously under strict surgical aseptic conditions. The initial dose is 1 pellet (125 mg) for each 0.5 mg of desoxycorticosterone acetate injectable required for in-hospital maintenance. Each 125 mg pellet releases an amount equivalent to approximately 0.5 mg Doca per day. The pellets are effective for a six- to ten-month period. Overdosage with Doca pellets, resulting in hypokalemia, has been observed. The author prefers to use fludrocortisone acetate tablets or desoxycorticosterone pivilate rather than pellet implantation, because the tablets are easy to administer and amenable to dosage correction.

Canine patients with adrenal insufficiency usually do well with oral sodium chloride tablets and mineralocorticoid treatment, which are required as lifelong therapy. Glucocorticoids usually are not required for home maintenance treatment. However, occasionally, the owner will report that the dog is sluggish and has a

---

†Florinef Acetate. Squibb and Sons, Princeton, New Jersey 08540.

‡Percorten Pivilate, CIBA Pharmaceutical Co., Summit, New Jersey 07901

§Percorten Acetate pellets, CIBA Pharmaceutical Co., Summit, NJ 07901

poor appetite despite normal serum electrolyte levels. When this situation arises, daily lifelong glucocorticoid treatment is also required. Cortisone acetate tablets (5 mg, 10 mg, and 25 mg)* at a dosage of 1 to 2 mg/kg body weight should be administered daily in the morning. Prednisolone or prednisone tablets at a rate of 0.2 to 0.4 mg/kg body weight/day can also be used.

During periods of surgical or traumatic stress or stress resulting from infections, clinicians should be aware that large supplemental doses of parenteral glucocorticoids are mandatory to avoid a precipitous addisonian crisis. The prognosis for a dog with Addison's disease is ex-

cellent. The patient can be expected to have a normal life span as long as its endocrine disorder is properly monitored and adequately treated.

---

*Cortisone Acetate tablets, Upjohn Co., Kalamazoo, Michigan 49001

SUPPLEMENTAL READINGS

Ettinger, P. O., et al.: Hyperkalemia, cardiac conduction, and the electrocardiogram: A review. Am. Heart J., 88:360, 1974.
Forsham, P. H.: The adrenal cortex. In Williams, R. H. (ed.): Textbook of Endocrinology, 5th ed. Philadelphia, W. B. Saunders Co., 1974.
Himathongkam, T., Newmark, S. R., Greenfield, M., et al.: Acute adrenal insufficiency. JAMA, 230:1317, 1974.
Levinsky, N. G.: Management of emergencies. VI. Hyperkalemia. N. Engl. J. Med., 274:1076, 1966.
Mulnix, J. A.: Hypoadrenocorticism in the dog. J. Am. Hosp. Assoc., 7:220, 1971.
Surawicz, B.: Electrolytes and the electrocardiogram. Postgrad. Med., 55:123, 1974.

SYSTEMIC GLUCOCORTICOID THERAPY

DANNY W. SCOTT, D.V.M.

Ithaca, New York

Glucocorticoids are probably the most used and abused drugs in veterinary medicine. The reasons for frequent use are readily understood. There is probably no organ system in the body that does not suffer from one or many diseases that require glucocorticoids for their proper management. On the other hand, abuse of these drugs is usually attributable to ignorance and neglect.

EFFECTS OF GLUCOCORTICOIDS

ANTI-INFLAMMATORY AND ANTIALLERGIC ACTIONS

Glucocorticoids non-specifically inhibit the inflammatory effects of many noxious agents, including microorganisms, chemical or thermal irritants, trauma, and allergens. The anti-inflammatory actions of glucocorticoids include (1) maintenance of cellular membrane integrity and (2) stabilization of the membranes of the intracellular lysosomes, which contain hydrolytic enzymes capable of cell digestion and extension of inflammatory tissue damage. The fibroblastic proliferation, which follows inflam-

mation as part of the reparative process and tends to localize infection, is greatly reduced and thus may potentiate the spread of an infection. However, this action is beneficial in preventing the adverse consequences of excessive fibrosis and scarring.

IMMUNOSUPPRESSIVE ACTIONS

Various facets of the immune system are affected by glucocorticoids: (1) macrophages and monocytes (because of depression of phagocytosis, chemotactic responses, processing of antigens, and influx from peripheral blood to sites of inflammation), (2) lymphocytes (because these drugs are lymphocytolytic), (3) neutrophils (because of depression of phagocytosis, intracellular killing, chemotactic responses, and influx from peripheral blood to sites of inflammation), (4) humoral antibodies (because of decreased synthesis), and (5) complement (through inhibition of several major subfractions of the complement system).

It is apparent that glucocorticoids suppress the specific and non-specific immune responses. It is not suprising, then, to find that humans and dogs with hyperadrenocorticism (naturally occurring or iatrogenic) have a high incidence of secondary bacterial infections (especially those of the urinary tract, respiratory tract, and skin). The critical consideration is that these infections can be present without any significant physical or laboratory abnormalities (e.g., without pyrexia, pain, or leukocytosis) because of the potent non-specific, anti-inflammatory properties of the glucocorticoids.

Another important consideration concerning the immunosuppressive side effects of glucocorticoids (in addition to the increased susceptibility to infection) is the possibility of increased incidence of neoplasia. People receiving long-term glucocorticoid therapy have a higher incidence of various types of cancer.

CARBOHYDRATE, PROTEIN, AND LIPID METABOLISM

Glucocorticoids promote gluconeogenesis through peripheral and hepatic actions. Physical and laboratory abnormalities that might be expected to arise from these actions include:

1. Skeletal muscle wasting and weakness (protein catabolism).
2. Hepatomegaly (fatty infiltration).
3. Fat redistribution (peripheral fat pads, liver, omentum).
4. Thin, hypotonic, alopecic skin, with poor wound healing and easy bruising (protein catabolism, inhibition of fibroblast proliferation and collagen deposition, increased vascular fragility).
5. Lameness, bone pain, and pathologic fractures (osteoporosis and osteomalacia due to protein catabolism, decreased intestinal absorption of calcium, inhibition of vitamin D activity, increased calcium resorption from bone, increased renal excretion of calcium, inhibition of osteoblast activity).
6. Lipemia and hypercholesterolemia (fat mobilization).
7. Hyperglycemia (rarely, overt diabetes mellitus, usually developing in patients with pre-existing latent diabetes).

WATER AND ELECTROLYTE BALANCE

In man practically all glucocorticoids tend to cause hypokalemia by increasing urinary losses of potassium. The author has not seen hypokalemia in dogs with naturally occurring or iatrogenic hyperadrenocorticism or in any dog treated with long-term glucocorticoid therapy.

Again in man, sodium retention is potentiated slightly or moderately by natural glucocorticoids (hydrocortisone, corticosterone) and negligibly by most synthetic glucocorticoids (prednisone, prednisolone, dexamethasone), while a few glucocorticoids actually enhance sodium excretion (triamcinolone, betamethasone, methylprednisolone). The author has not observed changes in serum sodium concentration in dogs with endogenous or exogenous hyperadrenocorticism.

Glucocorticoids increase free water clearance and promote water excretion in man and dog. This is recognized clinically as polyuria and polydipsia. The author has never recognized glucocorticoid-induced polydipsia and polyuria in cats and was unable to produce it in laboratory cats using either 5.5 mg/kg methylprednisolone acetate subcutaneously, once a week for four weeks, or 6.6 mg/kg prednisolone orally, once a day for eight weeks. Although the exact mechanisms of increased free water clearance and promotion of water excretion in man and dog are not completely understood, current knowledge suggests (1) increased glomerular filtration rate, (2) inhibition of antidiuretic hormone (ADH) release or action, and (3) direct action on the renal tubules.

GASTROINTESTINAL EFFECTS

Glucocorticoids (except for triamcinolone) enhance the appetite, which is manifested clinically as polyphagia and weight gain. The author has occasionally seen anorexia in association with glucocorticoid therapy. Glucocorticoids also increase gastric acid and pepsin secretion while decreasing the rate of gastric mucosal cell proliferation. This may predispose the animal to gastric ulcers. The author has also seen a few dogs and cats that were receiving prednisolone therapy develop diarrhea (often bloody, with large-bowel signs predominating). The diarrhea was resolved 48 to 72 hours after therapy was withdrawn.

An association between glucocorticoid therapy and pancreatitis in humans has long been appreciated. Glucocorticoids promote increased viscosity of pancreatic secretions and hyperplasia of pancreatic ductal epithelium. The author knows of four dogs (two of which later died) that developed acute pancreatitis while receiving glucocorticoid therapy.

Recently it has been reported that excessive amounts of endogenous or exogenous glucocorticoids may be associated with hepatopathy characterized by hepatomegaly, elevated serum enzyme levels, increased Bromsulphalein (BSP) retention, centrilobular vacuolization, perivacuolar glycogen accumulation within hepatocytes, and focal centrilobular necrosis.

NEUROLOGIC EFFECTS

Glucocorticoids are thought to promote a normal psyche. Psychologic abnormalities (behavioral and mood changes, psychoses, depression, mania, and others) are common in people receiving glucocorticoid therapy. The author has witnessed similar reactions in dogs and cats. Cats become depressed or prefer seclusion or both. Dogs may become irritable and sometimes vicious, or depressed and lethargic, or they may pant excessively. Dogs may also become "hair pullers" or "flank suckers." In man glucocorticoids also increase cerebral cortical irritability, especially in patients with underlying tendencies to a seizure disorder.

HEMATOLOGIC EFFECTS

Glucocorticoids classically produce leukocytosis (neutrophilia), eosinopenia, lymphopenia, and lesser degrees of erythrocytosis and thrombocytosis. These findings are inconsistent clinically in man, dog, and cat. The frequency of hematologic abnormalities in dogs with naturally occurring hyperadrenocorticism varies as follows: leukocytosis and neutrophilia (25 to 60 percent of cases), lymphopenia (33 to 70 percent), and eosinopenia (76 to 95 percent). The author has injected normal cats with 5.5 mg/kg methylprednisolone subcutaneously, once weekly, and then took hemograms. Neutrophilia, lymphopenia, and eosinopenia were noted in 50 percent, 25 percent, and 50 percent, respectively, of these cats.

BIOCHEMICAL EFFECTS

Serum chemistry abnormalities associated with exogenous or endogenous hyperglucocorticoidism in the dog may include mild to marked elevations in cholesterol (56 to 88 percent of cases), SGPT (52 to 90 percent), SGOT (30 to 50 percent), serum alkaline phosphatase (SAP) (80 to 95 percent), serum lactic dehydrogenase (SLDH) (50 percent), serum creatine phosphokinase (SCPK) (50 percent), and glucose (10 to 50 percent) and decreased BUN levels (30 percent). Serum electrolyte levels (sodium, potassium, chloride, calcium, phosphorus) are almost always normal. Cellulose acetate electrophoresis has demonstrated that the major isoenzyme of SAP that increased in canine hyperglucocorticoidism is steroid-induced and probably hepatic in origin.

In the methylprednisolone-treated cats referred to previously, serum glucose and cholesterol were elevated in 75 percent of cases, but the elevations were mild. Elevations in SAP were *not* seen in any cats.

ENDOCRINE EFFECTS

Baseline thyroid hormone levels are usually low in humans and dogs with exogenous or endogenous hyperglucocorticoidism. Thyroid hormone responses to exogenous thyrotropin (TSH) may be suppressed. High levels of glucocorticoids have been shown to induce a number of defects in thyroid physiology, including (1) suppression of hypothalamic thyrotropin-releasing hormone (TRH) and/or pituitary TSH release or action, (2) suppression of thyroid-binding globulin (TBG) synthesis, and (3) suppression of peripheral conversion of thyroxine (T_4) to triiodothyronine (T_3). It is therefore imperative to remember that "hypothyroid" thyroid function test results are to be expected in patients with hyperglucocorticoidism and that these patients are invariably euthyroid and require no thyroid hormone replacement therapy.

IATROGENIC HYPERADRENOCORTICISM (CUSHING'S SYNDROME)

Iatrogenic hyperadrenocorticism has been described frequently in both man and dog. The incidence of this unfortunate entity is definitely on the rise. Of 48 cases of canine hyperadrenocorticism managed by the author over a three-year period, 25 (52 percent) were iatrogenic in origin. The marked increase in incidence may be related to the emergence of newer, more potent glucocorticoids, especially the repositol injectable forms. The historoclinical findings are the same as those for naturally occurring hyperadrenocorticism (discussed elsewhere in this text). Apparently there is individual variation both in susceptibility to the adverse effects of glucocorticoid therapy and in the clinical signs manifested. The author has seen all combinations of clinical signs, from classic hyperadrenocorticism to calcinosis cutis. Cats appear to be more resistant to many of the various side effects of exogenous glucocorticoids than dogs and humans are. Iatrogenic hyperadrenocorticism has not been reported in the cat, and the author did not recognize physical signs of hyperadrenocorticism in the methylprednisolone-treated cats mentioned previously.

Laboratory findings in iatrogenic hyperadrenocorticism are quite variable. The classic findings of naturally occurring hyperadrenocorticism have already been described.

Diagnosis is based on historoclinical findings and the results of adrenocorticotropic hormone (ACTH) response tests. The ACTH response test *may* differentiate between naturally occurring hyperadrenocorticism due to adrenocortical hyperplasia (normal or elevated resting plasma cortisol level, with exaggerated response) or adrenocortical neoplasia (high normal to elevated resting plasma cortisol levels, with little or no response) and iatrogenic hyperadrenocorticism (low or normal resting plasma cortisol level, with no response). Frequently, adrenocortical tumors will give normal or hyperplastic ACTH responses. Table 1 includes the historoclinical data on seven cases of iatrogenic hyperadrenocorticism seen by the author in one year. Different glucocorticoids, given in varying doses by various routes and for varying periods of time, can cause disease. This emphasizes the individual differences that exist among dogs that have adverse reactions to glucocorticoids.

Treatment requires cessation of *excessive* glucocorticoids while continuing maintenance and stress therapy for the concomitant secondary adrenocortical insufficiency (see following discussion).

IATROGENIC SECONDARY ADRENOCORTICAL INSUFFICIENCY

The most occult yet most critical and life-threatening side effect of glucocorticoid therapy is *iatrogenic secondary adrenocortical insuffi-*

ciency. The primary abnormality is a lack of endogenous ACTH. The function of the zona glomerulosa of the adrenal cortex, which is dependent on the renin-angiotensin-aldosterone system and not on ACTH, is preserved. Thus the electrolyte disturbances associated with mineralocorticoid deficiency and classic hypoadrenocorticism (Addison's disease) are not seen. However, as long as glucocorticoid secretory capacity is suppressed the patient is extremely vulnerable to acute glucocorticoid insufficiency and circulatory collapse.

Patients receiving therapeutic doses of glucocorticoids develop ACTH insufficiency with secondary adrenocortical insufficiency in two ways: (1) when long-term exogenous glucocorticoid therapy is suddenly withdrawn and (2) when patients receiving long-term (low or high dose) glucocorticoid therapy are acutely stressed, e.g., by infection, trauma, surgery, or pregnancy. Thus, under normal conditions these patients usually do well, but under stress they cannot respond with adequate endogenous glucocorticoids.

All glucocorticoids suppress the release of corticotropin-releasing factor (CRF) from the

Table 1. *Historoclinical Data on 7 Dogs With Iatrogenic Hyperadrenocorticism and Secondary Adrenocortical Insufficiency*

BREED	AGE (Years)	SEX	STEROID THERAPY RECEIVED	HISTOROCLINICAL FINDINGS	LABORATORY ABNORMALITIES	ACTH RESPONSE TEST ($\mu g/dl$)°	
						Pre	*Post*
xer	8	M	40 mg repositol methylprednisolone IM, monthly for 7.5 years	Iatrogenic hyperadrenocorticism; acute collapse and shock	Eosinopenia and lymphopenia	4	6
ston errier	2	Fs	2.5 mg prednisolone PO, b.i.d. for 4 months	Polyuria, polydipsia, polyphagia, acute collapse and shock	—	0	2
g	6	Fs	2.5 mg prednisolone PO, s.i.d. for 3.5 years	Calcinosis cutis	—	2	4
sh etter	3	F	5 mg prednisolone PO, s.i.d. for 1 year	Iatrogenic hyperadrenocorticism; episodic weakness and lethargy	—	2	2
rman hepherd	9	Fs	40 mg repositol methylprednisolone IM every 1 to 2 months for 6 years	Iatrogenic hyperadrenocorticism, calcinosis cutis	—	4	5
sset ound	8	Fs	10 mg hydrocortisone PO, t.i.d. for 2 months	Calcinosis cutis	—	2	1
g	3	M	0.9 mg betamethasone IM, monthly for 3 months	Calcinosis cutis; iatrogenic hyperadrenocorticism; episodic weakness and anorexia	—	6	6

°ACTH response test: pre-ACTH blood sample, followed by 40 units ACTH gel IM, then post-ACTH blood sample in 2 hours. Plasma rtisol levels determined fluorimetric assay: normal dog = 5–10 $\mu g/dl$ resting and 10–20 $\mu g/dl$ post-ACTH.

hypothalamus and of ACTH from the pituitary. Suppression of the hypothalamic-pituitary-adrenal (HPA) axis is related to (1) the glucocorticoid being used, (2) the dose, (3) the duration of therapy, and (4) the route of administration (the parenteral route causes the greatest suppression, followed in order of decreasing action by the oral route and topical application).

Prolonged exposure to exogenous or endogenous glucocorticoids in quantities sufficient to cause signs of hyperadrenocorticism consistently causes suppression of CRF-ACTH release and consequent adrenocortical atrophy. So, ironically, an individual may simultaneously present with evidence of hyper- and hypo-adrenocorticism (see Table 1). The crucial factor to remember is that, if the dog has received enough glucocorticoids to show signs of hyperadrenocorticism, it must automatically have secondary adrenocortical insufficiency also. Even though cats are apparently quite resistant to the development of iatrogenic hyperadrenocorticism, they are quite susceptible to iatrogenic secondary adrenocortical insufficiency. In methylprednisolone-treated cats suppression of ACTH-responsiveness was detectable within one week and severe within four weeks.

Diagnosis is based on historoclinical findings, ACTH response test, plasma cortisol response to insulin-induced hypoglycemia, and radioimmunoassay for plasma ACTH (the last two tests are not being used at present in the dog). It should be emphasized that the characteristic serum electrolyte changes and resultant electrocardiographic abnormalities seen with naturally occurring hypoadrenocorticism are not found, because the mineralocorticoid secretion is intact.

When glucocorticoid therapy is withdrawn, patients will be susceptible to HPA insufficiency for several months. In man it is advisable to administer appropriate doses of glucocorticoids for daily maintenance and stress for at least *one year* after any course of glucocorticoid therapy that has lasted longer than three months.

From studies on carbohydrate metabolism in dogs after adrenalectomy it can be recommended that a daily maintenance dose of 0.2 to 0.5 mg/kg hydrocortisone be administered orally every morning between 7 and 10 A.M. Hydrocortisone is the glucocorticoid of choice for replacement therapy. For glucocorticoid replacement, it is necessary to mimic the normal diurnal or circadian cortisol secretory pattern (see following discussion).

During periods of stress it is necessary to increase the dose of hydrocortisone in order to mimic the normal patient with a normal HPA axis. Thus, for minor stresses cortisol production may increase two- to four-fold, whereas in major stresses cortisol production may increase 10- to 25-fold.

In treatment of secondary adrenocortical insufficiency due to exogenous glucocorticoids, one can anticipate the eventual return of normal HPA function. Only rarely is the adrenocortical atrophy irreversible. However, HPA insufficiency may persist more than a year. In man the return of HPA function is detected by evaluation of radioimmunoassay tests for plasma ACTH or by plasma cortisol response to insulin-induced hypoglycemia. However, these procedures are not available for animals at present. Thus, it is safest to follow the previously mentioned rule of thumb used in human medicine —continue maintenance and stress therapy with hydrocortisone for one year. The author has followed up several dogs with iatrogenic secondary adrenocortical insufficiency, using monthly ACTH response tests. In general, ACTH response tests have returned to normal in three months. Perhaps the biologically "faster-living" dog recovers HPA function more rapidly than humans do.

The usefulness of ACTH therapy, aimed at restoring the mass and functional capacity of the adrenal glands, has been widely debated and is open to considerable doubt, since the most obstinate block after prolonged glucocorticoid therapy is *not* at the level of the adrenocortical responses to ACTH but in the ability to the HP unit to resume release of adequate amounts of CRF-ACTH. This block cannot be corrected and, in fact, is probably worsened by the use of ACTH. Therefore, ACTH should *not* be used in secondary adrenocortical insufficiency.

ALTERNATE-DAY STEROID THERAPY

Many attempts have been made to decrease the side effects of glucocorticoid therapy. Changes in molecular structure, concomitant ACTH administration, the use of shorter-acting glucocorticoids, a reduction in total daily dose regimens, and modification of therapy to an intermittent basis have all been tried but have been unsuccessful. For instance, if oral prednisolone is given for three consecutive days of a week and then omitted for the remaining four days, the HPA axis will not be protected.

The critical factor in long-term glucocorticoid therapy is maintenance of the normal diurnal or circadian cortisol secretory pattern. This diurnal rhythm has been described for man and dog and appears to be determined by the hypothalamus. Plasma cortisol levels are highest in the morning (7 to 10 A.M.) and lowest at night (10 P.M. to 12 A.M.). Plasma ACTH levels vary inversely with plasma cortisol. Blood cortisol studies in the cat have revealed a circadian rhythm that is the reverse of that in humans and dogs; i.e., cortisol levels are highest at night and lowest in the morning.

The alternate-day steroid (ADS) regimen has been developed to preserve the normal diurnal cortisol rhythm and thus to avoid HPA suppression. It has been shown that certain oral glucocorticoids can be administered to dogs once every other morning, when plasma cortisol is normally highest and ACTH release is already inhibited by natural negative feedback. This usually still affords control of symptoms on the "off" days but allows the HPA axis to function normally. The only oral glucocorticoids that can be used in this manner are prednisone, prednisolone, and methylprednisolone. Hydrocortisone and cortisone allow HPA function on the off days but often do not control symptoms. ADS therapy in cats should be administered every other evening.

If long-term glucocorticoid therapy is indicated, the ADS regimen should be used whenever possible, since it is the only safe regimen available at present. The author has at this time about 300 dogs on ADS. Some have been medicated for periods of up to five years with no untoward side effects. These dogs have not developed signs or laboratory abnormalities suggestive of either iatrogenic hyperadrenocorticism or secondary adrenocortical insuffi-ciency. Occasional side effects noted by the owners have included polyphagia and/or polyuria on the day of glucocorticoid administration. Extreme polydispsia, polyuria, polyphagia, and weight gain have not been reported. Occasionally ADS will not be successful. This is particularly true in some autoimmune disorders (autoimmune hemolytic anemia, immune-mediated thrombocytopenia, systemic lupus erythematosus, pemphigus, pemphigoid). In man, some individuals will become cushingoid or develop HPA suppression on ADS. This is thought to reflect differences in the metabolism of glucocorticoids in the individuals. The author's present ADS regimen for the dog is as follows:

1. Five to seven days of induction (½ to 1 mg/kg prednisolone orally, twice daily). Daily induction therapy is recommended, because ADS is better at maintaining remissions than inducing them.

2. Then, 1 to 2 mg/kg prednisolone orally, every other morning between 7 and 10 A.M.

3. After that, the ADS dosage is reduced by 50 percent, at weekly intervals, until the lowest maintenance dose is determined. This maintenance dose varies considerably from dog to dog, but usually averages ½ mg/kg every other morning.

4. In cats ADS should be administered every other evening between 10 P.M. and midnight.

ADS is intended for maintenance therapy. Its purpose is to lessen side effects, especially HPA suppression, it is not intended to permit or

Table 2. *Characteristics of Pharmaceutical Derivatives of Adrenocorticosteroids for Oral Administration*

DRUG	GLUCOCORTICOID POTENCY*	MINERALOCORTICOID POTENCY	HPA-SUPPRESSIVE† ACTIVITY	SUITABLE FOR ADS‡	EQUIVALENT DOSE IN MG
Short-acting					
Hydrocortisone	1.0	++	+	No	20
Cortisone	0.8	++	+	No	25
Prednisolone	4.0	+	+	Yes	5
Prednisone	4.0	+	+	Yes	5
Methylprednisolone	5.0	0	+	Yes	4
Intermediate-acting					
Triamcinolone	5.0	0	++	No	4
Paramethasone	10.0	0	++	No	2
Fluprednisolone	10.0	0	++	No	2
Long-acting					
Dexamethasone	30.0	0	+++	No	0.75
Betamethasone	30.0	0	+++	No	0.60
Fludrocortisone	15.0	++++	+++	No	1.5

*Compared with hydrocortisone on a mg-for-mg basis
†HPA = Hypothalamic-pituitary-adrenal
‡ADS = Alternate-day steroid therapy

encourage indiscriminate use of glucocorticoids. The general principles of glucocorticoid therapy must *always* be enforced:

1. Use glucocorticoid therapy only when a diagnosis has been established and after less harmful forms of therapy have failed.

2. Use the smallest therapeutically effective dose.

Parentral sustained-release glucocorticoid preparations are unphysiologic, unnecessary, undesirable, and in most instances contraindicated in clinical medicine. These preparations are absolutely contraindicated when long-term symptomatic therapy is needed.

Table 2 summarizes the characteristics of some oral adrenocorticosteroids.

SUPPLEMENTAL READING

Axelrod, L.: Glucocorticoid therapy. Medicine, 55:39–65, 1976.
Berlinger, F.G.: Use and misuse of steroids. Postgrad. Med., 55:153–157, 1974.
Bondy, P.K.: The adrenal cortex. In Bondy, P.K., and Rosenburg, L.E. (eds.): *Duncan's Diseases of Metabolism*, 7th ed. Philadelphia, W.B. Saunders Co., 1974, pp. 1105–1180.
Fauci, A.S., Dale, D.C., and Balow, J.W.: Glucocorticoid therapy: Mechanisms of action and clinical consideration. Ann. Intern. Med., 84:304–315, 1976.
Fine, R.M.: Physiologic effects of systemic corticosteroids in dermatology. Cutis, 11:217–226, 1973.
Frawely, T.F.: Corticosteroid therapy: Updating of principles. Postgrad. Med., 56:123–129, 1974.
Liddle, G.W.: The adrenal steroids and their functions. In Beeson, P.B., and McDermott, W. (eds): *Textbook of Medicine*, 14th ed. Philadelphia, W.B. Saunders Co., 1975, pp. 1722–1752.
Sayers, G., and Travis, R.H.: Adrenocorticotropic hormone, adrenocortical steroids and their synthetic analogs. In Goodman, L.S. and Gilman, A. (eds.): *The Pharmacologic Basis of Therapeutics*, 4th ed. New York, Macmillan Co., 1970, pp. 1604–1642.
Scott, D.W.: Hyperadrenocorticism (hyperadrenocorticoidism, hyperadrenocorticalism, Cushing's disease, Cushing's syndrome). Vet. Clin. North Am. 9:3–28, 1979.
Scott, D.W., and Greene, C.E.: Iatrogenic secondary adrenocortical insufficiency in dogs. J. Am. Anim. Hosp. Assoc., 10:555–564, 1974.
Scott, D.W., Kirk, R.W., and Bentinck-Smith, J.: Some effects of short-term methylprednisolone therapy in normal cats. Cornell Vet., 69:104–115, 1979.
Streeten, D.H.P.: Corticosteroid therapy. I. Pharmacological properties and principles of corticosteroid use. JAMA, 232:944–947, 1975.
Streeten, D.H.P.: Corticosteroid therapy. II. Complications and therapeutic indications. JAMA, 232:1046–1049, 1975.

HYPOTHYROIDISM

BRUCE E. BELSHAW, D.V.M.,
and AD RIJNBERK, D.V.M.
Utrecht, the Netherlands

Hypothyroidism is the generalized metabolic disease resulting from deficiency of the thyroid hormones thyroxine (T_4) and triiodothyronine (T_3). This discussion is concerned with hypothyroidism in dogs, for we are aware of no convincingly documented reports of its spontaneous occurrence in cats. Canine hypothyroidism is usually primary, i.e., due to atrophy of the thyroid gland. In the majority of cases the atrophy is associated with lymphocytic thyroiditis, and in the remainder it is non-inflammatory and of as yet unknown etiology. Less than 10 percent of our cases of hypothyroidism are secondary, i.e., due to deficiency of thyroid-stimulating hormone (TSH). TSH deficiency may occur as a component of congenital hypopituitarism or as an acquired disorder in adult dogs, in which case it is invariably due to the growth of a pituitary tumor. Hypothyroidism due to congenital defects in thyroid hormone synthesis is quite rare in the dog, and severe iodine-deficiency hypothyroidism is now virtually unknown in countries in which commercial dog foods are used.

Primary hypothyroidism is rarely observed in dogs less than two years of age or in the toy breeds. The disease develops insidiously, and no consistent relationship to antecedent events or other diseases has been recognized. Both the number and severity of clinical signs increase as the disease remains untreated. Most hypothyroid dogs are presented for veterinary examination within six months to one year after the onset of the first signs, but the disease sometimes evades recognition by veterinarians for as long as two years.

CLINICAL SIGNS

It is misleading to speak of a "typical" case of hypothyroidism in the dog. The number and severity of signs vary with the duration of the disease, and almost any sign can constitute the principal problem in one patient and yet be of minor importance or lacking in another. The notable exception is diminished physical activity and endurance (lethargy, fatigue, increased sleeping). This is usually accompanied by a gradual slowing of mental activity (reduced alertness and excitability, lack of interest in familiar activities), but a highly trained police or guard dog may remain alert and willing although unable to perform long or strenuous exercise.

The clinical signs and relevant general laboratory findings are listed in Table 1, without regard to relative frequency or importance. In a given patient the most important sign or combination of signs is that which provides the impetus for tests that lead to the diagnosis. An example is the finding of low voltage on the electrocardiogram of a dog in which the only other notable findings are gradually increasing lethargy and a slow pulse rate, both of which are rather non-specific.

Some hypothyroid dogs gain as much as 30 to 40 percent in body weight, but others remain at or even below their normal weights. The dog with simple obesity is usually also lethargic and lacking in stamina but remains alert and displays no special preference for warmth.

Many hypothyroid dogs move with a very stiff and slow gait when they arise after sleeping, but the disability usually lessens or disappears after 15 to 20 minutes of activity. Slow or weak muscular action may cause dragging of the front feet, resulting in wearing of the anteriodorsal surfaces of the toenails. It is possible that the ineffective lifting of the front feet is partly due to a peripheral neuropathy, analogous to the carpal tunnel syndrome that sometimes occurs in human myxedema, but this has not been studied adequately. Quite infrequently there is lameness due to painful swelling of soft tissues

Table 1. *Signs of Hypothyroidism in Dogs*

Lethargy, lack of endurance, increased sleeping
Reduced interest, alertness, and excitability
Slow heart rate, weak apex beat and pulse, low
   voltage on ECG
Preference for warmth, low body temperature, cool skin
Increased body weight
Stiff and slow movements, dragging of front feet
Head tilt, disturbed balance, unilateral facial paralysis
Atrophy of epidermis, thickening of dermis
Surface and follicular hyperkeratosis, pigmentation
Puffy face, blepharoptosis, tragic expression
Dry, course, sparse coat; slow regrowth after clipping
Retarded turnover of hair (carpet coat of boxers)
Shortening or absence of estrus, lack of libido
Dry feces, occasional diarrhea
Hypercholesterolemia
Normochromic, normocytic anemia
Elevated serum creatinine phosphokinase

around one or more of the carpal and tarsal joints, with no involvement of the joint surfaces or increase in synovial fluid. The swelling decreases markedly or completely disappears after treatment of the hypothyroidism.

Slightly disturbed balance with tilting of the head may occur alone or in combination with slight facial paralysis on the same side. We do not yet know the exact cause of these disorders in the dog, but in man facial weakness is a rare complication of hypothyroidism and results from pressure on the facial nerve in the fallopian canal of the tenporal bone. Cerebellar ataxia has also been described in hypothyroidism in man, but the head tilt in hypothyroid dogs suggests involvement of the vestibular nerve, which is enclosed in a common dural sheath with the facial and cochlear nerves as they pass through the internal acoustic meatus. This relationship suggests the possibility of a concurrent unilateral diminution in hearing in affected hypothyroid dogs, but this is difficult to document. If they have not been of long duration both the disturbed balance and the facial paralysis can be reversed by treatment of the hypothyroidism.

The severity and extent of dermatologic changes are particularly dependent upon the duration of the hypothyroidism. Biopsies of affected skin reveal atrophy of the epidermis and sebaceous glands, with epidermal and follicular hyperkeratosis. Palpation of the skin reveals thickening of the dermis, but it is less common to find an appreciable increase in acid mucopolysaccharides (myxedema) histologically. However, we have not studied biopsies of face and forehead skin, where thickened folds are most prominent, giving the face a puffy appearance. This puffiness, together with slight blepharoptosis, accentuates the dull, uninterested attitude of some hypothyroid dogs, giving them a tragic expression. In boxers and some other short-haired dogs the retarded turnover of hair leads to a very thick coat that resembles a carpet, particularly on the temporal area. In some but by no means all hypothyroid dogs there are areas of frank alopecia, particularly on the chest, flanks, and thighs. The affected skin may be darkly pigmented and have the texture of emery paper.

One learns with experience to be alerted to the possibility of hypothyroidism less by dermatologic abnormalities and weight gain than by the dog's attitude. To appreciate this, one need only observe the dog's behavior while the history is being taken, before the dog is placed on the examination table. Most hypothyroid dogs sit or lie down rather than tugging nervously at the leash or attempting to investigate the room. It is unusual for a hypothyroid dog to pant or to develop tachycardia because of nervous excitement. The dog's general attitude and facial expression usually suggest fatigue, lack of interest in the surroundings, and a sense of discomfort; the lack of enthusiasm can be most impressive.

DIAGNOSIS

The clinical signs lead to consideration of hypothyroidism in the differential diagnosis, but diagnosis of this disease based on clinical signs alone is quite unreliable. In our clinic, where hypothyroidism has been a subject of particular interest, discussion, and investigation for several years, the diagnosis is subsequently confirmed in only about 10 percent of the canine patients in which there are sufficient signs to prompt specific diagnostic tests. The insidious development of the disease and the variability of its manifestations make a reliable screening procedure essential. In our experience, the most convenient and dependable method of screening is the radioimmunoassay (RIA) measurement of plasma T_4 concentration. As shown in Figure 1, plasma T_4 levels are consistently found to be subnormal in dogs with proved primary hypothyroidism. Further confirmation of the diagnosis is always required, however, for plasma T_4 concentration is frequently lowered by current or recent administration of certain drugs (including glucocorticoids, phenylbutazone, phenytoin, phenobarbital and o,p'-

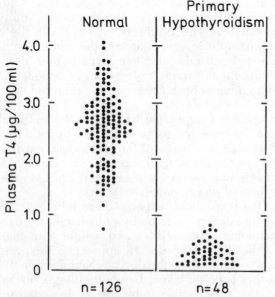

Figure 1. Basal plasma T_4(RIA) values in normal dogs and dogs with proved primary hypothyroidism. (Reproduced by permission of The Journal of the American Animal Hospital Association, *15*:17–23, 1979.)

DDD), by the corticosteroid excess of Cushing's disease, and probably by other factors.

Primary hypothyroidism can be distinguished from other causes of lowering of plasma T_4 concentration by measurement of the response to administration of TSH. For this purpose, 10 IU of TSH are injected intravenously, and plasma T_4 concentration is measured in samples obtained immediately before and four hours after the injection. In dogs with primary hypothyroidism there is virtually no increase in plasma T_4, whereas in those in which basal T_4 concentration is depressed by other causes the slope of the increase following administration of TSH is similar to that in normal dogs (Fig. 2).

The lowering of plasma T_4 concentration caused by drugs and Cushing's disease appears to occur primarily via interference with T_4 binding by plasma proteins. Thyroidal uptake of radioiodine or pertechnetate is normal, and such dogs do not require or benefit from administration of thyroid hormone. Furthermore, the plasma T_4 response to TSH stimulation remains intact even when the effect is sustained for months or years (e.g., by alternate-day corticosteroid therapy).

Plasma T_4 levels in normal dogs are considerably lower than those in man, and for clinical screening in dogs the measurement must be accurate at levels below 1 μg/100 ml. Methods established for use in man are invariably designed for measurement of levels up to 20 μg/100 ml or more, and this usually restricts the lower limit of accurate measurement to 1 to 2 μg/100 ml. This limit can readily be lowered to 0.1 μg/100 ml using RIA (with a proportional reduction of the upper limit of measurement), but regardless of the method of assay the procedure must be designed for this purpose. Hence, accurate measurement of subnormal plasma T_4 levels in dogs can seldom be obtained by submitting samples to laboratories that are essentially concerned with measurement in man or by using kit procedures.

Measurements of plasma T_3 concentration by RIA are equally useful for screening purposes but not for evaluating the response to TSH.

The diagnosis of secondary hypothyroidism poses additional problems. The clinical manifestations are indistinguishable from those of primary hypothyroidism, except that they do not ultimately reach the same degree of severity. Plasma T_4 levels are usually moderately depressed, but day-to-day fluctuations above and below the lower limit of normal are not unusual. The response to TSH stimulation is similar to that in dogs with drug-induced lowering of plasma T_4 (see Fig. 2). The plasma T_4 response to thyrotropin-releasing hormone

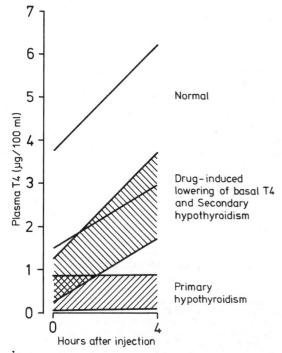

Figure 2. Plasma T₄(RIA) response to TSH stimulation in dogs, 4 hours after IV injection of 10 IU of TSH. The response line is essentially flat in dogs with primary hypothyroidism, whereas in dogs with secondary hypothyroidism or drug-induced lowering of basal T₄ concentration the response is roughly parallel to that in normal dogs. Drug-induced lowering of plasma T₄ is encountered quite frequently, while secondary hypothyroidism is relatively rare. See text for details.

(TRH) is rather small in normal dogs and, although a clearly diminished response is usually obtained in dogs with secondary hypothyroidism, the magnitude of the difference gives insufficient diagnostic assurance. The plasma T₃ response to TSH is even less helpful, for the same reason, and measurements of plasma TSH concentration, which might be more appropriate for this test, are not yet feasible in the dog. Thyroidal uptake of radioiodine is distinctly subnormal but increases after TSH stimulation (daily doses of 10 IU subcutaneously for three days), and this can be considered diagnostic if it can be ascertained that the initial low uptake was not caused by excessive intake of iodine (as may occur with some commercial dog foods). In our opinion, the most dependable means of confirming the diagnosis of secondary hypothyroidism in the dog is by thyroid biopsy. The distinctive histologic features of TSH deficiency are enlarged, colloid-filled follicles with flattened epithelium and few or no resorption vacuoles at the periphery of the colloid. These features are easily recognized within one month after hypophysectomy and are identical whether TSH deficiency is caused by the growth of a pituitary tumor or by administration of full replacement doses of L-thyroxine to normal dogs.

TREATMENT

The optimal method of treatment of canine hypothyroidism is the once-daily oral administration of L-thyroxine, in a dose of 20 μg/kg of normal body weight. When L-thyroxine is not available, desiccated thyroid is given in a once-daily oral dose of 15 to 20 mg/kg of normal body weight. We have found it necessary to crush or grind desiccated thyroid tablets before they are administered in a small amount of food. Even when this is done, the response in a small proportion of dogs reaches a plateau before complete restoration of clinical euthyroidism. Improvement is not obtained by increasing the dose of desiccated thyroid but is obtained by changing to L-thyroxine at the usual dose. We have as yet no satisfactory explanation for this difference.

A distinct increase in physical and mental activity is usually evident within the first seven to ten days of treatment. Most signs of the disease have decreased markedly within two months, but full regrowth of hair in areas of alopecia requires four to six months. Reactivation of the atrophic epidermis and adnexae leads to the shedding of old hair and the sloughing of excessive keratin, and this may be accompanied by transient pruritus. If this is explained in advance to the owner it will not be misinterpreted as a worsening of the condition. When necessary, the pruritus can be relieved by softening the dry skin with olive oil or by using a corticosteroid cream. Rather infrequently, the coat does not return completely to its original fullness and condition, even long after all other signs of hypothyroidism have disappeared. We do not know the reason for this, but increasing the dose of thyroid hormone has no beneficial effect.

Followup examinations are made at intervals of two months until we and the owner are satisfied with the dog's improvement; two or three such examinations usually suffice. Occasionally one or more of the original problems are not due to hypothyroidism (e.g., simple obesity) and thus require additional attention. Plasma T₄ concentration is measured at each followup examination until it is found to be stabilized within the normal range. For these measurements it is essential to instruct the owner to withhold medication on the day of examination until after the blood sample has been collected. When the dose of L-thyroxine is adequate, plasma T₄ concentration remains within the normal range for 24 hours, excluding a postabsorptive elevation that lasts four to six hours. It is not necessary to administer either L-thyroxine or dessicated thyroid in a divided daily dose.

We have never observed ill effects from beginning therapy at the full replacement dose, even in elderly dogs with hypothyroidism of long duration; we only advise beginning at a lower dose in the patient with clinically significant cardiac disease. It is not unusual for the owner to take the initiative in altering the dose slightly upward or downward, and we do not discourage this, since the owner's evaluation of and satisfaction with the dog's response will ultimately prevail. Nevertheless, the usual result is that the recommended doses are found to be optimal, and plasma T_4 levels are found to be in agreement with this. We do caution that some dogs recovering from hypothyroidism are paradoxically sensitive to even moderate overdosage. The most consistent signs are polyuria, polydipsia, restlessness, and panting, and upon their appearance the dose should be reduced promptly. The most serious effect is an increase in the rate and force of the heartbeat, with high voltage on the electrocardiogram. This may persist for weeks after the excessive dose of thyroxine has been lowered or even stopped.

Secondary hypothyroidism is treated in the same manner, but studies should always be performed to determine whether there is concurrent secondary adrenocortical insufficiency, which necessitates glucocorticoid substitution as well. Confirmation of the diagnosis of acquired secondary hypothyroidism in an adult dog is presumptive evidence of a pituitary tumor. There may be accompanying neurologic signs, but in some cases the growth of the tumor is rather slow, and with treatment of the hypothyroidism the dog may live comfortably for months or years.

SUPPLEMENTAL READING

Capen, C.C., Belshaw, B.E., and Martin, S.L.: Endocrine disorders. In Ettinger, S.J. (ed.): *Textbook of Veterinary Internal Medicine.* Philadelphia, W.B. Saunders Co., 1975.

Belshaw, B.E., and Rijnberk, A.: Radioimmunoassay of plasma T_4 and T_3 in the diagnosis of primary hypothyroidism in dogs. J. Am. Animal Hosp. Assoc. 15:17–23, 1979.

Nijhuis, A.H., Stokhof, A.A., Huisman, G.H., and Rijnberk, A.: ECG changes in dogs with hypothyroidism. Tijdschr. Diergeneesk., 103:735–741, 1978.

FELINE HYPERTHYROIDISM

PETER THERAN, V.M.D.,
and JEAN HOLZWORTH, D.V.M.*

Boston, Massachusetts

Hyperthyroidism develops in elderly cats (9 to 22 years) of both sexes as a result of hyperplasia or tumor of the thyroid gland. The clinical picture is so striking that perceptive owners have made the diagnosis and, once a veterinarian has encountered the condition, he or she will not easily fail to recognize it. Confirmation is by standard thyroid function tests, and treatment is surgical removal of the abnormal lobe(s).

Signs usually develop gradually: loss of weight despite increased appetite; stools that are frequent, abundant, soft, and sometimes loose; thirst and polyuria; restlessness, pacing, nervousness, wakefulness, and sometimes even panting. The haircoat may be matted and unkempt.

PHYSICAL EXAMINATION

The cat may be unusually tense or nervous and does not relax when fondled reassuringly. Mucous membranes and ear pinnae may be pinker than expected, suggesting hypertension. The heartbeat and pulse may be abnormally strong and also accelerated (200 to 300 beats per minute). Murmurs, premature beats, and gallop rhythms may be heard, and radiographs usually reveal cardiac enlargement. In advanced cases congestive heart failure may be present. The intestine may contain excessive gas, liquid, or soft stool. The rectal temperature is normal or

*With acknowledgment for the contributions of other Angell Memorial Animal Hospital staff members: Michael Bernstein, Susan Cotter, Neil Harpster, Gus Thornton, and Jeffery Todoroff

slightly elevated. Careful palpation just below the larynx reveals enlargement of one or, rarely, both thyroid lobes. Occasionally one lobe may be retrotracheal and difficult to palpate.

LABORATORY FINDINGS

The diagnosis of hyperthyroidism is confirmed by elevated serum thyroxine (T_4) or triiodothyronine (T_3) or both. Normal levels for the cat are considered to be 15 to 50 ng/ml for T_4 and 0.6 to 2 ng/ml for T_3[†]; T_4 values in hyperthyroid cats may be reported as high as 200 ng/ml and T_3 may exceed 4 ng/ml. SGPT, SGOT, and alkaline phospatase levels are usually significantly elevated as well. Normal blood and urine glucose values eliminate the possibility of diabetes mellitus, which is sometimes considered first when these cats are presented.

TREATMENT

Some cats have been treated preoperatively for a week or ten days with an empirical dose of propylthiouracil (50 mg b.i.d. or t.i.d.), but they did not seem to fare any better than those that did not receive such treatment. Cats in congestive heart failure must be stabilized before surgery.

A 5-cm midline incision is made from the hyoid region almost to the thoracic inlet. Hemostasis must be meticulous in order to identify all structures. The sternocephalicus and then the sternohyoideus muscles are separated on the midline and retracted to either side to expose the thyroid lobes. In most cases only one lobe is significantly enlarged, but the other, although smaller, usually appears grossly abnormal, too. Both should be carefully dissected free, the cranial and caudal thyroid vessels should be ligated and severed, and the recurrent laryngeal nerves, which course dorsomedially along the lobes, should be carefully isolated and spared. The parathyroid glands may be difficult to identify. If possible, one should be spared; however, if this cannot be done, ectopic parathyroid tissue is usually present in sufficient amounts to maintain function or to restore it within a few days.

In a minority of cases only one thyroid lobe is abnormal, whereas the opposite one may appear atrophied or cannot be found at all. Such

---

†Animal Health Diagnostic Laboratory, Endocrine Diagnostic Section, P.O. Box 30076, Lansing, MI 48909

a lobe has become reduced in size, presumably from inhibition of thyroid-stimulating hormone by the high serum concentration of thyroid hormones produced by the abnormal lobe. To judge from the postoperative courses, the atrophic lobe resumes function so efficiently and promptly that even temporary supplementation with thyroxine usually is not required.

Postoperatively, a minority of cats from which both thyroid lobes are removed may suffer transient hypocalcemia (two to three days) as a result of reduction in parathyroid tissue. These cats require careful monitoring and supplementation with intravenous or oral calcium and vitamin D_3. Most, however, recover uneventfully after bilateral removal and are discharged within several days, receiving lifetime supplementation with thyroxine (0.2 mg sodium L-thyroxine daily).

PATHOLOGY

Unlike dogs, in which hyperthyroidism has appeared invariably to be associated with thyroid cancers, cats with this condition have been found to have adenocarcinoma, adenomas, or simply adenomatous hyperplasia.

Recovery from the presenting signs is usually gratifyingly prompt and uncomplicated. The cat becomes relaxed and eats and defecates less but gains weight. The thirst and polyuria subside, and cardiac function improves. Thyroid function tests repeated three to four weeks after surgery indicate a decrease of hormone levels to the normal ranges.

Cats from which only one lobe is removed should be followed up for possible development of functional abnormality in the remaining lobe.

SUPPLEMENTAL READING

Clark, S.T., and Meier, H.: A clinicopathological study of thyroid disease in the dog and cat. Zentralbl. Veterinaermed. [A], 5:17–32, 1958.

Holzworth, J., et al.: Arterial thrombosis and thyroid carcinoma in a cat. Cornell Vet., 45:487–496, 1955.

Holzworth, J., et al.: Hyperthyroidism in cats. J. Am. Vet. Med. Assoc., February 15, 1980.

Leav, I., and Schiller, A.L.: Adenomas and carcinomas of the canine and feline thyroid. Am. J. Pathol., 83:61–122, 1976.

Lucke, V.M.: A histological study of thyroid abnormalities in the domestic cat. J. Small Anim. Pract., 5:351–358, 1964.

PRIMARY
HYPOPARATHYROIDISM*

DENNIS J. MEYER, D.V.M.
Gainesville, Florida

Hypoparathyroidism is a metabolic disturbance characterized by neuromuscular signs secondary to hypocalcemia. The decrease in serum calcium level results from a deficiency of parathyroid hormone. The two most common clinical types of primary hypoparathyroidism in the dog are postoperative and idiopathic.

Postoperative parathyroid deficiency can occur following cervial surgery in the area of the thyroid glands. The parathyroid glands may be inadvertently removed during thyroid surgery, or their blood supply may be compromised. The signs of hypoparathyroidism may occur soon after surgery (days) or may not be manifested for months. Transient hypoparathyroid deficiency may go unnoticed immediately postoperatively if the parathyroid glands are injured but recover or if a glandular remnant hypertrophies and returns the parathormone production to normal.

Idiopathic hypoparathyroidism in the dog is being recognized with increasing frequency, in part because of the more routine use of the biochemical profile. The hypocalcemia and hyperphosphatemia in the presence of normal renal function may be detected before clinical signs of tetany occur. The disease appears to be more common in the small breeds (terriers and schnauzers) but has been diagnosed in larger breeds. The dogs are frequently two to five years of age when the diagnosis is confirmed. An autoimmune process is implied by the histologic changes in the parathyroid gland in these dogs. The parathyroid gland parenchyma is replaced by an extensive lymphocytic-plasmocytic cellular infiltrate and connective tissue (Meyer and Terrell).

SIGNS

The clinical manifestations are the result of increased neuromuscular irritability due to the decreased serum concentration of ionized calcium. The predominant signs of the dog are

tetany and convulsions. Curling of the upper lip and spastic contractions of the muscles of the face and forelimbs frequently are noted early and may be elicited by handling the dog (latent tetany).

Two types of clinical presentation appear to define the clinical spectrum of the disease. The acute form (days) is characterized by an abrupt onset of tetany or convulsions or both, with no prodromal signs. The chronic type (weeks to months) is associated with recurrent disturbances, including mental depression, lethargy, restlessness, anorexia, vomiting, and latent tetany. Lethargy and generalized lymphadenopathy have been noted three weeks before the occurrence of mild, intermittent facial and foreleg spasms and hyperventilation (Meyer and Terrell). In one case the tetany became progressively more severe, and seizures developed during the following 11 weeks, at which time hypoparathyroidism was diagnosed. Acute death in dogs showing minimal clinical signs associated with hypocalcemia is not uncommon.

DIAGNOSIS AND DIFFERENTIAL DIAGNOSIS

Primary hypoparathyroidism is strongly suggested in a dog that has signs of hypocalcemia and that is documented as having both hypocalcemia and hyperphosphatemia in the presence of normal renal function. Neck surgery in the area of the thyroid glands days to months preceding the onset of hypocalcemia suggests postoperative hypoparathyroidism. The absence or relative absence of parathyroid hormone (as measured by radioimmunoassay) associated with hypocalcemia substantiates a diagnosis of primary hypoparathyroidism. However, the test is expensive and not routinely available.

Hypocalcemia may also be associated with hypoproteinemia, malabsorption, acute pancreatitis, and chronic renal failure. Hypoproteinemia is associated with a number of diseases that result in reduction of the total serum calcium because of reduced binding protein mass. Most of the remaining serum calcium is in

---

*The author expresses his gratitude to Drs. M. Schaer and G.E. Lees for their suggestions in the preparation of this article.

the physiologically active ionized form, thus preventing the signs of hypocalcemia in spite of decreased total serum calcium content. History, physical exmaination, and other clinical pathologic findings will differentiate the hypocalcemia associated with other diseases from primary hypoparathyroidism.

TREATMENT

The objective in the treatment of hypocalcemia secondary to postoperative thyroid surgery or idiopathic hypoparathyroidism is to re-establish a serum calcium concentration in the low normal range of 8.5 to 9.0 mg/dl. Hypoparathyroidism following thyroid surgery may be temporary or permanent. The persistence of low serum calcium and increased serum phosphorus levels six to eight weeks after thyroid surgery suggests permanent hypoparathyroidism.

Dihydrotachysterol and vitamin D_2 (ergocalciferol) are the pharmacologic agents currently recommended to overcome the absence of parathyroid hormone. Both drugs elevate serum calcium by stimulating intestinal calcium absorption and mobilizing bone calcium. Dihydrotachysterol has a more rapid rate of inactivation than vitamin D_2. Vitamin D_2 is stored in body fats and tends to be cumulative in its physiologic action. The metabolic advantages of dihydrotachysterol allow for greater ease of individual patient adjustment of the serum calcium concentration.

Dihydrotachysterol* and vitamin D_2† are available as capsules, tablets, and solutions. The solutions are recommended for smaller dogs because of the greater ease of adjusting the dose during the initiation of therapy. A tuberculin syringe rather than a dropper is suggested for the administration of the solution. A significant variation in the size of the dose from day to day has been shown to occur when a dropper is used.

Dogs showing signs of hypocalcemia (muscle twitching, tetany) are managed initially with the intravenous administration of 10 percent calcium gluconate at a dosage of 0.5 to 1.5 ml/kg body weight, up to 10 ml total, over a 15- to 30-minute period. An electrocardiogram is monitored, and the administration is stopped temporarily if bradycardia, elevation of the S–T segment, or shortening of the Q–T interval is observed. The intravenous dose can be repeated at six- to eight-hour intervals, if necessary, until the effect of the oral vitamin D supplement begin. Calcium solutions should never be given intramuscularly, and care must be taken to avoid extravascular infiltration, since severe necrosis can occur.

The management of chronic hypocalcemia is achieved by the use of dihydrotachysterol or vitamin D_2. The maintenance dose of dihydrotachysterol is 0.05 to 0.50 mg per day. A useful approximation for determining the maintenance dose of dihydrotachysterol is 0.01 mg/kg/day. The administration of the maintenance dose along with hospitalization is suggested as the initial treatment of hypoparathyroidism unless tetany is imminent.

The dose of vitamin D_2 is in the range of 25,000 to 100,000 units per day. An approximate starting dose of vitamin D_2 is 1000 to 2000 units/kg/day. Normocalcemia usually occurs in one to three weeks. A 15 to 20 percent adjustment of the previous dose is made if hypocalcemia persists.

Vitamin D therapy must be strictly individualized, with adjustment of the dose based on frequent determinations of serum calcium level. Dihydrotachysterol or vitamin D_2 should be instituted at the lower calculated dose, and changes should be made slowly. Approximately three to five days (for dihydrotachysterol) or five to ten days (for vitamin D_2) are required for a change in the serum calcium level following an adjustment of the dose. One mg of dihydrotachysterol is approximately equivalent to 120,000 units (3 mg) of vitamin D_2.

Limited observations indicate that the signs of hypocalcemia can be controlled in some dogs with hypoparathyroidism by weekly administration of vitamin D_2 along with oral calcium salt supplements, underscoring the need for an individualized approach to treatment. However, the consistency of the serum calcium levels in these dogs is unclear. The daily administration of dihydrotachysterol should allow for a more finely "tuned" calcium homeostasis.

Overdosage of vitamin D preparations causes hypercalcemia. Clinical signs of hypercalcemia in the dog include weakness, ataxia, depression, anorexia, and vomiting. Persistent hypercalcemia results in renal tubule toxicity, which manifests as polyuria-polydipsia. Renal failure then ensues.

Hypercalcemia is treated by discontinuing vitamin D and inducing a diuresis. Intravenous normal saline along with furosemide is given, and glucocorticoids (prednisolone, 10 to 30 mg daily) may be given orally.

The need for supplementary calcium salts in the diets of dogs with hypoparathyroidism is not

---

°Dihydrotachysterol Tablets USP: 0.125 mg, 0.2 mg, 0.4 mg; Hytakerol: 0.125 mg capsules or in oil, 0.25 mg/ml.

†Drisdol: 50,000 units (1.25 mg) per capsule or in oil, 10,000 units (0.25 mg)/ml; Calciferol: 50,000 units (1.25 mg) per tablet or in oil, 500,000 units (12.5 mg)/ml.

clearly established. A dog may be regulated with dihydrotachysterol or vitamin D_2 with a balanced commercial dog food diet that provides an adequate source of calcium. If the serum phosphorus content remains elevated, a calcium salt supplement is indicated to lower the serum phosphorus level by binding phosphorus in the intestinal tract. The dose of dihydrotachysterol or vitamin D_2 may have to be adjusted downward based on serum calcium determinations if calcium salts are added to the diet. Several calcium salts are available for the treatment of hypoparathyroidism. Calcium carbonate contains 40 percent calcium, whereas calcium lactate and calcium gluconate contain 13 and 9 percent calcium, respectively. A dose of 0.5 to 2.0 gm calcium carbonate or 1.0 to 4.0 gm calcium gluconate or calcium lactate is administered orally each day.

A novel approach to the treatment of hypoparathyroidism in human beings has recently been reported (Porter, et al.). Chlorthalidone, a pharmacologic agent similar to the thiazide diuretics, has been shown to return serum calcium levels to normal in hypoparathyroid patients. A concurrent low-salt diet is necessary for the calcium-evaluating effect of the drug. The advantage of this form of chronic therapy is the lack of potential hypercalcemic toxicity associated with the vitamin D preparations. However, reservations have been expressed in regard to the treatment. Further study must be completed before the traditional mode of therapy is discarded.

In man idiopathic hypoparathyroidism is occasionally associated with other endocrinopathies, notably adrenocortical insufficiency, hypothyroidism, and diabetes mellitus (Potts; Irvine and Barnes). Long-term experience with the spectrum of idiopathic hypoparathyroidism in the dog is limited. The possibility of a complicating endocrinopathy, either concurrent or occurring at a later time, should be considered.

One drug interaction should be mentioned because of its clinical significance. The administration of glucocorticoids to dogs being treated for hypoparathyroidism may increase the requirements for dihydrotachysterol or vitamin D_2 to maintain normocalcemia.

It cannot be overemphasized that the treatment for hypoparathyroidism must be tailored to the individual dog. The serum calcium concentration is initially determined every one to two days until normocalcemia (low normal) is attained. Serum calcium and phosphorus content is subsequently checked every one to four months. Reports in human patients on treatment for idiopathic hypoparathyroidism indicate that occasionally hypercalcemia develops after months to years of normocalcemia, necessitating a reduction in the dose of dihydrotachysterol or vitamin D_2. The reason for this phenomenon is unclear, but the observation emphasizes the need for continued periodic monitoring (every two to four months) of the serum calcium content and an individualized approach for the treatment of hypoparathyroidism.

SUPPLEMENTAL READING

Meyer, D.J., and Terrell, T.G.: Idiopathic hypoparathyroidism in a dog. J. Am. Vet. Med. Assoc., *169*:858–860, 1976.

Porter, R.H., Cox, B.G., Heaney, D., et al.: Treatment of hypoparathyroid patients with chlorthalidone. N. Engl. J. Med., 298:577–581, 1978.

Correspondence: Chlorthalidone for hypoparathyroidism. N. Engl. J. Med., 298:1478–1479, 1978.

Potts, J.T. Jr.: Disorders of parathyroid glands. In *Harrison's Principles of Internal Medicine*, 8th ed., New York, McGraw-Hill Book Co., 1977, 2014–2025.

Irvine, W.J., and Barnes, E.W.: Addison's disease, ovarian failure, and hypoparathyroidism. Clin. Endocrinol. Metabol., *4*:379–433, 1975.

PRIMARY HYPERPARATHYROIDISM

ALFRED M. LEGENDRE, D.V.M.
Knoxville, Tennessee

Primary hyperparathyroidism is a disease syndrome due to adenoma, adenocarcinoma, or hyperplasia of the parathyroid glands. Hypercalcemia is the hallmark of this condition and accounts for most of the clinical signs. Hypercalcemia appears to be uncommon in cats and dogs but may be one of the frequently undiagnosed conditions whose discovery is very likely to increase with the advent of routine use of multichannel autoanalyzers for biochemical screening of sick animals. In human medicine the use of routine biochemical screening and the increased awareness of hyperparathyroidism has resulted in a 10- to 15-fold increase in the recognition of primary hyperparathyroidism.

CLINICAL SIGNS

The clinical signs of hyperparathyroidism can be classified into three main categories: (1) effects of hypercalcemia on neuromuscular excitability; (2) demineralization of the skeleton with pathologic fractures of long bones and vertebrae and hyperostosis of the face; and (3) renal dysfunction associated with nephrocalcinosis.

Hypercalcemia causes decreased neuromuscular excitability, which results in skeletal muscle weakness. This results in vague signs of lethargy and exercise intolerance that clients usually fail to relate to the veterinarian until they are specifically questioned about it. Hypercalcemia also causes hypotonicity of the smooth muscles of the gastrointestinal tract. Anorexia, vomiting, and constipation result from the decreased motility of the GI tract. These may be the only signs noted in the early stages of the disease process; such signs warrant a biochemical screening profile to establish a cause for them.

The excessive levels of parathormone increase serum levels of calcium by increasing resorption of calcium from the renal tubules and by demineralization of the skeleton. This results in osteoporosis, which when severe results in loosening of the teeth and pathologic fractures of long bones. Demineralization of the vertebrae commonly produces compression fractures of the vertebral column, with paresis or paralysis as a presenting sign. If bone density of the cortex of a fractured bone appears to be inadequate, further radiographic evaluation and serum calcium and phosphorus levels should be determined. Radiographs of the mandible and the vertebral column are most useful in evaluating the patient for demineralization. Loss of bony density from the lamina dura around the tooth is an early finding in demineralization. The vertebrae are a prominent site of demineralization, and a pattern of relative increased density at the end plates with radiolucency of the vertebral body may be seen. In addition to fractures related to demineralization, a secondary effect is fibrous tissue proliferation, which occurs primarily in the face. This fibrous osteodystrophy may produce grotesque enlargement of the maxilla and facial bones and obliteration of the nasal passages. The teeth embedded in this fibrous tissue are loose, and eating produces pain.

Hypercalcemia may result in irreversible renal damage from calcium nephropathy. Calcium is deposited primarily in the basement membrane of the renal tubules and results in degeneration and necrosis of the renal tubular epithelium. Polyuria-polydipsia (Pu-Pd) is a prominent sign in hypercalcemia, and the evaluation of Pu-Pd should include serum calcium and phosphorus determinations. Dogs with significant renal damage may be azotemic and present with a variety of signs related to renal failure.

Many clinical signs can result from hypercalcemia, and any of them warrant investigation of serum calcium and phosphorus levels. This increased vigilance will result in early recognition when treatment is most effective.

DIFFERENTIAL DIAGNOSIS OF HYPERCALCEMIC STATES

The finding of an elevated serum calcium level (above 12 mg/dl) is not pathognomonic for primary hyperparathyroidism. The differential diagnosis of hypercalcemia must include pseu-

1003

dohyperparathyroidism, renal secondary hyperparathyroidism, neoplasms with bony metastasis, and hypervitaminosis D as well as primary hyperparathyroidism. It would appear that primary hyperparathyroidism is one of the least common causes of hypercalcemia.

Probably the most common cause of hypercalcemia is the pseudohyperparathyroidism of lymphosarcoma and other malignancies, e.g., mammary adenocarcinoma, multiple myeloma, and malignant perianal tumor. This occurs in dogs and cats as a result of the production of a parathormone-like substance by the tumor cells, which produces a condition similar to primary hyperparathyroidism. Parathormone, in addition to increasing serum calcium levels, inhibits renal tubular resorption of phosphate. This results in increased serum calcium (above 12 mg/dl) and decreased serum phosphorus (below 4 mg/dl). This pattern helps to separate primary and pseudohyperparathyroidism from the other causes of hypercalcemia, in which phosphorus levels are normal or elevated. The decrease in serum phosphorus can occur only if there is adequate renal function and will not occur if there is a significant increase in BUN. Ten to 40 percent of lymphosarcomas in dogs will have associated hypercalcemia; therefore, a diagnosis of lymphosarcoma must be eliminated through lymph node aspiration or biopsy, bone marrow examination, and thoracic radiographs (to identify mediastinal lymphosarcoma). In man parathormone (PTH) levels are useful in identifying cases of pseudohyperparathyroidism because the PTH-like substances are only partially reactive or nonreactive on radioimmunoassay, giving low PTH levels for the level of hypercalcemia. In the dog parathormone level determinations are expensive ($60 to $75), and the values for normal and disease states are not readily available. Because of the fulminating nature of lymphosarcoma, skeletal demineralization is uncommon in this condition; whereas in primary hyperparathyroidism it appears to be one of the most prominent features.

Other neoplastic conditions produce hypercalcemia by the direct osteolytic effects of skeletal metastasis. The biochemical parameters usually show a normal to elevated phosphorus level in addition to hypercalcemia. Radiography is useful in identifying bone metastasis in these cases. This appears to be an uncommon cause of hypercalcemia in dogs and cats.

Secondary hyperparathyroidism associated with renal failure is a common disease entity in the dog. Renal faulure results in phosphorus retention in the plasma. The increased phosphorus levels depress serum calcium, resulting in parathyroid stimulation, parathyroid hyper-

trophy, and a rise in parathormone levels. This mechanism attempts to maintain normal levels of calcium in the face of elevated phosphorus levels. Usually the calcium levels do not exceed normal values, but a recent article describes elevated calcium levels in secondary hyperparathyroidism (Finco and Rowland). In these conditions a greatly elevated phosphorus level and elevated BUN suggest that the condition is secondary to renal disease. Osteoporosis is a common feature of this condition and tends to be most severe in young animals. Secondary hyperparathyroidism may be difficult to differentiate from primary hyperparathyroidism with renal failure due to nephrocalcinosis. In both cases the prognosis is guarded.

Vitamin D intoxication will produce both hypercalcemia and hyperphosphatemia. There is no demineralization in this condition, and careful questioning will reveal overzealous supplementation of the diet with vitamin D.

The diagnosis of primary hyperparathyroidism is initially one of exclusion of other causes of hypercalcemia. Small tumors may produce pathologic amounts of parathormone, and the finding of a parathyroid tumor on palpation would be the exception rather than the rule. Demineralization of the skeleton is a prominent feature and is usually advanced at the time of diagnosis. A definitive diagnosis of primary hyperparathyroidism is made by histologically identifying a parathyroid adenoma or hyperplasia that is associated with appropriate clinical signs.

TREATMENT

The first priority in cases of primary hyperparathyroidism is to reduce blood calcium levels. Hypercalcemia, even of relatively short duration, may produce nephrocalcinosis and permanent renal damage. The polyuria-polydispsia, frequently accompanied by dehydration, tends to aggravate the hypercalcemic effect. Rehydration of the patient with saline solutions, which tend to promote excretion of calcium, is very beneficial. The use of furosemide also enhances calcium diuresis. Once the patient is stabilized, a thorough evaluation must be made to determine the cause of the hypercalcemia. When other causes of hypercalcemia are eliminated, exploratory surgery of the parathyroids is recommended. The majority of parathyroid tumors are adenomas and can be resected surgically. The anterior glands are more evident, whereas the posterior glands are hidden in the thyroid tissue. Meticulous technique is essential to prevent gross contamination of the surgical field with blood, which may obscure the tumor. Electrocautery to maintain a dry field is preferred. The neoplasm is usually found to be associated with the thyroid gland, but an ectopic neoplasm of parathyroid origin occasionally occurs in the mediastinum at the base of the heart in both dog and man. If cervical dissection fails to reveal a tumor and the diagnosis still appears firm, thoracic surgery should be considered.

POSTOPERATIVE COMPLICATIONS

In cases of primary hyperparathyroidism with severe demineralization, a guarded prognosis should be given because of the severe hypocalcemia that follows surgical removal of the neoplasm. The half-life of parathormone in the plasma is only 20 minutes; thus, severe hypocalcemia may occur within a few hours of surgery. Hypocalcemia following removal of a parathyroid tumor may be a life-threatening complication. In man postoperative hypocalcemia was shown to be related to low levels of parathormone in some patients, but many others developed hypocalcemia in spite of normal parathormone levels. In the latter patients hypocalcemia was attributed to bone deposition of calcium in an effort to remineralize the skeleton. Calcium levels may be sufficiently low to produce tetany. Postoperative management requires frequent monitoring of the patient for signs of hypocalcemia (tetany, muscular twitching, restlessness) and periodic evaluation of serum calcium. Blood calcium can be expected to drop to normal or subnormal levels two to twelve hours following surgery. At this time calcium should be added to the intravenous infusion of 5 per cent dextrose and water to produce a concentration of 1 mg/ml of calcium. An infusion rate of 0.5 to 2 mg calcium/kg/hour should be used as a starting point and then adjusted as necessary according to serum calci-

um levels. This may be supplemented by IV infusion of 10 percent calcium gluconate to effect if tetany develops. During rapid infusion of calcium the heart should be monitored for evidence of bradycardia and other arrhythmias that may occur. Oral calcium (2 to 3 grams three times a day) and vitamin D (10,000 to 25,000 IU per day) should be given to patients with persistent hypocalcemia. Magnesium levels may be low in these cases (normal is 1.8 to 2.4 mg/dl). Magnesium can be supplemented at a rate of 0.5 mg/kg in the IV drip slowly over a 24-hour period, using large-animal magnesium solutions. In spite of vigorous therapy, normocalcemia may be difficult to achieve in the severely demineralized animal.

Primary hyperparathyroidism offers a diagnostic challenge to the clinician, but with early recognition of the condition and surgical removal of the tumor a satisfactory outcome can be obtained. Recognition of the disease before severe demineralization and renal dysfunction have occurred will greatly reduce the severe postoperative problems that exist at present.

SUPPLEMENTAL READING

Capen, C. C., Belshaw, B. E., and Martin, S. L.: Endocrine disorders. In Ettinger, S. J. (ed.): *Textbook of Veterinary Internal Medicine*. Philadelphia, W. B. Saunders Co., 1975, pp. 1351–1378.

Finco, D. R., and Rowland, G. N.: Hypercalcemia secondary to chronic renal failure in the dog: A report of four cases. J. Am. Vet. Med. Assoc., *173*:990–994, 1978.

Legendre, A. M., Merkley, D. F., Carrig, C. B., and Krehbiel, J. D.: Primary hyperparathyroidism in a dog. J. Am. Vet. Med. Assoc., *168*:694–696, 1976.

MacEwen, E. G., and Siegel, S. D.: Hypercalcemia: A paraneoplastic syndrome in clinical veterinary oncology. Vet. Clin. North Am. 7:187–194, 1977.

Osborne, C. A., and Stevens, J. B. Pseudohyperparathyroidism in the dog. J. Am. Vet. Med. Assoc., 62:125–135, 1973.

Wilson, J. W., Harris, S. G., Moore, W. D., and Leipold, H. W.: Primary hyperparathyroidism in a dog. J. Am. Vet. Med. Assoc., *164*:942–946, 1974.

DIABETES INSIPIDUS

DOROTHEA SCHWARTZ-PORSCHE, D.Med.Vet.

Berlin, Germany

Diabetes insipidus (DI), a polyuria-polydipsia syndrome, is caused by a deficiency of antidiuretic hormone (ADH, vasopressin) or by non-responsiveness of the kidneys to the hormone.

ADH is synthesized in the supraoptic and paraventricular nuclei of the hypothalamus. It is transported along the axons of the tractus supraoptic-hypophyseus into the neurohypophysis, where it is stored. Synthesis and release of ADH is regulated by volume receptors and osmoreceptors. An increase of the plasma osmolality by 1 to 2 percent results in ADH release, thus causing antidiuresis. ADH secretion is inhibited by a decrease in plasma osmolality. The volume receptors cause ADH release only when the blood volume decreases.

In the kidneys ADH increases the water permeability of the distal tubules and collecting ducts. Through osmosis, free water passes passively from the hypotonic fluid within the tubules to the hypertonic interstitial tissue of the medulla and papillae. Depending on fluid requirements, isotonic or hypertonic urine is formed. The urine concentration, however, cannot exceed the level of osmotic pressure within the inner medullary tissue. The renal concentrating capacity thus depends on the amount of ADH in the blood and the degree of hypertonicity of the renal medulla.

ADH probably acts on the contraluminal side of the cells via a specific receptor. Adenyl cyclase is activated to catalyze the synthesis of cyclic adenosine 3',5'-monophosphate (cAMP) from adenosine triphosphate (ATP). cAMP stimulates a protein kinase to synthesize a phosphoprotein, aided by ATP, within the luminal cell membrane. This protein increases the number of pores of the cell membrane and allows movement of water along the osmotic gradient. The pores are occluded when a protein phosphatase removes inorganic phosphorus from the phosphoprotein.

ETIOLOGY

Central DI is caused by morphologic or functional damage to the hypothalamic-neurohypophyseal system. ADH secretion decreases or is completely inhibited. There are three forms of central DI: symptomatic, idiopathic, and hereditary (Table 1).

Table 1. *Classification, Etiology, and Pathophysiology of the Diabetes Insipidus (DI) Syndrome*

CLASSIFICATION	TYPE	ETIOLOGY	PATHOPHYSIOLOGY
DI centralis Hypothalamic-neurohypophyseal DI ADH-sensitive DI	Symptomatic	Tumors (primary or metastatic) Specific and non-specific inflammation in the brain Trauma Vascular disorders Hypophysectomy	Lack of ADH secretion: complete DI Insufficient ADH secretion: incomplete DI or partial DI
	Idiopathic	No detectable morphologic anomaly	Impaired osmoreceptor function: threshold adjusted to a hypernormal level
	Hereditary	Poorly defined or no morphologic anomaly detectable Not reported for dog and cat	Total lack of osmoreceptor function
DI renalis Peripheral DI ADH (pitressin, vasopressin)-resistant DI	Symptomatic	Pyelonephritis Interstitial nephritis Renal medullar fibrosis Tubular necrosis Hypokalemia Hypocalcemia	Reduction or lack of renal response to ADH
	Hereditary	No detectable morphologic anomaly Not proved for dog and cat	
Primary polydipsia Psychogenic polydipsia Potomania Compulsive water-drinking		Psychogenic origin Primary disorder of the thirst center	Functional lack of ADH due to artificial hyperhydration Reduced renal responsiveness to ADH (washing-out effect) Impaired osmoreceptor function = lowered threshold

Symptomatic DI (destroyed or degenerate supraoptic and paraventricular neurons) is caused by tumors, inflammation, trauma, vascular changes, surgical manipulation, and other conditions. Functional impairment of the osmoreceptors also results in central DI. ADH is released at much higher serum osmolality values than normal. Idiopathic DI is the most common form seen in the dog. No morphologic causes for the functional impairment can be found. Hereditary DI has not been reported in the dog and cat.

Nephrogenic DI, in contrast with central DI, is characterized by non-responsiveness of the kidneys to ADH. Acquired renal ADH resistance may be induced by structural changes in the kidneys, particularly in the cells of the distal tubules and collecting ducts, or by metabolic disorders (hypokalemia, hypocalcemia). Congenital renal DI has been described in a dog in which no morphologic renal anomalies could be found. In renal DI intracellular cAMP synthesis may be impaired, since ADH administration does not increase cAMP concentration in the urine, as it does in the normal subject.

Some authors include primary polydipsia in the DI syndrome. If hyperhydration is present for some time, a functionally based hyposynthesis of ADH may develop, as well as a relative ADH resistance of the kidneys due to a decrease of medullary hypertonicity (washing-out effect).

CLINICAL SIGNS

The main signs of DI are polyuria, polydipsia, and hyposthenuria. Nocturia and incontinence are also observed. Excessive thirst forces affected animals to drink any liquid within reach, including their own urine. Insufficient water intake induces rapid dehydration. Because they are constantly seeking water, most animals are restless, which causes inappetence and loss of weight. Signs may develop suddenly or occur gradually over several weeks. In the symptomatic form of DI, central nervous system signs (impaired vision and incoordination, disorientation, convulsions, and others) may appear at the same time as, shortly before, or after polyuria and polydipsia become prominent. These signs are caused by extension of morphologic changes to neighboring brain areas.

DIAGNOSIS

Normal urine output for the dog and cat is less than 50 ml/kg. Water intake is less than 100 ml/kg body weight per day. In DI the daily urine production may increase 5- to 20-fold; therefore, exact determination of daily water balance is important. In complete DI the specific gravity of the urine is 1.001 to 1.005 and urine osmolality is 40 to 200 mOsm/kg. In partial DI the specific gravity may reach 1.010 and the osmolality 300 mOsm/kg. The plasma osmolality in DI may be normal to slightly increased, but in primary polydipsia it is decreased.

The concentrating capacity of the kidneys and the hypothalamic-neurohypophyseal system must be tested in order to distinguish between ADH deficiency and non-responsiveness of the kidneys to ADH. If the osmoreceptors are intact, ADH secretion can be induced via an increase in plasma osmolality either by water deprivation or by infusion of a hypertonic NaCl solution. Responsiveness of the kidneys can be tested by administration of ADH.

During a water deprivation test the patient must be carefully supervised. The test should not last longer than 24 hours and should be discontinued if more than 5 percent of the body weight is lost or if plasma osmolality increases to 350 mOsm/kg or plasma sodium to 165 mmol/liter. The bladder must be emptied immediately before and at one- to two-hour intervals during the water deprivation test. Volume, specific gravity, and osmolality of the urine are evaluated. The test is terminated when consecutive urine osmolality values do not differ more than 5 to 10 percent or show a decrease. One hundred mU ADH per kg· body weight in an aqueous solution is injected subcutaneously. Urine is collected for two additional one-hour periods.

Plasma osmolality changes are insignificant in healthy dogs during water deprivation. The urine volume decreases markedly. After 24 hours, the specific gravity of urine reaches 1.028 to 1.042 and urine osmolality reaches 1200 to 1440 mOsm/kg. The ratio of urine osmolality to plasma osmolality ($U_{osm}:P_{osm}$) is 4.3 ± 0.5. Urine concentration is not increased or will increase only slightly following ADH administration.

In patients with central DI plasma osmolality rises after a short period of water deprivation, whereas urine osmolality values remain below those of plasma. Thus, $U_{osm}:P_{osm}$ is <1 and the specific gravity is <1.010, which is characteristic of central DI. The urine concentration increases two- to five-fold following ADH administration. In partial DI a certain amount of ADH is still being secreted, and urine concentration may be well above isotonic levels ($U_{osm}:P_{osm}$ >1). Characteristically, urine concentration reaches maximum values before the end of the dehydration test and then decreases significantly. This indicates an exhaustion of ADH secretion. Under the influence of exogenous ADH, urine concentration rises to normal values.

When congenital renal DI is present, neither endogenous ADH (thirst) nor exogenous ADH can induce a significant increase in concentration (U_{osm}:P_{osm} <1). In acquired renal ADH resistance manifestation varies greatly; under the influence of thirst, U_{osm}:P_{osm} may reach values up to 2.5, but exogenous ADH does not cause a further increase. In primary polydipsia the urine osmolality always increases above isotonic levels (U_{osm}:P_{osm} >1) but shows no further rise following ADH administration.

The ADH test is usually performed with a depot ADH preparation. Water balance is evaluated during a 24-hour period, then the bladder is completely emptied. Three to five units of Pitressin® Tannate in oil* are injected subcutaneously, and water balance is measured for an additional 24-hour period. During the first 12 hours, urine is collected every two hours. Volume, specific gravity, and osmolality of the urine are measured.

In healthy dogs depot ADH increases the urine concentration to maximal values (U_{osm}:P_{osm} >4). In central DI water intake and urine volume decrease markedly. Urine concentration always increases above isotonic levels. The response to the first ADH injection, however, may show considerable variation (Fig. 1). Therefore, it is advisable to collect the urine at shorter intervals; otherwise, the effect may be missed. In renal DI there is no response or only minimal response to exogenous ADH. In primary polydipsia the urine concentration rises and the plasma osmolality may be remarkably low. Since in most cases water intake continues despite ADH administration, water intoxication is possible. Only the responsiveness of the kidneys to ADH can be evaluated with the ADH test. A reliable diagnosis of central DI is not possible. For this reason, a water deprivation test must always be performed. In other diseases associated with polydipsia in which endogenous ADH still may be produced, exogenous ADH may induce a distinct antidiuresis.

DIFFERENTIAL DIAGNOSIS

All other diseases associated with an abnormality of water balance must be excluded. Besides primary polydipsia, these diseases are mainly those functional disorders of the renal concentrative capacity that make up the acquired renal DI group (see Table 1). The isothenuric polyuria of chronic renal insufficiency is caused by retention of obligate urinous substances. The tubules of the intact nephrons are flooded with a large amount of osmotically active substances because of the high concentration of these substances in the primary urine. An osmotic diuresis ensues that cannot be inhibited by ADH. An osmotic diuresis that is induced by elevated blood glucose levels is found in diabetes mellitus. Because of glucosuria, however, the specific gravity of the urine may be high. In hyperadrenocorticism renal concentrative capacity is reduced. Maximum U_{osm}:P_{osm} reaches 2 to 2.5 during water deprivation and administration of exogenous ADH. The concentrative disorder is thought to be induced by cortisol, which decreases the membrane permeability. In addition, the osmotic threshold stimulating ADH release possibly is elevated. In pyometra polyuria is induced by a reversible impairment of the tubular epithelium caused by bacteriotoxins.

THERAPY

The most effective treatment for ADH deficiency is hormone substitution. The most suitable form is the depot preparation Pitressin® Tannate in oil. In general, 2.5 units are not sufficient to reduce polyuria for 24 hours, except in very small dogs and cats. The action of 5 units usually lasts 24 to 72 hours, the extreme values being 12 hours to 7 days. The hormone should not be administered at fixed intervals but only after a new onset of polyuria.

The ADH response may not be sufficient when treatment begins, but Pitressin® Tannate in oil will produce the desired effect after repeated administration (see Figs. 1 and 3). Administration is by the subcutaneous or intramuscular route after *warming and vigorously shaking* of the ampule. To avoid water intoxication, the animals should not be allowed to consume large quantities of water immediately before or after hormone administration. In water intoxication the osmotic pressure of the extracellular fluid is lowered and water enters the cells. The cellular hyperhydration, especially within the brain, causes severe clinical signs, e.g., apathy, salivation, and nausea. The gait is staggering and incoordinated, consciousness is impaired, and there are muscular tremors or convulsions. Intravenous hypertonic NaCl solution is the treatment of choice in water intoxication.

Adverse side effects with Pitressin® Tannate are rarely seen. We have given it to dogs for up to 10 years. No clear signs of incompatibility or loss of activity have been observed, but occasional abdominal pain and hematuria have been seen. A disadvantage is the constant need for

---

*Pitressin® Tannate in oil, Parke-Davis, Detroit, Michigan.

Figure 1. Depot ADH test in two normal dogs and two dogs with central diabetes insipidus. Diagrams show the differences of reaction to initial injections of depot ADH. Urine volume (ml/hr) and the osmotic U/P ratio are plotted against time. In both patients with DI there was an immediate decline of diuresis in response to Pitressin® Tannate in oil (times of administration marked by arrows). In the first case (*top right*) the effect lasted longer than 24 hours. In the second case (*bottom right*) maximum effect was reached after 4 hours, and after 12 hours the effect has decreased significantly.

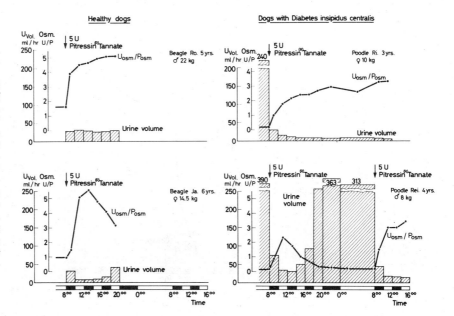

repeated injections. There is always the danger of local infection, inflammation, and subcutaneous induration, resulting in painful injections.

Analogs of vasopressin, which differ in structure and action from the natural hormone, have recently been synthesized. The most interesting of these compounds is 1-desamino-8-D-arginine vasopressin (DDAVP*). It differs from natural ADH by having a slower metabolic degradation time and probably a greater affinity for the renal ADH receptor. DDAVP acts nine times longer than vasopressin. The pressor activity is greatly lowered; therefore bowel movements are not increased, as may be seen in patients receiving vasopressin.

For long-term therapy, DDAVP is administered intranasally in man. This route of administration is difficult in animals because of sneezing or the passage of liquid into the pharynx. DDAVP should therefore be used as eye drops. DDAVP may also be administered into the prepuce or vagina but in a higher dose. One drop of solution corresponds to 1.5 to 4 μg of DDAVP. With two drops of DDAVP, given once or twice daily, polyuria is satisfactorily regulated. Maximum efficacy will be observed two to six hours after administration. Duration of action varies, even in the same individual, between 10 and 27 hours. This may be due to the variation in the drop size. DDAVP may induce a marked antidiuresis (Fig. 2) when administered twice daily. Since DDAVP is very expensive, it is recommended that it not be used before a new onset of polyuria or else only once daily, preferably at night to avoid nocturia.

We have used DDAVP for four years and have not observed any adverse side effects, irritation of the conjunctiva, loss of activity, or water intoxication.

Other drugs have been used for the treatment of DI. The most important of these is chlorpropamide,† an oral antidiabetic agent. It potentiates the renal ADH effects by increasing cAMP within the cells of the tubules and collecting ducts. Prerequisite for activity of this drug is the presence of minimum amounts of ADH, which by itself is without effect. It is of no value in renal DI or in some cases of severe central DI. We have tested chlorpropamide in several patients without success at doses of 10 to 40 mg/kg body weight/day. (Fig. 3). In one case severe hypoglycemia was observed. Successful treatment with chlorpropamide of a cat with partial DI has been reported.

Carbamazepine,‡ an antiepileptic agent, and clofibrate,§ an antihyperlipidemic drug, are also effective in some cases of central DI. Both drugs are ineffective in renal DI. They may potentiate residual ADH secretion but not the renal ADH action. Successful treatment with either drug of DI in dogs or cats has not been reported.

The only drugs, if any, that reduce the diuresis of renal DI are the thiazide diuretics, especially hydrochlorothiazide (HCT*). This paradoxical antidiuresis is due to their initial natriuretic action, which results in alleviation of

---

°Desmopressin® (Minrin® in many other countries)

†Diabinese®, Pfizer, New York, N.Y.
‡Tegretol®, Geigy Pharmaceuticals, Ardsley, N.Y.
§Atromid-S®, Ayerst Laboratories, New York, N.Y.
*Hydrodiuril®, Merck, Sharp & Dohme, West Point, Pa.

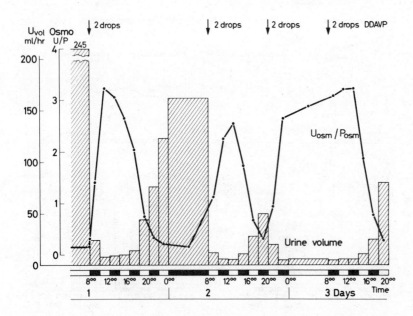

Figure 2. Response to DDAVP (Desmopressin® [Minrin®]) in central diabetes insipidus in the dog. Urine volume (ml/hr) and the osmotic U/P ratio are plotted against time. Two drops of DDAVP are sufficient to reduce diuresis for 16 hours or longer. Application twice daily is followed by a marked antidiuresis. (Poodle, male, 8 years old, weight 9 kg)

thirst. The reduced water intake decreases the extracellular fluid volume. This causes more sodium and water to be reabsorbed by the proximal tubules and probably causes a reduction of glomerular filtration. The urine volume decreases but the concentration does not reach isotonic levels.

In central DI the effects of HCT are not sufficient. Urine volume is reduced only by 10 to 40 percent (see Fig. 3). In some cases, however, an ADH-saving effect may be produced by combination therapy with Pitressin® Tannate and HCT. In acquired ADH-resistant polyuria we have had some therapeutic success using HCT. In these cases the daily fluid requirement is reduced by 50 to 85 percent. For each dog the dose must be estimated individually. The initial dose should be 2.5 to 5 mg/kg body weight. Since there is danger of hypokalemia with this therapy, serum potassium levels must be determined regularly and supplemented if necessary.

Polyuria may be decreased by a diet low in protein and salt, because a reduction in compounds obligatorily removed by the kidneys also reduces the amount of water needed for their excretion.

PROGNOSIS

In the symptomatic form of central DI the

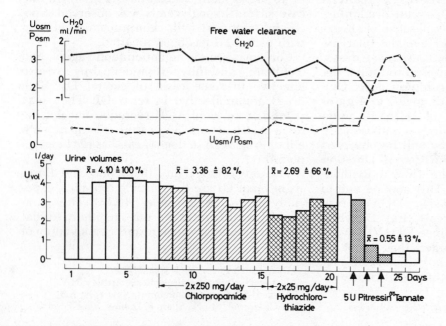

Figure 3. Effects of chlorpropamide, hydrochlorothiazide, and Pitressin® Tannate in oil on diuresis in central diabetes insipidus of the dog. Daily urine volumes, osmotic U/P ratios and free water clearance are plotted against time. The diet was standardized during the therapeutic tests. Successful treatment was not possible with chlorpropamide and hydrochlorothiazide. Only with Pitressin® Tannate was sufficient reduction of diuresis achieved from the second day on. U_{osm}/P_{osm} rose to values >1, and the C_{H2O} declined to negative values, indicating rediffusion of free water into hypertonic medulla tissue of the kidney. (Poodle, male, 5 years old, weight 13 kg).

prognosis is unfavorable. It depends on the basic disease and the nature and degree of impairment of the hypothalamic-neurohypophyseal region. In the idiopathic form prognosis is favorable, since such patients may survive for many years. With optimal substitution therapy, patients are asymptomatic. In cases of acquired renal ADH resistance prognosis depends on the nature and degree of the renal or metabolic disorders. In congenital renal DI there is no adequate treatment that will allow further maintenance of the animals.

SUPPLEMENTAL READING

Joles, J. A., and Mulnix, J. A.: Polyuria and polydipsia. In Kirk, R. W. (ed.): *Current Veterinary Therapy VI*. Philadelphia, W. B. Saunders Co., 1977, pp. 1050–1054.

Lage, A. L.: Nephrogenic diabetes insipidus in a dog. J. Am. Vet. Med. Assoc., *163*:251–253, 1973.

Mulnix, J. A., Rijnberk, A., and Hendricks, H. J.: Evaluation of a modified water deprivation test for diagnosis of polyuric disorders in dogs. J. Am. Vet. Med. Assoc., *169*:1327–1330, 1976.

Rogers, W. A., Valdez, H., Anderson, B. C., and Comella, C.: Partial deficiency of antidiuretic hormone in a cat. J. Am. Vet. Med. Assoc., *170*:545–548, 1977.

Schwartz-Porsche, D., and Müller, L. F.: Eine durch Hydrochlorothiazid zu beeinflussende Polydipsie beim Hund. Kleintier-Praxis, *12*:3–13, 1967.

DIABETES MELLITUS

EDWARD CHARLES FELDMAN, D.V.M.

Davis, California

Diabetes mellitus is a disorder of carbohydrate, protein, and lipid metabolism and is classically characterized by hyperglycemia and glycosuria. Central to this disturbance is a relative or absolute deficiency of insulin at the cellular level caused by an abnormality in the secretion or the effect of insulin. This concept does not ignore the established fact that counter-insulin substances, such as growth hormone, epinephrine, glucagon, and cortisol, may play contributory roles in the pathogenesis of this serious malady. The generalized chronic metabolic disturbances that develop can ultimately be life-threatening.

DIAGNOSIS

Diabetes mellitus is suspected whenever there is a history of polydipsia, polyuria, polyphagia, and weight loss. The diagnosis is confirmed by the finding of persistent fasting hyperglycemia. The normal fasting blood glucose concentration in the dog is 60 to 100 mg/dl, and the repeated finding of values above 150 mg/dl is usually considered diagnostic of overt diabetes in the absence of complicating factors. By "complicating factors" I mean hyperglycemia induced by stress (which can be quite dramatic in the feline), postprandial hyperglycemia, or hyperglycemia in an animal receiving certain medications. Glucocorticoids, ACTH, estrogens, progesterones, and numerous other drugs can cause diabetes mellitus. Dilantin® (phenytoin, Parke-Davis) and hydrochlorothiazide may

cause a reversible form of diabetes mellitus by inhibiting insulin secretion. Diabetes mellitus may also be associated with the hypercortisolemia of Cushing's syndrome.

When blood glucose concentration exceeds the renal threshold, glycosuria results. It is easily detected with Diastix® paper strips* or Clinitest® tablets.* Glycosuria without hyperglycemia can be caused by primary renal disease (most often noted in the Norwegian elkhound and basenji). Oral glucose tolerance tests (OGTT) should be used only when the diagnosis is in doubt. The most common indication for the OGTT is borderline hyperglycemia (120 to 175 mg/dl) without glycosuria. It is unnecessary to do glucose tolerance testing in patients that are overtly diabetic. Minimum laboratory evaluation in any candidate for long-term insulin therapy should include urinalysis, complete blood count (CBC), renal function test (BUN or creatinine), total serum protein, serum glutamic pyruvic transaminase (SGPT), alkaline phosphatase and fasting blood glucose. Stool testing for trypsin activity should be considered. The thorax and abdomen should be examined radiographically.

These studies are recommended in an attempt to evaluate the extent of expected changes from normal in any diabetic animal. We also want to recognize any active disease process that may be responsible for changing an

*Ames Company, Division of Miles Laboratory, Elkhart, Indiana 46514

asymptomatic borderline diabetic into one with obvious clinical signs. Any stress, such as boarding a dog or cat for some period of time, may be enough to push the borderline animal into full-blown diabetes mellitus.

As glucose utilization diminished in the diabetic, fat mobilization becomes excessive, and frank lipemia is often noted. SGPT and alkaline phosphatase levels are usually elevated in association with the resulting fatty metamorphosis of the liver seen with diabetes. The latter leads to hepatomegaly, which may be marked and which is the most common radiographic abnormality. Urine must be examined not only for glucose but also for signs of urinary tract infection. Proteinuria can occur secondary to damage of the glomerular basement membrane by hyperglycemia. Diabetes mellitus and pancreatic exocrine insufficiency can both be sequelae of pancreatitis, which explains the reasoning behind recommending fecal trypsin testing. Based on the history and physical examination, one may also elect to obtain other laboratory studies.

TREATMENT

Oral Hypoglycemics. These drugs are seldom used in veterinary medicine and should be reserved for the exceptional patient in which the glucose tolerance test is required to confirm the diagnosis of diabetes mellitus. Tolbutamide has severe hepatotoxic effects in the dog and hence should not be used. Other sulfonylureas, such as chlorpropamide and acetohexamide, have been used successfully in a few canine diabetics. However, they should never be used in the pregnant bitch because they are known to be teratogenic.

Insulin. By the time diabetes mellitus is diagnosed in the dog or cat, daily injections of insulin are usually required for control. NPH insulin is currently the most widely used form of insulin.

All insulins should be refrigerated, and the contents of the bottle must be mixed thoroughly before each dose is given. Following subcutaneous administration of NPH insulin, the onset of action is approximately three hours; peak blood levels occur in 6 to 10 hours, and the total duration of effect is 18 to 24 hours (Table 1). As the effect of insulin reaches its maximum, blood glucose concentration falls. To avoid the induction of possible hypoglycemic reactions, feeding must be timed to correspond with the period prior to insulin's greatest activity (Fig. 1).

NPH insulin, 100 units per ml (U100), is the preparation available to most veterinarians. Since cats and small dogs often require extremely small doses, the insulin is diluted to make administration of the correct amount easier for the owner. A 1:10 dilution is prepared so that a full "100-unit syringe" contains only 10 units of insulin.

Client Instruction. Diabetes mellitus is a serious disease and its treatment requires capable and willing owners. These owners must accept the responsibility for giving daily injections and feeding their pets at the proper time of day. Even though such a pet requires more care in comparison with a normal animal, it is unusual in this author's experience to have a client reject the responsibility and choose euthanasia for the animal.

This responsibility is important because of the serious consequences of improper care. Acute *overdosage* can result in a hypoglycemic episode, which may be seen as weakness and lethargy, changed behavior, or loss of consciousness and convulsions. Chronic *underdosage* can result in the cascade of metabolic changes that lead to a return of polydipsia, polyuria, polyphagia, and weight loss. Ultimately, ketoacidosis can occur. *Cataracts are a common sequela to mild insulin underdosage and hyperglycemia.* The time period between development of hyperglycemia and development of cataracts is unpredictable. For these reasons, daily monitoring of urine glucose and ketone levels provides better control of the diabetic. The goal of closer monitoring and insulin dose

Table 1. Commonly Used Insulin Preparations

		HOURS AFTER SUBCUTANEOUS INJECTION		
TYPE	FORM	*Effects Begin*	*Maximum Action*	*Duration of Effects*
Regular	Solution	$1/4$	2–4	6–8
NPH	Crystalline	3	6–10	18–24
Lente	30% Amorphous, 70% crystalline	3	8–12	18–24
PZI	Amorphous	3–4	14–20	24–36

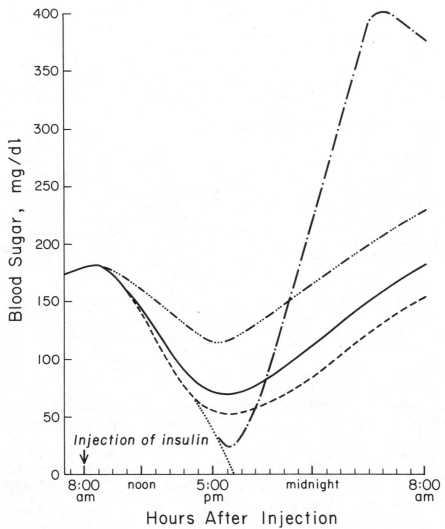

Figure 1. The changes seen in the blood sugar after an ideal amount of NPH insulin is administered at 8:00 AM to a dog fed approximately 9 hours later (———); poor control with too low a dose (– ····–); a mild overdosage (– – – –); a severe overdosage leading to convulsion (.........); and a severe overdosage resulting in the Somogyi overswing (· — · — ·).

adjustments is to maintain the blood glucose concentration as close to normal for as much of each 24-hour period as possible. The reported incidence of cataract development and blindness in poorly monitored diabetic dogs is much higher than that in the author's patients, in whom daily urine monitoring is imperative. This point should be emphasized to the owner/client. Day-to-day caloric intake and exercise are unavoidably variable and will affect the daily insulin requirement. Hence, the owner must understand that adjustments in insulin dosage must be based on the results of daily urine monitoring.

The owner is instructed to maintain a daily diary. This should include the results of morning urine glocuse and ketone measurements, the dose of insulin, whether the patient ate in the morning and evening, and the site of insulin injection (which should vary).

Method of Treatment. Exogenous insulin replacement is not as physiologic a process as one would hope. In contrast with the sensitively regulated endogenous secretion of insulin into the portal vein, exogenous insulin is given subcutaneously in one large dose. It is then absorbed continuously throughout the day. Food must be ingested at certain times and in specific amounts to avoid hyperglycemia or hypoglycemia. Each diabetic should be hospitalized until its metabolic condition is stabilized. The initial dose of insulin in the dog is approximately ½ unit (U)/kg body weight subcutaneously. In the cat, which is more sensitive to exogenous insulin, the initial dose is ¼ U/kg subcutaneously. It is preferable to begin therapy at a low dose, since it is easier to correct for hyperglycemia than to deal with an acute hypoglycemic crisis. In the hospital and at home a simple schedule is followed for monitoring and treating the diabetic (Table 2).

Each morning, the urine is tested for glucose and ketone levels by the use of Ketodiastix®.[°] The *corrected* dose of NPH insulin (see following discussion) is then administered subcutaneously, and the patient is given 10 to 25 percent of its daily food intake. The main meal is given approximately 8 to 10 hours later, to coincide with the peak in insulin action. During the initial in-hospital period, the afternoon blood glucose concentration must also be measured, seven to nine hours after insulin is administered. Such a determination allows the clinician to assess directly the insulin's effect and time of action in each patient. A blood glucose test should also be obtained once during hospitalization, four to six hours after insulin administration to document the individual variability of patient sensitivity to insulin. All afternoon blood glucose determinations must be performed prior to the evening meal. When animals are rechecked after their initial hospitalization, they must be seen late in the afternoon, prior to their evening meal, to best assess their response to insulin.

The basic objective of insulin therapy is to maintain the patient at $1/10$ to $1/4$ percent (trace to +) glycosuria in the morning. This goal avoids the precipitation of a severe hypoglycemic episode prior to the evening meal. No snacks are allowed. If the animal appears to be weak prior to the evening meal (suggesting hypoglycemia), the meal should be given earlier in the day.

The phrase *daily corrected insulin dose* refers to the change in insulin dosage determined by the morning urinalysis. The dosage adjustments (Table 3) shown are appropriate for a 10-kg dog. They should be reduced somewhat for smaller dogs and increased for larger ones. When a urine specimen cannot be obtained, the previous day's dose should be repeated.

Occasional ketonuria that is noticed by the owner in the Ketodiastix test is not worrisome if the dog is alert, eating, and not vomiting. Ketonuria on two consecutive days may signal the need for specific therapy for ketoacidosis, and in such cases the veterinarian should be notified.

Complications. The accepted renal threshold for glucose is 175 to 225 mg/dl, and therapy is dependent on this fact. Variable renal thresholds outside this range do occur, however. If a

*Ames Company, Division of Miles Laboratory, Elkhart, Indiana, 46514.

Table 2.   Recommended Treatment Schedule for Diabetics

8:00 AM:	Collect urine sample and determine level of glycosuria.
8:15 AM:	Administer insulin dose.
8:30 AM:	Feed $1/8$ to $1/4$ of the total daily food requirement.
6:00 PM:	Feed $3/4$ of the total daily food requirement.

patient is not reacting as expected during therapy one can attempt to determine the renal threshold by comparing urine glucose levels with blood glucose determinations obtained at the same time. A urine glucose level will be accurate if the bladder is emptied 15 to 30 minutes prior to obtaining the test sample. This procedure prevents misleading readings caused by urine mixing in the bladder over a prolonged period of time.

Rarely, marked glycosuria is observed each morning, even with increasing doses of insulin and proper renal thresholds for glucose. When the dose of insulin approaches 1.0 unit/lb of body weight (2.2 U/kg), there is an increased risk of significant hypoglycemia later in the day. Hence, the veterinarian must be consulted whenever high doses appear to be needed. The author has no canine or feline patients receiving more than 1.0 unit of insulin per pound of body weight.

The most common causes for an apparent increase in the dose requirement are (1) improper administration of the insulin by the owner, (2) inadequate mixing of the insulin prior to its withdrawal from the vial, (3) use of insulin that is outdated or inactivated by improper storage, and (4) use of Ketodiastix that are inaccurate. If these causes are eliminated, the possibility that the administered insulin is being metabolized too rapidly must be considered. When insulin levels in the blood are inadequate or absent, blood glucose levels will rise, and glycosuria occurs, resulting in the presence of large amounts of glucose in the morning urine specimen. This problem may often be resolved by the use of Lente insulin, which may have a slightly longer duration of effect (see Table 1). Thus, the early morning

Table 3   Daily Insulin Dose Adjustment for 10-kg Dog

GLYCOSURIA	ADJUSTMENT
2%	Increase 1 unit.
1%	Increase $1/2$ unit.
0 5%	Increase $1/2$ unit.
0.1–0 25%	Repeat previous day's dosage.
Negative	Decrease 1 unit.

absence of insulin in the blood is eliminated, and improved control can be achieved. It is not recommended that NPH insulin be administered twice daily, since both client compliance and urine monitoring become quite difficult. PZI insulin action overlaps from day to day and should not be used.

A phenomenon of hypoglycemia that induces counterregulatory mechanisms to raise the blood glucose to very high levels (see Fig. 1) is known as the "Somogyi effect." Epinephrine, glucagon, glucocorticoids, and growth hormone secretion participate in this response. The end result — hyperglycemia and glycosuria — may be misinterpreted as indicating the need for increased insulin dosage, when the dose actually should be decreased. Only close monitoring by owner and veterinarian, avoiding inordinately high insulin doses, will avoid such a complication.

Because the injected insulin is a foreign protein it consistently causes production of antibodies to insulin in man. Fortunately, production of antibodies sufficient to interfere with treatment is rare. Insulin products are constantly being made purer, reducing unwanted antigenic foreign protein. However, some patients develop insulin resistance because of the insulin-binding antibodies (which can be measured in man). This condition sometimes improves with the substitution of pork insulin, which is less antigenic than beef insulin.

The owner should be instructed to have a glucose-containing syrup, such as Karo Syrup®,* available at all times. If the animal appears to be weak or unusually tired, the syrup should be administered orally immediately. If convulsions occur, the syrup should be rubbed on the buccal mucosa and not poured into the mouth. The owner should be instructed to do this *immediately*, even before notifying the veterinarian. Hypoglycemia can produce coma as well as seizures.

Whenever a known diabetic is presented to the veterinarian because of an acute generalized central nervous system disturbance, a blood sample should be obtained for blood glucose determination and then a minimum of 5 to 10 ml of intravenous 50 percent dextrose should be given immediately unless ketoacidosis is obvious.

Diet. Once diabetes mellitus has been diagnosed, the patient's diet must be constant. The amount of food ingested will directly affect the amount of insulin required to maintain stability. Ideally, a palatable commercial canned food should be found, because it has a constant caloric value.

The patient should be fed according to its ideal body weight. A small dog should receive approximately 75 kcal/kg body weight, and large dogs should receive approximately 55 kcal/kg. If weight loss is deemed necessary to reach ideal body weight, total daily caloric intake should be reduced. The reducing diabetic must be monitored closely at home, since the daily insulin requirement will decrease as body weight decreases. In rare cases insulin will no longer be required once ideal body weight is achieved.

Exercise. The amount of daily exercise will greatly affect the daily insulin requirement and should therefore be as constant as possible. Working dogs require *less* insulin on working days. Although the cause is not well understood, the entry of glucose into skeletal muscle is increased during exercise even in the absence of insulin. Hence, diabetes is more difficult to manage in the working dog and requires close communication between the owner and the veterinarian. In our experience dogs exercise much more at home than in the hospital, but they also consume more food at home, so the insulin requirement usually increases after the animal is released from the hospital.

NONSPAYED BITCHES

Estrus, pseudopregnancy, and pregnancy complicate the management of diabetes, since they make the effect of insulin highly erratic. The hormones produced during pregnancy and pseudopregnancy antagonize the effects of insulin, and insulin is destroyed by an insulinase produced by the placenta. The increased energy needs associated with estrus, pseudopregnancy, and pregnancy often result in the onset of ketosis secondary to the bitch's chronic hyperglycemia, which stimulates fetal growth hormone. Fetuses of diabetic bitches tend to be large. In the neonate there is an increased risk of a hypoglycemic crisis due to beta-cell hyperplasia, which results again from chronic stimulation by high blood glucose concentrations *in utero*. Thus, for female diabetic patients ovariohysterectomy should be performed as soon as possible after their condition is stabilized.

ELECTIVE SURGERY

A simple protocol should be followed when any operation is performed on the diabetic dog or cat. Ketosis and hyperglycemia must be prevented during and immediately after surgery. Elective major operations should be delayed until the patient's clinical condition is stable. The day prior to surgery the patient receives

---

*Best Foods, Englewood Cliffs, New Jersey 07632

the normal dose of insulin and is fed as usual. No food is given after midnight. On the morning of the operation, half of the calculated dose of insulin for that day is given. During surgery the patient is maintained on an IV drip of 5 percent dextrose in water or 5 percent dextrose in saline until oral intake is re-established. The IV dextrose drip is important because it provides carbohydrate for response to the stress of surgery. Insulin must also be administered so that the diabetic animal can utilize the dextrose. A lower insulin dosage is administered, since the normal amount of food will not be consumed that day. It is easier to correct hyperglycemia than to treat a hypoglycemic crisis.

During and after surgery total urine output, urine ketones, and urine glucose must be monitored at frequent intervals. Measurements of blood glucose may also be required postopera-tively. If hyperglycemia and glycosuria occur, small amounts of regular insulin can be given at four- to six-hour intervals. The dose of regular insulin in this situation is approximately 20 percent of the total daily dose of NPH insulin for 4+ glycosuria. The dose is reduced further for lesser degrees of glycosuria or if long-acting insulin is expected to peak during the period.

On the day after surgery the diabetic can usually be returned to the routine schedule of insulin administration and feeding. A patient that is not eating can be maintained on IV dextrose and saline. Since the carbohydrate load in this situation is continuous, it is desirable to maintain a continuous supply of insulin. This is accomplished by giving half the usual dose subcutaneously at 12-hour intervals until the animal is eating regularly and can be returned to the normal schedule.

DIABETIC KETOACIDOSIS

WILLIAM D. SCHALL, D.V.M.
Lansing, Michigan

and LARRY M. CORNELIUS, D.V.M.
Athens, Georgia

Ketoacidosis and other complications of diabetes mellitus are a therapeutic challenge and are encountered with regularity in spite of the general trend toward early detection of diabetes. The clinician should suspect ketoacidosis and other complications when there is a history of anorexia, vomiting, diarrhea, lethargy, weakness, or increased depth and rate of respiration (Kussmaul's breathing). Physical findings that are suggestive of complications include depression or coma, weakness, dehydration, acetone breath odor, Kussmaul's breathing, fever, abdominal pain, icterus, or shock. When any of these abnormalities are identified in a diabetic dog or cat, the laboratory evaluation should include the following determinations: complete blood count, urinalysis, total serum protein, blood glucose, urea nitrogen, amylase and/or lipase, sodium, potassium, chloride, and blood gases (pH, P_{CO_2}, P_{O_2} and HCO_3). From these tests the serum osmolality (or tonicity) can be estimated and the anion gap calculated.

THERAPY OF DIABETIC KETOACIDOSIS

Therapy for diabetic ketoacidosis involves the simultaneous administration of fluids, electrolytes, regular (crystalline) insulin and, in many instances, alkalizing agents. Repeated laboratory assessment is important during therapy because the total quantity of each of the agents necessary for reversal of ketoacidosis can be determined only by titration.

IMMEDIATE CONSIDERATIONS

Patency of the airway should be established in comatose patients. Emesis with sluggish or absent reflexes necessitates endotracheal intubation. Aseptic catheterization of the cephalic vein provides a convenient means of fluid administration; however, if central venous pressure is to be monitored, jugular catheterization is needed. Patients with azotemia that are suspected of having impaired renal function should have an indwelling urinary catheter installed so that urine output can be monitored.

WATER

Dehydration can be estimated by combining the results of physical examination, packed cell volume test, and total plasma or serum protein concentration determination. Often, the extent of dehydration approaches an amount equivalent to 10 to 15 percent of body weight. Although rehydration is usually scheduled over 48 hours, rapid restoration of circulating blood volume is important, and fluids should be administered at the rate of 90 ml/kg body weight/hour for the first one or two hours, or until circulating volume is restored. At a slower rate of administration, one half of the total calculated deficit can be administered in the first 12 hours. Although some free water loss characterizes diabetic ketoacidosis, most clinicians prefer to use isotonic replacement fluids such as lactated Ringer's solution or 0.9 percent sodium chloride. Hypotonic fluids should be avoided, because cerebral edema may result from their administration.

ELECTROLYTES

The ketoacidotic diabetic is usually deficient in both sodium and potassium, but serum concentrations of these electrolytes may be normal because of free water loss. Moreover, the magnitude of potassium depletion is not reflected in the serum concentration, because addition of this cation to extracellular water occurs at the expense of intracellular concentration. In spite of these limitations it is important that serum sodium and potassium concentrations be determined before and during fluid and electrolyte therapy. Hypokalemia is occasionally detected prior to therapy but more often occurs as a result of insulin administration. The hypokalemia that results from insulin administration usually occurs as the blood glucose concentration decreases, but it may precede the decrease in glucose concentration on occasion because insulin may facilitate intracellular relocation of potassium independent of its action on glucose transport.

It is desirable to determine the serum potassium concentration every two hours during the first eight to 12 hours of insulin therapy, since the degree of hypokalemia may be sufficient to cause death and because uncertainty exists about the time of development of hypokalemia. Cautious potassium replacement is indicated if the serum concentration is determined to be less than 3 mEq/liter, especially if the patient is not fully hydrated. If serum potassium concentration cannot be determined, the clinician may assume that hypokalemia is present if obvious muscle weakness is observed at the same time that blood glucose concentration is decreasing rapidly. Potassium is usually administered intravenously to the ketoacidotic patient because oral intake is often precluded. Thirty to 40 mEq of potassium chloride or phosphate is usually added to each liter of fluids. The rate of potassium administration should not exceed 0.5 mEq/kg body weight/hour. In the case of a solution containing 35 mEq/liter, only 15 ml/kg body weight/hour should be administered.

Hypophosphatemia also occurs regularly during insulin therapy for diabetic ketoacidosis and tends to occur at the same time as hypokalemia. Hypophosphatemia is important, since it causes decreased intraerythrocytic 2,3-diphosphoglycerate (DPG) concentration, which results in decreased oxygen delivery to tissues. The effect of low serum inorganic phosphate concentration on DPG may be compounded by improved acid-base status of the patient, because alkalization also tends to decrease oxygen delivery to tissues (Bohr effect). If hypophosphatemia is detected, phosphate may be added to fluids at the rate of 15 to 20 mEq/liter.

ALKALIZING AGENTS

Neither clinical signs nor laboratory data (other than actual blood gas determinations or their equivalent) adequately predict the acid-base status of diabetic ketoacidotic cats and dogs. For this reason it is important that blood pH or bicarbonate level be determined so that severe metabolic acidosis can be identified and treated. It is ideal to measure P_{CO_2} and pH. Bicarbonate then can be estimated from a standard nomograph. If blood gas equipment is not available, other methods can be used. The CO_2 content of plasma can be measured rapidly, accurately, and relatively inexpensively using a commercially available total CO_2 apparatus.* The CO_2 content of plasma is largely composed of bicarbonate and therefore is a measure of the metabolic component of acid-base balance. If neither P_{CO_2} and pH nor total CO_2 can be determined, the clinician can only guess, although the dissipation of plasma and urine ketones and increases in urine pH generally can be interpreted as improvement in metabolic acidosis.

Consideration should be given to the selection of an alkalizing agent. Acetate may be

---

*Harleco CO_2 Apparatus, Harleco Division, American Hospital Supply, Philadelphia, Pennsylvania.

ketogenic and for this reason is not often used for diabetic acidosis. If lactic acidosis complicates diabetic ketoacidosis then the usual alkalizing effect of lactate will not occur. There is no evidence, however, that sodium lactate will contribute to lactic acidosis.

The total number of mEq of lactate or bicarbonate needed to correct the metabolic acidosis of diabetes can be estimated by multiplying the bicarbonate deficit (normal serum concentration minus measured value) times half the body weight in kg. The calculated quantity of base should be administered over 48 hours to avoid paradoxical cerebrospinal fluid (CSF) acidosis.

INSULIN

Regular (crystalline) insulin is used for treating diabetic ketoacidosis. All or part of the insulin is administered intravenously because absorption from subcutaneous sites is poor as a result of poor tissue perfusion secondary to dehydration. Two methods of intravenous insulin administration have evolved: the intermittent bolus method and the continuous infusion method. Both are described here, but we prefer the continuous intravenous infusion method.

INTRAVENOUS INTERMITTENT BOLUS METHOD

Regular insulin is administered intravenously as a bolus every two to six hours until the plasma glucose concentration reaches 200 mg/dl or less. Plasma glucose determinations are made every two hours, and subcutaneous NPH insulin is substituted for regular insulin after the plasma glucose concentration is 200 mg/dl or less. The initial dose of insulin is 1 to 2 units/kg (0.5 to 1.0 unit/lb) of body weight for dogs. Because cats are insulin-sensitive compared with dogs the recommended dose for them is 0.5 unit/kg body weight. Some clinicians have advocated the use of much higher initial insulin doses based on the notion that ketosis or low blood pH impairs tissue insulin responsiveness. However, there is no evidence to support this contention. Low doses of insulin have been documented to be just as effective as high doses in correcting ketoacidosis in man. In those rare instances in which the patient fails to respond to conventional doses, subcutaneous boluses of insulin can be increased.

INTRAVENOUS CONTINUOUS INFUSION METHOD

The advantages of low dose intravenous continuous insulin infusion in man have been reported, and we have been delighted with our successful use of the method for dogs. Both hypokalemia and hypoglycemia are less likely to occur and, if either of these complications should arise, stopping the insulin infusion will result in a rapid decline in blood insulin concentration. Another advantage is that the timing and dose calculations necessary in the bolus method are eliminated. The insulin infusion is simply continued until the plasma glucose concentration reaches 200 mg/dl. It is then stopped and NPH insulin is administered. The method is simple and inexpensive because the only special equipment needed is a pediatric drip set to regulate the drip rate more finely. We add 5 units of regular insulin to 500 ml of lactated Ringer's solution and, using a pediatric infusion set, administer insulin at the rate of 0.5 to 1.0 unit per hour. To achieve adequate rehydration, non-insulin–containing fluid is administered at an appropriate rate independently of the insulin-containing fluid. The plasma glucose concentration is determined every two hours and the infusion is stopped when the blood glucose is 200 mg/dl, which is usually six to eight hours after the infusion is started.

The low total doses of insulin that are effective in reversing diabetic ketoacidosis when administered by the intravenous continuous infusion method are even lower than calculated, because up to 75 percent of the insulin adheres to the fluid bottle and infusion apparatus.

The use of somatostatin to inhibit glucagon secretion in combination with insulin administration to our knowledge has not been attempted in dogs or cats with naturally occurring diabetic ketoacidosis, but some studies suggest that it may be a useful adjunct in man.

COMPLICATIONS

PANCREATITIS

Pancreatitis complicates diabetic ketoacidosis more frequently than any other disease and is the most common cause of death. Increased serum activity (greater than two times normal) of either amylase or lipase in a vomiting diabetic ketoacidotic dog is strongly suggestive of pancreatitis. Lesser increases in the serum activity of either enzyme may be the result of dehydration rather than pancreatic inflammation. Diabetic ketoacidotic patients should be treated for both diseases simultaneously, although none of the commonly used therapeutic maneuvers for pancreatitis is of established efficacy. We currently allow nothing per os to patients with pancreatitis until serum lipase and/or amylase activity approaches normal and the patient is no longer vomiting, usually an interval of three days. The effectiveness of atropine, antibiotics, analgesics, tranquilizers, and glucocorticoids is unproved and subject to debate. We do not administer them routinely. Hypocalcemia occurs rarely as a result of pancreatitis, and after it is documented we treat it with calcium gluconate.

DIABETIC COMA

Although not commonly encountered, animals in coma that is associated with diabetes mellitus are a medical challenge and require extensive laboratory monitoring. Ketoacidotic coma can apparently occur in diabetic ketoacidosis because of metabolic acidosis alone. The occurrence is not common because in metabolic acidosis cerebrospinal fluid (CSF) bicarbonate concentration is preserved, and CSF acidosis rarely occurs. The results of studies in human diabetics have shown that there may be little correlation between the level of acidosis and coma, but good correlation exists between serum osmolality and the state of consciousness.

HYPEROSMOLAR COMA

Stupor leading to coma can occur because of hyperosmolality. Patients with hyperosmolality often are not ketotic. The hyperosmolality occurs as a result of profound hyperglycemia or hypernatremia, or both. Serum osmolality can be measured or calculated in man from the following formula, and it may be accurate for the dog.

$$\text{Serum osmolality} = 2(\text{Na}^+ + \text{K}^+) + \frac{\text{Blood glucose}}{18}$$

The serum osmolality is expressed in mOsm/kg, the serum sodium and potassium in mEq/liter, and the blood glucose in mg/dl. The contribution to serum osmolality made by blood urea nitrogen (BUN) should not be included in the formula and should be subtracted from actual osmolality determinations because urea is freely diffusable. As a result, urea contributes to hyperosmolality but does not contribute to serum hypertonicity relative to the CNS. Normal serum osmolality (tonicity) is about 300 mOsm/kg. Signs referable to serum hypertonicity are not usually seen until the serum osmolality approaches 375 mOsm/kg, excluding the effect of urea. Treatment of serum hypertonicity must be approached with caution because cerebral edema can follow, particularly if hypotonic fluids are administered. For this reason either isotonic fluids or fluids no less hypotonic than half-strength saline should be administered.

CEREBRAL EDEMA

Cerebral edema can result from the administration of both isotonic and hypotonic fluids because of resultant serum hypotonicity relative to the CNS. In many instances the mechanism of cerebral edema remains obscure. One hypothesis involves the polyol pathway and a pathogenesis similar to that proposed for diabetic cataract formation.

PARADOXICAL CSF ACIDOSIS

Stupor progressing to coma can occur as a result of rapid correction of metabolic acidosis with intravenous alkalinizing agents. This phenomenon occurs because the CSF becomes acid during the time that blood pH is rapidly corrected to normal. In metabolic acidosis, CSF pH is better preserved than is blood pH, because of bicarbonate retention. If blood pH is rapidly corrected, blood bicarbonate and pH may exceed CSF concentrations. Blood CO_2 content then increases to a concentration greater than that of CSF and rapidly diffuses into the CSF, resulting in decreased CSF pH. For this reason correction of severe metabolic acidosis should be done over a 48-hour interval.

SUPPLEMENTAL READING

Fulop, M., Tannenbaum, H., and Dreyer, N.: Ketotic hyperosmolar coma. Lancet, 2:635, 1973.

Molnar, G. D., and Service, F. J.: Low-dosage continuous insulin infusion for diabetic coma. Ann. Intern. Med., *81*:853, 1974.

Schall, W. D., and Cornelius, L. M.: Diabetes mellitus. Vet. Clin. North Am., 6:687, 1976.

FUNCTIONAL PANCREATIC ISLET CELL ADENOCARCINOMA IN THE DOG

DENNIS D. CAYWOOD, D.V.M.
St. Paul, Minnesota

and JAMES W. WILSON, D.V.M.
Roseville, Minnesota

Functional islet cell tumors are rarely observed in the dog. The tumor, arising from beta cells in the islets of Langerhans, begins as a small, nodular mass in the pancreatic parenchyma. Unlike those in man, canine islet cell tumors are nearly always malignant. Although metastasis may become widespread, islet cell adenocarcinomas are often initially confined to the pancreas and regional lymph nodes. Therefore, early diagnosis is important when contemplating surgical or medical management.

CLINICAL FEATURES

All reported functional islet cell tumors have been in dogs older than four. Although seen in many breeds, the boxer, poodle, and terrier are most commonly affected. There is no sex predilection.

All clinical signs are attributable to hypoglycemia. They include muscle tremors, muscle weakness, ataxia, collapse, and convulsions. The onset of signs is generally precipitated by exercise or a stressful situation. Most dogs exhibit convulsions during the course of the disease; however, ataxia, muscle weakness, and muscle tremors are more common. Clinical signs often exist several months before initial clinical examination. Unfortunately, the disease is often misdiagnosed initially. As a result, seizures are commonly treated symptomatically with anticonvulsants. Clinical signs become more frequent and severe as the disease progresses. Dogs appear to adapt partially to chronic hypoglycemia. We have observed dogs late in the course of the disease with blood glucose concentrations of 20 to 30 mg/dl, which appear clinically normal. Hypoglycemia should be suspected when seizures are associated with a history of muscle weakness, muscle fascicula-

tion, and ataxia. Many owners report in the history that the dogs recover more quickly if they are fed following the onset of clinical signs. Hypoglycemia may cause a vast array of abnormal neurologic signs. Therefore, it is important to rule out other possible neurologic diseases. Differential diagnosis should include viral encephalitis, toxoplasmosis, brain tumor, trauma, cryptococcosis, idiopathic epilepsy, hydrocephalus, tetanus, hypocalcemia, and drug-induced seizures.

LABORATORY FEATURES

Tentative diagnosis of a functional pancreatic islet cell tumor is classically based on demonstration of Whipple's triad (neurologic disturbances associated with hypoglycemia, fasting plasma glucose concentration ≤40 mg/dl, and relief of neurologic disturbances by feeding or administration of glucose). Whipple's triad is characteristic of hypoglycemia, regardless of cause. It is often necessary to fast the dog for at least 24 hours to demonstrate Whipple's triad. We have had only one dog with a functional tumor in which the plasma glucose concentration remained > 40 mg/dl following a 24-hour fast. Although pancreatic islet cell tumors are the most common cause of hypoglycemia in the dog, it is important to rule out other possible diseases. Other causes of fasting hypoglycemia include hypopituitarism, Addison's disease, hypothyroidism, and disorders related to liver disease, such as glycogen storage disease and cirrhosis. Once the cause of neurologic disturbance is suspected to be hypoglycemia, additional laboratory data are needed to confirm a diagnosis of hyperinsulinism.

The high-dose intravenous glucose tolerance test (H-IVGTT) is useful for evaluating the

High Dose Intravenous Glucose Tolerance Test

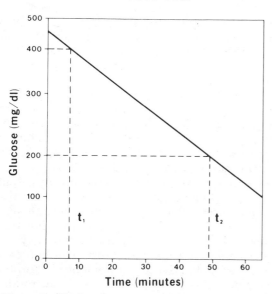

Figure 1. Plasma glucose response to intravenous glucose administration. Calculation of the K-value is done according to the formula $K = \dfrac{69.3}{T_2 - T_1}$ where T_1 and T_2 are arbitrarily chosen to correspond with a pair of glucose values that represents a 50 percent decrease in blood glucose concentration.

ability of an animal to shift glucose out of the plasma space. After a 24-hour fast, a zero-time blood sample is collected and then glucose (1 gm/kg body weight) is rapidly given intravenously (within 30 to 45 seconds). Blood samples are obtained 5, 15, 30, 45, and 60 minutes after infusion and analyzed for glucose concentration. In normal dogs plasma glucose concentration should return to normal in 30 to 60 minutes. A K-value is obtained from a semilog plot of glucose values. It reveals the percent rate of glucose disappearance per minute from a semi-

log plot (Fig. 1). The H-IVGTT checks the responsiveness of the islet cells to a massive glucose overload. Normal dogs have a K-value >2.5 and <3. Diabetic dogs, having a low population of islet cells or unreactive cells, have a K-value <2.0. All but one of our cases had K-values in the prediabetic range (Table 1). No cases showed an excessive response to glucose (K-value >3). These results suggest that the tumor is generally unresponsive to glucose overload and that the existing non-neoplastic islet cells are also unresponsive owing to constant negative feedback from insulin released by the tumor.

The glucagon tolerance test evaluates insulin because glucagon initiates insulinogenesis through direct tumor stimulation and insulin release and indirectly through glycogenolysis. We perform the test, following a 24-hour fast, by giving 0.03 mg/kg of glucagon USP intravenously. Plasma glucose concentrations are determined 0, 1, 5, 15, 30, 45, 60, and 120 minutes after administration of glucagon. In dogs with pancreatic islet cell tumors the blood glucose concentration does not exceed 150 mg/dl and returns to the hypoglycemic state within 60 minutes (Fig. 2).

Serum immunoreactive insulin (IRI) concentrations can be determined by commercial laboratories to confirm a diagnosis. Although elevated IRI concentrations do occur with islet cell tumors, many dogs have concentrations within the normal range (8 to 20 μU/ml). Failure to demonstrate elevated IRI concentrations does not exclude the diagnosis of a functional tumor, since some tumors secrete proinsulin predominantly. Clinical signs of hyperinsulinism associated with low IRI concentrations can occur in functional islet cell tumors. However, if the IRI concentration is compared with the plasma glucose concentration, the ratio is usually abnormal when compared to that of clinically normal

Table 1.   *Laboratory Values and Calculated Indices For 6 Fasted Dogs With Pancreatic Islet Cell Adenocarcinoma*

CASES	PLASMA GLUCOSE (mg/dl)	SERUM INSULIN (mμ/ml)	GLUCOSE: INSULIN RATIO	INSULIN: GLUCOSE RATIO	AMENDED INSULIN: GLUCOSE RATIO	K-VALUE
1	32	13	2.46	0.40	658	2.5
2	40	14	2.85	0.35	140	2.1
3	36	200	0.18	5.55	3333	—
4	52	8	6.5	0.15	36.3	2.1
5	40	—	—	—	—	2.1
6	40	14	2.86	0.35	240	2.04
Values Diagnostic of Islet Cell Tumor	<40	>20	<2.5	>0.3	>30	>3

Glucagon Tolerance Test

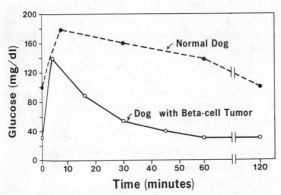

Figure 2. Plasma glucose response to intravenous glucagon in a normal dog and in a dog with a functional beta-cell tumor.

dogs. Essentially three ratios have been developed. The ratio of glucose to insulin (G/I) was first. Values <2.5 were considered diagnostic of an insulinoma. A second ratio was insulin to glucose (I/G). Values >0.3 were considered diagnostic. The third and most recent ratio was created following examination of reports of ethanol-induced hypoglycemia. Serum IRI concentrations were found to be near zero when plasma glucose concentrations were ≤30 mg/dl. The "amended insulin-glucose ratio" (AIGR) is obtained by evaluating the expression:

$$\frac{\text{Serum insulin } (\mu\text{U/ml}) \times 100}{\text{Plasma glucose (mg/dl)} - 30}$$

It is suggested that normal values are <30 μU/mg glucose.

We have compared all three ratios (see Table 1). The G/I ratio resulted in the highest percentage of false negative results. The I/G was more accurate, but one false negative was observed. The AIGR was correctly elevated in all cases and is truly diagnostic of hyperinsulinism. Rather than suggesting this disease, as the H-IVGTT and the glucagon tolerance test do, the AIGR confirms elevated insulin for the circulating glucose present.

SURGICAL FEATURES

Unfortunately, no laboratory test will predict widespread metastasis, nor does any test suggest a favorable prognosis. Exploratory celiotomy is suggested as the best prognostic tool available and the ideal choice of therapy. Animals should be prepared for surgery as for any other exploratory celiotomy. Some have suggested that postoperative pancreatitis is a frequent complication of partial pancreatectomy.

Although we suggest monitoring serum amylase and lipase activity, we have not observed postoperative pancreatitis in a single case. We do not recommend prophylactic therapy postoperatively, as some suggest. It has been our experience that, unlike in man, pancreatitis is extremely uncommon following partial pancreatectomy in the dog.

Many clinicians have also urged aggressive glucose administration during surgery to prevent possible hypoglycemic crises due to insulin release following tumor manipulation. In our experience intraoperative plasma glucose concentration rises to greater than normal values without glucose administration. Apparently, stress gluconeogenesis induced by anesthesia and surgery more than counteracts possible insulin release from the tumor resulting from manipulation. Glucose administration may still be advisable but not mandatory. We do recommend intraoperative measurement of the plasma glucose concentration as well as routine intraoperative fluid management.

Exploratory celiotomy should include a careful inspection of the liver, mesentery, and associated lymph nodes. These structures should be carefully palpated during surgical examination. If a mass is identified and is confined to the pancreas and mesenteric lymph nodes, it should be removed. Obviously, it should be considered operatively uncorrectable if there is liver or widespread abdominal metastasis. The plasma glucose concentration and serum amylase activity should be monitored closely for the first 12 to 24 hours postoperatively. Following recovery, these parameters should be monitored daily for a four- to five-day period.

PROGNOSIS

Surgery should be considered palliative. Several investigators have reported that removal of the neoplasm did not extend life; however, we have had three dogs with tumors involving both pancreas and mesenteric lymph nodes in which surgical excision was possible. As a result, they were asymptomatic for 270 days, 575 days, and 875 days, respectively. One dog was reoperated upon after recurrence of signs caused by lymph node metastasis at 270 days. This extended its asymptomatic life to 600 days. Life was thus prolonged for at least 575 days in each animal.

The mesenteric lymph nodes appear to be the first target organ, and their ability to prevent further metastasis appears to be considerable. Only after overwhelming the lymph nodes does widespread, surgically unresectable metastasis occur. If exploratory celiotomy indicates no hepatic or widespread metastasis and if the dog is not hypoglycemic following surgical excision of the tumor, then a good immediate postoperative recovery can be expected.

Temporary diabetes mellitus is frequently encountered postoperatively. This results from feedback inhibition caused by high levels of insulin or proinsulin produced by the tumor. We have observed persisting diabetes in one dog. Although the pancreatic islets appeared histologically normal, suppression of normal beta cells by tumor insulin may have resulted in irreversible loss of insulin production. Hypoglycemia appeared following recurrence of the tumor.

Temporary remission of hypoglycemia by treatment with streptozotocin has been reported in a dog with an islet cell tumor. The drug is associated with hepatic and nephrotoxicity, however, and should be used with caution.

SUPPLEMENTAL READING

Caywood, D.D., et al.: Pancreatic islet cell adenocarcinoma: Clinical and diagnostic features of 6 cases. J. Am. Vet. Med. Assoc., *174*: 714–717, 1979.
Johnson, R.K.: Insulinoma in the dog. Vet. Clin. North Am. 7:629–635, 1977.
Njoku, C.O., Strafuss, A.C., and Dennis, S.M.: Canine islet cell neoplasia: A review. J. Am. Anim. Hosp. Assoc., 8:284–290, 1972.

NON-NEOPLASTIC CAUSES
OF CANINE HYPOGLYCEMIA

ROGER K. JOHNSON, D.V.M.
Walnut Creek, California

and CLARKE E. ATKINS, D.V.M.
Stillwater, Oklahoma

Hypoglycemia is not a specific diagnosis but rather the manifestation of another disease or physiologic process. Extensive research in human medicine has resulted in the classification of hypoglycemia based on (1) age of onset: neonatal, juvenile, or mature; (2) occurrence: transient or persistent recurrent; and (3) hypoglycemic stimulus: reactive or fasting. Furthermore, in man a list of specific diagnoses has been defined for each classification. Relatively few disease processes characterized by hypoglycemia have been documented in the dog.

The regulation of normal blood glucose concentration is a complex process involving intestinal absorption, hepatic production, and peripheral utilization of glucose. In the early fasting state, glucose is derived mainly from liver glycogen. Later, glucose is formed in the liver via gluconeogenesis from amino acids (alanine being the most important), from glycerol derived from lipolysis, and from lactate. In prolonged fasting, ketones provide an alternate energy source for cerebral and other tissues. Normal function of liver enzyme pathways is essential to the hepatic regulation of the blood glucose concentration. In addition, profound influences on both hepatic production of glucose and peripheral glucose utilization are exerted by hormones such as insulin, glucagon, epinephrine, norepinephrine, cortisol, ACTH, and growth hormone.

CLINICAL MANIFESTATIONS

For the most part, the clinical manifestations of hypoglycemia are similar regardless of the etiology. The brain is largely dependent on glucose oxidation for energy and does not have readily available glycogen stores; in addition, glucose enters the neuron predominantly by diffusion rather than as an insulin-dependent process. Therefore, the blood glucose concentration is of prime importance to the brain, and the signs of hypoglycemia are understandably those of central nervous system dysfunction. The severity of clinical manifestations is related to the rate at which the blood glucose concentration declines and, to a lesser extent, to the degree of hypoglycemia.

We have observed nearly normal behavior in a dog whose blood glucose concentration decreased to 6 mg/dl over a 36-hour period. Conversely, we have observed a generalized seizure in a dog whose blood glucose concentration dropped from the normal range to 40 mg/dl over a 30-minute period.

Generalized or focal neurologic signs may be observed in dogs with hypoglycemia and include weakness of the rear legs or generalized weakness, muscular twitching, incoordination, amaurotic blindness, generalized siezures, and other bizarre neurologic aberrations. Pulmonary edema has recently been described as a possible sequela to hypoglycemia.

When hypoglycemia evolves rapidly there is a prompt increase in the concentrations of growth hormone, cortisol, pancreatic glucagon, epinephrine, and norepinephrine. The effect of these hormones is complex, but in general they serve to stabilize or elevate blood glucose concentrations and thus counteract hypoglycemia by increasing hepatic glucose release, inhibiting endogenous insulin release, or decreasing peripheral glucose utilization.

When the onset of hypoglycemia is slow, the counter-regulatory mechanism may not be triggered. Likewise, when acute hypoglycemia recurs frequently over a long period of time, the response mechanisms may become exhausted. Consequently, through either mechanism these recurrent episodes of hypoglycemia are marked by a lessened ability of the dog to restore blood glucose values to normal and may result in severe cerebral damage or so-called "irreversibe hypoglycemic brain damage."

NEONATAL HYPOGLYCEMIA

Owing to inefficient glucose homeostasis, the neonate is particularly susceptible to fasting and will become hypoglycemic in 24 to 48 hours, whereas the normal adult can fast for weeks. The reasons for this are that (1) the newborn pup requires two to three times the glucose per unit body weight as does the adult, (2) the pup's gluconeogenic enzymes are often "immature" and therefore do not function at peak capacity, (3) the protein mass to body mass ratio in the neonate and infant is far less than in the adult, thus minimizing hepatic gluconeogenesis from protein substrate, and (4) during the first five days of life the pup lacks a competent feedback mechanism between plasma concentration and hepatic production of glucose.

Premature or runted pups are quite often hypoglycemic. Hypothermic neonates are also often hypoglycemic, as are pups born to toxemic mothers. These pups should be maintained at a body temperature above 95 degrees and force-fed warmed bitch's replacement formula or dextrose in balanced electrolyte solution via gavage at frequent intervals.

JUVENILE-ONSET HYPOGLYCEMIA

TRANSIENT JUVENILE HYPOGLYCEMIA

This form of hypoglycemia, seen predominantly in puppies of the toy and miniature breeds that are less than three months of age, is usually precipitated by cold, starvation, or gastrointestinal disturbances. The signs of transient juvenile hypoglycemia are not dissimilar to those of other forms of hypoglycemia. In our experience, however, the puppies are more commonly presented comatose or severely depressed, with accompanying facial muscle twitching. The blood glucose concentration may be extremely low and is rarely above 30 mg/dl.

To prevent irreversible neuronal damage, prompt therapy is imperative. Initially, it should include a total of 1 to 2 ml of 50 percent glucose per kg body weight, administered intravenously as a bolus and diluted in equal parts of sterile water to avoid the possibility of hyperosmolarity.

If clinical signs are not ameliorated by repeated glucose administration, it can be assumed that cerebral edema is present. If the unresponsive signs include generalized seizures, sedation with diazepam is indicated prior to specific therapy for cerebral edema (mannitol and dexamethasone). Ten to 15 per cent glucose should then be administered in a balanced electrolyte solution at a rate sufficient to maintain normoglycemia until oral alimentation is possible. Pups should then be fed frequently, and oral sugar should be administered at regular intervals until normoglycemia is maintained. If the precipitating factors are adequately treated, recurrence of signs is uncommon.

PERSISTENT OR RECURRENT JUVENILE HYPOGLYCEMIA

In some puppies hypoglycemia may continue or recur despite therapy, and these puppies should be evaluated for other causes of hypoglycemia. Hereditary defects in carbohydrate metabolism, defects in amino acid metabolism, hormone deficiencies (growth hormone, glucagon, cortisol, and ACTH), and hyperinsulinism (beta-cell hyperplasia, leucine sensitivity, islet cell adenoma, and others) are known causes of persistent or recurrent hypoglycemia in children. Similar reports in the dog are limited to the glycogen storage diseases, and even these are incompletely documented.

Type I glycogen storage disease (von Gierke's disease) is caused by a deficiency of glucose-6-phosphatase, an enzyme necessary for the conversion of glucose-6-phosphate to free glucose. The end result of this enzyme deficiency is a visceral accumulation of glycogen and ensuing hypoglycemia. Children affected with type I glycogen storage disease are characterized by fasting hypoglycemia that responds poorly to glucagon and by growth retardation, hepatomegaly, renomegaly, ketosis and acidosis due to lactate accumulation, hyperlipidemia, and a bleeding diathesis.

Bardens described type I glycogen storage disease (GSD) in 6- to 12-week old puppies, characterized by symptomatic hypoglycemia with hepatomegaly and less than normal response to glucagon administration. Puppies that responded to initial therapy relapsed and eventually died, and autopsies were reported to reveal glycogen deposition in the liver, kidneys, and myocardium.

A tentative diagnosis of glycogen storage disease may be made if recurrent or persistent hypoglycemia is found in a puppy that also has hepatomegaly, acidosis, and ketosis. A negative glucagon tolerance test is strongly suggestive of but not diagnostic for a GSD, because a liver depleted of glycogen will also give a negative response to glucagon. To establish a definitive diagnosis, histologic evidence of glycogen accumulation should be provided and specific enzyme analysis performed. The prognosis for glycogen storage disease in the dog is grave; however, if treatment is attempted it should consist of frequent carbohydrate feedings, glucose supplementation, and avoidance of lactose, which may contribute to glycogen accumulation. Diazoxide, a benzothiazide derivative that causes elevations of blood glucose, may prove efficacious in the long-term treatment of type I glycogen storage disease in the dog.

Strombeck described persistent fasting hypoglycemia in an 11-week-old Pomeranian that manifested depression progressing to coma when fasted. It was postulated, based on subnormal blood ketone values, that the hepatic enzyme system — responsible for ketone production from fatty acids — was immature. This lack of ketones, an important energy source in the fasting dog, resulted in hypoglycemia and depressed levels of alanine and pyruvate (these precursors for gluconeogenesis were utilized in excess owing to the lack of ketones). An alternate theory, proposed by Meyer, is that this pup suffered from a glucagon deficiency. The pup was maintained with oral glucose supplementation, until 4½ months of age. At that time, normoglycemia could be maintained, and it was presumed that the enzyme immaturity had been outgrown.

Mosier has described hypoglycemic pups of the toy breeds with ketonuria and hepatic lipidosis at eight to nine weeks of age. He advises a high-protein diet and lipotrophic agents as the treatment of choice.

Both hypothyroidism and panhypopituitarism can cause hypoglycemia in children. However, to our knowledge this has not been recognized in the dog.

MATURE-ONSET HYPOGLYCEMIA

HEPATOGENOUS HYPOGLYCEMIA

Certain liver disease, when severe, may result in hypoglycemia as a result of destruction of hepatic enzyme systems responsible for storage or lysis of glycogen and for hepatic gluconeogenesis from amino acids. Cirrhosis, fatty degeneration, the glycogenoses (GSDs), neoplasia, vascular anomalies, and acute necrotic and other forms of hepatitis are notable examples.

Occasionally, dogs with severe liver disease are presented because of hypoglycemic signs, but more commonly the signs are those related to liver disease. Such an exception is an 11-year-old spayed female poodle that was eventually shown to have hepatic cirrhosis and whose history included recurrent hypoglycemic episodes over a 2½ year period. Late in the course of the disease when elevated serum alkaline phosphatase and SGPT concentrations were the only indications of liver disease, an intravenous glucagon tolerance test revealed an extremely flat curve. The fasting blood glucose concentration was 17 mg/dl and, following the administration of 0.03 mg glucagon IV, the peak blood glucose response was 28 mg/dl at 15 minutes, indicating insufficient glycogenolysis. Normal serum insulin levels were measured at 0 time (23.9 μU/ml) and one minute after injection (45.7 μU/ml). However, these concentrations were inappropriately high when compared with the corresponding glucose values of 17 mg/dl and 9 mg/dl, respectively. At laparotomy and necropsy, hepatic cirrhosis and portocaval shunting were noted, and careful examination of the pancreas revealed no evidence of an islet cell tumor. The conclusion was drawn that, since pancreatic portal blood was for the most part being shunted past the diseased and only partially functional liver, the usual hepatic destruction of insulin was lacking, and the result was inappropriately high levels of insulin in the circulation, which further depressed serum glucose concentrations.

ENDOCRINE HYPOGLYCEMIA

Hypoadrenocorticism. The presenting signs of hypoadrenocorticism are usually those of hypovolemia, hyperkalemia, and hyponatremia (refer to the article elsewhere in this section on primary adrenocortical insufficiency). Hypoglycemia occurs not uncommonly in severely ill dogs with hypoadrenocorticism, but what portion of the weakness associated with that disease is from hypoglycemia is debatable. We have observed generalized seizures associated with blood glucose concentrations of 45 mg/dl, 22 mg/dl, and and 30 mg/dl, resulting from a lack of glucocorticoid production in three dogs, proved to have very low cortisol levels both at rest and after ACTH stimulation. The direct cause in two of these dogs was most likely a primary cortisol deficiency or ACTH deficiency with secondary adrenal cortical atrophy, since these patients were controlled with glucocorticoids alone and showed no electrolyte imbalance. Feldman has recently described a dog suffering from ACTH deficiency proved by direct measurement of ACTH. The dog had low resting and post-ACTH cortisol levels but was not hypoglycemic.

HUNTING DOG HYPOGLYCEMIA

A hypoglycemia of hunting breeds has been described, usually affecting highly nervous dogs one to two hours after beginning a hunt. When afflicted these dogs appear dazed, then stagger and exhibit grand mal type seizures. Recovery generally occurs within minutes, but the dogs remain exhausted for the remainder of the day. Frequent feedings with protein-rich meals throughout the hunt have been recommended and found to be successful. Twice-daily feedings appear to be adequate on days when the dog is not working. Adrenocorticosteroids and tranquilizers have also been advocated. Bardens feels that this syndrome may represent a type III glycogen storage disease, but no evidence for this has been provided.

MISCELLANEOUS CAUSES OF HYPOGLYCEMIA

One of the most common causes of a low blood glucose report from the laboratory is simply the failure to remove the serum from the cells or utilize an agent such as sodium fluoride to preserve the sample. Whole blood at room temperature is said to oxidize glucose at the rate of 10 mg/dl/hour.

It is not uncommon to find a mild to severe hypoglycemia in a patient with a severely debilitating disease. If the underlying disease is adequately treated, blood glucose concentration usually returns to normal.

During routine screening of mature dogs it is not unusual, in our experience, to find blood glucose concentrations below normal. There is often no apparent cause for this finding, and normoglycemia is often found on retesting. The cause for this incidental finding of hypoglycemia is unclear.

Primary renal glycosuria, resulting from an enzymatic defect in the renal tubules, is known to occur in the dog. However, an associated hypoglycemia, which is found in this hereditary disease in man, has not been described in the dog. Extensive renal tubular damage can also result in glycosuria but generally not in hypoglycemia.

Other causes of hypoglycemia may include intestinal malassimilation, insulin overdosage, and ingestion of oral hypoglycemic drugs.

TESTS USED TO DIFFERENTIATE CAUSES OF HYPOGLYCEMIA

Endocrine causes of hypoglycemia can be substantiated by measurement of the appropriate hormone(s) — thyroxin, ACTH, cortisol, insulin, glucagon, or growth hormone. The glucagon tolerance test is useful to determine the availabilty of hepatic glycogen. In the fasting state a glycemic response to glucagon rules out the likelihood of a glycogen storage disease (this test is described in detail in *Current Veterinary Therapy VI*). Strombeck describes assaying for blood ketones, alanine, and pyruvate as useful means of determining the pathogenesis of hypoglycemia. A defect in gluconeogenic enzymes would be demonstrated, for example, by a marked elevation of the glucose precursors (lactate, pyruvate, alanine), whereas a subnormal blood ketone level in a hypogylcemic pup might suggest a defect in enzymes necessary for ketone production or possibly a glucagon deficiency. Challenge testing with various sugars, hormones, and amino acids may also be used to further differentiate causes of hypoglycemia. Hepatic enzyme quantitation can be performed on biopsy specimens if they are frozen immediately in liquid nitrogen and stored at −80 degrees C. Liver biopsy can also be utilized to determine the presence of glycogen or lipids.

SUPPLEMENTAL READING

Bardens, J.W.: Glycogen storage disease in puppies. Vet. Med. Small Anim. Clin., *61*:1174, 1966.
Bardens, J.W., Bardens, G.W., and Bardens, B.: Clinical observa-

tions of a von Gierke-like syndrome in puppies. Allied Vet., 32:4, 1961.

Bleicher, S.J.: Hypoglycemia. In Ellenberg, M., and Rifkin, H. (eds.): *Diabetes: Theory and Practice.* New York, McGraw-Hill Book Co., 1970.

Brady, L.J., et al.: Influence of prolonged fasting in the dog on glucose turnover and blood metabolites. J. Nutr., 107:1053–1061, 1977.

Feldman, E.C. and Tyrrell, J.B.: Hypoadrenocorticism. Vet. Clin. North Am., 7:555–581, 1977.

Hetenyi, G., Varma, S., and Cowan, J. S.: Relations between blood

glucose and hepatic glucose production in newborn dogs. Br. Med. J., 2:625–627, 1972.

Kogut, M.D.: Hypoglycemia: Pathogenesis, diagnosis, and treatment. Curr. Probl. Pediatr., 4:1–59, 1974.

Meyer, D.J.: Fasting hypoglycemia in a pup. (Letter) J. Am. Vet. Med. Assoc., 173:1286–1290, 1978.

Mosier, J.E.: Canine pediatrics. Vet. Clin. North Am., 8:106, 1978.

Pagliara, A.S., et al.: Hypoglycemia in infancy and childhood. J. Pediatr., 82:365–379, 558–557, 1973.

Strombeck, D.R., et al.: Fasting hypoglycemia in a pup. J. Am. Vet. Med. Assoc., 173:299–300, 1978.

PUERPERAL TETANY

S. L. MARTIN, D.V.M.
and C. C. CAPEN, D.V.M.
Columbus, Ohio

Puerperal tetany is encountered most frequently in small, excitable breeds of dogs, such as Chihuahuas, toy poodles, and small terriers, one to three weeks after parturition. This condition also occurs sporadically in larger dogs and in cats. The clinical course is rapid, with only an 8- to 12-hour interval between the onset of initial clinical signs and the development of tetany. Premonitory signs include restlessness, excessive panting, and excitable behavior. Within a few hours clinical signs may progress to ataxia, trembling, muscular tetany, and convulsive seizures. Hyperthermia frequently is associated with the increased muscular activity, and elevations of body temperatures to 107°C are not uncommon.

PATHOPHYSIOLOGY

Considerably more is known about the development of postparturient hypocalcemic syndromes in cattle than is known about the disease in other animal species. There is little evidence to suggest that puerperal tetany in lactating bitches is the result of an interference in parathyroid hormone secretion. The severe hypocalcemia and hypophosphatemia that develop near the time of peak lactation (one to three weeks postpartum) are probably the result of an imbalance between the rates of inflow and outflow from the extracellular calcium pool (Fig. 1). It is well known that feeding high-calcium diets to dairy cows in the prepartum period has a provocative effect on the development of hypocalcemic disorders following parturition because of diminished responsiveness of parathyroid hormone–mediated bone resorption (Fig. 2). The reduced availability of calcium from skeletal sources leads to an excessive reliance on intestinal calcium absorption.

Functional disturbances associated with hypocalcemia in the bitch are primarily the result of neuromuscular tetany (Fig. 3), in contrast with those in the cow, in which the clinical sign is mainly paresis. The occurrence of either tetany or paresis in response to hypocalcemia appears to be the result of basic physiologic differences between the bitch and cow in the function of the neuromuscular junction. The release of acetylcholine and transmission of nerve impulses across neuromuscular junctions are blocked by the severe hypocalcemia in

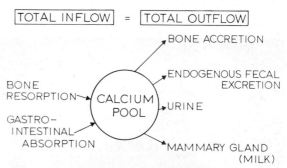

Figure 1. Relationship of inflow of calcium into the extracellular fluid pool (from bone resorption and gastrointestinal absorption) and outflow of calcium into milk, urine, feces, and bone. An imbalance between the rates of inflow and outflow from the extracellular fluid calcium pool because of the increased loss of milk appears to be an important factor in the pathogenesis of puerperal tetany in the bitch.

HIGH CALCIUM PREPARTAL DIET

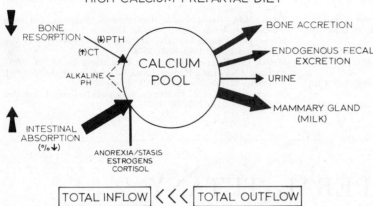

Figure 2. Calcium homeostasis in animals fed a high-calcium diet during the gestation period is primarily dependent upon intestinal calcium absorption. The rate of bone resorption is low, and parathyroid glands are inactive. Anorexia and gastrointestinal stasis that often occur near parturition interrupt the major inflow into the extracellular fluid calcium pool. Outflow of calcium at the peak of lactation exceeds the rate of inflow into the calcium pool and the animals develop a rapidly progressive hypocalcemia.

cows, leading to muscle paresis. The dog appears to have a higher margin of safety in neuromuscular transmission, in that the degree to which endplate potential exceeds the firing threshold is greater in the dog than the cow. Excitation-secretion coupling is maintained at the neuromuscular junction in the bitch with hypocalcemia. Tetany occurs in the bitch as a result of spontaneous repetitive firing of motor nerve fibers. As a result of the loss of stabilizing membrane-bound calcium, nerve membranes become more permeable to ions and require a stimulus of lesser magnitude to depolarize.

DIAGNOSIS AND TREATMENT

Diagnosis is based on history, clinical signs, and response to therapy in most cases. If laboratory facilities are readily available, demonstration of hypocalcemia with serum calcium levels less than 7 mg/dl confirms the clinical diagnosis. Serum phosphorus often is lowered to a comparable degree. Blood glucose is in the low normal range or decreased as a result of the intense muscular activity associated with tetany.

The slow intravenous administration of an organic calcium solution such as calcium gluconate should result in rapid clinical improvement and cessation of tetanic spasms within 15 minutes. In most bitches 5 to 10 ml of 10 percent calcium gluconate will provide sufficient calcium for a bitch weighing between 5 and 10 kg. Intravenous administration should proceed slowly to avoid inducing ventricular fibrillation and cardiac arrest.

Puppies should be removed from the bitch for 24 hours to reduce the lactational drain of calcium. During this period the puppies should be fed a milk substitute or other appropriate diet. If the puppies are mature enough, it is advisable to wean them; otherwise, they should be returned to the bitch after the 24-hour period. Supplemental dietary calcium and vitamin D

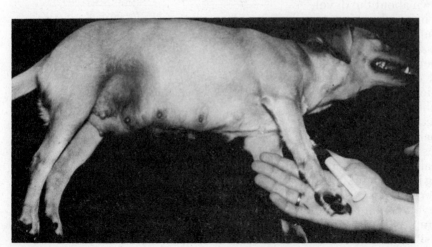

Figure 3. A bitch with puerperal tetany. Increased neuromuscular excitability occurs in the bitch with hypocalcemia, since excitation-secretion coupling is maintained at the motor endplate.

Figure 4. Calcium homeostasis in an animal fed a low-calcium prepartal diet. Bone resorption and intestinal absorption both contribute substantially to the inflow of calcium into the pool in extracellular fluids. The anorexia and gastrointestinal stasis that may occur near parturition can temporarily interrupt one inflow pathway. However, there is more likely to be an adequate pool of active bone-resorbing cells capable of responding to the increased parathyroid hormone secretion under these dietary conditions to maintain an approximate balance between calcium inflow and outflow, thereby preventing the development of progressive hypocalcemia.

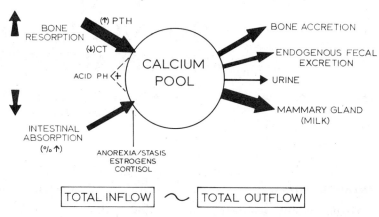

have proved useful in preventing relapses in certain bitches with puerperal tetany.

Although some clinicians advocate the use of corticosteroids in addition to calcium and vitamin D to prevent relapses after the original therapy, there is no logical basis for use of these drugs in such treatment regimens. Since these drugs may lower serum calcium by interfering with intestinal calcium transport, their real value in the treatment of eclampsia is uncertain.

PREVENTION

During gestation, a good-quality, balanced diet with a calcium-to-phosphorus ratio of 1:1 or less that provides the required (but not excessive) amounts of calcium may provide a more responsive calcium homeostatic mechanism to meet the markedly increased demands of lactation. Calcium homeostasis in animals fed balanced or relatively low-calcium diets during gestation appears to be under better control by parathyroid hormone secretion with the approach of parturition and initiation of the lactational drain (Fig. 4). The higher levels of parathyroid hormone secreted during the prepartal period by an expanded population of actively synthesizing chief cells results in a larger pool of active bone-resorbing cells to fulfill the increased needs for calcium mobilization at the critical time near parturition and initiation of lactation. These animals appear to be less susceptible to the influence of decreased calcium absorption and flow into the extracellular pool, which can occur in the immediate postpartum period.

Calcium homeostasis in animals fed a high-calcium diet during gestation appears to be maintained principally by intestinal calcium absorption (see Fig. 2). This greater reliance on intestinal absorption rather than on parathyroid hormone–stimulated bone resorption probably is a significant factor in the more frequent development of hypocalcemia near parturition in animals fed high-calcium diets prepartum. These animals are more susceptible to the decreased calcium available for absorption that results from the anorexia often associated with parturition and initiation of lactation.

SUPPLEMENTAL READING

Austad, R., and Bjerkas, E.: Eclampsia in the dog. J. Small Anim. Pract., *17*:795, 1976.

Bjerkas, E.: Eclampsia in the cat. J. Small Anim. Pract., *15*:411–414, 1974.

Black, H.E., Capen, C.C., and Arnaud, C.D.: Ultrastructure of parathyroid glands and plasma immunoreactive parathyroid hormone in pregnant cows fed normal and high-calcium diets. Lab. Invest., *29*:173–185, 1973.

Black, H.E., Capen, C.C., Yarrington, J.T., and Rowland, G.N.: Effect of a high-calcium prepartal diet on calcium homeostatic mechanisms in thyroid glands, bone, and intestine of cows. Lab. Invest., *29*:437–448, 1973.

Bowen, J.M., Blackman, D.M., and Heavner, J.E.: Effect of magnesium ions on neuromuscular transmission in the horse, steer, and dog. J. Am. Vet. Med. Assoc., *157*:164–173, 1970.

Capen, C.C., and Black, H.E.: Fine-structural evaluation of parathyroid glands of cows fed high-, normal-, and low-calcium diets. In Hess, M. (ed.): *Electron Microscopic Concepts of Secretion: Ultrastructure of Endocrinal and Reproductive Organs.* New York, John Wiley & Sons, 1975, pp. 379–398.

Yarrington, J.T., Capen, C.C., Black, H.E., Re, R., Potts, J.T., Jr., and Geho, W.B.: Experimental parturient hypocalcemia in cows following prepartal chemical inhibition of bone resorption. Am. J. Pathol., *83*:569–588, 1976.

Yarrington, J.T., Capen, C.C., Black, H.E., and Re, R.: Effects of a low-calcium prepartal diet on calcium homeostatic mechanisms in the cow: Morphologic and biochemical studies. J. Nutr., *107*:2244–2256, 1977.

THE OVARY, OVARIAN HORMONES, AND CONTRACEPTIVES

P. N. S. OLSON, D.V.M.
Fort Collins, Colorado

INTRODUCTION

Sexual receptivity (estrus) in the dog is dependent upon the ovary and its hormones. The many controlling factors of ovarian function are incompletely understood. The dog is unique in that, following estrus, the luteal phase of the estrous cycle (diestrus) remains for approximately the same length of time whether the bitch is pregnant or not. Following diestrus, the animal enters a reproductively quiescent stage (anestrus), and factors initiating a new estrus are, to date, only speculative.

Lengthening anestrus theoretically could solve the canine population problem. Shortening anestrus would enable researchers using the dog in heritability studies to save time and money. Shortening anestrus would also enable breeders to increase the number of offspring from valuable bitches.

THE OVARIES

The canine ovaries are located near the posterior poles of the kidneys. They are held close to the abdominal wall by the suspensory ligament of the ovary. The ovary is entirely within the ovarian bursa. A small bursal slit can be visualized. Occasionally a small amount of tissue, part of the fimbriated, everted mucosa of the infundibulum of the oviduct, will protrude from the bursal slit. Such tissue has been reported to protrude more frequently during estrus, but this can occur during any phase of the estrus cycle. Because the ovary is so completely covered with bursa, direct visualization of the ovary is usually impossible without incising the bursa. The amount of adipose tissue present within the bursal sheath is often abundant in older animals and may be so extensive that ovariohysterectomy is extremely difficult.

The size of the canine ovary varies with breed, stage of the estrual cycle, and pathologic conditions. Generally, larger dogs will have larger reproductive tracts. The quiescent ovary during anestrus usually is smaller than the estrual ovary. The size of the canine ovary can be greatly increased by ovarian tumors or cysts.

The normal ovary is usually smooth and pink in color. In beagles it becomes grayish with advancing age. During anestrus the ovary is small and has a slightly wrinkled surface. As estrus approaches the ovary enlarges and the surface becomes somewhat more smooth. Follicles do not protrude very much from the ovary's surface. During diestrus, salmon-colored corpora lutea protrude form the surface.

In pathologic states, the shape and size of the canine ovary can vary considerably. Cystadenocarcinomas of the ovary can greatly alter ovarian shape, with the smooth ovary being replaced by a rough proliferative tumor. Various cysts can also increase ovarian size. Follicular and luteal cysts occur in the dog and are a potential cause of infertility. More frequently, cysts of mesonephric duct remnants are seen in the canine reproductive tract but are usually not associated with infertility.

The ovaries of puppies contain more oocytes than do the ovaries of older animals. The ovaries of female puppies at birth contain approximately 700,000 oocytes; at puberty, 355,000; at five years of age, 34,000; and at ten years of age, only about 500 egg cells remain. After 12 years of age, follicle counts are usually extremely low, but generally ovaries are not afollicular. All factors contributing to reproductive failure in the aging bitch are not understood.

OVARIAN HORMONES — THE ESTROUS CYCLE

In the last few years the endocrine events controlling the estrous cycle have been partially delineated in the bitch. Validated radioimmunoassays for the determination of serum levels of LH, FSH, prolactin, estradiol, and progesterone in the bitch are now available.

The estrous cycle can be divided into proestrus, estrus, diestrus, and anestrus segments.

PROESTRUS

Proestrus is generally six to nine days in duration. The bitch begins to attract males but is generally not receptive to mating. A serosanguineous discharge drips from a swollen and turgid vulva. This discharge usually contains numerous red blood cells that are thought to come from diapedesis through uterine capillaries in response to increasing estrogen levels. The vaginal epithelium proliferates as blood estrogens rise. The uterine diapedesis and vaginal proliferation account for the many red blood cells and superficial vaginal epithelial cells seen on vaginal smears taken during proestrus. During proestrus an enlarging cervix can often be palpated abdominally.

Proestrus is the stage of the cycle during which estrogen concentrations are rising. Estrogen from the ovary increases in response to pituitary gonadotrophins. In late proestrus, plasma estradiol levels peak and subsequently decline, thereby initiating or potentiating the ovulatory surge of luteinizing hormone (LH). Serum progesterone starts to rise in proestrus (prior to ovulation) and later peaks in diestrus.

ESTRUS

Estrus is generally six to twelve days in duration and is the period of sexual receptivity. Often the serosanguineous discharge of proestrus clears in estrus, but occasionally it can persist into diestrus. When a male attempts to mount, the bitch will usually lift her tail off to the side of the perineum ("flagging") and stand to be bred. Some estrual bitches will not allow copulation even when no physical or endocrinologic abnormality can be identified.

Rising progesterone levels and declining estrogen levels have been observed with the onset of mating behavior. While the onset of receptivity is usually close to the time of LH peaking, it may lag two to four days behind the LH peak in puberal cycles. Thus, some puberal animals may have ovulated prior to their first acceptance of a male. Generally, LH peaks in early estrus and is followed by ovulation within 38 to 44 hours. Most ova are released over a 24-hour period and are primary oocytes. Maturation of ova must occur, with extrusion of the first polar body, before fertilization can take place. While the general recommendation is to breed bitches every other day during the receptive period, fertility reportedly has been high following a single mating on the first day of estrus. This is probably due to the longevity of canine spermatozoa in the estrual reproductive tract.

Vaginal smears during estrus contain superficial epithelial cells and cellular debris, but no neutrophils are found even when bacteria are present in considerable numbers.

DIESTRUS

Diestrus is defined as the period between the last acceptance of a male for mating and the cessation of luteal activity. The average length of diestrus is 60 to 90 days. Diestrus is characterized cytologically by intermediately cornified epithelial cells, non-cornified epithelial cells (parabasal cells), and neutrophils in vaginal swabbings.

Serum progesterone levels increase rapidly after ovulation and peak approximately 25 days after the LH peak. Serum progesterone concentrations are similar for pregnant, non-pregnant, and pseudopregnant bitches and are of no value in diagnosing pregnancy in the dog. The only difference detected between pregnant and non-pregnant bitches is that an acute drop in progesterone occurs immediately prior to whelping, whereas a gradually declining level occurs in the non-pregnant animal.

Corpora lutea are a bright salmon-pink color from the time of ovulation until ten days after ovulation. They then change to yellow and become a light tan color about 60 days after ovulation.

Metestrus is the period of rapid growth of the corpora lutea. In the canine this period lasts for three to five days and actually occurs during estrus. When referring to the luteal phase, it is probably better to use the term *diestrus* to avoid confusion.

ANESTRUS

Anestrus varies in length from two to ten months and is the period of sexual inactivity and ovarian quiescence. Anestrus accounts for the varying lengths of interestrous intervals (the intervals between periods of sexual receptivity), since the periods of proestrus, estrus, and diestrus are fairly constant. Breed differences in interestrous interval can vary from 149 ±28.5 days for the female German shepherd to 242 ±63.5 days for the Boston terrier. Therefore, little or no correlation between body weight per se and estrous cycle length has been determined.

Serum progesterone and estradiol are low during anestrus. It is hoped that fine hormone fluctuations during anestrus can be studied in the future, when newer methods in radioimmunoassay provide increased sensitivity.

CONTROL OF THE ESTROUS CYCLE

Theoretically, control of the canine estrous cycle would be possible if the length of anestrus could be controlled. Shortening anestrus is desirable to people with valuable breeding animals who want more puppies from a single bitch and to those researchers using the dog as a model for studying heritable diseases.

SHORTENING ANESTRUS (INDUCTION OF ESTRUS)

Methods for inducing estrus in the bitch have been reported (Bardens; Thun, et al.). Bardens describes a method of induction that employs follicle stimulating hormone (FSH). Thun's method utilizes pregnant mares' serum (PMS). It has been our experience that results are not always consistent when using FSH. Based on endocrinologic studies, animals showing some of the physical signs of estrus are not ovulating. We have not used PMS for induction of estrus because currently it is difficult to obtain. We are now studying different methods of estrus induction by varying dosages and times of administration of FSH. Commercially available preparations of FSH vary greatly in purity and actual FSH content. Generally, the induction of a fertile estrus in the dog seems more difficult than in some other species.

When owners request induction of estrus, it becomes extremely important to evaluate the animal's general health and to be satisfied that no systemic disease is causing the delayed estrus. Hypothyroidism, hypoadrenocorticism, and hyperadrenocorticism are examples of systemic diseases that can affect the reproductive cycle. It must also be stressed to the owner that, while hormones can be used in an attempt to induce estrus, many such hormones are glycoproteins and are potentially immunogenic. Repeated treatments with LH preparations potentially can render a subfertile animal totally infertile because of antibody production against exogenous LH, which may cross-react with her own LH.

SURGICAL LENGTHENING OF ANESTRUS

Ovariohysterectomy is an effective method of lengthening anestrus in the bitch. It is permanent and, with the newer methods and types of anesthesia, is quite safe. It eliminates uterine disease and, if done when the animal is young, significantly decreases the incidence of mammary neoplasia in later life.

Unfortunately, ovariohysterectomy has not been the total answer to pet population control in the United States. Cost is still a definite consideration to the pet-owning public. Even in communities implementing public clinics for spaying, the problem has not been totally alleviated. Ovariohysterectomy is not the answer for owners with breeding animals who desire a temporary means of contraception but want returned fertility at a later date.

PHARMACOLOGIC METHODS OF LENGTHENING ANESTRUS — CONTRACEPTIVES

Pharmacologic control of the pet population is currently receiving increasing publicity. Canine contraceptives that are now available to the public have generally been well accepted. Many steroid compounds can inhibit fertility but, because of the devastating side effects seen with some steroids, pharmaceutical companies have taken extreme care to market contraceptives that will prove safe and that will not render the animal permanently sterile. In the past many progestational compounds did indeed prove effective as contraceptive agents, but unfortunately they also significantly increased the risk of uterine disease and mammary hyperplasia.

CURRENTLY AVAILABLE CANINE CONTRACEPTIVES

MEGESTROL ACETATE

Megestrol acetate (Ovaban®, Schering) is a potent, orally effective synthetic progestogen. In the dog it is excreted mainly by the liver, with about 10 percent renal excretion, and has a half-life of about eight days. The mechanism of action is reportedly the suppression of estrus through inhibition of gonadotrophin release.

Megestrol acetate is given at dosages that depend on the reproductive stage of the bitch. If the animal is in early proestrus, estrus can be postponed by eight consecutive days of megestrol acetate given orally at a dosage of 2.2 mg/kg (1 mg/lb/day). It is important that the animals be started as close to day one of proestrus as possible to ensure the efficacy of the product and to minimize side effects. If given as recommended, the incidence of pyometra should be comparable to or lower than that in nontreated animals, according to the manufacturer.

If the bitch is in anestrus, megestrol acetate can be used in a 32-day administration schedule of 0.55 mg/kg (0.25 mg/lb/day) orally. For suppression, the drug must be initiated at least seven days prior to the expected onset of proestrus.

Megestrol acetate should not be used in animals experiencing their first estrus, because of the variability of results observed during the first cycle. Dogs with mammary tumors should not be given the contraceptive, since some canine mammary tumors may be stimulated by exogenous progestogens. Megestrol acetate is contraindicated in dogs in which there is evidence of uterine disease. Listed potential side effects of the drug are mammary enlargement, lactation, increased appetite, listlessness, and temperament change.

The next anticipated estrus may occur any time after cessation of treatment. If estrus occurs within 30 days of cessation of treatment with megestrol acetate, mating should not be allowed. In clinical studies most dogs returned to estrus in four to six months.

MIBOLERONE

Mibolerone (Cheque®, Upjohn Co.) is a nonprogestational steroid that has anabolic, androgenic, and antigonadotropic activity. Primary and secondary follicular development will still occur in the ovaries of animals receiving this drug, but follicles never mature to ovulatory size. Because LH surge is supposedly blocked, ovulation should not occur. Estrus, ovulation, and corpora lutea formation, therefore, should be prevented for as long as mibolerone is administered. Metabolites of mibolerone are excreted in approximately equal quantities via the urine and feces.

Mibolerone drops are administered orally once a day by adding the dose to a small portion of food or directly into the mouth. The daily dosage is determined by the weight of the animal and the breed; German shepherd females and German shepherd crosses require a higher dosage per unit of body weight. Mibolerone can be used continuously for 24 months. The drug should be initiated at least 30 days prior to an expected estrus. Estrus can occur during the first 30 days of treatment, and any animal showing signs of estrus should be monitored for pregnancy, since the drug can cause masculinization of female fetuses. In pregnant experimental animals receiving the drug, masculinization of female fetuses was seen as alterations in the patency of the vagina, multiple urethral openings into the vagina, a phallus-like structure in place of the clitoris, accumulations of fluid in the vagina or uterine body, and development of gross testes-like structures. Gross effects were not observed in male offspring.

Mibolerone should not be administered to any animal with prior history of liver or kidney disease. Elevations of liver serum enzymes may be encountered (e.g., SGPT) and are suggested as appropriate criteria for monitoring liver changes.

Mibolerone should be used with caution in the younger mature bitch because steroids with androgenic activity can result in early epiphyseal closure.

Clitoral hypertrophy, vaginitis, and epiphora have been reported in some dogs receiving the drug. Usually the signs are minimal.

Toxicologic studies over several years suggest that mibolerone, even at dosages much higher than those needed to suppress estrus, is relatively safe.

The efficacy of the drug in estrus prevention is reported to be 90 percent. After mibolerone treatment is discontinued, the animal may have the next estrus as soon as seven days or as long as 200 days after the last treatment. The average time to the next anticipated estrus is approximately 70 days.

CANINE CONTRACEPTION IN THE FUTURE

Research continues in an attempt to provide safer contraceptives that would also have good public acceptance. Currently testosterone implants are being studied. Such implants are inserted into the flank area of the bitch. Side effects are those of any androgen: clitoral enlargement, vaginal odor, and vaginitis. Animals return to cycle 34 to 291 days after removal of the implant. The advantage of such an implant is that it eliminates daily administration of a drug by the owner.

Immunization of an animal with luteinizing hormone (LH) has been studied with varying results. The theory is to produce cross-reacting antibodies against the animal's own LH, thereby preventing ovulation. Return of fertility has been variable; some animals become fertile soon after boostering with the gonadotropic hormone.

Intravaginal devices have been available in the past but are no longer marketed. Migration of the device and persistent vaginitis contributed to poor public acceptance of the device.

Intrauterine devices in the dog theoretically should inhibit fertility. However, cannulating the canine cervix and inserting a device via the vagina would be difficult, so the method is impractical.

SUPPLEMENTAL READING

Andersen, A.C., and Simpson, M.E.: *The Ovary and Reproductive Cycle of the Dog (Beagle)*. Los Altos, California, Geron-X, Inc., 1973.

Bardens, J.W.: Hormonal therapy for ovarian and testicular dysfunction in the dog. J. Am. Vet. Med. Assoc., *159*:1405, 1971.

Burke, T.J., and Reynolds, H.A.: Megestrol acetate for estrus postponement in the bitch. J. Am. Vet. Med. Assoc., *167*:286, 1975.

Concannon, P., Hansel, W., and McEntee, K.: Changes in LH, progesterone and sexual behavior associated with preovulatory luteinization in the bitch. Biol. Reprod., *17*:604, 1977.

Concannon, P., Cowan, R., and Hansel, W.: LH release in ovariectomized dogs in response to estrogen withdrawal and its facilitation by progesterone. Biol. Reprod., *20*:523, 1979.

Faulkner, L.C.: Prevention of estrus. In Kirk, R.W. (ed.): *Current Veterinary Therapy VI*. Philadelphia, W.B. Saunders Co., 1977.

Holst, P.A., and Phemister, R.D.: Onset of diestrus in the bitch: Definition and significance. Am. J. Vet. Res., 35:401, 1974.

Nett, T.M., Akbar, A.M., Phemister, R.D., Host, P.A., Reichert, L.E., and Niswender, G.D.: Levels of luteinizing hormone, estradiol, and progesterone in serum during the estrous cycle and pregnancy in the beagle bitch. Proc. Soc. Exp. Biol. Med., *148*:134–139, 1975.

Pineda, M.H., Kainer, R.A., and Faulkner, L.C.: Dorsal median postcervical folds in the canine vagina. Am. J. Vet. Res., *34*:1487, 1973.

Reimers, T.J., Phemister, R.D., and Niswender, G.D.: Radioimmunological measurement of follicle-stimulating hormone and prolactin in the dog. Biol. Reprod., *19*:673, 1978.

Sokolowski, J.H.: Reproductive patterns in the bitch. Vet. Clin. North Am., 7:653–666, 1977.

Sokolowski, J.H., and Geng, S.: Biological evaluation of mibolerone in the female beagle. Am. J. Vet. Res., 38:1371, 1977.

Thun, R., Watson, P., and Jackson, G.L.: Induction of estrus and ovulation using exogenous gonadotrophins. Am. J. Vet. Res., 38:483, 1977.

Upjohn Veterinary Report No. 9: Cheque®. Upjohn Veterinary Products, Kalamazoo, MI 49001.

OBESITY

GARY L. ANDERSEN, D.V.M.
San Antonio, Texas

and LON D. LEWIS, D.V.M.
Fort Collins, Colorado

Canine obesity is seen in most small animal practices on a daily basis. Occasionally an owner will recognize the overweight condition and present the dog in the hope of finding a reason for it. More often the animal is presented for a problem caused by obesity or for a routine visit, such as for annual vaccination. Frequently the owner is unaware of the overweight condition.

Even though a diagnosis of obesity is based upon a subjective evaluation, it is generally quite apparent. However, convincing the owner of the obese condition, of its potential for causing problems, and of the necessity for weight reduction can be very challenging. To meet this challenge a thorough knowledge of the causes and effects of obesity is essential. Client education is the foundation of any successful canine weight reduction program. Without full cooperation from the client any program is doomed to failure.

INCIDENCE

Canine obesity is an extremely common disease. An incidence of at least 25 percent has been reported in some studies, while in others nearly 50 percent of the dogs presented to small animal clinics were overweight. Dogs are more commonly overweight when owned by middle-aged and elderly people or by people who are overweight themselves and when home-cooked foods or table scraps are fed instead of commercial rations only (Mason). The higher incidence of obesity in these dogs may be because obese, middle-aged, and older owners get less exercise themselves and therefore exercise their pets less. These are also the types of owners who are more apt to submit to the demands of their pets for food and to pamper them with home-cooked meals and table scraps.

Cocker spaniels, Labradors, and collies have been found to have a higher incidence of obesity than other breeds, whereas boxers, fox terriers, and Sealyhams have a lower incidence (Mason). This may indicate a genetic predisposition for obesity.

As shown in Table 1, the incidence of obesity increases with age. This increase is most likely due to a decrease in both metabolic rate and physical activity. Except in very aged dogs, obesity is more common in females than in males (see Table 1). In addition, the incidence of obesity in spayed females is nearly twice that of the total population (Anderson).

Neutering has frequently been associated with an increase in body weight in both males and females. This usually results from a de-

Table 1. *Incidence of Obesity in Dogs According to Sex and Age** *

SEX	n	% OBESE AT VARIOUS AGES				
		All Ages	*1–4*	*5–7*	*8–11*	*Over 12*
Male	537	23	12	30	34	41
Female	463	32	21	37	41	40

*From: Mason, E.: Obesity in pet dogs. Vet. Rec. 86:612, 1970.

crease in physical activity with no compensatory decrease in food intake. As a result, a positive energy balance is established, with the excess energy being deposited as fat. In the castrated male the absence of the anabolic hormone testosterone may also play a role in inducing obesity as a result of decreased amino acid deposition into muscle protein, with more energy going into fat. High FSH levels in the spayed female may also play a role in causing the higher incidence of obesity that occurs in this group.

Many feel that the incidence of obesity in dogs is increasing. If this is true there are a number of factors that may be responsible. In today's affluent society better quality and larger quantities of human and pet foods are available to initiate and perpetuate obesity. The marked popularity of health spas has also served to take pet owners away from home for their exercise, thereby leaving the pets in an environment that is devoid of opportunities for needed exercise. The urbanization of our society has also led to more apartment-type living, more leash laws, and more neutering of pets. All these factors lead to decreased pet activity, which results in a positive energy balance and obesity.

EVALUATION

All attempts to evaluate the degree of obesity in dogs objectively have been unsuccessful because of the large number of breeds involved, the variation of normal within a given breed, the large mixed-breed population, and other factors. As a result, the degree of obesity must be determined on a subjective basis, e.g., by observing and palpating the amount of tissue overlying the rib cage. By this method, a dog may be considered too thin if the ribs are easily seen, normal if they are barely seen and easily felt, and too fat if they cannot be seen and an appreciable layer of fat is felt. If the ribs cannot be palpated at all the dog is grossly obese. This method, although not as scientific as may be desired, is practical and adequate for diagnosing the degree of obesity in a given animal.

EFFECTS

It has been shown that mortality is markedly increased in people who are overweight. If the same is true in dogs, then obesity reduces the animal's life span and general enjoyment of life and the owner's enjoyment of the animal.

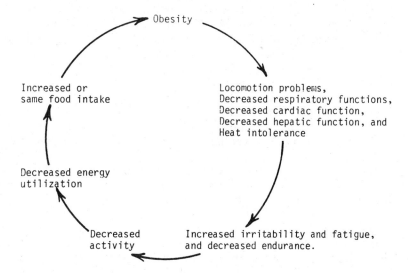

Figure 1. Vicious circle resulting from and in turn causing obesity.

The following problems can occur in the dog as a result of obesity:

1. Increased irritability.

2. Joint or locomotion problems caused by carrying excessive weight.

3. Respiratory distress, especially with exercise, due to the increased amount of tissue that requires oxygenation and the increased weight placed upon the thoracic cavity by excessive fat accumulation.

4. Congestive heart problems due to the increased workload required to provide circulation to the excess tissue imposed on a heart already weakened by fatty infiltration.

5. Decreased hepatic function as a result of a fatty liver.

6. Increased dystocia.

7. Diabetes mellitus due to the beta cell's inability to provide the extra insulin required for the excess tissue and the higher fasting blood glucose levels seen in the obese state.

8. Heat intolerance caused by the insulating properties of excess fat.

9. Increased surgical difficulty and anesthetic risk. Many anesthetics are absorbed by the excess fat, resulting in the need for higher doses and prolonged recovery periods.

10. Lowered resistance to infectious diseases.

11. Impaired gastrointestinal function, resulting in increased constipation and flatulence.

12. Dermatologic problems.

A number of these problems are not only caused or predisposed by obesity but in turn may cause or predispose the animal to obesity, resulting in the vicious circle shown in Figure 1.

CAUSES

Emotional trauma, hypopituitarism, and cerebral, cortical, or hypothalamic lesions can predispose to canine obesity. Endocrine imbalances, including insulinoma, hypothyroidism, pituitary chromophobe adenoma, diffuse hyperplasia of the pancreatic islets, and hypercorticosteroidism from various causes, also can result in canine obesity. Obesity in the dog, however, is only occasionally predisposed to by any of these factors. It is most frequently caused by eating too much, exercising too little, or both.

There are usually two stages of canine obesity — an initial phase and a static phase. The initial phase is that period when energy intake exceeds utilization, and the excess calories are deposited as fat. This is the phase when the dog gains excess weight. During the static phase that follows, dietary intake is reduced to equal utilization. This phase is the result of several "feedback mechanisms," the most important of which is the direct effect that high plasma insulin levels in the obese state exert on the satiety center, thereby causing the obese individual to eat less (Woods, et al.).

Adipocyte size and number as well as taste and awareness of satiation have been shown to predispose some individuals to obesity. These factors may be involved in genetic predisposition to obesity in dogs. This work has been done primarily in humans and rats, and, although it has not been confirmed in dogs, it is probable that it is also true for them.

TREATMENT

Prior to initiating therapy, the animal should receive a thorough physical examination to determine if there is an endocrine or metabolic factor responsible for the obesity. Hypothyroidism and hyperadrenocorticism, the two most common endocrine abnormalities associated with canine obesity, can usually be ruled out with history, physical examination, and basic laboratory tests. If there is any doubt, adrenal and thyroid function studies should be conducted.

Intensive client education is essential for the successful treatment of simple canine obesity. Without complete cooperation from all associated with the dog prior to initiating therapy, the results will be poor. The client should realize that some type of diet and exercise control will probably be needed for the life of the animal, even after the initial treatment phase when the animal is at a near-normal weight.

There are two major methods of treating canine obesity: pharmacologic weight reduction and control of diet and exercise. Anorexigenics and thyroid hormones are the two types of drugs that have been used to the greatest extent for weight reduction in the obese dog. The most common anorexigenic used has been amphetamine. It is not recommended because of the number of undesirable side effects, its potential for abuse by people, and its ineffectiveness in obese spayed bitches as determined in one study (Bomson and Parker).

Thyroid hormones given at pharmacologic doses will result in weight loss in the obese canine but should not be used unless hypothyroidism is present. Thyroid hormone at pharmacologic doses in a dog with normal thyroid function has the potential of disrupting the endogenous feedback mechanism, thereby subjecting that animal to future hormonal imbalances. In addition, thyroid hormone causes weight reduction not from fat mobilization but from protein breakdown, which is of no long-term benefit and may be harmful.

The control of diet and exercise is the recommended treatment of canine obesity. To achieve weight reduction, caloric intake must be less than calories expended. An energy deficit of 3500 kcal is needed to lose one pound of fat. This deficit can be accomplished by reducing food intake, increasing exercise, or both.

There are two approaches to reducing food intake: partial caloric restriction and total caloric restriction (starvation). When used correctly each is successful. The method used will depend on the circumstances and the clinician's and owner's preferences.

When food intake is to be reduced by partial caloric restriction, exercise generally is indicated. A certain minimal amount of exercise reduces appetite. Some owners, however, may not be able to exercise their dogs, or the animal may not be able to exercise because of joint problems, cardiac disease, or another condition. Such animals are often good candidates for total caloric restriction where exercise is not recommended owing to the potential for inducing ketoacidosis.

PARTIAL CALORIC RESTRICTION

Weight reduction by partial caloric restriction may be accomplished as follows:

1. Obtain complete client cooperation.
2. Provide the owner with written instructions and explanations to take home.
3. Weigh the dog accurately and establish a realistic goal for weight reduction.
4. Give an estimate of the time required. This can be quite variable, but Table 2 will help give an approximation.
5. Decrease caloric intake to 60 percent of that required for maintenance of the dog at its optimum body weight (not at its obese weight), as given in Table 3.
6. Feed the daily ration in several small feedings rather than one or two large ones.

Table 2. *Time Required for Weight Reduction*

OPTIMUM BODY WEIGHT *(lb)*	LB LOST/WEEK
Less than 20	0.5
20–40	1.0
More than 40	1.5

7. Instruct the client to keep the dog out of the room in which food is prepared and eaten by the family.
8. Change the dog's diet. Success is rarely obtained if the dog is kept on its present diet. Table scraps, snacks, and sweets are absolutely forbidden. A diet specifically formulated for weight reduction is usually the best. Such a diet is available commercially as Prescription Diet R/D®, or a similar diet can be made at home using the following recipe (Morris):

¼ lb lean ground beef
½ cup cottage cheese, uncreamed
2 cups carrots, canned solids
2 cups green beans, canned solids
1½ tsp dicalcium phosphate

Cook beef, drain fat, cool, and add remaining ingredients. Yield: 1.75 lb providing 300 kcal/lb. Table 4 shows the amount of the reducing diets to be fed. It must be made explicitly clear to the owner that he or she is to feed only the prescribed amount.

9. The dog should be seen on a weekly basis for weighing. The frequency with which obese patients are seen has a direct relationship to the success of weight reduction. If there is no weight loss, decrease the amount being fed by 20 percent.
10. Whenever possible, get the owner involved in monitoring the dog's progress. Having owners keep a graph of daily weight versus time helps keep their interest in the program. This is essential for success.
11. Put the dog on the proper maintenance diet once a satisfactory weight has been reached. Instruct the owner to weigh the dog

Table 3. *Caloric Requirements for Maintenance and Weight Reduction*

OPTIMUM BODY WEIGHT *(lb)*	KCAL/LB BODY WT/DAY NEEDED FOR:*	
	Maintenance	*Weight Reduction*
5	50	30
10	40	24
20	35	21
30	30	18
75	25	15
200	20	12

*Interpolation between these values will give the amount needed for any size dog.

Table 4. *Reducing Diet and* R/D
*Feeding Guide**

OPTIMUM BODY WEIGHT *(lb)*	LB OF FEED/DAY
5	1/3
10	1/3
20	1
40	1¾
60	2½
80	2¾
100	3¼

*From: Morris, M. L., Jr : Index of dietetic management. In Kirk, R. W. (ed.): *Current Veterinary Therapy VI.* Philadelphia, W. B. Saunders Co., 1977, p.

weekly and record the weight on the graph. If the animal begins to gain weight again, decrease the amount fed by 10 to 20 percent until the weight stabilizes. Occasionally a dog's caloric requirements will be so low that the reducing diet can be used for maintenance, with the amount being fed adjusted to what is needed for weight stabilization. With a home-prepared diet, multiple vitamins should be given daily.

12. Continue frequent followup examinations to monitor the animal's weight until it stabilizes with the maintenance diet.

Success with partial caloric restriction is often poor for the following reasons: (1) It often takes three to six months to achieve the desired weight loss. (2) It is usually difficult to get complete owner cooperation for that long. (3) Many trips to the veterinarian are necessary. (4) The ability of many owners to incorporate exercise in the program is limited for various reasons. (5) Much veterinary staff time is required. Total caloric restriction in a hospital environment is often the answer to these problems.

TOTAL CALORIC RESTRICTION

We, as well as others (de Bruijne and Lubberink), have found total caloric restriction to be a safe and effective method for achieving weight reduction in the dog. Some may feel that this method is inhumane. To the contrary, we have found that dogs undergoing total caloric restriction exhibited less hunger after the first few days of the diet than dogs with partial caloric restriction. Numerous human therapeutic starvation diets have also been found to result in less hunger misery than do conventional partial calorie-restricted diets.

Close monitoring of six dogs revealed that no adverse clinical or biochemical changes occurred during or after the periods of starvation, which ranged from 24 to 42 days. Ketoacidosis was not observed, weight reduction goals were reached in less time than would be expected with other diets, and each client was more than pleased with the results. Total caloric restriction in many instances is a simpler, easier, and more reliable method of treatment.

The only disadvantage to total caloric restriction is the need for and cost of hospitalization. Owners cannot be expected to accomplish the regimen themselves. However, even with hospitalization, much less veterinary staff time is required than with a properly instituted and supervised weight reduction regimen by partial caloric restriction conducted at home. Because of this, the cost for weight reduction by total caloric restriction may not be substantially more than that for weight reduction by partial caloric restriction at home. In addition, the cost of weight reduction by total caloric restriction is reduced if it is possible to schedule it at a time when the owner plans to be out of town and would otherwise be boarding the dog.

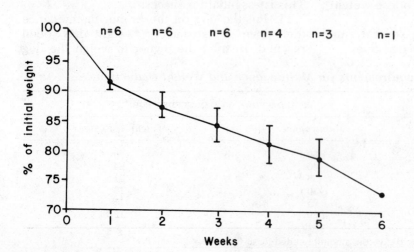

Figure 2. Weight loss during total caloric restriction in the dog. Brackets indicate range. These results are from a clinical study conducted at Colorado State University.

As shown in Figure 2, obese dogs lost 8 percent of their body weight by the end of the first week of starvation, 5 percent more during the second week, and 3 to 4 percent per week thereafter. The initial rapid weight loss is primarily a result of excess sodium and water losses. However, within a few days sodium and water excretion decreases to very low levels. The majority of dogs in this study showed polydipsia and polyuria during starvation. This may have been a compensatory mechanism to satisfy hunger, because all dogs resumed normal patterns upon refeeding. Because much of the weight loss in the obese dog is fat, which has a higher energy density than that of other tissues, this loss is slower than that which will occur as a result of starvation of non-obese or less obese dogs.

The procedures used for total caloric restriction are:

1. Provide extensive client education.
2. Hospitalize the animal.
3. Perform a complete examination to eliminate any endocrine or metabolic disorders. A complete blood count, urinalysis, and chemistry panel should also be done to rule out any subclinical condition that might be aggravated by the diet.
4. Completely withdraw all food.
5. Give vitamin and mineral supplements daily to meet most of the dog's requirements and provide water on a free-choice basis.
6. Observe the dog on a daily basis and record its weight twice weekly.
7. When the desired weight is reached give the dog gradually (over a two- to three-day period) a balanced commercial dog food in the amount needed for maintenance. The dog is sent home on this diet. A 3 to 4 percent weight gain is expected upon refeeding because of sodium and water retention.
8. Examine and weigh the animal weekly for several weeks and adjust the amount fed accordingly. Some animals may have such low caloric requirements that the use of a reducing diet may be desirable for maintenance in order to prevent weight gain.

The results using this procedure to date have been very successful and gratifying for the client, the animal, and the veterinarian. The frustrating and often unsuccessful experiences encountered with a home weight reduction program are eliminated. The client receives a livelier, happier, and friendlier dog in exchange for the previously lethargic, irritable animal that was left at the hospital.

SUPPLEMENTAL READING

Anderson, R.S.: Obesity in the dog and cat. The Vet. Ann., 186, 1973.

Bomson, L., and Parker, C.H.L.: Effect of fenfluramine on overweight spayed bitches. Vet. Rec., 96:202, 1975.

de Bruijne, J., and Lubberink, A.M.M.E.: Obesity. In Kirk, R.W. (ed.): *Current Veterinary Therapy VI.* Philadelphia, W. B. Saunders Co., 1977, pp. 1068–1070.

Lewis, L.D.: Obesity in the dog. J. Am. Anim. Hosp. Assoc., *14*:402, 1978.

Mason, E.: Obesity in pet dogs. Vet. Rec., 86:612, 1970.

Morris, M.L., Jr.: Index of dietetic management. In Kirk, R.W. (ed.): *Current Veterinary Therapy VI.* Philadelphia, W. B. Saunders Co., 1977, pp. 59–73.

Woods, S.C., Decke, E., and Vasselli, J.R.: Metabolic hormones and regulation of body weight. Psycholog. Rev., *81*:26, 1974.

Section 12

GENITOURINARY DISORDERS

CARL A. OSBORNE, D.V.M.
Consulting Editor

The Kidneys
Urinary System Emergencies 1042
Toxic Nephropathy 1047
Glomerulonephropathy and the Nephrotic
    Syndrome 1053
Renal Amyloidosis 1063
Hypercalcemic Nephropathy and Associated
    Disorders 1067
Hydronephrosis 1073
Fanconi Syndrome in the Dog 1075
Chronic Tubular-interstitial Disease of the Kidney 1076
Overview of the Uremic Syndrome 1079
Water Deprivation and Vasopressin Concentration Tests in the
    Differentiation of Polyuric Syndromes 1080
Neonatal Clinical Nephrology 1085
Management of Oliguric and Anuric Renal Failure 1087
Intensive Diuresis in Polyuric Renal Failure 1091
Medical Management of Polyuric Renal Failure:
    Salt and Sodium Bicarbonate 1094
Conservative Management of Polyuric Primary Renal
    Failure: Diet Therapy 1097
Medical Management of Polyuric Renal Failure:
    Anabolic Agents 1102
Medical Management of Chronic Renal Failure:
    Control of Hyperphosphatemia 1103
Nutrition During the Uremic Crisis 1104
Current Status of Peritoneal Dialysis 1106
Current Status of Veterinary Hemodialysis 1111
Drug Therapy in Renal Disorders 1114
Anesthesia in Renal Failure 1117

The Urinary Tract
Neurogenic Urinary Incontinence 1122
Non-neurogenic Urinary Incontinence 1128
Canine Polypoid Cystitis 1137
Rupture of the Canine Urinary Bladder 1139
Parasites of the Canine Urinary Tract 1141

Continued

Congenital Diseases of the Urachus.. 1143
Medical Management of Prostatic Disease............................... 1146
Cystocentesis... 1150
Screening Tests for the Detection of Significant
    Bacteriuria.. 1154
Urinary Tract Infections.. 1158
Choice of Antimicrobial Agents in the Treatment of Urinary
    Tract Infections.. 1162
Ancillary Treatment of Urinary Tract Infections...................... 1164
Struvite Urolithiasis.. 1168
Urate Urolithiasis... 1172
Cystinuria and Cystine Urolithiasis.................................... 1175
Calcium Oxalate Urolithiasis.. 1177
Canine Silica Urolithiasis... 1184
Feline Cystic Calculi.. 1187
Feline Urologic Syndrome: Management of the
    Critically Ill Patient.. 1188
Feline Urologic Syndrome: Removal of Urethral Obstructions
    and Use of Indwelling Urethral Catheters.......................... 1191
Feline Urologic Syndrome: Medical Aspects of Prophylaxis........ 1196
Feline Urologic Syndrome: Surgical Aspects of Prophylaxis........ 1201
Neoplasms of the Canine and Feline Urinary Tracts.................. 1203

The Genital System
Dystocia... 1212
Acute Metritis... 1214
Canine Pyometra.. 1216
Canine Vaginitis... 1219
Vaginal Hyperplasia and Uterine Prolapse............................ 1222
Non-neoplastic Disorders of the Mammary Glands.................... 1224
Management of Canine Infertility....................................... 1226
Prognosis and Management of Feline Infertility....................... 1231
Prevention of Estrus.. 1237
Pregnancy Prevention and Termination............................... 1239
Pseudohermaphroditism... 1241
Canine Cryptorchidism.. 1244

Additional Pertinent Information, Still Current, Found in
Current Veterinary Therapy VI:

Barrett, R. E., and Theilen, G. H.: Neoplasms of the canine
  and feline reproductive tracts, p. 1263.
Hart, B. L.: Urine spraying in cats, p. 1259.

Lein, D. H.: Canine orchitis, p. 1255.
Seager, S. W. J.: Semen collection and artificial insemination of dogs, p. 1245.
Seager, S. W. J.: Semen collection, evaluation, and artificial
  insemination of the domestic cat, p. 1252.

The Kidneys

URINARY SYSTEM EMERGENCIES

JAMES J. BRACE, D.V.M.
Knoxville, Tennessee

and DENNIS J. CHEW, D.V.M.
Columbus, Ohio

RENAL FAILURE

A number of disease processes can alter renal function and lead to profound changes in fluid and electrolyte balance. These changes can result in death within a few hours to a few days. Any abnormality that causes the functional destruction of three fourths or more of the nephrons of both kidneys will result in renal failure and may be characterized by the clinical signs of uremia (see article in this section on the uremic syndrome). Renal failure may be due to prerenal, primary renal, or postrenal disorders.

PRERENAL RENAL FAILURE

Prerenal renal failure is caused by disorders that decrease renal function by decreasing renal perfusion (e.g., cardiac failure, hypovolemia, and others). Prerenal renal failure implies the presence of structurally normal kidneys. However, if the cause of prerenal renal failure is not corrected rapidly, the kidneys may develop primary ischemic changes. Prerenal renal failure does not usually result in symptoms of the uremic syndrome unless it occurs in conjunction with pre-existing primary renal failure. Prerenal renal failure is treated by correcting the cause of poor renal perfusion.

PRIMARY RENAL FAILURE

Primary renal failure can have many causes (e.g., infection, ischemia, toxins, congenital anomalies, and others), all of which result in the destruction of three-fourths or more of the nephrons of both kidneys. Depending on the severity of the underlying cause, primary renal failure may be acute or chronic and reversible or irreversible. Primary renal failure, if not resolved quickly, may result in the clinical signs of uremia. The spectrum and severity of signs are dependent upon the degree of nephron damage, the ability of damaged nephrons to heal, and the ability of remaining viable nephrons to undergo compensatory hypertrophy and hyperplasia. Therapy for primary renal failure is aimed at eliminating the underlying cause and supporting the patient until damaged nephrons can heal or until remaining viable nephrons can undergo sufficient compensatory adaptation to re-establish adequate body fluid volume and composition. Supportive care requires careful regulation of fluid, electrolyte, and acid-base balance.

POSTRENAL RENAL FAILURE

Postrenal renal failure is caused by disease processes that result in failure of excretion of urine from the body. Accumulation of urine in the body may lead to the clinical signs of uremia even though the kidneys may be structurally and functionally normal. General causes of postrenal renal failure include rupture of the excretory pathway and urinary tract obstruction.

Obstruction of urine flow may be caused by a variety of lesions throughout the urinary tract, from the renal pelves to the tip of the urethra. The most common site of urinary tract obstruction in dogs and cats is the urethra, and obstruction is seen most often in males of both species. Urolithiasis is the most common cause of urethral obstruction in the dog, whereas in the cat the usual cause is material composed of magnesium ammonium phosphate hexahydrate (struvite), mucus, and cellular debris. Other causes of urethral obstruction include imperforate urethra, congenital or acquired urethral strictures, urethritis, traumatic injuries, primary urethral neoplasms or neoplasms of periurethral tissues, prostatic disease, and abnormal locations of the urinary bladder (e.g., entrapment of the bladder in perineal or traumatic hernias). Lesions of the urinary bladder that may obstruct urine flow through either the urethra or the ureters include calculi, bladder neoplasms, blood clots, and uterine stump granulomas. Lesions of the ureters or renal pelves that result in postrenal renal failure are uncommon, since both kidneys must be affected. Such lesions include renal or ureteral calculi, blood clots, ureteral strictures, ureteritis, inflammatory or neoplastic abdominal masses that compress the ureters, and accidental ligation of the ureters during abdominal surgery.

Complete obstruction of urine outflow from one kidney is not life-threatening as long as the opposite kidney is capable of adequate function. Complete obstruction of urine outflow from both kidneys for approximately 24 hours will usually result in postrenal renal failure. Death from uremia may occur in three to six days.

Therapy for postrenal renal failure should be aimed at re-establishing urine flow, correcting fluid, electrolyte, and acid-base abnormalities, and eliminating the underlying cause (see "Management of Oliguric and Anuric Renal Failure," "Rupture of the Canine Urinary Bladder," and articles on the feline urologic syndrome elsewhere in this section).

If urethral obstruction is present, catheterization of the urethra and reverse flushing with sterile isotonic solutions may relieve the obstruction. If this is not effective and a small catheter cannot bypass the obstruction, temporary decompression of the bladder may be accomplished by cystocentesis (see article on cystocentesis). Following cystocentesis, reverse flushing may dislodge the obstruction and should be repeated.

If non-surgical methods of relieving urethral obstruction are unsuccessful, a urethrostomy or urethrotomy should be performed. Obstruction of the ureters or renal pelves should also be treated surgically.

Following relief of complete or severe partial obstruction of urine outflow from both kidneys, there may be a moderate to severe postobstructive diuresis. This may develop within a few hours following relief of obstruction and may last for several days. Postobstructive diuresis may lead to dehydration, hyponatremia, and hypokalemia because of massive loss of water and electrolytes.

ABNORMAL BODY FLUID COMPOSITION IN RENAL FAILURE

WATER IMBALANCE

DEHYDRATION

Dehydration is commonly encountered in uremic animals as a result of varying combinations of prerenal, primary renal, and postrenal azotemia. Fluid deficit occurs because of an imbalance between intake and loss of water. Vomiting, diarrhea, and diuresis cause excessive loss of fluid. Diuresis (polyuria) may be seen in animals with chronic renal failure or in animals recovering from oliguric acute renal failure. Diminished intake of food and water as a result of anorexia and vomiting contributes to the fluid deficit. Obligatory loss of fluid through ventilation (insensible loss) occurs in all animals.

Clinical dehydration is detected on physical examination by loss of skin elasticity, sunken globes, and dry mucous membranes. Physical examination, however, will not reveal dehydration until at least 5 percent of body weight has been lost because of water deficit. In patients with severe dehydration tachycardia may be present as a compensatory mechanism for volume depletion. Increases in both the packed cell volume (PCV) and the total protein (TP) support a clinical diagnosis of intravascular dehydration. It should be noted that in cases with pre-existing anemia or hypoproteinemia hemoconcentration may not be reflected in elevated PCV and TP even though dehydration exists. Acute loss of body weight is indicative of water loss, although some catabolism of body tissues may also contribute to the weight loss.

Rapid correction of dehydration regardless of the underlying cause is important to prevent ischemic renal damage. Consequently, correction of dehydration in the uremic animal is attempted within six to eight hours unless complicating factors such as congestive heart failure are involved. A polyionic isotonic fluid such as lactated Ringer's solution is usually chosen for rehydration. This fluid may be modified after evaluation of the animal's serum electrolyte and acid-base status. The volume of fluid to be administered for rehydration is estimated by the formula:

% clinical dehydration × body wt (lb) × 500 = ml of fluid to be replaced

The intravenous route for fluid administration should be used initially in severely dehydrated patients, since poor peripheral perfusion may delay absorption of fluid from subcutaneous tissue.

Once dehydration has been corrected, additional fluid volumes are required to replace insensible loss, urinary loss, and additional losses from vomiting and diarrhea. Measuring urine output volume via an indwelling urinary catheter connected to a bottle collection system facilitates more accurate estimates of these fluid requirements, but it is associated with the risk of iatrogenic urinary tract infection.

OVERHYDRATION

Overhydration in animals with renal failure usually occurs as a result of overzealous fluid administration to patients with persisting oliguria or anuria. Peripheral pitting edema, pulmonary edema with tachypnea and rales, and congestive heart failure may be seen as a result of the circulatory volume overload. Administration of parenteral fluids should be stopped while an attempt to mobilize excess body water is made, utilizing potent non-osmotic diuretics such as furosemide (Lasix®, Hoescht, 2 to 4 mg/kg intravenously). This dose of diuretic may be doubled and repeated after 30 minutes if diuresis does not occur. Osmotic diuretics (mannitol and glucose) should not be used. Peritoneal dialysis may be necessary to control life-threatening edema if diuretics are not effective (see "Current Status of Peritoneal Dialysis" and "Management of Oliguric and Anuric Renal Failure").

Spontaneous edema may be encountered in animals with nephrotic syndrome, with or without accompanying renal failure. Natriuretic diuretics are usually helpful in controlling this edema but may cause further depletion of intravascular volume (see "Glomerulonephropathy and the Nephrotic Syndrome").

ELECTROLYTE ABNORMALITIES

POTASSIUM

Hyperkalemia (potassium > 5.5 mEq/liter) can be a life-threatening complication of oliguric or anuric renal failure. The magnitude of potassium elevation is influenced by the degree of remaining renal function and by potassium input into the body from food, tissue catabolism, and potassium-containing parenteral fluid. Metabolic acidosis may result in hyperkalemia or may increase the magnitude of hyperkalemia. This occurs as excess hydrogen ions enter the cells in exchange for potassium ions leaving the cells.

The cardiotoxic effects of hyperkalemia are clinically most important. Electrocardiographic changes may consist of tall, peaked T waves, decreased amplitude of P waves, atrial standstill, and sinoventricular rhythms. Bradycardia with a heart rate less than 60 beats per minute may be detected.

The initial treatment of hyperkalemia usually consists of an intravenous bolus infusion of 2–4 mEq/kg of sodium bicarbonate, because correction of acidosis with bicarbonate enhances the return of potassium into cells. The effects of this infusion can be monitored via electrocardiography. Supplemental bicarbonate in the IV drip will help to maintain lower serum potassium values temporarily. In hyperkalemic crisis that is accompanied by severe arrhythmias and imminent death, treatment with intravenous dextrose and regular insulin may be life-saving. Regular insulin is given intravenously at a dose of approximately 0.5 to 1.0 unit per kg. Dextrose is given at a dose of 1 gm/unit of insulin administered as an intravenous bolus to prevent hypoglycemia. An additional 1 gm dextrose/unit of insulin is added to the intravenous drip, also to prevent hypoglycemia. This treatment is not often necessary but does utilize the principle of insulin-enhanced intracellular transport of potassium.

As the initial oliguric or anuric renal failure enters a diuretic phase, the hyperkalemia will resolve without further medical treatment. If the oliguria or anuria persists, alternate routes for potassium removal should be considered, including oral or rectal ionic exchange resins (Kayexalate®, Winthrop) and peritoneal dialysis (see "Management of Oliguric and Anuric Renal Failure").

Hypokalemia (potassium < 3.5 mEq/liter) may be detected in animals that have excessive urinary losses in polyuric renal failure, particularly if there has been no intake of foods containing potassium. Clinical signs related to weakness and depression become increasingly obvious as serum potassium values become less than 3.0 mEq/liter. Parenteral fluids may be supplemented with potassium chloride, but potassium infusion should not exceed a rate of 0.5 mEq/kg/hr. Oral potassium supplementation may be given if the animal is not vomiting. The dosage is determined by serial evaluation of serum potassium values.

SODIUM AND CHLORIDE

Serum sodium and chloride values are often normal in dehydrated uremic animals because of isotonic loss of body fluid. Hyponatremia can occur in animals undergoing water and salt diuresis if replacement fluids are limited to water alone. Hyponatremia may also occur if dehydration is corrected through the use of sodium-poor fluids such as 5 percent dextrose in water. Hyponatremia can usually be corrected by administration of 0.9 percent sodium chloride. Hypernatremic dehydration from loss of more water than salt is most likely to be seen in cases of prerenal azotemia. Hypernatremia can be managed initially by administration of 5 percent dextrose in water or 2½ percent dextrose in 0.45 percent sodium chloride until serum sodium values return to normal.

Hypochloremia may be caused by the same disorders that cause hyponatremia. Additionally, chloride loss from gastric losses in vomiting may be extensive. Hypochloremia may be corrected by the intravenous infusion of 0.9 percent sodium chloride.

The extremes of sodium chloride deficits or relative excesses generally cause weakness and depression. Death due to these abnormalities alone is unlikely.

CALCIUM

Serum calcium values in renal failure generally are normal or low. The ionized fraction of serum calcium is biologically active. Hypocalcemic tetany in renal failure is rare, possibly because the protective effect of metabolic acidosis increases the amount of ionized calcium. Tetany may be precipitated by rapid infusion of sodium bicarbonate, which removes the protective effect of acidosis by reducing the amount of ionized calcium. Acute renal failure due to ethylene glycol poisoning may chelate calcium from the serum, causing hypocalcemic tetany. Intravenous infusion of calcium gluconate is given to control tetany or seizures due to hypocalcemia.

Hypercalcemia may be a cause of renal failure and severe depression (see "Hypercalcemic Nephropathy"). Treatment with IV 0.9 percent sodium chloride, furosemide, and possibly corticosteroids should be started while a search for the cause of the hypercalcemia is undertaken.

PHOSPHORUS

Hyperphosphatemia of varying magnitude is often encountered in uremic animals. Signs directly attributable to elevated serum phosphorus are minimal. A reciprocal effect of hyperphosphatemia on serum ionized calcium may contribute to hypocalcemia. Soft-tissue mineralization may also be a consequence of hyperphosphatemia. Intestinal binding agents such as aluminum hydroxide have been effective in lowering levels of serum phosphorus (see "Medical Management of Polyuric Renal Failure: Control of Hyperphosphatemia").

ACID-BASE IMBALANCE

Metabolic acidosis usually develops in uremic animals as a consequence of impaired renal excretion of hydrogen ion and titratable acid. The magnitude of acidosis is not directly related to the degree of serum urea nitrogen or creatinine elevation. Respiratory mechanisms may partially or fully compensate for the reduction in serum bicarbonate values encountered in metabolic acidosis and therefore minimize changes in blood pH. Progressive reduction in blood pH results in increasing depression, coma, and eventually death. Blood pH values < 7.0 represent critical acidosis, and pH values < 6.8 are not compatible with life. Alkali replacement with sodium bicarbonate in parenteral fluids should be based on blood gas values or estimated by the severity of clinical signs. (See article in Section 1 on fluid and electrolyte therapy.) Rarely, metabolic alkalosis may be present if extensive loss of acid gastric contents has occurred through vomiting.

TRAUMA

KIDNEYS

Blunt abdominal trauma may damage renal tissue by direct compression, hemorrhage into the tissue, or both. Rarely, penetrating wounds may injure the kidneys. Serious traumatic injury is not common because the kidneys are protected by the rib cage, vertebrae, and lumbar muscles. The kidneys of dogs and cats are also loosely attached to the body wall and are further protected by a tough fibrous capsule.

Severe trauma may rupture the renal capsule and parenchyma. This may be associated with severe hemorrhage into the retroperitoneal space or into the abdominal cavity. Avulsion of the renal artery or renal vein poses an immediate threat to life because of massive blood loss. Communicating tears in the renal pelvis may allow urine to accumulate in the retroperitoneal space or abdomen. Less severe trauma may cause perirenal or subcapsular hematomas and contusions that are of minimal clinical consequence. Blood clots within the collecting system, renal pelvis, and ureter may obstruct urine flow.

Clinical signs of renal trauma are often related to blood loss and shock. Pain may be elicited by palpation or a tucked-up "guarded" posture may be maintained by the animal. An enlarging mass in the area of the kidney may be palpated. Gross or microscopic hematuria will be present if urine flow from the damaged kidney(s) continues. Occasionally red blood cell casts may be seen indicating renal involvement. Elevations in serum urea nitrogen or creatinine concentrations due to prerenal shock may be seen. In this instance the urine specific gravity will be > 1.025. Primary renal azotemia may be seen if both kidneys have been extensively damaged; then urine specific gravity will be < 1.025.

Emergency treatment should first be directed toward correction of hemorrhage and shock using intravenous infusions of whole blood, isotonic fluids, corticosteroids, and antibiotics. Only the most severely traumatized kidneys require emergency surgical intervention. Criteria for surgery include uncontrolled hemorrhage and radiographic evidence of severe renal trauma.

Various radiographic abnormalities may be seen, depending upon the type of renal trauma. Inability to visualize the kidney(s) on plain radiographs may indicate accumulation of fluid (urine, blood) around the kidney(s) in the retroperitoneal space. Irregularity or enlargement of the renal shadow may also be detected. Further evaluation requires excretory urography (IVP). The IVP may reveal extravasation of contrast material into the renal parenchyma or surrounding structures in addition to an irregular nephrogram. In cases that have extensive renal damage and poor renal perfusion, high-dose excretory urographic techniques will be needed to visualize the anatomic structures adequately.

Unilateral nephrectomy is performed if extensive renal injury such as pulpefaction or "shattered kidney" has occurred. Adequate function of the remaining kidney should be established preoperatively, as monitored by determination of BUN or creatinine concentration, urinalysis, and IVP. Uncontrollable hemorrhage and avulsion of the renal artery are also indications for unilateral nephrectomy. Partial nephrectomy is recommended if less than 50 percent of the traumatized kidney is involved. Large subcapsular hematomas should be decompressed, but small hematomas and contusions do not require surgical intervention. Postoperative management includes continued fluid therapy, antibiotics, and supportive care.

URETER

Severe abdominal trauma may cause rupture of the ureter, usually in the area of the bladder or renal pelvis. Clinical signs and radiographic features will be similar to those discussed under renal trauma, although less severe blood loss is usually detected. Azotemia may be encountered if a sufficient volume of extravasated urine has accumulated and sufficient time has

elapsed to allow reabsorption of urine from the peritoneal cavity. Microscopic hematuria is often seen.

In ureteral rupture surgery is indicated after stabilization of the patient. Nephrectomy may be performed if damage to the ureter is extensive, provided that adequate function of the other kidney remains. Partial tears of the ureter can be handled by stenting alone or by stenting and suturing (DeHoff, et al.). Complete tears of the ureter may be handled by débridement and anastomosis; however, the incidence of postoperative stricture is high. If the ureter is torn near the bladder, transplantation of the ureter into the bladder is recommended. Postoperative management includes fluid therapy, urinary antibiotics, and supportive measures.

BLADDER

Rupture of the bladder may occur following abdominal trauma or urethral obstruction. Overzealous palpation or poor catheterization technique may also result in bladder rupture. Severe inflammatory disease may weaken the bladder wall and predispose to rupture.

Initial signs of bladder rupture are usually related to the traumatic event. The animal may initially respond to treatment for shock and then steadily deteriorate. Posterior abdominal tenderness, depression, vomiting, and fluid distention of the abdomen may be detected. Some urine may be voided, even though most of the urine is accumulating within the abdomen. Gross hematuria of variable degree is often seen. Abdominocentesis often will yield a serosanguineous fluid, with cytologic evidence of inflammation. Analysis of the abdominal fluid for urea or, preferably, for creatinine content will confirm that it is urine. Elevation in blood urea nitrogen and serum creatinine concentration occurs as a form of postrenal azotemia when urea and creatinine in the abdominal fluid are reabsorbed into the blood. Other biochemical abnormalities may include hyponatremia, hypochloremia, hyperkalemia, and metabolic acidosis.

Positive-contrast cystography is the preferred procedure in documenting a bladder tear. Extravasation of radiopaque dye into the peritoneal cavity is seen more readily than free air in the peritoneal cavity on pneumocystography. An IVP should also be performed if significant injury to the kidneys or ureters is suspected.

Correction of fluid deficits, electrolyte imbalances, and metabolic acidosis should be attempted prior to surgical intervention. Simultaneously, an indwelling urinary catheter that will serve to drain urine from the bladder and possibly from the peritoneal cavity should be inserted. Once stabilized, the tear should be repaired surgically. Postoperatively, appropriate fluid and antibiotic therapy should be continued.

URETHRA

Rupture of the urethra in dogs and cats may follow abdominal trauma, bite wounds, urethral obstruction, and improper catheterization technique. Often traumatic urethral ruptures are associated with a fractured pelvis. Rupture may occur anywhere along the length of the urethra. Clinical signs depend on the location of the rupture and whether or not obstruction of urine outflow occurs. Rupture of the pelvic urethra will result in accumulation of urine in the abdominal cavity, and signs will be identical to those of ruptured bladder. Rupture of the urethra at more distal sites will cause soft-tissue swelling, pain, and dysuria due to cellulitis from extravasated urine. Tissue necrosis and urinary fistulas may develop in cases with distal urethral rupture if the animal survives.

Diagnosis of ruptured urethra is confirmed by demonstration of a rent with positive-contrast urethrography. Varying degrees of azotemia typically occur as a result of reabsorption of extravasated urine or obstructive uropathy, or both. Hematuria is usually seen if urine is voided.

Repair of the ruptured urethra depends on the location and severity of the rent. Parial tears in the pelvic urethra can be sutured in an interrupted pattern but may require symphysiotomy for exposure. Complete tears in the pelvic urethra require anastomosis and an indwelling urinary catheter. Very small urethral tears may heal without surgery if an indwelling catheter is used for five to seven days. Rupture of the urethra in distal locations may be managed by performing a urethrostomy proximal to the point of rupture. Urinary antibiotics and fluid therapy should be continued postoperatively in all cases of urethral rupture.

SUPPLEMENTAL READING

Bovée, K.: The uremic syndrome. J. Am. Anim. Hosp. Assoc., 12:189–196, 1976.
DeHoff, W., Greene, R., and Greiner, T.: Surgical management of abdominal emergencies. Vet. Clin. North Am., 2:301–330, 1972.
Fluid therapy in small animal practice. J. Am. Anim. Hosp. Assoc., 8:147–241, 1972.
Osborne, C.: Urinary tract emergencies. In Kirk, R. W. (ed.): Current Veterinary Therapy V. Philadelphia, W. B. Saunders Co., 1974, pp. 829–837.
Osborne, C., and Finco, D.: Urinary tract emergencies and renal care following trauma. Vet. Clin. North Am., 2:259–292, 1972.
Scott, R., and Greene, R.: Urinary tract emergencies. In Kirk, R. W. (ed.): Current Veterinary Therapy VI. Philadelphia, W. B. Saunders Co., 1977, pp. 1073–1077.

TOXIC NEPHROPATHY

JERRY A. THORNHILL, D.V.M.
West Lafayette, Indiana

Toxic nephropathy is the term used to describe any adverse functional or structural change in the kidney resulting from drugs, chemicals, or biologic products that are inhaled, ingested, injected, or absorbed (Schreiner, et al.). The renal abnormality may be caused by compounds in their unchanged form or by their metabolites. This syndrome may be expanded to include nephrotoxic effects of physiologic substances circulating in abnormal concentrations, as occurs in hypercalcemic and hypokalemic nephropathy.

The incidence of drug-induced renal failure in animals with functionally normal kidneys and the incidence of adverse toxic drug effects in host animals with varying degrees of renal dysfunction are unknown (Osborne and Klausner). In veterinary medicine, therefore, the importance of nephrotoxicity in the genesis of renal failure and the contribution of certain nephrotoxic drugs or compounds (Table 1) to the clinical deterioration of patients with existing renal insufficiency have heretofore played minor roles. This has been caused partly by the paucity of information in veterinary literature on the pharmacokinetics of different potentially nephrotoxic drugs for varying levels of renal function and partly by the imprudent extrapola-

Table 1. Nephrotoxin Inventory

THERAPEUTIC AGENTS	METALS
Antimicrobials	Antimony
Gentamicin	Arsenic
Kanamycin	Beryllium
Neomycin	Bismuth
Streptomycin	Cadmium
Cephalosporins	Copper
Sulfonamides	Gold
Penicillin	Iron
Methicillin	Lead
Tetracycline	Mercury
Antifungals	Silver
Amphotericin B	Thallium
Analgesics	Uranium
Phenacetin	
Phenylbutazone	PESTICIDES
Salicylates	Chlorinated hydrocarbons
Anticonvulsants	Phosphorus
Phencurone	
Trimethadione	PHYSIOLOGIC SUBSTANCES
	Hypercalcemia
INHALED ANESTHETICS	Hypokalemia
Methoxyflurane	
	OSMOTIC AGENTS
GLYCOLS	Sucrose
Notably, ethylene glycol	Mannitol
	Dextran
ORGANIC SOLVENTS	
Carbon tetrachloride	MISCELLANEOUS
Methanol	Hemolysins
Tetrachlorethylene	Mushroom poison
	Snake venom
	Cyclophosphamide
	Penicillamine
	Thiacetarsamide

tion and application of dosage recommendations and precautions designed for human beings.

PATHOPHYSIOLOGY

SUSCEPTIBILITY OF THE KIDNEY TO TOXINS

The vulnerability of the kidney to drugs and biologically active materials stems from factors outlined in Table 2. In dogs and cats both kidneys have a combined weight of less than 1 percent of the body weight, yet approximately 20 percent of the cardiac output is delivered to the kidneys every minute. This high blood flow/tissue ratio is greatly pronounced in the

Table 2. Pathophysiologic Factors Affecting Renal Susceptibility to Toxins

Blood flow
Capillary endothelial surface area
Oxygen supply
Countercurrent multiplier system
Tubular secretion
Tubular fluid acidification
Uncoupling of protein-bound toxins
Enzyme suppression

renal cortex, which receives more than 90 percent of the renal blood flow. Renal cortical tissue, therefore, may receive a high concentration of circulating toxins. The voluminous blood flow of the kidneys is associated with the unique glomerular capillary system, which contains the largest endothelial vascular surface area per weight of any body organ. This predisposes the kidneys to precipitation of immune deposits and other noxious solutes. The kidney consumes oxygen at a great rate, especially in the cortex, and is susceptible to compounds that can produce cellular hypoxia. The renal countercurrent multiplier system may predispose the medullary interstitium to toxicity by progressively increasing tissue concentrations of drugs in the renal parenchyma. Tubular secretion of drugs into the luminal fluid can greatly increase the concentration of these substances. Tubular epithelial cells, in turn, are exposed to levels of drugs that may be toxic. These cells are more vulnerable to nephrotoxicity than other renal cells because they are metabolically active and have relatively rapid rates of turnover. Tubular fluid acidification may influence ionization characteristics of certain solutes in the luminal fluid, increasing their local concentration and solubility. Renal tubular cells may uncouple protein-bound toxins too large for glomerular filtration that are delivered by peritubular capillaries (Roxe). Finally, nephrotoxins can interfere with many enzymatic reactions in renal epithelial cells, especially those of oxidative respiratory enzymes in mitochondria (Maher, 1970).

MECHANISMS OF NEPHROTOXICITY

The morphologic changes induced by nephrotoxins include a wide range of lesions, varying with etiologic agents and their concentration. Histologically, cloudy swelling, fatty change, tubular and interstitial edema, interstitial inflammation and/or fibrosis, intranephron obstruction, glomerulonephritis, and cortical necrosis may be seen. Although the pathogenesis of these lesions is often obscure, drugs can be directly toxic by suppressing intracellular enzymes, resulting in cell death. They may also initiate hypersensitivity reactions, resulting in glomerular infiltration and may cause indirect toxicity by crystal formation, resulting in obstructive nephropathy (Maher, 1976).

MECHANISMS OF DRUG INTOLERANCE

See "Drug Therapy in Renal Disorders," elsewhere in Section 12, for specific information related to the pathophysiology of drug intolerance.

The following discussion summarizes the pathogenicity of some important nephrotoxic drugs, agents, and physical substances used in clinical veterinary medicine.

ANTIMICROBIAL AGENTS

AMINOGLYCOSIDES

Aminoglycoside antibiotics (i.e., gentamicin, streptomycin, kanamycin, neomycin, tobramicin, and vancomycin) are nephrotoxic; their toxicity is dose-related. They may also cause ototoxicity. Glomerular filtration is the major route of excretion for the group. In animals (Falco, et al.) neomycin is the most nephrotoxic, streptomycin is the least, and kanamycin and gentamicin are in between. Toxicity is manifested initially by proteinuria, cylindruria, and azotemia. The ensuing renal failure may be oliguric or non-oliguric. Microscopic lesions consist of varying degrees of glomerular or tubular edema, tubular cloudy swelling, proximal convoluted tubular vacuolation, and intracellular organelle damage. These lesions are potentially reversible following drug withdrawal; however, oliguric failure associated with acute tubular necrosis may result in death if appropriate therapy is not administered.

TETRACYCLINES

Tetracyclines have been shown experimentally to be intrinsically nephrotoxic (Obek, et al.); however, kidney damage appears primarily following administration of large intravenous doses (Czerwinski, et al.). Administration of tetracyclines to normal individuals or to patients with impaired renal function causes an increase in blood urea nitrogen concentration; serum creatinine levels remain stable. The mechanism of this increase has been hypothesized to be an antianabolic effect of tetracyclines that induces negative nitrogen balance. Liver synthesis of protein from amino acid precursors is suppressed, resulting in metabolism of amino acids for energy. Production of nitrogenous waste products is increased; these must be excreted by the kidneys (Osborne and Klausner). Normal kidneys can readily excrete this increased metabolic waste load, whereas functionally impaired kidneys cannot. Thus, excretory products accumulate, leading to azotemia and eventual clinical uremia. The increase in blood urea nitrogen concentration following tetracycline administration to human beings appears to be most marked in patients with underlying renal impairment and can lead to clinical renal failure in otherwise compensated patients. Administration of outdated tetracycline has initiated a multiple luminal membrane defect in the proximal tubule, resulting in a Fanconi syndrome characterized by proteinuria, bicarbonaturia (inducing a metabolic acidosis), glycosuria, phosphaturia, aminoaciduria, and potassium wasting.

CEPHALOSPORINS

Cephalosporins are eliminated primarily by the kidneys. At therapeutic dosages, cephalosporins are relatively non-toxic; however, in human patients with impaired renal function drug levels may be attained that become nephrotoxic. Proximal tubular cell damage, interstitial edema, mononuclear cell infiltration, and tubular necrosis may be seen histologically. In man toxicity of cephalosporins appears to be enhanced by concomitant use of other nephrotoxic agents, such as gentamicin, or potent diuretics, such as furosemide. In animal studies (Silverblatt, et al.) cephaloridine and, to a lesser extent, cephalothin and cefazolin, produced proximal tubular abnormalities and renal failure. In a recent study on cephaloridine administration to dogs with reduced renal function (Klausner, et al.) abnormal drug retention was circumvented by adjusting the dosage interval to various degrees of renal insufficiency.

SULFONAMIDES

In man sulfonamide therapy has resulted in a variety of nephrotoxic reactions, including hypersensitivity glomerulonephritis and vasculitis, interstitial nephritis, tubular cell edema and necrosis, and obstructive nephropathy from crystallization (Weinstein, et al.). Crystal formation occurs as the drug passes down the nephron, becoming progressively more concentrated as water is abstracted and more precipitous as the filtrate becomes more acidic. Sulfapyridine, sulfathiazole, and sulfadiazine tend to crystallize, whereas newer short-acting sulfonamides (i.e., sulfisoxazole and sulfamethoxazole) tend to be more soluble and associated with less risk of toxicity. The combination of trimethoprim and sulfamethoxazole has advanced sulfonamide therapy. The mixture provides a potent antimicrobial combination; trimethoprim does not appear to alter the solubility or renal excretion of sulfamethoxazole. Trimethoprim has been shown to alter excretion of creatinine in man, thus allowing patients receiving therapy to develop elevated serum creatinine concentrations and reduced creatinine clearance without actual reduction in glomerular filtration (Berglund, et al.).

PENICILLINS

The penicillins are excreted primarily by the kidneys. The elimination of the isoxazolyl penicillins (cloxacillin, dicloxacillin, oxacillin, and nafcillin) is virtually unchanged with renal impairment. Penicillin G, methicillin, ampicillin, amoxicillin, and carbenicillin, however, require modification in dosage regimens with renal impairment. Although penicillin G is relatively non-toxic in dogs and cats, its use has produced three patterns of renal damage in man: (1) hypersensitivity glomerulonephritis, (2) acute renal insufficiency, and (3) acute interstitial nephritis. The third condition has been described most often when penicillins (particularly methicillin) were used but also with ampicillin, nafcillin, oxacillin, and carbenicillin. Acute interstitial nephritis appears to be an immune-mediated disorder with antibodies directed against methicillin — renal structure protein conjugates. Although penicillin G excretion is prolonged in dogs with renal insufficiency, the apparent lack of toxicity allows normal therapeutic dosages to be administered. Large doses of potassium penicillin G should be avoided in oliguric or anuric uremic patients, however, since they are prone to hyperkalemia (unlike renal failure patients with polyuria).

ANTIFUNGAL AGENTS

AMPHOTERICIN B

In dogs intravenous amphotericin administration induces a dose-related renal vasoconstriction, creating a profound fall in both renal plasma flow and glomerular filtration rate and a progressive nitrogen retention (Butler, et al.). Early lesions are characterized by intracellular deposition of calcium, followed by necrosis and degeneration of proximal and distal convoluted tubules, flattening of epithelial surfaces, and thickening of tubular basement membranes. Cylindruria may be the first sign of toxicity, followed closely by hematuria, pyuria, and proteinuria. If therapy is continued at existing levels, blood urea nitrogen retention soon develops. The development of moderate to severe azotemia calls for a reduction in dosage or cessation of therapy. Lesions of the kidneys induced by amphotericin are potentially reversible if appropriate adjustments in dosage are made. If patients are monitored for renal dysfunction and dosed accordingly, amphotericin B

therapy rarely is associated with progressive, irreversible kidney failure. However, the drug may cause a membrane defect in the distal tubule that suppresses luminal secretion of hydrogen ion from within the cell to the tubular fluid. The distal renal tubular acidosis (RTA) induced is usually mild, producing slight bicarbonate and potassium loss in urine.

GLYCOLS

ETHYLENE GLYCOL

Renal lesions produced by glycol are considered to be due to its metabolic product, oxalic acid. When ingested, 3 to 10 percent of ethylene glycol is converted in the liver to oxalic acid. Renal involvement is usually the third and last metabolic consequence of ethylene glycol intoxication. Central nervous system and cardiopulmonary system dysfunction are thought to occur before the parent compound is partially converted to a nephrotoxin. Whether oxalic acid titrates calcium in the plasma or combines with calcium in tubular cells is unknown. In any event, calcium oxalate is formed, which induces tubular cell calcification. Degenerated calcified oxalate crystals and plaques slough into tubular lumina. Microscopic changes are characterized by marked destruction of renal tubular epithelial cells, tubular degeneration, obstruction of tubular lumina with masses of birefringent calcium oxalate crystals, interstitial edema, and mononuclear cell infiltration. Basement membranes are usually preserved and provide a foundation for tubular cell regeneration. Nephrotoxicity is thought to be due to direct effects of calcium oxalate on tubular cells, rather than to subsequent tubular obstruction. Once intoxication has surpassed the ability of conservative therapy to minimize oliguric uremia, peritoneal or hemodialysis is indicated for patient support until regeneration of renal tubules permits return of adequate renal function.

INHALANT ANESTHETICS

METHOXYFLURANE

Metabolism of methoxyflurane yields two potentially nephrotoxic products, inorganic fluoride and oxalic acid. Animal studies (Mazze, et al.) have demonstrated that the toxicity of methoxyflurane is dose-related and that the extent of renal impairment correlates with the amount of inorganic fluoride and oxalate in the urine. Factors that contribute to nephrotoxicity in man include prolonged exposure to methoxyflurane during an operative procedure, concomitant use of tetracycline, kanamycin, or gentamicin medication, underlying renal impairment, dehydration, and obesity. Calcium oxalate crystallization, proximal tubular epithelial necrosis, tubular degeneration, and interstitial fibrosis may occur. Human patients develop polyuric (high output) renal failure following surgery; it may persist for weeks or may develop into oliguric renal failure. In a recent study on the effects of methoxyflurane in dogs (Pedersoli) mild nephrogenic diabetes insipidus developed. However, renal failure due to tubular destruction (as found in man) could not be induced. Consult the article on anesthesia in renal failure for further details.

PHYSIOLOGIC SUBSTANCES

HYPERCALCEMIA

Primary and tertiary hyperparathyroidism (Finco, et al.), and pseudohyperparathyroidism all are associated with excessive secretion of parathyroid hormone (PTH). In these diseases PTH secretion is not sensitive to ionized calcium, and there is no negative feedback. Therefore, hypercalcemia develops. Studies in dogs (Epstein) have revealed that hypercalcemia initially causes intratubular cell calcification, ADH resistance, and polyuria. Tubular cells eventually undergo necrosis and slough into the lumen, becoming lodged in nephrons. When more than 75 percent of the nephrons become obstructed, azotemia develops. As a rule renal failure does not cause hypercalcemia, but hypercalcemia can cause renal failure. Therefore, the serum calcium concentration of patients with primary renal failure should be evaluated routinely.

MISCELLANEOUS NEPHROTOXINS

PENICILLAMINE

Penicillamine is used clinically in veterinary medicine to promote excretion of chelated lead in the urine and to bind precursors of cystine (penicillamine-cystine disulfide) in attempt to prevent cystine urolithiasis. Hypersensitive nephrotoxicity (glomerulonephritis and/or acute interstitial nephritis) induced by penicillamine has been reported in man. Thus, patients receiving long-term penicillamine therapy should be periodically evaluated for renal dysfunction.

THIACETARSAMIDE SODIUM

This arsenical compound is used to kill adult *Dirofilaria immitis*. Besides being hepatotoxic, thiacetarsamide sodium is potentially nephrotoxic, especially in patients with underlying renal impairment. The drug can initially cause glomerulonephritis, with proteinuria, hematuria, and cylindruria. Varying degrees of tubular degeneration or necrosis may follow and may be associated with nephrotoxic renal failure.

PREVENTION

"It is better to avert a malady with care than to use physic after it has appeared" (Shao Tze). The best therapy for toxic nephropathy is prevention of its occurrence. Knowledge of the biochemical mechanisms of drugs and agents used in clinical medicine will assist practitioners in properly evaluating body functions adversely affected. See the article entitled "Drug Therapy in Renal Disorders," elsewhere in Section 12, for specific recommendations about modification of drugs given to patients with primary renal failure.

When applicable, protective measures should be taken with the administration of nephrotoxic agents to assist in prevention of adverse functional or structural renal changes. The concentrations of blood urea nitrogen, serum creatinine, and serum electrolytes and the results of urinalyses and complete blood counts should be re-evaluated periodically in patients with varying degrees of renal insufficiency who are receiving medications that require minimal or moderate adjustments in dosage. Since blood urea nitrogen and serum creatinine concentrations may be within the normal range until more than 75 percent of functional tissue is lost, the initial evaluation ideally should include evaluation of endogenous creatinine clearance, since this procedure is a better index of renal function (Bovee, et al.). After drug therapy has been initiated, evaluation of serum creatinine concentration usually provides an adequate measure of renal performance (except with trimethoprim therapy, which may suppress creatinine clearance). Protective measures that can be taken during therapy include concomitant administration of mannitol with amphotericin B, alkalinization of urine with sulfonamides, limited if any combined use of synergistic or potentiating nephrotoxic drugs, and maintenance of fluid balance.

DIAGNOSIS

Diagnosis of nephrotoxicity begins with the history, followed by a thorough physical examination and laboratory confirmation of renal dysfunction. It must be determined whether the ill patient has been or is being treated with a nephrotoxic drug, has been exposed to a nephrotoxic agent, or has an underlying disorder that is creating metabolic toxic substances.

Signs of toxic nephropathy usually appear suddenly after kidney damage has occurred. Patients often develop vomiting, diarrhea or constipation, depression, anorexia, and oliguria. Body temperatures are often depressed, mucous membranes appear reddened, heart rate may be slow (as a result of hyperkalemia), and patients may be dehydrated and weak. Examination of urine may reveal casts, red blood cells, white blood cells, renal epithelial cells, and protein. The urinary sediment may show specific etiologic parent compounds or metabolites, such as sulfonamde crystals or birefringent calcium oxalate crystals from ethylene glycol intoxication. Elevated urea nitrogen and creatinine concentrations associated with increased levels of phosphorus and potassium may also be detected. If serum calcium concentration is elevated and serum protein concentration is normal, hypercalcemic nephropathy may be present. Radiographic examination of the abdomen will often reveal large, swollen kidneys.

THERAPY

The cornerstone of therapy for toxic nephropathy is elimination of the offending toxin by cessation of drug therapy and/or by *in vivo* binding of the toxin with specific substances to increase elimination. If the patient is not oliguric, withdrawal of the nephrotoxic agent followed by adequate replacement of fluid volume and stimulation of diuresis may be associated with amelioration of clinical and laboratory abnormalities.

If the patient develops oliguric renal failure, peritoneal dialysis or hemodialysis will be required to maintain life until the renal damage can be repaired. Long-term dialysis has not been very successful in veterinary medicine; however, in one uremic canine patient (Thorn-

hill, et al., in preparation) hemodialysis therapy supported life for 17 days.

If renal function does not return to normal following toxic nephropathy, a renal biopsy should be performed to evaluate renal structure.

SUPPLEMENTAL READING

Anderson, R.J., Gambertoglio, J.G., and Schrier, R.W.: Fate of drugs in renal failure. In Brenner, B.M., and Rector, F.C., Jr. (eds.): *The Kidney*, vol. 2. Philadelphia, W.B. Saunders Co., 1976.

Appel, G.B. and Nen, H.C.: The nephrotoxicity of antimicrobial agents. N. Engl. J. Med., 296:663–670, 772–778, 784–787; 1977.

Berglund, F., Killander, J., and Pompeius, R.: The effect of trimethoprim-sulfamethoxazole on the renal excretion of creatinine in man. J. Urol., 114:802–808, 1975.

Bovée, K.C., and Joyce, T.: Clinical evaluation of glomerular function: 24-hour creatinine clearance in dogs. J. Am. Vet. Med. Assoc., 174:488–491, 1979.

Butler, W.T., Hill, G.J., II, Szwed, C.F., et al.: Amphotericin B renal toxicity in the dog. J. Pharmacol. Exp. Ther., 143:47–56, 1964.

Czerwinski, A.W., and Pederson, J.A.: Drug-induced renal disease. Kidney, 8:20–23, 1975.

Epstein, F.H.: Calcium and the kidney. In Becker, E.C., Heinemann, H.D., and Sherman, R.L. (eds.): *Nephrology*. Cornell seminars. Baltimore, Williams & Wilkins Co., 1971.

Falco, F.G., Smith, H.M., and Arcieri, G.M.: Nephrotoxicity of the aminoglycosides and gentamicin. J. Infect. Dis., 119:406–409, 1969.

Finco, D.R., and Rowland, G.N.: Hypercalcemia secondary to chronic renal failure in the dog: A report of four cases. J. Am. Vet. Med. Assoc., 173:990–994, 1978.

Klausner, J.S., Meunier, P.C., Osborne, C.A., et al.: Half-life of cephaloridine in dogs with reduced renal function. Am. J. Vet. Res., 38:1191–1195, 1977.

Maher, J.F.: Nephrotoxicity of drugs and chemicals. Rational Drug Ther., 4:1–5, 1970.

Maher, J.F.: Toxic nephropathy. In Brenner, B.M., and Rector, F.C., Jr. (eds.): *The Kidney*, vol. 2. Philadelphia, W.B. Saunders Co., 1976.

Mazze, R.I., Cousins, M.J., and Kosek, J.C.: Dose-related methoxyflurane nephrotoxicity in rats. Anesthesiology, 36:571–587, 1972.

Obek, A., Petorak, I., Erogler, L., and Gurkon, A.: Effects of tetracycline on the dog kidney. A functional and ultrastructural study. Isr. J. Med. Sci., 10:765–771, 1974.

Osborne, C.A., and Klausner, J.S.: Drug therapy in renal failure: Cause or cure. I. Overview. Vet. Med. Reporter (Univ. of Minn.), No. 102, 1977, pp. 2–3.

Osborne, C.A., and Klausner, J.S.: Drug therapy in renal failure: Cause or cure. II. Recommendations for veterinary medicine. Vet. Med. Reporter (Univ. of Minn.), No. 103, 1977, pp. 1–3.

Pedersoli, W.M.: Serum fluoride concentration, renal and hepatic function test results in dogs with methoxyflurane anesthesia. Am. J. Vet. Res., 38:949–953, 1977.

Reidenberg, M.M.: *Renal Function and Drug Action*. Philadelphia, W.B. Saunders Co., 1971.

Roxe, D.M.: Toxic nephropathy due to drugs. Rational Drug Ther., 9:1–5, 1975.

Schreiner, G.E. and Maher, J.F.: Toxic nephropathy. Am. J. Med., 38:409–449, 1965.

Silverblatt, F., Harrison, W., and Turek, M.: Nephrotoxicity of cephalosporin antibiotics in experimental animals. J. Infect. Dis., 128:367–372, 1973.

Thornhill, J.A., Crabtree, B.J., and Ash, S.R.: Hemodialysis support of an oliguric ethylene glycol intoxicated dog. (In preparation)

Weinstein, L., Madoff, M.A., and Samet, C.M.: The sulfonamides. N. Engl. J. Med., 263:793–800, 952–957, 1960.

GLOMERULONEPHROPATHY AND THE NEPHROTIC SYNDROME

CARL A. OSBORNE, D.V.M.,
and KARIM JERAJ, B.V.Sc.
St. Paul, Minnesota

INTRODUCTION

The terms *glomerulonephropathy* and *glomerulonephritis*, with various qualifying prefixes (*proliferative, membranous, membranoproliferative,* and others), are commonly used to describe the variable response of different cells and structures within glomeruli to injury. Because glomerular lesions in many patients are not associated with an inflammatory response, the less specific term *glomerulonephropathy* provides a more accurate collective description than *glomerulonephritis*. These terms are analogous to the terms *enteritis* and *dermatitis*, in that lesions of a specific anatomic area are implied without reference to a specific cause or pathogenic mechanism. Since the etiopathogenesis as well as the clinicopathologic and immunologic manifestations of this disorder are highly variable, a diagnosis of glomerulonephritis (-opathy) does not imply a specific diagnosis. Glomerulonephropathy is a disease process characterized by morphologic and functional abnormalities in glomeruli that, if progressive, may induce changes in the renal tubules, interstitial tissue, and blood vessels. Primary glomerulonephropathy is distinguished from other types of primary renal disease (i.e., tubular disease, pyelonephritis, interstitial disease) by changes that initially and predominantly affect glomeruli. Consult other articles in Section 12 for specific information about other forms of primary renal disease.

The nephrotic syndrome is characterized by severe proteinuria, hypoproteinemia, hypoalbuminemia, hypercholesterolemia and, frequently, edema. These abnormalities occur as a result of increased permeability of glomerular capillaries to plasma protein, especially albumin. It is commonly observed in dogs and cats with membranous or membranoproliferative glomerulonephropathy and in dogs with renal amyloidosis. See "Renal Amyloidosis," elsewhere in this section, for specific details.

ETIOPATHOGENESIS

Knowledge of glomerular anatomy and physiology is an essential prerequisite to understanding the pathophysiology of glomerular disorders, which in turn is essential to establishment of diagnoses and prognoses and formulation of specific, supportive, symptomatic, or palliative therapy. Since this information has been reviewed in detail in previous editions and elsewhere, the following discussion consists of a brief overview of the etiopathogenesis of glomerulonephropathy. For specific details consult material cited in the reference list.

Investigation of naturally occurring renal diseases in domestic animals has undergone major change in the past decade. Widespread use of renal biopsy techniques, increased knowledge about the pathogenesis of kidney disease, and the use of immunofluorescent and electron microscopy have revealed that clinically significant "primary" glomerulonephropathy (glomerulonephritis) is relatively common in dogs, cats, and horses. Glomerulonephropathy has also been observed in association with polysystemic diseases, including amyloidosis, canine systemic lupus erythematosus, feline leukemia, canine pyometra, a variety of canine malignancies, canine *Dirofilaria immitis* infection, hog cholera, and equine infectious anemia. In some cases the severity of glomerular disease has been sufficient to cause the nephrotic syndrome, renal failure, or both.

Although correction of the erroneous but almost universal conception that glomerulonephropathy does not occur in domestic animals has received widespread attention during recent years, we still know painfully little about its underlying cause(s) and its natural course. Currently it appears that many forms of glomerular disease are initiated or perpetuated, or both, by abnormalities in humoral and possibly in cellular immunity. Tissue damage rather than host protection is sometimes the result of participation of cellular and humoral components of the immune system in attempts to maintain normalcy. Immunologic injury may be associated with one or any combination of four basic humoral and cellular mechanisms. Immediate, or antibody-mediated, hypersensitivity may be classified as (1) local or systemic anaphylactic reactions, (2) cytotoxic reactions, or (3) local (Arthus reaction) or systemic (serum sickness–like) immune-complex reactions. The fourth mechanism, delayed hypersensitivity, is mediated by the cellular immune system.

Cytotoxic reactions are involved in a form of glomerulonephritis called antiglomerular basement membrane (anti-GBM) glomerulonephritis. They may also induce a form of nephritis called antitubular basement membrane (anti-TBM) nephritis. Immune-complex reactions play a major role in the pathogenesis of immune-complex, or immune-deposit, glomerulonephritis.

Although components of cellular immunity (so-called T lymphocytes) must cooperate with components of humoral immunity (so-called B lymphocytes) for maximal antibody production, there is little experimental or clinical evidence in man or animals that cellular immune mechanisms play a direct role in the pathogenesis of anti-GBM or immune-complex glomerulonephritis. Lack of direct participation of cellular immunity in these forms of immune-mediated glomerular disease is in distinct contrast with renal transplant rejection, in which cellular immunity plays a prominent role. It is of interest that recent studies of minimal lesion glomerulopathy in man indicate that cellular immunity and lymphokines may play a role in the etiopathogenesis of this common disorder.

Results of experimental studies in animals and clinical studies in human beings and domestic animals suggest that spontaneously occurring glomerular lesions in animals may be mediated by *at least* two distinct immunologic mechanisms. The most common is similar to serum sickness in that soluble, *circulating, nonglomerular* antigen-antibody-complement complexes become localized in glomeruli (capillary walls and/or the mesangium). This type of glomerulonephropathy is commonly called "immune-complex" or "immune-deposit" glomerulonephropathy. Unfortunately, most antigens associated with immune-complex glomerulonephropathy have not yet been identified. However, it is thought to occur in association with diseases such as *Dirofilaria immitis* infection, feline leukemia, systemic lupus erythematosus, hog cholera, equine infectious anemia, neoplasia, and possibly infectious canine hepatitis.

The other type of glomerulonephropathy is characterized by localization of antiglomerular basement membrane (anti-GBM) antibodies produced by the host in glomerular capillary walls. It is commonly called anti-GBM glomerulonephropathy. Although anti-GBM glomerulonephropathy has been experimentally produced in domestic animals (especially dogs) by injecting material containing glomerular basement membrane, naturally occurring forms appear to be much less common than immune-complex glomerulonephropathy. Isolated naturally occurring cases have been reported in horses and dogs. Immune-complex glomerulonephropathy differs from anti-GBM glomerulonephropathy in that neither the antigen nor the antibody has any direct immunologic relationship to antigen determinants in glomeruli. Anti-GBM glomerulonephropathy is not associated with circulating antigen-antibody complexes.

Results of experimental studies performed in laboratory animals in recent months suggest that another mechanism characterized by *local* formation of immune complexes in glomeruli may represent a variant of immune-complex glomerulonephropathy. As previously mentioned, recent observations in human beings suggest that cellular immunity may also play an important role in the etiopathogenesis of some forms of glomerular disease, most notably minimal change glomerulonephropathy.

Certain characteristics of glomeruli may predispose them to immune injury. Because glomeruli are perfused with a large proportion of blood derived from cardiac output and because glomerular capillary blood is subjected to relatively high hydrostatic pressure, glomeruli are more likely to be exposed to large quantities of molecules that are products of immune interactions than are capillaries elsewhere in the body. The phagocytic function of mesangial cells adjacent to glomerular capillaries also may concentrate biologically active immune reactants in glomeruli. Studies in dogs, rats, and man have revealed that glycoproteins in the GBM are highly antigenic and are capable of inducing an immune response under appropriate conditions. Glomerular basement membrane antigens also are cross-reactive with antigens in lung and placenta and to a lesser degree with heart, intestine, liver stroma, and muscle.

One of the major unsolved problems concerning the etiopathogenesis of most cases of naturally occurring immune-complex glomerulonephropathy is identification of the nature and source of antigens that induce the immune response. Experimental models of immune-complex glomerulonephropathy have revealed that a wide variety of unrelated exogenous and endogenous antigens may cause immune-complex disease and that more than one antigen may be present in glomerular immune deposits. As exemplified by systemic lupus erythematosus, it is probable that a similar situation occurs in domestic animals and man. Any infection of low pathogenicity that does not kill the host and in which organisms (bacteria, parasites, viruses, protozoa, and so on), their antigens, or altered host antigens are present in the circulation for relatively long periods of time have the potential to cause immune-complex glomerular disease.

Each variant of glomerular injury results from the interaction of similar immunologic mediators. Interaction of antibodies with specific antigens *initiates* immunologic injury under appropriate conditions and represents a "first-order phenomenon" in the genesis of glomerular damage. A series of complicated and partially defined mediator systems appears to be subsequently associated with *production* of glomerular damage induced by anti-GBM antibody or immune-complex deposition. Activation of complement and the inflammatory and coagulation disorders that follow often result in development of destructive glomerular lesions. Leukocytes, vasoactive materials, platelets, and fibrin deposition play an active role in producing damage characterized by varying degrees of proteinuria and impaired renal clearance. Unfortunately, current knowledge of immunologic mechanisms and host factors does not provide a satisfactory explanation of all variants of clinical and morphologic abnormalities associated with glomerulonephropathy. It is clear that glomerulonephropathy encompasses a clinically complex and heterogeneous group of disorders.

NEPHROTIC SYNDROME

Most forms of glomerulonephropathy are associated with a variable degree of increased permeability of glomerular capillary walls to protein molecules. A characteristic indication (occasionally the only one) of glomerular disease is persistent proteinuria, which is often unassociated with significant hematuria or pyuria. Since the quantity of plasma proteins excreted in urine correlates inversely with their molecular weight, albumin (molecular weight 68,000) is the principal protein found in urine. Depending on the severity of damage to glomerular capillary walls, varying quantities of plasma globulins having higher molecular weights may also be excreted. Hyaline, granular, or waxy casts may be observed in urine sediment but are not a constant finding. Except

during later stages of progressive membranous glomerular disease, renal clearance of substances normally present in glomerular filtrate is not significantly impaired, and signs of renal failure are usually absent.

In dogs, cats, and human beings prolonged severe proteinuria and resultant hypoproteinemia that occur secondary to damage to glomerular capillary walls initiate physiologic, metabolic, and nutritional defects associated with the nephrotic syndrome (Fig. 1). If the proteinuria that occurs secondary to damage of filtration barrier(s) in capillary walls is persistent and severe, urine protein loss (especially of albumin) may exceed the capacity of the liver to maintain normal plasma protein concentration. In uremic patients an increase in the rate of endogenous catabolism of albumin and a decreased dietary intake of protein may also contribute to hypoproteinemia. Since albumin molecules account for approximately 75 per cent of plasma colloidal osmotic pressure, progressive hypoalbuminemia is associated with a proportionate decrease in plasma colloidal osmotic pressure. According to the Starling-Landis cycle of capillary-interstitial fluid exchange, a marked decrease in colloidal osmotic pressure will initiate an abnormal shift of fluid from the vascular compartment to the extravascular compartment, resulting in hypovolemia and edema.

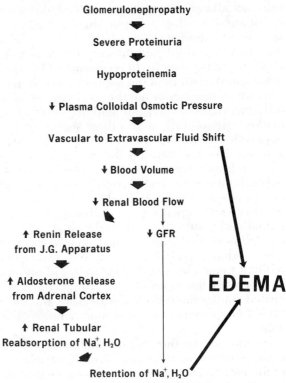

Figure 1. Pathophysiology of the nephrotic syndrome.

In addition to reduction in colloidal osmotic pressure that occurs as a result of glomerular loss of plasma protein, body compensatory mechanisms play a role in the development and maintenance of edema. As a result of loss of vascular fluid into extravascular tissue spaces, vascular volume is reduced. Reduction of renal blood flow associated with decreased vascular volume is thought to initiate the compensatory release of aldosterone through the renin-angiotensin system. (Recent studies of nephrotic human beings revealed that plasma aldosterone concentration was often normal, however.) Reduction in vascular volume may also stimulate the release of antidiuretic hormone. These hormones promote reabsorption of sodium and water from glomerular filtrate by the renal tubules. Because the reabsorbed sodium and water molecules are not large enough to be retained selectively in the vascular compartment by capillary walls, they rapidly equilibrate with extravascular fluid compartments. The pharmacologic effects of these hormones tend to perpetuate and aggravate edema in addition to expanding vascular volume. Impaired glomerular filtration that occurs as a consequence of decreased vascular volume and reduced renal blood flow may also promote retention of sodium and thus of water.

Although the nephrotic syndrome is a well-established complication of generalized glomerular disease in dogs, cats, monkeys, and man, not all patients with generalized glomerular disease develop a nephrotic syndrome. A specific glomerular disease in its mildest form may result in mild proteinuria that is insufficient to cause severe hypoalbuminemia and other manifestations of the nephrotic syndrome. The same disease in another patient, or at a different stage in the same patient, may cause marked proteinuria and other signs of the nephrotic syndrome. Glomerulonephritic dogs and cats may develop all features of the nephrotic syndrome (proteinuria, hypoproteinemia, hypoalbuminemia, and hypercholesterolemia) except edema. Even when edema is present its severity varies greatly from individual to individual and within the same individual. In fact, the clinical and biochemical manifestations may undergo partial or complete remission without treatment. Long-term studies of human beings with the nephrotic syndrome have revealed similar findings. Unfortunately, the likelihood of spontaneous remissions is unpredictable.

In addition to the biologic behavior of the underlying cause, the unpredictable variability of the natural course of the nephrotic syndrome is related to fluctuations in aldosterone, antidiuretic hormone, electrolytes, colloids, water within the body, and perhaps other factors. Of these factors, the severity of proteinuria and hypoalbuminemia is probably the most significant. In general, subcutaneous edema does not develop unless serum albumin concentration is less than about 0.8 gm/dl. However, because of variations in the capacity of the body to compensate for increased protein loss by increased hepatic protein synthesis and because of fluctuations in the concentrations of these hormones and electrolytes, not all patients with hypoalbuminemia of this magnitude develop edema.

With progression of glomerular lesions and onset of primary renal failure, the severity of proteinuria, hypoproteinemia, and edema may decrease. This decrease occurs when reduction in glomerular perfusion with plasma is of sufficient magnitude that it results in a significant reduction in the clearance of protein. In contrast with patients who have remission of glomerular lesions, however, uremic nephrotic patients have a progressive increase in the concentration of serum creatinine and urea nitrogen and a progressive loss of ability to concentrate and dilute urine.

RECOGNITION OF GLOMERULONEPHROPATHY

Persistent proteinuria indicates generalized glomerular disease. Care must be used in interpreting the significance of proteinuria, however, since it may be of renal or non-renal origin. A mild degree of proteinuria may occasionally be associated with fever or generalized passive congestion due to heart failure. Marked hematuria, regardless of cause, will be associated with moderate to severe proteinuria because of concomitant loss of plasma proteins. Slight to large quantities of protein may appear in urine as a result of inflammatory exudate (hematuria, pyuria, proteinuria) from any location in the urinary tract or contamination of voided urine and exudate from the genital tract. Proliferative glomerulonephropathy associated with exudation of inflammatory cells may result in proteinuria, hematuria, and pyuria that is difficult to distinguish from inflammatory lesions of the lower urinary tract. Concomitant hypoproteinemia and hypoalbuminemia provide support for the conclusion that persistent proteinuria is of glomerular origin. Hypercholesterolemia also appears to be a consistent finding in most species with marked albuminuria of glomerular origin.

Since protein-losing glomerulopathies are not the only potential cause of ascites and pitting edema of subcutaneous tissue, other non-renal causes of abnormal fluid accumulation, including congestive heart failure, hepatic cirrhosis, and malabsorption syndrome, should be considered. Distinction among these disorders can readily be based on associated clinical and laboratory findings.

Renal biopsies must be employed to establish the underlying cause of glomerular disease, because clinical and laboratory findings are not sufficiently specific to allow a diagnosis other than renal disease. Light microscopy and the use of special stains will usually suffice to differentiate amyloidosis from other types of glomerular disease.

Both immune-complex disease and anti-GBM disease focus antigen-antibody reactions in glomeruli. Since both immunologic mechanisms have the potential to stimulate an inflammatory response by activation of complement and other mediators of injury (kinins, vasoactive amines, coagulation factors) and since both may induce many morphologic forms of glomerular disease, they cannot be differentiated with certainty on the basis of clinical or laboratory findings or by light microscopic examination of kidneys. Depending on the amount and duration of antigen-antibody interaction and the types and quantities of mediators involved, either type of immune glomerular injury may be associated with severe, rapidly progressive disease or mild, slowly progressive disease. Each, however, has characteristic immunofluorescent and ultrastructural patterns.

The hallmark of immune-complex glomerulonephropathy consists of randomly distributed discrete, irregular, granular immune deposits within or adjacent to the GBM when kidney sections stained with fluorescein-tagged antibody specific for antibody, antigen, or complement are evaluated by immunofluorescent microscopy. Simultaneous presence of albumin associated with immunoglobulins and complement suggests non-selective deposition of plasma proteins. Immune complexes appear as electron-dense granular deposits in subepithelial, intramembranous, or subendothelial portions of glomerular capillary walls when evaluated by electron microscopy.

Anti-GBM glomerulonephropathy is characterized by smooth, diffuse, uniformly linear deposition of antibody and usually of complement along the inner surface of the GBM when evaluated by immunofluorescent microscopy. There are no characteristic electron microscopic findings other than the conspicuous absence of electron-dense deposits typical of immune-complex disease. Inconspicuous dense deposits may be observed along the subendothelial side of the GBM. Although anti-GBM glomerulonephritis can be tentatively diagnosed by detection of linear immunofluorescent deposits of immunoglobulins along the GBM, the specificity of the immunoglobulins should be confirmed by washing cortical homogenates with reagents that dissociate antigen-antibody complexes and by subsequently demonstrating fixation of the immunoglobulin(s) to normal homologous kidney *in vitro* or to homologous or heterologous kidneys *in vivo*. It may also be possible to transfer anti-GBM antibody by incubation of sections of homologous normal kidney with patient's serum followed by indirect immunofluorescent techniques. Non-specific linear GBM deposits of immunoglobulin have been identified in human kidneys at autopsy and also in kidneys obtained from human beings with diabetes mellitus.

In either form of glomerulonephropathy there may be irregular deposition of electron-dense or immunofluorescent material containing immunoglobulin, complement, fibrinogen, and other plasma proteins within glomerular capillary lumina, beneath the endothelium, and in the mesangium. Varying quantities of this material may represent non-specific adherence of plasma proteins to previously damaged glomeruli.

SPECIFIC THERAPY

OVERVIEW

Current therapeutic measures are empirical by nature, frequently ineffective, and too often potentially hazardous. Caution must be used in selecting potentially harmful drugs for treating patients with glomerulonephropathies, because the prognosis is not so uniformly poor in all patients that any type of treatment is warranted. In man guidelines for therapy are based on knowledge of specific types of glomerular disease (i.e., minimal-change glomerular disease, focal glomerulosclerosis, membranous glomerulonephropathy, proliferative glomerulonephropathy, membranoproliferative glomerulonephropathy, poststreptococcal glomerulonephritis, IgA nephropathy, rapidly progressive glomerulonephritis, anti-GBM glomerulonephritis, and others). Similar diagnostic and therapeutic classifications have not yet been developed for naturally occurring glomerulonephropathy in domestic animals.

On the basis of current knowledge, it seems reasonable to formulate therapy for immune-complex glomerulonephritis in dogs and cats on the basis of (1) removal of antigens, (2) correction of immunologic disturbances, (3) inhibition of inflammation, and (4) inhibition of coagulation. We have no experience with treatment of anti-GBM glomerulonephritis. Consult the article on amyloidosis for recommendations of therapy for that glomerular disorder.

REMOVAL OF ANTIGENS

Efforts to identify infectious and non-infectious agents in animals suspected of having immune-complex glomerulonephropathy are recommended, since knowledge of the antigens involved is of therapeutic significance. Eradication of exogenous antigens (bacteria, viruses, parasites, hapten drugs) may halt the progression of glomerular disease or induce its remission. The potential value of this recommendation is exemplified by the reversible nature of poststreptococcal glomerulonephritis. Likewise, withdrawal of D-penicillamine (used to treat Wilson's disease) or gold salts (used to treat rheumatoid arthritis) from human beings with drug-induced immune-complex glomerulonephropathy is often associated with remission of glomerular lesions and their clinical and biochemical sequelae. We have observed significant improvement in the severity of proteinuria and hypoalbuminemia in some glomerulonephritic dogs with *Dirofilaria immitis* infection following elimination of adult organisms and microfilaria by medical therapy. Removal of the uterus from dogs with pyometra may be associated with improvement in the subclinical glomerular lesions occasionally associated with that disorder.

Although we have no documented proof, it is reasonable to hypothesize that extirpation or destruction of neoplastic lesions (and their associated antigens) in patients with concomitant immune-complex glomerulonephropathy may halt the progression of, or induce the remission of, glomerular lesions. The frequency with which naturally occurring canine glomerulonephropathy is associated with malignancies is exemplified by the results of one survey in which 17 of 42 glomerulonephritic dogs had concomitant neoplasia.

Although dogs with lupus erythematosus and cats with feline leukemia may develop immune-complex glomerular disease, unfortunately it is not yet possible to eliminate the antigen(s) associated with these disorders.

Results of experimental studies have suggested the possibility of altering the size and biologic activity of immune-complexes by administration of large doses of specific antigen. Immune-complexes formed in extreme antigen excess are often soluble, do not activate comple-

ment, and are biologically inactive. The fact that more than one antigen may play a role in the genesis of immune-complexes, however, would appear to limit the potential value of this mode of therapy.

Attempts to formulate specific therapy for immune-mediated glomerulonephropathy often involve more than identification and elimination of antigens that stimulate a harmful immune response. It is now recognized that basic genetic and immunologic aberrations play an important role in the susceptibility of animals to immune-mediated glomerular disease and also influence the intensity and duration of glomerular lesions. Although elimination of antigens may result in temporary remission of the disease, long-term control and prevention may require manipulations that correct the predisposition to formation of biologically active immune reactants. Unfortunately, nothing is known about immunologically specific forms of therapy or modification of host factors that predispose to immunologic damage.

CORRECTION OF IMMUNOLOGIC DISTURBANCES

Experimental and clinical evidence implicating an immunologic basis for anti-GBM and immune-complex glomerulonephropathy and the success of corticosteroids and immunosuppressive drugs in controlling homograft rejections of renal transplants provide a logical basis for considering the use of various combinations of corticosteroids and immunosuppressants (cyclophosphamide, azathioprine, methotrexate, and others) in the treatment of immunologic glomerulonephropathy. Drugs of this type have been used in the treatment of immune-mediated glomerular disease with the expectation that they will inhibit the production of pathogenic antibodies or suppress the inflammatory response thought to be initiated by antigen-antibody-complement reactions. However, there has been no documentation that naturally occurring immune-mediated glomerulonephropathy is consistently associated with hyperactivity of the immune system. In addition, inflammatory reactions apparently are not always an integral part of the evolution of the disease process.

One of the most significant hypotheses regarding the pathogenesis of immune-complex disease that has been developed on the basis of experimental studies is that *some* patients with immune-complex disease may have a suppressed rather than hyperactive immune system. This concept is of fundamental therapeutic significance, since it suggests that administration of corticosteroids and the more potent immunosuppressant agents may be of no benefit. In fact, they may potentiate the underlying disorder of immunocompetence. Administration of a variety of types and combinations of immunosuppressant drugs to experimental animals, dogs, and human beings supports this hypothesis. Results of prospective studies of the administration of corticosteroids to human beings with several variants of glomerulonephropathy indicate that this form of treatment is not a cure-all.

In one study in which azathioprine and prednisone were administered to human patients with proliferative glomerulonephritis, responses were favorable only in patients with clinical and morphologic findings similar to those observed in patients who often recovered without treatment. Although remissions of clinical and laboratory manifestations have been observed in some patients (especially those with lupus erythematosus), it has often been difficult to demonstrate a clear temporal relationship between therapy and remissions. Even though the rate of progression of glomerulonephropathy has sometimes been delayed, the disorder has not been eradicated. In summary, the beneficial effect of corticosteroid and immunosuppressant therapy in human beings with immunologic glomerulonephropathy remains unsubstantiated. In general, the results of such therapy have been disappointing.

Establishment of meaningful generalities about the therapeutic benefit of corticosteroid therapy of glomerular disease in domestic animals is difficult, since published results have been limited to isolated case reports. In our limited clinical experience with canine and feline glomerulonephropathy, beneficial results from administration of corticosteroids (when they occurred) were transient and often associated with unwanted side effects. The fact that clinical and laboratory manifestations of glomerulonephropathy were associated with unpredictable remissions and exacerbations has complicated attempts to evaluate the effects of therapy. We remain skeptical of reports that indicate that corticosteroid and immunosuppressant therapy were successful in inducing remission of clinical signs of the nephrotic syndrome in dogs with generalized glomerular disease. The conclusions of these investigators have been based on the evaluation of a limited number of patients and apparently have not taken into account the possibility that clinical remission could have occurred without any therapy. Although corticosteroid therapy frequently is effective in suppressing hematologic and serologic manifestations of systemic lupus erythematosus in dogs, it appears to be ineffective in the treatment of canine lupus nephritis.

We maintain our recommendation that widespread use of corticosteroids and more potent immunosuppressant therapy in domestic animals with immune-mediated glomerulonephropathy should be withheld (1) until the natural course of the disease has been evaluated in a larger number of patients and (2) until results of carefully monitored and — where possible — controlled clinical trials confirm or deny their value. This recommendation is based on the following: (1) Corticosteroids and immunosuppressant drugs have the potential to inhibit beneficial as well as harmful immune and inflammatory responses. (2) These drugs may precipitate or aggravate renal failure by inducing gluconeogenesis. (3) These drugs have the potential to perpetuate immunologic imbalances that favor the production of biologically active immune complexes. (4) Patients in renal failure typically have varying degrees of immunodeficiency.

Experimental studies of long-term effects of administration of corticosteroids to rabbits with immune-complex glomerulonephropathy have revealed that corticosteroid therapy may augment the incidence of glomerulonephritis. Cortisone-induced depression of antibody production resulted in the formation of large quantities of circulating pathogenic, soluble immune complexes in rabbits that otherwise might have produced non-pathogenic, insoluble immune complexes if their capacity to produce antibody had not been suppressed.

If the characteristics of individual cases or the psychological pressure imposed by clients to "do something" results in consideration of steroid therapy, differentiation via renal biopsy of glomerular disease caused by amyloidosis from that caused by immune-complex disease is essential. Currently available evidence suggests that corticosteroids should be avoided in patients with amyloidosis, since these drugs have enhanced experimental production of amyloidosis in animals and have been of no benefit in human patients with renal amyloidosis.

In the absence of results of experimental and clinical trials, it is necessary to make the unproved assumption that commonly used therapeutic dosages of steroids should be used when formulating trial therapy. The magnitude of proteinuria (preferably determined by 24-hour collections) and the status of serum albumin and globulin concentrations should be serially monitored. In addition, the serum concentration of urea nitrogen and creatinine should be monitored so that augmented production of urea associated with steroid-induced gluconeogenesis can be distinguished from changes in glomerular filtration rate (GFR). Steroid-induced azotemia, lack of improvement in GFR, and lack of change in urine protein loss after a suitable period of therapy (four to six weeks?) are indicators that steroid therapy should be withdrawn. If remission of clinical and laboratory signs is associated with steroid therapy, we suggest that the dosage be reduced and finally discontinued. Recurrence following withdrawal of steroids should prompt consideration of longer-term administration of steroids in dosages sufficient to induce remission of clinical abnormalities. In human beings alternate-day steroid therapy has usually been associated with fewer adverse side effects than daily steroid therapy. Encouraging results should be viewed critically against the unpredictable nature of the natural history of many glomerular diseases.

Whether it is of benefit to initiate therapy in patients with subclinical persistent proteinuria caused by immune complexes is unknown. However, if laboratory and biopsy data suggest that renal lesions are generalized, irreversible, and associated with renal failure or uremia, we recommend that steroid therapy be withheld. Steroids will not reverse established lesions and may potentiate uremia by their catabolic effects.

Although the use of combinations of steroids with more potent immunosuppressant drugs has been reported to interfere with immune responses without producing intolerable toxicity in human glomerulonephritic patients, we have had no experience with this mode of therapy.

Future efforts must be directed toward defining types of glomerulonephropathy that are steroid-responsive and finding alternative forms of therapy for those that are steroid-resistant. Perhaps immunostimulant therapy with drugs such as levamisole may prove to be more effective for some patients than immunosuppressant therapy.

INHIBITION OF INFLAMMATION AND COAGULATION

Evaluation of experimentally induced immune-complex glomerulonephropathy in laboratory animals has revealed that inflammation may be an important component in the pathogenesis of glomerular damage. Activation of complement (an enzymatic system of plasma proteins) by immune complexes (or by the so-called alternate pathway of complement activation) is associated with several reactions, including release of chemotactic substances that attract polymorphonuclear leukocytes (PMNs) and the phenomenon of immune adherence,

which promotes the retention of PMNs in glomeruli. This mechanism is called neutrophil-dependent injury of the glomerular basement membrane. The PMNs may displace the endothelial cells lining the glomerular capillaries and approximate themselves along the GBM, presumably in an attempt to engulf immune complexes. If proteolytic enzymes (cathepsins, collagenase, and elastase, for example) and other lysosomal proteins are released from PMNs, the GBM and glomerular cells may be damaged. Glomerular damage results in nonselective renal clearance of plasma proteins and proteinuria. If the immune response is severe or prolonged, it may be associated with the formation and deposition of fibrin. This may interfere with resolution of the lesion and result in healing by replacement fibrosis. Fibrin deposition in Bowman's space may stimulate the formation of epithelial crescents.

In neutrophil-dependent injury of the GBM, neutrophils are the effectors of injury. Depletion of either complement or neutrophils from experimental animals will prevent the development of injury in this form of glomerulonephropathy, even though immune complexes are deposited in glomeruli. Use of anti-inflammatory agents (including corticosteroids, cytotoxic agents, and indomethacin) in the treatment of glomerulonephritis has been defended on the basis of neutrophil-dependent glomerulonephritic models.

A neutrophil-independent form of immune-complex glomerulonephropathy has been observed in experimental animals in which removal of complement and neutrophils will not prevent the development of glomerular injury. Few neutrophils have been found in the glomeruli of dogs, cats, and other species with naturally occurring immune-complex glomerulopathy associated with clinical signs. This observation suggests that neutrophil-independent injury of the GBM does occur and that the use of corticosteroids to suppress neutrophil-mediated damage to glomeruli is illogical. The mechanisms that cause neutrophil-independent glomerulonephritis have not been defined.

Activation of the clotting mechanism by immune reactants has led to the use of anticoagulants (including heparin and warfarin) and antiplatelet drugs (including indomethacin and dipyridamole) in the treatment of some forms of glomerulonephropathy in human beings, especially those with rapidly progressive glomerulonephritis. The rationale for their use is to minimize intraglomerular coagulation and fibrin deposition despite the persistence of underlying immunologic abnormalities. We have had no experience with the use of these agents in the treatment of naturally occurring glomerular disease of animals.

SUPPORTIVE AND SYMPTOMATIC THERAPY

Despite vast voids in knowledge and the unavailability of specific therapy for most forms of glomerulonephropathy, the situation is far from hopeless. Although uncommon, prolonged remission of glomerulonephropathy associated with the nephrotic syndrome has been observed in dogs without the benefit of any therapy. It is emphasized that nephrotic patients may tolerate a mild to moderate degree of edema without obvious ill effect. Elimination of subcutaneous transudative edema and mild ascites with potent diuretics such as furosemide may provide some psychological relief to the owner and veterinarian but may further compromise reduction in vascular volume caused by hypoproteinemia. In this instance treatment of the effect may aggravate other consequences of the cause.

The following recommendations concerning symptomatic and supportive therapy of different manifestations of generalized glomerular disease are intended as generalities only. The method used and the vigor with which it is pursued should be formulated according to the needs of each patient.

1. *Proteinuric, non-edematous, non-uremic:* Provide unlimited access to water. If the protein loss is severe, formulate a diet with a sufficient quantity of high-quality protein to help compensate for protein loss in urine. Monitor serum protein concentration. Administer B-complex vitamins orally. Consider the use of anabolic agents such as Winstrol-V® (Winthrop), according to the manufacturer's recommended dosage.

2. *Proteinuric, non-edematous, polyuric, uremic:* Avoid stress-inducing factors such as changes in home environment (hospitalization, boarding in kennels, and so on). Provide unlimited access to water unless the patient is vomiting, in which case fluids should be administered parenterally. Administer anabolic agents. Cautiously supply additional high-quality protein in the diet to balance protein loss in urine. Do not provide excessive amounts of protein, since it will be deaminated and metabolized for energy and will increase the quantity of metabolic waste to be excreted by failing kidneys. Monitor serum urea nitrogen, creatinine, and albumin concentrations. Administer B-complex vitamins orally. Administer sodium bicarbonate with caution, since the addition of excessive sodium may precipitate edema. Consult the articles elsewhere in Section 12 on management of renal failure for dosage recommendations. Reduce the dosage or discontinue sodium bicarbonate therapy if

edema develops. Oral calcium lactate may be used in lieu of sodium bicarbonate to combat metabolic acidosis.

3. *Proteinuric, edematous, non-uremic:* Provide unlimited access to water. Provide a diet with a sufficient quantity of high-quality protein to help compensate for protein loss in urine. Monitor serum urea nitrogen, creatinine, and albumin concentrations. Avoid stress and administer anabolic agents. Administer B-complex vitamins orally. Cosmetic improvement is not an indication for diuretic therapy because diuresis may aggravate subnormal vascular volume caused by hypoalbuminemia. For moderate to severe edema, administer saliuretic diuretics such as furosemide (Lasix®, National) or ethacrynic acid (Edecrin®, Merck). These diuretics are so effective that removal of fluid by paracentesis is rarely necessary. Thoracocentesis should be considered only if pleural fluid is impairing respiration. Repeated paracentesis should be avoided, if possible, since it will deplete the patient of fluids and metabolites. Prevent diuresis-induced fluid and electrolyte depletion by proper control of diuretic dosage and by replacement therapy with fluids and electrolytes when necessary. Depending on the biologic behavior of the underlying cause of the nephrotic syndrome, control of edema may necessitate administration of low dosages of oral diuretics for the life of the patient. Drug-induced hypokalemia has not been observed in nephrotic dogs receiving long-term therapy with low doses of furosemide at the University of Minnesota. Intravenous administration of solutions containing protein is of potential value for patients in circulatory collapse caused by hypovolemia and for initiating diuresis in patients with refractory edema. It will produce only a transient effect and therefore is impractical for long-term therapy. Administration of excessive quantities of plasma protein may result in azotemia if significant quantities are metabolized for energy.

4. *Proteinuric, edematous, polyuric, uremic:* Avoid stress, administer anabolic agents and B-complex vitamins, and cautiously supply additional high-quality protein in the diet with the objective of minimizing urine protein loss. Do not provide excessive protein, since some may be deaminated and metabolized for energy. Monitor serum urea nitrogen, creatinine, and albumin concentrations. Provide unlimited access to water unless the patient is vomiting, in which case fluids should be administered parenterally. Administer sodium bicarbonate with caution. Reduce the dosage or discontinue use of this drug if the edema increases in severity. Oral calcium lactate may be provided in lieu of sodium bicarbonate to combat meta-

bolic acidosis. Consider the use of furosemide or ethacrynic acid to control or eliminate the edema. Alternatively, aldosterone antagonists such as spironolactone (Aldactone®, Searle) may be used to control edema. We have had no experience with the use of aldosterone-antagonizing agents.

5. *Proteinuric, edematous, oliguric, uremic* (oliguria caused by primary renal failure and not prerenal azotemia): Avoid stress and administer anabolic agents and vitamins parenterally. Consider the use of furosemide or ethacrynic acid to control edema and to induce diuresis. Correct deficits or excesses of fluids and electrolytes; avoid overhydration. Avoid administration of potassium if the patient is hyperkalemic. Supply adequate calories to minimize endogenous protein catabolism. Consider peritoneal dialysis with 4.25 per cent dextrose dialysate solutions to control or eliminate the edema and to remove body excesses of electrolytes, protein breakdown products, and other substances. Return to therapy designed for polyuria as soon as the patient can sustain urine output.

PROGNOSIS

The glomerulus has good capacity to repair acute inflammatory lesions, as exemplified by studies of experimentally induced anti-GBM glomerulonephritis in dogs. In this study widespread glomerular damage and capillary occlusion were present during early stages of the disease. Within three weeks, however, there was marked resolution of lesions, and by 60 days the only consistent finding was excess mesangial matrix and focal mesangial proliferation.

Repair of severe or chronic lesions seldom results in normal glomeruli. The fact that new glomeruli and tubules cannot be formed following maturation in order to replace irreversibly damaged nephrons is an important event related to the evolution of progressive glomerulonephropathy. Progressive irreversible lesions initially localized to glomeruli are eventually responsible for development of lesions in remaining, but initially unaffected, portions of the nephron and are ultimately associated with healing by replacement fibrosis and scarring.

Pending controlled studies that elucidate the cause, pathogenesis, natural clinical course, and therapeutic response of various types of glomerular disease, forecasts of the future course of events for glomerulonephritic patients will remain unpredictable. These generalities should not be interpreted to indicate that all glomerular diseases are clinically irreversible. Several types of glomerulonephropathy, as exemplified by acute poststreptococcal proliferative glomerulonephritis in man and mixed membranoproliferative glomerulonephropathy in dogs with pyometra, may be associated with complete functional recovery. Others may be associated with irreversible but non-progressive lesions. For example, membranous glomerulonephropathy associated with the nephrotic syndrome in a four-year-old dog was associated with complete spontaneous functional recovery despite persistent non-progressive glomerular lesions of more than three years' duration. Functional recovery may be complete even when considerable nephron destruction has occurred, since remaining viable nephrons may increase their functional capacity by compensatory hypertrophy. Progressive renal failure results only if continued nephron destruction exceeds the capacity of viable nephrons to compensate.

SUPPLEMENTAL READING

Brenner, B.M., and Rector, F.C.: *The Kidney*, vols. 1 and 2. Philadelphia, W.B. Saunders Co., 1976.

Cameron, J.S.: Drug treatment of chronic glomerulonephritis. National Kidney Foundation. 8(4):14–19, 1975.

Donadio, J.V., et al.: Treatment of diffuse proliferative lupus nephritis with prednisone and combined prednisone and cyclophosphamide. N. Engl. J. Med., 299:1151–1155, 1978.

Ehrenreich, T., et al.: Treatment of idiopathic membranous nephropathy. N. Engl. J. Med., 295:741–746, 1976.

Fauci, A.S.: Alternate-day corticosteroid therapy. Am. J. Med., 64:729–731, 1978.

Friend, P.S., and Michael, A.F.: Hypothesis: Immunologic rationale for the therapy of membranous lupus nephropathy. Clin. Immunol. Immunopathol., 10:35–40, 1978.

Gelfand, M.C., et al.: Therapeutic studies in NZB/W mice. Arthritis Rheum., 15:239–246, 1972.

Hahn, B.H., et al.: Comparison of therapeutic and immunosuppressive effects of azathioprine, prednisolone, and combined therapy in NZP/NZW mice. Arthritis Rheum., 16:163–170, 1973.

Lindeman, R.D.: Drug treatment of chronic idiopathic glomerulopathies. Postgrad. Med., 62:135–143, 1977.

McIntosch, R.M., Kaufman, D.B., Griswold, W., Urizar, R., Smith, F.G., and Vernier, R.L.: Azathioprine in glomerulonephritis: A long-term study. Lancet, 1:1085–1089, 1972.

Murray, M., and Wright, H.G.: A morphologic study of canine glomerulonephritis. Lab. Invest., 30:213–221, 1974.

Osborne, C.A., Stevens, J.B., McLean, R., and Vernier, R.L.: Membranous lupus glomerulonephritis in a dog. J. Am. Anim. Hosp. Assoc., 9:295–300, 1973.

Osborne, C.A., Hammer, R.F., Resnick, J.S., Stevens, J.B., Yano, B.L., and Vernier, R.L.: Natural remission of nephrotic syndrome in a dog with immune-complex glomerular disease. J. Am. Vet. Med. Assoc., 168:129–137, 1976.

Osborne, C.A., Hammer, R.F., Stevens, J.B., O'Leary, T.P., and Resnick, J.S.: Immunologic aspects of glomerular disease in the dog and cat. Gaines Veterinary Symposium, 26:15–32, 1976.

Osborne, C.A., Hammer, R.F., Stevens, J.B., Resnick, J.S., and Michael, A.F.: The glomerulus in health and disease: A comparative review of domestic animals and man. Adv. Vet. Sci. Comp. Med., 21:207–285, 1977.

Simon, N.M., and Rosenberg, M.J.: Medical treatment of glomerular diseases: Symposium on renal therapeutics. Med. Clin. North Am., 62:1157–1181, 1978.

Stuart, B.P., Phemister, R.D., and Thomassen, R.W.: Glomerular lesions associated with proteinuria in clinically healthy dogs. Vet. Pathol., 12:125–144, 1975.

Willkens, R.F.: The use of nonsteroidal anti-inflammatory agents. JAMA, 240:1632–1635, 1978.

RENAL AMYLOIDOSIS

J. A. BARSANTI, D.V.M.,
and WAYNE CROWELL, D.V.M.
Athens, Georgia

Amyloidosis is a disease in which organ function is disturbed by the physical presence of amyloid, an extracellular glycoprotein. No inflammatory response is present. In dogs clinical signs are related to the deposition of amyloid in the renal glomeruli, resulting initially in proteinuria and later in generalized renal failure. Other organs in affected animals may contain amyloid, but associated clinical signs are uncommon.

Amyloid has been characterized by many different techniques, including light microscopy, immunofluorescent microscopy, electron microscopy, x-ray diffraction, and histochemical studies. By light microscopy it is an amorphous, homogeneous, eosinophilic substance closely associated with basement membranes, vessel walls, and stromal connective tissue. When stained with congo red and examined under polarized light, it has an apple-green birefringence due to its fibrillar nature. The nonbranching, randomly arranged fibrils can be visualized with electron microscopy. Amyloid is mainly protein with only a small quantity of neutral sugars. It contains no gamma globulin. In human patients two different types of amyloid have been identified, based on differences in amino acid composition. Amyloid from patients with multiple myeloma or from those with no identifiable predisposing disease (primary amyloidosis) has a composition similar to light chains of immunoglobulins. Amyloid from patients with an identifiable predisposing disease (secondary amyloidosis) has as its major constituent a previously undescribed glycoprotein of 8500 daltons molecular weight (protein A) that has no relation to immunoglobulins. Whether both immunoglobulin light chains and protein A can occur in the same patient is unknown. The composition of amyloid in spontaneous cases in dogs and cats has not been investigated.

The etiology of amyloid is unknown. Its production can be induced experimentally with numerous antigens, including bacterial toxins, antitoxins, serum, plasma globulins, gamma irradiation, and casein. No consistent immunoglobulin abnormalities have been found in animals with spontaneous or experimentally induced disease or in humans with secondary amyloidosis. One theory of amyloid formation suggests an aberration in the immune system that develops after prolonged antigenic stimulation or in association with abnormal plasma cells. According to this theory, reticuloendothelial (RE) cells produce amyloid, an insoluble inactive protein, or its precursor and deposit this extracellularly. In primary amyloidosis the RE cells produce amyloid from immunoglobulin light chains derived from abnormal plasma cells. In support of this theory, Bence Jones proteins have been digested *in vitro* to produce amyloid. In secondary amyloidosis RE cells produce protein A, perhaps from an antigenically related protein present in the serum of normal people and in increased concentration in serum from people with chronic diseases and secondary amyloidosis. The RE cell has a dual role in amyloidosis, since it can also phagocytize and digest amyloid. It is not known whether the disease is due to increased production, decreased degradation, or both. Other cells that have been implicated in the production of amyloid include glomerular mesangial cells (considered to be RE cells), glomerular epithelial and endothelial cells, histiocytes, fibroblasts, pancreatic acinar cells, and thyroid carcinoma cells.

PATHOGENESIS

Chronic suppurative or necrotic diseases and neoplasia are predisposing causes for amyloidosis in small animals. Such conditions as abscesses, osteomyelitis, dirofilariasis, pyometra, empyema, tuberculosis, systemic fungal infections, multiple myeloma, lymphosarcoma, and immunologic diseases (such as systemic lupus erythematosus) have been associated with amyloidosis in dogs. All experimental dogs over six months of age with hereditary cyclic hematopoiesis (grey collie cyclic neutropenia) have generalized amyloidosis. This may be related to abnormal development of lymphoid organs or to the repeated infections these dogs suffer. In many spontaneous cases in dogs no predisposing cause is identifiable. In cats chronic hypervitaminosis A has been associated with amyloidosis. Marked stimulation of the RE system has been postulated as the reason for amyloid production. The exact relationship between the duration and severity of any underlying disease and the development and progression of amyloidosis is unknown.

In dogs deposition of amyloid in the glomerulus first disrupts glomerular basement membrane function, resulting in persistent proteinuria. The protein lost is mainly albumin. If the albuminuria is of sufficient magnitude hypoalbuminemia may result, lowering intravascular colloidal pressure. This decrease can result in edema and reduced intravascular volume. The reduction in intravascular volume will stimulate the compensatory release of antidiuretic hormone and aldosterone, which perpetuate fluid accumulation and edema through the retention of sodium and water. Proteinuria with hypoalbuminemia and edema in association with hypercholesterolemia are classic findings associated with the nephrotic syndrome. Renal tubular function at this stage of the disease process may be normal, as indicated by ability to concentrate urine or excrete phenolsulfonphthalein (PSP) dye. If amyloid is rapidly and massively deposited the kidneys may increase in size.

As amyloid continues to be deposited it encroaches on glomerular capillary lumen size, reducing blood flow through glomeruli. This results in a decreased glomerular filtration rate (GFR). When the GFR reaches approximately 25 percent of normal, serum urea nitrogen (SUN), creatinine, and phosphorus (P) concentrations begin to rise. Reduction in blood flow through glomeruli also reduces peritubular blood flow, leading to ischemia and dysfunction of the rest of the nephrons. If the disease progresses slowly, damaged nephrons are replaced by connective tissue, resulting in small, scarred, fibrotic, or "end-stage" kidneys. Decreased tubular function below approximately 33 percent of normal leads to inability to concentrate urine. As the disease renders more nephrons non-functional, the number of remaining nephrons becomes too small to maintain normal homeostasis, and signs of uremia develop. The rate of development of clinical signs depends on the rate of deposition, the quantity of amyloid deposited, and concomitant renal disease. Amyloid may also be deposited in larger renal blood vessels, the interstitium, and tubular basement membranes, but these are usually not as severely affected as glomeruli.

Renal amyloidosis has been rarely reported in cats. Pathologic studies have revealed the greatest accumulation of amyloid in the renal medulla, in capillary walls, and in the interstitium, although glomeruli are also affected in varying degrees (Clark and Seawright). In one case report in which the animal was evaluated clinically prior to death, proteinuria and mild azotemia were found (Crowell, et al.). Further details about amyloidosis in cats must await additional reports of clinical and necropsy findings.

Large vessel thrombosis has been reported in association with canine renal amyloidosis. Since it has been reported only in cases of renal amyloidosis, it has been associated with renal failure rather than with the presence of amyloid. However, in one study the incidence of thrombosis was much higher in dogs with renal amyloidosis (20/52) than in azotemic dogs without amyloid (7/150) (Slauson and Gribble). The major vessels, in order of frequency involved, were the pulmonary arteries, splenic arteries, coronary arteries, intrarenal arteries, portal vein, mesenteric arteries, iliac arteries, and brachial artery. The cause of thrombosis is unknown. It has been suggested that decreased fibrinolytic activity exists because of decreased renal production of fibrinolysins and that hyperfibrinogenemia causes increased ADP-mediated platelet aggregation. Paradoxically, a few human cases of amyloidosis have been associated with acquired factor X deficiency and bleeding problems. It is theorized that factor X is adsorbed by amyloid in the vascular endothelium.

CLINICAL HISTORY

No breed or sex predisposition has been reported in dogs. However, 10 of the 24 cases of renal amyloidosis diagnosed in dogs at the University of Georgia over the last eight years were in pointers. This is much higher than the percentage of pointers in the hospital population (1.3 percent for 1977). In humans, males are more often affected. The mean age of affected dogs is eight to nine years, but the age range is broad (one to 18 years). The presenting complaint may be related to the predisposing cause, chronic infection, or neoplasia. It may be dependent edema secondary to proteinuria or it may be related to renal failure with polyuria, polydipsia, and weight loss. In later stages of the disease signs may be related to uremia, with weakness, depression, anorexia, and vomiting. The presenting complaint may be due to sudden thrombosis causing acute dyspnea or limb dysfunction. Since no clinical signs may be present during the early stages of the disease, the dog may be evaluated for unrelated reasons.

PHYSICAL EXAMINATION

If serum albumin concentration is markedly decreased, dependent edema will be present. Edema may be generalized or localized to one area such as one limb. Transudative ascites has been reported in cases with severe hypoalbuminemia. Pleural and pericardial effusions may also develop.

If amyloid deposition is rapid and massive, the kidneys may be increased in size and smooth in contour. Since amyloid can be deposited in other organs, the size of the liver and spleen may also be increased. If amyloid deposition is gradual, renal size may be normal. If ischemia, necrosis, and fibrosis occur, renal size will decrease and the contour will become slightly irregular.

If the disease has progressed to renal failure, signs related to uremia — stomatitis, anemia, emaciation, dehydration, depression, weakness, and renal osteodystrophy — may be detected.

In some cases signs will be related to vascular thrombosis. Pulmonary arterial thrombosis causes acute dyspnea and cyanosis. Progressive limb dysfunction with decreased temperature and absent arterial pulse indicates arterial thrombosis. Severe abdominal pain has occurred secondary to mesenteric arterial thrombosis with bowel infarction.

There is no specific order in which clinical signs develop. Either the nephrotic syndrome or signs of uremia may occur alone. The nephrotic syndrome may precede signs of uremia, or both may occur simultaneously.

LABORATORY EVALUATION

Clinical laboratory tests indicate a glomerulopathy characterized by persistent proteinuria in the absence of pyuria or hematuria. Microscopic hematuria has been reported in a few cases in man in association with proteinuria. The degree of proteinuria can be quantitated by measuring loss for at least 24 hours using a metabolism cage. If the animal does not urinate in its cage, quantification of protein loss can be accomplished by collecting all urine voided voluntarily when the animal is exercised. If it is not feasible to collect 24-hour specimens, repeated random samples should be obtained. Random samples must be interpreted in association with specific gravity, since concentration is dependent on urine volume. Large quantities of protein in urine will raise specific gravity at the rate of 0.003 unit per gm/dl. Hyaline casts, if present, also suggest glomerular protein loss.

The nature of the protein being lost can be further evaluated by urine electrophoresis. Albumin is the predominant protection lost in any glomerulopathy, although various globulins are often also identified. Serum electrophoresis should be performed concomitantly for comparison.

Loss of albumin may result in hypoalbuminemia. This may not be reflected in total serum protein concentration, since serum globulin levels may be increased, normal, or decreased. Results of serum electrophoresis usually indicate a decrease in albumin and α_1-globulins, an increase in α_2-globulins, and variable changes in β- and γ-globulins. Serum calcium concentration may be decreased secondary to hypoalbuminemia. Hypercholesterolemia is associated with glomerulopathies and is one of the characteristics of the nephrotic syndrome. The cause of the hypercholesterolemia is unknown. Hyperfibrinogenemia and an increase in erythrocyte sedimentation rate, which are present in some cases, may reflect an associated chronic infection.

Changes in renal size can be evaluated with intravenous urography or renal angiography.

When the GFR is reduced to 25 percent of normal, SUN, serum creatinine, and serum P concentrations rise. The quantity of proteinuria may decrease at this point owing to the decrease in GFR. When tubular function is reduced to 33 percent of normal secondary to the glomerulopathy, the ability to concentrate urine is lost. Loss of tubular function may proceed more slowly than loss of glomerular function. This may lead to a stage of the disease in which azotemia is present and the ability to concentrate urine is retained to some degree. This stage is referred to as "glomerulotubular imbalance." The presence of proteinuria helps differentiate this stage of glomerular disease from prerenal azotemia. As renal failure progresses, non-regenerative anemia and metabolic acidosis may develop.

None of these findings are diagnostic of amyloidosis. Detection of amyloid fibrils in the urine of a human patient by electron microscopy was interpreted as a possible diagnostic test, but similar fibrils have been described recently in urine from normal people as well as from people with proteinuria unassociated with amyloidosis. The congo red dye retention test has not been reliable in the few cases in dogs in which its use is reported.

DIAGNOSIS

The diagnosis of renal amyloidosis in dogs can be made only by histologic or electron microscopic examination of kidney tissue obtained by renal biopsy or necropsy. Rectal or gingival biopsies are used in humans, since there is a high correlation between amyloid in these locations and renal amyloidosis. This has not been evaluated in dogs.

Glomeruli appear as dark-staining dots when the cut surface of the renal cortex at necropsy is bathed successively with 2 percent iodine and dilute sulfuric acid. This reaction with iodine resulted in the name *amyloid* being applied by Virchow in 1854. Although this test is rapid and simple, it has been found to be unreliable because it yields both false positive and false negative results.

Microscopic evaluation is necessary to confirm the diagnosis. Congo red staining followed by examination for green birefringence with polarized light is the standard histologic test. Electron microscopy provides the definitive diagnosis.

TREATMENT

There is no proved, specific treatment for amyloidosis. Theoretically, there are four potential treatments based on the stage of disease: (1) removing the stimulus for amyloid production, (2) inhibiting synthesis, (3) preventing extracellular deposition, and (4) mobilizing existing deposits. The single most effective treatment in human medicine has been control of the underlying disease. When this has been accomplished, clinical signs of the nephrotic syndrome have resolved and amyloid deposits in the glomeruli have gradually regressed over periods of years. None of the successfully treated people had progressed to renal failure prior to the initiation of therapy. The underlying disease must be corrected as soon as possible or renal disease may progress to the point at which reversal is not possible. Reported canine cases have been progressive.

When no predisposing disease is evident, treatment in humans is still experimental. Melphalan has been used to decrease amyloid synthesis, based on its use in multiple myeloma to decrease plasma cell production. It has been ineffective in many cases. D-Penicillamine has been used to mobilize amyloid. Corticosteroids have been used in combination with these two drugs. Corticosteroids alone are ineffective and are contraindicated once renal failure occurs, since they induce gluconeogenesis, causing the deamination of amino acids and increasing the amount of metabolic waste products that must be excreted. None of these drugs have been evaluated in spontaneous canine cases of amyloidosis.

Treatment of canine amyloidosis remains largely symptomatic and supportive. High quality and quantity protein diets have been recommended to compensate for urinary loss, although high protein diets may chiefly increase proteinuria, with little rise in serum albumin (Dock). Diuretics are indicated to control edema or ascites. Chronic polyuric renal failure should be managed medically as described in other articles. Sodium chloride and sodium bicarbonate must be used cautiously if hypoalbuminemia is present, since sodium may enhance development of edema. Whether anticoagulants such as aspirin should be used to prevent thrombotic episodes has not been evaluated.

PROGNOSIS

The long-term (years) prognosis for dogs is poor unless the underlying disease can be identified and controlled or eliminated. The short-term (months) prognosis depends on the dog's condition at the time of diagnosis and the response to symptomatic therapy. Some dogs have been managed for a year. Dogs may die acutely at any stage of the disease from thrombosis or the consequences of renal failure.

SUPPLEMENTAL READING

Clark, L., and Seawright, A.A.: Generalized amyloidosis in seven cats. Pathol. Vet., 6:117–134, 1969.
Crowell, W.A., Goldston, R.T., Schall, W.D., and Finco, D.R.: Generalized amyloidosis in a cat. J. Am. Vet. Med. Assoc., 161:1127–1132, 1972.
Dock, W.: Proteinuria: The story of 280 years of trials, errors, and rectifications. Bull. N.Y. Acad. Sci, 50:659–666, 1974.
Kyle, R.A., and Bayrd, E.D.: Amyloidosis: Review of 236 cases. Medicine, 54:271–299, 1975.
Osborne, C.A., Johnson, K.H., Perman, V., Fangmann, G.M., and Riis, R.C.: Clinicopathologic progression of renal amyloidosis in a dog. J. Am. Vet. Med. Assoc., 157:203–219, 1971.
Slauson, D.O., and Gribble, D.H.: Thrombosis complicating renal amyloidosis in dogs. Vet. Pathol., 8:352–363, 1971.

HYPERCALCEMIC NEPHROPATHY AND ASSOCIATED DISORDERS

DENNIS J. CHEW, D.V.M.
and CHARLES C. CAPEN, D.V.M.
Columbus, Ohio

INTRODUCTION

Hypercalcemia exists when serum consistently contains in excess of 12.0 mg/dl calcium. The age of the animal, however, must be considered when defining hypercalcemia, because young growing dogs normally may have calcium values greater than 12.0 mg/dl. Normal calcium values for mature dogs should be near 10.0 mg/dl with some variation caused by diet and analytical method employed.

Standard laboratory measurements determine total calcium in blood, which consists of ionized, complexed, and protein-bound fractions. It is the ionized calcium fraction that is biologically active; in most states of hypercalcemia there is a parallel increase in both the ionized and non-ionized fractions. Assay procedures to determine ionized calcium are available, but they are too difficult to justify for routine use and generally are not necessary for successful clinical diagnosis and management of hypercalcemic disorders. Detection of hypercalcemia has become more common in veterinary medicine with increased utilization of automated biochemical profiles in sick animals.

Hypercalcemia can be the result of many different disorders (Table 1). Increased resorption of calcium from bone, increased gastrointestinal absorption of calcium, increased protein binding of calcium in serum, increased complexing of calcium to anions, and decreased removal of calcium from serum by the kidney and intestine are all possible pathogenic mechanisms of hypercalcemia.

CLINICAL SIGNS

Many clinical signs of hypercalcemia are similar regardless of underlying cause. Hypercalcemia affects primarily the urinary, gastrointestinal, and nervous systems, although other systems may also be affected.

Anorexia, vomiting, and constipation may result from the decreased excitability of gastrointestinal smooth muscle caused by hypercalcemia. Generalized weakness of skeletal muscle develops as a result of decreased neuromuscular excitability. Decreased neuromuscular excitability may also cause depression of lower motor neuron reflexes (e.g., hyporeflexia of patellar, gastrocnemius, and triceps reflexes). Behavioral changes, depression, stupor, coma, seizures, and muscle twitching have been observed in dogs with hypercalcemia. Lameness and bone pain from demineralization of bone or pathologic fractures may be major signs. Cardiac arrhythmia, shortening of the Q–T interval, and prolongation of the P–R interval (first-degree heart block) may be detected by electrocardiographic evaluation. Ventricular fibrillation can develop in extreme hypercalcemia.

Polyuria and polydipsia are encountered early in the course of most diseases characterized by hypercalcemia and often are major reasons causing client concern. Initially the polyuria and polydipsia are independent of uremic signs from primary renal failure; however, the syndrome of uremia may develop as a result of the toxic effects of persistent hypercalcemia on the kidney. Severe dehydration often occurs from the combined effects of polyuria, emesis, and lack of oral water intake.

The severity of clinical signs often is related to the magnitude of the hypercalcemia and the rapidity of elevation in blood calcium. Animals with serum calcium values in excess of 16.0 mg/dl generally have the most severe clinical signs. Exceptions to this rule occur. We have observed markedly hypercalcemic animals with minimal clinical signs and animals with mild to moderate hypercalcemia with dramatic functional disturbances. Concomitant electrolyte and acid-base imbalances may modulate the severity of clinical signs. Most notably, metabolic acidosis will increase the ionized fraction

Table 1. *Diseases Characterized by Hypercalcemia*

Pseudohyperparathyroidism
    Lymphosarcoma
    Perirectal apocrine gland carcinoma
Osteolytic lesions
    Primary or metastatic tumors of bone
    Septic osteomyelitis
Primary hyperparathyroidism
Hypervitaminosis D
Primary renal disease
    Chronic renal failure
    Diuretic phase of acute renal failure
Hemoconcentration (hyperproteinemia)
Hypoadrenocorticism (Addison's-like disease)
Disuse osteoporosis (immobilization)
Laboratory error

of serum calcium and may magnify the severity of clinical signs. The magnitude of simultaneous phosphorus retention appears to influence the degree of soft-tissue mineralization in the kidney and elsewhere.

Other clinical signs not directly attributable to hypercalcemia may be associated with the underlying cause of the elevation in blood calcium concentration. Since neoplasms of several types are commonly associated with hypercalcemia, tumor growth in lymph nodes and various organs may be detected as enlargement or dysfunction of the particular organ involved.

LABORATORY EVALUATION

Hypercalcemic animals should be further evaluated by serum phosphorus and alkaline phosphatase determinations, since these tests provide information that helps establish a definite diagnosis (Table 2). Hypophosphatemia or normal blood phosphorus values are likely to be found in dogs with primary hyperparathyroidism or pseudohyperparathyroidism, if renal failure has not become a feature of the disease.

Since hypercalcemia is known to be detrimental to renal function, blood urea nitrogen (BUN) or serum creatinine determination and urinalysis are indicated. Polyuria, compensatory polydipsia, and dilute urine often are encountered because hypercalcemia impairs renal concentrating ability. Urine specific gravity is often hyposthenuric (1.001 to 1.007) and will not change in response to exogenous antidiuretic hormone (ADH). Postulated mechanisms for hypercalcemia-induced hyposthenuria are (1) calcium damage to receptors for ADH in the collecting tubules, (2) interruption in cyclic 3',5'-AMP production in the collecting tubule due to inactivation of adenylate cyclase, (3) inactivation of sodium-potassium ATPase required for active transport of sodium or chloride into the renal medullary interstitium, and (4) mineralization of renal tubular epithelial cells. It is emphasized that dilute urine may appear without concurrent BUN or creatinine elevation. Glucosuria usually attributable to proximal tubular injury and failure to reabsorb glucose is seen occasionally in dogs with experimental and naturally occurring hypercalcemia. Urine sediment may contain varying numbers of leukocytes, erythrocytes, and casts. Renal epithelial cells, epithelial casts, and coarsely granular casts may be seen in acute stages of renal tubular cell injury as a result of hypercalcemia.

Elevations in BUN and creatinine may occur in animals with hypercalcemia as a result of prerenal and primary renal failure. Dehydration from anorexia, vomiting, and water diuresis often occur. Early in the course of the hypercalcemia, the azotemia may be predominantly prerenal in origin, even though the urine is dilute (< 1.025 specific gravity). However, the BUN and creatinine values rapidly return to normal following intravenous fluid therapy. In more advanced cases calcium injury to the kidney can be substantial and the azotemia will not

Table 2. *Differential Diagnosis of Hypercalcemia*

DISEASE	SERUM CALCIUM	SERUM PHOSPHORUS	SERUM ALKALINE PHOSPHATASE	BONE LESION	SOFT-TISSUE MINERALIZATION	PARATHYROID LESION
Primary hyperparathyroidism	High	Low	Elevated	Severe, generalized	Moderate	Adenoma Carcinoma
Pseudohyperparathyroidism	High	Low	Normal or slight elevation	Mild, generalized	Moderate	Inactivity or atrophy
Osteolytic bone tumor	High	Normal or high	Moderate elevation	Focal, multifocal	Moderate	Inactivity or atrophy
Vitamin D intoxication	High	High	Normal	Mild or absent	Severe	Atrophy

immediately resolve in response to replacement fluid therapy.

Aspiration biopsy of lymph nodes or bone marrow is often useful in detecting neoplasia (lymphosarcoma, multiple myeloma) or an infectious agent such as a fungal organism causing extensive osteolysis. Excisional biopsy of lymph nodes should be undertaken if results of aspiration biopsy are inconclusive.

Abnormalities of liver function often are encountered in cases in which the process causing hypercalcemia (e.g., neoplasia, mycotic infection) has extensively infiltrated the liver. Elevations may be detected in serum glutamic oxaloacetic transaminase (SGOT), glutamic pyruvic transaminase (SGPT), and alkaline phosphatase activity, and possibly in total bilirubin concentration. A liver biopsy may be necessary to establish a diagnosis if other, more accessible, tissue cannot be evaluated.

RENAL LESIONS OF HYPERCALCEMIA

Injury to renal tubular epithelium may be a direct toxic effect of the elevated concentration of calcium in serum and filtered tubular fluid. Tubular injury may also be sustained from ischemia resulting from vasoconstriction of renal vessels induced by hypercalcemia. Initial injury consists of focal degeneration in the ascending loops of Henle, distal convoluted tubules, and collecting tubules. The lesions are most severe and extensive in the collecting system. Cell injury occurs with or without histopathologic evidence of calcium deposition. Mineralization begins as an intracellular deposition of amorphous calcium-phosphorus complexes in mitochondria that disrupt vital cell function, leading to necrosis. Thickening and mineralization of basement membranes of proximal tubules occurs concomitantly. Calcium deposition is most extensive in dead and dying tissues. In severe and prolonged hypercalcemia mineralization may extend throughout the kidney. Desquamation of necrotic epithelial cells results in the formation of obstructing casts that also may become mineralized. Cast formation usually occurs in the distal nephrons and can result in intrarenal hydronephrosis. Varying degrees of tubular atrophy may occur in association with interstitial infiltration of mononuclear inflammatory cells. Regenerating tubular epithelial cells may be observed along denuded tubular basement membranes, if these membranes have not been disrupted. Shrunken and collapsed glomeruli with a hyperplastic juxtaglomerular apparatus have been reported in dogs with experimentally induced hypercalcemia.

In some animals the extent of light microscopic renal injury seems insufficient to account for the degree of primary renal failure observed clinically. Renal failure in such cases may be explained by vasoconstriction of renal vessels or by altered electrophysical forces of the glomerular filter, resulting in decreased glomerular filtration rate (GFR). Altered forces affecting the glomerular filter may occur with hypercalcemia and with elevations in circulating parathyroid hormone.

Extensive mineral deposition in renal tubular epithelium and tubular basement membranes has been observed frequently in the population of dogs with hypercalcemia associated with lymphosarcoma that we have studied. However, a recent report on long-standing and severe hypercalcemia in dogs with perirectal apocrine gland adenocarcinomas failed to demonstrate renal mineralization.

DISORDERS ASSOCIATED WITH HYPERCALCEMIA IN SMALL ANIMALS

PSEUDOHYPERPARATHYROIDISM

This syndrome is caused by malignant tumors of non-parathyroid origin without bone metastasis that secrete parathyroid hormone–like polypeptides. Consequently, many of the clinical and biochemical features of pseudohyperparathyroidism closely resemble those of primary hyperparathyroidism. Hypercalcemia, hypophosphatemia (in the absence of renal failure), and minimal elevations in serum alkaline phosphatase are present in animals with pseudohyperparathyroidism (see Table 2). Demineralization of the skeleton is mild compared with the severe changes observed in primary hyperparathyroidism.

Lymphosarcoma is the most common neoplasm associated with hypercalcemia in dogs. Estimates of the prevalence of hypercalcemia in lymphoma dogs vary from 10 to 40 percent. Peripheral lymph node enlargement may or may not be detected, but there usually is evidence of anterior mediastinal or visceral involvement. It is uncertain whether the hypercalcemia develops from the production of humoral substances by neoplastic cells (e.g., PTH-like polypeptides, prostaglandins, osteoclast-activating factor) or from physical disruption of trabecular bone due to frequent marrow involvement, or both.

Pseudohyperparathyroidism has been reported in dogs with polydipsia, polyuria, hypercalcemia, hypophosphatemia, and a mass in the perirectal region. All affected dogs were elderly females. Additional cases have been evaluated at our hospital with identical findings. The perirectal masses in these cases were adenocarcinomas that appeared to arise from the apocrine glands of the anal sac. Metastases to the internal iliac lymph nodes occurred most frequently but were also observed in the lungs. Hypercalcemia abated following surgical excision of the perirectal masses and metastases in inguinal lymph nodes, if the lungs were free of metastatic lesions.

Adenocarcinoma and squamous carcinoma of the mammary gland, gastric squamous carcinoma, thyroid carcinoma, and testicular interstitial cell tumors have been reported as isolated examples of other tumors associated with the syndrome of pseudohyperparathyroidism in dogs and horses.

OSTEOLYSIS ASSOCIATED WITH TUMOR METASTASES OR SEPTIC OSTEOMYELITIS

The degree and rate of bone destruction will determine whether multifocal osteolytic lesions will result in hypercalcemia. Tumor metastases in bone may result in hypercalcemia from direct physical destruction by proliferating neoplastic cells, or by substances elaborated by neoplastic tissue that results in bone dissolution. Osteoclast-activating factor (OAF) and prostaglandins have been reported as possible humoral substances mediating the bone dissolution associated with tumor metastases in man and laboratory animals. Multiple myeloma and lymphosarcoma with widespread bone marrow infiltration have been associated with hypercalcemia. Myeloma patients with hypercalcemia may have increased binding of calcium to an abnormal quantity of globulin in addition to the increased amount of ionized calcium from bone dissolution.

Metastatic tumors to bone are not commonly encountered in dogs or cats with malignant neoplasms but may be associated with hypercalcemia at certain stages of tumor growth. Primary bone tumors occasionally may be associated with hypercalcemia.

Bacterial or fungal osteomyelitis and neonatal septicemia in puppies with septic emboli and lysis of bone are sporadic causes of hypercalcemia in dogs.

Osteolysis associated with tumor metastases or septic osteomyelitis may result in normal or moderately elevated serum phosphorus concentration and alkaline phosphatase activity, in addition to hypercalcemia. Skeletal radiographs are indicated to document the sites and severity of multifocal bone lesions.

PRIMARY HYPERPARATHYROIDISM

This metabolic disorder is encountered occasionally in older dogs, and arises as a consequence of a functional lesion in the parathyroid gland that produces an excessive amount of parathyroid hormone (PTH). The lesion usually is a single adenoma in the cervical region associated with the thyroid gland. Ectopic parathyroid tissue displaced during embryogenesis may be found at the heart base in the anterior mediastinum; a functional tumor of this tissue could result in hyperparathyroidism. Chief cell carcinomas have been encountered rarely as a cause of primary hyperparathyroidism in dogs.

The parathyroid glands are usually not large enough to be detected by palpation, even when they are neoplastic. Therefore, a definitive diagnosis usually depends upon surgical exploration of the parathyroid region and excisional biopsy. The excess parathyroid hormone mobilizes calcium and phosphorus from bone, enhances intestinal absorption of calcium (probably by increasing the production of 1,25-dihydroxycholecalciferol in the kidneys), increases the renal tubular reabsorption of calcium, and decreases renal tubular reabsorption of phosphorus. A marked elevation in serum calcium concentration , decrease in serum phosphorus concentration, and elevation in serum alkaline phosphatase activity are the characteristic biochemical alterations of primary hyperparathyroidism (see Table 2). Normal or slightly elevated serum phosphorus levels may be detected if a significant degree of azotemia has developed from primary renal damage. Radiographs of the skeleton may reveal severe and generalized demineralization, subperiosteal areas of cortical bone resorption, loss of lamina dura dentes, soft-tissue mineralization, and bone cysts.

Removal of the parathyroid adenoma typically results in a rapid decline in serum calcium values. Postoperative hypocalcemia may result within 12 to 24 hours because of the rapid influx of plasma calcium into bone. Intravenous infusion of calcium gluconate may be necessary to prevent the development of hypocalcemic tetany.

HYPERVITAMINOSIS D

Excessive vitamin D administration to dogs, cats, and other animals will result in hypercalcemia. Dietary oversupplementation with potent mineral–vitamin D preparations by breeders or veterinarians often is the cause of the excess, particularly in young pups of the larger breeds. Dogs with hypocalcemia associated with hypoparathyroidism may inadvertently be overdosed with vitamin D in an attempt to raise serum calcium values, since large doses of the parent compound (25,000 to 50,000 international units) are required to elevate blood calcium concentration in the absence of the trophic effects of parathyroid hormone on production of the active metabolites of vitamin D. It is emphasized that vitamin D therapy is cumulative in effect, and it may be seven to ten days before its maximum effect in elevating serum calcium concentration occurs.

Cestrum diurnum (day-blooming jessamine) is a popular house plant that should be considered as a possible source of vitamin D intoxication, since it contains very high concentrations of the principal active metabolite of vitamin D (1,25-dihydroxycholecalciferol). Ingestion of this plant could be a clinical problem in cats because of their tendency to eat plant leaves.

The magnitude of hypercalcemia in vitamin D intoxication is dose-related. Hypercalcemia is usually accompanied by hyperphosphatemia (see Table 2). Since the source of elevated calcium and phosphorus is primarily from vitamin D–enhanced gastrointestinal absorption, demineralization of bone is not seen radiographically and serum alkaline phosphatase activity is within normal limits.

PRIMARY RENAL DISEASE

Chronic Renal Failure. Most cases of chronic renal failure have either a normal or low serum calcium concentration with varying degrees of elevation in blood phosphorus concentration. However, 5 to 10 percent of dogs with chronic renal failure have serum calcium values of 12.0 mg/dl or greater. Postulated pathogenic mechanisms to explain the development of hypercalcemia in certain cases of chronic renal failure include (1) decreased excretion of calcium by the diseased kidney, (2) decreased renal tubular degradation of parathyroid hormone, (3) PTH-induced hypercitricemia with a consequent increase in complexed calcium, (4) autonomous transformation or overcompensation by the parathyroid gland, and (5) an exaggerated response to vitamin D, with increased intestinal calcium absorption. In our experience, microscopic evaluation has failed to reveal evidence of "autonomous" or "overcompensated" parathyroid glands in dogs with hypercalcemia associated with chronic renal disease

A transient and mild hypercalcemia has been observed with chronic renal failure in dogs following a precipitous decline in blood phosphorus value through intestinal binding treatments (e.g., aluminum hydroxide) and fluid therapy. This may be a consequence of a reciprocal movement of calcium from the bone fluid to the extracellular fluid space in response to the rapid lowering of circulating phosphorus levels.

Acute Renal Failure. Persistent hypercalcemia has been reported in human patients during the diuretic phase of acute renal failure associated with rhabdomyolysis and is thought to be caused by mobilization of calcium from soft tissues, where it was initially deposited during oliguria. Recently, we observed a dog recovering from the oliguric phase of acute primary renal failure that developed hypercalcemia during diuresis. The hypercalcemia resolved without specific treatment.

HEMOCONCENTRATION

Occasionally hypercalcemia may be detected in dehydrated animals. The magnitude of elevation in blood is usually mild and is attributed to fluid volume contraction that results in hyperproteinemia and an increased relative concentration of ionized and non-ionized calcium. The hypercalcemia rapidly resolves following fluid therapy. The majority of dehydrated animals do not develop hypercalcemia.

HYPOADRENOCORTICISM (ADDISON'S-LIKE DISEASE)

Hypercalcemia is observed in experimentally adrenalectomized dogs and in some cases of naturally occurring Addison's-like disease in dogs. The magnitude of elevation in serum calcium values may exceed 16 mg/dl under experimental conditons, whereas dogs with Addison's-like disease evaluated in our hospital have had values up to 15 mg/dl calcium. Experimental evidence suggests that the type of hypercalcemia associated with hypoadrenocorticism is unusual, in that ionized calcium fraction remains normal whereas non-ionized calcium fraction increases. If the ionized calcium does indeed remain normal, it follows that this type of hypercalcemia should not be deleterious to the animal. The elevated calcium value rapidly returns to normal following treatment for hypoadrenocorticism.

DISUSE OSTEOPOROSIS

Prolonged immobilization may lead to hypercalcemia as a consequence of continued bone resorption associated with diminished bone accretion. Hypercalcemia of this type occurs infrequently in animals that cannot move around freely because of extensive musculoskeletal or neurologic injury.

LABORATORY ERROR

Although technical error is unlikely with quality control standards on automated biochemical profiles, it is wise to make certain that elevation in serum calcium is a repeatable finding.

TREATMENT

SYMPTOMATIC TREATMENT FOR HYPERCALCEMIA

Since many of the severe effects of hypercalcemia are accentuated by dehydration, disturbances in fluid balance should be corrected in all instances. Replacement fluids such as isotonic solutions, lactated Ringer's, or 0.9 percent sodium chloride should be administered intravenously. Calciuresis may be enhanced by administering 0.9 percent sodium chloride I.V., because the additional sodium presented to the renal tubules diminishes calcium reabsorption. If the serum concentration of calcium is only moderately increased (12 to 14 mg/dl), these therapeutic measures alone may result in adequate initial lowering of serum calcium. Additional measures to combat hypercalcemia may be necessary when the calcium elevation and clinical signs are more severe (> 15 mg/dl). Furosemide, ethacrynic acid, and sodium sulfate are calciuretic agents that may be used. It is important to maintain adequate extracellular fluid volume by proper administration of intravenous fluids while using these diuretics. Furosemide given to dogs with experimental hypercalcemia at 5 mg/kg intravenously has been reported to be effective in reducing serum calcium concentration. Thiazide diuretics reduce the urinary excretion of calcium and therefore are contraindicated in cases of hypercalcemia. Peritoneal dialysis is an alternative method of removing calcium from the body, particularly in uremic animals. Intravenous and oral phosphate solutions are used in human patients to promote calcium movement into the tissues; however, there is little data available concerning their use in dogs or cats with hypercalcemia.

Glucocorticoids are effective in some instances in lowering serum calcium concentration. Their effects are thought to be mediated by inhibiting intestinal absorption of calcium and increasing urinary calcium excretion. In addition, direct antitumor activity may be responsible for reduction of serum calcium concentration, most notably in cases of lymphosarcoma. Mithramycin and calcitonin are agents sometimes used in the therapy of hypercalcemia in human patients, but clinical experience in dogs, cats, and other animals with hypercalcemia is lacking at present.

In cases of hypercalcemic crises, intravenous administration of sodium bicarbonate may be of value in temporarily reducing the toxic effects of elevated ionized calcium concentration. The beneficial effect is related to diminution in the level of ionized calcium associated with alkalosis induced by sodium bicarbonate.

TREATMENT OF RENAL FAILURE

Since prerenal factors are commonly associated with hypercalcemia, proper attention to fluid therapy will help to maintain renal perfusion, thereby minimizing progressive ischemic damage to nephrons. No therapeutic regimen will eliminate the renal lesions already present; however, if the hypercalcemia can be controlled and the patient kept alive long enough, tubular lesions may be repaired by regeneration and functional adaptation. Dissolution of mineral deposits may also occur, although this is a slow process.

TREATMENT OF UNDERLYING CAUSE OF HYPERCALCEMIA

Since neoplasia is most commonly found to be the underlying cause of hypercalcemia, total surgical extirpation of the tumor is indicated. When this is not possible because malignant neoplasms have infiltrated locally or metastasized, radiotherapy, chemotherapy, and immunotherapy may be of value in reducing tumor mass and concomitant hypercalcemia. Remission of neoplasia is usually accompanied by remission of hypercalcemia.

SUPPLEMENTAL READING

Capen, C.C., and Martin, S.L.: Calcium metabolism and disorders of parathyroid glands. 7:513–548, 1977.

Epstein, F.H.: Calcium nephropathy. In Strauss, M.B., and Welt, L.G. (eds.): *Diseases of the Kidney,* 2nd ed. Boston, Little, Brown and Co., 1971.

Finco, D.R., and Rowland, G.N.: Hypercalcemia secondary to renal failure in the dog: A report of four cases. J. Am. Vet. Med. Assoc., 173:990–994, 1978.

MacEwen, E.G., and Siegel, S.D.: Hypercalcemia: A paraneoplastic disease. Vet. Clin. North Am. 7:187–194, 1977.

Ong, S.O., et al.: Effect of furosemide on experimental hypercalcemia in dogs. Proc. Soc. Exp. Biol. Med., 145:227–233, 1974.

Osborne, C.A., and Stevens, J.B.: Pseudohyperparathyroidism in the dog. J. Am. Vet. Med. Assoc. 162:125–135, 1973.

Rijnberk, A., et al.: Pseudohyperparathyroidism associated with perirectal adenocarcinomas in elderly female dogs. Tijdschr. Diergeneeskd., 103:1069–1075, 1978.

Walser, M., et al.: The hypercalcemia of adrenal insufficiency. J. Clin. Invest., 42:456–465, 1963.

HYDRONEPHROSIS

JAMES J. BRACE, D.V.M.
Knoxville, Tennessee

Hydronephrosis is an abnormality of the kidney characterized by progressive dilation of the renal pelvis and progressive atrophy of renal parenchyma. It occurs more commonly in dogs than cats. It may be unilateral or bilateral and occurs as a result of obstruction of urine outflow anywhere from the renal pelvis to the external urethral orifice.

ETIOLOGY

Obstruction of urine outflow may be complete or partial and is usually due to congenital or acquired mechanical abnormalities. Congenital causes of hydronephrosis include aberrant renal vessels that constrict the ureters, torsion or kinking of the ureters due to abnormal position of the kidneys, stenosis or atresia of the ureters or urethra, ureteroceles, and ectopic ureters. Acquired causes of hydronephrosis include urinary calculi, neoplastic or inflammatory abdominal or pelvic masses that compress the urinary outflow tract, neoplasia or inflammation of the bladder, accidental ligation of the urinary outflow tract during surgery, prostatic enlargement, inflammation and stricture of the ureters or urethra, displacement of the bladder in perineal hernias, and *Dioctophyma renale* organisms. Occasionally, hydronephrosis is seen in dogs and cats in which mechanical obstruction cannot be identified. In these cases hydronephrosis may be a congenital anomaly or may be associated with ureteral aperistalsis or a neurogenic bladder. A unique type of "hydronephrosis," in which a large quantity of fluid collects between the renal cortex and the renal capsule, has been reported in cats. This condition has been referred to as a "capsulogenic renal cyst" or "capsular hydronephrosis." This is not true hydronephrosis because the kidney is usually small and shrunken rather than dilated. The etiology is unknown, but it may be associated with obstruction of the lymphatic drainage of the renal capsule.

PATHOPHYSIOLOGY

Continued production of urine following obstruction will increase both volume and pressure in those parts of the urinary tract proximal to the obstruction. Complete obstruction of urine outflow from both kidneys for approximately 24 hours will usually result in postrenal azotemia. Death from uremia may occur in three to six days. If a lesion results in partial chronic obstruction of urine outflow from one or both kidneys, varying degrees of hydronephrosis will develop. Structural changes seen in the kidney are usually more severe if the hydronephrosis is unilateral. If not treated successfully, bilateral hydronephrosis usually results in death of the animal before extensive structural changes develop. These structural changes are due to increased back pressure within the kidney, resulting in dilation of the renal pelvis, collapse of portions of the renal vasculature, renal ischemia, and atrophy. Fibrous tissue eventually replaces necrotic tubular epithelium, and in the end stage only a thin rim of renal parenchyma surrounding a large, dilated pelvis may be seen.

Complete obstruction of urine outflow from one kidney is not life-threatening as long as the opposite kidney is capable of adequate function. The degree of structural and functional change that occurs in complete unilateral obstruction depends on the duration of obstruction. In the dog, if the obstruction is of short duration (5 to 60 minutes), the glomerular filtration rate (GFR) will quickly return to normal. If the obstruction is corrected within six to seven days, GFR will return to normal and permanent structural abnormalities will not occur. If the obstruction is present for 14 days before being corrected, GFR may return to 50 to 65 per cent of normal over several months, indicating permanent structural damage. If the obstruction is present for 30 days, GFR may eventually return to 30 per cent of normal. Obstruction of more than 30 days' duration usually results in complete destruction of the kidney.

CLINICAL FINDINGS

Clinical findings associated with hydronephrosis are variable. Early signs are often related to the underlying cause of urine outflow obstruction and include dysuria, hematuria, a distended bladder, a palpable abdominal mass, urinary calculi, and others. If the hydronephrosis is unilateral and the opposite kidney is capable of adequate function, the animal may be asymptomatic for long periods. When clinical signs do not occur, abdominal enlargement and non-specific gastrointestinal signs may be seen. An enlarged, smooth kidney distended with fluid may be noted on abdominal palpation. Fever, depression, vomiting, anorexia, and a neutrophilic leukocytosis with a left shift may occur if infection complicates hydronephrosis. Hematuria, pyuria, proteinuria and bacteruria may also be seen if obstruction of urine outflow is incomplete. If hydronephrosis is bilateral and severe or if it is unilateral and the opposite kidney is not capable of adequate function, signs of uremia may be seen.

DIAGNOSIS

A diagnosis of hydronephrosis may be suggested by history, physical examination, and laboratory data. Survey radiographs may show one or both kidneys to be enlarged and smooth, with rounded borders, and may reveal the cause of the obstruction. Intravenous urography may allow visualization and assessment of the degree of renal dilation in early cases of hydronephrosis. In chronic hydronephrosis either no functional tissue or only a cortical rim of functional tissue may be seen. A definitive diagnosis can also be made by percutaneous aspiration of hydronephrotic fluid from a suspected hydronephrotic kidney or by exploratory laparotomy.

THERAPY

Treatment of hydronephrosis should be aimed at eliminating the underlying cause of obstruction before irreversible renal lesions have developed. Surgery is therefore the treatment of choice in most cases of hydronephrosis. Nephrotomy, ureterotomy, ureteral anastomosis, cystotomy, or other procedures may be necessary to eliminate the underlying cause of obstruction. In severe unilateral hydronephrosis associated with a kidney that has little or no function, nephrectomy is indicated if the oppo-

site kidney is capable of adequate function. If hydronephrosis is complicated by bacterial infection, appropriate antimicrobial agents should be administered, based on bacterial culture and sensitivity tests. Long-term therapy may be necessary if the underlying cause of the hydronephrosis cannot be eliminated. Because severe bilateral hydronephrosis is associated with irreversible renal damage, no effective therapy is available. Symptomatic and supportive management of renal failure (dietary management, vitamin supplements, anabolic steroids, and so on) may provide a comfortable life for the patient for variable periods.

PROGNOSIS

The prognosis of hydronephrosis depends upon the underlying cause of obstruction of urine outflow, the length of time the obstruction has been present, and whether it is unilateral or bilateral. If the cause of obstruction can be eliminated before significant renal damage occurs, or if the obstruction is unilateral and the opposite kidney is capable of adequate function, the prognosis is good. The prognosis in severe bilateral hydronephrosis is guarded to poor. If hydronephrosis is due to a neoplasm, the prognosis will depend on the degree of urinary tract involvement as well as the biologic behavior of the neoplasm.

SUPPLEMENTAL READING

Biery, D.N.: Upper urinary tract. In O'Brien, T.R. (ed.): *Radiographic Diagnosis of Abdominal Disorders in the Dog and Cat.* Philadelphia, W.B. Saunders Co., 1978, p. 481.
Howards, S.S., and Wright, F.S.: Obstructive injury. In Brenner, B.M., and Rector, S.C. (eds.): *Diseases of the Kidney.* Philadelphia, W.B. Saunders Co., 1976, p. 1297.
North, D.C.: Hydronephrosis and hydroureter in a kitten: A case report. J. Small Anim. Pract., *19*:237, 1978.
Osborne, C.A., Finco, D.R., and Low, I.G.: Renal failure: Diagnosis, treatment and prognosis. In Ettinger, S.J. (ed.): *Textbook of Veterinary Internal Medicine.* Philadelphia, W.B. Saunders Co., 1975, p. 1465.
Osborne, C.A., Low, D.G., and Finco, D.R.: *Canine and Feline Urology.* Philadelphia, W.B. Saunders Co., 1972.
Ticer, J.W.: Capsulogenic renal cyst in a cat. J. Am. Vet. Med. Assoc., *143*:613, 1963.

FANCONI SYNDROME IN THE DOG

K. C. BOVÉE, D.V.M.
Philadelphia, Pennsylvania

The Fanconi syndrome is a constellation of abnormalities associated with renal tubular reabsorption defects. The defects may lead to excessive urinary loss of water, glucose, phosphate, sodium, potassium, amino acids, and other solutes. While the disease has been characterized in man for many years, it has only recently been described in dogs (Bovée, et al., 1978a).

The syndrome has been reported in several breeds but appears most commonly in Basenjis (Bovée et al., 1978b; Easley and Breitschwerdt, 1976). While the syndrome is suspected to be an inherited metabolic disease, symptoms do not develop until dogs become adults or reach middle age.

Clinical signs include persistent polydipsia and polyuria. Physical examination is usually normal, with the exception of slight dehydration and weight loss. Glycosuria associated with normal blood glucose concentrations is usually found. Renal function, as measured by BUN and plasma creatinine concentration and creatinine clearance, is normal or slightly reduced.

Glycosuria and dilute urine (specific gravity 1.005 to 1.018) are the only abnormalities found by routine urinalysis. Several grams of glucose may be excreted in 24 hours. Urinary albumin excretion is normal or slightly increased. Complete blood counts, plasma electrolytes, plasma chemistries and enzymes are generally normal. Only after a prolonged symptomatic period and development of renal failure do plasma electrolytes become abnormal.

Renal clearance studies performed in affected dogs to measure the fractional reabsorption of several solutes revealed defects in the reabsorption of glucose, sodium, phosphate, potassium, and urate (Bovée, et al., 1978b). At least two patterns of aminoaciduria were also found in these dogs. Some dogs had generalized aminoaciduria, whereas others had a pattern similar to canine cystinuria. Some dogs also had tubular defects for chloride and calcium reabsorption.

Some dogs with the Fanconi syndrome develop moderate metabolic acidosis many months or years after detection of initial signs. It is likely that the acidosis is due to renal tubular acidosis associated with inability to reabsorb bicarbonate or to excrete hydrogen ion. However, studies that might characterize this possible defect clearly are as yet incomplete.

The course of the disease may be several months or years. The clinical signs — severe dehydration, marked polyuria, weight loss, and anorexia — become more profound and eventually result in death. During the terminal episode moderate azotemia, hypophosphatemia, hypokalemia, hyperglycemia, and metabolic acidosis may be present. While the histology of the kidneys is not remarkable during early stages of the disease, papillary necrosis may occur as the terminal event. Urinary tract infection does not occur as a part of the syndrome.

Therapy to control progression of the disease has not been undertaken. The mode of genetic transmission of the disease is unknown.

SUPPLEMENTAL READING

Bovée, K.C., Joyce, T., Reynolds, R., and Segal, S.: Spontaneous Fanconi syndrome in the dog. Metabolism, 27:45–52, 1978a.

Bovée, K.C., Joyce, T., Reynolds, R., and Segal, S.: The Fanconi syndrome in basenji dogs: A new model for renal transport defects. Science, 201:1129–1131, 1978b.

Easley, J.R., and Breitschwerdt, E.B.: Glycosuria associated with renal tubular dysfunction in three basenji dogs. 168:938, 1976.

CHRONIC TUBULAR-INTERSTITIAL DISEASE OF THE KIDNEY

RICHARD C. SCOTT, D.V.M.
New York, New York

The term *chronic interstitial nephritis* (CIN) may require greater definition as a consequence of increased knowledge and understanding of renal disease. The term implies that this disease has a specific cause that produces pathologic changes associated with diffuse interstitial fibrosis, tubular atrophy, focal mononuclear cell infiltration, and glomerulosclerosis. However, this pathologic description may be associated with many different diseases that originally caused more specific and diagnostic pathologic changes but that progressed to an end stage. The clinical signs of renal disease at this advanced stage will be similar and collectively constitute the chronic uremic syndrome.

DISEASES THAT CAN PROGRESS TO CHRONIC TUBULAR AND INTERSTITIAL RENAL DISEASE

PYELONEPHRITIS

Lower urinary tract infections that ascend to the kidneys are thought to be the most common cause of pyelonephritis. Early in the disease there may be patchy involvement of the renal medulla and cortex, progressing to more diffuse tubular-interstitial disease. Infiltrates of inflammatory cells, including neutrophils, initially suggest pyelonephritis; however, the end stage is indistinguishable from other diseases associated with fibrosis, tubular atrophy, and glomerulosclerosis. The disease may progress to an end stage if bacterial resistance develops or inadequate antibiotic therapy is provided. Slowly progressive cases may be unassociated with recognizable signs of urinary tract infection until uremia has occurred.

Early signs of pyelonephritis include periodic hematuria, pyuria, frequency of urination, and strangury. Radiography may reveal kidneys of unequal but reduced size as a result of fibrosis. Urinalysis may contain white cell casts if fresh sediments are performed; however, they are uncommon.

GLOMERULONEPHRITIS

Progressive lesions that initially and primarily affect glomeruli may induce progressive lesions in remaining portions of the nephrons and interstitial tissue. Consult the article entitled "Glomerulonephropathy and the Nephrotic Syndrome" for additional details.

LEPTOSPIROSIS

Although unconfirmed clinical reports suggest that leptospirosis can cause chronic tubular interstitial disease (CTID) as a sequelae to acute interstitial nephritis or as a chronic infection unassociated with serious clinical illness until uremia appears, these impressions have not been supported by studies of experimentally produced leptospirosis in dogs. The most common organism involved is *Leptospira canicola*, but others have been found, including *L. icterohaemorrhagiae*, *L. pomona*, and *L. sejroe*. Clinical signs of acute infection are anorexia, depression, vomition and diarrhea, high fever, myositis associated with muscle pain, iritis, and icterus. Laboratory tests may reveal leukocytosis with a left shift, azotemia, and anemia. Definitive diagnosis is made by identifying *Leptospira* organisms in the urine by dark field microscopy and positive serologic tests.

ACUTE RENAL FAILURE WITH INCOMPLETE RECOVERY

The causes of acute renal failure are numerous and include nephrotoxic agents (e.g., various antibiotics, ethylene glycol, calcium, heavy metals), severe protracted dehydration, shock resulting in acute tubular necrosis, and diseases causing hypercalcemia. Functional recovery following any of these disorders is possible with proper therapy, yet complete recovery is not invariable. If irreversible damage initially associated with adequate renal function is present when a subsequent disease develops, progression to end stage is possible. Associated le-

1076

sions may be identical to other diseases reaching end stage.

The history usually includes an incident of acute illness with incomplete recovery, followed by the onset of renal failure or a uremic crisis at a variable time later.

IMMUNE-MEDIATED TUBULAR-INTERSTITIAL DISEASES

Immune complex tubular-interstitial lesions have been produced experimentally in animals and have been identified in man (Brentjens et al.; Klassen et al., 1972; Lehman et al.). Rabbits injected for several weeks with a soluble extract of homologous renal cortex in adjuvant developed renal lesions consistent with tubular-interstitial disease (Klassen et al., 1971). Glomerular morphology was normal. Immune-complex deposits were found, but no antitubular basement membrane antibodies were detected (Klassen et al., 1971). Immune-complex deposits have been described in rats after sensitization with homologous renal tissue in adjuvant (Klassen and Milgrom, 1969). Rats immunized with Tamm-Horsfall protein have also been reported to have immune complex deposits in various regions of the tubules (Hoyer). Damage to the tubules is thought to result from mononuclear cell infiltration, but immune complexes may also cause damage directly.

Tubular and interstitial lesions have also been reported after experimental production of antitubular basement membrane antibodies (Steblay and Rudofsky, 1971). Guinea pigs immunized with heterologous renal tissue rich in tubules developed fatal tubular-interstitial nephritis associated with linear tubular basement membrane immunofluorescence and antitubular basement membrane antibodies (Steblay and Rudofsky). How these antibodies mediated damage was not determined.

These experiments suggest a role for immune-mediated mechanisms as a cause of CTID unexplained by any other disease processes.

CLINICAL SIGNS AND THERAPY OF CHRONIC TUBULAR-INTERSTITIAL DISEASE

POLYURIA AND POLYDIPSIA

Polyuria and polydipsia are typically associated with tubular-interstitial diseases at some phase. They are caused by loss of nephrons to the extent that each intact nephron is presented with more solute and water than is normal. Excretion of this solute and water maintains homeostasis for a time but eventually results in polyuria. Ensuing volume contraction stimulates compensatory polydipsia. Another pathogenic mechanism is destruction of the countercurrent system in the renal medulla (loops of Henle and vasa recta) responsible for normal urine concentrating ability together with antidiuretic hormone. Production of a natriuretic substance in chronic renal failure also results in partial loss of active sodium transport by nephrons (Bourgoignie et al.). This maintains sodium homeostasis initially by inducing natriuresis and polyuria.

The underlying renal disease must be eliminated, and the body must repair diseased nephrons if polyuria and polydipsia are to be eliminated.

GASTROINTESTINAL SYMPTOMS

Vomition, anorexia, and diarrhea predominate as the gastrointestinal signs of uremia. The causes of these signs are still being investigated. Vomiting and anorexia are thought to result from local irritation of the stomach by ammonia, a bacterial breakdown product of excessive urea accumulation characteristic of the uremic syndrome. The uremic environment is also thought to stimulate the emetic center of the medulla oblongata. Diarrhea may be caused by abnormal formation of keto-bile acids (especially urodeoxycholic acid) in the intestine (Gordon et al.). This is a result of decreased deoxycholic acid formation in uremia, which then initiates anaerobic bacterial overgrowth in the gut.

Bowel emollients may be used to decrease vomition and diarrhea if they arise. In addition, antiemetics may be used periodically to control vomition.

ANEMIA

Non-regenerative anemia of variable severity is common in advanced renal disease. Clinical signs may include pale mucous membranes and lethargy. Anemia is associated with suppression of red cell precursors in bone marrow secondary to lack of production of erythropoietin by diseased kidneys. The uremic environment has also been shown to suppress bone marrow directly by as yet unindentified mechanisms. Anemia can also result from altered red blood cell membrane or normal osmotic relationships (e.g., lack of sodium, pumping edema to increase intracellular water), which induces shortened red blood cell survival. Altered red cells are removed by the reticuloendothelial system. The severity of anemia may also be enhanced by gastrointestinal hemorrhage. Bleeding is largely the result of abnormal platelet function. Delayed release of platelet factor 3 is thought to be a consequence of a uremic toxin, possibly guanidinosuccinic acid (Horowitz et al.).

Treatment of anemia associated with advanced uremia is difficult. Hematinics and bone marrow stimulants such as the anabolic steroids may be given in an attempt to increase production of red blood cells. If severe anemia persists, periodic transfusions of whole blood may be necessary. These provide only transient remission, however, and therefore are not recommended as routine therapy.

UREMIC BONE DISEASE

Progressive reduction in glomerular filtration rate due to diseases affecting the kidneys result in retention of phosphate, which reciprocally causes a decrease in ionized calcium. Low levels of serum calcium stimulate parathormone (Aurbach et al.), which causes resorption of bone and release of calcium. This phenomenon helps to minimize the altered calcium:phosphorus ratio. Further reduction in glomerular filtration rate ultimately leads to osteodystrophy.

The kidneys normally convert vitamin D metabolites into the active form, vitamin D_3 (Bilezikian et al.) via stimuli including parathormone and phosphorus levels. Vitamin D aids the transfer of calcium from the intestine into the circulation (DeLuca). Vitamin D_3 also functions with parathormone to mobilize calcium from bone. Thus, deficiency of vitamin D_3 associated with generalized renal disease reduces ionized calcium, leading to hyperparathyroidism and osteodystrophy. Renal osteodystrophy is usually manifested by poor bone radiographic density but may become so severe that it results in pathologic fractures, dystrophic soft-tissue calcification, "rubber jaw," and rarely bone pain.

Severe hyperparathyroidism may be treated with orally administered phosphate binding gels, which may decrease serum phosphate concentrations and thus minimize hypocalcemia. Provided that serum phosphorus concentration can be reduced to normal values, cautious oral administration of synthetic vitamin D_3 may be attempted to increase serum calcium levels. Careful monitoring of serum calcium concentration is indicated initially to avoid hypercalcemia. Thereafter, serum calcium and phosphorus concentrations should be periodically evaluated to adjust the dosage of vitamin D_3 in order to maintain a normal level of serum calcium.

CARDIOVASCULAR-RESPIRATORY SYSTEM

Cardiopulmonary dysfunction can result from overhydration at the final phase of end-stage renal disease. Although uncommon, overhydration may be caused by excess water intake at a time when the kidney can no longer excrete a water load; more frequently, it is a complication of overzealous fluid therapy. Clinical signs may include pulmonary edema with dyspnea and possibly also a gelatinous appearance to the skin as a result of higher-than-normal amounts of interstitial and cellular water. Therapy includes appropriate adjustments in fluid administration, and diuretics if severe. If these measures fail or if overhydration is life-threatening, peritoneal dialysis should be performed to remove excess body water.

IMMUNE SYSTEM

The uremic environment suppresses primarily B lymphocyte functions (humoral immunity), but T lymphocytes (cellular immunity) are also suppressed (Boulton-Jones et al.). The combination results in delayed responsiveness by the immune system, which can potentially result in increased susceptibility to infections. Treatment with broad-spectrum antibiotics is indicated when infections occur during the course of uremia. Consult the article entitled "Drug Therapy in Renal Disorders" for specific details.

NEUROLOGIC SIGNS

Encephalopathy associated with lethargy, malaise, and confusion frequently occurs in severe anemia. Ultimately seizures, stupor, and coma ensue. Cranial nerve abnormalities and peripheral neuropathies, which have been reported in man, have been reported rarely in animals. The pathogenesis of these signs is still under investigation, but they may be due to diminished oxidation of myoinositol to D-glucoronate by diseased kidneys (Clements). Abnormally high levels of myoinositol result in demyelination (Clements). Recently, high levels of parathormone in uremic patients have been implicated in demyelination (Avram et al.).

Seizures may be treated with anticonvulsants if they complicate uremia. Other neurologic manifestations cannot be managed adequately unless the renal disease is successfully treated or unless dialysis is performed.

SUPPLEMENTAL READING

Avram, M.M., Feinfeld, D.A., and Huatuco, A.H.: Search for the uremic toxin: Decreased motor-nerve conduction velocity and elevated parathyroid hormone in uremia. N. Engl. J. Med., 298:1000–1003, 1978.

Aurbach, G.D., Potts, J.T., Jr., Chase, L.R., et al.: Polypeptide hormones and calcium metabolism. Ann. Intern. Med., 70:1243–1265, 1969.

Bilezikian, J.P., Canfield, R.E., Jacobs, T.P., et al.: Response of 1-alpha, 25-dihydroxyvitamin D₃ to hypocalcemia in human subjects. N. Engl. J. Med., 299:437–441, 1978.

Boulton-Jones, J.M., Vick, R., Cameron, J.S., and Black, P.J.: Immune responses in uremia. Clin. Nephrol., 1:351–360, 1973.

Bourgoignie, J.J., Hwang, K.H., Espinel, C., et al.: A natriuretic factor in the serum of patients with chronic uremia. J. Clin. Invest., 51:1514–1527, 1972.

Brentjens, J.R., Sepulveda, M., Baliah, T., et al.: Interstitial immune complex nephritis in patients with systemic lupus erythematosus. Kidney Int., 7:342–350, 1975.

Clements, R. S., DeJesus, P.U., Jr., and Winegrad, A.I.: Raised plasma myoinositol levels in uremia and experimental neuropathy. Lancet, 1:1137–1141, 1973.

DeLuca, H.F.: Vitamin D endocrinology. Ann. Intern. Med., 85:367–377, 1976.

Gordon, S.J., Miller, L. J., Haefner, L.J., et al.: Abnormal intestinal bile acid distribution in azotemic man: A possible role in the pathogenesis of uremic diarrhea. Gut, 17:58–67, 1976.

Horowitz, H.I., Stein, I.M., and Cohen, B.D.: Further studies on the platelet inhibitory effect of guanidinosuccinic acid and its role in uremic bleeding. Am. J. Med., 49:336–345, 1970.

Hoyer, J.R.: Autoimmune tubulointestinal nephritis induced in rats by immunization with rat Tamm-Horsfall urinary glycoprotein. Kidney Int., 10:544, 1975.

Klassen, J., Andres, G.A., Brennan, J.C., et al.: An immunologic renal tubular lesion in man. Clin. Immunol. Immunopathol., 1:69–83, 1972.

Klassen, J., McCluskey, R.T., and Milgrom, F.: Nonglomerular renal disease produced in rabbits by immunization with homologous kidney. Am. J. Pathol., 63:333–350, 1971.

Klassen, J., and Milgrom, F.: Autoimmune concomitants of renal allografts. Transplant. Proc., 1:605–608, 1969.

Lehman, D.H., Wilson, C.B., and Dixon, F.J.: Extraglomerular immunoglobulin deposits in human nephritis. Am. J. Med., 58:765–786, 1975.

Steblay, R.W., and Rudofsky, U.: Renal tubular disease and autoantibodies against tubular basement membrane induced in guinea pigs. J. Immunol., 107:589–594, 1971.

OVERVIEW OF THE UREMIC SYNDROME

K.C. BOVÉE, D.V.M.
Philadelphia, Pennsylvania

The uremic syndrome is defined as a group of biochemical changes caused by loss of a critical number of functioning nephrons. Uremia may result from either acute or chronic renal failure. In acute renal failure uremic changes are somewhat attenuated because of the shortened time course. In chronic failure the uremic syndrome is more fully developed. These comments will deal primarily with changes associated with chronic renal failure.

The pathophysiology of chronic renal failure is similar regardless of cause. Therefore, one would not expect a different form of renal failure to appear in a case of pyelonephritis compared with that seen in congenital renal dysplasia. Clinical manifestations are determined by multiple factors, including excretory defects, altered catabolic load of metabolites, integrity of cell membranes and their transport potency, and altered production of humoral agents by the kidney.

The fundamental pathophysiologic disorder of chronic renal failure is loss of functioning nephrons. Destructive morphologic changes cause a fall in renal blood flow, glomerular filtration rate, and tubular transport capacity and lead to compensatory morphologic and functional responses. In order for the animal to survive, remaining nephrons must undergo appropriate and adaptive functional changes. These changes include increased glomerular capillary size with increased glomerular filtration per nephron, hypertrophy of proximal tubular cells, increased absorptive rate per cell, increased secretory rate of specific ions, and others. A recent review describes the functional adaptations of chronically diseased kidneys (Gottschalk).

Adaptive changes mask the presence of chronic renal failure for prolonged periods. However, as adaptive changes are gradually exhausted, surviving nephrons lose their ability to maintain physiologic balance, and symptoms of uremia develop. In effect, surviving nephrons expend their compensatory properties and become confined to a limited range of physiologic activities. Because of the multiple functions of the kidneys, it is not surprising that the end-stage kidney does not display a programmed or uniform group of functional dis-

Table 1. *Components of the Uremic Syndrome*

Sodium and water balance
Renal osteodystrophy—calcium and phosphorus metabolism
Anemia
Carbohydrate intolerance
Neurologic disorders
Acid-base balance
Cardiopulmonary abnormalities
Gastrointestinal dysfunction
Disturbances in the immunologic system
Endocrine abnormalities

turbances. Gastrointestinal signs, bone disease, neurologic manifestations, and other problems appear in a non-uniform fashion.

Toxins of uremia and their mechanism of action have been sought for many years. No one toxic substance or group of substances has been shown to produce the uremic syndrome. A recent review describes the possible toxicity of urea, creatinine, ammonia, guanidine, uric acid, and other substances (Bovée).

Major components of the uremic syndrome are summarized in Table 1. Because some of these metabolic disturbances are well understood, it has been possible to formulate specific therapy to alleviate them or reduce their severity. For metabolic disturbances that are poorly understood, specific therapy is not available. Consult articles dealing with specific abnormalities for specific therapeutic recommendations.

SUPPLEMENTAL READING

Bovée, K.C.: The uremic syndrome. J. Am. Anim. Hosp. Assoc., 12:189–197, 1976.
Gottschalk, C.W.: The function of the chronically diseased kidney. Circ. Res., 28–29, Suppl. II, May 1971, pp. 1–13.

WATER DEPRIVATION AND VASOPRESSIN CONCENTRATION TESTS IN THE DIFFERENTIATION OF POLYURIC SYNDROMES

ROBERT M. HARDY, D.V.M.
and CARL A. OSBORNE, D.V.M
St. Paul, Minnesota

Polyuria is a common clinical sign in veterinary practice. The cause of polyuria may be readily determined in many cases by combining a limited amount of historical and laboratory data. However, polyuric patients may become major diagnostic challenges when the cause of their polyuria is not immediately established. An algorithm has been formulated to simplify the diagnostic approach to polyuric patients (Fig. 1). By combining appropriate laboratory data with results of complete or gradual water deprivation and ADH response tests, one can determine the cause of polyuric syndromes in nearly all cases.

VERIFICATION OF POLYURIA

In the evaluation of patients with suspected polyuria, it is recommended that the following procedure be used. First, the polyuria should be verified by observation or by quantitation of 24-hour urine output from the patient. Determining the urine specific gravity may also be of value in verification of polyuria. If the specific gravity of the initial urinalysis of non-glucosuric, non-dehydrated dogs is greater than 1.025, either the assumption that polyuria exists is erroneous or the presence of large quantities of abnormal solutes (protein, radiographic contrast agents, and so on) in the sample should be

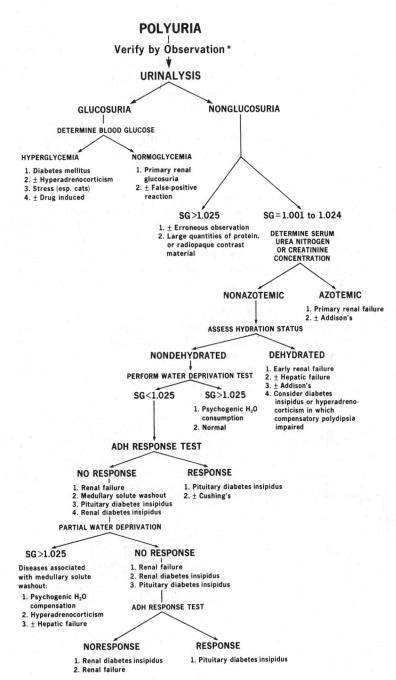

Figure 1. Diagnostic algorithm for patients with polyuria and polydipsia.

suspected. If the urine specific gravity is significantly below 1.025, any of the following might be true: (1) The patient could have physiologic polyuria. (2) The patient could have pathologic polyuria. (3) The patient could have pathologic oliguria. Pathologic oliguria usually occurs during the early phase of acute primary renal failure caused by generalized ischemic or nephrotoxic tubular disease. An oliguric state may also occur in a patient with primary polyuric renal failure if some prerenal abnormality (vomiting, decreased water consumption, cardiac decompensation, or other problem) develops. If the prerenal cause is removed or if proper fluid balance is restored, or both, polyuria will resume. In addition, oliguria may develop as a terminal event in patients with chronic progressive primary renal failure.

ADDITIONAL DIAGNOSTIC CONSIDERATIONS

For non-glucosuric patients in which polyuria is verified or in which the initial urine specific gravity is between 1.001 and 1.024, or both, additional diagnostic data should be collected before proceeding with renal concentration tests. Such information may establish the cause of the polyuria and eliminate the need for water deprivation or vasopressin concentration tests. Diagnostic information obtained from polyuric patients prior to initiating water deprivation should include a complete blood count, urinalysis, serum concentrations of urea nitrogen (SUN), creatinine, potassium, calcium, glutamic-pyruvic transaminase, alkaline phosphatase, and total plasma or serum proteins (TPP). If these data are normal and the patient is not dehydrated, a water deprivation test should be performed to establish the patient's renal concentrating ability. Water deprivation tests should never be performed on azotemic patients and are unnecessary for dehydrated patients.

WATER DEPRIVATION TEST

The purpose of the water deprivation test is to induce a sufficient degree of dehydration to cause a mild increase in serum osmolality (2 to 5 percent), which in normal dogs will stimulate the release of antidiuretic hormone (ADH) from the posterior pituitary gland. ADH normally promotes water reabsorption from the renal distal tubules and collecting ducts and induces formation of concentrated urine.

Prior to beginning the test, the patient's body weight, urine specific gravity, packed cell volume (PCV), total plasma protein concentration, skin elasticity, and SUN should be determined. We recommend construction of a water deprivation flow chart for reference throughout the testing period (Fig. 2). If laboratory facilities exist for obtaining osmolality determinations, aliquots of serum and urine should be saved at each sampling interval for potential use later.

The patient should be deprived of water until it is determined that the kidneys can or cannot significantly concentrate urine. Significant urine concentration will normally occur when

Time (Hours)	Body Weight (kg)	Skin Pliability (Normal → decreased)	PCV* (%)	TPP* (gm/dl)	U_{sg}*	U_{Osm}* (mOsm/kg)	S_{Osm}* (mOsm/kg)	SUN* (mg/dl)
0								
2								
4								
8								
12								
16								
20								
24								
28								
32								
36								

Figure 2.   Flow chart of physiologic parameters monitored during water deprivation tests.

*PCV = packed cell volume, TPP = total plasma protein, U_{sg} = urine specific gravity, U_{Osm} = urine osmolality, S_{Osm} = serum osmolality, SUN = serum urea nitrogen.

the patient has lost approximately 5 percent of its body weight and has a corresponding increase in serum osmolality of 2 to 5 percent. These changes are usually associated with early signs of clinical dehydration. Commercial dry dog food may be fed during the test because it is low in moisture content while providing urea and other solutes important for maximal renal concentration. Since the weight of food consumed and of feces eliminated may significantly affect non-fluid–related weight changes, these weights should be estimated, particularly in small patients. To obtain the most accurate assessment of the patient's hydration status, it is best to correlate changes in body weight with changes in PCV, TPP, SUN, and skin elasticity.

Patients need not always be taken to states of clinical dehydration. Many dogs with normal renal concentrating ability will concentrate urine to a specific gravity of 1.025 or greater with no signs of dehydration. Once the urine specific gravity is 1.025 or higher, the test may be stopped. Conversely, patients with impaired renal concentrating ability may never attain such an "optimal" specific gravity even though they are clinically dehydrated. In the latter situation the test is stopped as soon as the patient becomes dehydrated or the urine specific gravity reaches a plateau (i.e., is unchanged on two successive determinations spaced at intervals four or more hours apart).

The duration of water deprivation necessary to attain significant urine concentration is highly variable. The endpoint of the test is determined by formation of significantly concentrated urine or by dehydration, rather than by an arbitrarily established time interval such as 24 hours. In dogs with significantly impaired renal concentrating ability characterized by obligatory water or solute diuresis, dehydration may occur within hours following water restriction. In clinically normal dogs, however, water deprivation for 24 hours or longer may be necessary before maximal urine concentration is achieved.

Sampling intervals should be between 4 and 12 hours, the exact duration being determined by the severity of polyuria and status of the patient. Extreme caution must be exercised when subjecting severely polyuric dogs to extended periods of water deprivation (i.e., 12 hours or longer). Polyuric dogs with water diuresis induced by pituitary diabetes insipidus, renal diabetes insipidus, or medullary solute washout often become clinically dehydrated quite rapidly. In such patients water deprivation for 18 to 24 hours may result in death. Therefore, the initial sampling interval should be 8 to 12 hours. Urine should be re-

moved from the bladder and discarded approximately one hour prior to collecting diagnostic samples. This procedure will ensure that the specific gravity obtained represents recently formed urine, rather than a composite of dilute and more concentrated urine formed during the previous 8 to 12 hours. The specific gravity of the composite sample should be determined, however, since it may be greater than 1.025. In this situation the test may be discontinued because formation of concentrated urine indicates the presence of an adequate population of functioning nephrons.

If the urine specific gravity following the first sampling interval is 1.025 or greater, the test should be stopped. The patient may be assumed to have adequate renal concentrating ability and the polyuria is most likely due to non-renal causes. If the urine specific gravity is less than 1.025 and the patient is not dehydrated or azotemic, the test should be continued for an additional 4 to 18 hours, depending on the patient's clinical status (as determined by changes in baseline data). The test should be stopped when (1) urine specific gravity reaches or exceeds 1.025, (2) the patient becomes clinically dehydrated, regardless of the urine specific gravity, or (3) the SUN or serum creatinine concentration becomes abnormally elevated, regardless of urine specific gravity value.

Results of water deprivation do not always permit clear-cut interpretations. Animals thought to be polyuric that concentrate their urine to a specific gravity of 1.025 or higher have adequate renal concentrating ability. Assuming that the observation of polyuria is accurate, a diagnosis of psychogenic water consumption (primary polydipsia) should be considered. Animals with a maximal urine specific gravity between 1.008 to 1.019 following water deprivation most likely have generalized renal disease or partial pituitary diabetes insipidus. An exogenous ADH test may be of diagnostic usefulness in such animals. Patients that elaborate persistently dilute urine (1.001 to 1.007) following water deprivation most likely have pituitary diabetes insipidus, renal diabetes insipidus, or severe renal medullary solute washout. Of this group, pituitary diabetes insipidus patients are most likely to respond dramatically to ADH administration, and an exogenous aqueous or repositol ADH test should be the next diagnostic consideration.

VASOPRESSIN CONCENTRATION TEST

The exogenous ADH test is performed as follows: A short indwelling venous catheter should be placed in the dog, and the urinary bladder should be catheterized and emptied. Next, a fresh solution of aqueous ADH* should be added to 5 percent dextrose in water. Vasopressin should be administered intravenously at a dosage of 10 milliunits per kg over a 60-minute period. Adding 5 units of aqueous vasopressin to one liter of 5 percent dextrose in water results in a vasopressin concentration of 5 milliunits per milliliter. Thus, 2 milliliters per kg are administered slowly over a 60-minute period. Urine samples should be collected at 30, 60, and 90 minutes following the start of vasopressin infusion. The bladder should be emptied completely at each collection period.

When water-loaded normal dogs were subjected to the described procedure, they achieved a mean maximal urine specific gravity of 1.021 with a range of 1.012 to 1.033. We have obtained similar results with this test on a limited number of dogs with spontaneous pituitary diabetes insipidus.

A "significant" response to exogenous ADH may be less dramatic than that observed following water deprivation. Hyposthenuric patients (SG = 1.001 to 1.007) that increase their urine specific gravity to 1.012 or higher following ADH infusion have a significant response indicative of either partial or complete pituitary diabetes insipidus. Hyposthenuric patients that have no response to intravenous ADH have either renal diabetes insipidus or severe medullary solute washout. Patients with isosthenuric or mildly hypertonic urine that have no response to ADH most likely have generalized renal disease.

As an alternative to the use of aqueous antidiuretic hormone, repositol ADH may also be administered to assess renal concentrating ability. The test is conducted as follows: Five units of repositol ADH† should be administered by intramuscular injection. Urine samples should be collected at 9 and 12 hours following ADH administration, if possible. Experimental results utilizing water-loaded normal dogs indicated that maximal renal response to repositol ADH occurs 9 to 12 hours after administration; urine specific gravity values ranging from 1.028 to 1.057 were obtained. Specific gravity values for dogs with long-standing pituitary diabetes insipidus may not reach the magnitude of those in normal experimental dogs because of prolonged water diuresis and associated medullary washout. In such cases, however, repeated repositol ADH administration at 24- to 36-hour intervals for several days may be associated with progressively increasing urine specific gravity values if medullary solute concentration is replenished.

PARTIAL WATER DEPRIVATION

Occasionally, dogs have persistently hyposthenuric urine after both water deprivation and exogenous ADH administration. These patients most likely have either renal diabetes insipidus, pituitary diabetes insipidus with severe medullary solute washout, or medullary solute washout caused by other diseases, such as primary polydipsia, hyperadrenocorticism, or hepatic failure. Partial water deprivation tests may be used to differentiate these syndromes.

Partial water deprivation involves gradual daily reduction in total water intake along with daily monitoring of renal concentrating ability and hydration status. Because of the time required, this procedure may be conducted on an outpatient basis. The dog's unrestricted water intake should be quantitated by the owner for two to four days. Once the dog's daily intake is known, the owner should be instructed to decrease this amount by 5 to 10 percent per day for several days (three to five initially). The total volume of water administered over a 24-hour period should never be less than the amount needed for daily maintenance in normal dogs (approximately 40 ml/kg/day). Additionally, each day a morning urine sample should be collected and the dog should be weighed carefully. Clients can be instructed in methods used to assess the presence of clinical dehydration so that severe iatrogenic dehydration does not occur. The total volume of water allowed over 24 hours should be divided during the day in order to prevent the patient from drinking the entire amount early in the day and having no water available for the remainder.

Patients that have medullary solute washout but functionally normal ADH production will gradually increase urine concentration as water intake is restricted over several days. Patients with renal diabetes insipidus will have no response to gradual water restriction and usually become rapidly dehydrated. Patients with pituitary diabetes insipidus and medullary solute washout usually respond to gradual water deprivation combined with repeated repositol ADH administration.

TECHNICAL DO'S AND DON'TS

1. DO obtain baseline clinical and laboratory data prior to administration of diagnostic or therapeutic agents.

---

*Pitressin, Parke-Davis Co., Detroit, Michigan
†Pitressin Tannate in oil, Parke-Davis Co., Detroit, Michigan

2. DO remove urine that has accumulated in the bladder lumen after initiation of water deprivation tests before obtaining a urine sample indicative of urine concentration at that time. This step will eliminate errors induced by mixture of residual dilute urine formed during early periods with urine formed under conditions of more prolonged water deprivation.

3. DO continue water deprivation tests until it is established that the patient can or cannot concentrate urine.

4. DO save aliquots of urine and serum throughout water deprivation and urine concentration tests for potential osmolality determination.

5. DO shake the ampule of vasopressin thoroughly prior to injection of ADH.

6. DON'T withhold water for prolonged periods in patients with profound polyuria.

7. DON'T use outdated antidiuretic hormone.

SUPPLEMENTAL READING

Balazs, T., Sekella, R., and Pauls, J.F.: Renal concentration test in beagle dogs. Lab. Anim. Sci., 21:546–548, 1971.

Hardy, R.M.: Renal function tests in the normal dog: Water deprivation test and exogenous vasopressin test. (M.S. Thesis) University of Minnesota, August 1975.

Hardy, R.M., and Osborne, C.A.: Water deprivation test in the dog: Maximal normal values. J. Am. Vet. Med. Assoc., 174:479–484, 1979.

Madewell, B.R., Osborne, C.A., Norrdin, R.A., Stevens, J.B., and Hardy, R.M.: Clinicopathologic aspects of diabetes insipidus in the dog. J. Am. Anim. Hosp. Assoc., 2:497–506, 1975.

Page, L.B., and Reem, G.H.: Urinary concentrating mechanism in the dog. Am. J. Physiol., 171:572–577, 1952.

NEONATAL CLINICAL NEPHROLOGY

ARTHUR L. LAGE, D.V.M.
South Weymouth, Massachusetts

The kidneys of neonatal dogs and cats should be considered in a different light than kidneys of animals of older ages and body states. Neonatal kidneys have not developed to the same degree as those of older animals and consequently function differently and react to noxious and stressful situations in a different manner.

APPLIED ANATOMY AND PHYSIOLOGY OF NEONATAL KIDNEYS

New nephrons do not develop after approximately the half-way point of embryonic life. Thus, the neonatal puppy and kitten have a full complement of nephrons. For several weeks following birth, cells of the nephrons (especially the tubules) develop morphologically and enzymatically so that they can begin to function fully in response to their internal and external environments.

Neonatal glomerular lobulation approaches the adult glomeruli in complexity, although the glomerulus will continue to increase in cross-sectional area until about the first quarter of the normal life span. Glomerular and tubular maturation proceeds through developmental stages. Interstitial tissue is more abundant in fetal kidneys than in immature neonatal kidneys. Extramedullary blood formation is present in the renal interstitium of the fetus but is not normally present in neonates.

Age definitely has an influence on renal function. Although there is renal function *in utero*, the glomerular filtration rate (GFR) of neonates is only about one-fourth to one-third of mature levels. This low GFR has been attributed to reduced permeability of immature glomerular epithelium; however, it may result from the decreased glomerular capillary bed available for filtration or from the lower systemic blood pressure in neonates, or both. Despite the low GFR, glomerular function is greater than tubular function in neonates. Many tests of tubular function suggest tubular immaturity. All levels of tubular function have not been studied in neonatal dogs and cats; but in humans adult levels of tubular function are not reached until the end of the first year of life. In general there is a progressive decline in GFR, renal plasma flow (RPF), tubular maximum reabsorption of glucose (TmG) and concentrating ability after the middle years of life. In addition to reduction in renal function, results of a number of experiments indicate decreased ability to recover from renal insult in aged dogs and cats. There are many differences in tubular function between neonates and adults; however, the relative inability of neonates to concentrate urine has received the greatest attention thus far. Neonatal kidneys can concentrate urine only to approximately 1½ times plasma osmolality compared with urine concentrations of three to four times that of plasma in adults. Fluid balance (intake and excretion) in neonates is five to seven times as great in relation to weight compared with adult dogs and cats. This means that slight changes in fluid balance may cause rapidly developing problems for the newborn. The metabolic rate of neonates is 2 to 2½ times as great in relation to body mass as that in adults. This means that at least two times as much acid is normally formed, easily resulting in acidosis in neonates if fluid balance and/or renal function are affected.

In summary, because of the immaturity of the kidneys, the great turnover in water balance, and increased acid formation, neonates are very susceptible to problems of dehydration, therapeutic overhydration, acidosis, and endogenous and exogenous toxicosis.

APPLIED NEONATAL CLINICAL NEPHROLOGY

The special homeostatic problems of neonates in relation to renal function have been summarized. The renal physiology of the newborn has unique characteristics because of the progressive maturation of the kidney. When disease is ecnountered at this period of life, the need for diagnosis is urgent. Formulation of treatment must be influenced by the special demands of neonatal kidneys. Renal or lower urinary tract disorders may be complicated by metabolic problems, neurologic disorders, or respiratory distress.

Micturition begins in the first 24 hours of life in most neonatal dogs and cats. Evaluation of volume is nearly impossible because of maternal hygiene of the puppy or kitten, unless the neonate is orphaned. Although crystalluria is quite common in neonates, it does not commonly cause obstruction of the lower urinary tract. Palpation of a large, distended bladder is indicative of urethral obstruction. Neonatal renal function studies are nearly impossible to perform in clinical cases because of safety and technical errors. The time of maturation of each renal function is not well documented in the newborn dog and cat; however, some points to consider are (1) the low GFR, which increases the risk of a possible uremic crisis, (2) the easy production and frequent appearance of glycosuria, (3) frequent hyperphosphatemia, and (4) decreased concentrating ability.

Acute dehydration is perhaps the single most dangerous problem of neonates and may quickly lead to serious functional renal failure. Acute renal failure of the newborn usually results from dystocia-related problems (anoxia) or postpartum dehydration, septicemia, or hemolytic problems. Gentamycin and other therapeutic drugs and heavy metals such as lead have produced acute tubular necrosis in the newborn. For an unexplained reason the most common signs of acute renal failure of the newborn are diarrhea and abdominal distention. Respiratory, circulatory, or metabolic disorders can easily lead to renal failure in the neonate. The only evidence of early organic disturbance of the kidneys may be hematuria or proteinuria.

Canine herpesvirus infection in puppies usually causes death in the first one to three weeks of life. The renal lesions consist of focal necrosis and hemorrhages.

Urinary infection is characterized by large numbers of bacteria and leukocytes in urine. The newborn should be examined for anatomic predisposing causes to urinary tract infections. Examination should include the external genitalia and the perianal region for the presence of malformation, infections, parasitic infestations, and foreign bodies. Obvious abnormalities of the kidneys and urinary tract such as tumors, hydronephrosis, cysts, and calculi should be noted. General predisposing causes of urinary tract infection of the newborn include (1) acute respiratory or intestinal infections, (2) metabolic disorders, and (3) malnutrition.

Diagnosis depends on finding significant numbers of bacteria and leukocytes in the urine on direct or centrifuged sediment examination. Bacteriuria may exist without leukocytes, and leukocyturia may exist without urinary infection (as in some forms of glomerulonephritis or reproductive tract infection).

The urine should be cultured to identify the organism(s), and antibiotic sensitivity tests should also be performed. In neonatal dogs and cats urine for culture should be collected by cystocentesis. Antibiotics chosen for neonatal urinary infections should be of low toxicity and high concentration in urine. Selection should be based on sensitivity tests. Furadantin, chloramphenicol, ampicillin, and sulfonamides are recommended.

It is often difficult if not impossible to distinguish between infection localized to the lower urinary tract and infection involving the kidneys. The diagnosis of pyelonephritis may remain only a probable diagnosis. Signs and symptoms suggesting a diagnosis of pyelonephritis include pyuria associated with any combination of hyperthermia, fever, bacteremia, leukocytosis, painful abdomen, and gastrointestinal upsets. The treatment of urinary infections of the newborn should continue for two weeks after the elimination of the signs and symptoms. Production of sterile urine should be verified by culture after the antibiotic has been withdrawn for an appropriate period.

POINTS TO REMEMBER

1. Alarm signals include (a) delay in the onset of micturition, (b) an abnormal urine stream, (c) a large, palpably distended bladder, and (d) a large, palpable kidney.
2. Renal insufficiency should be considered whenever a serious illness exists or whenever there are signs of respiratory or gastrointestinal disorders or convulsions.

3. Avoid urethral cateterization; perform sterile suprapubic cystocentesis.
4. Avoid intravenous perfusion to start diuresis if dehydration has not been proved.
5. During treatment for dehydration, carefully monitor urine output to prevent water intoxication. Weigh the patient accurately.
6. If acute renal failure is diagnosed, and if BUN concentration is higher than 200 mg/dl or potassium level is above 7.5 mEq/liter, or if signs of vascular overload are present, use peritoneal dialysis.

SUPPLEMENTAL READING

Heptinstall, R.H.: *Pathology of the Kidney.* Boston, Little, Brown & Co., 1966.
Latimer, H.B.: The growth of the kidneys and the bladder in the fetal dog. Anat. Rec., *109*:1–12, 1951.
Osborne, C.A., Low, D.G., and Finco, D.R.: *Canine and Feline Urology.* Philadelphia, W.B. Saunders Co., 1972.
Papper, S: *Clinical Nephrology.* Boston, Little, Brown & Co., 1971.
Royer, P., Habib, R., Mathieu, H., and Broyer, M.: *Pediatric Nephrology.* Philadelphia, W.B. Saunders Co., 1974.
Strauss, M.B., and Welt, L.G.: *Diseases of the Kidney,* Vols. 1 and 2. Boston, Little, Brown & Co., 1971.

MANAGEMENT OF OLIGURIC AND ANURIC RENAL FAILURE

LARRY D. COWGILL, D.V.M.
Davis, California

Treatment of acute oligoanuric renal parenchymal failure demands an understanding of the scope and the nature of the critical complications of acute uremia. Because of the necessity of initiating therapeutic measures early in the course of the disease, it is also important to recognize clinical manifestations and circumstances in which acute renal failure might occur.

Because the kidneys play a key role in regulating the volume and composition of the extracellular fluid (ECF), acute impairment of renal function is associated with alterations in ECF. Disturbances of greatest consequence are (1) alterations in the volume of ECF, resulting in dehydration or overhydration, (2) hyperkalemia, (3) acid-base disorders, and (4) uremic intoxications.

DIAGNOSIS

Oliguric or anuric renal failure can result from prerenal or postrenal disorders in addition to primary renal parenchymal diseases. Extrarenal problems can be managed readily by proper fluid therapy or surgery and are not typically associated with intrinsic morphologic damage to the kidney.

Intrinsic renal disease should be suspected in any azotemic hydrated patient with a structurally intact and patent lower urinary system. The diagnosis of acute parenchymal renal failure requires careful evaluation of clinical and laboratory information. Of prime importance in early diagnosis is recognition of potential settings for the development of acute renal failure (ARF). Exposure to nephrotoxic chemicals or drugs is a common cause of ARF in dogs.

Ingestion of antifreeze (ethylene glycol) or heavy metals, or administration of gentamicin, kanamycin, or amphotericin B should prompt consideration of acute nephrosis as a tentative diagnosis. Renal hypoperfusion and subsequent acute tubular necrosis should be anticipated when oliguria follows surgery, sepsis, hemorrhage, dehydration, or hypotension. Acute oliguric renal failure may also occur as a complication of generalized diseases, including decompensated polyuric renal insufficiency, sepsis, hypercalcemia, bacterial endocarditis, acute vascular disease, intravascular hemolysis, and leptospirosis.

LABORATORY EVALUATION

A tentative diagnosis of ARF must be confirmed by laboratory testing. The minimum data base should include a complete blood count, a complete urinalysis, serum urea nitrogen or creatinine concentration, serum sodium, potassium, and chloride concentrations, and bicarbonate or blood gas determinations. Microscopic examination of urine sediment can be of great help in establishing a diagnosis of acute parenchymal disease if granular and cellular casts are present. The sediment may also provide clues to the etiology if oxalate crystals, heme-pigment casts, or RBC casts are present. The patient's laboratory status is dynamic and subject to considerable variation, depending on the severity of the disease and response to therapy. Accordingly, many or all of the parameters in the initial data base will require at least daily surveillance.

Distinction between potentially reversible acute renal failure and chronic, end-stage renal disease is necessary for proper management, prognosis, and client communication. If a clear distinction between the two states cannot be obtained from the history, physical examination, and laboratory data, a renal biopsy is often indicated for histologic confirmation of the nature and severity of the disease. Radiographic evaluation of kidney size may also provide useful prognostic information.

THERAPY

Therapy for oliguric or anuric renal failure may be separated into conservative measures and dialysis. Conservative measures are designed to promote renal blood flow and urine formation and to correct metabolic and biochemical disturbances associated with acute uremia. It is important that conservative measures be formulated with knowledge of specific clinical and biochemical abnormalities of the patient and be initiated at the earliest indication of renal failure.

VOLUME STATUS

As one of the critical complications of ARF, disorders of the patient's body fluid volume must be initially assessed and corrected. Patients with oliguric or anuric renal failure are characteristically hypovolemic and dehydrated. The volume deficit should be estimated by clinical parameters (skin turgor, central venous pressure, hematocrit, and plasma protein), and a replacement volume should be calculated on the basis of the patient's body weight. Volume deficits are primarily caused by ionic fluid losses from vomiting and diarrhea and should therefore be replaced with ionic, sodium-containing fluids (balanced electrolyte solutions). Five percent dextrose in water is not an adequate replacement solution and should be reserved for insensible maintenance losses. The initial volume deficit should be replaced intravenously over two to six hours, depending upon the severity of the dehydration. This will generally require infusion rates of 10 to 20 ml/kg/hr, but faster rates may be utilized if severe dehydration or hypotension exists. At faster infusion rates or if impaired cardiovascular function is present, central venous pressure may serve as a useful indicator of volume expansion and the ability of the heart to accept the fluid load. Failure to induce significant urine flow after volume replacement indicates that either parenchymal damage is severe or the fluid deficit was initially underestimated. Additional fluid may be administered, but care should be taken to prevent overhydration and the severe consequences of pulmonary edema. The animal's weight following rehydration should be used as the baseline against which future changes are compared.

The volume status of the patient should be subsequently evaluated by clinical parameters and regular determinations of body weight. Gross fluctuations in body weight usually reflect alterations in the fluid volume and are reflective of dehydration or overhydration. Maintenance fluids should be limited to 5 percent dextrose in water for insensible losses (20 to 25 ml/kg/day) and balanced electrolyte solutions to replace urine output and gastrointestinal losses.

Overhydration or hypervolemia can be as detrimental to oliguric uremic patients as hypovolemia. Hypervolemia is a common result of overzealous initial therapeutic efforts or improper monitoring of fluid balance. Overhydration can precipitate peripheral and pulmonary edema, congestive heart failure, and hypertension. Once administered, an excessive volume load represents a serious therapeutic error because it can be corrected only by dialysis.

During development of the polyuric recovery phase of acute renal failure, urine volume may increase to several times normal and may be associated with a large sodium loss. In this stage it is important to adjust fluid requirements to meet urinary losses in order to prevent dehydration and further renal injury.

HYPERKALEMIA

Hyperkalemia is a serious consequence of oliguric primary renal failure and must be quickly and effectively managed. The cardiotoxicity of high serum potassium concentrations are largely responsible for the early mortality associated with ARF. Hyperkalemia can be recognized by measuring the serum concentration of potassium or by recognition of characteristic electrocardiographic (ECG) abnormalities. The type of therapy initiated depends on the severity of ECG disturbances and the degree of hyperkalemia. When the serum potassium is greater than 8 mEq/liter, parenteral calcium is indicated. As a specific antagonist of the cardiotoxic effects of potassium, 10 percent calcium gluconate should be administered as a slow intravenous bolus in sufficient quantity to correct the ECG abnormalities. A dosage of 0.5 ml/kg is a useful estimate of the required amount. Although the effects of calcium gluconate are rapid, they are short-lived. For this reason, administration of calcium is primarily used to correct life-threatening situations until longer-lasting therapy can be initiated.

Management of moderate hyperkalemia (serum potassium between 5.5 and 8.0 mEq/liter) is based on measures to promote movement of extracellular potassium to the intracellular compartment. In non-alkalemic patients this is effected by the intravenous administration of sodium bicarbonate at 0.5 to 1.0 mEq/kg body weight. A 20 to 30 percent glucose solution administered intravenously, with or without insulin at one unit per 3 grams glucose, is similarly effective. The benefits of bicarbonate or glucose-insulin therapy occur within a few minutes but are relatively short in duration. Therefore, therapy with a more prolonged effect should be considered.

Prolonged control of hyperkalemia can be effected by use of the cationic exchange resin sodium polystyrene suphonate*, given at 25 to

---

*Kayexate®, Winthrop Laboratories, New York, New York

50 grams in three divided doses daily. However, peritoneal dialysis or hemodialysis is the most effective long-term approach to potassium regulation in oliguric or anuric renal failure.

ACID-BASE DISTURBANCES

Most patients with acute primary oliguric renal failure develop metabolic acidosis that parallels the severity of the uremia. Although this is the rule, patients may manifest a variety of acid-base disturbances and be acidemic, alkalemic, or have a normal blood pH. For this reason it is desirable to measure the bicarbonate deficit or to perform a complete blood gas analysis before empirically treating suspected acidosis. If the bicarbonate deficit is known, the required sodium bicarbonate replacement can be calculated from the formula: Bicarbonate replacement (mEq) = body weight (kg) × 0.3 × bicarbonate deficit. If the bicarbonate deficit is not determined, an estimate based on the clinical status of the patient can be utilized. Mild uremic states are often characterized by a bicarbonate deficit of 5, whereas the typical bicarbonate deficit in moderate and advanced uremic states is 10 and 15, respectively. The calculated bicarbonate replacement should not be administered rapidly in an attempt to correct the acidosis quickly. Half the calculated replacement should be administered in the first hour and the remainder given during the next five to six hours. The acid-base status should be re-evaluated at six hours, and at least daily on subsequent days, to monitor the adequacy of replacement therapy and to detect changes or ongoing disturbances. Sodium bicarbonate should be used only to manage the metabolic component of a simple or mixed acid-base disorder and could be inappropriate or contraindicated if other acid-base disturbances (i.e., respiratory acidosis or metabolic alkalosis) are present.

DIURETICS

Osmotic (hypertonic mannitol or glucose) or loop (furosemide, ethacrynic acid) diuretics have been advocated for the management of oliguric renal failure. The benefits of hyperosmotic agents in prophylaxis or the early stages of ARF have been well documented in both clinical and experimental settings. The precise manner in which these agents act is not clearly established, but they appear to alter early mechanisms that initiate ARF. These agents are often of little benefit in established ARF of greater than 12 hours' duration, although successful diuresis has been reported in a few cases with more prolonged oliguria. In a referral practice, however, the duration of oliguria or anuria has usually been sufficiently long that these agents are ineffective. In posttraumatic or surgical patients or in cases in which the onset of oliguria is early and clearly established, osmotic diuresis may be beneficial. In these situations a trial infusion of mannitol or dextrose (as 20 to 25 percent solutions) at 0.25 to 0.5 gm/kg can be given to well-hydrated patients. If significant diuresis develops, a maintenance infusion of 8 to 10 percent mannitol in normal saline or in a balanced electrolyte solution can be continued to promote the diuresis for the next 12 to 24 hours. If diuresis is not established within 30 to 45 minutes of the trial infusion, additional doses should be withheld to prevent serious vascular overload.

Loop diuretics are also purported to initiate diuresis effectively in oliguric patients. Although they may promote diuresis in the early stages of ARF, proof that they are beneficial in the treatment of oliguric renal failure is scanty. Loop diuretics may induce diuresis without measurable improvements in the glomerular filtration rate, renal blood flow, or intrarenal distribution of renal blood flow. While an increase in water turnover by loop diuretics may prevent intratubular obstruction, the increase in urine flow may not be associated with demonstrable clinical improvement. Therefore, their use may be detrimental unless strict fluid volume supervision is maintained. Loop diuretics are perhaps most beneficial when administered to hypervolemic or hypertensive patients to promote increased fluid and sodium excretion. Because of the limited risks of a single dose of furosemide, a routine trial in patients who fail to have diuresis with initial fluid therapy is often advocated. Under these circumstances, furosemide is given intravenously at 2 to 4 mg/kg of body weight. This dose may be doubled or tripled if the initial dose does not induce a significant diuretic response within an hour. If this regimen fails to promote diuresis, continued administration of these drugs is pointless. Dialysis must be considered as the only alternative therapy.

If these initial measures are ineffective in promoting and sustaining an increase in urine production or in controlling the metabolic and biochemical disturbances of uremia, therapeutic efforts must be quickly directed toward either peritoneal dialysis or hemodialysis. Consult the articles on peritoneal dialysis and hemodialysis for further details.

Nutrition and drug administration are two additional areas of concern in the therapy of acute renal failure. The caloric requirements of uremic patients must be satisfied in order to prevent marked tissue catabolism and the accumulation of nitrogenous metabolic waste products. The calories provided, however, should be restricted in or devoid of protein and supplied mainly as high-caloric-density fats and carbohydrates (see the article entitled "Nutrition During the Uremic Crisis"). Caloric mixtures should contain a minimum of water and be administered in frequent small feedings in order to prevent vomiting. More protein can be provided if therapy is supplemented with dialysis.

Caution must be exercised in administering drugs to uremic animals. See the article "Drug Therapy in Renal Disorders" for further information.

PROGNOSIS

A good recovery can be anticipated for patients with prerenal oliguria. The prognosis for patients with primary acute oliguric renal failure, however, is initially guarded to unfavorable. The duration of oliguria, concurrent medical or surgical problems, and the extent of nephron destruction affect the response to therapy. Establishment of a sustained diuresis can be considered a favorable response to therapy. Failure to sustain diuresis with conservative therapeutics indicates severe or advanced disease and suggests an unfavorable outcome.

SUPPLEMENTAL READING

Bennett, W.M., et al.: Guidelines for drug therapy in renal failure. Ann. Intern. Med., 86:754–783, 1977.

Osborne, C.A., and Klausner, I.S.: Adverse drug reactions in the uremic patient. In Kirk, R.W. (ed.): *Current Veterinary Therapy VI.* Philadelphia, W.B. Saunders Co., 1977.

INTENSIVE DIURESIS IN POLYURIC RENAL FAILURE

DELMAR R. FINCO, D.V.M.
Athens, Georgia,

and DONALD G. LOW, D.V.M.
Davis, California

Diuresis can be caused by water loss secondary to loss of an osmotic agent or by primary water loss. All diuretics used at present in dogs and cats, except glucocorticoids, act by causing water loss secondary to loss of osmotic agents. Glucocorticoids seem to act as water diuretics. Osmotic agents cause diuresis by remaining in the lumen of renal tubules and preventing passive water reabsorption. Many diuretics, including furosemide, have diuretic action because of impairment of normal NaCl reabsorption by the kidney. Unabsorbed NaCl acts as the diuretic agent. Mannitol and glucose act directly as osmotic agents. Mannitol is restricted to the extracellular space but freely passes the glomerular filter. It is not reabsorbed by the renal tubules and thus is a potent diuretic agent. Glucose enters cells for metabolism but also freely passes the glomerular filter. Tubular reabsorption of glucose occurs, but renal tubules have a limited capacity for glucose reabsorption. When a quantity of glucose in excess of tubular reabsorptive capacity is presented to the kidney, glucose remaining in the tubules prevents water reabsorption and diuresis ensues. Although more glucose than mannitol is required to induce diuresis, the same intensity of diuresis can be achieved with either compound.

In addition to effects on tubular reabsorption of water, some studies indicate that osmotic diuretics may affect systemic circulation or renal circulation and glomerular filtration. Studies reveal that furosemide has effects on pulmonary congestion unrelated to its diuretic properties. Glomerular filtration rate and renal blood flow are apparently increased moderately by furosemide and mannitol, although some conflicting data are reported on this point.

Osmotic diuretics have been used widely in human medicine for prophylaxis of renal shutdown during surgical procedures and after known exposure to nephrotoxic agents. They have also been used in anuric renal failure in attempts to induce urine flow. The efficacy of these agents for prophylaxis of renal failure seems to be well established in man. Osmotic diuresis also has been advocated for use in the treatment of polyuric renal failure in the dog and cat. The subsequent discussion outlines rationale, desirable effects, potential complications, and preferred method for this procedure.

CHARACTERISTICS OF POLYURIC RENAL FAILURE

Most cases of renal failure in the dog and cat have a fixed urine specific gravity and polyuria. This indicates that at least two-thirds of the nephrons are non-functional and that renal concentrating ability is lost (isosthenuria). If the progression of disease is slow, patients may have no signs other than polydipsia and polyuria for indefinite periods of time. With progression of disease, however, additional signs referable to renal dysfunction eventually appear. Abrupt onset of depression, anorexia, and vomiting herald the onset of a uremic crisis.

Patients in uremic crisis are markedly dehydrated because of polyuria, inadequate water intake, and vomiting. Dehydration results in hypovolemia and impaired renal perfusion. Thus, one prerenal factor is superimposed on primary renal failure. A second prerenal factor that is likely during the uremic crisis is an increase in production of nitrogenous wastes as a consequence of the catabolic state brought about by anorexia and uremia. Degradation of body proteins for calories results in production of these wastes (see the article "Nutrition During the Uremic Crisis").

Although serum sodium concentration is usually normal, existing dehydration indicates an isotonic contraction of the extracellular space and a sodium deficit. There probably are deficits in chloride and potassium as well, although serum potassium concentration is usually normal in polyuric failure. These deficits are probably due to losses associated with renal dysfunction and vomiting. Hyperphosphatemia is characteristic of polyuric renal failure.

Acid-base status may range from normal to severe metabolic acidosis. Acidosis is caused by impaired renal excretion of hydrogen ions. Patients that are vomiting severely may lose hydrogen ions; acid-base status in these patients depends on the balance between hydrogen ion loss due to vomiting and hydrogen ion retention due to renal failure.

Uremia is associated with retention of nitrogen wastes. Urea or creatinine is used as an index of this retention, but specific uremic toxins have not been identified. At present, even hemodialysis is an empirical form of therapy because of the lack of knowledge regarding uremic toxins. However, signs of uremia are fairly well correlated with BUN, and dietary approaches that decrease BUN seem to result in clinical improvement of the patient.

OSMOTIC DIURESIS IN POLYURIC RENAL FAILURE

RESPONSE OF DISEASED KIDNEYS TO DIURETICS

Evidence based on experimental studies in dogs indicates that urine flow rate is enhanced by furosemide even when azotemia is present. Similar increases can be expected with glucose or mannitol. Thus, natural osmotic diuresis of renal failure can be augmented. Although diuresis may even be induced in dehydrated patients, it is to the disadvantage of the patient to do so because of accentuation of pre-existing hypovolemia. Consequently, osmotic diuresis in the dog and cat should not be undertaken until dehydration has been corrected with a multiple electrolyte solution such as lactated Ringer's solution.

BENEFITS OF OSMOTIC DIURESIS

The increase in renal blood flow and glomerular filtration rate that occurs with osmotic diuretics is small but may be beneficial to the patient. More important are immediate diuretic effects of osmotic agents. Diuresis is induced minutes after administration of the agent and persists until it is inactivated or excreted. In contrast, volume expansion by administration of electrolyte solutions does not initiate diuresis for hours after administration, and thus the same intensity of diuresis is not achieved.

Since the toxins of uremia are not defined, the benefit of diuresis can be judged only clinically or by the advantageous biochemical alterations that diuresis induces. Mannitol osmotic diuresis in chronic renal failure in humans produces significant increases in excretion of water and chloride and variable increases in urea excretion. Rehydration of dogs with multiple electrolyte solutions and subsequent diuresis cause a significant decrease in BUN and clinical improvement.

The apparent benefits of osmotic diuresis may relate to inhibition of tubular reabsorption of solutes. Many compounds that pass through renal glomeruli subsequently are partially or totally reabsorbed by the tubules. With osmotic diuresis, inhibition of reabsorption results in their loss in urine. Fluid with the composition of blood, minus cells and materials with molecular weight greater than 70,000, can theoretically be removed from the body by this technique. The actual efficiency is even greater than indicated because the concentration of most nitrogenous wastes in the urine is much greater than in the blood in renal disease as well as in health. Therefore, the quantity of nitrogenous wastes in the additional urine flow induced by osmotic diuresis (above the existing urine flow) is greater than in the same quantity of fluid used for exchange by peritoneal dialysis. This point is important in putting diuresis and peritoneal dialysis in perspective as alternate forms of therapy. It indicates, for example, that inducing a diuresis of 2 liters (above normal urine flow) is more efficient than an exchange of dialysate of 2 liters.

CHOICE OF THE DIURETIC AGENT

The same degree of diuresis can be achieved with glucose, mannitol, or furosemide, and thus other factors must be considered in choosing among these agents.

Mannitol has no advantages over other agents but has the disadvantage of greater cost than glucose. Besides low cost, glucose is preferable to mannitol because glucose can be metabolized for energy. The patient in uremic crisis is in a catabolic state. Body fats and protein are being used to fulfill caloric needs, and protein catabolism accentuates the uremia (see the chapter entitled "Nutrition During the Uremic Crisis").

In addition to inducing diuresis, parenteral administration of 10 to 20 percent glucose provides some calories to the patient in uremic crisis and thus is protein-sparing. This nutritional advantage of glucose over mannitol is extremely important.

Furosemide administration is technically simple but has major disadvantages. It depends on chloride for diuretic action and may result in considerably more NaCl loss than does glucose or mannitol. Since polyuric renal failure is a salt-losing disease, the potential exists for massive salt depletion. In addition, there is probably more likelihood of development of water deficits with the use of furosemide than with glucose, since glucose is given as an aqueous solution. Most important is the fact that furosemide has no effect on the negative caloric balance.

MECHANICS OF OSMOTIC DIURESIS

1. As previously indicated, restoration of fluid deficit with lactated Ringer's or a comparable solution is necessary prior to inducing diuresis. If clinical evidence of dehydration is not apparent, it is still advisable to give a quantity of fluid equal to 3 to 5 percent of body weight. The fluid deficit should be administered intravenously over a period of about one hour.

2. After deficit therapy, accurately weigh the patient. This baseline weight is used to assess underhydration or overhydration during subsequent therapy.

3. Administer 20 percent dextrose intravenously at a total dose of 25 to 65 ml/kg and at a rate of 2 ml/min for 10 to 15 minutes. Then reduce the infusion rate to 1 ml/min.

4. As soon as the IV infusion of glucose is begun, catheterize the patient and empty the bladder.

5. Test newly formed urine (if any) for glucose.

6. If the test is positive, sufficient glucose to exceed the renal threshold has been administered, and anuria does not exist. Urine volume should increase if the procedure can be safely continued. A urine volume of 1 to 4 ml/min should be obtained, depending on body size.

7. If adequate urine flow is not obtained by the time half the dose of glucose is given, the procedure must be discontinued, since overhydration and hyperosmolality will occur and may be accompanied by pulmonary edema.

8. If adequate urine flow is obtained, the entire calculated dosage of osmotic agent is given. Lactated Ringer's (3 to 5 percent of body weight) followed by hypertonic glucose is repeated as described previously. Fluid input and urine output are measured so that reasonable balance is maintained. Two or three cycles of

dextrose and lactated Ringer's solution are administered every 24 hours.

9. After 24 hours, the patient is re-evaluated by physical examination, BUN concentration, and body weight.

10. If necessary, the entire procedure is repeated. Weight gain indicates fluid retention and contraindicates lactated Ringer's prior to the osmotic agent. Weight loss indicates fluid deficit; lactated Ringer's should be administered in sufficient quantity to rectify the deficit.

11. Extreme weakness suggests potassium deficiency. If serum potassium concentration is less than 3.0 mEq/liter, solutions containing 25 to 35 mEq/liter of potassium should be administered at a rate of 0.5 mEq/kg/hr.

12. Initially, all fluids should be given intravenously. Lactated Ringer's to maintain hydration can be given subcutaneously if it is absorbed well. Generally, response to therapy as indicated by a decrease in BUN concentration, will occur within two to four days. Failure to respond indicates severe functional impairment and dictates the use of supplementary techniques such as peritoneal dialysis.

13. If diuresis with dextrose fails, furosemide may be used at the recommended dosage to attempt to induce diuresis. If no urine forms after one hour, the dosage can be doubled. If this is not successful in inducing urine output, it can generally be assumed that the patient must be treated for anuria.

14. In instances in which clinical and laboratory response occurs, oral alimentation and medication are gradually resumed as the parenteral routes of therapy are abandoned. Oral medications (salt, bicarbonate, anabolic steroids, B vitamins) are continued indefinitely in chronic disease. After acute polyuric disease they are continued until renal function has improved sufficiently so that the patient can concentrate urine above 1.025 SG.

SUPPLEMENTAL READING

Gennari, F.J., and Fassirer, J.P.: Osmotic diuresis. N. Engl. J. Med., *291*:714–720, 1974.

Gutmann, F.D.: Altered effect of furosemide upon the unilateral experimentally diseased kidney of the dog. J. Lab. Clin. Med., 77:14–22, 1971.

Krishna, D. et al.: Renal and extrarenal hemodynamic effects of furosemide in congestive heart failure after acute myocardial infarction. N. Engl. J. Med., 288:1087–1090, 1973.

Shelp, W.D., and Rieselbach, R.E.: The effect of furosemide on residual nephrons of the chronically diseased kidney in man. Nephron, 8:427–439, 1971.

MEDICAL MANAGEMENT OF POLYURIC RENAL FAILURE: SALT AND SODIUM BICARBONATE

LARRY D. COWGILL, D.V.M.,
and DONALD G. LOW, D.V.M.
Davis, California

In the past, use of sodium chloride in the conservative management of progressive renal insufficiency has been based on the concept that uremic dogs have an obligatory urinary sodium loss and are therefore prone to significant negative balances of sodium and chloride (Bovee; Osborne et al., 1975; Osborne et al., 1972). In therapeutic terms this is translated into liberal dietary supplementation with sodium chloride and sodium bicarbonate. In recent years the pathophysiologic events in adaptation to progressive renal insufficiency have become more clearly defined. The regulation of sodium excretion is one area in which substantial advances have been made. A series of investigations in both dogs and man over the past ten years have provided considerable support for the concept that the observed increase in salt excretion per unit of surviving renal mass is a physiologic adaptation of the patient in renal failure to maintain salt balance (Danovitch et al.; Schmidt et al.; Schultze et al.).

The concept of salt balance suggests that during a steady state salt excretion must equal salt intake. If the input (i.e., from the diet and parenteral fluids) exceeds the capacity of the patient to excrete an equivalent amount, the balance of sodium will be positive, resulting in sodium retention and extracellular fluid (ECF) volume expansion until a new steady state is achieved. If, on the other hand, sodium losses are greater than dietary intake, sodium balance will be negative, resulting in ECF volume contraction and dehydration.

The exact mechanisms regulating this adaptive natriuresis in renal failure are not completely characterized but appear to involve a combination of physical forces and a humoral natriuretic factor that inhibits tubular reabsorption of sodium. Patients in renal failure can vary renal sodium excretion and maintain sodium balance within the normal range of dietary sodium intake, but the capacity to adjust sodium excretion rapidly to accommodate sudden changes in intake is severely limited. Sudden reductions in sodium intake could therefore be associated with marked decreases in total body sodium content and dehydration, while sudden increases in sodium intake could result in increases in total body sodium content and ECF volume expansion. Additionally, adaptations in sodium excretion may occur as a "trade off" for the establishment of other physiologic or pathologic states. ECF volume expansion that is manifested as hypertension or edema is a potential "trade off" for patients in advanced renal failure who have maintained sodium balance on normal or high-salt diets. Hypertension as a clinical entity has been virtually ignored in veterinary medicine, yet the incidence of significant hypertension may be as great as 75 percent in dogs with progressive renal insufficiency (Weiser, et al.). Degenerative vascular changes and nephrosclerosis have been found in dogs with hypertension just as these lesions are found in man. Whether hypertension is a significant factor in the establishment or progression of chronic renal failure in dogs or not remains to be evaluated.

An additional complication or "trade off" for sodium balance may be the aggravation of metabolic acidosis in a general relationship to the level of dietary sodium intake. In this setting supplementation with salt may exacerbate the development of metabolic acidosis and renal osteodystrophy as bone buffer reserves are consumed to maintain hydrogen ion homeostasis.

On the other hand, subtle increases in ECF volume, when unaccompanied by hypertension, may be beneficial by increasing glomerular filtration rate and urea clearance and lowering plasma urea concentration through greater urine flow. In many cases salt supplementation will promote clinical improvement in patients in renal failure.

The recommendations for the use of sodium chloride and sodium bicarbonate in uremic animals therefore need re-evaluation. The objective of therapy with these agents is to supply a level of dietary sodium that will promote clinical benefits without producing serious complications.

CLINICAL EVALUATION

Rational therapy for any problem associated with renal insufficiency cannot be formulated without a complete clinical and biochemical evaluation of the patient. In considering sodium chloride and sodium bicarbonate for therapy, clinical evaluation of the patient should include initial and subsequent determinations of body weight, assessment of edema, ascites, jugular pulse, dehydration, and a complete cardiovascular evaluation including, if possible, blood pressure measurements (Weiser, et al.). The biochemical profile should include measurement of blood urea nitrogen, creatinine, inorganic phosphorus, sodium, potassium, chloride, and bicarbonate concentrations and a complete urinalysis.

Congestive heart failure, glomerulonephritis, amyloidosis, nephrotic syndrome, salt-losing nephropathy, and hypertension are clinical syndromes that require special considerations in dietary salt management and should be carefully evaluated in uremic patients. In many such patients sodium supplementation is relatively or absolutely contraindicated.

THERAPEUTIC CONSIDERATIONS

DECOMPENSATED UREMIC CRISIS

Many patients who have stable polyuric renal insufficiency will develop uremic episodes following mild disease or environmental stress. Attempts should be made to correct volume deficits and increase renal blood flow in these patients (see the article entitled "Intensive Diuresis in Renal Failure"). ECF volume deficits will be due primarily to ionic fluid losses, and replacement therapy should therefore contain sodium (i.e., saline or a balanced electrolyte solution) and be administered intravenously at an appropriate rate to replace the estimated deficit in four to six hours. After correcting fluid deficits, maintenance fluids should be provided orally or parenterally to maintain normal fluid volume. The route and choice of fluids will depend upon the clinical status of the patient and concurrent therapy.

Osmotic diuretics (i.e., hypertonic glucose or mannitol) will usually promote a diuresis as well as a natriuresis. Fluid balance should therefore be maintained by administering balanced electrolyte solutions as well as electrolyte-free solutions to cover insensible water loss. This can be accomplished by alternating a balanced electrolyte solution with 5 percent dextrose.

Concurrent with fluid volume replacement, the acid-base status of the patient should be evaluated by determining serum bicarbonate or blood gas concentrations. Existing bicarbonate deficits should be corrected by parenteral administration of sodium bicarbonate. From the unknown or estimated bicarbonate deficit, the approximate replacement dose of bicarbonate can be calculated from the formula: Bicarbonate replacement (mEq) = body weight (kg) × 0.6 × bicarbonate deficit. This value represents the calculated bicarbonate replacement, but the total amount should *not* be administered rapidly in an attempt to correct the acidosis quickly. Half the calculated bicarbonate should be given in the first few hours and the remainder during the next 12 to 24 hours. The acid-base status of the patient should re-evaluated at that time to manage ongoing disturbances. When the uremic crisis is under control, the patient can be treated as described in the next category.

STABLE POLYURIC RENAL INSUFFICIENCY

Specific recommendations for salt and sodium bicarbonate supplementation are difficult to formulate for patients in this group. Previous recommendations have stressed the importance of liberally increasing dietary salt (Bovee; Osborne, et al., 1975; Osborne et al., 1972). The rationale of this approach was to ensure that urinary sodium loss was matched by dietary intake and to promote an augmented urine flow and, therefore, increased urea clearance. Recent investigations suggest that sodium balance can be maintained when dietary sodium is reduced in proportion to the reduction in functional renal mass. The relative intolerance of these patients to sudden alterations in sodium intake and the potential "trade offs" associated with liberal sodium intake in uremic patients must also be considered. Therefore, the relative merits of high sodium intake need to be re-evaluated. Until further information is accumulated from patients with naturally occurring renal disease, the following general guidelines are suggested: Severe alterations in sodium intake should not be implemented suddenly. The kidney is adapted to a level of sodium excretion equal to the existing sodium intake and may not be able to make sudden adjustments to change. Increases or decreases in sodium may precipitate sodium retention or sodium depletion, respectively. If a protein-restricted diet is formulated for the patient, the sodium content should be adjusted to match the estimated previous intake. If the patient has been eating a commercial diet, the sodium intake can be estimated from the nutritional analysis of the food and the quantity of food consumed. As a guide, commercial diets provide the following approximate sodium chloride loads: dry dog food, 4500 mg/lb; semi-moist food, 5300 mg/lb; and canned food, 2600 mg/lb.

If the patient is neither hypertensive nor edematous, a trial program of moderate sodium loading may be instituted in an effort to promote increased urine flow. Fifty mg sodium chloride/kg body weight in three daily doses have been recommended for this purpose (Osborne, et al., 1975). In addition, 25 mg sodium bicarbonate/kg body weight/day in three divided doses should be given. During administration, changes in the patient's weight, blood pressure, and acid-base status should be monitored. In patients with pre-existing hypertension, moderate acidosis, cardiac insufficiency, or nephrotic syndrome, such therapy must be monitored very carefully, and discontinued if complications occur.

Moderate to severe metabolic acidosis is a consistent abnormality in uremic patients. Metabolic acidosis contributes substantially to the clinical signs of uremia and therefore should be corrected with appropriate therapy. Serum bicarbonate concentrations may be increased by administering sodium bicarbonate or metabolically equivalent agents such as sodium lactate or sodium citrate. The dosage of these drugs is variable and depends upon the severity of acidosis. Sufficient sodium bicarbonate should be given to maintain serum bicarbonate concentra-

tions above 18 mEq/liter. The initial dosage of 25 to 35 mg/kg body weight per day can be modified as based on knowledge of serial determinations of serum bicarbonate concentration.

NEPHROTIC SYNDROME, CONGESTIVE HEART FAILURE, AND EDEMATOUS STATES

The nephrotic syndrome and congestive heart failure are clinical states associated with sodium retention and excess total body sodium content. Treatment in these situations should consist of sodium restriction to reduce ECF volume and careful use of diuretic agents as needed. Oral furosemide at a dosage of 3 to 5 mg/kg body weight once or twice daily is usually satisfactory. Care must be exercised to avoid hypotension or hypovolemia in these patients. Diuretics should be used cautiously in patients with profound hypoalbuminemia and marked reductions in "effective arterial blood volume" in order to prevent precipitous reductions in blood pressure and renal perfusion.

SUPPLEMENTAL READING

Bovée, K.: Medical management of polyuric primary renal failure. In Kirk, R.W. (ed.): *Current Veterinary Therapy VI*. Philadelphia, W.B. Saunders Co., 1977.

Danovitch, F.M., Bourgoignie, J., and Bricker, N.S.: Reversibility of the "salt-losing" tendency of chronic renal failure. N. Engl. J. Med., *296*:14–19, 1977.

Osborne, C.A., Finco, D.R., and Low, D.G.: Renal failure: Diagnosis, treatment, and prognosis. In Ettinger, S.J. (ed.): *Textbook of Veterinary Internal Medicine*. Philadelphia, W.B. Saunders Co., 1975.

Osborne, C. A., Low, D.G., and Finco, D.R.: *Canine and Feline Urology*. Philadelphia, W.B. Saunders Co., 1972.

Schmidt, R.W., Bourgoignie, J.J., and Bricker, N.S.: On the adaptation in sodium excretion in chronic uremia. The effect of "proportional reduction" of sodium. J. Clin. Invest., *53*:1736–1741, 1974.

Schultze, R.G., Shapiro, H.S., and Bricker, N.S.: Studies on the control of sodium excretion in experimental uremia. J. Clin. Invest., *48*:869–877, 1969.

Weiser, M.G., Spangler, W. L., and Gribble, D.H.: Blood pressure measurements in the dog. J. Am. Vet. Med. Assoc., *171*:364–368, 1977.

CONSERVATIVE MANAGEMENT OF POLYURIC PRIMARY RENAL FAILURE: DIET THERAPY

DAVID J. POLZIN, D.V.M.
and CARL A. OSBORNE, D.V.M.
St. Paul, Minnesota

OVERVIEW

Uremia is not directly caused by renal lesions but rather is a syndrome associated with fluid, electrolyte, acid-base, and nutritional imbalances, vitamin and endocrine alterations, and retention of protein catabolites that develop as a result of reduced renal function. At present, conservative medical management of companion animals with primary polyuric renal failure consists of variable combinations of the following: (1) oral administration of sodium chloride and sodium bicarbonate, (2) oral administration of multiple vitamins, (3) oral administration of phosphate-binding compounds when appropriate, (4) unlimited access to water, (5) administration of anabolic agents, (6) dietary regulation, (7) administration of vitamin D when appropriate, and (8) avoidance of conditions associated with body stress. While conservative management of renal failure does not reverse or eliminate renal lesions, it does minimize metabolic, biochemical, endocrine, and nutritional abnormalities associated with the uremic state. In addition, clinical evidence in man and experimental evidence in rats and dogs suggests that conservative management initiated early in the course of chronic renal failure may delay its progression significantly.

The objective of this discussion is to provide the rationale and objectives of diet therapy in the management of dogs with primary polyuric renal failure. While the major emphasis of dietary regulation in renal failure has historically been placed on the quantity and quality of protein ingested, formulation of therapeutic diets also includes: (1) non-protein calories, (2) minerals (including calcium, phosphorus, sodium, and potassium), and (3) vitamins (including B-complex vitamins and, when appropriate, vitamin D). Failure to consider these components of the diet may result in a suboptimal therapeutic response.

APPLIED BIOCHEMISTRY

Understanding the rationale and formulation of therapeutic diets for patients with renal failure requires conceptual knowledge of the biochemistry of protein, fat, and carbohydrate metabolism. Proteins are composed principally of amino acids, which in turn are composed of hydrogen, oxygen, carbon, nitrogen, and sometimes sulfur. Some amino acids can be manufactured from these basic elements by the body in sufficient quantities to meet daily needs, and therefore they are commonly called "non-essential amino acids." "Essential amino acids" are those that cannot be manufactured by the body rapidly enough to meet the body's needs. For nitrogen balance to be maintained they must be provided by the diet. The nine essential amino acids required by dogs are tryptophan, threonine, histidine, lysine, leucine, isoleucine, methionine, valine, and phenylalanine. Arginine becomes an essential amino acid in dogs during growth periods.

Each body protein is composed of a unique combination of essential and non-essential amino acids. If one or more essential amino acids are deficient or missing from the diet, or if inadequate amounts are absorbed from the gastrointestinal tract, proteins requiring these amino acids cannot be manufactured. Remaining unused amino acids are not stored for times of deficiency but are excreted unchanged in urine and catabolized for energy as carbohydrates and fats are. The non-nitrogenous portions of amino acids are converted to energy, whereas amino groups are converted to non-protein nitrogenous waste products. These metabolic waste products are eliminated from the body primarily in urine.

Biologic value or biologic index rating is an expression of protein quality and is measured as the quantity of nutrient absorbed compared with the quantity retained in the body. The

1097

biologic value of a protein is rated by the percentage of absorbed nitrogen retained in the body after ingestion and digestion. It is based on a scale of 0 to 100. Proteins of high biologic value contain the nine or ten essential amino acids in proportions similar to those required for protein anabolism. Examples of proteins of high biologic value (BV) include eggs (BV = 94), milk (BV = 84), and lean meats (BV = 70 to 80). Proteins of low biologic value do not contain all the essential amino acids in optimum quantities and ratios. In general, vegetable proteins have a lower biologic value than animal proteins because they are often deficient in one or more essential amino acids. Additionally, digestion of vegetable proteins is frequently less complete.

A significantly reduced intake of high-biologic-value proteins is required to produce nitrogen equilibrium, compared with consumption of proteins with a suboptimum amount of essential amino acids. As biologic value is reduced, daily requirements of essential amino acids can be met only by ingesting greater quantities of protein. Alternatively, the diet may be supplemented with the deficient amino acids. Consumption of excess quantities of essential and non-essential amino acids results in their catabolism for energy and production of an increased quantity of metabolic waste products that must be eliminated from the body by the kidneys. Waste products of protein catabolism include urea, creatinine, guanidinoacetic acid, methylguanidine, hydrogen ions, potassium, phosphate, sulfate, and many others.

While a direct cause-and-effect relationship has not been proved in many instances, it is a well-accepted fact that protein catabolites contribute significantly to the production of uremic signs in patients with renal failure. Patients with primary renal failure have an impaired ability to excrete protein catabolites because of marked reduction in glomerular filtration rate. Retention of metabolic waste may be further aggravated by alterations in tubular reabsorption and tubular secretion and by extrarenal factors that cause reduction in renal perfusion or increased catabolism of body tissue, or both. Metabolism of carbohydrates and fats for energy results in the production of carbon dioxide and water. Since these metabolites may be excreted via non-renal routes, they are not likely to contribute to abnormalities associated with uremia.

The body's demand for energy has a higher priority than protein anabolism. When carbohydrates and fats are not available in sufficient quantities to meet caloric requirements, proteins will be catabolized as a source of energy.

Catabolism of large quantities of protein for energy results in retention of protein catabolites and thus causes associated clinical signs. Therefore, provision of adequate quantities of non-protein calories (carbohydrates and fats) is important in the determination of protein requirements because they have a protein-sparing effect. In states of caloric deficit amino acids will be metabolized for energy, regardless of the body's need to maintain nitrogen balance.

RATIONALE OF DIET THERAPY

The rationale of nutritional management of patients with primary renal failure is based on the premise that controlled reduction of non-essential proteins will result in decreased production of nitrogenous wastes, with consequent amelioration of some clinical signs. By formulating diets that contain the minimum quantity of high-biologic-value protein that will maintain nitrogen balance and by providing adequate quantities of non-protein calories, many of the signs associated with uremia may be reduced in severity or eliminated, even though renal function remains unchanged.

THERAPEUTIC GOALS AND IMPLEMENTATION

GOALS

The goals of diet therapy in the management of patients with chronic primary renal failure are summarized in Table 1. Modification of

Table 1. *Goals of Long-Term Dietary Therapy of Chronic Polyuric Renal Failure*

1. Ameliorate clinical signs of uremia by reducing production of protein catabolites, including:
   a. urea　　　　　　　　d. methylguanidine
   b. creatinine　　　　　e. others
   c. guanidinoacetic acid
2. Minimize electrolyte, vitamin, and mineral disturbances associated with consumption of excessive or reduced quantities of protein in patients with renal failure, including:
   a. hydrogen　　　　　　f. calcium
   b. sulfate　　　　　　　g. B vitamins
   c. phosphate　　　　　h. vitamin D
   d. potassium　　　　　i. others
   e. sodium
3. Supply daily protein and caloric requirements.
   a. Protein and caloric requirements for uremic patients are unknown but are probably variable.
   b. We currently recommend 1.25 gm/kg (0.57 gm/lb) high-biologic-value protein.
   c. We currently recommend 70 to 110 kcal/kg body weight (30 to 50 kcal/lb). A minimum of 1.3 gm/kg (0.6 gm/lb) fat and 10.1 gm/kg (4.6 gm/lb) carbohydrates may be used in formulating this requirement.

diets to minimize deficits and excesses of metabolites associated with generalized renal dysfunction is not an all-or-nothing phenomenon, however. In our experience the best results associated with proper modification of diets have been achieved when other components of conservative medical management are also included in therapy. Consult other articles and reference material for specific details. While diet therapy is often of value in controlling some of the polysystemic disturbances associated with uremia, it is not a panacea that can be expected to control or modify all dysfunctions associated with primary renal failure.

PROTEIN REQUIREMENTS

The minimum requirement for high-biologic-value protein for normal dogs has been reported to be approximately 1.25 gm/kg body weight/day (Rice, et al.; Corbin, et al.). In one study in dogs, however, it was reported that the daily requirement for high-biologic-value protein varied from 1.25 to 1.75 gm/kg body weight/day (Morris and Doering).

Optimal protein and amino acid requirements for uremic dogs have not been established. Based on the assumption that non-essential amino acids could be synthesized using ammonium derived from protein degradation in the intestines, it has been suggested that patients with renal failure might have reduced dietary protein requirements. However, recent data indicate that urea nitrogen is not significantly utilized for protein synthesis in uremic human patients.

Reducing high-quality protein intake to levels below those required by normal dogs for maintenance of nitrogen balance may be harmful, unless the minimum protein requirement for uremic dogs is substantially less than that required for normal dogs. Recent evidence obtained from studies in rats and human beings with chronic renal failure suggests that consumption of ultralow-protein diets may result in malnourishment. There is convincing evidence that protein requirements for *some* human patients with chronic renal failure may be higher than normal (as much as double).

Protein and amino acid requirements of uremic patients may be altered by pathophysiologic disturbances associated with the uremic syndrome, including (1) glucose intolerance, (2) impaired intestinal absorption of amino acids, (3) impaired tubular reabsorption of amino acids, (4) decreased activity of intestinal dipeptidases and disaccharidases that may result in impaired digestion of carbohydrates, and (5) elevated serum concentration of some hormones, such as glycogen and insulin. In addition, acidosis has been reported to stimulate urea production. Both total-body potassium depletion and hyperkalemia have been reported to promote protein catabolism. Protein requirements may also be increased as a result of albuminuria, hematuria, gastrointestinal hemorrhage, and other conditions.

Considering the intrinsic variability in normal dogs and the multifactorial influences of uremia on protein requirements, it is probable that protein requirements of uremic dogs are variable. Because of this variability, attempts should be made to individualize dietary protein requirements according to patient needs.

CALORIC REQUIREMENTS

Minimum daily requirements for calories (carbohydrates and fats) in dogs have not been established under conditions of renal failure. Because this information is unavailable, it has been necessary to make the unproved assumption that the minimum requirement for these nutrients in uremic animals is the same as that required for normal animals. Accordingly, most investigators have recommended that dogs receive 70 to 110 kcal/kg body weight/day. A minimum of 1.3 gm/kg fat and 10.1 gm/kg carbohydrate may be used in formulating this requirement. Since carbohydrate, fat, and caloric requirements for uremic dogs may be affected by pathophysiologic disturbances associated with uremia (including glucose intolerance, decreased intestinal peptidases and disaccharidases, and elevated serum insulin and glycogen concentrations), these values should be used as guidelines only. Determination of caloric requirements must be individualized on the basis of serial body weight determinations. Unless the patient is markedly obese and weight reduction is deemed necessary, an attempt should be made to maintain stable body weight. If the animal is malnourished, caloric intake should be increased for an appropriate period.

VITAMIN AND MINERAL REQUIREMENTS

Minimum daily requirements for vitamins and minerals have not been established under conditions of renal failure. It has been assumed that the minimum requirements for these nutrients is the same as that required for normal animals; however, studies in other species suggest that this assumption may be incorrect. For example, human patients with renal failure often develop hypervitaminosis A and therefore do not require dietary supplementation with this vitamin. Excess vitamin A may directly or indirectly increase parathormone release and therefore enhance the development of renal osteodystrophy and acidosis.

It has been recommended that dietary intake of B-complex vitamins and vitamin C be supplemented because of their inadequate renal conservation. When possible, dietary calcium, phosphorus, and vitamin D requirements should also be considered.

PRODUCTS FOR THERAPY

COMMERCIAL PREPARATIONS (PRESCRIPTION DIETS)

During the past few years, several investigators have questioned the therapeutic value of prescription diets formulated especially for dogs with primary renal failure. Specifically, they have stated that many prescription diets may contain amounts of protein in excess of the minimum daily requirement for high-biologic-value protein required by normal adult dogs and therefore have not been formulated to achieve maximum therapeutic benefit. Prescription diets with a reduced quantity of high-biologic-value protein (U/D) having been marketed recently. Studies of comparative feeding trials utilizing dogs with a known degree of primary renal dysfunction are currently in progress at the University of Minnesota to answer questions about the therapeutic efficacy of prescription diets. Although a more ideal "homemade" diet may be formulated to meet an individual patient's needs, prescription diets are often superior to "regular" commercially prepared dog foods in minimizing signs of primary renal failure. Advantages of prescription diets include convenience and elimination of client error in preparation of the diet. A disadvantage of prescription diets is that individualization of the diet to suit the patient's need is more difficult. Failure to adapt the diet to a patient's needs may result in suboptimum therapeutic response.

HOMEMADE DIETS

Formulation of diets for use in patients with polyuric renal failure should be based on the recommendations and goals stated earlier. The advantage of formulating diets from natural sources is that it permits individualization of the diet to suit an individual patient's needs and taste. Natural proteins of high biologic value include cooked eggs, lean meats, chicken, and dairy products. Proteins of low biologic value that should be avoided include most plant proteins, meat byproducts, gelatin, and dehydrated meat and fish meal. Sources of non-protein calories include commercially prepared products, butter, margarine, vegetable oils, jellies, sugar, honey, and candy. High-caloric-value foods with a minimum quantity of protein include spaghetti, macaroni, pancakes, rice, cake, bread, cookies, crackers, potato chips, and pretzels.

SUMMARY OF RECOMMENDATIONS

Until additional information based on controlled diet trials utilizing dogs with a known degree of renal dysfunction becomes available, it is recommended that dogs with primary polyuric renal failure be given diets formulated according to the following guidelines:

INITIATION OF THERAPY

There are no controlled studies that indicate when initiation of dietary therapy is beneficial. Therefore, the decision about when to begin using low-protein diets remains a matter of personal opinion. Formulation of high-quality, low-quantity protein diets will not prevent renal failure or reverse established renal lesions. Recent information derived from experimental studies in rats suggests that long-term control of hyperphosphatemia and hyperparathormonemia — abnormalities that occur during early phases of progressive renal failure — may be of value in minimizing the development of polysystemic clinical signs and perhaps the progression of generalized renal disease.

PROTEIN

Approximately 1.25 gm/kg body weight (0.6 gm/lb) high-biologic-value protein (egg or its equivalent)/day should be provided. The amount of protein given should be the maximum that the patient can tolerate at its given degree of renal dysfunction. Ideally, none of the protein should be catabolized for energy. Additional amounts of high-quality protein may be required to balance protein loss caused by severe proteinuria (e.g., addition of 1 gram of protein in the diet for each gram of protein lost in urine per day). This recommendation is especially applicable to patients with hypoproteinemia. The number of grams of protein lost in urine per unit of time may be determined with the aid of a metabolism cage and should be correlated with serum protein concentration.

CALORIES

Approximately 70 to 110 kcal/kg body weight/day (30 to 50 kcal/lb/day) should be provided. Since the caloric requirement per pound of body weight tends to vary inversely with total body weight, small adult dogs (approximately 2 to 5 kg) should receive approximately 110 kcal/kg body weight, whereas large dogs (more than 25 kg) should receive approximately 65 to 70 kcal/kg body weight. At least 1.3 gm/kg body weight/day should consist of fat. At least 10.1 gm/kg body weight/day should consist of carbohydrate. Additional modifications of caloric intake may be required to compensate for the nutritional status and activity of the patient. Steady weight over a period of weeks or months is usually a reliable index of adequate caloric intake.

VITAMINS

Therapeutic supplements of B-complex vitamins and vitamin C should be provided. A single high-potency capsule containing these water-soluble vitamins given daily is probably sufficient for most patients.

PALATABILITY

Loss of palatability may be associated with restricted-protein diets. Palatability may be enhanced by (1) warming the food to create an appetizing odor, (2) flavoring the food with small quantities of meat or animal fat (e.g., gravy or butter), and (3) dividing the diet into three to four meals daily.

MONITORING RESPONSE

Patient re-evaluation at regular intervals is necessary to assess response to therapy. Diet formulation may be altered on the basis of these re-evaluations. Routine physical examination, evaluation of hydration, determination of body weight, and evaluation of the owner's impressions of therapeutic response are essential. Certain laboratory evaluations should also be considered. Because restriction of dietary protein may reduce the concentration of serum urea nitrogen without any significant improvement in renal function, it is recommended that both serum urea nitrogen and creatinine concentrations be evaluated as indices of therapeutic response. Reduction of urea nitrogen concentration associated with a stable creatinine concentration usually suggests a favorable therapeutic response.

Periodic evaluation of the serum concentration of phosphorus and determination of blood pH and plasma bicarbonate (or total CO_2 or CO_2 content) may indicate the need for supplemental forms of therapy to control hyperphosphatemia and metabolic acidosis.

SUPPLEMENTAL READING

Bovée, K.C.: What constitutes a low protein diet for dogs with chronic renal failure? J. Am. Anim. Hosp. Assoc., 8:246, 1972.

Corbin, J.E., Lehrer, W.P., Newberne, P.M., Visek, W.J., and Wiese, H.F.: Nutrient requirements of domestic animals: Nutritional requirements of dogs. Publ. No. 8. Washington, D.C., National Academy of Science/National Research Council, 1972.

Ibels, L.S., et al.: Preservation of function in experimental renal disease by dietary restriction of phosphate. N. Engl. J. Med., 298:122–126, 1978.

Morris, M.L., and Doering, G.G.: Dietary management of renal failure in dogs. Canine Pract., 5:46–52, 1978.

Osborne, C.A., and Polzin, D.J.: Strategy in the diagnosis, prognosis, and management of renal disease, renal failure, and uremia. In Scientific Proceedings of the 46th Annual Meeting of the American Animal Hospital Association, South Bend, Indiana, 1979.

Osborne, C.A., Stevens, J.B., and Polzin, D.J.: Gastrointestinal manifestations of urinary diseases. In Anderson, N.V. (ed.): *Veterinary Gastroenterology*. Philadelphia, Lea & Febiger (in press.).

Rice, E.E., Allison, J.B., Corbin, J.E., Engel, R.W., and Herman, V.: Nutrient requirements of domestic animals: Nutrient requirements of dogs. Publ. No. 989. Washington, D.C. National Academy of Science/National Research Council, 1962.

Walser, M.: The conservative management of the uremic patient. In Brenner, B.M., and Rector, F.C. (eds.): *The Kidney*. Philadelphia, W.B. Saunders Co., 1976.

Walser, M., and Mitch, W.: Dietary management of renal failure. Kidney, *10*:13, 1977.

MEDICAL MANAGEMENT OF POLYURIC RENAL FAILURE: ANABOLIC AGENTS

DONALD G. LOW, D.V.M.

Davis, California

Some of the physiologic effects of androgens have been known since prehistoric times, but it has been only in the past 25 years that accepted, well-documented pharmacologic uses of anabolic steroids, which essentially are structural modifications of testosterone, have been established. These molecular alterations have been made in an attempt to maximize their beneficial effects while minimizing their undesirable virilizing effects. The physiologic and pharmacologic effects of anabolic steroids, which are of interest in the medical management of polyuric renal failure, are promotion of positive nitrogen balance and stimulation of production of erythropoietin and erythropoiesis.

Definitive studies on the use of anabolic steroids in the treatment of chronic progressive renal failure have not been made in clinical veterinary medicine. Clinical impressions among some veterinarians are that the response of dogs and cats in chronic renal failure is similar, in a qualitative sense, to that of man. The recommendations made here are tentative. They are based largely on uncontrolled clinical observations in dogs and cats with primary renal failure and on information transferred from studies done in man and experimental animals.

Anabolic steroids have been shown in man and experimental animals to stimulate the production or release, or both, of erythropoietin from the kidneys. The erythropoietic response of patients to administration of anabolic steroids is better when the kidneys are present than it is when administered to anephric patients. It has been shown in experimental animals that increased production of erythropoietin occurs at least 48 hours following administration of anabolic steroids. The magnitude of the erythropoietic response is roughly proportional to the amount of erythropoietin available, and the amount of erythropoietin available bears a relationship to the quantity of functional renal tissue present.

Anabolic steroids also stimulate undifferentiated stem cells in bone marrow to enter an erythroid-critical stage. This permits the maximum possible red cell response by the marrow to a limited amount of erythropoietin. Carefully controlled experiments in experimental animals indicate that nandrolone decanoate* is the most effective of the currently available anabolic steroids for moving stem cells into the erythroid-critical stage. Increased incorporation of ^{59}Fe into red cells occurs about 48 hours after the increase in erythropoietin concentration or about 96 to 120 hours after administration of nandrolone decanoate. The dose of nandrolone decanoate used in man is 200 mg weekly. Because of the lack of an established veterinary dose, it is suggested that 5 mg per kg per week, with a maximum dose of 200 mg, be used in dogs for an indefinite time.

Maximum nitrogen retention occurs about five days after administration of the anabolic steroid, plateaus after 15 to 20 days, and is maintained during continued administration. Cessation of administration results in rebound nitrogen excretion and a return to baseline levels after about ten days.

Subjective benefits from nandrolone decanoate reported in man include an improved sense of well-being, improved strength, and increased physical activity. Such observations are harder to make in animals, but the changes may very well occur.

Contraindications that have been established for anabolic steroids include use in patients with prostatic cancer (an unusual disease in dogs and cats), nephrosis or edematous states, and liver disease. If anabolic steroids are used continuously over a long period, liver function should be monitored periodically.

SUPPLEMENTAL READING

Gorschein, D., Murphy, S., and Gardner, F.H.: Comparative study on the erythropoietic effects of androgens and their mode of action. J. Appl. Physiol., 35:376–378, 1973.

Doane, B.D., Fried, W., and Schwartz, F.: Response of uremic patients to nandrolone decanoate. Arch. Intern. Med., 135:972–975, 1975.

*Decadurabolin, Organon, Inc., Orange, N.J.

MEDICAL MANAGEMENT OF CHRONIC RENAL FAILURE: CONTROL OF HYPERPHOSPHATEMIA

K. C. BOVÉE, D.V.M.
Philadelphia, Pennsylvania

Elevated serum inorganic phosphate levels occur during moderate and severe chronic renal failure. Serum phosphate concentration usually ranges from 6 to 20 mg/dl. Dogs with serum phosphate elevations of less than 10 mg/dl can usually be treated successfully.

Hyperphosphatemia is associated with a group of metabolic disturbances that includes osteodystrophy, hyperparathyroidism, and reduced intestinal calcium absorption. These disturbances are very important in the pathogenesis of chronic renal failure. Since hyperphosphatemia is one of the initiators and co-factors in the perpetuation of these metabolic disturbances, reduction of phosphate retention may result in an amelioration of these defects. The objective of therapy is to reduce the severity of hyperparathyroidism, soft-tissue calcification, and bicarbonate loss in the urine and to increase calcium absorption from the intestine by reducing serum inorganic phosphate concentration to normal or near-normal levels.

DIETARY RESTRICTION

Long-term dietary phosphate restriction may help to reduce phosphate retention. Low phosphate intake occurs with the extremely low-protein diets used in renal failure, since meats and dairy products contain high levels of phosphate. Therefore, a low-protein diet will generally be a reduced-phosphate diet. Commercial dog foods, including most special products for dogs with renal disease, deliver more than 100 mg of phosphate/kg body weight/day. Although the exact quantity of dietary phosphate required to control hyperphosphatemia in dogs has not been determined, experimental evidence suggests that it would be approximately 10 percent of the standard intake (Slatopolsky, et al.). Therefore, it is recommended that usual commercial diets be avoided. Home-prepared diets using foodstuffs shown in Table 1 are recom-

Table 1. Foods Recommended for Use in Renal Failure

FOOD	PROTEIN (Grams)	ENERGY (Kcal)
Bread or toast, 1 slice	2.0	60
Butter or margarine, 1 tsp	–	40
Cake or cupcake	2.6	130
pound, 1 slice 2 × 3 × 5	2.1	130
sponge, 2″ slice	3.2	120
Candy: caramel, 1 oz	0.8	120
chocolate, sweetened, 1 oz	2.0	140
Cream cheese, 1 oz	2.6	106
Cream, light, 1 oz	–	50
Doughnut, 1	2.1	130
Eggs, cooked, 1	7.0	120
Gravy, 1 tbsp	–	80
Ice cream, 1 oz	1.2	62
Jelly, 1 tsp	–	60
Milk, whole, 2 oz	2.0	40
Pancakes, wheat, 4″ diameter	1.8	60
Sweet roll, 4 × 1″, 50 gm	4.2	160
Rice, cooked, 1 cup	4.2	200
Soups:		
bouillon or consomme, 1 cup	2.0	9
chicken, 1 cup	3.5	75
Spaghetti, cooked, 1 cup	7.4	220
Sugar or honey, 1 tsp	–	20

mended. The diets should be designed to deliver 0.6 gm of protein/kg body weight and approximately 70 kcal/kg body weight/day. These foods consist principally of carbohydrates and lipids. In addition, an increased calcium intake may be helpful to depress the effects of hyperparathyroidism and osteodystrophy. Supplementation with approximately 50 mg/kg body weight of calcium carbonate or calcium gluconate is recommended each day. Vitamin D therapy has also been recommended, but dosages for dogs have not been established. Vitamin D therapy should not be used if the serum calcium-phosphate product is greater than 70; otherwise, soft-tissue calcification may occur. In some cases a reduced dietary phosphate intake is inadequate to lower or maintain plasma phosphate concentration. In these cases orally administered intestinal phosphate binders in addition to restriction of phosphate may be used.

INTESTINAL PHOSPHATE BINDERS

Phosphate binders administered orally before meals may be helpful to minimize hyperphosphatemia. These aluminum salts combine with phosphate in the intestinal lumen and result in elimination of aluminum phosphate in the stool. These products are available as aluminum hydroxide suspensions or aluminum carbonate capsules. Our experience with the aluminum

hydroxide suspensions is that 5 to 10 ml given orally three times per day before meals will control hyperphosphatemia. Most aluminum hydroxide suspensions contain approximately 900 mg of aluminum hydroxide/15 ml. Since the severity of hyperphosphatemia is dependent on the degree of renal failure and dietary phosphate intake, the dosage of these products must be individualized for each case.

SUPPLEMENTAL READING

Slatopolsky, E., et al.: On the pathogenesis of hyperparathyroidism in chronic experimental renal insufficiency in the dog. J. Clin. Invest., 50:492–499, 1971.

NUTRITION DURING THE UREMIC CRISIS

DELMAR R. FINCO, D.V.M.
Athens, Georgia

Considerable attention has been given to dietary management of renal failure in the dog. This attention has been motivated by the belief that a diet is beneficial to the azotemic dog if it (1) fulfills the dog's need for calories from non-protein sources, (2) contains "adequate" vitamins, minerals, and essential fatty acids, and (3) has a protein content that maintains nitrogen balance in the dog without leading to catabolism of ingested amino acids (i.e., protein) to nitrogenous wastes. The character, formulation, and controversy concerning such diets is discussed elsewhere (see article entitled "Conservative Management of Polyuric Renal Failure: Diet Therapy").

Paradoxically, nutrition in the azotemic dog during periods of anorexia and vomiting (i.e., a uremic crisis) has received little attention. Because of lack of oral intake, this patient requires nutritional therapy by parenteral means.

In order to evaluate the benefits and limitations of parenteral nutritional therapy during a uremic crisis, knowledge of some background information on metabolism during uremia and starvation is required.

DELETERIOUS EFFECTS OF ANOREXIA ON THE UREMIC DOG

The uremic crisis is usually characterized by a severe catabolic state. Because of lack of intake, body tissues must be degraded to provide calories for maintenance of function. Muscle and hepatic stores of glycogen probably are depleted within 48 hours. Thereafter, calories are provided by breakdown of lipid stores and body proteins. Unfortunately, lipid stores are not preferentially utilized. Proteins of body tissues (especially muscle because of its large mass) are catabolized to provide the calories required to sustain life. Dogs with chronic azotemia are especially vulnerable to catabolic events of the uremic crisis, since a decrease in their lipid stores often precedes the onset of the crisis.

Breakdown of lean body tissue is more important in uremic patients than in patients with simple starvation because of the biochemical products of catabolism. Catabolism of tissues with a high protein content has the same effect on production of nitrogenous wastes as oral intake of a diet of meat. The obvious difference is that the tissue in the case of the uremic crisis is a component of the patient's own body. The toxins of uremia have not been biochemically defined but appear to be produced in association with protein catabolism. Consequently, the end result of anorexia in uremic dogs is an increase in production of uremic toxins during the period of catabolism. A phenomenon occurs in which uremic toxin production, anorexia, and catabolism create a self-perpetuating cycle.

CAPABILITIES OF THE UREMIC PATIENT TO REVERSE THE CATABOLIC STATE

Since catabolism manifested as weight loss is known to occur prior to anorexia and vomiting associated with uremic crises, it is reasonable to question whether reversal of catabolism can be achieved even when appropriate nutrients are supplied. It is known that certain metabolic alterations exist during the uremic state. These include glucose intolerance and altered lipid and amino acid metabolism. Despite these formidable adversities, nutritional treatment of uremic human beings has resulted not only in a reversal of catabolism but also in the production of an anabolic state. During therapy, BUN values have decreased coincident with the administration of amino acids. An experimental study in nephrectomized dogs revealed that life could be prolonged by providing nutritional therapy with dextrose and amino acids. Dogs given food and water *ad lib.* survived 4 ± 1 days. Dogs infused with 50 ml/kg/24 hr of 5 percent dextrose survived 5 ± 1 days. Dogs that received 50 ml/kg/24 hr of 56 percent dextrose survived 8 ± 3 days. Dogs given 50 ml/kg/24 hr of a solution containing 56 percent dextrose and 0.525 gm/kg of essential L-amino acids survived 10 ± 4 days. Serum creatinine levels increased at the same rate in dogs on all regimens of therapy, but dogs receiving amino acids had markedly lower BUN values than the other three groups. These data clearly demonstrate the benefits of nutritional therapy during uremia and emphasize the deleterious effects if nutritional therapy is ignored.

METHODS OF CORRECTING NUTRITIONAL DEFICIENCIES DURING THE UREMIC CRISIS

OBJECTIVES

The objectives of parenteral nutritional therapy are nearly the same as those for oral therapy prior to the uremic crisis. Fulfillment of the maintenance caloric requirements of the dog from non-protein sources is probably the most important step. In addition, it is beneficial to provide just enough amino acids in the correct proportion for nitrogen balance or anabolism. Administration of water-soluble vitamins is also important, but giving fatty acids and trace minerals is indicated only if therapy is conducted for several weeks.

SOURCES OF NON-PROTEIN CALORIES

Dextrose solutions are available for use from numerous manufacturers. Five percent dextrose is an inadequate source of calories unless massive volumes of fluid are used (see *Current Veterinary Therapy VI*, pp. 3–12). Twenty to 25 percent solutions are sufficiently concentrated to fulfill caloric requirements in reasonable volumes of fluid.

A lipid emulsion is now available in the United States for use in humans.* This product is apparently safe for dogs, although other lipid emulsions sold in Europe have caused fatalities in dogs. Lipid emulsions have the advantage of being a concentrated source of calories that do not have the hyperosmotic property of concentrated glucose solutions. Their current cost prohibits their routine use in veterinary medicine.

SOURCES OF AMINO ACIDS

Solutions of protein (casein, fibrin) hydrolysates have been available for years.† The hydrolyzed solution is supplemented with essential amino acids to provide a reasonably balanced product. Because hydrolysis of the protein is not complete, however, only about 75 percent of the contents are actually retained for anabolism after injection.

More recently, parenteral preparations of "semisynthetic" amino acids have become available.‡ These products are devoid of unutilizable polypeptide chains, but their cost is nearly twice that of protein hydrolysates. It has been stated that administration of essential amino acids alone is advantageous since the non-essential amino acids can be synthesized by the body.

Keto acids and hydroxyacids have recently attracted considerable attention for use in uremic human beings. Studies revealed that some

---

*Intralipid 10%, Cutter Laboratories, Berkeley, California

†Aminosol 5, 10%, Abbott Laboratories, Chicago, Illinois; Amigen 5, 10%, Baxter Laboratories, Morton Grove, Illinois

‡Aminosyn, Abbott Laboratories, Chicago, Illinois; Freamine, McGaw Laboratories, Glendale, California

analogs of essential amino acids that are devoid of nitrogen could be converted to amino acids in uremic individuals. Species variation in the ability to make the conversion and the efficiency of conversion exists. These compounds have potential advantages over amino acids, since nitrogen that would otherwise be excreted as harmful wastes is used to convert the keto or hydroxy acid to an amino acid, which can then be used for anabolism. BUN values even lower than those obtained with amino acid solutions result from use of these compounds. An additional benefit appears to be a stimulation of anabolism to levels beyond those attainable by amino acids and with a residual effect once the analogs are no longer administered. These compounds are not available for commerical use at the present time. Specific studies in dogs are required in order to assess their efficacy.

PROGRAMS FEASIBLE FOR THE DOG

The first priority for nutrition of dogs during uremic crises is to provide non-protein calories in adequate quantities to minimize catabolism. The daily caloric requirements of dogs are determined; 20 or 25 percent dextrose is used to provide these calories. The solution is given slowly via jugular catheter in order to avoid complications of extracellular hyperosmolality. The program can be conveniently combined with that of intensive diuresis (see the article entitled "Intensive Diuresis in Renal Failure"). Since about 20 percent of the glucose may be lost during the diuresis program, daily requirements should be increased by this increment. Precautions listed for intensive diuresis should be strictly followed. Since dextrose is relatively inexpensive, this procedure is economically feasible. A minor negative nitrogen balance will exist with this program because nitrogen losses are inevitable.

Use of amino acids in addition to dextrose increases the cost of the procedure but provides potential for establishing nitrogen balance. Data are not available in the dog concerning the superiority of semisynthetic preparations over hydrolysates. Likewise, the amino acid requirements of the uremic dog are not known. Until more specific data are available, it is recommended that 0.3 gm/kg/24 hr of a balanced amino acid solution be provided to dogs in a uremic crisis. Thus, for a 20-kg dog 6 gm, or 125 ml, of an amino acid solution would be required each day. Since amino acids may spill over in the urine, slow administration over the course of each day is advisable.

SUPPLEMENTAL READING

Abel, R.M., et al.: Improved survival from acute renal failure after treatment with intravenous essential L-amino acids and glucose. N. Engl. J. Med., 288:696–699, 1973.
Kopple, J.D., and Swendseid, M.E.: Amino acids and keto acid diets for therapy in renal failure. Nephron, 18:1–12, 1972.
Van Buren, C.T., et al.: Effects of intravenous essential L-amino acids and hypertonic dextrose on anephric beagles. Surg. Forum, 23:83–84, 1972.
Walzer, M.: Keto acid therapy in chronic renal failure. Nephron, 21:57–75, 1978.

CURRENT STATUS OF PERITONEAL DIALYSIS

HAROLD R. PARKER, D.V.M.
Davis, California

Peritoneal dialysis has proved to be a valuable aid in treatment of acute renal failure, decompensated chronic renal failure, and certain fluid and electrolyte imbalances. It can also be useful in acute peritonitis and pancreatitis. By using hyperosmotic dialysate solutions containing 4.25 percent or 7 percent glucose to reduce plasma volume, fluid overload and pulmonary edema have been improved. Rationale for its use is not to cure renal failure but to prevent death from uremia while allowing reversible renal lesions a chance to heal. For economic reasons one should not anticipate its use as a long-term substitute for kidney function in end-stage renal disease.

PHYSICAL ASPECTS

The process of dialysis depends on diffusion of small particles and water through a semipermeable membrane. Larger particles are restricted in their movements, whereas ions and small molecules rapidly migrate down a concentration gradient and establish equilibrium on either side of the membrane. The peritoneal membrane permits rapid equilibration between plasma on one side and dialysis fluid in the peritoneal space on the other. The peritoneal membrane consists of four layers: capillary endothelium, basement membrane and epithelium, interstitial space, and peritoneal mesothelium. The ultrastructure of peritoneal mesothelium is similar to capillary endothelium, in which intercellular spaces permit transfer of fluid and small particles. The capillary wall basement membrane is probably the ultimate barrier to transfer of larger solutes of blood.

Several factors influence clearance of various solutes by peritoneal dialysis, including volume of blood flow to the peritoneal membranes, total surface area being utilized, and permeability of peritoneal membranes. Blood flow to splanchnic and peritoneal membranes of dogs is sufficient to permit maximum diffusion of solute, even during mild hypotension. During peritoneal dialysis the rate at which solute is removed depends upon the volume of fluid instilled into the peritoneal space (the surface area used) and the length of time it remains there. Diffusable solutes eventually reach equilibrium between dialysate and extracellular fluid. To a certain point, the larger the volume the greater the dialyzing area. Larger volumes require longer equilibration times, however. On the other hand, larger volumes remove more solute. Filling the peritoneal cavity with fluid has important hemodynamic implications. Abdominal fluid reduces left heart and lung volumes, increases peripheral vascular resistance, and has a tendency to reduce cardiac output. The effects are probably related to interference with venous return. Therefore, coexisting cardiovascular or pulmonary disease must be considered when determining the volume to be used. Thus, a balance must be reached between volumes to be used and time allowed for equilibration (dwell time). Figure 1 graphically depicts rates of diffusion of some substances commonly removed during peritoneal dialysis. Small molecules (like urea and potassium) attained 85

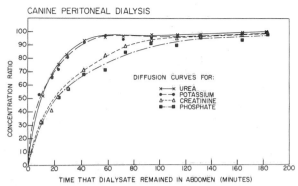

CANINE PERITONEAL DIALYSIS

DIFFUSION CURVES FOR:
×—× UREA
●—● POTASSIUM
△---△ CREATININE
■—■ PHOSPHATE

Figure 1. Fractional approach to equilibrium for urea, potassium, creatinine, and phosphate. Urea and potassium diffused rapidly and reached 85 percent of equilibrium in 40 minutes, while creatinine and phosphate were only 65 percent equilibrated. The flattening shapes of diffusion curves indicate that equilibration periods (dwell times) of 40 minutes or less were most efficient.

percent and larger molecules (like creatinine and phosphate) attained 65 percent of equilibration within 40 minutes. The most rapid diffusion occurred in the first 30 minutes; therefore, there is little advantage to leaving fluid in the abdomen longer than 40 minutes. Leaving fluid in the peritoneal space for extended periods has no deleterious effects other than to prolong the process.

Osmotic forces play an important role in movement of water from plasma to peritoneal fluid. Smaller molecules (like urea) move by bulk flow along with water, thus enhancing the clearance rate for metabolites of uremia. Because water moves from plasma more freely than sodium does, a tendency for hypernatremia exists, especially when hypertonic dialysis fluids are used. Any fluid used for peritoneal dialysis must have at least 1.5 percent glucose to prevent rapid water absorption caused by the hyperosmotic state of uremic plasma. Dialysate should also be warmed several degrees above body temperature to induce vasodilation, which facilitates diffusion and osmotic exchange.

Even though dogs and cats have slightly higher plasma sodium and chloride concentrations than humans, commercial fluids prepared for human peritoneal dialysis are satisfactory for small animals. Most dialysis fluids have a composition and osmolality similar to those summarized in Table 1. Raising glucose concentration increases osmotic movement of water. Dialysis fluids with 4.25 percent or 7 percent glucose can effectively be used to reduce plasma volume to control pulmonary edema or other forms of fluid overload.

Table 1. *Composition of Commercial Peritoneal Dialysis Solutions**

	A	B	C
Sodium (*mEq/liter*)	141	141	141
Calcium (*mEq/liter*)	3.5	3.5	3.5
Magnesium (*mEq/liter*)	1.5	1.5	1.5
Potassium† (*mEq/liter*)	0	0	0
Chloride (*mEq/liter*)	101	101	101
Lactate (*mEq/liter*)	45	45	45
Dextrose‡ (*gm/liter*)	15	42.5	70.0
Osmolality (*mOsm/liter*)	366	505	644

°Dianeal® Peritoneal Dialysis Solution, Travenol Laboratories, Inc., Morton Grove, Illinois 60053

†Potassium is added to 4.0 mEq/liter when the patient's plasma potassium status is known to be safe, or after three or four exchanges that will reduce plasma potassium to a safe concentration.

‡Standard peritoneal dialysis solutions contain 15 gm/liter (1.5%) dextrose (solution A). When ultrafiltration (removal of excess water) is desired, a solution with 42.5 (4.25%) (B) or 70.0 gm/liter (7.0%) (C) dextrose is used.

TECHNICAL ASPECTS

Peritoneal dialysis has been used frequently by veterinarians with variable success. The major deterrent has been the difficulty with which fluids can be removed from the peritoneal cavity. A variety of techniques have been tried. Some clinicians have used the repeated-puncture technique with some success, especially since the development of cannulas-around-a-needle such as the Medicut®* (Fig. 2A) and Angiocath®† (Fig. 2B). Sometimes these have been secured in place for repeated use. Techniques utilizing repeated puncture of the abdominal wall are hazardous because of the increased chance of visceral perforation. Other veterinarians have used commercial cannulas developed for human use, such as the Trocath®‡ (Fig. 2C). These have the disadvantage of being too large for cats and small dogs, and they are hard to seal at the incision site to control leakage. In addition, there is always danger of ascending infection producing peritonitis because of leakage when the catheter is left for use on subsequent days.

The Parker peritoneal dialysis cannula (Fig. 3) has proved to be unusually effective and safe because both ends are secured in a transabdominal position. This feature holds it away from the omentum. The incision site is sealed by a Dacron cuff. Once it has been aseptically placed in the abdominal cavity, it can be used for extended periods. This cannula allows rapid infusion of fluid and quick withdrawal of the

*Ole Medical, St. Louis, Missouri 63103
†Deseret Pharmaceutical Co., Sandy, Utah 84070
‡McGaw Laboratories, Irvine, California 92714

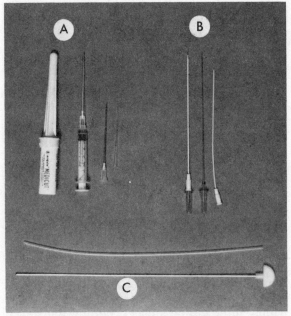

Figure 2. The Medicut® catheter (*A*) comes complete with a syringe and has been used in small dogs and cats. The Angiocath® catheter (*B*) is available with longer cannullae. Both of these over-the-needle type cannulas are available in a variety of lumen sizes. The Trochath® cannula (*C*) is available in adult and pediatric sizes and comes complete with a metal stylet.

total volume. A complete exchange can usually be made in less than one hour, utilizing a dwell time of 30 minutes. Because the cannula is inserted into the flank rather than the ventral abdomen, animals can be dialyzed in their cages (Fig. 4).

Whatever technique is utilized, there is an absolute requirement for strict asepsis. Uremic animals are usually depressed sufficiently to tolerate cannulation under local anesthesia. The body wall must be scrubbed and draped as if for abdominal surgery. A common site for

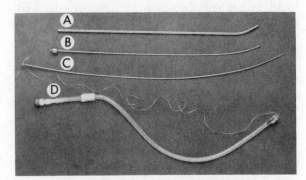

Figure 3. The Parker peritoneal dialysis cannula. From top to bottom, the stainless steel needle guide (*A*), the trochar (*B*), the stainless steel needle (armed with Vetafil suture) (*C*), and the silicone rubber cannula (*D*). The cannula is closed with a tapered plastic adapter and a B-D diaphragm cap Luer-loc plug.

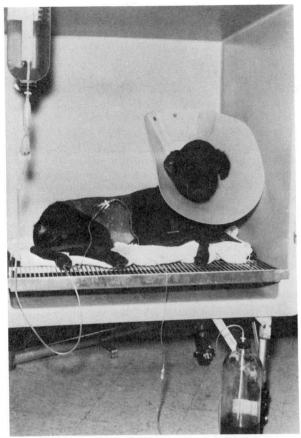

Figure 4. A dog fitted with a Parker Peritoneal Dialysis Cannula protruding from the right flank. The high location of this cannula minimizes leakage and allows the patient to lie comfortably in its cage while being dialyzed. A closed system is essential to prevent ascending infection. A three-way stopcock permits control of fluid flow. The Elizabethan collar prevents the dog from chewing the cannula and tubing. An abdominal wrap between dialyses provides additional protection to the cannula and further reduces chances of contamination.

cannulation is 3 to 4 cm caudal and slightly to the right of the umbilicus. The cannula, whether it is a human peritoneal dialysis type or some other form, should be directed toward a point between the bladder and body wall at the caudal apex of the abdominal cavity (called the pelvic gutter in humans). This location is most distant from the omentum, the usual cause of plugged cannulas. Infusing several hundred ml of dialysate when the abdomen is first entered will permit easier placement of the cannula. Use of as small an incision as possible is recommended. The incision should be closed about the cannula with a purse-string suture to prevent escape of fluid and entrance of bacteria. Between dialyses the cannula must be flushed with heparinized saline and firmly plugged. It is advisable to instill 100 to 500 mg of ampicillin or other low-toxicity antibiotic into the perito-

neal cavity between dialyses to help prevent peritonitis.

During dialysis the cannula plug is replaced with a three-way stopcock. One opening of the stopcock is connected by a sterile infusion tube to the dialysate bottle, and the other opening is connected by a second sterile tube to a sterile drainage container (usually an empty dialysate bottle). A closed system is essential to prevent ascending infection caused by respiration or other movements that create negative abdominal pressure.

Uremic animals have difficulty maintaining body temperature and usually are hypothermic. Therefore, the dialysate fluid should be warmed several degrees higher than normal body temperature (40 to 42°C). Infusing warmed dialysate provides heat and helps dilate visceral vascular beds to augment exchange across the peritoneum.

Instillation of a volume of 40 ml/kg body weight has given the most satisfactory results. This dosage may be modified downward in animals with cardiovascular or respiratory disease. After 30 minutes the fluid is drained from the peritoneal cavity by switching the stopcock. On the first exchange, up to 20 percent of the dialysate may be lost to the interspaces of intestines. The first few exchanges may also be blood-tinged as a result of minor hemorrhage during cannula insertion. On subsequent exchanges most of the infused dialysate should be recovered within 15 minutes and should be free of blood. With some of the smaller or less efficient cannulas a longer drainage period will be necessary. To prevent vascular overload it is essential to remove at least 90 percent of the fluids infused before filling the abdomen again.

Because uremic patients are usually lethargic, they can usually be dialyzed with minimal restraint while lying on a table or resting in a cage (Fig. 4). An extension tube from the cannula to the cage door permits switching inflow and outflow from outside the cage without disturbing the patient. Cats respond particularly well to this type of dialysis. Dogs have been dialyzed while confined to an oxygen cage. For less easily restrained patients a supportive stand with a canvas sling allows easy management during dialysis.

CLINICAL CONSIDERATIONS

Although peritoneal dialysis is a readily available life-saving procedure, it must never be performed casually. Certain physiologic principles and strict asepsis must be used routinely. Accurate records must be kept, including the

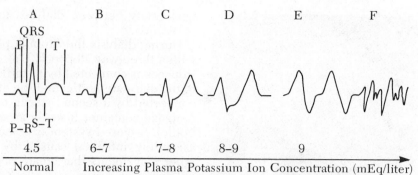

Figure 5. Changes in the electrocardiogram (ECG) that occur with increasing concentrations of plasma potassium ion above normal levels. *A.* The normal ECG showing the P, QRS, and T waves, the P–R interval, and the S–T segment. *B.* As potassium ion concentration increases, the T wave becomes elevated ("tenting"). *C.* With potassium ion concentrations of 7.0 to 8.0 mEq/liter the P wave diminishes, the P–R interval lengthens, the R wave may have reduced amplitude, and the S–T segment becomes depressed. *D.* At more toxic levels of potassium ion there is atrial asystole (no P waves), prolonged QRS waves associated with intraventricular block, and further depression of the S–T segment. *E.* Concentrations of potassium ion higher than 9 mEq/liter usually produce a sinusoidal pattern that often progresses to fatal ventricular fibrillation (*F*).

animal's weight "on" and "off" dialysis, volumes of dialysate infused and removed, and other pertinent data such as vital signs. Serial measurement of body weight provides a reliable index of fluid gain or loss. One pound equals 1 pint (473 ml or about 0.5 kg).

Proper formulation of dialysis fluids will permit normalization of plasma electrolytes. Because oliguric uremic animals are frequently hyperkalemic, potassium-free dialysate is used for the first few (three to four) exchanges. Potassium is added at 4 to 5 mEq/liter (as KCl) for subsequent exchanges. Plasma potassium status can be monitored easily by electrocardiography. Hyperkalemia can be detected by typical ECG changes, including first, an increased vertical height of the T wave (tenting), followed by S–T segment depression, low amplitude or loss of the P wave (atrial arrest), lengthened QRS interval, and eventually a sinusoidal S–T wave that precedes ventricular fibrillation (Fig. 5).

Uremic animals usually have metabolic acidosis. In acidosis plasma potassium is abnormally high because of displacement of intracellular potassium by hydrogen ions. Lactate (or acetate) in dialysis fluid will quickly correct acidosis. This may improve the patient's sense of well-being. Correcting acid-base balance will also promote return of plasma potassium to cells. Symptoms of hypokalemia may be seen after successful dialysis, especially if sufficient potassium was not added to the dialysate.

Commercial dialysis solutions are recommended (Table 1). In an emergency one can use lactated Ringer's solution by adding 1.5 percent (30 ml of 50 percent) dextrose per liter. Lactated Ringer's solution contains 4 mEq/liter of potassium.

Frequency of dialysis is important. In severely azotemic animals the severity of acidosis, hyperkalemia, and azotemia will be significant-

ly reduced by six to eight hours of intense dialysis (one exchange per hour). However, they rebound rapidly as plasma solute equilibrates with interstitial and intracellular fluid. Therefore, these patients must receive at least six exchanges daily for the first three days. Then six exchanges given on alternate days are recommended until uremia is controlled and the patient's clinical condition improves.

Because peritoneal dialysis removes significant quantities of protein, plasma proteins must be monitored during prolonged dialysis (four to five days). Infusion of canine plasma is helpful in anorectic dogs. Provision of high-quality protein such as egg white (1 gm/kg body weight/day) will help maintain plasma protein in uremic animals that can ingest and absorb food.

Prevention of peritonitis must be of prime concern. Infusing 100 to 500 mg of ampicillin through the cannula following dialysis has been a helpful prophylactic measure because of its broad bactericidal spectrum and low toxicity.

If peritoneal lavage is used to manage peritonitis, a dwell time is not necessary. It is more important to perform frequent exchanges to remove tissue debris rapidly and control infection. Ampicillin is also useful in this procedure and should be included in the lavage fluid at a concentration of 50 mg/liter. The same considerations apply for management of pancreatitis associated with peritonitis. Use of antibiotics will depend upon the presence or absence of infection. During treatment of peritonitis and pancreatitis with peritoneal lavage, the principles of peritoneal dialysis apply. The fluid must be at least at body temperature and must equal or slightly exceed the osmolality of plasma. The latter is best achieved by adding 1.5 percent dextrose to the lavage solution or by using peritoneal dialysate solutions for lavage.

SUPPLEMENTAL READING

Peritoneal dialysis: An update — 1976. Dialysis and Transplantation, 6(2):11–74, 1977.

Vaamonde, C.A., and Perez, G.O.: Peritoneal dialysis today. Kidney, 10:31–35, 1977.

Parker, H.R., Gourley, I.M. and Bell, R.L.: Current developments in peritoneal and hemodialysis. Gaines 22nd Veterinary Symposium. Stillwater, Oklahoma, September 17, 1972, pp. 3–15.

Henderson, L.W.: Peritoneal dialysis. In Massry, S.G., and Sellers, A.L. (eds.): Clinical Aspects of Uremia and Dialysis. Springfield, Ill., Charles C Thomas, 1976, pp. 555–582.

Boen, S.T.: Peritoneal Dialysis in Clinical Medicine. Springfield, Ill., Charles C Thomas, 1964.

Nolph, K.D., Stoltz, M.L. and Maher, J.F.: Altered peritoneal permeability in patients with systemic vasculitis. Ann. Intern. Med., 75:753, 1971.

Erbe, R.W., Green, J.A., Jr., and Weller, J.M.: Peritoneal dialysis during hemorrhagic shock. J. Appl. Physiol., 22:131, 1967.

Goldschmidt, Z.H., Pote, H.H., Katz, M.A. and Shear, L.: Effect of dialysate volume on peritoneal dialysis kinetics. Kidney Int., 5:240, 1974.

Nolph, K.D., Hano, J.E. and Teschan, P.E.: Peritoneal sodium transport during hypertonic peritoneal dialysis. Physiologic mechanisms and clinical implications. Ann. Intern. Med., 70:931, 1969.

Hirszel, P., Maher, J.F., Tempel, G.E. and Mengel, C.E.: Influence of peritoneal dialysis on factors affecting oxygen transport. Nephron, 15:438, 1975.

Vidt, D.G.: Recommendations on choice of peritoneal dialysis solutions. Ann. Intern. Med., 78:144, 1973.

CURRENT STATUS OF VETERINARY HEMODIALYSIS

LARRY D. COWGILL, D.V.M.

Davis, California

Hemodialysis is one of the few available forms of therapy useful in the management of acute renal failure in patients unresponsive to general conservative measures. It is an efficient and effective way to normalize or regulate fluid volume, electrolyte composition, and acid-base status of patients with little or no renal function. In addition, hemodialysis provides a means to effectively clear or remove metabolic waste products and solutes that are retained in uremia and that contribute to the clinical abnormalities of renal failure.

Despite its clinical efficacy and frequent use in advanced renal insufficiency and acute renal failure in humans, hemodialysis has had little use in veterinary patients (Butler; Cowgill and Bovee, 1977; Cowgill and Bovee, 1975; Gourley, et al.; Parker et al.). The availability of pediatric artificial kidneys and extracorporeal equipment and the development of safe procedures for dialysis in dogs should stimulate more widespread application and demand for veterinary hemodialysis in the future.

Hemodialysis is similar in principle to peritoneal dialysis. Alterations in the volume and composition of the extracellular fluid (ECF) are adjusted by regulating osmotic and diffusion gradients between the plasma and dialysate across a selective membrane. Plasma protein and formed elements of blood (RBCs, WBCs, thrombocytes) are restricted to the vascular compartment by the membrane, but water and low-molecular-weight solutes are freely permeable and therefore are subject to dialysis equilibrium. Solutes in higher concentration in plasma water (such as urea, creatinine, phosphorus, and potassium) pass through the membrane into the dialysate, where the concentration is lower or zero, and therefore are removed from the patient. If the concentrations of a solute (i.e., sodium, calcium chloride, or glucose) in the dialysate and in plasma are the same, no net solute exchange occurs, and the ECF concentration remains unchanged.

With hemodialysis, the exchange of solutes occurs across a thin, semipermeable artificial membrane of cellulose or regenerated cellulose. The artificial membrane allows a more efficient exchange between the blood and the dialysate than does the peritoneum. Because the exchange occurs outside the patient's body, extracorporeal circulation of blood is required. The combination of a large surface area in the dialyser, thin and highly permeable exchange membranes, and a high extracorporeal blood flow accounts for the fact that hemodialysis is more efficient than peritoneal dialysis. Because of comparatively short treatment periods, patient fatigue and manipulation are minimized (Fig. 1). Patients are rapidly returned to a physi-

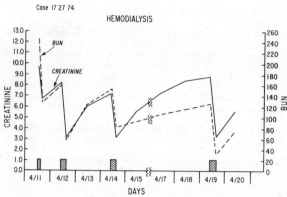

Figure 1. Responsiveness of plasma creatinine (mg/dl) and blood urea nitrogen (BUN) (mg/dl) to hemodialysis treatment (cross-hatched bars) in a dog with acute renal failure following elective surgery for septic prostatitis. The postdialysis increases in both solutes are a result of redistribution from intracellular and extracellular fluid compartments. The patient was maintained in a stable condition for two weeks with intermittent but suboptimal hemodialysis (see text).

ologic state that requires fewer dietary and drug restrictions than that seen with peritoneal dialysis.

INDICATIONS

The principal indication for hemodialysis in veterinary medicine is acute reversible renal failure in patients whose fluid, electrolyte, and metabolic disturbances are unresponsive to or unmanageable by conservative supportive measures. It is important to establish before or early in the course of dialysis that the diseased kidneys have the potential for repair and regeneration of a life-sustaining critical mass. This judgment is difficult and requires careful evaluation of the patient's prior health status, history of the current disease, and all available clinical, biochemical, histopathologic, and radiographic parameters. The most meaningful information for distinguishing acute, potentially reversible renal failure from end-stage disease is obtained from microscopic evaluation of renal biopsy specimens.

The indications for maintenance hemodialysis in chronic progressive renal insufficiency are debatable. Although the challenge and potential are clear, economic and technical limitations overshadow potential benefits. Possible exceptions include patients with compensated renal insufficiency that periodically become decompensated as a result of environmental stresses, infection, or dietary fluctuations and patients with decompensated renal insufficiency that could be stabilized by proper dietary and medical management. In these situations intermittent or limited courses of hemodialysis are

indicated to establish a better baseline for continued conservative management.

PROCEDURES AND EQUIPMENT

Many different types of artificial kidneys and dialysate delivery systems are currently available for human use. Of these, the hollow fiber artificial kidney (HFAK) is well suited to veterinary needs and has been the type most frequently utilized by the author. The HFAK is composed of thousands of capillary fiber membranes sealed in a plastic holder. As blood flows through the fibers, dialysate circulates continuously around them in a counter-current direction within the holder. The HFAK provides a large dialysing surface area, requires a low priming blood volume, provides efficient solute clearances, has a noncompliant blood compartment, and may be reused.

Vascular access is gained through Teflon®-Silastic arteriovenous shunts that are surgically placed in the femoral or cervical vessels and exteriorized through the skin. For hemodialysis the shunt is disconnected, and the arterial and the venous ends are attached to the artificial kidney via pediatric blood lines. Arterial blood supplied to the artificial kidney is dialysed and returned to the patient via the venous blood line. During nondialysis periods the arterial and venous limbs of the shunt are connected together to re-establish the shunt and provide ready vascular access for the next dialysis.

The dialysate is supplied by a dialysis delivery system in which a concentrated solution is properly diluted, warmed to body temperature, degassed, monitored for ionic conductivity, and pumped through the artificial kidney. Commercial delivery equipment also provides monitors and alarm systems to inform the clinician of blood leaks, alterations in dialysate composition, and changes in blood pressure. These devices make the dialysis procedure relatively free of complications.

EXPERIENCE

In acute experimental renal failure induced by nephrotoxins or nephrectomy, hemodialysis is an effective and efficient means of controlling many of the associated metabolic disturbances. (Cowgill and Bovee, 1977, 1975). Plasma creatinine, urea nitrogen, phosphorus, potassium and osmolality concentrations can be returned to normal ranges following five hours of therapy with an adult-sized artificial kidney. Electrocardiographic abnormalities of hyperkalemia are normalized within an hour, and hydration can be selectively regulated to correct volume deficits or overloads. Similar experience has been encountered in patients with acute renal failure secondary to sepsis, antifreeze nephrosis, nephrotoxic antibiotic administration, and postoperative complications (see Fig. 1). In addition to regulating the biochemical abnormalities, hemodialysis can keep patients alert, responsive, and ambulatory. Unlike experimental dogs, however, these patients often die as a result of their primary disease in spite of the fact that their uremia is well controlled through hemodialysis. Similar experience has been reported in man, in whom the mortality may approach 60 percent in acute renal failure following trauma or infection. Figure 1 depicts the response of plasma creatinine and urea nitrogen to hemodialysis using a pediatric HFAK in a patient with acute renal failure following elective surgery for septic prostatitis. Hemodialysis effectively lowered plasma creatinine and urea nitrogen concentrations to acceptable levels and was associated with marked clinical improvement. Following dialysis there is a typically rapid increase in the plasma concentrations of solutes secondary to redistribution from intracellular and extracellular compartments. Longer dialysis periods or shorter intervals between dialyses will prevent extremes of azotemia that seem to correlate with the patient's clinical condition.

In acute renal failure it is important to initiate hemodialysis as soon as possible. Previous experience suggests that initial treatments should be longer and more frequent than depicted in Figure 1. A more effective approach would be to dialyze the patient aggressively for six to eight hours on the first three days of therapy, followed by alternate days of dialysis as necessary to control the uremic disturbances. It may be necessary to manage a patient for three or more weeks with intermittent hemodialysis until the diseased kidneys regain adequate renal function to maintain homeostasis.

Experimentally nephrectomized dogs have been maintained in satisfactory health for one month with alternate-day hemodialysis. Clinical cases have been managed similarly but often died of complications unrelated to their renal disease or hemodialysis.

Any procedure requiring extracorporeal circulation of blood is subject to technical difficulties and patient risks. Hemodialysis is a clinically challenging and technically demanding procedure that requires highly skilled personnel. Risks to the patient include internal and external hemorrhage, hypotension, hemolysis, embolization, and infection. Establishment of standard veterinary procedures and the availability of pediatric equipment and good patient monitoring and alarm systems, however, have significantly reduced these risks.

Because of the need for specialized technical personnel, versatile clinical laboratory procedures and intensive care facilities and because of economic considerations, hemodialysis is limited at present to veterinary teaching hospitals. With the growing interest in nephrology as a veterinary speciality, however, hemodialysis should become available on a more widespread basis to service the needs of clinical practices.

SUPPLEMENTAL READING

Butler, H.C.: Renal support systems and transplantations. Proceedings of the 38th Annual Meeting, Am. Anim. Hosp. Assoc., 1971, pp. 162–164.

Cowgill, L.D., and Bovée, K.C.: Current status of hemodialysis and renal transplantation. In Kirk, R.W. (ed.): *Current Veterinary Therapy VI*. Philadelphia, W.B. Saunders Co., 1977.

Cowgill, L.D., and Bovée, K.C.: The feasibility and efficiency of hemodialysis in acutely uremic dogs. Proceedings of the 42nd Annual Meeting, Am. Anim. Hosp. Assoc., 2:165, 1975.

Gourley, I.M., Parker, H.R., Bell, R.L., and Ishizaki, G: Reponses of nephrectomized dogs during hemodialysis. Am. J. Vet. Res., 34:1421–1425, 1973.

Parker, H.R., Gourley, I.M., and Bell, R.L.: Current developments in peritoneal and hemodialysis. Gaines 22nd Veterinary Symposium, Stillwater, Oklahoma, September 17, 1972, pp. 3–15.

DRUG THERAPY IN RENAL DISORDERS

LLOYD E. DAVIS, D.V.M.

Urbana, Illinois

Drugs must occasionally be used for the treatment of a patient with renal dysfunction. Commonly recommended dosage regimens are predicated on the assumption that pathways for elimination are normal and, therefore, that the pharmacokinetics of the drug in the patient are the same as in experimental subjects. If the influence of modified renal excretion of the drug were ignored, drug toxicity might result. Data are not available to assess the incidence of drug intoxication occurring in animal patients as a result of impaired renal function. It has been inferred from studies of human patients that the rate of occurrence of adverse drug reactions in patients with a BUN level higher than 40 mg/dl was two and a half times that observed in subjects with normal BUN values. A number of other studies have shown that drug toxicity is a major hazard for patients with renal insufficiency. It is logical to assume that the same will hold true in veterinary medicine. Because of increased risks, it is wise to avoid drug therapy in patients with impaired renal function unless absolutely necessary. Then it is important to have a conceptual understanding of the pathophysiology of disordered renal function and of the disposition and pharmacodynamics of the drug intended for use. Furthermore, because of the increased risks it is unwise to prescribe multiple-drug therapy or fixed-dose combination products in patients with poor renal function. Such therapy would make the clinical situation extraordinarily complex.

The information in this article provides a summary of (1) the influence of the kidneys on drug disposition in the body, (2) disorders in drug disposition in renal insufficiency that may act to increase drug toxicity, and (3) general recommendations for modification of dosage regimens for patients with impaired renal function.

ROLE OF THE KIDNEYS IN DRUG ELIMINATION

Drug elimination occurs by processes of excretion and biotransformation. The kidneys subserve both of these functions, although the liver is the principal organ for drug biotransformation. The contribution of the kidneys to biotransformation of foreign chemicals is largely unknown. The kidney of the dog is known to conjugate salicylate with glycine and to metabolize insulin, catecholamines, morphine, serotonin, Prontosil, and other substances. The kidneys are the principal route of excretion for many drugs and their metabolites.

Normal physiologic processes occurring within the kidney mediate the excretion of drugs. These include filtration by the glomerulus and active or passive transport across the tubular epithelium. Many pharmacologic agents are small molecules that pass readily through the sieve-like structure of glomeruli into glomerular filtrate. The main features determining the rate of elimination of drugs by this mechanism are glomerular filtration rate, integrity of glomeruli, and extent of protein binding of the drug in plasma. Only the free (unbound) fraction of the drug is filtered, whereas that bound to albumin is retained within the plasma. This is why drugs that are excreted by glomerular filtration and are extensively protein-bound (e.g., sulfadimethoxine) have prolonged half-lives in the body.

A number of drugs diffuse passively from the tubular fluid into blood that perfuses peritubular capillaries. The extent of reabsorption of a drug from the distal tubules is dependent on urine flow rate, lipid solubility of the drug, and urine pH. At low flow rates there is a greater opportunity for drug molecules to diffuse from the tubules back into blood. Un-ionized drug molecules are more lipid-soluble than charged ions and diffuse more readily. The ratio of ionized to un-ionized molecules is expressed by the familiar Henderson-Hasselbalch equation. The clinical significance of this relationship for weak acids is that, as the urine pH increases, the fraction of ionized molecules increases, and more is excreted. Conversely, as the urine pH increases, the fraction of weak bases ionized becomes less, and the excretion rate diminishes. This principle is employed in management of canine and feline salicylate intoxication. We institute a brisk alkaline diuresis by infusing mannitol and sodium bicarbonate solutions. The increase in urine flow rate together with the alkaline pH of urine greatly increases renal clearance of the salicylate. On the other hand, alkalinization of the urine may prolong the action of basic drugs and enhance their pharmacologic effects or toxicity. This may be of particular significance with procainamide or quinidine, because these drugs are commonly employed in a critical patient care setting, where intensive bicarbonate therapy is common.

Acidic and basic drugs are excreted by separate active transport mechanisms in the proximal tubule. Unlike glomerular filtration, active secretion of drugs is not affected by the extent of protein binding of the drug in plasma. A number of drugs that are rather highly protein-bound (e.g., penicillins, salicylate, furosemide, and chlorothiazide) are efficiently excreted by active tubular secretion. An important point to remember is that two drugs can compete for the same transport system and mutually delay excretion. Thus, probenicid will prolong the half-life of penicillin in the plasma. Penicillin may diminish the response to chlorothiazide or furosemide, because these drugs must be secreted to reach their sites of action in the kidney. Some drugs known to be secreted by active transport mechanisms in the kidney are listed in Table 1.

Table 1. Drugs Excreted by Active Tubular Secretion*

ACIDS	BASES
Acetazolamide	Choline
p-Aminohippurate	Hexamethonium
Chlorothiazide	Histamine
Chlorpropamide	Mecamylamine
Dapsone	Procainamide
Diodrast	Procaine
Ethereal sulfates	Quinacrine
Furosemide	Tetraethylammonium
Glucuronides	Tolazoline
Indomethacin	
Methotrexate	
Oxalate	
Penicillins	
Phenolsulfonphthalein	
Phenylbutazone	
Probenicid	
Salicylic acid	
Sulfonamides	

*Adapted from: Prescott, L. F.: Mechanisms of renal excreation of drugs. Br. J. Anaesth., *44*:246, 1972.

DISORDERS IN DRUG DISPOSITION IN RENAL INSUFFICIENCY

Renal failure can modify drug disposition directly by altering mechanisms for their renal excretion and indirectly by affecting absorption, biotransformation, distribution, or protein binding. Uremia can change the sensitivity of various tissues to the action of certain drugs. Collectively, these changes create a situation in which the patient may be more susceptible to adverse drug reactions. Accordingly, modification of dosage regimens will frequently be required.

Severe glomerular diseases, such as amyloidosis and immune-mediated glomerulonephropathy, are accompanied by alterations in glomerular blood flow and permeability of the glomerular basement membrane. Decreases in glomerular filtration rate lead to retention of drugs and their metabolites and have a significant effect on the pharmacokinetics of many drugs. One might expect that losses of protein in the nephrotic syndrome might increase the rate of elimination of highly protein-bound drugs. This was investigated for phenytoin (Gugler, et al.). The excretion of the drug was increased, but there was a parallel decrease in the extent of protein binding of the drug, with the result that the amount of free drug in the serum was unchanged.

Extensive damage to renal tubules from toxins, interstitial nephritis, hypercalcemic nephropathy, and other causes will impair the kidneys' ability to secrete drugs and polar conjugates of drugs. Conditions such as renal tubular acidosis and the Fanconi syndrome can modify the rate of elimination of drugs by enhancing the reabsorption of acidic drugs and decreasing reabsorption of basic drugs by the distal tubules.

Renal disorders may impair drug absorption from alimentary, muscular, and subcutaneous sites by means of diminished perfusion associated with dehydration. Potassium wasting can affect gastrointestinal motility and therefore the rate and extent of drug absorption from the gut. While these effects have not been well-characterized in patients, the therapist should consider the possibility of altered drug absorption and observe the patient carefully for signs of effective drug action or toxicity.

Disordered renal function can affect drug distribution in the body by several mechanisms. Acidosis, changes in fluid compartments, and altered binding of drugs to macromolecules will all act to modify drug distribution. By altering the dissociation of some acidic drugs, acidemia will increase their ability to permeate cellular membranes. Salicylate and phenobarbital concentrations will increase in the brain and thereby accentuate their CNS effects. Uremia will decrease the extent of protein binding of some drugs (e.g., phenytoin) and increase the unbound fraction that is free to diffuse into tissues. The volume of distribution of digoxin is decreased in uremia, necessitating use of smaller loading and maintenance dosages.

The effect of uremia on the biotransformation of drugs has been studied extensively. Uremia appears to have little effect on oxidation, reduction, glucuronide synthesis, sulfate conjugation, or methylation of the drugs studied. Glycine conjugation, acetylation, and hydrolysis were all slowed by uremia. Thus, it is important to know the normal pathways for the biotransformation of a particular drug to be employed in a uremic patient. Biotransformation of drugs such as procaine, salicylate, succinylcholine, isoniazid, and insulin is impaired in uremia and thus would require adjustments in dosage. Drugs that are metabolized extensively by the liver by pathways known not to be affected by uremia should be selected whenever possible. For example, we have shown that the half-life of pentobarbital was unchanged in bilaterally nephrectomized and uremic dogs as compared with intact controls (Davis, et al.).

The sensitivity of various tissues to certain drugs may be modified by uremia and may be associated with several factors. Increased sensitivity to CNS depressants is related to a decrease in plasma protein binding, which increases the concentration of free, diffusible drug. This effect is augmented by an increase in the permeability of the "blood-brain barrier." For these reasons the effective dose of opiates, barbiturates, and tranquilizers should be reduced in uremia. In one study erythrocytes from uremic patients had a greater sensitivity to cephalothin as evidence by development of a positive Coombs' test at lower cephalothin concentrations (Molthan, et al.). Delayed elimination of many drugs caused by impaired renal excretion or biotransformation will enhance their toxicity and duration of action. Sensitivity of tissues to insulin is decreased in uremic patients, as shown by high plasma insulin:blood glucose ratios following glucose administration and slow decline in blood glucose concentrations following administration of insulin (Westervelt).

DRUG THERAPY IN RENAL FAILURE

Patients with renal failure present a challenge to the understanding, ingenuity, and skills of veterinarians. Because of uncertainty about the extent of modification of drug disposition and receptor sensitivity, even the most sophisticated, experienced clinician can produce severe drug reactions in such patients with drugs used routinely and safely in other patients. The treatment of each patient with renal failure is an experiment in itself that demands careful assessment of benefit vs. risk, precise diagnosis, establishment of therapeutic objectives, and careful evaluation of the effects (good or bad) of the drug in the patient.

Drugs must not be administered to patients with decreased renal function for trivial reasons (to please the client, to do "something," to correct a minor but not life-threatening ailment, to make diagnosis by therapy, or other such reasons). When it has been determined that the patient has a condition requiring therapy that is likely to preserve life, there are several considerations that may improve the benefit:risk ratio. Try to select a drug that is metabolized by the liver or excreted in the bile rather than one that is excreted unchanged by the kidneys (Table 2). In congestive heart failure one might select digitoxin in preference to digoxin. In gram-negative sepsis chloramphenicol might be preferred to gentamicin. For anesthesia, a barbiturate or an inhalant agent, or both, would be used in place of ketamine. This is not always possi-

Table 2. *Dosage Modification in Renal Insufficiency*

DRUGS THAT REQUIRE DOSAGE MODIFICATION OR THAT ARE CONTRAINDICATED IN RENAL INSUFFICIENCY

Acetazolamide	Mannitol
Antimonials	Mercurials
Aspirin	Methenamine
Atropine	Methotrexate
Barbital	Neomycin
Bendroflumethiazide	Neostigmine
Cephalothins	Nitrofurantoin
Chelating agents	Ouabain
Chlorothiazide	Penicillins
Colistin and polymyxin	Phenazopyridine
Digoxin	Procainamide
Erythromycin	Spironolactone
Furosemide (increased	Streptomycin
dose)	Sulfonamides
Gentamicin	TEA
Iodide	Tetracyclines
Kanamycin	Tubocurarine, gallamine, dec-
Lincomycin and clinda-	amethonium
mycin	Vancomycin

DRUGS THAT DO NOT REQUIRE DOSAGE MODIFICATION IN RENAL INSUFFICIENCY

Acetaminophen	Phenobarbital
Chloramphenicol	Phenothiazines
Diazepam	Phenytoin
Narcotic analgesics	Procaine
Novobiocin	Propranolol
Pentobarbital	

ble, particularly when dealing with severe infections. In this case one must select the best drug available based on culture and sensitivity data and adjust the dosage regimen for impaired renal function.

Dosage adjustments must often be formulated empirically, since in most clinical settings it is impractical to determine plasma concentrations of drugs in the patient. The two basic approaches to adjusting the dosage regimen are (1) maintaining the same dose as recommended for a normal animal of the same species and lengthen the interval between doses and (2) administering smaller doses at the recommended maintenance interval. There are advantages and disadvantages to each alternative. Increasing the dosage interval will cause greater swings between peak and trough concentrations and a greater likelihood of the concentration being subtherapeutic for varying times between doses. It has the advantage of being less time-consuming for the practitioner. The most effective means of maintaining a constant plasma concentration of a drug is by continuous infusion at a constant rate. This is not usually practical in clinical situations because it is very time-consuming. Giving small doses frequently can approximate the advantages of continuous infusion, because plateau concentrations will eventually occur and the variations between high and low plasma concentrations will be minimized. This approach is still time-consuming, but it has the advantage of providing an imperative for frequent observation of the patient's progress. As an example, consider the use of an aminoglycoside with a half-life of about 100 minutes in an animal with healthy kidneys. If the clearance of this drug (which is filtered by the glomerulus) were reduced to 10 percent of normal in a patient with a glomerulonephropathy, the half-life would be increased to about 17 hours. If one normally gave a dose of 10 mg/kg every six hours, it might now be necessary to give the 10 mg/kg only once every 24 hours. Alternatively, one might give 2.5 mg/kg every six hours or 1.25 mg/kg every three hours. If the patient were completely anuric, it would be necessary to give only a single 10 mg/kg dose.

SUGGESTED READING

Bennett, W.M.: Principles of drug therapy in patients with renal disease. West. J. Med., 123:372, 1975.

Davis, L.E., Baggot, J.D., Neff-Davis, C.A., and Powers, T.E.: Elimination kinetics of pentobarbital in nephrectomized dogs. Am. J. Vet. Res., 34:231, 1973.

Dettli, L.C.: Drug dosage in patients with renal disease. Clin. Pharmacol. Ther., 16:274, 1974.

Gugler, R., Shoeman, D.W., Huffman, D.H., Cohlmia, J.B., and Azarnoff, D.L.: Pharmacokinetics of drugs in patients with the nephrotic syndrome. J. Clin. Invest., 55:1182, 1975.

Hollenberg, N.K., and Epstein, M.: The use of drugs in the patient with uremia. Mod. Treatm., 6:1011, 1969.

Molthan, L., Reidenberg, M.M., and Eichman, M.: Positive direct Coombs' tests due to cephalothin. N. Engl. J. Med., 277:123, 1967.

Prescott, L.F.: Mechanisms of renal excretion of drugs. Br. J. Anaesth., 44:246, 1972.

Reidenberg, M.M.: Renal Function and Drug Action. Philadelphia, W.B. Saunders Co., 1971.

Rennick, B.R.: Renal excretion of drugs: Tubular transport and metabolism. Ann. Rev. Pharmacol., 12:141, 1972.

Schreiner, G.E., and Maher, J.F.: Drugs and the kidney. Ann. N. Y. Acad. Sci., 123:326, 1965.

Smith, J.W., Seidl, L.G., and Cluff, L.E.: Studies on the epidemiology of adverse drug reactions. V. Clinical factors influencing susceptibility. Ann. Intern. Med., 65:629, 1966.

Westervelt, F.B.: Insulin effect in uremia. J. Lab. Clin. Med., 74:79, 1969.

ANESTHESIA IN RENAL FAILURE

DAVID B. BRUNSON, D.V.M.

East Lansing, Michigan

INTRODUCTION

Dogs and cats with renal failure that require emergency surgery must be considered to be high anesthetic risks. Anesthetic management of these patients is difficult, since renal failure cannot be treated prior to surgery, and concurrent problems often exist in other major organ systems. In order to anesthetize renal failure patients the patient's condition and the resulting effects of anesthetic drugs must be considered.

The type of renal failure must be determined

(i.e., prerenal, postrenal, and/or primary renal failure). Prerenal azotemia is caused by conditions such as hypovolemia, shock, hypoadrenalism, and cardiac disease, which diminish renal function by decreasing perfusion of the kidneys (Osborne et al.). Treatment of prerenal causes should be initiated prior to anesthesia. Causes of postrenal azotemia include obstruction of urine flow that prevents elimination of waste products by the kidneys and rupture of the excretory pathway. Patients with prerenal and postrenal azotemia have structurally normal kidneys. Rapid correction of underlying conditions allows the patient's kidneys to respond appropriately to elimination of waste products and drugs.

Uremia caused by primary renal failure is the most serious form of renal failure, because it signifies the dysfunction of at least three-fourths of the renal parenchyma. Although many different diseases can cause primary kidney damage, the functional changes that occur are similar. Therefore, anesthetic management is similar no matter what the cause. This article deals primarily with anesthetic management of primary renal failure.

DRUG EFFECTS ON RENAL FUNCTION

Before considering the anesthetic management of patients with renal failure, it is important to consider the effects that anesthetics have on normal renal function. All general anesthetics decrease renal function by reducing urine production, glomerular filtration rate (GFR), renal blood flow (BRF), and electrolyte excretion (Mazze and Cousins). The causes of these changes include the depth of anesthesia, length of surgery, vascular volume during anesthesia, physical status of the patient, and anesthetics administered. Normally, changes in renal function during anesthesia are only slight and are reversible.

Reduction of renal function during anesthesia occurs secondary to changes in the patient's circulatory, sympathetic nervous, and endocrine systems. Circulatory changes caused by anesthetics include peripheral vasodilation and decreased cardiac output due to myocardial depression. These secondarily increase renal vascular resistance. Inhalation anesthetics also increase the tone of sympathetic constrictor fibers in renal blood vessels. This neuronal activity disrupts the normal autoregulation of blood flow through the kidneys.

Antidiuretic hormone (ADH) and aldosterone frequently are released during anesthesia. Increased blood levels of ADH cause increased reabsorption of water from the renal tubules. Aldosterone, which controls the kidney's regulation of sodium excretion, is elaborated secondary to blood volume changes in the baroreceptors of the carotid sinus. Halothane anesthesia, dehydration, and blood loss stimulate aldosterone secretion and water conservation by the kidneys.

In healthy dogs and cats these anesthetic-induced changes in renal function are well tolerated and reversible. However, when renal disease limits the ability of the kidneys to maintain normal fluid and electrolyte homeostasis, the added stress of surgery and anesthesia may precipitate serious kidney dysfunction.

EFFECTS OF UREMIA ON ANESTHETIC DRUG ACTION

Once dysfunction of three-fourths of the nephrons of both kidneys has occurred, a consistent pattern of symptoms develops. Several of these characteristic signs of uremia affect the action of anesthetic-related agents. It is important, therefore, to identify these changes and consider their relationships with anesthetics to be employed.

In chronic renal failure a non-regenerative anemia may develop, caused at least in part by loss of renal erythropoietin production. If red blood cell numbers become markedly depressed, blood transfusions should be administered prior to anesthesia to ensure adequate oxygen-carrying capacity during the stress of the operation and to counteract the potential intra-operative blood loss or hemodilution caused by fluid administration. Dehydration often occurs in patients with polyuric renal failure if compensatory polydipsia is blocked by vomiting. Correction of fluid deficits is necessary because anesthetic-induced peripheral vasodilation and myocardial depression accentuate pre-existing fluid deficits and may cause profound hypotension.

Overhydration may develop if oliguric or anuric renal failure exists. When present, it usually is caused by overzealous fluid therapy. Correction of hypervolemia should precede anesthesia because overhydration and potassium retention may precipitate cardiac failure.

Acid-base disturbances are frequently associated with renal failure. Metabolic acidosis occurs when the kidneys become unable to excrete hydrogen ion or conserve bicarbonate ions. The lower pH is responsible for increased myocardial irritability, altered membrane polarity, and drug ionization. Restoration of blood pH to acceptable limits of 7.35 to 7.45 is preferred before administration of anesthetics. Other electrolytes also are affected when renal function is severely reduced. In addition to hydrogen and bicarbonate ion changes, hyponatremia, hypochloremia and hyperkalemia can develop during oliguria.

ANESTHETIC AGENTS

All drugs are potentially toxic if given to patients that are unable to eliminate them normally. Because of the depressive effects of anesthetic agents, they must be given to renal failure patients with caution. Reductions in dosage of approximately 25 to 50 percent should be expected. This reduction is important because the effects of anesthetics often act synergistically with existing CNS depression or previously administered drugs.

Atropine. Approximately 50 percent of the administered dose of atropine is excreted unchanged by the kidneys. If severe renal failure is present, the dose should be reduced.

Phenothiazine, Butyrophenones, and Benzodiazepines. These tranquilizers, including acetylpromazine, droperidol, and Valium, are almost completely metabolized by the liver prior to excretion. Renal failure only minimally prolongs their effects. However, these agents should be used cautiously, since uremic animals often are depressed and require minimal (if any) sedation. Phenothiazines and butyrophenones are alpha-adrenergic blockers and may accentuate hypotension caused by hypovolemia.

Several advantages are associated with the use of preanesthetic tranquilizers. The antiemetic action of these drugs may help to reduce the amount of vomiting caused by uremia. Another benefit of these drugs is their antiarrhythmic effect during halothane anesthesia. Electrolyte changes, acidosis, and increased blood levels of catecholamines frequently predispose uremic patients to arrhythmias. In addition, preinduction administration of tranquilizers may diminish induction and maintenance dosages of other anesthetics.

Narcotics. In severe renal failure the effects of standard dosages of narcotics are intensified and prolonged primarily because of pre-existing depression of the patient. In healthy humans approximately 35 percent of the total plasma morphine is bound to proteins (Olsen, et al.). In patients with glomerulonephropathy, plasma proteins and albumin may be lost in urine. As plasma protein levels diminish, less binding of morphine occurs and the narcotic activity of a given dose is increased. The increased unbound morphine is another reason for prolonged narcosis. The same phenomenon probably applies to all narcotic analgesics. Narcotics

such as Demerol, fentanyl, oxymorphone, and pentazocine are almost entirely metabolized by the liver prior to excretion. No known depressive effects are attributed to their metabolites. Narcotic tranquilizer combinations (neuroleptanalgesics) are the least depressive anesthetic agents in humans with renal failure (Mazze and Cousins). Innovar (fentanyl and droperidol) is a readily available neuroleptanalgesic for use in dogs. Narcotics have an additional advantage in that their effects can be antagonized with pharmacologic agents if complications occur.

Barbiturates. The short-acting barbiturates most commonly used in veterinary practice — pentobarbital, sodium thiamylal, thiopenthal — are initially redistributed and metabolized before being excreted by the kidneys. Therefore, renal dysfunction does not greatly affect the duration of their anesthetic action. If renal failure has resulted in a metabolic acidosis, however, more of the barbiturate is in an un-ionized or active form. In addition, loss of serum albumin diminishes available binding sites for the barbiturate and results in an increase in the level of pharmacologically active drug (Ghoneim and Pandya). Uremic patients may also have greater sensitivity to these agents caused by alterations in their blood-brain barrier.

Long-acting barbiturates like phenobarbital should not be used in renal failure patients, since they are primarily excreted unchanged by the kidneys.

Inhalation Anesthetics. When inhalation anesthetics first became available it was believed that they were eliminated entirely through the lungs without endogenous metabolism. It is now known that ether, halothane, and especially methoxyflurane undergo extensive metabolism. Studies have shown that as much as 40 percent of halothane and 70 percent of methoxyflurane may be metabolized. Many of the metabolites of these agents are excreted in urine. With the exception of methoxyflurane, none of the metabolites of inhalation anesthetics have been shown to be deleterious to renal function.

Two of the six metabolites of methoxyflurane are known to cause renal dysfunction. These are fluoride ion and oxalic acid. Although clinical evidence of methoxyflurane-related renal failure has not been documented in dogs or cats, several research studies in dogs have produced evidence of renal function impairment following methoxyflurane administration. Fluoride ion has been identified as a cause of a high-volume diuresis in dogs (Frascino). The diuresis was similar to the syndrome known to occur in man following methoxyflurane anesthesia. Recent studies in dogs have proved that serum fluoride, urine fluoride, and urine oxalate levels markedly increased following exposure to methoxyflurane (Brunson, et al.).

Because methoxyflurane is metabolized to a large extent and its metabolites have the potential to induce renal dysfunction, the use of this inhalation anesthetic should be avoided in patients with renal disease.

Since patients with renal failure may already have conditions predisposing them to arrhythmias (e.g., hyperkalemia, hypocalcemia, and metabolic acidosis), inhalation anesthetics (like halothane) that increase myocardial sensitivity should be administered cautiously.

In anemic patients, nitrous oxide administration should not exceed 50 percent in order to ensure adequate oxygenation. Nitrous oxide is a valuable adjuvant to many other anesthetics, since it is only slightly metabolized and has few cardiovascular or respiratory depressive effects.

Muscle Relaxants. Depolarizing and non-depolarizing muscle relaxants are a useful addition to neuroleptanalgesic techniques. The addition of paralyzing agents to prevent involuntary muscle movement during use of narcotic analgesics allows maintenance of lighter anesthetic planes for surgery on critical patients.

Succinylcholine, a depolarizing muscle relaxant, can be used in renal failure patients. The total dosage should be kept minimal because one of its metabolites, succinylmonocholine, is excreted by the kidneys. If large amounts of succinylmonocholine accumulate, a non-depolarizing neuromuscular block can be produced.

D-tubocurare should not be used in dogs because it produces severe hypotension, even in healthy animals. Gallamine, a reversible non-depolarizing muscle relaxant, is almost entirely excreted unchanged in urine. Gallamine should not be used in uremic patients because prolongation of the blockade will occur. Pancuronium, a steroid-based non-depolarizing muscle relaxant, can be used in patients with renal failure because it is metabolized by the liver and the blockade can be antagonized by neostigmine.

Other Drugs. Xylazine is a potent sedative that should not be used in uremic patients. The frequent arrhythmias associated with xylazine and the myocardial irritability associated with renal failure increase the risk of cardiovascular problems. In addition, xylazine stimulates the chemoceptor trigger zone in the brain and frequently causes vomition. Dissociative anesthesia is commonly used for minor procedures on cats. Ketamine is partially metabolized by the liver but primarily excreted by the kidneys. Prolongation of ketamine anesthesia will occur in uremic cats.

Urinary obstruction causing postrenal uremia in male cats is a frequent problem. Small intramuscular dosages of ketamine (4.4 mg/kg) combined with acetylpromazine (0.1 mg/kg) can safely be given to facilitate unblocking of the urethral obstruction. Caution should be taken to ensure that the obstruction has not caused primary renal damage before using ketamine. Furthermore, the obstruction must be removed and maintenance of urine production and elimination ensured if the dissociative agent is to be used.

RECOMMENDATIONS

Dogs and cats suspected of having renal failure should be evaluated by appropriate history, physical, and laboratory examinations. It should be determined whether the renal failure is acute or chronic and reversible or irreversible and whether the uremia is due to prerenal, primary renal, or postrenal causes.

Laboratory tests useful in classifying renal failure include a complete urinalysis, determination of serum urea nitrogen (SUN) or creatinine concentration, a complete blood count (CBC) and, if possible, serum electrolytes and blood gases. All abnormal test results should be analyzed and appropriate treatments given to improve the patient's condition prior to the beginning of surgery. Special attention should be directed toward correcting existing metabolic acidosis. If results of serum electrolyte concentration and blood gas value determinations are not available, extreme care must be used in the selection and administration of anesthetic agents. When anesthetic drugs are dependent upon renal excretion, or when their effects are likely to be enhanced by the uremic syndrome, the administered dose should be reduced by approximately 50 percent. Additional amounts may be given cautiously after the initial effects have been observed. Dosages of drugs minimally affected by renal failure should be decreased by 25 percent. Anesthetic agents that are excreted primarily by the kidneys should be avoided (e.g., phenobarbital, gallamine, and ketamine). Drugs known to be nephrotoxic must also be avoided in uremic patients. Included in this group are aminoglycoside antibiotics and the nephrotoxic metabolites of the tetracyclines and methoxyflurane.

During induction and maintenance of anesthesia, particular care must be taken to keep mean arterial blood pressure above 60 mm Hg. Below this pressure glomerular filtration is severely limited. Parenteral fluids are usually indicated in these patients to maintain adequate vascular volume, tissue perfusion, and blood pressure. Fluids are especially necessary in renal failure patients because deficits often exist before surgery and patients are often unable to conserve body water. For dogs intravenous administration of lactated Ringer's solution in a quantity of 20 to 40 ml/kg during the first hour of anesthesia is recommended. Half of this amount should then be administered in the next hour if surgery continues and if urine output is satisfactory. Cats should receive half the amount recommended for dogs. If hypervolemia of left ventricular failure exists concurrently with the renal failure, fluid administration must be carefully monitored.

Recent innovations in indirect blood pressure monitoring have resulted in monitors that are applicable to veterinary medicine. Unfortunately, these instruments are not widely used for dogs and cats because they are expensive. Direct blood pressure measurements are possible but require catheterization of a peripheral artery. At present, most practitioners rely on digital palpation of an artery to detect general trends in pulse strength. Urine production can also be utilized as a crude index of blood pressure. When mean arterial blood pressure drops below 60 mm Hg, urine formation ceases. The continual excretion of 1.0 ml/kg/hr of urine indicates that blood pressure is above 60 mm Hg. Use of vasopressors to maintain systemic arterial pressure should be used only if fluid administration and reduction of anesthetic levels have failed, because most vasopressors decrease renal blood flow. However, dopamine hydrochloride (Intropin) is a potent beta-adrenergic stimulator known to enhance renal blood flow (Innes and Nickerson). I have used dopamine successfully to increase mean arterial pressure and restore urine production in an-esthetized dogs. Adequate vascular volume is necessary prior to dopamine administration; dosages should be kept low (2 to 5 μg/kg/minute) so that total system vascular resistance remains stable. Dopamine should be diluted in a liter of lactated Ringer's or other suitable diluent before administration.

In addition to use of blood pressure monitoring, cardiovascular function is best monitored by electrocardiography (ECG). Electrolyte changes, myocardial hypoxia, and potentially lethal arrhythmias are readily detected with ECGs. Ventilation must also be supported during general anesthesia so that hypercardia or hypoxemia do not occur. Cardiac arrhythmias are more frequent and more severe if respiratory acidosis is present.

SUPPLEMENTAL READING

Brunson, D.B., Stowe, C.M., and McGrath, C.J.: Serum and urine inorganic fluoride concentrations and urine oxalate concentrations following methoxyflurane anesthesia in the dog. Am. J. Vet. Res., 40:197–203, 1979.

Deutsch, S.: Anesthetic management in acute and chronic renal failure. Vet. Clin. North Am., 3:57–64, 1973.

Frascino, J.A.: Effects of inorganic fluoride on the renal concentration mechanism. Possible nephrotoxicity in man. J. Lab. Clin. Med., 79:192–203, 1972.

Ghoneim, M.M., and Pandya, H.: Plasma protein binding of thiopental in patients with impaired renal or hepatic function. Anesthesiology, 42:535–549, 1975.

Innes, I.R., and Nickerson, M.: Norepinephrine, epinephrine and the sympathomimetic amines. In Goodman, L.S., and Gilman, A. (eds.): *The Pharmacologic Basis of Therapeutics*, 5th ed. New York, Macmillan, 1975, pp. 477–513.

Mazze, R.I., and Cousins, M.J.: Renal diseases in relation to anesthesia. In Katz, J., and Kadis, L.B. (eds.): *Anesthesia and Uncommon Diseases*. Philadelphia, W.B. Saunders Co., 1973.

Olsen, G.D., Bennett, W.M., and Porter, G.A.: Morphine and phenytoin binding to plasma proteins in renal and hepatic failure. Clin. Pharmacol. Ther., 17:677–684, 1975.

Osborne, C.A., Low, D.G., and Finco, D.R.: *Canine and Feline Urology*. Philadelphia, W.B. Saunders Co., 1972.

The Urinary Tract

NEUROGENIC URINARY INCONTINENCE

JOHN E. OLIVER, JR., D.V.M.

Athens, Georgia

and CARL A. OSBORNE, D.V.M.

St. Paul, Minnesota

Micturition is the physiologic process of storage and complete voiding of urine. Abnormalities of the nervous system may cause inappropriate voiding, inadequate storage of urine, incomplete voiding, or absence of voiding. All these abnormalities may be considered as forms of incontinence, which is defined as the loss of voluntary control of micturition. Behavioral disorders resulting in inappropriate micturition and abnormalities of the urinary tract resulting in incontinence are discussed in other articles.

ANATOMY AND PHYSIOLOGY OF MICTURITION

The neural organization of micturition is a complex integration of parasympathetic, sympathetic, and somatic components involving all levels of the nervous system. A simplified description applicable to understanding most clinical problems is presented in Figure 1. Filling of the urinary bladder is accommodated by gradual stretching of smooth muscle called the detrusor. Sensory endings of the pelvic (parasympathetic) nerve detect changes in the amount of stretch. When capacity is reached these afferent fibers discharge impulses to the sacral segments of the spinal cord (S1, 2, and 3). The signals are relayed through spinoreticular pathways to the pons (brain stem). Reflex integration occurs at this level, with a resultant efferent discharge down reticulospinal pathways to the sacral parasympathetic nucleus. Preganglionic parasympathetic neurons are activated, sending impulses through the pelvic nerve. Ganglia are located along the course of the pelvic nerve and in the bladder wall. Postganglionic neurons are activated, sending impulses to the detrusor muscle. Each muscle

fiber in the detrusor does not receive direct innervation; rather, "pacemaker" fibers scattered through the detrusor are depolarized, with subsequent spread of excitation to adjoining muscle fibers through "tight junctions." Tight junctions are areas of fusion of the outer components of the cell membranes. The resulting wave of excitation causes contraction of the detrusor, which pulls the neck of the bladder open like a funnel and squeezes out urine. Simultaneously, inhibitory interneurons that synapse on pudendal motor neurons are activated in the sacral spinal cord. The pudendal neurons are silenced, resulting in a relaxation of the external urethral sphincter. When the bladder is empty, afferent discharge in the pelvic nerve subsides and is followed by cessation of discharge in the pelvic motor neurons. The detrusor muscle relaxes, the inhibitory interneurons no longer block pudendal motor activity, and the external urethral sphincter returns to its normal state of contraction.

The external urethral sphincter (skeletal muscle) maintains a low level of tonus through spinal stretch reflexes. Sudden changes in intra-abdominal pressure (from coughing or sneezing, for example) cause a rapid increase in tone in the sphincter and permit maintenance of urinary continence. Continence in the relaxed animal is maintained at the neck of the bladder ("internal sphincter") by the relaxation of the spiraling detrusor fibers.

The sympathetic nervous system has input to the bladder from spinal segments L1 to 4 through the caudal mesenteric ganglion and the hypogastric nerve. Sympathetic neurons have both alpha-adrenergic synapses (excitatory) and beta-adrenergic synapses (inhibitory) on ganglia in the pelvic plexus, detrusor muscle fibers,

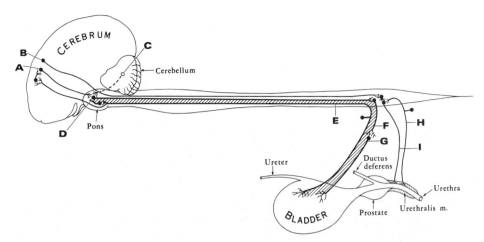

Figure 1. Anatomic organization of micturition. *A*. Cortical neurons for voluntary control of micturition. *B*. Cortical neurons for voluntary control of sphincters. *C*. Cerebellar neurons that have inhibitory influence on micturition. *D*. Pontine reticular neurons that are necessary for detrusor reflex. *E*. Afferent (sensory) pathway for detrusor reflex. *F*. Preganglionic pelvic (parasympathetic) neuron to detrusor. *G*. Postganglionic pelvic (parasympathetic) neuron to detrusor. *H*. Afferent (sensory) neuron from urethral sphincter, pudendal nerve. *I*. Efferent (motor) neuron to urethral sphincter, pudendal nerve.

and blood vessels. The physiologic significance of these fibers is not clear, since ablation of the hypogastric nerve does not significantly alter micturition. There appears to be an increased influence of the sympathetic pathways following lesions of the parasympathetic nerves (Sundin et al.). Patients with neurogenic bladder dysfunction complicated by narrowing of the bladder neck or spasms of the urethra may be helped by alpha-adrenergic blockade (McGuire et al.).

Voluntary control of micturition is mediated from the cerebral cortex to the pontine micturition center. Voluntary control of sphincters is derived from the cerebral cortex and is relayed to the sacral spinal cord nucleus of the pudendal nerve. Micturition can occur without cerebral cortex input, but there is no voluntary control.

The cerebellum has an inhibitory effect on the pontine neurons of micturition.

Abnormalities of micturition associated with lesions of the nervous system are outlined in Table 1.

DIAGNOSIS OF URINARY INCONTINENCE

Consult the article entitled "Non-neurogenic Urinary Incontinence" for a problem-specific data base for urinary incontinence.

History. Evaluation of the onset and chronologic course of the problem will allow construction of a sign-time graph that is useful for determining the etiology of the disease (Oliver, 1972). The ability of the animal to control micturition voluntarily is an important differentiat-

ing feature (Fig. 2). In this context, voluntary control means that the animal is able to initiate voiding at appropriate times.

Associated problems such as paresis, fecal incontinence, pain, and other problems are important criteria for differentiating neurogenic from non-neurogenic incontinence and for localizing lesions in neurogenic incontinence.

Physical Examination. Observation of voiding may help determine whether voluntary control is present, whether the detrusor reflex is present, and whether the sphincter relaxes during voiding. Reflex dyssynergia (usually a result of partial spinal cord lesions) is characterized by voluntary initiation of voiding but is associated with a small urine stream that stops abruptly before the bladder is empty. Small spurts of urine may be produced intermittently as the animal strains to urinate against a closed sphincter. Absence of voiding or dribbling of urine when the urinary bladder is distended suggests absence of a detrusor reflex or obstruction of the urethra.

Palpation of the bladder before and after voiding will usually permit a flaccid atonic bladder to be differentiated from a small contracted bladder with thickened walls. Calculi or tumor masses may also be palpated. Manual expression of the bladder provides an evaluation of sphincter tone. Tone will be decreased when lesions are present in the sacral spinal cord, roots, or pudendal nerve (lower motor neuron) and will be increased when lesions are present between the brain stem and L7 (upper motor neuron).

Catheterization   immediately   after   voiding

Table 1. Effect of Lesions of the Neuromuscular System

LOCATION OF LESION	NORMAL FUNCTION	BLADDER					SPHINCTER			
		Voluntary Control	Sustained Detrusor Reflex	Tone	Volume	Residual Urine	Voluntary Control	Reflexes (Perineal, Bulbourethral)	Tone	Synergy with Detrusor
Cerebral cortex to brain stem	Voluntary control to detrusor and sphincter	Absent	Normal	Normal	May be greater or smaller than normal	None	Absent	Normal to hyperreflexic	Normal to increased	Normal
Cerebellum	Modulation (inhibition) of detrusor reflex	Normal, but increased frequency	Possible hyperreflexic	Normal	Small	None	Normal	Normal	Normal	Normal
Brain stem (pons) to sacral spinal cord	Sustained detrusor reflex	Absent	Lost early; small unsynchronized contractions late	Atonic early; possibly increased late	Large	Large	Absent	Normal to hyperreflexic	Normal to increased	Absent
Partial lesions (reflex dyssynergia)	Sustained detrusor reflex	May be present	May be present	Normal to atonic	Large	Small to large	May be normal	Normal	Normal to increased	Absent
Sacral spinal cord or roots	LMN° to detrusor and sphincter	Absent	Absent	Atonic	Large	Large	Absent	Absent	Flaccid	Absent
Disruption of tight junctions of detrusor	Spread of excitation in detrusor	Absent	Absent	Atonic	Large	Large	Normal	Normal	Normal	Normal (cannot evaluate, however)

°LMN = lower motor neuron

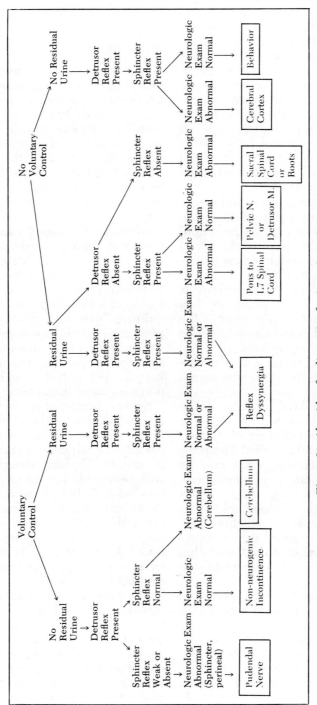

Figure 2. Algorithm for diagnosis of urinary incontinence

allows an accurate measurement of residual urine, which should be less than 10 ml in normal dogs. Most urethral obstructions can be localized when a catheter is passed through the urethral lumen.

Neurologic Examination. In addition to a complete neurologic examination for localization of abnormalities in the nervous system, it is imperative that reflexes through the sacral spinal cord also be evaluated. The tone of the external anal sphincter may be observed or palpated with a gloved finger. Reflex contraction of the sphincter can be elicited by squeezing the bulb of the penis or the vulva (bulbocavernosus reflex) or by pricking with a pin or pinching the perineum (perineal reflex). Both reflexes are dependent on the integrity of the pudendal nerve (afferents and efferents) and sacral segments of the spinal cord.

The history, physical examination, and neurologic examination should provide adequate information to differentiate neurogenic from nonneurogenic disorders and to localize the site of the lesion in the nervous system when neurogenic disorders are present (Fig. 2).

Electrophysiology. Electrophysiologic tests have not been included in the minimum data base because they are not widely used at the present time. They will, however, provide more objective evidence of abnormalities detected during the general examination and may disclose subtle abnormalities that otherwise would not be recognized.

The cystometrogram (CMG) measures intravesical pressure during a micturition reflex. It provides information about bladder tone, bladder capacity, and the detrusor reflex. The presence or absence of a detrusor reflex may be difficult to evaluate without a cystometrogram in some cases.

Electromyography of the skeletal sphincters may detect partial denervation, which is difficult to assess clinically. Urethral pressure profiles show promise for evaluation of the urethra but have not yet been evaluated adequately in animals.

Laboratory Examination. Hematology, blood chemistries, and urinalyses provide information that may help one to detect non-neurogenic causes of abnormal micturition. They are essential if a meaningful prognosis is to be formulated. Disorders of micturition are frequently complicated by cystitis, ureteral reflux, pyelonephritis, and uremia.

Radiologic Examination. Survey radiographs provide information about kidney and bladder size, shape, and position. Calculi or masses may be seen. A pneumocystogram,

double-contrast cystogram, or urethrogram may be necessary to detect bladder and urethral masses or calculi. Intravenous urography (IVU) must be used to detect ureteral dilation caused by reflux. A voiding cystourethrogram is useful for assessing the coordinated function of the bladder and urethra.

TREATMENT

Abnormalities of the nervous system causing disorders of micturition may be reversible or irreversible. Reversible lesions include spinal cord or peripheral nerve compressions (from vertebral discs or trauma, for example). Treatment should be directed toward correction of the primary cause of the disease (Hoerlein). Although management of the micturition problem may be only temporary in these cases, it may mean the difference between success and failure.

Irreversible lesions include congenital defects and injuries or diseases associated with neuronal destruction. Management of these patients is dependent on the underlying problem. Behavior problems or cerebral cortex lesions that lead to inappropriate voiding (loss of house training, "marking" inside the house, and other problems) may be managed by behavior modification or the use of anticonvulsants or tranquilizers, or the problem may be avoided by housing the pet outside. Such cases are often a diagnostic and therapeutic challenge.

Severe brain stem or spinal cord lesions (above S1) are characterized by detrusor areflexia and hypertonus of the sphincter. Most paraplegics fall into this category. Management of urinary bladder abnormalities in patients with reversible lesions of this type is critical if success is to be achieved. Management of patients with irreversible deficits of this type is often difficult and discouraging. Removal of urine by intermittent aseptic catheterization (t.i.d.) is imperative. If the sphincter is not excessively hypertonic (especially in females), expulsion of urine by manual expression of the bladder may be possible. The patient should be catheterized periodically following manual expression of the bladder to be certain that adequate emptying is achieved. After the first few weeks (one to three), reflex bladder contractions may partially empty the bladder. Complete evacuation of the bladder is *rarely* accomplished by these segmental reflexes, and serious complications usually develop if assistance is not provided. If the animal appears to be voiding completely, this observation should be verified by catheterization immediately after micturition. If a residual urine volume of more than 10 ml is present, assistance must be continued.

Cystitis is a frequent complication of detrusor areflexia. Urinalyses, bacterial culture, and antibiotic sensitivity tests are indicated to detect abnormalities at an early stage. Appropriate antibiotics should be administered (consult article entitled "Urinary Tract Infections").

Partial lesions of the spinal cord may produce reflex dyssynergia (contraction of the bladder without relaxation of the sphincter). Trials with neuromuscular relaxants such as diazepam and alpha-adrenergic blocking agents such as phenoxybenzamine have not resulted in long-lasting benefits. Partial rhizotomy of the sacral dorsal roots has been used with some success in man. Pudendal neurectomy will allow complete voiding but will also induce urinary incontinence.

Human beings with detrusor hyper-reflexia caused by cerebellar or partial spinal cord lesions have been reported to respond to anticholinergic medication. Propantheline (Pro-Banthine®, Searle) has been used at dosages ranging from 7.5 to 30 mg t.i.d. in dogs.

Lesions of the sacral spinal cord or roots cause detrusor areflexia and sphincter areflexia. The same type of management as described for spinal cord lesions is suggested. Catheterization may not be required, since manual expression of the bladder is usually easy. Since nerve roots are peripheral nerves with the capability of regeneration, traumatic lesions at the lumbosacral junction that compress the cauda equina are much more likely to respond to decompression than similar lesions affecting the spinal cord. Chronic compression of the cauda equina from a malformation or malarticulation of the L7–S1 vertebrae may cause neurogenic incontinence (Oliver, et al., 1978). Decompression of the nerve roots by dorsal laminectomy and foraminotomy has restored normal micturition in some cases.

Overdistention of the bladder that disrupts the tight junctions between smooth muscle fibers results in detrusor areflexia. Function will be restored in one to two weeks if the bladder is maintained in a decompressed state by the methods just described, provided that infection has not caused a proliferation of fibrous tissue in the bladder wall.

Prosthetic devices for control of micturition, such as bladder stimulators and artificial sphincters, have been used to a limited extent in experimental animals and in man. Frequent complications and prohibitive cost prevent their widespread use in veterinary medicine at the present time.

Recently, trigonal-colonic anastomosis for diversion of urine into the colon was used with varying degrees of success to salvage dogs with irreversible urinary incontinence. This procedure should be considered only when other methods of management prove unsatisfactory, however, since it is associated with a high incidence of pyelonephritis, reduction in renal function, and gastrointestinal disturbances (Bovée et al.).

SUPPLEMENTAL READING

Bovée, K.C., Pass, M.A., Wardley, R., Biery, D., and Allen, H.L.: Trigonal-colonic anastomosis: A urinary diversion procedure in dogs. J. Am. Vet. Med. Assoc., *174*:184–191, 1979.

DeGroat, W.C.: Nervous control of the urinary bladder of the cat. Brain Res., *87*:201, 1975.

Hoerlein, B.F.: *Canine Neurology*, 3rd ed. Philadelphia, W. B. Saunders Co., 1978.

McGuire, E.J., Wagner, F.M., and Weiss, R.M.: Treatment of autonomic dysreflexia with phenoxybenzamine. J. Urol., *115*:53, 1976.

Oliver, J.E., Jr.: Neurologic examination: Taking the history. Vet. Med. Small Anim. Clin., *67*:433, 1972.

Oliver, J.E., Jr.: Neurology of visceral function. Vet. Clin. North Am., *4*:517, 1974.

Oliver, J.E., Jr., and Young, W.O.: Air cystometry in dogs under xylazine-induced restraint. Am. J. Vet. Res., *34*:1433, 1973.

Oliver, J.E., Jr., Selcer, R.R., and Simpson, S.: Cauda equina compression from lumbosacral malarticulation and malformation in the dog. J. Am. Vet. Med. Assoc., *173*:207, 1978.

Osborne, C.A., and Oliver, J.E., Jr.: Non-neurogenic urinary incontinence. In Kirk, R.W. (ed.): *Current Veterinary Therapy VI.* Philadelphia, W.B. Saunders Co., 1977, pp. 1165–1172.

Sundin, T., Dahlstrom, A., Norlen, L., and Svedmyr, N.: The sympathetic innervation and adrenoreceptor function of the human lower urinary tract in the normal state and after parasympathetic denervation. Invest. Urol., *14*:322, 1977.

NON-NEUROGENIC URINARY INCONTINENCE

CARL A. OSBORNE, D.V.M.,
St. Paul, Minnesota

JOHN E. OLIVER, Jr., D.V.M.,
Athens, Georgia

and DAVID E. POLZIN, D.V.M.
St. Paul, Minnesota

Urinary incontinence in dogs and cats may result from several fundamentally different disease mechanisms. Because formulation of specific treatment and an accurate forecast of the probable future course of the disease process are primarily dependent on the underlying cause of urinary incontinence, every attempt should be made to localize the source of the incontinence and to establish its underlying cause. We have found a problem-specific data base useful in this regard (Table 1). Consult the article entitled "Neurogenic Urinary Incontinence" for details concerning the etiopathogenesis, diagnosis, and treatment of this form of incontinence. This article is concerned with ectopic ureters, patent urachus, pseudohermaphrodites, urethrorectal fistulas, estrogen-responsive urinary incontinence, obstructive (paradoxical) incontinence, urge incontinence, iatrogenic incontinence, and inappropriate micturition.

ECTOPIC URETERS

APPLIED ANATOMY AND PHYSIOLOGY

The ureters are primarily muscular tubes that actively transport urine produced in the kidney and stored in the renal pelvis to the urinary bladder. Urine that accumulates in the renal pelvis initiates peristaltic movement of pelvic and then of ureteral smooth muscle. As a result, elongated boluses of urine are propelled through the ureteral lumen by unilateral peristalsis to the urinary bladder (Weiss).

Anatomic ureterovesical sphincters are not present; however, the oblique course of the ureters through the bladder wall at the trigone forms a one-way flap valve that normally pre-vents retrograde flow of urine from the bladder. The ureterovesical valves protect the kidneys from abnormal retrograde pressure and from contamination with infected bladder urine.

INCIDENCE

Dogs. Ureteral ectopia is a common cause of urinary incontinence in female dogs. In one survey of 54 dogs with ectopic ureters Siberian huskies, West Highland white terriers, fox terriers, and miniature and toy poodles had a higher risk for this anomaly than other breeds of dogs (Hayes). A familial tendency has been reported in Siberian huskies (Johnston, et al., 1977b). We have the clinical impression that black Labrador retrievers also have a higher-than-expected incidence of the disorder.

Cats. Four cases of ectopic ureters have been reported in cats, suggesting that it is more common in this species than previously recognized (Bebko, et al.; Biewenga, et al.; Reis).

Sex. Although the incidence of ectopic ureters in dogs is unknown, it has been more frequently recognized in females than in males. In a recent survey of the world literature, 35 of 36 reported cases were in females (Owen, 1973a). One investigator reported a female-to-male ratio of 21:1 (Hayes).

In the past the consensus of opinion has been that the frequency with which ectopic ureters are recognized in female dogs was associated with the almost invariable occurrence of urinary incontinence in females. The lack of urinary incontinence in human males with ectopic ureters has been used as additional support for this generality. Urinary incontinence does not occur in association with urethral termination of one or both ureters in human males because all wolffian duct derivative structures are located

Table 1. Problem-specific Data Base for Urinary Incontinence

1. Owner's definition of incontinence
2. Duration of incontinence
3. Status of reproductive tract and relationship to incontinence
4. Hemogram
5. Urinalysis
6. Observation of micturition
7. Evaluation of bladder size
    a. Before micturition
    b. After micturition
8. Verification of incontinence
9. Appropriate neurologic examination
10. Catheterization to evaluate patency of urethral lumen if patient is dysuric or if urine cannot be expelled readily from the bladder by manual compression
11. Contrast radiography
    a. High-dose intravenous urography
    b. Retrograde contrast vaginogram or urethrogram if intravenous urography is not diagnostic

proximal to the external urethral sphincter. When a ureter empties into the urethra, the urine flows back into the lumen of the urinary bladder because the proximal urethra is less resistant to urine flow than more distal portions.

Although the first reported case of an ectopic ureter in a male dog was not associated with urinary incontinence, two subsequent cases in male dogs in which ectopic ureters terminated in the urethra were associated with urinary incontinence (Osborne, et al., 1975a). Male cats with ectopic ureters also had urinary incontinence (Biewenga, et al.).

Age. Since ureteral ectopia is a congenital anomaly, the incidence in young dogs and cats is high. In one survey 58 percent of the female dogs with ectopic ureters were diagnosed before they were one year old (Hayes).

ETIOLOGY

Termination of one or both ureters outside the urinary bladder occurs as a result of faulty differentiation of the mesonephric and metanephric ducts (Owen, 1973a). The underlying cause of faulty differentiation of these structures in the dog has not been established. Familial aggregations of ectopic ureters have been reported in black Labrador retrievers and Siberian huskies (Holt and Kievit; Johnston, et al., 1977b). The finding of certain breeds at high risk, coupled with the probable low risk of dogs of mixed breeding, suggests genetic involvement (Hayes). Ectopic ureters have been produced experimentally in the offspring of pregnant rats by altering their diet during certain stages of gestation.

PATHOPHYSIOLOGY

Location. In female dogs and cats either or both ureters may terminate in the vagina, urethra, bladder neck, or uterus. In a survey of the world literature the vagina was the most common site of ureteral termination (70 percent), with the urethra (20 percent), neck of the bladder (8 percent) and uterus (3 percent) being less common sites (Owen, 1973a). Although there is no apparent predisposition of either the right or left ureter, unilateral ectopia has been encountered far more frequently (approximately 80 percent) than bilateral ureteral ectopia (approximately 20 percent) (Owen, 1973a). In male dogs and cats with urinary incontinence the ureters must terminate in the urethra.

Associated Diseases. Ectopic ureters often are associated with other congenital anomalies of the urinary system and with acquired diseases that develop as a sequel to ureteral ectopia.

MEGAURETER. Megaureter (ureteroectasia) characterized by dilation of the ureteral lumen and abnormal peristalsis is a very common finding in dogs with ectopic ureters but has been detected less frequently in cats. Megaureter was reported in 16 of 36 canine cases of ectopic ureters evaluated in one large survey (Owen, 1973a). Varying degrees of megaureter (two to ten times normal) were observed in all 20 ectopic ureters present in 17 dogs (14 with unilateral ectopia and three with bilateral ureteral ectopia) studied at the University of Minnesota. Some patients had concomitant dilation of the renal pelvis (pyelectasis).

The cause of megaureter has not been established. Although stricture of the ureter associated with hydroureter and hydronephrosis has been reported in a few patients, total obstruction of urine outflow would not be a plausible explanation because of the presence of urinary incontinence. In our series gross anatomic obstruction of the ureters was observed in only one male dog with unilateral ureteral ectopia.

The possibility that impaired development of the distal portion of ectopic ureters might be the cause of megaureter has not been investigated. Developmental abnormalities in the distal portion of the ureter have been cited as a cause of so-called megaureter in human beings (Belman).

The pathogenesis of megaureters might also be related, at least in part, to the fact that the distal end of an ectopic ureter has no functional valve and permits reflux of urine. Megaureters may also be associated with urinary tract infection caused by *Escherichia coli* or *Pseudomonas* spp., organisms known to impair or inhibit ureteral peristalsis in the dog by release of bacterial products or stimulation of biologically active products by the host, or both (Boyarsky, et al.). Developmental abnormalities of the ureters in human beings are known to be associated with decreased or absent peristaltic activity (Hutch and Tanagho; McLaughlin, et al.). Impaired or inhibited peristalsis is associated with functional obstruction characterized by decreased emptying of affected ureters and resultant megaureter.

DECREASED RENAL SIZE. Reduction in renal size is often associated with an ectopic ureter. Although the observation that kidneys associated with ectopic ureters are sometimes smaller than normal is beyond question, the interpretation that reduction in size is always caused by congenital hypoplasia is erroneous. Since there is no functional sphincter at the distal end of an ectopic ureter, the potential for reflux predisposes the associated kidney to ascending bacterial infection. We have encountered small, contracted kidneys in patients with ectopic ureters in which gross, microscopic, and bacteriologic findings were typical of chronic generalized pyelonephritis. Reduction of renal size in human beings with ectopic ureters has been attributed to pyelonephritis, dysplasia, or obstructive atrophy, or a combination of these.

DECREASED BLADDER SIZE. In one large survey of ectopic ureters in dogs, bilateral ectopic ureters frequently were associated with an abnormally small urinary bladder (Owen, 1973a). Many investigators have stated that such bladders are hypoplastic, implying that their reduction in size was also caused by embryologic maldevelopment.

We are of the opinion that reduction in the size of the urinary bladder in patients with bilateral ureteral ectopia may also be associated with disuse. Our conclusion is based on experimental studies in laboratory animals (Goss and Singleton) and dogs (Schmaelzle, et al.) and clinical studies in dogs (Owen, 1973a, 1973b, 1973c) and man (Tanagho) that indicate that natural or surgically induced defunctionalization of the urinary bladder may be associated with a potentially reversible reduction in bladder capacity. Bilateral ureteral ectopia was observed in an incontinent two-year-old female Siberian husky at the University of Minnesota. Both ureters terminated in the urethra. Despite the fact that neither ureter entered the urinary bladder, the dog could micturate in a normal fashion. The urinary bladder was normal in size. Apparently, a significant quantity of urine expelled from the ureters into the urethra passed into the urinary bladder before being voided.

URETHRAL ABNORMALITIES. Dogs with ectopic ureters that terminate in the urethra may continue to have urinary incontinence following transplantation or extirpation of the affected ureter. Although less severe, urinary incontinence persisted in four of five female dogs with urethral ectopic ureters following surgical correction at the University of Minnesota. In contrast, all four dogs with vaginal ectopic ureters became continent following surgery.

MISCELLANEOUS PROBLEMS. Other congenital anomalies that have been observed in dogs with ectopic ureters include agenesis of the urinary bladder and urethra, persistent hymen, and abnormalities of the urethra (Osborne, et al., 1972; Pearson and Gibbs).

CLINICAL SIGNS

Clinical signs associated with ectopic ureters are dependent upon their site of termination and upon the presence or absence of other congenital or acquired abnormalities.

Female Dogs and Cats. In female dogs and cats ectopic ureters are usually associated with varying degrees of urinary incontinence. Affected dogs usually have a history of urinary incontinence since birth or weaning. Urine may drip from the vulva continuously or pool in the vagina and gravitate out of the vulva when body position is changed. Because the nerve supply and functional capacity of the urinary bladder are normal, the bladder does not become overdistended with urine. Patients with one ectopic ureter are typically able to micturate normally, since urine continues to pass into the urinary bladder through the unaffected ureter. Patients with bilateral ectopic ureters may be unable to micturate normally.

We have observed a progressive decrease in the severity of urinary incontinence in some female dogs that also had chronic generalized progressive disease of the associated kidney. The disease was thought to be caused by pyelonephritis. It is hypothesized that progressive destruction of the majority of functioning nephrons caused by ascending bacterial infection ultimately causes a progressive decrease in the total volume of urine produced by the kidney (even though remaining viable nephrons were producing an increased volume of urine).

Male Dogs and Cats. Only three cases of ectopic ureters have been reported in male dogs and only two have been reported in male cats. In all cases the ureters terminated in the urethra. Two of the three canine cases had urinary incontinence that was corrected surgically. Both feline cases had urinary incontinence. One was completely corrected by surgery and the other was partially corrected by surgery.

ENDOSCOPIC FINDINGS

Detection of abnormal openings in the vagina via endoscopy provides strong support for a diagnosis of ureteral ectopia. The opening of an ectopic ureter may be difficult to find, however. Satisfactory visualization of the entire mucosal surface of the vagina is dependent on the use of a vaginoscope that eliminates mucosal infoldings by distention of the vaginal wall. Glass (Pyrex) test tubes from which the bottoms have been removed and the ends fire-polished, pediatric proctoscopes, disposable plastic syringe cases from which a large rectangular section has been removed from the wall, and fiberoptic endoscopes are preferred over otoscopic cones and nasal specula for dogs. Injection of air into the vaginal lumen may enhance visualization by causing distention of the vaginal wall.

Many female dogs with ectopic ureters have a persistent hymen. Visual inspection of the vagina of such patients often reveals a fleshy piece of tissue that is attached to the dorsal and ventral walls of the vagina. The lateral aspects of the structure often form slitlike openings with the vaginal wall and may be mistaken for ectopic ureteral orifices.

RADIOGRAPHIC FINDINGS

Evaluation of the entire urinary tract by intravenous urography is indicated to confirm the presence of ectopic ureter(s) and to determine whether other abnormalities of the kidneys, ureters, urinary bladder, or urethra are present. Although intravenous urography is an important diagnostic aid, visualization of the exact site of termination of the distal ureter may be difficult or impossible. Poor visualization may occur if the ectopic ureter tunnels through the bladder wall before terminating at an ectopic site. Poor visualization may also occur because of lack of sufficient contrast medium in the lumen of the distal ureter. This may result from impaired ability of poorly functioning renal tissue to excrete a sufficient quantity of radiopaque medium to opacify the ureter. This problem may be minimized by the use of high-dose urography (Osborne, et al., 1972). Accumulation of contrast medium in the lumen of the urinary bladder may also interfere with visualization of the distal portion of the ureter. This problem may be minimized by exposure of films before the bladder becomes distended with radiopaque contrast material or by a combination of pneumocystography with intravenous urography.

As mentioned previously, ectopic ureters frequently are dilated and often are associated with dilation of the renal pelvis. The degree of megaureter detected by intravenous urography is dependent on the amount of radiopaque medium in the ureter and therefore on the amount administered (McLaughlin, et al.). The fact that there has been no uniformity in radiographic techniques performed in cases of ureteral ectopia reported in the literature may explain why megaureter has been a more consistent finding in cases evaluated by high-dose urography at the University of Minnesota than in other studies. When evaluated by high-dose urography, enlarged ureters frequently are filled with radiopaque medium throughout their entire length and are often tortuous, and their diameter in some portions may be two to ten times normal. In contrast, the entire length of normal ureters rarely is filled with radiopaque medium because peristaltic contractions normally constrict the ureteral lumen.

When an abnormal orifice is detected in the vagina or suspected to be in the urethra, catheterization of the orifice with a radiopaque catheter* followed by retrograde ureterography may be performed. This technique should not be used as a substitute for intravenous urography, however, since it may not reveal other abnormalities of the urinary system, including the presence of bilateral ureteral ectopia. We have had excellent results in detecting the site of termination of ectopic ureters utilizing retrograde contrast urethrography, retrograde contrast vaginography (Fig. 1), or both. Either pediatric Foley catheters† or Swan-Ganz flow-directed balloon catheters‡ may be used (Johnston, et al., 1977a). Care must be used so as not to occlude the opening of the ectopic ureteral orifice with inflated balloons of these catheters.

DIAGNOSIS

A history of urinary incontinence that has been present since birth or weaning in cats or dogs (especially females) should stimulate a high index of suspicion of ectopic ureter(s).

---

*American Cystoscope Makers, Inc., Pelham Manor, New York 10803

†American Cystoscope Makers, Inc., Pelham Manor, New York 10803

‡Edwards Laboratories, 17221 Red Hill Avenue, Santa Ana, California 92705

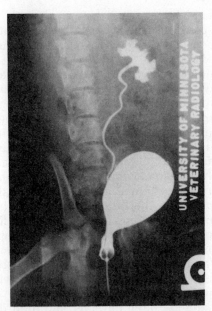

Figure 1. Dorsoventral oblique view of a retrograde urethrogram of an incontinent immature female Siberian husky with a unilateral left ectopic ureter. The distal end of the ectopic ureter entered the urethra. (Courtesy of Dr. Gary R. Johnston, University of Minnesota.)

Observation of an abnormal orifice in the vagina or failure to observe ureteral orifices at the trigone by cystoscopy provides supportive evidence. Additional support for the diagnosis may be obtained by injecting sterilized, colored dye into the urinary bladder. Normal-colored urine should appear at the vulva or tip of the penis in patients with urinary incontinence caused by an ectopic ureter.

Radiographic detection of megaureter, especially when associated with pyelectasis and reduction in renal size, provides strong supportive diagnostic evidence. Retrograde ureterography via direct catheterization with radiopaque catheters, retrograde contrast urethrography, or retrograde contrast vaginography provides definitive information concerning the ureter being studied.

In the event that endoscopic and radiographic studies fail to provide diagnostic information, an ectopic ureter may be confirmed by exploratory laparotomy. Lack of termination of one or both ureters at the trigone of the urinary bladder confirms the diagnosis. If the pathway of the distal ureter cannot be evaluated because it tunnels through surrounding tissue, a cystotomy may be performed to determine whether the ureteral orifices are in their normal location in the mucosal surface of the bladder. Alternatively, injection of a sufficient quantity of saline or other sterilized liquid into the lumen of an ectopic ureter should result in its immediate appearance at the vulva or tip of the penis rather than in the bladder lumen. The tip of a small catheter inserted into the lumen of an ectopic ureter should also pass through the vulva or external urethral orifice of the penis.

Treatment

There is no effective medical treatment for urinary incontinence caused by an ectopic ureter.

Proper surgical management of a patient with urinary incontinence caused by ureteral ectopia is dependent on (1) the functional capacity of associated and contralateral kidneys, (2) the presence or absence of infection or other pathologic changes in the urinary tract (an attempt to eliminate or control infection of the urinary system with appropriate antimicrobial drugs should be made prior to surgery), (3) whether one or both ureters are ectopic, and (4) the site of termination of the anomalous ureter. Dogs with ureters that terminate in the urethra may continue to have urinary incontinence despite surgical correction of the affected ureter(s).

We have been successful with transplantation of ectopic ureters when a submucosal antireflux tunnel has been made in the bladder (Archibald and Owen). Dilation of transplanted ureters has not interferred with the success of this technique. In fact, it often reduces the difficulty of reimplanting the distal ureter into the bladder. A technique of ureterovesical anastomosis without transection of the distal ureter has also been successfully used in dogs (Dingwall, et al.). Transplantation of the ureter into the urinary bladder is the procedure of choice if any of the following conditions exist: (1) normal function of the kidney drained by the ectopic ureter, (2) extravesical termination of both ureters, or (3) reduced functional capacity of both kidneys. In the last situation, extirpation of a kidney may result in removal of a sufficient quantity of renal parenchyma to precipitate renal failure.

Nephrectomy and removal of as much of the anomalous ureter as possible should be performed when the kidney attached to the ectopic ureter is affected by generalized disease or when intractable infection is present in the affected ureter or kidney, or both. When the ureter opens into the vagina it should be resected to as low a level as can be conveniently reached by a lower abdominal incision. Care must be taken not to damage the vesicourethral sphincter by dissection of ectopic ureters that become buried in the wall of the urinary bladder. Tracing the ureter to its precise termination is not necessary, since in our experience the unresected distal portion rarely is a source of further trouble. If one or both ureters empty into the urethra, incomplete excision may result in the formation of a diverticulum, urinary stasis, and persistent infection. Because of difficulties in operative exposure and the risk of damaging the vesicoureteral sphincter, however, it is usually preferable to perform distal ureterectomy at a later time if the need arises.

PROGNOSIS

If surgical correction of a unilateral ectopic ureter that terminates in the vagina or uterus is feasible, a guarded to good prognosis should be offered. If one or both ectopic ureters terminate in the urethra, the owner should be advised that some degree of urinary incontinence may continue following surgical correction of the problem.

Transplantation of dilated ureters into the urinary bladder may be followed by varying degrees of vesicoureteral reflux. Vesicoureteral reflux in turn predisposes the patient to ascending infection of the kidney. A better long-term result may be obtained when the ureters have some degree of peristalsis and are not extremely dilated. We have obtained satisfactory results by transplanting dilated ureters without radiographic evidence of peristalsis into the urinary bladder in several patients, however.

PATENT URACHUS

The urachus functions in the fetus to provide a channel of communication between the urinary bladder and the allantoic sac. The urachus is normally non-functional at birth.

COMPLETELY PATENT URACHUS

If the urachal canal remains completely patent following birth, urine will be voided through the umbilicus. Urine-scald dermatitis of the abdomen is common, as is secondary bacterial infection of the urinary bladder and umbilicus (omphalitis). Affected animals maintain the capacity to micturate normally.

The diagnosis may be confirmed by intravenous urography or retrograde cystography. Treatment consists of complete excision of the urachus and elimination of secondary bacterial infection with appropriate antibiotics.

PARTIALLY PATENT URACHUS

The urachal canal may remain partially patent. If the patent portion of the urachal canal communicated with the bladder lumen, a blind diverticulum frequently is present. Urachal di-

verticula frequently are associated with recurrent cystitis. Diagnosis and treatment are the same as those described for a completely patent urachus. Consult the article entitled "Congenital Diseases of the Urachus" for specific details.

Clinical signs are apparently uncommon in patients with a partially patent urachus that communicates with the umbilicus. Urachal cysts may form at any point between the umbilicus and the urinary bladder as a result of persistence of secreting urachal epithelium in isolated stretches of patent lumen. Urachal cysts may become infected with bacteria, necessitating surgical excision.

URETHRORECTAL FISTULAS

Fistulas that connect the lumina of the urogenital tract and the intestine may be congenital or acquired. Although relatively uncommon, they may be associated with signs related to the urinary, reproductive, or gastrointestinal system.

In dogs urethrorectal fistulas most commonly have been congenital and have been associated with passage of urine from the anus and penis (male) or vulva (female) at the time of micturition (Osborne, et al., 1975b). The disorder is commonly associated with urinary tract infections. Treatment by surgical correction following localization of the fistula by retrograde contrast urethrography is recommended. Consult the article entitled "Urinary Tract Infections" for details concerning eradication of secondary bacterial pathogens.

PSEUDOHERMAPHRODITISM

Non-neurogenic incontinence has been a common finding in canine pseudohermaphrodites with abnormalities of the vagina or urethra, or both (Jackson, et al.). In our experience the pathogenesis of incontinence associated with this disorder has been retention of urine in anomalous communications with the genital tract and subsequent leakage into the urethra, resulting in involuntary escape of urine. Consult the article entitled "Pseudohermaphroditism" for further information about cause, diagnosis, and treatment.

ESTROGEN-RESPONSIVE URINARY INCONTINENCE

An as yet poorly understood type of urinary incontinence occasionally develops after a variable postoperative period in dogs that have had ovariohysterectomy. Although the incidence of the problem is unknown, there is a general consensus of opinion that it is an uncommon sequela to ovariohysterectomy. The disease has apparently not been observed in cats. In a retrospective survey of 47 canine cases at the University of Minnesota there was no age or breed predisposition. The mean age at the time of reported owner recognition of urinary incontinence was 8.3 years (range = 1 to 15 years). In some dogs the onset and severity of incontinence coincided with concomitant but apparently unrelated disorders associated with polyuria.

ETIOPATHOGENESIS

The etiology and pathophysiology of this syndrome have not yet been determined. The fact that affected dogs can micturate normally suggests that the nerve supply and detrusor muscle are normal. Signs of urinary tract infection and inflammation typically are absent.

Whether removal of the ovaries or uterus (or both) is important in the etiopathogenesis of this disorder has not been determined, since a complete ovariohysterectomy is the surgical technique almost invariably employed to prevent estrus and unwanted pregnancies. One theory is that the uterine stump of affected animals adheres to the bladder neck following ovariohysterectomy and that subsequent retraction of the stump associated with senescence results in mechanical interference with physiologic sphincter activity. This hypothesis, however, does not provide an obvious explanation of the observation that exogenous administratino of estrogens induces remission of urinary incontinence.

The fact that administration of relatively low doses of estrogens to affected dogs is frequently associated with remission of incontinence, whereas withdrawal of estrogen therapy is associated with recurrence of incontinence, has been interpreted by some to indicate that the disease is caused by hypoestrogenism. Similar observations made in postmenopausal women with stress incontinence have been used to support this hypothesis (Musiani). It is theorized that the mucosal lining of the trigone of women is dependent on estrogens, as is vesicourethral sphincter tone. The popularity of this theory in veterinary medicine is associated with the commonly used term *hypoestrogenic urinary incontinence*.

Although logical, the hypoestrogenism theory has not yet been substantiated, inasmuch as the estrogen concentration in the plasma and urine of affected dogs (and human beings) has not been measured and compared with that of nonaffected ovariohysterectomized or normal dogs. This theory also does not offer an obvious explanation as to why urinary incontinence occurs only in a small percentage of dogs that undergo ovariohysterectomy.

Recent experimental studies performed in rabbits indicate that estrogens can influence the response of the urethra and urinary bladder to alpha-adrenergic stimulation. Ovariectomy of rabbits was associated with decreased sensitivity to stimulation of alpha-adrenergic receptors in the bladder and urethra (Hodgson, et al.). These observations are of great interest, since alpha-adrenergic receptors in the bladder neck and urethra are important in the maintenance of urine continence (Khanna).

DIAGNOSIS

Estrogen-responsive urinary incontinence in dogs that have had ovariohysterectomies is frequently an exclusion diagnosis that is established after other causes of urinary incontinence have been eliminated. Remission of urinary incontinence following therapy with appropriate dosages of estrogens is required to confirm the diagnosis.

TREATMENT

Administration of low doses of estrogens usually results in remission of urinary incontinence. In the past, we have recommended oral administration of diethylstilbestrol at a dose of 0.1 to 1.0 mg/day for three to five days, followed by a maintenance dosage of approximately 1.0 mg/week. Alternatively, 0.1 to 1.0 mg of estradiol cypionate* may be administered parenterally at intervals of weeks to months. It must be emphasized that these dosages and maintenance intervals have been established on the basis of uncontrolled clinical observations and therefore are empirical.

More recently, we have observed patients that required larger doses of estrogens to become continent. In one, incontinence had previously been controlled successfully with lower dosages, whereas in others higher doses were required to ameliorate incontinence at the onset of therapy. Although the reason for these differences has not been determined, in some patients return or onset of urinary incontinence has been associated with polyuria due to apparently unrelated causes. Although cases available for evaluation have been too few in

---

*ECP, The Upjohn Co., Kalamazoo, Michigan 49002

number to permit establishment of meaningful generalities, it appears that spontaneous or therapeutic remission of the severity of polyuria was associated with decreased severity or remission of urinary incontinence in some patients. On the basis of these limited observations we are cautiously suggesting that the dosage of estrogens required to maintain urine continence may be influenced by polyuria. However, we are not suggesting that water be withheld in an attempt to control this type of urinary incontinence.

We emphasize the fact that excessive quantities of estrogens may induce signs of estrus and may be toxic to bone marrow. Myelotoxicity induced by estrogens in dogs is characterized initially by leukocytosis associated with increased granulopoiesis and thrombocytopenia associated with decreased megakaryocytopoiesis. In severe cases total suppression of hematopoiesis may result in a normocytic, normochromic anemia, marked neutropenia, and persistent thrombocytopenia. Death may occur as a result of hemorrhagic diathesis (Schalm).

OBSTRUCTIVE (PARADOXICAL) INCONTINENCE

ETIOPATHOGENESIS

Paradoxical incontinence may occur in patients with partial obstruction of the urethra due to organic or functional causes. Consult the article "Neurogenic Urinary Incontinence" for details concerning reflex dyssynergia, an example of neurogenic functional paradoxical incontinence (Khanna). Paradoxical incontinence has been encountered most often in male dogs, presumably because of the length of their urethras and because the os penis restricts the degree to which the urethra passing through its ventral groove can dilate. The obstructive lesion in the urethra (calculus, neoplasm, stricture, space-occupying mass in periurethral tissue) must be of such a nature that it prevents normal micturition but not so severe that it completely obstructs urine outflow. When the bladder becomes overdistended with urine, intravesical pressure exceeds the resistance imparted by the urethral lesion, and urinary incontinence results. Prolonged overdistention of the bladder may induce a variable degree of damage to structures in the bladder wall. If this occurs, the pathogenesis becomes complicated by neuromuscular deficit (consult "Neurogenic Urinary Incontinence"). The paradox of this syndrome is that urinary incontinence occurs in a patient with obstruction of urine outflow.

DIAGNOSIS

Paradoxical incontinence should be suspected in patients with abnormal micturition characterized by voluntary or involuntary dribbling of urine and by dysuria. The urinary bladder is usually overdistended with urine, and difficulty is encountered in expelling urine from the bladder by digital palpation. Insertion of a catheter through the urethral lumen may be difficult or impossible. Localization of the urethral lesion may be established with the aid of a catheter or, preferably, by contrast urethrography. The presence or absence of postrenal uremia should be determined by evaluating serum creatinine or urea nitrogen concentration.

TREATMENT

Specific. Specific treatment is dependent on the nature of the underlying cause. Urethral calculi may be removed by urohydropropulsion, by means of a Mitchell stone basket,* or by urethrotomy. In dogs with irreversible urethral strictures a permanent urethrostomy proximal to the site of obstruction may be required. In cats perineal, preputial, or antepubic urethrostomy may be considered. Neoplasms that have not metastasized should be extirpated surgically. In our experience, by the time transitional cell carcinomas of the urethra were of sufficient size to induce clinical signs, they were usually inoperable because of local invasion and metastases.

Supportive. The urinary bladder of patients with postrenal uremia should be decompressed as soon as possible by catheterization or, if necessary, cystocentesis. Abnormalities in fluid, acid-base, and electrolyte balances associated with renal failure should also be corrected (consult articles on treatment of renal failure).

If the urinary bladder is hypotonic or atonic because of prolonged overdistention, it should be maintained in a non-distended state by manual compression, intermittent aseptic catheterization, or via an indwelling catheter. If neuromuscular structures have not been damaged irreversibly, normal bladder function may return (see "Neurogenic Urinary Incontinence").

URGE INCONTINENCE

Urge incontinence is defined as uncontrollable desire to micturate, resulting in involun-

---

*Bard Hospital Division, C. R. Bard Inc., Murray Hill, New Jersey 07974

tary loss of urine. Incontinence occurs soon after the sensation of bladder fullness. It is characterized by inability to control micturition between the time of the urge to micturate and the actual time of bladder evacuation. Micturition usually occurs at a low volume of bladder filling. Apparently there is no damage to the sphincter mechanism, since continuous loss of urine is not observed. It is often caused by bacterial inflammation or trauma of the urinary bladder and urethral mucosa. Consult the article entitled "Urinary Tract Infections" for additional information about etiopathogenesis, diagnosis, and treatment.

Cystitis may develop in patients with small, hyperactive neurogenic bladders as a result of retention of residual urine in the bladder lumen. In such patients abnormal patterns of micturition may not be caused by bacterial inflammation. Diagnosis, prognosis, and therapy are dependent on the underlying cause of neurogenic dysfunction (consult the article, "Neurogenic Urinary Incontinence").

IATROGENIC INCONTINENCE

Urinary incontinence may occur following cystotomy or prostatectomy in dogs, presumably as a result of damage to the intricate arrangement of smooth muscle fibers at the junction of the bladder with the urethra. It may also be associated with damage to regional nerves and thus may have a neurogenic component. In order to minimize postoperative incontinence, care should be used in manipulating the bladder during surgery. In addition, incisions should not involve the junction of the bladder neck and urethra or the bladder trigone unless absolutely essential.

INAPPROPRIATE MICTURITION

Puppies, nervous adult dogs, and animals with CNS lesions that cause psychomotor disturbances may have uncontrollable (or inappropriate) patterns of micturition. In some cases inappropriate micturition may be confused with other causes of urinary incontinence. Inappropriate micturition associated with behavioral patterns (sometimes called "submissive micturition") usually is intermittent and initiated by stress or fright. It may undergo remission as the animal matures or may be controlled by conditioning and training. The prognosis and therapy of psychomotor disturbances induced by CNS lesions is dependent on the biologic behavior of the underlying cause.

SUPPLEMENTAL READING

Archibald, J., and Owen, R.R.: Urinary system. In Archibald, J. (ed.): *Canine Surgery*, 2nd ed. Santa Barbara, California, American Veterinary Publications, 1974.

Bebko, R.L., Prier, J.E., and Biery, D.N.: Ectopic ureters in a male cat. J. Am. Vet. Med. Assoc., *171*:738–740, 1977.

Belman, A.B.: Megaureter: Classification, etiology, and management. Urol. Clin. North Am., *1*:497–513, 1974.

Biewenga, W.J., Rothuizen, J., and Voorhout, G.: Ectopic ureters in the cat: A report of two cases. J. Small Anim. Pract., *19*:531–537, 1978.

Boyarsky, S. et al.: *Urodynamics: Hydrodynamics of the Ureter and Renal Pelvis.* New York, Academic Press, 1971.

Dingwall, J.S., Eger, C.E., and Owen, R.R.: Clinical experiences with the combined technique of ureterovesicular anastomosis for treatment of ectopic ureters. J. Am. Anim. Hosp. Assoc., *12*:406–410, 1976.

Goss, R.J., and Singleton, S.D.: Disuse atrophy of the bladder after bilateral nephrectomy. Proc. Soc. Exp. Biol. Med., *138*:861–864, 1971.

Hayes, H.M.: Ectopic ureter in dogs: Epidemiologic features. Teratology, *10*:129–132, 1974.

Hodgson, B.J., Dumas, S., Bolling, D.R., and Heesch, C.M.: Effect of estrogen on sensitivity of rabbit bladder and urethra to phenylephrine. Invest. Urol., *16*:67–69, 1978.

Holt, J.C., and Kievit, T.: Correction of ectopic ureter. Aust. Vet. Practitioner, *1*:19–21, 1971.

Hutch, J.A., and Tanagho, E.A.: Etiology of nonocclusive ureteral dilatation. J. Urol., *93*:177–184, 1965.

Jackson, D.A., Osborne, C.A., Brasmer, T.H., and Jessen, C.R.: Non-neurogenic urinary incontinence in a canine female pseudohermaphrodite. J. Am. Vet. Med. Assoc., *172*:926–930, 1978.

Johnston, G.R., Jessen, C.R., and Osborne, C.A.: Retrograde contrast urethrography. In Kirk, R.W. (ed.): *Current Veterinary Therapy VI.* Philadelphia, W.B. Saunders Co., 1977a.

Johnston, G.R., Osborne, C.A., Wilson, J.W., and Yano, B.L.: Familial renal ectopia in the dog. J. Am. Anim. Hosp. Assoc., *13*:168–170, 1977b.

Khanna, O.P.: Disorders of micturition: Neuropharmacologic basis and results of drug therapy. Urology, *8*:316–328, 1976.

McLaughlin, A.P., Pfister, R.C., Leadbetter, W.F., Salzstein, S.L., and Kessler, W.O.: The pathophysiology of primary megaloureter. J. Urol., *109*:805–811, 1973.

Musiani, U.: A partially successful attempt at medical treatment of urinary stress incontinence in women. Urol. Int., *27*:405–410, 1972.

Osborne, C.A., Dieterich, H.F., Hanlon, G.F., and Anderson, L.D.: Urinary incontinence due to ectopic ureter in a male dog. J. Am. Vet. Med. Assoc., *166*:911–914, 1975a.

Osborne, C.A., Engen, M.H., Yano, B.L., Brasmer, T.H., Jessen, C.R., and Blevins, W.E.: Congenital urethrorectal fistula in two dogs. J. Am. Vet. Med. Assoc., *166*:999–1002, 1975b.

Osborne, C.A., Low, D.G., and Finco, D.R.: *Canine and Feline Urology.* Philadelphia, W.B. Saunders Co., 1972.

Owen, R.R.: Canine ureteral ectopia: A review. I. Embryology and etiology. J. Small Anim. Pract., *14*:407–417, 1973a.

Owen, R.R.: Canine ureteral ectopia: A review. II. Incidence, diagnosis and treatment. J. Small Anim. Pract., *14*:419–427, 1973b.

Owen, R.R.: Three case reports of ectopic ureters in bitches. Vet. Rec., *93*:2–10, 1973c.

Pearson, H., and Gibbs, C.: Urinary tract abnormalities in the dog. J. Small Anim. Pract., *12*:67–84, 1971.

Reis, R.H.: Renal aplasia, ectopic ureter, and vascular abnormalities in domestic cats. Anat. Rec., *135*:105–107, 1959.

Schalm, O.W.: Exogenous estrogen toxicity in the dog. Canine Pract., *5*:57–61, 1978.

Schmaelzle, J.F., Cass, A.S., and Hinman, F.: Effect of disuse and restoration of function on vesical capacity. J. Urol., *101*:700–705, 1969.

Tanagho, E.A.: Congenitally obstructed bladders: Fate after prolonged defunctionalization. J. Urol., *111*:102–109, 1974.

Weiss, R.M.: Ureteral function. Urology, *12*:114–133, 1978.

CANINE POLYPOID CYSTITIS

SHIRLEY D. JOHNSTON, D.V.M.,
CARL A. OSBORNE, D.V.M.,
and JERRY B. STEVENS, D.V.M.
St. Paul, Minnesota

Polypoid cystitis is an uncommon inflammatory disease of the urinary bladder of dogs that is characterized by growth of one or more nonneoplastic space-occupying lesions into its lumen. This disorder is of importance to veterinarians because it exemplifies the fact that all polypoid lesions of the bladder are not neoplastic (Table 1). In our experience polypoid cystitis has often been associated with chronic recurrent bacterial infection of the urinary tract. It has not been determined whether bacteria cause or complicate the underlying lesion.

CLINICAL FINDINGS

Affected dogs usually develop constant or intermittent chronic hematuria that may persist throughout micturition or occur predominantly at the end of micturition. Dysuria, pollakiuria, and other signs of lower urinary tract disease are also common. These signs may temporarily undergo remission following antimicrobial therapy.

Palpation of the bladder may not reveal abnormalities or detect non-grating masses within the bladder lumen. The bladder wall may or may not be detectably thickened.

Urinalysis often reveals a disproportionate number of red cells to white cells, findings indicative of hemorrhage. Typical inflammatory signs (pyuria, hematuria, and proteinuria) may also be observed. Examination of urine sediment may reveal hyperplastic transitional epithelial cells and bacteria. Care must be taken not to confuse hyperplastic transitional epithelial cells with neoplastic transitional epithelial cells.

Quantitative urine culture often reveals significant bacteriuria. In our experience *Proteus* spp. have been isolated most frequently, although it is logical to assume that other bacteria commonly associated with urinary tract infections may also be found.

Polypoid cystitis is usually not associated with systemic illness. Results of a hemogram are usually normal. Unless both ureters or the urethral lumen is obstructed by the space-occupying lesions or unless ascending infection leads to generalized pyelonephritis, the serum concentration of urea and creatinine will be normal. In our experience these complications have not occurred.

Survey and contrast urography typically reveal one or more space-occupying lesions protruding into the bladder lumen. Visualization of small lesions may be enhanced by double-contrast cystography. Intravenous urography combined with pneumocystography offers the advantage of evaluation of the kidneys and ureters in addition to the urinary bladder. Survey radiographs of the thorax are recommended to rule out metastatic neoplastic pulmonary lesions.

Because the radiographic appearance of inflammatory polyps is similar to urothelial neoplasms, attempts to obtain a diagnostic sample by catheter biopsy (or cystoscopy when feasible) is recommended. Although detection of cells typical of inflammation does not exclude the possibility of neoplasia, detection of malignant urothelial cells will affect prognosis and may influence the surgical technique used (if any).

Exploratory surgery often reveals numerous distended blood vessels on the serosal surface of the bladder. The bladder wall may or may not be thickened. The mucosal surface of the bladder may contain one or more raised, sometimes friable, lesions that have a congested or hemorrhagic appearance. Gross examination will not permit distinction among inflammatory polyps, benign urothelial polyps (papillomas), and malignant urothelial polyps.

A definitive diagnosis of polypoid cystitis must be based on careful microscopic examination of polypoid lesions and adjacent portions of bladder wall removed during surgery. Because inflammatory lesions may coexist with neoplastic lesions, all growths removed should be preserved for microscopic evaluation. Conventional formalin-fixed tissue sections and impression smears for cytologic study are recommended. The microscopic appearance of inflammatory polyps is variable, but often they are covered by

Table 1. *Similarities and Differences of Inflammatory Polyps and Urothelial Neoplasms*

ABNORMALITY	POLYPOID CYSTITIS	NEOPLASIA
Dysuria, pollakiuria, and hematuria	++++	++++
Hematuria, pyuria, and proteinuria	++++	++++
Bacteriuria	++++	++++
Neoplastic cells in urine sediment	–	±
Catheter biopsy	Inflammation	Inflammation and/or neoplasia
Radiographic findings indicative of lung metastasis	–	±
Radiographic and macroscopic appearance	Single or multiple raised polypoid mucosal lesions; bladder wall may be thickened	Single or multiple raised polypoid mucosal lesions; bladder wall may be thickened
Microscopic appearance	Inflammation	Neoplasia often associated with inflammation

hyperplastic transitional epithelium that may be ulcerated. Vascular congestion is often a prominent feature of macroscopically reddened lesions. The mucosa, submucosa, and muscularis coat may contain varying quantities of lymphocytes, plasma cells, and eosinophils. Polymorphonuclear leukocytes may be prominent in patients with significant bacteriuria. Varying quantities of connective tissue may also be present.

THERAPY

Solitary lesions should be removed by partial cystectomy if they are not located near the trigone or bladder neck. Multiple polypoid lesions that involve large quantities of the bladder mucosa should be resected down to the level of the submucosa with the aid of an electrocautery unit.

Choice of therapeutic agents should be based on antimicrobial sensitivity tests. Patients should be treated with appropriate drugs for at least four to six weeks following surgery. In our experience prolonged antimicrobial therapy has been necessary to prevent recurrence of urinary tract infection. This may be related to persistence of an as yet unrecognized alteration in local host defense mechanisms. Therapy for an indefinite period may be required to prevent recurrence of urinary tract infection in some patients.

SUPPLEMENTAL READING

Johnston, S.D., Osborne, C.A., and Stevens, J.B.: Canine polypoid cystitis. J. Am. Vet. Med. Assoc., *166*:1155–1160, 1975.
Kessler, W.O., Clark, P.L., and Kaplan, G.W.: Eosinophilic cystitis. Urology, 6:499–501, 1975.
Melhoff, T., and Osborne, C.A.: Catheter biopsy of the urethra, urinary bladder, and prostate gland. In Kirk, R.W. (ed.): Current Veterinary Therapy. VI. Philadelphia, W.B. Saunders Co., 1977.
Osborne, C.A., and Finco, D.R.: Urinary tract infections: New solutions to old problems. In Scientific Proceedings of the AAHA Annual Meeting, American Animal Hosp. Assoc., South Bend, Indiana, 1977.
Osborne, C.A., Low, D.G., and Perman, V.: Neoplasms of the canine and feline urinary bladder: Clinical findings, diagnosis and treatment. J. Am. Vet. Med. Assoc., *152*:247–259, 1968.

RUPTURE OF THE CANINE URINARY BLADDER

COLIN F. BURROWS, B. Vet. Med.

Philadelphia, Pennsylvania

and RONALD J. KOLATA, D.V.M.

Athens, Georgia

Release of urine into the peritoneal cavity initiates a unique series of pathophysiologic changes that, if untreated, result in death from a combination of acute uremia, hypovolemia, and endotoxemia in about 60 hours. Abnormal physical findings and changes in blood chemistry can be subtle in the first 12 to 24 hours after rupture, however, making early diagnosis difficult unless the disorder is suspected.

The most common cause of urinary bladder rupture is external abdominal trauma, but traumatic palpation or catheterization may also rupture the organ, particularly if it is diseased. Spontaneous rupture is rare but may occur in association with atony, necrotizing cystitis, and bladder tumors.

The incidence of bladder injury in cases of abdominal trauma is not clear, but in a study of motor vehicle accidents 29 per cent of dogs with confirmed intra-abdominal injuries had ruptured bladders (Kolata and Johnston). A study of urinary tract trauma found that 65 per cent of injuries to that system involved the bladder (Kleine and Thornton). Ruptured bladders occur more frequently in male dogs, as does physical trauma in general.

Rupture commonly occurs when sudden compression of the distended bladder increases intraluminal pressure beyond a critical limit. The wall bursts, usually along the greater curvature near the apex. The bladder may also be punctured by fragments of the ileum and pubis when the pelvis is fractured. In some cases the bladder has been found to be avulsed from the urethra at the level of the prostate when the pelvis has been severely crushed. In contrast to man, extraperitoneal rupture is rare in the dog because of the anatomic location of the urinary bladder.

Urine in the peritoneal cavity causes chemical peritonitis associated with vomiting, paralytic ileus, and sequestration of peritoneal fluid. Hypertonic urine accentuates fluid sequestration by drawing fluid into the peritoneal cavity to establish osmotic equilibrium. Diffusion of urinary solutes into the blood results in uremia. The combination of intraperitoneal fluid sequestration and fluid lost as vomitus results in rapid and severe hypovolemia and dehydration. In some cases secondary bacterial infection occurs, which increases fluid sequestration and causes endotoxemia.

Since uroperitoneum is a form of postrenal azotemia, acidosis would be expected to develop. However, loss of hydrogen and chloride ions in the vomitus prevents acidosis in most animals. In fact, hydrogen and potassium loss may be so severe that some patients have a metabolic alkalosis and may be normokalemic or even hypokalemic (Burrows and Bovee).

HISTORY AND PHYSICAL FINDINGS

There are two distinct categories of urinary bladder rupture in dogs. Both are usually associated with external trauma and have the same sequence of pathophysiologic changes, but they differ in the period of time from rupture to diagnosis.

The "early diagnosis" category is usually associated with multisystem trauma sufficiently severe to require veterinary care immediately following the accident. Many of these patients have pelvic fractures and a tense, painful abdomen but are not uremic or dehydrated. Bladder rupture usually is diagnosed as part of the post-trauma evaluation.

The "late diagnosis" category is usually associated with milder trauma, and diagnosis is seldom made until signs directly associated with ruptured bladder are evident. These animals are seldom presented for evaluation immediately after the accident but, if they are, they may appear normal or have abdominal discomfort detectable by palpation. More overt signs usually do not become apparent until 12 to 24 hours after trauma. Progressive central nervous system depression, increasing polydipsia, and increasing frequency of vomiting are the predominant signs. Clients may also notice an increasing reluctance on the part of the animal to move about as toxemia and peritonitis worsen.

Although many animals with a ruptured bladder are able to urinate, urination frequently is associated with tenesmus and passage of small quantities of bloody urine.

If untreated, most dogs with urinary bladder rupture live about 60 hours, the exact time varying with the nature and severity of concomitant injuries. Following rupture, physical findings, including depression and dehydration, become progressively abnormal. Abdominal palpation gradually becomes more painful, a fluid wave may be detected on percussion of the abdominal wall, and the breath may develop a uremic odor. Many animals are hypothermic, but fever may develop if secondary bacterial infection is present.

Diagnostic Studies

Diagnosis is best made from a combination of radiographic and blood chemistry studies. Abdominal radiographs may reveal a homogeneous appearance, with obliteration of the normal viscera, ileus, and sometimes signs of trauma to other tissues. Contrast cystography is the most specific diagnostic procedure; the diagnosis can be confirmed by injection of 50 to 100 ml of a 50 per cent solution of iodinated radiopaque material into the bladder. The catheter must be inserted gently; if resistance is met it should be withdrawn a short distance and a urethrogram should be performed to rule out urethral injury. If the bladder is ruptured the contrast material will escape into the abdominal cavity. A film of the lateral abdomen, exposed as the solution is injected, usually reveals the size and location of the rupture. Small tears have a tendency to seal spontaneously as the bladder contracts and reopen as it distends. To make a diagnosis in these cases it may be necessary to distend the bladder with larger volumes of contrast material.

Injection of 50 to 100 ml of air into the bladder through a urinary catheter is another useful diagnostic procedure. If the ear is placed close to the abdominal wall during injection, air can be heard bubbling into the abdomen if the bladder is ruptured. A survey radiograph exposed immediately after injection reveals lack of distention of the bladder with air and accumulation of air in the uppermost portion of the abdominal cavity.

Abdominocentesis facilitates diagnosis in cases presented soon after injury when fluid is present within the abdomen (Kolata). Abdominal fluid typically has a packed cell volume (PCV) less than that of peripheral blood. In cases examined more than 12 hours after rupture the fluid is turbid and blood-tinged. Cytologic study reveals changes typical of an inflammatory exudate or, more often, of a modified transudate. The fluid contains urea nitrogen concentrations similar to, and creatinine concentrations higher than, those of peripheral blood. Detection of this difference is a useful diagnostic aid. The difference most likely is a result of differences in the sizes of urea and creatinine molecules (Burrows and Bovee).

The combination of prerenal and postrenal azotemia, together with changes induced by sepsis and prolonged vomiting, leads to marked changes in blood chemistry that become of increasing diagnostic and therapeutic importance as the disease progresses. Changes in the hemogram and plasma chemistries are compatible with hemoconcentration, inflammation, and azotemia. Provided that excessive hemorrhage has not occurred, the packed cell volume, total solids, and red cell count will be elevated to a degree proportional to the extent of dehydration. The PCV increases rapidly to a maximum of about 60 per cent after rupture. In most cases a leukocytosis characterized by a steadily rising neutrophilia is also present (Burrows and Bovee).

After 24 hours serum creatinine, potassium, inorganic phosphorus, and urea nitrogen concentrations are increased, whereas serum sodium and chloride concentrations are decreased. All these changes become progressively worse with time.

The differential diagnosis includes other causes of uroperitoneum and Addison's disease. Contrast radiography usually differentiates ruptured bladder from other causes of uroperitoneum. The severe vomiting, weakness, hyponatremia, and hyperkalemia that occur more than 48 hours after bladder rupture are similar to signs associated with Addison's disease. Differentiation is made on the basis of ascites, abdominal tenderness, and the difference in creatinine concentrations of plasma and abdominal fluid of dogs with ruptured bladders. Once the diagnosis of ruptured bladder is suspected, confirmation is made by contrast radiography.

Treatment

Surgical repair is the specific treatment for rupture of the urinary bladder; however, the timing of surgical intervention is of critical importance. In cases in which the diagnosis is made early (i.e., less than 12 hours after rupture) repair is undertaken as soon as shock has been adequately treated. Repair should not be undertaken in a hemodynamically unstable or toxemic patient until appropriate supportive steps have been taken to ensure a good surgical candidate. In cases of delayed diagnosis, repair best awaits correction of metabolic, fluid, and electrolyte imbalances.

Supportive measures should be instituted immediately. Parenteral fluid therapy consisting of physiologic saline to replace sodium, chloride, and water lost by vomiting and fluid sequestration should be initiated and continued until the deficit is replaced. Response to therapy is indicated by return of vital signs toward normal and improvement of the overall state of the patient. At this time the replacement fluid is best changed to a polyionic fluid administered at a rate of about 80 ml/kg/day.

A urinary catheter should be inserted to drain the urine and abdominal fluid. If a catheter cannot be inserted because of urethral or pelvic trauma or if a free flow of urine is not obtained, a peritoneal dialysis catheter should be inserted into the abdomen and closed drainage maintained by this means.

Prophylactic doses of a broad-spectrum antibiotic should be given parenterally to reduce the chance of infection. Drainage of urine coupled with appropriate fluid replacement allows rapid return of blood chemistries toward normal in about 12 to 16 hours.

These procedures result in a significant improvement in the physiologic state of the patient and are indicated in all severely depressed and uremic animals.

The surgical approach consists of a routine caudal midventral incision. Provisions should be made to extend the incision cranially if other intra-abdominal injuries are suspected. Repair of the ruptured bladder is the same as for cystotomy, except that the wound edges should be debrided before closure.

Synthetic absorbable suture materials are recommended for suturing the bladder because they have the advantages of predictable absorption and minimal tissue reaction (Laufman and Rabel). Chromic gut or one of the monofilament non-absorbable materials may also be used.

Once the bladder is repaired the abdomen should be lavaged with a copious volume (1 to 3 liters) of warm polyionic solution. The addition of an antibacterial agent such as Betadine® solution (Purdue Frederick) may be advantageous. Unless there is a nidus of infection or necrosis that cannot be debrided adequately, surgical drains are contraindicated because of the risk of ascending peritonitis.

SUPPLEMENTAL READING

Kolata, R.J., and Johnston, D.E.: Motor vehicle accidents in urban dogs: A study of 600 cases. J. Am. Vet. Med. Assoc., 167:938–941, 1975.

Kleine, L.J., and Thornton, G.W.: Radiographic diagnosis of urinary tract trauma. J. Am. Anim. Hosp. Assoc., 7:318–327, 1971.

Burrows, C.F., and Bovee, K.C.: Metabolic changes due to experimentally induced rupture of the canine urinary bladder. Am. J. Vet. Res., 35:1083–1088, 1974.

Kolata, R.J.: Diagnostic abdominal paracentesis and lavage: Experimental and clinical evaluations in the dog. 168:697–705, 1976.

Laufman, H., and Rabel, T.: Synthetic absorbable sutures. Surg. Gynecol. Obstet., 145:597–608, 1977.

PARASITES OF THE CANINE URINARY TRACT

DAVID F. SENIOR, B.V.Sc.

Gainesville, Florida

Two nematode parasites, *Dioctophyma renale* and *Capillaria plica*, infect the urinary tracts of dogs. Both infections are readily recognized by identification of parasite eggs in urine and, although these infections are not of major significance, the clinician must be aware of the implications and management in each case.

DIOCTOPHYMA RENALE

Dioctophyma renale, the giant kidney worm of the dog, is the largest known nematode. In dogs, female worms can be 100 cm and male worms 45 cm in length; however, there is variation in size among different definitive hosts.

The parasite has been reported in Europe, North and South America, Russia, Africa, South Vietnam, China, and Japan. In North America it has been reported in Manitoba, Ontario, and Quebec in Canada, in most of the East Coast states except Florida, in the midwestern states except Missouri, and in Kentucky, Louisiana, California, and Hawaii.

The principal definitive hosts probably are wild, fish-eating carnivores. The highest prevalence has been recorded in minks, in which renal infection with parasites of both sexes ensures perpetuation of the life cycle. The prevalence in dogs in the United States is very low.

In the definitive host, gravid females shed eggs in the urine. In an aqueous environment first-stage larvae develop within the egg in one to seven months. The embryonated eggs can remain viable for up to two years if they are protected from desiccation or freezing. After ingestion by *Lumbricus variegatus,* an aquatic oligochaete annelid, the eggs hatch and develop into infective third-stage larvae. The rate of embryonation and larval development are temperature-dependent. Although third-stage larvae are infective for minks, when crayfish are ingested by various species of frogs and fish (commonly bullheads) the larvae can re-encyst and remain infective in the liver and mesentery of these paratenic hosts. The definitive host becomes infected by eating uncooked infected frogs or fish.

The larvae are thought to penetrate the stomach or duodenum of the definitive host, enter the abdominal cavity, and migrate toward the kidney. In dogs the majority (60 percent) fail to penetrate the kidney and remain in the abdominal cavity. The prepatent period in dogs is 135 days, and the entire life cycle can take up to two years to complete.

Although *D. renale* organisms have been recovered from various locations in the abdomen and thorax, in dogs they are most commonly found free in the abdomen (60 percent) or within the right kidney (32 percent). Abdominal parasites and hepatic migration may cause peritonitis, ascites, and hemorrhage, but clinical signs are rarely seen. In the kidney parasitic renal destruction can cause renal fibrosis and contraction or dilation, with the parasite enclosed in a fluid-filled sac surrounded by a thin layer of remaining cortex and outer capsule.

D. renale infection is often a chance discovery, because most infections are asymptomatic. When both kidneys are parasitized, or when the uninfected kidney has reduced renal function, clinical signs of uremia may occur. Enlarged, hydronephrotic kidneys may be evident on abdominal palpation and radiographically, and urine sediment may contain numerous red and white blood cells. Occasionally, gross hematuria may be seen.

The diagnosis can be confirmed by radiographic signs of an enlarged kidney, typical *D. renale* eggs in the urine sediment or abdominal fluid, and discovery of mature parasites and eggs with granulomas at exploratory laparotomy and autopsy.

Renal enlargement due to *D. renale* must be differentiated from renal cysts, abscess, carcinoma, and hydronephrosis secondary to ureteral obstruction.

Treatment of renal infection by nephrotomy and nephrectomy is used after intravenous pyelography to estimate the magnitude of residual function in the involved kidney. Renal function should also be evaluated by determination of urine specific gravity and measurement of serum urea nitrogen or creatinine concentration. Infection can be prevented by avoiding consumption of raw or improperly cooked fish.

Although it is a zoonosis, *D. renale* infection very rarely involves man, even in areas in which the prevalence in fish-eating mammals is high. Pathology and signs are similar to those seen in the dog.

CAPILLARIA PLICA

The trichurid nematode *Capillaria plica* is parasitic in the urinary tracts of dogs, foxes, and wolves. The thin, fragile adult worms may be up to 60 mm long and can only be detected microscopically. The parasite is thought to be widespread and has been reported in England, Europe, and the United States. A similar species, *C. felis cati,* has been reported in Egypt and Australia.

The prevalence of *C. plica* infection in dogs is unclear because most infections are asymptomatic; however, 75 percent of mature dogs can be infected when dogs are exercised on soil runs under crowded conditions.

The exact life cycle is unknown. After passage in urine, the typical oval eggs with bipolar caps embryonate. When ingested by earthworms the larvae develop to the infective stage in the coelomic cavity of the earthworm. Experimentally, earthworms from contaminated exercise yards can infect dogs. The larvae migrate to the urinary tract via an unknown route. They localize in the renal pelvis, ureter, and bladder and cause a mild inflammatory reaction and submucosal edema. The prepatent period in dogs after ingestion of infected earthworms is 60 to 88 days.

It is unlikely that the definitive host becomes infected by direct ingestion of live earthworms, because they are unpalatable. There may be other intermediate hosts, or infection may occur by ingestion of larvae in mud when dogs groom themselves.

Eggs cannot be found in urine until puppies are five months old. There is no age, breed, or sex predilection in mature dogs. The infection is self-limiting, and egg output becomes negative after confinement from infected areas for 80 days.

In most infected dogs clinical signs are not apparent, and infection can be determined only by detection of eggs or fragmented worms in urine sediment. The sediment of infected dogs often contain numerous clumps of epithelial cells; red blood cells can be seen in more extreme cases. With heavy infections, gross hematuria, dysuria, and pollakiuria occur. In foxes retarded growth and difficulty in mating in males have been recorded in addition to the other signs. Although *C. plica* may predispose dogs to secondary bacterial infection, this is a rare occurrence.

At present, a safe effective treatment is not known. Control can be achieved by preventing access to earthworms by means of sand or gravel runs or by raising dogs on wire mesh.

Clinicians should be aware of management conditions that predispose to heavy infection and include *C. plica* infection in the differential diagnosis of hematuria, dysuria, and pollakiuria.

SUPPLEMENTAL READING

Osborne, C.A., Stevens, J.B., Hanlon, G.F., Rosin, E., and Bernrick, W.J.: *Dioctophyma renale* in the dog. J. Am. Vet. Med. Assoc., *155*:605–620, 1969.

Senior, D.F., Solomon, G.B., Goldschmidt, M.H., Joyce, T., and Bovée, K.C.: *Capillaria plica* infection in dogs. J. Am. Vet. Med. Assoc. (in press).

CONGENITAL DISEASES OF THE URACHUS

JEFFREY S. KLAUSNER, D.V.M.,
CARL A. OSBORNE, D.V.M.,
JERRY B. STEVENS, D.V.M.,
and JAMES W. WILSON, D.V.M.

St. Paul, Minnesota

The urachus is an embryologic structure that arises from the urinary bladder and provides a channel of communication between the urinary bladder and allantoic sac. In most animals the urachus closes and atrophies after birth, leaving only a scar at the bladder apex. In man, however, the urachus persists as a non-functional, fibromuscular cord — the middle umbilical ligament — that connects the bladder apex to the umbilicus. Although it is normally not patent, the middle umbilical ligament has a small lumen lined by transitional cell epithelium. In dogs and cats the middle umbilical ligament is a double fold of peritoneum that connects the ventral wall of the bladder (not the apex) to the ventral abdominal wall.

Congenital anomalies of the urachus occasionally cause disease in man and domestic animals. Urachal disease results from failure of the urachus to undergo complete atrophy following birth. Four variations of urachal anomalies have been described (Fig. 1). Persistent urachus results if the entire urachal canal remains patent between the bladder and umbilicus and is characterized by voiding of urine to the exterior by this route. Vesicourachal diverticula result if the urachus near the bladder fails to close. The result is a blind diverticulum that protrudes from the bladder vertex. A urachal cyst may develop if secreting urachal epithelium persists in isolated segments of a persistent urachus. A urachal sinus results if the distal urachus remains patent and communicates with the exterior at the umbilicus.

PERSISTENT URACHUS

Although apparently rare, persistent urachus has been described in dogs (Osborne, et al., 1966), cats (Greene, et al.), foals (Jamder, 1956),

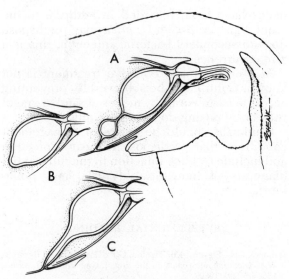

Figure 1. Congential urachal anomalies. *A.* Urachal cyst. *B.* Vesicourachal diverticulum. *C.* Persistent urachus.

cattle (Jamder, 1955), and man (Hinman). If the urachus is patent, clinical signs include leakage of urine from the umbilicus and secondary omphalitis and urine scalding of the skin. Signs are usually noted in young animals. Typically the animal can micturate normally through the urethra. Animals in which the urachal canal is non-patent may remain asymptomatic. In some instances signs have developed following obstruction of bladder outflow. Increased intravesicular pressure apparently can convert a closed urachal canal into a patent urachus.

Persistent patent urachus is a predisposition to bacterial urinary tract infection. The urachal canal provides an abnormal communication directly from the external environment to the bladder. By ascending the urachus, bacteria bypass normal urethral host defenses, such as the urethral high-pressure zone and specialized urethral epithelial cells. In addition, a persistent urachus may interfere with normal bladder contraction, resulting in incomplete emptying of the bladder. Residual urine in the bladder also predisposes to urinary tract infection.

Urinalyses from patients with persistent urachus and urinary tract infections usually reveal varying degrees of hematuria, pyuria, proteinuria, and bacteriuria. Significant numbers of bacteria ($\geq 10^5$/ml) can be isolated from quantitative urine cultures. Laboratory findings would be normal if urinary tract infection were not present.

Diagnosis of persistent urachus should be confirmed by radiographic studies. Abdominal radiographs reveal an elongated urinary bladder with a pointed vertex (Park). The urinary bladder may be displaced in a cranioventral direction. Intravenous urography or positive-contrast cystography may demonstrate the communication from the bladder apex to the umbilicus. Injection of positive-contrast medium through the umbilical opening into the bladder may also be possible.

A persistent urachus should be removed surgically by making an elliptical incision around the umbilical opening and dissecting the urachus free to the apex of the bladder, where it is excised. The urinary bladder wall should be closed in a routine fashion. If urinary tract infection is present, an antibiotic chosen by sensitivity testing should be administered for at least 14 days following surgery. Response to treatment should be evaluated by urine culture obtained approximately five days after termination of antibiotic therapy.

VESICOURACHAL DIVERTICULUM

Vesicourachal diverticula have been reported in dogs (Park), cats (Hansen), and man (Hinman). They result from failure of the urachus just distal to the urinary bladder to undergo complete atrophy. The diverticula vary in diameter from a few millimeters to a centimeter or more. A small diverticulum may not protrude beyond the serosal margin of the bladder.

Vesicourachal diverticula are significant because they are a frequent predisposing factor to recurrent urinary tract infections, especially in young animals. Retention of urine and bacteria within the diverticulum probably alters normal host defense mechanisms by reducing bacterial clearance from the urinary tract. Although urine may be sterilized by administration of an appropriate antibiotic, urinary tract infection often recurs soon after the antibiotic is discontinued. Recurrences typically continue until the diverticulum is removed.

By predisposing to urinary tract infections, vesicourachal diverticula may indirectly contribute to the formation of magnesium ammonium phosphate uroliths. Failure to remove a diverticulum at the time of calculus removal may result in recurrence of infection and subsequent recurrence of calculi. Magnesium ammonium phosphate calculi, especially in young animals, should alert one to possible vesicourachal diverticula.

In our experience vesicourachal diverticula have produced no clinical signs unless lower urinary tract infection is present. Dysuria, hematuria, and increased frequency of urination are associated with bacterial cystitis. Signs are generally (but not invariably) observed in animals less than two years of age. Occasionally a vesicourachal diverticulum develops because of increased intravesicular pressure due to obstruction of urine outflow, in which case signs can occur at any age.

Urinalyses from animals with infected diverticula usually reveal varying degrees of pyuria, hematuria, proteinuria, and bacteriuria. Significant numbers of bacteria may be isolated by quantitative urine culture. Urinalyses will be normal and urine cultures sterile from patients that have diverticula without urinary tract infection.

The diagnosis of vesicourachal diverticulum should be based on typical radiographic findings, observations of the diverticulum at the time of laporatomy, or both. Diverticula are best identified by positive-contrast cystography and appear as convex or triangular protrusions from the vertex of the bladder. One must be careful not to overdistend the bladder with contrast material, thus obscuring small diverticula that may not extend beyond the serosal margin. To prevent overdistention, radiographs should be taken at different degrees of bladder distention with contrast material.

Vesicourachal diverticula should be removed surgically. Visualization of the diverticulum at the time of surgery can sometimes be improved by applying pressure to the bladder and forcing urine into the bladder vertex, distending the diverticulum. The diverticulum may be excised by making an elliptical incision through the bladder wall around the margin of the diverticulum.

Microscopic examination of bladder tissue located near the diverticulum usually reveals evidence of inflammation, including accumulations of mononuclear cells and lymphoid follicles.

Postoperative therapy should include a 14-day course of an antibiotic chosen by sensitivity testing. Response to therapy should be evaluated by urine cultures approximately five days after treatment. Recurrent infections following removal of the diverticulum are uncommon.

URACHAL CYST

Urachal cysts have been reported in dogs (Osborne, et al., 1972) and man (Hinman). They result from persistence of secreting urachial epithelium in isolated segments of patent lumen that exist in one or more places between the bladder and umbilicus. Urachal cysts are usually filled with viscous fluid and are small, but they may become quite large. If the cyst does not become infected or extremely large, it may remain undetected until discovered at surgery or necropsy. Infected urachal cysts may be associated with abdominal pain and fever; rupture of an infected cyst may cause peritonitis. Urachal cysts associated with clinical signs or fortuitously discovered during laparotomy should be removed surgically.

URACHAL SINUS

Urachal sinus, a condition in which the distal urachus remains patent and communicates with the umbilicus, has been reported only in human beings (Hinman). It is associated with omphalitis. Treatment includes surgical excision of the urachus.

SUPPLEMENTAL READING

Greene, R.W., and Bohning, R.H.: Patent urachus associated with urolithiasis in a cat. J. Am. Vet. Med. Assoc., *158*:489–491, 1971.
Hansen, J.S.: Urachal reminant in the cat: Occurrence and relationship to feline urological syndrome. Vet. Med. Small Anim. Clin., *72*:1735–1741, 1977.
Hinman, F., Jr.: Surgical disorders of the bladder and umbilicus of urachal origin. Surg. Gynecol. Obstet., *113*:605–614, 1961.
Jamder, M.N.: Urachus. Indian Vet. J., *32*:19, 1955.
Jamder, M.N.: Urachal remnant of domestic animals as compared to that of man and two cases of partially involuted urachus in equines. Indian Vet. J., *33*:143–145, 1956.
Osborne, C.A., Low, D.G., and Finco, D.R.: *Canine and Feline Urology.* Philadelphia, W. B. Saunders Co., 1972.
Osborne, C.A., Rhodes, J.D., and Hanlon, G.F.: Patent urachus in the dog. Anim. Hosp., *2*:245–250, 1966.
Park, R.D.: Radiology of the urinary bladder and urethra. In O'Brien, T.R. (ed.): *Radiologic Diagnosis of Abdominal Disorders in the Dog and Cat.* Philadelphia, W. B. Saunders Co., 1978, pp. 543–614.

MEDICAL MANAGEMENT OF PROSTATIC DISEASE

WILLIAM E. HORNBUCKLE, D.V.M.
Ithaca, New York

and LAWRENCE J. KLEINE, D.V.M.
Boston, Massachusetts

The primary forms of prostatic disease diagnosed in dogs at the Angell Memorial Animal Hospital (AMAH) and the New York State College of Veterinary Medicine are acute prostatitis, chronic active prostatitis, abscesses, large retention cysts or paraprostatic cysts, adenocarcinomas, and a group of cases identified as "complicated" benign prostatic hyperplasia (BPH) (Hornbuckle, et al.). This last group often has clinical features of prostatitis. Uncomplicated BPH is regarded as a normal aging change in dogs. Other neoplasms include hemangiosarcoma and leiomyosarcoma; two cases of prostatic adenocarcinoma have been diagnosed in domestic cats.

HISTORY

Prostatic disease has no breed incidence; the majority of dogs affected are older than five years. Three cases of prostatic hematocyst were diagnosed in Doberman pinschers less than two years of age at AMAH. Seventy-five percent of dogs with prostatic neoplasia are at least 10 years old.

Four primary signs observed in dogs with prostatic disease, in decreasing order of frequency, are lower urinary tract signs (59.3 per cent), systemic signs (47.9 per cent), defecation abnormalities (36.4 per cent), and locomotion problems (8.3 per cent) (Hornbuckle, et al.). Occasionally infertility problems or prostatic injury are encountered. The predominant signs of dogs with various types of prostatic disease are listed in Table 1. Table 2 lists systemic signs of illness. If lameness or paresis is the predominant sign, adenocarcinoma should be suspected. Nine of 13 dogs with ambulatory problems due to prostatic adenocarcinoma had metastasis to muscle, bone, or both (eight cases) or hypertrophic osteoarthropathy (one case) (Hornbuckle, et al.).

The history should include a search for previous urinary tract disease, the treatment given, and the attractiveness of the dog to other males. Dogs with chronic prostatitis, abscesses, cysts and, rarely, neoplasms often have prior histories of urinary tract disease. There is an apparent association with excessive estrogen therapy in the first three conditions and a modest association with Sertoli cell tumors.

Although the prostate is commonly the focus of chronic or recurrent urinary tract infections (urethritis, cystitis, pyelonephritis), prostatitis can exist as a subclinical problem. In many dogs BPH may be associated with varying degrees of enlargement, cystic changes, and/or inflammatory infiltrates without apparent complications, although they are the underlying cause of clinical disease in others. Cysts can attain huge proportions before detection. A diagnosis of prostatic neoplasia is usually associated with a poor prognosis if clinical signs are apparent, an observation that emphasizes the importance of periodic physical examination throughout the dog's life.

PHYSICAL EXAMINATION

Examination of the prostate gland should be interpreted in light of an inspection of the entire body because systemic or metastatic findings may have diagnostic importance. Evaluation of accessible parts of the urogenital system, perineum, anorectal area, pelvic canal, and sublumbar area is also important. Prostatic disease and testicular tumors often are concomitant findings in dogs with perineal hernias. Estrogen-induced prostate disease can result from functional testicular tumors. Prostatic cysts or abscesses occasionally drain at the perineum; peritonitis can result if they drain into the peritoneum. Palpable sublumbar masses can result from tumor-induced lymph node enlargement or vertebral proliferation.

The prostate gland is best examined by simultaneous caudal abdominal palpation and rectal palpation. It is sometimes advantageous

Table 1. *Predominant Signs of Canine Prostatic Disease**

SIGN	ACUTE PROSTATITIS OR PROSTATIC ABSCESS	CHRONIC PROSTATITIS	COMPLICATED BPH†	PROSTATIC CYST	ADENOCARCINOMA
Urinary	+	++++	++++	++	
Systemic-urinary	++++	+	+	+	+
Systemic	++++	+	+		+
Defecation			++++	+	++
Urinary-defecation	++++	++	++++	++++	+++
Systemic-defecation	++++		+		+
Locomotion-mixed‡	+	+	+		++++
Systemic-urinary-defecation	++	+++		+	++++
Locomotion					++++

+ = Least common compared with others
++++ = Very common compared with others
*From: Hornbuckle, W.E., MacCoy, D.M., Allan, G.S., Kleine, L.J., and Gunther, R.: Prostatic disease in the dog, Cornell Vet., 68(7):284–305, 1978.
†BPH = benign prostatic hyperplasia
‡Combinations of systemic, urinary, or defecation signs

to elevate the dog's forequarters and to encourage prior urination to facilitate rectal palpation. The prostate should be examined for mobility, symmetry, prominence of the dorsal raphe, texture, pain, size, and location within the pelvic canal relative to the rectum. Size alone is a relative assessment. Pertinent history and other physical alterations are necessary to add credibility to a presumptive diagnosis of prostatic disease.

Compression or stricture of the prostatic urethra can be assessed by gentle urethral catheterization. Paraprostatic cysts can be differentiated from the urinary bladder by urethral catheterization and careful abdominal palpation. If reduction of urine volume via catheterization does not help, injection of air into the bladder concomitant with abdominal palpation may permit localization of the bladder. This method can also be applied to cases in which the enlarged prostate has encroached sufficient-

ly on the neck of the bladder to cause it to be mistaken for the bladder.

Prostatic massage can result in rupture of an abscess or can contribute to epididymitis, orchitis, or both. Circulating neoplastic cells in peripheral blood have been observed following prostate massage in men with adenocarcinomas (Alsaker and Stevens).

RADIOLOGY

Radiographic techniques are useful in determining the size, shape, and location of the prostate gland. Radiographically visualized lesions are non-specific; there is no indication of whether the changes are due to hyperplasia, infection, or neoplasia. However, when the radiographic interpretation is combined with the clinical data the differential diagnoses can be narrowed. Furthermore, since radiographs are permanent records, they may form a basis for

Table 2. *Systemic Signs of Canine Prostatic Disease**

SIGN	ACUTE PROSTATITIS OR PROSTATIC ABSCESS	CHRONIC PROSTATITIS, COMPLICATED BPH, OR LARGE CYSTS	ADENOCARCINOMA
Fever	++++	+	+
Prostatic pain	++++	+	+
Depression	++++	+	+
Inappetence	++++	+	+
Vomiting	++++	++	+
Polydipsia	++++	+++	++
Weight loss	+++	++	++++

+ = Least common compared with others
++++ = Very common compared with others
*From: Hornbuckle, W.E., et al.: Prostatic disease in the dog. Cornell Vet., 68(7):284–305, 1978.

progress checks throughout the course of therapy. The average size of the prostate gland in a mature 30-kg dog is 1.7 cm long by 2.5 cm in diameter, but considerable variation is encountered because of age-related changes and breed differences (Miller, et al.). In lateral radiographs the prostate gland is usually in the pelvic canal at the brim of the pelvis, although its position varies with the degree of distention of the urinary bladder and colon. In ventrodorsal views it usually lies within the pelvic canal on or near the midline. The margin of the gland and its density are normally uniform. Survey radiographs usually permit an estimation of the size and location of the gland, but overlapping of soft tissues of the rear limbs upon the pelvic canal sometimes reduces radiographic detail in this area. When a paraprostatic cyst is present, differentiation of the prostate gland from the urinary bladder may be difficult. In such cases, cystourethrography may provide a more thorough evaluation. We perform cystourethrography by passing a urinary catheter to the level of the prostatic urethra and infusing between 5 and 15 ml of positive-contrast medium,* which contains approximately 200 mg of organically bound iodide per ml of solution. Ventrodorsal and lateral radiographs are exposed at the end of the infusion. This procedure defines the urethral silhouette and any reflux into the prostate gland that may have occurred. The urinary bladder should not be evacuated before performing cystourethrography because the resistance to flow of contrast medium provided by the distended bladder helps to outline the urethra. The urinary bladder should be emptied if cystography is to be performed.

When the prostate gland is affected with benign hypertrophy of prostatitis it is often symmetrically enlarged, whereas prostatic cysts, neoplasms, and abscesses cause asymmetric enlargement (Stone, et al.). Encasement of the urinary bladder with cellulitis may occur following rupture of a prostatic abscess. In such cases the urinary bladder may become circular or even tubular rather than its normal tear-drop shape. Neoplastic, inflammatory, or even hyperplastic prostatic disease may encroach upon the bladder neck and reduce the capacity of the urinary bladder, causing it to have a circular appearance in the cystogram and occasionally causing partial obstruction of the ureters. Rarely, a prostatic abscess may erode and rupture into the abdominal cavity, producing loss of radiographic detail. Mineralization may occur

within the prostate or its associated lymph nodes secondary to long-standing hemorrhage or necrosis, or both. The medial iliac or sacral lymph nodes (dorsal to the rectum at the pelvic canal) may be enlarged in patients with any type of prostatic disease. When the lymph nodes and the prostate gland are both enlarged, the rectum is narrowed by pressure exerted dorsally by the lymph nodes and ventrally by the prostate gland.

LABORATORY EXAMINATION

The hemogram seldom has diagnostic specificity, but it is important in evaluating and monitoring dogs with systemic manifestations of prostatic disease. Blood urea nitrogen levels should be evaluated. A number of prerenal factors (vomiting, dehydration), concomitant renal disease, and obstructive uropathy can contribute to azotemia. Hydronephrosis and hydroureter can be complications associated with prostatic abscesses, cysts, or neoplasia.

The urinalysis is an important screening test for urinary tract disease. Gram stains and urine cultures may indicate extension of infection from the prostate gland. Aspirates or washings of the urethra following prostatic massage or ejaculation specimens are preferred for cytologic examinations and culture. Bacterial cultures taken from prostatic tissue have higher yield (85.7 percent) compared with those from bladder urine (63.6 percent) in cases of prostatic abscesses (Hornbuckle, et al.). Gram-negative bacteria (especially *Escherichia coli*) are cultured more often than gram-positive bacteria.

Exfoliative cytology and microscopic examination of biopsy samples of diseased prostate glands are important diagnostic procedures in a select group of cases (Finco). Justification for biopsy is based on initial history and physical findings in some cases. Failure to resolve prostatic disease by castration or medication, or both, is the reason for biopsy in others. Metastatic neoplastic disease should be ruled out by radiography prior to biopsy procedures. If surgery is being performed for an obvious abscess or cyst, prostatic tissue should still be submitted for microscopic examination, since concomitant neoplasia or metaplasia could be the underlying cause of these abnormalities.

The need for additional diagnostic tests is variable. The workup for infertility might include a brucellosis titer and hormone assays. Hormone assays might result in recognition of estrogen-induced prostatitis. The value of serum acid phosphatase determination in the diagnosis of prostatic adenocarcinoma is equivocal and therefore is not recommended.

---

*Renografin-60, Squibb Pharmaceutical Company, Princeton, New Jersey 08540.

TREATMENT

Treatment of prostatic disease involves surgery, medical management, or both. Prudent hormone and/or antimicrobial therapy will resolve most cases of BPH and prostatitis. Castration can simplify medical management, and if done early it can reduce susceptibility to prostatic disease. Some diseases of the prostate cannot be resolved solely by medication or castration, including abscesses with or without peritonitis, cysts, neoplasia, and urethral strictures. These disorders usually require specific surgery (e.g., marsupialization or prostatectomy) (Hornbuckle, et al.). Justification for surgery should take into account the value of the dog as an intact male, metastatic or systemic effects of disease, prognosis with and without surgery, and cost.

The primary indications for medical management of prostatic disease are systemic illness, symptomatic enlargement of the prostate, bacterial infection, and neoplasia. Systemic signs, including dehydration, require appropriate treatment. Stool softeners and gentle enemas may be necessary in patients with constipation. Compromised bladder function infrequently requires special management. The following general considerations often influence therapy for prostatic enlargement:

1. BPH (acinar or glandular hyperplasia) is the most common cause of prostatic enlargement. Its concomitant prevalence with other forms of prostatic disease approaches 80 percent.

2. Estrogen-induced prostatic disease (fibromuscular hyperplasia, squamous metaplasia) should be suspected in patients with feminization or testicular tumor(s), abdominal masses and/or absence of scrotal testicle(s), or a history of excessive hormone therapy. Prostatic infection is a common sequela to excessive estrogen.

3. Large discrete cysts of the uterus masculinus are rare. The more common paraprostatic or large retention cysts are usually unresponsive to both estrogen therapy and castration (Weaver). Inadequate drainage and peritonitis are potential sequelae to needle aspiration of cysts or abscesses, and therefore surgery is preferred in their management. If an abscess has adequate urethral drainage, surgery may not be necessary.

4. Prostatic adenocarcinomas of dogs are not responsive to estrogen therapy or castration. Any palliative effect is due to atrophy of normal or hyperplastic prostatic tissue around tumor cells.

5. If castration does not cause significant and permanent atrophy of an enlarged prostate within one week, abscesses or neoplasms should be considered.

6. If estrogen therapy does not cause significant prostatic atrophy, an abscess, pre-existing estrogen-induced disease, or neoplasia should be suspected. Excessive estrogen therapy can cause prostatic enlargement, feminization, and bone marrow toxicity.

7. Hormones can suppress spermatogenesis.

If enlargement of the prostate is uniform and asymptomatic, the assumed diagnosis is uncomplicated BPH. Unless a survey urinalysis is abnormal, further testing or treatment is usually unnecessary. Occasionally BPH is the cause of constipation or tenesmus; prior to hormone therapy or castration, urinalysis should be done to rule out subclinical infection. Symptomatic enlargement or more complicated prostatic disease requires careful examination before treatment. If a reasonable presumptive diagnosis cannot be made from history, physical examination, and laboratory tests, radiography and biopsy are indicated.

Estradiol cypionate or diethylstilbestrol will cause significant atrophy of BPH wihtin one week. If prostatic palpation and remission of clinical signs do not indicate response, further estrogen therapy is not advised without a definitive diagnosis. Though a single intramuscular injection of 0.25 to 2.0 mg of estradiol is recommended, we do not exceed a total dose of 1.0 mg in dogs. Dogs under 13.6 kg (e.g., dachshunds) are treated with 0.25 to 0.50 mg of estradiol. An alternative treatment is oral administration of diethylstilbestrol (DES) at a dosage schedule of 5.0 mg the first day followed by 1.0 mg daily for 4 treatments. Other investigators recommend 1.0 mg DES orally every other day.

Progesterones and cyproterone acetate (an antiandrogen) have been used in animal experiments to cause regression in prostate size (Marberger, et al.). The New York State College of Veterinary Medicine has had favorable experience with dithiazone (a zinc-chelating agent) in reducing prostate size; however, its efficacy must be weighed against evidence that zinc is an important antimicrobial factor in prostatic fluid (Marberger, et al.). In addition, the potential toxic effects of dithiazone on the retina and pancreas — tissues also high in zinc — is a factor to be considered. Candicidin and amphotericin-B have been used experimentally to reduce the volume and texture of prostatic tissue (Gordon, et al.).

Chloramphenicol or trimethoprim-sulfadiazine is preferred for treatment of bacterial prostatitis with or without urinary tract infection (Granato, et al.; Stamey, et al.). Selection of other antibiotics should be based on culture and sensitivity studies or clinical re-

sponse. Although erythromycin and oleando-
mycin attain high concentrations in the prostate
gland, their antimicrobial efficacy within prostatic tissue is suspect. Experimental studies
indicate that intravenous tetracycline also attains high prostatic tissue levels. In spite of the
results of studies using normal canine prostate
glands, we have successfully treated prostatitis
with ampicillin and the cephalosporins.

Effective antibiotic therapy should be sustained for a minimum of three weeks. Five to
seven days following the last administration,
culture and sensitivity studies should be repeated. If infection persists or recurs more than
three times, and if no further benefits are gained
from culture-sensitivity studies and antibiotic
changes, the dog should be maintained on continuous antimicrobial therapy to produce "bactericidal" bladder urine. This technique is designed to isolate the infection to the prostate
gland and prevent generalized urinary tract
infection. If severe prostatic infection remains
refractory to antimicrobial treatment, surgical
evaluation is indicated.

Continuous antimicrobial therapy involves a
minimum of three to six months. Drug selection
is usually a compromise based on several factors, including bacterial susceptibility, urinary
tract or prostatic tissue specificity, form, toxicity, and cost. Periodic physical and laboratory
examinations should be performed to monitor
treatment response and avoid undesirable drug
effects. Long-term daily administration of
trimethoprim-sulfadiazine (one-quarter of the
daily dose given at bedtime) or perhaps oral
tetracycline is compatible with prostatic specificity. Daily maintenance dosages of sulfisoxazole or a urinary antiseptic such as Mandelamine are commonly used for chronic bacteriuria
when sensitivity studies are not helpful. A uri-

nary acidifier (e.g., ascorbic acid) should be
used with Mandelamine to enhance its activity.

With some notable exceptions, most cases of
prostatic neoplasia are inoperable because of
local tissue invasion or metastasis. For patients
with debilitating signs, euthanasia is usually
recommended. Castration or estrogen therapy is
ineffectual or gives only short-term palliative
effect. In man chemotherapy (e.g., cyclophosphamide, Adriamycin, 5-fluorouracil) and immunotherapy have been sufficiently promising
to be worthy of more clinical study (Marberger,
et al.) In selected human cases of adenocarcinoma, irradiation therapy has been of some value;
the same is true of cryosurgery (Marberger, et
al.).

SUPPLEMENTAL READING

Alsaker, R.D., and Stevens, J.B.: Neoplastic cells in the blood of a
dog with prostatic adenocarcinoma. J. Am. Anim. Hosp. Assoc.,
13:486–488, 1977.
Evans, H.E., and Christensen, G.C.: *Miller's Anatomy of the Dog*,
2nd ed. Philadelphia, W.B. Saunders Co., 1979.
Finco, D.R.: Prostate gland biopsy. Vet. Clin. North Am., 4:367–375,
1974.
Gordon, H.W., et al.: The effect of polyene macrolides on the
prostate gland and canine prostatic hyperplasia. Appl. Biol.,
60:1201–1208, 1968.
Granato, J., et al.: Trimethoprim diffusion into prostatic and salivary
secretions of the dog. Invest. Urol., 2(3):205–210, 1973–74.
Hornbuckle, W.E., MacCoy, D.M., Allan, G.S., Kleine, L.J., and
Gunther, R.: Prostatic disease in the dog. Cornell Vet., 68:284–
305, 1978.
Marberger, H., Haschek, H., Schirmer, H.K.A., Colston, J.A.C., and
Witkin, E.: *Prostatic Disease. Proceedings.* (Volume 6 of the
Progress in Clinical and Biological Research Series). New York,
Alan R. Liss, Inc., 1976.
Stamey, T.A., Mearles, E.M., and Winningham, D.G.: Chronic
bacterial prostatitis and the diffusion of drugs into prostatic fluid.
J. Urol., 103:187–194, 1970.
Stone, E.A., Thrall, D.E., and Barber, D.L.: Radiographic interpreta-
tion of prostatic disease in the dog. J. Am. Anim. Hosp. Assoc.,
14:115–118, 1978.
Weaver, A.D.: Discrete prostatic (paraprostatic) cysts in the dog. Vet.
Rec., 102:425–440, 1978.

CYSTOCENTESIS

CARL A. OSBORNE, D.V.M.,
GEORGE E. LEES, D.V.M.,
and GARY R. JOHNSTON, D.V.M.
St. Paul, Minnesota

Cystocentesis is a form of paracentesis that
consists of needle puncture of the urinary bladder for the purpose of removing a variable
quantity of urine by aspiration. Although tech-

niques and complications of cystocentesis have
not been evaluated by controlled studies, clinical experience has revealed that properly performed cystocentesis is of great diagnostic and

therapeutic value. It is usually associated with a smaller risk of iatrogenic infection than catheterization and is often better tolerated by patients (especially cats and female dogs) than catheterization.

INDICATIONS

Diagnostic. A resident population of bacteria normally is present in progressively increasing numbers from the mid-zone of the urethra to the distal urethra in humans and dogs and probably in cats. Resident bacteria are also present in the vagina and prepuce. In contrast, urine in the kidneys, ureters, and urinary bladder of normal animals typically is sterile. In addition to systemic natural defense mechanisms, the following local defense mechanisms are thought to prevent urinary tract infection in animals: normal micturition, normal anatomy, mucosal defense barriers, antibacterial properties of urine, and renal defense mechanisms (Klausner and Osborne; Osborne and Finco; Osborne and Lees).

Collection of urine during natural micturition is very satisfactory for routine urinalyses performed to screen patients for abnormalities of the urinary tract and other body systems. Contamination of urine with bacteria, cells, and other debris from the urethra, genital tract, and integument, however, sometimes makes it necessary to repeat analysis of urine collected by catheterization or cystocentesis. Urine samples obtained by catheterization may also be contaminated with resident urethral bacteria. In addition, catheterization — no matter how carefully executed — is always associated with the hazard of iatrogenic urinary tract infection caused by carrying resident urethral bacteria into the bladder (Osborne and Schenk). The risk of bacterial infection caused by catheterization is dependent on the integrity of systemic and local host defenses and is therefore higher in patients with pre-existing diseases of the urethra or urinary bladder.

Potential problems associated with collection of urine samples by normal micturition, manual compression of the urinary bladder, and catheterization may be avoided by cystocentesis. Diagnostic cystocentesis is indicated to (1) prevent contamination of urine samples with bacteria, cells, and debris from the lower urogenital tract; (2) aid in localization of hematuria, pyuria, and bacteriuria; and (3) minimize iatrogenic urinary tract infection caused by catheterization, especially in patients with pre-existing diseases of the urethra or urinary bladder.

Therapeutic. Therapeutic cystocentesis may be employed to provide temporary decompression of the excretory pathway of the urinary system when urethral obstruction or herniation of the urinary bladder prevents normal micturition. It is frequently used in male cats when reverse flushing or other non-surgical techniques have failed to dislodge urethral plugs. Following cystocentesis, attempts to dislodge urethral plugs by reverse flushing are frequently successful. This may be related to the fact that the patient has less discomfort and the skeletal muscle surrounding the distal urethra has relaxed.

CONTRAINDICATIONS

The main contraindications to cystocentesis are an insufficient volume of urine in the urinary bladder and patient resistance to restraint and abdominal palpation. Blind cystocentesis performed without digital localization and immobilization of the urinary bladder is usually unsuccessful, and it may be associated with damage to the bladder or adjacent structures.

In our experience collection of urine by cystocentesis from patients with bacterial urinary tract infection has not been associated with detectable spread of infection outside the urinary tract. In fact, collection of a urine sample for bacterial culture that has not been contaminated by passage through the urethra and genital tract is a frequent reason for performing cystocentesis.

EQUIPMENT

We routinely use 22-gauge needles. Depending on the size of the patient and the distance of the ventral bladder wall from the ventral abdominal wall, 1.5-inch hypodermic or 3-inch spinal needles* may be selected.

Small-capacity (2½ to 12 ml) syringes are usually employed for diagnostic cystocentesis, whereas large-capacity (20 to 60 ml) syringes are used for therapeutic cystocentesis. Alternatively, therapeutic cystocentesis may be performed with 6- to 12-ml syringes and a two-way or three-way valve.† If desirable, a 22-gauge needle may be transected midway between its tip and hub and reconnected with a section of flexible polyethylene tubing (PE 60).‡

---

*Yale Spinal Needles. Becton, Dickenson Co., Rutherford, New Jersey 07070

†Pharmaseal, Inc., Toa Alta, Puerto Rico 00758

‡PE 60. Clay Adams, Inc., Parsippany, New Jersey 07054

SITE

Careful planning of the site and direction of needle puncture of the bladder wall is recommended. Although some clinicians recommend insertion of the needle into the dorsal wall of the bladder to minimize gravity-dependent leakage of urine into the peritoneal cavity following withdrawal of the needle, we recommend that the needle be inserted in the ventral or ventrolateral wall of the bladder in order to minimize the chance of trauma to the ureters and major abdominal vessels (Fig. 1). If therapeutic cystocentesis is to be performed, we recommend insertion of the needle a short distance cranial to the junction of the bladder with the urethra rather than at the vertex of the bladder (Fig. 1). This will permit removal of urine and decompression of the bladder without requiring reinsertion of the needle into the bladder lumen (Fig. 1). If the needle is placed in or adjacent to the vertex of the bladder it may not remain within the bladder lumen, because the bladder progressively decreases in size following aspiration of urine.

We also recommend that the needle be directed through the bladder wall at approximately a 45-degree angle so that an oblique needle tract will be created (Fig. 1). By directing the needle through the bladder wall in an oblique fashion, the elasticity of the vesical musculature and the interlacing arrangement of individual muscle fibers will provide a better seal for the small pathway created by the needle when it is removed. In addition, subsequent distention of the bladder wall as the lumen refills with urine will tend to force the walls of the needle tract into apposition in a fashion somewhat analogous to the flap valve of the ureterovesical junction.

PREBIOPSY CONSIDERATIONS

Because insertion and withdrawal of a 22-gauge needle through the walls of the abdomen and bladder are associated with little discomfort, tranquilization, general anesthesia, and local anesthesia are rarely required for diagnostic or therapeutic cystocentesis. If the urinary bladder does not contain a sufficient volume of urine to permit digital localization and immobilization, the patient may be given oral fluids or a diuretic. Although diuretics such as furosemide may be used to facilitate collection of urine samples by increasing urine formation, alteration of urine specific gravity and urine pH are notable drawbacks of this procedure. Even the quantity of bacteria per milliliter of urine may be significantly reduced, altering the results of quantitative urine cultures. Use of diuretics to enhance urine collection by augmenting urine flow is therefore best suited for serial urine sample collections when information about urine specific gravity, urine pH, and semiquantitative evaluation of routine test components are not significant.

TECHNIQUE

In order to perform cystocentesis without risk to the patient, adequate localization and immobilization of the urinary bladder together with planning of the site and direction of needle puncture are essential. The ventral abdominal skin penetrated by the needle should be cleansed with an antiseptic solution each time cystocentesis is performed. Appropriate caution should be used to avoid iatrogenic trauma to or infection of the urinary bladder and surrounding structures.

In cats it is usually easiest to perform the procedure with the patient in lateral or dorsal recumbency. In dogs the procedure may also be performed when the patient is standing. Following localization and immobilization of the urinary bladder, the needle should be inserted through the ventral abdominal wall and advanced to the caudoventral aspect of the bladder. The needle should be inserted through the bladder wall at an oblique angle. If a large quantity of urine is to be aspirated, the needle

Correct   Incorrect

Figure 1. Schematic drawing illustrating correct and incorrect sites of insertion of a needle into the bladder for the purpose of evacuating urine. The needle should be inserted in the ventral or ventrolateral surface of the wall a short distance cranial to the junction of the bladder with the urethra rather than at the vertex of the bladder. This will permit removal of urine and decompression of the bladder without need for reinsertion of the needle into the bladder lumen. (Medical illustrations by Michael P. Schenk, College of Veterinary Medicine, University of Minnesota.)

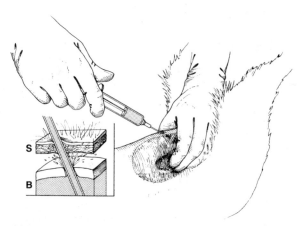

Figure 2. Schematic drawing illustrating escape of urine through the bladder wall adjacent to the needle tract as a result of excessive digital pressure used to localize and immobilize the bladder. S = skin of abdominal wall; B = wall of urinary bladder.

should be directed so that it will enter the bladder lumen a short distance cranial to the junction of the bladder with the urethra. While the needle and bladder are immobilized, urine should be gently aspirated into the syringe. If a large quantity of urine is to be evacuated from the bladder, a two-way or three-way valve may be used.

Excessive digital pressure should not be applied to the bladder wall while the needle is in its lumen. This will prevent urine from being forced around the needle into the peritoneal cavity (Fig. 2). Use of a 3-inch spinal needle rather than a 1.5-inch hypodermic needle when the ventral surface of the bladder wall is more than 1 to 1.25 inches from the ventral abdominal wall permits immobilization of the urinary bladder without pulling it toward the ventral abdominal wall.

If disease of the bladder wall or virulence of urinary pathogens is a likely cause of complications associated with loss of urine into the peritoneal cavity, the bladder should be emptied as completely as is consistent with atraumatic technique. These potential complications have not been a problem in our patients.

POSTBIOPSY CARE

The need for prophylactic antibacterial therapy following cystocentesis must be determined on the basis of the status of the patient and retrospective evaluation of technique. In most instances it is not required.

In order to minimize contamination of the peritoneal cavity with urine, unnecessary digital pressure on the urinary bladder following cystocentesis should be avoided.

POSTBIOPSY COMPLICATIONS

Patient. We have not observed antemortem postbiopsy complications in experimental or clinical studies in cats. Potential complications include damage to the bladder wall or adjacent structures with the needle, local or generalized peritonitis, vesicoperitoneal fistulas, and adhesion of adjacent structures to the bladder wall.

Laboratory. We have encountered a few instances in which penetration of a loop of intestine by the needle resulted in false positive significant bacteriuria. Varying degrees of microscopic hematuria might be expected for a short time following cystocentesis but are of little consequence, since samples for laboratory analysis are rarely collected at this time.

SUPPLEMENTAL READING

Klausner, J.S., and Osborne, C.A.: Bacterial infections of the urinary tract. In Kirk, R. W. (ed.): *Current Veterinary Therapy VI.* Philadelphia, W. B. Saunders Co., 1977.

Osborne, C.A., and Finco, D.R.: Urinary tract infections: New solutions to old problems. In Scientific Presentations and Seminar Synopses of the 44th Annual Meeting of the American Animal Hospital Association, South Bend, Indiana, 1977.

Osborne, C.A., and Lees, G.E.: Feline cystitis, urethritis, urethral obstruction syndrome. I. Etiopathogenesis and clinical manifestations. Mod. Vet. Pract., 59:173–180, 1978.

Osborne, C.A., and Schenk, M.P.: Techniques of urine collection. In Scientific Presentations and Seminar Synopses of the 44th Annual Meeting of the American Animal Hospital Association, South Bend, Indiana, 1977.

SCREENING TESTS FOR THE DETECTION OF SIGNIFICANT BACTERIURIA

JEFFREY S. KLAUSNER, D.V.M.,
CARL A. OSBORNE, D.V.M.,
and JERRY B. STEVENS, D.V.M.
St. Paul, Minnesota

Urine culture is essential for evaluation of animals with urinary tract disease. If performed and evaluated correctly, urine cultures aid in the solution of diagnostic and therapeutic problems. Failure to perform urine cultures or failure to interpret the results of urine cultures correctly may lead to diagnostic errors and therapeutic failures.

INFLAMMATION VS. INFECTION

It is essential to distinguish between inflammation and infection as related to urinary tract disease. Many diverse disease processes, including bacterial infection, neoplasia, and urolithiasis, result in inflammatory lesions of the urinary tract leading to exudation of red blood cells, white blood cells, and protein into urine. The resultant hematuria, pyuria, and proteinuria suggest inflammatory urinary tract disease but do not indicate its etiology or location within the urinary tract. Urine culture, radiographic studies, and biopsy procedures often provide the additional information necessary to localize the disease process and establish its etiology.

Bacterial urinary tract infection is a common cause of urinary tract disease in dogs, but it is uncommon in cats. Detection of infection should be established by urine culture, since diagnosis based solely on recognition of inflammatory change in urinalyses will result in overdiagnosis of infection. Conversely, absence of hematuria, pyuria, and proteinuria does not rule out the existence of infection, since it may occur without stimulating detectable inflammatory response. Positive urine culture results indicate that bacterial infection is either the cause of the disease process or a secondary complication of another process, such as neoplasia, metabolic stone disease, and perhaps immune-mediated disease.

SIGNIFICANT BACTERIURIA

Although urine contained in the urinary bladder is normally sterile, urine that passes through the urethra and genital tract may become contaminated with resident bacteria normally present in these locations. Therefore the significance of bacteria in midstream or catheterized samples may be difficult to interpret because they may represent pathogens or contaminants.

The concept of significant bacteriuria was introduced to aid in the differentiation between contaminants and bacteria causing urinary tract infection. This concept was based on the observation that a high bacterial count in a properly collected and cultured midstream or catheterized urine sample is indicative of urinary tract infection. In human beings urine bacterial counts in excess of 100,000 organisms of a single species per milliliter of urine are considered to be significant (Kass). Isolation of 10,000 to 100,000 bacteria of a single species per milliliter is interpreted as being suggestive of bacterial infection. If the same organism is isolated from a second culture at a similar or higher concentration, bacterial infection is confirmed. It is highly unlikely that the same contaminant organism would be isolated in high numbers from consecutive cultures. Detection of fewer than 10,000 bacteria per milliliter usually represents contamination. Similar criteria have been applied to interpretation of canine quantitative urine culture results (Klausner, et al.). In a recent report, midstream or catheterized urine samples from dogs without urinary tract infection usually contained fewer than 10,000 bacteria per milliliter (Carter, et al.). The concentration of organisms that indicates significant bacteriuria in feline urine cultures has not been determined, but it may be less than those in human beings and dogs because feline urine may be less conducive to bacterial growth.

1154

QUALITATIVE VS. QUANTITATIVE URINE CULTURE

Qualitative urine culture includes isolation and identification of bacteria present in urine. As noted previously, the results of qualitative culture may be misleading in urine samples collected by voluntary voiding or by catheterization, even if midstream aliquots are used. Since urine contamination is usually not significant in samples collected by cytocentesis, qualitative culture results of samples obtained by this technique are more reliable.

Quantitative urine culture includes determination of the number of bacteria per unit volume in addition to isolation and identification of bacteria. It is the preferred method of diagnostic culture for urine samples obtained by any collection method.

The generalities listed in the preceding section regarding interpretation of results of quantitative culture will be valid only if urine samples are properly collected and processed. The external genitalia of males and females must be rinsed with an appropriate cleansing solution before urine is obtained. It may be necessary to clip the hair surrounding the vulva of some long haired female dogs. Only sterilized catheters and collection containers should be used, and the containers should have tight-fitting lids. Sterile containers may be obtained by sterilizing Dixie cups in ethylene oxide gas, or they may be purchased from commercial manufacturers.*

Because urine may support bacterial growth or destroy bacteria following collection, we recommend that it be cultured within 30 minutes from the time of collection if significant results are to be obtained. If this is not possible, the sample should be refrigerated immediately. Refrigerated samples may be stored for several hours without significant increase in bacterial numbers. It is also emphasized that fastidious organisms may be killed in the urine environment if storage time is prolonged, resulting in a decreased concentration of organisms.

LABORATORY METHODS FOR QUANTITATIVE URINE CULTURE

The most accurate results of quantitative bacterial cultures of urine are obtained by dilution pour-plate methods and surface streaking of media plates with calibrated loops. Pour plates are prepared by mixing a diluted aliquot of urine with a measured volume of molten agar. After incubation, bacterial colonies that appear deep in the agar can be counted. The pour-plate technique must be combined with surface streaking for organism identification.

A less time-consuming technique involves the use of calibrated bacteriologic loops† that deliver exactly 0.01 or 0.001 milliliters of urine to culture plates. Urine is streaked over the surface of both blood agar and MacConkey's agar by conventional methods. The plates are then incubated at 37° C for 24 hours. Bacterial colonies are counted and the total numbers of colonies on each plate are multiplied by the dilution factor to obtain the quantitative bacterial count.

SCREENING METHODS FOR QUANTITATIVE URINE CULTURE

Although pour-plate and loop-dilution techniques provide accurate results, they have several disadvantages. Because they are time-consuming they are not well suited for most "in-office" laboratories. Transport of urine specimens to a commercial microbiology laboratory results in an increase in time between urine collections and culture and therefore adds a potential source of erroneous results. Delay in obtaining results from a commercial laboratory may delay initiation of appropriate therapy. In addition, the cost of laboratory-performed quantitative urine cultures may be significant, especially in those cases in which serial cultures from the same patient are required.

Screening techniques of quantitative urine culture have been developed to minimize these technical problems. In general, screening culture techniques can be done as office procedures, are rapidly performed, require little special equipment other than a 37° C incubator, and are relatively inexpensive.

Screening culture techniques are of two basic types: those based on bacterial growth on bacteriologic culture media and those based on bacteria-induced chemical reactions.

DIP-SLIDES

Dip-slides consist of a plastic slide or paddle coated on each side with a layer of culture medium (Guttman and Naylor). One side is usually coated with a medium (e.g., eosin–methylene blue or MacConkey's agar) that supports growth of gram-negative bacteria. A medium designed to support gram-negative and

---

*Falcon Company, 1950 William Drive, Oxnard, California 93030

---

†Scientific Products, McGraw Park, Illinois

Table 1. *Causes of False-Negative and False-Positive Results with Screening Tests for Quantitative Urine Culture*

TEST	FALSE-POSITIVE RESULTS	FALSE-NEGATIVE RESULTS
Dip-slide	Delay in culturing specimen Slide incubation at room temperature (?)	Patient receiving antibiotic therapy Contamination of collection container with antiseptic solution Decreased bacterial count associated with diuresis Outdated media Incubation at room temperature
Pad culture	Delay in culturing specimen Rapidly spreading strains of *E. coli, Proteus mirabilis* and *Enterobacter aerogenes* Hematuria	Patients receiving antibiotic therapy Contamination of collection container with antiseptic solution Decreased bacterial count associated with diuresis Outdated culture pads Slow-growing streptococci Blood, bilirubin, and methylene blue may interfere with reading the test
Nitrite test	Delay in testing specimen Administration of phenazopyridine or other dyes that impart red color to urine	Ascorbic acid in urine Urine specific gravity > 1.020 Bacteria that do not convert nitrate to nitrite Inadequate bacterial incubation time in bladder
Glucose consumption test	Delay in testing specimen	Presence of diabetes mellitus or other causes of glucosuria Infection with bacteria that do not utilize glucose
Urinary catalase test	Renal epithelial cells, red blood cells, or white blood cells in urine samples	Bacteria without catalase

gram-positive bacteria (e.g., tryptase soy agar) is coated on the other side. To use, the dip-slide is removed from its sterile housing and dipped into the urine specimen. The slide is then replaced in its housing and incubated for 18 to 24 hours at 37° C. Quantitation is based on the principle that a small but constant volume of urine will adhere to the surface of the agar medium. Quantitative bacterial counts are obtained by comparing the density of bacterial colonies on the paddles to a standard supplied by the manufacturer. Results obtained with dip-slides are generally similar to those obtained by laboratory quantitative culture methods, but false-negative and false-positive reactions occasionally occur (Table 1) (Adelman). Two dip-slide systems (Culturia,* Bacteriuria Screening Test†) have been evaluated at the University of Minnesota Veterinary Hospital and found to be effective screening tests in dogs.

PAD CULTURE TEST

The pad culture test‡ combines both microbiologic and chemical techniques for detec-

tion of significant bacteriuria. The reagent strip contains a nitrite test reagent pad and two dehydrated culture medium pads. One pad permits growth of gram-negative and gram-positive bacteria, whereas the other permits only growth of gram-negative bacteria. Since a constant quantity of urine is absorbed by the culture medium pads, the bacterial count can be estimated by comparing the density of the bacterial growth on the pads to a standard chart supplied by the manufacturer. Detection of bacterial colonies is enhanced by the addition of triphenyltetrazolium to the pads by the manufacturer. After incubation, most bacteria reduce triphenyltetrazolium to formazan, a reaction that is associated with the production of an easily identifiable magenta-colored spot around the bacterial colonies growing on the culture pads.

The nitrite test is dependant on the conversion of nitrate (a metabolite normally present in urine) to nitrite by certain species of bacteria. In the acid environment of the reagent pad, urinary nitrite reacts with *p*-arsenilic acid to form a diazonium compound. The diazonium compound in turn reacts with an indicator dye in the pad to form a pink color. The appearance of a pink color, regardless of intensity, is reported by the manufacturer to indicate 100,000 or more bacteria per milliliter of urine.

*Clinical Convenience Products, Inc., Madison, Wisconsin 53701
†Balitmore Biologics Laboratory, Cockeysville, Maryland 21030
‡Microstix, Ames Company, Elkhart, Indiana 46514

The pad culture technique is almost as sensitive as the calibrated loop technique in identifying significant bacteriuria in canine and feline urine samples (Klausner, et al.). As with other screening tests, however, false-negative and false-positive results have occurred in a small percentage of cases (see Table 1). If gross hematuria masks the color change in the reagent pads the test is unreliable.

The nitrite portion of the reagent strip will not detect significant bacteriuria in canine or feline urine samples (Klausner, et al.). Ascorbic acid, a metabolite normally present in dog and cat urine, inhibits the nitrite test reaction.

GLUCOSE CONSUMPTION TEST

Since most bacteria utilize glucose, the absence of glucose in urine is sometimes used as an indicator of significant bacteriuria (Schersten, et al.). A test strip§ has been developed that is sufficiently sensitive to detect the normal glucose concentration of 2 to 10 mg/dl. Absence of normal quantities of glucose in urine suggests the presence of bacterial infections. Results of clinical studies of this test in human beings with urinary tract infections revealed a significant number of false-positive reactions (Kunin). The test has not been evaluated in dogs or cats.

CATALASE TEST

Most bacteria contain the enzyme catalase. If urine containing catalase is mixed with hydrogen peroxide, oxygen is released. Since renal epithelial cells, erythrocytes, and leukocytes also contain catalase, a positive catalase test does not necessarily indicate bacterial urinary tract infection (Kunin). The catalase test is

therefore not recommended as a screening test for detection of urinary tract infections.

GUIDE LINES FOR USE OF SCREENING TESTS

1. Screening tests may be used to monitor patients with previous histories of urinary tract infection.

2. Screening tests performed while a patient is receiving antibiotic therapy are often effective in detecting therapeutic failures.

3. Screening tests are an inexpensive method to evaluate urine samples from patients in which there is a low index of suspicion of urinary tract infection.

4. Urine samples should be collected and handled in a manner similar to that described for laboratory culture techniques.

5. Positive results obtained with screening tests should be verified by laboratory quantitative cultures when possible.

6. Negative results obtained with screening tests should be verified by laboratory quantitative cultures if clinical or laboratory data suggest urinary tract infection.

SUPPLEMENTAL READING

Adelman, R.D.: The dip slide in diagnosis of urinary tract infections. J. Family Pract., 3:647–649, 1976.

Carter, J.M., Klausner, J.S., Osborne, C.A., and Bates, F.Y.: Comparison of collection techniques for quantitative urine culture in dogs. J. Am. Vet. Med. Assoc., 173:296–298, 1978.

Guttmann, D., and Naylor, G. R.: Dip-slide: An aid to quantitative urine culture in general practice. Br. Med. J., 3:343–346, 1967.

Kass, E.M.: The role of asymptomatic bacteriuria in the pathogenesis of pyelonephritis. In Quin, E.L., and Kass, E.M. (eds.): *Biology of Pyelonephritis*. Boston, Little, Brown and Co., 1960.

Klausner, J.S., Osborne, C.A., and Stevens, J.B.: Clinical evaluation of commercial reagent strips for detection of significant bacteriuria in dogs and cats. Am. J. Vet. Res., 37:714–722, 1976.

Kunin, C.M.: New methods in detecting urinary tract infections. Urol. Clin. North Am., 12:423–432, 1975.

Schersten, B., Dahlquist, A., Fritz, H., Kohler, L., and Westlund, L.: Screening for bacteriuria with a test paper for glucose. JAMA, 204:205–208, 1968.

---

§Uriglox, KABI Laboratories, Stockholm, Sweden

URINARY TRACT INFECTIONS

DELMAR R. FINCO, D.V.M.

Athens, Georgia

INTRODUCTION

This discussion of urinary tract infection (UTI) is limited to bacterial agents isolated by common culture procedures. Insufficient study of viral agents in both the dog and cat prevents an assessment of their role in UTI. Fastidious bacterial organisms that may escape detection by common culture techniques have likewise not been studied very thoroughly as causes of UTI in the dog and cat. Mycotic agents are uncommon urinary pathogens. Non-bacterial or fastidious bacterial agents should be suspected when conventional culture results are negative but evidence of UTI exists. This situation occurs commonly in cats but rarely in dogs.

A survey of cases of UTI in the dog diagnosed by quantitative urine culture at the University of Georgia revealed that of 187 urine samples, *E. coli* was isolated from 68, *Proteus* spp. from 59, *Staphylococcus aureus* from 35, *Streptococcus* from 16, *Enterobacter* spp. from 11, *Klebsiella* spp. from 9, *Pseudomonas* spp. from 5, and *Staphylococcus epidermidis* from 3. These data indicate that gram-negative organisms accounted for roughly 75 percent of the isolations. The cultures also revealed that a single infecting organism was isolated in 92 percent of the cultures. These data provide a perspective for causes of UTI in one hospital population and emphasize the diversity of organisms that may be encountered.

PATHOGENESIS

Organisms causing UTI are ubiquitous, and thus the potential for development of UTI seems great. It is believed that infection most likely develops as a consequence of the ascent of organisms via the urethra. The hematogenous route of infection is also possible. Studies have shown that the distal urethra of the normal dog contains bacteria. The number of bacteria decreases progressively as the urethra ascends, and the bladder contents are sterile.

Factors that seem relevant in preventing infections include the flushing action of micturition when bladder emptying is complete, the physical barrier of the mucosa, local antibody production by cells in the mucosa or submucosa, and antibacterial properties of urine associated predominantly with high osmolality and acid pH. Knowledge of these factors is relevant in cases of persistent or recurrent UTI, since any correctable defects in these mechanisms should be a part of the therapy that is employed.

DIAGNOSIS

Diagnosis of UTI is made by identifying bacteria at a site in the urinary tract in which they normally do not exist. While this statement may appear trite, it seems to be ignored frequently in veterinary practice. Infection is often diagnosed when it does not exist and ignored when it is present. Since accurate diagnosis of UTI must precede its treatment, it is imperative that reliable and unreliable methods of diagnosis be differentiated.

Clinical signs provide a basis for suspicion of UTI but do not reliably allow its diagnosis. Signs referable to lower tract infection (dysuria or dysuria combined with hematuria) may be caused by non-bacterial factors as well as UTI. This is amply demonstrated by failure to isolate common bacteria from cases of the feline urologic syndrome. Signs referable to the upper urinary tract that have been reported in association with UTI include fever, renal pain, and possibly polyuria. Likewise these signs are non-specific and do not provide a reliable diagnosis of UTI. Equally important, absence of clinical signs does not rule out the possibility of UTI in either the kidneys or the lower urinary tract. The incidence of asymptomatic bacteriuria in small animals is unknown, but documented cases are commonplace.

Urinalysis findings consistent with infection (bacteriuria, pyuria) are relevant to diagnosis of UTI only if the method of collection of the sample is considered. Voided samples may be contaminated with these elements as normal constituents of the urethra and genitalia. Catheterized samples are superior to voided speci-

1158

mens, but the catheterization procedure imposes the risk of infecting the patient, and samples still may be contaminated. Cystocentesis is the best method of obtaining urine for diagnosis of UTI. The procedure is simple, safe, and completely bypasses lower tract contamination (see the article "Cystocentesis").

Urinalysis must include a competent examination of urinary sediment to provide meaningful results regarding UTI. If urinalysis is normal on a specimen obtained by cystocentesis, UTI usually can be ruled out. Exceptions may exist because cocci sometimes are difficult to identify in sediment. The absence of WBCs in sediment does not rule out UTI in human beings; it is likely that the same interpretation should be applied in small animals. Urine pH changes alone are not sufficient for diagnosis of UTI; alkaline urine may exist without infection and acid urine may often exist with infection.

Urine culture provides the best data for diagnosing UTI, but certain precautions are necessary. Without these precautions, data reveal that UTI may be erroneously diagnosed in 75 percent of dogs and 50 percent of cats in which UTI is absent. As with urinalysis, these data are due to contamination of sterile bladder urine by normal urethral or genital flora. The precautions that are required include consideration of both the method and conditions of procurement of urine and the method of handling the sample at the time of culture. To distinguish bacterial infection from contamination, quantitative bacterial culture is performed on the assumption that small numbers of organisms indicate contamination and large numbers of organisms indicate infection. See the article "Screening Tests for the Detection of Significant Bacteriuria" for methods of estimating bacterial counts.

As for urinalysis, cystocentesis is the best method of collecting urine for culture. Midstream voided samples are the worst. Overall recommendations for urine culture in the dog and cat are as follows:

1. Obtain culture samples by cystocentesis if possible.

2. Obtain a midstream urine specimen from the dog by catheterization as a second choice. The dog's genitalia should be thoroughly cleaned with soap and water, and sterile technique and equipment should be used for catheterization.

3. Obtain urine from the cat by manually expressing the bladder as an alternative to cystocentesis. Catheterization of the female cat is difficult, and routine catheterization of the male is to be avoided because of potential urethral trauma.

4. Routinely use quantitative urine culture

procedures. Although any bacterial growth in samples collected by cystocentesis is indicative of an abnormality, the large numbers of organisms that are usually present with infection remove doubt concerning the possibility of contamination of sterile urine during procurement or handling. Quantitative urine culture is essential for midstream specimens obtained by catheterization.

5. Interpret 10^5 or more organisms per ml in catheterized samples and 10^3 or more organisms in cystocentesis samples as evidence of infection. Interpret 10^3 or fewer organisms in midstream catheterized or expressed specimens as contamination. Intermediate values require re-evaluation of the patient. Values of 10^2 to 10^3 in cystocentesis samples also require re-evaluation.

Urine for quantitative culture should be used for enumeration studies soon after procurement so that numbers reflect *in vivo* conditions rather than bacterial growth subsequent to urine collection.

LOCALIZATION

Localization of UTI may be beneficial for both treatment and prognosis. Renal and prostate infection may be more difficult to eradicate than bladder infection. In the case of renal infection, intrarenal retention of urine may not be correctable, and the defense response of the renal medulla is known to be inferior to that of the cortex. In addition, renal interstitial concentrations of antibiotics may be less than urine concentrations. Prognostically, renal infection is serious, inasmuch as progressive destruction of renal parenchyma could lead to death from uremia. With chronic infection of the prostate gland, difficulty in eradicating the infection is often encountered. This may be due to the failure of most antibiotics to appear in prostate fluid despite adequate blood concentrations.

Unfortunately, simple and reliable methods of localizing UTI are not available for the dog and cat. Lower tract signs (dysuria, hematuria) do not eliminate the possibility of coexisting renal infection. Renal infection may be present in the absence of renal pain, fever, or leukocytosis. Urinalyses may aid in identifying renal infections if casts and low urine specific gravity are present, but the absence of these findings does not rule out renal infection. Likewise, excretory urography may aid in identifying renal abnormalities that are believed to be consistent with pyelonephritis (dilated pelvis, dilated ureters). However, absence of these signs does not eliminate the possibility of renal infection.

Bladder washout procedures and antibody

coating of bacteria have been used in human beings for localization of UTI. However, these methods have proved unreliable in experimental UTI in the dog.

If recurrent or persistent UTI occurs in male dogs, consideration should be given to prostate infection that extends to the urinary tract. Treatment may eradicate urinary infection but fail to eliminate prostatic infection. Localization of infection to the prostate gland may be achieved by culture procedures that are discussed elsewhere. Physical examination may be helpful in localization if prostate palpation reveals abnormalities, but a prostate gland considered normal by physical examination may nevertheless be infected.

MANAGEMENT OF URINARY INFECTIONS

The economic factors that face the veterinary practitioner dictate that an overall knowledge and understanding of UTI be combined with logic and common sense in the formulation of programs for its management.

Single Episodes of Dysuria or Dysuriahematuria. Dysuria and hematuria are suggestive, but not diagnostic, of UTI. The following are recommended as the minimum data base for such cases:

1. Subjective data should include questions to establish if such signs have occurred previously. If so, the time(s) of occurrence should be related to the present episode. If the same signs have been present previously, the case is handled as one of persistent or recurrent infection, as subsequently discussed. The presence or absence of other relevant signs pertaining to the genitourinary tract (discharge, lethargy, polyuria) should also be ascertained.

2. Objective data should include rectal temperature determination, rectal examination of the prostate of male dogs, and careful palpation of the bladder by abdominal and rectal examination for abnormalities such as calculi, masses, or diffuse thickening. Since these patients have dysuria, the bladder usually is empty. Finding moderate or large quantities of urine in the bladder should lead one to question the presence of dysuria caused by lower tract irritation and seek other explanations for the owner's complaints. The kidneys should be palpated when possible, and the external genitalia should be examined.

If the signs represent the only instance of dysuria and/or hematuria and if physical findings are normal when accurately assessed, UTI is presumed to exist and the patient is treated. It is important that both the veterinarian and the client recognize the presumptive nature of the diagnosis so that persistence of signs despite

treatment can be put in the proper perspective.

Antibiotics (or sulfonamides or nitrofurantoin) alone are usually adequate for therapy. Urinary acidifiers are necessary only for modification of urine pH for optimal antibiotic activity and should not be used as a bacteriostatic or bactericidal form of treatment because of their lack of efficacy. Sensitivity testing of organisms isolated from dogs with UTI presented to the University of Georgia indicated that Furadantin, gentamicin, chloramphenicol, and ampicillin were good choices for empirical treatment of UTI. Sulfadiazine-trimethoprim was not included in the study. Treatment should be continued for ten days despite prior resolution of signs. This point should be emphasized to the owner.

PERSISTENT OR RECURRENT SIGNS OF UTI

Failure to respond to symptomatic therapy, recurrence following response to therapy, or a history of previous episodes of signs compatible with UTI warrants a more exhaustive evaluation of the patient. The timing of these studies in relation to the duration or frequency of recurrence of signs is at the discretion of the clinician, but at some time all such cases require these studies. The objective is to establish whether UTI actually exists and to determine whether factors exist that predispose the patient to UTI. The data base for such cases includes careful evaluation of the process of micturition. The patient is evaluated for urine retention by bladder palpation or catheterization following efforts at voiding. The patency of the urethra can be judged if catheterization is performed. Micturition is evaluated in this manner to check the history of dysuria and to investigate the possibility of urine retention as a predisposing factor to UTI. Urinalysis, urine culture (organism identification, quantitation, and sensitivity testing), and survey radiographic examination of the urinary tract are also conducted. In male dogs procurement of an ejaculate sample for cytologic examination and culture should be performed. In preparation for obtaining the ejaculate, the dog should be allowed to urinate so as to clean the urethra mechanically. The tip of the penis is gently cleansed with warm water as it extrudes from the sheath during erection. If an ejaculate cannot be obtained, a second method of identifying bacterial prostatitis may be attempted. A urinary catheter is passed aseptically, and the bladder is emptied. Five ml of sterile saline is used to rinse the bladder. The sample (P-1) is saved. The catheter is retracted so that the tip is just caudal to the prostate gland, and the gland is massaged for one minute. The catheter is held carefully in place, and 5 ml of sterile saline is injected to push any material forced into the urethra back into the bladder. The catheter is then advanced into the bladder and the rinse retrieved (P-2). Samples P-1 and P-2 may be compared by cytologic examination and culture procedures on the noncentrifuged specimens. Higher content of bacteria or inflammatory cells in P-2 implies a prostatic source of the infection.

A further method of identifying bacterial prostatitis as a predisposing factor in recurring UTI in the male dog takes advantage of lack of penetration of antibiotics into the prostate. A dog with lower tract signs is treated for 48 hours with an appropriate antibiotic other than chloramphenicol, trimethoprim, or erythromycin. This should diminish the number of organisms in the bladder but should have little effect on numbers in the prostate fluids. Quantitative culture of either urine and ejaculate or P-1 and P-2 samples may aid in distinguishing primary prostate infection from primary bladder infection.

Special radiologic procedures (contrast cystography, urethrography, excretory urography) are chosen by the clinician based on the patient's signs. I prefer to have both contrast cystography and excretory urography performed on these patients, since clinical signs are not accurate in localizing abnormalities. Negative-contrast cystography with CO_2 seems superior to positive-contrast agents in most instances.

Patients with correctable predisposing factors (e.g., calculi, bladder diverticula) should have these factors resolved by surgery that is performed coincident with initiation of antibacterial therapy. The choice of antibacterial agent should be made on the basis of culture and sensitivity testing. However, *in vitro* sensitivity as determined by the Kirby-Bauer method may not accurately reflect *in vivo* sensitivity. Discs used for *in vitro* studies have quantities of antibiotic that are roughly comparable to blood levels, while urine levels of antibiotic are often 10 to 100 times that of blood. As a result, some drugs with *in vitro* resistance will have *in vivo* sensitivity. Antibacterial therapy should be continued for about 30 days. It is advisable to perform a urinalysis after a week of therapy in order to assess efficacy. At least five days after cessation of therapy and again one and two months later, urine cultures are advised to assure that infection has been eradicated and has not recurred. In problem cases in which infection with urea-splitting organisms causes alkaline urine, pH paper is dispensed to the owner for monitoring urine pH as an early

indication of reinfection. The owner is advised to determine the pH once weekly on midstream urine from the first voiding of the day. If the pH is above 7.5, daily readings are made. If the pH is above 7.5 for three days, reinfection is likely and the patient is evaluated by urinalysis and culture. The surveillance program with pH paper is of no value for detecting infection by acid-forming bacteria.

In some cases of persistent or recurrent UTI it is not possible to identify predisposing factors. Persistent infection may exist because of inadequate treatment without follow-up to see if eradication occurred. Recurrent infection may reflect undetectable defects in the host's defense mechanism for which there is no solution. Persistence of infection may be suspected when the same organism is isolated on urine cultures taken over an extended interval. Such circumstances warrant an intensive program of treatment and post-treatment evaluation, since eradication of infection may not be followed by recurrence. Recurrent infection is documented when pure cultures of different organisms are isolated on different occasions. Prospects for solution of this patient's problems are slim, and treatment of episodes is necessary as they recur.

Some cases of UTI will have predisposing factors identified that cannot be solved. Dogs with bladder dysfunction and an inability to empty the bladder completely are included in this category. These cases may require constant antibacterial therapy to control infection. Since many antibacterial agents have undesirable effects when used for extended periods, the choices of drugs for these patients are restricted. Nitrofurantoin, triple sulfas, and ampicillin are some agents that may be used. Urinary antiseptics such as methenamine are often effective when urine pH is kept sufficiently acid (see the chapter entitled "Ancillary Treatment of Urinary Tract Infections"). These products are superior to acidifiers alone and should be used in preference to them.

Persistent or recurrent signs of UTI with sterile urine or non-significant numbers of bacteria in the urine are commonplace in the cat. This entity is not appropriately referred to as UTI, and its method of management differs from that described herein. See "Feline Urologic Syndrome: Medical Aspects of Prophylaxis" for further details concerning this syndrome.

SUPPLMENTAL READING

Osborne, C.A., and Finco, D.R.: Urinary tract infections: New solutions to old problems. Proc. 44th Annual Meeting, American Animal Hospital Association, 1977.

Stamey, T.A.: *Urinary Infections.* Baltimore, Williams & Wilkins Co., 1972.

CHOICE OF ANTIMICROBIAL AGENTS IN THE TREATMENT OF URINARY TRACT INFECTIONS

GERALD V. LING, D.V.M.
Davis, California

It is generally accepted that urine concentrations of antimicrobial agents are more important than blood concentrations in the successful treatment of urinary tract infections (UTI). All of the antimicrobials commonly used in the treatment of UTI are present in the urine in active form at concentrations that exceed up to 100 times their peak blood concentrations. The critical antimicrobial concentration in the treatment of any UTI is called the *minimum inhibitory concentration* (MIC), which may be defined as the least amount of an antimicrobial agent that causes complete inhibition of growth of the infecting species or strain of bacteria under controlled and reproducible laboratory conditions. The relationship of bacterial MIC to the concentration of antimicrobial in the urine is of prime importance, since it is the reason that drugs such as penicillin can be used to treat successfully many gram-negative infections encountered in the urinary tract (*E. coli, Proteus* spp., and others).

The major therapeutic goal in the treatment of UTI is to use an antimicrobial agent that is easy to administer, has few (if any) undesirable side effects, is relatively inexpensive, and will result in urine concentrations that exceed the MIC for the infecting species or strain of bacteria at least four-fold. The drug should be administered frequently enough to maintain inhibitory urine concentrations (usually three times daily for oral antimicrobials) and long enough to rid the urinary tract of the infecting agent (usually 7 to 14 days).

It is usually not possible to obtain reliable susceptibility test results to aid in the selection of an appropriate antimicrobial agent for the treatment of UTI in animals. The information obtained from the Kirby-Bauer test, available from most commercial laboratories, is of limited value since only those agents that test in the sensitive (S) or intermediate (I) ranges may be considered appropriate choices. Antimicrobics

that test resistant (R) by this method may or may not actually be effective at easily attainable urine concentrations, since the test is standardized to blood concentrations.

It is often possible, however, to select an appropriate antimicrobial agent if the species of the infecting bacteria is known. Common bacterial isolates from canine UTI and their susceptibility, based on the results of clinical trials in dogs, are presented in Table 1.

The MIC of oral penicillin G and ampicillin for virtually all urinary streptococcal and staphylococcal isolates, including penicillinase-producing strains, are less than 10 μg/ml, whereas the mean six-hour urine concentrations of both of these antimicrobials are about 350 μg/ml at recommended urinary dosages. It may be assumed with almost 100 percent confidence, therefore, that either of these antimicrobials will be effective in the treatment of urinary infections caused by *Streptococcus* spp. and *Staphylococcus* spp. Approximately 80 percent of urinary infections caused by *E. coli* may be treated successfully with oral trimethoprim-sulfa, a prediction based on information obtained by testing the drug against urinary tract isolates of *E. coli*. Using similar information, oral penicillin G or ampicillin may be used to treat successfully about 80 percent of canine UTI caused by *Proteus mirabilis*, and oral tetracycline has been used in the treatment of UTI caused by *Pseudomonas* spp. with a success rate of about 80 percent. The surprising success of oral tetracycline is due to the fact that the MIC of tetracycline for most canine urinary isolates of *Pseudomonas* spp. is less than 40 μg/ml, whereas the mean eight-hour urine concentration of tetracycline given orally at standard dosages to dogs is about 150 μg/ml. Among the common bacterial genera isolated from the urine of dogs with UTI, only the successful oral treatment of *Klebsiella* spp. cannot be predicted with ≥ 80 percent confidence. Trimethoprim-

1162

Table 1. In Vivo *Susceptibility of Common Canine Urinary Tract Pathogens to Selected Oral Antimicrobial Agents*

ORGANISM	SUSCEPTIBILITY		
	100%	*80%*	*<80%*
Escherichia coli		Trimethoprim/sulfa†	
Proteus mirabilis		Trimethoprim/sulfa	
Staphylococcus aureus	Penicillin G, ampicillin°		
Streptococcus spp.	Penicillin G, ampicillin		
Klebsiella pneumoniae			Trimethoprim/sulfa
Pseudomonas spp.		Tetracycline‡	

°Penicillin G: Given orally at the rate of 110,000 U/kg (50,000 U/lb) of body weight in 3 divided doses daily. Ampicillin: Given orally at the rate of 77 mg/kg (35 mg/lb) of body weight in 3 divided doses daily.

†Tribrissen: Given orally at the rate of 26.4 mg/kg (12 mg/lb) of body weight in 2 divided doses daily.

‡Tetracycline: given orally at the rate of 55 mg/kg (25 mg/lb) of body weight in 3 divided doses daily.

sulfa has been used in canine UTI caused by *Klebsiella* spp. with a success rate of approximately 65 percent.

The daily doses and recommended frequency of administration of penicillin G, ampicillin, tetracycline, and trimethoprim-sulfa are listed in Table 1. There are many other antimicrobial agents available for the treatment of UTI in animals. These four drugs are mentioned specifically because they seem to offer the best chance of therapeutic success at the least cost to the client and risk to the patient and because clinical trials substantiating their efficacy have been conducted in dogs.

It may be temping at times to initiate treatment by administering two or more antimicrobials simultaneously, especially when two or more causative bacterial species are isolated or in cases of infection caused by a single bacterial species that is resistant to several antimicrobial agents. When two antimicrobials are administered simultaneously, the effect of the combination on the infecting bacterial population may be additive, synergistic, antagonistic, or one of indifference and may vary with the antimicrobial agents administered, the bacterial species involved, and the site of the infection. Combining two or more antimicrobials without in-depth knowledge of the results of such a combination in the specific set of circumstances for which therapy is being given is inappropriate at best. Mixtures of antimicrobial agents have been shown to be superior to a single agent on the basis of controlled clinical trials in only a few instances.

Aminoglycoside antimicrobials (e.g., gentamicin, tobramycin, and amikacin) should be limited in their use in UTI to those situations in which an infection has persisted in spite of appropriate therapy with other antimicrobials or when two or more bacterial species with widely differing antimicrobial susceptibilities are present in a single episode (e.g., *Streptococcus* spp. and *Klebsiella* spp. in combination). In this example the bacterial species have such widely differing susceptibilities that only a broad-spectrum agent such as gentamicin or tobramycin will be effective against both species.

SUPPLEMENTAL READING

Klastersky J., Daneau, D., Swings, G., and Weerts, D.: Antibacterial activity in serum and urine as a therapeutic guide in bacterial infections. J. Infect. Dis., *129*:187–193, 1974.

Musher, D.M., Minuth, J.N., Thorsteinsson, S.B., and Holmes, T.: Effectiveness of achievable urinary concentrations of tetracyclines against "tetracycline resistant" pathogenic bacteria. J. Infect. Dis., *131* (Suppl.):S40–S44, 1975.

Stamey, T.A.: *Urinary Infections.* Baltimore, The Williams & Wilkins Co., 1972, Chapter 10.

Stamey, T.A., Fair, W.R., Timothy, M.M., Millar, M.A., Mihara, G., and Lowery, Y.C.: Serum versus urinary antimicrobial concentrations in cure of urinary tract infections. N. Engl. J. Med., *291*:1159–1163, 1974.

ANCILLARY TREATMENT OF URINARY TRACT INFECTIONS

CARL A. OSBORNE, D.V.M.,
JEFFREY S. KLAUSNER, D.V.M.,
ROBERT M. HARDY, D.V.M.
and GEORGE E. LEES, D.V.M.
St. Paul, Minnesota

In the not-too-distant past, conceptual understanding of urinary tract infections was limited primarily to detection and eradication of pathogenic bacteria thought to be their primary cause. It has become apparent, however, that interaction of abnormal host defense mechanisms and pathogenic bacteria must be considered in the diagnosis, prognosis, and management of urinary tract infections. Although pathogenic bacteria must gain access to the urinary tract to induce infection, entrance of bacteria into the urinary tract is not synonymous with infection. Current evidence indicates that host mechanisms must be transiently or persistently abnormal for bacterial colonization to occur. In other words, abnormalities in host defense mechanisms that permit time-honored bacterial villains to produce their "dirty work" appear to be a more basic cause of urinary tract infections. See the article entitled "Urinary Tract Infections" and consult reference material for specific details.

Therapeutic recommendations summarized in this chapter are designed to (1) enhance the effectiveness of antimicrobial drugs, (2) minimize abnormalities caused by abnormal host defense mechanisms, (3) create an environment that is unfavorable for bacterial survival or growth, and (4) reduce the severity of clinical signs. Many forms of ancillary therapy for urinary tract infections have been developed and evaluated on an empirical basis. In terms of value to the patient, they usually rank behind antimicrobial therapy and correction of predisposing factors of urinary tract infections. Although antimicrobial drugs currently remain the cornerstone of treatment and although their effectiveness may be augmented by ancillary forms of therapy, we predict that the development of consistently effective methods of management of recurrent and resistant urinary tract infections will not be forthcoming until methods to detect and correct host abnormalities are perfected.

URINARY ACIDIFIERS

Although urine is capable of supporting bacterial growth under certain circumstances, urine from dogs, cats, and human beings may also be inhibitory and sometimes bactericidal to pathogens that cause urinary tract infections. The antibacterial properties of urine are influenced by its composition. Unfavorable physiologic factors for bacterial growth include low (or extremely high) pH, high osmolality, high concentration of urea, and certain weak organic acids derived primarily from the diet.

Urinary acidifiers have been commonly advocated as adjunctive therapy for urinary tract infections because in man most aerobic bacteria found in urine grow well at a neutral or mildly alkaline pH. Comparable studies have not been performed in dogs or cats. While unproved, the general consensus has been that the same conclusions derived from studies in man apply to these species.

The efficacy of acidifiers in suppressing bacterial growth is dependent on several factors, including (1) susceptibility of pathogenic organisms to acid pH, (2) urine pH obtained, and (3) contact of acid urine with pathogenic bacteria. Because the antimicrobial activity of urinary acidifiers is inferior to that of most antibiotic and chemotherapeutic agents, acidifiers should not be expected to eradicate urinary tract infections. They should be used only when the urine produced is not persistently acid (frequent evaluation of urine pH may be needed to determine this) and in conjunction with other modes of therapy. Although urinary acidifiers alone may not be capable of sterilizing urine, reduction of bacterial numbers caused by the unfavorable environment they create may permit host defense mechanisms to become more effective. Consult the article entitled "Choice of Antimicrobial Agents in the Treatment of Urinary Tract Infections" for specific recommendations.

Urinary acidifiers may be ineffective in some patients with urinary tract infections caused by urease-producing bacteria (*Proteus* spp., staphylococci, and others) because therapeutic dosages may be insufficient to overcome the continuous production of ammonia from urea by bacterial urease. Urinary tract infections in such patients should be treated with antibacterial agents that are effective at an alkaline pH. Once infection is controlled the need for acidifiers may be eliminated. If deemed beneficial, however, combined use of antibiotics effective in an acid environment with urinary acidifiers may be employed.

One of the major benefits of urinary acidifiers is adjustment of urine pH to an optimum for antibiotic activity. In one study of 204 human patients with urinary tract infections treated with appropriate antimicrobial agents, 102 had their urine pH adjusted and 102 had no pH adjustment (Brumfitt and Reaves). The cure rate was 67 percent in the unadjusted group, but the rate increased to 87 percent in pH-adjusted patients. These and other results indicate that failure to adjust urine pH to the optimum value for certain chemotherapeutic agents (especially aminoglycoside antibiotics) or to select antimicrobial agents on the basis of knowledge of the patient's urine pH may result in therapeutic failures. According to Kunin penicillin, carbenicillin, chlortetracycline, tetracycline, nitrofurantoin, and methenamine have optimal activity in acid urine. Neomycin, streptomycin, gentamicin, kanamycin, erythromycin, and polymyxin B have optimal activity in alkaline urine. Urine pH does not influence significantly the effectiveness of chloramphenicol, sulfonamides, cephalosporins, and nalidixic acid. Reports concerning the optimum urine pH for activity of ampicillin are contradictory.

Urinary acidifiers commonly recommended for use in dogs and cats include DL-methionine (Pedameth, Durst; Methigel, EVSCO; Odortrol, Haver-Lockhart), ascorbic acid, ethylene diamine dihydrochloride (Chlorethamine, Pitman-Moore), and ammonium chloride. Consult the article entitled "Feline Urologic Syndrome: Medical Aspects of Prophylaxis" for specific information regarding the use of these drugs to acidify the urine of cats. The advantages and disadvantages of these agents in dogs have been reviewed (Hardy and Osborne). The relative ineffectiveness of ascorbic acid as a urinary acidifier in man (Nahata et al.) and the inability of some acidifiers to induce an acid pH in the urine of dogs and cats indicate the need for careful evaluation of these products.

It has been reported that ascorbic acid in urine may inhibit bacterial growth irrespective of its action as a urine acidifier (Gnarp, et al.). In man the maximum effect occurred with concentrations of 100 to 200 mg/dl of urine, but some inhibition occurred at concentrations of 25 to 50 mg/dl. Since the concentration of urinary ascorbic acids in dogs and cats ranges from 0 to 90 mg/dl, it has been hypothesized that inhibitory levels may normally be present in canine and feline urine (Osborne, et al.)

Dosage of urinary acidifiers should be individualized for each patient. Urine should be maintained at a pH of 6.5 or less when possible and should be monitored until it has been established that acidification has been achieved and maintained. The effectiveness of urinary acidifiers increases as urine pH decreases. Administration of divided daily doses has been suggested to maintain a consistently acid environment in the urinary tract. Owners may participate in monitoring urine pH with pH paper (pHydrion, Microessential Laboratory, Brooklyn). Evaluation of the pH of the first voided urine in the morning has been advocated on the basis that it is least likely to be influenced by dietary "alkaline tide."

URINARY ANTISEPTICS

There is a general consensus that urinary antiseptics are useful as adjunctive agents in the treatment, control and prevention of urinary tract infections of dogs and cats, but studies that substantiate this belief have not been reported. Empirical clinical observations suggest that they are less effective than specific antibacterial therapy in eradication of infection but are probably more effective than urinary acidifiers. They cannot be used to treat systemic infections, because when sufficient quantities are administered to attain effective serum concentrations systemic toxicity results.

METHENAMINE

Methenamine is a cyclic hydrocarbon that is one of the most popular urinary antiseptics used in man. In an acid environment (pH less than 6.0) methenamine hydrolyzes to form formaldehyde (Musher, et al., 1976). Enteric tablets are usually administered to prevent degradation in the acid environment of the stomach. Antimicrobial sensitivity tests are not required.

Because of the necessity of acid urine for the formation of formaldehyde, methenamine is usually given in combination with an acidifier such as mandelic acid* or hippuric acid.† It is often necessary to administer more potent acidifiers in addition to these combined drugs to acidify urine of patients infected with urease-producing bacteria. In patients infected with urease-producing pathogens (especially *Proteus* spp. and staphylococci) urinary acidifiers may be ineffective in producing acid urine. Recent studies have revealed that acetohydroxamic acid, a potent inhibitor of urease, potentiates the action of methenamine by favoring production of acid urine (Musher, et al., 1974). Acetohydroxamic acid is not yet commercially available to the veterinary profession.

Methenamine may be of value in the management of patients with antibiotic-resistant organisms. It may also be used as prophylactic therapy for patients having recurrent urinary tract infections. It is best to sterilize the urine with an antimicrobial agent prior to prophylactic therapy with methenamine (Stamey).

CRANBERRY JUICE

Hippuric acid, a conjugate of benzoic acid and glycine, is bacteriostatic at an acid pH. Benzoic acid may be ingested or formed in the intestines from quinic acid, absorbed, conjugated in the liver, and excreted as hippuric acid. Quinic acid is a constituent of cranberry juice, a common home remedy for urinary tract infections (Bodel, et al.).

METHYLENE BLUE

Administration of methylene blue as a urinary antiseptic was first reported in 1891. Although it is commonly included in "shotgun" remedies for UTI (Urised, Uritin, Urilax, and others), its role in the management of UTI is unclear.

As reviewed elsewhere (Osborne and Lees), methylene blue and other oxidant drugs such as phenazopyridine (an azo dye commonly used as a urinary analgesic) have the potential to cause methemoglobinemia and irreversible oxidative changes in hemoglobin, resulting in Heinz body formation and anemia. Cats are very susceptible to the dose-related effects of these agents. Extremely high doses have also been reported to induce hemolytic anemia in dogs (Schalm). Use of products containing methy-

lene blue in cats is contraindicated since these drugs may induce severe and potentially fatal anemia.

IRRIGATION OF THE URINARY BLADDER

Although commonly used, this technique is of unproved and doubtful value. Controlled studies of the value of local instillation of fluids and antibiotics into the bladder lumen of dogs and cats have not been reported, but intermittent irrigation of human urinary bladders with antibacterial solutions (neomycin, furacin, polymyxin, and other agents) has resulted in only a transient antibacterial effect (Warren, et al.). Suboptimal results are thought to be related, at least in part, to the fact that patients with lower urinary tract infection frequently void the medication soon after it is instilled into the bladder lumen. In addition, local instillation of antimicrobial agents would not be expected to be of benefit in therapy of concomitant infection elsewhere in the urinary tract.

Because of the normal resident population of bacteria in the lumen of the distal urethra and genital tract, a philosophy of "it may not help but can do little harm" is not appropriate for this procedure. Catheterization, no matter how carefully executed, is always associated with the hazard of iatrogenic urinary tract infection because bacteria normally residing in these locations are carried into the bladder. Because of abnormalities in local host defense mechanisms, catheterization of patients with pre-existing disease in the urethra or bladder is much more likely to be associated with iatrogenic infection. Thus, catheterization for the sole purpose of instilling medications is not recommended.

This procedure may be justified as a prophylactic measure following catheterization for diagnostic purposes or intermittent catheterization of patients with bladder atony to remove residual urine (Hachen). In patients with atonic bladders the medication will remain within the lumen of the bladder until it is removed during the next catheterization. Since the efficacy of this form of therapy is questionable and at best transient, however, it should not be used in lieu of meticulous "feather-touch" technique designed to prevent iatrogenic trauma and infection.

If this method is employed, only solutions known to be sterile should be injected into the bladder. The volume of solution should be sufficient to permit contact with all portions of the bladder mucosa (Zinner, et al.). Caution in

---

*Mandelamine (methenamine mandelate), Warner-Chilcott Labs., Morris Plains, New Jersey 07950

†Hiprex (methenamine hippurate), Merrell-National Labs, Cincinnati, Ohio 45215

the use of solutions is recommended, since accumulation of large quantities of acid, anesthetic, or antimicrobial solutions within an inflamed bladder lumen may result in absorption and systemic toxicity (Weinstein, et al.).

ALTERING URINE VOLUME

As resolved elsewhere, studies in animals have revealed some findings that appear paradoxical (Osborne, et al.). Rats may become resistant to attempts to induce pyelonephritis via intravenous injection of a large dose of certain bacteria (staphylococci and enterococci) by inducing an intense water diuresis. In contrast, dilution of urine increases the susceptibility of animals to urinary colonization with certain bacteria following their instillation into the urinary bladder. As summarized in the article entitled "Feline Urologic Syndrome: Removal of Urethral Obstructions and Use of Indwelling Urethral Catheters," administration of parenteral fluids to normal cats with indwelling urethral catheters increased the severity of UTI. These observations suggest differences in renal and urinary bladder host defense mechanisms.

A logical but as yet untested hypothesis based on these observations is that diuresis might benefit patients with urinary tract infections primarily involving the kidneys but would be less advantageous to patients with infection of the lower urinary tract. Until further information becomes available, however, meaningful generalizations cannot be established. Because most antibiotics are excreted in high concentrations in patients with normal renal function, we do *not* recommend restriction of oral intake of water to promote antidiuresis and increased concentration of antimicrobial agents in urine. A fresh supply of water should be available at all times.

ANALGESICS AND ANTISPASMODICS

Phenazopyridine (Pyridium, Warner Chilcott) is a red azo dye that is rapidly excreted in urine. It is reported to have properties as a urinary analgesic but has no antiseptic properties. The mechanism(s) of action by which it relieves pain and other irritative signs of the lower urinary tract is unknown. Like methylene blue, phenazopyridine may produce a severe and potentially fatal anemia in cats.

Atropine, scopolamine, methantheline (Banthine, Searle & Co.), and propantheline (Pro-Banthine, Searle & Co.) are anticholinergic agents commonly used to alleviate detrusor muscle spasm and to increase bladder capacity. The value of these agents in providing comfort to dogs and cats with urinary tract infections is unknown. We rarely use them.

ENCOURAGING MICTURITION

Voluntary Micturition

The hydrodynamics associated with voiding urine are thought to represent one of the most important natural defense mechanisms against infection of the urinary tract. Mechanical washout induced by unimpeded, frequent, and complete voiding of urine inhibits bacterial colonization of the urinary tract by rapidly eliminating organisms in the lumen of the proximal urethra and urinary bladder. Micturition also reduces the population of bacteria lining the urethral mucosa by flushing the urethral lumen. For these reasons, dogs and cats with UTI should be provided with the opportunity to micturate freely in order to minimize stasis of urine within the bladder and to enhance washout of bacteria and their toxins. Allowing an animal to empty its bladder completely prior to forced confinement (overnight, for example) is emphasized. The duration of periods of forced confinement without the opportunity to micturate should be kept as short as feasible.

Urine Stasis

If a patient with urinary tract infection has a hypotonic or atonic bladder detrusor muscle, urine may be removed by manual compression of the bladder, by catheterization, or by administration of parasympathomimetic drugs. Provided it is effective and not associated with trauma to the bladder wall, manual compression of the bladder is acceptable. The efficacy of this technique may be evaluated by catheterizing the bladder lumen and determining how much urine remains following its use. If more than 5 to 10 milliliters remain, alternative methods should be considered.

Parasympathomimetic drugs such as bethanechol chloride (Urecholine, Merck, Sharp & Dohme) may be used in combination with manual compression or catheterization to stimulate postganglionic cells of the detrusor muscle. Parasympathomimetic drugs have no known value in promoting repair of lesions in the detrusor muscle. They should not be given unless the urethra is patent, since contraction of the bladder associated with an obstructed urethra may cause patient discomfort, reflux of infected urine into ureters and renal pelves and, conceivably, rupture of the excretory pathway.

Since the likelihood of iatrogenic catheter-induced infection is increased in patients with diseases of the urinary tract, intermittent and especially indwelling catheterization to manage patients with detrusor dysfunction should be performed with appropriate caution (Lees and Osborne).

SUPPLEMENTAL READINGS

Bodel, P.T., Cotran, A.R., and Kass, E.H.: Cranberry juice and the antibacterial action of hippuric acid. J. Lab. Clin. Med., 54:881, 1959.

Brumfitt, W., and Reaves, D.S.: Recent developments in treatment of urinary tract infection. J. Infect. Dis., 120:61–81, 1969.

Gnarp, H., Michaelson, M., and Dreborg, S.: The in vitro effect of ascorbic acid on bacterial growth in urine. Acta Pathol. Microbiol. Scand., 74:41, 1968.

Hachen, H.J.: Bladder instillations with trimethoprim-sulfamethoxazole in the treatment of urinary infection. Chemotherapy, 24:55–60, 1978.

Hardy, R.M., and Osborne, C.A.: The use and misuse of urinary acidifiers. In Scientific Proceedings of the 40th Annual Meeting of the American Animal Hospital Association, South Bend, Indiana, 1973.

Kunin, C.M.: Detection, Prevention and Management of Urinary Tract Infections, 2nd ed. Philadelphia, Lea & Febiger, 1974.

Lees, G.E., and Osborne, C.A.: Urinary tract infections associated with use and misuse of urinary catheters. Vet. Clin. North Am., 9: 713–727, 1979.

Musher, D.M., Griffith, D.P., and Richie, Y.: The generation of formaldehyde from methenamine. Invest. Urol., 13:380, 1976.

Musher, D.M., Griffith, D.P., Tyler, M., and Woelfel, A.: Potentiation of antibacterial effect of methenamine by acetohydroxamic acid. Antimicrob. Agents Chemother., 5:101–105, 1974.

Nahata, M.C., Shimp, L., Lampman, T., and McLeod, D.C.: Effect of ascorbic acid on urine pH in man. Am. J. Hosp. Pharm., 34:1234–1237, 1977.

Osborne, C.A., Klausner, J.S., and Lees, G.E.: Urinary tract infections: Normal and abnormal host defense mechanisms. Vet. Clin. North Am., 9:587–609, 1979.

Osborne, C.A., and Lees, G.E.: Feline cystitis, urethritis, and urethral obstruction syndrome. II. Therapy of disorders of the upper and lower urinary tract. Mod. Vet. Pract., 59:349–347, 1978.

Schalm, O.W.: Methylene blue–induced Heinz body hemolytic anemia in a dog. Canine Pract., 5:20–25, 1978.

Stamey, T.A.: Urinary Infections. Baltimore, The Williams & Wilkins Co., 1972.

Warren, J.W., et al.: Antibiotic irrigation and catheter-associated urinary-tract infections. N. Engl. J. Med., 299:570–573, 1978.

Weinstein, A.J., McHenry, M.C., and Gavan, T.L.: Systemic absorption of neomycin irrigating solution. JAMA, 238:152–153, 1977.

Zinner, N.R., Kenny, G.M., and Weinstein, S.: Effect of bladder irrigations during indwelling urethral catheterization. J. Urol., 104:538–541, 1970.

STRUVITE UROLITHIASIS

JEFFREY S. KLAUSNER, D.V.M.,
and CARL A. OSBORNE, D.V.M.
St. Paul, Minnesota

Uroliths of which the predominant inorganic component is struvite ($NH_4MgPO_4 \cdot 6H_2O$) are the most frequently encountered calculi in dogs. Other names for struvite calculi include magnesium ammonium phosphate (MAP) calculi, phosphate calculi, "infection stones," "urease stones," and triple phosphate calculi. The term *triple phosphate* is a misnomer, since struvite does not contain calcium. However, struvite calculi often contain small quantities of calcium phosphate ($Ca_{10}[PO_4]_6[OH]_2$).

INCIDENCE

Struvite calculi are found more frequently in the urinary tract of dogs and cats than other types of uroliths. Although they may occur in any breed of dog, they have been observed most commonly in miniature schnauzers, Welsh corgis, dachshunds, poodles, beagles, and Scottish terriers. Dogs of any age (one month to 15 years or older) may develop struvite calculi; the mean age of occurrence is approximately six years (Brown, et al.). In one survey of reported cases of urolithiasis in dogs less than one year of age, 90 percent had MAP uroliths (Hardy, et al.).

Female dogs develop struvite urolithiasis more frequently than male dogs. This may be related to the higher incidence of urinary tract infections in females.

ETIOPATHOGENESIS

Bacterial urinary tract infections (UTI), alkaline urine, and genetic factors are thought to play a role in the development of struvite uroliths.

Bacterial Urinary Tract Infection. Urine must be supersaturated with struvite before calculi will form. Struvite concentration is influenced primarily by urine pH, although the urine concentrations of magnesium, ammonium, and phosphate are also important (Elliot, et al.). Since struvite concentration is markedly increased in alkaline urine, factors that induce persistent urine alkalinity predispose to formation and growth of struvite uroliths.

Urea-splitting bacterial urinary tract infections are a frequent cause of alkaline urine. Urease produced by bacteria catalyzes the formation of ammonia and carbon dioxide from urea and water, resulting in an elevated urine pH. Staphylococci and *Proteus* spp. are potent urease producers; *E. coli, Klebsiella* spp. and *Pseudomonas* spp. are usually urease-negative, although an occasional strain may be positive.

Most dogs with struvite urolithiasis have concomitant infection of the urinary tract (Brown, et al.). Urease-positive staphylococci are the most commonly isolated pathogens. In contrast with dogs that have struvite uroliths, dogs with non-struvite calculi (urate, cystine, oxalate, and silica calculi) may have UTI, but its frequency is comparatively low and causative bacteria usually do not produce urease. While bacteria can frequently be isolated from the center of MAP uroliths (indicating that bacteria were present at the time the stone began to develop), bacteria have rarely been cultured from the center of non-struvite calculi (Weaver). In a study performed at the University of Minnesota, 8 of 13 dogs with experimentally induced staphylococcal UTI developed cystic and/or urethral struvite calculi. Urinary tract infections were induced by injection of urease-positive *Staphylococcus aureus* into cauterized and non-cauterized bladders. The average time prior to radiographic detection of calculi following establishment of UTI was 4.5 weeks (range was two to eight weeks).

A small percentage of dogs with phosphate urolithiasis have had sterile urine. In some of these cases, however, bacteria have been isolated from the center of calculi. This observation indicates that bacterial infection of the urinary tract may undergo spontaneous remission after initiating calculi formation in some patients.

On occasion, both the centers of calculi and the urine obtained from dogs with struvite urolithiasis have been sterile (Weaver). The significance of this observation and its relationship to the hypothesis that struvite calculi are caused by bacterial infection are unknown.

Alkaline Urine. As noted previously, factors that produce persistently alkaline urine decrease the solubility of struvite. Although it is improbable that alkaline urine per se causes struvite urolithiasis, it appears to predispose to calculi formation. Factors that may produce persistently alkaline urine include (1) bacterial urease, (2) administration of medications such as sodium bicarbonate and sodium lactate, and (3) disorders associated with alkalosis, such as renal tubular acidosis.

Genetic Factors. The high incidence of struvite uroliths in miniature schnauzers suggests a familial tendency. We are currently exploring the hypothesis that susceptible miniature schnauzers inherit some abnormality of local host defenses of the urinary tract that increases their susceptibility to urinary tract infections.

Other Factors. Hyperexcretory rates of minerals similar to those associated with urate, cystine, and oxalate calculi appear to play an insignificant role in the initiation and growth of struvite uroliths. Currently no data exist to support the hypothesis that diet is a factor in the formation of struvite calculi in dogs or cats.

CLINICAL FINDINGS

Clinical findings are dependent, at least in part, on the location of calculi in the urinary system. Urethral calculi originate from the urinary bladder and may be associated with any combination of the following: frequent attempts to micturate or inability to micturate, signs of renal failure that occur secondary to obstruction of urine outflow (postrenal azotemia), and overdistention of the bladder with urine. Urethral calculi may be detected by palpation, catheterization, or radiography.

Calculi in the urinary bladder are frequently associated with dysuria and hematuria. They may be detected by palpation or radiography. If the bladder is distended with urine it may be impossible to palpate calculi until most of the urine is voided or removed.

Ureteral calculi are uncommonly encountered in dogs and cats, but they may occur. Ureteral calculi originate from the renal pelves. The infrequent occurrence of ureteral calculi is probably related to the relative infrequency with which renal calculi occur in these species. Ureteral uroliths may be associated with severe pain or obstruction of urine outflow and hydronephrosis. Ureteral uroliths can be detected only by radiography or exploratory surgery.

Renal calculi account for approximately 10 percent of the uroliths encountered in dogs. They may be associated with calculi elsewhere in the urinary tract. Renal uroliths may be associated with any combination of the following: renal pain caused by stimulation of pain receptors in the renal capsule, signs of uremia if bilateral renal involvement is present and three-fourths or more of the parenchyma of both kidneys has been altered, and enlargement of affected kidneys as a result of obstruction of urine outflow and hydronephrosis. Renal calculi may be detected by radiography or exploratory surgery.

Abnormalities detected by urinalysis are

usually consistent with inflammation (i.e., pyuria, hematuria, and proteinuria). Bacteria can usually be detected in the urine sediment.

Significant numbers of bacteria (more than 100,000 organisms per milliliter of urine) can usually be cultured from the urine (see "Urinary Tract Infections"). Bacteria may also be cultured from the center of struvite calculi. Isolation of staphylococci should always alert one to the possible presence of struvite urolithiasis.

Although the radiopacity of calculi is dependent on their size and composition, struvite calculi typically are radiopaque. Visualization of small calculi may require contrast radiography, however. Uroliths found in one portion of the urinary tract dictate radiographic evaluation of other portions for additional calculi. Two anatomic views that are at right angles to each other should always be obtained. Interposition of skeletal bone between uroliths and film is a common cause of failure to visualize calculi.

DIAGNOSIS

Uroliths are usually suspected on the basis of typical findings obtained by history and physical examination. Urinalyses, urine culture, and radiography may be required to eliminate urinary tract infection, diverticula of the bladder, and neoplasia. Urolith analysis is required to establish a diagnosis of struvite urolithiasis once the calculi have been removed from the patient. Bacterial culture of the centers of calculi may also be of value.

Since therapy formulated to prevent recurrence of struvite, urate, oxalate, and cystine calculi is dependent on knowledge of the mineral composition of uroliths, analysis of uroliths by qualitative or quantitative methods is essential. Commerical kits* for qualitative urolith analysis utilize chemical reagents to identify constituent radicals of calculi such as ammonium, carbonate, calcium, magnesium, phosphate, cystine, and urate. They are relatively inexpensive and simple to use. Since uroliths that are predominantly composed of one mineral type often contain traces of other minerals, it is important to sample representative areas. The center of the urolith is especially important, since it is most likely to provide clues regarding the abnormality that initiated stone formation. Representative samples of uroliths may be obtained by cutting them with a jeweler's saw, a bone saw, or White toenail clippers.

Although somewhat more expensive, quantitative analyses† of uroliths provide more information about the type and quantity of compounds present (apatite, calcium oxalate dihydrate, struvite, and so on). They eliminate confusion caused by qualitative identification of traces of one mineral type in stones composed predominantly of another mineral type (for example, identification of phosphates in urate calculi).

TREATMENT

Therapeutic plans for patients with struvite urolithiasis should include relief of obstruction, removal of existing calculi, eradication of urinary tract infection, and prevention of recurrent calculi.

RELIEF OF OBSTRUCTION

In patients with renal failure due to obstructive uropathy, every effort should be made to re-establish urine flow. Calculi lodged in the urethra of male dogs may be removed by urohydropropulsion (Piermattei and Osborne). If urohydropropulsion is unsuccessful, a well-lubricated, small-diameter catheter may be used to bypass the calculi. Cystocentesis may provide immediate but temporary decompression of an obstructed urinary system. If all else fails, an emergency urethrotomy may be performed. If urine flow cannot readily be re-established in uremic patients by use of the aforementioned techniques, alterations in fluid, electrolyte, and acid-base balances may be minimized by appropriate fluid therapy and peritoneal dialysis.

REMOVAL OF CALCULI

Surgical removal of struvite calculi is the preferred treatment for most cases of struvite urolithiasis, because restoration of urine hydrodynamics is rapid and pathogenic bacteria harbored within calculi are removed. In addition, if an underlying cause of UTI can be identified before surgery, it may be possible to correct it at the time of calculus removal. For example, diverticula on the anterior ventral aspect of the urinary bladder wall predispose to recurrent UTI, especially in young dogs. Struvite calculi may develop as a result of the urinary tract infection. Contrast cystograms performed during diagnostic evaluation usually reveal the diverticula, which can be excised at the time of calculi removal.

In those instances in which economic or medical circumstances make surgery unaccept-

---

*Oxford Stone Analysis Set for Urinary Calculi, Oxford Laboratories, 1149 Chess Drive, Foster City, California 94404

†Urolithiasis Laboratory, P.O. Box 25375, Houston, Texas 77005

able, medical therapy aimed at calculus dissolution may be attempted. Calculus dissolution will occur if urine can be maintained in a state of undersaturation with respect to calculus-forming solutes. A struvite urolith can be expected to dissolve if urinary struvite concentration can be reduced below that concentration at which crystallization occurs. Because urine acidification dramatically reduces urinary struvite crystallization it is essential for the dissolution of struvite calculi.

Since it may be impossible to acidify urine with acidifiers because of the large quantity of urease produced by bacteria, control of UTI with antibiotic therapy is a prerequisite to successful medical therapy. Temporary urine sterilization may be achieved with antibiotic therapy; however, eradication of UTI is often impossible until calculi have been removed from the urinary tract.

Urine acidification and urolith dissolution were induced by administration of acetohydroxamic acid (a urease inhibitor) to rats with foreign body–induced struvite uroliths and *Proteus* spp. UTI (Griffith and Musher). Combination therapy, including antibiotics, urinary acidifiers, and acetohydroxamic acid, resulted in struvite calculi dissolution in three human beings (Griffith, et al.). Similar therapy has not yet been evaluated in canine patients. Spontaneous dissolution of struvite uroliths has been observed in dogs, however.

ERADICATION OF UTI

Once calculi have been removed, UTI can usually be eliminated. An appropriate antibiotic selected on the basis of sensitivity or minimum inhibitory concentration (MIC) testing should be used at therapeutic levels for at least two weeks to allow time for repair of urinary tract epithelium. Quantitative urine cultures should be performed during therapy and five to seven days following therapy. Persistence of urinary tract infection while the patient is receiving antibiotics suggests the presence of a resistant organism. Rapid recurrence of UTI following withdrawal of therapy may indicate residual calculi in the urinary tract or other abnormalities in local host defense mechanisms. Radiographic studies should be performed to determine whether a predisposing cause for reinfection exists.

PREVENTION OF RECURRENCE

The recurrence rate following surgical removal of struvite uroliths has been reported to be approximately 21 percent (Brown, et al.). Most recurrences were associated with staphy-lococcal UTI and occurred within one year of initial surgery.

Maintaining urine in a persistent state of undersaturation with struvite is the goal of preventive therapy. Prevention of UTI, administration of urinary acidifiers, and induction of polyuria should reduce urine struvite concentration.

Any factor that alters normal host defense mechanisms may predispose to UTI. Since UTI with urease-producing bacteria is an important factor in the initiation of struvite calculi, attention should be directed toward identification and elimination of predispositions to infection. Permanent eradication of infection often is impossible unless a predisposing factor is identified and removed.

Following calculus removal and initial antibiotic therapy, a schedule of urine cultures at appropriate intervals should be established. Once UTI develops, struvite urolith formation may occur rapidly (within two weeks). It is emphasized that remission of clinical signs is not a reliable indicator of UTI, since many infections are asymptomatic. Recurrent UTI should be treated for at least two weeks with an antibiotic selected on the basis of sensitivity or MIC testing.

In patients experiencing frequent recurrences of UTI it may be necessary to provide continuous antibacterial therapy to prevent urolith formation. Initial antimicrobial therapy should be selected on the basis of results of sensitivity or MIC tests and is aimed at sterilization of urine. Response to therapy should be determined by urine culture performed 48 to 72 hours after initiation of therapy. A positive culture indicates treatment failure, and another antibiotic should be selected. Following at least ten days of effective preliminary treatment, consideration should be given to the use of drugs suitable for long-term therapy. Trimethoprim-sulfa and nitrofurantoin are effective for long-term prophylaxis, since these drugs are not likely to cause emergence of resistant organisms. It may be possible to reduce the amount of the maintenance drug to less than the usual dosage, but urine cultures should be monitored for evidence of lack of therapeutic effectiveness.

Since struvite concentration is reduced in acid urine and since acid urine is somewhat bacteriostatic, the administration of urine acidifiers should help prevent recurrence of struvite uroliths. The dosage of urine acidifiers should be adjusted on the basis of urine pH. The pH of the first voided morning sample is least likely to be altered by postprandial alkaline tide. Acidifiers should not be administered to uremic animals, since these drugs will aggravate the metabolic acidosis that is associated with renal failure. Ideally, acidifiers should be administered three to four times a day to maintain persistent urine acidity.

Induction of polyuria by oral administration of sodium chloride may interfere with the formation of struvite calculi by decreasing the concentration of calculogenic material in urine. Polyuria may also enhance elimination of bacteria from the urinary tract. Depending on the size of the patient, a dose of 0.5 to 10 grams of salt should be administered orally. Urine specific gravity should be monitored and maintained below approximately 1.025. An ample supply of water must be available at all times.

SUPPLEMENTAL READING

Brown, N.O., Parks, J.L., and Greene, R.W.: Canine urolithiasis: Retrospective analysis of 438 cases. J. Am. Vet. Med. Assoc., 170:414, 1977a.

Brown, N.O., Parks, J.L., and Greene, R.W.: Recurrence of canine urolithiasis. J. Am. Vet. Med. Assoc., 170:419, 1977b.

Elliot, J.S., Sharp, R.F., and Lewis, L.: The solubility of struvite in urine. J. Urol., 81:366, 1959.

Griffith, D.P., and Musher, D.M.: Prevention of infected urinary stones by urease inhibition. Invest. Urol., 11:228, 1973.

Griffith, D.P., Bargin, S., and Musher, D.M.: Dissolution of struvite urinary stones. Invest. Urol., 13:351, 1976.

Hardy, R.M. et al.: Urolithiasis in immature dogs. Vet. Med. Small Anim. Clin., 67:1205, 1972

Piermattei, D.L., and Osborne, C.A.: Nonsurgical removal of urethral calculi from male dogs. J. Am. Vet. Med. Assoc., 159:1755, 1971.

Weaver, A.D.: Relationship of bacterial infection in urine and calculi to canine urolithiasis. Vet. Record, 97:48, 1975.

URATE UROLITHIASIS

JERRY A. THORNHILL, D.V.M.
West Lafayette, Indiana

PATHOGENESIS

Uric acid is the end product of purine metabolism (Fig. 1). The formation of urate calculi is dependent on the concentration of free uric acid in urine and the concentration of its salts, sodium urate and potassium urate. The solubility of uric acid is less than that of the salts of uric acid. Therefore, urine pH is a major determinant of the fraction of urate excreted in its poorly soluble undissociated form. The pK of the N-9 position of the uric acid molecule, which accounts for the majority of its acidic properties, is 5.75. At this pH, uric acid is half-undissociated and half-ionized. Urine pH less than 5.75 increases the concentration of undissociated uric acid, and urine pH greater than 5.75 increases the concentration of ionized uric acid. At a urine pH of 7.0 there is greater than 20-fold increase in the solubility of urate in urine.

There is a remarkable divergence of purine metabolism among various animal species. In man uric acid is the end product of purine metabolism and must be excreted via the gastrointestinal tract (15 to 40 percent) and kidneys (60 to 85 percent). In non-Dalmatian dogs little uric acid is excreted because it is converted in the liver by uricase to allantoin, a metabolite that is quite soluble and easily metabolized (see Fig. 1). The liver of Dalmatians contains adequate amounts of uricase but, apparently, hepatic cellular membranes are only partially impermeable to uric acid uptake. Therefore, conversion of uric acid to allantoin in this breed is incomplete. As in man, uric acid must be excreted primarily by the kidneys.

Another membrane transport defect of uric acid uptake is apparently present in the proximal renal tubules of Dalmatians. Unlike non-Dalmatian breeds, in which more than 98 percent of uric acid in glomerular filtrate is reabsorbed in this portion of the nephron, proximal tubular reabsorption in Dalmatians is suppressed, resulting in excretion of large quantities of urate in urine. Dalmatian dogs excrete approximately 400 to 600 mg of uric acid in their urine per day. Non-Dalmatian dogs excrete approximately 10 to 60 mg per day, while human beings excrete approximately 500 to 700 mg per day.

Urate exists as a colloid suspension in urine and can be flocculated by an increase in ammonium ion or an increase in hydrogen ion. Flocculation with ammonium ion appears to be a signficant predisposition to canine urate urolithiasis, inasmuch as the majority of urate calculi in the Dalmatian are composed of ammonium urate. In man, uric acid is precipitated primarily by hydrogen ion. Since alkaline urine is commonly found in Dalmatian dogs with urate calculi, phosphates may also be incorporated into urate calculi.

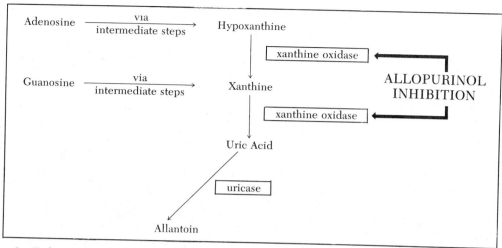

Figure 1. Pathway of uric acid and subsequent allantoin synthesis and the sites of inhibitory action of allopurinol on xanthine oxidase.

DIAGNOSIS

Dalmatians have the highest incidence of urate calculi, but these uroliths have also been recovered from airedales, boxers, English bulldogs, Chihuahuas, dachshunds, fox terriers, Irish terriers, cocker spaniels, Welsh corgis, mongrels, and cats. Dalmatian dogs may also develop other types of calculi, including struvite calculi.

Urate calculi are usually small and smooth and may be flattened, round, spherical, or ellipsoidal. They may be radiolucent but are often radiopaque. They may appear yellow, orange, or reddish-brown as a result of urinary pigments. They probably occur with equal frequency in males and females but are reported more often in males because of urethral lodgement.

Urate calculi should be suspected in Dalmatian dogs with dysuria, painful hematuria, pollakiuria, urge incontinence, overdistended bladders due to partial or complete obstruction, small and painful bladders due to inflammation, or voiding of uroliths during micturition. Since multiple sites of deposition in the urethra of males may occur, every effort should be made to determine the sites of uroliths. Digital palpation of the entire urethra should be performed and should include evaluation by rectal examination. Because urate calculi may not be remarkably radiodense, survey radiographs followed by negative- or positive-contrast radiography, or both, should be performed on all suspected cases.

Analysis of calculi for mineral content is the only reliable method of urolith classification. Commercially available kits* may provide qualitative identification of the mineral composition of calculi. Uroliths should be prepared for analysis by cutting into sections with a bone saw or jeweler's saw. If they are too small to cut they may be crushed into small peices. It is important to evaluate the mineral content of the center and outer portions of calculi, since the composition in these areas may differ. The mineral composition of the center of a calculus most likely represents the cause of urolithiasis.

Although urate calculi characteristically are not initiated by urinary tract infection, urine cultures should be performed on all patients. A phosphate layer added to urate stones is suggestive of previous or active urinary tract infection.

TREATMENT

Following surgical removal of uroliths in the bladder or urethra, the stones should be analyzed for mineral composition, since this information is required to formulate prophylactic therapy. Clients should be informed that urate calculi may recur despite prophylaxis. The likelihood of recurrence in individual patients is unpredictable.

Recommendations for prophylaxis of urate urolithiasis include:

1. Administration of sodium chloride. Induction of polyuria by administration of sodium chloride is the cornerstone of prevention of urate uroliths. Increasing urine volume dilutes the concentration of urate and ammonium ions, thus suppressing flocculation. Sodium chloride should be given orally at a dosage range of from 0.5 to 10 grams daily, depending on the size of the patient and clinical response. Ideally, a specific gravity of the urine less than 1.025 should be maintained. Table salt (½ tsp equals

---

*Oxford Stone Analysis Kit, Oxford Laboratories, 107 North Bayshore Blvd., San Mateo, California 94401

approximately 3½ grams NaCl) can be used, but it should be mixed well with food to prevent gastric irritation.

2. Administration of allopurinol.† Allopurinol is a synthetic isomer of hypoxanthine and interferes with the enzymatic action of xanthine oxidase. In this way it suppresses conversion of hypoxanthine to xanthine and of xanthine to uric acid (see Fig. 1). Hypoxanthine, xanthine and, to a lesser extent, uric acid are all excreted in the urine of patients receiving allopurinol. Although xanthine uroliths have developed in humans receiving long-term therapy with allopurinol, this complication has not been reported in dogs. The oral dosage of allopurinol commonly administered to dogs is 30 mg/kg/day divided b.i.d. or t.i.d. for one month, then reduced to 10 mg/kg/day. Since alloxanthine and oxypurinol (byproducts of allopurinol) are excreted by the kidneys, dosage of allopurinol should be reduced in patients with renal failure.

3. Administration of sodium bicarbonate. Alkalinization of urine to a pH greater than 5.75 favors formation of soluble ionized uric acid as sodium urate or potassium urate. Because ammonium urate crystals in dog urine can be flocculated by ammonium ion and hydrogen ion, administration of oral sodium bicarbonate as an alkalinizing agent prevents acid urine from increasing renal tubular production of ammonia. Sodium bicarbonate ($NaHCO_3$) should be administered to maintain a urine pH of 6.5 to 7.0. An oral dose of 2 gm/day may be required as tablets or powder (½ tsp baking soda equals approximately 2 gm $NaHCO_3$).

4. Administration of a low-purine diet. As an adjunct to prevention of urate uroliths, dietary purine precursors of uric acid synthesis may be reduced. Lean meats and glandular organs such as liver and kidney have a high purine content and should be avoided if possible. It is recommended that dogs predisposed to urate calculi be fed dry dog foods containing vegetable sources of protein.

5. Administration of antibiotics. The incorporation of phosphates into ammonium urate uroliths is suggestive of existing urinary tract infection. Proper long-term antibiotic therapy based on results of quantitative urine bacterial culture and specific antimicrobial sensitivity testing is recommended.

The efficacy of sodium bicarbonate administration for prevention of ammonium urate calculi in the dog is questionable. Since alkaline urine has been detected in Dalmatians with ammonium urate uroliths, the value of modifying urine pH to control flocculation of ammonium urate is debatable. Continuous administration of sodium bicarbonate may help to minimize daily fluctuations in urine pH and thus suppress ammonia secretion. Without sodium bicarbonate therapy, greater daily ammonia secretion would occur when urine pH is acid. Perhaps ammonium urates only flocculate in acid urine, and the finding of alkaline urine in association with these calculi in Dalmatian dogs does not represent the urine pH when the calculi were initiated. For this reason, alkalinization of urine with sodium bicarbonate is recommended as a prophylactic measure for ammonium urate calculi.

SUPPLEMENTAL READING

Finco, D.R.: Urate urolithiasis. In Kirk, R.W. (ed.): *Current Veterinary Therapy VI.* Philadelphia, W.B. Saunders Co., 1977, pp. 1214–1216.

Osborne, C.A., and Klausner, J.S.: War on canine urolithiasis: Problems and solutions. AAHA Scientific Proceedings, 1978, pp. 569–620.

---

†Zyloprin,® Burroughs Wellcome, 3030 Cornwallis Road, Research Triangle Park, North Carolina 27709

CYSTINURIA AND CYSTINE UROLITHIASIS

ARTHUR L. LAGE, D.V.M.
South Weymouth, Massachusetts

Cystinuria is a disorder of proximal tubular transport of the amino acid cystine and, to varying degrees, other dibasic amino acids (lysine, arginine, and ornithine). In dogs it is considered an inherited metabolic disease. Urinary loss of amino acids in cystinuria is of minor nutritional significance, but it is of clinical importance because of the insolubility of cystine in urine. This insolubility predisposes affected dogs to formation of cystine calculi anywhere in the urinary tract. The symptoms and clinical signs are dependent on the location of calculi in the excretory pathway and the presence or absence of obstruction of urine outflow. The symptoms of cystine urolithiasis are similar to those seen in other types of urolithic disease of the urinary tract.

Although cystinuria may occur in both male and female dogs, cystine calculi have been recognized only in males. Cystine calculi have been reported in many purebred dogs, in mixed breeds, and in the maned wolf. As reported in the literature and as seen in our practice, the dachshund is the most commonly affected breed.

The usual signs — hematuria, pollakiuria, strangury and urinary obstruction — usually begin at a relatively young age (one to three years). In general, cystine calculi are small, smooth, and yellow-brown to yellow-green in color; however, we have seen large (6 cm) cystine stones with brain-like convolutions on the surface. Although cystine stones are radiopaque because of their sulfur content, occasionally very small cystine calculi cannot be detected by survey radiographic examination.

Cystinuria may be detected by several laboratory methods, including (1) finding hexagonal cystine crystals in the urine sediment, (2) testing the urine with cyanide-nitroprusside, and (3) measuring the amount of cystine excreted in urine by means of an amino acid analyzer or quantitative urinary amino acid chromatography.

All calculi removed from the urinary tract should be analyzed to determine their chemical composition, since formulation of prophylactic therapy is based on this information. Infrared spectrometry is recommended for its accuracy and economic advantages.

The solubility of cystine is dependent on pH and is about 300 mg/liter in an acid solution. The solubility changes very little from pH 4.5 to 7.0 but increases to about 500 mg/liter at pH 7.5. It is even higher at pH 8.0. The solubility in urine is higher than in water. Most concentrated urine samples will dissolve about 150 mg/liter more cystine than the figures just mentioned. In adult humans the normal daily output of cystine is 40 to 80 mg. Stones usually will not form if less than 300 mg of cystine is excreted daily in urine.

TREATMENT

Following surgical removal of calculi, the goal of prophylactic management is to prevent supersaturation of urine with cystine in order to prevent cystine crystallization and urolith formation. This may be accomplished by (1) reducing the amount of cystine excreted into urine, (2) increasing the volume of urine in which cystine is excreted, and (3) increasing the solubility of cystine in urine.

Reducing the amount of cystine excreted in urine is difficult to accomplish, and it has not proved to be useful in man or dogs. A protein-restricted diet that is low in methionine is needed, but such a diet is not palatable and may be detrimental. I do not recommend its use in the management of canine cystinuria.

The cornerstone of therapy is to maintain a high urine volume by increasing the fluid intake, especially at night. At night the urine is more likely to become supersaturated with cystine because it is more concentrated and usually more acid than during the day. One of the most reliable methods of achieving increased fluid intake in veterinary practice is to add extra water to the food. In general, animals do not seem to like an abrupt change in the consistency of their food, especially a change from dry or semimoist to soupy consistency. I start gradually increasing the patient's water intake in food that already contains 70 percent water by weight by adding up to 4 to 6 oz of water per 30 lb (14 kg) of body weight at each feeding. If only one meal is given, it should be at night, and the amount of water added should be doubled.

There are two methods used to increase the solubility of cystine in urine. One method is alkalinization of urine. Alkalinization is probably of little value unless the urine formed at night can be kept at a pH higher than 7.5. Obviously, the client and clinician must check the urine pH to make sure that the desired effect is reached following use of an alkalinizer like sodium bicarbonate. The usual dosage for dogs is about 2 gm/30 lb (2 gm/14 kg) body weight daily in divided doses; however, the amount used must be determined on the basis of urine pH. Most conventional color-reaction pH papers may be used to check the success of urine alkalinization. The potential advantage of alkalinizing therapy may be offset by the possibility of precipitation of calcium phosphate or other phosphate calculi in an alkaline medium. This has not been well documented in cystinuric dogs, however.

The second method of increasing the solubility of cystine in urine is changing cystine to a more soluble form. D-Penicillamine (Cuprimine®, Merck) has been used for many years to accomplish this. The dosage recommended by various investigators is 30 mg/kg of body weight, divided into two daily doses. I have found this doage level to be intolerable in about half of canine patients. The major toxic reaction in dogs is vomiting; however, anorexia has also been noted in a number of cases. If the dosage seems to be tolerated in the dog and the patient is receiving continuous medication, it is recommended that hemograms and urinalysis be performed every four to six months and that a blood chemistry profile be performed every eight to ten months, since the drug has produced bone marrow, liver, and renal complications in man. If vomiting is a problem, I recommend that the drug be administered only in the evening at a dosage of 10 mg/kg body weight. In combination with augmentation of fluid intake and urine output, this dosage has been successful.

Alpha-mercaptopropionylglycine (MPG) (Thiola, Santen Pharmaceutical Co.) is a promising, newly developed drug that seems to be more effective than D-penicillamine and is associated with fewer toxic side effects in man. Like D-penicillamine, this drug is a mercaptan or thiol. Its beneficial action is based on the thiol disulfide exchange reaction. Thiols dissociate to yield active anions that undergo exchange reactions with disulfides. Using a water-soluble thiol, it is possible to transform the less soluble cystine into a water-soluble disulfide derivative. Use of this drug has been associated with remarkable success in human cystinuric patients in Japan and Germany. By adjusting the dose of MPG (600 to 2000 mg/day) so that the urine cystine level remains below 100 mg/day, cystine calculus formation can be prevented. The drug has not been approved for use in dogs; however, results of pilot tests have been very promising.

In summary, I recommend that cystine urolithiasis in dogs be controlled by using increased fluid intake, D-penicillamine therapy, and urine alkalinization. Urinary tract infections should be treated and controlled in a conventionally accepted manner. Because cystine stones may form within four to six months, I recommend routine abdominal radiographic examination of cystinuric dogs at yearly intervals. Suspicious findings should be further evaluated by intravenous urography. Routine urinalyses should be performed every six months.

SUPPLEMENTAL READING

Bovée, K.C., Thier, S.O., Rea, C, et al.: Renal clearance of amino acids in canine cystinuria. Metabolism, 23:51–58, 1974.

Brand, E., and Cahill, G.F.: Canine cystinuria III. J. Biol. Chem., 114:XV, 1936.

Bush, M. and Bovée, K.C.,: Cystinuria in a maned wolf. J. Am. Vet. Med. Assoc., 173:1159–1162, 1978.

Frimpter, G.W., Thouin, P., and Ewald, B.: Penicillamine in canine cystinuria. J. Am. Vet. Med. Assoc., 151:1084, 1967.

Hautmann, R., Terhorst, B., Stuhlsatz, H.W., and Lutzezer, W.: Mercaptopropionylglycine: a progress in cystine stone therapy. J. Urol., 117:628–630, 1977.

Segal, S., and Thier, S.O.: Cystinuria. In Stanburg, J.B., Wyngaarden, J.B., and Fredrickson, D.S., (eds.): *The Metabolic Basis of Inherited Disease*, 4th ed. New York, McGraw-Hill, 1978.

CALCIUM OXALATE UROLITHIASIS

CARL A. OSBORNE, D. V. M.,
and JEFFREY S. KLAUSNER, D. V. M.
St. Paul, Minnesota

ETIOPATHOGENESIS

OVERVIEW

Conceptual understanding of the etiopathogenesis of urolithiasis is an essential prerequisite to medical therapy and prevention of calcium oxalate calculi.

Calculi formation is associated with two phases: initiation and growth. The initial step in the development of a urolith is the formation of a crystal nidus (or crystal embryo). This phase of initiation of urolith formation, called nucleation, is dependent on supersaturation of urine with calculogenic crystalloids. The degree of supersaturation may be influenced by the magnitude of renal excretion of the crystalloid, the urine pH, and the presence of crystallization inhibitors in urine. Further growth of the crystal nidus is dependent on (1) its ability to remain in the urinary system, (2) the degree and duration of supersaturation of urine with crystalloids identical or different from that of the nidus, and (3) physical characteristics of the crystal nidus.

Several theories have been proposed to explain the initiation of calculogenesis. Each theory emphasizes a single factor. On the basis of current knowledge, the most popular hypotheses are (1) precipitation-crystallization theory, (2) matrix-nucleation theory, and (3) crystallization-inhibition theory.

Precipitation-crystallization Theory. This hypothesis incriminates excessive supersaturation of urine with stone-forming crystalloids as the primary event in calculogenesis. In this hypothesis nucleation (initiation of urolith formation) is considered to be a physiochemical process of precipitation of crystalloids from a supersaturated solution. Calculus formation is thought to occur independently of preformed matrix or inhibitors of crystallization.

According to this hypothesis, production of urine excessively saturated with one or more urolith-forming crystalloids leads to spontaneous nucleation of the crystalloid. If nucleated crystalloids become trapped in the urinary system in the presence of continued supersaturation, urolith growth will occur. Protein matrix is thought to be nonspecifically incorporated into the urolith as calculus growth proceeds.

Supersaturation of urine with urolith-forming crystalloids may be associated with (1) increased renal excretion of crystalloids as a result of increased glomerular filtration, increased tubular secretion, or decreased tubular reabsorption (examples include hypercalciuria, hyperuricosuria, hyperoxaluria, cystinuria, and xanthinuria), (2) negative body water balance associated with increased tubular reabsorption of water and subsequent urine concentration (examples include excessive water loss via other routes, lack of water consumption, and living in a hot, dry climate), and (3) urine pH favoring crystallization (examples include formation of alkaline urine by urease-producing bacteria, formation of alkaline urine as a result of renal tubular acidosis, and administration of alkalinizing or acidifying drugs).

The precipitation-crystallization hypothesis provides a plausible explanation for the formation of cystine, urate, and magnesium ammonium phosphate calculi. It is also applicable to those patients with oxalate calculi in which hypercalciuria, hyperoxaluria, hyperuricosuria, or a combination of these, can be detected.

Matrix-nucleation Theory. This hypothesis incriminates preformed organic matrix (thought to be a mucoprotein with calcium-binding properties) as the primary determinant in calculogenesis. It is based on the assumption that preformed organic matrix forms an initial nucleus that subsequently permits urolith growth by precipitation of crystalloids. The role of organic matrix in calculogenesis has not been defined with certainty; however, the similarity of the overall composition of matrix from human uroliths of various mineral composition has been used to support this hypothesis. Opponents of the matrix nucleation theory cite data indicating that uroliths can acquire a large portion of organic matrix by physical adsorption during urolith growth.

Crystallization-inhibition Theory. This hypothesis incriminates reduction or absence of organic and inorganic inhibitors of crystallization as the primary determinant of calcium oxalate and calcium phosphate calculogenesis. This theory is based on the fact that several crystalloids, including calcium, are maintained in solution at concentrations significantly higher than is possible in water (i.e., urine is a metastable supersaturated solution). The following substances have been reported to inhibit calcium salt crystallization: (1) organic acids (especially citrates) that form soluble chelates with calcium; (2) magnesium, which is thought to attach non-specifically to crystal surfaces and thereby interfere with migration of the solute to crystal growth sites; (3) inorganic pyrophosphates (products of intermediary metabolism) that inhibit crystallization of calcium salts; however, the role that pyrophosphates play in the pathogenesis of urolithiasis has not been determined because similar quantities are excreted in normal and urolith-forming human patients; and (4) a variety of other substances, including urea, mucopolysaccharides, and some that are not yet identified.

Summary. To date, several lines of evidence have been reported to support each hypothesis. None has been completely accepted, however. The balance of evidence suggests that the most likely cause of nucleation and formation of a crystal embryo is precipitation from a supersaturated solution. An organic matrix is not required for precipitation, and inhibitors may be more important in growth than in initiation of urolith formation.

Irrespective of the theory proposed for nucleation and nidus formation, an essential requirement is supersaturation of urine with a urolith-forming crystalloid. A crystal nidus cannot be formed if urine is undersaturated with the crystalloid in question. The matrix-nucleation theory implies that only a low degree of supersaturation is required to initiate urolith formation. The precipitation-crystallization and crystallization-inhibition theories are based on the supposition that a greater degree of supersaturation is required to initiate urolith formation. Thus, the greater the degree of urine supersaturation the greater the predisposition to urolith formation.

Following initiation, calculi appear to grow in an orderly fashion. Mechanisms of urolith growth include (1) crystal growth, (2) epitaxial growth, and (3) crystal aggregation. Consult reference material for further details.

CALCIUM OXALATE UROLITHS

Most of the currently available information pertaining to the etiopathogenesis of calcium oxalate uroliths is based on studies in man and laboratory animals. Caution must be used in extrapolating this information for use in companion animals. The reason for the high incidence of calcium oxalate uroliths in man and the comparatively low incidence of calcium oxalate uroliths in dogs and cats is unknown.

Applied Biochemistry. Oxalate is a salt of oxalic acid. Oxalic acid is usually synthesized in small quantities from glyoxylic acid (which may be derived from glycine) and ascorbic acid. Oxalic acid is also commonly found in green leafy vegetables, including rhubarb, spinach, celery, and cabbage. Oxalic acid is poorly absorbed from the gastrointestinal tract, however, and under normal conditions does not contribute significantly to urinary oxalate. In man most of the oxalic acid excreted in urine is produced endogenously by the liver.

Following excretion in urine, oxalic acid combines with calcium to form an insoluble salt of calcium oxalate. The specific condition or conditions that govern crystallization of calcium oxalate (whewellite and weddellite) remain undetermined. Urine pH within physiologic range (4.5 to 8.0) does not appear to affect the solubility of calcium oxalate significantly. Factors incriminated in the etiopathogenesis of calcium oxalate urolithiasis include (1) hypercalciuria, (2) hyperoxaluria, and (3) hyperuricosuria.

Hypercalciuria. Hypercalcemic hypercalciuria appears to be a relatively infrequent cause of oxalate uroliths in man and dogs. Potential causes include primary hyperparathyroidism, pseudohyperparathyroidism, vitamin D intoxication, osteolytic neoplasia, and hyperthyroidism.

Normocalcemic hypercalciuria is a much more common finding in human beings with oxalate uroliths. Renal tubular acidosis is a potential cause. In most patients, however, the specific cause of normocalcemic hypercalciuria is unknown. The underlying cause appears to be related to either (1) increased intestinal absorption of calcium (so-called intestinal hyperabsorption) or (2) decreased renal tubular reabsorption of calcium from glomerular filtrate (renal tubular defect). Current studies involve the complex interrelationships between hypercalciuria, hypophosphatemia, hyperparathormonemia, and vitamin D metabolism.

Hyperoxaluria. Most human beings with oxalate calculi have no detectable abnormality of oxalate metabolism and excrete normal quantities of oxalate in their urine. Causes of hyperoxaluria in man that may predispose to oxalate urolithiasis include (1) increased ingestion of oxalates, (2) primary hyperoxaluria (an inherited enzyme deficiency in which glycine cannot be metabolized beyond oxalate), (3) ileal disease, and (4) jejunal bypass procedures used to correct obesity.

Potential causes of enhanced *in vivo* production of oxalate include pyridoxine deficiency, ethylene glycol intoxication and methoxyflurane anesthesia. These mechanisms do not appear to be significant in the etiology of naturally occurring oxalate urolithiasis.

Oxalate uroliths have been produced experimentally in rats by feeding them glycolic acid or ethylene glycol and by depriving them of pyridoxine.

Hyperuricosuria. Because of similarities in the physical characteristics of calcium oxalate monohydrate and sodium hydrogen urate, it appears that hyperuricosuria may play a role in the formation of calcium oxalate uroliths. Crystals of sodium hydrogen urate are thought to serve as seed nuclei that initiate calcium oxalate crystallization from oversaturated urine. The cause of hyperuricosuria may be excessive consumption of purines. Preliminary studies showing that administration of allopurinol is associated with reduced formation of calcium oxalate uroliths in hyperuricosuric-hypercalciuric human patients support this hypothesis.

Summary. Increased urinary concentration of calcium, oxalate, or urates appears to play a role in initiating calcium oxalate urolith formation and also in promoting their growth. Urinary tract infection is a sequela rather than a cause of oxalate urolithiasis. Consult the article entitled "Struvite Urolithiasis" for further details about the role of bacterial infection in initiating urolith formation. See Table 1 for more information about calcium oxalate uroliths.

CLINICAL FINDINGS

Clinical findings associated with calcium oxalate uroliths vary but are similar to those associated with other types of calculi. Clinical findings are dependent on (1) anatomic location(s) of uroliths, (2) duration of uroliths in specific location(s), (3) physical characteristics of uroliths (size, shape, number), (4) secondary urinary tract infection and virulence of infecting

Table 1. *Characteristics of Calcium Oxalate Uroliths*

TERMINOLOGY

Chemical Name	Crystal Name	Formula
Calcium oxalate monohydrate	Whewellite	$CaC_2O_4 \cdot H_2O$
Calcium oxalate dihydrate	Weddellite	$CaC_2O_4 \cdot 2H_2O$

COMPOSITION
  Whewellite only
  Weddellite only
  Whewellite and weddellite
  Calcium oxalate nucleus surrounded by struvite

PHYSICAL CHARACTERISTICS
  Color: White or cream
  Shape: Frequently have rough, jagged, quartz-like appearance. In man uroliths composed of whewellite frequently
        have the shape of hempseeds, mulberries, or jackstones. The jackstone type is apparently rare in dogs and cats.
        Weddellite crystals have a characteristic envelope shape and may occur in normal or abnormal urine at any pH.
  Number: Often single, may be multiple
  Laminations: Uncommon
  Density: Typically dense and hard to cut; on survey radiographs, very dense compared with soft tissues
  Location: Usually the bladder; occasionally, bladder and urethra; uncommonly, renal; rarely, renal and ureteral.

INCIDENCE
  0 to 32% of canine uroliths; uncommon in cats
  More common in Europe than in the United States
  Reported to recur in approximately 25% of affected dogs

PREDISPOSING FACTORS (HUMAN BEINGS)
  Hypercalciuria
    Hypercalcemic
    Normocalcemic
  Hyperoxaluria
  Hyperuricosuria

CHARACTERISTICS OF AFFECTED CANINE PATIENTS
  Mean age = 8 years
  Reported to occur more frequently in males

Table 2. *Radiographic Characteristics of Common Uroliths**

PREDOMINANT MINERAL TYPE	DEGREE OF RADIOPACITY	SHAPE
Cystine	+ to ++	Smooth; usually small; round to oval
Oxalate	++++	Rough; round or oval
Phosphate (struvite)	++ to ++++	Smooth; round or faceted; sometimes assume shape of renal pelvis, ureter, bladder, or urethra
Phosphate (apatite)	++++	Smooth, round, or faceted
Urate	+ to ++	Smooth, round, or oval
Silica	++ to ++++	Typically jackstone

*From Osborne, C. A., and Klausner, J. S.: War on urolithiasis: Problems and solutions, 1978. Scientific Proceedings of the American Animal Hospital Association (AAHA), South Bend, Indiana, 1978.

organism(s), and (5) presence of concomitant diseases in the urinary tract and other body systems.

The pH of urine obtained from patients with oxalate uroliths is variable; however, it may become persistently alkaline if secondary infection with urease-producing bacteria occurs. Abnormalities typical of inflammation (pyuria, proteinuria, and hematuria) are common. Calcium oxalate crystals have a characteristic octahedral or envelope shape. They may occur in normal or abnormal urine and may be absent even though calcium oxalate uroliths are present. Other types of crystals normally found in urine (phosphate, urate, and others) may also be detected.

Hemograms are usually normal, unless there is concomitant generalized infection of the kidneys or prostate gland. With the possible exception of hypercalcemia, serum chemistry values are usually normal. Obstruction of urine outflow or generalized renal infection may lead to changes characteristic of renal failure.

Most canine uroliths have varying degrees of radiodensity and therefore can be detected by survey abdominal radiography (Table 2). Oxalate and phosphate uroliths are typically but not invariably more radiodense than cystine, urate, and silica calculi. This may be related to their calcium content. Because of significant variation, the radiodensity of uroliths is not a reliable index of their mineral composition. Calculi that appear radiodense by survey radiography may appear to be radiolucent when evaluated by positive-contrast urography. This phenomenon is related to the fact that many calculi are more radiodense than soft tissue but less radiodense than positive-contrast media.

ANALYSIS OF CALCULI

A definitive diagnosis of calcium oxalate urolithiasis is dependent on analysis of the compo-

sition of calculi. The mineral composition of uroliths may be determined by qualitative* or quantitative† techniques, or both. Because many uroliths contain more than one mineral component, it is important to examine representative sections. The nucleus or center of the urolith should be analyzed separately from its outer zones when possible, because the underlying cause of its presence may be suggested by the mineral composition of the nucleus (Table 3). Consult reference material for further details.

PROGNOSIS

Variables that influence the prognosis for patients with urolithiasis include the (1) composition of the urolith, (2) presence of predisposing factors that are correctable, controllable, or uncontrollable, (3) number, size, and location of uroliths, (4) degree of reversible or irreversible damage to adjacent renal, ureteral, bladder, and urethral parenchyma, (5) presence and duration of partial or complete obstruction of urine outflow, (6) rate of urolith growth, and (7) presence of concomitant but unrelated diseases of the urinary system and other body systems.

The *short-term prognosis* for alleviation of clinical signs following surgical removal of most uroliths is favorable, provided that associated urinary tract infection is controlled. The *long-term prognosis* for prevention of recurrence of oxalate uroliths is unpredictable (see Table 1). Because the etiopathogenesis of oxalate uroliths is unknown, prophylactic therapy is largely empirical.

---

*Oxford Stone Analysis Set, Oxford Laboratories, 107 North Bayshore Blvd., San Mateo, California 94401

†Urolithiasis Laboratory, P. O. Box 23375, Houston, Texas 77005

Table 3. *Summary of Steps for Urolith Analysis*

1. Harvest all uroliths and place them in a sterilized container with a tight-fitting lid.
2. Compare the number of uroliths removed with the number identified by radiography.
3. If multiple samples are available, place one or more in buffered formalin for potential microscopic evaluation.
4. Record the location, number, size, shape, color, and consistency of uroliths.
5. Submit one or more samples for qualitative analysis. Specify analysis of nucleus and periphery.
6. If only one urolith is available:
   a. Cut it in half and submit half for a qualitative analysis. Save the remaining half for potential quantitative analysis.
   b. If only one small stone is available, submit it for quantitative analysis.
7. If the results of qualitative analysis are equivocal, submit appropriate samples for quantitative analysis.
8. Culture the inside of the urolith, if necessary.
9. Consider microscopic examination of the urolith, if necessary.

THERAPY

OVERVIEW

Therapy of calcium oxalate urolithiasis encompasses (1) reestablishment of urine flow, (2) medical management, (3) surgical management, and (4) prevention of recurrence.

Surgery has been a time-honored approach to therapy of urolithiasis in veterinary medicine. Although this has obvious short-term benefits, it does not always remove the underlying cause, may not remove all the uroliths, and may be hazardous in some patients. Furthermore, it may not be required if uroliths are inactive and not causing clinical signs. Surgery appears to play a much less prominent role in the management of non-obstructing calcium oxalate, calcium phosphate, and uric acid uroliths in man than in dogs and cats. These uroliths may be managed successfully with carefully formulated medical therapy. As with all forms of therapy, however, cautious and careful judgment is in order. The unpredictable and erratic rate at which uroliths form, grow, recur following removal, and undergo spontaneous dissolution mandates carefully designed and controlled experimental trials before a particular regimen of therapy is judged to be of benefit.

Consult standard textbooks of veterinary surgery and reference material for details about surgical and non-surgical methods of reestablishing urine flow and surgical removal of uroliths.

GENERAL PRINCIPLES OF MEDICAL THERAPY

The objective of medical management is to arrest further stone growth and if possible to promote stone dissolution by correcting or controlling underlying abnormalities, including dietary factors, metabolic disorders, and urinary tract infections.

Most effective forms of therapy create an undersaturated state of calculogenic crystalloids in urine by (1) reducing the quantity of calculogenic crystalloids in urine, (2) increasing the solubility of crystalloids in urine, or (3) increasing the volume of urine in which crystalloids are dissolved or suspended.

Knowledge of the mineral composition of the urolith is of paramount importance to formulation of effective therapy. For example, administration of D-penicillamine would be of no benefit to patients with oxalate uroliths. Administration of ascorbic acid, a commonly used acidifier, might potentiate oxalate urolithiasis, since it is a precursor of oxalic acid. In situations in which uroliths are not available for analysis and consideration is being given to medical therapy, one may be forced to make an educated guess about their mineral composition (Table 4).

MEDICAL MANAGEMENT OF CALCIUM OXALATE UROLITHS

As summarized previously, medical therapy often plays an important role in the manage-

Table 4. *Factors in the "Guesstimate" of the Mineral Composition of Uroliths*

1. Radiographic density and physical characteristics of urolith(s) (see Tables 1 and 2)
2. Crystalluria, especially cystine
3. Type of bacteria (if any) isolated from urine:
   a. Urease-producing bacteria, especially staphylococci, are commonly associated with struvite uroliths.
   b. Urinary tract infections may not be present in patients with calcium oxalate, cystine, ammonium urate, and silica uroliths.
   c. Remember: urinary tract infection can be initiated by calcium oxalate and other metabolic uroliths, with subsequent formation of struvite around them.
4. Serum chemistries:
   a. Hypercalcemia may be associated with calcium-containing uroliths.
   b. Hyperuricemia may be associated with urate and, less commonly, with calcium oxalate uroliths.
5. Species and breed of animals with uroliths and history of occurrence of uroliths in their ancestors or littermates
6. Analysis of uroliths fortuitously passed and collected during micturition

ment of non-obstructing oxalate uroliths in man. The common denominator of such therapy is reduction of the degree of supersaturation of urine with calcium, oxalate, and/or urate.

Diuresis. Increasing the volume of urine produced by increasing water consumption appears to be a logical recommendation. Depending on the size of the patient, we recommend oral administration of 0.5 to 10 grams of salt per day to stimulate thirst. Obviously, the success of this procedure implies the availability of a fresh water supply at all times. Alternatively, water, gravy, or other liquids could be mashed into food with a fork. It appears desirable to encourage water consumption throughout the day. A satisfactory compensatory increase in urine volume is indicated by formation of urine with a specific gravity <1.030. Provided that these recommendations are effective in augmenting water consumption and formation of less concentrated urine, we currently recommend that they be continued indefinitely, unless it is certain that the underlying cause of urolithiasis has been eliminated.

Diet. Diets may be formulated to minimize consumption of calcium, oxalate, or purines (Smith, et al.). Although this approach sounds logical, its effectiveness has not been evaluated.

Urine pH. It is questionable whether alteration of urine pH will alter the occurrence, growth, or dissolution of calcium oxalate stones, because the solubility of calcium oxalate is not appreciably altered in the range 4.5 to 7.5. Since ascorbic acid is a precursor of oxalic acid, it appears logical to recommend that it be avoided in patients with oxalate uroliths.

By using an ethylene glycol–pyridoxine-deficient diet to induce oxalate uroliths in rats, it was shown that alkalization of urine decreased and acidification of urine increased the rate of urolith production (Borden and Lyon).

Thiazide Diuretics. Thiazide diuretics (hydrochlorothiazide and bendroflumethiazide) decrease renal excretion of calcium. Thiazides are thought to lower urine concentration of calcium by (1) reducing extracellular fluid volume and thus glomerular filtration rate, (2) increasing renal tubular reabsorption of calcium, and (3) perhaps contributing a parathormone-like action. In man thiazides are recommended for use in calcium oxalate urolith patients with idiopathic renal hypercalciuria (Pylypchuk, et al.). They are not used in patients with idiopathic intestinal hypercalciuria because they may cause hypercalcemia.

Cellulose Phosphate. Cellulose phosphate is an orally administered calcium-binding agent. It has been recommended to reduce hypercalciuria in patients with idiopathic intestinal absorptive hypercalciuria and recurrent calcium oxalate or calcium phosphate urolithiasis. Cellulose phosphate is not recommended for patients with idiopathic renal hypercalciuria because it may induce hypocalcemia. The precise dosage is dependent on urine calcium excretion, but the approximate recommendation for human beings is 5 grams three times per day immediately following meals (Pak, et al.). Supplementation with magnesium may be required.

Inorganic Phosphates. Oral administration of inorganic phosphates (potassium acid phosphate and its metabolic products) has been advocated to increase the concentration of crystallization inhibitors in urine. Their mechanism of action is unclear, but it has been hypothesized that they compete with pyrophosphates (potent crystal solubilizers) for renal tubular reabsorption and thereby increase the urine concentration of pyrophosphates. Studies in human beings with recurrent oxalate urolithiasis have failed to demonstrate that inorganic phosphates retard calcium oxalate crystallization in urine (Ettinger). Administration of inorganic phosphates might enhance formation of magesium ammonium phosphate and calcium phosphate uroliths.

Methylene Blue. Methylene blue is an inorganic cationic dye that is excreted unchanged into urine following gastrointestinal absorption. Prior to the advent of antibiotics it was popularly used in the treatment of urinary tract infections. Use of methylene blue in the medical management of uroliths in man was prompted by experimental studies in which it was observed that oral administration of methylene blue to rats with zinc pellet–induced vesical concretions resulted in inhibition and dissolution of calculi (Van't Reit et al.). Since that time evidence has been accumulated that both supports and denies its effectiveness in the treatment of urolithiasis. In uncontrolled studies in man it was concluded that methylene blue was an effective inhibitor of nucleation and growth rate of calcium oxalate crystals (Sutor). Methylene blue has been used effectively to prevent incrustation of indwelling urinary drainage tubes. Administration of methylene blue to patients with oxalate and struvite calculi was thought to promote urolith dissolution and prevent new stone formation (Boyce, et al.). In another study, however, administration of methylene blue to human beings resulted in as many patients with increased urolith size and new urolith formation as there were with decreased stone size (Wein, et al.). *In vitro* addition of methylene blue to a standardized test system for growing struvite crystals did not inhibit struvite crystal formation (Miller and Opher).

The mechanism or mechanisms of action of

methylene blue are unknown. The dosage commonly recommended for human beings is 65 mg given t.i.d. Neither effectiveness nor dosages have been established for domestic animals. Methylene blue should not be administered to cats because it may induce a severe, potentially fatal Heinz-body anemia.

Magnesium Oxide. By using an ethylene glycol–pyridoxine-deficient diet to produce oxalate uroliths in rats, it was shown that oral administration of magnesium, especially as an alkaline salt (magnesium oxide), decreased the incidence of urinary calculi (Borden and Lyon). Administration of magnesium oxide (100 mg t.i.d.) in combination with pyridoxine has been reported to prevent recurrence of idiopathic calcium oxalate uroliths in man (Prien and Gershoff). Although administration of magnesium markedly exaggerates hypercalciuria, it is presumed to exert a beneficial effect by forming a complex with oxalate to increase its solubility. Because of its hypercalciuric effect, it has been recommended that it be used only as prophylactic therapy in patients that are recurrent urolith-formers.

Pyridoxine (Vitamin B$_6$). Administration of vitamin B$_6$ has been shown to reduce the magnitude of oxaluria caused by its deficiency in rats. Administration of pyridoxine is of questionable value in the medical therapy of oxalate uroliths in man and domestic animals (Revusova, et al.).

Alanine and Pyruvate. Addition of DL-alanine or pyruvate to the diet of rats with experimentally induced oxalate urolithiasis promoted urolith dissolution and prevented urolith formation (Chow, et al.). The mechanism of action was not specified.

Allopurinol. Combined oral therapy with thiazide diuretics and allopurinol in hypercalciuric, hyperuricosuric human urolith-formers resulted in a substantial reduction in the rate of new urolith formation (Coe, 1977, 1978).

PREVENTION OF UROLITH RECURRENCE

Because of the potential for recurrence of all types of calculi, long-term success is usually dependent on prophylactic therapy. As was the case for formulation of medical therapy, knowledge of etiopathogenic mechanisms of urolith formation is an essential prerequisite for formulation of effective prophylactic therapy. Knowledge of mineral composition of uroliths is also essential.

Methods to reduce the degree of supersaturation of urine with calcium oxalate are identical to those described in the section on medical management and include (1) inducing diuresis, (2) reducing urinary excretion of calcium, oxalate, and uric acid, and (3) increasing the solubility of calcium oxalate in urine. In addition to these measures, control of secondary urinary tract infection (when present) is also important. Consult the article on urinary tract infections for specific details.

PROBLEM-SPECIFIC DATA BASE

The problem-specific data base for urinary calculi includes:

1. Appropriate history and physical examination, including rectal examination of the urethra.
2. Complete urinalysis.
3. Hemogram.
4. Freezing of serum collected at the time of venipuncture to obtain a hemogram for possible future determination of serum calcium, urea, or creatinine concentration.
5. Quantitative urine culture (no antimicrobial therapy for three to five days).
6. Survey radiograph of entire urinary system.
7. Intravenous urogram for renal and/or ureteral calculi.
8. Intravenous urography or contrast cystography for bladder calculi.
9. Possibly contrast urethrography for urethral calculi.
10. Removal of appropriate bladder or kidney biopsy samples during nephrotomy or cystotomy for microscopic examination.
11. Correction of anatomic defects during same surgical procedure performed to remove uroliths.
12. Comparison of number of uroliths removed at surgery with number of uroliths identified radiographically. (Postoperative radiographs should be obtained to evaluate completeness of urolith removal, if necessary.)
13. Retention of all uroliths for qualitative and/or quantitative analysis.
14. Initiation of appropriate therapy to eradicate urinary tract infection.
15. Initiation of therapy to prevent recurrence of uroliths and/or to dissolve remaining uroliths.
16. Formulation of follow-up protocol with clients.

SUPPLEMENTAL READING

Bohonowych, R.O., Parks, J.L., and Greene, R.W.: Features of cystic calculi in cats in a hospital population. J. Am. Vet. Med. Assoc., 173:301–303, 1978.

Borden, T.A., and Lyon, E.S.: The effects of magnesium and pH on experimental calcium oxalate stone disease. Invest. Urol., 6:412–422, 1969.

Boyce, W.H., McKinney, W.M., Long, T.T., and Drach, G.W.: Oral administration of methylene blue to patients with renal calculi. J. Urol., 97:783–789, 1967.

Brown, N.O., Parks, J.L., and Greene, R.W.: Canine urolithiasis: Retrospective analysis of 438 cases. J. Am. Vet. Med. Assoc., 170:415–418, 1977.

Chow, F.C., Hamar, D.W., Boulay, J.P., and Lewis, L.D.: Prevention of oxalate urolithiasis by some compounds. Invest. Urol., 15:493–495, 1978.

Clark, W.F.: The distribution of canine urinary calculi and their recurrence following treatment. J. Small Anim. Pract., 15:437–444, 1974.

Coe, F.L.: Treated and untreated recurrent calcium nephrolithiasis in patients with idiopathic hypercalciuria, hyperuricosuria, or no metabolic disorder. Ann. Intern. Med., 87:404–410, 1977.

Coe, F.L.: Calcium–uric acid nephrolithiasis. Arch. Intern. Med., 138:1090–1093, 1978.

Ettinger, B.: Recurrent nephrolithiasis: Natural history and effect of phosphate therapy. A double-blind controlled study. Am. J. Med., 61:200–206, 1976.

Finco, D.R.: Current studies of urolithiasis. J. Am. Vet. Med. Assoc., 158:327–334, 1971.

Miller, J.M., and Opher, A.W.: The lack of effect of methylene blue on struvite crystal formation. J. Urol., 112:390–392, 1974.

Osborne, C.A., and Klausner, J.S.: War on urolithiasis: Problems and solutions. Scientific proceedings of the 45th annual meeting of the American Animal Hospital Association, South Bend, Indiana, 1978.

Pak, C.Y.C., Delea, C.S., and Bartter, F.C.: Successful treatment of recurrent nephrolithiasis (calcium stones) with cellulose phosphate. N. Engl. J. Med., 290:175–180, 1974.

Piermattei, D.L., and Osborne, C.A.: Nonsurgical removal of calculi from the urethra of male dogs. J. Am. Vet. Med. Assoc., 159:1755–1757, 1971.

Prien, E.L., and Gershoff, S.F.: Magnesium oxide–pyridoxine therapy for recurrent calcium oxalate calculi. J. Urol., 112:509–512, 1974.

Pylypchuk, G., Ehrig, U., and Wilson, D.R.: Effect of hydrochlorothiazide on urine saturation with brushite, in vitro collagen calcification in urine, and urinary inhibitors of collagen calcification. Can. Med. Assoc. J., 118:792–797, 1978.

Revusova, V., Gratzlova, J., et al.: The evaluation of some biochemical parameters in pyridoxine-treated calcium oxalate renal stone formers. Urol. Int., 32:348–352, 1977.

Smith, L.H., Van Den Berg, C.J., and Wilson, D.M.: Nutrition and urolithiasis. N. Engl. J. Med., 298:87–89, 1978.

Sutor, D.J.: The possible use of methylene blue in the treatment of primary hyperoxaluria. Br. J. Urol., 42:389–392, 1970.

Van't-Riet, B., McKinney, W.M., et al.: Dye effects on inhibition and dissolution of urinary calculi. Invest. Urol., 1:446–456, 1964.

Weaver, A.D.: Canine urolithiasis: Incidence, chemical composition, and outcome of 100 cases. J. Small Anim. Pract., 11:93, 1970.

Wein, A.J., Benson, G.S., Raezer, D.M., and Mulholland, S.G.: Oral methylene blue and the dissolution of renal calculi. J. Urol., 116:140–141, 1976.

White, E.G.: Symposium on urolithiasis in the dog. I. Introduction and incidence. J. Small Anim. Pract., 7:529–535, 1966.

CANINE SILICA UROLITHIASIS

CARL A. OSBORNE, D.V.M.,
ROBERT F. HAMMER, D.V.M.,
and JEFFREY S. KLAUSNER, D.V.M.

St. Paul, Minnesota

In recent years a unique type of urolith has been encountered in the lower urinary tract of dogs in the United States. These calculi have a characteristic "jackstone" shape and are composed primarily of amorphous silica (Fig. 1). Perusal of the literature reveals a conspicuous absence of these calculi in the past. Naturally occurring canine silica urolithiasis was first reported in a four-year-old male German shepherd in 1976 (Legendre). These uroliths were not encountered in patients admitted to the University of Minnesota Veterinary Hospital until approximately three years ago (Osborne, et al.). Since that time we have had the opportunity to evaluate silica uroliths removed from the urinary bladders and urethras of 48 dogs. Calculi in this series were obtained from patients evaluated at our hospital and from veterinarians in 18 of the 48 continental United States and Hawaii. All geographic regions were represented.

BREED, SEX, AND AGE

German shepherds constituted 20 of the 48 affected dogs. The remainder comprised 19 different breeds, including Doberman pinschers (4), Irish setters (4), Staffordshire terriers (2), great Danes (2), springer spaniels (2), and mixed breeds (2).

For as yet undetermined reasons, 47 dogs in our series were males and only one was female.

The mean age of 48 dogs evaluated in our series was 6.4 years, with a range of 2 to 10 years.

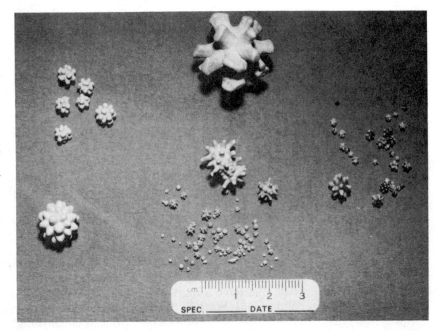

Figure 1. Characteristic jackstones composed primarily of silica removed from the urethras and/or the urinary bladders of several different breeds of dogs.

LOCATION IN THE URINARY TRACT

All uroliths in our series were removed from the urinary bladder or urethra. They were usually but not invariably multiple. Some were small; others were large (see Fig. 1). Uroliths were not detected by survey or contrast radiography of the entire urinary tract of 11 Minnesota dogs.

Silica uroliths were detected in a high percentage of native Kenyan dogs (125 of 241) (Brodey, et al.). Both males and females were affected, and the mean age was three years. With one exception, all uroliths observed in native Kenyan dogs were present in the renal pelves. Fifty percent of the renoliths were bilateral; none had a jackstone shape.

Silica uroliths have been detected throughout the urinary tracts of dogs fed an experimental atherogenic diet containing a high percentage of silicic acid (Ehrhart and McCullagh; McCullagh and Ehrhart).

CHARACTERISTICS OF UROLITHS

Most silica uroliths had a characteristic jackstone appearance (see Fig. 1). Not all silica uroliths had this configuration, however, and not all jackstones were composed of silica. One jackstone obtained from the urinary bladder of a bulldog was composed of ammonium urate. We have also analyzed canine jackstones composed of magnesium ammonium phosphate (struvite).

Silica uroliths are radiodense. They are not associated with characteristic crystals in urine sediment, however, presumably because they are composed of amorphous silica.

To date, jackstones containing silica have not been observed in cats. However, silica was identified as one of several components in a urolith removed from a cat (Sutor, et al.). We have observed an ammonium-urate jackstone in a cat.

Silica will not be detected by analysis of uroliths using the commercially prepared qualitative stone analysis kits in common use.* Since silica calculi may contain small quantities of magnesium, calcium, and other minerals, however, these substances may be detected by qualitative analysis. Caution must be used so as not to conclude that small quantities of mineral contaminants detected by qualitative analysis compose the primary mineral portion of the urolith. This problem may be prevented by appropriate methods of mineral analysis, especially of jackstones.

BIOLOGIC BEHAVIOR OF SILICA UROLITHS

Silica uroliths may recur following surgical removal. Since factors associated with initiation and growth of these uroliths have not been determined, specific recommendations for prophylactic therapy cannot be formulated.

---

*Oxford Stone Analysis Set For Urinary Calculi, Oxford Laboratories, 1149 Chess Drive, Foster City, California 94404

Urinary tract infections, when they occur, appear to be a sequela of silica urolithiasis.

RELATIONSHIP TO DIET

Silica uroliths developed in male dogs fed experimental diets containing a high concentration of silicic acid for several months (Ehrhart and McCullagh; McCullagh and Ehrhart). Elimination of silicic acid from the diet prevented further urolith development. It was hypothesized that the high incidence of silica uroliths in native Kenyan dogs might be related to consumption of corn, a common ingredient in their diet (Brodey, et al.). Experimental studies in normal dogs revealed that, once absorbed into the body, silica is rapidly cleared from plasma by the kidneys (King, et al.).

Silica uroliths are common in range cattle consuming forage grasses that have a high concentration of silica (White and Porter). Silica uroliths have also been produced experimentally in rats fed diets containing a large quantity of tetraethylorthosilicate (Emerick, et al.). Silica uroliths have been reported in human beings who consume large quantities of magnesium trisilicate to alleviate signs of peptic ulcers (Herman and Goldberg; Joekes, et al.).

Whether or not diet is associated with the current "outbreak" of silica uroliths in dogs is unknown. However, the apparent role of diet in experimental silica urolithiasis in dogs and rats and in spontaneously occurring silica urolithiasis in cattle and man prompts speculation that diet may be a causative factor.

MANAGEMENT

Therapy for silica urolithiasis, as for all types of uroliths, should encompass (1) reestablishment of urine flow, (2) medical management, (3) surgical management, and (4) prevention of recurrence. A comprehensive outline of these components of the management of uroliths has been reviewed elsewhere and therefore will not be repeated here (Osborne and Klausner).

Provided that affected patients are suitable candidates, silica uroliths in the urinary bladder (and those in the urethra, if necessary) should be removed surgically. Calculi in the urethra may be removed or returned to the urinary bladder by urohydropropulsion. Consult the article on urinary tract infections for recommendations regarding eradication or control of secondary bacterial infections of the urinary tract.

Since initiating and perpetuating causes of silica urolithiasis are unknown, only nonspecific measures can be recommended for prophylaxis. Increasing the volume of urine produced by increasing water consumption appears to be a logical recommendation, in that it will increase the volume of urine in which calculogenic substances are dissolved or suspended. Depending on the size of the patient, we recommend oral administration of 0.5 to 10 grams of salt per day to stimulate thirst. A satisfactory increase in urine volume is indicated by a urine specific gravity below approximately 1.030.

Since information regarding the solubility of calculogenic silica substances at acid, neutral, and alkaline urine pH values is unavailable, no recommendations regarding alteration of urine pH can be formulated.

Although the role of diet in the genesis of silica uroliths is speculative, it seems reasonable to recommend a change in diet if the problem is recurrent. Although empirical, this maneuver is unlikely to be harmful and may be helpful.

SUPPLEMENTAL READING

Brodey, R.S., et al.: Silicate renal calculi in Kenyan dogs. J. Small Anim. Pract., *18*:523–528.

Ehrhart, L.A., and McCullagh, K.G.: Silica uroliths in dogs fed an atherogenic diet. Proc. Soc. Exp. Biol. Med., *143*:131–132, 1973.

Emerick, R.J., Kugel, E.E., and Wallace, V.: Urinary excretion of silica and the production of siliceous urinary calculi in rats. Am. J. Vet. Res., *24*:610–613, 1963.

Herman, J.R., and Goldberg, A.S.: New type of urinary calculus caused by antacid therapy. JAMA, *174*:1206–1207, 1960.

Joekes, A.M., Rose, G.A., and Sutor, J.: Multiple renal silica calculi. Br. Med. J., *1*:146, 1973

King, E.J., Stantial, H., and Dolan, M.: The biochemistry of silicic acid. III. Excretion of administered silica. Biochem. J., *27*:1007–1014, 1973.

Legendre, A.M.: Silica urolithiasis in a dog. J. Am. Vet. Med. Assoc., *168*:418–419, 1976.

McCullagh, K.G., and Ehrhart, L.A.: Silica urolithiasis in dogs fed semisynthetic diets. J. Am. Vet. Med. Assoc., *164*:712–714, 1974.

Osborne, C.A., Hammer, R.F., and Klausner, J.S.: Canine silica urolithiasis: A report of preliminary findings. Minnesota Vet., *18*:15–20, 1978.

Osborne, C.A., and Klausner, J.S.: War on urolithiasis: Problems and solutions. In 1978 Scientific Proceedings of the AAHA. Am. Animal Hosp. Assoc., South Bend, Indiana, 1978.

Sutor, D.J., Wooley, S.E., and Jackson, O.F.: Crystalline material from the feline bladder. Res. Vet. Sci., *11*:298–299, 1970

White, E.G., and Porter, P.: Urinary calculi. In Medway, W., et al. (eds.): *A Textbook of Veterinary Clinical Pathology*. Baltimore, Williams & Wilkins Co., 1969.

FELINE CYSTIC CALCULI

RICHARD W. GREENE, D.V.M.

New York, New York

Very few cases of cystic calculi in cats have been reported in the veterinary literature. In a recent study at The Animal Medical Center (New York, NY) the case records of 131 cats undergoing surgery for cystic calculi during a 5½-year period were reviewed (Bohonowych, et al.). The mean annual rate of occurrence of cystic calculi in our hospital population of cats was approximately 0.08 percent. The greatest number of first episodes appeared during the third year of life, whereas the mean age for all first occurrences was 4.9 years. Calculi were found in intact females, spayed females, intact males, and castrated males, but there seemed to be a higher incidence of calculi in spayed females. There did not seem to be any particular breed predisposition.

The cause of cystic calculi in cats is unknown but is probably multifactorial. More research on etiology is necessary for this disease as well as for the "feline urologic syndrome." In fact, cystic calculi in the cat may be a part of this syndrome.

Cats with cystic calculi usually develop signs similar to those associated with cystitis (i.e., hematuria, strangury, and pollakiuria). Some cats may have a history of little or no response to previous antibiotic therapy. Since the bladder wall often is thickened, the calculi may be difficult to palpate. In our experience radiography has been the best method of confirming the diagnosis because 96 percent of the calculi in our series were radiopaque. Contrast radiography or exploratory cystotomy was used to confirm the existence of radiolucent calculi. Radiodense and radiolucent calculi have been both large and very small, singular and multiple.

TREATMENT

Removal of calculi by surgery, followed by proper medical therapy, is recommended. The mineral composition of calculi should be analyzed to aid in formulation of prophylactic therapy. Bacterial cultures and antibiotic sensitivity tests should be performed on swabs taken directly from the bladder wall. In our study 96.8 percent of the calculi were phosphate, 1.6 percent were urate, and 1.6 percent were oxalate. Only 3.2 percent of the cultures were positive for bacteria. *Staphylococcus* spp. were the most common organisms isolated.

Antibiotics selected on the basis of culture and sensitivity tests should be used postoperatively. They should be administered for 14 to 21 days. In cases with a positive postoperative culture the culture should be repeated after antibiotic therapy has been discontinued. Chloramphenicol, cephalothin, nitrofurantoin, and gentamicin are the antibiotics we use most often. The clinician should be aware of the side effects of various antibiotics in cats. The use of urinary acidifiers is a debatable issue, however. Long-term therapy with DL-methionine is indicated in cats with a urinary pH over 6.8.

Addition of salt to the diet will increase water intake and, thus, urine output. Diuresis in turn will decrease the concentration of calculogenic crystalloids in urine. Cold drinking water should always be available.

SUPPLEMENTAL READING

Bohonowych, R.O., Greene, R.W., and Parks, J.L.: Features of cystic calculi in cats in a hospital population. J. Am. Vet. Med. Assoc., *173*:301–303, 1978.

FELINE UROLOGIC SYNDROME: MANAGEMENT OF THE CRITICALLY ILL PATIENT

DELMAR R. FINCO, D.V.M.

Athens, Georgia

INTRODUCTION

Feline urologic syndrome (FUS) is an appropriate name for the condition in cats of unknown etiology that is characterized by dysuria, hematuria, and sometimes urethral obstruction. Dysuria and hematuria are a nuisance to the cat and its owner but do not constitute a threat to the cat's life. Urethral obstruction, in contrast, is potentially fatal because of the body abnormalities associated with anuria. The severity of signs in cats with urethral obstruction is dependent on several factors, subsequently discussed. For the purposes of this article, the designation of critical illness in cats with FUS is made on the basis of moderate to severe depression that is detected on initial examination. Although specific data are not available, it is estimated that less than 10 percent of cases of urethral obstruction fall into this category. The remaining 90 percent or more are presented in better physical condition and require less intensive therapy than described herein. However, if errors are to be made in the assessment of the patient, they should be made in the direction of applying intensive treatment to the patient with questionable need rather than withholding such therapy. Application of therapy entails little, if any, risk whereas depriving the patient that is actually in need may have dire consequences.

PATHOGENESIS OF ABNORMALITIES

Several abnormalities have been identified in cats obstructed by both artificial means and naturally occurring disease. The abnormalities in both groups seem identical. They include hypothermia, azotemia, dehydration, electrolyte abnormalities, acidosis, and a catabolic state. These alterations reflect the consequences of abrupt cessation of renal function.

With obstruction, bladder distention occurs at a rate dependent on urine flow rate. Bladder expansion in a cat with a concentrating defect that produces high volumes of low specific gravity (1.010) urine would occur seven times faster than in a cat with urine specific gravity of 1.070. The degree of distention that the bladder is capable of undergoing seems to vary from one cat to another. Cats with previous episodes of obstruction may have a larger bladder capacity because of lack of bladder muscle tone.

With extreme bladder distention, propulsion of urine from the ureters into the bladder ceases. This causes intraureteral and intratubular pressure to increase. When intratubular pressure rises to equal net glomerular filtration pressure, urine formation ceases.

Products of metabolism that would normally be excreted are restricted to two sites: the body itself and the intravesicular urine. Although the bladder contents are normally considered to be functionally outside the body, the situation with FUS may be different. Marked distention and epithelial trauma may destroy the bladder lumen–blood barrier. Thus, compounds such as nitrogenous wastes and potassium that are more concentrated in urine than in blood may diffuse to the blood from the urinary bladder.

From this discussion it is apparent that, following total obstruction, the degree of bladder distention and the permeability of bladder mucosa are two factors that influence the rate of onset of signs. Cats with experimental obstruction remained normal for about 48 hours following obstruction but had rapid progression of disease thereafter. Deaths occurred prior to 72 hours of obstruction.

As a result of impaired excretory function of the kidneys, ionic imbalances occur. Retention of hydrogen ions leads to development of mild to severe metabolic acidosis. In addition to affecting cell metabolism more diversely, acidosis complicates the regulation of extracellular potassium concentration. Potassium is shifted from within cells to interstitial fluid and blood. Because of anuria, this potassium is not excreted. The overall consequence of the two factors (anuria and acidosis) is hyperkalemia, which may be life-threatening because of its effects on cell membrane potential. Anuria is also associated with hyperphosphatemia. Because of the solubility product constant of calcium phosphate, the increase in phosphorus causes a decrease in serum calcium concentration. Mild hyponatremia, hypermagnesemia, hyperglycemia, hyperproteinemia, and azotemia are also found in cats with experimental obstruction.

Dehydration occurs despite lack of urine outflow because of sequestration of fluid in the bladder, lack of oral intake, and continued water loss by non-renal routes.

The pathogenesis of the catabolic state and of hypothermia associated with urethral obstruction has not been studied adequately. It is likely that azotemia and its consequences play a role in both. The severity of the catabolic state was demonstrated in experimental obstruction, in which cats lost an average of 15 percent of body weight after obstruction despite adequate rehydration.

Overall, the more significant abnormalities for which therapy is employed are the obstruction itself, dehydration, hyperkalemia, acidosis, and hypothermia.

In some cats, postobstruction diuresis that can lead to dehydration and electrolyte deficits may occur. The pathogenesis of these abnormalities is related to solute diuresis associated with urinary loss of urea and other particles. Cats may also suffer renal damage as a consequence of the obstruction, which interferes with urine concentrating ability and conservation of electrolytes. Water and electrolyte balance in cats during the postobstructive period should receive careful attention by the clinician.

EMERGENCY TREATMENT OF FUS

The markedly depressed, moribund cat with urethral obstruction must be treated quickly and effectively. The physical condition of the cat reflects the abnormalities previously described. Although case-to-case variation in the magnitude of abnormalities may exist, general principles of therapy can be applied to all. Priority must be given to therapy rather than to diagnostic gymnastics.

The objectives are to reduce hyperkalemia, restore fluid and acid-base balance, and correct hypothermia. The following are logical approaches to achieving these goals. They are listed in the order in which they should be performed.

1. Place an indwelling catheter in a peripheral vein and begin administration of a warmed alkalizing solution. Multisol-R° was used successfully in experimental cats. A blood sample may be obtained at the time of venous catheterization if pretreatment laboratory values are desired. Administer fluids at a rate of 90 ml/kg/hr until the deficit has been replaced. The fluid deficit is calculated by multiplying body weight (kg) by percent dehydration. Thus, a three-kg cat with 7 percent dehydration would require 210 ml of fluid. Since the maximal rate of administration recommended is 90 ml/hr/kg, the entire deficit in this case can be given in 50 minutes.

2. As soon as administration of fluids has been started, obtain the cat's rectal temperature and place the cat on a heating pad if hypothermia exists or develops.

3. Restore urine formation by emptying the bladder. Removal of the urethral obstruction is the preferred method, but if this cannot be achieved within five minutes, cystocentesis should be performed. Removal of obstructing material is often facilitated by decompression of the urinary bladder by cystocentesis.

4. Place an indwelling catheter in the urinary bladder once obstruction has been removed.

RATIONALE OF EMERGENCY TREATMENT

As previously indicated, the primary objective of therapy is to correct dehydration, acidosis, and hyperkalemia that are likely to exist. The previous regimen of therapy is successful in achieving these goals by the following mechanisms:

1. Rapid correction of dehydration restores circulatory volume. Thus, renal perfusion should be adequate so that renal excretion of wastes can resume once the bladder is emptied.

2. Administration of alkalizing agents corrects the acidosis. This treatment not only has general beneficial effects on cell metabolism but also specifically causes cell uptake of potassium to aid in alleviation of hyperkalemia.

3. Emptying of the bladder removes renal back-pressure and facilitates resumption of urine flow. The kidney is able to resume its homeostatic role with regard to body water and electrolyte balance. Studies in obstructed cats have demonstrated that a marked increase in urinary potassium excretion follows removal of obstruction.

The type of fluid initially used for therapy in

---

*Abbott Laboratories, Chicago, Illinois.

obstructed cats is probably not too relevant, except that it should be alkalizing and should decrease hyperkalemia by dilution. Several preparations can be used with equal efficacy. For example, lactated Ringer's solution with 25 mEq of sodium bicarbonate added per liter, or saline with 50 mEq of sodium bicarbonate per liter, could be used. The potassium content of some solutions may seem to contraindicate them, but their use should be kept in perspective. Administration of solutions containing 4.0 mEq of potassium per liter, when compared with the elevated blood potassium levels in obstructed cats, will still cause a decrease in serum potassium. The decrease could be expected to be less rapid, however, than when saline with 50 mEq of added sodium bicarbonate per liter is used.

The cat's urine production should be monitored. Once flow is resumed, renal excretion of potassium will occur. For maintenance and contemporary loss therapy, a more balanced electrolyte solution (i.e., lactated Ringer's or Multisol-R) should be used.

Glucose and insulin have been used for treatment of hyperkalemia in other species, since these compounds are associated with cellular uptake of potassium. Although these compounds have been advocated for use in the cat, they have been used only in combination with fluid therapy and relief of obstruction. Thus, proof of efficacy for the dose of insulin-glucose recommended for the cat has not been reported. In view of the success of removal of obstruction and fluid therapy alone, glucose-insulin does not seem to be indicated or required for the postrenal failure associated with FUS.

OTHER CONSIDERATIONS IN THERAPY

Studies in experimental cats indicated that urethral obstruction caused a severe catabolic state. Catabolism and anorexia associated with disease should receive attention. Force-feeding and gavage should be initiated after the initial 24 hours of therapy and should be continued unless voluntary eating or vomiting occurs.

Postobstruction diuresis, as previously discussed, should be considered as a possible occurrence, although it does not occur in all cats. Diuresis may be associated with water and electrolyte loss. Oral administration is the best approach to providing water and electrolytes, but parenteral fluid therapy using lactated Ringer's solution may be required to supplement fluid needs.

The azotemia of urethral obstruction resolves in about 72 hours if renal damage has not occurred because of obstruction.

SUPPLEMENTAL READING

Burrows, C.F., and Bovée, K.C.: Characterization and treatment of acid-base and renal defects due to urethral obstruction of cats. J. Am. Vet. Med. Assoc., *172*:801–805, 1978.

Finco, D.R.: Induced feline urethral obstruction: Response of hyperkalemia to relief of obstruction and administration of parenteral electrolyte solution. J. Am. Anim. Hosp. Assoc., *12*:198–201, 1976.

Finco, D.R., and Cornelius, L.M.: Characterization and treatment of water, electrolyte, and acid-base imbalances of induced urethral obstruction in the cat. Am. J. Vet. Res., *38*:823–830, 1977.

FELINE UROLOGIC SYNDROME: REMOVAL OF URETHRAL OBSTRUCTIONS AND USE OF INDWELLING URETHRAL CATHETERS

GEORGE E. LEES, D.V.M.,
and CARL A. OSBORNE, D.V.M.
St. Paul, Minnesota

RELIEF OF URETHRAL OBSTRUCTION

Since peristence of complete obstruction of the urethra will eventually kill the patient, re-establishment of urine outflow should receive emergency priority. Several non-surgical techniques have been advocated to relieve urethral obstructions. Any procedure that is effective in removing the obstruction rapidly and maintaining patency of the urethral lumen while inducing a minimum of trauma and minimizing the risk of iatrogenic urinary tract infection is acceptable. During initial treatment every effort should be made to prevent short-term recurrence (i.e., within hours to days) of urethral obstruction as a result of iatrogenic trauma or infection. We do not depend routinely on indwelling urethral catheterization for maintenance of urethral patency because of its undesirable consequences.

MASSAGE OF URETHRA

Gentle massage of the penis between the thumb and fingers may help to dislodge plugs located in the penile urethra. Plugs located in the preprostatic (abdominal) or membranous (pelvic) urethra may occasionally be dislodged by massaging the urethra through the rectum. Although these modes of therapy are often ineffective, their simplicity and occasional success make them worth trying.

RETROGRADE URETHRAL IRRIGATION

Flushing the urethral lumen with sterilized solutions following catheterization may dislodge urethral plugs or calculi. Various solutions have been recommended, including steril-

ized water or saline, local anesthetics, and solutions intended to dissolve or inhibit the formation of crystals. Walpole's buffered acetic acid solution is an example of the third type and may be prepared by mixing 57 ml 0.2 molar acetic acid with 43 ml 0.2 molar sodium acetate. Prior to its use, this solution should be filtered to remove debris and then sterilized, because it may support bacterial growth. Weak, non-buffered acetic acid should not be used, since it may damage the mucosa of the urethra and bladder.

Reverse flushing solutions should be used cautiously, since accumulation and absorption of large quantities of acid or anesthetic solutions from an inflamed urinary bladder may cause systemic toxicity. Solutions under pressure, such as anesthetic sprays, are not recommended because they could cause damage to the urethra or rupture of the bladder wall. We prefer lactated Ringer's solution or isotonic saline because they are sterilized, non-toxic, non-irritating, economical, and readily available.

A variety of catheters may be used, including disposable polypropylene,[*][†] polyvinyl,[‡] or nylon[§] catheters manufactured for this purpose, intravenous catheters[||][¶] and catheters fabricated from polyethylene tubing.[**] Silver abscess cannulas[††] are also useful, especially when the urethral obstruction is so far anterior that insertion of other catheters cannot be accomplished. Metal lacrimal cannulas and other instruments that can easily damage the urethral mucosa should be avoided.

Every effort should be made to protect the patient from iatrogenic complications associated with catheterization, including trauma to the urinary tract and urinary tract infection. Since the urine of most affected cats is bacteriologic-

---

All footnotes are on page 1196.

ally sterile and since inflammation of the urethra and bladder together with stagnation of urine within the bladder predispose the patient to bacterial urinary tract infection, appropriate precautions must be taken to prevent iatrogenic infection. Only catheters that have been sterilized should be used. In addition, the penis should be cleaned with an appropriate solution prior to catheterization.

Regardless of the technique employed, meticulous aseptic and feather-touch technique should be used to prevent damage to delicate tissue of the urethra and urinary bladder. Use of careful technique during initial efforts to remove obstructing material from the urethra will minimize the likelihood of recurrent urethral obstruction and may eliminate the need for an indwelling urethral catheter. Physical restraint alone or in combination with topical anesthesia may be sufficient for patients that are particularly docile or severely depressed. Because of an increased risk of adverse drug reactions associated with azotemia, pharmacologic restraint should be avoided when possible. Wrapping the cat in a bath towel may help to protect the patient and the assistant. The potential risk of adverse drug reactions must be weighed against the possibility of iatrogenic trauma to the urethra, however. If the disposition of the patient is such that attempts to dislodge the urethral obstruction are likely to be associated with additional damage to the urethra or iatrogenic urinary tract infection, some form of pharmacologic restraint should be used. Short-acting barbiturate anesthetic agents (thiamylal) that are metabolized by the liver or inhalant anesthetics, or both, are recommended if general anesthesia is required. Anesthetic agents must be given cautiously, since dosages less than those recommended by the manufacturer are often required in azotemic patients. Administration of ketamine hydrochloride at the manufacturer's recommended dose is not advised because it is excreted in active form by the kidneys. In patients with renal dysfunction its effect may be enhanced or prolonged.

Following cleaning of the penis with warm water, a catheter coated with sterilized aqueous lubricant should be advanced carefully to the site of the obstruction. The distance the catheter can be inserted indicates the level of the urethral obstruction. This information should be recorded, since it may be of value when considering use of smooth muscle relaxants and when considering urethral surgery to prevent recurrent obstructions. A large quantity of lactated Ringer's solution (as much as several hundred milliliters) should then be flushed into the urethral lumen and allowed to flow out of the external urethral orifice. When possible the catheter should be advanced toward the bladder. As a result of this maneuver, the obstructing material may gradually be dislodged and flushed out of the urethra around the catheter.

In some instances it may be necessary to propel the material back into the bladder by occluding the distal end of the urethra around the catheter prior to injection of fluid into the urethra. This will prevent reflux of solution from the urethra and will dilate the urethral lumen. If the plug does not advance into the urinary bladder, it may be *gently* advanced with the catheter. Excessive force should *not* be used. Prior to advancement of the catheter the extended penis should be displaced in a dorsal direction until the long axis of the urethra is approximately parallel to the vertebral column. This maneuver will facilitate atraumatic catheterization by reducing the natural curvature of the caudal portion of the urethra.

Alternatively, application of steady but gentle digital pressure to the bladder wall after the urethra has been flushed with lactated Ringer's solution may force the plug out of the urethra. Excessive pressure should not be used because it may result in (1) trauma to the bladder, (2) reflux of potentially infected urine into the ureters and renal pelves, and (3) rupture of the bladder wall.

Use of smooth muscle relaxants has been advocated as an aid in relief of urethral obstruction. Subjective clinical evaluation of these drugs suggests that they are not consistently effective. Lack of response may be related to the fact that the preprostatic urethra is surrounded by smooth muscle, whereas the portion of the urethra distal to the prostate gland is surrounded by an inner layer of smooth muscle and an outer layer of skeletal muscle.

CYSTOCENTESIS

In situations in which urethral obstructions cannot be removed by non-surgical methods, cystocentesis should be considered to provide immediate but temporary decompression of the urinary system. Following cystocentesis, attempts to dislodge urethral plugs by reverse flushing frequently are successful. This may be related to the fact that the patient is in less discomfort and has relaxed the skeletal muscle surrounding the distal urethra. Consult the article entitled "Cystocentesis" for technical details.

SURGICAL TECHNIQUES

In the unusual circumstance that the urethral obstruction cannot be removed by non-surgical techniques and the patient is severely uremic, intermittent cystocentesis and peritoneal dialysis should be considered with the objective of improving the patient's anesthetic risk. Surgical techniques to remove the obstruction, including cystotomy, flushing of the urethra, or urethrostomy, may then be performed. We do not recommend surgical intervention in severely uremic patients unless no alternatives exist.

Amputation of the distal portion of the penis or placement of a longitudinal incision in the distal portion of the urethra have been advocated to provide immediate relief of urethral obstruction. Although these barbaric techniques may provide immediate relief they should not be performed, since they may be associated with urethral strictures during healing.

IMMEDIATE AFTERCARE

After urine flow has been re-established by non-surgical techniques, the bladder should be emptied via manual compression or a syringe and catheter. It is unnecessary and usually inadvisable to attempt to remove all of the urine from the bladder by manual compression through the abdominal wall, since the associated trauma may aggravate the severity of bladder lesions. If insoluble material is found in the urine it may be advisable to flush the bladder lumen with a sterilized non-irritating solution in an attempt to minimize reobstruction.

The bladder should be evaluated periodically following removal of the urethral plug to ensure that urethral obstruction has not recurred and that the detrusor muscle is not hypotonic. Micturition induced by gentle digital compression of the bladder facilitates evaluation of the diameter of the urine stream.

THE INDWELLING CATHETER CONTROVERSY

Because of the frequency with which urethral obstruction recurs shortly after urethral patency has been established, some clinicians prefer to use indwelling urethral catheters routinely. Indwelling urethral catheterization has several advantages, including (1) prevention of injury to the lower urinary tract produced by repeated efforts to relieve recurrent urethral obstructions, (2) maintenance of urine outflow, and (3) prevention of trauma to the urinary bladder caused by manual compression used to assess urethral patency or empty the bladder lumen.

We have recommended more restricted use of indwelling urethral catheters in all situations, including urethral obstruction associated with the feline urologic syndrome, because of the substantial risk of iatrogenic ascending urinary tract infection associated with the procedure. In order to verify our suspicions, experimental studies were performed in normal cats utilizing commercially manufactured urethral catheters of different composition and lengths.*†‡ The duration of catheterization in different groups of cats varied from one to five days. In some experimental groups, broad-spectrum antibiotics (ampicillin) or parenteral fluids, or both, were administered in an effort to prevent iatrogenic infection. A summary of the results of these studies follows:

1. Gross hematuria that was sometimes severe usually developed within 24 hours following insertion of long polypropylene catheters* whose tips protruded into the bladder lumen. The hematuria was induced by catheter-tip trauma to the epithelial surface. Examination of the bladder wall after three days of catheterization typically revealed substantial edema and hemorrhage.

2. Long polyvinyl catheters‡ that protruded into the bladder lumen generally produced less bladder injury than long polypropylene catheters;* however, in some cats the degree of bladder wall injury was also severe.

3. Shorter catheters† did not reach the bladder lumen and generally did not produce gross hematuria. In the absence of infection, the urinary bladders were normal. Even though the bladder was spared, short polypropylene catheters consistently produced urethritis, which appeared to be a foreign-body reaction. Microscopic urethral lesions were apparent within 24 hours of indwelling catheterization and were characterized by mild to moderate degrees of inflammation and varying degrees of mucosal loss.

4. Many catheterized cats developed bacteriuria. Some bacteriuric cats developed severe gross and microscopic lesions of the bladder, even when the catheter did not enter the bladder lumen. Concomitant urinary tract infection typically enhanced the severity of urethral inflammation associated with the catheter. In a few cats with suppurative urethritis, the inflammatory response extended into the prostate gland.

5. The most severe catheter-induced urinary tract infections consistently occurred in cats with diuresis produced by parenteral polyionic fluid administration.

6. Parenteral administration of ampicillin reduced the frequency and severity of catheter-induced urinary tract infection. Infections developed in some cats treated with ampicillin, however, and were even more common in cats

given both ampicillin and fluids. Bacteria isolated from these cats had *in vitro* resistance to ampicillin.

Although these studies were not designed to assess the reversibility of iatrogenic inflammation and infection induced by indwelling catheters, the results indicate that indwelling urethral catheters may be associated with complications of clinical significance. The fact that significant catheter-induced disease developed in normal cats suggests that the susceptibility and severity of complications would be even greater in cats with the feline urologic syndrome (FUS).

In addition to the results of these studies, other factors indicate that a selective approach to the use of indwelling urethral catheters for management of urethral obstruction is beneficial. They include the facts that many cats do not become reobstructed following initial removal of obstructing material and that the urine of most cats with FUS is bacteriologically sterile. Therefore, we recommend that use of indwelling catheters to be limited to the following situations: (1) persistence of a poor urine stream as a result of partial urethral obstruction caused by tissue swelling and/or obstructing material, (2) repeated reobstruction associated with the current episode, (3) impaired ability to micturate associated with dysfunction of the bladder destrusor muscle, and (4) in the measurement of urine output as a guide for the administration of intravenous fluids to critically ill cats in intensive care settings. We again emphasize the use of adequate restraint, feather-touch technique, and appropriate flushing procedures from the outset of attempts to remove urethral plugs in order to minimize the likelihood of urethral reobstruction.

Increasing urine volume with the objective of diluting the concentration of materials that contribute to urethral plug formation appears to be a logical recommendation for cats *without* indwelling urethral catheters. It has been our experience that hospitalized cats often do not consume much water, especially if they are ill. Although fluids given by mouth may induce diuresis, we routinely augment urine output by giving an appropriate quantity of isotonic polyionic solution subcutaneously. A satisfactory response is suggested by formation of an increased volume of urine with a specific gravity less than 1.030. We emphasize, however, that induction of diuresis in normal cats with indwelling urethral catheters increased the severity of catheter-induced infection. Pending results of further studies, induction of diuresis with parenteral fluids in FUS cats with indwelling catheters must be considered with appropriate caution. Similarly, diuresis caused by obstructive nephropathy or produced in the treatment of azotemia may unavoidably increase the risk of iatrogenic urinary tract infection in cats with indwelling urinary catheters.

INDWELLING CATHETERIZATION TECHNIQUES

Iatrogenic complications associated with the use of indwelling catheters may be minimized by selection of appropriate catheters (Table 1). Commercially manufactured polypropylene catheters are often longer than optimum (14.5 cm)* or too short (8 cm)† to reach the bladder lumen. Commercially manufactured nylon catheters§ are intermediate in length (11 cm) compared with the polypropylene catheters just described. Commercially manufactured polyvinyl catheters‡ are designed for use at variable lengths. Because of their lengths, either polyvinyl or nylon catheters appear to be better suited for constant bladder drainage than short or long polypropylene catheters. It is emphasized, however, that all catheters with side openings must project more than a centimeter into the bladder lumen to be functional. Only the polyvinyl catheter is soft and flexible enough to minimize trauma to the epithelium

Table 1. *Features of Commercially Manufactured Feline Urethral Catheters*

| | | LENGTH | | CATHETER TIP | | |
| | | | | | LENGTH BEYOND SIDE OPENINGS | |
TYPE	DIAMETER (French Units)	OVERALL (cm)	MAXIMUM INSERTABLE (cm)	TYPE	(cm)	FLEXIBILITY
Long polypropylene	3.5	17.3	14.5	2 side openings	1.5	poor
Short polypropylene	3.5	10.2	8.0	open-end	—	poor
Polyvinyl	3.5 or 5.0	39.0	variable	2 side openings	1.4	good
Nylon	3.0 or 4.0	13.5	11.0	2 side openings	1.1	poor

that is produced as the bladder contracts around the catheter tip. Despite the fact that it is provided with a stylet, the nylon catheter§ is slightly less flexible than the polypropylene catheters at room temperature.

Based on these observations, we recommend the use of polyvinyl catheters when the goal of indwelling catheterization is continuous drainage of the bladder lumen (e.g., in cats with hypotonic bladders). Regardless of the type of catheter selected, insertion of an excessive length of catheter into the bladder lumen should be avoided. Not only does protrusion of an excessive length of catheter into the bladder lumen commonly result in epithelial trauma as the bladder contracts, but contraction of the bladder may also force a sufficient length of catheter beyond the external urethral orifice to permit the cat to remove it. The catheter tip is properly positioned when the catheter is inserted no further than necessary to recover readily a small volume of air or sterilized fluid injected into an otherwise empty bladder with a syringe.

If the objective of indwelling catheterization is only to maintain patency of the penile or postprostatic urethra in order to prevent reobstruction, short catheters with an open end may be selected. That they are not in direct communication with the bladder lumen should not be a problem, since obstructions rarely occur in the preprostatic urethra. Patency of this system can be ensured by manual compression of the bladder or reverse flushing with the aid of a syringe. Although unproved, it seems logical to expect that urethral catheters that do not reach the bladder lumen might actually increase resistance to urine flow (and thus decrease ability to micturate effectively) in some circumstances, since the internal caliber of the catheter is necessarily smaller than that of the urethra.

Indwelling urethral catheters are generally secured in position by suturing them to the prepuce. One catheter§ is manufactured with a perforated flange at its distal end for this purpose. For other catheters adhesive tape may be wrapped around the distal end, or suture material may be passed through the catheter wall with a needle in order to facilitate transfixation to the prepuce. Tape sometimes has the disadvantage of slipping on the catheter when it becomes saturated with urine or irrigating solutions.

Indwelling catheters should be used for as short a time as possible. In most instances 24 to 72 hours is sufficient. The cat should be observed for about 24 hours following removal of the catheter to ensure that patency of the urethra is sustained.

In man infections associated with indwelling urethral catheterization may be minimized by routine use of closed sterile urine drainage. Although difficult to accomplish in cats in most clinical circumstances, this technique should be used whenever possible. To be maximally effective the entire collection system must be sterilized initially and kept sealed to prevent contamination. It is emphasized, however, that even meticulous attention to principles of aseptic management of indwelling urinary catheters reduce the incidence of but does not prevent iatrogenic infections.

Oral or parenteral administration of antimicrobial agents during indwelling catheterization should not be expected to prevent bacterial infections consistently. Because infections that develop are typically caused by organisms resistant to the drug being used, the practice of continuing therapy (started during catheterization) for a period following catheter removal may not be effective. Routine use of bacterial urine cultures following indwelling catheterization is recommended prior to selection of antimicrobial agents.

MANAGEMENT OF HYPOTONIC URINARY BLADDERS

Severe or prolonged overdistention of the urinary bladder caused by obstruction of urine outflow may cause the detrusor muscle to become hypotonic or atonic. Many clinicians prefer to manage this problem with an indwelling urinary catheter. Provided that the bladder lumen is kept relatively empty, the detrusor muscle often will regain normal function. Alternatively, manual compression may be applied at appropriate intervals to expel urine. Gentle but steady digital pressure should be used rather than forceful intermittent squeezing motions in order to prevent trauma to the bladder wall. Parasympathomimetic drugs such as bethanechol chloride‡‡ may also be used in combination with these techniques to stimulate the bladder wall to contract. By promoting voiding of residual urine from the bladder, they prevent distention of the bladder wall and minimize further predisposition of the patient to bacterial urinary tract infection. Parasympathomimetic drugs are of no known value in promoting repair of lesions in the detrusor muscle. They should not be administered unless the urethra is patent, since contraction against an obstructed urethra may cause patient discomfort, reflux of infected urine into the ureters and renal pelves and, conceivably, rupture of the excretory pathway.

Because stasis of urine is a well-established predisposition to bacterial urinary tract infection, antimicrobial agents should be administered systemically. Irrigation of the bladder lumen with antimicrobial solutions may also be justified, especially if a sufficient quantity of the agent will remain in the bladder long enough to have a beneficial effect. Catheterization for the sole purpose of instilling medications is not recommended, since patients with disease of the urinary tract are predisposed to iatrogenic catheter-induced infection. If this method is used, only sterilized solutions should be injected into the bladder. The volume of solution should be sufficient to allow contact with all portions of the bladder mucosa.

ADDENDUM

Following preparation of this article, lengths of some feline urinary catheters described here were changed by their manufacturer. Polypropylene catheters with side openings* are now only 5.5 inches long (instead of 6.5 inches). Open-ended polypropylene catheterst are now available in two lengths, the original 4.5 inches and 5.5 inches.

SUPPLEMENTAL READING

Lees, G.E., and Osborne, C.A.: Urinary tract infections associated with use and misuse of urinary catheters. Vet. Clin. North Am., 9:713–727, 1979.

Osborne, C.A., and Lees, G.E.: Feline cystitis, urethritis, urethral obstruction syndrome. II. Therapy of disorders of the upper and lower urinary tract. Mod. Vet. Pract., 59:349–357, 1978.

FOOTNOTES

*Sovereign® Tom Cat Catheter, Sherwood Medical Industries, St. Louis, Missouri 63103

†Sovereign® Open End Tom Cat Catheter, Sherwood Medical Industries, St. Louis, Missouri 63103

‡Sovereign® Sterile Disposable Feeding Tube and Urethral Catheter, Sherwood Medical Industries, St. Louis, Missouri 63103

§Jackson Cat Catheter, Arnold's Veterinary Products, Ltd., Reading RGI 8NF, England. Distr. by Portex Division, Wilmington, Massachusetts 01887

‖Argyle® Medicut® Intravenous Cannula, Sherwood Medical Industries, St. Louis, Missouri 63103

¶Sovereign® Indwelling Catheter, Sherwood Medical Industries, St. Louis, Missouri 63103

**Intramedic polyethylene tubing, PE60 to PE90, Clay Adams, Parsippany, New Jersey 07054

††Becton, Dickenson & Co., East Rutherford, New Jersey 07070

‡‡Urecholine; Merck, Sharp, & Dohme, West Point, Pennsylvania 19486

FELINE UROLOGIC SYNDROME: MEDICAL ASPECTS OF PROPHYLAXIS

CARL A. OSBORNE, D.V.M.,
and GEORGE E. LEES, D.V.M.
St. Paul, Minnesota

INTRODUCTION

Because of a significant potential for recurrence and because the likelihood of recurrence in each affected patient is unpredictable, prophylactic therapy is an important aspect of management of the feline urologic syndrome (FUS). Unfortunately, lack of understanding of the underlying causes of FUS has resulted in recommendations of therapeutic maneuvers that are based largely on uncontrolled clinical observations and personal opinion rather than on controlled clinical and experimental studies. With-

out knowledge of the interrelationship of various events that lead to FUS, medical or surgical attempts to eliminate or control predisposing and perpetuating factors thought to be associated with the disorder appear to be the only logical alternative (Table 1). Our decision to use surgical or medical therapy is based on the cause and frequency of recurrence of signs of FUS.

As with evaluation of all forms of therapy, cautious and reasoned judgment is in order. The following generalities are intended as

Table 1. Predisposing and Perpetuating Factors Thought to be Associated with the Feline Urologic Syndrome

PREDISPOSING FACTORS	PERPETUATING FACTORS
Struvite Crystals	Narrowing of urethral lumen
Urine pH	Acute inflammation
Urine volume	Connective tissue
Diet	Struvite crystals
Obesity and inactivity ?	Others ?
Seasonal variation ?	
Others ?	

guidelines in formulating non-surgical prophylactic therapy for patients with FUS. For further information on management of recurrent urethral obstruction in male cats, consult the article on surgical aspects of prophylaxis.

ALTERATION OF URINE STRUVITE SUPERSATURATION

OVERVIEW

Initiation of urolith formation (sometimes called nucleation) is dependent on the degree of supersaturation of urine with calculogenic crystalloids (Osborne and Klausner). The degree of supersaturation may in turn be influenced by (1) the magnitude of renal excretion of the crystalloid, (2) urine pH, and (3) substances in urine that inhibit crystallization (sometimes called crystallization inhibitors or crystal poisons). It follows that uroliths may be prevented or even dissolved by creating an undersaturated state of calculogenic crystalloid(s) in urine (Osborne and Klausner). This might be achieved by (1) reducing the quantity of crystalloids in urine (for example, by altering the diet or administering oral agents that prevent gastrointestinal absorption of calculogenic crystalloids), (2) increasing the solubility of crystalloids in urine (e.g., by administering agents that alter urine pH to create a less favorable environment for crystallization), and (3) increasing the volume of urine in which crystals are dissolved or suspended.

REDUCTION OF THE QUANTITY OF CRYSTALLOIDS IN URINE

To date, the only plausible relationship that could be hypothesized to relate urinary excretion of calculogenic crystalloids to the etiopathogenesis of the feline urologic syndrome involves the diet. Excessive production of endogenous calculogenic substances and impaired tubular reabsorption of calculogenic substances from glomerular filtrate both seem unlikely causes. Diet has been incriminated as a causal factor on the basis of (1) ash content, (2) moisture content, and (3) mineral imbalances.

Dietary Ash Content. The long-held supposition that the ash content of the diet (especially of dry cat foods) plays a role in FUS has not been supported by experimental studies. In these studies cats fed up to 30 percent ash diets did not develop uroliths (Dickensen and Scott; Gershoff).

Dietary Moisture Content. Several investigators have documented a relationship between consumption of large quantities of dry cat food and the occurrence of feline urologic syndrome (Reif, et al.; Willeberg). One hypothesis advanced to explain the relationship between consumption of large quantities of dry food and FUS is the resultant decrease in water consumed in dry food and the subsequent production of a reduced volume of highly concentrated urine (Barker and Povey; Jackson). It was reasoned that production of highly concentrated urine would increase the quantity of calculogenic substances per unit volume of urine, thus favoring supersaturation of urine with struvite crystals and the formation of urethral plugs. This hypothesis has been supported by results of two experimental studies in which water consumption and urine volume were monitored in cats consuming dry cat foods (Holme; Jackson and Tovey), but it was refuted by another (Thrall and Miller). In one of the aforementioned studies it was concluded that cats consuming expanded dry cat foods lost a greater quantity of water in their feces than cats consuming moist foods or non-expanded dry foods (Jackson and Tovey). Pending further studies on the relationship of dry food to the feline urologic syndrome, it seems reasonable to recommend the addition of moisture to dry cat foods consumed by cats with a history of recurrent urethral obstruction. This may be accomplished by mashing milk, water, gravy, or other liquids into the food with a fork. Alternatively, these cats may be fed moist foods.

Dietary Mineral Imbalances. Use of experimental calculogenic diets containing high concentrations of magnesium (0.75 to 1.0 percent) to produce magnesium phosphate uroliths leaves little doubt that dietary minerals may play a role in the initiation and growth of some calculi (Chow, 1977; Chow, et al., 1976; Lewis, et al.; Rich, et al.). The significance of studies based on use of these diets in relation to naturally occurring feline cystitis, urethritis, and urethral obstruction must be considered carefully, however, since the type of urolith produced (magnesium phosphate) is different from most naturally occurring urethral plugs (magnesium ammonium phosphate). In addition, the quantity of magnesium in calculogenic diets was significantly in excess of that present in most commercially prepared cat foods (Feldman, et al.).

Other experimental studies using calculogenic diets in cats indicate that the relative quantities of minerals (including magnesium, phosphorus, and calcium) may also be of significance in initiating calculus formation or promoting calculus growth (Chow, 1977; Lewis, et al.). Further studies are required before meaningful generalities can be established.

Summary. It seems logical to us that cats should be fed properly balanced moist or dry diets. We can see little harm in the recommendation that water be added to dry cat food when it constitutes a large proportion of the diet, and we are willing to speculate that it may be beneficial. We are opposed to the recommendations of some clinicians that in effect make their patients dietary cripples for life.

INCREASING URINE CRYSTALLOID SOLUBILITY

Since struvite crystals often constitute a substantial portion of urethral plugs, procedures designed to minimize or inhibit struvite crystallization and urine supersaturation would be expected to be beneficial as prophylactic therapy (Carbone; Rich and Kirk, 1968, 1969). Crystals of struvite have a greater tendency to form when urine pH is greater than 6.8 (Carbone), but they may be observed in acid urine. Increased solubility of struvite crystals in acid urine has led to the widespread use of urine acidifiers in an attempt to prevent recurrence of the feline urologic syndrome. Uremic cats should not be given acidifiers, since these drugs will aggravate the severity of metabolic acidosis that consistently is associated with renal failure.

The rationale for use of acidifiers as prophylactic therapy for this syndrome is supported by clinical and experimental studies. Using a model of struvite calculus formation on zinc discs implanted in rat urinary bladders, urine acidification resulted in complete dissolution of calculi in 14 of 20 animals in six weeks (Vermuelen, et al.). Small uroliths were dissolved in three humans by inducing a state of struvite undersaturation following urine sterilization and acidification (Griffith, et al.). Studies in normal cats revealed that the amount of measurable struvite crystals in urine decreased by mixing 1 gram of DL-methionine in their food each day (Rich, et al.). Addition of 1 percent methionine to calculogenic diets high in mag-

nesium delayed but did not prevent the onset of urethral obstruction (Chow, et al., 1976).

Since the urine pH of cats with feline urologic syndrome is often acid (Osbaldiston and Taussig; Schechter), the value of urine acidification has been questioned. In one study administration of DL-methionine decreased urine struvite crystalluria, even though urine pH was acid (Rich and Kirk, 1968).

Acidifiers commonly recommended include ascorbic acid, ethylenediamine dihydrochloride (Chlorethamine, Pitman-Moore), ammonium chloride, and DL-methionine (Pedameth, Durst; Methigel, EVSCO; Odortrol, Haver-Lockhart). The advantages and disadvantages of these agents have been reviewed (Hardy and Osborne). The relative ineffectiveness of ascorbic acid as a urinary acidifier in man (Nahata, et al.) and the inability of some acidifiers to induce an acid pH in the urine of cats indicate the need for careful evaluation of these products. Although the ability of ethylenediamine dihydrochloride to acidify the urine of guinea pigs, rabbits, and rats has been reported (Boyd and Dorrance), similar studies have not been reported for normal cats or cats with feline urologic syndrome. Pilot studies performed at the University of Minnesota and the University of Pennsylvania revealed that ethylenediamine dihydrochloride did not consistently acidify the urine of cats when administered at dosages equal to or in excess of that recommended by the manufacturer (Bovee, et al.). The observation that intact tablets were passed with feces suggests that the enteric coating of these tablets may inhibit their digestion and absorption from the gastrointestinal tract. Results of studies of consumption of a constant amount of ammonium chloride, DL-methionine, sodium phosphate, or ascorbic acid in a diet fed to normal cats once per day were interpreted to indicate that ammonium chloride produced the most consistent results in terms of urine acidification (Chow, et al., 1978). A dosage of 15 grains of ammonium chloride for six- to eight-pound (three- to four-kg) cat was subsequently recommended (Chow, 1978).

Dosage of urine acidifiers should be individualized for each patient. Urine should be maintained at a pH of 6.5 or less and should be monitored until it has been established that acidification has been achieved and maintained. Examination of urine sediment for struvite crystalluria may be used in conjunction with urine pH as an index of clinical effectiveness. Administration of divided daily doses has been suggested to maintain a consistently acid environment in the urinary tract. Owners may participate in monitoring urine pH with pH paper (pHydrion, Microessential Laboratory, Brooklyn). Evaluation of the pH of the first voided urine in the morning has been advocated on the basis that it is least likely to be influenced by dietary "alkaline tide."

Although acidification of urine has not always prevented recurrence of urethral obstruction, subjective clinical evaluation at our hospital indicates that it reduces the rate of recurrence in many cats. We recommend that acidifiers be continued indefinitely in cats with a history of recurrent obstruction and a urine pH greater than 6.8.

Another method to increase the solubility of calculogenic crystalloids in urine is administration of substances that are excreted in urine as crystallization inhibitors (Osborne and Klausner). Although administration of crystallization inhibitors (including citrates and inorganic pyrophosphates) to human beings and laboratory animals with calcium-containing uroliths has been reported to be beneficial, specific inhibitors of struvite crystallization have not been identified. A commercially manufactured product (Curecal, Albion) alleged to contain a crystallization inhibitor (sodium tripolyphosphate) and an agent that chelates calcium and magnesium has been advertised to be effective in prevention of the feline urologic syndrome. Unfortunately, no controlled or long-term studies of the efficacy of this drug in cats with FUS have been documented. It is not clear whether the action (if any) of this product occurs in the gastrointestinal or the urinary tract, or both.

Administration of 15 percent alanine to calculogenic diets prevented the formation of magnesium phosphate uroliths in cats (Chow, et al., 1976). It has been suggested that a high concentration of alanine in urine increases the solubility of magnesium phosphate (Hamar, et al., 1974) and impairs aggregation of proteinaceous material hypothesized to be a calculogenic matrix (Chow, et al., 1973).

AUGMENTATION OF URINE VOLUME

The urine of cats is typically more concentrated than the urine of other companion animals and man. In a survey of 424 urinalyses obtained from cats admitted to the University of Minnesota Veterinary Teaching Hospital during 1976 and 1977, the median specific gravity was 1.044 and the mean was 1.042 (range was 1.005 to 1.087). Evaluation of 98 urinalyses obtained from normal cats in conjunction with experimental studies in progress at the University of Minnesota revealed a mean specific gravity of 1.057 and a median of 1.059 (range was 1.023 to 1.084).

Because of the tendency of cats to produce concentrated urine, increasing the volume of urine produced by enhancing water consumption appears to be a logical recommendation, regardless of the type of diet that cats with recurrent FUS are consuming. It is the time-honored recommendation for the prevention and dissolution of uroliths in dogs and human beings (Osborne and Klausner). Chronic diuresis was effective in promoting dissolution of foreign body uroliths in rats, presumably by decreasing urine concentration of calculogenic substances and maintaining a state of struvite undersaturation and possibly by minimizing urine stagnation by increasing the frequency of micturition (Grove, et al.). Increased water consumption and increased urine volume induced almost complete amelioration of hematuria that was induced experimentally in cats by feeding them a calculogenic diet high in magnesium (Holme).

Oral salt has long been used to stimulate water consumption and compensatory polyuria. We recommend oral administration of 0.25 to 1.0 grams of salt per day in the form of tablets. Alternatively, salt may be mixed with food. Obviously, the success of this procedure implies the availability of a fresh water supply at all times. It would appear to be desirable to encourage water consumption throughout the day. A satisfactory compensatory increase in urine volume is suggested by formation of urine with a specific gravity of 1.035 or less. Provided that addition of salt is effective in augmenting water consumption and the formation of less concentrated urine, we currently recommend that it be continued indefinitely for patients with recurrent FUS.

Inability of the addition of 4 percent NaCl to a calculogenic diet to prevent the formation of magnesium phosphate uroliths in cats has prompted speculation that salt may not be an effective prophylactic agent for the feline urologic syndrome (Hamar, et al., 1976). Caution must be used in accepting this hypothesis, however, since both the calculogenic diet and the type of uroliths were dissimilar to diets and urethral plugs observed in naturally occurring FUS. In addition, the significance of the results is clouded because urine specific gravity and urine volume apparently were not monitored. More recent experimental studies in cats revealed that addition of salt to dry food resulted in increased water consumption and urine volume (Holme).

OTHER CONSIDERATIONS

The association of FUS in cats that are inactive and overweight (Willeberg and Priester) and its significance in formulating prophylactic measures are unknown. Recommendations that testosterone, caster oil, progesterone, vitamin A, and hyaluronidase be given appear to be based on supposition rather than fact. We do not recommend them.

Although struvite has been the primary component of urethral plugs evaluated by all investigators, there has not been a large survey of plugs evaluated from cats with naturally occurring FUS. It is well known that crystals identified in urine sediment are not a reliable index of the mineral composition of uroliths in other species. Because of the importance of knowledge of mineral composition in the formulation of prophylactic therapy for various types of uroliths, it seems reasonable to suggest that the mineral composition of urethral plugs obtained from cats with recurrent urethral obstruction be determined at least once during the course of the disease.

Methenamine (Mandelamine, Warner Chilcott) is a cyclic hydrocarbon that is one of the most popular urinary tract antiseptics in man. In the presence of an acid environment (pH less than 6.0) methenamine hydrolyzes to form formaldehyde. Because of the necessity of acid urine for the formation of formaldehyde, methenamine is usually given in combination with acidifiers such as mandelic acid or hippuric acid. It is often necessary to administer more potent acidifiers in addition to these combination drugs to acidify urine, especially if infection with urease-producing bacteria is present. The unproved suggestion that methenamine may have virocidal action in addition to bactericidal action is of considerable interest (Jackson).

Products (Urised, Uritin, Urilax, and others) that contain methylene blue and products (Azo-Gantrisin, Pyridium, and others) that contain phenazopyridine (a mucosal analgesic) should not be administered to cats. As reviewed elsewhere, these drugs have the potential to cause methemoglobinemia and irreversible oxidative changes in hemoglobin that result in the formation of Heinz bodies and anemia (Osborne and Lees).

Consult the article on urinary tract infections for recommendations concerning treatment and prevention of bacterial urinary tract infection.

SUMMARY

The following suggestions summarize the recommendations we routinely discuss with owners of cats that have a history of the feline urologic syndrome:

1. Provide the cat with the opportunity to micturate frequently in order to minimize prolonged retention of urine. The duration of forced periods of confinement without an opportunity to micturate should be kept as short as possible. Fastidious cats may avoid using a dirty litterbox, but we are skeptical that the box needs to be changed daily.

2. Observe the cat's micturation habits and urine color when possible in order to detect abnormalities early in the course of recurrence. The signs and consequences of urethral obstruction are emphasized to owners of male cats. Some clients may become adept at evaluating bladder size by abdominal palpation.

3. Provide a readily available source of clean water. Encourage water consumption and urine formation by administering salt tablets, mixing salt with food, and/or mashing water, milk, gravy, and other liquids into dry food.

4. Continue medications as directed. Periodically monitor urine pH with pH paper. Record results for future reference.

5. Return the cat for radiographic evaluation of the urinary tract for anatomic abnormalities or classic uroliths if signs persist for several weeks.

6. Submit a urine sample for analysis if recurrence is suspected.

SUPPLEMENTAL READING

Barker, J., and Povey, R.C.: The feline urolithiasis syndrome: A review and inquiry into the alleged role of dry cat foods in its etiology. J. Small Anim. Pract., 14:445–457, 1973.
Bovée, K.C., et al.: Recurrence of feline urethral obstruction. J. Am. Vet. Med. Assoc., 174:93–96, 1979.
Boyd, E.M., and Dorrance, J.A.S.: Ethylenediamine dihydrochloride or chlorethamine. I. As a urinary acidifier. Exp. Med. Surg., 4:212–222, 1946.
Carbone, M.G.: Phosphocrystalluria and urethral obstruction in the cat. J. Am. Vet. Med. Assoc., 147:1195–1200, 1965.
Chow, F.H.C.: Dietary mineral effects on feline urolithiasis. Proceedings of Kal Kan symposium, Kal Kan Foods Inc., Vernon, California, 1977.
Chow, F.H.C.: Urinary acidifiers. Feline Pract., 8:4, 1978.
Chow, F.H.C., et al.: Effect of dietary additives on experimentally produced feline urolithiasis. Feline Pract., 6:51–56, 1976.
Chow, F.H.C., et al.: Effect of dietary ammonium chloride, DL-methionine, sodium phosphate and ascorbic acid on urinary pH and electrolyte concentrations of male cats. Feline Pract., 8:30–34, 1978.
Chow, F.H.C., Hamar, D.W., and Udall, R.H.: Effect of alanine on urinary calculi. Invest. Urol., 11:38–40, 1973.
Dickensen, C.D., and Scott, P.P.: Failure to produce urinary calculi in kittens by the addition of mineral salts derived from bone meal to the diet. Vet. Rec., 68:858–859, 1956.
Feldman, B.M., Kennedy, B.M., and Schelstraete, M.: Dietary minerals and the feline urologic syndrome. Feline Pract., 7:39–45, 1977.
Gershoff, S.N.: Nutritional problems in household cats. J. Am. Vet. Med. Assoc., 166:455–458, 1975.
Griffith, D.P., Bragin, S., and Musher, D.M.: Dissolution of struvite urinary stones. Experimental studies *in vitro.* Invest. Urol., 13:351–353, 1976.
Grove, W.L., Vermeulen, C.W., Goetz, R., and Ragins, H.D.: Experimental urolithiasis. II. Influence of urine volume upon calculi experimentally produced by foreign bodies. J. Urol., 64:549–554, 1950.
Hamar, D., Chow, F.H.C., Dysart, M.I., and Rich, L.J.: Effect of

sodium chloride in prevention of experimentally produced phosphate uroliths in male cats. J. Am. Anim. Hosp. Assoc., 12:514–517, 1976.

Hamar, D.W., Huang, S., and Chow, F.H.C.: Effect of alanine and dimethyl sulfoxide on the solubility of calcium phosphate, magnesium phosphate, and calcium oxalate. Biochem. Med., 11:98–102, 1974.

Hardy, R.M., and Osborne, C.A.: Use and misuse of urinary acidifiers. Proceedings of the 40th annual meeting of the American Animal Hospital Assoc., South Bend, Indiana, 1973.

Holme, D.W.: Research into feline urologic syndrome. Proceedings of the Kal Kan symposium, Kal Kan Foods Inc., Vernon, California, 1977.

Jackson, J.W.: Methenamine mandelate in feline urologic syndrome. Feline Pract., 6:10, 1976.

Jackson, O.F., and Tovey, J.D.: Water balance studies in domestic cats. Feline Pract., 7:30–33, 1977.

Lewis, L.D., et al.: Effect of various dietary mineral concentrations on the occurrence of feline urolithiasis. J. Am. Vet. Med. Assoc., 172:559–563, 1978.

Nahata, M.C., Shimp, L., Lampman, T., and McLeod, D.C.: Effect of ascorbic acid on urine pH in man. Am. J. Hosp. Pharm., 34:1234–1237, 1977.

Osbaldiston, G.W., and Taussig, R.A.: Clinical report on 46 cases of feline urologic syndrome. Vet. Med. Small Anim. Clin., 65:461–468, 1970.

Osborne, C.A., and Klausner, J.S.: War on urolithiasis: Problems and solutions. Proceedings of the 45th annual meeting of the American Animal Hospital Assoc., South Bend, Indiana, 1978.

Osborne, C.A., and Lees, G.E.: Feline cystitis, urethritis, and urethral obstruction syndrome. Mod. Vet. Pract., 59:173–180, 349–357, 513–518, 669–673; 1978.

Reif, J.S., et al.: Feline urethral obstruction: A case control study. J. Am. Vet. Med. Assoc., 170:1320–1324, 1977.

Rich, L.J., et al.: Urethral obstruction in male cats: Experimental production by addition of magnesium and phosphate to the diet. Feline Pract., 4:44–47, 1974.

Rich, L.J., and Kirk, R.W.: Feline urethral obstruction: Mineral aspects. Am. J. Vet. Res., 29:2149–2156, 1968.

Rich, L.J., and Kirk, R.W.: The relationship of struvite crystals to urethral obstruction in cats. J. Am. Vet. Med. Assoc., 154:153–157, 1969.

Schechter, R.D.: The significance of bacteria in feline cystitis and urolithiasis. J. Am. Vet. Med. Assoc., 156:1567–1573, 1970.

Thrall, B.E., and Miller, L.G.: Water turnover in cats fed dry rations. Feline Pract., 6:10–17, 1976.

Vermuelen, C.W., et al.: Experimental urolithiasis. III. Prevention and dissolution of calculi by alteration of urinary pH. J. Urol., 66:1, 1951.

Willeberg, P.: Diets and feline urologic syndrome: A retrospective case control study. Nord. Vet. Med., 27:15–19, 1975.

Willeberg, P., and Priester, W.A.: Feline urologic syndrome. Associations with some time, space and individual patient factors. Am. J. Vet. Res., 37:975–978, 1976.

FELINE UROLOGIC SYNDROME: SURGICAL ASPECTS OF PROPHYLAXIS

TERESA L. TOMCHICK, D.V.M.,
Puyallop, Washington

and RICHARD W. GREENE, D.V.M.
New York, New York

Medical management of the chronically obstructed cat is variably successful. Until the etiology of the feline urologic syndrome is defined precisely, medical management will continue to be only partially effective. Surgical treatment in the form of perineal and occasionally antepubic urethrostomies has become increasingly effective in preventing recurrent obstruction (Smith and Schiller).

Many urethrostomy techniques have been described in the veterinary literature (Carbone, 1963, 1967, 1971; Manziano and Manziano; Blake; Ford; Mendham; Johnston; Wilson and Harrison; Richards, et al.). The primary goal of each of these techniques is to bypass the penile urethra and create a larger urethral stoma by anchoring the pelvic urethra to the skin. In perineal and preputial urethrostomies the pelvic urethra just cranial to the bulbourethral glands is sutured to the skin; in the antepubic urethrostomy the abdominal urethra caudal to the prostate gland is sutured to the skin. The perineal urethrostomy described by Wilson and Harrison has been performed successfully by many surgeons. A perineal urethrostomy should be the first choice, but an antepubic urethrostomy may be performed in cases of pelvic urethral rupture or irreversible obstructions in the pelvic urethra.

INDICATIONS FOR SURGERY

Clinical judgment must be used in selecting candidates for surgery because many cats experience only one obstructive episode in a lifetime. The cat that has two or more occurrences of urinary obstruction within a relatively short period (approximately one year) is an obvious candidate. Cats with penile urethral stricture from previous urinary obstruction or prolonged catheterization should undergo surgery. Those with iatrogenic urethral tears and those whose obstruction cannot be relieved by retrograde flushing are treated as emergency surgical cases. Less obvious candidates for elective perineal urethrostomy are cats that become extremely ill during urethral obstruction. In these animals surgery must be delayed until all signs of hyperkalemia, uremia, and cardiac arrhythmia have disappeared.

For the cat and its owner, surgery may prove to be less expensive and less inconvenient than constant vigilance for obstruction, repeated medical rechecks, and a lifetime of oral medication.

PREOPERATIVE CONSIDERATIONS

Dehydration, uremia, and hyperkalemia often occur in obstructed cats. Prior to surgery the cat should be rehydrated with the objective of enhancing the return of serum urea nitrogen, creatinine, and electrolyte concentrations to normal. In cats with chronic cystitis, radiography should be performed to rule out cystic calculi.

Exceptions to this preoperative routine are patients with urethral tears or urethral obstructions that cannot be relieved. If a urethral tear is thought to be present surgery should be performed immediately, since periurethral extravasation of urine is potentially life-threatening. In the rare instance in which the urethral obstruction cannot be removed by back-flushing or bypassed by a catheter, perineal urethrostomy should be considered as an emergency procedure. Operative risk in these cases can be reduced by (1) immediate intravenous fluid, antibiotic, and corticosteroid therapy, (2) induction and maintenance of halothane gas anesthesia, and (3) cardiac monitoring before and during surgery (consult the article "Drug Therapy in Renal Disorders" regarding risks associated with the use of corticosteroids and antibiotics in uremic patients). During a 15-month period at The Animal Medical Center, nine cats with irreversible urethral obstructions were treated in this manner. All cats survived the operation and, in a follow-up period that ranged from three months to two years, had no postoperative complications.

It is important to evaluate the neurologic status of affected cats prior to surgery. Some Manx cats and occasionally other breeds develop neurologically induced urinary signs, including strangury and incontinence. These signs are caused by anatomic abnormalities of the lumbar or sacral vertebrae, which result in "tiedown" or compression of the cauda equina. In these cases decompressive dorsal laminectomy is the surgical treatment of choice.

Cat owners should be made aware that, although perineal urethrostomy may prevent recurrent obstruction by providing a larger opening for urination, the major postoperative problem is cystitis.

URETHROSTOMY

Surgical techniques for urethrostomy have been adequately described elsewhere. Because it can be successfully performed by surgeons of variable experience, the Wilson perineal urethrostomy is highly recommended. Consideration of the following details will help to ensure good results. The surgeon should (1) have a working knowledge of perineal anatomy and be able to recognize anatomic structures, (2) correctly position the cat on a perineal stand, (3) empty the cat's bladder at the time of surgery to lessen tension on sutures as they are placed, (4) open the urethra up to or slightly beyond the bulbourethral glands to ensure the largest possible urethral stoma, and (5) use care in suturing urethral mucosa directly to the skin.

POSTOPERATIVE CARE

Correct postoperative management is essential for success. Because cats instinctively groom themselves, an Elizabethan collar is necessary to prevent them from mutilating the operative site. The collar should be used for two to four weeks postoperatively. It can usually be removed at the time of suture removal.

Each cat should be given an effective urinary tract antibiotic for two to three weeks following surgery. Sulfisoxazole* (10 mg/kg body weight t.i.d. per os), cephalexin† (2.5 to 3.5 mg/kg body weight t.i.d. per os), and chloramphenicol‡ (10 mg/kg body weight t.i.d. per os) are excellent choices. Alternatively, a preparation§ that includes an antispasmodic agent and a sulfa drug may be used instead.

---

*Gantrisin, Roche Laboratories, Nutley, New Jersey

†Keflex suspension, Eli Lilly & Co., Indianapolis, Indiana

‡Mychel-Vet, Rochelle Laboratories, Long Beach, California

§Urisoxole, EVSCO Pharmaceutical Corp.

Hemorrhage from the vascular urethral tissue has occasionally been a problem immediately after surgery. It may be controlled by applying epinephrine or cold packs to the area. If this fails, a tranquilizer (acepromazine at 0.025 to 0.05 mg/kg body weight IM or SQ) may be given. This calms the animal, lowers blood pressure, and facilitates local treatment of the hemorrhage.

Routine use of indwelling urinary catheters postoperatively should be avoided, since they may induce urethritis and inflammatory strictures of the surgical site. If the operation is performed correctly, catheters are not necessary.

We recommend that the sutures be removed two weeks postoperatively. Although most cats will tolerate this procedure well, a small amount of ketamine (5 to 10 mg) may be given intravenously to minimize discomfort.

Because most strictures of the surgical site tend to occur between four and eight weeks after surgery, the cat's progress should be monitored during this time interval. Stricture formation should be considered if strangury or reobstruction occurs. A no. 8 French male catheter should pass easily through the urethral opening and into the bladder. If it does not, a stricture of the surgical site probably is present. Strictures are most successfully treated by repeating the Wilson perineal urethrostomy. Dilating the surgical site with forceps has not been successful in relieving postoperative strictures at The An-imal Medical Center. During a 15-month period, Wilson perineal urethrostomies were performed on 128 cats for the first time. The procedures were performed by staff, surgeons, surgical residents, and interns. Of the 128 patients that had primary operations, only 12 (9 percent) developed strictures of the surgical site. Follow-up evaluation ranging from three months to two years indicated that 90 percent of these strictures were treated successfully by a second Wilson perineal urethrostomy.

SUPPLEMENTAL READING

Blake, J.A.: Perineal urethrostomy in cats. J. Am. Vet. Med. Assoc., 152:1499, 1968.

Carbone, M.G.: Perineal urethrostomy to relieve urethral obstruction in the male cat. J. Am. Vet. Med. Assoc., 143:34, 1963.

Carbone, M.G.: A multiple technique for peripheral urethrostomy in the male cat. J. Am. Vet. Med. Assoc., 151:301, 1967.

Carbone, M.G.: Urethral surgery in the cat. Vet. Clin. North Am., 1:281, 1971.

Ford, D.C.: Antepubic urethrostomy in the cat. J. Am. Anim. Hosp. Assoc., 4:415, 1968.

Johnston, D.E.: Feline urethrostomy: A critique and new method. J. Am. Anim. Hosp. Assoc., 15:421, 1974.

Manziano, C.F., and Manziano, T.R.: Perineal urethrostomy for relief of urethral blockage in the male cat. J. Am. Vet. Med. Assoc., 149:1312, 1966.

Mendham, J.H.: A description and evaluation of antepubic urethrostomy in the male cat. J. Small Anim. Pract., 11:709, 1970.

Richards, D.A., Hinko, P.J., and Morse, E.M.: Feline perineal urethrostomy: A new technique for an old problem. J. Am. Anim. Hosp. Assoc., 8:66, 1972.

Smith, C.W., and Schiller, A.G.: Perineal urethrostomy in the cat: A retrospective study of complications. J. Am. Anim. Hosp. Assoc., 14:225, 1978.

Wilson, G.P., and Harrison, J.W.: Perineal urethrostomy in cats. J. Am. Vet. Med. Assoc., 159:1789, 1971.

NEOPLASMS OF THE CANINE AND FELINE URINARY TRACTS

DENNIS D. CAYWOOD, D.V.M.,
CARL A. OSBORNE, D.V.M.,
and GARY R. JOHNSTON, D.V.M.
St. Paul, Minnesota

NEOPLASMS OF THE KIDNEY

TYPES

Benign. Benign renal tumors are less common in dogs and cats than malignant renal neoplasms (Tables 1 and 2). They are rarely of clinical significance and are usually incidental necropsy findings. An exception is renal hemangioma of dogs. This tumor has been the most commonly encountered benign canine renal tumor (Table 1) and is frequently associated with constant or intermittent gross hematuria and varying degrees of enlargement of the affected kidney.

Table 1. *Neoplasm Type, Age, and Sex Characteristics of 175 Dogs with Primary Renal Neoplasms**

TUMOR TYPE	NO. OF CASES	SEX			AGE (*Years*)		
		MALE	FEMALE	NOT DETERMINED	MEAN	RANGE	NOT DETERMINED
Epithelial tissue							
Adenoma	3	1	1	1	8.5	8–9	1
Renal carcinoma	113	57	27	29	8.2	1–15	34
Squamous cell carcinoma	9	6	3	–	8.7	4–14	–
Connective tissue							
Fibroma	2	1	1	–	8.5	5–12	–
Fibrosarcoma	2	1	1	–	6.5	5–8	–
Rhabdomyosarcoma	1	1	0	–	12	12	–
Leiomyoma	1	1	0	–	–	–	1
Leiomyosarcoma	1	–	–	1	–	–	1
Lipoma	1	0	1	–	8	8	–
Liposarcoma	1	0	1	–	5	–	–
Reticulum cell sarcoma	1	1	0	–	3	3	–
Unclassified sarcoma	4	1	3	–	7.2	6 mo–12 yr	1
Vascular tissue							
Hemangioma	7	4	3	–	11.3	8–15	–
Hemangiosarcoma	3	3	0	–	10.6	9–12	–
Mixed tissue							
Nephroblastoma	26	11	10	5	4.2	2 mo–11 yr	4
Teratoma	1	0	1	–	2	2	–
TOTAL	176	88	52	36	7.4	2 mo–15 yr	42

*Data from the University of Minnesota Veterinary Teaching Hospital, the Veterinary Medical Data Program sponsored by the National Cancer Institute, and the literature.

Malignant. Renal carcinomas (hypernephroma, renal adenocarcinoma, clear cell carcinoma, malignant nephroma) are the most common primary malignant neoplasm of the kidneys of dogs and cats. As in man, there is a higher incidence of these tumors in male dogs (Table 1). It has been suggested that this tumor may be hormonally induced. No sex predisposition has been identified in cats (Table 2). The incidence of the tumor increases with age in cats and dogs (Tables 1 and 2).

Renal carcinomas originate from renal tubular epithelial cells. Whether renal carcinomas arise *de novo* from renal tubular cells, by evolution through adenomatous hyperplasia, or from renal cortical adenomas has not been resolved. Renal carcinomas are typically composed of cells that are clear or granular, depending on the cellular content of glycogen, lipids, and cytoplasmic organelles. They may develop in solid, cystic, trabecular, tubular, or papillary patterns. In man and animals correlation between histologic patterns and survival is poor.

The natural history of renal carcinomas is ill-defined and unpredictable. In general, however, they have a highly malignant potential. Their growth may be characterized by an explosive increase in size with widespread metastases, or it may be slow and asymptomatic. Late metastases have been reported in dogs.

Renal carcinomas spread by direct extension through the renal capsule or renal pelvis and by invasion of intrarenal veins and lymphatics. Invasion and growth of renal carcinomas into renal veins can occur and is thought to account for the high incidence of lung metastases. Invasion of the renal vein has been reported to be less common in dogs than in man. The most common sites of metastases in dogs and cats are the lungs, lymph nodes, liver, brain, and bone. Any tissue of the body may be affected, however, and metastases to unusual sites are common. Many dogs have been reported to have metastatic lesions at the time of diagnosis of renal carcinoma. Metastasis may occur prior to the onset of signs related to the urinary system.

Embryonal nephroma (Wilms' tumor, nephroblastoma, congenital mixed tumor) is considered to be a congenital neoplasm derived from the pleuripotential metanephrogenic blastema, which allows production of epithelial and connective tissue elements. It is regarded as part of the developing kidney and is associated with continued growth but abnormal differentiation. The neoplasm occurs more often in young dogs and cats, although many cases have been observed in dogs and cats four or more years old (Tables 1 and 2). No breed or sex predilection is apparent (Tables 1 and 2).

Embryonal nephromas are usually unilateral;

Table 2. *Neoplasm Type, Age, and Sex Characteristics of 43 Cats with Primary Renal Neoplasms**

TUMOR TYPE	NO. OF CASES	SEX			AGE (Years)		
		MALE	FEMALE	NOT DETERMINED	MEAN	RANGE	NOT DETERMINED
Epithelial tissue							
Adenoma	2	1	1	–	–	–	2
Renal carcinoma	17	3	4	10	9	2–15	6
Transitional cell carcinoma	3	2	1	–	8	6–9	1
Squamous cell carcinoma	2	2	–	–	–	–	2
Connective tissue?							
Unclassified sarcoma	8	–	1	7	–	–	8
Muscle tissue							
Leiomyosarcoma	2	–	1	1	–	22	1
Mixed							
Nephroblastoma	9	2	–	7	6	2–8	5
TOTAL	43	10	8	25	7	2–22	25

*Data from the University of Minnesota Veterinary Teaching Hospital, the Veterinary Medical Data Program sponsored by the National Cancer Institute, and the literature.

however, bilateral involvement has been reported. They may be microscopic or grow to an enormous size. Microscopic evaluation of tissue sections typically reveals generalized replacement of normal renal parenchyma with gland-like acini or tubules dispersed within large masses of fibroblastic cells. As the tumor grows, the kidney is destroyed partly by neoplastic invasion and partly by compression. A pseudocapsule may develop, separating the growth from the remaining renal tissue.

If the tumor penetrates the renal capsule, local invasion of perinephric fat, posterior abdominal muscles, the diaphragm, and neighboring organs may occur. Distant metastases occur via the lymphatics into pararenal and para-aortic lymph nodes or, more commonly, by venous metastasis from the renal vein into the vena cava. The most common site of metastasis is the lung, followed by the liver, mesentery, and lymph nodes.

Transitional cell and squamous cell carcinomas of the canine renal pelvis are much less common than the same type of tumor in the urinary bladder (Table 1) and are rare in cats (Table 2). They may invade the kidney or ureter or metastasize to more distant sites. Because of their location within the renal pelvis, they may be expected to cause hydronephrosis before attaining a large size. The fact that urothelium maintains the embryonic potential to produce mucus-secreting glandular epithelium and squamous epithelium in addition to transitional epithelium accounts for the occurrence of different morphologic varieties of urothelial carcinomas, including transitional cell carcinomas and squamous cell carcinomas. It appears that the sequence of events leading to development of transitional cell and squamous cell neoplasms is similar in all species. Studies in man, dogs, and laboratory animals have revealed that urothelial cellular hyperplasia precedes formation of many malignant transitional cell neoplasms.

Metastases usually occur via the lymphatics to regional lymph nodes. The lungs and liver are the most common sites of distant metastases, but any organ or tissue may be involved, especially in terminal stages.

Sarcomas (fibrosarcomas, leiomyosarcomas, rhabdomyosarcomas, undifferentiated sarcomas) of the kidneys of dogs and cats are less common than epithelial neoplasms or nephroblastomas (Tables 1 and 2). They frequently penetrate adjacent tissue and are associated with widespread metastases.

Metastatic. Metastatic neoplasms are commonly found in the kidneys. This may be related, at least in part, to the large blood volume that the kidneys receive and their abundant supply of capillaries. Focal accumulations of malignant cells in the kidneys usually are not associated with clinical signs of renal disease. Most patients succumb as a result of neoplastic destruction of some other body organ or tissue before signs referable to renal disease have time to develop.

Malignant lymphoma is the most common renal neoplasm of cats (Table 3), but it is less frequently encountered in the kidneys of dogs (Table 4). Dogs with malignant lymphomas have renal involvement in less than 50 percent of cases. Even fewer cases are associated with renal failure secondary to generalized neoplas-

Table 3. *Age and Sex Characteristics of 40 Cats with Malignant Lymphoma Involving the Kidneys*[*]

AGE			SEX		
MEAN	RANGE	NOT DETERMINED	MALE	FEMALE	NOT DETERMINED
6	1–15	6	20	12	8

[*]Data from the University of Minnesota Veterinary Teaching Hospital, the Veterinary Medical Data Program sponsored by the National Cancer Institute, and the literature.

tic renal destruction. In cats the abdominal form of malignant lymphoma is usually associated with extensive renal involvement. Both kidneys are usually affected and may be palpated as enlarged asymmetric structures in the abdominal cavity. Renal failure caused by bilateral renal lymphoma occurs more commonly in cats than in dogs. Non-specific clinical signs include progressive weight loss, depression, anorexia, vomiting, and diarrhea. Cachexia, fever, anemia, and secondary infections occur during terminal phases.

CLINICAL SIGNS AND DIAGNOSIS

Clinical signs vary with location, size, and duration of neoplasia. Neoplasms of the renal pelvis are usually associated with local signs (hematuria, hydronephrosis, and others) that precede polysystemic signs. This pattern is often opposite to that observed in patients with renal parenchymal neoplasms.

Clinical signs of renal cell carcinomas are non-specific and may not indicate involvement of the urinary system initially. Local signs include persistent or intermittent gross or microscopic hematuria and abdominal distention with an associated palpable mass. Enlarged kidneys caused by neoplasia must be differentiated from enlarged kidneys caused by hydronephrosis or polycystic disease. In addition, neoplastic enlargement of the kidneys must be differentiated from neoplastic enlargement of one or both adrenal glands and the ovaries,

spleen, liver, pancreas, and intestine. Even though both kidneys are involved, a sufficient quantity of functional renal parenchyma may persist to prevent signs of renal failure. Extensive bilateral involvement of the kidneys that destroys 70 to 75 percent or more of the nephrons will be associated with signs of progressive renal insufficiency.

Polysystemic signs unrelated to the urinary tract are common and may be the first clinical manifestation of renal carcinomas. Anemia, pyrexia, anorexia, and weight loss have been commonly reported. Polysystemic clinical signs may be related to production of excessive quantities of erythrocyte-stimulating factor, renin, parathormone, prostaglandins, and other hormones by these neoplasms. Polycythemia has been reported in dogs with renal cell carcinomas that elaborated excessive quantities of erythrocyte-stimulating factor. Clinical signs may be caused by metastatic lesions and on occasion may be the first evidence of their presence.

Clinical signs associated with nephroblastomas are similar to those associated with renal cell carcinomas. Hypertrophic osteoarthropathy has been observed in dogs with renal tumors. In one case characteristic bony lesions of this syndrome developed in the absence of detectable pulmonary metastases.

Intravenous urography (IVU) will often help to localize the site of neoplasia and may permit estimation of the extent of renal parenchymal involvement. Distortion in the shape of the

Table 4. *Age and Sex Characteristics of 10 Dogs with Malignant Lymphoma Involving the Kidney*[*]

AGE			SEX		
MEAN	RANGE	NOT DETERMINED	MALE	FEMALE	NOT DETERMINED
5.5	6 mo–15 yr	1	3	5	2

[*]Data from the University of Minnesota Veterinary Teaching Hospital, the Veterinary Medical Data Program sponsored by the National Cancer Institute, and the literature.

renal pelvis and diverticula and retention of contrast medium are generally seen in the neoplastic kidney. Lack of excretion of detectable quantities of radiopaque contrast material suggests severe hydronephrosis. Selective angiography may also be performed to delineate the precise location and extent of renal destruction. Renal neoplasms associated with enlargement of the kidneys must be differentiated from hydronephrosis and polycystic disease.

The only means by which a definitive antemortem diagnosis may be established is by microscopic identification of neoplastic cells. This may be accomplished by biopsy of the kidney or by detection of neoplastic cells in urine sediment. Needle biopsy of a unilateral renal neoplasm may be inadvisable if treatment by surgical extirpation is contemplated, since the potential for iatrogenic metastasis exists. An exploratory celiotomy is advised in such cases because a biopsy may be obtained with less risk of metastasis, the abdomen may be explored for metastases, and nephrectomy can be performed for treatment. In cases with suspected bilateral involvement the risk of iatrogenic metastasis should not preclude percutaneous needle biopsy, since the neoplasm is inoperable.

TREATMENT

If the neoplasm has not metastasized and if the opposite kidney is not neoplastic and has adequate function, nephrectomy and partial ureterectomy are indicated. We suggest that preoperative abdominal palpation be restricted to prevent rupture of the tumor and seeding of the abdomen with neoplastic cells. Adequate surgical exposure, careful manipulation of the affected kidney, and ligation of the renal vein are advised prior to mobilizing the tumor so as to prevent release of neoplastic cells into the blood stream. In addition to complete removal of the tumor, the associated ureter should be removed, since metastasis may occur anywhere along its length. Systematic dissection and excision of regional lymph nodes are advised in order to prevent inadvertent incomplete removal of tumor cells within lymphatics. We have had no experience with the use of irradiation and chemotherapeutic agents in the treatment of renal cell carcinomas, primary renal tumors arising from the urothelium, or sarcomas. Clinical and experimental studies in man suggest limited success.

Chemotherapy has offered great advances in the management of embryonal nephroma in man. Use of actinomycin D has been associated with prevention of metastasis. In addition to laboratory evidence for a direct tumoricidal effect, this drug also appears to be a radiosensitizer that augments the effect of radiation on embryonal nephromas. The drug acts by binding the guanine moiety of deoxyribonucleic acid, thereby preventing the formation of ribonucleic acid polymerase. As a result of suppressed ribonucleic acid and protein synthesis, cellular damage occurs. It has been shown that repeated doses of actinomycin D are much more effective than a single dose in preventing relapse of metastatic disease. Unfortunately, actinomycin D has many toxic side effects, including depression of bone marrow, liver damage, interference with wound healing, alopecia, depression of immune response, and ulceration of the alimentary tract. Serial monitoring of packed cell volume (PCV), white blood count (WBC) and platelet count are recommended during therapy to evaluate the degree of toxicity.

Although we have not used vincristine in the management of nephroblastomas, it is a chemotherapeutic agent that has been used with success in the treatment of nephroblastomas in man. It is much less toxic than actinomycin D and has a synergistic effect when combined with that drug. Its use in combined therapy may greatly decrease risks of toxic side effects encountered with actinomycin D.

The use of irradiation following surgery was introduced in man in the 1940's and significantly improved survival rates. It is probable that cancer cells dislodged during surgery or left behind because of incomplete excision are destroyed by irradiation. Radiotherapy should be initiated shortly after surgery. Generally 3000 to 4000 rads should be delivered to the midline of the tumor bed at the rate of 1000 rads/week.

We have successfully controlled a unilateral nephroblastoma with metastases in a one-year-old female mixed-breed dog by surgical extirpation of the right kidney, local irradiation of tissue adjacent to the right kidney, and periodic administration of actinomycin D (Cosmegen) (0.015 mg/kg daily for five days). Combination therapy, incorporating principles of surgical management, radiotherapy, and chemotherapy, has been extremely effective in management of embryonal nephromas in man. Cure rates of 70 to 80 percent have been reported, even in patients with metastatic disease.

PROGNOSIS

The prognosis is dependent on the type, location and extent of neoplastic involvement, the presence or absence of metastases, and the biologic behavior of the neoplasm. A guarded to good prognosis is justified following complete surgical extirpation of a unilateral malignant neoplasm. Unfortunately, early diagnosis is not the rule and metastasis is often present, particularly with parenchymal tumors. In cases in which there is bilateral renal involvement or metastases or in which treatment is not provided, a guarded to poor prognosis should be offered.

NEOPLASMS OF THE URETER

Primary neoplasms of the ureter of dogs are rare (Table 5). Limited clinical experience suggests that a good prognosis is associated with nephroureterectomy of benign and malignant neoplasms confined to the ureter. Clinical signs are usually associated with hydronephrosis. On occasion, neoplasms originating from abdominal organs or tissues encroach upon ureters, occlude their lumina, and cause hydronephrosis. Occlusion of the distal ends of ureters by bladder neoplasms invading the trigone is the most common cause of neoplastic involvement of the ureters. Primary neoplasms of the ureter have not been reported in cats.

NEOPLASMS OF THE URINARY BLADDER

ETIOPATHOGENESIS

Benign and malignant neoplasms of the epithelial lining of the urinary bladder are more common than epithelial neoplasms of the renal pelves, ureters, and urethra (Tables 1,2,6 and 7). The higher incidence of primary epithelial neoplasms in the urinary bladder may be associated with storage of urine. Storage of urine in the bladder may enhance the action of carcinogenic agents by allowing increased contact time with tissue. Neoplasms of the urinary bladder are less common in cats than in dogs. This may result from a difference in the metabolism of potentially carcinogenic agents, including tryptophan.

Unlike those in humans, canine and feline urothelial neoplasms of the bladder are more common in females (Tables 6 and 7). In all species studied, most epithelial and connective tissue tumors of the bladder were associated with advancing age (Tables 6 and 7). An exception is rhabdomyosarcoma of the urinary bladder. This neoplasm is typically encountered at a young age in dogs; it has not been reported in cats.

TYPES

Benign. Papillomas of the canine and feline urinary bladder have been encountered less frequently than carcinomas of the urinary bladder (Tables 6 and 7). Although papillomas may occur at any age, they are more common in older dogs. The biologic behavior of naturally occurring urothelial papillomas of dogs and cats is unknown, although they have been removed from patients without recurrence. The size of papillomas is variable (microscopic to several centimeters); they may be single or multiple. As papillomas enlarge they tend to become ulcerated. Ulceration, which frequently is aggravated by bacterial infection, is commonly associated with persistent hematuria.

Fibromas and leiomyomas may be single or multiple. They often grow slowly and therefore are usually asymptomatic. Larger tumors may protrude into the lumen of the urinary bladder but usually do not produce clinical signs until they become large enough to cause mechanical interference with micturition.

Malignant. Carcinomas are the most common primary malignant tumor of the urinary bladder of dogs and cats (Tables 6 and 7).

Table 5. *Neoplasm Type, Age, and Sex Characteristics of 5 Dogs with Primary Ureter Neoplasms**

TUMOR TYPE	NO. OF CASES	SEX		AGE (Years)	
		MALE	FEMALE	MEAN	RANGE
Epithelial tissue					
Papilloma	1	1	0	2	2
Transitional cell carcinoma	3	0	3	10.6	8–15
Muscle tissue					
Leiomyoma	1	0	1	11	11
TOTAL	5	1	4	7.8	2–15

*Data from the University of Minnesota Veterinary Teaching Hospital, the Veterinary Medical Data Program sponsored by the National Cancer Institute, and the literature.

Table 6. *Neoplasm Type, Age, and Sex Characteristics of 297 Dogs with Primary Neoplasms of the Urinary Bladder**

TUMOR TYPE	NO. OF CASES	SEX			AGE (Years)		
		MALE	FEMALE	NOT DETERMINED	MEAN	RANGE	NOT DETERMINED
Epithelial tissue							
Papilloma	7	0	3	4	11.1	10–12.5	3
Fibroadenoma	1	1	–	–	10	10	–
Adenocarcinoma	15	9	6	–	10	2–15	–
Squamous cell carcinoma	19	10	8	1	9.9	5–15	1
Transitional cell carcinoma	143	60	81	2	10.2	2–15	–
Unclassified carcinoma	42	8	13	21	8.9	4–13	15
Muscle tissue							
Leiomyoma	12	1	2	9	12.7	12–13	7
Leiomyosarcoma	12	4	8	–	6.7	2–13	1
Botryoid rhabdomyosarcoma	11	3	5	3	1.7	1–5	4
Connective tissue							
Fibroma	12	0	2	10	7	4–11	7
Fibrosarcoma	8	4	3	1	6.3	1–15	1
Unclassified sarcoma	7	3	2	2	3.6	1–5	–
Vascular tissue							
Hemangioma	2	1	0	1	10	10	1
Hemangiosarcoma	6	5	1	–	9.3	2–15	–
TOTAL	297	109	134	54	8.3	1–15	40

*Data from the University of Minnesota Veterinary Teaching Hospital, the Veterinary Medical Data Program sponsored by the National Cancer Institute, and the literature.

Although transitional cell carcinomas have been observed most frequently, squamous cell carcinomas, adenocarcinomas, and undifferentiated carcinomas are potential morphologic varieties arising from bladder urothelium.

Carcinomas may occur as solitary or multiple papillary projections that involve the bladder mucosa or as local or diffuse swellings of the bladder wall, or both. The non-papillary variety has been encountered most frequently in dogs. Invasion of the bladder wall is common, especially with non-papillary varieties. The mucosa and underlying muscle layers may be completely destroyed and replaced with neoplastic cells. Neoplastic tissue may occlude the urethra or ureters (or both) and cause hydronephrosis. Metastases occur frequently and most commonly involve the lungs and lymph nodes.

Table 7. *Neoplasm Type, Age, and Sex Characteristics of 24 Cats with Primary Neoplasms of the Urinary Bladder**

TUMOR TYPE	NO. OF CASES	SEX			AGE (Years)		
		MALE	FEMALE	NOT DETERMINED	MEAN	RANGE	NOT DETERMINED
Epithelial tissue							
Papilloma	2	–	1	1	1.2	0.33–2	–
Cystadenoma	1	–	1	–	12	12	–
Transitional cell carcinoma	10	1	6	3	10.6	3–15	1
Squamous cell carcinoma	1	–	–	1	–	–	1
Adenocarcinoma	1	–	–	1	–	–	1
Unclassified carcinoma	5	3	–	2	13.3	13–14	2
Connective tissue							
Myxosarcoma	1	1	–	–	6	6	–
Muscular tissue							
Leiomyoma	1	–	1	–	12	12	–
Leiomyosarcoma	2	–	2	–	9.8	8.5–11	–
TOTAL	24	5	11	8	9.3	0.33–15	5

*Data from the University of Minnesota Veterinary Teaching Hospital, the Veterinary Medical Data Program sponsored by the National Cancer Institute, and the literature.

Sarcomas have been encountered much less commonly than carcinomas, but when present they are usually characterized by diffuse invasive growth into the bladder wall and metastases.

Metastatic tumors of the urinary bladder have been observed infrequently and were usually not associated with clinical signs.

CLINICAL SIGNS AND DIAGNOSIS

Signs referable to the urinary tract induced by benign or malignant urothelial or connective tissue bladder neoplasms are similar. Intermittent hematuria is frequently observed by owners. Owners often indicate that a wide variety of medications have been used to treat hematuria without success. Increased frequency of urination, a less common complaint, occurs as a result of associated cystitis or reduction in bladder capacity, or both, because of the large size of the neoplasm. On occasion, urinary incontinence may be observed. Urinary incontinence may be caused by partial obstruction of urine outflow (so-called paradoxical incontinence) or destruction of the detrusor muscle. Anorexia and depression are less common complaints.

Neoplasms that are at an early and potentially curable stage usually do not produce abnormalities detectable by physical examination alone. Later, after tumor growth, clinical signs are similar to those associated with cystitis. Cystitis is a frequent complication of bladder neoplasia because bacteria readily invade the necrotic and ulcerated surface of neoplasms and stimulate an inflammatory response. Partial or complete obstruction of the urethra may cause dysuria, urinary incontinence, a decrease in the size of the urine stream, overdistention of the bladder with urine, hydronephrosis, signs referable to renal failure, or a combination of these. Obstruction of the ureters at the bladder trigone may also cause signs referable to obstructive uropathy.

Signs referable to metastatic lesions may occur but are uncommon until advanced stages of neoplasia. Hypertrophic pulmonary osteoarthropathy has been observed in several dogs with malignant bladder neoplasia.

Urinalysis may be of value when investigating possible neoplastic diseases of the urinary bladder. Renal function tests will be normal unless there is obstruction of urine flow from both kidneys. The results of urinalysis may be indicative of cystitis (i.e., proteinuria, hematuria, pyuria, and bacteriuria). In uninfected or treated patients red blood cells may dominate the microscopic findings in urine sediment.

Neoplastic cells may also be found in urine sediment, especially in patients that have carcinoma.

Evaluation of the morphology of various types of cells (especially transitional epithelial cells) in urine sediment is of proven value in the investigation of neoplastic diseases of the bladder. A diagnosis of neoplasia following examination of cytologic preparations is based on multiple criteria, including abnormal changes in the nuclei and cytoplasm of individual cells and modification of normal intercellular architecture. Recognition of benign or well-differentiated malignant neoplasms on the basis of cytologic preparations may be difficult, since exfoliated cells may differ little from hyperplastic or normal transitional epithelial cells. Regardless of the type and degree of differentiation of the underlying neoplasm, secondary bacterial infection of neoplastic lesions may result in collection of samples that are composed primarily of inflammatory cells and that contain relatively few neoplastic cells. Thus, a negative result does not exclude neoplasia. Because of difficulties sometimes encountered in evaluating the significance of biopsy findings, results should always be interpreted in association with other clinical, laboratory, and radiographic findings.

Bladder neoplasms are sometimes difficult to demonstrate radiographically, especially if they are diffuse. Radiographic findings are not pathognomonic, as they may be the same as those associated with chronic cystitis. Neoplasms that protrude into the lumen of the bladder may be visualized as space-occupying masses. Pneumocystography, positive-contrast cystography, or double-contrast cystography may be used to enhance visualization of such masses.

A definitive diagnosis of bladder neoplasia must be based on microscopic detection and evaluation of neoplastic cells in urine sediment or in biopsy samples obtained via catheter biopsy, cystoscopy, or exploratory celiotomy. Even when the bladder is examined visually at the time of surgery, differentiation between diffuse neoplasia and cystitis may be difficult because the tissue may be necrotic, inflamed, ulcerated, and thickened in either condition. In such circumstances the lesions should be biopsied, preferably by complete excision, so that a histopathologic diagnosis can be established. When excision biopsy is impossible, multiple specimens should be obtained from large solitary lesions, or several lesions should be sampled if many smaller growths are present. The internal iliac and lumbar lymph nodes should be examined and, if necessary, biopsied at the time of celiotomy in order to confirm or eliminate the possibility of metastasis.

TREATMENT

Therapy for bladder neoplasms may be curative or palliative. Therapeutic results are related to the type of tumor, its location, and the presence or absence of metastasis. Untreated, the majority of animals with malignant bladder neoplasms will succumb from direct or indirect manifestations of the disease. Current methods available to treat bladder neoplasia include surgery and radiation.

Neoplasms located in accessible areas of the bladder should be removed by partial cystectomy. The neoplastic tissue and a wide zone of healthy tissue, including the entire depth of the bladder wall, should be removed. Ureteral transplantation may be necessary. Tumors that occupy the neck of the bladder, the trigone, or a great portion of the bladder surface and wall cannot be removed by partial cystectomy. Total cystectomy and transplantation of the ureters into the intestines or an ileal conduit may be considered, but postoperative complications and loss of normal function make such an approach impractical for most household pets.

Adjunctive radiotherapy may be of benefit following partial cystectomy of malignant neoplasms of the bladder. Irradiation may destroy neoplastic tissue not removed by surgery and may also be of value in cases in which total excision is impossible. Radiotherapy techniques involve local application of radon packs or radon seeds.

It is usually necessary to treat the patient for cystitis following surgery. Because of the possibility of postoperative recurrence of the neoplasm, periodic examination of the patient, including radiography and examination of the urine sediment for neoplastic cells, is recommended.

PROGNOSIS

The location, extent, histologic appearance, and depth of penetration are important factors to be considered when establishing a prognosis. The site of the neoplasm is often as closely related to the future course of events as is the histopathologic type. In cases in which complete surgical extirpation of solitary non-infiltrating benign tumors has been performed, a fair to good prognosis is justified. In cases in which malignant neoplasms have been surgically removed, a guarded to fair prognosis should be offered because of the tendency of these tumors to recur and metastasize. In general, tumors that have penetrated the mucosa are more likely to recur and become metastatic than are non-invasive neoplasms. In cases in which no treatment is given or in which the neoplasm has metastasized, a guarded to poor prognosis should be offered. The poor results generally reported in the treatment of urinary bladder neoplasms of dogs and cats are partially related to the fact that the initial diagnosis is usually not established until the condition is inoperable.

NEOPLASMS OF THE URETHRA

Primary neoplasms of the urethra are uncommon in dogs and rare in cats. Canine urethral neoplasms have been observed predominately in females (Table 8); there is increased risk

Table 8. *Neoplasm Type, Age, and Sex Characteristics of 43 Dogs with Primary Neoplasms of the Urethra**

| TUMOR TYPE | NO. OF CASES | SEX | | | AGE (Years) | | |
		MALE	FEMALE	NOT DETERMINED	MEAN	RANGE	NOT DETERMINED
Epithelial tissue							
Adenoma	4	–	–	4	–	–	4
Adenosarcoma	4	1	2	1	10.6	6–14	1
Squamous cell carcinoma	13	0	13	–	11	8–13	–
Transitional cell carcinoma	17	2	15	–	10.5	6 mo–15 yr	1
Unclassified carcinoma	1	0	1	–	15	15	–
Connective tissue							
Myxosarcoma	1	0	1	–	9	9	–
Muscle tissue							
Rhabdomyosarcoma	1	1	0	–	3	3	–
Vascular tissue							
Hemangiosarcoma	2	0	2	–	9.5	9–10	–
TOTAL	43	4	34	5	9.8	6 mo–15 yr	6

*Data from the University of Minnesota Veterinary Teaching Hospital, the Veterinary Medical Data Program sponsored by the National Cancer Institute, and the literature.

associated with increased age. Although unproved, it has been suggested that these neoplasms may arise from hyperplastic tissue resulting from irritation associated with chronic urethritis. Epithelial tumors have been the most common type encountered and include squamous cell carcinomas, transitional cell carcinomas, and adenocarcinomas. Other tumor types have rarely been observed. Metastasis to regional lymph nodes has been observed frequently at necropsy. A non-metastatic transitional cell carcinoma has been reported in the urethra of a six-year-old male domestic shorthaired cat.

Dysuria is a constant sign and presumably occurs as a result of obstruction of the urethral lumen and irritation of the urethral mucosa. Hematuria is a common but not invariable sign and may occur independent of micturition. Urinary incontinence may develop as a result of damage to the urethral sphincter mechanism or partial obstruction of urine outflow (so-called paradoxical incontinence). If urethral obstruction is severe or prolonged, varying degrees of postrenal azotemia or hydronephrosis may develop. In the latter instance a distended, turgid urinary bladder may be detected by abdominal palpation. If the neoplasm is extensive, rectal palpation may reveal thickening and irregularity of the urethra.

Localization of urethral neoplasms may be aided by palpation, catheterization, retrograde contrast urethrography, cystoscopy, or exploratory surgery. Inability to pass the catheter through the urethral lumen or abnormal resistance during insertion of the catheter may be detected. Retrograde positive-contrast urethrography is extremely valuable in tumor localization. Biopsy of mucosal neoplasms may be obtained with the aid of a urinary catheter.

Treatment is usually limited to surgical excision of operable lesions. Radiation therapy and chemotherapeutic measures are unproved as effective therapeutic modalities.

SUPPLEMENTAL READING

Baskin, G.B., and DePaoli, A.: Primary renal neoplasms of the dog. Vet. Pathol., 14:591–605, 1977.
Caywood, D.D., Osborne, C.A., Stevens, J.B., Jessen, C.R., and O'Leary, T.P.: Hypertrophic osteoarthropathy associated with an atypical nephroblastoma in a dog. (In preparation)
Hayes, H.M., and Fraumeni, J.F.: Epidemiological features of canine renal neoplasms. Cancer Res., 37:2553–2556, 1977.
Hayes, H.M.: Canine bladder cancer: Epidemiologic features. Am. J. Epidemiol. 104:673–677, 1976.
Melhoff, T., and Osborne, C.A.: Catheter biopsy of the urethra, urinary bladder and prostate gland. In Kirk, R.W. (ed.): Current Veterinary Therapy VI. Philadelphia, W.B. Saunders Co., 1977, pp. 1173–1175.
Osborne, C.A., et al.: Rental lymphoma in the dog and cat. J. Am. Vet. Med. Assoc., 158:2058–2070, 1971.
Osborne, C.A., Low, D.G., and Finco, D.R.: Canine and Feline Urology. Philadelphia, W.B. Saunders Co., 1972.
Osborne, C.A., et al.: Neoplasms of the canine and feline urinary bladder: Incidence, etiologic factors, occurence and pathologic features. Am. J. Vet. Res., 29:2041–2055, 1968.
Tarvin, G., Patnaik, A., and Greene, R.: Primary urethral tumors in dogs. J. Am. Vet. Med. Assoc., 172:931–933, 1978.

The Genital System

DYSTOCIA

EDWARD F. DONOVAN, D.V.M.
Columbus, Ohio

Abnormal or difficult parturition, or dystocia, is a common and challenging problem. Each veterinarian must develop a philosophy for solving dystocia that is best suited to his or her technical and diagnostic skills. The most difficult problem is often the choice among drug therapy manual delivery, and cesarean section. Factors that must be considered include the nature of the dystocia, physical condition of the bitch, available equipment, and time. In addition, the utility of the bitch and the economic value of the puppies should be considered.

Many cases of dystocia can be prevented by proper care during the gestation period. The bitch should have regular exercise and her diet should be regulated to prevent obesity. As a guidline, her postwhelping body weight should not exceed her normal pregestational body weight by more than 5 to 10 percent. Blood hemoglobin, hematocrit, and total serum protein values should be measured during the fourth and seventh week of gestation to evaluate the bitch's general health and nutritional state. Classification of dystocia as maternal, fetal, or due to uterine inertia helps in the decision-making process.

Maternal dystocia may occur in any breed, but it is more common in Scottish terriers, Boston terriers, English bulldogs, Sealyhams, and Pekingese. Maternal dystocia can be subdivided by cause into anatomic, endocrine, and psychologic (behavioral) types. Anatomic causes include (1) pelvic structure that has a tendency to be flattened dorsoventrally, which occurs in breeds such as Scottish terriers and Sealyhams, (2) fractures or other injuries that compromise the lumen of the pelvic canal, and (3) torsion of the gravid uterus. Endocrine dysfunction is characterized by (1) small litter size for the breed, (2) minimal labial and mammary enlargement, (3) lack of amniotic fluid, or (4) prolonged gestation. Psychologic stress is seen in pampered house pets and some toy breeds.

Fetal dystocia is associated with oversize puppies, brachycephalic puppies, fetal hydrocephalus, abnormal position of the head or buttocks at the pelvic inlet, and fetal edema, as seen in English bulldogs. Irregular limb posture is rarely of consequence in dogs or cats.

Uterine inertia may be primary or secondary. Primary uterine inertia is caused by a lack of tone or degenerative (geriatric) changes in the uterine musculature. It may occur in any breed. Lack of exercise, obesity, and excessive stretching of the uterus by fluid and/or fetuses are factors that cause or contribute to uterine inertia. Secondary uterine inertia is primarily a result of exhaustion and is the most common problem we are called upon to handle. It is most often seen in animals with large litters, older bitches with normal litters, or obese bitches. It is often followed by retained fetal membranes, prolonged postpartum hemorrhage, or subinvolution of the uterus.

Clinical signs of dystocia vary considerably. Bitches with uterine inertia may have few signs. As a rule, they are often depressed, make frequent attempts to urinate, and labor with their heads extended dorsally and their mouths open. If this is allowed to persist, they may go into shock and should be treated for that before attempting delivery of the puppies. A greenish-black discharge indicating placental separation is normal in most whelping bitches; however, its presence without evidence of approaching labor is indication for intervention.

All cases of dystocia should receive immediate medical attention. A good history (particularly of previous whelpings), a quick but thorough physical examination (including abdominal palpation for pregnancy, approximate number of fetuses, fetal movement, and fetal heart beat), and a vaginal examination should be performed. If time is available before the vaginal examination, the bladder should be emptied and an enema administered. The vulvar area should be clipped, if necessary, and thoroughly disinfected. The examination should include evaluation of pelvic size, feathering (linear pressure on the dorsal vaginal wall) to determine the presence or absence of uterine contractions, evaluation of the condition of the cervix, and determination of the location and position of the fetuses. If the fetuses cannot be palpated through the vagina, instrument delivery would be highly questionable because of the trauma involved in probing for the puppies.

Maternal dystocia is best handled by cesarean section or manual delivery. The latter is reserved for those cases in which there are one or two puppies and economic considerations do not warrant a cesarean section. In those in which it is felt that psychologic factors are delaying parturition, small doses of tranquilizers (Sparine®, Wyeth, 1 mg/kg) in a quiet home environment may be tried.

Primary and secondary uterine inertia should be considered medical problems initially. A combination of calcium lactate and oxytocin is used in an attempt to stimulate uterine contractions. The animal is first given 2.5 to 10 ml of calcium lactate intravenously to sensitize the uterus to the action of oxytocin. Ten minutes later, 5 to 20 units of oxytocin are given intramuscularly. The bitch is placed in a quiet environment and the oxytocin may be repeated at 20-minute intervals. If active labor is not initiated within one to one and one-half hours, further medical therapy is not indicated. Instrument delivery using clam-shell forceps should be attempted if the puppies (one or two) can be moved to the pelvic inlet. Failing this, surgical intervention is indicated. It is important that the bitch's condition not be allowed to deteriorate to such a point that surgical intervention is unduly hazardous.

With the exception of grossly oversized puppies, fetal dystocia can usually be handled by manual extraction. Episiotomy may be necessary when the puppies have large heads or the bitch has a small vulva. When either the head or buttocks can be grasped, gentle traction may be applied to coincide with uterine contractions. Traction should be on a horizontal plane until the head or buttocks are delivered, then directed ventrally at a 45-degree angle until the delivery is completed. Lubrication of the vaginal canal with K-Y® jelly is a must prior to forced extraction. Postural abnormalities are best handled by grasping the head or buttocks with clam-shell forceps, repelling the puppy by abdominal manipulation, and directing it into the pelvic canal. The bitch should be allowed to expel the puppy normally or with slight traction. If secondary uterine inertia is present as a result of prolonged labor, it may be necessary to administer calcium and oxytocin, as mentioned previously. Slightly oversized puppies may become locked in the pelvic canal at either the shoulders or buttocks. They should be manipulated in a side-to-side manner to facilitate delivery.

In summary, dystocia presents a particularly complex problem for the clinician. However, careful consideration of the type of dystocia, condition of the bitch and puppies, and experience of the veterinarian will usually result in successful management of the condition. If in doubt, prompt cesarean section is recommended.

ACUTE METRITIS

ALAN J. LIPOWITZ, D.V.M.,
and ROLF E. LARSEN, D.V.M.
St. Paul, Minnesota

Acute metritis is a uterine bacterial disease of the immediate postpartum period. It is most common following dystocia, especially those cases attended by obstetrical manipulations, and is often associated with retained placental or fetal tissues. However, it can also occur following natural or artificial insemination or natural delivery. Uterine involution is delayed, resulting in an enlarged flaccid uterus, thus creating a favorable environment for bacterial growth. Gram-negative bacilli are the most common causative agents. All uterine layers are affected by the acute inflammatory process and, although the uterine wall may be thickened, it can be quite friable, especially at areas of placental attachment.

CLINICAL SIGNS AND LABORATORY FINDINGS

Clinical signs may include pyrexia, depression, loss of maternal instincts, and a foul-smelling vaginal discharge. In advanced cases affected animals may be hypothermic, dehydrated, and weak.

Following an uncomplicated delivery the normal vaginal discharge is dark green to brown in color and odorless. Within 12 hours following complete passage of the fetal membranes the discharge becomes more mucoid and clear, although it may be blood-tinged. Persistence of a dark-green to reddish-brown, thick, and usually foul-smelling discharge 12 to 24 hours following delivery is indicative of acute metritis.

Physical examination usually reveals an elevated body temperature and increased heart and respiratory rates. The enlarged uterus can usually be delineated by abdominal palpation, and radiography will verify the presence of retained fetuses.

An immature neutrophilic leukocytosis is usually seen on the hemogram, although a normal count with hypersegmented neutrophils may be found. Packed cell volume and serum protein values may be elevated as a result of the hemoconcentration of dehydration. Hepatic and renal function test results may be altered as well.

Microscopic examination of the vaginal discharge usually reveals clusters of endometrial cells, hypersegmented and degenerating neutrophils, cellular debris, mucus, and bacteria. Organisms may be seen both inside and outside cells.

THERAPY

Therapeutic success depends on the duration of illness. Because of the acute progressive nature of the condition, any sign of developing metritis is cause for immediate treatment.

Initial treatment should consist of administration of broad-spectrum antibiotics and intravenous fluid replacement if dehydration is evident. Material for bacterial culture and antibiotic sensitivity should be obtained from the region of the cervix, and further antibiotic administration should be based on the results. Treatment of acute metritis uncomplicated by retained placental tissues in breeding animals consists of uterine drainage, antibacterial medication, and supportive fluid therapy. Nitrofurazone, soluble tetracyclines, gentamicin, or other broad-spectrum antibiotics may be used for uterine infusion until results of antimicrobial sensitivity tests are available.

A plastic insemination pipette with a smooth tip that can be manipulated through a vaginoscope or speculum is satisfactory for uterine infusion. A vaginoscope or speculum 5 to 6 inches in length may be needed even in small bitches. The tip of the pipette should be placed against the folds of the cervix at the external os. Because of the fragile nature of the uterine wall, infusion should be done without actually passing the pipette into the uterus. If the cervix is not immediately recognized, the folds of the fornix may be probed gently with the infusion pipette until the opening is found. Several attempts at proper placement of the pipette are often necessary. Once the uterine opening is identified, a soft rubber catheter may be passed for infusion of the antibiotic solution. In some bitches gentle ventral traction of the uterine body by external abdominal manipulation will align the cervix with the vagina and allow easy identification of the external os and passage of the catheter.

Uterine involution and evacuation can be hastened by intramuscular administration of oxytocin (0.5 units/kg body weight). This dosage can be repeated within one to two hours. Estrogens enhance the effects of oxytocin. They may be given intramuscularly one time only in the form of ECP (estradiol 17β-cypionate) at a dosage of 0.02 mg/kg or repositol diethylstilbestrol, 0.5 mg/kg, 25 mg maximum. Estrogens may reduce lactation and can cause suppression of bone marrow function. Therefore, they must be used with caution. Ergonovine has a more intense effect on myometrial activity than does oxytocin. It may be given intramuscularly at a dose of 0.2 mg/15 kg body weight only after repeated administration of oxytocin has proved inadequate.

Prostaglandin $F_{2\alpha}$ is now being investigated to promote uterine evacuation. When given subcutaneously in proper doses it will cause dilation of the uterine cervix and uterine contractions. As yet, prostaglandin $F_{2\alpha}$ is not approved for use in dogs, except as an experimental drug.

Surgical procedures used to augment medical management of acute metritis include ovariohysterectomy, intra-abdominal uterine massage, and hysterotomy and uterine lavage. Ovariohysterectomy is recommended only in situations of retained fetal tissues or when severe infection and uterine erosions threaten the animal's life. Ovariohysterectomy has also been recommended when the bitch or queen is no longer desired by the owner as a breeding animal. A generous abdominal incision should be made to allow easy manipulation of the friable uterus and to give adequate exposure of both ovaries, the uterine horns, and the cervix. Use of laparotomy sponges is recommended to pack off other abdominal viscera and to prevent contamination should uterine rupture occur. In the compromised or debilitated patient aggressive medical management should be combined with surgery.

A technique of uterine massage and lavage has been successful in several longer-standing cases of postpartum metritis in which medical management did not control the uterine infection. After a catheter is placed through the cervix into the uterus, the uterus is examined through a ventral midline abdominal incision. Lavage solution is passed into the uterus by the catheter while the uterine horns are gently massaged to break up accumulated debris. The uterine contents are drained and the lavage and massage regime repeated two or three more times. Antibiotics are then instilled in the uterus, the catheter is removed, and the abdomen is closed routinely.

A hysterotomy at the uterine bifurcation has been recommended to remove intrauterine debris in cases in which a catheter could not be passed through the cervix. Prior to uterine manipulation and lavage or hysterotomy, the uterus must be carefully examined. Dark, swollen, discolored areas and palpable crater-like defects or swellings in the uterine wall are indicative of endometritis. Because manipulation may rupture such a uterus and cause severe peritonitis ovariohysterectomy should be performed instead.

SUPPLEMENTAL READING

Burke, T.J.: Acute metritis. In Kirk, R.W. (ed.): *Current Veterinary Therapy* V. Philadelphia, W.B. Saunders, 1974, pp. 923–924.

Burke, T.J.: Postparturient problems in the bitch. Vet. Clin. North Am., 7:693–698, 1977.

Durfee, P.T.: Surgical treatment of postparturient metritis in the bitch. J. Am. Vet. Med. Assoc., 153:40–42, 1968.

Herron, M.R., and Herron, M.A.: Surgery of the uterus. Vet. Clin. North Am., 5:471–476, 1975.

Larsen, R.E., and Wilson, J.W.: Acute metritis. In Kirk, R.W. (ed.): *Current Veterinary Therapy* VI. Philadelphia, W.B. Saunders, 1977, pp. 1227–1229.

CANINE PYOMETRA

ROBERT M. HARDY, D.V.M.
St. Paul, Minnesota,

and DAVID F. SENIOR, B.V.Sc.
Gainesville, Florida

Canine pyometra is an acute or chronic diestral disease of the mature bitch with systemic signs related to both genital and extragenital lesions.

PATHOGENESIS OF GENITAL LESIONS

Pyometra is a complication of cystic endometrial hyperplasia (CEH), which develops during diestrus. The diestral period of the normal, non-pregnant bitch lasts approximately 70 days when the uterus is under the influence of progesterone produced by ovarian corpora lutea. Progesterone induces proliferation of endometrial glands and secretion of "uterine milk" to sustain embyonic development prior to implantation. Endometrial hyperplasia also occurs in preparation for placental attachment. The uterus becomes relatively atonic and the cervix functionally closed.

Cystic endometrial hyperplasia is an abnormal uterine response to progesterone with excessive proliferation of mucus-producing glands and infiltration of lymphocytes and plasma cells. Because the uterus becomes unsuitable for embryonic development, infertility may occur. Often a reddish, mucoid vulval discharge is seen. At the end of diestrus, when progesterone levels decline, CEH resolves. Although not firmly established, CEH may become progressively worse during subsequent diestral periods. Pyometra occurs when excessive mucus and inflammatory exudate accumulate in the uterus as a result of the functionally closed cervix; the condition is further exacerbated by secondary bacterial infection.

Cystic endometrial hyperplasia can be produced experimentally by administration of exogenous progesterone; this response is enhanced by previous estrogen treatment. Long-acting progestins, once used to prevent signs of estrus, were frequently associated with the development of CEH and pyometra. This has led to the belief that excessive or prolonged endogenous progesterone production from retained or cystic corpora lutea may be the cause of spontaneous CEH and pyometra. However, in those cases in which progesterone levels have been measured, the levels were neither excessive nor prolonged in duration. Although it is unclear at present, it is tempting to speculate that the enhanced uterine response may be due to other hormonal factors or altered uterine sensitivity to progesterone, or both.

The low prevalence of infertility and pyometra in commercial breeding kennels suggests that pregnancy may be protective; however, available statistical data are contradictory. Pseudopregnancy and irregular estrous cycles do not appear to predispose dogs to pyometra.

PATHOGENESIS OF RENAL MANIFESTATIONS

Dehydration in pyometra may be of sufficient magnitude to cause poor renal perfusion and prerenal azotemia. A mixed membranoproliferative glomerulonephropathy may also be associated with pyometra and is thought to be due to deposition of immune complexes in glomerular capillary walls. Glomerular lesions are not sufficiently severe to cause primary renal failure and are reversible after the uterine disease is resolved.

Obligatory polyuria and compensatory polydipsia that result from impaired capacity to concentrate urine are commonly observed. Reduced renal concentrating capacity occurs despite adequate levels of circulating antidiuretic hormone. Renal medullary hypertonicity is lost, and the urine becomes hyposthenuric (specific gravity less than 1.010). Like glomerular lesions, impaired ability to concentrate urine is a reversible condition if the uterine disease is corrected.

PATHOPHYSIOLOGY OF DISEASE IN OTHER SYSTEMS

Accumulation of neutrophils in the uterus causes massive production of leukocytes with a

tive in decreasing the viscosity of inspissated uterine exudate. In animals with a closed cervix, catheters may be inserted following dilation of the cervical lumen via a hysterotomy incision.

Surgical removal of the corpora lutea has been advocated as part of a combined medical-surgical approach to pyometra. The objective is to promote regression of pathologic uterine changes by eliminating the major source of endogenous progesterone. At present, the risk-benefit ratio of this procedure is unknown. Luteolysis is probably best achieved in the bitch with prostaglandins.

In all cases systemic and intrauterine broad-spectrum antibiotics, chosen on the basis of culture and sensitivity testing of uterine exudate, should be given to control secondary bacterial infections.

SUPPLEMENTAL READING

Asheim, A.: Pathogenesis of renal damage and polydipsia in dogs with pyometra. J. Am. Vet. Med. Assoc., 147:1736, 1965.
Dow, C.: The cystic hyperplasia-pyometra complex in the bitch. J. Comp. Pathol., 69:237–250, 1959.
Ewing, G.D., Schecter, R.D., Whitney, R.C., and Wind, A.P.: The therapy of canine pyometra. J. Am. Anim. Hosp. Assoc., 6:218, 1970.
Gourley, I.M.: Treatment of canine pyometra without ovariohysterectomy. In Bojrab, M.J. (ed.): Current Techniques in Small Animal Surgery. Philadelphia, Lea & Febiger, 1975.
Hardy, R.M., and Osborne, C.A.: Canine pyometra: Pathophysiology, diagnosis and treatment of uterine and extra-uterine lesions. J. Am. Anim. Hosp. Assoc., 10:245, 1974.
Sandholm, M., Vasenius, H., and Kivisto, A.K.: Pathogenesis of canine pyometra. J. Am. Vet. Med. Assoc., 167:1006, 1975.

CANINE VAGINITIS

PATRICIA N. S. OLSON, D.V.M.
Fort Collins, Colorado

Clinical evaluation of canine vaginitis can be a difficult problem. The etiology and pathogenesis of infectious vaginitis often are obscure, because many microorganisms associated with vaginitis are also present in the vaginas of otherwsie normal animals. Because the pathogenesis of infectious vaginitis is not fully understood, diagnosis is often tenuous and treatments empirically administered. A thorough workup should be performed on any animal presented with a vaginal discharge and congested vaginal mucosa. Non-infectious inciting factors, such as vaginal tumors or clitoral hypertrophy, can lead to secondary vaginitis. Clinically normal dogs may have slight vaginal discharges in early diestrus. On the other hand, purulent accumulations of material within the vaginal canal can be associated with pathologic conditions elsewhere in the genitourinary tract.

CLINICAL FINDINGS

Dogs presented with a vaginal discharge and inflamed vaginal mucosa should be suspected of having vaginitis (colpitis). The discharge should not be confused with normal proestrual bleeding, the discharge occasionally seen in early diestrus, the lochia immediately following parturition, or abnormal uterine discharges.

Proestrual bleeding is normal in the bitch and is usually associated with swelling of the vulva. A slight vaginal discharge without congested vaginal mucosa may occasionally be observed as a result of the leukocytic response in early diestrus. Lochia, a green-colored material seen following parturition, rapidly diminishes in quantity within a few days after whelping and completely subsides within a few weeks. Uterine discharges may be associated with metritis, pyometra, or subinvolution of placental sites (SIPS). Metritis and pyometra are usually associated with fever and signs of systemic illness. The onset of discharges caused by SIPS is usually associated with a history of previous parturition. The condition has been observed in "nulliparous" animals, but may in fact follow resorption of fetuses or unobserved abortions. The discharge seen with SIPS is frequently hemorrhagic. Although the bloody discharge frequently is noticed by the owner, signs of systemic illness are not. A thorough history, complete blood count, abdominal palpation, and radiographs usually permit differentiation of vaginal discharges from uterine discharges. It should be recognized, however, that animals with uterine discharges could have concomitant vaginitis.

Non-infectious factors, such as vaginal tumors

or clitoral hypertrophy, can lead to secondary vaginitis. Hemorrhagic discharges can be associated with vascular tumors of the vagina, whereas purulent discharges can be associated with any vaginal tumor if mechanical irritation or secondary infection is present. Animals receiving androgenic steroids occasionally develop clitoral hypertrophy and mechanical vaginitis.

Puppies often are presented with vaginitis prior to their first estrus. Although juvenile vaginitis is not normal, it usually subsides without treatment following the first estrus. If the vaginal discharge persists for several weeks or causes the animal discomfort, therapy should be considered.

DIAGNOSIS

The posterior vagina can be evaluated by palpation with a well-lubricated, gloved index finger. This will usually reveal tumors, foreign bodies, vaginal hyperplasia, vestibular-vaginal strictures, and lacerations in the posterior vagina. Examination of the posterior vaginal lumen may be performed by using a sterilized vaginal endoscope or an otoscopic cone for small breeds or young animals. Because of the length of the canine vagina, anterior portions can be evaluated only with fiberoptic equipment or a modified human anoscope of sufficient length (Pineda, et al.). A pediatric proctoscope can also be used to provide visualization of the anterior vagina (Lein). Cranial portions of the vagina should be evaluated for inflammation and other abnormalities. A urine sample should be obtained and cultured quantitatively to rule out concomitant urinary tract infections.

Vaginal smears can be obtained by rubbing or rolling saline-moistened cotton-tipped applicators against the vaginal mucosa and transferring the cells to a glass slide for cytologic examination. Large numbers of leukocytes typically are present in smears obtained from dogs with clinical signs of vaginitis. The significance of leukocytes must be interpreted with the animal's estrual stage in mind, since numerous leukocytes can also be present in early diestrual smears. Bacteria can be present in vaginal smears obtained both from dogs with vaginitis and from normal dogs. If large numbers of degenerative-appearing neutrophils are observed on the vaginal smear, acute vaginitis should be considered. Differentiation of early diestrus from chronic vaginitis may be more difficult.

Vaginal swabs from dogs with clinical signs of vaginitis should be cultured. It is recommended that the anterior vagina of larger dogs be cul-

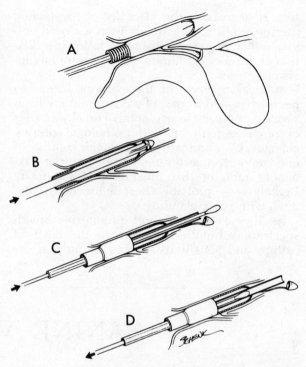

Figure 1. Sampling technique for anterior vaginal swabbing, using a plastic applicator glide. *A.* Insertion of plastic applicator glide. *B.* Passage of the guarded culture instrument (arrow indicates direction). *C.* Passage of a sterile swab through the instrument (arrow indicates direction). *D.* After the swab is rotated 360 degrees, it is retracted (*arrow*) into the glide prior to removal of the entire system from the vagina. (From Olson, P.N.S., and Mather, E.C.: Canine vaginal and uterine bacterial flora. J. Am. Vet. Med. Assoc., *172*:709, 1978. Used with permission.)

tured by first placing a glide* in the posterior vagina and then passing a guarded culture instrument† through the glide to the cranial vagina (Fig. 1). The posterior vagina can be cultured by passing a sterile culturette‡ or sterilized cotton-tipped applicator through a vaginal speculum or otoscope cone at the time of vaginal examination. Bacteria isolated should be identified if possible, and antimicrobial sensitivities of minimal inhibitory concentrations (MIC) should be determined. Although not yet evaluated in the dog, quantitation of vaginal isolates in humans appears to be more rewarding than qualitative identification of microbial types in cases of suspected vaginitis.

The aerobic bacterial flora of the vagina has been studied in dogs historically free of reproductive diseases (Table 1). The types of bacteria found in clinically normal females are

*Playtex Gentle Glide, Playtex Inc., Dover, Delaware
†Guarded Culture Instrument, Kalayjian Industries, Long Beach, California
‡Securline, MH-100 Culture System, Precision Dynamics Corp., Burbank, California

Table 1. *Classification of Vaginal Isolates from 81 Postpuberal Bitches**

TYPE OF ISOLATE	ANTERIOR VAGINAL SWABBINGS			POSTERIOR VAGINAL SWABBINGS		
	NO. OF ISOLATES	TOTAL ISOLATES (%)	BITCHES WITH ISOLATE (%)	NO. OF ISOLATES	TOTAL ISOLATES (%)	BITCHES WITH ISOLATE (%)
E. coli	15	19.0	18.5	25	13.2	30.9
Coagulase + staphylococci	5	6.3	6.2	15	7.9	18.5
Coagulase − staphylococci	5	6.3	6.2	16	8.4	19.8
α-hemolytic streptococci	8	10.1	9.9	18	9.5	22.2
β-hemolytic streptococci	12	15.2	14.8	15	7.9	18.5
Non-hemolytic streptococci	3	3.8	3.7	10	5.3	12.3
Pasteurella sp	8	10.1	9.9	26	13.7	32.1
Proteus sp	4	5.1	4.9	5	2.6	6.2
Bacillus sp	3	3.8	3.7	13	6.8	16.0
Hemophilus sp	1	1.3	1.2	0	0	0
Corynebacterium sp	2	2.5	2.5	12	6.3	14.8
Pseudomonas sp	0	0	0	2	1.1	2.5
Moraxella sp	1	1.3	1.2	7	3.7	8.6
Acinetobacter sp	0	0	0	3	1.6	3.7
Flavobacterium sp	1	1.3	1.2	4	2.1	4.9
Lactobacillus sp	0	0	0	1	0.5	1.2
Micrococcus sp	1	1.3	1.2	3	1.6	3.7
Neisseria sp	2	2.5	2.5	7	3.7	8.6
Enterobacter sp	1	1.3	1.2	1	0.5	1.2
Klebsiella sp	0	0	0	0	0	0
Nonclassified	7	8.9	8.6	7	3.7	8.6
Total	79 (0.975 isolate/bitch)			190 (2.35 isolates/bitch)		
No Growth	30			7		

*From: Olson, P.N.S., and Mather, E.C.: Canine vaginal and uterine bacterial flora. J. Am. Vet. Med. Assoc., *172*:710, 1978. Used with permission.

similar to those isolated from dogs with vaginitis. In one study there was a tendency to isolate fewer species of bacteria from vaginas containing exudates (Hirsh and Wiger). The vaginal flora in prepuberal dogs is different from that in adult bitches. Puppies tend to harbor staphylococcal organisms more frequently than mature dogs do (Table 2). It is unknown whether the higher incidence of staphylococcal organisms isolated from prepuberal vaginas contributes to the pathogenesis of juvenile vaginitis. Staphylococcal organisms have not been isolated from all puppies with vaginitis. In fact, smears taken from puppies with juvenile vaginitis often contain few bacteria in relation to the tremendous leukocytic response. Non-classified gram-negative bacteria have been isolated from the canine vagina (Olson; Osbaldiston), but their significance is unknown. It is emphasized that the vaginal flora is a dynamic ecosystem in which the predominant organisms isolated at one time are often not present at a later time.

Table 2. *Classification of Vaginal Isolates from 21 Pups, 12 Weeks to 6 Months Old**

TYPE OF ISOLATE	NO. OF ISOLATES	TOTAL ISOLATES (%)	PUPS WITH ISOLATE (%)
E. coli	8	17.0	38.1
Coagulase + staphylococci	14	29.8	66.7
Coagulase − staphylococci	5	10.6	23.8
α-hemolytic streptococci	4	8.5	19.0
β-hemolytic streptococci	3	6.4	14.3
Non-hemolytic streptococci	2	4.3	9.5
Proteus sp	1	2.1	4.8
Bacillus sp	3	6.4	14.3
Corynebacterium sp	2	4.3	9.5
Micrococcus sp	3	6.4	14.3
Neisseria sp	1	2.1	4.8
Klebsiella sp	1	2.1	4.8
Total	47 (2.2 isolates/pup)		

*From: Olson, P. N. S., and Mather, E. C.: Canine vaginal and uterine bacterial flora. J. Am. Vet. Med. Assoc., *172*:709, 1978. Used with permission.

Herpesvirus infection should be considered any time vesicular vaginitis is observed. Although herpesvirus rarely causes clinical signs in adults, its potential pathogenicity to puppies passing through the birth canal should be stressed to clients with pregnant bitches.

In some cases of persistent vaginitis the posterior vagina contains raised areas that resemble follicular hypertrophy of the glans penis. The etiology of these lesions is unknown.

Varying strains of mycoplasma have been isolated from dogs with vaginitis, but these have also been identified in clinically normal animals (Rosendal and Laber).

TREATMENT

Because the diagnosis of primary bacterial vaginitis is often tenuous, treatment is frequently empirical. If primary bacterial infection is suspected, treatment is generally dependent on antimicrobial sensitivity results or MIC. Antibiotics may be infused directly into the vagina or applied as vaginal suppositories. Systemic antibiotics may be used in combination with intravaginal infusions or suppositories. Pharmacologic studies have not been performed to determine which antibiotics become concentrated optimally in the canine reproductive tract. If pregnant dogs with vaginitis are encountered, systemic antibiotics must be evaluated critically for possible teratogenic effects.

The owner should be advised not to breed a dog during the first estrus following a diagnosis of infectious vaginitis. Some breeders may not follow this advice, especially if the vaginitis is a recurring problem. In such cases rigorous treatment is necessary if the infection is to be eradicated prior to breeding. Since little information is available concerning which antibiotics are spermicidal, those used prior to breeding must be chosen discriminately.

Estrogenic steroids have reportedly been used to control infections. The use of long-lasting estrogens for prolonged periods may be associated with deleterious side effects. Administration of estrogens should be avoided when possible (Jochle).

Treatment of secondary vaginitis should include removal or control of the inciting cause (neoplasia, foreign bodies, vestibular-vaginal strictures, vaginal hyperplasia, and other causes). If clitoral hypertrophy and secondary vaginitis are observed in animals receiving androgenic steroids, withdrawal of the drug usually results in remission of the condition.

SUPPLEMENTAL READING

Barton, C.L.: Canine vaginitis. Vet. Clin. North Am., 7:711–714, 1977.
Hirsh, D.C., and Wiger, N.: The bacterial flora of the normal canine vagina compared with that of vaginal exudates. J. Small Anim. Pract., 18:25, 1977.
Jochle, W.: Hormones in canine gynecology: A review. Theriogenology, 3(4), April 1975.
Lein, D.H.: Personal communication. New York State Veterinary Hospital, Ithaca, N.Y., August 1978.
Olson, P.N.S., and Mather, E.C.: Canine vaginal and uterine bacterial flora. J. Am. Vet. Med. Assoc., 172:708–711, 1978.
Osbaldiston, G.W.: Bacteriological studies of reproductive disorders of bitches. J. Am. Anim. Hosp. Assoc., 14:363–367, 1978.
Pineda, M.H., Kainer, R.A., and Faulkner, L.C.: Dorsal median post-cervical fold in the canine vagina. Am. J. Vet. Res., 34:1487–1491, 1973.
Rosendal, S., and Laber, G.: Identification of 38 mycoplasma strains isolated from the vagina of dogs. Zentralbl. Bakteriol. [Orig. A], 225:346, 1973.

VAGINAL HYPERPLASIA AND UTERINE PROLAPSE

R. ALLEN RUSHMER, V.M.D.
Kennett Square, Pennsylvania

INTRODUCTION

These two conditions are associated with a common clinical sign: a protruding vaginal mass. The conditions are easily differentiated on the basis of historical and physical findings. The remaining differential diagnostic considerations for a protruding vaginal mass are vulvovaginal leiomyoma and transmissible venereal tumor.

VAGINAL HYPERPLASIA

Vaginal hyperplasia (vaginal prolapse, estral eversion, estral hypertrophy) is an occasional condition of young large-breed bitches (not queens). The condition occurs during proestrus or estrus and regresses during diestrus. The problem is usually recognized when the bitches are in one of their first three heats, because the problem is characteristically most severe at these times.

The exact cause or causes of vaginal hyperplasia are not known. Apparently the normal effects of estrogen on the vaginal mucosa (hyperemia, edema, keratinization) are very pronounced in those bitches with hyperplasia. One or more folds of edematous tissue anterior to the urethral meatus protrude into the uterine lumen. When the tissue expansion reaches the limits of accommodation within the lumen, it expands posteriorly over the urethral meatus. The mucosa of the floor of the vagina is most commonly involved; it gives rise to a broad, tongue-shaped mass with a narrow base that protrudes through the lips of the vulva. Very occasionally, the entire circumference of the vagina is affected, giving rise to a large, doughnut-shaped mass.

The protruding mass should be examined carefully to determine its origin, size at the base, location of the vaginal lumen and the urethral meatus, and extent of any damage (ulceration, hemorrhage, infection) to the tissue. The stage of the estrous cycle may be determined by vaginal cytology. The owners should also be asked for information about the stage of the estrous cycle. In addition, they may have noted a pronounced swelling of the vulva or perineum prior to observing the mass. Intermittent protrusion of the mass during urination or sleep may have been noted, and the bitch may have mild polyuria or dysuria.

The choice of treatment for each case is determined by several specific considerations, including underlying cause of the hyperplastic tissue, breeding potential of the bitch, and size and condition of the hyperplastic tissue. The tissue will regress during the luteal phase of the cycle unless the entire circumference of the vagina is involved. Approximately two thirds of untreated bitches will develop a hyperplastic mass during a subsequent heat; this tissue may be larger or smaller than the initial condition. Approximately one quarter of surgically treated cases will also recur.

If the bitch is not intended for breeding, ovariohysterectomy is the treatment of choice. It will eliminate the current problem and the possibility of recurrence, and has the additional benefits of effective contraception and reduced risk of mammary tumors. The tissue may be managed medically (see following discussion) until the bitch enters diestrus to reduce the problems of hemorrhage associated with estrus.

If the bitch is intended for breeding, the treatment depends on the size and condition of the mass. If the mass is small to moderate in size and tissue damage is not extensive, it should be managed medically. The tissue should be kept clean and protected from drying by liberal application of an antibiotic ointment. Elizabethan collars and tranquilization may be required to reduce self-mutilation of the mass. Exogenous progestins should be avoided because they may induce cystic endometrial hyperplasia of the estrogen-primed uterus. Hormone therapy designed to shorten estrus (human chorionic gonadotropin, gonadotropin-releasing hormone) has had limited success. Artificial insemination may be used to impregnate the bitch.

If the hyperplastic mass is large or circumferential or if there is extensive mucosal damage, a submucous resection is indicated. The operation should be performed using general anesthesia and with the bitch positioned with the perineum elevated. The perineal area should be prepared for surgery, and a purse-string suture should be placed in the anus. The urethra should be catheterized to avoid iatrogenic trauma and urine contamination of the operative field. An episiotomy may be necessary to expose the base of the mass. Extensive bleeding of the hyperplastic tissue can be anticipated. It may be controlled with electrocautery, extensive ligation, or post-operative vaginal packing. An elliptical incision is made around the base of the mass, and the edematous mucosa is then excised. The mucosal edges should be reapposed with simple interrupted sutures of 2–0 chromic gut (cutting edge needle). When the entire vaginal circumference is involved, two circular incisions, one on the luminal and the other on the antiluminal surface of the doughnut-shaped mass, are required. Excision and closure are otherwise similar. The anal purse-string suture must be removed. The incisions generally heal rapidly with little or no infection. The owners should always be cautioned about the possibility of recurrence.

UTERINE PROLAPSE

Uterine prolapse is an uncommon condition in both the bitch and the queen. It occurs in the immediate postpartum period when the cervix is dilated. Prolapse may occur in either primiparous or multiparous animals; there is no distinct age at risk. There is no known specific cause or predisposing factor(s).

In a complete or true prolapse one or both uterine horns protrude from the vagina. A partial prolapse may also occur, in which one horn or the body of the uterus is prolapsed into the anterior vagina. Animals with partial prolapse may develop restlessness, straining, abnormal posture, and abdominal pain. A thorough (digital and speculum) vaginal examination will reveal a partial prolapse.

The physical status of the bitch or queen with any degree of prolapse must be assessed carefully. Prolapse may be associated with rupture of the uterus or ovarian artery and subsequent complications (hemorrhage, shock, peritonitis). The prolapsed tissue must also be examined to determine the extent of tissue damage (hemorrhage, edema, necrosis).

The choice of treatment and technique depends on the status of the bitch or queen and the extent of damage to the prolapsed tissue. If there is little or no damage to the tissue, the bitch or queen is in good condition, and the prolapse is recent, the tissue should be replaced. The patient should be anesthetized and placed in a head-down position. The tissue should be thoroughly cleaned and the prolapsed part gently manipulated into its correct position. A probe (syringe plunger, test tube) may be helpful to ensure complete eversion of the uterus. In difficult cases celiotomy and bimanual manipulation of the uterus may be required. Hysteropexy or vaginal suturing may

be elected in specific cases. The bitch or queen should be treated with local and systemic antibiotics and oxytocin. The animal should be monitored carefully 24 hours for signs of hemorrhage or shock. The uterus probably will not prolapse again this time or after a subsequent pregnancy.

If the patient has signs of internal hemorrhage or shock, if the tissue is traumatized, or if the condition is of long duration, the prolapsed tissue should be removed. An abdominal ovariohysterectomy following reduction of the prolapse is the technique of choice, because it offers the best visualization of the ovarian vasculature, uterus, and ovaries. Direct amputation of the prolapsed tissue is also possible. Shock and hemorrhage must be treated appropriately.

SUPPLEMENTAL READING

Schutte, A.P.: Vaginal prolapse in the bitch. J. South African Vet. Med. Assoc., 38:197–203, 1967.
Smith, K.W.: Female genital system. In Archibald, J. (ed.): Canine Surgery. Wheaton, Illinois, American Veterinary Publications, Inc., 1965.
Troger, C.P.: Vaginal prolapse in the bitch. Mod. Vet. Pract., 51:38–41, 1970.

NON-NEOPLASTIC DISORDERS OF THE MAMMARY GLANDS

SHIRLEY D. JOHNSTON, D.V.M.,
and DAVID W. HAYDEN, D.V.M.
St. Paul, Minnesota

MASTITIS

Inflammation of the mammary glands of the bitch and queen is caused by bacterial infection of the lactating gland post partum or during pseudopregnancy. Enterobacteria, streptococci, and staphylococci are commonly cultured from mastitic milk; routes of infection have not been well examined but may be assumed to occur by ascending or hematogenous routes. There is no evidence at present to indicate that mastitis occurs with greater frequency in previously affected animals.

Clinically, the dam shows one or more warm,

painful mammary glands and elevated rectal temperature (103.5 to 106.0°F). Because elevated temperature may be an early sign of both mastitis and metritis, owners of lactating companion animals should be encouraged to monitor rectal temperature twice daily throughout lactation. The dam may show depression, anorexia, and reluctance to care for her offspring. Her hemogram reveals an immature leukocytosis. Quantitative culture of the mastitic milk usually reveals a pure culture of a large number of bacteria that are resistant to commonly used antibiotics.

Therapeutically, the affected bitch or queen

should be given broad-spectrum antibiotics immediately; specific antibiotics are selected when culture results become known. If signs of septicemia or septic shock (tachycardia, hypotension, increased capillary refill time, muscle weakness, hyperventilation) are present, immediate intravenous fluid, antibiotic, and steroid therapy are warranted.

When acute mastitis is diagnosed and treated early and when mammary abscessation is absent, the offspring may be allowed to continue nursing. Offspring ingest antibiotics in milk, and frequent nursing helps drain the mastitic gland, preventing galactostasis. In addition, nursing offspring may themselves be the source of the mammary infection, as has been documented in the human disease. Human mothers under therapy for acute mastitis in absence of abscessation continue to nurse without difficulty or infant illness; our experience with bitches indicates that early and aggressive treatment of acute mastitis need not interrupt lactation.

Acute mastitis may progress to abscessation or gangrenous mastitis or both. In either condition surgical drainage followed by immersion of the glands in a dilute povidone-iodine solution* and warm water three times daily is effective. Specific parenteral antibiotic therapy is given, and offspring are not allowed to nurse from the affected glands.

Very little glandular tissue is present in non-lactating glands, so inflammation of them due to trauma or laceration may be treated in the same way as simple skin wounds.

Galactostasis

Stasis of milk in mammary glands resulting in hard, painful engorgement occurs when secreted milk is not removed from the glands. This may occur when puppies are removed abruptly at birth or at weaning. It may also occur in mastitic glands.

If possible, the condition should be avoided by weaning puppies gradually. Their time with the mother should be decreased each day for a week. In addition, the dam's food and water intake should be reduced by half. When puppies are removed at birth, the bitch should be given an injection of oxytocin (5 to 20 units intramuscularly) to promote uterine involution and should be fed only half her normal adult maintenance ration of calories and water for the next two to three days.

Galactostasis of the mastitic gland is treated with mild diuretics and analgesics in addition to specific mastitis therapy. Nursing is encouraged in the absence of abscessation or gangrenous mastitis.

Galactorrhea (inappropriate lactation)

Lactation is observed in bitches and queens following abrupt decline of serum progesterone. This occurs normally at parturition in pregnant females. An abrupt decline in serum progesterone level may also occur at the end of diestrus in bitches, because they maintain functional corpora lutea for approximately 60 days whether or not they are pregnant. The female cat is induced to ovulate by cervical stimulation. If she ovulates but does not conceive, she will produce corpora lutea that persist for approximately 40 days before progesterone levels drop. Inappropriate lactation is also observed occasionally after ovariohysterectomy performed during diestrus, when the serum progesterone level drops sharply after removal of corpora lutea–bearing ovaries. Finally, inappropriate lactation may also occur following cessation of progestogen therapy with products such as megestrol acetate (MGA)† in intact or neutered animals.

Inappropriate lactation will undergo spontaneous remission without treatment. If the animal is extremely uncomfortable, light sedation and alternating hot and cold compresses to the glands are indicated. Hormone therapy with mibolerone,‡ a synthetic androgen, has been reported to alleviate signs of false pregnancy, although this drug is not yet approved for that use. Alternatively, injection of 1 to 2 mg/kg testosterone (not to exceed 30 mg) intramuscularly is also effective.

Agalactia

True agalactia is rare in bitches and queens. Its cause is unknown, and no effective treatment has been reported.

More often, females with mammary development who lack appropriate nutrition for good milk production or who psychologically impair milk letdown are encountered. When the dam is in good physical condition at breeding, we recommend that food intake be increased gradually during the last half of pregnancy. At whelping caloric intake should be approximately 125 to 150 per cent of that required for maintenance. High-quality commercial diets

---

*Betadine Surgical Scrub, Purdue Frederick Co., Norwalk, Connecticut 06856

†Ovaban, Schering Corporation, Kenilworth, New Jersey 07033

‡Cheque, The Upjohn Company, Kalamazoo, Michigan 49001

are recommended. If supplements must be fed they should be limited to milk products, fortified meat, or small quantities of cooked eggs. Calcium supplements are given to dams with a history of puerperal hypocalcemia.

The primiparous bitch or queen who is reluctant to nurse may be treated with an oral tranquilizer once daily. Oxytocin nasal spray§ is effective in promoting milk letdown in bitches and queens. It can be used 5 to 10 minutes before nursing three times daily.

MAMMARY HYPERTROPHY

Mammary hypertrophy (mammary fibroadenomatosis, fibroglandular mammary hypertrophy) has been well documented in cats and is observed occasionally in bitches. The feline condition occurs primarily in young intact females following estrus. It has also been observed in male and female cats receiving long-term therapy with progestogens such as MGA.

Animals develop diffuse or localized non-painful firm swellings of one or more mammary glands. The masses in young females consist of benign fibroglandular proliferation. There is no evidence of necrosis or inflammation. In animals that have received MGA therapy, gross and histologic appearance differs slightly, in

§Syntocinon, Sandoz Pharmaceuticals, East Hanover, New Jersey 07936

that papillary outgrowth into the ducts is present.

Tentative diagnosis is based on gross appearance, patient signalment, and history. Because of the highly malignant nature of most feline mammary neoplasms, biopsy of all localized swellings is recommended.

Mammary hypertrophy in diestrous cats will regress spontaneously if untreated. Ovariohysterectomy will also effect a cure. Surgical removal of masses and cessation of therapy are effective in MGA-treated animals.

SUPPLEMENTAL READING

Allen, H.L.: Feline mammary hypertrophy. Vet. Pathol., 10:501–508, 1973.
Concannon, P.W., Hansel, W., and Visek, W.J.: The ovarian cycle of the bitch: Plasma estrogen, LH and progesterone. Biol. Reprod., 13:112–121, 1975.
Devereux, W.P.: Acute puerperal mastitis. Am. J. Obstet. Gynecol., 108:78–81, 1970.
Hinton, M., and Gaskell, C.J.: Non-neoplastic mammary hypertrophy in the cat associated with pregnancy or with oral progestogen therapy. Vet. Rec., 100:277–280, 1977.
Hosek, J.J.: Syntocinon: A treatment for agalactia in the dog. Vet. Med. Small Anim. Clin., 67:405, 1972.
Mandel, M.: Spontaneous regression of feline benign mammary hypertrophy. Vet. Med. Small Anim. Clin. 70:846–847, 1975.
Marshall, B.R., Hepper, J.K., and Zirbel, C.C.: Sporadic puerperal mastitis: An infection that need not interrupt lactation. JAMA, 233:1377–1379, 1975.
Sheffy, B.E.: Nutrition and nutritional disorders. Vet. Clin. North Am., 8:7–29, 1978.
Silver, I.A.: The anatomy of the mammary gland of the dog and cat. J. Small Anim. Pract., 7:689–696, 1966.
Verhage, H.G., Beamer, N.B., and Brenner, R.M.: Plamsa level of estradiol and progesterone in the cat during polyestrus, pregnancy and pseudopregnancy. Biol. Reprod., 14:579–585, 1976.

MANAGEMENT OF CANINE INFERTILITY

ROLF E. LARSEN, D.V.M.
Gainesville, Florida

and SHIRLEY D. JOHNSTON, D.V.M.
St. Paul, Minnesota

Causes of canine infertility are poorly defined. In our experience the majority of conception failures result from poor breeding management. The bitch should be bred early in standing heat, and the breeding should be repeated. Because proestrus (the period of blood-tinged vaginal discharge, vulvar swelling, and refusal to mate) may vary from one to 15 days, the owner cannot reliably count days from the onset of vaginal discharge when choosing the best breeding date. Instead, the owner should be counseled to identify the first day of estrus when the bitch will stand for mounting by the male and deflect her tail off to the side of the perineum ("flagging"). A male must be present in order to detect the first day of estrus; the bitch can be teased by a local dog before being shipped to a stud dog. Evaluation of vaginal smear reveals complete cornification of squamous epithelial cells toward the end of proestrus and more than 50 percent anuclear squamous cells in the completely cornified smear early in estrus. Vaginal cytology is a valuable prognostic tool in planning shipping dates, but it should not be used in place of behavior to identify the first day of estrus. Vaginal cytology need not be performed on normal bitches as long as behavioral estrus can be identified.

The normal bitch should be bred every other day for a total of three breedings, starting with the onset of standing heat. Some stud dog owners permit only two breedings, in which case the goal is to accomplish them early in standing heat.

If conception failure occurs after these breedings, the semen of the stud dog should be evaluated before the more time-consuming and costly evaluation of the bitch is done. If the dog is not accessible but has sired recent litters, the bitch should be examined.

MALE INFERTILITY

Infertility in stud dogs may occur in association with infections, endocrine deficits, anomalies, and neoplasia of the male genital tract. Bacterial orchitis, epididymitis (including that caused by *Brucella canis*), and prostatitis may be associated with morphologic changes in sperm. Low serum thyroxine levels have been observed in many cases of infertility in stud dogs, but administration of exogenous thyroxine does not uniformly cause a return to normal (in contrast with hypothyroid infertile bitches). Enlargement of the spermatic cord due to inguinal hernia may cause infertility. Segmental aplasia of the epididymis, bilateral spermatocele or, less commonly, tumors of the male genital tract may prevent sperm from reaching the ejaculate even with normal spermatogenesis. Intersex states, such as Klinefelter's syndrome (XXY sex chromosome complement), are causes of infertility in a variety of species. Klinefelter's syndrome has been associated with testicular hypoplasia in dogs.

Infertile males may be azoospermic (no sperm present in the ejaculate), oligospermic (fewer than 100×10^6 sperm present), or have a high percentage of immotile or morphologically abnormal sperm, even though the number of sperm is normal.

DIAGNOSIS

Males should be examined as soon as possible after conception failure in a bitch is recognized. The owner should be asked for a complete medical and breeding history and for a proestrous or estrous bitch for use as a mount animal during semen collection. Alternatively, an anestrous bitch may be used if the male has previously demonstrated good libido. It is often wise to collect semen before performing a complete physical examination or manipulations that cause anxiety to owners or patients.

Semen should be collected via a rubber cone artificial vagina* into a warm plastic tube. The presperm and sperm-rich fractions should be collected together; the tube should then be changed for collection of a portion of the prostatic fluid. The prostatic fraction should be collected aseptically so that a portion can be submitted for quantitative bacteriologic culture. The remainder should be centrifuged for cytologic examination.

Volume and color of the sperm-rich fraction should be recorded. Sperm motility should be assessed at $100\times$ magnification on a warm, coverslipped slide after 1:10 dilution with 2.9 percent sodium citrate. Sperm motility below 70 percent is uncommon and is usually associated with disease (such as canine brucellosis) or poor handling technique. Even at room temperature, normal canine semen will retain high motility. Spermatozoa from this species are relatively resistant to cold shock but sensitive to heat. Slide warmers and baths should not exceed 37° C.

Sperm concentration is determined by diluting semen in commercially available blood cell dilutors† and counting an aliquot in a hemocytometer. Alternatively, a Coulter Counter or calibrated spectrophotometer may be used. Concentration is multiplied by volume, and the final number of sperm per ejaculate is recorded. Total sperm numbers should exceed 200×10^6 per ejaculate. Numbers below 100×10^6 are usually associated with infertility.

Sperm morphology is assessed using an eosin-nigrosin stain.‡ Head shape, proximal droplets, distal droplets, and midpiece and tail defects should be quantitated by percent incidence. Head shape and acrosome defects or proximal cytoplasmic droplets in more than 20 per cent of the sperm are generally associated with reduced conception rates. Kinked tails and detached heads are the earliest and most common abnormalities seen following inflammation

---

*Artificial vagina, Davol Latex End Cone, FarVet, 1821 University Avenue, St. Paul, Minnesota

†Unopette White Blood Cell Dilutor (Becton-Dickinson), Scientific Products, 13505 Industrial Park Blvd, Minneapolis, Minnesota

‡Morphology Stain, American Veterinary Society for the Study of Breeding Soundness, Association Building, 9th and Minnesota, Hastings, Nebraska

and heating of the scrotum. Cases of infertility characterized by high numbers of morphologically defective sperm should be pursued by bacterial culture of prostatic fluid; diagnostic numbers of the inflammatory cells are not always present in ejaculates when bacterial infection is present. Males infected with *B. canis* have high percentages of sperm abnormalities (30 to 80 per cent), severe reduction in motility, neutrophils and monocytes in the ejaculate, and occasionally head-to-head sperm agglutination.

Semen evaluation will help to define the problem as one of azoospermia, oligospermia, low motility, or abnormal morphology with possible infection. It is rare to find an infertile dog with normal sperm numbers and morphology.

The physical examination should include careful palpation to determine size and consistency of the testes, epididymides, inguinal rings and spermatic cords, prepuce, and penis (the penis in the erect state following semen collection). Excess fluid within the scrotum should be aspirated and examined cytologically. The prostate should be palpated rectally and may be examined radiographically if signs of benign prostatic hypertrophy or prostatitis (blood dripping from the penis, hematuria, constipation) are present.

Laboratory tests that may be of value include serum thyroxine concentration and *B. canis* antibody titer. Reproductive sequelae to hypothyroidism in males are not as well defined as in females. Although infertile studs often have low serum thyroxine concentrations, caution should be exercised before ruling out other etiologies. Although the slide and tube agglutination tests for *B. canis* have been reported to be sensitive, a recent report of an infected male dog with a negative slide agglutination titer and a low tube agglutination titer should lead the clinician to pursue brucellosis as a cause of infertility when clinical signs are consistent with that disease.

Serum testosterone concentrations in the dog range from 0.4 to 10.0 ng/ml. Dogs with normal libido and ability to mate rarely have less than that range, regardless of fertility. Variation in serum testosterone concentrations may be 2 to 3 ng/ml within a few hours in the same dog, making single samples useless in diagnosing male infertility. Follicle stimulating hormone (FSH) levels are often elevated in infertile men, and FSH response to gonadotropin-releasing hormone (GnRH) or clomiphene citrate (a synthetic estrogen) has been used to localize endocrine lesions in men. With the development of a canine FSH assay, critical assessment of the hormonal nature of canine infertility may become possible.

Testicular biopsy is of value in establishing a diagnosis of efferent duct obstruction or abnormal testicular function in dogs with azoospermia. Normal histology of seminiferous epithelium obtained from azoospermic dogs confirms a diagnosis of obstruction. In man a microsurgical technique for anastomosis of the vas deferens to an epididymal duct distal to the obstruction is successful in restoring fertility. There have been no reports of the use of this procedure in dogs. Results of testicular biopsy may be of prognostic significance if they define the extent and nature of pathology within the seminiferous tubules. In man, however, testicular biopsy has been of limited help in selecting proper therapy. Surgical exploration of the scrotum should include visualization of one complete testis and epididymis for gross assessment of obstructive lesions. Biopsy results are of greatest value in establishing a diagnosis and indicating the feasibility of corrective surgery for obstruction.

Chromosome analysis may be of value in patients with congenital infertility characterized by hypoplastic testicles or penis or other evidence of an intersex state. Unfortunately, the canine karyotype is difficult to analyze, and the cost of cytogenetic evaluation is often prohibitive.

TREATMENT

Treatments for canine male infertility have not been subjected to controlled studies. Virtually all reports of successful therapy have been anecdotal. Although sperm production may return spontaneously following azoospermia due to overuse, environmental stress, or systemic disease, the majority of dogs with azoospermia neither recover spontaneously nor respond to treatment.

Oligospermic dogs have been reported to respond to injections of pregnant mare serum gonadotropin (PMSG) and FSH. Doses used have been 200 to 500 IU PMSG SQ twice weekly and 25 mg FSH SQ once weekly for five weeks. Use of gonadotropic hormones has not reached its full potential in canine andrology because of failure to continue therapy through a number of seminiferous production cycles, which take approximately eight weeks each. Administration of a gonadotropin with luteinizing hormone (LH) activity for a minimum of three months is of value in man; however, dose, frequency, and effectiveness have not been established in dogs. Use of GnRH injected daily may also be useful if continued for a period of months. A number of synthetic analogues of GnRH are currently being tested. The advantages of GnRH over the gonadotropins include lack of immune reaction and release of endogenous FSH and LH.

Androgens have been used in oligospermic men to obtain two responses. Testosterone rebound therapy is a classic treatment involving administration of testosterone for six to ten weeks or until azoospermia is induced. When therapy is withdrawn, sperm numbers often rebound to higher levels than those seen before therapy. Two synthetic androgens are also used for their direct effects on sperm production and motility. Mesterolone (1α-methyl-17β-hydroxy-5α-androstan-3-one) is an orally active androgen that can increase sperm output in selected patients when given at the proper dose. Halotestin (fluoxymesterone) is an orally active androgen used to increase sperm motility.

In congenitally azoospermic animals, prognosis is poor. Congenital oligospermic animals occasionally may sire small litters if the total sperm number in the ejaculate exceeds 20×10^6. In general, ejaculates with fewer than 100×10^6 sperm have high percentages of spermatozoal defects. It may be possible for an oligospermic male to produce offspring by repeated matings. The prognosis for development of normal fertility as measured by conception rate is poor.

When infertility is acquired as a result of systemic or local infection, aggressive therapy is indicated. Diagnosis of the severity of the lesion is usually made on the basis of semen evaluation, culture, and palpation during the physical examination. Inflammation and infection of the epididymis and testis is often due to retrograde movement of infectious material into the vas deferens during acute or chronic prostatitis. In any case of local bacterial infection of the genital tract it is best to assume that prostatitis and epididymitis are also present. Intensive specific antibacterial therapy should be instituted. Antibiotics should be chosen on the basis of their ability to enter prostatic secretions. Blockage of the epididymis may lead to testicular degeneration regardless of whether the testicular parenchyma is involved. Severity and irreversibility of the lesion due to blockage is related to the site of the obstruction — the nearer to the testis, the greater the severity. Obstructions of the epididymal tail and vas deferens may be followed by complete regeneration of the seminiferous tissue. Mycoplasmas and strains of *Escherichia coli* with a sperm-immobilizing factor have been blamed for lowered fertility associated with normal spermatozoa in a number of species. In this instance it appears that bacteria exert an effect on the sperm rather than on testicular or epididymal tissue.

Epididymal obstruction due to spermatocele is difficult to identify by physical examination. Abscesses are often associated with enlargement and induration of the body or tail of the epididymis. Unilateral orchiectomy is indicated when abscessation involves one side only. In our practice, infertility due to omental-inguinal hernia has been resolved by herniorrhaphy and 10 weeks of sexual rest.

The cause of most cases of canine male infertility remains unknown. Few dogs have responded to non-specific therapy. However, there are studs that become temporarily infertile or even azoospermic because of systemic disease, overuse, or unknown causes. They may subsequently return to normal without treatment. Prognosis for congenital or acquired idiopathic azoospermia or oligospermia is guarded, at best. Clients should be advised that treatment is usually unsuccessful.

FEMALE INFERTILITY

An ideal time to examine infertile bitches is 28 to 30 days after breeding. At this time the uterus can be palpated for fetal vesicles. If they are absent and the male is thought to be fertile, evaluation of serum progesterone concentration will allow assessment of whether normal ovulation has occurred. In the normal spontaneously ovulating bitch, serum progesterone concentration peaks 20 to 30 days after the onset of standing heat. Serum concentrations greater than 5 ng/ml indicate functional corpora lutea. Additional diagnostic work (other than vaginal culture) can be performed at this visit, and the bitch can be given therapy before the onset of her next season. Vaginal culture should be performed early in proestrus, a time when the cervix normally is open.

DIAGNOSIS

The medical and breeding history should include duration of interestrous intervals, lengths of cycles and standing behavior, days of the cycle and of standing when bred, and dates of pregnancies (if any). Normal interestrous intervals range from five to eight months. German shepherds have been reported to have a relatively short cycle (149 ± 28 days). Although most bitches have their first cycle between 9 and 12 months of age, females of large breeds may not show onset of estrus until nearly two years of age. Acyclic bitches probably should not be evaluated until then. The first cycle often is irregular and therefore should not be used to assess fertility. "Split" or "false" heats occur for the most part in puberal bitches, but they are also seen in adults. These cycles are characterized by vulvar swelling and discharge for a few days. Proestrus signs then disappear for four to six weeks before the bitch enters a true heat. They are not associated with infertility. A cycling female may induce an anestrous bitch to come into proestrus early. Inability or failure to mate may be caused by vaginal or vestibular strictures, psychologic objection to a particular male, or use of older bitches with virgin males. Muzzled restraint or artificial insemination may be used in these bitches. Reproductive efficiency, as measured by conception rate, litter size, and number of puppies whelped per corpus luteum, declines after age six in most breeds.

The physical examination should include abdominal palpation of the uterus, rectal palpation of the vagina and bony pelvis, inspection of the vulva for size, conformation, and discharge, digital examination of the vagina, and vaginoscopy. If vaginal culture is to be performed it should be done with a guarded swab* introduced to the external cervical os prior to digital or vaginoscopic examination. Use of a human anoscope will permit inspection of structure, color, and texture of the vaginal mucosa and evaluation of discharges. Urethral catheterization can be performed during this procedure if a urine sample is desired but should be avoided if vaginitis is suspected. (Consult the article entitled "Cystocentesis.")

Initial laboratory data should include a complete blood count, urinalysis, *B. canis* serologic study, and serum thyroxine measurement.

TREATMENT

Normal Cycles. Normal cycling implies some function of the reproductive endocrine organs. When a normally cycling bitch has failed to conceive after properly managed breeding with a fertile male, the female tubular tract should be investigated. Structural abnormalities of the vagina and vestibule may be recognized with the aid of an endoscope.

Infectious causes of infertility include bacterial infections of the female tract caused by streptococci, *Pseudomonas* spp., *E. coli*, and a variety of other bacteria. Infertile bitches or those with history of abortion, reabsorption, uterine discharge (with cytologic evidence of inflammation), or vaginitis should be cultured during proestrus. Specific antibacterial therapy from the time of proestrus to whelping has been successful in maintaining pregnancies provided that non-toxic antibiotics selected on the basis

of sensitivity testing have been used. Although bacterial uterine infections have been documented to cause infertility in bitches, the same types of bacteria have been isolated from clinically normal bitches and those with infertility or vaginal discharges. Therefore, a diagnosis of infectious infertility may require evaluation of response to therapy.

Hysterosalpingography has been used routinely for diagnosis of occlusion of the oviduct in women for more than 50 years. Unfortunately, contrast radiography of the reproductive tract of the bitch has rarely been performed, despite the usefulness of this technique in detecting obstruction, intrauterine filling defects, ovarian or adnexal masses, congenital deformity, and dysplasia. Hysterosalpingography should be performed using general anesthesia early in proestrus. Even though cervical catheterization is difficult at this stage of the cycle, contrast medium can be introduced into the uterus if the catheter tip is placed in the anterior vagina.

Abnormal Cycles. 1. *Prolonged standing heat* is associated with failure of ovulation. Bitches that stand for longer than ten days often have decreased fertility. Human chorionic gonadotropin (HCG) at a dose of 500 IU IV and 500 IU IM or 100 μg GnRH may be given to induce ovulation and luteinization of follicles. If the bitch shows prolonged standing at more than one cycle, this therapy may be given early in standing heat, followed by insemination 24 hours later.

2. *Short interestrous intervals* are less than 4½ months from the onset of the first day of proestrus to the onset of the next proestrus. Potential therapy for these animals is suppression of estrus for six months with mibolerone* (an androgenic steroid), followed by breeding on the first cycle following cessation of therapy.

3. *Long interestrous intervals* exceed eight months except in basenjis, which normally cycle only once annually. In our practice the most common cause of long intervals has been hypothyroidism. Serum thyroxine concentration should be determined at a laboratory in which precision in the 2.0 to 2.5 μg/dl range can be demonstrated. (The useful part of the standard curve in assays of human thyroxine is in the range of 5 to 11 μg/dl.) Treatment should be instituted when thyroxine values are less than 2.0 or when other clinical signs of hypothyroidism are present. Because dogs metabolize thyroxine rapidly, replacement therapy must be given at least twice daily.

---

*Teigland Swab (modified), Haver-Lockhart Labs, 12707 W. 63rd Street, Shawnee, Kansas

*Cheque, The Upjohn Company, Kalamazoo, Michigan

4. *Failure to cycle*, like long interestrous intervals, may be a manifestation of hypothyroidism. Previous ovariohysterectomy, pseudohermaphroditism, and other intersex states should also be ruled out. Chromosome analysis of affected bitches is desirable. Other endocrine disorders, including adrenocortical insufficiency and hyperfunction, have also been observed in association with failure to cycle. In the absence of other abnormalities, the clinician may consider inducing heat by giving 25 mg FSH weekly until signs of vulvar enlargement and blood-tinged vaginal discharge occur. The vaginal smear should be examined periodically and 1000 units HCG (half IM and half IV) should be given when cornification approaches 100 per cent. The bitch should be bred during standing heat; the breeding should be repeated twice.

SUPPLEMENTAL READING

Andersen, A.C., and Simpson, M.E.: *The Ovary and Reproductive Cycle of the Dog.* Los Altos, California, Geron-X, 1973.

Bardens, J.W.: Management of sterility and obstetrical problems in the bitch. AAHA Proc, South Bend, Indiana, Am. Anim. Hosp. Assoc. 1973, pp. 264–267.

Carmichael, L.E.: Canine brucellosis: An annotated review with selected cautionary comments. Theriogenology, 6(2):105–116, 1976.

Cobb, L.M.: The radiographic outline of the genital system of the bitch. Vet. Rec., 71:66–68, 1959.

Concannon, P.W., Hansel, W., and Visek, W.J.: The ovarian cycle of the bitch: Plasma estrogen, LH and progesterone. Bio. Reprod., 13:112–121, 1975.

Hirsch, D.C., and Wiger, N.: The bacterial flora of the normal canine vagina compared with that of vaginal exudates. J. Small Anim. Pract., 18:25–30, 1977.

Holst, P.A., and Phemister, R.D.: Onset of diestrus in the beagle bitch: Definition and significance. Am. J. Vet. Res., 35:401–406, 1974.

Holst, P.A., and Phemister, R.D.: Temporal sequence of events in the estrous cycle of the bitch. Am. J. Vet. Res., 36:705–706, 1975.

Larsen, R.E.: Testicular biopsy in the dog. Vet. Clin. North Am., 7:747–755, 1977.

Olson, P.N.S., and Mather, E.C.: Canine vaginal and uterine bacterial flora. J. Am. Vet. Med. Assoc., 172:708–711, 1978.

Osbaldiston, G.W., Nuru, S., and Mosier, J.E.: Vaginal cytology and microflora of infertile bitches. J. Am. Anim. Hosp. Assoc., 8:93–101, 1972.

Sokolowski, J.H., Stover, D.G., and VanRavenswaay, F.: Seasonal incidence of estrus and interestrous interval for bitches of seven breeds. J. Am. Vet. Med. Assoc., 171:271–273, 1977.

Wooley, R.E., Hitchcock, P.L., Blue, J.L., Neuman, M.A., Brown, J., and Shotts, E.B.: Isolation of *Brucella canis* from a dog seronegative for brucellosis. J. Am. Vet. Med. Assoc., 173:387–388, 1978.

PROGNOSIS AND MANAGEMENT OF FELINE INFERTILITY

MARY A. HERRON, D.V.M.

College Station, Texas

and BARBARA STEIN, D.V.M.

Chicago, Illinois

ANOMALIES

Genital anomalies are rare but warrant inclusion in the differential diagnosis of infertility in young animals. Two intersex conditions, hermaphroditism and male pseudohermaphroditism, have been reported in cats. Hermaphroditism is characterized by ovarian and testicular tissues as separate gonads or ovotestes. The external genitalia may appear immature or sexually intermediate. Male pseudohermaphrodites have only testicular tissue. In dogs external signs of male pseudohermaphroditism include an enlarged clitoris containing an os clitoris and abnormal location of the vulvar opening. In cats external alterations may be less dramatic, but affected cats have been reported to behave as females. These animals may attract males and even permit mounting. The owner might believe that the animal is a normal female. Intersex animals are sterile.

Laparotomy and observation of gonads and internal organs may confirm the diagnosis of intersex. In lieu of surgery, microscopic examination of cells for Barr bodies or karyotyping may be useful in detecting genotypes. Karyotyping is more precise and will detect chimeras or mosaics.

Sterility in male cats with tri-colored coats is a well-known genetic abnormality. These males, nearly all of which are sterile, have diploid-triploid chimerism, with the sex chromosomes of at least a part of the cell population represented by XXY.

Ovarian hypoplasia may be the underlying cause of females that never cycle. Small, fibrous, inactive ovaries are observed at ovariohysterectomy or necropsy. When knowledge concerning serum steroid levels is better defined in cats, serum estrogen levels could be helpful in diagnosis. Treatment has never been reported for this condition, but administration of gonadotropins using the regimen suggested for treatment of anestrus is a logical recommendation. If the ovary can be stimulated, pregnancy might be possible.

Cryptorchidism produces infertility only when both testes are retained. Unilaterally cryptorchid males are fertile, but use of these animals for breeding is discouraged because the condition is probably heritable. There is no proved medical treatment that will consistently induce the descent of retained testicles.

Uterus unicornis and segmental aplasia of the uterus are common anomalies in cats. In uterus unicornis only one normal uterine horn is present. The contralateral uterine horn, and in some instances the contralateral ovary and kidney, is absent. Absence of one or more portions of the uterine horn constitutes segmental aplasia. If normal portions of the horn are isolated from the cervix, mucometra may occur, resulting in abdominal distention and a palpable mass. These dilated portions of the uterus may be removed surgically. Both of the anomalies may be detected incidentally at necropsy, since infertility is expressed only in cases in which neither horn has a normal connection to the cervix. Normal pregnancies may occur if a single anatomically normal horn is present.

COPULATORY FAILURE AND LOSS OF LIBIDO

Knowledge of feline mating behavior is an important prerequisite to diagnosis of infertility resulting from copulatory failure. In most cases copulatory failure is not serious and can be corrected or prevented by good breeding management. Most males prefer to mate in their established territory — a cage, room, or yard. Males forced to breed in unfamiliar environments may spend minutes to hours investigating and marking new surroundings while ignoring the estrous female. Simply waiting for the tom to adjust will probably result in eventual mating, but to expedite matters the female is customarily taken to the male's territory.

Proper mounting ensures the proper alignment of the male and female genitalia, which is mandatory for copulation. For proper positioning, the tom learns to grasp the dorsum of the female's neck. If the tom grasps the skin over the thoracic vertebrae, copulation is impossible. Malpositioning may also result from the pairing of a short-bodied tom with a long-bodied female. Trial and error may correct the malposition, or an assistant may encourage the male to grasp the correct place. The assistant should be familiar to the tom, since intervention by strangers may terminate the breeding attempt.

Copulation may be clumsy or incomplete when two novice breeders are paired. Pairing novices with experienced breeders may be helpful, but the experienced animal should be selected with care. If a novice is initially exposed to an overly aggressive or brutal animal, the experience may make a lasting impression that inhibits future performance.

Queens with timid personalities or infrequent exposure to other cats may cease behavioral estrus when placed abruptly with the tom. The simplest solution is to leave the queen in the new environment with periodic exposure to the male. In some cases behavioral estrus returns in 24 to 48 hours. To eliminate rapid environmental change during estrus, the queen may be moved to the breeding environment for a period of adjustment prior to estrus. Occasionally a queen may reject a specific tom but will breed readily with an alternative mate. Capriciousness is certainly one explanation for such rejection. A more credible explanation, however, is that the male's color, size, or odor plays a role in rejection.

Since ovulation in the cat is induced by the stimulus of copulation, ovulation failure would seem to be an unlikely cause of infertility. However, ovulation may require varying levels of stimulation. The stimulus of a single copulation may be insufficient to induce ovulation in some queens. Multiple matings are suggested if anovulation is suspected.

Lack of libido in males may account for breeding failure. In older males with little or no opportunity to breed, libido may be stimulated by testosterone (0.25 to 0.50 mg/kg). Excessive doses or chronic use, however, could lead to suppression of spermatogenesis through pituitary inhibition. In some cases of depressed libido thyroid function tests may prove useful. If deficiencies are corrected, breeding enthusiasm is favorably affected. Urethral irritation associated with feline urologic syndrome in males may also inhibit breeding performance. Medical treatment of the syndrome followed by one to two months of sexual rest is advised.

In all cases of copulation failure not solved by ordinary measures, artificial insemination is an alternative.

ENDOCRINE DISORDERS

Infertility caused by hormone imbalance is frequently an exclusion diagnosis. Serum hormone levels could be a helpful diagnostic tool, but normal feline serum hormone levels have not been well established. Reports of hormone levels in cases of suspected imbalance are nonexistent. Until these levels are determined and tests become available to the practitioner, endocrine disorders will continue to be diagnosed by elimination.

Anestrus, cystic follicles, and hypoluteoidism are three syndromes that are probably caused by endocrine dysfunction. Anestrus may occur in adolescent and adult females. In young cats that have apparently never cycled, ovarian hypoplasia might be suspected, but the cause of cessation of estrus in adults in which no infection is present is difficult to explain. Silent heats are a plausible explanation of some cases, since vaginal cornification and follicular development may occur cyclically in the absence of behavioral estrus. A logical approach to treatment of anestrus is stimulation of follicular growth. Follicle stimulating hormone (FSH) and pregnant mare serum gonadotropin (PMSG) have been used in research colonies to induce estrus during seasonal anestrus or at will. These drugs have been successful in normal animals; the same dosages may be applied to queens with clinical anestrus. Two milligrams of FSH are administered intramuscularly each day for five days. Alternatively PMSG is administered for eight days with an initial dose of 100 IU, followed by 50 IU for two days, then 25 IU for five days. Close observation and evaluation of vaginal smears help to assess the success of treatment. If estrus is stimulated, an injection of 250 to 500 IU of human chorionic gonadotropin (HCG) may be necessary to ensure ovulation, although natural mating may be sufficient. Breeding should begin on the day of injection. Treatment with hormones carries the risk of superovulation and induction of cystic ovaries.

Clinical signs of cystic ovaries in cats are clearly indicative of hyperestrogenism. The queen may roll on the ground, rub against furniture, call, and assume breeding postures.

Males are attracted, but the queen resists mounting. Many queens become ill-tempered and unsuitable as pets. The overall prognosis for return to fertility is poor but not hopeless. Attempts to induce ovulation with HCG have not been successful. Either the injection fails to stimulate abnormal follicles or excessive endometrial proliferation produced by estrogens prevents implantation. Laparotomy and manual removal of follicles and corpora lutea may be attempted to salvage valuable queens. These queens should be bred at the first postoperative estrus by an aggressive male.

Hypoluteoidism is manifested by repeated abortion at about the same time late in gestation. Since the corpus luteum of the cat ceases to function close to day 40 of gestation, the combination of declining progesterone production by the corpus luteum and the inability of the placenta to produce progesterone might result in insufficient hormone to maintain pregnancy. Although this seems logical, there are no published reports of circulating hormone levels in these queens. However, the condition has been treated with repositol progesterone (0.25 to 0.5 mg/kg) at weekly intervals, starting seven to ten days before the expected abortion. Since exogenous progesterone inhibits relaxation of the cervix, treatment should be terminated about one week before expected parturition. Orally administered progesterone would also be suitable, but there are no published dosages. The diagnosis of hypoluteoidism should not be made before considering bacterial endometritis, feline leukemia, and feline infectious peritonitis, all of which may result in late abortion.

GENITAL INFECTIONS

The cat has no recognized species-specific venereal disease, but bacterial infections are well established as contributors to feline infertility. *E. coli*, staphylococci, and streptococci commonly invade the genital tract and may cause acute metritis, chronic endometritis, pyometra, orchitis, or epididymitis. Viral agents affect feline fertility to an undefined extent. Feline leukemia virus has been implicated in fetal resorption, abortion, and increased numbers of stillborn or weak kittens. Feline infectious peritonitis may cause similar signs. The viruses of feline panleukopenia and feline viral rhinotracheitis are known to cross the placenta to infect fetuses, but the relationship of these viruses to subsequent breedings, pregnancies, and spermatogenesis has not been established. Infertility related to virus infections has been readily observed in catteries and colonies. Colonies experiencing abnormally high rates of resorptions, abortions, stillbirths, or conception failures should prompt collection of a detailed history and laboratory tests to identify the specific virus. If a vaccine is available for the specific virus, improvement in the vaccination program with improved management practices may save the colony. If no vaccine is available, identification and elimination of infected animals is the only method of salvaging the colony.

ACUTE METRITIS

In addition to the following discussion, articles devoted to acute canine metritis and pyometra should be consulted for specific details.

The uterus is exposed to ascending bacterial infection when the cervix is open. Therefore, acute metritis is a frequent occurrence in the wake of parturition, particularly when there has been fetal manipulation without full attention to aseptic procedures or when placentas are retained. Less commonly, ascending infections follow breeding. In these cases the infection may be spread from the vagina of the female or from the prepuce or genital organs of the male.

Early signs include lack of interest in nursing and caring for the kittens, depression, and fever. The vaginal discharge may be the same color as normal postpartum discharge, but often it has a foul odor and persists longer. Untreated cases progress rapidly to dehydration and toxemia.

Although palpation of the uterus may be painful and resisted by the queen, it may reveal retained placentas or an enlarged, distended uterus. The uterus may also be evaluated radiographically. Vaginal smears are characterized by large numbers of neutrophils, bacteria, and uterine cells. Hemograms may reveal an immature neutrophilic leukocytosis or mature leukocytosis with hypersegmentation of nuclei.

Kittens should be removed for raising by hand because of the potential for bacterial contamination from concomitant mastitis or vaginal discharge. Immediate treatment is vital, since the severity of uterine damage is proportional to the duration of infection. The condition may advance rapidly to a toxemic state.

In early cases systemic antibiotics and supportive therapy may be successful. If maintenance of breeding capacity is of major concern, uterine infusion or surgical intervention may be necessary to maintain a functional uterus. Regardless of the severity of the case, the immediate priority is to obtain a cervical or high vaginal swab for culture and sensitivity tests. Wide-spectrum antibiotic treatment and supportive therapy should not be delayed until sensitivity reports are available. In some cases expression of uterine contents may be facilitated by intramuscular administration of 0.1 mg ergonovine maleate followed by oral administration of 0.05 mg b.i.d. for two or three days. In more advanced cases uterine infusion of antibiotic solutions may also be useful. Utonex®* has been used with good results. Great caution should be exercised in placement of catheters, since visualization of the feline cervix is difficult. A pliable catheter should be passed through the cervix and directed into each horn for a thorough, gentle washing. External uterine massage may aid distribution of the fluid; however, there is risk of uterine perforation with the catheter as a result of overzealous massage.

Surgical intervention offers some prognostic and treatment advantages. If the animal is a suitable candidate for surgery, laparotomy allows visual examination of the uterus for tissue damage, biopsies, and manipulation of tissues for lavage. By manipulating them through the laparotomy incision, catheters are easier to guide through the cervix, and the horns may be manipulated with reduced risk of perforation.

Antibiotic therapy should be continued for two to three weeks. In all cases breeding should be delayed for at least three months. The prognosis for recovery of reproductive function is good if acute metritis is diagnosed early and treated correctly. Queens with this condition should be observed carefully for several months for signs of chronic endometritis.

CHRONIC ENDOMETRITIS

Chronic endometritis is characterized by low-grade bacterial infection of the endometrium and is likely to become established in uteri with cystic endometrial changes. It may also be the sequela of acute metritis. It is less life-threatening than acute metritis, but detection is more difficult. The animal usually has no clinical signs, and routine laboratory tests are often inconclusive. The only clue may be a history of infertility. The owner may complain of chronic conception failure, fetal resorptions, or abortions. Small litters from a queen or vague estrus irregularities may also be associated with chronic endometritis.

Systemic antibiotic therapy is the most conservative treatment for chronic endometritis. Treated queens require monitoring, since less than 30 per cent of the cases will respond to this method. A cervical culture should be taken

---

*Schering Corp., Kenilworth, N.J.

during or immediately following estrus to help select an antibiotic. Light anesthesia may aid sample collection. Post-treatment cultures collected during estrus may be helpful in evaluating therapy.

Surgical intervention is another option for clients who wish a positive diagnosis and rigorous, immediate treatment. Laparotomy affords direct visualization of the genital organs, direct culture, biopsy of the endometrium, and lavage of the uterine horns.

The degree of endometrial damage will determine whether pregnancy is possible. Return to full function after prolonged endometritis is unlikely. A more optimistic prognosis can be given for cats treated after a short-duration infection. In all cases of cystic endometrial hyperplasia the prognosis must be guarded. Although the infection may be eliminated by proper treatment, the underlying cystic disorder may prevent successful pregnancies.

PYOMETRA

Of all uterine infections, pyometra is the most devastating and least responsive to treatment. This disease is complex, originating with progesterone-induced cystic endometrial hyperplasia and concomitant infection. Before bacterial invasion, the appropriate term descriptive of the lesions is *mycometra*. However, since infection is the final stage of this disease complex, preinfection stages are often termed *sterile pyometra*. E. coli is the most common invader. Early during the onset of cystic endometrial hyperplasia, the cat may cycle but will not conceive. If the cervix is open and permits drainage, the disease may exist for weeks or months with few systemic signs until the condition is well advanced. Later signs include anestrus, anorexia, and depression, accompanied by a decline in body condition. Polydipsia, polyuria, and non-painful abdominal distention also develop. There is generally no fever. If the cervix is open, the perineal area may be wet or soiled. The discharge may vary in color from brown to white. If the cervix is closed, the cat is more seriously ill and body condition declines rapidly.

The uterus may be segmentally enlarged or evenly distended. It may be palpated or visualized radiographically. Hemograms and renal function tests aid in the diagnosis and prognosis and should be routinely obtained in all suspected cases of pyometra. Leukocyte counts are excessive (often 30,000 to 90,000/mm³) with absolute neutrophilia. In advanced cases with severe toxemia, leukocytes may decrease to normal numbers but are often toxic and hyper-

segmented. Many affected cats have a normocytic, normochromic anemia. Renal function may be impaired, as indicated by urinalysis, serum urea nitrogen concentration, and creatinine concentration. Renal function assessment is important in selecting supportive therapy. Consult the article on canine pyometra for further information about laboratory findings.

As with other uterine infections bacterial culture, systemic antibiotics, and support therapy should be initiated immediately. Although some patients with pyometra are poor surgical risks, ovariohysterectomy is the treatment of choice to save the life of the cat. In valuable breeding animals an attempt may be made to salvage the uterus. Uterine infusion is probably inadequate, since the tissues are extremely friable and the exudate is thick and tenacious. Hysterotomy may be considered for patients diagnosed prior to development of severe toxicity. Laboratory tests should be carefully scrutinized, however. Even after determining that the cat is a candidate for hysterotomy, the surgeon should retain the option to perform ovariohysterectomy during surgery.

During surgery a portion of one uterine horn should be exteriorized, incised, and drained. A moist sponge may be passed carefully over the endometrial surface to remove thick exudate. The entire horn should be washed with an antibiotic solution. A catheter may be positioned in the cervix for external lavage the day after surgery. The uterus should be closed with 00 surgical gut in an inverting pattern. The other horn should be treated in the same manner. During the procedure care should be taken to avoid contamination of the peritoneal cavity. If the condition is unilateral, the affected horn and accompanying ovary may be removed and the contralateral horn salvaged.

Since pyometra is a sequela of progesterone secretion by retained corpora lutea (CL), removal of the CL has been suggested in surgical treatment of pyometra in dogs. CL removal has also been used in cats with positive results. Excessive manipulation of the ovary and bursa should be avoided if possible, since it may create adhesions that interfere with ovulation and transport of ova. Postoperative care includes continuation of supportive therapy and systemic administration of antibiotics. Even with successful recovery from surgery, fewer than half of these patients will conceive again. If the condition is unilateral, the prognosis is better.

Prostaglandins have been used experimentally in dogs for luteolysis and to aid uterine evacuation if the cervix is open. Evacuation of uterine contents is desirable to facilitate ovariohysterectomy or hysterotomy. Combination of prostaglandins with other therapy may be successful in treating pyometra. When adapted for use in cats, this drug will be a valuable adjunct to other treatments.

INFECTIONS OF THE MALE GENITAL TRACT

Systemic disease associated with elevated body temperatures or local infections of the scrotum or perineum may suppress spermatogenesis by elevating testicular temperature. The suppression is generally temporary and spermatogenesis returns after the systemic illness or local infection is corrected. Infections of the testis or epididymis are potentially more devastating to fertility. They are often secondary to bite or scratch wounds. In addition to the detrimental effects of heat on spermatogenesis, infection stimulates fibrosis, which damages seminiferous tubules. Since the epididymis is a single tube, fibrosis at any point is likely to result in blockage of sperm flow, whereas focal testicular lesions will not necessarily interrupt function totally. The degree of tissue damage determines the degree of functional loss. Trauma to the testicle also interrupts the blood-testis barrier, allowing development of antisperm antibodies. Although this type of autoimmunization has not been reported in cats, it is logical to assume that it occurs, as it does in other species.

Local infections are treated with systemic and local antibiotics and good nursing. Postinfection assessment of the genital tract should include examination of the penis and prepuce for adhesions and palpation of the gonads and epididymides. The size and texture of the organs should indicate the extent of fibrosis. Semen quality may be evaluated in two ways. The most time-consuming is performance testing three to six months following injury. If this method is selected, companion queens should be proved and have no history of reproductive failures. Alternatively, postinfection semen samples may be collected and evaluated. Two or more samples collected at two to three month intervals may be necessary to appraise functional improvement correctly.

Microscopic observation of postbreeding vaginal fluids may allow a cursory appraisal of sperm motility and concentration. This method is not specific but is useful in detecting cases of azoospermia. Oligospermia is detectable but difficult to monitor by this method. Evaluation of semen collected by electroejaculation is superior but not generally available to practitioners.

If only one testis or epididymis is involved, fertility may be maintained by the opposite intact organs, although semen concentration may be reduced. The prognosis for fertility in unilateral destruction is good if the breeding program is well managed. The prognosis for fertility is poor if azoospermia follows infection. Males with oligospermia should also be given a poor prognosis; however, some reproductive capacity may be salvaged through pooled semen samples and artificial insemination.

NON-INFECTIOUS OLIGOSPERMIA AND AZOOSPERMIA

Potential causes of oligospermia and azoospermia other than infection include scrotal hernias, sexual overuse, genetic defects, hormonal imbalances, and toxins. The first two conditions may be corrected by surgery and breeding management, respectively. Other potential causes have not been recognized in cats. Feline semen evaluation is useful for detecting abnormal sperm numbers or abnormal sperm morphology but does not define the underlying cause. A definitive diagnosis usually requires detailed study of individual clinical cases and well-structured research. At present, toms with oligospermia or azoospermia are often culled from breeding programs after a series of nonproductive matings.

A high number of services per conception or multiple conception failures suggest oligospermia or azoospermia. Palpation of the gonads for size and texture is an important part of the physical examination. Semen should also be collected and evaluated. Even though there is risk of stimulating antisperm antibodies, testicular biopsy should not be omitted from the diagnostic armamentarium, particularly in cases of azoospermia and selected cases of oligospermia. Knowledge of the histology of the seminiferous tubules allows a prognosis to be made with confidence.

Gonadotropin therapy may be of value in some cases, but therapeutic guidelines are not available. Since no other treatments have been suggested for either azoospermia or oligospermia of unknown cause, only a grim prognosis for return to fertility can be given.

GENERAL CAUSES OF INFERTILITY

The impact of obesity, poor nutrition, inbreeding, genital neoplasia, and advanced age on feline infertility is unknown. Of these factors, inbreeding poses the greatest potential threat. Intensive inbreeding in other species, particularly cattle, has resulted in genetically based infertility characterized by abnormal sperm motility and morphology, hypogonadism, and decreased conception rates. Although a thorough family history may indicate a genetic problem, positive diagnosis can be made only with sophisticated and expensive testing procedures. To eliminate the problem, entire breeding lines may have to be terminated if the defect itself does not terminate the line.

Obesity does not play a role in feline infertility, since the condition is rare in this species. Thyroid malfunction is known to affect reproduction in other species; depressed libido in male cats may not be the only expression of hypothyroidism. While deficiencies of vitamin A, B complex vitamins, copper, iron, and phosphorus have been related to infertility in other domestic species, only vitamin A deficiency has been related to infertility in cats. Classic signs of vitamin A deficiency include hair loss, night blindness, weight loss, and abnormal bone growth. The deficiency may also cause conception failure or production of kittens with an increased proportion of anomalies such as cleft palates, hydrocephalus, and spina bifida. Hypervitaminosis A is also a potential cause of infertility and is produced by feeding large quantities of liver. Periarticular exostoses is the primary sign of chronic disease. Bony changes cause painful locomotion in males and females and testicular degeneration in males. Correction of the diet can reverse testicular degeneration, but bony changes persist.

With the exception of mammary neoplasia, genital neoplasms are extremely rare in cats. Even mammary tumors, which have a high malignancy rate in cats, may not terminate fertility if diagnosed and treated early in the disease process.

No age limit for fertility is established for the cat, although aging animals may tend to produce smaller litters. One age-related syndrome is recognized in female cats (particularly exhibition cats) that are allowed to cycle for several years before breeding is attempted. A combination of aging and hormones may produce endometrial changes. Depending upon the degree of change, these females may not conceive. If they do conceive, they may bear small litters and have an increased frequency of stillbirths. Since there is no proposed medical treatment for the condition, females being held as potential breeders should be permitted to bear some litters in their early adult years in hope of avoiding endometrial changes.

SUPPLEMENTAL READING

Colby, E. D.: Induced estrus and timed pregnancies in cats. Lab. Anim. Care, 20:1075–1080, 1970.
Herron, M. A.: Feline reproduction. Vet. Clin. North Am., 7:715–720, 1977.
Herron, M. A.: Feline vaginal cytologic examination. Feline Pract., 7:36–39, 1977.
Stein, B.: Feline Medicine and Surgery. Santa Barbara, California, American Veterinary Publications, 1975, pp. 303–354.
Wildt, D. E., and Seager, W. J.: Ovarian response in the estrual cat receiving varying dosages of HCG. Hormone Res., 9:144–150, 1978.
Wildt, D. E., Kinney, G. M., and Seager, S. W. J.: Gonadotropin-induced reproductive cyclicity in the domestic cat. Lab. Anim. Sci., 28:301–302, 1978.

PREVENTION OF ESTRUS

THOMAS J. BURKE, D.V.M.
Urbana, Illinois

INTRODUCTION

Although surgical methods are the most reliable means of fertility control in dogs and cats, they are also permanent. Methods of temporary control of fertility currently available consist of pharmacologic prevention or postponement of estrus, prevention of conception (mismating treatment), and interruption of established pregnancies. Only the first method will be discussed here.

PROGESTOGENS

Progesterone was the first hormone used to prevent estrus successfully in the bitch. Oral and parenteral progestogenic compounds have been and are being used in the bitch and queen for estrous control.

Use of long-term oral or repositol parenteral progestogens has been shown to cause or predispose to development of sterile inflammatory or non-inflammatory uterine disease, pyometra, mammary neoplasia, and several other organic dysfunctions. For these reasons neither the bitch nor queen should be subjected to continual long-term progestogenic therapy.

Intermittent short-term therapy with oral progestins has been shown to have a high safety:efficacy ratio. Currently, only one compound — megestrol acetate (Ovaban, Schering Corp.) — is cleared for this indication in the bitch in the United States. It is eliminated from the dog mainly via the liver, with total excretion in 22 days.

Megestrol may be used to postpone an anticipated estrous cycle in the bitch at a dose of approximately 0.25 mg/lb (0.55 mg/kg) daily for 32 days, beginning at least a week prior to the onset of proestrus. If administration is properly timed, efficacy exceeds 97 percent. If the owner is unsure of the dog's cycle but wishes to avoid a heat for a particular purpose at a given time, this method is excellent. In these cases I perform a vaginal cytologic examination. If no erythrocytes (RBCs) are seen (they commonly precede the visible onset of proestrus by about a week), therapy is initiated. If RBCs are seen, the owner is told that proestrus probably is imminent and is advised to wait until prevention therapy can be initiated.

Return to cyclicity is highly variable, but most patients will cycle four to six months after treatment unless the timing of therapy was incorrect.

In Europe the anestrus period is commonly prolonged by administration of 0.05 to 0.1 mg/lb (0.1 to 0.2 mg/kg) twice weekly for another four months after the initial 32-day treatment period. No treatment is given during the first post-treatment cycle.

Megestrol also is indicated for prevention of estrus while the bitch is in proestrus. A daily dose of 1.0 mg/lb (2.2 mg/kg) is given for eight days, commencing during the first three days after proestral bleeding *and* vulvar swelling are noted. If started too early, an abbreviated interestrus period should be expected. If initiated too late, treatment may be ineffective. Since this treatment obviates formation of corpora lutea (i.e., ovulation does not occur), the normal interestrus period commonly is shortened by the period of time that luteal function predominates (60 to 90 days). Thus, the next proestrus often occurs three to five months after treatment.

European practitioners commonly prolong the return to the next proestrus by giving megestrol for four days at 1.0 mg/lb (2.2 mg/kg), followed by 0.25 mg/lb (0.55 mg/kg) for 16 days.

If mating occurs during the first three days of the eight-day treatment period, megestrol administration should cease and mismating therapy should be discussed with the owner. If four or more doses have been given the rest of the treatment should be administered, because megestrol apparently exerts a contraceptive effect in virtually all these cases.

Megestrol is not approved for use in cats in the United States. Unpublished studies by the author showed that 5 mg/cat/week kept queens out of heat for the ten-week treatment period. Significant drug-related lesions were not found at necropsy. British studies indicate that 5 mg/cat/day will stop estrus in three to five days. Postponement doses depend upon whether the cat is in a breeding season but between estrus periods (diestrus) or is in actual anestrus. For the former, 2.5 mg/cat/day is given for up to two months. For maintaining anestrus, 2.5 mg/cat is given weekly for up to 18 months. In either case an unmedicated cycle is recommended prior to beginning another course of therapy.

In both the bitch and queen the temporary side effects of megestrol usually reported are weight gain from water retention, increased appetite, less aggressive behavior and other related behavioral changes, and general decrease in activity. As with all progestogens, megestrol may cause the exogenous insulin requirements of diabetics to fluctuate markedly.

ANDROGENS

Testosterone propionate and methyltestosterone have been used for estrus prevention. This practice currently is most prevalent in racing greyhounds. Return to cyclicity generally occurs after withdrawal of therapy, but some bitches have experienced difficulties in attaining normal cyclicity and fertility. The major side effect is clitoral hypertrophy, which is sometimes irreversible, and associated vulvovaginitis.

Recently, a potent, orally active synthetic androgen — mibolerone (Cheque, The Upjohn Company) — was approved for long-term estrus prevention in the bitch. Dose depends upon body weight, except in German shepherds and German shepherd crosses, which require comparatively higher doses (Table 1). For maximum efficacy, therapy should be begun at least 30 days prior to proestrus. Daily administration is required. Label indications are for a two-year maximum treatment period, although extension of this time is anticipated by the manufacturer. Return to cyclicity and fertility is unimpaired, and normal conception rates are attained by the second post-treatment heat in mature bitches.

Side effects associated with administration of

Table 1. *Dose of Mibolerone for Estrus Prevention*

BODY WEIGHT *(lb)*	DAILY DOSE *(μg)*
1–25	30
26–50	60
51–100	120
100+	180
Shepherd dogs	180

mibolerone are minimal and include clitoral hypertrophy that is at least partially reversible, associated vulvovaginitis, and deepening of the voice. Vaginitis seems to be more severe in prepuberal bitches. Patients with seborrhea oleosa may experience a worsening of symptoms. A musky odor also has been reported by some owners, apparently a result of increased sebaceous gland activity. Decreased serum cholesterol and microscopic hepatic changes (intranuclear hyaline bodies) have been observed in treated bitches. Increased kidney weight without microscopic renal pathology also has been reported. Alterations in routine hepatic and renal function tests have not been observed. If administered to pregnant bitches, severe masculinization of female fetuses, resulting in multiple urogenital anomalies, will occur.

Mibolerone is not approved for use in queens. Daily doses of 50 μg/cat will prevent estrus but result in thyroid dysfunction, thickening of the cervical dermis, and clitoral hypertrophy and formation of os clitorides in some cases. At 60 μg/cat/day hepatic dysfunction is seen, and mortality occurs at doses as low as 120 μg/cat/day. Therefore, the drug should not be used in cats because the efficacy:safety ratio is very low.

PILOCARPINE

The German literature refers to the use of oral pilocarpine to suppress estrus in bitches and queens. Two to 4 drops of 1 percent pilocarpine solution stopped estrus within two days. The author has not used this treatment, but perhaps it should be investigated. A mechanism of action was not proposed.

SUPPLEMENTAL READING

A Glaxo Guide to Ovarid. Greenford, Middlesex, England, Glaxo Laboratories Ltd., 1976.
Lauderdale, J.W., and Sokolowski, J.H. (eds.): Proceedings of the symposium on Cheque for canine estrus prevention. Kalamazoo, Michigan, The Upjohn Co., 1978.

PREGNANCY PREVENTION AND TERMINATION

WILLIAM F. JACKSON, D.V.M.
Lakeland, Florida,

and SHIRLEY D. JOHNSTON, D.V.M.
St. Paul, Minnesota

Prevention of pregnancy in the bitch and queen is often a challenge to the companion animal owner. Preventing contact between an eager female and one or more overeager males is a contest between human and animal minds. Tall fences, screen doors, and britches are rarely dependable. Chlorophyll tablets used to control the odor of pheromones produced by the female are not much of a challenge to most males.

PREGNANCY PREVENTION

For the pet-owning public, ovariohysterectomy (OHE) is the most reliable method of preventing estrus and pregnancy and, if performed before or shortly after the first estrus, the procedure confers protection against later mammary neoplasia in both dogs and cats. Laparoscopic tubal ligation is reported to be easier and safer than OHE, but it still requires general anesthesia and expensive equipment while failing to prevent cycling or later mammary and uterine disease. Medical suppression of cycling is discussed in the article entitled "Prevention of Estrus."

Sterilization of the male may be useful in preventing pregnancy in some situations; castration is the preferred method. Low numbers of sperm may be present in the ejaculate of vasectomized dogs for as long as three weeks following surgery, suggesting that fertile sperm may also survive in the vasa deferentia in castrated males for this period of time. If surgical sterilization is opposed, percutaneous injection of 0.5 ml of a sclerosing agent (1.5 percent chlorhexidine gluconate in 50 percent dimethyl sulfoxide) into each cauda epididymis of sedated males has been reported to induce long-lasting azoospermia. Immunization of dogs against luteinizing hormone (LH) is feasible and effective, although there is great individual variation in antibody titer response, time of onset of azoospermia, and return to fertility.

PREGNANCY TERMINATION

An accurate history is needed to ascertain whether copulation actually has occurred. Vaginal cytology can be used to estimate the stage of the cycle. Presence of sperm in a vaginal wash or bite marks at the nape of the neck may help to confirm breeding. The bitch ovulates approximately three days after the onset of standing behavior; the cat is induced to ovulate 24 to 36 hours after coitus or cervical stimulation. Even though ova can be fertilized only for 12 to 24 hours, canine sperm are motile for ten days and fertile for as long as five to six days in the female reproductive tract. Morulae enter the uterus six to ten days following ovulation in dogs and four to five days after coitus in cats. Implantation in both species occurs approximately 16 to 18 days following first acceptance of the male.

OVARIOHYSTERECTOMY

OHE performed during the first month of pregnancy in the bitch and queen is safe and is preferred to medical means of pregnancy termination when reproductive function need not be preserved.

MISMATING INJECTIONS

The relatively long process (six to ten days) of ova transport through canine oviducts and the characteristic of queens to ovulate 24 to 36 hours after coitus make these species especially vulnerable to postcoital contraceptive agents that affect tubal transport. Estrogens delay ova transport through canine and feline oviducts, probably by causing contraction of isthmal musculature or of the uterotubal sphincter. They may also exert direct degenerative effects on ova and alter the histologic character of endometrial implantation sites.

Optimum time of administration of drugs following mismating is three to five days after onset of standing heat in bitches and two to three days after coitus in queens. Suggested doses are 2 mg/kg (not to exceed 25 mg) of repositol diethylstilbestrol given intramuscularly or 0.125 to 1 mg of estradiol cypionate given intramuscularly in dogs. Intramuscular injections of 2 mg of repositol diethylstilbestrol or 0.25 mg of estradiol cypionate have been reported to be effective in cats, but these products are not approved for that use.

Undesirable side effects include persistence of estrual behavior for seven to ten days after therapy, myelosuppression leading to thrombocytopenia and aplastic anemia. Although there is great individual variation among dogs in their response to toxic effects of estrogens, most cases of estrogen toxicity reported following mismating therapy have occurred after administration of doses much greater than those just described. A third undesirable side effect of mismating therapy is the tendency to induce open-cervix pyometra one to six weeks after administration. Although the exact mechanism of this complication is unclear, estrogen is known to stimulate synthesis of progesterone receptors in target tissues such as the endometrium. It may therefore potentiate the effect of endogenous progesterone, which the bitch normally secretes for two months after estrus. Dow demonstrated that cystic endometrial hyperplasia that occurs after progesterone treatment in dogs that undergo ovariectomy developed more rapidly, or at lower dose, when dogs were pretreated with estrogen. When administering estrogens following mismating, the clinician is repeating Dow's experiment by treating with estrogen before a 60-day period of endogenous progesterone influence on the endometrium.

CORTICOSTEROIDS

A ten-day course of intramuscular injections of dexamethasone (5 mg b.i.d.) to a small number of bitches has been shown to cause intrauterine death followed by fetal resorption (when started at day 30 of pregnancy) or abortion (when started at day 45). Subsequent fertility of treated bitches was not evaluated.

PROSTAGLANDINS

Prostaglandin $F_{2\alpha}$ is luteolytic in bitches. Because bitches require functional corpora lutea for pregnancy maintenance throughout gestation, this compound has been tested as an abortifacient. Four of seven pregnant bitches aborted between days 31 and 53 of gestation when given 60 μg/kg prostaglandin $F_{2\alpha}$ divided b.i.d. or t.i.d. for three days. The single reliable luteolytic dose, however, is 1 mg/kg, which is very near the LD_{50} of 5.13 mg/kg and which also induces severe side effects. Two subcutaneous injections of prostaglandin $F_{2\alpha}$ (0.5 to 1.0 mg/kg) 24 hours apart have been shown to induce abortion in pregnant cats after day 40 of pregnancy; no postpartum complications were observed at this dosage. Abortion could not be induced prior to day 40 in cats, even though ovariectomy prior to (but not after) this time induced abortion. Signs of prostaglandin toxicosis in dogs include hyperpnea, excessive salivation, vomiting, diarrhea, ataxia, and possible death 90 to 120 minutes after treatment. At present, prostaglandins are not approved for use in companion animals.

SUPPLEMENTAL READING

Austad, R., Lunde, A., and Sjaastad, O.V.: Peripheral plasma levels of oestradiol-17β and progesterone in the bitch during the oestrous cycle, in normal pregnancy and after dexamethasone treatment. J. Reprod. Fertil., 46:129–136, 1976.

Clark, J.H., Peck, E.J., and Glasser, S.R.: Mechanism of action of sex steroid hormones in the female. In Cole, H.H., and Cupps, P.T. (eds.): Reproduction in Domestic Animals. New York, Academic Press, 1977, pp. 143–173.

Colby, E.D.: Feline reproduction. AAHA Proceedings, Boston, 1977.

Concannon, P.W., and Hansel, W.: Prostaglandin $F_{2\alpha}$-induced luteolysis, hypothermia and abortions in beagle bitches. Prostaglandins, 13:533–542, 1977.

Concannon, P.W., Powers, M.E., Holder, W., and Hansel, W.: Pregnancy and parturition in the bitch. Biol. Reprod., 16:517–526, 1977.

Dow, C.: Production of the cystic hyperplasia–pyometra complex in the bitch. J. Pathol. Bacteriol., 78:267, 1959.

Herron, M.A., and Sis, R.F.: Ovum transport in the cat and the effect of estrogen administration. Am. J. Vet. Res., 35:1277–1279, 1974.

Holst, P.A., and Phemister, R.D.: The prenatal development of the dog: Preimplantation events. Biol. Reprod., 5:194–206, 1971.

Jackson, W.F.: Management of canine mismating with diethylstilbestrol. Calif. Vet., 22:29, 1953.

Jöchle, W., Lamond, D.R., and Andersen, A.C.: Mestranol as an abortifacient in the bitch. Theriogenology, 4:1–9, 1975.

Kennelly, J.J.: The effect of mestranol on canine reproduction. Biol. Reprod., 1:282–288, 1969.

Legendre, A.M.: Estrogen-induced bone marrow hypoplasia in a dog. J. Am. Anim. Hosp. Assoc., 12:525–527, 1976.

Lowenstine, L.J., Ling, G.V., and Schalm, O.W.: Exogenous estrogen toxicity in the dog. Calif. Vet., 41:14–19, 1972.

McDonald, L.E.: Veterinary Endocrinology and Reproduction. Philadelphia, Lea & Febiger, 1975, pp. 408–423.

Mulligan, R.M.: Mammary cancer in the dog: A study of 120 cases. Am. J. Vet. Res., 36:1391–1396, 1975.

Nachreiner, R.F., and Marple, D.N.: Termination of pregnancy in cats with prostaglandin $F_{2\alpha}$. Prostaglandins, 7:303–308, 1974.

Pineda, M.H., and Faulkner, L.C.: Immunologic control of reproduction in dogs. Canine Pract., 1:11–23, 1974.

Pineda, M.H., Reimers, T.J., and Faulkner, L.C.: Disappearance of spermatozoa from the ejaculates of vasectomized dogs. J. Am. Vet. Med. Assoc., 168:502–503, 1976.

Pineda, M.H., Reimers, T.J., Faulkner, L.C., Hopwood, M.L., and Seidel, G.E.: Azoospermia in dogs induced by infection of sclerosing agents into the caudae of the epididymides. Am. J. Vet. Res., 38:831–838, 1977.

Sokolowski, J.H.: The effects of ovariectomy on pregnancy maintenance. Lab. Anim. Sci., 21:696–699, 1971.

Sokolowski, J.H.: Effect of prostaglandin $F_{2\alpha}$-THAM in the bitch. J. Am. Vet. Med. Assoc., 170 536–537, 1977.

PSEUDOHERMAPHRODITISM

DENNIS A. JACKSON, D.V.M.
Urbana, Illinois

INTRODUCTION

Hermaphrodite or intersex animals have genitalia with some characteristics of both sexes. They are classified by the type of gonadal tissue present. True hermaphrodites have both testicular and ovarian tissue. Pseudohermaphrodites have testes or ovaries and possess external genitalia resembling the opposite sex. Two types of pseudohermaphrodites have been described. Male pseudohermaphrodites have testes and genitalia with some female characteristics, whereas female pseudohermaphrodites have ovaries with genitalia resembling that of males. In dogs male pseudohermaphrodites are encountered more frequently than true hermaphrodites or female pseudohermaphrodites. True hermaphrodites and pseudohermaphrodites have been reported in cats, but apparently occur infrequently.

ETIOPATHOGENESIS

An understanding of the pathogenesis of pseudohermaphroditism requires knowledge of the normal process of sex differentiation. The genetic sex of animals is determined at the time of fertilization. Normal mammalian sex differentiation involves a sequence of events that occurs before birth and at puberty (Hare; Jackson et al.). The initial event involves differentiation of the fetal indifferent gonad into a testis or ovary. The controlling mechanism is not fully understood, but appears to be under the influence of sex chromosomes. The indifferent gonad in zygotes with the XY genotype develops into a testis. In zygotes lacking the Y chromosome and possessing the XX genotype, the indifferent gonad develops into an ovary.

Development of the male (wolffian) or female (müllerian) duct system occurs next. In males the wolffian duct develops as the epididymus and ductus deferens. In females the müllerian duct develops as the oviduct, uterus, and part of the vagina. These events are controlled by hormones secreted by the fetal testis (Jost). These hormones include an androgen-like substance that stimulates development of the male duct and an inhibitory substance that suppresses development of the female duct. The fetal ovary does not secrete controlling hormones and has no known effect on differentiation of the duct systems.

The final event of sex differentiation involves formation of the phenotypic sex by organogenesis of the urogenital sinus and external genitalia. In males the androgen-like hormone from the fetal testis controls this event. In the absence of this hormone, the urogenital sinus and external genitalia take the female form.

Hermaphrodites arise when the fetal gonads experience abnormal differentiation or function, or both. The resulting deficiency of male-stimulating or female-inhibiting hormones causes faulty hormonal control during organogenesis (Jost). Hermaphrodites may also arise from lack of sensitivity by the receptor organ to normal amounts of controlling hormones (Burns) or from excessive endogenous androgens (i.e., congenital adrenogenital syndrome) or exogenous androgens (Hare; Shane).

CLINICAL FINDINGS

Male pseudohermaphrodites may appear to be females with an enlarged clitoris containing an os. They may also appear as males with an underdeveloped prepuce and penis. Hypospadias may be a finding in some cases. The testes are usually abdominal, but may also be found in the inguinal canal or scrotum. Some development of the müllerian duct is seen in most cases, but internal sex organ development can be variable. These animals are thought to be sterile, since spermatogonia found in the testes

are usually inactive. Male pseudohermaphrodites have normal micturation but may assume the male stance when voiding. All reported cases of canine male pseudohermaphroditism with genotype determination have been XX or XY.

Female pseudohermaphrodites appear as males, but have marked underdevelopment of the prepuce and penis and may lack a scrotum. In some cases the penile urethra may show hypospadias and possess an os penis. A normal vulva is absent, as are other vestiges of the female external genitalia. The ovaries are intraabdominal and may be functional, causing periodic estrus with attraction of males. Müllerian duct development is complete; however, a rudimentary prostate may be the only wolffian remnant found. Dogs with female pseudohermaphroditism have normal micturation, but squat in female fashion when voiding. The genetic sex has been female (XX) in all dogs whose genotype has been determined.

Owners of dogs with pseudohermaphroditism may frequently complain of involuntary urine dribbling. Non-neurogenic urinary incontinence caused by an anomalous communication of the urethra and genital tract has been reported in female pseudohermaphrodite dogs (Jackson et al.) Formation of a urethrovaginal fistula in these animals may have resulted from faulty differentiation of the urogenital sinus. A similar developmental anomaly causing urinary incontinence may exist in some male pseudohermaphrodites. Urinary incontinence is caused by retention of urine in the genital tract, with subsequent leakage into the urethra through the anomalous communication that results in involuntary escape of urine.

RADIOGRAPHIC FINDINGS

Anomalies of the genitourinary tract of pseudohermaphrodites usually cannot be demonstrated by standard radiographic methods. Special diagnostic procedures such as retrograde contrast urethrography and intravenous urography are important for detecting such anomalies. The technique for retrograde contrast urethrography has been described and is best performed using a balloon catheter to prevent reflux of contrast material from the distal end of the urethra (Johnston et al.). As contrast material is injected in dogs with urethrovaginal fistulas, a direct communication is seen between the pelvic urethra and distal vagina (Jackson et al.). Intravenous urograms are indicated in animals with suspected anomalies of the genitourinary tract to detect co-existing abnormalities of the kidneys, ureters, or bladder.

Urinalyses, urine cultures, and, occasionally,

vaginal cultures should be submitted for evaluation of pseudohermaphrodite animals, since urinary or genital infections may be associated with the genitourinary anomaly.

Evaluation of hermaphrodite animals may contribute significantly to the elucidation of sex determination and differentiation in mammals. For this reason, complete documentation of cases is needed, including pedigree studies, hormonal evaluation, and sex determination. Whenever possible, sex determination should be made, using cells from several tissues, by sex chromosome analysis (i.e., karyotyping) and sex chromatin techniques (i.e., Barr body determination).

DIAGNOSIS

Intersexuality may be suspected from information obtained in the history. Pseudohermaphrodites frequently are evaluated because their sex is undetermined. Assistance may be sought because males have signs of estrus, including attraction of other males. Owners may request evaluation of females because they have an enlarged, protruding clitoris. A common complaint is that males or females assume the stance of the opposite sex when voiding. Intermittent involuntary urine dribbling present since birth but associated with normal micturation may also be observed by owners.

The usual finding on physical examination is a female with an enlarged clitoris or a male with an underdeveloped prepuce and penis. Hypospadias and lack of scrotal development may be noted.

Genitourinary anomalies are detected best by retrograde contrast urethrography. A definitive diagnosis of pseudohermaphroditism requires exploratory celiotomy, microscopic examination of the gonads, and sex determination by karyotyping and sex chromatin determination.

PROGNOSIS

Non-neurogenic urinary incontinence in pseudohermaphrodites may be a reversible condition. Successful surgical correction of non-neurogenic urinary incontinence has been reported in a one-year-old female pseudohermaphrodite dog with a urethrovaginal fistula (Jackson et al.) Recently, at the University of Illinois, non-neurogenic urinary incontinence caused by urethrovaginal fistulas in three female pseudohermaphrodite Lhasa apso dogs was corrected surgically.

THERAPY

Surgical correction of non-neurogenic urinary incontinence in female pseudohermaphrodites involves transection and closure of urethrovaginal fistulas. Exploratory celiotomy usually reveals the vagina to be filled with urine and terminated at the pelvic urethra. The ovarian stumps and uterine arteries should be ligated, and the fistula adjacent to the vagina should be isolated by careful dissection. Placement of a sterile urethral catheter often aids in identifying and preserving the pelvic urethra. Once isolated, the fistula is cross-clamped and severed, and the opening into the urethra is sutured. The ovaries, uterus, and vagina are removed and submitted for microscopic evaluation.

Pseudohermaphrodites may have an enlarged clitoris that is esthetically objectionable to the owner. In these cases clitoridectomy can be performed through an episiotomy. Surgical removal involves simple incision, with control of hemorrhage, dissection of the clitoris, and closure of the mucosal defect. Care must be taken not to damage the distal urethra or external urethral meatus.

Neoplasia of the retained testis is reported in male pseudohermaphrodites, with development of a feminization syndrome or cystic endometrial hyperplasia, or both (Brown et al.). Surgical removal of the reproductive tract is recommended in these individuals to prevent potential neoplasia or torsion of the gonads and development of pyometra.

SUPPLEMENTAL READING

Brown, T.T., et al.: Male pseudohermaphroditism, cryptorchidism, and Sertoli cell neoplasia in three miniature schnauzers. J. Am. Vet. Med. Assoc., *169*:821–825, 1976.

Burns, R.K.: Hormones versus constitutional factors in the growth of embryonic sex primordia in the oppossum. Am. J. Anat., 98:35–59, 1956.

Hare, W.C.D.: Intersexuality in the dog. Can. Vet. J., *17*:7–15, 1976.

Jackson, D.A., et al.: Non-neurogenic urinary incontinence in a canine female pseudohermaphrodite. J. Am. Vet. Med. Assoc., *172*:926–930, 1978.

Johnston, G.R., et al.: Retrograde contrast urethrography. In Kirk, R.W. (ed.): *Current Veterinary Therapy VI.* Philadelphia, W.B. Saunders Co., 1977, pp. 1189–1194.

Jost, A.: Gonadal hormones in the sex differentiation of the mammalian fetus. In Dehaan, R.L., and Ursprung, H. (eds.): *Organogenesis.* New York, Holt, Rhinhart and Winston, 1965, pp. 611–628.

Shane, B.S., et al.: Methyl testosterone-induced female pseudohermaphroditism in dogs. Biol. Reprod., *1*:41–48, 1969.

CANINE CRYPTORCHIDISM

LARRY J. WALLACE, D.V.M.
and VICTOR S. COX, D.V.M.
St. Paul, Minnesota

INTRODUCTION

Cryptorchidism has been defined as that condition in the male animal in which one or both testicles do not descend into the scrotum at the usual time. The retained testicle(s) of a cryptorchid animal are usually located somewhere along the normal pathway of testicular descent. Retained testicles are found with a higher frequency in the abdominal location as compared with the inguinal region. Testicles are infrequently retained in the prescrotal position. Ectopic testicles are rare in dogs. A unilaterally cryptorchid animal will have one scrotal and one retained testicle. Such animals have often been incorrectly referred to as monorchid, which refers to the extremely rare condition of unilateral testicular agenesis. Bilateral cryptorchidism is less common than unilateral cryptorchidism. Testicles in the bilaterally cryptorchid dog are often located in the abdomen somewhere between the kidney and the vaginal ring. Since cryptorchidism involves the arrest of a normal development process, it is not surprising that abdominal cryptorchidism is often associated with male pseudohermaphrodites. (Consult the article on pseudohermaphroditism.)

The age at which testicular descent is complete in many species is just prior to or shortly after birth. In dogs the normal age at which testicular descent is complete is difficult to establish, because the process is apparently very gradual. Therefore, it is not surprising that reported data on the age at which the canine testicles should be in the scrotal position are variable. One can find data stating that the testicles should be in the scrotal position at birth or sometime during the first 14 weeks after birth. It rarely occurs after three and one-half months and never after six months of age. Tension of the cremaster muscle may hold the testicles near the external inguinal ring during early life. It has been stated that the small size of prepuberal testicles often makes them difficult to locate. However, by the time a dog is six to eight weeks of age, the testicles can be palpated without much difficulty.

INCIDENCE

Cryptorchidism is common in dogs. The incidence is higher in purebred than in mixed-breed dogs; it has been found in at least 68 breeds. This may reflect the more common occurrence of inbreeding in purebred dogs. The incidence is significantly higher in small breeds as compared with large breeds. In one study utilizing the Veterinary Medical Data Program (VMDP), a sample of 1266 dogs with the defect was obtained from 12 veterinary colleges. In that study the eight breeds with the highest incidence of cryptorchidism were, in descending order, the Yorkshire terrier, Pomeranian, poodle (miniature or toy), Siberian husky, miniature schnauzer, Shetland sheepdog, Chihuahua, and standard poodle. In another study conducted in a private practice, 1494 male dogs of all ages were palpated manually to determine the frequency of cryptorchidism. In that study poodles were affected in the majority of cases, followed by mixed breeds, German shepherds, and dachshunds. The high incidence of cryptorchidism in poodles found in this study was partially attributed to the popularity of this breed in that geographic area at the time the study was conducted. Other reports include many of these breeds as well as various brachycephalic breeds (i.e., Boston terriers and boxers) as having a high incidence of cryptorchidism. The study utilizing the VMDP reflects a wide geographic area and should be more representative of the actual breed incidence. In analyzing the VMDP study the number of cases reported for each breed may have been low if some dogs with cryptorchid testicles were missed or failed to be recorded when examined. The study conducted in the private practice was a prospective one, and each of the 1494 male dogs were palpated specifically to detect cryptorchidism. In that study the diagnosis was accurate; however, the breed incidence was biased by geographic breed popularity. Cryptorchidism is reported to occur in about 10 percent of all adult dogs. One can find reports from university hospitals and private practices with overall incidences ranging from 9.7 to 12.9 percent. The incidence of cryptorchidism reported from experimental dog colonies has been higher. In a large beagle colony the incidence of cryptorchidism in males at least six months old was 85/556 (15.3 percent) and in a miniature schnauzer colony the incidence was 8/12 (67 percent). In summary, it is obvious that actual figures that are without serious bias regarding the overall incidence of cryptorchidism in dogs are not available.

HERITABILITY

Cryptorchidism in dogs is usually considered to be an autosomal recessive trait. Although it is not sex-linked, it is sex-limited, since expression of the trait occurs only in males. The recessive nature of the trait and the fact that unilaterally cryptorchid males have nearly normal fertility account for the widespread distribution of the trait in the general population. Elimination of the trait is possible only if both the affected animal and its parents are removed from breeding programs. It is incumbent upon the veterinarian when certifying the soundness of dogs to palpate their scrota to assure that the animals are not unilaterally or bilaterally cryptorchid. Since unilaterally cryptorchid animals are fertile, it is especially important to detect them by physical examination.

Bilaterally cryptorchid males have been shown to have a higher coefficient of inbreeding than unilaterally cryptorchid animals. These differences may be indicative of a multiple gene basis for the defect.

ANATOMY AND PATHOLOGY

Testicular descent is induced by contraction (shrinkage) of the gubernaculum testis, causing the testis to be pulled caudally through the inguinal ring and into the scrotum. As the testis procedes caudally the epididymis becomes organized around it, and the gubernaculum eventually condenses to become the caudal ligament of the testis. Bilaterally cryptorchid males usually have more primitive-appearing epididymides. The tail of the epididymis is far from the testis, indicating that the process of descent was arrested at an earlier stage. In addition, these testes tend to be quite small and lie close to the kidneys rather than near the vaginal ring, where unilateral abdominal testicles are usually found.

Contrary to the widespread notion that testicular descent is a retroperitoneal process, cryptorchid testicles hang free in the abdominal cavity and therefore are vulnerable to torsion.

Most cases of torsion, however, are associated with neoplasia, indicating that greater inertia plays a role in torsion.

Cryptorchid testicles are predisposed to neoplasia. In one large sample, the risk of neoplasia was found to be 13.6 times greater for cryptorchid testicles. Abdominal testicles are predisposed to Sertoli cell tumors, whereas inguinal testicles are predisposed to seminomas. The incidence of interstitial cell tumors is unrelated to cryptorchidism. The differential tumor incidence at various locations is best explained by the effect of temperature differences on the major cell types of the testis. Interstitial cells are not affected by temperature, and therefore tumors of this cell type and libido are not affected by cryptorchidism. The small size of the abdominal testis is due to the loss of most tubule cells except the Sertoli cells. Therefore, it is not surprising that such testes are prone to Sertoli cell neoplasia. Although abdominal temperature tends to destroy spermatogenic cells, the inguinal position apparently has a transitional temperature that encourages neoplasia of the spermatogenic cell line. Both abdominal and inguinal testicles are usually sterile.

PHYSICAL FINDINGS

It is important to palpate the scrotum of every male dog, regardless of age, to determine whether both testicles are in the scrotum and whether they have a normal consistency. A palpable non-neoplastic cryptorchid testicle in the inguinal region typically is flaccid, softer, and smaller than the contralateral scrotal testicle in a unilaterally cryptorchid animal. The cryptorchid testicle can also be identified by its prominent epididymis. In most instances the descent canal feels normal. The gubernaculum is usually intact and attached in the scrotum. The cremaster muscle generally is shortened and usually resists attempts at stretching.

In unilaterally cryptorchid males the right testicle is retained more frequently than the left. In one study of 55 dogs with non-neoplastic cryptorchid testicles, it was found that the right testis was affected in 27, the left testis in 14, and both testicles in 14 dogs. Thus, the right-to-left ratio was 1.9:1. In direct correlation with this statement, it has been reported that Sertoli cell tumors and seminomas occur more frequently in the right testicle; the right-to-left ratio for both tumor types was 1.8:1. Testicular neoplasia generally occurs two to two and one-half years earlier in cryptorchid dogs as compared with non-cryptorchid dogs. Controlled prospective studies are needed to determine the risk of testicular neoplasia in cryptorchid dogs.

TREATMENT

Medical treatment of cryptorchidism is generally of no value in dogs. Testosterone and human chorionic gonadotropin (HCG) have been used to induce testicular descent in young dogs with relatively little success. The primary effect of HCG is on interstitial cells, but unpublished studies of dogs revealed no difference in testosterone levels in normal and cryptorchid animals, in response to HCG challenge. High doses of HCG can actually damage the tubular epithelium by inhibiting endogenous gonadotropin release. Even if successful, hormone therapy does not correct the genetic defect and therefore should not be considered. For the same ethical reasons, plastic surgical procedures to bring the testicle into the scrotum should not be performed.

The owner of a cryptorchid dog should be informed about the genetic nature of the condition and urged not to use the dog for breeding. In addition, owners should be informed of the increased risk of testicular neoplasia and associated effects (i.e., feminization and skin changes, potential changes in temperament, and the possibility of testicular torsion). In view of these considerations, we recommend orchiectomy for cryptorchid dogs.

SUPPLEMENTAL READING

Ashdown, R.R.: The diagnosis of cryptorchidism in young dogs: A review of the problem. J. Small Anim. Pract., 4:261–263, 1963.

Bierich, J.R., Rager, K., and Ranke, M.B.: Maldescensus testis. Colloquium at Tubingen, Feb. 14, 1976. Baltimore, Urban and Schwarzenberg, 1977, pp. 165–176.

Bloom, F.: *Pathology of the Dog and Cat*. Evanston, Illinois, American Veterinary Publications, 1954, pp. 215–218.

Brown, T.T., Burek, J.D., and McEntee, K.: Male pseudohermaphroditism, cryptorchidism and Sertoli cell neoplasia in three miniature schnauzers. J. Am. Vet. Med. Assoc., 169:821–825, 1976.

Burns, M., and Fraser, M.N.: *Genetics of the Dog*. Philadelphia, J.B. Lippincott, 1966, pp. 20–23.

Cox, V.S., Wallace, L.J., and Jessen, C.R.: An anatomic and genetic study of canine cryptorchidism. Teratology, 18:233–240, 1978.

Dunn, M.L., Foster, W.J., and Goddard, K.M.: Cryptorchidism in the dog: A clinical survey. J. Am. Anim. Hosp. Assoc., 4:180–182, 1968.

Gier, H.T., and Marion, G.B.: Development of mammalian testes and genital ducts. Biol. Reprod., 1:1–23, 1969.

Green, E.L.: Mutant stocks of cats and dogs offered for research. J. Hered., 48:56–57, 1957.

Hayes, H.M., and Pendergrass, T.W.: Canine testicular tumors: Epidemiologic features of 410 dogs. Int. J. Cancer, 18:482–487, 1976.

Huber, W., and Schmid, E.: Ein Kryptorchidenstammbaum biem St. Bernardshund. Arch. Genet. (Zur.), 34:252–256, 1959.

Mattheeuws, D.R.G., and Comhaire, F.H.: Tumors of the testes. In Kirk, R.W. (ed.): *Current Veterinary Therapy VI*. Philadelphia, W.B. Saunders Co., 1977, pp. 1054–1058.

Pearson, H., and Kelly, D.F.: Testicular torsion in the dog: A review of 13 cases. Vet. Rec., 97:200–204, 1975.

Priester, W.A., Glass, A.G., and Waggoner, N.S.: Congenital defects in domesticated animals. General considerations. Am. J. Vet. Res., 31:1871–1879, 1970.

Pullig, T.: Cryptorchidism in cocker spaniels. J. Hered., 44:250–264, 1953.

Rehfeld, C.E.: Cryptorchidism in a large beagle colony. J. Am. Vet. Med. Assoc., 158:1864, 1971.

Reif, J.S., and Brodey, R.S.: The relationship between cryptorchidism and canine testicular neoplasia. J. Am. Vet. Med. Assoc., 155:2005–2010, 1969.

Rhoades, J.D., and Foley, C.W.: Cryptorchidism and intersexuality. Vet. Clin. North Am., 7:789–794, 1977.

Willis, M.B.: Abnormalities and defects in pedigree dogs. V. Cryptorchidism. J. Small Anim. Pract., 4:469–474, 1963.

Section
13

INFECTIOUS DISEASES

FREDRIC W. SCOTT, D.V.M.
Consulting Editor

Theory and Practice of Immunization 1248
Update on Canine Immunization.. 1252
Update on Feline Immunization 1256
Immunization of Exotic Cats... 1258
Rabies: Immunization and Public Health Aspects 1261
Pet-associated Zoonoses 1265
Control of Canine Infectious Diseases in Adoption Shelters........ 1268
Control of Feline Infectious Diseases in Catteries and
    Adoption Shelters... 1270
Control of Infectious Diseases in Aviaries and Pet Shops........... 1273
Canine Respiratory Disease Complex 1276
Feline Respiratory Disease Complex 1279
Canine Distemper.. 1284
Feline Panleukopenia... 1286
Feline Infectious Peritonitis 1288
Canine Viral Enteritis 1292
Pseudorabies in Dogs and Cats 1296
Feline Pneumonitis 1299
Canine Brucellosis... 1303
Feline Salmonellosis.. 1305
Toxoplasmosis – Feline Infections and Their Zoonotic
    Potential.. 1307
Feline Cytauxzoonosis 1312
Kitten Mortality Complex 1313
Shipping Regulations for Small Animals................................. 1316

THEORY AND PRACTICE OF IMMUNIZATION

RONALD D. SCHULTZ, Ph.D.

Auburn, Alabama

One of the most significant advances in veterinary medicine in the last 50 years has been the prevention of many infectious diseases that once killed large numbers of dogs and cats. Prevention is possible because it has become technologically feasible to develop safe and efficacious vaccines that are easily administered and offer long-term protection.

The purpose of a vaccination program is to prevent the development of overt clinical disease, either by preventing or limiting infection. If planned properly, vaccine programs can improve animal care by providing a convenient time for a routine health examination. This aspect of the vaccination program has been abandoned by many clinicians but should be considered an important feature of a sound animal health program. The mechanisms by which dogs and cats are protected from infection and disease after vaccination have been and still are the subject of numerous studies by veterinary researchers and clinicians.

It is currently accepted that there are two parts of the specific host defense system: (1) the humoral (antibody) system, consisting of B lymphocytes and the four immunoglobulin classes (IgG, IgM, IgA, and IgE), plus helper cells and, to assist this sytem, K cells, phagocytic cells, and effector molecules such as complement and properdin and (2) the cell-mediated immune (CMI) system, consisting of T lymphocytes, macrophages, and a number of products of these cells called lymphokines and monokines. Available information would suggest that vaccine protection is regulated primarily by humoral immunity and secondarily by cell-mediated immunity. This finding would be particularly true if vaccination is known to prevent reinfection, which occurs with effective vaccination and protection against canine distemper, infectious canine hepatitis, and feline panleukopenia. However, when vaccination protects against the development of clinical disease but not against reinfection (which is often the case with feline viral rhinotracheitis, a herpesvirus), cell-mediated immunity and local antibodies play important and perhaps primary roles in preventing disease.

FACTORS INFLUENCING THE HOST DEFENSE SYSTEM

Numerous factors can influence the host defense system and thus affect the immune response to the vaccine. Factors to be considered in designing an effective vaccination program for dogs and cats include the specific immunosuppressive or blocking effect of colostral antibody, the nature of the vaccine, the route of vaccination, the age of the animal, its general nutritional condition, concurrent infections, and drug treatments. These factors will be discussed briefly with respect to the possible influences that each may have on the success of an immunization program.

COLOSTRUM

It is known that approximately 95 percent of immunoglobulin in puppies and kittens comes from absorption of colostrum shortly after birth. Following absorption from the gut, specific colostral antibodies — particularly the IgG antibodies — have the ability to prevent most vaccine antigens from reaching the lymphocytes and macrophages, which are responsible for the genesis of active immunity. It is necessary, therefore, for this acquired antibody of colostral origin to reach low levels before active immunization is possible. For puppies born to bitches that are immune to canine distemper and infectious canine hepatitis (CAV-1), this period of uncertain response to vaccination may be as long as 14 to 16 weeks after birth. A method of circumventing this blocking effect is to use measles vaccine to protect against canine distemper. In addition, vaccines that contain high titers or large antigenic doses of the vaccine viruses or bacterial antigens may be more effective in overcoming low levels of passive antibody than are vaccines with low titers. As will be mentioned later, these methods of overcoming the effects of colostral immunity are not absolute.

This situation presents an immunologic paradox, in that colostral antibody is extremely important for protection of the neonate against a multitude of potentially harmful antigens during the first few weeks of life. Therefore, no consideration should be given to preventing puppies and kittens from getting colostrum.

NATURE OF THE VACCINE

Certain questions must be considered if the most effective vaccination program is to be achieved. Is the vaccine virus a modified live or an inactivated virus? If live virus vaccine is used, the vaccine should be handled according to directions supplied by the manufacturer so that it does not become inactive and non-antigenic. Live virus vaccines do not contain enough antigen to immunize the animal unless the virus can infect and replicate in the host. Inactivated vaccines, on the other hand, have a large antigenic mass but in general must be administered several times in order to get an adequate and protective immune response. The question of modified live versus inactivated virus vaccines is often raised. Currently, there are no absolute answers; however, modified live virus vaccines in general are more efficacious and provide a longer period of immunity that inactivated vaccines, but there are notable exceptions. It should be kept in mind that both modified live and inactivated products have a place in the immunization schedule. Does the vaccine contain adjuvant? Adjuvants are added only to killed products to help stimulate protective immunity. Some of the most effective adjuvants cannot be used in vaccines because of the severe reactions they cause.

To achieve maximum success the entire dose of vaccine should be given as recommended; it should not be divided and given to more than one animal.

ROUTE OF VACCINATION

The directions specified by the manufacturer should be followed; for example, if an intramuscular route is recommended, do not give the vaccine subcutaneously. Significant differences in host response to certain vaccines exist and are dependent on the route of administration of vaccine. For rabies vaccine it has been reported that the intramuscular route is much more effective than the subcutaneous route. We have also found that the intramuscular route is more effective than the subcutaneous route for measles virus. For canine distemper and panleukopenia both the subcutaneous and intramuscular routes are effective. These findings would suggest that the combined canine distemper and measles virus vaccine should be administered intramuscularly and not subcutaneously.

The question of parenteral versus local immunization is one requiring a thorough understanding of the pathogenesis of the disease. Intranasal immunization has the advantage of inducing local antibody as well as local cell-mediated immunity in the respiratory tract. However, if the specific agent replicates in the systemic tissue and not at the local level of the epithelial cells lining the respiratory tract, there is no obvious advantage to local versus parenteral immunization. An example is canine distemper virus, frequently considered to be a respiratory infection but known to replicate initially in lymphoid tissue. In this case there is no advantage to an intranasal product. Panleukopenia is similar, in that the disease is frequently considered an enteric infection, but the virus replicates first in the lymphoid tissue and later infects cells of the gastrointestinal tract. Oral immunization is not only less efficacious than parenteral immunization, but we have also found oral administration to be without effect unless there is simultaneous intranasal immunization. One should attempt to protect the site of infection; therefore, local immunization may be more efficacious when the primary site of replication is the respiratory or gastrointestinal tract.

The practice of administering panleukopenia vaccine in food to wild cats maintained in zoos cannot be recommended, since we have found the oral route to be ineffective both for the development of antibody and for protection against challenge with feline panleukopenia virus.

AGE OF THE ANIMAL

Age is important not only because of persistence of colostral antibody but also because the relative hypothermia that exists during the first week or two of life can cause a state of CMI unresponsiveness. Optimum body temperatures between 38 and 39°C are very critical for T cell as well as macrophage function in dogs and possibly in cats. Body temperatures less than 37°C are not uncommon in puppies during the first week or so of life, and this lower body temperature is capable of suppressing the CMI system. Because of the interdependence of the B cell system for helper T cells, the antibody response could also be affected by the lowered body temperature. Vaccination during this early period (less than two weeks of age) with live attenuated vaccines is not recommended. Orphaned pups or kittens could receive immune serum in their formula or parenterally to aid in resistance against infection.

There also is evidence to suggest that certain

older dogs (seven years of age or more) may have a decreased ability to produce antibody as well as a decreased CMI response. Annual revaccination during these later years, therefore, is particularly important to maintain an active state of immunity. It is assumed that a similar situation exists for cats, but no information is available.

NUTRITIONAL STATE OF THE ANIMAL

A severely debilitated animal may not respond adequately to a vaccine. The general state of nutrition should meet minimal recommended standards to ensure that nutritional factors do not interfere with immune responsiveness. If a debilitated dog or cat is vaccinated, vaccination should be repeated when the animal's general condition has improved in order to ensure adequate immunity. In addition, some caution should be exercised when using modified live viruses in a severely debilitated animal, since attenuation is dependent on the host as well as the parasite.

CONCURRENT INFECTIONS

It is important to ensure that animals presented for vaccination are not already incubating the disease. This possibility frequently motivates owners to present their animals for vaccination and may lead to so-called "vaccination breakdowns." A detailed history about the possibility of exposure to infected animals should be obtained and a thorough physical examination should be performed for every patient presented for vaccination in order to minimize this risk.

Other diseases may also be associated with immunosuppression and may potentially interfere with successful vaccination. For example, the general state of T cell suppression present in cases of generalized demodectic mange may interfere with the response to vaccination or, at worst, may contraindicate use of live attenuated vaccines. Likewise, dogs infected with distemper virus develop a generalized T cell suppression four days after infection, and vaccination with other antigens during this period may result in an inadequate immune response.

Feline leukemia virus is also known to cause immunosuppression in some cats. The immunosuppression may interfere with protective immunity and may increase the apparent virulence of certain attenuated vaccines.

DRUG TREATMENTS

Vaccines should not be given concurrently with immunosuppressive drugs such as cyclo-phosphamide, azathioprine, methotrexate, and corticosteroids. Corticosteroid treatment of dogs at therapeutic levels does not appear to influence antibody responses to vaccine viruses. However, primary vaccination with modified live virus vaccine cannot be highly recommended in dogs receiving steroid therapy. Attenuated viruses should be harmless in a normal host but may produce clinical disease in an immunologically compromised host.

High doses of steroid are known to reactivate canine herpesvirus and feline viral rhinotracheitis virus and potentially could cause infection in susceptible contacts.

IMMUNE SERUM

Hyperimmune serum, immune serum, or gamma globulin has been described by some in the medical community as "the miracle worker that isn't." The potential of gamma globulin should be re-evaluated and considered for what it is. It must be understood that for gamma globulin to be effective it must contain high levels of antibody to the specific organism (e.g., canine distemper or feline panleukopenia) one wants to protect the animal against.

Immune serum or gamma globulin will be of little or no value after the clinical signs of disease are present. However, it will be effective if given immediately after contact exposure with a diseased animal. The situations in which immune serum can be recommended are (1) when an animal enters a shelter, pet store, or veterinary clinic; (2) newborn, orphaned pups (give immune serum orally or parenterally); and (3) newborn pups from a bitch without canine herpesvirus antibody but experiencing herpesvirus infection.

IMMUNIZATION SCHEDULE

There probably is no perfect schedule; however, certain recommendations can be made. The following should be considered for minimal disease prevention in dogs and cats:

1. Give the first immunization when the animal is between 6 and 10 weeks of age.

2. Revaccinate at 14 to 16 weeks of age.

3. Revaccinate on an annual basis or every three years to coincide with rabies vaccination.

Annual revaccination is of questionable importance for some vaccines, but for others it is essential. (See specific recommendations in the articles on canine and feline immunization, elsewhere in Section 13.)

FUTURE TRENDS IN VETERINARY VACCINES AND IMMUNOPROPHYLACTICS

Currently, research and development are being done for a number of new products. Recently, a new vaccine to prevent infectious canine hepatitis (ICH) was released. The vaccine, which in part follows the heterotypic concept of immunization, is a canine adenovirus type 2 (CAV-2) vaccine that is antigenically similar to canine adenovirus type 1 (ICH) but does not cause the immunologically mediated reactions (e.g., uveitis) sometimes associated with the ICH vaccines. This product has the added potential of providing protection against ICH as well as CAV-2, a virus known to be associated with "kennel cough," or the respiratory disease complex (RCD), in dogs. It is anticipated that the CAV-2 product will be a safe and effective vaccine.

A very recent development in canine biologics is a *Bordetella bronchiseptica* bacterin. *Bordetella bronchiseptica* has been demonstrated to be an important agent, along with others, in causing kennel cough, or RCD, in dogs. Of the agents now known to be associated with infectious RCD, there are vaccines for most, with the notable exception of mycoplasma. Proving efficacy or the ability to eliminate RCD by any or all of these products will be difficult. Experience will determine the most useful combination of products and the ones that will provide the best immunization program.

Recent outbreaks of infectious enteric disease in dogs, presumably caused by coronavirus, rota-like virus, and/or parvovirus, have led to research and potential development of vaccines to reduce or prevent future outbreaks of disease caused by these agents. Research continues on parasitic vaccines, particularly a vaccine effective against heartworm (*Dirofilaria immitis*). Products, both man-made and natural, that act as immune-modulating or immunopotentiating agents are being developed and tested and may hold some promise for future treatment of immunodepressed or immune-compromised patients.

To reiterate, there is no perfect immunization schedule and there are no limits to the numbers and types of vaccines that can be employed. One must, however, weigh the value of and need for certain vaccines and adopt a minimal disease prevention program satisfactory to both practitioner and client.

SUPPLEMENTAL READING

Bellanti, J.: *Immunology II.* Philadelphia, W. B. Saunders Co., 1978.

Osburn, B., and Schultz, R.D. (eds.): Veterinary immunology. *In Veterinary Science and Comparative Medicine*, vol. 23, New York, Academic Press, 1979.

Tizard, I.R.: *An Introduction to Veterinary Immunology.* Philadelphia, W. B. Saunders Co., 1977.

UPDATE ON CANINE IMMUNIZATION

RONALD D. SCHULTZ, Ph.D.,
Auburn, Alabama

MAX APPEL, D.V.M.,
LELAND E. CARMICHAEL, D.V.M.,
Ithaca, New York

and BRIAN FARROW, B.V.Sc.
Sydney, Australia

The following recommendations are based on the Panel Report of the Symposium on Immunity to Selected Canine Infectious Diseases, Rabies Subcommittee, Animal Health Committee, National Research Council, National Academy of Science, and on recent research reports (Table 1).

RABIES VACCINES

The two types of rabies vaccines available are modified live virus and inactivated virus. Live virus vaccines are of chicken embryo or cell culture origin. It is recommended that the first vaccination be administered at three or four months of age, again at one year, and then at least once every three years after the vaccination at one year. If the first vaccination occurs after four months of age, the second vaccination is given one year later and then again at least every three years.

Inactivated virus vaccine is available with and without adjuvant. It is required that this vaccine be given more frequently than modified live virus vaccine because there is a more rapid decline in immunity. If the first vaccination is given at three months of age or older, the second vaccination should follow in three to four weeks, and annual revaccination is recommended thereafter.

No rabies vaccine is licensed in the United States for wild animals; however, when it is necessary to vaccinate them only inactivated vaccine should be used, and the procedure recommended for dogs should be followed.

CANINE DISTEMPER VIRUS

Modified live virus vaccines of chicken embryo or cell culture origin are recommended. In pups of unknown immune status that are older than three months, one dose of modified live virus vaccine should be given. For animals less than three months old when first presented, two or more doses should be administered; the first dose should be given at weaning and the last dose at 12 to 16 weeks of age. Vaccination at two-week intervals during this critical time of diminishing maternally acquired immunity more nearly approaches the ideal method but is not necessary. Annual revaccination is recommended but probably is not essential in most instances. It is suggested that pregnant bitches not be vaccinated. This suggestion is made because of our lack of information about possible side effects of the virus on fetuses, not from any results indicating that vaccine virus can damage the canine fetus.

Vaccines that incorporate viral or bacterial antigens, or both, with the canine distemper component are available and provide the advantages of protection against the component antigens with one injection. These vaccines incorporate modified CAV-1 or CAV-2, modified canine parainfluenza virus, and *Leptospira* bacterins in various combinations. The use of measles virus vaccines to provide protection against canine distemper is discussed in the next section of this article.

Passive immunization using antiserum or concentrated antiserum in pups exposed to canine distemper virus is not recommended, since it will delay subsequent active immunization and seems to have less merit in most cases than multiple doses of attenuated live virus vaccine.

MEASLES VIRUS

Measles virus has been used with a variable degree of success for more than 20 years to

Table 1. Canine Immunization

DISEASE	VACCINE	TYPE OF VACCINE	AGE OF VACCINATION
Distemper	Canine distemper virus (CDV) and/or	Modified live virus	First vaccination at 6 to 8 weeks of age; second vaccination at 12 to 16 weeks; revaccinate annually.
	Measles virus (MV)		Vaccinate at 6 weeks of age, then vaccinate with CDV vaccine at 12 to 16 weeks. Do not use in bitches of breeding age.
Hepatitis	Infectious canine hepatitis (ICH)	Modified live (CAV-1 or CAV-2) virus	Vaccination schedule is same as for CDV vaccine and is commonly given with CDV in a combined vaccine.
Rabies	Rabies virus	Modified live virus	First vaccination at 3 to 4 months of age; revaccinate at 1 year and at least every 3 years thereafter; if dog is over 4 months of age at first vaccination, revaccinate in 1 year, then once every 3 years.
		Inactivated virus	First vaccination at 3 to 4 months; second vaccination in 3 to 4 weeks; revaccinate annually.
Respiratory disease complex	Canine parainfluenza virus (CPI)	Modified live virus	Manufacturer's recommendation: Give as combined vaccine with canine distemper and infectious canine hepatitis vaccines.
	Canine adenovirus 2 (CAV-2)	Modified live virus	Vaccination schedule is same as for CDV vaccine and is commonly given with CDV in a combined vaccine.
	Bordetella bronchiseptica	Killed bacteria (bacterin)	First inoculation after 3 weeks of age; second inoculation 3 to 4 weeks later; annual revaccination recommended by manufacturer.
Enteric disease complex	Canine parvovirus	None licensed	Two doses of inactivated panleukopenia virus vaccine may protect against disease.
	Canine coronavirus	None available	
	Canine rota-like or reo-like virus	None available	
Herpes	Canine herpesvirus	None available	
Brucellosis	Canine brucellosis	None available	

protect young puppies from canine distemper. When first introduced, measles vaccine was given alone as the first vaccine to puppies four weeks of age or older. Recently, a combination of canine distemper virus and measles virus has become available commercially, and the manufacturers recommend that it be used at six weeks of age. The manufacturers claim that this combination protects a higher percentage of animals against distemper than when measles virus is given alone. Although it was originally thought that canine distemper antibody received from colostrum did not interfere with measles virus vaccination, we have recently found that high levels (approximate titers of 1:300 to 1:500) can interfere with measles vaccination. Measles virus is not as sensitive to the blocking effects of colostral canine distemper virus antibody as is canine distemper vaccine virus, and it is unlikely that any six-week-old puppy has enough canine distemper virus antibody to interfere with measles vaccination. This is unlike vaccination with canine dis-

temper virus at this age, in which case 50 percent or more of the puppies do not respond to canine distemper virus vaccine.

Measles vaccine can be used successfully to protect dogs from developing disease with canine distemper virus, but it will not protect against infection with canine distemper virus. Measles vaccination should be considered a temporary method of preventing canine distemper until canine distemper vaccine can be effectively administered. There are no indications for the use of vaccines containing measles antigen in dogs over 16 weeks of age, and their use is contraindicated in breeding bitches. There are no known human health hazards associated with these vaccines. It should be emphasized that human measles vaccines are not recommended for dogs.

INFECTIOUS CANINE HEPATITIS (CAV-1)

Immunizing agents include only modified live virus vaccines. Vaccination with live

CAV-1 virus vaccine is not without its problems, since a small percentage of dogs receiving it may develop uveitis and corneal edema ("blue eye"). Although certain vaccine manufacturers advertise that their vaccine does not cause uveitis, we are not aware of any strain of CAV-1 virus that does not cause uveitis in a small percentage of dogs.

We have found that CAV-1 virus vaccine will cause disease when inoculated into term fetuses (58 days of age). This does not imply that vaccination of the bitch causes disease in the fetus, but it does suggest that vaccines with attenuated CAV-1 virus should not be given to pregnant bitches until more is known about their possible effects on fetuses.

CAV-1 vaccine may be given in combination with other viral and bacterial vaccine antigens. The use of suitably attenuated CAV-2 as an alternative to vaccinal CAV-1 strains has been recommended to avoid the ocular and renal lesions associated with CAV-1 and to provide protection against systemic CAV-1 infection. CAV-2 vaccine was recently made available commercially. The safety and efficacy of CAV-2 vaccines have been field-tested for years at the Baker Institute, Cornell University. It is suggested that CAV-2 has the added advantage of providing optimal protection against the respiratory pathogen CAV-2 in addition to protection against infectious canine hepatitis. The necessity for annual revaccination against CAV-1 is questionable.

CANINE PARAINFLUENZA VIRUS (CPI OR SV₅)

A modified live canine parainfluenza virus vaccine in combination with canine distemper virus and CAV-1, with or without *Leptospira* bacterin, has been available commercially for several years. The role of canine parainfluenza virus as a cause of contagious respiratory disease in dogs is well established. In addition, infections with other viruses, bacteria, and mycoplasms may complicate this disease complex. When contagious respiratory disease as a result of canine parainfluenza infection is a problem among dogs, incorporation of attenuated canine parainfluenza virus in the vaccination program is indicated.

Direct inoculation of term fetuses with canine parainfluenza virus (wild type) resulted in puppies that were weak at birth and that survived for variable periods of time up to nine days of age. As with CAV-1, these results do not necessarily indicate that canine parainfluenza virus infects the fetus during natural infection or after vaccination of the bitch; however, the results do

suggest that bitches should not be vaccinated until further research about this possibility has been performed.

CANINE HERPESVIRUS

An attenuated (small plaque variant) canine herpesvirus with vaccine potential has been developed; however, there appears to be no critical need for such a vaccine at present. Adult dogs that are exposed to the virulent virus do not develop disease but do develop immunity and adequately protect their pups via colostrum from the neonatal disease, which frequently is lethal. Immune serum appears to be protective against clinical disease if given to the pups before or shortly after infection.

CANINE CORONAVIRUS

Recently, scattered episodes of a contagious and occasionally fatal gastrointestinal disease of dogs was reported. Coronavirus was identified in the feces of these dogs, and the virus fulfilled Koch's postulates, at least partially, by causing a milder form of the disease in experimental animals than that reported from the field. This disease, although more widespread and more severe in 1978 than reported previously in the U.S., was originally recognized in 1971, and its association with coronavirus was reported by Binn and co-workers at Walter Reed Army Institute for Research. Fortunately, death from this disease is rare; however, the most recent outbreaks appeared to be caused by a more virulent strain of the virus than was recognized previously, or else secondary factors caused the death of a significant number of dogs.

Currently, no vaccine is available for this disease; however, future research with the coronavirus should provide information on the feasibility of developing an efficacious vaccine.

CANINE PARVOVIRUS

Recently, by means of electron microscopy, a parvovirus was found in the feces of a dog with enteritis. Further studies revealed the virus to be very similar to panleukopenia virus of cats, and they have found the disease in dogs to be characterized by enteritis, leukopenia and, in youngs pups, occasional myocarditis. This virus may be found in association with the coronavirus discussed previously, but it is most often found alone and may be more important in causing infectious enteritis of dogs than any other agent. The virus is believed to be a new virus; current evidence suggests its recent emergence in the dog population. It was found that dogs experimentally immunized with two doses of inactivated panleukopenia virus were temporarily resistant to infection with the canine parvovirus. However, it should be emphasized that panleukopenia vaccines are not licensed for dogs.

CANINE ROTA-LIKE OR REO-LIKE VIRUS

A rota- or reo-like virus has also been recognized in fecal and intestinal samples submitted from dogs with enteritis and from some very young puppies (less than one week old) dying from enteric disease. It would not be surprising to find a rotavirus associated with enteric disease in the dog, since viruses of this group are associated with enteric diseases in a variety of species. The relationship between its presence and disease in dogs has not been established. Currently, no vaccine is available to prevent disease caused by this virus.

CANINE LEPTOSPIROSIS

If leptospirosis is endemic, vaccination with appropriate bacterin should be considered. Vaccination is recommended when the pup is nine weeks of age or older. The second dose is given two to three weeks later, and a third is recommended after a similar period or when the final vaccination for canine distemper virus and CAV-1 is given. For effective immunity, revaccination should occur at least annually.

Anaphylactoid reactions have occurred as a result of vaccination with this bacterin, and provisions to treat such a patient should be readily available when this vaccine is given.

CANINE BORDETELLA

Bordetella, along with mycoplasma and a number of viruses, are involved in the canine respiratory disease complex commonly called "kennel cough." With the exception of mycoplasma, vaccines are now available for the major pathogens associated with kennel cough. *B. bronchiseptica* alone or in combination is reported to cause respiratory disease, and it is anticipated that use of vaccine will reduce disease associated with this bacteria. The efficacy of this new product awaits critical field-testing. It should be recognized that this product may cause some swelling and pain at the site of injection. The manufacturer recommends two or more vaccinations initially, followed by annual revaccination.

An intranasal product has recently been licensed and is now available for use. This product has the advantage of inducing local immunity and does not cause the unwanted reactions seen with the parenteral product. Currently there are no substantiated claims for greater efficacy with the intranasal product.

CANINE BRUCELLOSIS

A vaccine against canine brucellosis is not available. Although dogs infected with *Brucella canis* eventually become immune, the period necessary for immunity to develop is measured in terms of months or years. Methods to reduce the time needed for dogs to develop protective immunity are being considered and tested.

SUPPLEMENTAL READING

Appel, M.J., Scott, F.W., and Carmichael, L.E.: Isolation and immunization studies of canine parvo-like virus in dogs with hemorrhagic enteritis. Vet. Rec., *105*:151–159, 1979.

Binn, L.N., et al.: Recovery and characterization of a coronavirus from military dogs with diarrhea. Proc. 78th Annual Meeting Am. Anim. Hosp. Assoc., 78:359–366, 1974.

Schultz, R.D., et al.: Canine vaccines and immunity. In Kirk, R.W. (ed.) *Current Veterinary Therapy VI.* Philadelphia, W. B. Saunders Co., 1977.

Schultz, R.D., and Scott, F.W.: Canine and feline immunization. Vet. Clin. North Am., 8:755–768, 1978.

UPDATE ON FELINE IMMUNIZATION

FREDRIC W. SCOTT, D.V.M.

Ithaca, N.Y.

Most of the basic parameters of immunization and the basic immune response outlined in the previous article hold true for cats as well as dogs. The type of vaccine used, the route of vaccination, the effect of maternal antibody derived from colostrum, and the age of the cat vaccinated can affect the immune response (or lack of it) that occurs in cats following vaccination.

NATURE OF THE VACCINE

Both inactivated and modified live virus (MLV) vaccines are available. The MLV vaccines must be handled and stored according to the manufacturer's instructions in order to maintain potency. MLV vaccines should not be administered to pregnant cats.

ROUTE OF VACCINATION

The route by which the vaccine is administered may affect the degree of protection provided. Feline panleukopenia (FPL) vaccine can be given IM or SC with equal effect. The MLV-FPL vaccines can also be given by the intranasal or aerosol route, but they will not result in immunization if administered orally.

Rabies vaccine must be given by the IM route. Although extensive studies on the route of rabies vaccination in cats have not been reported, studies in dogs have shown that the IM route is at least 100 times more effective than the SC route. The same should hold true for the cat.

The MLV respiratory vaccines appear to be slightly more effective by the IM route, but they can be given SC. Aerosol vaccination with injectable vaccines may result in mild signs of illness.

The intranasal (IN) respiratory vaccines are administered by allowing the cat to inhale drops of recently reconstituted lyophilized FVR-FCV or FVR-FCV-FPL vaccine into the nostrils. One or two drops are also placed in each conjunctival sac. These vaccines produce rapid local as well as systemic immunity. Clients should be warned that vaccinated cats may sneeze and develop mild ocular and/or nasal discharge four to seven days after vaccination. Occasionally, ulcers develop on the tongue. Vaccinated cats shed FVR and FCV viruses for long periods after IN vaccination.

AGE OF THE CAT

The most frequent cause of vaccine failure with FPL vaccines is interference caused by maternally derived immunity. These cats become susceptible later, after the passive immunity wanes. The level and duration of passive immunity following nursing are determined by the antibody titer of the queen at parturition, assuming that the kitten nurses. Although the majority of cats can be immunized successfully at 9 to 10 weeks of age, occasional kittens may not be susceptible to vaccination until 12 weeks of age. Therefore, if FPL vaccines are given at ages less than 12 weeks, they should be repeated at four-week intervals until the cat is at least 12 weeks old.

Little is known about maternal antibody interference in feline viral rhinotracheitis (FVR) and feline calicivirus (FCV) disease vaccines. The same principles of colostral transfer, antibody half-life, and vaccine virus neutralization should apply to these viruses as well as FPL. Therefore, we can predict that there will be interference if the maternal titers are high enough. Generally the FVR and FCV titers are much lower than the FPL titer, and therefore the duration of interference (and passive protection) should be much shorter. It is doubtful that this will be longer than five to six weeks for the FVR and seven to eight weeks for the FCV. By nine to ten weeks of age, the vast majority of cats should be susceptible to FVR and FCV vaccination.

FELINE PANLEUKOPENIA VACCINES

There are many excellent vaccines available for immunization of cats against panleukopenia (Scott and Gillespie). If these are used correctly and at the proper age, cats should be completely protected against this very severe viral infection. It behooves veterinarians to immunize as many cats as possible in their practices.

Several slightly different programs for the immunization of cats against panleukopenia have been presented during the past few years. The safest recommendation is to start the immunization program at an early age and to vaccinate kittens at frequent intervals until they are at least 16 weeks of age. This might prove beneficial in certain circumstances, such as in catteries or colonies, in which kittens could be vaccinated at six weeks of age, followed by repeated vaccinations at two-week intervals until the cats are 16 weeks old. However, most kittens presented to the practitioner must be immunized with a minimum of two or possibly three vaccinations. Therefore, the clinician must attempt to immunize the maximum number of cats with a reasonable number of vaccinations per cat.

Most recommendations indicate that the kittens should be vaccinated starting at eight, nine or ten weeks of age. A single vaccination will immunize the cats if they are susceptible at the time of vaccination. If interference occurred at the time of the first vaccination, chances are much greater that the cat will be susceptible to vaccination four weeks later, instead of seven to ten days later. If the first vaccination was successful, the increase in titer following the second vaccination will be comparable whether it is given at four weeks or two weeks if inactivated vaccines are used. For MLV vaccines the second vaccination would have no effect in a previously immunized kitten, owing to the high titer.

In reviewing the different programs for immunization of cats, the Panel for the Colloquium on Selected Feline Infectious Diseases preferred a two-week interval to a four-week interval, since fewer cats would be returned for revaccination four weeks later. After evaluating all the available information, the Panel recommended that two doses of inactivated vaccine be given at two-week intervals, starting at 9 to 10 weeks of age. For maximum protection, especially in areas of high concentration of street virus, a third vaccination is recommended at 16 weeks of age. For the modified live virus vaccines, the first dose should be administered at 9 to 10 weeks of age, followed by a second dose of vaccine between 14 and 16 weeks of age. If the cat is older than 12 weeks at the time of the first vaccination with MLV vaccine, a repeat vaccination is not indicated.

With the advent of respiratory vaccines, for which there is good evidence for revaccination at a three- to four-week interval instead of a two-week interval, and since one should try to immunize the maximum number of cats with the least number of office visits, it now seems advisable to recommend the four-week interval between vaccinations, as outlined in Table 1.

FELINE VIRAL RHINOTRACHEITIS (FVR) VACCINES

FVR vaccines may be obtained as a single vaccine, in combination with calicivirus vaccine, or as a triple FPL-FVR-FCV vaccine. The FVR vaccines produce significant protection following vaccination and, as such, should be part of the routine vaccination program, as outlined in Table 1. As a result of local viral replication, vaccinated cats develop a rapid anamnestic response when exposed to virulent virus. Some vaccinated cats may sneeze, and an occasional one may have watery eyes for one to two days. Severe systemic disease does not occur in properly immunized cats, as it does in unvaccinated cats.

FELINE CALICIVIRUS (FCV) VACCINE

Until recently, it was thought that multiple serotypes of FCV existed and thus that an effec-

Table 1. *Feline Vaccine Recommendations*

DISEASE	TYPE OF VACCINE	AGE AT FIRST VACCINATION (*weeks*)	AGE AT SECOND VACCINATION (*weeks*)	REVACCINATION	ROUTE OF ADMINISTRATION
Panleukopenia	(1) Inactivated	8	12	Annual	SC or IM
(FPL)	(2) MLV°	8	12	Annual	SC or IM
	(3) MLV-IN	8	12	Annual	IN
Viral rhinotracheitis	(1) MLV	8 (or earlier)	12	Annual	IM
(FVR)	(2) MLV-IN	8	—	Annual	IN
Caliciviral disease	(1) MLV	8 (or earlier)	12	Annual	IM
(FCV)	(2) MLV-IN	8	—	Annual	IN
Pneumonitis	MLV	8	—	Annual	SC or IM
Rabies	(1) Inactivated	12	—	Annual	IM
	(2) MLV	12	—	Annual	IM

°Modified live virus

tive vaccine would not be possible. Studies have shown that there is a single serotype of FCV with multiple strains. The strains of FCV tested exhibit good protection against other strains of FCV. The same parameters (i.e., route of vaccination, anamnestic response when challenged, and good clinical protection against virulent virus exposure but not protection against local viral replication) apply to FCV vaccines as to FVR vaccines. These vaccines are produced in combination with FVR vaccine and recommendations are the same as for FVR (see Table 1).

FELINE PNEUMONITIS (FPN) VACCINE

Although FPN is not as prevalent as FVR or FCV disease, it is evident that in some cat populations a severe, chronic respiratory disease is produced by the FPN agent, a chlamydial organism. According to recent studies, the one vaccine currently available appears to produce significant protection following a single IM vaccination. As with other respiratory vaccines, complete protection is not afforded, but clinical signs, if they do occur, are restricted to a very short course and are mild and local. Chronic disease (characteristic of natural infection in susceptible cats) apparently does not occur in vaccinated cats.

Although there are many basic parameters concerning immunity to FPN that are not known, it appears that, if FPN is a problem in a particular area, the FPN vaccine should be part of the routine vaccination program. The age at which to vaccinate is not critical, since there appears to be little interference with maternal antibody by the time kittens would normally be old enough to be vaccinated. A single injection appears to afford adequate protection.

RABIES VACCINES

The latest rabies vaccine recommendations are included in the 1980 Compendium of Animal Rabies Vaccines (see the article entitled "Rabies: Immunization and Public Health Aspects").

SUPPLEMENTAL READING

Mitzel, J.R., and Strating, A.: Evaluation of a feline chlamydial pneumonitis vaccine in cats. Proc. Am. Soc. Microbiol., 76:72, 1976.
Practitioner's guide to feline vaccines and serums, 1976–1977. Feline Pract., March 1976, pp. 23–30.
Report of the Panel for the Colloquium on Selected Feline Infectious Diseases. J. Am. Vet. Med. Assoc., 158:835–843, 1971.
Scott, F.W.: Evaluation of an experimental vaccine against feline viral rhinotracheitis and feline calicivirus disease. Am. J. Vet. Res., 38:229–234, 1977.
Scott, F.W., and Gillespie, J.H.: Immunization for feline panleukopenia. Vet. Clin. North Am., 1:231–240, 1971.

IMMUNIZATION OF EXOTIC CATS

DANIEL C. LAUGHLIN, D.V.M.
Riverside, Illinois

The principles set forth in previous articles regarding immunization and immune response in domestic cats are applicable to exotic cats as well. The nature of the vaccine, the route of vaccination, the age of the cat, and the presence of maternal antibody all affect the integrity of the immune response following vaccination (Scott, 1977b).

NATURE OF THE VACCINE

Several inactivated and modified live virus (MLV) vaccines are available for utilization in domestic cats. Most of these have not been evaluated adequately in exotic cats. However, one commercially available vaccine (Pitman-Moore's FVRC-P) was evaluated recently for safety and efficacy in exotic cats. That study involved 224 exotic cats representing 19 species and subspecies; the results are summarized later in this article.

Vaccines, especially MLV vaccines, should be handled and stored in accordance with the manufacturer's instructions. Modified live virus vaccines should not be administered to pregnant exotic cats.

ROUTE AND METHOD OF VACCINATION

The route and method used in the administration of vaccines to exotic cats may affect the degree of protection provided. While feline panleukopenia (FPL) vaccine may be administered to domestic cats either intramuscularly or subcutaneously with equally good results (Scott, 1977b), there is no evidence to support the efficacy of subcutaneous administration in exotic cats. It is likely that the feline viral rhinotracheitis (FVR) and feline calicivirus (FCV) disease vaccines are more effective when administered intramuscularly. The modified live virus vaccines that are given intranasally to domestic cats are not desirable for use in exotic cats because of the difficulty in administration.

Vaccination of exotic cats should be accomplished with a minimum amount of restraint and trauma to the patient but with consideration for the safety of the handler and veterinarian. Smaller exotic cats may be restrained manually in a squeeze cage or a net. This can best be accomplished if the cat is first induced into a holding cage, den box, or other confined enclosure. Because exotic cats are more susceptible to the effects of stress than domestic cats, it is undesirable to make repeated attempts to catch them. Manual restraint of smaller exotic cats should be performed quickly and assertively. When the cat is appropriately restrained, the vaccine should be administered intramuscularly in the posterior thigh muscles with a 20- or 21-gauge one-inch needle.

The immunization of larger exotic cats may be accomplished by restraint in an appropriate squeeze cage or, if the enclosure design permits, the cat can be backed momentarily against one side by a handler working with a pole on the side opposite the veterinarian. At the moment the cat is against the side of the enclosure, the vaccine may be administered quickly by manual injection. This method is satisfactory for the vaccination of many larger exotic cats, and the amount of stress and trauma to the cat is minimal.

A less desirable method of vaccinating larger exotic cats is utilization of gas-powered or powder-charged projectors with dart-syringes. While this is the method most frequently used to vaccinate larger exotic cats in zoological parks, traumatic injury to the cat may result from excessive impact of the dart-syringe, inappropriate choice of the dart needle, and/or improper placement of the dart-syringe. To utilize this method safely and effectively the veterinarian must be a skilled marksman. An additional disadvantage of this method is that associated tissue trauma at the dart-syringe entry point often results in the seepage of vaccine through the injection site.

Another less-utilized method of vaccinating larger exotic cats involves the use of a blow-gun and dart-syringe. This method also requires experience and skill but reduces the risk of impact trauma associated with the use of the gas-powered and powder-charged projectors.

AGE OF THE CAT

In exotic cats as well as domestic cats, failure of FPL vaccines is often the result of interference by maternally derived antibody. The FVR and FCV titers are usually much lower than the FPL titers, and therefore passive protection from these two diseases in the young cat exists for a shorter time. Clinical experience with exotic cats suggests that passive protection may not extend past four to six weeks for FVR and FCV, depending on the level of maternal antibody. The principles of vaccine virus neutralization, antibody half-life, and colostral transfer (as discussed in previous articles) appear to be as applicable to exotic cats as to domestic cats.

FELINE PANLEUKOPENIA VACCINES

Feline panleukopenia has been diagnosed definitively in several species of exotic cats, including the African leopard (*Panthera pardus*), jaguar (*Panthera onca*), Bengal tiger (*Panthera tigris tigris*), cheetah (*Acinonyx jubatus*), African lion (*Panthera leo*), and mountain lion (*Puma concolor*). It should be presumed that all species of exotic cats are susceptible to this serious viral disease. Data from the study mentioned earlier suggest that several of the currently available FPL vaccines are safe and effective when utilized on exotic cats (Felocine and Felocell, Norden; Panagen, Pitman-Moore).

An immunization program begun at 8 weeks of age, followed by vaccinations at 12 and 16 weeks, has proved to be effective in providing protective antibody titers against FPL in exotic cats. Such a vaccination program allows for the appropriate utilization of a triple FPL-FVR-FCV vaccine.

FELINE VIRAL RHINOTRACHEITIS VACCINES

FVR vaccines may be obtained as a single vaccine, combined with FCV vaccine, or combined with both FPL and FCV vaccines. FVR can be a serious problem in exotic cats, and the FVR agent (a herpesvirus) has been identified in several species of exotic cats afflicted with the clinical disease. FVR has been diagnosed in the Pallas' cat (*Otocolobus manul*), African leopard (*Panthera pardus*), ocelot (*Leopardus pardalis*), mountain lion (*Puma concolor*), leopard cat (*Prionailurus bengalensis*), fishing cat (*Prionailurus viverrinus*), and cheetah (*Acinonyx jubatus*). It should be assumed that all species of exotic cats are susceptible to FVR. In the study referred to earlier, a commercially available vaccine produced significant protection against FVR when used according to the manufacturer's recommendations.

FELINE CALICIVIRUS VACCINES

It is now known that there is a single serotype of FCV that has multiple strains. Some strains, including the one utilized in the recently evaluated combined FVR-FCV vaccine, have shown good protection against other strains of FCV (Scott, 1977a). Recommendations regarding vaccination against FCV are the same as for FVR.

FELINE PNEUMONITIS VACCINE (FPN)

Feline pneumonitis is apparently not as prevalent in exotic cats as FVR and FCV disease, and documented cases of FPN in exotic cats do not appear in the literature. However, some instances of chronic respiratory disease in exotic cats that have protective antibody titers to FVR and FCV are most likely the result of the FPN agent (a chlamydial organism). Studies on the safety and efficacy of the FPN vaccine in exotic cats have not been reported. The one vaccine currently available (Fromm) appears to produce significant protection in domestic cats following a single intramuscular inoculation (Mitzel and Strating). The vaccine has been utilized in a wide variety of exotic cats without any untoward effects. It is probable that a single vaccination, administered after eight weeks of age, provides adequate protection and should be incorporated in a routine vaccination program for exotic cats if FPN is a problem in the area.

RABIES VACCINES

Although no reports exist regarding the safety and efficacy of rabies vaccines when utilized on exotic cats, at least one commercially available killed vaccine (Trimune, Ft. Dodge) has been utilized in many species of exotic cats without adverse reaction. However, it should be remembered that data regarding efficacy of the vaccine are not yet available, and this fact may affect decisions regarding the handling, quarantine, and disposition of cats suspected of having rabies.

SUMMARY

Between 1974 and 1978 an attenuated vaccine against FVR, FCV, and FPL (FVRC/P, Pitman-Moore) was administered to 224 healthy exotic cats representing 19 different species and subspecies (Table 1). All 224 cats were vaccinated at least twice intramuscularly, with approximately four-week intervals between vaccinations. In several species unvaccinated cats were used as contact controls. The entire study group was utilized in the evaluation of the vaccine's safety, and approximately one third (76 cats) were utilized in the evaluation of the vaccine's efficacy. Blood samples were taken from the latter group at the time of the first and second vaccinations and at varied times thereafter. Determination of the presence and level of serum-neutralizing titers to FPL, FVR, and FCV was performed on the serial blood samples by Dr. F.W. Scott, Cornell Feline Research Laboratory. Mean serum-neutralizing titers against FVR, FCV strain F9, and FPL were 1.7, 12.3, and 652, respectively, after the first vaccination. These titers increased to 21.6, 55.4, and 3920 respectively, after the second vaccination. Adverse reactions were not noted after vaccination, and the vaccinal virus did not spread to contact

Table 1. *Species of Exotic Cats Utilized in an Evaluation of a FVR-FCV-FPL Vaccine**

COMMON NAME	SCIENTIFIC NAME
European wild cat	*Felis silvestris*
Sand cat	*Felis margarita thinobia*
Pallas' cat	*Otocolobus manul*
Canada lynx	*Lynx lynx canadensis*
Bobcat	*Lynx rufus*
Golden cat	*Profelis temmincki*
Indian leopard cat	*Prionailurus bengalensis*
Amur leopard cat	*Prionailurus bengalensis euptilura*
Fishing cat	*Prionailurus viverrinas*
Margay	*Leopardus wiedi*
Jaguarundi	*Herpailurus jagouaroundi*
Mountain lion	*Puma concolor*
Snow leopard	*Uncia uncia*
African leopard	*Panthera pardus*
Jaguar	*Panthera onca*
Bengal tiger	*Panthera tigris tigris*
White Bengal tiger	*Panthera tigris tigris*
Siberian tiger	*Panthera tigris altaica*
African lion	*Panthera leo*
Cheetah	*Acinonyx jubatus*

*FVRC-P, Pitman-Moore, Inc., Washington Crossing, New Jersey

control cats. Because of the value of the cats in the study group, postvaccination challenge with virulent virus was not planned or performed.

Results of this study indicate that the combined FVR-FCV-FPL vaccine utilized (FVRC-P) is safe for intramuscular vaccination of exotic cats and, additionally, the data suggest that the vaccine is effective in protecting exotic cats against FPL, FVR, and serious FCV disease. Because of these results and the seriousness of the three diseases to susceptible exotic cats, vaccination against FPL, FVR, and FCV disease should be part of a routine exotic cat immunization program. Initial vaccination can be at 8 weeks of age (or earlier) but should be followed by vaccinations at 12 and 16 weeks, and a single

annual revaccination should be given thereafter.

SUPPLEMENTAL READING

Mitzel, J.R., and Strating, A.: Evaluation of a feline chlamydial pneumonitis vaccine in cats. Proc. Am. Soc. Microbiol., 76:72, 1976.

Practitioner's guide to feline vaccines and serums,1976–77. Feline Pract., March 1976, pp. 23–30.

Report of the Panel for the Colloquium on Selected Feline Infectious Diseases. J. Am. Vet. Med. Assoc., 158:835–843, 1971.

Scott, F.W.: Evaluation of an experimental vaccine against feline viral rhinotracheitis and feline calicivirus disease. Am. J. Vet. Res., 38:229–234, 1977a.

Scott, F.W.: Feline immunization. In Kirk, R.W. (ed.): *Current Veterinary Therapy VI.* 1977b, pp. 1276–1281.

Scott, F.W., and Gillespie, J.H.: Immunization for feline panleukopenia. Vet. Clin. North Am., 1:231–240, 1971.

RABIES: IMMUNIZATION AND PUBLIC HEALTH ASPECTS

MELVIN K. ABELSETH, D.V.M.
Albany, New York

The history of rabies dates back at least 2000 years, and the disease has been the subject of many reviews (Baer). Although some countries have been successful in remaining rabies-free and others have eliminated the disease, many countries continue their efforts to keep it under control and prevent human mortality. The purpose of this article is primarily to review methods efficacious for the prevention and treatment of rabies.

PATHOGENESIS

Rabies virus travels centripetally via the neurons from the site of exposure to the spinal cord and brain (Murphy, et al., 1973a). It then travels centrifugally to most tissues of the body, with a predilection for the salivary gland (Murphy, et al., 1973b). Although the virus has not been demonstrated in the salivary glands of every rabid animal, the infection can be spread by exposing another animal or man to virus-laden saliva. Since the virus is present in most tissues of infected animals, all body discharges should be considered a potential source of infection.

Bats have been incriminated as asymptomatic carriers. However, it is likely that they become infected and maintain the cycle by being bitten, as occurs in other animals. The virus may also spread in bats by the respiratory route, since they tend to live in close contact with one another.

IMMUNIZATION

Animals. The National Association of State Public Health Veterinarians has developed the Compendium of Animal Rabies Vaccines — a complete list of all licensed vaccines, together with recommendations for their use (Table 1).

Excellent vaccines are available that will provide immunity for three years under specified conditions. If a dog less than one year old is vaccinated, it should be revaccinated when it turns one and then triannually. However, yearly vaccination is recommended for other species. No vaccine is currently licensed for use in wildlife. In several instances vaccine-induced rabies has occurred in skunks, and exposed humans had to be treated. Veterinarians should be aware of the legal implications of such cases

Table 1. Compendium of Animal Rabies Vaccines, 1980*
VACCINES MARKETED IN THE U.S. (1980)

VACCINE: GENERIC NAME	PRODUCED BY	MARKETED BY (PRODUCT NAME)	FOR USE IN	DOSAGE†	AGE AT PRIMARY VACCINATION‡	BOOSTER RECOMMENDED
Modified live virus						
Canine cell line origin	Norden License No. 189	Norden (Endurall-R)	Dogs	1 ml	3 mo and 1 yr later	Triennially
High egg passage, Flury strain			Cats	1 ml	3 months	Annually
			Dogs	1 ml	3 mo and 1 yr later	Triennially
Porcine tissue culture origin	Jensen-Salsbery License No. 107	Jensen-Salsbery (ERA Strain Rabies Vaccine)	Cattle	1 ml	4 months	Annually
High cell passage, SAD strain			Horses	1 ml	4 months	Annually
			Sheep	1 ml	4 months	Annually
			Goats	1 ml	4 months	Annually
Canine tissue culture origin	Philips Roxane License No. 124	Bio-Ceutic (Neurogen-T-C)	Dogs	1 ml	3 mo and 1 yr later	Triennially
High cell passage, SAD strain						
Canine tissue culture origin	Philips Roxane License No. 124	Bio-Ceutic (Unirab)	Dogs	1 ml	3 months	Annually
High cell passage, SAD strain						
Canine tissue culture origin	Philips Roxane License No. 124	Pitman-Moore (Rabvax)	Dogs	1 ml	3 mo and 1 yr later	Triennially
High cell passage, SAD strain						
Bovine kidney tissue culture origin	Pitman-Moore License No. 264	Pitman-Moore (Rabies Vaccine)	Dogs	1 ml	3 months	Annually
High cell passage, SAD strain						
Hamster cell line origin	Beecham License No. 225	Beecham (Rabtect)	Dogs	1 ml	3 months	Annually
High cell passage, Kissling strain						
Inactivated vaccines						
Murine origin	Rolynn License No. 266	Ft. Dodge (Trimune)	Dogs	1 ml	3 mo and 1 yr later	Triennially
			Cats	1 ml	3 months	Annually
Murine origin	Rolynn License No. 266	Ft. Dodge (Annumune)	Dogs	1 ml	3 months	Annually
			Cats	1 ml	3 months	Annually
Murine origin	Douglas License No. 266	Douglas (SMBV)	Dogs	1 ml	3 months	Annually
			Cats	1 ml	3 months	Annually
Murine origin§	Douglas License No. 266	Douglas (Pan-Rab)	Cats	1 ml	3 months	Annually
Hamster cell line origin	Beecham License No. 225	Beecham (Rabcine)	Dogs	1 ml	3 months	Annually
High cell passage, Kissling strain			Cats	1 ml	3 months	Annually
Hamster cell line origin	Beecham License No. 225	Beecham (Rabcine-Feline)	Cats	1 ml	3 months	Annually
High cell passage, Kissling strain						
Hamster cell line origin	Vaccines, Inc. License No. 227	Bandy (Rabies Vacc)	Dogs	1 ml	3 months	Annually

*Prepared by the National Association of State Public Health Veterinarians, Inc., P.O. Box 13528, Baltimore, Maryland 21203
†All vaccine must be administered intramuscularly at one site in the thigh.
‡Three months is the earliest age recommended. Dogs vaccinated between 3 and 12 months of age should be revaccinated one year later.
§Combination vaccine.

RECOMMENDATIONS FOR IMMUNIZATION PROCEDURES

The purpose of these recommendations is to provide information on rabies vaccines to practicing veterinarians, public health officials, and others concerned with rabies control. This document will serve as the basis for animal rabies vaccination programs throughout the United States. Its adoption by cooperating organizations will result in standardization of recommendations and requirements among jurisdictions, which is necessary for an effective national rabies control program. These recommendations shall be reviewed and revised as necessary prior to the beginning of each calendar year. (All animal rabies vaccines licensed by the USDA and marketed in the United States are listed in the Compendium.)

VACCINE ADMINISTRATION: It is recommended that all animal rabies vaccines be restricted to use by or under the supervision of a veterinarian.

VACCINE SELECTION: While recognizing the efficacy of vaccines with the shorter durations of immunity, the Committee recommends the use of vaccines with the three-year duration of immunity, since they offer the least expensive and most effective method of community rabies control.

ROUTE OF INOCULATION: All rabies vaccines must be administered intramuscularly at one (1) site in the thigh.

HIGH-RISK RABIES AREA: Revaccination schedules may be altered from stated recommendations in high-risk rabies areas, herein defined for the purpose of canine rabies vaccination to mean any area (County, City, or Town) wherein indigenous dog-to-dog rabies transmission is occurring, as identified by the State health department.

WILDLIFE VACCINATION: Since data on efficacy and duration of immunity are generally lacking, no vaccine is licensed for use in wildlife in the United States. It is recommended that neither wild nor exotic animals be kept as household pets.

ACCIDENTAL HUMAN EXPOSURE TO VACCINE: Accidental inoculation may occur in individuals during the administration of animal rabies vaccines. Such exposure to inactivated vaccines constitutes no known rabies hazard. There have been no cases of rabies resulting from needle or other exposure to a licensed modified live virus vaccine in the United States. However, because of its relatedness to the Challenge Virus Standard (CVS) strain, the United States Public Health Service and most state health departments recommend post-exposure treatment for any individual with exposure to the Kissling strain modified live virus vaccine.

IMPLEMENTATION OF COMPENDIUM: In order to implement a more meaningful and manageable program of rabies vaccination for dogs and cats in the United States, the NASPHV recommends that all states promptly adopt the following standard certificate and tag system. This will aid the administration of local, state, national and international procedures. Veterinary practitioners and rabies control authorities are encouraged to specify the supplying of the standardized tags and certificates when rabies vaccine is ordered. Standardized tags can help a bite victim identify the vaccination status of an animal that cannot be apprehended. Such information is valuable to the attending physician. Committee recommendations for tag colors and shapes by year as well as a standardized certificate are:

RABIES TAGS

Calendar Year	Color	Shape
1980	Red	Heart
1981	Blue	Rosette
1982	Orange	Fireplug
1983	Green	Bell

License tags should not conflict in shape and color with rabies tags. The schedule for shapes and colors will be repeated commencing in 1984. It is suggested that two-hole attachments be provided in tags of 0.064-inch thickness or greater.

RABIES CERTIFICATE: 4″ × 6″ printer's ready proofs and samples are available from NASPHV and state public health veterinarians. Since the form is standardized for administrative and computerization purposes, changes cannot be permitted without approval by the NASPHV. Biologic manufacturers may submit "logo" inserts for approval. Agencies, biologics manufacturers, or corporations may print and adopt the form by reference to NASPHV Form #50. Provide owner's copy, agency copy, and veterinarian's copy.

Flexibility has been created by allowing two spaces: The "other data" can be used if vaccine lot numbers are required by jurisdictions. The space labeled "other" (in Licensing Block) may be used for special licensing information such as neutered status and county of residence, etc.

It is essential that biologics manufacturers routinely supply this form when distributing rabies vaccines, since it allows for effective nationwide rabies control procedures.

When this form is printed in other than the English language, the form must remain unchanged except for the translation so as to facilitate international travel.

RABIES VACCINATION CERTIFICATE
NASPHV Form #50

Owner's Name & Address — Print-use ball point pen or type

PRINT–Last		First		M.I.	Telephone

No.	Street	City		State	Zip

Species:	Sex:	Age:	Size:	Predominant Breed:	Colors:
Dog ☐	Male ☐	3 mo to 12 mo ☐	Under 20 lbs. ☐		
Cat ☐	Female ☐	12 mo. or older ☐	20-50 lbs. ☐		
			Over 50 lbs. ☐		

Name

Producer: ▢ ▢ ▢ (First 3 letters)

☐ 1 yr. Lic./Vacc.
☐ 3 yr. Lic./Vacc.

Other

Modified — Killed

☐ ☐ ☐   ☐ Murine
CEO TCO CLO   ☐ Caprine
              ☐ Hamster

For Licensing Agency Use

License No.   Year
_____ 19____
_____ 19____
_____ 19____

Other _____
Change ☐ Add ☐
Control No. _____

DATE VACCINATED:
_____ 19__
Month   Day
Rabies Tag No. _____

VACCINATION EXPIRES:
_____ . 19___
Month   Day

Veterinarian's: # _____
License No.

Signature

Address

THE NASPHV COMPENDIUM COMMITTEE FOR 1980: Melvin K. Abelseth, DVM, DVPH, PhD; Kenneth L. Crawford, DVM, MPH, Chairman; John I. Freeman, DVM, MPH; Grayson B. Miller, Jr., MD; James M. Shuler, DVM, MPH; R. Keith Sikes, DVM, MPH; CONSULTANTS TO THE COMMITTEE: Luther E. Fredrickson, DVM, MPH, AVMA Council on Public Health and Regulatory Medicine; Robert J. Price, DVM, Biologics Licensing and Standards Staff, APHIS, USDA; William G. Winkler, DVM, MS: CDC, PHS, DHEW; Rick Zehr, Vet., Biological License Committee, Animal Health Inst.; ENDORSERS: U.S. Animal Health Assn., Rabies Comm.; AVMA, Council on Public Health and Regulatory Veterinary Medicine; Conference of State and Territorial Epidemiologists.

and refuse to vaccinate any animal for which the vaccine is not licensed. However, veterinarians should advise vaccination of pets, especially in areas in which rabies is enzootic.

A few dogs have acquired vaccine-induced rabies from some modified live virus rabies vaccines. Many of these cases were associated with vaccination immediately after trauma or surgery or during corticosteroid therapy — a practice that should be discouraged with any live virus vaccine and especially with live rabies virus vaccine.

Humans. Pre-exposure immunization is a necessity for practicing veterinarians, rabies laboratory personnel, and others working with and around wildlife. Duck embryo vaccine (DEV) is the only product now available in the United States. Three doses at ten-day intervals, followed by a booster six months later, should provide an acceptable antibody titer of 1:16 or higher. However, this cannot be assumed. A serum sample should be submitted to the appropriate state health department for testing. If the titer is low, boosters and testing should be continued until the acceptable titer is attained.

If an individual with an acceptable antibody level is exposed, three to four injections of vaccine at daily intervals should provide protection. If the antibody level has not been determined, the full treatment course must be considered.

A new rabies vaccine, produced in human diploid cell culture (WI-38), has been developed for humans. Field tests indicate that this vaccine is antigenically more potent and has caused fewer allergic reactions. Although not yet licensed for general use, it is available through the Center for Disease Control for exposed individuals who are allergic to the egg proteins in DEV, who fail to respond to DEV, or who are exposed to a laboratory-confirmed rabid animal. The treatment regimen for WI-38 vaccine is one intramuscular injection on days 0, 3, 7, 14, and 28. Day 0 is the first day of vaccine therapy.

TREATMENT OF SUSPECTED CASES

Animals. If a dog or cat has been exposed to a rabid animal but can be shown to be adequately immunized, a booster dose of vaccine will confer adequate protection. If it has not been vaccinated, it should either be destroyed or isolated for at least four months in such a manner that it cannot be in contact with human beings and other animals.

If a non-vaccinated animal has bitten a human or another animal and if rabies is suspected, there are two alternatives. If the owner agrees or the animal is unowned, it should be killed immediately, and its head should be submitted to a laboratory for detection of virus by the fluorescent antibody test. If virus is not in the brain it will not be in the salivary gland either, and the bitten individual will not have been exposed. The other alternative is to isolate the animal for ten days in such a manner that it cannot have contact with people or other animals. If it develops signs of rabies during that period, it should be destroyed. If not, it may be released.

Before examining a "choking" bovine, the veterinarian should investigate all aspects of the case. If possible, he or she should wear gloves. A veterinarian in Europe recently died of rabies after such an exposure.[*]

Humans. When human exposure occurs, wash the site of exposure with copious amounts of soap and water. Rinse well and apply a quaternary ammonium compound or tincture of iodine.

A good diagnostic service is essential. The fluorescent antibody technique, in competent hands, will determine whether treatment should be started. When immediate diagnosis is not available, treatment should begin promptly. Should the specimen be diagnosed negative, treatment can be suspended. If treatment is being withheld pending laboratory examination, the specimens should be delivered directly to the laboratory, and arrangements should be made for examination.

The initial treatment should consist of human rabies immune globulin (HRIG), 20 international units per kilogram body weight (9 IU/lb). As much as possible should be infiltrated around the bite, and the remainder should be given by deep intramuscular injection. This is followed by 21 daily 1-ml doses of DEV starting on day 0, with boosters on days 30 and 40. After this treatment the antibody level should be determined by submitting a serum sample to the state health department. If the antibody level is insufficient, further boosters should be given at the physician's discretion until adequate antibody titer is elicited.

PUBLIC HEALTH ASPECTS

Although the incidence of rabies, especially

---

[*]Dr. George Baer, Center for Disease Control: Personal communication.

in dogs (the main route of exposure to man), has been reduced, the threat of disease still exists worldwide. In Central and South America loss of bovines due to rabies carried by the vampire bat is an economic hardship. Veterinarians can play an important public health role by maintaining an immunized animal population and by helping to keep the public informed about the continuing danger of this disease.

SUPPLEMENTAL READING

Baer, G.M. (ed.): *The Natural History of Rabies*, vol. I and II. New York, Academic Press, 1975.
Murphy, F.A., Bauer, S.P., Harrison, A.K., and Winn, W.C.: Comparative pathogenesis of rabies and rabies-like viruses. Viral infection and transit from inoculation site to the central nervous system. Lab. Invest. 28:361–376, 1973a.
Murphy, F.A., Harrison, A.K., Winn, W.C., and Bauer, S.P.: Comparative pathogenesis of rabies and rabies-like viruses: Infection of the central nervous system and centrifugal spread of virus to peripheral tissues. Lab. Invest., 29:1–16, 1973b.

PET-ASSOCIATED ZOONOSES

DOROTHY N. HOLMES, D.V.M.
Ithaca, New York

New concerns about pet involvement in human disease have arisen from such findings as (1) cats are definitive hosts for *Toxoplasma gondii*, (2) feline leukemia virus may be involved in human cancer, and (3) multiple sclerosis may be associated with prolonged contact with small house pets. As a community authority on animal health, the veterinarian must be prepared to address these issues and provide knowledgeable advice for pet owners and community officials. There are over 200 zoonoses (animal diseases transmissible to man), and of these only a few are associated with pets. It is not the intent of this article to discuss all of them in great detail. The reader is referred to the definitive textbook on the subject (Hubbert, et al.) for comprehensive coverage of zoonotic diseases and to *Current Veterinary Therapy VI* for a presentation of the salient features of pet-associated zoonoses in concise table form. Our purpose is to discuss briefly some of the recent information regarding diseases of pets transmitted to man. The zoonotic aspects of toxoplasmosis and canine brucellosis will be covered elsewhere in this text.

PSITTACOSIS

The number of cases of psittacosis in man reported to the Center for Disease Control (CDC) increased steadily from 23 in 1976 and 33 in 1977 to 55 in the first six months of 1978. A corresponding increase in the number of psittacosis-positive psittacine birds has been noted in several states. Psittacosis in man is usually an acute, generalized disease manifested by an influenza-like illness or a more serious pneumonic disease with high fever, chills, severe headache, nausea and vomiting, unproductive cough, chest pains, pulmonary infiltrates, myalgia, and malaise. The incubation period is 4 to 15 days, and infection is usually acquired by inhalation of dust from the droppings of infected birds. The infected birds may have no signs of illness. Diagnosis is confirmed by isolation of the causative agent, *Chlamydia psittaci*, or by a significant increase in the complement-fixing antibody titer. The U.S. Department of Agriculture requires that imported psittacine birds be quarantined for 30 days and fed a mash medicated to achieve 1.5 micrograms of chlortetracycline per milliliter of blood for that period of time in order to eliminate psittacosis. However, more effective control is needed to ensure adequate levels of the antibiotic, since psittacosis has been diagnosed in birds recently released from quarantine. One of the real health hazards associated with psittacine birds is the apparently large number of untreated birds being smuggled into the country. As a precautionary measure, owners acquiring psittacine birds from any source would be well advised to feed a chlortetracycline-medicated seed for at least 15 days. Diagnosis of psittacosis is a specialized laboratory procedure and is dependent on the proper submission of the specimens to be tested. Suspect birds should be killed, put in air-tight plastic bags, frozen, and shipped frozen with enough dry ice to ensure that they reach the laboratory in a frozen state. Clients should be advised by their veterinarians of the possibility of human infection after exposure to infected birds.

PLAGUE

Sylvatic plague (*Yersinia pestis* infection) is endemic in the southwestern United States, where sporadic cases of bubonic plague in man are associated with exposure to rabbits or rodents or their fleas. It is of interest that in 1977 two cases of human plague infection were apparently acquired from pet cats. In one case the patient had been bitten and scratched by a kitten that was later found dead. *Yersinia pestis* was isolated from its tissues. In the second instance the patient had examined the mouth of a pet cat that was incoordinated, drooling, and coughing up blood. This cat also died and had tissues positive for *Y. pestis*. Other cases of plague in cats without human spread have been reported in California. Signs in the sick animals included submandibular lymphadenopathy, swelling beneath the eyes, sluggishness, fever (107°F), and sneezing that produced purulent material. Cultures of aspirates from the cervical lymph nodes were positive for *Y. pestis*. Treatment with tetracyclines resulted in the cat's recovery. The people exposed to the sneezing cat were treated prophylactically with antibiotics and remained well. While it is undoubtedly not a zoonotic disease of national importance, plague should be kept in mind in dealing with cats from areas in which the disease is endemic in rodents.

ANIMAL BITES

Animal bites are the most common pet-associated human health problem in the United States, with an annual attack rate estimated at one in every 170 people. Because of their small size and greater tendency to engage in bite-provoking behavior, children are the most frequent victims. While rarely fatal, animal bites are painful and expensive (the Maryland State Department of Health and Hygiene reports an average cost to the victim of $150 per bite), and they elicit considerable anxiety about rabies and tetanus. Bites by wild animals such as raccoons, foxes, skunks, and monkeys that are kept as pets are a particular problem. Skunks are especially dangerous; in three separate instances during 1978 a total of 78 people received antirabies treatment after exposure to rabid skunks that had been kept as pets. Rabies has a long incubation period in skunks, and virus is shed in the saliva for an extended period, making these animals particularly risky. Clinical rabies has developed in some wild animal species after vaccination with modified live virus rabies vaccines. It should be re-emphasized that *no* rabies vaccine is licensed for use in wildlife in the United States. If wild animals must be vaccinated, only inactivated vaccines should be used.

Bites by dogs and cats may result in *Pasteurella* wound infection, a painful and disabling condition. Other diseases, less common but still occasionally associated with animal bites, include tetanus, tularemia, and erysipeloid. Infection of bite wounds with anaerobic species of bacteria such as *Sphaerophorus* and *Bacteroides* is undoubtedly of importance but is probably under-reported because of the difficulty in isolating these organisms from clinical specimens.

An additional bite-transmitted disease of concern is monkey B-virus encephalitis. The agent, *Herpesvirus simiae*, is carried by Old World monkeys that may or may not show signs of disease. When they do occur, signs may be limited to formation of vesicles similar to human cold sores in and around the mouth or tongue. After a bite by an infected monkey, there can be vesicle formation at the wound site. Frequently this is followed by regional lymphadenopathy, with signs of encephalitis occurring within one to five weeks of exposure. These signs are accompanied by fever, headache, and nausea and are followed by ataxia, ascending paralysis, and death. Since there is no specific treatment or protective vaccination for this disease, control rests entirely with proper handling techniques and use of protective clothing when working with monkeys. In addition to *Herpesvirus simiae* infection, monkeys can carry tuberculosis, human infectious hepatitis, salmonellosis, shigellosis, and Marburg virus, a rare systemic infection that is sometimes fatal to man.

Veterinarians have the opportunity to reduce the numbers of animal bites by educating the public on how to avoid bite-provoking behavior and by encouraging clients to heed the American Veterinary Medical Association's recommendation against the keeping of wild animals as pets. This job will demand the best persuasive powers.

Q FEVER

A small outbreak of Q fever (*Coxiella burnetii*), a rickettsial disease characterized in man by fever, headache, chills, malaise, and vomiting, was reported in 1978 among employees of an exotic bird and reptile importing company. Disease was related to contact with a shipment of imported, tick-infested ball pythons (*Python regius*). Seven of the 11 people who had been in contact with the pythons, their ticks, or the excreta from ticks or pythons had had a febrile illness, and 8 of the 11 were serologically confirmed as having had a recent Q fever infection. Reptiles have rarely been documented as potential hosts for *C. burnetii*. Most human infection has been related to contact with cattle, sheep, and goats, in which exposure takes place by inhalation of air-borne particles containing the organism or by drinking unpasteurized milk from infected cows. In view of this recent report, however, reptiles may have to be considered a potential reservoir host for man.

LYMPHOCYTIC CHORIOMENINGITIS

Lymphocytic choriomeningitis (LCM) is a virus frequently found in the house mouse, in which it produces inapparent infection. During the 1970's numerous instances of human infection associated with laboratory and pet Syrian hamsters (*Mesocricetus auratus*) were reported. Hamsters may excrete LCM virus for months or may become lifelong carriers, as mice do. Man becomes infected by contamination with excrement or by the aerosol route, often after minimal exposure. The clinical disease in man is usually biphasic. The first phase is a flu-like illness, which may be followed in one to two weeks by a recurrence of flu-like signs or by onset of meningitis or encephalomyelitis with fever, myalgia, headache, and cough. The disease is seldom fatal but tends to be more severe in older patients. Control of this infection may be effected by using only serologically negative animals for breeding stock. The complement-fixation test is used for screening.

CAMPYLOBACTER FETUS INFECTION

Campylobacter (Vibrio) fetus ss. *jejuni* appears to be emerging as an enteric pathogen of importance in man. *Campylobacter* sp. are associated with many animal species (cattle, sheep, fowl, and swine), but a recent study in the Denver area revealed a group of *Campylobacter* enteritis patients who had histories of contact with puppies showing diarrhea. The affected puppies or their littermates were culture-positive for *C. fetus*. The puppies were reported to have developed diarrhea soon after their arrival in a household, and the onset of human illness was closely related to the onset of illness in the dogs. A survey of four kennels revealed a 5 per cent prevalence of infection in dogs more than six months of age and a 13 to 33 percent prevalence in dogs younger than three months. Prevalence in cats younger than three months ranged from 4 to 10 percent. The data, although preliminary, indicate that young dogs and cats can be a reservoir for human *Campylobacter* infection.

FELINE PNEUMONITIS

There is at least one case reported in the literature of infection in man by the chlamydial agent of feline pneumonitis. The organism was isolated from conjunctival scrapings of a man with acute follicular keratoconjunctivitis. Investigation of the source of his infection revealed that his two pet cats, which had recent histories of rhinitis and sneezing, were culturally positive for the agent of feline pneumonitis. Additionally, the isolate from the human patient produced in experimental cats eye disease similar to that described as resulting from natural feline infection.

SARCOPTIC MANGE

The canine sarcoptic mange mite, *Sarcoptes scabiei* var. *canis*, may occasionally infect humans, where it produces papulovesicular eruptions on the lower cheeks, abdomen, and forearms. The lesion is called "puppy-dog dermatitis" and is usually acquired when children fondle puppies with sarcoptic mange. When treating cases of mange in pets, veterinarians should warn owners that the possibility of transmission exists. Another skin problem in pet owners is the occasional development of an acute, primary-irritant, contact dermatitis after exposure to flea collars, especially when the collars are wet. Most collars now carry a warning to users about this possibility.

FELINE LEUKEMIA

There is still no substantive evidence that feline leukemia virus infects man or causes human neoplasms. The virus can, however, infect cell cultures of human origin and has produced leukemias and sarcomas in dogs and monkeys when inoculated into them on or before the day of birth. These findings make it difficult to dismiss completely concern about its potential for human infection. However, without condemning feline pets in general, it would seem reasonable to recommend that pregnant women and young infants avoid close contact with cats, especially those that are known carriers of feline leukemia virus.

CANINE DISTEMPER AND MULTIPLE SCLEROSIS

In the same category as the feline leukemia situation is the concern generated by recent reports of a possible association between exposure to house dogs and subsequent development of multiple sclerosis (MS). MS is a demyelinating disease of major importance in man. Its cause is still unknown, in spite of the extensive research effort it has received for years. Some authors have suggested that intimate contact with small house dogs and, thereby, contact with canine distemper virus may be of etiologic significance in MS. Such an association in light of today's evidence is unsubstantiated, although it would be foolhardy to ignore the *possibility* of such a relationship. Until such time as valid evidence is available, pet owners should be advised not to be alarmed by these reports but rather to practice hygienic pet care and to follow vaccination programs as recommended by their veterinarians.

The transmission of pet-borne zoonoses is complex and generally requires close contact between susceptible humans and animals or animal excretions. Children are more commonly affected because transmission usually reflects both poor hygienic practice (hand-to-mouth behavior patterns) and intimate contact with animals. As veterinarians we should be able to answer questions about potential hazards of disease transmission from pets to man in a realistic manner that places the danger in reasonable perspective and to make well-informed recommendations for avoiding problems.

Veterinarians can keep up to date on developments in the field of pet-borne zoonoses by reading *Veterinary Public Health Notes* and *Morbidity and Mortality Weekly Reports,* which are obtainable from the Center for Dis-

ease Control (CDC) in Atlanta, Georgia. CDC also maintains supplies of rabies vaccine for use in the postexposure treatment of rabies in people. Requests for the vaccine can be made by calling the CDC at (404) 329–3727. Supplies of antirabies immune globulin of human origin are available from Cutter Laboratories for use in rabies postexposure prophylaxis. The company maintains an emergency phone by which this product can be ordered at any time. The number is (214) 661–5850.

SUPPLEMENTAL READING

Benenson, A. (ed.): *Control of Communicable Diseases in Man,* 12th ed. Washington, D.C., American Public Health Association, 1975.

Blaser, M.J., et al.: *Campylobacter* enteritis associated with canine infection. Lancet, 2:979–981, 1978.

Burridge, M.J.: Multiple sclerosis, house pets, and canine distemper: Critical review of recent reports. J. Am. Vet. Med. Assoc., 173:1439–1444, 1978.

Center for Disease Control: *Morbidity and Mortality Weekly Report.* Atlanta, Georgia, U.S. Department of Health, Education and Welfare, Public Health Service, Center for Disease Control.

Center for Disease Control: *Veterinary Public Health Notes.* Atlanta, Georgia, U.S. Department of Health Education and Welfare, Public Health Service, Center for Disease Control.

Hirsch, M.S., et al: Lymphocytic-choriomeningitis-virus infection traced to a pet hamster. N. Engl. J. Med., 291:610–612, 1974.

Hubbert, W.T., McCullock, W.P., and Schnurrenberger, P.R. (eds.): *Diseases Transmitted from Animals to Man,* 6th ed. Springfield, Illinois, Charles C Thomas, 1975.

Kahrs, R.F., Holmes, D.H., and Poppensiek, G.C.: Diseases transmitted from pets to man: An evolving concern for veterinarians. Cornell Vet., 68:442–459, 1978.

Norins, A.L.: Canine scabies in children. Am. J. Dis. Child., 117:239–242, 1969.

Post, J.E.: Feline leukemia and related viruses. Feline Information Bulletin (Cornell Feline Research Laboratory), 1:1–5, 1976.

Schachter, J., Ostler, H.B., and Meyer, K.F.: Human infection with the agent of feline pneumonitis. Lancet, 1:1063–1065, 1969.

CONTROL OF CANINE INFECTIOUS DISEASES IN ADOPTION SHELTERS

DAVID H. TAYLOR, D.V.M.
Syracuse, New York

The control of canine infectious diseases in shelters presents many unique problems. Veterinarians must be acquainted with them and become active in shelter operations. These unique circumstances begin with the admission procedures. Because of the nature and purpose of shelters, all animals are accepted. Failure to

accept them results in the ruthless abandonment of pets by irresponsible owners. The entering animals' health status ranges from normal to clinically ill to those that are incubating diseases.

Most personnel are involved in a shelter because of their emotional concern for animals.

This makes rational decision-making difficult. Employees often work on a voluntary basis, and controlling their actions presents problems. Most shelters have financial problems and do not have proper funds to function in an ideal way.

Infectious canine diseases of most concern are distemper, hepatitis, leptospirosis, tracheobronchitis, intestinal infections, internal parasites, external parasites, and fungal diseases. The key to control of these conditions lies in careful personnel management and implementation of rigid procedural policies. This should be augmented by a realistic vaccination program.

The shelter must be constructed properly. It is essential to have controlled air circulation, humidity, and lighting. All surfaces must be easy to clean, including walls, floors and, most important, the animal compartments, which should also be positioned so as to be convenient to clean. These criteria should exist for all types of housing within the shelter — individual compartments, indoor runs, outdoor runs, and puppy pens. If non-disposable food and water dishes are used, they must also be easy to clean and disinfect.

Another important aspect of disease control within the shelter involves personnel. Employees must be aware of the absolute necessity of good sanitation. They must realize the reasons for proper procedures to control disease because, if they do not know, it is unlikely that they will do an adequate job. They must know the common signs of infectious diseases, how they are transmitted, and the significance of "incubation" periods.

Operational procedures must be posted and followed. Because of the high turnover in shelter personnel, these procedures must be referred to frequently.

The flow of pets through a shelter is important. The most serious disease problems are encountered in puppies, and these constitute the largest number of dogs entering most shelters. Unfortunately, only 10 to 20 percent of incoming puppies will be adopted. It is important that employees realize this fact, because it means that 80 to 90 percent of incoming puppies will be destroyed. Sick animals, particularly puppies showing signs of disease, should be euthanatized promptly. Keeping the smallest possible number of dogs within the shelter makes disease control easier.

Five general areas of shelters should be identified. These can be designated as a holding area, a pre-adoption area, an adoption area, a euthanasia area, and a "quarantine" area. The quarantine area is optional and should be used only for suspiciously ill animals being held while a determination of their fate is being made. Personnel must determine the approximate number of puppies being adopted and move into the pre-adoption area only enough healthy puppies to satisfy this demand. The rest must go to the euthanasia area. In the pre-adoption area the pups should be examined thoroughly, preferably by a veterinarian, and vaccinated for distemper, hepatitis, leptospirosis, and tracheobronchitis. The sooner this can be done, the sooner the protection process can begin. In our experience the use of the distemper-measles vaccine gives the best protection for distemper. After vaccination, the pups should be placed in the adoption area. Pups should be observed constantly for signs of disease and removed immediately if illness is noted. They should go to the euthanasia area, but if a judgment must be made by a supervisor, a quarantine area should be available.

Shelter cleaning is very important in controlling disease. The most disease-free area (i.e., the adoption area) should be cleaned first, followed in order by the holding, quarantine, and euthanasia areas. Cleaning materials used are those that are most effective against the common viruses and bacteria found in shelter conditions. The use of disposable food and water dishes helps eliminate the spread of disease.

If disease occurs in the adoption area, several steps can be taken. The most effective procedure and, in most instances, the most efficient involves euthanasia of all exposed puppies, thorough cleaning and drying of the area, and starting again. In shelters in which both puppies and kittens are handled, alternation of the "kitten" and "puppy" rooms helps break disease cycles.

Controlling infectious diseases in shelter puppies is difficult, and one must be able to select and eliminate immediately any animals showing signs of disease. This may not be possible with adult dogs, since many must be held for specific periods according to state and local regulations.

It is important to be familiar with the law, since some localities permit euthanasia of diseased dogs even during the holding period, if disease is verified by a veterinarian or by shelter personnel. The sooner a sick pet can be eliminated, the fewer problems the remaining animals will have. If sick dogs must be held in a shelter, they should be isolated and cared for after the healthy ones have been attended to.

Controlling canine infectious diseases under shelter conditions can be challenging. Implementation of sound shelter management procedures combined with vaccination is the way to control infectious diseases.

CONTROL OF FELINE INFECTIOUS DISEASES IN CATTERIES AND ADOPTION SHELTERS

JEAN HOLZWORTH, D.V.M.
Boston, Massachusetts

Control of infectious diseases in catteries and adoption shelters primarily involves measures against panleukopenia, upper respiratory infections, leukemia, infectious peritonitis, and ringworm. Toxoplasmosis is endemic in some catteries. With the exception of panleukopenia, all these diseases may exist in and be passed from apparently healthy carriers to susceptible cats, virtually assuring that, despite the most rigorous and indeed ruthless measures, no shelter and very few catteries can be completely free of disease.

CATTERIES

The chief causes of the high incidence of infectious diseases in many catteries are (1) shipment of cats among catteries for breeding purposes and (2) exposure to carrier cats at shows. The ideal cattery is a "closed" one, limited strictly to its own breeding stock. The fewer cats the better; they can be observed and tended more closely, and litters can be spaced so that only a few young kittens are in a cattery at one time.

PANLEUKOPENIA

The panleukopenia (FPL) vaccines, particularly if administered at four-week intervals from 8 to 16 weeks of age (for maximum protection), are so effective that this disease is seldom a problem. In the rare instance in which a queen fails to transmit FPL antibodies in colostrum, homologous feline serum (now available only from Fromm) given at birth and again at three to four weeks of age provides protection until vaccinations are started. In the uncommon situation in which panleukopenia is a persistent cattery problem, the safest course is vaccination repeated every two weeks from age 6 to 16 weeks. FPL vaccination should be repeated yearly for all cats.

UPPER RESPIRATORY INFECTIONS

Vaccines against upper respiratory infections — viral rhinotracheitis (FVR, herpes), calcivirus (formerly, picornavirus) infection (FCV), and pneumonitis (FPN, caused by *Chlamydia psittaci*) — do not produce immunity as solid or as lasting as that given by FPL vaccine, but nonetheless they contribute greatly toward preventing or lessening the incidence of "colds." These vaccines may be given separately or in various combinations with FPL vaccine. It is recommended that FVR-FCV vaccinations be given initially at 8 and 12 weeks of age and then repeated yearly. One FPN vaccination given at 8 weeks is believed to suffice and is certainly advisable for cats that will travel extensively on the show circuit.

If upper respiratory illness develops, infection may be transmitted through the air as well as by contact between cats and also by contaminated bedding, dishes, and clothing of personnel. It is therefore advisable to move affected cats to separate quarters, where they can receive the painstaking nursing and hand-feeding that are essential for their physical needs and morale.

In catteries in which these upper respiratory infections are a serious endemic problem it may be necessary to eliminate carrier queens that repeatedly infect their kittens. Another extreme measure is to wean kittens early (perhaps at three to four weeks of age) before their passive maternal immunity has waned, hand-rear them separately, and start vaccinations early (at five weeks). Finally, it may be helpful for the veterinarian supervising such a cattery to take throat swabs and obtain the assistance of a virologist in determining which agent or agents may be involved in an outbreak. Frequently more than one is involved, and the severity of illness may be aggravated further if the cats' resistance is impaired by their being carriers of FIP virus or FeLV.

LEUKEMIA

Conscientious breeders have by now made great progress in eliminating the virus of leukemia (FeLV) from their cats by using the immunofluorescence test and then either destroying all cats with positive results or placing apparently healthy carriers as indoor pets in "only cat" homes, where they will not endanger other cats. Knowledgeable buyers, particularly breeders, who do not wish to gamble about receiving a carrier, require as a condition of purchase that a cat have had a negative test result within the previous month.

INFECTIOUS PERITONITIS

Feline infectious peritonitis (FIP) is now the most troublesome and insidious infectious disease among cats in general and particularly among cattery-raised purebreds. Making its appearance in the 1950's as a rather uncommon but uniformly fatal disease, it has now been shown by serologic testing to be widespread in the cat population. Primary infection is either asymptomatic or manifested as an extremely mild, transient upper respiratory infection that is indistinguishable from mild forms of other upper respiratory infections. Weeks or months later, less than 1 percent of such cats may develop the effusive or granulomatous secondary form of the disease.

Any cat having a positive titer, whether low or high, is presumed to be a carrier and shedder of the virus and, hence, a threat to test-negative, susceptible cats. Rather impressive circumstantial and serologic evidence also suggests that FIP, as well as FPL and the upper respiratory infections, may be involved in the reproductive failure of queens, abortions, stillbirths, and mortality of kittens.

To establish whether a cattery is infected it is advised that 10 to 20 percent of the cats over one year old be tested. Once a cattery has tested negative, no cat should enter it unless the animal has tested negative within the previous month, and even these cats should be quarantined for two weeks. Cats from the cattery should not have contact with FIP-positive cats for breeding or any other purpose. Cats returning from breeding or shows should be quarantined for at least two weeks, and if they develop signs of upper respiratory infection they should be tested for FIP after three or four weeks (Scott, et al.).

Testing a kitten before about three months of age could provide difficulties in interpretation. It might actually be infected or merely be carrying remnants of maternal antibody (Scott, 1979).

Breeders with cats suffering a high incidence of clinical FIP or with FIP-associated kitten losses may well decide to test at intervals and eliminate all cats with positive results. Breeders willing to "live with" the disease face at least occasional losses in the cattery and also among kittens and young cats some time after sale. In these catteries good general care is especially important in order to avoid any stress that could convert a carrier into a clinically ill cat. Ample space, good sanitation and nutrition, warmth with low humidity, and protection against intercurrent diseases are needed.

TOXOPLASMOSIS

Toxoplasmosis is endemic in some catteries. If clinical disease is identified microscopically by biopsy or autopsy, this infection should be considered among the possible causes of any undiagnosed febrile illness, reproductive failure, or kitten mortality. Serologic testing helps to define the extent of infection in such a cattery.

RINGWORM

Ringworm (dermatomycosis, sometimes referred to by breeders as "fungus") is endemic in many catteries that raise long-haired breeds. Kittens are often treated with enough griseofulvin to eliminate gross lesions but not to prevent the carrier state. Within a couple of weeks after purchase, humans and dogs or cats in contact with the newcomer may develop tell-tale lesions. Veterinarians should check newly purchased long-haired cats with a Wood's ultraviolet lamp at least; some clinicians also brush out and culture samples of fur.

As a precaution against infections generally, catteries should hold newly purchased cats and cats returning from shows or mating in separate quarters for from two to four weeks. Any cats within the cattery should be similarly isolated at the first sign of infectious disease. Cats that appear abnormally quiet or fail to eat should have their temperatures checked.

No death, whether of an older cat or newborn kitten, should go uninvestigated. A thorough autopsy should be performed, preferably by or in consultation with an experienced veterinary pathologist. More often than not, microscopic or microbiologic studies are necessary to make such a diagnosis; therefore, ample tissue specimens must be taken, preserved or frozen properly, and shipped so as to reach their destination promptly and in good condition. Shipping perishable materials over weekends and at holiday periods is risky.

SHELTERS

Although infectious diseases are more likely to be endemic or virulent in the concentrated environment of a cattery, it is inevitable that cats carrying or ill with infectious agents frequently find their way into shelters and expose healthy cats to disease.

Shelters require constant and rigorous veterinary supervision and alert and experienced attendants. Ideally, a shelter should have a holding or quarantine area, and any cat showing the slightest evidence of infectious disease should never enter the main "display" area.

Shelters are legally bound to hold all strays for a certain period, and the majority also hold all possible adoptees for several days, giving FPL-FVR-FCV vaccinations only when an animal is actually adopted. Inevitably some of these cats, exposed to infection during the waiting period, develop disease shortly after entering their new homes. In the case of panleukopenia, homologous serum provides somewhat better protection for delayed inoculation than vaccine, but FPL vaccination is, of course, then required three to four weeks later.

Since only a small proportion of all potential adoptees actually find homes, some shelters estimate realistically how many and which cats or kittens are likely to attract new owners and vaccinate them immediately upon entrance to the shelter, destroying all others at the outset. Such a course is indeed ruthless but reduces disease problems and provides the best protection for the cats that will actually be adopted.

One exceptional shelter tests adoptees for FeLV before placing them.

Sanitation and management for catteries and shelters are similar: ten changes of fresh air per minute, humidity on the low side (35 percent) and, above all, cleanliness. Clorox® is the disinfectant most effective against feline viruses, including the highly resistant agent of panleukopenia. To enhance its cleaning properties it may be combined with a detergent such as A-33®* (4 oz of Clorox and 2 oz of A-33 per gallon of water). All cage surfaces, including the inner and outer sides of cage doors, should be scrubbed frequently and thoroughly, particularly after a change of occupants. Food and water dishes should be cleaned, disinfected, and rinsed well daily unless, as is preferable, disposable dishes are used. Sanitary pans must be cleaned and disinfected frequently.

Ideally, attendants should wash their hands or gloves after handling each cat or litter of kittens. They should change frequently into clean uniforms, and separate garments, gloves, and shoes should be used for working in areas in which cats are quarantined or ill.

Although having a varied assortment of kittens disporting themselves in a large display cage with toys, perches, a tree, and other items is an attractive feature of a shelter, such "pooling" of kittens from different litters may predispose to the spread of infectious disease and should be avoided.

The experience of a number of small animal hospitals suggests that, for shelters or catteries that can afford it, round-the-clock ultraviolet lighting (to which the animals are not directly exposed) could well pay for itself in controlling infectious disease. Such lighting must be professionally installed and regularly monitored, and even then the results are varied.

SUPPLEMENTAL READING

Hardy, W.D., Jr.: Management of lymphosarcoma. In Kirk, R.W. (ed.): *Current Veterinary Therapy V*. Philadelphia, W.B. Saunders Co., 1974, pp. 381–387.

Scott, F.W., Hoshino, Y., and Weiss, R.C.: Feline infectious peritonitis. Feline Information Bulletin (Cornell Feline Research Laboratory), Number 4, October 1978.

Scott, F.W.: Feline immunization. In Kirk, R.W. (ed.): *Current Veterinary Therapy VI*. Philadelphia, W.B. Saunders Co., 1977, pp. 1276–1281.

Scott, F.W.: Personal communication, 1979.

---

*Airkem, Airwick Industries, Carlstadt, New Jersey 07072

CONTROL OF INFECTIOUS DISEASES IN AVIARIES AND PET SHOPS

STEPHEN B. HITCHNER, V.M.D.
Ithaca, New York

Birds are becoming increasingly popular as companions, as objects of interest and beauty in aviary collections, and as hobbies. The satisfaction birds impart to their owners can be achieved only when the birds are in good health. Therefore, in the breeding, marketing, and management of birds every effort should be made to prevent contact with infectious agents. Whenever animals are drawn from various sources and congregated in a small enclosure the risk of exposure to disease agents is multiplied. This is equally true when we confine birds in aviary collections, pet shops, breeding colonies, or any other situation in which numerous species are in proximity.

It may be impossible to eliminate all risk of exposure to infectious agents when operating under these conditions, but the risks can be greatly reduced by applying sound procedures of disease prevention to the care and handling of birds. A little investment of time in planning disease prevention will pay dividends in healthier birds and more satisfied owners.

GENERAL SANITATION

Cleanliness around the holding area should be maintained at all times. It is preferable that the holding rooms be such that they can be hosed down daily. When this is not feasible, wet-mopping of the floor is the next-best thing. Dry sweeping of floors raises so much dust that it is counterproductive in controlling infections unless the floor is first sprinkled liberally with a moist sweeping compound. Holding cages and food and water cups should not be exchanged among birds without thorough washing, followed by soaking in hypochlorite solution (household bleach used according to directions), with a final rinse in clear water.

Disease agents generally are shed from carrier or actively infected birds by respiratory droplets or in the feces. The risk of disease transmission to other residents in the colony can be reduced by providing good ventilation and by removing droppings frequently. Ventilation dilutes infectious agents in the air and removes them from the holding area. Droppings frequently are dry when removed, and careless handling can disperse infected particles through the air. When droppings are collected on paper, they should be folded up carefully inside the paper. If shavings or other litter is used to catch droppings, the litter should be moistened with water before removal.

PARASITES

External parasites (lice, mites, fleas, ticks, and mosquitoes) cause skin irritation by their presence, and heavy infestations can debilitate birds. Blood-sucking parasites, in particular, can be responsible for the transmission of infectious agents. Pox of birds, transmitted by mosquitoes, is a good example of a viral disease spread by blood-sucking insects.

Frequent examination of birds and their perching areas should be made to detect parasites. The red mite (*Dermanyssus gallinae*) and ticks (*Argas persicus*) are usually not seen on birds and can be detected only by careful examination of perches, cages, and nearby surroundings. There are insecticides that are safe and effective for use on and around birds. However, one should avoid contamination of food and water. Mites and lice on birds may be controlled by applying a mist spray of a 0.5 percent carbaryl (Sevin) suspension in water. Do not spray in a confined, unventilated area; ventilate the room while spraying. Repeat after four weeks if necessary.

Malathion in a 4 percent dust also may be applied to birds for the control of lice and mites. A 2 percent malathion emulsion used as a spray for the inside of a house gives effective control of insects harbored in cracks and crevices of walls or floors.

Another control for lice and mites is pyrethrum in the form of a dust applied directly to the birds. It also may be used as a space spray of a 0.02 percent pyrethrin mixture with piperonyl butoxide. If no birds are present at the time of fogging, close the room for 15 minutes, then ventilate. If birds are present, ventilate the room during application. The small passerine birds are often affected by the presence of tracheal mites, *Sternostoma tracheacolum*, which cause dyspnea, open-mouth breathing, and sometimes rales. Individually affected birds may be successfully treated by five or six weekly exposures to 5 percent malathion dust. One-half gram of dust is placed in a small plastic bag with the bird. The fluttering of the bird distributes the dust. Five-minute exposure is sufficient per treatment. When several birds in a colony are infested with tracheal mites, apply one of the space sprays at weekly intervals until the infestation is controlled.

BACTERIAL INFECTIONS

Bacteria may be responsible for eye infections, nasal discharge, joint swellings, central nervous system signs, diarrhea, acute systemic infection, and death. Some of these problems are confined to individual birds and may not be contagious. However, when any of these signs appear in a colony of birds the course of the infection is unpredictable. Therefore, at the first sign of drooping or illness a bird should be removed from the colony and kept isolated.

Many bacterial diseases can be treated with antibiotics, but for effective treatment one needs to know the type of organism involved and its sensitivity to various antibiotics. Before treatment is started swabs should be taken from the affected birds and cultured on blood agar. In the live bird, swab the palatine cleft for upper respiratory infections and the cloaca for intestinal infections. If necropsy is performed, culture the affected organs. If a bacterial cause is evident, antibiotic sensitivity tests should determine the treatment of choice. *Pasteurella*, *Salmonella*, *Staphylococcus*, *Streptococcus*, *Pseudomonas*, and *E. coli* are a few of the bacterial agents found in birds. Intramuscular injections in the breast or leg offer the quickest response to treatment. Oral administration of drugs in the drinking water or feed is an alternative route that can be used, provided that the bird is eating and drinking. Antibiotics and dosages that have been found useful in treating birds are listed in Table 1.

Vaccines are available for a few of the bacterial infections of birds. These could be useful in situations in which the disease is endemic. Preventive vaccination can be helpful in controlling fowl cholera (pasteurellosis), infectious coryza, and erysipelas (see Table 2).

Avian tuberculosis is found frequently in long-established aviaries. Affected birds become extremely emaciated, and necropsy reveals tuberculous lesions in the intestine or visceral organs. Infected birds may be detected by the tuberculin test, which is performed by injecting 0.05 ml of avian tuberculin into the skin of one wattle with a 25-gauge needle. The test is read in 48 hours. A positive reaction is indicated by edema of the wattle of up to five times normal thickness.

Another test procedure, which is more applicable for species without well-defined wattles, is the rapid plate agglutination test. This test is performed by mixing a drop of blood with the antigen, composed of a 10 percent suspension of avian tubercle bacilli. If agglutination occurs within one minute, the bird is considered a positive reactor (Thoen and Karlson).

Birds that have a positive reaction to the tuberculin test should be eliminated from the

Table 1. *Antibiotics for Birds*

ANTIBIOTIC	IM° DOSAGE (per gm body weight)	COMMENT
Erythromycin (50 mg/ml)	0.045 mg	Once daily or divided b.i.d.
Potassium penicillin	100 units	IM or oral
Ampicillin	0.055–0.11 mg	Administer b.i.d. or t.i.d.; same dosage may be given orally.
Gentamicin	0.00015–0.00035 ml	
Tetracycline (100 mg/ml)	0.00035 ml	Can cause tissue reaction and shock. Reduce dosage by 1/3 in larger species.
Chloramphenicol (chloromycetin succinate) (100 mg/ml)	0.00035–0.0005 ml	Reduce dosage by 1/3 in larger species.

°Intramuscular

Table 2. Avian Vaccines*

DISEASE	VACCINE TYPE	ROUTE OF ADMINISTRATION	SOURCES†
Newcastle disease	Live virus	Eye drop or intramuscular	Sterwin Laboratories, Millsboro, Del. 19966 and Vineland Laboratories Vineland, N.J. 08360
	Killed virus	Intramuscular	Vineland Laboratories and Salsbury Laboratories Charles City, Iowa 50616
Duck virus enteritis (duck plague)	Live virus	Subcutaneous	Duck Research Laboratory Eastport, N.Y. 11941
Duck virus hepatitis	Live virus	Subcutaneous	Duck Research Laboratory
Equine encephalitis	Killed virus	Intradermal	Fort Dodge Laboratories Fort Dodge, Iowa 50501 and Jensen-Salsbery Kansas City, Mo. 64141
Erysipelas	Killed bacterin	Subcutaneous	Salsbury Laboratories and American Scientific Laboratories Madison, Wis. 53701
Infectious coryza	Killed bacterin	Subcutaneous	Salsbury Laboratories
Fowl cholera	Killed bacterin	Subcutaneous	Salsbury Laboratories and Abbott Biological Laboratories Berlin, Md. 21811

*Aviary collections containing gallinaceous birds may need other vaccines not included in this list. Other vaccines (available from most laboratories that market poultry vaccines) are for Marek's disease, infectious bronchitis, avian encephalomyelitis, coccidiosis, laryngotracheitis, infectious bursal disease, fowl pox, and tenosynovitis. (*Note:* The fowl pox vaccine will *not* prevent canary pox.)

†Not all sources are listed here. Check with the nearest poultry vaccine laboratory about available vaccines.

flock, and the remaining birds should be moved to a new location. Once the premises become contaminated with *Mycobacterium avium* it is difficult to decontaminate the soil satisfactorily.

Chlamydial infection (ornithosis-psittacosis) of birds is of special concern to bird handlers. *C. psittaci* varies greatly in its pathogenicity, but infection in psittacine birds is particularly contagious for humans. Dust from dried excrement is highly infectious. The signs — respiratory distress, lethargy, depression, and diarrhea — are common to several infections and are not diagnostic of chlamydial infection. Therefore, the disease may not be easily recognized, and facilities for isolation and identification of the agent are not always available.

When the disease is suspected, treatment with chlortetracycline gives a positive response. For parakeets, a convenient and effective treatment is to feed millet impregnated with 0.5 mg chlortetracycline/gm of seed (Keet-Life). This should be fed exclusively for 15 days to birds that have been exposed but appear well or for 30 days if the birds are sick. Clinically sick birds that are not eating well may be given chlortetracycline injections in the pectoral muscles, 5 to 10 mg daily in 0.5 ml inoculum for five days, followed by 15 days of feeding the medicated millet.

Larger birds need a more varied diet than millet for subsistence. For more detailed information on the preparation of chlortetracycline-treated diets, see Bankowski et al. and page 681.

VIRAL INFECTIONS

There is considerable knowledge about viral infections of domesticated birds, and effective vaccines have been developed against many of them. Some of the viruses that affect domestic flocks, such as Newcastle disease, also infect pet and aviary birds. However, because of the diversity of species in pet and aviary collections it is becoming apparent that there are additional viral infections in these species that are not found in domestic poultry (Hitchner and Hirai). Unfortunately, research has not been carried out on these diseases to the point of developing preventive vaccines. Until vaccines are available the best control we have is prevention by the measures outlined previously.

Commercially available vaccines that could be useful in pet and aviary collections are listed in Table 2. Please note that the pox vaccine mentioned in the footnote of Table 2 will not prevent canary pox. Unfortunately, a commercial canary pox vaccine is not available in the United States, but experimental vaccines are being developed.

SUPPLEMENTAL READING

Bankowski, R.A., Arnstein, P., and Meyer, K.F.: Psittacosis-ornithosis. In Kirk, R.W. (ed.): *Current Veterinary Therapy VI.* Philadelphia, W.B. Saunders Co., 1977, pp. 698–703.

Hitchner, S.B., and Hirai, K.: Isolation and growth characteristics of psittacine viruses in chicken embryos. Avian Dis., 23:139–147. 1979.

Thoen, C.O., and Karlson, A.: Tuberculosis. In Hofstad, M.S., et al. (eds.): *Diseases of Poultry.* Ames, Iowa, Iowa State University Press, 1978, pp. 209–224.

CANINE RESPIRATORY DISEASE COMPLEX

GLEN L. SPAULDING, D.V.M.
Ithaca, New York

INTRODUCTION

The canine upper respiratory disease complex commonly referred to as "kennel cough" or "infectious tracheobronchitis" incorporates a number of different disease processes. Etiologic factors include both viral and bacterial infectious diseases, as well as environmental and iatrogenic causes. They may occur singly or in combination. The diagnosis of canine upper respiratory disease complex is usually made on the basis of historical and physical findings. Ancillary tests usually are not necessary or beneficial unless complications arise. The problem is usually self-limiting. It responds to supportive care and has a good prognosis. Appropriate husbandry practices and immunoprophylaxis can decrease the incidence and severity of the disease.

ETIOLOGY

Numerous viruses, bacteria, mycoplasmas, and environmental factors have been incriminated, either singly or in combination, as the cause of "infectious tracheobronchitis." Canine distemper virus infection is a frequent cause of severe respiratory disease in dogs and is discussed elsewhere in this volume.

The SV-5 parainfluenza virus (an RNA virus) is most frequently incriminated as a cause of "infectious tracheobronchitis." This is documented by virus isolation and serologic evaluations. In a majority of the cases the clinical signs associated with parainfluenza infections include low-grade fever, serous nasal discharge, and a mild, unproductive cough. The clinical course lasts one to three weeks. The clinical signs are more severe when concurrent *Bordetella bronchiseptica* and mycoplasma infections occur. Subclinical infections can also occur. Stress and environmental factors predispose animals to the infection, and transmission is rapid to susceptible dogs. The virus is shed early and heavily in respiratory secretions for eight to nine days. There is evidence suggesting that the virus may cause infections in cats and humans. Commercially available vaccines are effective in controlling clinical diseases associated with parainfluenza virus infections.

Two different adenoviruses (DNA viruses) can cause respiratory infections in dogs. The CAV-2 virus (Toronto A-26/61), or infectious canine laryngotracheitis virus, is a more significant cause of respiratory disease than the CAV-1 virus (the canine hepatitis virus). Infections with the CAV-2 virus result in clinical signs similar to those of parainfluenza virus infections. Concurrent bacterial and mycoplasma infections result in a more severe clinical state. The virus is shed for eight to nine days and spreads rapidly to susceptible dogs. There is no apparent seasonal predilection or documented spread to other species. Effective commercial vaccines are available for CAV-2 that also offer protection against CAV-1 infections. This is extremely advantageous, since CAV-2 does not replicate in endothelial cells and thus does not produce ocular, hepatic, or persistent renal disease. A minor concern about its potential oncogenicity seems to have been resolved.

Three serotypically different reoviruses (respiratory-enteric-orphan) can cause respiratory infections in dogs. Titers against reovirus type I are more frequently demonstrated in the United States, whereas reovirus type III predominates in western Europe. Natural and experimental infections frequently are asymptomatic. However, infections may also result in a low-grade fever, mucoid nasal discharge, and occasionally a cough. The virus is shed only for several days because immunity develops rapidly. There is a potential for zoonotic infections. Commercial vaccines against reovirus type III are available in Germany. They are not available in the United States and are probably not needed.

Canine herpesvirus infections can cause severe pneumonia in puppies, especially those less than two weeks of age. The virus has been isolated from the respiratory tracts of asymptomatic adult dogs, and carrier states can occur. The virus is not transmitted rapidly between dogs.

Several human respiratory viruses can cause experimental and natural infections in dogs, as determined by virus isolation and serologic studies. They include several myxoviruses (influenza) and the respiratory syncytial virus. Some commercial vaccines produced in Germany contain influenza A_2 (Hong Kong) virus. However, the need for it is questionable.

Numerous bacteria have been isolated from dogs with canine respiratory disease complex. Most frequently isolated organisms include *Escherichia coli*, *Pseudomonas* spp., *Klebsiella* spp., and *Bordetella bronchiseptica*. They usually represent opportunistic infections secondary to viral disease. Their presence contributes significantly to the severity of the clinical signs and may result in bacterial bronchopneumonia. Appropriate antibiotic therapy is indicated.

In certain instances *Bordetella bronchiseptica* can cause primary infections and outbreaks of respiratory disease, especially in puppies. There is no apparent seasonal prevalence. Clinical signs develop approximately ten days following exposure, and usually include a moist cough and frequently a purulent nasal discharge. The clinical course usually lasts for one to two weeks. However, the infection may persist and bacteria may be shed for several months until adequate immunity develops. Following infection the animals are immune for approximately one year. The disease can spread fairly rapidly to other susceptible dogs as well as potentially to other species, including cats and (rarely) humans. Varying sensitivity to antibiotics is reported. Nebulization of gentamicin or kanamycin may be necessary to control some infections. Commercial bacterins are now available. Adverse reactions to the vaccines occur in a significant percentage of animals and include pain and swelling at the injection site and sterile abscess formation. Vaccination may best be restricted to animals at high risk of infection.

Ten different species of mycoplasma have been isolated from both clinically normal and affected dogs. Infections spread rapidly, with more than 80 percent of all dogs affected. Organisms may be shed for several weeks. Experimental infections fail to produce clinical signs; however, mycoplasmas are suspected of contributing to the severity of viral respiratory infections.

Environmental factors and poor husbandry practices may predispose susceptible animals to canine respiratory disease complex. These include rapid changes in environmental temperatures and humidity, overcrowding, and poor nutrition. Coughing may result from inhalation of smoke, gasses, and chemicals such as volatile disinfectants, including ammonia and Clorox. Excessive barking and tracheal intubation may also contribute to tracheal irritation.

HISTORY

Affected dogs are presented with a history of a dry, hacking, unproductive cough of relatively sudden onset. The paroxysms may be terminated when the patient retches phlegm. Serous ocular and nasal discharge and partial anorexia may also be present.

Although the problem occurs throughout the year, there is a significantly increased incidence in the fall. A history of stress or exposure from boarding, grooming or participation in dog shows or field trials is common. The incubation period is eight to ten days. Pet stores, dog pounds, and veterinary hospitals are frequently involved because they house many stressed, unimmunized puppies of diverse backgrounds.

PHYSICAL EXAMINATION

Fever is an inconsistent finding. When accompanied by signs such as serous or mucopurulent ocular and nasal discharge, depression, and anorexia, complications such as bacterial bronchopneumonia or canine distemper should be considered. Pharyngeal examination may reveal enlarged tonsils and excessive phlegm in the pharynx and larynx. A paroxysm of coughing may be initiated by laryngeal or tracheal palpation but is not pathognomonic for this disease syndrome. Auscultation of the thorax gives unremarkable results. Increased lung sounds may be auscultated and are suggestive of concurrent viral interstitial pneumonia or bacterial bronchopneumonia, or both. If canine distemper is involved, a fundoscopic examination may reveal active chorioretinitis.

LABORATORY EVALUATION

Ancillary laboratory tests are not often useful for making the diagnosis, formulating or monitoring therapy, or providing an accurate prognosis. A complete blood count usually is normal, or a stress-induced leukocytosis and neutrophilia may be observed. Thoracic radiographs may reveal changes referable to viral interstitial pneumonia or bacterial bronchopneumonia. Cytologic studies of tracheal washes may reveal neutrophils, bacteria, and occasional epithelial cells containing viral inclusion bodies. Bacterial cultures are not performed routinely, but if done at all they should be obtained from the trachea or bronchi rather than the pharynx. Serologic evaluation is of little importance, but in some cases paired acute and convalescent serum samples may be evaluated for the previously described viruses.

TREATMENT

Treatment involves nursing care and correction of any predisposing environmental factors. The animal should be kept in a warm, well-ventilated area that is free of drafts and should be fed a highly palatable diet. Only exhausting dry coughs should be suppressed with cough medications such as dextromethorphan or codeine derivatives. Codeine-derivative cough suppressants may cause depression and anorexia if administered in excessive doses. Placing the animal in a steam-filled room or using cold-mist vaporizers several times daily may provide symptomatic relief.

Treatment with antibiotics is usually not necessary and should be restricted to animals showing systemic signs of disease, such as fever. Antibiotics, when used, should be given at full therapeutic levels for 10 to 14 days. If bacterial cultures and sensitivity test results are not available, chloramphenicol or tetracycline is usually efficacious. Tetracycline should not be used in puppies because it may stain their teeth. Aminoglycoside antibiotics are not indicated because inadequate levels are obtained in the bronchial secretions. They require parenteral administration, are potentially nephrotoxic, and are relatively expensive. Sulfonamides and the penicillins frequently are ineffective. The use of products containing a combination of antibiotics and corticosteroids is of questionable efficacy. Intratracheal injection of such products may result in some respiratory distress and occasionally may induce transient dramatic bradycardia. Nebulization of antibiotics, especially gentamicin or kanamycin, is usually unnecessary but may be beneficial in refractory cases.

PROGNOSIS

The prognosis is good unless canine distemper infection or bacterial bronchopneumonia complicates the problem. The disease syndrome is usually self-limiting within one to three weeks and has no permanent effects. Stressed, debilitated puppies and older dogs with congestive heart failure or chronic bronchitis may develop complications secondary to the disease.

CONTROL

Once infections occur in a kennel, control is difficult without appropriate preventive measures and depopulation of the area for approximately two weeks. Commonly used disinfectants, such as chlorhexidine (Novalsan®, Fort Dodge) and benzalkonium (Roccal®, Winthrop), effectively kill the causative viruses and bacteria.

PREVENTION

Natural immunity develops in many dogs and is maintained by constant re-exposure to the infectious agents. Effective biologic products are available against the important infectious agents. All of these products can be used in dogs as young as six to eight weeks of age. They should be administered at least ten days prior to anticipated exposure. Yearly revaccination is recommended.

SUPPLEMENTAL READING

Appel, M., and Bemis, D.A.: The canine contagious respiratory disease complex. Cornell Vet., 68:70–75, 1978.

Appel, M., Picherill, P., Menegus, M., Percy, D.H., Parsonson, I.M., and Sheffu, B.: Current status of canine respiratory disease. 20th Gaines Veterinary Symposium, 1970, pp. 15–23.

Bibrach, B., and Gass, H.: Praxiserfahrungen nut eiver neuen Zwinger husten-Kombinations vaccine. Berl. Munch. Tieraerztl. Wochenschr., 91:81–94, 1978.

Head, J.R., Suter, P.F., and Ettinger, S.J.: Lower respiratory tract disease. In Ettinger, S.J. (ed.): *Textbook of Veterinary Internal Medicine*, vol. 1. Philadelphia, W.B. Saunders Company, 1975.

Scatozza, F.: Virus infections of the respiratory tract of dogs. Folia Vet. Lat. 5:254–295, 1975.

FELINE RESPIRATORY DISEASE COMPLEX

BARBARA S. STEIN, D.V.M.
Chicago, Illinois

The feline respiratory disease complex consists primarily of feline viral rhinotracheitis and feline calicivirus. Secondary agents such as feline reovirus, feline pneumonitis (*Chlamydia psittaci*), mycoplasma, and various bacteria (*Staphylococcus* spp., *Bordetella bronchiseptica*, and *Pasteurella multocida*) are incriminated in less than 20 percent of respiratory cases. *Salmonella* and feline infectious peritonitis virus have also been cited as causes of feline respiratory disease.

CLINICAL SIGNS

Feline viral rhinotracheitis (FVR) virus, or feline herpesvirus infection, exhibits tropism for the respiratory tract, conjunctiva, and genital tract. Epithelial necrosis of the nasal turbinates, conjunctiva, and trachea produces clinical signs. In addition to fever, paroxysmal sneezing, coughing, and ropy hypersalivation are common in the early stages. As the disease progresses, serous nasal discharges become mucopurulent and may occlude the nares, resulting in mouth-breathing. Lacrimation and chemosis may precede ulcerative keratitis, and heavy fibrinous discharges may paste the eyelids closed. Oral ulcers or pulmonary lesions are uncommon with FVR infection.

As an enveloped DNA virus, FVR has a short incubation period of two to four days; the primary disease may persist for 10 to 14 days.

Feline calicivirus (FCV), formerly known as picornavirus, is considered a "tongue and lung" disease. Although there is only one FCV serotype, manifestations of disease caused by FCV vary because of the wide difference in pathogenicity among strains. In its mildest form FCV results in epithelial ulceration of the tongue, hard palate, and nasal commissure. Initially, vesicles may appear in these areas. The vesicles then rupture and show evidence of necrosis. More virulent strains of FCV cause pneumonia, with acute alveolar edema and purulent bronchial exudate. Unfortunately, this interstitial pneumonia often exists undetected by auscultation until secondary bacterial pathogens result in audible bronchopneumonia. Rhinitis, conjunctivitis, and tracheitis are not commonly seen with FCV infection.

Incubation of FCV may take less than 48 hours, but rarely does the primary disease persist more than five to seven days.

In both diseases the morbidity and mortality are highest in young, non-vaccinated cats (less than one year old) and kittens. Some degree of natural immunity is likely after one year of age.

The severity of pathogenicity associated with each virus may vary widely and is dependent on many factors, including (1) the amount and strain of virus exposure, (2) the overall health and immune status of the exposed cat, (3) the age of the cat, and (4) the promptness of symptomatic treatment.

Unfortunately, differentiation between FVR and FCV is not always as simple as descriptions might suggest. Concurrent infection with other diseases, atypical manifestations of either FVR or FCV, or secondary infection with feline pneumonitis or bacteria may cloud the diagnosis. Although much of the treatment for FVR and FCV is similar, the clinician's ability to establish a definite diagnosis will allow a better assessment of prognosis in terms of sequelae.

Positive confirmation of FVR or FCV is obtained through pharyngeal swab virus isolation by cell culture propagation or detection of virus-neutralizing antibody. Unfortunately, the cost and delay involved in these tests preclude their everyday use. However, for catteries in which chronic respiratory disease is a problem, intensive laboratory evaluation should be considered.

TREATMENT

The intensity of treatment of viral respiratory diseases is dependent on the severity of clinical signs. In some cases viral manifestations are so mild and the cat so relatively unaffected that no treatment is required.

In contrast with panleukopenia, FVR and

FCV are primarily responsible for the majority of clinical signs associated with each disease, and secondary bacterial infection is usually of lesser significance. It is imperative that this fact be understood by both the veterinarian and the client so that the limited role of antibiotics in treatment of the feline respiratory disease complex is clarified. It is also interesting to note that the antibiotic that seems helpful in control of secondary invaders in one episode of respiratory diseases may appear ineffective in another outbreak.

ANTIBIOTIC THERAPY

A variety of broad-spectrum antibiotics may be used to treat secondary bacterial pathogens associated with viral respiratory disease. These include ampicillin (20 mg/kg q 12 hours orally, IM, or IV), gentamicin (4 mg/kg IM every 12 hours for two days, then once every 24 hours), tylosin (10 mg/kg q 8 hours orally, 2 mg/kg q 12 hours IM or IV), kanamycin (6 mg/kg q 12 hours IM), and chloramphenicol (20 mg/kg q 12 hours orally, 10 mg/kg q 12 hours IM or IV). Chloramphenicol is contraindicated if anemia has developed. The route of administration of any antibiotic is determined by the cat's acceptance and overall condition and the owner's ability to medicate. Liquid forms of antibiotics are often easier to administer, especially if oral ulceration exists.

HOME CARE VERSUS HOSPITALIZATION

Whenever possible, the affected cat should be treated as an outpatient, with intensive home care provided. The degree of stress created in a hospital environment may be detrimental to a sick cat that requires frequent nursing care. If the cat is hospitalized, owner visitation is helpful and to be encouraged.

The owner should be instructed that nursing care includes frequent gentle cleaning to remove any nasal or ocular discharges, occasional brushing and combing, and gentle reassurance. Warm humidification is helpful and may be provided easily at home, either by a room vaporizer or by placing the cat in a steamy bathroom. If the nares are kept clear the cat is more apt to retain its appetite and to breathe easier.

The owner should cater to the cat's whims regarding food in order to maintain its appetite. Strong-flavored or odorous foods are especially preferred by cats whose taste and sense of smell are marginal. Such foods include bacon, smoked turkey, baked ham, cooked chicken, and sardines. Often baby-food meats are highly palatable to the anorectic cat.

If a veterinarian is considering hospitalization of a feline with infectious respiratory disease, the object must be to provide a necessary form of therapy that cannot be met at home, e.g., nebulization and oxygen therapy, blood transfusion, or IV fluid replacement. Obviously, strict isolation procedures must be used when treating a hospitalized cat with infectious respiratory disease.

FLUID THERAPY

Because early inanition is seen in both diseases and because copious amounts of fluid are lost through hypersalivation and the nasal and ocular discharges of FVR, affected cats rapidly become dehydrated. Subcutaneous isotonic or hypotonic fluid therapy (lactated Ringer's solution, 2½ percent dextrose with half-strength saline) often is adequate, provided that substantial replacement amounts are given. In cats with severe dehydration, however, intravenous fluid therapy is necessary and may be required for several days.

BLOOD TRANSFUSION

After basic fluid replacement, blood transfusion should be considered in profoundly sick cats. This is especially beneficial if the donor is a well-exposed hospital cat that might be expected to have excellent immunity to respiratory infections. The donor should previously be determined to be negative to FeLV and *Haemobartonella felis* tests. If the recipient is not anemic, a transfusion of 4 to 6 ml/kg is sufficient. Often within hours of the transfusion a severely debilitated cat will respond by moving around, grooming itself, and even eating. The blood should not be cold when slowly administered intravenously; if vomiting occurs it is a result of too-rapid administration. An elevation of body temperature (1 to 2°F) may be expected following transfusion and lasts up to 24 hours.

PHARYNGOSTOMY

Cats with severe infectious respiratory disease usually die of starvation and dehydration rather than from the direct effects of the virus. Repeated syringe feeding, force feeding, and stomach-tube alimentation are all difficult in the depressed cat. Furthermore, the presence of oral ulcers may make forced feeding not only painful but harmful. Both calorie and fluid replacement may be achieved easily by means of a pharyngostomy tube. This minor surgical procedure is indicated if complete anorexia has persisted for a few days and if the condition of the cat is deteriorating.

Local anesthesia may be all that is required if the cat is severely debilitated; in most instances, intravenous ketamine hydrochloride (1 to 4 mg/kg) will provide a sufficient level of anesthesia for manipulation. Inhalation anesthesia of cats with respiratory infections is contraindicated. With an oral speculum in place, a natural retropharyngeal pouch located posterior to the base of the tongue and lateral to the hyoid apparatus may be palpated with the index finger inside the cat's mouth. The gloved finger should be easily palpable by the other hand, separated only by skin, subcutaneous tissue, and mucous membrane. Outward pressure with the flexed finger will indicate the position externally for the skin incision on the lateral neck surface.

The immediately surrounding area is prepared for surgery. A large curved artery forceps is substituted in the position of the gloved finger, and pressure is applied from within the pharynx outward. A small skin incision is made over the outward bulge, and the artery forceps is then jabbed carefully through the mucous membrane of the pharyngeal pouch, through the subcutaneous tissues, and out through the skin incision. The tip of the indwelling esophageal feeding tube (size 12 French)* is then grasped with the forceps, and the feeding tube is introduced into the pharynx and directed a predetermined distance down the esophagus so as just to enter the stomach. The length of the tube from the stoma to the last rib should be measured and marked for correct placement into the stomach. The remaining external portion of the tube is attached to the cat by applying a purse-string suture around the skin opening and suturing a butterfly tape anchor placed around the tube to the skin. The feeding tube is positioned dorsolateral to the neck, and a light Kling (Johnson & Johnson) bandage is applied around the neck and fastened with a strip of surgical tape. If the cat is still anesthetized, it may be safer to bandage after the animal is awake.

The external tip of the feeding tube should be kept capped or closed to prevent excess air from entering the stomach and possible leakage of stomach contents. Frequent feedings (six to ten times daily) should be followed by a 5-ml flush of warm water or broth to clear the tube. Liquid antibiotics, anabolic agents, and vitamins may be administered easily in addition to food. For the average-size cat, a maximum volume of 30 ml is administered at each feeding. Calorie replacement may be in the form of strained

baby-food meats and egg yolk or canned cat food processed in a blender. High-calorie concentrates (Nutrical, Evsco Pharmaceutical; Lipomul, Upjohn) may also be included in esophageal tube feedings. The caloric needs of an adult cat or kitten (70 and 200 kcal/kg daily, respectively) increase by 10 percent for each degree F above normal body temperature.

Once the ill cat begins to respond, it will be able to eat and drink on its own with the tube in place. A cat can usually vomit with the tube in place, although a pharyngostomy tube should not be applied to a cat known to vomit frequently. When the cat is eating on its own and the tube is to be removed, the sutures are cut and the tube is simply withdrawn. Antibiotic ointment applied to the stoma will ensure healing by granulation within a few days.

VITAMIN THERAPY

Multiple vitamins are indicated in the presence of any severely debilitating disease; in the feline, vitamins A and B-complex are important additions to therapy. The use of vitamin C has been both proclaimed and condemned. The cat synthesizes this vitamin itself; however, whether higher needs exist in the presence of repiratory disease is unknown. Because no serious side effects are reported, many clinicians advocate the use of 1000 mg ascorbic acid intravenously daily.

OCULAR CARE

Ocular therapy, especially in FVR, is critical to avoid corneal damage, panophthalmitis, and even blindness. Under no circumstances should corticosteroids be used in the eye if there is any indication of infectious respiratory disease. Unfortunately, in the earliest and mildest stages of many respiratory diseases, including pneumonitis, the cat may exhibit only a mild unilateral conjunctivitis with serous lacrimation. Even in these instances steroids should be excluded from therapy. Any broad-spectrum ocular antibiotic may be initiated but, if pneumonitis is suspected, tetracycline ophthalmic ointment is the treatment of choice. Ointments are preferred to ophthalmic drops because administration need not be as frequent.

Because of the tropism FVR displays for the cornea, viral keratitis with dendritic ulceration is a common problem. Specific antiviral drugs for ophthalmic use are available and effective. Idoxuridine ointment (Stoxil, Smith Kline & French) or vidarabine 3 percent ointment (Vira-A, Parke-Davis) instilled every four to six hours

---

*Sovereign Disposable Feeding Tube and Urethral Catheter, Sherwood Medical.

interferes with viral replication and may effect a dramatic improvement within 72 hours. Antibiotic ointment should be used concurrently.

Ophthalmic mucolytic agents are indicated when thick, ropy, fibrinous discharges prevent penetration of therapeutic agents. Often collagen-type material will lie in the lower conjunctival sac and eventually cause the eyelids to adhere to each other. A 50-50 mixture of acetylcysteine 20 percent (Mucomyst, Mead Johnson) with Adapt solution (Burton, Parsons & Co.) as a carrier may be instilled frequently in the eye as a cleaning agent. The anticollagenase activity of acetylcysteine allows antiviral and antibiotic ointments to penetrate deeply into the cornea and thus may be of primary importance in dealing with deep keratitic ulcers.

INHALATION THERAPY

Oxygen and nebulization therapy should be provided to any cat exhibiting severe open-mouth breathing, dyspnea, or pneumonic signs. In contrast with warm humidification, in which steam carries large mist particles to the level of the nasopharynx, nebulization results in fine mist particles, which are carried to the alveolar level. In severe cases of FCV and bronchopneumonia, nebulization with oxygen therapy may be life-saving.

Bronchodilating drugs such as isoproterenol 1:200 should be used in conjunction with other forms of nebulization therapy, because most drugs will result in some degree of bronchial irritation and constriction. Antibiotics such as gentamicin (4 mg/kg/day) and kanamycin (10 mg/kg/day), which are poorly absorbed from the respiratory mucosa but are topically effective, have good application in aerosol therapy. Mucolytics are indicated if bronchial secretions are viscous and inspissated. Acetylcysteine 20 percent (Mucomyst, Mead Johnson) in a ratio of 1:8 with saline may be added to the nebulization formula.

QUESTIONABLE AIDS TO THERAPY

Questionable aids to therapy include antihistamines, decongestants, diuretics, and atropine. Both antihistamines and decongestants are variable in their effect on cats with viral respiratory disease. Some cats with copious serous discharges appear more comfortable after these drugs are given. However, when thick, mucopurulent discharges are present there is some controversy about whether these drugs might cause the viscous material to dry and become more difficult to expel.

Atropine is contraindicated in cats with infectious respiratory disease because the effect of the drug is transitory in decreasing nasal and oral secretions, and it may cause the bronchial secretions to become too thick for the cat to cough up. Because dehydration is often a part of the respiratory complex, the use of diuretics to diminish secretions is more harmful than helpful.

CONTRAINDICATIONS

In the presence of acute viral respiratory disease, corticosteroids are contraindicated. If debilitation lasts for more than two weeks, their use may help to promote appetite and a sense of well-being, but this is still controversial.

IMMUNOSUPPRESSION

Failure of a cat to respond to intensive supportive therapy should lead the clinician to suspect the presence of other underlying diseases causing immunosuppression. The feline leukemia and infectious peritonitis viruses, toxoplasmosis, and glomerulonephritis may all be responsible for previously asymptomatic conditions that cause the severely challenged cat to become immunologically incompetent. The presence of secondary disease should be considered when one cat in a group of affected animals is more seriously ill for a longer period of time than the others.

TRANSMISSION

Direct cat-to-cat contact is the most common means of virus transmission. Although aerosol transmission is considered to be the classic form of disease passage, it is probably only of significance for a distance of six to eight feet. The primary source of infection in catteries, laboratories, and hospitals is fomite transmission via hands, clothing, water and food containers, and litter boxes.

The envelope of the FVR virus is sensitive to lipid solvents such as detergents and alcohol and becomes inactivated by desiccation in less than 24 hours at room temperature. Caliciviruses, however, are much less sensitive to environmental factors and may persist after ten days of ambient exposure. They are sensitive to hypochlorite disinfection.

Carrier animals are an important aspect of FVR and FCV epidemiology, although each virus differs in its behavior. Recovered FVR cats may shed the virus intermittently for at least one year; stress factors such as boarding, hospitalization, breeding, and cat shows or the administration of corticosteroids may exacerbate the carrier state, and cats may develop mild signs of respiratory infection. In contrast with the intermittent shedding seen with FVR, cats recovered from FCV shed virus continuously from the pharynx and in the feces for as long as a year.

Kittens of queens previously infected with FVR or FCV may be exposed readily at the time of weaning. Because FVR displays tropism for the female genital tract, neonates may be exposed at the time of queening and die within two weeks. Experimentally, FVR infection has caused placental lesions and fetal deaths.

SEQUELAE

One of the most serious aspects of viral respiratory disease is not just the treatment of the infected cat but the sequelae that often follow apparent recovery. Cats that are difficult to handle and must endure weeks of force feeding, nursing, and medication may recover from the disease but be so affected psychologically that their value as pets is diminished.

By far the most serious result of viral respiratory infections in homes with more than one cat and in catteries is the development of a carrier state that may well prove dangerous to other cats. Reproductive problems, including infertility of the queen, abortion, and neonatal deaths, may be expected in catteries if normal queens are allowed contact with recovered animals.

Frontal sinusitis is another serious and common sequela to viral respiratory infections, particularly FVR. The problem may be seen in all breeds, but Persians, Siamese, and Burmese are commonly affected. Frequent humidification is helpful in the early stages of frontal sinusitis, along with bacterial culturing and sensitivity tests. The more chronic the condition becomes, the more unlikely conservative therapy will help. Ultimately, frontal sinus surgery in the form of an autogenous fat implantation with an osteoplastic flap may be required.

Chronic ocular discharges may follow feline respiratory disease. In these cases the patency of the tear ducts should be determined and the conjunctiva cultured. Permanent corneal damage and even blindness may follow FVR infection if ocular treatment is not aggressive at the time of illness.

Pyothorax has often been incriminated as a sequela to viral respiratory infection but, in fact, it is usually due to bacteremia or subsequent to penetrating chest wounds.

PROPHYLAXIS

The development of vaccines against FVR and FCV is potentially the most effective means of controlling the known viral respiratory diseases of felines. At present, two forms of vaccination are available: (1) parenteral and (2) intranasal. The parenteral FVR/FCV vaccines are often combined with modified live or killed panleukopenia vaccine and are highly effective. In the rare instances in which the vaccines do not protect the exposed cat totally, they will ensure a much milder form of the disease. The intranasal vaccines may produce mild to moderate upper respiratory signs in 50 to 75 percent of inoculated cats four to seven days after administration. The possibility of these symptomatic cats acting as carriers during this stage should be considered.

Within a veterinary hospital, many factors can be controlled to prevent iatrogenic contagion. Adequate ventilation is probably the most effective means of disease prevention; twelve air exchanges per hour are desirable, and each ward should be ventilated separately with no carry-over or mixture of air with that from other parts of the hospital. The humidity should be maintained at 30 to 50 percent. Disposable food dishes and litter pans and water bowls that can be steam-sterilized are part of basic hospital hygiene.

The role of human vectors should be stressed to all hospital personnel. When known exposure occurs, outer smocks should be changed and hands washed thoroughly. Prolonged hospitalization and boarding of cats are to be avoided. Cats should not be moved from one cage to another unless absolutely necessary, and thorough cage cleaning procedures should be practiced.

In the cattery, in addition to vaccination, isolation becomes an important aspect of disease control. Although two weeks' quarantine is recommended whenever a new cat is brought into a cattery or returns from a show, from breeding, or from a veterinary hospital, this practice will not totally prevent introduction of respiratory disease into a cattery. That is, the very long period (up to one year) during which an asymptomatic carrier cat may be infectious renders the quarantine period effective only against blatant disease.

Kittens borns to carrier queens should be separated from their mothers at four weeks of age and vaccinated promptly. Feline vaccination is discussed in greater detail in the article entitled "Update on Feline Immunization."

SUPPLEMENTAL READING

Böhning, R.H., Jr., et al.: Pharyngostomy for maintenance of the anorectic animal. J. Am. Vet. Med. Assoc., 156:611–615, 1970.
Bolton, G.: Aerosol therapy. In Kirk, R.W. (ed.): Current Veterinary Therapy V. Philadelphia, W.B. Saunders Co., 1974, pp. 12–15.
Gaskell, R.M., and Wardley, R.C.: Feline viral respiratory disease: A review with particular reference to its epizootiology and control. J. Small Anim. Pract., 19:1–16, 1977.
Kahn, D.E., and Hoover, E.A.: Infectious respiratory diseases of cats. Vet. Clin. North Am. 6:399–413, 1976.
Tomlinson, M.J., and Schenck, N.L.: Autogenous fat implantation as a treatment for chronic frontal sinusitis in a cat. J. Am. Vet. Med. Assoc., 167:927–930, 1975.

CANINE DISTEMPER

BRIAN R. H. FARROW, B.V.Sc.
Sydney, Australia

Distemper is a highly contagious viral disease of dogs and other members of the Canidae family. The natural host range also includes members of the Mustelidae family (e.g., ferrets, minks, skunks, and badgers) and the Procyonidae family (e.g., raccoons and pandas). It is an important disease because of its worldwide occurrence and the severity of clinical disease that may follow infection. The etiologic agent is a paramyxovirus closely related to the viruses of human measles and rinderpest of cattle. Although different isolates of canine distemper (CD) virus are serologically indistinguishable, various strains are capable of producing consistently different patterns of disease. In addition, the response of individual dogs to a particular strain also varies markedly. These two factors account for the extreme variability in the response to infection, ranging from a transient subclinical illness to a severe fulminating disease with involvement of many body systems.

CLINICAL SIGNS

Following infection of susceptible animals, which usually occurs by inhalation of air-borne organisms, the virus spreads to local lymphatic tissue. During the first week after exposure viremia occurs with widespread dissemination of the virus to lymphoid organs, bone marrow, and the lamina propria of epithelial structures. This phase is associated with temperature elevation and transient anorexia, depression, and mild serous conjunctivitis. There are no localizing signs evident at this stage. In dogs that develop a rapid antibody response to the virus, further extension to epithelial structures is minimal, and the virus is cleared from the body.

In dogs that fail to develop an adequate immune response, virus spreads rapidly to epithelial cells and the central nervous system. These animals develop a second temperature rise associated with depression, anorexia, ocular and nasal discharges, and signs related to disease of the respiratory and gastrointestinal tracts. The ocular and nasal discharges initially are serous and later become mucopurulent. Coughing is a frequent manifestation of the respiratory diseases and, upon examination, a mild dyspnea and harsh, dry rales may be detected. Diarrhea and occasional vomiting reflect gastrointestinal tract involvement. The condition almost invariably deteriorates from this point, and weight loss and dehydration develop. Eventually, animals become moribund and die with or without convulsions or other evidence of neurologic disease.

Some affected dogs show improvement of the severe systemic signs, but weeks or months later they develop neurologic disturbances that terminate in death or necessitate euthanasia. A few dogs recover from the systemic signs and are left with residual neurologic dysfunction that is non-progressive and, in many cases, compatible with a reasonable existence. Still others may be presented with neurologic signs only and no history of systemic illness. In these cases careful examination will usually indicate multifocal neurologic disease, of which the most common cause in dogs is distemper.

Rhythmic clonic contraction of muscle groups is often seen with CD and is considered by many to be pathognomonic for the disease. Visual disturbances are sometimes observed and may result from damage at various levels of the nervous system. Non-granulomatous focal or diffuse retinitis, optic neuritis, or lesions affecting the optic tracts or central visual pathways have all been observed in CD. The underlying neuropathology in CD is a non-suppurative encephalomyelitis with demyelination. The clinical expressions of this are varied and depend on the areas of the nervous system involved. It is not possible to predict the outcome with certainty in individual cases, and owners should be warned of the possible development or progression of neurologic signs.

Hyperkeratosis of the footpads is observed rarely and is a more chronic manifestation of CD.

Neonatal infections can occur in pups born with inadequate levels of maternally derived antibody. The fatality rate with such infections is high. Transplacental transmission of CD virus may also occur, resulting in neonatal deaths in the absence of clinical signs of CD in the bitch.

DIAGNOSTIC AIDS

The clinical picture of the generalized systemic disease is fairly characteristic, and laboratory support for the diagnosis is usually unnecessary. Hematologic evaluation of these cases usually reveals lymphopenia, mild neutrophilia, and occasionally monocytosis. Inclusion bodies can sometimes be seen in blood cells, particularly lymphocytes, during routine examination of blood smears. Smears from buffy coat preparations may facilitate their detection. Smears of conjunctival or tonsillar scrapings may also be examined for inclusion bodies and, when available, fluorescence techniques can be utilized to detect viral antigen in these samples. Viral antigen may also be present in footpad biopsy specimens or cells from cerebrospinal fluid.

Difficulty can be encountered with antemortem confirmation of CD in animals presented with neurologic disease only. In these dogs the virus has normally been cleared from all other tissues except the nervous system, where isolated foci of intracellular viral material remain. Cerebrospinal fluid examination may reveal an increase in protein or mononuclear cells, or both, changes consistent with viral disease. Immunoelectrophoretic examination of CSF proteins shows the presence of IgM and high concentrations of IgG in many patients with CD encephalitis. Specific neutralizing antibody to CD can also be present in the CSF of these dogs. These CSF antibodies are not present in dogs following vaccination, in those animals that develop circulating antibodies quickly and remain asymptomatic after exposure, or in those that die from acute CD infection.

Interpretation of levels of CD antibodies in serum is difficult because levels may be lowest in animals with the severest disease.

TREATMENT

No specific antiviral agents are available for use in treating CD. There is no evidence that high doses of ascorbic acid, ether inhalations, or any of the countless other "remedies" advocated for treating CD are effective in any way. In addition, once clinical signs are established the administration of specific CD antiserum does not appear to influence the course of the disease. If given during the initial febrile phase, before epithelial localization has occurred, large doses of antiserum may boost the immune response sufficiently to prevent the development of clinical signs. There is some experimental evidence that intravenous injection of modified live virus vaccine, given within four days of initial infection (i.e., before characteristic clinical signs have developed), may confer protection by inducing the production of interferon and neutralizing antibody. Administration after this time, when characteristic clinical signs are apparent, does not influence the course of the disease and may in fact be deleterious.

Considerable evidence now exists that immunosuppression results from CD infection and persists for some weeks, favoring the establishment of secondary infections from bacteria and mycoplasmata. Protozoal infections, such as toxoplasmosis, may also be facilitated by CD viral immunosuppression. Antibiotic therapy should be instituted in order to minimize the effects of secondary bacterial infections, and full symptomatic and supportive therapy should be offered.

PREVENTION

Canine distemper can be prevented by appropriate vaccination procedures. The majority of pups have lost their maternally acquired passive immunity by 14 weeks of age and are capable of active immunologic response to vaccine. In younger animals passively acquired maternal antibodies may interfere with successful active immunization. In neonatal pups physiologic immaturity of the immune system may interfere with their ability to respond to vaccination, in addition to rendering them more susceptible to severe disease following CD infection. Details of the various immunization procedures are presented in the article entitled "Update on Canine Immunization."

SUPPLEMENTAL READING

Appel, M.J.G.: Pathogenesis of canine distemper. Am. J. Vet. Res., 30:1167, 1969.

Krakowka, S., and Koestner, A.: Comparison of canine distemper virus strains in gnotobiotic dogs: Effects on lymphoid tissues. Am. J. Vet. Res., 38:1919, 1977.

Krakowka, S., Hoover, E.A., Koestner, A., and Ketring, K.: Experimental and naturally occurring transplacental transmission of canine distemper virus. Am. J. Vet. Res., 38:912, 1977.

Watson, A.D.J., and Wright, R.G.: The ultrastructure of inclusions in blood cells of dogs with distemper. J. Comp. Pathol., 84:417, 1974.

Wright, N.G., Cornwell, H.J.C., Thompson, H., and Lauder, I.M.: Canine distemper: Current concepts in laboratory and clinical diagnosis. Vet. Rec., 94:86, 1974.

FELINE PANLEUKOPENIA

SUSAN M. COTTER, D.V.M.

Boston, Massachusetts

Panleukopenia is a contagious viral disease that affects all members of the cat family as well as raccoons, coatimundis, minks, and ferrets. The virus is a small (18 to 22 nm), non-enveloped, single-stranded DNA virus of the parvovirus group. It is quite stable in the environment, and suspensions held at room temperature have remained viable for more than one year. The virus is resistant to alcohol, phenol, ether, quaternary ammonium compounds, iodine, and increased temperature. It is killed by formalin, ethylene oxide, and some chlorine products and by boiling. Transmission occurs via feces, vomitus, and urine, and shedding of virus has been reported in some recovered animals. Replication of virus requires cells in active mitosis, such as marrow, intestine, thymus, developing cerebellum, and lymphoid tissue. This requirement explains why the pathogenesis of the naturally occurring disease differs from that induced experimentally in gnotobiotic kittens. Germ-free kittens develop moderate to severe lymphopenia and neutropenia with fever and anorexia. There is no enteritis, and the only detectable lesions are thymic atrophy and lymphoid depletion. These lesions induce temporary immune suppression that is not reflected in clinical signs because the immune system is never challenged in a sterile environment. The cell turnover time in the intestine is low in gnotobiotic animals that have no intestinal flora, hence the absence of intestinal lesions.

Clinical signs in the natural infection follow an incubation period of two to nine days and usually consist of anorexia and vomiting. Physical findings are fever, dehydration, a dry, congested oropharynx, evidence of pain on abdominal palpation, and sometimes enlarged mesenteric lymph nodes. Diarrhea often occurs later in the clinical course, and gas or fluid may be palpable in the intestines. An owner may present a kitten for worming because ascarids have been vomited, or exacerbation of another infection such as otitis or respiratory viral infections may be the presenting complaint. Profound leukopenia, sometimes with a degenerative left shift or relative lymphocytosis, is the typical laboratory finding.

Panleukopenia typically is an acute disease, with death or recovery within the first week. Occasionally, diarrhea persists until the lining of the intestine has completely recovered its absorptive capacity. Recovery of the white blood cell count begins with a left shift rapidly followed by leukocytosis, which may be substantial. Most adult cats are immune because of previous exposure and subclinical disease, although occasional older cats may develop clinical disease. Prenatal infection may result in fetal resorption or abortion. Infection in late gestation or the first three weeks after birth results in cerebellar ataxia, since the external granular layer of the cerebellum is not fully developed until about three weeks of age. Antibodies develop seven days after inoculation in experimental infections. This is usually three to four days after the onset of signs and coincides with the end of viremia. Lesions seen at necropsy of cats that die of panleukopenia include enteritis, with mucosal necrosis primarily in the ileum and jejunum; cryptitis, with dilated crypts often containing cellular debris; lymphoid depletions, primarily in B cell–dependent areas; and decreased myelopoiesis. Intranuclear inclusions, present early in the disease, are best seen when tissues are fixed with Zenker's or Bouin's solutions, since they are less well preserved in formalin.

DISEASES THAT MAY BE CONFUSED WITH PANLEUKOPENIA

Few clinicians would fail to diagnose panleukopenia in an unvaccinated, febrile kitten that has vomiting, evidence of pain on abdominal palpation, and profound leukopenia. However, when any of these findings is missing one must consider the possibility that another disease is present. Feline leukemia virus can suppress the bone marrow; the erythroid or myeloid series, or both, could be affected. If myeloid hypoplasia occurs severe leukopenia, predisposing the cat to secondary bacterial (usually gram-negative) sepsis, can develop. Cats that die of panleukopenia usually die of gram-negative infection, so one can readily see how the two disorders could be confused. Some differences that may allow the clinician to differentiate them are that the feline leukemia virus–induced "panleukopenia-like syndrome" arises most readily in stressed or debilitated cats and is not uncommonly associated wuth anemia and thrombocytopenia. Recovery of the white blood cell count, if it does occur, is slower than in panleukopenia. Thrombocytopenia and anemia are not usual signs in panleukopenia, except in some cats that fail to improve quickly and then become debilitated by secondary infection. Some of these cats are thrombocytopenic because of disseminated intravascular coagulation. These animals seldom recover. A history of vaccination against panleukopenia and the fluorescent antibody (FA) test for FeLV are of value, although there is no reason to assume that panleukopenia cannot occur in the FeLV-positive cat.

Primary bacterial enteritis resulting in septicemia may also occur, apparently as a primary disease. The species of bacteria most likely to be involved is *E. coli*, which is the most common secondary invader in panleukopenia as well. The treatment for panleukopenia is the same as for the FeLV-associated syndrome and bacterial sepsis.

Salmonellosis usually occurs in young cats with signs of gastroenteritis and fever. Leukopenia occurs more frequently than leukocytosis, and the white blood cell count may be low enough to cause confusion with panleukopenia. Diagnosis is made by stool culture. Recovered cats may continue to shed organisms for two to four weeks. Chloramphenicol is the treatment of choice. Tyzzer's disease, caused by *Bacillus piliformis*, has been reported in cats. The clinical disease was quite similar to panleukopenia and can result in septicemia. The organisms can be stained in tissues by silver stains.

One condition that resembles penleukopenia superficially is enteritis caused by string or another soft foreign body. A string or thread under the tongue should never be missed. A routine physical examination of the cat should include examination of the under surface of the tongue, since the area is easily seen by pushing the thumb from under the rami of the mandible.

TREATMENT

Cats that die of panleukopenia generally die of bacterial sepsis, primarily due to *E. coli*. Treatment is directed toward bacterial infection, maintenance of fluid and electrolyte balance, and prevention of further fluid loss. Because of impaired host defenses and gastrointestinal absorption, bactericidal injectable antibiotics such as gentamicin or cephaloridine can be used. Subcutaneous fluids should be used only in mild cases or in kittens too small for practical IV administration. Other cats should have an intravenous catheter placed aseptically for fluid administration. Lactated Ringer's solution with 5 percent dextrose is a reasonable choice, although plain lactated Ringer's can be substituted for subcutaneous administration when an isotonic fluid is needed. B-complex vitamins can be added to the fluids. No oral feeding or medication should be given initially because it might stimulate vomiting. In the presence of diarrhea an oral protectant and antispasmodic agent may be indicated. Oral non-absorbable antibiotics are probably of little value either in prophylaxis or treatment of bacterial sepsis. Immune (homologous) serum is also probably of no value once signs of illness have developed, although it is strongly indicated after exposure but before signs develop. Blood transfusions have traditionally been recommended, probably in the hope of supplying white cells or immune factors. There is no experimental evidence that transfusions are more effective than good fluid and electrolyte support. White cells cannot be supplied in numbers high enough to have any effect, even in fresh blood. The half-life of white cells in the circulation is only six to eight hours, so even if large numbers could be supplied, any effect would be transient. Cats with panleukopenia usually do not have anemia or thrombocytopenia, so erythrocytes and platelets are not needed. However, in patients with severe hemorrhagic enteritis and associated thrombocytopenia or anemia, transfusions appear to be helpful. As improvement is noted, a bland diet can be offered. Antibiotics and fluids can be discontinued when the cat is afebrile, has an adequate white blood cell count, is eating, and is not losing excessive fluid in diarrhea.

Except for peracute panleukopenia, which occurs in young kittens, the majority of cats can be saved with adequate therapy. The advent of practical intravenous fluid therapy and newer broad-spectrum antibiotics has improved the prognosis significantly. Cats with panleukopenia associated with persistent leukopenia or chronic illness probably should be checked for feline leukemia virus infection, since this may explain the failure of some cats to respond.

SUPPLEMENTAL READING

Carlson, J.H.: Feline panleukopenia. In Kirk, R.W. (ed.): *Current Veterinary Therapy VI*. Philadelphia, W.B. Saunders Co., 1976, pp. 1292–1296.

Cotter, S.M.: Some uncommon diseases in the cat. Proceedings of the American Animal Hospital Association, 1979, pp. 115–117.

Feline infectious diseases report. Proceedings of a Colloquium on Selected Feline Infectious Diseases. J. Am. Vet. Med. Assoc., 58:857–915, 1971.

Scott, F.: Panleukopenia. In Kirk, R.W. (ed.): *Current Veterinary Therapy IV*. Philadelphia, W.B. Saunders Co., 1972, pp. 644–649.

FELINE INFECTIOUS PERITONITIS

RICHARD C. WEISS, V.M.D.,

and FREDRIC W. SCOTT, D.V.M.

Ithaca, New York

Feline infectious peritonitis (FIP) is one of the most important and complex infectious diseases affecting domestic and wild cats today. In the past FIP was thought to be (1) a sporadic and highly fatal disease with a mortality of nearly 100 percent, (2) a disease with no cure or effective treatment, and (3) a presumably viral disease, moderately contagious, for which there was no preventive vaccine.

Recent research and epidemiologic studies, however, now indicate that these concepts represent merely the "tip of the FIP iceberg." FIP virus (FIPV) appears to be widespread in the general feline population, and at present it is estimated that 25 percent or more of cats in the U.S. are actually infected.

In addition to the classic effusive ("wet") and non-effusive ("dry" or granulomatous) clinical forms of FIP, the virus may also be involved in a variety of previously undiagnosed reproductive and neonatal disorders. These syndromes frequently plague breeding catteries and include fetal resorptions, stillbirths, abortions, "fading kittens," metritis, chronic upper respiratory disease, and possibly certain gastrointestinal infections and acute congestive cardiomyopathy.

ETIOLOGY

The causative agent of FIP is a coronavirus, a pleomorphic RNA virus with a lipoprotein envelope surrounded by numerous spike-like projections resembling the corona around the sun. FIPV is quite labile as a result of its lipoprotein envelope and probably does not survive more than several days outside the host. Most disinfectants (e.g., quaternary ammonium compounds or a 1:32 dilution of household bleach) should inactivate the virus, but apparently there is some resistance to phenol (Lysol) and chlorhexidine (Nolvasan).

FIPV is antigenically related to and will serologically cross-react with certain other animal and human coronaviruses, including transmissible gastroenteritis (TGE) virus of swine, canine coronavirus, and human bronchitis virus 229-E. Serum antibodies against FIPV in cats will therefore cross-react with TGE virus, and this phenomenon is utilized diagnostically in the indirect fluorescent antibody test (IFAT) for determination of FIP antibody titers.

Some but not all cases of FIP produce neutralizing antibody against TGE virus; this suggests that perhaps more than one serotype of FIPV exists.

Despite extensive attempts by many investigators during the past decade to cultivate FIPV in tissue cultures, the virus still has not been isolated in conventional monolayer cell cultures. Breakthroughs in FIP research have recently occurred, following the first successful isolation and propagation of FIPV in intestinal ring organ cultures (Hoshino and Scott) and in newborn mouse brain (Osterhaus).

EPIZOOTIOLOGY

The results of IFAT surveys on random and selected groups of cats indicate that at least 25 percent or more of cats in the U.S. are serologically positive for FIPV. The relative number of cats in this exposed population that actually develop the fatal clinical form of FIP is, in contrast, remarkably small when compared with the total number of infected cats; perhaps 1 to 5 percent or less of FIP-positive cats will eventually die from the disease.

These percentages may be somewhat misleading from an epidemiologic viewpoint, since the incidence of infection and death in catteries and multiple-cat households exposed to FIP is dramatically increased. In these situations the overall infection rate usually exceeds 90 percent and may even reach 100 percent, and the death rate in some catteries may be 20 percent or more. The factors responsible for these increases are not known but probably reflect certain predisposing stress factors, overcrowding, and conditions favoring repeated or prolonged exposure of susceptible cats to infectious virus.

The natural means of transmission of FIPV are not known. Recent experiments at the Cornell Feline Research Laboratory have produced severe respiratory and systemic disease in kittens following aerosol exposure to FIPV, and there is considerable opinion at present that initial exposure to FIPV may result in mild respiratory infection, especially in neonates. Other possible natural means of transmission include the oral-fecal route (cats with FIP may have lesions involving the intestine, liver, and gallbladder), urine, bites from blood-sucking parasites, and maternal transmission from *in utero* or perinatal infection.

Natural transmission frequently occurs within several weeks after susceptible kittens are housed with asymptomatic, serologically positive carrier cats. Cats with high antibody titers (1:400 to 1:1600 or greater) are probably more efficient at infecting and seroconverting susceptible kittens than are cats with low antibody titers (1:25 or less).

The incubation period for FIP (the interval between initial exposure and seroconversion) is generally two to six weeks. The latent period (the interval between seroconversion and the onset of the fatal forms of FIP) is extremely variable and may be prolonged several weeks to many years.

PATHOGENESIS AND IMMUNITY

Studies by Pederson have shown that FIP may initially produce localized upper respiratory disease in about 25 percent of cats two weeks following natural exposure. This "primary disease" is a mild chronic infection characterized by a slight ocular or nasal discharge, or both, which persists for one to four weeks. Approximately 75 percent of exposed cats will develop an inapparent infection. Although the vast majority of cats undergoing the primary infection recover uneventfully, most will remain persistently infected (i.e., they will be virus carriers). A very small number (probably less than 1 to 5 percent of all infected cats) will develop the fatal "secondary disease" weeks to years later. The "secondary disease" refers to classic effusive and non-effusive (granulomatous) FIP, the lethal disseminated forms of the disease.

Currently, very little is understood regarding immunity to FIP. Many factors, including stress, age, physical condition, genetic background, concurrent infections (e.g., respiratory viruses or FeLV), immunosuppression (by FeLV, immunosuppressive drugs, or radiotherapy), and virus factors (strain, dose, route, duration of exposure), may influence individual susceptibility to the secondary disease. The initiating factors are not known specifically but probably involve altered or deficient immunologic mechanisms.

If the initial exposure to virus is not too great and the cat is not immunosuppressed, the host's body defenses will contain the localized infection, and disseminated disease does not occur. However, if the virus overwhelms the local immune response and invades blood vessels and lymphatics, viremia and systemic disease may result and produce pyogranulomatous inflammatory lesions, necrosis, and vasculitis in abdominal and thoracic viscera, lymph nodes, eyes, or brain. These lesions are believed to be the result of immunologically mediated inflammatory reactions in response to antigen-antibody complexes.

There is an increasing amount of experimental evidence that the secondary disease is immune-mediated and the result of complement-mediated inflammation and tissue injury. Activation of complement might occur following intravascular and perivascular deposition of immune complexes or possibly from the action of a cytotoxic complement-fixing antibody directed against virus or virus-infected target cells. Intravascular activation of complement may result in endothelial damage, microthrombus formation, vasculitis, and disseminated intravascular coagulation (DIC). Several cases of DIC with vasculitis in multiple organs have been produced experimentally in our laboratory following intraperitoneal inoculation of FIPV in antibody-positive cats.

CLINICAL SYNDROMES

There are two distinct clinical manifestations of the secondary or disseminated forms of FIP: (1) effusive peritonitis or pleuritis ("wet" FIP or non-parenchymatous FIP) and (2) chronic granulomatous disease ("dry" FIP, granulomatous FIP, or parenchymatous FIP). Both forms occur with almost equal frequency and invariably lead to the death of the animal. A third variant of FIPV infection is an acute necrotizing hepatitis, which is frequently observed under experimental conditions.

Effusive FIP is characterized by chronic weight loss, depression, fever, and progressive abdominal enlargement caused by ascites. Pleural effusion occurs in less than one third of cases. Pyogranulomatous inflammatory lesions associated with a fibrinous exudate are present over wide areas of the omentum, visceral serosa, pleura, and other organs.

The onset of dry FIP is also insidious, and it has a progressive and invariably fatal course. In addition to weight loss, chronic, non-responsive fever, and lethargy, frequently there are organ-specific symptoms resulting from disseminated granulomatous lesions in one or several organs. These lesions may involve liver, kidney, mesenteric lymph nodes, pancreas, eyes, brain, spinal cord, pleura, heart, and lungs. Clinical signs of renal insufficiency, liver failure, pancreatic disease, and CNS disease may be observed in patients with severe organ impairment. Ocular lesions may be observed in 25 percent or more of cases of dry FIP and include iritis, hyphema, keratic precipitates, retinal hemorrhage or detachment, chorioretinitis, and panophthalmitis.

In addition to the classic secondary forms of FIP, a variety of FIPV-related reproductive and neonatal diseases frequently affect breeding catteries. Often occurring in FIP-positive catteries experiencing sporadic outbreaks of FIP, significant neonatal losses, and breeding problems, these disorders typically include (1) fetal resorptions occurring at four to six weeks' gestation, (2) metritis, (3) "fading kittens" immediately after birth or at one to six weeks of age, (4) acute effusive or granulomatous FIP, (5) mild, chronic, recurrent upper respiratory infection in kittens and older cats, (6) abortion at mid- to late gestation, and (7) stillbirths. Other less frequently reported problems are fetal malformations, non-specific diarrheas with severe leukopenia (in FPL-negative and FeLV-negative kittens), and acute congestive cardiomyopathy characterized by sudden respiratory distress, cyanosis, and death in previously "healthy" kittens one to eight weeks of age; necropsy reveals severe cardiac dilatation and hydrothorax. Although not all of these syndromes will occur in any one cattery, several usually occur together. Virologic studies in several "problem" catteries have consistently failed to isolate FPL, FVR, FCV, reovirus, FPN, or other cytopathic feline viruses, and most of the catteries are FeLV-negative. However, all catteries tested to date are positive for FIPV.

To date, none of the disorders (with the exception of classic FIP) in this "kitten mortality complex" has been proved to be caused by FIPV. However, the circumstantial evidence is striking, and further research is needed to clarify the role of FIPV.

DIAGNOSIS

The diagnosis of FIP is not difficult in classic cases, in which extensive accumulations of the characteristic fluid are demonstrated in the peritoneal or pleural cavity by paracentesis. Interestingly, there is little evidence of abdominal pain upon palpation in these cases. Cats that lack detectable amounts of fluid (particularly in dry FIP) may present a more formidable diagnostic challenge.

The presence of the typical effusion in association with a positive serum or fluid FIP antibody titer supports a diagnosis of effusive FIP. The fluid is characteristically clear, straw-colored, and viscous, contains fibrin flakes, and may clot on exposure to air. It is an exudate with a high specific gravity (1.017 to 1.047), high protein content (5 to 8 gm/dl), and a variable cell count that consists of neutrophils (predominantly), macrophages, mesothelial cells, and lymphocytes.

In addition to the non-specific clinical signs associated with development of dry FIP (e.g., depression, weight loss, and chronic, recurrent high fevers not responsive to antibiotic therapy), there are several categories of clinical and clinicopathologic abnormalities that, when found in combination with elevated FIP serum antibody titers, support a diagnosis by dry FIP (Pedersen). These changes include

1. Hematologic   disturbances   frequently

showing leukocytosis (predominantly, an absolute and relative neutrophilia), profound lymphopenia, and mild normochromic anemia. Cats in terminal stages or with fulminating disease may show a marked leukopenia, and animals co-infected with FeLV or *Haemobartonella felis* may suffer severe anemia.

2. Total plasma protein elevations (above 8 gm/dl) with hyperglobulinemia (more than 4.60 gm/dl) and serum protein electrophoretic abnormalities, including hypergammaglobulinemia and polyclonal gammopathies reflecting variable increases in IgG_1 and/or IgG_2 antibody subclasses. Other globulins, including alpha$_2$ and beta$_2$ globulins, may also be elevated.

3. Elevations in serum fibrinogen (more than 400 mg/dl).

4. Neurologic signs (posterior ataxia, incoordination, convulsions, hyperesthesia), often with increased levels of protein and white blood cells (mostly neutrophils) in CSF.

5. Ocular lesions (see previous discussion).

6. Marked mesenteric lymphadenopathy.

7. Irregular enlargement of kidneys, frequently associated with proteinuria and elevation of blood urea nitrogen.

8. Clinical signs of liver disease (icterus, malaise, fever, with or without hepatomegaly), with elevation of serum enzymes (SGPT, SGOT, LDH, SDH), hyperbilirubinemia, and urobilinogenuria.

It may be necessary to examine biopsy specimens of visceral organs (liver, kidney, enlarged mesenteric nodes, omentum) taken during exploratory laparotomy to differentiate dry FIP from other infectious, granulomatous, or neoplastic conditions. Histopathologic examination typically reveals perivascular pyogranulomatous or fibrinonecrotic inflammatory lesions and vasculitis.

Diagnosis of clinical FIP has recently been aided by the development and use of the IFAT. The FIP antibody titer, when used in conjunction with anamnesis, physical examination, clinicopathologic tests (CBC, total protein, serum protein electrophoresis, abdominal or thoracic paracentesis), and biopsy, is useful in diagnosis. Clinically ill cats usually have elevated serum antibody titers ranging from 1:400 to 1:25,000 or greater; asymptomatic normal cats may also have positive titers, but these are usually less than 1:400 (Pederson). Peritoneal fluid from affected cats also shows positive anti-FIP antibody titers, but frequently they are lower in magnitude then the serum titer.

At present there is no *in vitro* diagnostic test that measurss specific neutralizing activity of cat serum to FIPV; indeed, it is not even known whether systemic FIPV infection produces protective antibody. Considering that the present FIP test measures only the magnitude of a previous immune response to FIPV and not neutralizing antibody per se, it does not by itself indicate active disease or resistance. It may, however, have some prognostic value, since cats with very high antibody titers may be more susceptible to the fatal disease than cats with a low level of antibody. The IFAT may also be used to monitor response to therapy, since the antibody titer may decline temporarily in cats undergoing remission and remains elevated or increases in cats unresponsive to treatment (see following discussion).

TREATMENT

Currently there is no cure for the disseminated forms of FIP. However, various therapeutic regimens have been effective in inducing remissions for up to several months in about one quarter to one third of carefully screened patients. The best candidates for therapy are cats in good physical condition that have good appetite and do not show significant organ damage, severe anemia, or neurologic symptoms.

The basic rationale of therapy is to minimize the intense inflammatory reactions resulting from deposition of antigen-antibody complexes. The most effective treatments consist of combinations of immunosuppressive drugs, high levels of corticosteroids, broad-spectrum antibiotics, and good supportive care. Prednisolone, 4 mg/kg/day, cyclophosphamide (Cytoxan),* 2 mg/kg/day for four consecutive days of each week, and ampicillin, 100 mg t.i.d., is an effective combination. Melphalan (Alkeran),† 1 mg every third day, is an alkylating agent of the nitrogen mustard group that has been used quite successfully in place of cyclophosphamide. Abdominocentesis or thoracocentesis, or both, followed by instillation of fibrinolytic enzymes (e.g., Varizyme,‡ 10,000 units) twice daily, is beneficial in cases of effusive FIP. Anabolic steroids such as Winstrol-V,§ 1 mg b.i.d., should be used to counteract the marked catabolic effects of the disease and the immunosuppressive therapy.

If the patient shows a positive response to therapy over the first few weeks, treatment should continue for three months. If the cat is in complete remission at this time, therapy may be

---

*Cytoxan, Mead Johnson Pharmaceutical, Evansville, Indiana

†Alkeran, Burroughs Wellcome Co., Research Triangle Park, North Carolina

‡Varizyme, American Cyanamid Co., Princeton, New Jersey

§Winstrol-V, Winthrop Laboratories, New York, New York

discontinued. Treatment should be reinstituted when symptoms recur or when the antibody titer rises. Progressive deterioration of condition and persistence of high antibody levels in the face of treatment indicate treatment failure, and euthanasia is best advised.

It must be emphasized that the use of immunosuppressive drugs is not without risk, and the hemogram should be routinely monitored for evidence of myelosuppression. Serious side effects, including leukopenia, thrombocytopenia, secondary malignancies, and hemorrhagic cystitis, are reported in man following the use of immunosuppressive drugs, and there is a report describing myeloproliferative disease in a cat receiving immunosuppressive therapy for FIP (Madewell, et al.).

Co-infection with FeLV occurs in about 50 percent of cases of FIP, and cats treated successfully for FIP may rapidly succumb instead to one of the FeLV-related diseases.

CONTROL

At present, no preventive vaccine against FIP is available. Experiments with crude inactivated virus have so far failed to produce active immunity capable of resisting virus challenge. Attenuation of present strains of FIPV awaits large-scale production of virus in cell cultures and subsequent virus purification. Further research is also required to investigate the feasibility of intranasal or oral vaccines capable of establishing effective local immunity in the respiratory and gastrointestinal tracts, since parenteral FIPV immunization with existing virus strains may paradoxically predispose the cat to severe systemic disease.

Thorough disinfection of contaminated premises with quaternary ammonium compounds or a 1:32 dilution of household bleach is necessary for proper control. The bleach may be added to A-33 (Airchem) (4 oz of bleach and 2 oz of A-33 per gallon of water) to increase its cleaning properties. Since the virus probably does not persist for more than several days outside the host, new animals should not be introduced into such disinfected premises for at least one week following removal of all infected and dead cats.

It is highly recommended that catteries and multiple-cat households routinely test all cats. FIPV-negative catteries should not introduce any new animals, including studs for breeding, unless a negative FIP antibody titer is demonstrated in the cat within 10 to 14 days of entry. FIPV-negative cats newly introduced into the cattery should be isolated for two weeks and retested. Catteries with both FIPV-positive and FIPV-negative cats should house the two groups in separate facilities.

SUPPLEMENTAL READING

Gaskin, J.G.: Feline infectious peritonitis. In Kirk, R.W. (ed.): *Current Veterinary Therapy VI.* Philadelphia, W.B. Saunders Co., 1977, pp. 1305–1308.

Hoshino, Y., and Scott, F.W.: Brief communication: Replication of feline infectious peritonitis virus in organ cultures of feline tissue. Cornell Vet., 68:411–417, 1978.

Loeffler, D.G., Ott, R.L., Evermann, J.F., and Alexander, J.E.: The incidence of naturally occurring antibodies against feline infectious peritonitis in selected cat populations. Feline Pract., 8:43–47, 1978.

Madewell, B.R., Crow, S.E., and Nickerson, T.R.: Infectious peritonitis in a cat that subsequently developed a myeloproliferative disorder. J. Am. Vet. Med. Assoc., 172:169–172, 1978.

Osterhaus, A.D.M.E., Horzinek, M.C., and Wirahadiredja, R.M.S.: Feline infectious peritonitis virus. II. Propagation in suckling mouse brain. Zentralbl. Veterinaermed. [B], 25:301–307, 1978.

Pedersen, N.C.: Feline infectious peritonitis. Feline Pract., 5:42–51, 1976.

Pedersen, N.C.: Feline infectious peritonitis. In AAHA Proceedings, 45:142–146, 1978.

CANINE VIRAL ENTERITIS

LELAND E. CARMICHAEL, D.V.M.,

and MAX J. APPEL, D.V.M.

Ithaca, New York

Widespread outbreaks of contagious vomiting and diarrhea, sometimes hemorrhagic, first were reported to us in February 1978 by veterinarians and breeders of purebred dogs in the East and Southeast. Initial outbreaks were reported in collies that had attended specialty shows in the South and southern Midwestern states. Some animals had died. Later (March through May 1978), outbreaks in other breeds were reported in various locations throughout the United States. Several strains of a virus were isolated from stool and fresh intestinal specimens in canine kidney cell cultures. The isolates had morphologic features of coronaviruses. The virus is not a newly recognized one, for in 1970 Binn and associates isolated a canine coronavirus from fecal samples of military dogs stationed in Germany that were suffering from suspected "viral gastroenteritis." Preliminary serologic comparisons indicate that the 1978 North American isolates are very similar to those recovered by Binn. Reasons for the failure to associate this virus with diarrheal disease in the United States until now are unclear, although retrospective evidence leaves no doubt that it has been present.

Then, in the summer of 1978, a second series of outbreaks of contagious diarrheal disease, sometimes associated with sudden death in puppies, was observed in Southwestern and Midwestern states. These outbreaks were more severe, with higher morbidity (sometimes reaching 100 percent) and mortality. Especially affected were pups, but deaths also occurred in adults. Particularly severe outbreaks were reported from Texas by Eugster and co-workers, who had earlier observed a very small virus in feces from puppies with non-fatal diarrhea. The virus had characteristics of the parvovirus group. A similar virus ("minute virus of canines," or MVC) was isolated in 1970 from feces of normal dogs, and antibody prevalence was found to be very high. It now is known that the MVC is distinct from the pathogenic parvoviral isolates.

Starting in August 1978, very small (20-nm) parvovirus-like particles, often in aggregates, began to be seen in fecal specimens submitted to our laboratory from suspected outbreaks of "coronavirus diarrhea." Although epidemiologic information is limited, outbreaks of parvoviral disease initially seemed more prevalent in the West, Southwest, and Midwest of the United States, but by September 1978 they were occurring throughout the country. Samples of random collected sera from dogs in Northeastern states maintained for reference failed to reveal parvoviral antibody prior to 1978. Similar viruses, associated with a "feline panleukopenia-like" disease of dogs, have been observed in the feces of dogs with enteritis in Australia, Canada, Holland, and Belgium.* Particularly severe outbreaks have occurred in veterinary hospitals, boarding kennels, and commercial or research kennels, as well as in family dogs, especially if they had been boarded or

hospitalized in close confinement with ill animals. In two instances both the coronavirus and the parvo-like virus were identified in the same stool sample. In some cases a rota-like virus also has been observed. The pathogenicity of this virus is unknown at present.

At this writing, information is incomplete; however, the following descriptions attempt to assist veterinarians in diagnosing these two newly recognized viral diseases.

CLINICAL SIGNS

The diseases caused by the canine coronavirus (CCV) and the canine parvovirus (CPV) may be difficult to differentiate clinically; however, there are certain important distinguishing characteristics. Signs in individual animals vary greatly and may be influenced by age, environmental circumstances, and resident gut organisms.

Canine Coronaviral Gastroenteritis. Typical signs in field cases are lethargy, decreased appetite, and a loose ("mushy") stool. The onset of illness is often sudden, with diarrhea preceded by or simultaneous with vomiting. Typically, vomiting is less frequent after the first day or two of illness. There may be mucus and variable amounts of blood in the feces. Stools often are somewhat orange in color, and the smell is characteristically fetid. Owners often comment on the particularly foul and offensive fecal odor. The diarrhea may continue as a loose stool or as an oozing of frothy, yellow-orange, semisolid material. Projectile diarrhea sometimes is seen, either as a watery or sanguineous fluid. Young puppies may become dehydrated rapidly, even when fluid therapy is instituted early in the course of illness. Animals generally recovered spontaneously after a week to ten days, but dogs that receive early symptomatic treatment and are kept warm and quiet seem to recover more rapidly. Persistent diarrhea, even with treatment, has been observed. Young pups may die suddenly, with a thin yellowish or frankly hemorrhagic stool. Stress seems to be related to increased severity of signs. Some animals in contact with diseased dogs fail to have symptoms, or else the signs are very mild, consisting only of a slightly loose, foul-smelling stool. Elevated temperatures are not a feature of coronaviral gastroenteritis. Leukopenia has not been observed in dogs with this viral disease. The coronavirus is highly contagious and spreads rapidly through kennels of susceptible dogs.

Experimental CCV infection in laboratory beagles was, without exception, mild. The incubation period in experimentally infected animals was about 24 to 36 hours. Diarrhea or soft

---

*Personal communications, 1978: R. H. Johnson, James Cook University, Townsville, Australia; and G. Burtonboy, Universite Catholique de Louvain, Brussels.

stools often persisted for one to two weeks but was not observed in all animals.

Canine Parvoviral Enteritis. As with CCV gastroenteritis, signs vary greatly. Dogs of all ages may be afflicted, with deaths in both adults and pups. Mortality seems highest in puppies. Sudden deaths may occur without signs of enteritis or shortly after the onset of enteritis. In such cases labored breathing, anorexia, depression, or convulsive movements have been observed shortly before death. Common clinical signs are vomiting (which is often severe and protracted), anorexia, depression, diarrhea, and rapid dehydration, especially in pups. In several cases myocarditis with pulmonary congestion was prominent. In cases in which enteritis is the principal sign the feces are often grayish or yellow-gray in color at the onset of illness; however, fluid stools that are either streaked with blood or frankly hemorrhagic may be the initial sign and may persist until recovery or death. Some cases initially were regarded by veterinarians as "atypical distemper." Temperatures ranging from 104 to 106° F may be observed in some animals, especially pups; however, affected older dogs may have normal or only slightly elevated (103° F) temperatures. Some animals continue to vomit at frequent intervals and have diarrhea, sometimes projectile and frankly hemorrhagic in nature, until they die; others have only a loose ("pancake") stool and recover uneventfully. Occasionally, pups die suddenly in a shock-like syndrome as early as two days after onset of illness. A very common feature of the parvovirus infection is leukopenia (often a relative lymphopenia), especially during the first four to five days of illness. White cell counts less than 100 cells/mm³ have been recorded; however, available information suggests that counts of 1000/mm³ through 4000/mm³ are more common at the peak of illness. Leukopenia often is accompanied by fever. Both of these signs were prominent in experimentally infected laboratory beagles. The incubation period varied between four and eight days.

LESIONS

Canine Coronavirus. Lesions in experimentally infected beagle pups are characteristically mild. Macroscopic changes consist of dilated intestinal loops filled with thin, watery, green-yellow fecal material. In contrast, several field cases with strongly suspicious viral etiology, based on isolation or demonstration of virus by electron microscopy, had lesions ranging from those just described to more severe changes consisting of mild to moderate congestion or

frank hemorrhage of the intestinal mucosa, with enlarged and congested mesenteric lymph nodes. Microscopic changes in the experimental disease were modest, characterized by atrophy and fusion of intestinal villi and deepening of crypts, increase in cellularity of the lamina propria, flattening of epithelial cells, and discharge of goblet cells. Changes were remarkably similar to those described in gnotobiotic calves infected with the calf coronavirus.

As in other viral infections, the bacterial and parasitic populations of the gut may alter the course of the disease greatly and suppress the restoration of damaged epithelium.

Canine Parvovirus (CPV). The experimental disease has not been adequately studied at this writing; however, field outbreaks with proved viral etiology have provided valuable case material. In contrast with the lesions of coronavirus enteritis, CPV infection is characterized by necrosis of the epithelium of the rapidly dividing crypt cells in the small intestine. Often there is extensive loss of epithelial cells and dilatation of remaining crypts. In more advanced cases regeneration of epithelium occurs, and the lamina propria may be infiltrated by inflammatory cells. Intranuclear inclusion bodies may be present in epithelial cells, especially in dogs that died following a short course of illness. Necrosis or depletion of lymphoid tissue is often present. Heart lesions are characterized by focal lymphocytic infiltration, edema, and hemorrhage. Cardiac myofibers with intranuclear inclusions also may be found, but they are not numerous. The lesions of CPV infection are remarkably similar to those of feline panleukopenia (FPL), which also is caused by a parvovirus. Most pathologists agree that CPV infection is a novel, emerging disease. Seroepidemiologic studies support this view.

DIAGNOSIS

Both viruses have been isolated and propagated in cell cultures, but they are fastidious. A presumptive diagnosis may be based on clinical signs and postmortem findings when the history suggests contagious enteritis. Dual or sequential infections with both viruses have been observed. When fresh fecal material is available for study, rapid diagnosis may be obtained by observing characteristic viral particles via electron microscope examination (negative-stain) of prepared stool samples. Since artifacts are common, especially with the coronavirus, caution must be observed in interpreting results. It is expected that diagnostic laboratories will shortly have available immunofluorescent reagents for both viruses. Inhibition of hemagglutination

(HA) by CPV antibody provides a rapid sero-diagnostic test. Antibody is generally present at high levels at the onset of intestinal signs. The CPV agglutinates swine and rhesus monkey erythrocytes at 4° C. Fecal extracts made in saline from acutely ill dogs usually have high titers of HA activity. CPV hemagglutination is inhibited by specific antiserum.

Since there are many causes of vomiting and diarrhea in the dog, including bacterial and parasitic diseases, acute pancreatitis, poisoning, and "canine hemorrhagic gastroenteritis (HGE)," it is important to consider each possibility. Viral gastroenteritis should be given special consideration when several animals are involved or if other evidence suggests a contagious disease.

TREATMENT

Prompt symptomatic treatment is essential in severely ill animals, especially pups. Treatment is similar for both viral diseases; the objective is control of diarrhea, vomiting, and dehydration. It is extremely important to attempt to restore lost body fluids as early as possible following the onset of illness. Whole-blood transfusions are indicated.

Although experimental studies are lacking, the use of corticosteroids or other immunosuppressive drugs in animals with suspected viral enteritis seems to be contraindicated.

CONTROL

Vaccines are not commercially available for either disease at this writing; but studies in our laboratories on experimental inactivated and attenuated-live CPV vaccines encourage us to expect an immunizing agent for the canine parvovirus shortly.

The canine parvovirus and feline panleukopenia virus (FPLV) are antigenically indistinguishable by serologic tests (SN, H-I). Experimental protection of dogs against CPV disease was engendered by live (one dose) and inactivated (two feline doses given seven to ten days apart) FPLV vaccines. However, FPL vaccines presently are licensed only for use in cats. A formal recommendation therefore cannot be made at this time.

Experimental studies have shown that homotypic (CPV) and heterotypic (FPLV) inactivated vaccines require at least seven days before adequate immunity is engendered. Laboratory and field studies also indicate interference with the development of immunity by maternally transferred CPV antibody. Dogs immunized with inactivated vaccines shed virulent CPV after challenge inoculation; i.e., viral spread is not interrupted in dogs that have been inoculated with inactivated vaccines and are then challenged orally with virulent virus.

SUPPLEMENTAL READING

Appel, M.J.G., Cooper, B.J., Greisen, H., Scott, F., and Carmichael, L.E.: Canine viral enteritis. I. Status report on corona- and parvo-like enteritides. Cornell Vet., 69:123–133, 1979.

Binn, L.N., Lazar, E.C., Eddy, G.A., and Kajina, M.: Recovery and characterization of a minute virus of canines. Infect. Immun., 1:503–508, 1970.

Binn, L.N., Lazar, E.C., Keenan, K.P., Huxsoll, D.L., Marchwicki, R.H., and Strano, A.J.: Recovery and characterization of a coronavirus from military dogs with diarrhea. Proc. 78th Meeting, U.S. Animal Health Assoc. (October 1974), 1975, pp. 359–366.

Carmichael, L.E.: Infectious canine enteritis caused by a corona-like virus. Laboratory Report (The James A. Baker Institute for Animal Health, Cornell University), 2(9):1978.

Cooper, B.J., Carmichael, L.E., Appel, M.J.G., and Greisen, H.: Canine viral enteritis. II. Morphologic lesions in naturally occuring parvovirus infection. Cornell Vet., 69:134–144, 1979.

Csiza, C.K., deLahunta, A., Scott, F.W., and Gillespie, J.H. Pathogenesis of feline panleukopenia virus in susceptible newborn kittens. II. Pathology and immunofluorescence. Infect. Immun., 3:838–846, 1971.

Eugster, A.K., Bendele, R.A., and Jones, L.P.: Parvovirus infection in dogs. J. Am. Vet. Med. Assoc., 173:1340–1341, 1978.

Keenan, K.P., Jervis, H.R., Marchwicki, R.H., and Binn, L.N.: Intestinal infection of neonatal dogs with canine coronavirus 1-71: Studies by virologic, histologic, histochemical, and immunofluorescent technics. Am. J. Vet. Res., 37:247–256, 1976.

Thomson, G.W., and Gagnon, A.N.: Canine gastroenteritis associated with a parvovirus-like agent. (Letter to the editor.) Can. Vet. J., 19:346, 1978.

PSEUDORABIES IN DOGS AND CATS

D. P. GUSTAFSON, D.V.M.
West Lafayette, Indiana

In 1902, while investigating a case of fatal encephalopathy in an ox, Dr. Aladar Aujeszky of Budapest inoculated material from the ox's brain into two rabbits, with lethal results. In the same report a similar syndrome in a dog and a cat were briefly described. Thus, the first publication on the infectious nature of what was to be named pseudorabies virus (PrV) included a description of the disease in dogs and cats. The literature contains reports of PrV infections in dogs and cats from both urban and rural communities on all of the continents of the world, except Australia. The disease occurs more commonly among dogs and cats in areas in which swine are raised or consumed.

Pseudorabies, or Aujeszky's disease, is caused by a herpesvirus and is infectious for a broad spectrum of animal life. The disease is apparently invariably fatal for dogs, cats, cattle, sheep, goats, deer, foxes, minks, badgers, opossums, rats, and mice. Swine are much more resistant; therefore, variations in the virulence of PrV strains may be observed. These animals have resistance related to age that is not well defined in other species; in some episodes all very young swine die, whereas losses among shoats and mature animals are less than 50 percent. Successful experimental infections have been achieved in other mammals, including some subhuman primates, and in many species of birds. Natural infections of birds have not been reported.

MODES OF INFECTION

Dogs and cats can be infected by a variety of routes, as has been demonstrated under laboratory conditions. The disease has been initiated by feeding infectious material and by subcutaneous, intramuscular, intracranial, and intraocular routes. Since the oral route leads to infection, it might be assumed (with good reason) that infection could be established by inhalation of air-borne virus. Under natural conditions an overwhelming number of reports find the source of infection to be virus-contaminated flesh of swine and sometimes of cattle or rats

that was consumed by the affected dog or cat. That rural dogs and cats might eat infected flesh available on farms and thus become infected themselves seems clear. In urban areas dogs and cats may be given raw pork from a refrigerated carcass. The source animal may have been an asymptomatic carrier, which ordinary inspection could not identify. A tragic infection in a kennel was reported in Sweden. In a building housing about 45 dogs, 14 dogs died of pseudorabies. Evidence presented strongly suggests that uncooked infected pork from a packing house was the source of the virus. The construction of fences permitted contact between dogs. However, some dogs kept in or adjacent to pens in which deaths had occurred survived and were serologically negative. The report suggests that 31 of the 45 were not susceptible to oral exposure. However, since they did not develop antibodies, it is evident that they did not react to the virus. One explanation is that gastric acidity denatured the virus. Similar results in swine can be achieved by placing the virus into the stomach. Indeed, it has been found in a recent study that less than half of a series of virus feedings to dogs led to infection. In those instances in which the disease did not ensue, antibodies did not develop either. However, when the dogs were exposed to the virus parenterally, all died of the disease.

On the other hand, it has been found that feeding virus-contaminated food to domestic cats invariably leads to fatal disease. One develops the impression that cats are among the most susceptible species to pseudorabies infection. In every instance in which the means of infection of cats has been described in the available literature and from experience, ingestion of virus-contaminated food has been noted. However, it must be recognized that other modes of access to the virus are possible.

Since 1962, the number of PrV infections among swine in the United States has gradually been increasing and, as an expected corollary, the number of cases in other susceptible species has increased too. Thus, the number of

1296

infections among dogs and cats has increased in a rather dramatic fashion but is essentially confined to rural areas.

CANINE PSEUDORABIES

Once a dog has become infected, the natural course of the disease proceeds to death in a short time. The incubation period ranges from about two to ten days, and most cases take between three and six days under natural conditions. Experimental intracerebral, subcutaneous, or intramuscular exposures reduce the prodromal period and the course of the disease. As the infecting dose of virus is increased, the duration of the disease is somewhat shortened. After signs appear, death occurs in a relatively short period — 24 to 48 hours. Thus, from infection to termination the natural disease usually lasts five to eight days.

The syndrome runs a rather constant course, but there are exceptions. In a typical case there is an excitement phase followed by dullness, coma, and death. In the excitement phase the dog is febrile and restless and may vomit bilious fluid. The saliva is usually copious and viscid. Clonic spasms of facial muscles, paralysis of an eyelid or the lower lip, incoordination of movement, and difficult breathing often signal the onset of intense pruritus somewhere about the head. The dog rubs the area incessantly, and it becomes raw and often edematous. Vocal expressions of discomfort often accompany the progress of the syndrome, yet aggressive behavior toward objects or people has not been observed or reported. The course of the encephalopathy deepens into depression, followed by coma and death. Exceptions to this syndrome lie in the abbreviation or apparent absence of the excitement phase, in which case the disease course is also shortened.

The physiology of this pruritus has been studied. Itching is apparently caused by functional dissociation of the afferent nerve system between receptor and motor nerve elements. As a result of depression in cholinergic processes in the cerebral cortex by the virus and the toxic products of its presence, the analyzing function of the cortex becomes altered, leading to a disturbance in esthesic perception.

FELINE PSEUDORABIES

The usual clinical syndrome in cats begins about four days after infection and generally parallels the canine syndrome but is less consistent. The excitement phase is somewhat different, in that cats first appear to be sluggish and then become agitated. Their movements suggest discomfort just prior to the onset of salivation, which in turn signals the approach of a variety of signs. At about this time the fur becomes matted with saliva, and the cat appears to have something caught in its throat or an esophageal obstruction. The cat resists being caught and mewing is persistent. In many cases an intense pruritus is localized on one side of the head, and when this occurs anisocoria is often present. In a lesser number of cases pruritus and irritability are absent. The response to pruritus is strong, and the area is often scratched raw. Late in the syndrome respiration becomes difficult and the pulse rate is increased, sometimes becoming uncountable. The qualitative blood picture is normal, but because of dehydration the blood is concentrated. When the cat is picked up, often it will void urine immediately from a full bladder, and the penis of males may become erect. On palpation the intestines may be distended with gas. The signs soon diminish as the encephalopathy progresses to convulsive spasms, exhaustion, and death. Cats usually die within 24 hours of the onset of symptoms. In less typical cases the clinical signs are more difficult to interpret. In such instances the cats become feeble and salivate excessively, making frequent attempts to swallow. The head may be canted to one side, and the tail flagellates in a horizontal plane, but there are no signs of agitation, mewing, or pruritus. These cats have been observed to live at least 36 hours after the onset of symptoms.

DIAGNOSIS

The clinical signs of the disease, especially when pruritus is well pronounced, provide the basis for a presumptive diagnosis of pseudorabies. The course of the syndrome in both species is short and fatal.

Laboratory diagnosis is made through fluorescent antibody tests. The tissue of choice is the mesencephalon, that portion of the brain stem containing the gasserian ganglion of the trigeminal nerve. Almost as valuable is tonsillar tissue. Both tissues contain high virus concentrations early in the disease, and they persist until after death. The persistence of the virus after death is related to the speed of tissue denaturation, which is essentially a function of temperature. The lower the carcass temperature, the longer the virus will remain viable.

Diagnosis can also be made by isolation of the virus in cell cultures. Extracts of tissues are inoculated into media bathing cell cultures. High-titered preparations will cause cytopathic effects in 18 hours, and very low-titered material needs to be held a maximum of 120 hours before discarding. The test is made specific for PrV through virus neutralization tests with reference antiserum.

Tissue extracts may be inoculated into a variety of laboratory animals for diagnosis on the basis of their response. Rabbits are highly sensitive to the virus and are commonly used. They are inoculated subcutaneously in the flank with tissue extracts suspected of containing PrV. Mice are less sensitive but are often used. They are inoculated intracranially with similar material. The death of any laboratory animal used to establish a diagnosis requires familiarity with the syndrome, close observation, and adequate control procedures.

TREATMENT

There is no known treatment that will change the course of events once signs of the disease are present. However, to reduce expression of reaction to the virus, sedation is recommended.

PROGNOSIS

Once the syndrome has begun, the prognosis in dogs and cats is death.

PROPHYLAXIS

Both attenuated and inactivated immunizing biologicals are commercially available for swine. They are not recommended for use in other species.

Antiserum is not commercially available but is often present in research organizations. Its use in cats and dogs has not been encouraging. Timing is of the essence; it is unlikely to be of value if administered more than eight hours after exposure to the virus. Antiserum of at least 5×10^2 titer against 300 tissue culture doses of PrV should be given IP. Finite doses have not been established for dogs and cats. However, it seems likely that a minimum dose for a puppy is 15 ml and a maximum dose for a 30-kg animal is about 100 ml.

Antiviral chemicals that have value in emergency situations are available for use in human beings infected with herpes simplex. Pseudorabies infections in swine are also amenable to treatment with adenine arabinoside monophosphate (Ara AMP) given IP.

MANAGEMENT IN INFECTED ENVIRONMENTS

If an outbreak occurs in swine or other susceptible species on a farm, it would be wise to exclude dogs and cats from the virus-contaminated area until the threat of transmission has passed. It is most important to prevent cats or dogs from eating infected flesh and to avoid their being nipped by an infected animal, for the virus is likely to be in the oral fluids.

Infected dogs and cats have the virus in their oral secretions and tonsils during the prodromal period and the clinical course of the disease. While lateral spread among dogs or cats has not been widely recognized, it seems quite possible.

PUBLIC HEALTH

The reports of human infections describe rather mild disease manifested by itching of a few days' duration. The descriptions and proof are not very convincing but, because some subhuman primates have been shown to be susceptible, caution is needed. The threshold of infection for man seems high, since among people working in our laboratory or in the field with many strains of PrV the record of seroconversion has remained consistently negative for 16 years.

SUPPLEMENTAL READING

Gustafson, D.P.: Pseudorabies. Dunne, H.W., and Leman, A.D. (eds.): In *Diseases of Swine*, 4th ed. Ames, Iowa, Iowa State University Press, 1975, pp. 391–410.

Horvath, Z., and Papp, L.: Clinical manifestations of Aujeszky's disease in the cat. Acta Vet. Acad. Sci. Hung., 17:49–54, 1967.

Hugoson, G., and Rockborn, G.: On the occurrence of pseudorabies in Sweden. II. An outbreak in dogs caused by feeding abattoir offal. Zentralbl. Veterinaermed. [B], 19:641–645, 1972.

FELINE PNEUMONITIS

EDWARD A. HOOVER, D.V.M.

Columbus, Ohio

INTRODUCTION

The feline pneumonitis agent was the first respiratory pathogen isolated from cats, and feline pneumonitis was the first respiratory disease described in cats. Because feline respiratory viruses were not identified until 15 years later, all respiratory infections in cats once were called "pneumonitis." The causative agent of feline pneumonitis is a feline strain of *Chlamydia psittaci*, a gram-negative bacterium that replicates intracellularly and resembles the prototype avian strain of *C. psittaci*, the cause of avian and human psittacosis. Like other members of the psittacosis group, feline *C. psittaci* is sensitive to antibiotics.

Currently available experimental and clinical observations indicate that feline pneumonitis agent (feline *Chlamydia psittaci*) is primarily a conjunctival rather than a pulmonary pathogen and that feline pneumonitis is a disease characterized principally by chronic follicular conjunctivitis. Present information also indicates that the overall significance of feline pneumonitis infection in the etiology of feline respiratory disease is relatively minor when compared with that of feline rhinotracheitis and calicivirus infections. However, since diagnostic procedures to identify feline chlamydial infections are not widely employed and clinical signs overlap with those of other infections, the actual incidence of feline pneumonitis infection is difficult to estimate. Most experimental studies have employed various passages of the one isolate of feline *C. psittaci*, and the extent of variation in pathogenicity among feline chlamydial isolates is not known. At least two cases of zoonotic human conjunctival infection with the feline pneumonitis agent have been identified.

ETIOLOGY AND PATHOGENESIS

The feline pneumonitis agent is a cat-adapted strain of *Chlamydia psittaci*. The organism formerly was known as *Miyagawanella felis*. *Chlamydia* are bacteria-like organisms that are obligate intracellular parasites. They are gram-negative and non-motile, have cell walls, contain both DNA and RNA, and replicate in the cytoplasm of cells by binary fission. *Chlamydia* organisms require the energy-generating mechanisms of a host cell for their replication. They can be propagated in yolk-sac membranes of chick embryos, in the lungs of mice, and in certain cell culture systems.

Two species of *Chlamydia* are recognized — *C. trachomatis* and *C. psittaci*. They are distinguished by their capacity to form iodine-staining intracytoplasmic inclusions and by their sensitivity to sulfonamides. *C. psittaci* strains are sensitive to sulfonamides and their inclusions do not stain with iodine; the reverse is true for *C. trachomatis*. *C. psittaci* isolates include many animal pathogens that have zoonotic potential. *C. trachomatis* is a human conjunctival and genital pathogen.

The infectious form of *Chlamydia psittaci*, the elementary body, is a coccoid organism 0.3 to 0.5μ in diameter and is the only form capable of extracellular survival. Elementary bodies attach to host cell membranes and induce their own entry into the cell by phagocytosis. Intracellular elementary bodies within membrane-bound phagocytic vacuoles in the cytoplasm undergo reorganization into larger forms 0.7 to 0.9μ in diameter that are called initial bodies. The initial bodies undergo binary fission and subsequently differentiate into a new generation of smaller, more condensed elementary bodies. The entire developmental cycle takes approximately 48 hours. Intracytoplasmic colonies of proliferating *Chlamydia* organisms can be detected by microscopic examination of infected cells stained with Giemsa or Wright stain (Fig. 1).

Chlamydial replication interferes with cell metabolism and prevents cell division, but the process is substantially less cytopathic than that of feline respiratory viruses. Nevertheless, substantial numbers of parasitized cells undergo degeneration, detach, and liberate the infectious elementary bodies from cytoplasmic vacuoles.

Feline *C. psittaci* infection probably is transmitted among cats by direct contact or short-distance aerosolization of infectious conjunctival and nasopharyngeal secretions. Adherence of elementary bodies to host cells and their subsequent phagocytosis have been shown to

1299

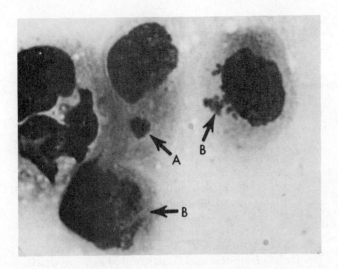

Figure 1. Conjunctival epithelial cells in a Giemsa-stained conjunctival smear from a cat infected with *Chlamydia psittaci.* Intracytoplasmic developmental forms (initial bodies) are evident as either *(A)* a solitary aggregate of tightly packed organisms or *(B)* numerous distinct organisms dispersed throughout the cytoplasm.

be dependent on specific receptors on the surface of both parasites and host cells. The same receptor system probably is responsible for the species and tissue tropisms of chlamydiae.

Conjunctival epithelium appears to be the chief target for feline chlamydial infection. Replication of chlamydiae in conjunctival cells results in cellular degeneration, necrosis, and sloughing. The associated inflammatory response includes hyperemia, edema, and leukocytic infiltration, which is dominated initially by neutrophils and subsequently by lymphocytes and plasma cells. Maximal replication of chlamydiae in conjunctival cells occurs seven to ten days after experimental aerosol infection of cats. Chlamydiae also replicate in the mucosae of the nasal passages, trachea, and bronchioles; however, it appears that proportionately fewer numbers of cells are infected. *C. psittaci* also has been isolated from spleen and liver of experimentally infected cats.

Chlamydiae persist in certain tissues of infected cats for weeks after clinical signs have subsided. In experimental studies, chlamydial infectivity has been demonstrated in conjunctiva, spleen, or liver from four to seven weeks after inoculation. Persistent latent infection is recognized as a general feature of chlamydial diseases.

CLINICAL SIGNS

Experimental studies in which concomitant viral infections could be excluded have shown that feline *C. psittaci* induces a disease characterized by chronic conjunctivitis and mild rhinitis. Lower respiratory disease does not appear to be a significant feature of feline pneumonitis. Signs of conjunctivitis appear five to ten days after aerosol exposure and persist for up to 45 days. Conjunctivitis often is unilateral initially.

Bilateral involvement usually follows; however, the severity of the conjunctival disease commonly varies between eyes. Early conjunctival signs are blepharospasm, congestion, chemosis, and increased lacrimation. Mucopurulent exudates occur in three to five days, and follicular (nodular) hyperplasia of lymphoid tissue in the nictitating membrane and palpebral conjunctiva is evident by ten days after exposure. It can become a prominent and persistent feature of chlamydial conjunctivitis (Fig. 2). Anorexia, decreased alertness, and inactivity occur in cats with severe conjunctivitis. Corneal lesions have not been associated with feline chlamydial infections.

Intermittent sneezing and a mild to moderate serous nasal discharge also occur in cats infected with the feline pneumonitis agent. However, neither severe rhinitis with copious mucopurulent exudates nor ulcers of the oral mucosae or nostrils are characteristic of the disease.

Fever in cats with chlamydial infection occurs several days after the onset of conjunctivitis. In experimental infections pyrexia appeared between days 11 and 15 and persisted for three to eight days.

Hematologic changes in chlamydial disease are minimal. Erythrocyte parameters are unaffected, and leukocyte counts may reveal either no deviation from normal or moderate neutrophilic leukocytosis.

LESIONS

Conjunctival lesions include degeneration, necrosis, and loss of epithelium accompanied by early marked neutrophilic exudation and followed by lymphocytic and plasmacytic infiltration. Nodular accumulations of lymphoid tissue are common in cats with well-established conjunctivitis. Regeneration of conjunctival epithelium occurs from surviving basilar epithelial cells, which attenuate and spread over areas of epithelial loss as well as undergo regenerative hyperplasia. Chlamydiae are relatively inconspicuous and difficult to detect in histologic sections. Consequently, histologic examination is an insensitive method of identifying the feline pneumonitis agent. Giemsa staining of tissue sections is necessary; hematoxylin-eosin staining is inadequate. The greatest number of intracytoplasmic organisms in the superficial conjunctival epithelial cells of experimentally infected cats appear five to ten days after exposure (see Fig. 1).

Mild to moderate neutrophilic rhinitis without mucosal ulceration has been demonstrated in cats with experimentally induced feline pneumonitis. Mild focal lesions of interstitial pneumonia, characterized by mild alveolar infiltration of macrophages, interstitial infiltration of mixed leukocytes, and mild hyperplasia of pneumocytes, also have been detected histologically in cats exposed to aerosol preparations of *C. psittaci*. Splenic lymphoid hyperplasia has been detected in cats two to seven weeks after exposure to *Chlamydia* but is not of diagnostic significance. It appears that specific visceral lesions are not produced by feline *C. psittaci* infection, although the organism has been isolated from spleen and liver of some experimentally infected cats as long as 27 days after aerosol inoculation.

DIAGNOSIS

Chronic follicular conjunctivitis that originates unilaterally and is responsive to antibiotic therapy in cats without concomitant severe rhinitis or oral ulcers may represent feline chlamydial infection. Because these diagnostic features do not permit exclusion of other feline bacterial or viral infections, isolation or cytologic demonstration of *C. psittaci* is required for definitive diagnosis. *C. psittaci* can be cultured from conjunctival swabs transferred to a sterile fluid medium. These specimens can be preserved for days by refrigeration and for longer periods by freezing. Inoculation of the yolk-sac membrane of embryonated hen's eggs is the chief method used for isolation. In other chlamydial systems isolation by inoculation of cell cultures has been shown to be more sensitive than isolation in embryonated eggs.

Examination of conjunctival smears represents a more readily available, if somewhat less sensitive, means of identification of feline *C. psittaci* infection. Conjunctival epithelium can be collected by rotating a moistened Dacron, cotton, or calcium alginate swab against the palpebral mucosa and the inner surface of the nictitating membrane. The swab is then rolled over a glass slide to deposit the cells, and the preparation is stained by either the Wright or Giemsa method. *Chlamydia* are identified as clusters of basophilic coccoid bodies (0.5 to 1.0 μ in diameter) in the cytoplasm of epithelial cells. Oil immersion examination ($\mu1000\times$) usually is necessary. Many neutrophils, lymphocytes, and other leukocytes from conjunctival exudate may be in the smear preparation. Examination of these cells for *C. psittaci* is not rewarding.

Feline conjunctival epithelial cells have large, round nuclei and abundant, lightly staining cytoplasm. Conjunctival epithelial cells may contain melanin granules, which appear as green or brown bodies dispersed throughout the cytoplasm. Melanin granules usually are smaller than chlamydiae and are never basophilic. Bacterial rods or cocci may also be present in conjunctival smear preparations. Bacteria usually are extracellular or else occur within the cytoplasm of leukocytes rather than epithelial cells. The period of maximal occurrence of chlamydiae in conjunctival smear preparations is one to seven days after the onset of conjuncti-

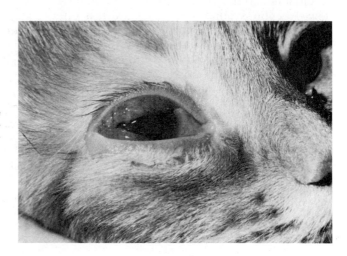

Figure 2. Conjunctivitis characterized by severe congestion, chemosis and nodular (follicular) lymphoid hyperplasia in a cat 20 days after aerosol exposure to feline *Chlamydia psittaci*.

vitis. After this period, the lower incidence of infected cells in conjunctival smears reduces the sensitivity of cytologic examination as a diagnostic procedure. Although not yet applied to feline chlamydial infection, immunofluorescent staining of conjunctival smears has been shown to be more sensitive than Giemsa staining for detecting human *C. trachomatis* infections.

Determination of complement-fixing antibody titers to group-reactive chlamydial antigen (from avian *C. psittaci*) has been unreliable and difficult to interpret as a diagnostic procedure. Determination of neutralizing antibody in paired serum samples theoretically could be employed to detect feline chlamydial infection, but it has substantial technical limitations and has not been employed on a diagnostic basis. Moreover, humoral antibody titers in chalmydial infections generally do not correlate with resistance to challenge. Therefore, these serologic assays often have limited usefulness as diagnostic tests and indicators of chlamydial immunity.

TREATMENT

Tetracyclines are the drugs of choice for the treatment of chlamydial infections. *C. psittaci* also is sensitive to sulfonamides but is much less sensitive to penicillin, ampicillin, and streptomycin. Tetracycline therapy should be continued for 14 days to eliminate the organism and to minimize the occurrence of the latent carrier state and possible exacerbations of clinical disease. These recommendations are based primarily on experiences with avian and human psittacosis and with human trachoma. With chlamydial infections in general, previous infection does not convey immunity to reinfection, although subsequent infection is more likely to produce mild or asymptomatic infection. Tetracycline (chlortetracycline) resistance in chlamydiae has not been observed, and with few exceptions other antibiotics are less effective or more toxic, or both. There is no evidence that topical tetracycline therapy is more effective than systemic administration. Systemic treatment is recommended.

VACCINATION

Modified live virus feline pneumonitis vaccines produced in embryonated eggs have been available for twenty years. Both the specific efficacy of these products and their relevance to the prevention of respiratory disease in cats have been controversial since the recognition of the major role of viruses as feline respiratory pathogens. A recent controlled evaluation of a commercial feline pneumonitis vaccine has indicated that the average severity and duration of clinical disease (conjunctivitis, serous rhinitis) were reduced in vaccinated cats as compared with controls after both groups were exposed to aerosols of virulent feline *C. psittaci* (Cello strain). Vaccination did not prevent conjunctival infection or shedding. The incidence of chlamydial infection in vaccinated and control cats was similar for the first 11 days after virulent challenge; thereafter, the incidence of chlamydial isolations from conjunctival swabs was significantly lower in the vaccinated cats. It can be concluded, therefore, that intramuscular administration of feline pneumonitis vaccine does help to ameliorate the clinical disease resulting from exposure to virulent *C. psittaci*. Complete protection from clinical disease and infection cannot be anticipated. Similar relationships between immunization and incomplete resistance to virulent challenge exist with the feline viral respiratory infections and with chlamydial infections of other species. In implementing immunization programs for feline pneumonitis it should be recognized that the overall impact of feline pneumonitis in the etiology of feline respiratory disease appears to be minor in comparison with that of feline viruses. The rationale for immunization against feline pneumonitis, therefore, may be less compelling than that for vaccination against the feline respiratory viruses.

SUPPLEMENTAL READING

Baker, J.A.: A virus causing pneumonia in cats and producing elementary bodies. J. Exp. Med., *79*:159–171, 1944.
Cello, R. M.: Microbiological and immunologic aspects of feline pneumonitis. J. AM. Vet. Med. Assoc., *158*:932–938, 1971.
Hoover, E.A., Kahn, D.E., and Langloss, J.M.: Experimentally induced feline chlamydial infection (feline pneumonitis). Am. J. Vet. Res., *39*:541–547, 1978.
Mitzel, J.R., and Strating, A.: Vaccination against feline pneumonitis. Am. J. Vet. Res., 38:1361–1363, 1977.
Schacter, J.: Chlamydial infections. N. Engl. J. Med., *298*:428–434, 490–495, 540–549, 1978.
Schacter, J., Ostler, H.B., and Meyer, K.F.: Human infection with the agent of feline pneumonitis. Lancet, *1*:1063—1065, 1969.

CANINE BRUCELLOSIS

RICARDO FLORES-CASTRO, D.V.M.
Mexico City, Mexico

and LELAND E. CARMICHAEL, D.V.M.
Ithaca, New York

Canine brucellosis, due to *Brucella canis,* has been recognized since 1966, when widespread abortions were observed in colonies of beagles. Since that time, the disease has been diagnosed in various breeds, and its occurrence has been recorded on several continents. Although the disease is widespread in the United States, the reported prevalence rates vary from approximately 1 to 6 percent, depending on the area sampled and the type of diagnostic test employed. Prevalence is highest where dogs are not controlled. For example, recent studies in Mexico revealed an infection rate greater than 10 percent, based on results of culture.

The recent availability of a rapid slide test has made presumptive diagnosis of this disease relatively simple. However, the occurrence of non-specific agglutination when the stained antigen (Canine Brucellosis Diagnostic Test, Pitman-Moore) is mixed with a patient's serum emphasizes that the plate (slide) test should never be the only criterion applied in the diagnosis of this disease. Further tests are necessary, requiring laboratory assistance.

Since no treatment for the disease is certain, and the implications are very serious for dogs proved to be infected, vigorous attempts to establish a diagnosis by all available means should be made before an animal is declared infected. Unfortunately, there have been many instances in which inadequate diagnostic procedures were applied and dogs were needlessly destroyed. Each case deserves extensive study. A basic knowledge of the general nature of brucellosis and the insidious nature of the disease in dogs, especially non-pregnant females and apparently normal males, is important. Many fundamental questions about the *Brucella*-host interaction remain unanswered. The supplemental reading list includes references that should be consulted to amplify the brief description presented here.

CLINICAL SIGNS

Clinical signs in bitches include abortion after day 30 of gestation, most commonly between days 45 and 55. Occasional litters may be born with some pups alive and some dead. Early embryonic deaths with termination of pregnancy may occur, suggesting to the owner that the bitch had failed to conceive. Generalized lymph node enlargement, principally due to reticular cell hyperplasia, is common in both sexes.

Brucella canis can be isolated readily from the blood or vaginal discharges of infected animals and from the fetal and placental tissues. Prolonged bacteremia, often lasting more than two years, is a notable feature of the canine disease. After several months' infection, bacteremia may be intermittent.

An important aspect of the disease in males is infertility. Between the second and fifth weeks after infection, abnormal sperm (30 to 80 percent) with bent tails, swollen midpieces, and distal protoplasmic droplets are evident; by 20 weeks after infection by the oral route, more than 90 percent of the sperm may be abnormal and have severely reduced motility. Neutrophils and monocytes are common in the ejaculate, and detached heads are evident. Clumps of spermatozoa with head-to-head agglutination are readily observed. Spermagglutinins have been found in both serum and seminal fluid samples from infected males. *Brucella* organisms may be isolated from ejaculated semen in abundance during the second month after infection; however, the number of organisms decreases rapidly after this time. Shedding is sporadic thereafter; however, organisms have been recovered from semen of infected dogs for as long as 60 weeks. The prostate gland is an abundant source of the organisms. In males epididymitis and orchitis, often followed by testicular atrophy, are common.

It is important to recognize that many infected animals appear normal, even though they may have bacteremia. There is no fever. Agglutinins appear in the serum approximately three weeks following oral infection and persist at high levels (titer value will depend on the particular test system employed) until recovery commences, typically one year or longer. Recovered animals are immune to reinfection.

1303

Diagnosis

A diagnosis should not be made until adequate clinical, serologic, and bacterial examinations are carried out. A history of abortions, infertility, testicular abnormalities (epididymitis, atrophy), poor semen quality, or lymph node enlargement with or without these signs should lead to consideration of *B. canis* infection.

A rapid slide agglutination test that produces presumptive diagnostic information in a few minutes is now available (Pitman-Moore). This test is rapid and has proved to be accurate in identifying non-infected animals, for false negative reactions are extremely rare. However, false positive reactions are not uncommon, and a positive slide test should always be followed by additional examination. Several laboratories offer diagnostic assistance; however, there is no standardized procedure, and interpretation of tube agglutination test results varies.* Serum samples must be clear and uncontaminated. It is not possible to intrepret agglutination test results on sera from dogs that have received antibiotic treatment for brucellosis, unless an interval of at least four weeks has elapsed since cessation of treatment. One test requires incubation of serum dilutions and antigen for 48 hours at 52° C; another test uses 2-mercaptoethanol. The latter gives slightly lower titers (about twofold), but non-specific reactions are reduced. Recently, an immunodiffusion test using a *B. canis* cell wall antigen has been found to be particularly useful in detecting non-specific reactions (cross-reacting antibodies) that confound the serodiagnosis of canine brucellosis.

Serologic evidence of infection (generally indicated by tube agglutination test titers in excess of 1:200 or 2-mercaptoethanol titers in excess of 1:100) should always be followed by attempts to isolate the organism by blood cultures or culture of lymph node or bone marrow biopsy specimens. Because of the serious prognosis, especially in dogs used for breeding purposes, all available aids should be employed before a diagnosis is confirmed.

Treatment

There is no certain treatment, although some success has been achieved experimentally. Evaluation of any treatment regimen must be followed by periodic bacteriologic and serologic tests. Early apparent success in treating the

---

*The Diagnostic Laboratory, New York State College of Veterinary Medicine, Ithaca, New York 14853, offers a *B. canis* diagnostic service. Diagnostic assistance also may be obtained from the Veterinary Services Diagnostic Laboratory, USDA, Ames, Iowa 50010.

disease has proved disappointing, even though a period of abacteremia may have occurred for a few weeks after cessation of a course of antibiotic therapy. The goal of treatment is to eliminate the organism from the infected animal — a difficult task for all *Brucella* infections. Treatment may be considered in cases in which it is made clear to the owner that the procedure is expensive in both cost and time and that success cannot be assured. Follow-up blood cultures and serologic tests are essential. These should be performed six to eight weeks after cessation of any treatment.

Several treatment schedules have been tried, and most have been unsuccessful; however, the following have been claimed to be successful in some instances:

1. Tetracycline hydrochloride given orally (t.i.d.) for three weeks at 60 mg/kg body weight/day. Treatment is then discontinued for three to four weeks. Following this, a second course of tetracycline hydrochloride is given, together with streptomycin 20 mg/kg, b.i.d.).

2. Minocycline hydrochloride given orally (b.i.d.) for 14 days at 50 mg/kg body weight/day. Simultaneous IM administration of astreptomycin (20 mg/kg/day, b.i.d.) is given for the first seven days and then discontinued. This treatment resulted in complete clearance of *B. canis* from the tissues of 17 of 21 treated animals.

Only intensive treatment schedules such as those just described have proved successful. Additional trials using newer antibiotics found to be inhibitory for *B. canis* in *in vitro* tests are under study. Eradication of organisms from the prostate tissue of infected males generally has been unsuccessful.

Control

Control and prophylactic measures should include the use of serum agglutination tests, blood cultures, isolation and removal of infected animals, good sanitation, and common sense.

All females that have aborted or failed to conceive after successive matings and males with genital disease should be considered as possibly infected. Such dogs should be isolated immediately, and a serum sample should be taken and tested by the slide or tube agglutination test. Blood should be cultured. Dogs with positive blood cultures in a breeding kennel should be destroyed. Treatment may be considered for valuable pets and working dogs; however, owners should be advised of the cost and the uncertain outcome. Control within a breeding kennel consists of serologic testing and, if possible, blood cultures, with elimination of all positive animals. Repeated tests at monthly intervals should be performed on all dogs in a colony that has infected animals. Animals found to be positive should be removed, and at least three negative monthly tests should be obtained on all dogs before a kennel can be considered negative. All dogs introduced into a kennel, especially if they are to be used for breeding, should be maintained in separate quarters until at least two negative tests, done at monthly intervals, are obtained. The entire kennel should be cleaned and disinfected daily. Roccal® (Winthrop) solution and Wescodyne® (West Chemical) have proved to be bactericidal. Animal handlers should wear disposable gloves. Hands should be rinsed in disinfectant before each animal is examined for heat. Animals with titers that arouse suspicion should not be introduced into a kennel unless repeated tests indicate non-specific agglutinins.

Bacterins are not available for prophylaxis.

PUBLIC HEALTH ASPECTS

Human infections have been observed. At the present time, 16 human cases have been reported. Six were laboratory workers. All have been relatively mild, and infected individuals responded well to tetracycline therapy. Headache, sore throat, fatigue, enlarged regional lymph nodes without splenomegaly, and mild fever were the principal signs. The owners of infected dogs should be informed of the public health risk but should not be alarmed since man, like other non-canine species, appears to be relatively resistant.

SUPPLEMENTAL READING

Carmichael, L.E., and Kenney, R.M.: Canine brucellosis: The clinical disease and immune response. J. Am. Vet. Med. Assoc., 156:1726–1734, 1970.
Flores-Castro, R., and Carmichael, L.E.: Canine brucellosis: Current status of methods for diagnosis and treatment. Gaines Veterinary Symposium, 27:17–24, 1978.
Fredrickson, L.E., and Barton, C.E.: A serologic survey for canine brucellosis in a metropolitan area. J. Am. Vet. Med. Assoc., 165:987–989, 1974.
Moore, J.A., and Gupta, B.N.: Epizootiology, diagnosis, and control of Brucella canis. J. Am. Vet. Med. Assoc., 156:1737–1740, 1970.
Pickerill, P.A., and Carmichael, L.E.: Canine brucellosis: Control programs in commercial kennels and effects on reproduction. J. Am. Vet. Med. Assoc., 160:1607–1615, 1972.

FELINE SALMONELLOSIS

JAMES G. FOX, D.V.M.
Cambridge, Massachusetts

Salmonella, a ubiquitous organism, is found in both wild and domestic animals, including pet cats and dogs. Until recently, the disease was diagnosed infrequently in cats, and only scattered reports of the disease were documented in the literature. However, it is now recognized that infections, including nosocomial infections, caused by *Salmonella* can occur in cats stressed by hospitalization, concurrent disease, or surgery. There has been a dramatic increase in the number of animal shelters and pounds that care for stray pets and pets placed there for adoption. In these facilities animals may become carriers of *Salmonella* through contact with infected animals.

ETIOLOGIC AGENT

Salmonella, a gram-negative organism of the family Enterobacteriaceae, can be isolated on selective enteric media from infected tissues, feces, and oral and conjunctival membranes.

Investigations of the incidence of salmonellosis in cats have been conducted infrequently, although incidences ranging from 0.5 to 13.6 percent have been reported in the U.S. and other countries (Fox and Beaucage; Borland). Although there are approximately 1200 serotypes of *Salmonella, S. typhimurium* is the serotype usually isolated from cats with clinical disease, as well as from asymptomatic carriers (Timoney, 1976; Fox and Beaucage). Other serotypes that have been isolated include *S. arizonae, S. derby, S. anatum, S. enteritidis, S. bredeney, S. cholerae-suis, S. paratyphi, S. newport,* and *S. oranienburg* (Wilkinson).

TRANSMISSION

The mode of transmission is usually ingestion of the organism in food contaminated by infected feces. Pet animal foods may also contain *Salmonella* organisms (Galton, et al.; Thornton). Cats can also be infected by grooming a haircoat contaminated with *Salmonella*. Infection via the conjunctival route is also possible (Fox and Gallus).

In nosocomial infections the outbreak may be initiated by a cat with active infection, a carrier animal shedding the organism, or a clinical infection in a previously normal carrier animal subjected to the stress of hospitalization or surgery. Contaminated caging, or water and food dishes can serve as a nidus for spread of the infection. Because of the highly contagious nature of the infection, strict attention must be focused on disinfection of the premises and on the personal hygiene of employees so as to preclude spread of the disease when cats are housed in a hospital environment. Clinically ill cats or cats that are transient carriers of *Salmonella* without clinical signs of disease may serve as primary sources of infection to man.

CLINICAL SYNDROME

The disease occurs most frequently in kittens and in cats less than one year old (Buxton). The endotoxins produced by *Salmonella* organisms are responsible for the clinical alterations and laboratory changes found in infected animals (Schalm, et al.). The typical presenting clinical signs are those of acute gastroenteritis, manifested by diarrhea and vomiting. Accompanying signs can include dehydration, moderately elevated temperature, partial to complete anorexia, pale mucous membranes, and malaise. Conjunctivitis and abortion can also be primary signs associated with salmonellosis (Fox and Gallus; Hemsley). In a recent nosocomial outbreak in cats housed at a veterinary hospital, mortality was 61 percent (13 of 21 cats) (Timoney, et al.).

The hemogram from an acutely ill cat can include a lowered white blood cell count with marked neutropenia and lymphopenia. Cats with an acute septicemia can also have thrombocytopenia and a non-regenerative anemia (Krum, et al.). Serum protein levels may be decreased to levels as low as 3.5 gm/dl.

The vaccination history, a careful examination of the hemogram, and a thorough bacteriologic examination of rectal cultures can help in differentiating feline salmonellosis from feline distemper and enterocolitis due to *Escherichia coli*. The neutropenia seen with salmonellosis and coliform infections is not as profound as that seen in feline viral panleukopenia.

NECROPSY FINDINGS

The gross and microscopic findings are compatible with those described in other animals with *Salmonella* infections. If the cat has had a protracted clinical illness, it will be emaciated and dehydrated. The mucosa of the small intestine may be congested or have petechial hemorrhages, and mucus and occasionally blood may be present in the liquid intestinal contents. The liver, spleen, and mesenteric lymph nodes may contain areas of necrosis, which can be detected grossly as yellowish-white foci of varying size. Although not pathognomonic, the necrotic foci (the so-called "paratyphoid nodules") are often visible on the surface or in cut sections of the liver.

Thrombosis of abdominal vessels is sometimes encountered and may be consistent with the syndrome of disseminated intravascular coagulation. In cases of septicemia ecchymoses and petechiae can be noted on the visceral and parietal pleura, peritoneum, endocardium, epicardium, and meninges.

TREATMENT

It is important not only to recognize the clinical syndrome of feline salmonellosis but also to isolate, identify, and establish antibiotic sensitivities to the *Salmonella* serotype causing the disease. It is common for *Salmonella* isolates from cats to be resistant to a number of the antibiotics routinely used in veterinary medicine. The serotypes recovered from clinically ill or asymptomatic cats have been resistant to streptomycin, ampicillin, cephaloridine, tetracycline, neomycin, and kanamycin (Timoney, 1976; Beaucage and Fox). Fortunately, chloramphenicol resistance is not common, and at present it is the drug of choice for either asymptomatic or clinical infection in cats. *Salmonella* isolates from cats are often capable of transferring part or all of the antibiotic resistance pattern present on plasmids to susceptible *E. coli* (Beaucage and Fox). Resistance to chloramphenicol in species other than *S. typhi* has been rare in North America until recently. However, resistance to chloramphenicol of *Salmonella* recovered from animals and man has been reported increasingly in the last several years. (Grant, et al.; Timoney, 1978). The improper selection and utilization of an antibiotic will limit the success of clinical treatment and may also increase the amount, duration, and antibiotic resistance pattern of shedding *Salmonella* organisms (Wilcock and Olander; Aserkoff and Bennett).

Careful attention to the management of fluid and electrolyte balance will aid in successful recovery of clinically affected cats. Of particular importance is the treatment of the hypoglycemia that can result from endotoxemia. To counteract intestinal vasoconstriction, acepromazine (1 mg/kg) has been recommended (Timoney, et al.). Glucocorticoids and, in selected cases, blood therapy are also recommended for treatment of endotoxic shock. Elimination of stress, treatment of concurrent diseases, and supportive therapy with nutrients and vitamins are also essential.

SUPPLEMENTAL READING

Aserkoff, B., and Bennett J.V.: Effect of antibiotic therapy in acute salmonellosis on the fecal excretion of salmonellae. N. Engl. J. Med., 281:636–640, 1969.

Beaucage, C.M., and Fox, J.G.: Transmissible antibiotic resistance in Salmonella isolated from random-source cats purchased for use in research. Am. J. Vet. Res., 40:849–851, 1979.

Borland, E.C.: Salmonella infection in dogs, cats, tortoises, and terrapins. Vet. Rec., 96:401–402, 1975.

Buxton, A.: Salmonellosis in animals — A review. Commonwealth Agricultural Bureaux, Farnham Royal, Bucks., England, 101:48–49, 1957.

Fox, J.G., and Beaucage, C.M.: The incidence of Salmonella in random-source cats purchased for use in research. J. Infect. Dis. 139:362–365, 1979.

Fox, J.G., and Gallus, C.M.: Salmonella-associated conjunctivitis in a cat. J. Am. Vet. Med. Assoc., 171:845–847, 1977.

Galton, M.M., Harless, M., and Hardy, A.V.: Salmonella isolations from dehydrated dog meals. J. Am. Vet. Med. Assoc., 126:57–58, 1955.

Grant, R.B., Bannatyne, R.M., and Shapiey, A.J.: Resistance to chloramphenicol and ampicillin of Salmonella typhimurium in Ontario, Canada. J. Infect. Dis., 134:354–361, 1976.

Hemsley, L.A.: Abortion in two cats, with the isolation of Salmonella choleraesuis from one case. Vet Rec., 68:152, 1956.

Krum, S.H., Stevens, D.R., and Hirsh, D.C.: Salmonella arizonae bacteremia in a cat. J. Am. Vet. Med. Assoc., 170:42–44, 1977.

Schalm, O.W., Jain, N.C., and Carroll, E.J.: Veterinary Hematology.Philadelphia, Lea & Febiger, 1975, pp. 524–526.

Thornton, H.: The public health danger of unsanitized foods. Vet. Rec., 91:430–432, 1972.

Timoney, J.F.: Feline salmonellosis. Vet. Clin. North Am., 6:395–398, 1976.

Timoney, J.G.: The epidemiology and genetics of antibiotic resistance of Salmonella typhimurium isolated from diseased animals in New York. J. Infect. Dis., 137:67–73, 1978.

Timoney, J.F., Niebert, H.C., and Scott, F.W.: Feline salmonellosis. A nosocomial outbreak and experimental studies. Cornell Vet., 68:211–219, 1975.

Wilcock, B., and Olander, H.: Influence of oral antibiotic feeding on the duration and severity of clinical disease, growth performance, and pattern of shedding in swine inoculated with Salmonella typhimurium. J. Am. Vet. Med. Assoc., 172:472–477, 1978.

Wilkinson, G.T.: Diseases of the Cat. Oxford, England, Pergamon Press, 1966, p. 275.

TOXOPLASMOSIS — FELINE INFECTIONS AND THEIR ZOONOTIC POTENTIAL

RICHARD H. JACOBSON, Ph.D.
Ithaca, New York

Although the prevalence of toxoplasmosis among humans has probably not changed significantly during the last several years, an increased awareness and concern about the disease has been precipitated by the discovery that members of the cat family can serve as a source of human infection. It is estimated that approximately 50 percent of the human population in the United States harbors the asymptomatic chronic form of *Toxoplasma gondii*. The disease is important because it is responsible for over 3000 congenitally infected infants each year, is known to become symptomatic and often lethal in immunosuppressed patients, and is responsible for lymphadenopathy that is easily confused with Hodgkin's disease. For these reasons, veterinarians are frequently asked to clarify the role cats play in human toxoplasmosis.

In addition to humans, this coccidian parasite infects virtually all species of warm-blooded animals throughout the world. Variable seroprevalence rates of from 20 percent to greater than 80 percent have been reported in surveys of toxoplasmosis in domestic animals. These serologic studies and a large volume of necropsy data indicate that *T. gondii* ranks as one of the few zoonotic infectious agents that are endemic in a wide variety of birds and mammals. The wide host range of *T. gondii*, coupled with high prevalence rates and the ability of this agent to localize in a variety of host tissues, compels one to consider toxoplasmosis in the differential diagnosis of several conditions having veterinary medical importance.

In order to evaluate the clinical manifestations of toxoplasmosis and to prescribe preventive and control measures for the disease, it is essential to understand fully the life cycle of the causative organism.

LIFE CYCLE

The life cycle of *T. gondii* consists of two phases, the enteroepithelial phase and the systemic, or generalized, phase (Fig. 1). In members of the cat family, the only known definitive hosts of *T. gondii*, asexual and sexual stages occur in the intestinal mucosa (enteroepithelial phase of infection) and result in oocyst formation. Concurrently, other asexual stages of the organism are spread hematogenously or via the lymphatics and are responsible for the generalized or systemic form of toxoplasmosis; these stages localize in a variety of tissues of the intermediate host. It is this more familiar form of the disease that occurs in humans and many other host species in addition to felids. Thus, cats are the only definitive host but also serve, along with many other species, as intermediate hosts.

ENTEROEPITHELIAL PHASE OF INFECTION

The coccidial nature of *T. gondii* is reflected in the enteroepithelial phase of infection, which results in production of oocysts that have typical isosporan morphologic characteristics. Oocyst production is probably initiated most frequently in cats by their ingestion of intermediate host tissue that contains infective zoites; cats can also become infected by accidental ingestion of sporulated (infective) oocysts from fecal sources.

Oocyst production commences about 5 days after ingestion of tissue cysts or 20 days after ingestion of sporulated oocysts. Oocyst production lasts approximately 14 days and can result in shedding of millions of oocysts in a single stool. The cessation of oocyst production is generally concurrent with development of immunity to *T. gondii*.

GENERALIZED TOXOPLASMOSIS

While the process of oocyst production is occurring, other forms of *T. gondii* concurrently undergo asexual reproduction and either localize in the intestinal mucosa or are spread to other organs of the cat. Similarly, ingestion of tissue cysts or sporulated oocysts by many species of mammals (including humans) and birds results in release of zoites (sporozoites from oocysts and specialized trophozoites from cysts), which spread systemically to all organs. In non-immune hosts, the zoites may proliferate rapidly and result in acute infection. Such tachyzoites (rapidly proliferating zoites) repro-

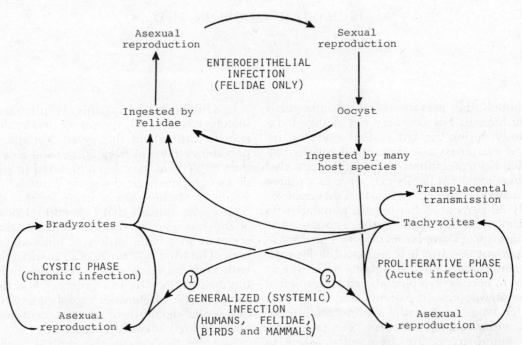

Figure 1. Life cycle of *Toxoplasma gondii.* (*1*) Tachyzoites encyst as bradyzoites concurrent with development of immunity. (*2*) Upon ingestion of tissues containing cysts, proliferation of *T. gondii* occurs. If immunity wanes or is depleted by immunosuppressive agents, a chronic latent infection may enter the proliferative phase.

duce asexually until they rupture the host cell; they then either infect neighboring cells or are carried to other tissues, where the process is repeated. As immunity to *T. gondii* develops, the organisms enter a resting stage and become encysted, particularly in the brain, heart muscle, and skeletal muscle. These encysted bradyzoites (slowly dividing zoites) are long-lived organisms of chronic infections and also are the highly infective form of *Toxoplasma* for hosts ingesting such cyst-laden tissue.

CLINICAL MANIFESTATIONS OF DISEASE

ASYMPTOMATIC AND CHRONIC TOXOPLASMOSIS

Toxoplasmosis in cats is usually asymptomatic, resulting in oocyst production, development of few focal necrotic lesions in varying extraintestinal sites, and encystment of viable bradyzoites. Acute disease with clinical manifestations is rare in felids. When it occurs, the enteroepithelial phase of the disease may be accompanied, albeit infrequently, by a mucoid or sanguineous diarrhea.

The most important manifestations of acute feline toxoplasmosis are fever, interstitial and alveolar pneumonia accompanied by dyspnea, hepatitis and associated bilirubinemia, adenitis (mainly of mesenteric lymph nodes), and sometimes myositis and myocarditis. Although the disease can be fatal, it more frequently leads to an unremarkable recovery that is associated with development of a strong specific immunity.

In subacute and chronic infections leukopenia, anemia, retinochoroiditis, iritis, and encephalitis may appear. Oocyst shedding has usually ceased by the time these signs appear; tissue cysts containing viable and persistent bradyzoites have also developed. Periodically cysts rupture, releasing bradyzoites that rapidly elicit a hypersensitivity response that leads to tissue necrosis. These lesions occur most frequently in the brain, retina, and heart.

Intestinal smooth muscle granulomata are occasionally seen in older cats experiencing recurrent toxoplasmosis. This condition may result in intestinal obstruction and has been attributed to a decline in immunity associated with aging.

THE ROLE OF IMMUNITY

Immunity plays a crucial role in the regulation of toxoplasmosis. As indicated previously, cessation of oocyst production by cats is concur-

rent with development of immunity to *T. gondii*. The containment of chronic infection and reinfection is also a function of the immune response. Once immunity to an initial infection develops and oocyst shedding has ceased, cats normally do not show evidence of oocyst recrudescence and are usually refractory to a challenge *T. gondii* infection. In some isolated instances, however, a second infection may result in production of a few oocysts over an abbreviated patent period. Additionally, immunosuppressive factors may allow oocyst recrudescence of a primary infection. When immunity is severely depressed as a consequence of immunosuppressive therapy or when aged animals lose immunocompetence, bradyzoites of a chronic latent infection may be released from cysts and enter a rapid proliferative phase as tachyzoites. Fulminant myocarditis and retinochoroiditis or fatal encephalitis or pneumonia may then occur.

Although reports of peracute toxoplasmosis in immunocompromised hosts relate principally to human cases, similar veterinary clinical problems should be expected as a result of the current increased usage of corticosteroid therapy in veterinary medicine.

TRANSMISSION AND PREVENTION

Toxoplasmosis is transmitted principally by carnivorism, fecal contamination, and the transplacental route. It is generally accepted that cats and other non-human carnivores are probably infected most frequently by ingestion of mammals, birds, or other raw meat containing *T. gondii* cysts. Cyst-bearing reservoir hosts apparently can remain infected and thus are capable of transmitting the disease throughout their lifetime. Epidemiologic evidence indicates that human infection also occurs by ingestion of raw or grossly undercooked meat.

Prevention of such infections is achieved by cooking meat to an internal temperature of at least 66°C, which kills cysts. Although one report indicates that cysts are killed at −20°C, others suggest that freezing is not a reliable means of killing *T. gondii* tissue cysts. Restricting cats from access to birds and rodents and offering them only cooked meat or commercially prepared canned or dry food should preclude transmission of toxoplasmosis by carnivorism.

Another important means of transmission of toxoplasmosis to any host is the ingestion of sporulated (infective) oocysts originating from feline feces. Unsporulated oocysts deposited at the time of defecation are not infective; however, sporulation occurs rapidly under optimal conditions, and oocysts can become infective in one to five days. Oocysts are highly resistant to environmental extremes and thus can remain infective in moist soil for more than a year. Since millions of oocysts may be present in one stool, it is obvious that sand boxes, flower beds, gardens, and other areas of loose soil where cats defecate frequently are subject to gross contamination with oocysts. Another means of infection by oocysts is suggested by a recent outbreak of toxoplasmosis that occurred in people who frequented a riding stable. The epidemiologic data strongly suggest that inhalation of dust particles carrying oocysts or of aerosolized oocysts alone was the method of transmission.

Prevention of toxoplasmosis acquired via oocysts obviously requires eliminating contact with contaminated soil, covering sandboxes to preclude fecal contamination by cats, and washing hands thoroughly after possible oocyst exposure. Daily disposal of feces from cat litter boxes will eliminate this potential source of infection, since oocysts would be destroyed before sporulation is complete. However, if litter boxes are suspected to contain infective oocysts, boiling water or dry heat (55°C for 30 minutes) is an effective disinfectant.

Transplacental transmission of toxoplasmosis is important in humans and sheep but has not been reported in cats. Because of the zoonotic importance of feline toxoplasmosis and its relationship to pregnant women, it is important to know the conditions under which a human fetus is susceptible to infection. Twenty-five to 45 percent of women of child-bearing age (20 to 39 years of age) in the United States have chronic asymptomatic toxoplasmosis and are immune to reinfection. A chronically infected woman who becomes pregnant will deliver a child that is *not* infected; also, there is no proof that spontaneous abortion occurs in women chronically infected with toxoplasmosis. However, toxoplasmosis acquired during pregnancy by women serologically negative for toxoplasmosis may result in an infected fetus (two to six cases per 1000 pregnancies per year in the U.S.). To endanger the fetus, initial *T. gondii* infection must occur at the time of or after conception.

These observations are the basis for a rational approach to cat management in a household occupied by a pregnant woman or one who contemplates pregnancy: (1) Cats should be tested serologically. If titers are significant, the animal is most likely immune and not passing oocysts and thus would most probably not be a source of human infection. If cats are seronegative, they are generally susceptible to infection and are potential oocyst shedders. (2) Even if the cat is negative on fecal analysis and is serologically positive for *T. gondii* (thus, most likely immune), a possibility exists for recrudescence of oocyst shedding. Therefore, pregnant women should not handle cat litter boxes. The litter box should be changed daily by some other person to eliminate any potential for inadvertent infection. (3) Cats should be prevented from exposure to *T. gondii* by precluding their access to birds, small mammals, and uncooked meat. (4) We also suggest that direct contact with cats by pregnant women be limited. It is theoretically possible for an acutely infected cat that is experiencing *Toxoplasma*-induced pneumonitis to aerosolize tachyzoites via sneezing. Tachyzoites are infective to humans. Additionally, free-roaming cats may be contaminated externally with oocysts from other infected cats that use common defecation sites. Human hand-to-mouth infection following petting of such animals is possible. (5) Hands should be washed after handling the animal.

Transmission of *T. gondii* was clarified considerably by the discovery of *Toxoplasma* oocysts in feline feces. However, transmission is still not fully understood. Various reports indicate that cats can be infected by cockroaches that harbor oocysts ingested from feces. Flies are known to carry oocysts mechanically. Trophozoites of *T. gondii* have been isolated in eggs, milk and, most recently, the semen of rams. Aerosolization of oocysts on dust particles must now be considered a potential hazard. Clearly, more work is required to define the role of birds and mammals in the transmission of toxoplasmosis.

DIAGNOSIS

Because the clinical picture for toxoplasmosis is variable and not necessarily pathognomonic, identification of oocysts in cat feces, rising antibody titers, and isolation of the organisms histologically or by animal inoculation are useful adjuncts to clinical diagnosis.

Oocyst Identification

Early in infections, oocysts can be detected in cat feces before serum antibody appears. Subjection of feces to a typical parasitologic flotation technique allows for concentration of oocysts and microscopic examination of the preparation. Oocysts of *T. gondii* are very small, measuring only $12 \times 10\ \mu$, and must be distinguished from *Isospora rivolta* ($25 \times 20\ \mu$) and *I. felis* ($40 \times 30\ \mu$).

SEROLOGY

Serodiagnosis of feline toxoplasmosis is presumptive only when a significant (fourfold) rise in titer occurs in serum samples drawn at two to three week intervals. Because antibodies to *T. gondii* appear relatively slowly in cats and do not rise to levels comparable with those of man and other animals, it is not advisable to attempt correlation of single titers with the degree of clinical illness. For instance, a negative titer may not indicate a lack of infection in a clinically ill cat but may reflect an early acute infection that will be confirmed upon serologic retesting two to three weeks hence. Additionally, retinochoroiditis is associated with a high and stable antibody titer. Conversely, we have observed cats that have remained at relatively high titers (1:2048 on the indirect hemagglutination assay) for over three months with no evidence of associated clinical disease.

Thus, antibody titers indicate infection but may not necessarily correlate with clinical illness. The presence of significant antibody titers, however, does suggest strongly that the cat is immune; the lack of antibodies indicates that the cat is susceptible to infection and associated oocyst shedding.

ISOLATION OF T. GONDII

Suspected tissue can be inoculated intraperitoneally into mice, which are then observed for development of tachyzoites or serum antibody titers to *T. gondii*. Alternatively, histologic examination may reveal cysts or tachyzoites of chronic or acute infections, respectively.

TREATMENT

Because *T. gondii* cannot utilize exogenous folinic acid and must synthesize its own, the organism differs from mammals, which are able to incorporate folinic acid directly from exogenous sources. Thus, inhibitors of the folic acid biosynthetic pathway, pyrimethamine (Daraprim) and sulfadiazine, act synergistically against *T. gondii*, while toxic side effects are alleviated by administration of folinic acid (leucovorin). The recommended treatment regimen is to administer the drugs in food as follows: sulfadiazine (four to six divided doses daily) at 60 mg/kg/day and pyrimethamine (one dose daily) at 0.5 mg/kg/day. Because these drugs are not toxoplasmacidal but rather are inhibitory, the rationale is to treat the animal until its immune response is capable of controlling the disease. This requires that treatment be started as soon as possible after symptoms appear and be continued for about two weeks even if symptoms subside. If clinical improvement is not detected in two or three days, the diagnosis of toxoplasmosis is doubtful.

An antagonist may be required to prevent toxic side effects. Folinic acid (1 mg/kg/day) can be given concurrent with treatment or when the WBC or platelet level drops to 25 to 50 percent of normal value. It is also advisable to administer baker's yeast (100 mg/kg/day). Because the folinic acid inhibitors are toxic to fetuses, pregnant animals should always be given the antagonists. If animals are to be given pharmacologic doses of corticosteroids, immunity may wane, and a relapse of latent toxoplasmosis may occur. Thus, prophylactic chemotherapy should be considered in such cases.

SUPPLEMENTAL READING

Frenkel, J.K.: Toxoplasmosis: Parasite life cycle, pathology, and immunology. In Hammond, D.M., and Long, P.L. (eds.): *The Coccidia: Eimeria, Isosopora, Toxoplasma, and Related Genera.* Baltimore, University Park Press, 1973, pp. 343–410.

Frenkel, J.K.: Toxoplasmosis in cats: Diagnosis, treatment and prevention. Comp. Immunol. Microbiol. Infect. Dis., *1*:15–20, 1978.

Krick, J.A., and Remington, J.S.: Toxoplasmosis in the adult. N. Engl. J. Med., *298*:550–553, 1978.

Turner, G.V.S.: Toxoplasmosis as a public health hazard. J. S. Afr. Vet. Assoc., *47*:227–231, 1976.

FELINE CYTAUXZOONOSIS

STEPHEN R. WIGHTMAN, D.V.M.

Greenfield, Indiana

Feline cytauxzoonosis has recently been recognized as an acute, uniformly fatal parasitic disease of domestic cats. The etiologic agent manifests itself as an intraerythrocytic piroplasm (blood phase) and as a schizont developing in reticuloendothelial (RE) cells in many organs (tissue phase). Following the original report of the disease in Missouri and Arkansas, several additional cases have been identified in Texas, Florida, and Georgia. For the most part, cytauxzoonosis has been seen in cats that are free to roam in rural, heavily wooded areas. Cytauxzoonosis had previously been diagnosed only in ungulates in Africa; however, there is as yet no evidence to indicate that the feline disease represents an introduction of an exotic animal disease.

ETIOLOGIC AGENT AND HOST RANGE

There remains some question as to the etiology of cytauxzoonosis of cats. Based on the morphologic appearance of the blood and tissue phases of the agent, Wagner (1976) suggested that the causative agent is a protozoan parasite resembling *Cytauxzoon* sp. (family Theileriidae). He declined to assign the parasite to that genus, however, preferring to await further clarification of both the feline disease and the taxonomy of the Theileriidae. The classification of the piroplasms has been the subject of repeated revision. It is possible that in the next few years the genus *Cytauxzoon* will be incorporated into the genus *Theileria*. Members of the genus *Cytauxzoon* are characterized as being relatively small, round to ovoid parasites with minimal internal structure; they undergo schizogony in RE cells and then invade erythrocytes, where they appear to reproduce by binary and cruciform division.

Since feline cytauxzoonosis is an infrequently seen disease and since all known infected cats have succumbed to the infection following a short course of illness, it seems probable that another animal may be involved in the epizootiology of the condition. Attempts to infect numerous domestic, laboratory, and wildlife species with *Cytauxzoon* have, with one exception, been unsuccessful. Cytauxzoonosis has been experimentally transmitted to the bobcat, *Lynx*

rufus. Studies conducted on two animals resulted in a fatal infection typical of that seen naturally in domestic cats in one bobcat and a non-fatal parasitemic state in the other. It has not been determined whether the bobcat is a biologic reservoir of cytauxzoonosis in nature.

TRANSMISSION

The mechanism of natural transmission is unknown. Experimentally, cytauxzoonosis can easily be transmitted by parenteral injection of blood or tissue homogenates from an infected cat. Direct contact or oral gavage are ineffectual. Other members of the Theileriidae have been shown to be transmitted by Ixodid ticks and, although preliminary attempts to transmit feline cytauxzoonosis by ticks have failed, an arthropod vector remains the most logical mechanism of transmission.

CLINICAL SIGNS

The first clinical signs observed in naturally occurring cases of cytauxzoonosis are lassitude and loss of appetite. The body temperature increases markedly over a period of three to six days, reaching a peak of 105 to 106° F or more. During this period, depression becomes profound and anorexia complete. Anemia, icterus, and dehydration develop rapidly during the febrile period. Dyspnea is usually seen late in the course of illness. Body temperature begins a precipitous decline about one day before death. Total duration of illness seldom exceeds one week. Because of the non-specific nature of the early signs and the rapid course of illness, many cats are moribund or dead by the time they are presented to the veterinarian.

DIAGNOSIS

In enzootic areas cytauxzoonosis should be considered in the differential diagnosis when a cat shows anemia or icterus and high fever that has developed acutely. Hemograms and blood chemistry profiles will reflect the clinical picture but will not provide additional diagnostic information. Diagnosis is made by observing the piroplasms in Wright- or Giemsa-stained thin blood smears. The organisms appear in erythrocytes as rounded "signet ring" bodies 1 to 1.5 μ in diameter or as bipolar oval "safety pin" forms measuring 1 by 2 μ. Both forms are seen in the same animal; however, the "signet ring" form is predominant. The cytoplasm of the organism stains light blue, whereas the nucleus is dark red to purple. Parasite numbers vary greatly among individual cats and with the stage of disease. Piroplasms first appear in the erythrocytes at, or shortly after, the onset of fever; their numbers increase slowly during the febrile period and then dramatically in the final day before death. Near the time of death, 25 percent or more of the erythrocytes may contain piroplasms. A single erythrocyte usually contains a solitary piroplasm; however, pairs and tetrads are sometimes encountered.

Further confirmation of cytauxzoonosis is obtained by necropsy and histopathologic evaluation. Veins in the abdominal cavity are distended with blood; the spleen is darkened and enlarged; the lungs show diffuse reddening and multiple petechial hemorrhages; and lymph nodes are enlarged, reddened, and edematous. Additional necropsy findings may include petechial hemorrhages on most internal organs and small amounts of fluid in the peritoneal, pleural, and pericardial cavities. The characteristic histologic lesion is the accumulation of large numbers of hypertrophic, parasitized RE cells lining the lumina of veins and venous channels in virtually all organs. Spleen, lungs, and lymph nodes are most heavily parasitized

and are the organs of choice for histopathologic evaluation.

TREATMENT AND CONTROL

Attempts to treat cats with cytauxzoonosis have failed. Tetracyclines have been used to arrest theilerial infections, but they are ineffective once a parasitemia is manifest. Rapid multiplication of the parasites causes mechanical obstruction of blood flow, especially through the lungs. Byproducts of the parasites' metabolic activity are presumed to be toxic, pyrogenic, and vasoactive. The piroplasms may be responsible for erythrocyte lysis and erythrophagocytosis. Infected cats die from a shock-like state, the inciting cause of which (the schizont) is reproducing logarithmically and cannot be removed. Supportive therapy may prolong the course of illness but will not effect a cure.

It is reasonable to assume that a conscientiously applied ectoparasite control program would be beneficial in reducing the incidence of cytauxzoonosis in enzootic areas.

SUPPLEMENTAL READING

Barnett, S.F.: Theileria. In Kreier, J.P.: *Parasitic Protozoa*, vol. 4. New York, Academic Press, 1977, pp. 77–113.
Bendele, R.A., Schwartz, W.L., and Jones, L.P.: Cytauxzoonosis-like disease in Texas cats. Southwest Vet., 29:244–246, 1976.
Wagner, J.E.: A fatal cytauxzoonosis-like disease in cats. J. Am. Vet. Med. Assoc., 168:585–588, 1976.
Wightman, S.R., Kier, A.B., and Wagner, J.E.: Feline cytauxzoonosis: Clinical features of a newly described blood parasite disease. Feline Pract., 7:23–28, 1977.

KITTEN MORTALITY COMPLEX

FREDRIC W. SCOTT, D.V.M.
Ithaca, New York

Kitten mortality complex (KMC) is an apparently new disease entity that results in unusually high reproductive failure and kitten deaths in catteries and feline breeding colonies. Recent reports describe KMC in more than 35 catteries and three breeding colonies throughout the United States (Norsworthy, 1979; Scott, et al., 1979). Continued inquiries to the Cornell Feline Research Laboratory indicate that nu-

merous breeders are experiencing similar problems. The severity and consistency of the problems clearly indicate that a specific disease complex is occurring throughout the U.S.

The etiology of KMC is not known. However, all catteries and colonies investigated either have lost cats with clinical feline infectious peritonitis (FIP) or have a high incidence of FIP antibody–positive cats. This includes a large breeding colony maintained as a strict barrier facility that is free of all known viral pathogens other than FIP. Studies are in progress to ascertain the possible role of FIP in KMC.

THE DISEASE COMPLEX

The usual complaint by the breeder is a large number of reproductive failures and deaths of young kittens. Queens usually experience repeated problems with subsequent litters for two or three years, although some have losses only in one litter. Owners become concerned and frustrated because of the losses and the uncertainty of the cause. Most are convinced that there is a specific cause and may blame genetics, nutrition, toxic chemicals, or the new respiratory vaccines.

KMC has been reported in several breeds, including Abyssinians, domestic shorthairs, Burmese, Himalayans, Persians, and Siamese. The greatest problem has been in Himalayans, which agrees with a recent breed survey of kitten mortality reported from our laboratory, in which Himalayans had the highest kitten losses (40 percent compared with average mortality of 27.1 percent for all breeds) (Scott, et al., 1978). There appears to be no age incidence, since problems occur in young queens in their first pregnancy and in older, experienced queens that have had several successful litters before encountering problems.

The diets reported were varied and include several commercial diets and home-formulated diets.

The feline leukemia virus (FeLV) status of most problem catteries has been negative, although there have been a few with FeLV-positive cats. Most catteries routinely vaccinate for panleukopenia (FPL), viral rhinotracheitis (FVR), and calicivirus (FCV). Some have used the intranasal respiratory vaccine but most use parenteral vaccines.

The complex can be broken down into several problems:

REPRODUCTIVE FAILURE

Repeat Breeders. Some queens have a history of one or several breedings without apparent conception. Of course, cases of early embryonic death with resorption are not detected, and such queens appear to the owner to be repeat breeders.

Fetal Resorption. Queens may appear to have a normal pregnancy for about four weeks of gestation, when pregnancy is confirmed by palpation. Between four and six weeks queens fail to develop or fill out normally, and pregnancy rechecks at six weeks reveal no evidence of pregnancy. Some queens that abort during the last half of gestation may abort one or more partially resorbed fetuses.

Abortion. Queens may abort during the last half of gestation, most often during the last two weeks. Fetuses may appear in various stages of development and resorption. Some aborted fetuses have been reported to have areas of hemorrhage under the skin, and some queens apparently have passed an unusually large quantity of "blood."

Stillbirths. A frequent complaint is stillbirths, with one or two kittens or the entire litter being born dead. The condition of the stillborn kittens would indicate that death may have occurred either shortly before birth or several days prepartum. A few mummified fetuses have been reported.

Congenital Birth Defects. Although it is not a consistent finding, a few breeders have reported a number of malformed fetuses. The breeders' reports include skull malformations ("open top fontanelles"), schistosomus ("open stomachs"), atresia ani, septal heart defects, and several single-incidence malformations.

KITTEN MORTALITY

Fading Kittens. A common complaint of most breeders is "fading" kittens. Kittens may be born emaciated and weak and die within one or two days. Queens frequently reject these kittens. Kittens may appear healthy for a few days or weeks and then gradually fade, becoming depressed and anorectic and losing weight. Specific signs or lesions, except evidence of emaciation and malnutrition, are usually absent.

Acute Congestive Cardiomyopathy. Several breeders have reported kittens that developed acute attacks of severe dyspnea. These kittens gasp for breath, sometimes become cyanotic, and die within a few hours. Stress, such as transporting the animal to the veterinarian's office, frequently precipitates death. Owners have described the kittens as "suffocating." One veterinarian described several of these kittens as having an extremely anxious appearance as they attempted to breathe. Radiographic examination reveals an enlarged heart and hydrothorax.

Necropsy of these kittens reveals greatly dilated, thin-walled hearts. The thoracic cavities and lungs are usually filled with fluid, and there may be ascites and edema in tissues. Histologic examination of heart muscle reveals acute muscle fiber degeneration and subendocardial fibroelastosis.

Feline Infectious Peritonitis. Several catteries have experienced kitten losses that were diagnosed clinically or histopathologically as FIP. A few cases of typical effusive ("wet") FIP have occurred, but most have been the granulomatous ("dry") form. Histologic lesions are suggestive of FIP and include multifocal necrotizing hepatitis, granulomatous interstitial pneumonia, and non-suppurative meningitis (sometimes with petechial hemorrhages).

DISEASES IN ADULTS

Respiratory Disease. A highly consistent finding in nearly every cattery is chronic mild upper respiratory disease. Sneezing is the most common symptom, but watery ocular and nasal discharges may be present. Signs wax and wane for several weeks. Occasional low-grade fevers have been reported, but cats are usually not seriously ill. The histopathologic findings of mild granulomatous interstitial pneumonia in some fading kittens would indicate lower respiratory disease as well; however, clinical signs of pneumonia have not been reported.

Endometritis. A common complaint is the presence of either bloody or white vaginal discharge in one or more queens. Culture, clinical examination, or necropsy of these queens usually reveals endometritis or pyometra. The bloody vaginal discharge in some queens four to six weeks after breeding may be an indication of abortion rather than metritis. However, these same queens frequently develop metritis later. Forty-four cases occurred in one research colony of 102 queens, and one cattery had 12 cases (41.4 percent of the queens).

Fever Spikes. Adults and older kittens may have intermittent fevers. These usually are low-grade (103 to 104° F), although fevers of 106 to 108° F have been reported. Cats usually do not appear ill, or they may be "a little off."

Acute Congestive Cardiomyopathy and Cardiovascular Disease. In at least two catteries cases of acute congestive cardiomyopathy occurred in adults as well as kittens. Deaths were sudden, with few clinical signs. A few cases of endocarditis and vascular disease, including thrombosis, have been reported.

DISCUSSION

The cause of KMC has not been determined. It would appear to be an infectious agent, probably a virus. In our own breeding colony (a barrier, or SPF, colony) all known viruses other than FIP and endogenous C-type virus were ruled out. In other catteries FIP was present, but no information about the presence of endogenous C-type virus was obtained. Thus, the possibility remains that either or both of these viruses could be the cause. There is also the possibility that an as yet unknown virus or agent could be the primary cause of KMC with FIP virus only an incidental finding. Although the number of FIP antibody–positive catteries in the U.S. is not known, the existence of more than 35 consecutive KMC catteries positive for FIP virus would seem to be significant.

It is obvious from recent studies and antibody assays that FIP virus infection is far more prevalent than previously suspected. We now believe that the initial infection with FIP virus is either a subclinical or mild respiratory disease. After a period of weeks or months, a small percentage of infected cats develop a secondary disease — typical effusive or granulomatous FIP. From the high incidence of FIP antibody–positive cats in catteries, it appears that many cats remain persistently infected and shedders of virus. It is not known whether this virus can be transmitted to offspring *in utero* or only horizontally, by contact after birth.

It is obvious from the serious effects on embryos and fetuses that the etiologic agent of KMC is acting *in utero*. It is also obvious that queens experiencing problems in one litter are prone to repeated problems in subsequent litters, probably carrying the agent of KMC for months or years.

The role of stud cats in KMC is not known. Illnesses in males have not been reported from most catteries. However, a few males have died from cardiomyopathy. One stud had a period of not settling queens during a KMC outbreak. However, it was not ascertained whether the stud was at fault or whether endometritis and early embryonic deaths were the problem.

It has been ascertained that not all cats with cardiomyopathy have positive FIP antibody titers. In fact, most chronic cases of cardiomyopathy in older cats that have been tested have been FIP antibody–negative. It has been suggested that acute congestive cardiomyopathy might be of viral origin, whereas hypertrophic cardiomyopathy was not virus-induced (Tilley and Liu). There have been no reports of the hypertrophic form of cardiomyopathy associated with KMC.

The occurrence of neonatal FIP has been reported previously in the literature (Norsworthy, 1974). Our observations of typical FIP in young neonatal kittens is consistent with this report.

There is little question that KMC is a specific disease complex that is widespread in the U.S.

Only further research will establish conclusively the etiology of this important disease.

SUPPLEMENTAL READING

Norsworthy, G.D.: Neonatal feline infectious peritonitis. Feline Pract., 4:34, 1974.
Norsworthy, G.D.: Kitten mortality complex. Feline Pract., 9:57–60, 1979.

Scott, F.W., Geissinger, C., and Peltz, R.: Kitten mortality survey. Feline Pract., 8:31–34, 1978.
Scott, F.W., Hoshino, Y., and Weiss, R.C.: Feline infectious peritonitis. Feline Information Bulletin (Cornell Feline Research Lab.), No. 4, Oct. 1978.
Scott, F.W., Weiss, R.C., Post, J.E., Gilmartin, J.E., and Hoshino, Y.: Kitten mortality complex (neonatal FIP?). Feline Pract., 9:44–56, 1979.
Tilley, L.P., and Liu, S.K.: Feline cardiology. Feline Pract., 5:32–44, 1975.
Weiss, R.C.: Feline infectious peritonitis: An update. Mod. Vet. Pract., 59:832–836, 1978.

SHIPPING REGULATIONS FOR SMALL ANIMALS

ROBERT W. KIRK, D.V.M.
Ithaca, New York

INTERSTATE REGULATIONS

The regulations regarding the entry of dogs and cats into the various states of the United States and Puerto Rico are summarized in Table 1. The regulations summarized, insofar as they are known, are current to January 1979. No responsibility is accepted for their complete accuracy. For the exact requirements for each state, inquiry should be made to the State Veterinarian in the state of destination.

Under most circumstances, no animal that is affected with or has recently been exposed to any infectious, contagious, or communicable disease or that originates from a rabies-quarantined area shall be shipped or, in any manner, transported or moved into any state until written permission for such entry is first obtained from the State Veterinarian or chief animal health official of the state to which the animal is to be transported.

Common carriers will usually not accept dogs or cats for interstate movement without health certificates; thus, it would seem advisable, even if not specifically required, that such certificates be issued by the accredited practicing veterinarian in the state of origin.

INTERNATIONAL REGULATIONS

Travelers from the United States to foreign countries on vacations and duty assignments frequently desire to take their pets with them. Similarly, people returning from abroad need to make arrangements for the re-entry of their pets and for animals acquired in other countries. For both importations and exportations, there are usually health requirements with which one must comply.

MOVEMENT INTO FOREIGN COUNTRIES

There are no United States regulations governing the movement of dogs and cats to any foreign country. The regulations that must be complied with are those of the receiving country. These regulations are many, varied, and subject to change. If pets are to be moved to any foreign country except Canada, the owner should obtain from the nearest consulate of the country of destination that country's regulations governing the import of pets and procedural instructions, such as the number of copies to be furnished, an indication of whether the health certificate must be validated by the consulate, or whether certified copies of the pedigree or photograph of the pet must accompany the health certificate.

Dogs from the United States may be imported into Canada through any Canadian customs port of entry when accompanied by a certificate signed by a veterinarian licensed in Canada or the United States. The certificate must show

Table 1. *Regulations for Shipping of Small Animals*

STATE OF DESTINATION	RABIES VACCINATION		TYPE (KV)	TIME LIMIT (MLV)	AGE EXEMPTION (MONTHS)	HEALTH CERTIFICATE REQUIRED
	Dogs	Cats				
Alabama	Yes	No	Within 6 mo. of entry		3	X
Alaska	Yes	No	Within 6 mo. of entry		4	X
Arizona	Yes	No	KV (12 mo.); MLV (36 mo.)		4	
Arkansas	Yes	No	Within 12 mo. of entry		3	
California	Yes	No	Current rabies vac.		4	X
Colorado	Yes	No	Within 12 mo. of entry		3	
Connecticut	No	No				X
Delaware	Yes	No			4	X
Florida	Yes	No	Within 6 mo. of entry			X
Georgia	Yes	No	Within 6 mo. of entry		3	
Hawaii	No	No	120 days quarantine			
Idaho	Yes	No	NT (6 mo.); CE (24 mo.)		4	X
Illinois	Yes	No	KV (6 mo.); MLV (12 mo.)		4	X
Indiana	Yes	Yes	Within 12 mo. of entry		3	X
Iowa	Yes	No	KV (12 mo.); MLV (24 mo.)		3	X
Kansas	Yes	No	Within 12 mo. of entry		3	X
Kentucky	Yes	Yes	KV (12 mo.); MLV (24 mo.)		4	X
Louisiana	Yes	No	NT (12 mo.); CE (24 mo.)		2	X
Maine	No	No				X
Maryland	Yes	No	Within 12 mo. of entry		4	X
Massachusetts	Yes	No	Within 12 mo. of entry			X
Michigan	No	No				X
Minnesota	Yes	No	KV (12 mo.); MLV (24 mo.)		6	X
Mississippi	Yes	No	Within 6 mo. of entry		3	X
Missouri	Yes	No	KV (12 mo.); MLV (24 mo.)		4	X
Montana	Yes	No	MLV (24 mo.)		3	X
Nebraska	Yes	No	KV (12 mo.); MLV (24 mo.)		4	X
Nevada	Yes	No	NT (12 mo.); CE (24 mo.)		4	X
New Hampshire	Yes	No	KV (12 mo.); MLV (36 mo.)		3	X
New Jersey	No	No				X
New Mexico	Yes	No	Within 12 mo. of entry		4	X
New York	No	No				X
North Carolina	Yes	No	Within 12 mo. of entry		4	X
North Dakota	Yes	No	Within 36 mo. of entry		4	X
Ohio	Yes	No	KV (12 mo.), CE (36 mo.)		6	X
Oklahoma	Yes	No	NT (12 mo.); MLV (24 mo.)		4	
Oregon	Yes	Yes	KV (6 mo.); MLV (24 mo.)		4	X
Pennsylvania	No	No				X
Puerto Rico	Yes	Yes	Within 6 mo. of entry		2	
Rhode Island	Yes	No	KV (6 mo.); MLV (24 mo.)		4	X
South Carolina	Yes	No	Within 12 mo. of entry		4	X
South Dakota	Yes	Yes	Within 12 mo. of entry		3	X
Tennessee	Yes	No	Within 12 mo. of entry		No exemption	X
Texas	Yes	No	Within 6 mo. of entry		No exemption	X
Utah	Yes	Yes	KV (12 mo.); MLV (24 mo.)		4	X
Vermont	Yes	Yes	MLV (12 mo.)		4	X
Virginia	Yes	No	Within 12 mo. of entry		4	X
Washington	Yes	No	KV (12 mo.); MLV (24 mo.)		4	X
West Virginia	Yes	Yes	Within 12 mo. of entry		6	X
Wisconsin	Yes	No	KV (12 mo.); CE (36 mo.)		6	X
Wyoming	Yes	No	Within 24 mo. of entry		4	X

NT, Nerve tissue; CE, chick embryo; KV, killed vaccine; MLV, modified vaccine.

that the dog has been vaccinated against rabies during the preceding 12 months.

IMPORTATION OR RE-ENTRY OF DOGS INTO THE UNITED STATES

The entry of dogs into the United States from all foreign countries is under the jurisdiction of the Public Health Service of the United States Department of Health, Education, and Welfare.

SUPPLEMENTAL READING

Traveling With Your Pet. New York, American Society for the Prevention of Cruelty to Animals, 1972.

APPENDICES

ROBERT W. KIRK, D.V.M.
Consulting Editor

Tables of Normal Physiological Data: Electrocardiography.......... 1319
Tables for Conversion of Weight to Body-surface Area in
    Square Meters for Dogs...................................... 1320
A Roster of Normal Values for Dogs and Cats 1321
Table of Common Drugs: Approximate Doses 1331

TABLES OF NORMAL PHYSIOLOGICAL DATA

ELECTROCARDIOGRAPHY[*]

It is recognized that normal and abnormal electrocardiographic measurements overlap and that the criteria for the normal electrocardiogram serve only as a guide for the clinician. Deviations from normal in an individual electrocardiogram suggest but are not always diagnostic of heart disease. As additional statistical data become available for the electrocardiograms of dogs of each breed, body type, age and sex, the data herein may require revision and "normal" may be more precisely defined. The *value of serial electrocardiograms* from an individual cannot be overemphasized, since serial changes best demonstrate electrocardiographic abnormalities.

Criteria for the Normal Canine Electrocardiogram[†]

Heart rate—70 to 160 beats per minute for adult dogs; up to 180 beats per minute in toy breeds, and 220 beats per minute for puppies.

Heart rhythm—Normal sinus rhythm; sinus arrhythmia; and wandering sinoatrial pacemaker.

P wave—Up to 0.4 millivolt in amplitude; up to 0.04 second in duration; always positive in leads II and aVF; positive or isoelectric in lead I.

P-R interval—0.06 to 0.13 second duration.

QRS complex—Mean electric axis, frontal plane, 40 to 100 degrees.

Amplitude—Maximum amplitude of R wave 2.5 to 3.0 millivolts in leads II, III, and aVF. Complex positive in leads II, III, and aVF; negative in lead V_{10}.

Duration—To 0.05 second (0.06 second in large breeds).

S-T segment and T wave—S-T segment free of marked coving (repolarization changes).

S-T segment depression not greater than 0.2 millivolt in leads II and III and not greater than 0.3 millivolt in lead CV_6LL.

S-T segment elevation not greater than 0.15 millivolt in leads II and III.

T wave negative in leads V_{10} and T wave positive in CV_5RL (except in the Chihuahua).

T wave amplitude not greater than 25 per cent of amplitude of R wave.

Criteria for the Normal Feline Electrocardiogram[‡]

Heart rate—240 beats per minute maximum.

Heart rhythm—Normal sinus rhythm or, infrequently, sinus arrhythmia.

P wave—Positive in leads II and AVF: may be isoelectric or positive in lead I; should not exceed 0.04 second in duration.

P-R interval—0.04 to 0.10 second duration (inversely related to the heart rate).

QRS complex—More variable than in the canine; the mean electric axis in the frontal plane is often insignificant. Often the QRS complex is nearly isoelectric in all frontal plane limb leads (so-called horizontal heart).

Amplitude—The amplitude of the R wave is usually low; marked amplitude of R waves (over 1.0 millivolt) in the frontal plane leads may suggest ventricular hypertrophy.

Duration—Less than 0.04 second.

S-T segment and T wave—S-T segment and T wave should be small and free of repolarization changes as well as marked depression of elevation.

---

[*]From Ettinger, S. J., and Suter, P. F.: *Canine Cardiology.* Philadelphia, W. B. Saunders Co., 1970, pp. 102–169.

[†]Derived from personal observations and from sources gratefully acknowledged in the bibliography and cited in the text of *Canine Cardiology,* Chapter 4, pp. 102–169.

[‡]From Ettinger, S. J.: *Textbook of Veterinary Internal Medicine,* vol. 2. Philadelphia, W. B. Saunders Co., 1975, p. 922.

TABLES FOR CONVERSION OF WEIGHT TO BODY-SURFACE AREA IN SQUARE METERS FOR DOGS

KG.	M.²	KG.	M.²
0.5	0.06	26.0	0.88
1.0	0.10	27.0	0.90
2.0	0.15	28.0	0.92
3.0	0.20	29.0	0.94
4.0	0.25	30.0	0.96
5.0	0.29	31.0	0.99
6.0	0.33	32.0	1.01
7.0	0.36	33.0	1.03
8.0	0.40	34.0	1.05
9.0	0.43	35.0	1.07
10.0	0.46	36.0	1.09
11.0	0.49	37.0	1.11
12.0	0.52	38.0	1.13
13.0	0.55	39.0	1.15
14.0	0.58	40.0	1.17
15.0	0.60	41.0	1.19
16.0	0.63	42.0	1.21
17.0	0.66	43.0	1.23
18.0	0.69	44.0	1.25
19.0	0.71	45.0	1.26
20.0	0.74	46.0	1.28
21.0	0.76	47.0	1.30
22.0	0.78	48.0	1.32
23.0	0.81	49.0	1.34
24.0	0.83	50.0	1.36
25.0	0.85		

(From Ettinger, S. J.: Textbook of Veterinary Internal Medicine. Philadelphia, W. B. Saunders Co., 1975.)

*Nomogram for the Estimation of Surface Area of the Dog**

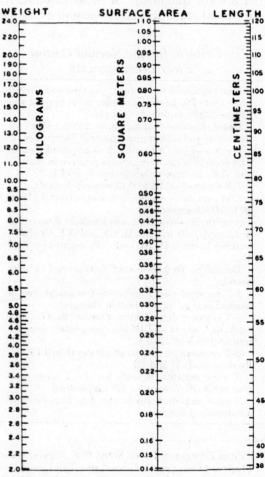

*Length = Nose to anus measured along abdomen.
From Smith, H. W.: Principles of Renal Physiology.
3rd ed. New York, Oxford University Press, 1957.

A ROSTER OF NORMAL VALUES FOR DOGS AND CATS

JOHN BENTINCK-SMITH, D.V.M.

Ithaca, New York

Age, sex, breed, diurnal periodicity, and emotional stress at the time of sampling can be expected to cause variation in normal values. The methodology will also affect the biologic parameters.

For these reasons practitioners are well advised to employ the normal values supplied by the laboratory that they patronize. However, this laboratory must have determined their normal ranges and means by a sufficient number of normal samples to provide statistical validity. The laboratory should run control serum samples and provide other means of quality control.

Since biochemical results are most frequently determined on Technicon SMA, equipment values for this method are provided (through the courtesy of Dr. A. I. Hurvitz and Dr. Robert J. Wilkins of the Animal Medical Center). Other data are derived from the New York State College of Veterinary Medicine, the Ralston Purina Corp., Biozyme Veterinary Laboratory (a division of Biozyme Medical Laboratories, Inc.), standard texts, and the literature. References are cited as footnotes within the tables and appear in full at the end of this appendix. Values for reptiles and exotic animals can be found on pages 748 and 749 and also in *Current Veterinary Therapy VI*, page 795.

Inappropriate collection and preparation, prolonged storage, hemolysis, lipemia, and hyperbilirubinemia may invalidate the laboratory results.

NORMAL BLOOD VALUES[31]

ERYTHROCYTES	ADULT DOG	AVERAGE	ADULT CAT	AVERAGE
Erythrocytes (millions/μl.)	5.5–8.5	6.8	5.5–10.0	7.5
Hemoglobin (g./dl.)	12.0–18.0	14.9	8.0–14.0	12.0
Packed Cell Volume (vol. %)	37.0–55.0	45.5	24.0–45.0	37.0
Mean Corpuscular Volume (femtoliters)	66.0–77.0	69.8	40.0–55.0	45.0
Mean Corpuscular Hemoglobin (picograms)	19.9–24.5	22.8	13.0–17.0	15.0
Mean Corpuscular Hemoglobin Concentration (g./dl.)				
Wintrobe	31.0–34.0	33.0	31.0–35.0	33.0
Microhematocrit	32.0–36.0	34.0	30.0–36.0	33.2
Reticulocytes (%) (excludes punctate retics.)	0.0–1.5	0.8	0.2–1.6	0.6
Resistance to hypotonic saline (% saline solution producing) Minimum	0.40–0.50	0.46	0.66–0.72	0.69
initial and complete hemolysis Maximum	0.32–0.42	0.33	0.46–0.54	0.50
Erythrocyte Sedimentation Rate (mm. at 60 min.)	PCV 37 PCV 50	13 0	PCV 35–40	7–27
RBC life span (days)	100–120		66–78	
RBC diameter (μ)	6.7–7.2	7.0	5.5–6.3	5.8

LEUKOCYTES	ADULT DOG	AVERAGE	ADULT CAT	AVERAGE
Leukocytes (no./μl.)	6,000–17,000	11,500	5,500–19,500	12,500
Neutrophils—Bands(%)	0–3	0.8	0–3	0.5
Neutrophils—Mature (%)	60–77	70.0	35–75	59.0
Lymphocyte (%)	12–30	20.0	20–55	32.0
Monocyte (%)	3–10	5.2	1–4	3.0
Eosinophil (%)	2–10	4.0	2–12	5.5
Basophil (%)	Rare	0.0	Rare	0.0
Neutrophils—Bands (no./μl.)	0–300	70	0–300	100
Neutrophils—Mature (no./μl.)	3,000–11,500	7,000	2,500–12,500	7,500
Lymphocytes (no./μl.)	1,000–4,800	2,800	1,500–7,000	4,000
Monocytes (no./μl.)	150–1,350	750	0–850	350
Eosinophils (no./μl.)	100–1,250	550	0–1,500	650
Basophils	Rare	0	Rare	0

CANINE BLOOD PARAMETERS AT DIFFERENT AGES—AVERAGE VALUES[1]

Age	millions/μl. RBC	Retic. % *	Nucl. RBC/ 100 WBC *	g./dl. Hb	Vol. % PCV	/dl. WBC	/dl. Neut.	/dl. Bands	/dl. Lymph.	/dl. Eos.
Birth	5.75	7.1	1.8	16.70	50	16,500	1,300	400	2,500	600
2 weeks	3.92	7.1	1.8	9.76	32	11,000	6,500	100	3,000	300
4 weeks	4.20	7.1	1.8	9.60	33	13,000	8,600	0	4,000	40
6 weeks	4.91	3.6	1.8	9.59	34	15,000	10,000	0	4,500	100
8 weeks	5.13	3.9	0.3	11.00	37	18,000	11,000	234	6,000	270
12 weeks	5.27	3.9	Rare	11.60	36	15,300	9,400	115	4,600	322

*See reference 13.

CANINE BLOOD PARAMETERS AT DIFFERENT AGES[26]

	Sex	Birth to 12 mo.	Average	1–7 yr.	Average	7 yr. and Older	Average
Erythrocytes (million/μl)	Male	2.99–8.52	5.09	5.26–6.57	5.92	3.33–7.76	5.28
	Female	2.76–8.42	5.06	5.13–8.6	6.47	3.34–9.19	5.17
Hemoglobin (gm/dl)	Male	6.9–16.5	10.7	12.7–16.3	15.5	14.7–21.2	17.9
	Female	6.4–18.9	11.2	11.5–17.9	14.7	11.0–22.5	16.1
Packed Cell Volume (vol. %)	Male	22.0–45.0	33.9	35.2–52.8	44.0	44.2–62.8	52.3
	Female	25.8–55.2	36.0	34.8–52.4	43.6	35.8–67.0	49.8
Leukocytes (thousands/μl)	Male	9.9–27.7	17.1	8.3–19.5	11.9	7.9–35.3	15.5
	Female	8.8–26.8	15.9	7.5–17.5	11.5	5.2–34.0	13.4
Neutrophils	Male	63–73	68	65–73	69	55–80	66
Mature (%)	Female	64–74	69	58–76	67	40–80	64
Lymphocytes (%)	Male	18–30	24	9–26	18	15–40	29
	Female	13–28	21	11–29	20	13–45	29
Monocytes (%)	Male	1–10	6	2–10	6	0–4	1
	Female	1–10	7	0–10	5	0–4	1
Eosinophils (%)	Male	2–11	3	1–8	4	1–11	4
	Female	1–9	5	1–10	6	0–19	6

FELINE BLOOD PARAMETERS AT DIFFERENT AGES[31]

Age	millions/μl. RBC	g./dl. Hb	Vol. % PCV	/dl. WBC	/dl. Neut.	/dl. Lymph.
Birth	4.95	12.2	44.7	7,500		
2 weeks	4.76	9.7	31.1	8,080		
5 weeks	5.84	8.4	29.9	8,550		
Average*	4.80	7.5	26.2	11,770	4,600	6,970
Range*	3.90–5.70	6.6–8.4	21.0–33.5	7,500–14,500		4,500–9,400
6 weeks	6.75	9.0	35.4	8,420		
8 weeks	7.10	9.4	35.6	8,420		
Average*	5.90	7.5	26.2	12,400	7,500	4,900
Range*	3.30–7.30	7.6–15.0	22–38	6,900–23,100		1,925–10,100

*See reference 2.

FELINE BLOOD PARAMETERS AT DIFFERENT AGES[25]

	Sex	Birth to 12 mo.	Average	1–5 yr.	Average	6 yr. and Older	Average
Erythrocytes (millions/μl)	Male	5.43–10.22	6.96	4.48–10.27	7.34	5.26–8.89	6.79
	Female	4.46–11.34	6.90	4.45–9.42	6.17	4.10–7.38	5.84
Hemoglobin (gm/dl)	Male	6.0–12.9	9.9	8.9–17.0	12.9	9.0–14.5	11.8
	Female	6.0–15.0	9.9	7.9–15.5	10.3	7.5–13.7	10.3
Packed Cell Volume (vol. %)	Male	24.0–37.5	31	26.9–48.2	37.6	28.0–43.8	34.6
	Female	23.0–46.8	31.5	25.3–37.5	31.4	22.5–40.5	30.8
Leukocytes (thousands/μl)	Male	7.8–25.0	15.8	9.1–28.2	15.1	6.4–30.4	17.6
	Female	11.0–26.9	17.7	13.7–23.7	19.9	5.2–30.1	14.8
Neutrophils	Male	16–75	60	37–92	65	33–75	61
Mature (%)	Female	51–83	69	42–93	69	25–89	71
Lymphocytes (%)	Male	10–81	30	7–48	23	16–54	30
	Female	8–37	23	12–58	30	9–63	22
Monocytes (%)	Male	1–5	2	1–5	2	0–2	1
	Female	0–7	2	0–5	2	0–4	1
Eosinophils (%)	Male	2–21	8	1–22	7	1–15	8
	Female	0–15	6	0–13	5	0–15	6

EFFECT OF PREGNANCY AND LACTATION ON BLOOD PARAMETERS OF THE DOG[1]

	GESTATION				TERM	LACTATION		
	2 Weeks	4 Weeks	6 Weeks	8 Weeks	0 Weeks	2 Weeks	4 Weeks	6 Weeks
RBC (millions/dl.)	8.85	7.48	6.73	6.26	4.53	5.13	5.65	6.15
PCV (Vol. %)	53	47	44	37	32	34	38	42
Hb (g./dl.)	19.6	16.4	14.7	13.8	11.0	11.7	12.8	13.4
Sedimentation Rate (mm. at 60 min.)	0.6	11.0	31.0	14.0	12.0	14.0	14.0	13.0
WBC (thousands/dl.)	12.0	12.2	15.7	19.0	18.9	16.9	17.1	15.9

EFFECT OF PREGNANCY AND LACTATION ON BLOOD PARAMETERS OF THE CAT[6]

	1 Day Past Conception	GESTATION				TERM	LACTATION	
		2 Weeks	4 Weeks	6 Weeks	8 Weeks	0 Weeks	2 Weeks	4 Weeks
RBC (millions/dl.)	8.0	7.9	7.1	6.7	6.2	6.2	7.4	7.4
PCV (Vol. %)	36.1	37.0	33.0	32.0	28.0	29.0	33.0	33.0
Hb (g./100 ml.)	12.5	12.0	11.0	10.8	9.5	10.0	11.5	11.2
Reticulocytes (%) (includes punctate retics.)	9	11	9	10	20.1	15	9	6

	ADULT DOG	AVERAGE	ADULT CAT	AVERAGE[31]
Thrombocytes $\times$ 10^5/μl.	2–5	3–4	3–8	4.5
Icterus Index	2–5 units		2–5 units	
Plasma Fibrinogen (g./l.)	2.0–4.0		0.50–3.00	

NORMAL BONE MARROW (Percentage)

ERYTHROCYTIC CELLS	DOG[31]	CAT[23]
Rubriblasts	0.2	1.71
Prorubricytes	3.9	12.50
Rubricytes	27.0	
Metarubricytes	15.3	11.68
Total Erythrocytic Cells	46.4	25.89
GRANULOCYTIC CELLS		
Myeloblasts	0.0	1.74
Progranulocytes	1.3	0.88
Neutrophilic Myelocytes	9.0	9.76
Eosinophilic Myelocytes	0.0	1.47
Neutrophilic Metamyelocytes	7.5	7.32
Eosinophilic Metamyelocytes	2.4	1.52
Band Neutrophils	13.6	25.80
Band Eosinophils	0.9	—
Neutrophils	18.4	9.24
Eosinophils	0.3	0.81
Basophils	0.0	0.002
Total Granulocytic Cells	53.4	58.542
M:E Ratio—Average	1.15:1.0	2.47:1.0
M:E Ratio—Range (Schalm)	0.75–2.50:1.0	0.60–3.90:1.0
OTHER CELLS		
Lymphocytes	0.2	7.63
Plasma Cells	0	1.61
Reticulum Cells	0	0.13
Mitotic Cells	0	0.61
Unclassified	0	1.62
Disintegrated Cells	0	4.60

BLOOD, PLASMA, OR SERUM CHEMICAL CONSTITUENTS
(B) = Blood, (P) = Plasma, (S) = Serum

Chemical constituents are liable to show markedly different values, depending on the methodology employed.

CONSTITUENT	ADULT DOG		ADULT CAT	
	Coulter Chemistry[34]	*Technicon SMA*[36]	*Coulter Chemistry*[34]	*Technicon SMA*[36]
Urea N(S) (mg/dl)	8–23	10–22	18–32	5–30
Glucose (S) (mg/dl)	71–115	50–120	66–95	70–150
Total bilirubin (S) (mg/dl)	0.1–0.6	0–0.6	0.15–0.3	0–0.8
Total protein (S) (gm/dl)	5.2–7.0	5.4–7.8	5.9–7.3	5.5–7.5
Albumin (S) (gm/dl)	2.7–3.8	2.2–3.4	2.2–3.0	2.2–3.5
Alkaline phosphatase (S) (IU/l)	10–82	20–120	7–30	10–80
Calcium (S) (mg/dl)	9.8–11.4	9–11.6	8.9–10.6	7.6–11.0
Inorganic phosphorus (S) (mg/dl)	2.8–5.1	3.9–6.3	4.3–6.6	3.2–6.3
LDH (S) (IU/l)	8–89	40–200	33–99	10–200
AST or SGOT (S)	13–93°	5–80†	32–58°	10–60†
ALT or SGPT (S)(IU/l)	15–70	5–25	10–50	10–60
Total CO_2 (S) (mEq/l)	18–25	17–25‡	18–25	16–25‡
Creatinine (S) (mg/dl)	0.5–1.2	0.4–1.5‡	0.5–1.7	1.3–2.1‡
Uric acid (S) (mg/dl)		0.2–0.8‡		0.1–0.7‡
Total cholesterol (S) (mg/dl)	82–282	156–294‡	41–225	116–126‡
Triglycerides (S) (mg/dl)		10–42‡		6–58‡
CPK (S) (IU/l)	12–84	27–93‡	6–130	62–262‡

CHEMICAL PARAMETERS AFFECTED BY AGE	DOG < 6 MO–SMA[36]	CAT < 6 MO–SMA[36]
Inorganic phosphorus (S) (mg/dl)	3.9–9.0	3.9–8.1
Calcium (S) (mg/dl)	7.0–11.6	7.0–11.0
Alkaline phosphatase (S) (IU/l)	20–200	10–120
LDH (S) (IU/l)	40–400	10–300

	SEX	DOGS[26] AND CATS[25]					
		Birth to 12 mo.	*Average*	*1–5 yr.*	*Average*	*6 yr. and Older*	*Average*
Total Protein (S) (gm/dl)	Male	3.90–5.90	5.15	4.90–9.60	6.33	5.5–7.3	6.4
(Dogs)	Female	4.00–6.40	5.58	5.50–7.80	6.34	4.7–7.5	6.2
Total Protein (S) (gm/dl)	Male	4.3–10.0	6.4	6.8–10.0	8.1	6.2–8.5	7.2
(Cats)	Female	4.8–9.1	6.4	6.6–8.9	7.4	6.0–9.0	7.3

ELECTROPHORESIS	DOG	CAT
Albumin (S) (gm/dl)	2.3–3.4	2.3–3.5
Globulin (S) (gm/dl)	3.0–4.7	2.6–5.0
Alpha 1 (S) (gm/dl)	0.3–0.8	0.3–0.5
Alpha 2 (S) (gm/dl)	0.5–1.3	0.4–1.0
Beta (S) (gm/dl)	0.7–1.8	0.6–1.9
Gamma (S) (gm/dl)	0.4–1.0	0.5–1.5
Albumin/globulin ratio, A/G (S)	0.7–1.1	0.5–1.0

° Trans Act Units/liter (General Diagnostics). 1 Trans Act Unit of GOT activity is the amount of enzyme in 1 liter of sample that will form 1 mM of oxalic acid in 1 minute under specified conditions.

† IU/liter.

‡ See reference 7

BLOOD, PLASMA OR SERUM CHEMICAL CONSTITUENTS—*Continued*
(B) = Blood, (P) = Plasma, (S) = Serum

Chemical constituents are liable to show markedly different values depending on the methodology employed.

OTHER CONSTITUENTS	ADULT DOG	ADULT CAT
Lipase (S)		
(Sigma Tietz Units/ml)	0–1	0–1
Roe Byler Units (5)	0.8–12	0–5
IU (5)	13–200	0–83
Amylase (S)		
Harleco Units/dl	0–800	0–800
Harding Units/dl	1600–2400	0–2700 (5)
Dy Amyl (General Diagnostics)	<3200 (5)	0–2600 (5)
Caraway Units/dl[24]	330–1530	170–1170
Lactic acid (S) (mg/dl)	3–15	
Pyruvate (B) (mEq/l)	0.1–0.2	
Cholesterol esters (S) (mg/dl)	84–168	45–120
Free cholesterol (S) (mg/dl)	28–84	15–60
Total lipid (P) (mg/dl)	47–725	145–607
Free glycerol (S) 24-hr fast (mg/dl)[28]	14.2–23.2	
Bromsulfalein retention test (P) (%)	<5	
Iron (S) (μg/dl)	94–122	68–215
Total iron-binding capacity (S) (μg/dl)	280–340	170–400
Lead (B) (μg/dl)	0–35	0–35

	DOGS		CATS	
ELECTROLYTES	Coulter[34]	Technicon[7]	Coulter[34]	Technicon[7]
Sodium (S) (mEq/l)	143–151	144–154	150–162	147–161
Potassium (S) (mEq/l)	4.1–5.7	3.8–5.8	3.7–5.5	3.7–4.9
Magnesium (S) (mEq/l)	1.4–2.4	1.07–1.73	2.2	1.92–2.28
Chloride (S) (mEq/l)	103–115	93–121	114–124	80–158
Sulfate (S) (mEq/l)	2.0			
Osmolality (S) (mOsm/kg)	280–310		280–310	
pH (Corning)	7.31–7.42		7.24–7.40	

BLOOD GASES	ADULT DOG	ADULT CAT
PO_2 (B) mm Hg (arterial)*	85–95	—
(B) mm Hg (venous)*	40–60	—
PCO_2 (B) mm Hg (arterial)*	29–36	—
(B) mm Hg (venous)*	29–42	—
Base excess (B) (mEq/l)	±2.5	±2.5
Bicarbonate (P) (mEq/l)	17–24	17–24

*Standard temperature and pressure.

	ADULT DOG		ADULT CAT	
ENDOCRINE SECRETIONS	Resting Level	Post-ACTH*	Resting Level	Post-ACTH*
Cortisol (S) (RIA) (μg/dl)[27]	1.8–4	3–4× Pretreatment	1–3	3–4× Pretreatment
Cortisol (S) (CPB) (μg/dl)[35]	2–6	3–4× Pretreatment[32]	2–5	3–4× Pretreatment[32]
Cortisol (S) (fluorometric) (μg/dl)	5–10	10–20		
	Resting Level	Post-TSH†	Resting Level	Post-TSH
T_4 (P) (RIA) (μg/dl)[4]	1.52–3.60	At least 3–4 fold	1.2–3.8	
T_3 (P) (RIA) (ng/dl)[4]	48–154	More than 10 ng increase		
Protein-bound iodine[3] (μg/dl)	1.6–3.0	Increase of 3 μg/dl (mean)		

BLOOD, PLASMA OR SERUM CHEMICAL CONSTITUENTS—*Continued*
(B) = Blood, (P) = Plasma, (S) = Serum

Chemical constituents are liable to show markedly different values depending on the methodology employed.

T_4 CHANGES WITH AGE	DOG	CAT
T_4 (S) (RIA)	Decrease of 0.07 μg/dl per year of age[4]	No values for cat
T_4 (S) (CPB) (μg/dl)		
10–12 wk[1, 16]	3 24 ± 0 51	2 82 ± 0 73
1 yr[1, 16]	2 25 ± 0 33	2 43 ± 0 55
	Adult Dog	*Adult Cat*
Thyroid uptake of radioiodine (^{131}I) (%)[1, 16]	17–30	
Insulin (S) (RIA) (μU/ml)[37]	0–30	0–50

*2 μ ACTH gel IM 2 hours after injection
†5 μ TSH IV 4–6 hours after injection.

HEMOSTATIC PARAMETERS (No test should be interpreted without an accompanying normal control.)

	ADULT DOG	ADULT CAT
Bleeding time		
Dorsum of nose (min)	2–4	1–5[33]
Lip (sec)	85–110	
Ear (min)	2.5–3	
Abdomen (min)	1–2	
Whole blood coagulation time		
Glass (Lee and White) (min)	6–7 5	8[33]
Silicone (Lee and White) (min)	12–15	
Capillary tube (min)[11]	3–4	5 2 ± 0 2[41]
Activated coagulation time of whole blood		
Room temp. (sec)	60–125[10]; 83–129[19]	A limited number of cats have shown a range similar to that of the dog.
37°C (sec)	64–95[19]	
Prothrombin time (sec)[11]	6–10	8 6 ± 0 5[41]
Puppies 1–4 hours old (sec)[5]	42 2	
6–12 hours old (sec)	49 1	
16–48 hours old (sec)	36 8	
48 hours old (sec)	24 5	
Russell's viper venom time (sec)[29]	11	9
Partial thromboplastin time (sec)	15–25	
Prothrombin consumption (sec)[29]	20 5	20
Fibrin degradation products (μg/ml)	<10	

BASENJI DOGS[13]		CATS[31]	
Plasma Proteins (g./dl.)		*Plasma Proteins (g./dl.)*	
6–8 weeks	5.33 ± 0.29	Lower values for younger animals	
9–12 weeks	5.87 ± 0.46	Adults 6–8	
4–6 months	6.6 ± 0.25		
1–2 years	7.03 ± 0.33		

NORMAL RENAL FUNCTION AND URINE PARAMETERS

Urine[22]	Adult Dog	Adult Cat
Specific Gravity		
Minimum	1.001	1.001
Maximum	1.060	1.080
Usual Limits (normal water and food intake)	1.018–1.050	1.018–1.050
Volume (ml./kg. body weight/day)	24–41	22–30
Osmolality Urine (m osm./kg.)		
Usual Range	500–1200	
Maximal Limits	2000–2400	
Osmolality Plasma	300	

Urine Constituents[37] (Values markedly affected by degree of concentration.)	Adult Dog	Adult Cat
Creatinine (mg/dl)	100–300	110–280
Urea (gm/dl)	1.0–2.5	1.0–3.0
Protein (mg/dl)	0–30	0–20
Amylase (Somogyi units)	50–150	30–120
Sodium (mEq/l)	20–165	
Potassium (mEq/l)	20–120	
Calcium (mEq/l)	2–10	
Inorganic phosphorus (mEq/l)	50–180	

Urinalysis—Semiquantitative Values	Adult Dog	Adult Cat
Protein	0–trace	0–trace
Glucose	0	0
Ketones	0	0
Bilirubin	0	0
10–20% Dogs—high specific gravity	1+	
5% Cats—high specific gravity		1+
Urobilinogen (Ehrlich unit)	0–1	0–1
(Wallace and Diamond)	<1:32	<1:32

Renal Function—Dog[22]	
Effective renal plasma flow	266 ± 66 ml/min/m² body surface
	13.5 ± 3.3 ml/min/kg body weight
Glomerular filtration rate	84.4 ± 19 ml/min/m² body surface
	4 ml/min/kg body weight

Renal Function Tests—Dog	
Phenolsulfonphthalein	
Excretion in urine at 20 min, 6-mg dose[11]	21–66%
Clearance (P) 1 mg/kg at 60 min[17]	$<80\mu$/ml
$T_{1/2}$ clearance 5 mg/kg[9]	19.6 min
Creatinine, endogenous clearance[22]	60 ± 22 ml/min/m² body surface
	2.98 ± 0.96 ml/min/kg body weight

CEREBROSPINAL FLUID AND SYNOVIAL FLUID

CEREBROSPINAL FLUID[12]	ADULT DOG	ADULT CAT
Color	Clear, colorless	Clear, colorless
Pressure (mm H_2O)	<170	<100
Cells/μl	<5 lymphocytes	<5 lymphocytes
Protein (ml/dl)	<25	<20
Glucose (mg/dl)	61–116	85

CEREBROSPINAL FLUID AND SYNOVIAL FLUID—*Continued*

NORMAL SYNOVIAL FLUID—CARPAL, ELBOW, SHOULDER, HIP, STIFLE, AND HOCK JOINTS[30]	ADULT DOG	
	Range	Mean
Amount (ml)	0.01–1.00	0.24
pH	7–7.8	7.33
Leukocytes ($\times 10^3/\mu l$)	0–2.9	0.43
Erythrocytes ($\times 10^3 \mu l$)	0.320.0	12.15
Neutrophils/μl	0–32	3.63
Neutrophils(%)[20]	10	
Monocytes/μl	0–838	230.77
Lymphocytes/μl	0–2436	245.6
Clasmatocytes/μl	0–166	14.69
Mononuclear cells(%)[20]	90	
Mucin clot	Tight ropy clump Clear supernate	

CANINE SEMEN[14]

Regular collection by hand manipulation with a teaser (125 ejaculates from small dogs, mostly beagles).[8]

	Mean	Standard Deviation	Range
Volume (ml.)	5	4.3	0.5-20.4
% Motile Sperm	75	7.5	30-90
% Normal Sperm	86	14.7	34-97
pH	6.72	0.19	6.49-7.10
Concentration/cu. mm. (10^3)	148	84.6	27.2-388.8
Total Sperm per Ejaculate (10^6)	528	321.0	94-1428

FRACTIONATED EJACULATES (BASED ON 65 EJACULATES)

	Mean	Range	pH
1st Fraction	0.8 ml.	0.25-2.00	6.37
2nd Fraction	0.6 ml.	0.40-2.00	6.10
3rd Fraction	0.4 ml.	1.0-16.3	7.20

PUREBRED LABRADOR RETRIEVERS, 18 TO 48 MONTHS OLD[33]

	Mean	Range
Volume (ml.)	2.2*	0.5-6.5
% Motile Sperm	93	75-99
% Unstained Sperm (Eosin Nigrosin)	84	61-99
Concentration/cu. mm. (10^3)	564	103-708

*Only the first two fractions were collected, resulting in smaller volume and higher concentration of sperm/cu. mm. than would result if all the prostatic fluid (3rd fraction) were obtained.

SUPPLEMENTAL READING AND REFERENCES

1. Andersen, A. C., and Gee, W.: Normal values in the beagle. Vet. Med., 53:135–138, 156; 1958.
2. Anderson, L., Wilson, R., and Hay, D.: Haematological values in normal cats from four weeks to one year of age. Res. Vet. Sci., 12:579–583, 1971.
3. Baker, H. J.: Laboratory evaluation of thyroid function. In Kirk, R. W. (ed.): *Current Veterinary Therapy IV.* Philadelphia, W. B. Saunders Co., 1971.
4. Belshaw, B. E., and Rijnberk, A.: Radioimmunoassay of plasma T_4 and T_3 in the diagnosis of primary hypothyroidism in dogs. J. Am. Anim. Hosp. Assoc., 15:17–23, 1979.
5. Benjamin, M.: *An Outline of Veterinary Clinical Pathology,* 3rd ed. Ames, Iowa, Iowa State University Press, 1978.

6. Berman, E.: Hemogram of the cat during pregnancy and lactation and after lactation. Am. J. Vet. Res., 35:457–460, 1974.
7. Biozyme Veterinary Laboratory (a division of Biozyme Medical Laboratories, Inc.): *Normal Ranges Chemistry.* Olean, N.Y., Bioenzyme Vet. Lab., 1978.
8. Boucher, J. H.: Evaluation of semen quality in the dog and the effects of frequency of ejaculation upon semen quality, libido and restoration of sperm reserves. M.S. Thesis, Cornell University, Ithaca, N.Y., 1957.
9. Brobst, D. F., Carter, J. M., and Horron, M.: Plasma phenolsulfonphthalein determination as a measure of renal function in the dog. 17th Gaines Veterinary Symposium, University of Minnesota, 1967, p. 15.
10. Byars, T. D., Ling, G. V., Ferris, N. A., and Keeton, K. S.: Activated coagulation time (ACT) of whole blood in normal dogs. Am. J. Vet. Res., 37:1359–1361, 1976.

11. Coles, E. H.: *Veterinary Clinical Pathology,* 2nd ed. Philadelphia, W. B. Saunders Co., 1974.
12. deLahunta, A.: New York State College of Veterinary Medicine, Cornell University, Ithaca, New York 14853. Personal communication.
13. Ewing, G. O., Schalm, O. W., and Smith, R. S.: Hematologic values of normal Basenji dogs. J. Am. Vet. Med. Assoc., *161:* 1661, 1972.
14. Revisions and corrections courtesy of Dr. R. H. Foote, Professor of Animal Physiology, Department of Animal Science, New York State College of Life Sciences, Cornell University, Ithaca, New York 14853.
15. Kallfelz, F. A.: Associate Professor of Clinical Nutrition, Department of Large Animal Medicine, Obstetrics and Surgery, New York State College of Veterinary Medicine, Ithaca, New York 14853. Personal communication.
16. Kallfelz, F. A., and Erali, R. P.: Thyroid function tests on domesticated animals. Am. J. Vet. Res., *34:*1449, 1973.
17. Kaufman, C. F., and Kirk, R. W.: The 60-minute plasma phenolsulfonphthalein concentration as a test of renal function in the dog. J. Am. Anim. Hosp. Assoc., 9:66, 1973.
18. Kraft, W.: Schielddrusenfunktionsstörungen beim Hund. (Thyroid function disturbances in the dog.) Thesis, Justus Liebig University, Giessen, West Germany, 1964. (Cited by Belshaw.)
19. Middleton, D. J., and Watson, A. D. J.: Activated coagulation times of whole blood in normal dogs and dogs with coagulopathies. J. Small Anim. Pract., *19:*417–422, 1978.
20. Miller, J. B., Perman, V., Osborne, C. A., Hammer, R. F., and Gambardella, P. C.: Synovial fluid analysis in canine arthritis. J. Am. Anim. Hosp. Assoc., 10:392, 1974.
21. Osbaldiston, G. W., Stowe, E. C., and Griffith, P. R.: Blood coagulation: Comparative studies in dogs, cats, horses and cattle. Br. Vet. J., *126:*512, 1970.
22. Osborne, C. A., Low, D. G., and Finco, D. R.: *Canine and Feline Urology.* Philadelphia, W. B. Saunders Co., 1972.
23. Penny, R. H. C., Carlisle, C. H., and Davidson, H. A.: The blood and marrow picture of the cat. Br. Vet. J. *126:*459–464, 1970.
24. *Chemassay Amylase.* Pitman-Moore, Inc., Washington Crossing, N.J. 08560
25. *1975 Normal Blood Values for Cats.* Ralston Purina Co., Professional Marketing Services, Checkerboard Square, St. Louis, Missouri 63188.
26. *1975 Normal Blood Values for Dogs.* Ralston Purina Co., Professional Marketing Services, Checkerboard Square, St. Louis, Missouri 63188.
27. Reimers, Thomas J.: Assistant Professor and Director of the Endocrinology Laboratory, New York State College of Veterinary Medicine, Cornell University, Ithaca, N.Y. 14853. Personal communication.
28. Rogers, U. A., Donovan, E. F., and Kociba, G. J.: Lipids and lipoproteins in normal dogs and dogs with secondary hyperlipoproteinemia. J. Am. Vet. Med. Assoc., *166:*1092–1100, 1975.
29. Rowsell, H. C.: Blood coagulation and hemorrhagic disorders. In: Medway, W., Prier, J. E., and Wilkinson, J. S. (eds.): *Textbook of Veterinary Clinical Pathology.* Baltimore, Williams & Wilkins Co., 1969, p. 247.
30. Sawyer, D. C.: Synovial fluid analysis of canine joints. J. Am. Vet. Med. Assoc., *143:*609, 1963.
31. Schalm, O. W., Jain, N. C., and Carroll, E. J.: *Veterinary Hematology,* 3rd ed. Philadelphia, Lea & Febiger, 1975.
32. Scott, D. W.: Assistant Professor of Medicine, Dept. of Clinical Sciences, New York State College of Veterinary Medicine, Cornell University, Ithaca, N.Y. 14853. Personal communication.
33. Seager, S. W. J., and Fletcher, W. S.: Collection, storage, and insemination of canine semen. Lab. Anim. Sci., *22:*177–182, 1972.
34. Tasker, J. B.: Reference values for clinical chemistry using the Coulter Chemistry System. Cornell Vet. *68:*460–479, 1978.
35. Wallace, R.: Research Support Specialist, New York State College of Veterinary Medicine, Cornell University, Ithaca, N.Y. 14853. Personal communication.
36. Wilkins, R. J. and Hurvitz, A. I.: *Profiling in Veterinary Clinical Pathology.* Tarrytown, New York, Technicon Instruments Corp., 1978, pp. 17, 19.
37. Wilkins, R. J.: Animal Medical Center, 510 East 62nd St., New York, New York 10021. Personal communication.

TABLE OF COMMON DRUGS: APPROXIMATE DOSES [*]

DRUG NAME	DOG	CAT
Acetazolamide	10 mg/kg q6h PO	Same
Acetylcysteine (Mucomyst)	*Eye*: Dilute to 2% soln with artificial tears and apply topically q2h to eye for maximum of 48 hours *Respiratory*: 50 ml/hr for 30–60 min every 12 hr by nebulization	Same
Acetylpromazine (acepromazine)	0.55–2.2 mg/kg PO 0.55–1.1 mg/kg IV, IM, SC	1.1–2.2 mg/kg PO, IV, IM, SC
Acetylsalicylic acid (aspirin)	*Analgesia*: 10 mg/kg PO q12h *Antirheumatic*: 40 mg/kg PO q18h or 25 mg/kg q8h	*Analgesia*: 10 mg/kg PO q52h *Antirheumatic*: 40 mg/kg q72h
ACTH	2 units/kg/day IM (therapeutic) or 40 units/dog IM (response test; take post sample in 2 hr)	Same
Actinomycin D (Cosmegan)	0.015 mg/kg/once daily for 5 days	None
Aldactone (spironolactone)	1–2 mg/kg q12h	Same
Alevaire	50–60 ml/hr for 30–60 minutes q12h by nebulization	Same
Allopurinol (Zyloprim)	10 mg/kg PO q8h, then reduce to 10 mg/kg PO daily	None
Amforol	2–6 tablets/9 kg initially. Maintenance: 1–3 tabs/9 kg q8h	None
Aminophylline	10 mg/kg q8h PO, IM, IV	Same
Ammonium chloride	100 mg/kg q12h PO	20 mg/kg q12h PO
Amoxicillin	11 mg/kg q12h PO for 5–7 days	11–22 mg/kg q24h PO for 5–7 days
Amphetamine	4.4 mg/kg IV, IM	Same
Amphotericin B	0.15–1.0 mg/kg dissolved in 5–20 ml 5% dextrose and water given rapidly IV 3× weekly for 2–4 mo. Do not exceed 2.0 mg/kg. Pretreat with antiemetics if needed. Monitor BUN.	Same
Ampicillin (Polyflex, Princillin)	10–20 mg/kg q6h PO, or 5–10 mg/kg q6h IV, IM, SC	Same
Amprolium	100–200 mg/kg/day in food or water for 7–10 days	None
Anterior pituitary gonadotropin	*Bitches*: 100–500 units once daily to effect	None
Apomorphine	0.02 mg/kg IV or 0.04 mg/kg SC	None
Aqua-B (vitamin B complex)	0.5–2.0 ml q24h IV, IM, SC	0.5–1.0 ml q24h IV, IM, SC
Aquamephyton (vitamin K_1)	5–20 mg q12h IV, IM, SC	1–5 mg q12h IV, IM, SC
Ascorbic acid (vitamin C)	100–500 mg/day (maintenance) or 100–500 mg q8h (urine acidifier)	100 mg/day (maintenance) or 100 mg q8h (urine acidifier)
L-Asparginase	10,000–20,000 IU/M² weekly IP or 400 IU/kg weekly	Same
Atropine	0.05 mg/kg q6h IV, SC, IM or 1% soln in eye *Organophosphate poisoning*: 0.2–2.0 mg/kg IV, SC, IM. Give ¼ dose IV and remainder IM or SC prn.	Same
BAL	4 mg/kg q4h IM until recovered	None
Betamethasone (Betasone®)	0.028–0.055 ml/kg IM. Give only once.	None
Bethanechol (Urecholine)	5–25 mg q8h PO	2.5–5.0 mg q8h PO
Bismuth, milk of	10–30 ml q4h PO	Same
Bismuth (subnitrate, subgallate, or subcarbonate)	0.3–3.0 gm q4h PO	Same
Bleomycin (Blenoxane®)	10 mg/M² daily IV or SC for 4 days, then 10 mg/M² weekly to a maximum total dose of 200 mg/M²	None
Blood	20 ml/kg IV or IP or to effect	Same
Brewer's yeast	0.2 gm/kg once daily PO	Same

[*]See page 1320 for Tables for Conversion of Weight to Body-surface Area in Square Meters for Dogs.

DRUG NAME	DOG	CAT
Bromsulphalein (BSP) (5% solution)	*Test only*: 5 ml/kg IV; post sample in 30 min	None
Bunamidine (Scolaban)	25–50 mg/kg PO. Fast 3 hr before and after administration.	Same
Busulfan (Myleran®)	4.0 mg/M² daily PO or 0.1 mg/kg daily	None
Caffeine	0.1–0.5 gm IM	None
Calcium	500 mg/kg/day PO	150 mg/kg/day PO
Calcium carbonate	1–4 gm/day PO	Same
Calcium EDTA	100 mg/kg diluted to 10 mg/ml in 5% dextrose and given SC in 4 divided doses; continue for 5 days	Same
Calcium gluconate (10% solution)	10–30 ml IV (slowly)	5–15 ml IV (slowly)
Calcium lactate	0.5–2.0 gm PO	0.2–0.5 gm PO
Canine distemper-hepatitis vaccine	1 vial SC at 8, 12, and 16 weeks of age; annual booster	None
Canopar	500 mg PO for dogs heavier than 4.55 kg; 250 mg bid for those 2.27–4.55 kg. Repeat in 2–3 weeks.	None
Carbenicillin	15 mg/kg q8h IV	Same
Cardioquin	10–20 mg/kg q8h PO	Same
Castor oil	8–30 ml PO	4–10 ml PO
Cephalexin (Keflex)	30 mg/kg q12h PO	Same
Cephaloridine	10 mg/kg q8–12h IM, SC	Same
Cephalothin sodium	35 mg/kg q8h IM, SC	Same
Charcoal, activated (Requa)	0.3–5 gm q8–12h PO	Half the canine dose
	Poisoning: 1–2 tsp/10–15 kg in 200 ml tap water. Administer by stomach tube.	
Cheracol	5 ml q4h PO	3 ml q4h PO
Chlorambucil (Leukeran)	0.2 mg/kg PO once daily	Same
	1.5 mg/M² PO as single dose; decrease for repeated dosage	
Chloramphenicol	50 mg/kg q8h PO, IV, IM, SC	Same, except q12h
Chlordane	0.5% solution on dog or premises	None
Chlorethamine	0.2–1.0 gm q8h PO	100 mg q8h PO
Chlorpheniramine	4–8 mg q12h PO	2 mg q12h PO
Chlorpromazine (Thorazine)	3.3 mg/kg PO sid to qid;	Same
	1.1–6.6 mg/kg IM sid to qid;	
	0.55–4.4 mg/kg IV sid to qid	
Chlortetracycline	20 mg/kg q8h PO	Same
Chlorthiazide (Diuril)	20–40 mg/kg q 12h PO	Same
Cimetidine (Tagamet)	5–10 mg/kg q6h	None
Cloxacillin	10 mg/kg q6h PO, IV, IM	Same
Cod liver oil	1 tsp/10 kg once daily PO	Same
Codeine	*Pain*: 2 mg/kg q6h SC	None
	Cough: 5 mg/dose q6h PO	
Colistimethate (Coly-Mycin)	1.1 mg/kg q6h IM	Same
Colistin	1 mg/kg q6h IM	Same
Cyclophosphamide (Cytoxan)	6.6 mg/kg PO for 3 days, then 2.2 mg/kg PO once daily;	Same
	10 mg/kg q7–10 days IV;	
	50 mg/M² PO, IV once daily for 3–4 days/wk; repeat prn.	
Cyclothiazide	0.5–1.0 mg/PO once daily	None
Cytarabine (Cytosar)	5–10 mg/kg once daily for 2 wk, or 30–50 mg/kg IV, IM, SC once/wk; 100 mg/M² once daily IV, IM for 4 days, then 150 mg/M².	Same
Darbazine	0.14–0.22 ml/kg q12h SC	0.14–0.22 ml/kg q12h SC
	2–7 kg: 1 #1 capsule q12h PO	
	7–14 kg: 1–2 #1 capsules q12h PO	
	Over 14 kg: 1 #3 capsule q12h PO	
Delta albaplex	3–7 kg: 1–2 tablets/day PO	1 tablet q12h PO
	7–14 kg: 2–4 tablets/day PO	
	14–27 kg: 4–6 tablets/day PO	
	Over 27 kg: 6–8 tablets/day PO	
Depo-penicillin	15,000–30,000 units/kg q48h IM, SC	Same
Desoxycorticosterone acetate (Doca)	1–5 mg q24h IM	0.5–1.0 mg q24h IM

DRUG NAME	DOG	CAT
Desoxycorticosterone pivalate	Each 25 mg releases 1 mg Doca/day for 1 month. IM dose: 5–50 mg once/month to effect.	Same
Dexamethasone (Azium)	0.25–1.0 mg IV, IM once daily; 0.25–1.25 mg PO once daily *Shock*: 5 mg/kg IV	0.125–0.5 mg once daily PO, IV, IM *Shock*: same
Dextran	20 ml/kg IV to effect	Same
Dextrose solutions (5% in water, saline, or Ringer's)	40–50 ml/kg q24h IV, SC, IP	Same
D.F.P. (Floropryl)	0.1% solution for eyes, topically	Same
Diazepam (Valium)	2.5–20 mg IV, PO; 10-mg bolus IV (slowly) if in status epilepticus; repeat if no effect	2.5–5.0 mg IV, PO
Dichlorphenamide	50 mg/15 kg tid PO	10–25 mg tid PO
Dichlorvos (Task)	26.4–33 mg/kg PO; in risk animals divide dose; give remaining half 8–24 hr later	None
Dicloxacillin (Dicloxin)	11–55 mg/kg q8h PO	Same
Diethylcarbamazine (Caricide, Cypip, Filaribits)	*Treatment of ascarids:* 55–110 mg/kg PO *Prevention of ascarids* (Cypip): 3.3 mg/kg PO once daily *Prevention of heartworms* (Caricide, Filaribits): 6.6 mg/kg PO once daily	*Treatment of ascarids:* 55–110 mg/kg PO
Diethylstilbestrol (DES)	0.1–1.0 mg/day PO or 2 mg/kg up to 25 mg total IM (repositol) *once*.	0.05–0.10 mg/day PO (Caution)
Di-Gel (liquid)	30–60 ml PO	Half the canine dose
Digitoxin (Foxalin-Vet)	0.033–0.11 mg/kg PO, divided bid	None
Digoxin (Lanoxin, Cardoxin)	*Digitalization*: 0.028–0.055 mg/kg q12h PO for 2 days *Maintenance*: 0.0055–0.011 mg/kg q12h PO 0.044 mg/kg IV to digitalize, then switch to oral maintenance; *or* 0.01–0.02 mg/kg IV q1h to digitalize, then switch to oral maintenance	0.0055 mg/kg q12h (tablet only)
Dihydrocodeinone	5 mg q6h PO	None
Dihydrostreptomycin	20 mg/kg q6h PO; 10 mg/kg q8h IM, SC	Same
Diphenhydramine (Benadryl)	2–4 mg/kg q8h PO; 5–50 mg q12h IV	Same
Dimenhydrinate (Dramamine)	25–50 mg q8h PO	12.5 mg q8h PO
Dioctyl sulfosuccinate (Surfak, Permeatrate)	10–15 ml of 5% soln with 100 ml water q12h PO, per rectum prn; 1 or 2 50-mg capsules q12–24h PO	2 ml of 5% soln with 50 ml water q12h PO, per rectum prn 1 50-mg capsule q12h–24h PO
Diphenthane 70	200 mg/kg PO after 12-hr fast; repeat in 3 weeks	Same
Diphenylhydantoin (Dilantin). See *Phenytoin*		
Diphenylthiocarbazone	60 mg/kg q8h PO for 5 days beyond recovery	None
Disophenol (D.N.P.)	10 mg/kg SC; may be repeated in 2–3 weeks	None
Dithiazanine (Dizan)	6.6–11 mg/kg PO once daily for 7–10 days	None
Dobutamine HCl (Dobutrex®)	250 mg in 500 ml saline; give IV to effect	None
Domeboro's solution	1–2 tablets/pint water; apply topically q8h; store soln no longer than 7 days	Same
Dopamine HCl (Intropin®)	200 mg in 500 ml saline; give IV to effect	Same
Doxapram (Dopram)	5–10 mg/kg IV *Neonate*: 1–5 mg SC, sublingual or umbilical vein	5–10 mg/kg IV *Neonate*: 1–2 mg SC, sublingual vein
Doxorubicin (Adriamycin)	30 mg/M² IV q 3 weeks	None
Doxylamine succinate	1–2 mg/kg q8h IM	Same
D-Penicillamine (Cuprimine)	10–15 mg/kg q12h	None

DRUG NAME	DOG	CAT
Emetrol	4–12 ml q 15 min PO until emesis ceases	Same
Enflurane (Ethrane)	*Induction*: 2–3% *Maintenance*: 1.5–3%	Same
Ephedrine	5–15 mg PO	2–5 mg PO
Epinephrine (1:1000 soln)	0.1–0.5 ml SC, IM, IV, or intracardiac	0.1–0.2 ml SC, IM, IV, or intracardiac
Erythromycin	10 mg/kg q8h PO	Same
Estradiol cyclopentyl propionate (ECP)	0.25–2.0 mg IM *once*	0.25–0.5 mg IM *once*
Ether	0.5–4.0 ml (Induction: 8%; maintenance: 4%) Inhalant to effect.	Same
Ethoxzolamide (Cardrase)	4 mg/kg q12h PO	Same
Feline panleukopenia vaccine	Used, but not FDA-approved	1 vial SC at 8, 12, and 16 weeks of age; annual booster
Fentanyl (Sublimaze)	0.02–0.04 mg/kg (preanesthetic) IM, IV, SC	Same, but use with tranquilizer to prevent excitation
Ferrous sulfate	100–300 mg q24h PO	50–100 mg q24h PO
Festal	1–2 tablets PO with or immediately after feeding	1 tablet PO with or immediately after feeding
Flucytosine (Ancobon)	100 mg/kg q12h PO	Same
Fludrocortisone (Florinef)	0.2–0.8 mg once daily PO	0.1–0.2 mg once daily PO
Flumethasone (Flucort)	0.06–0.25 mg once daily PO, IV, IM, SC	0.03–0.125 mg once daily PO, IV, IM, SC
5-Fluorouracil	5 mg/kg IV q 5–7 days; 200 mg/M² IV once daily for 3 days followed by 100 mg/M² IV on alternate days until signs of toxicity appear; then 200–400 mg/M² IV weekly	None
Folic acid	5 mg/day PO	2.5 mg/day PO
Framycetin	20 mg/kg q6h PO	Same
Furosemide (Lasix)	2–4 mg/kg q8–12h PO; no more than 40–50 mg total IV to any dog, q12h	2–3 mg/kg bid or tid IV, IM (5–10 mg total IV); 2–4 mg/kg q8–12h PO
Gentamicin	4 mg/kg IM, SC q12h first day, then q24h	Same
Glucagon	*Tolerance test*: 0.03 mg/kg IV	None
Glycerin	0.6 ml/kg q8h PO	Same
Glycobiarsol (Milibis-V)	220 mg/kg PO once daily for 5 days with food; repeat in 3 months	None
Glycopyrrolate	0.01 mg/kg IM or SC	None
Griseofulvin	50 mg/kg PO once daily with fat for 6 weeks	Same
Halothane (Fluothane)	*Induction*: 3% *Maintenance*: 0.5–1.5%	Same
Heparin	Initial IV dose: 200 units/kg; continue by SC administration q8h	Same
Hetacillin (Hetacin)	10–20 mg/kg q8h PO	Same
Hydrochlorothiazide (Hydrodiuril)	2–4 mg/kg q12h PO	Same
Hydrocortisone (Solu-Cortef)	4.4 mg/kg q12h PO *Shock*: 50 mg/kg IV	Same
Hydrogen peroxide (3%)	5–10 ml q 15 min PO until emesis occurs	Same
Hydroxyurea (Hydrea)	80 mg/kg q 3 days PO; 40–50 mg/kg divided twice daily PO; 20–30 mg/kg PO as a single daily dose	Same
Imidazole (DTIC)	200 mg/M² for 5 days IV; repeat 5-day cycle q 3 weeks	None
Innovar-Vet	0.1–0.14 ml/kg IM; 0.04–0.09 ml/kg IV; Administer with atropine to minimize bradycardia and salivation	CNS excitation Do not use.
Insulin (regular)	2 units/kg q2–6h IV (ketoacidosis), modified to effect *Hyperkalemia*: 0.5–1.0 units/kg with 2 gm dextrose per unit of insulin	3–5 units SC q6h, modified to effect

DRUG NAME	DOG	CAT
Insulin (intermediate)	0.5–1.0 units/kg q24h SC, modified as needed	3–5 units q24h SC, modified as needed
Isuprel	0.1–0.2 mg q6h IM, SC; 15–30 mg q4h PO; 1 mg in 200 ml 5% dextrose IV to effect Elixir: 0.2 ml q8h PO	Same
Jenotone	2 mg/kg q12h IM, SC	Same
Kanamycin (Kantrim)	10 mg/kg q6h PO; 7 mg/kg q6h IM, SC	Same
Kaobiotic	1 tablet/4 kg/day in 2 or 3 divided doses	Same
Kaopectate	1–2 ml/kg q2–6h	Same
Ketamine (Vetalar)	None	*Restraint*: 11 mg/kg IM *Anesthesia*: 22–33 mg/kg IM; 2.2–4.4 mg/kg IV
Ketaset Plus	None	33–44 mg/kg IM (ketamine content); do not exceed 20 mg/kg for initial dose
Lactated Ringer's solution	40–50 ml/kg/day IV, SC, IP	Same
Laxatol	0.11–0.15 ml/kg q12h SC	Same
Laxatone	*Laxative*: 2–4 ml PO 2–3 days/week	*Laxative*: 1–2 ml PO 2–3 days/week *Hairballs*: 2–4 ml/day PO for 2–3 days; then 1–2 ml 2–3 days/week
Levallorphan (Lorfan)	0.02–0.2 mg/kg IV prn	1 mg/kg IV prn
Levamisole (L-tetramisole)	*Microfilariae*: 10 mg/kg once daily PO for 6–10 days	*Lungworms*: 20–40 mg/kg PO every other day for 5–6 treatments
Lidocaine (without epinephrine) (Xylocaine)	1–2 mg/kg IV bolus, followed by IV drip, 0.1% soln at 30–50 μg/kg/min	Do *not* use as antiarrhythmic.
Lime sulfur (Vlem-Dome) (1:16–1:40 dilution of concentrate)	Topical	Same
Lincomycin	15 mg/kg q8h PO; 10 mg/kg q12h IV, IM	Same
Lindane	0.025–0.1% aqueous soln topically	None
Lomotil	2.5 mg q8h PO	None
Magnesium hydroxide (milk of magnesia)	*Antacid*: 5–30 ml PO *Cathartic*: 3–5 times the antacid dose	*Antacid*: 5–15 ml PO
Magnesium sulfate (Epsom salts)	8–25 gm PO	2–4 gm PO
Mannitol (20% soln)	1.0–2.0 gm/kg q6h IV	Same
Measles vaccine	1 vial SC to dogs between 6 and 8 weeks of age	None
Mebendazole (Telmintic)	0.5 gm/kg with food q24h for 5 days	None
Meclizine (Bonine)	25 mg once daily PO	12.5 mg once daily PO
Megestrol acetate (Ovaban®)	*Skin*: 1 mg/kg/day PO	*Skin:* 5 mg/day PO for one week, then twice weekly.
	Behavior: 2–4 mg/kg once daily; reduce to half dose at 8 days for maintenance	*Behavior*: 2–4 mg/kg once daily; reduce to half dose at 8 days for maintenance.
	To postpone estrus: In proestrus: 2 mg/kg PO daily for 8 days In anestrus: 0.5 mg/kg PO daily for 32 days False pregnancy: 2.0 mg/kg PO daily for 8 days	None
Melatonin	1–2 mg once daily SC for 3 days; repeat monthly as needed	None
Melphalan (Alkeran)	0.05–0.1 mg/kg PO once daily; 1.5 mg/M² PO once daily for 7–10 days, then no therapy for 2–3 weeks	Same
Meperidine (Demerol)	10 mg/kg IM prn	3 mg/kg IM prn
6-Mercaptopurine (6-MP)	50 mg/M² daily PO or 2 mg/kg daily	None
Mercuhydrin	2 mg/kg IM, SC, IV	Same
Metaraminol (Aramine)	2–10 mg SC, IM; 10–50 mg/500 ml saline infused IV to effect	None
Methenamine mandelate (Mandelamine)	10 mg/kg q6h PO to effect	None
Methicillin	20 mg/kg q6h IV, IM	Same

DRUG NAME	DOG	CAT
DL-Methionine	0.2–1.0 gm q8h PO	0.2 gm q8h PO
Methischol	1 capsule/15 kg q8h PO	1 capsule q12h PO
Methohexital (Brevital)	11 mg/kg IV (2.5% soln)	Same
Methotrexate	0.06 mg/kg once daily PO; 0.3–0.8 mg/kg IV weekly; 2.5 mg/M² once daily PO, IV, IM	Same
Methoxyflurane (Metofane)	*Induction*: 3% *Maintenance*: 0.5–1.5%	Same
Methylprednisolone (Medrol®)	See *prednisolone*	Same
(Depomedrol®)	1.0 mg/kg IM every 2 weeks	20 mg/cat IM once
Methyltestosterone	0.5 mg/kg q24h PO	Same
Metronidazole	60 mg/kg q24h PO for 5 days	Same
Metropine	0.5–1.0 mg q8h PO	None
Milk of magnesia. See *Magnesium hydroxide*		
Mineral oil	2–60 ml PO	2–10 ml PO
Mithramycin	2 μg/kg IV once daily for 2 days	Same
Morphine	1 mg/kg SC, IM prn	0.1 mg/kg SC, IM prn
Nafcillin	10 mg/kg q6h PO, IM	Same
Nalorphine	1.0 mg/kg IV, IM, SC	None
Naloxone (Narcan)	0.04 mg/kg IV, IM, SC	None

Neo-Darbazine	1 #1 capsule q12h PO (4.5 to 9 kg)
	2 #1 capsules q12h PO (9 to 13.6 kg)
	3 #1 capsules or 1 #3 capsule q12h PO
	  (13.6 to 27.3 kg)
	1 or 2 #3 capsules q12h PO
	  (over 27.3 kg)
		None

Neomycin (Biosol)	20 mg/kg q6h PO; 3.5 mg/kg q8h IV, IM, SC	Same
Neostigmine (Stiglyn)	1–2 mg IM prn; 5–15 mg PO prn	None
Nikethimide (Coramine)	7.8–31.2 mg/kg IV, IM, SC	Same
Nitrofurantoin (Dantefur)	4 mg/kg q8h PO; 3 mg/kg q12h IM	Same
Novobiocin	10 mg/kg q8h PO	Same
Nystatin	100,000 units q6h PO	Same
Octin	0.5–1.0 ml IM; 1 tablet q8–12h PO	0.25–0.5 ml IM; ½ to 1 tablet q12h PO

o,p-DDD(Lysodren)	50 mg/kg once daily PO to effect
	  (approx. 5–10 days), then once
	  every 2 weeks
		None

Ouabain	0.04 mg/kg total dose IV; give half of
	  dose stat, ⅛ of dose q 30 min
	  (maintenance dose: ¼ of total q3h)
		Same

Oxacillin	10 mg/kg q6h PO, IV, IM	Same
Oxymorphone (Numorphan)	0.1–0.2 mg/kg SC, IM, IV prn	Same
Oxytetracycline	20 mg/kg q8h PO; 7 mg/kg q12h IV, IM	Same
Oxytocin	5–10 units IM, IV; repeats q 15–30 min	0.5–3.0 units IM, IV

2-PAM	40 mg/kg IV over 2-minute period,
	  q12h as needed (may be given IM
	  or SC)
		None

Pancreatin	2–10 tablets with food	1–2 tablets with food
Paregoric	3–5 ml q6h PO	None
Penicillin G, benzathine	40,000 units/kg q 5 days IM	Same
Penicillin G (Na or K)	40,000 units/kg q6h PO (not with food); 20,000 units/kg q4h IV, IM, SC	Same
Penicillin G, procaine	20,000 units/kg q12–24h IM, SC	Same
Penicillin V	10 mg/kg q8h PO	Same
Pentazocine (Talwin)	0.5–1.0 mg/kg IM maximum. **Never IV.**	None
Pentobarbital	*Sedation*: 2–4 mg/kg IV *Anesthesia*: 30 mg/kg IV to effect	Same
Phenethicillin	10 mg/kg q8h PO	Same

DRUG NAME	DOG	CAT
Phenobarbital	*Status epilepticus*: 6 mg/kg q6–12h IM, IV prn *Less severe conditions*: 2 mg/kg PO bid	Same
Phenylbutazone (Butazolidin)	22 mg/kg q8h IV; total dose not to exceed 0.8 gm/day	None
Phenylephrine (Neo-Synephrine)	0.15 mg/kg IV; 10% soln topically in eye	Same
Phenytoin (Dilantin)	*Antiepileptic*: 2–6 mg/kg q8–12h PO *Antiarrhythmic*: 24 mg/kg PO stat, then 3–5 mg/kg q6–8h	None
Phthalofyne (Whipcide)	180 mg/kg PO after 24-hr fast; repeat in 3 months	None
Phthalylsulfathiazole (Sulfathaladine)	50 mg/kg q6h PO; 100 mg/kg q12h PO	Same
Phytonadione. See *Aquamephyton*		
Piperacetazine (Psymod)	*Tranquilization*: 0.11 mg/kg PO bid to qid; 0.11 mg/kg IV, IM, SC *Sedation*: 0.44 mg/kg IV, IM, SC	Same
Piperazine	62 mg/kg PO; may be repeated in 30 days	Same
Pitressin (ADH)	10 units IV, IM (aqueous) or 0.5–1.0 ml IM every other day (oil)	Same
Polymyxin B	2 mg/kg q12h IM; 1–2 mg/kg q12h PO Aerosol: Nebulize 300,000 units in 2.5 ml saline q8–12h	Same
Potassium chloride	1–3 gm/day PO IV: maximum 10 mEq/hr and 40 mEq/day/dog	0.2 gm/day PO
Prednisolone	*Allergy*: 0.5 mg/kg bid PO or IM	1.0 mg/kg bid PO or IM
	Immune suppression: 2.0 mg/kg bid PO or IM	3.0 mg/kg bid PO or IM
	Prolonged use: 0.5–2.0 mg/kg every other morning PO	2.0–4.0 mg/kg every other evening PO
(Solu-Delta-Cortef®)	*Shock*: 5.5–11.0 mg/kg IV, then q 1,3,6, or 10 hours prn	Same
Primidone	55 mg/kg PO sid	None
Procainamide (Pronestyl)	50 mg/kg/day *total* PO q3–6h; 11–22 mg/kg IM q3–6h; 100-mg bolus IV, followed by IV drip at 10–40 µg/kg/min	Not recommended
Promazine (Sparine)	2.2–4.4 mg/kg IV, IM	Same
Promethazine (Phenergan)	0.2–1.0 mg/kg q8–12h PO, SC	None
Propantheline (Pro-Banthine)	Small: 5–7.5 mg q8h PO Medium: 15 mg q8h PO Large: 30 mg q8h PO	5–7.5 mg q8h PO
Propiopromazine (Tranvet)	1.1–4.4 mg/kg PO sid to bid	None
Propranolol (Inderal)	5–40 mg PO tid; 1–3 mg IV (1 mg q 1–2 min); total dose not to exceed 1.5 mg/kg	None
Prussian blue	0.1 gm/kg/day PO q8h	None
Pyrimethamine	1 mg/kg q24h PO for 3 days, then 0.5 mg/kg q24h PO	Same
Quadrinal	¼ to ½ tablet q4–6h PO	¼ tablet q4–6h PO
Quibron	1–3 capsules q8h PO Elixir: 5 ml/15 kg q8h PO	½ capsule q8h PO Elixir: 2 ml q8h PO
Quinacrine (Atabrine)	50–100 mg q12h PO for 3 days; repeat in 3 days	None
Quinaglute	6–20 mg/kg q8–12h PO	Same
Quinidine (Cardioquin, Quinaglute)	10–20 mg/kg PO, IM tid to qid	Not recommended
Rabies vaccine (CEO)	1 vial IM (as per state regulations)	Same
Rabies vaccine (TCO)	1 vial IM (as per state regulations)	Same
Renzol	1 tablet/10 kg q8h PO	Same
Respireze	1 tablet q6–8h PO (up to 12 kg) 2 tablets q6–8h PO (over 12 kg)	None

DRUG NAME	DOG	CAT
Riboflavin	10–20 mg/day PO	5–10 mg/day PO
Ringer's solution	40–50 ml/kg/day IV, IP, SC	Same
Rompun. See *Xylazine*		
Ronnel (Ectoral)	*Sarcoptic mange*: 1% solution q 7–10 days for 3 applications	Not for cats
	Demodectic mange: Mix 180 ml Ectoral with 1000 ml propylene glycol. Shake well. Apply to 1/3 of body daily or every other day for 6–8 weeks or until skin scrapings are negative.	
Septra	30 mg (combined)/kg q24h PO or 15 mg/kg q12h	None
Sodium bicarbonate	50 mg/kg q8–12h PO (1 tsp powder equals 2 gm)	Same
Sodium chloride (0.9% soln)	40–50 ml/kg/day IV, IP, SC	Same
Sodium dioctyl sulfosuccinate	100–300 mg q12h PO	100 mg q12–24h PO
Sodium iodine (20% soln)	1 ml/5 kg q8–12h PO, IV	Same
Sodium levothyroxine	0.1–0.6 mg PO once daily or 0.05–0.3 mg PO bid	0.05–0.1 mg PO once daily
Sodium sulfate (Glauber's salt)	*Purgative*: 10–25 gm PO *Laxative*: 1/5 the purgative dose	*Purgative*: 2–4 gm PO
Spectinomycin	5.5–11 mg/kg q12h IM	None
Stanozolol (Winstrol-V)	1/2 to 2 tablets q12h PO	1/2 tablet q12h PO
Streptomycin	20 mg/kg q6h PO; 10 mg/kg q8h IM, SC	Same
Styrid-Caricide	1 ml/10 kg once daily PO for heartworm prevention	None
Sulfonamides:		
Phthalylsulfathiazole	100 mg/kg q12h PO (not absorbed)	Same
Sulfadiazine	220 mg/kg initial dose, then 110 mg/kg q12h	Same
Sulfadimethoxine	25 mg/kg q24h PO, IV, IM	Same
Sulfamethazine, sulfamerazine, sulfadiazine	50 mg/kg q12h PO, IV	Same
Sulfasalazine (Azulfidine)	10–15 mg/kg q6h PO	None
Sulfathalidine	100 mg/kg q12h PO (not absorbed)	Same
Sulfisoxazole, sulfamethizole	50 mg/kg q8h PO	Same
Tannic acid (Tannalbin)	1 tablet/5 kg q12h PO; decrease dose for several days after diarrhea is under control	Same
Tan-Sal (5% tannic acid, 5% salicylic acid, and 70% ethyl alcohol)	Topical, q8h; no more than 2 treatments	Same
Temaril-P	1 capsule PO q24h (up to 5 kg) 2 capsules PO q24h (5–10 kg) 4 capsules PO q24h (10–20 kg) 6 capsules PO q24h (over 20 kg)	Same
Testosterone	2 mg/kg once daily q 2–3 days PO up to 30 mg total; 2 mg/kg (up to 30 mg total) IM (repositol) q 10 days	Same
Tetracycline	20 mg/kg q8h PO; 7 mg/kg q12h IV, IM	Same
Thiabendazole	50 mg/kg once daily PO for 3 days; repeat in 1 month	None
Thiarcetamide (Caparsolate)	2.2 mg/kg IV bid for 2 days	None
Thiamine	10–100 mg/day PO	5–30 mg/day PO
Thiamylal (Suritol, Bio-Tal)	17.5 mg/kg IV (4% soln)	Same, but use 2% soln
6-Thioguanine (6-TG)	1 mg/kg/day PO	Same
ThioTEPA	0.5 mg/kg once daily for 10 days IV or intralesionally; 9 mg/M² as single dose or in 2–4 divided doses on successive days IV or intracavitary	Same
Thyroid (desiccated)	10 mg/kg/day PO	Same
Toluene (methylbenzene)	200 mg/kg PO	Same
Tresaderm	Topically, q12h; maximum duration of treatment 7 days	Same

DRUG NAME	DOG	CAT
Triamcinolone (Vetalog)	0.25–2 mg once daily PO for 7 days; 0.11–0.22 mg/kg IM, SC	0.25–0.5 mg once daily PO for 7 days; 0.11–0.22 mg/kg IM, SC
Trifluomeprazine (Nortran)	0.55–2.2 mg/kg PO, sid to bid	Same
Trimethobenzamide (Tigan)	For dogs over 15 kg only. 10 mg IM or 100-mg suppository	None
Trimethoprim plus sulfadiazine (Tribrissen)	15 mg (combined)/kg q12h PO or 30 mg (combined)/kg q24h	None
Trimethoprim plus sulfadoxine	15 mg (combined)/kg q24h IM, IV	Same
Tripelennamine	1.0 mg/kg q12h PO; 1 ml/20 kg IM	Same
Trisulfapyrimidine	50 mg/kg q12h PO	None
TSH (thyroid-stimulating hormone)	5 units IV (response test); post sample in 4 hours	5 units IM or SC
Tylosin	10 mg/kg q8h PO; 5 mg/kg q12h IV, IM	Same
Vermiplex	*Single-dose Method:* 1 #000 capsule/0.23 kg 1 #00 capsule/0.57 kg 1 #0 capsule/1.14 kg 1 #1 capsule/2.27 kg 1 #2 capsule/4.55 kg 1 #3 capsule/9.1 kg 1 #4 capsule/18.2 kg Can be repeated in 2–4 weeks. *Divided-dose Method:* Divide body weight by 5 and administer appropriate size capsule once daily for 5 days. Can be repeated in 2–4 weeks.	Same Same
Vinblastine (Velban)	3.0 mg/M² weekly IV or 0.1–0.5 mg/kg weekly	Same
Vincristine (Oncovin)	0.025–0.05 mg/kg q 7–10 days; 0.5 mg/M² IV weekly or biweekly	Same
Viokase	Mix into food 20 minutes prior to feeding; 1–3 tsp/lb of food	Same
Vi-Sorbin	1–3 tsp/day PO	½ tsp/day PO
Vitamin A	400 units/kg/day PO for 10 days	Same
Vitamin B₁₂	100–200 μg/day	50–100 μg/day
Vitamin D	30 units/kg/day PO for 10 days	Same
Vitamin E	500 mg/day PO	100 mg/day PO
Vitamin K₁ (phytonadione)	5–20 mg IV, IM, or SC q12h	1–5 mg IV, IM, or SC q12h
Xylazine (Rompun)	1.1 mg/kg IV; 1.1–2.2 mg/kg IM, SC	Same
Yomesan	157 mg/kg PO. Overnight fast. Repeat in 2–3 weeks.	Same

INDEX

Note: Page numbers in *italic* refer to illustrations; page numbers followed by (t) refer to tables. Additional pertinent information, still current, found in *Current Veterinary Therapy V* or *VI*, is designated within brackets by the edition and page number.

Abdominal paracentesis, cytologic specimen from, 18
Abscess, carnassial tooth, 870
  retro-orbital, 583
Absorption, of poison, delaying of, 106
Acanthocephala, of aquatic turtles, 645
  of fish, 614
Accidental hypothermia, 197–199
  rewarming techniques for, 198, 198(t)
Acid-base disturbances, fluid therapy for, 41
  in poisoning, 113
  in renal failure, 1045, 1089
Acidifiers, urinary, 1164–1165, 1198
Acidosis
  metabolic, in diabetic ketoacidosis, 1017
    in poisoning, 113
    in renal failure, 1045
  paradoxical cerebrospinal fluid, 1019
ACTH, measurement of, in hyperadrenocorticism, 979
Actinomycin D, for embryonal nephroma, 1207
Actinomycosis, 485
Addison's disease, 983–988
  chronic, treatment of, 987
  home therapy for, 987
  laboratory findings in, 985(t)
Addisonian crisis, acute, treatment of, 985
Adenocarcinoma, functional pancreatic islet cell, canine, 1020–1023
  of ciliary body, 585
Adenoma, of ciliary body, 585
Adenovirus, canine, 229, 1251, 1253(t), 1254, 1276
ADH, exogenous, 1083
  in diabetes insipidus, 1005–1011

Adoption shelters, control of infectious diseases in, canine, 1268–1269
  feline, 1272
Adrenal gland imaging, 979
Adrenal insufficiency, causes of, 984(t)
  physical findings in, 985(t)
  primary, 983–988
Adrenalectomy, 981
Adrenergic drugs, 211(t)
  decongestant, 212
  effects of, 210(t)
Adrenocortical function, evaluation of, in hyperadrenocorticism, 976–977
Adrenocortical insufficiency, episodic weakness and, 792(t), 795
  secondary, iatrogenic, 991–992, 991(t)
Adrenocortical tumor, hyperadrenocorticism due to, 976
  therapy of, 983
Adrenocorticosteroids, 497–500, 499(t). See also *Corticosteroids; Steroids.*
  characteristics of, 993(t)
Adrenocorticotropic hormone, measurement of, in hyperadrenocorticism, 979
Adsorbents, in poisoning, 107
Aelurostrongylus abstrusus, 264
Aerodynamic filtration, in bronchopulmonary clearance, 209
Aerosol therapy, [VI:12]
  in bacterial pneumonia, 238
Aflatoxicosis, 123
African green monkey disease, 737
Agalactia, 1225
Aggression, 841–844
  interspecies, 842–843
  intraspecies, 841–842
  normal development of, 845

Aggression *(Continued)*
  territorial, 847
  therapy of, 843–844
    progestin, 845, 847–853, 848–849(t)
Air bronchograms, 285, *285*
Airway, collapse of, 283
  lower, disease of, radiographic diagnosis of, 283–284
  obstructed, cardiopulmonary resuscitation for, 295, 295(t), *296*
  patency of, in shock, 39
Airway resistance, modification of, 210
Alanine, in calcium oxalate urolithiasis, 1183
Aldosterone, 498
Algae infection, of fish, 613
Alimentation, artificial, of laboratory animals, 762
Alkalizing agents, for diabetic ketoacidosis, 1017
Alkalosis, in poisoning, 113
  respiratory, in heat stroke, 195
Alkylamine, 501(t)
Allergens, inhalant, skin tests for, 207
Allergic bronchitis, 230
Allergic dermatitis, 438
  contact, 447(t)
  in cats, 471, 471(t)
Allergic diseases, of cats, 471
Allergic pneumonia, 240, 287
Allergy, alopecia and, 492
  fleabite, in cats, 471
  food, in cats, 471
Alligators, infectious agents in, 628
Allopurinol, in urolithiasis, calcium oxalate, 1183
  urate, *1173,* 1174
Alopecia
  canine breeds with, 489
  color mutant, 489
  congenital, 489
  feline, 490–493

Alopecia (*Continued*)
    feline, endocrine, 492
        universalis, 489
    of pinna, 489
    psychogenic, 491
Aluminum hydroxide, for diarrhea, 918
Alveolar edema, pulmonary, *286*
Amino acids, sources of, 1105
Aminoglycosides, 14
    properties of, 6(t)
    nephrotoxicity of, 1049
Aminopterin, teratogenicity of, 170
Ammonia, toxicity of, to tropical fish, 608, 610, 610(t), 611(t)
Amphibians, diseases of, 616–617, 616(t)
    environmental considerations for, 617(t)
    treatment and care of, 617, 618(t)
Amphotericin B, in mycotic pneumonia therapy, 240, 240(t)
    nephrotoxicity of, 1050
    properties of, 7(t)
Amputations, in captive reptiles, 624–625
Amyloidosis, renal, 1063–1066
Anabolic agents, in polyuric renal failure, 1102
Anal area, anatomy of, 952
Analgesics, for birds, 655(t)
    narcotic, in diarrhea, 916, 916(t)
    urinary, 1167
Anamnesis, 505–506
Anconeal process, un-united, 810, *810*
Ancylostoma caninum, 266
Androgens, for estrus prevention, 1238
    for male canine infertility, 1229
Anemia, 414
    aplastic, 415
    chronic, effect on heart, 346
    hemolytic, autoimmune, 390, *391*, [VI:431]
        Heinz body, 417–418
    in chronic interstitial nephritis, 1077
    management of, [VI:421]
Anesthesia
    in heart disease, canine, [VI:388]
    in laboratory animals, 767
    in renal failure, 1117–1121
    of caged birds, 653–656, 655(t)
    of non-domestic carnivores, 719, 730–732(t)
    of rabbits and rodents, 706–710, 707–709(t)
    of reptiles, 618–620
Anesthetics
    inhalation, in renal failure, 1119
        nephrotoxicity of, 1050
    local, 501–503, 502(t)
    topical ophthalmic, 519
Anestrus, 1031
    lengthening of, pharmacologic methods of, 1032–1033
        surgical, 1032
    shortening of, 1032
Angiography, in canine heartworm disease, 328
Angiostrongylus vasorum, 267
Anisocoria, 511, 539

Anorexia, effects of, on uremic dog, 1104
Anorexia nervosa, 851
Ant bites, 177
Antacids, for diarrhea, 918
Anthelmintics, 938–940(t)
    benzimidazole, for heartworm prophylaxis, 333
    for carnivores, 728(t)
Antiallergic properties of glucocorticoids, 988
Antiarrhythmic drugs, 387
    pharmacodynamics of, 357–359
Antibiotics
    for birds, 1274(t)
    in feline respiratory disease, 1280
    in gastric dilation, acute, 900
    in hepatitis, chronic active, 888
    in ocular therapy, 521, 524(t), 525(t)
    in prostatitis, 1149
    in reptiles, 647–649
    in shock, 42
    in ulcerative colitis, 950
    teratogenicity of, 171
Anticholinergic drugs, in diarrhea, 917, 917(t)
Anticholinesterase therapy, in myasthenia gravis, 793(t)
Anticoagulant poisoning, 125(t), 131–134, 132(t)
Anticonvulsants, in epilepsy, 836, 837
Antidiuretic hormone, exogenous, 1083
    in diabetes insipidus, 1005–1011
Antidotes, against poisoning, 107, 108–112(t)
Antifreeze poisoning, 125(t), 126, 144–146
Antifungal agents, in ocular disease, 526, 526(t)
    nephrotoxicity of, 1050
Antigens
    dog leukocyte and erythrocyte, histocompatibility tests for, 401
    removal of, in glomerulonephropathy, 1058
    selection of, in canine atopic disease, diagnosis of, 451, 452(t)
        treatment of, 455, 456(t), 457(t)
Antiglobulin (Coombs') test, 390, *391*
Antihistamines, 500–501, 501(t)
    in canine atopic disease, 455
Anti-inflammatory drugs, 988
Antimicrobial agents
    conventional regimens for, 9(t)
    failure of, causes of, 10, 12(t)
    nephrotoxicity of, 1049
    newer, 14–16
    pharmacokinetic data for, 10(t)
    pharmacologic hazards of, 12
    properties of, 6–8(t)
    selection of, 2–13, 4–5(t)
    tissue distribution of, 11(t)
Antimicrobial therapy, 2–16, 4–5(t)
Antinuclear antibody test, 393
Antipruritic drugs, pharmacology of, 497–503
Antiseptics, urinary, 1165–1166
Antispasmodics, urinary, 1167
Antitussives, 232, 232(t)
Antivenins, 181(t)

Antiviral agents, in ocular disease, 526
ANTU poisoning, 125, 125(t), [VI:117]
Aortic arch, persistent right, [VI:398]
Aortic stenosis, 303–305, [VI:392]
Aortic thromboembolism, feline, and acquired heart disease, [V:305]
Aplastic anemia, 415
Aquarium, conditioning of, 608, *609*
Aqueous dynamics, 576
Arboviral arboreal disease cycles, 739–740, 740(t)
Arboviruses, infectious viral diseases caused by, 740(t)
Arrhythmia, cardiac, control of, 375
    digitalis-induced, diphenylhydantoin for, 381
    episodic weakness and, 792(t), 794
Arsenic poisoning, 125(t), [VI:134]
Arthritis, canine, synovial fluid in, 801(t)
    rheumatoid, 392, *392*
    canine, 800–802
Arthropods, nasal, 266
Arthus reaction, skin tests for, 401
Artificial ventilation, in pulmonary edema, 248
Ascarids, 937, 941
Ascites, in chronic active hepatitis, 889
Aspergillosis, 479
    in captive wildfowl, 691
    nasal, 479
    serology of, 208
Aspiration, transtracheal, 207
Aspiration pneumonia, 241
Asteroid hyalosis, 579
Asthma, feline, 230
    radiographic diagnosis of, 283
Atarax, teratogenicity of, 170
Atelectasis, radiographic diagnosis of, 284
Atopic disease, 447(t)
    canine, diagnosis of, 450–453
        treatment of, 453–458
Atrial fibrillation, 384, *385*
Atrial premature beats, 382, *383*
Atrial septal defect, 316, [VI:394]
Atrial standstill, 377, *379*, 380
Atrial tachycardia, 383, *384*
Atrioventricular heart block, 377, 378, 379
Atropine, in insecticide poisoning, 148
    in renal failure, 1119
Auscultation, of chest, pneumonia, 236
    of respiratory sounds, 205
Australia, tick paralysis in, 777–779
Australian elapid venoms, pathogenesis of, 179–182
Autoimmune diseases, of skin, 432–436, 433(t)
Autoimmune hemolytic anemia, 390, *391*, [VI:431]
Autoimmune thyroiditis (lymphocytic), 394
Avian herpesvirus infections, acute, 704–706
Avian influenza, 675
Avian pox, 702

Aviaries, control of infectious
  diseases in, 1273–1276
Azoospermia, canine, 1228
  feline, 1236
Azulfidine, in ulcerative colitis, 950

B cells, 909
  erythrocyte-antibody-complement
    rosettes for, 400
  membrane immunoglobulin assay
    for, 400
B-cell system, deficiencies of, 397
Bacterial conjunctivitis, 551
Bacterial diseases, of captive reptiles,
  [VI:787]
  of imported birds, 676
Bacterial folliculitis-furunculosis, 436
Bacterial infection, control of, in
    aviaries, 1274
  of respiratory tract, in psittacine
    birds, 700
Bacterial pneumonia, 237–239
Bacterial polyarthritis, canine, 797
Bactericidal function test, 396
Bacteriuria, significant, screening
  tests for, 1154–1157, 1156(t)
Barbiturate anesthetics, for rabbits
    and rodents, 706–707, 707(t)
  use of, in renal failure, 1119
Barium sulfate, for diarrhea, 919
Basal cell carcinoma, cryotherapy of,
  496
Basenjis, plasma proteins in, 1327(t)
Bedlington liver disease, 885,
  [VI:995]
Bee stings, 177
Behavior
  aggressive. See Aggression.
  control of, with progestin, 845–853
  development of, normal and
    abnormal, [V:703]
  physiology of, 845–846
Bence Jones protein, thermal
  solubility test for, 396
Benzimidazole anthelmintics, for
  heartworm prophylaxis, 333
Benzodiazepines, use of, in renal
  failure, 1119
Bicarbonate therapy, in urate
    urolithiasis, 1174
  of polyuric renal failure, 1094–1096
Bilirubin, 876
  in diagnosis of jaundice, 877(t)
Biologic carcinogens, 173
Biopsy
  endoscopic, 955
    gastric, 959
  gastrointestinal, 962–969
  intestinal, in malassimilation
    syndrome, 932
  liver, 883, 894
  of colon, 966
  of esophagus, 965
  of rectum, 967
  of small intestine, 966
  of stomach, 965
Birds
  antibiotics for, 1274(t)
  caged, anesthesia of, 653–656,
    655(t)

Birds (Continued)
  caged, clinical laboratory examina-
      tion of [V:543]
    diseases of, 599, 649–706
    feather disorders of, [VI:675]
    lead poisoning in, 143
    neoplasia in, [V:585]
    parasitic diseases of, [VI:682]
    psittacosis in, 677–686
  captive wild, care and treatment of,
    692–696
    husbandry of, [VI:687]
  fractures of, 663–667, 664–666,
    669–672, 669–671
    of extremities, [VI:717]
  imported, foreign diseases and,
    674–676
  infectious disease control in, in
      aviaries and pet shops,
      1273–1276
  laparoscopy in, diagnostic, 659–661,
    660, 661
  oil-soaked, management of,
    687–692
  orthopedic diseases of, 662–673,
    664–673
  psittacine. See Psittacine birds.
  radiographs of, in respiratory
      disease, 698
    technique and interpretation for,
      649–653, 651, 652(t)
  sexing of, by laparoscopy, 659
    otoscope technique for, 656, 657,
      658
  surgery of, [VI:711]
  urinary system of, diseases of,
    [VI:703]
  vaccines for, 1275(t)
Bitch, nonspayed, diabetes mellitus
  in, 1015
Biters, hereditary, 850
Bites, animal, 1266
  venomous, 174–178
Bladder
  calculi in, 1169
  decreased size of, 1130
  hypotonic, management of,
    1195–1196
  irrigation of, 1166–1167
  neoplasms of, 1208–1211, 1209(t)
  rupture of, 1139–1141
    traumatic, 1046
Blastomycosis, 239, 482
Blepharitis, 548
Blepharoedema, 542
Blindness, 505
Blood
  chemical constituents of,
    1325–1327(t)
  in shock, monitoring of, 48
  coagulation defects in, acquired,
    879, 879(t)
  collection of, in laboratory animals,
    746–749(t), 749–750
    sites for, in carnivores, 724(t)
  genetic disorders of, 83–84(t)
  replacement of, in shock, 40
Blood flow, regional, in shock state,
  34–35
Blood gases, analysis of, in
    pulmonary edema, 246
  exchange improvement of, in
    pulmonary edema, 247

Blood gases (Continued)
  normal, 1326(t)
Blood pressure, in shock, monitoring
  of, 47
Blood replacement, in shock, 40
Blood transfusion, in feline
  respiratory disease, 1280
Blood values, normal, 1321–1330(t)
  canine, 1321(t), 1322(t)
  feline, 1321(t), 1322–1323(t)
"Blue-eye," 564
Blue irides, genetic etiology of, 590
Body fluid, abnormalities of, in renal
    failure, 1043–1045, 1089
  volume disorders of, 1043, 1088
Body lumps and swellings, in aquatic
  turtles, 643
Body-surface area, conversion of
  weight to, 1320(t)
Bone disease, genetic, 85–86(t)
  uremic, 1078
Bone marrow, normal values in,
  1324(t)
Bone marrow failure, 413–416
Bordetella bronchiseptica infection
  canine, 229
    respiratory disease and, 1277
    vaccine for, 1251, 1253(t), 1255
  in non-domestic carnivores, 714
Botfly, rodent, 266
Botulism, 773–776
Bouvier, young, laryngeal paralysis
  in, 290–291
Brachial plexus, avulsion of, in dogs,
  [VI:828]
Brachycephalic dogs, upper
  respiratory disease in, 221
Bradycardia, 376–381, 378–380
  atropine non-responsive, 380
  atropine-responsive, 377
Brain injury, 815–820, 819
Brain stem damage, 816, 816(t), 818,
  818(t)
Breath sounds, classification of, 236,
  236(t)
Breathing, positive pressure, 277
Breeding stock, selection of, 75
Bronchial breath sounds, 236, 236(t)
Bronchial collapse, 282, 283
Bronchial washings, 207
Bronchiectasis, 232–233, 283
Bronchiolitis, obstructing, 283
Bronchitis, 229–232
  allergic, 230
  chronic, 283
  cycle of, 230, 231
Bronchograms, air, 285, 285
Bronchopneumonia, 283, 285
Bronchopulmonary clearance, 209
Bronchoscopy, 206
Bronchospasm, due to adverse drug
  reaction, 213
Bronchovesicular breath sounds, 236,
  236(t)
Brucella canis, in kennels, 75
Brucellosis, canine, 1303–1305
  neonatal death and, 80
  vaccine for, 1255
Budgerigars, enlargement of thyroid
  glands of, 704
Burns, 191–192
  classification of, 192
  pathophysiology of, 192–193

Burns (*Continued*)
  treatment of, 193–194
Butyrophenones, use of, in renal
    failure, 1119

C3 component, quantitation of, by
    RID, 397
CaEDTA, in lead poisoning, 139, 142
Caimans, infectious agents in, 628
Calcium, abnormalities of, in renal
    failure, 1045
  metabolism of, [VI:1038]
Calcium oxalate urolithiasis,
    1177–1184, 1179–1181(t)
Calculus(i). See also *Urolithiasis*.
  analysis of, 1180, 1181(t)
  formation of, theories of, 1177
  prevention of recurrence of, 183
  problem-specific data base for, 1183
  subgingival, 863, *864*
    scaling technique for, 866, *866,
      867*
  supragingival, 863, *864*
Calicivirus, feline, 224, 225(t), 229,
    1279–1284
  control of, in catteries, 1270
  vaccine for, 1257, 1257(t), 1260,
    1283
Calories
  in parenteral hyperalimentation,
    927, 928(t)
  non-protein, sources of, 1105
  requirements of, in renal failure,
    1099, 1101
  restriction of, partial, 1037, 1037(t),
    1038(t)
  total, 1038, *1038*
Campylobacter fetus infection, in
    humans, 1267
Canary, physical examination,
    laboratory and medication
    techniques and hospitalization
    procedures for, [V:533]
Cancer. See also *Carcinoma;
    Neoplasia; Tumors;* and under
    individual types of tumors.
  chemotherapy of, 423–426,
    425–426(t)
Canine hereditary black hair follicle
    dysplasia, 488
Canine upper respiratory disease,
    214–223
  acute, 214–219
  chronic, 219–223
  localization of clinical signs in,
    215(t)
Cannulas, for peritoneal dialysis,
    1108, *1108, 1109*
Capillaria aerophila, 265
Capillaria plica, 1142–1143
Capillary hematocrit technique, for
    microfilariae, 329
Capillary hydrostatic pressure,
    reduction of, in acute heart
    failure, 364(t), 365, *366*
  in pulmonary edema, 247
Capillary refill time, in shock, 45
Carbamate poisoning, 126, 147–148
Carbamazepine, for diabetes
    insipidus, 1009

Carbohydrate metabolism, effect of
    glucocorticoids on, 989
  measurements of, as liver test, 883
Carbonic anhydrase inhibitors, 527
Carcinogenesis, 172–173
Carcinoma
  basal cell, cryotherapy of, 496
  cytology of, 22, *22*
  hepatocellular, primary, 883, 883(t)
  of urethra, 1211(t), 1212
  of urinary bladder, 1208, 1209(t)
  renal, 1204, 1204–1205(t), 1206
Cardiac arrest, 297
Cardiac arrhythmias, control of, 375
Cardiac catheterization, [V:251]
Cardiac output, measures to increase,
    364(t), 365
Cardiac workload, reduction of, 372
Cardiomyopathy, 307–315, *308*
  canine dilated, 312, *312*
    therapy of, 315
  canine hypertrophic, 311
  clinical findings in, 308(t)
  dilated, 307, *308*, 308(t)
    therapy of, 314
  feline dilated, 311, *311*
  feline hypertrophic, 307, *309, 310*
  hypertrophic, 307, *308*, 308(t)
    therapy of, 312
Cardiopulmonary resuscitation,
    human, 293–296, 293(t), *294*, 295(t),
    296
Cardiorespiratory system, obesity
    and, 341
Cardiovascular diseases, 292–388
  episodic weakness and, 792(t), 794
  genetic, 87(t)
  ocular signs of, 596(t)
Cardiovascular support, in poisoning,
    113
Cardiovascular system, in large
    animals, clinical examination of,
    [VI:410]
  of racing dog, 347–351
Carnivores, 710, 710(t)
  disease susceptibility of, 710, 711(t)
  non-domestic, anesthesia and
    chemical restraint of, 719,
    730–732(t)
    blood collection sites in, 724(t)
    dentition of, 726(t)
    hematologic data for, 720–723(t)
    immunization of, 711–713, 712(t)
    infectious diseases of, 713–715,
      713(t)
    medical care of, 710–732
    nutrition of, 718–719, 719(t)
    parasites of, 719
      treatment of, 726–729(t)
    pediatrics of, 715–717
    reproductive physiology of,
      724–725(t)
    surgery of, 728–733
Castration, 731
Catabolism, reversal of, in uremia,
    1105
Catalase test, urinary, 1156(t), 1157
Cataplexy, 838, *838*
  drug levels for, 840
Cataracts, 532, 567–569
  classification of, 566(t)
  development of, 568

Cataracts (*Continued*)
  genetic etiology of, 591, 592(t)
  heredity of, 567(t)
  progression of, based on location,
    568(t)
  sugar, 568
Catecholamines, for acute heart
    failure, 364(t), 365
Cathartics, in poisoning, 107
Catheter
  indwelling urethral, in feline
    urologic syndrome, 1193–1195,
    1194(t)
  intravenous, for fluid therapy, 49
  for oxygen therapy, 43
  for peritoneal dialysis, 1108, *1108*
Catheterization, cardiac, [V:251]
  jejunal, for portography, 826, *826*
Catteries, control of infectious
    diseases in, 1270–1271
CAV-1, 1276
  vaccine for, 1253, 1253(t)
CAV-2, 1276
  vaccine for, 1251, 1253(t), 1254
Caval syndrome, posterior, 328
Cavities, 856–861, *861*
Celiotomy, in reptiles, 623–624
Cell kinetics, and chemotherapeutic
    agents, 423, *424*
Cell-mediated immunity, deficiencies
    of, 397–400
Cell migration, inhibition of, 399
Cellulose acetate electrophoresis, 395
Cellulose phosphate, in calcium
    oxalate urolithiasis, 1182
Central nervous system, disorders of,
    in poisoning, 114
  effect of steroid hormones on,
    846–847
Central venous pressure, in shock,
    monitoring of, 46
Cephalosporins, 14
  nephrotoxicity of, 1049
  properties of, 6(t)
Cerebral circulation, in shock, 34
Cerebral edema, 818, 1019
  in heat stroke, 196
Cerebral infarction syndrome, feline,
    [VI:906]
Cerebral toxins, hepatic
    encephalopathy and, 823, 824(t)
Cerebrospinal fluid
  acidosis of, paradoxical, 1019
  analysis of, 769–772
  changes in, with disease, 772–773
  contaminated, correction formula
    for, 770(t)
  normal values in, 1328(t)
Cestodes, of aquatic turtles, 645
  of fish, 614
Chalazion, 548
Chelonia, infectious agents in,
    626–628
  shell repair of, 621–623
Chemical agents, carcinogenic, 172
  teratogenetic, 168, 169(t)
Chemical analysis of tissues, in
    poisoning, 115–121, 117–118(t)
Chemical constituents, of blood,
    1325–1327(t)
  in shock, monitoring of, 48
Chemical disorders, 104–201

Chemical injury, inhalation, 187. See also *Inhalation injury.*

Chemical products, hazardous, 151–153(t)

Chemical restraint, of non-domestic carnivores, 719, 730–732(t)

Chemosis, 551

Chemotherapy
adjuvant, rationale for, 424
cancer, 423–426, 425–426(t)
combination, 423
induction-remission, of feline lymphosarcoma, 409, 409(t)
of canine heartworm disease, 331, 331(t)
of renal tumors, 1207
with *o,p'*-DDD, in hyperadrenocorticism, 982

Chest
auscultation of, in pneumonia, 236
drainage of, 255
in pneumothorax, 271, 272
flail, 274

Cheyletiellosis, 470

Chickenpox, in non-human primates, 739

Chikingunya, 740, 740(t)

Chlamydia psittaci, 677
feline pneumonitis and, 1299–1302, *1300, 1301*

Chlamydial conjunctivitis, 552
feline, 1300–1302, *1301*

Chlamydial infection, control of, in aviaries, 1275
of caged birds, 677
of imported birds, 676

Chloramphenicol, properties of, 7(t)

Chloride, serum, abnormalities of, in renal failure, 1044
alterations of, effect on heart, 345

Chlorinated hydrocarbon insecticide toxicosis, 125(t), [VI:141]

Chlorpropamide, for diabetes insipidus, 1009

Cholera, fowl, vaccine for, 1275(t)

Cholestasis, 876–878

Cholesterol, radiolabeled, for adrenal gland imaging, 979

Cholesterol fractionation, in liver disease in man, 882(t)

Cholinergic drugs, 519

Cholinomimetic agents, 519

Choriomeningitis, lymphocytic, 738
human infection with, 1267

Choroidal disease, 579–582

Choroidal hypoplasia, focal, genetic etiology of, 592

Choroiditis, 580

Chow, myotonia in, 787–790, *788, 789*

Chromolyn, 212

Chromosomal abnormalities, canine, 87(t)

Chylothorax, 259(t), 260

Chylous effusions, 259(t), 260

Cilia, abnormalities of, 546, 547
genetic etiology of, 589

Ciliary body, adenomas and adenocarcinomas of, 585
cysts of, 575

Cirrhosis, of liver, laboratory findings in, 884

Clindamycin, properties of, 7(t)

Cloaca, impactions of, in oil-soaked birds, 691

Clofibrate, for diabetes insipidus, 1009

Coagulants, in snake venom, 179

Coagulation
defects acquired, 879, 879(t)
with chronic active hepatitis, 890
disseminated intravascular, [VI:448]
from chronic liver disease, 879, 879(t)
in heat stroke, 196
inhibition of, in glomerulonephropathy, 1060

Coccidia infections, 944–946, 945(t)

Coccidioidomycosis, 240, 482

Colchicine, for resolution of liver fibrosis, 887

Cold, common, 738

Cold injury, 199–201

Colitis, acute, 948–949
management of, 948–952
ulcerative, 949–952

Collie dogs, gray, cyclic neutropenia in, 415

Collie eye anomaly, 592

Collie nose, 438

Colloids, in shock, 41

Coloboma, of iris, 571

Colon, biopsy of, 966
polyps of, 960
spastic syndrome of, 952

Colonoscopy, 960

Colostrum, immunity and, 1248

Coma, diabetic, 1019
hyperosmolar, 1019

Communicable diseases, in laboratory animals, 767

Complement, quantitation of C3 component by RID, 397
total hemolytic assay, 397

Compound 1080 poisoning, 125, 125(t), [VI:119]

Congenital anomalies, neonatal kennel deaths and, 73
potential causes of, 164–171, 167(t), 169(t)

Congestive heart failure. See *Heart failure, congestive.*

Conjunctiva
cytology of, 509
diseases of, 550–553
foreign bodies in, 543
lacerations of, 543
microbiologic cultures of, 506
plasma cell infiltration of, 553
tumors of, 553

Conjunctivitis
bacterial, 551
chlamydial, 552
feline, 1300–1302, *1301*
chronic, 551
follicular, 552
mycoplasma-associated, 552

Contraceptives, 1032–1033

Contact allergic dermatitis, 447(t)
in cats, 471, 471(t)

Coombs' test, 390, *391*

Coonhound paralysis, 773–776

Copepod parasites, 614

Copulatory failure, feline, 1232–1233

Cor pulmonale, 335–337

Cornea
anatomy and physiology of, 559
cytology of, 509
diseases of, 558–565
congenital, 559
genetic etiology of, 590
foreign bodies in, 543
microbiologic cultures of, 506
perforated, 544
ulcers and abrasions of, 543

Corneal degeneration, 561
genetic etiology of, 590

Corneal dystrophy, 560
genetic etiology of, 590

Corneal edema, genetic etiology of, 590

Corneal endothelialitis, 564

Corneal sequestrum, 563

Corneal ulcers, *533*, 543, 561

Corneal wounds, traumatic, 564

Coronary circulation, in shock, 34

Coronavirus, canine, 1293, 1294
vaccine for, 1254

Coronoid process, of ulna, fragmentation of, 811–813, *811, 812*

Corticosteroids
anti-inflammatory, 497–500, 499(t)
for management of pulmonary diseases, 212
for pregnancy termination, 1240
in allergic pneumonia, 241
in canine atopic disease, 454
in chronic active hepatitis, 885, 886(t)
in flea allergy dermatitis, 448
in gastric dilation, acute, 900
in ocular therapy, 520, 522(t)
in ulcerative colitis, 951
teratogenicity of, 170
topical, 442

Cortisol, 498

Coryza, infectious, avian vaccine for, 1275(t)

Cough
in tracheobronchial disease, 231
kennel, 229, 1276–1278
in non-domestic carnivores, 714
vaccine for, 1251, 1255
non-productive, 209

Cough reflex, common causes for, 230(t)

Cough suppressants, 209

Coulter chemistry, 1325(t), 1326(t)

Crackles, 236, 236(t), 237

Creatine phosphokinase, in cerebrospinal fluid, 772, 772(t)

Crenosoma vulpis, 264

Crocodiles, infectious agents in, 628

Crusting dermatosis, in cats, 469–472

Cryosurgery, 65–66
in small animal dermatology, 495–497
of captive reptiles, 625
of epidermal cyst, 496
of eyelid tumors, 549
of mastocytoma, 496
of perianal fistula, 954

Cryptococcosis, 483
nasal, feline, 227, 228

Cryptorchidism, canine, 1244–1246

Crystallization-inhibition theory, of calculogenesis, 1177
Crystalloids, in volume replacement, 39
Curet, for dental debriding and scaling, 866, 867
Cushing's syndrome, 990–991, 991(t)
  effect on heart, 340
  myopathy with, 790, 791
Cutaneous lymphoma, canine, 493–495
Cutaneous lymphosarcoma, 494
Cuterebra maculata, 266
Cyclic-AMP, pathway to, 211, 211
Cyst
  capsulogenic renal, 1073
  epidermal, cryotherapy of, 496
  of ciliary body, 575
  of iris, 575
  urachal, 1144, 1145
Cystic calculi, feline, 1187
Cystine urolithiasis, 1175–1176
Cystinuria, 1175–1176
Cystitis, canine polypoid, 1137–1138, 1138(t)
Cystocentesis, 1150–1153, 1152, 1153, 1192
Cystourethrography, in prostatic disease, 1148
Cytauxzoonosis, feline, 1312–1313
Cytologic specimen, collection and preparation of, 17–19
  in respiratory disease, 207
  interpretation of, 17, 19–24
Cytology, diagnostic, 16–27
  of cerebrospinal fluid, 770
Cytotoxicity tests, 399
Cytotoxics, in snake venom, 179

Dacryocystitis, 551
DDAVP, in diabetes insipidus, 1009, 1010
Death, neonatal, 79–82
  causes and treatment of, [VI:44]
  congenital anomalies and, 73
Deciduous teeth, development and retention of, 855–858
Declawing, 728
Decongestion, 212
Dehydration, in renal failure, 1043
Demodectic mange, 437
Demodicosis, 437
Dermatitis
  allergic, 438
  canine nasal solar, 438, 440–443
  contact allergic, 447(t)
    in cats, 471, 471(t)
  facial, differential diagnosis of, 436–440, 437(t)
  flea allergy, 446–450, 447(t)
  flea-collar, 126
  fungal, 437
  "puppy-dog," human infection with, 1267
  pustular, of neonate, 73
  seborrheic, 438
  zinc-responsive, 439
Dermatitis herpetiformis, 443–445
Dermatophilosis, 436, 486

Dermatophytosis, 437
Dermatosis, crusting, in cats, 469–472
  subcorneal pustular, 438, 443–445
  zinc-responsive, 472–476
Dermoids, ocular, genetic etiology of, 588
De-scenting, 728
Desmopressin, in diabetes insipidus, 1009, 1010
Desoxycorticosterone acetate, 986, 987
Dexamethasone tests, in diagnosis of canine hyperadrenocorticism, 977–978, 977(t)
Diabetes insipidus, 1005–1011, 1006(t), [V:805]
Diabetes mellitus, 1011–1016
  diet in, 1015
  elective surgery in, 1015
  in nonspayed bitches, 1015
Diabetic ketoacidosis, 1016–1019, [V:822]
Diagnostic cytology, 16–27
Dialysate solutions, 1107, 1108(t)
Dialysis, peritoneal, current status of, 1106–1111
  in hypothermia, 199, 200
Diaphragmatic hernia, 273, 273
Diarrhea
  chronic, diagnostic approach to, [VI:971]
  intestinal motility in, 914–916
  locally acting drugs for, 918–919
  management of, 914–919
  motility modifiers in, 916–918, 916(t), 917(t)
Diazepam, in epilepsy, 836, 837
Diestrus, 1031
Diet
  calculi formation and, 1197
  commercial controlled, 925
  commercial defined, 925–929
  elemental, 925, 926(t)
  in calcium oxalate urolithiasis, 1182
  in cardiomyopathy, 315
  in congenital maldevelopment, 167
  in diabetes mellitus, 1015
  in management of gastrointestinal problems, 919–929
    formulation of, 922–924
    principles of, 920–922, 920(t), 921(t)
  in hepatitis, chronic active, 886
  in hyperphosphatemia, 1103, 1103(t)
  in physical fitness and training for dogs, 62–64
  in polyuric primary renal failure, 1097–1101, 1100(t)
  management of, [VI:59]
  zinc requirements in, 474
Dietary disorders, of aquatic turtles, 641
Diethylcarbamazine, for heartworm prophylaxis, 332
Diethylstilbestrol, for benign prostatic hyperplasia, 1149
Digestive system, genetic disorders of, 88(t)
Digitalis, in chronic congestive heart failure, 373
  pharmacodynamics of, 352

Digitalis glycosides, 352–355
  in heart failure, acute, 364(t), 365, 366
  chronic congestive, 373
Digitalis intoxication, 355, 374
  with heart failure, 347
Digitalization, in chronic congestive heart failure, 373
Digitoxin, pharmacodynamics of, 353, 353(t)
Digoxin, in chronic congestive heart failure, 373
  in dilated cardiomyopathy, 314
  pharmacodynamics of, 353, 353(t)
Dihydrotachysterol, in hypoparathyroidism, 1001
Dimple, myotonic, 788, 788
Dioctophyma renale, 1141–1142
Dipetalonema reconditum, 326, 326(t), 327, 330(t)
Diphenylhydantoin, for tachyarrhythmia, 381
  teratogenicity of, 170
Dip-slides, for urine culture, 1155
Dirofilaria immitis, 267
  immunity and, 333
  infection by, 326–335
  life cycle of, 327
Dirofilariasis, zoonotic, 334
Disk disease, intervertebral, canine, [VI:841]
Disseminated intravascular coagulation, [VI:448]
  from chronic liver disease, 879, 879(t)
  in heat stroke, 196
Dissociative anesthetics, for rabbits and rodents, 707–708, 708(t)
Distemper virus, canine, 1284–1286
  multiple sclerosis and, 1267
  vaccines for, 1252, 1253(t)
  feline, 712, 713
Distichiasis, 546
  genetic etiology of, 589
Diuresis
  in calcium oxalate urolithiasis, 1182
  in polyuric renal failure, 1091–1093
  osmotic, mechanics of, 1093
Diuretics
  in congestive heart failure, 374
  in oliguric renal failure, 1089
  loop, 1090
  mercurial, 357
  osmotic, 1089, 1091
    in intracranial injury, 818
  pharmacodynamics of, 356–357
  thiazide, 357
    for renal diabetes insipidus, 1009
    in calcium oxalate urolithiasis, 1182
    in congestive heart failure, 375
Diverticulum, vesicourachal, 1144, 1144
Doca, 986, 987
Droperidol-fentanyl anesthesia, for rabbits and rodents, 708, 709(t)
Drug(s)
  adrenergic, 210(t), 211(t), 212
  adverse reactions to, 155–160, 156–158(t)
    effect on lungs, 213
  antiarrhythmic, 357–359, 387

Drug(s) (*Continued*)
antibacterial, for tropical fish, 615
anticonvulsant, 836, 837
antifungal, in ocular disease, 526, 526(t)
nephrotoxicity of, 1050
anti-inflammatory, 988
antimicrobial. See *Antimicrobial agents.*
antipruritic, 497–503
antiviral, in ocular disease, 526
cholinergic, 519
common, approximate doses of, 1331–1339(t)
elimination of, role of kidneys in, 1114, 1115(t)
for laboratory animals, 764–766(t), 767
for turtles, 642(t)
hypoglycemics, oral, 1012
immunosuppressive, in ulcerative colitis, 951
vaccination and, 1250
in cancer treatment, 425–426(t)
in diarrhea, 916–919, 916(t), 917(t)
in gastric dilation, acute, 900
in glaucoma, 520(t), 578(t)
in renal disorders, 1114–1117, 1115(t), 1116(t)
nephrotoxic, 1048(t), 1049–1051
ophthalmic, 517–527
Drug eruption, 458–461, 459(t), 460(t)
Drug intolerance, mechanisms of, 1048–1050
Drug resistance, in cancer chemotherapy, 424
Drug toxicity, anemia secondary to, 414
Dysplasia, elbow, 810, *810*
hip, canine, 802–806, *803, 804*
retinal, 591
Dyspnea, causes of, in small animals, 362(t)
evaluation of patient with, 363(t)
Dysrhythmia, vagal, 377, *378*
Dystocia, 1212–1214
Dysuria, 1160
Dysuria-hematuria, 1160

EAC rosettes, for B cells, 400
Ear, genetic disorders of, 88(t)
Eclampsia, in kennels, 75
Ectoparasites, in kennels, 71
in laboratory animals, 751
Ectropion, 548
Edema
cardiogenic, 369, *369, 370*
cerebral, 818, 1019
in heat stroke, 196
corneal, 590
pulmonary. See *Pulmonary edema.*
Effusions
chylous, 259(t), 260
hemorrhagic, 257, 259(t)
inflammatory, 258, 258(t)
neoplastic, 259(t), 261
obstructive, 258(t), 260
pyogranulomatous, 259(t), 261
Egg binding, in aquatic turtles, 644
Ehrlichia canis infection, aplastic anemia of, 415

Elapids, Australian, venoms of, pathogenesis of, 179–182
Elbow dysplasia, 810, *810*
Elbow joint, osteochondrosis in, 809–813, *810–812*
Electrocardiography
in Addison's disease, 984, *986*
in dirofilariasis, 329
in pulmonary edema, 246
in shock, 46
normal criteria in, 1319(t)
Electrolyte(s)
abnormalities of, effect on heart, 342–345
in diabetic ketoacidosis, 1017
in renal failure, 1044
balance of, effect of glucocorticoids on, 989
imbalance of, in chronic active hepatitis, 889
in parenteral hyperalimentation, 928
serum, normal, 51(t), 1326(t)
Electrolyte therapy, 49–53
in heat stroke, 197
in shock, 39–41, 40(t)
Electromyography, in myotonia, 788, 789
Electrophoresis, cellulose acetate, 395
normal values in, 1325(t)
serum protein, in liver disease, 881, 881(t)
Emesis, induction of, in poisoning, 106
Emphysema, subcutaneous, of psittacine birds, 703
Encephalitis, equine, avian vaccine for, 1275(t)
monkey B-virus, 1266
Encephalopathy, hepatic, 888
canine, 822–829, 823–826(t)
ischemic, feline, [VI:906]
Endocarditis, mural, 305–307
valvular, 305–307
Endocrine disorders, 974–1039
effect on heart, 340
feline infertility and, 1233
genetic, 89(t)
Endocrine effects, of glucocorticoids, 990
Endocrine factors, in teratogenesis, 168
Endocrine secretions, normal, 1326(t)
Endometritis, chronic, feline, 1234
Endometrium, cystic hyperplasia of, 1216
Endoparasites, in kennels, 71
Endophthalmitis, antibiotic treatment of, 525(t)
Endoscopy, gastrointestinal fiberoptic, 954–961
in respiratory disease, 206
Endothelialitis, corneal, 564
Endotracheal intubation, of rabbit, 709–710
Enophthalmos, 584
Enteritis
canine parvoviral, 1294
canine viral, 1292–1295
vaccines for, 1253(t), 1254
duck virus, vaccine for, 1275(t)

Enterocolitis, acute, adjunctive therapy in, 917(t)
Entropion, 547
Eosinophilic granuloma, of cats, 872
Eosinophilic ulcer, cryotherapy of, 496
Epidermal cysts, cryotherapy of, 496
Epidermolysis bullosa simplex, 439
Epilepsy, 830, [VI:853]
treatment of, 835–837
types of, 831–833
Epiphora, 557
genetic etiology of, 598
Episodic weakness, 791–795, 792(t)
Epistaxis, 214
differential diagnosis of, *216*
Erysipelas, avian vaccine for, 1275(t)
Erythrocyte(s), normal values for, 1321(t)
Erythrocyte-antibody-complement rosettes, for B cells, 400
Erythrocyte antigens, dog, histocompatibility test for, 401
Erythron disorders, in burns, 193
Eserine test, 515
Esophageal worm, of dogs, 267
Esophagitis, acute, 956
Esophagoscopy, 206, 956
Esophagus
biopsy of, 965
dilation of, 957
diseases of, [VI:931]
foreign bodies in, 957
Estradiol cypionate, for benign prostatic hyperplasia, 1149
Estrogen, and urinary incontinence, 1133–1135
for pyometra, 1218
toxicity of, thrombocytopenia and, 415
Estrous cycle, 1030–1031
control of, 1032
Estrus, 1031
induction of, 1032
prevention of, 1237–1239
Ethanolamines, 501(t)
Ethylene glycol, nephrotoxicity of, 1050
poisoning with, 125(t), 126, 144–146
Ethylenediamines, 501(t)
Exercise, 347
energy sources for, 348
insulin requirement and, 1015
restriction of, in dilated cardiomyopathy, 315
Exostoses, multiple cartilaginous, in dogs, [VI:886]
Exotic pets
diseases of, 599–649, 706–767
feline, immunization of, 1258–1261
hematology of, [VI:765]
radiology of, [VI:756]
Expectorants, 209
Eye. See also *Ocular* and *Ophthalmic* entries.
bulging, 505
care of, in feline respiratory disease, 1281
cloudy, *531*
examination of, 506–510
genetic disorders of, 90–91(t)

Eye (*Continued*)
  opacities over, 505
  prolapse of, 545
  red, 535
  surgical preparation of skin of, 527
  systemic disease and, 593,
    594–598(t)
Eyelids
  conformation abnormalities of,
    genetic etiology of, 589
  diseases of, 546–550
  double eversion of, 508
  ecchymoses in, 542
  edema of, 542
  lacerations of, 542
  third. See *Nictitating membrane.*

Facial dermatitis, differential
  diagnosis of, 436–440, 437(t)
Fading kitten syndrome, 81, 1314
Fading puppy syndrome, 72, 80
Fanconi syndrome, in dogs, 1075
Fat absorption test, 931
Fat balance studies, 931
Fatty liver, laboratory findings in, 884
FCV. See *Calicivirus, feline.*
Feathers, broken, repair of, 672, 673
  disorders of, in common caged
    birds, [VI:675]
  oil-soaked, 688
Fecal trypsin activity, 931
Feces, analysis of, in laboratory
    animals, 751
  microscopic examination of, in
    malassimilation syndrome, 931
Feline calicivirus. See *Calicivirus,
  feline.*
Feline infectious peritonitis, 299,
    713, 1288–1292
  control of, in catteries, 1271
Feline leukemia virus, 713
  control of, in catteries, 1271
  disease complex of, 404–410
  human infection with, 1267
Feline oncornavirus-associated cell
    membrane antigen
    (FOCMA)-antibody test, 407, 427
Feline upper respiratory disease,
    224–228, 714
  acute infectious, 224
  acute non-infectious, 226
  chronic infectious, 226
  chronic non-infectious, 227
Feline urologic syndrome
  management of, 1188–1190
    of hypotonic bladder, 1195–196
  prophylaxis of, medical, 1196–1201
    surgical, 1201–1203
  urethral obstruction in, relief of,
    1191–1193
  use of indwelling urethral catheters
    in, 1193–1195, 1194(t)
Feline viral rhinotracheitis, 224,
    225(t), 229, 872, 1279–1284
  control of, in catteries, 1270
  vaccines for, 1257, 1257(t), 1259,
    1283
FeLV. See *Feline leukemia virus.*
Fevers of unknown origin, 28–31,
    28(t), 29(t)

Fiberoptic endoscopy,
    gastrointestinal, 954–961
Fibrinogenolysis, primary, with
    chronic liver disease, 879, 879(t)
Fibrosis, resolution of, in hepatitis,
    chronic active, 887
Filarioid nematodes, 326, 326(t)
Filaroides hirthi, 263
Filaroides milksi, 263
Filaroides osleri, 229, 262
Filter technique, for microfilariae,
    329
Fish, tropical, infectious diseases of,
    611–615
  medical care of, 606–615
Fistula, perianal, 952–954
  urethrorectal, 1133
Flagellates, 944
Flail chest, 274
Flea allergy dermatitis, 446–450,
    447(t)
Flea-collar dermatitis, 126
Flea control, 448
Flea infestation, in cats, 469
Fleabite allergy, in cats, 471
Fluid(s), body, normal distribution of,
    51(t)
  intravenous, contents of, 51(t)
  stomach, abnormal production of,
    897
Fluid therapy, 49–53, [VI:3]
  determination of volume needed
    in, 50
  for acid-base disturbances, 41
  in acute gastric dilation, 899
  in captive wild birds, 693
  in feline viral respiratory disease,
    1280
  in heat stroke, 197
  in shock, 39–41, 40(t)
  monitoring of, 52
  placement of catheters for, 49
  rate of administration of, 51
  selection of catheters for, 49
  special considerations in, 52
Fluorescein dye test, 508, 527
Fluorescent antibody technique, 395,
    395(t)
FOCMA, 407, 427
Follicular conjunctivitis, 552
Folliculitis-furunculosis, bacterial,
    436
Food allergy, in cats, 471
Food-borne intoxication, [VI:176]
Food poisoning, 124
Foreign body pneumonia, 213
Fowl plague variant, 675
Fractures
  in captive reptiles, repair of, 624
  of birds, 663–667, *664–666,*
    669–672, *669–671*
  of extremities, [VI:717]
  rib, 274, 275
Freezing injury, 200–201
Frostbite, 200–201
Fundus, pigmentation variations of,
    genetic etiology of, 591
Fungal dermatitis, 437
Fungal disease
  of captive reptiles, [VI:787]
  of imported birds, 676
  of fish, 613

Fungal disease (*Continued*)
  of respiratory tract, in psittacine
    birds, 702
  systemic, 239
    processing clinical specimens for,
      478
    serology of, 208
Fungicides, for tropical fish, 615
  poisoning with, [VI:143]
  teratogenic, 169, 169(t)
Furosemide, 313, 314, 357
  in congestive heart failure, 375
FVR. See *Rhinotracheitis, feline
  viral.*

Galactorrhea, 1225
Galactostasis, 1225
Gammopathies, 395–396, [VI:451]
Garbage intoxication, [VI:176]
Gas, stomach, abnormal production
  of, 897
Gas exchange, improvement of, in
  acute heart failure, 364(t), 365
Gastric biopsy, 965
  endoscopic, 959
Gastric decompression, 898
Gastric dilation, 896–901
Gastric lavage, in poisoning, 106
Gastritis, giant hypertrophic, 959
Gastroenteritis, canine coronaviral,
  1293
Gastroesophageal junction, abnormal,
  896
Gastroesophageal sphincter,
  abnormal, 896
Gastrointestinal biopsy, techniques
  of, 962–969
Gastrointestinal disorders, 854–973
  antimicrobial agents in, 913–914
  diet and nutrition in management
    of, 919–929
  of puppy, in kennels, 73
Gastrointestinal fiberoptic endoscopy,
  954–961
Gastrointestinal parasitism, 935–948
Gastrointestinal tract, immunity of,
  907–912
  microbiology of, 901–912
  microflora of, 901–907, 902(t), 903(t)
Gastroscopy, 957–960
Genetic defects, canine, 82–96
Genetic disorders, 78–79
  ophthalmic, 587–593
Genital anomalies and infections,
  feline infertility and, 1233–1236
Genital system, 1212–1246
Genitourinary disorders, 1040–1246
Genodermatoses, 487–490
Gerbils, diseases of, 761(t)
  physiologic data on, 742(t)
  sexing of, *745,* 745(t)
Gestation, 76
Gingivectomy, 867, *868*
Gingivitis, 864, *865*
  role of complement in, 863, *864*
Glaucoma, 576–578
  acute, 546
  congenital, 576
  drugs and dosages for, 578(t)
  genetic etiology of, 591

Glaucoma (*Continued*)
  primary, 576
  secondary, 577
  topical miotics for, 520(t)
Globe, proptosis of, 545
Glomerulonephritis, 1076
  immune-complex, 394
  membranous, in heartworm
    disease, 328
Glomerulonephropathy, 1053–1062
  anti-GBM, 1054, 1057
  immune-complex, 1054, 1057
    therapy of, 1057–1060
Glossopharyngitis, feline, 871
Glucocorticoids, 498
  effects of, 988–990
  in Addisonian crisis, acute, 986
  in ocular therapy, 522(t)
  in shock, 41
  in tracheobronchitis, 232
  relative potencies and average
    systemic dosage of, 499(t)
  systemic, 988–994
Glucocorticoid-induced hepatopathy,
    laboratory findings in, 884, 884(t)
Glucose consumption test, for urine
    culture, 1156(t), 1157
Glucose tolerance test, intravenous,
    in pancreatic islet cell tumor,
    1020, *1021, 1022*
  oral, in malassimilation syndrome,
    932
Glycogen storage disease, type I,
    1024
Glycogenoses, 821(t)
Glycols, nephrotoxicity of, 1050
  poisoning with, 125(t), 126,
    144–146
Glycosides, digitalis, 352–355
    in heart failure, acute, 364(t), 365,
    366
    chronic congestive, 373
Glycosuria, 1011, 1014
Gonadotropic hormones, in male
    canine infertility, 1228
Gonioscopy, 509
Granuloma, eosinophilic, of cats, 872
Greyhounds, behavior problems in,
    851
  cardiovascular system of, 349–351
  racing, exertional rhabdomyolysis
    in, 783–787
Griseofulvin, properties of, 7(t)
  teratogenesis and, 169
Guinea pigs, diseases of, 754–755(t)
  physiologic data on, 742(t)
  sexing of, *745*, 745(t)

Haemobartonella felis, 410, *411*
Hair, hereditary abnormalities of,
    487–490
Hamsters, diseases of, 756–757(t)
  physiologic data on, 742(t)
  sexing of, *745*, 745(t)
Heart, influence of non-cardiac
    diseases on, 340–347
  traumatic injury to, 345, *346*
Heart block, atrioventricular, 377,
    378, 379

Heart disease. See also *Cardio-
    myopathy* and *Myocardial
    disease.*
  acquired, and aortic thrombo-
    embolism, feline, [V:305]
  canine, anesthesia in, [VI:388]
  diagnosis and management of,
    [VI:313]
  valvular, 297–307
Heart failure
  acute, 359–367, *360*
    causes of, 360, 360(t)
    diagnosis of, 361–364
    management of, 364–367, 364(t)
  chronic congestive, long-term
      therapy of, 368–376
    management of, 371–376
  congestive, 1096
    episodic weakness and, 792(t),
      794
    pathophysiology of, 369–371
  low-output, management of, 367
  management of, chronic, 367
  prevention of, 372
Heartworm(s), canine, 267
Heartworm disease, canine, 326–335
  episodic weakness and, 792(t), 794
  occult, serology of, 207
Heat, detection of, 76. See also
    Estrus.
Heat stress, 195–197
Heat stroke, 195–197
Heinz body hemolytic anemia,
    417–418
Helminth infection, prevalence of, in
    dogs, 935, 936(t)
Helminth parasites, preventive and
    control measures for, 947–948
Hematocrit, in shock, monitoring of,
    46
Hematology, of captive reptiles,
    [VI:792]
  of non-domestic carnivores,
    720–723(t)
  of zoo animals and exotic pets,
    [VI:765]
Hemeralopia, genetic etiology of, 592
Hemobartonellosis, feline, 410–413
Hemoconcentration, 1071
Hemodialysis, current status of,
    1111–1113
Hemogram parameters, in liver
    disease, 876(t)
Hemolymphatic disorders, 389–430
Hemolysins, in snake venom, 179
Hemolytic complement, C3
    component, quantitation by RID,
    397
  total, assay of, 397
Hemorrhage, control of, in shock, 39
Hemorrhagic defects, inherited,
    [VI:438]
Hemorrhagic effusions, 257, 259(t)
Hemostasis, disorders of, in burns,
    193
  normal parameters of, 1327(t)
Hemothorax, 275, *276*
Hepatic. See also *Liver.*
Hepatic encephalopathy, 888
  canine, 822–829, 823–826(t)
  ischemic, feline, [VI:906]

Hepatic mass, reduced functional,
    879–882
Hepatitis
  canine infectious, 1276
    vaccine for, 1251, 1253, 1253(t)
  chronic active, canine, 885–891
    laboratory findings in, 883, 883(t)
  chronic progressive, in Bedlington
      terriers, [VI:995]
  duck virus, vaccine for, 1275(t)
  infectious (simian), 737
Hepatocellular carcinoma, primary,
    laboratory findings in, 883, 883(t)
Hepatocellular disease, 878–879
Hepatopathy, glucocorticoid-induced,
    laboratory findings in, 884, 884(t)
Herbicides, poisoning with, 126,
    [VI:143]
  teratogenic, 169, 169(t)
Hermaphroditism, feline, 1231
Hernia(s), 94(t)
  diaphragmatic, 273, *273*
Herniation, tentorial, 816, 817(t), *818,*
    818(t)
Herpes B, 734
Herpesvirus hominis type I, in
    non-human primates, 739
Herpesvirus infections
  avian acute, 704–706
  canine, vaccine for, 1254
  in neonate, 80
    in kennels, 73
  in raptors, 705–706
  parrot, 704–705
  pigeon, 705
  psittacine, 675
Herpesvirus platyrrhinae, 736
Herpesvirus simiae, 734, 1266
Herpesvirus T, 736
Herpesvirus tamarinus, 736
Herpetic keratoconjunctivitis, 522
Heterochromia irides, 571
  genetic etiology of, 590
Hip dysplasia, canine, 802–806, *803,*
    804
Histocompatibility tests, for dog
    leukocyte and erythrocyte antigens,
    401
Histoplasmosis, 239, 483
Hock, osteochondritis dissecans of,
    813–814, *814*
Hookworms, 935–937
Hordeolum, 548
Hormones
  adrenocorticotropic, measurement
      of, 979
  antidiuretic, exogenous, 1083
    in diabetes insipidus, 1005–1011
  ectopic production of, by
      nonendocrine neoplasms,
      [VI:1061]
  luteinizing, immunization with, for
      canine contraception, 1033
  ovarian, 1030–1031
  steroid, effect on central nervous
      system, 846–847
  teratogenicity of, 170
Horner's syndrome, 515
  clinical features of, 516
  pharmacologic localization of, 516,
      516(t)

Hornet stings, 177
Howling, night, canine, 851
Humerus, osteochondritis dissecans of medial condyle of, 811–813, *812*
Hunting dog hypoglycemia, 1026
Hyalitis, 579
Hyaloid vasculature, persistence of, 579
Hyalosis, asteroid, 579
Hyaluronidase, in snake venom, 180
Hydrocarbons, chlorinated, poisoning with, 125(t), [VI:141]
Hydronephrosis, 1073–1074
    capsular, 1073
Hydroxyurea, teratogenicity of, 170
Hydroxyzine, teratogenicity of, 170
Hymenoptera, stings of, 177
Hyperadrenocorticism
    canine, 975–979
        dexamethasone tests in diagnosis of, 977–978, 977(t)
        due to adrenocortical tumor, 976
        effect on heart, 340
        evaluation of pituitary-adrenocortical function in, 976–977
        iatrogenic, 990–991, 991(t)
        pituitary-dependent, 975–976, 975(t)
        therapy of, 979–983, *980, 981*
    spontaneous, therapy for, 979–983
Hyperalimentation, parenteral, 926–929, 926–929(t)
Hypercalcemia
    and nephropathy, 1051, 1067–1072
    differential diagnosis of, 1003, 1068(t)
    diseases characterized by, 1068(t)
    disorders associated with, in small animals, 1069–1072
    effect on heart, 345
    in lymphosarcoma, 422
    in renal failure, 1045
    primary hyperparathyroidism and, 1003
    renal lesions of, 1069
    treatment of, 1072
Hypercalcitoninism, nutritional, [VI:1048]
Hypercalciuria, oxalate uroliths and, 1178
Hyperinsulinism, hypoglycemia and, 794
Hyperkalemia
    effects of, 984(t)
        on heart, 343, *344*
    myocardial toxicity due to, treatment of, 986
    renal failure and, 1044
        oliguric, 1089
    sinoventricular rhythm due to, 377, *379, 380*
        treatment of, 381(t)
Hyperkinesis, 850
Hypernatremia, in renal failure, 1045
Hyperoxaluria, 1178
Hyperparathyroidism, primary, 1003–1005, 1068(t), 1070
    secondary, with renal failure, 1004
Hyperphosphatemia, control of, 1103–1104

Hyperphosphatemia (*Continued*)
    in renal failure, 1045
Hyperplasia, reactive, cytology of, 23, 24(t), *25*
Hyperpotassemia, effect on heart, 343, *344*
Hyperpyrexia, 195–197
Hypersensitivity, delayed, 401
    immediate, 401
Hyperthermia, in poisoning, 113
Hyperthyroidism, feline, 998–999
Hyperuricosuria, oxalate uroliths and, 1179
Hypervitaminosis D, 1068(t), 1070
Hyphema, 545, 574, 575(t)
Hypoadrenocorticism, 983–988. See also *Addison's disease.*
    effect on heart, 341
    hypercalcemia in, 1071
    hypoglycemia and, 1025
Hypoalbuminemia, with liver disease, 880, 881
Hypocalcemia, effect on heart, 345, *345*
    puerperal tetany and, 1027–1029, *1027–1029*, 1045
Hypochloremia, in renal failure, 1045
Hypoglycemia
    canine, non-neoplastic causes of, 1023–1027
    causes of, 1026
    clinical manifestations of, 1023
    endocrine, 1025
    episodic weakness and, 792(t), 794
    hepatogenous, 1025
    hunting dog, 1026
    in functional pancreatic islet cell tumor, 1020
    juvenile-onset, 1024–1025
    mature-onset, 1025–1026
    neonatal, 1024
Hypoglycemics, oral, 1012
Hypokalemia, effect on heart, 342, *343*
    in diabetic ketoacidosis, 1017
    in renal failure, 1044
Hyponatremia, effects of, 984(t)
    in renal failure, 1044
Hypoparathyroidism, primary, 1000–1002
Hypophosphatemia, in diabetic ketoacidosis, 1017
    in heat stroke, 196
Hypophysectomy, 979–981, *980, 981*
Hypopigmentation, 488
Hyposensitization, in canine atopic disease, 455–458, 456–458(t)
    in flea allergy dermatitis, 449
Hypothermia, 199–200
    accidental, 197–199
    in poisoning, 113
    rewarming techniques for, 198, 198(t), 200
Hypothyroidism, 994–998, 995(t), *996, 997*
    effect on heart, 341
Hypovitaminosis A, vs. respiratory disease, in psittacine birds, 700
    in reptiles, 636, 636(t)
Hypovolemia, in poisoning, 113

Ichthyosis, canine, 490
Imipramine, in cataplexy, 840
Immune system
    cell-mediated, 1248
    factors influencing, 1248–1250
    humoral, 1248
    uremia and, 1078
Immune-complex glomerulonephritis, 394
Immune-complex glomerulo-nephropathy, 1054, 1057
    therapy of, 1057–1060
Immune-mediated disorders, 390–395
Immunity
    active, 908
        intestinal, 910–912
    cell-mediated, deficiencies of, 397–400
    humoral, deficiencies of, 397
    non-specific, disorders of, 396
    of gastrointestinal tract, 907–912
    restoration of, 429
    specific, disorders of, 397–403
Immunization
    canine, 1252–1255, 1253(t)
    feline, 1256–1261, 1257)t), 1260(t)
    of exotic cats, 1258–1261
    of non-domestic carnivores, 711–713, 712(t)
    schedule of, in kennels, 70, 71(t)
    theory and practice of, 1248–1251
Immunodeficiency disorders, 396–403
Immunodiffusion, radial, 396, 397, 400
Immunoelectrophoresis, 395
Immunofluorescence test, 395, 395(t)
Immunoglobulin assay, membrane, for B cells, 400
Immunologic disorders
    autoimmune responses in, percentage of positive tests for, 402(t)
    correction of, in glomerulone-phropathy, 1058–1060
    in burns, 193
    laboratory diagnosis of, 390–403, *391*
Immunologic surveillance, 426–428
Immunologic thrombocytopenic purpura, 393
Immunomodulators, non-specific, 429(t)
Immunoproliferative disorders, 395–396
Immunoprophylactics, 1251
Immunosuppression, effect of glucocorticoids on, 988
Immunosuppressive agents, in ulcerative colitis, 951
    vaccination and, 1250
Immunotherapy, 428
    active, 428
    of malignant disease, 426–430
    passive, 429
Impactions, intestinal, in aquatic turtles, 644
Imping, 672, *673*
Incontinence. See *Urinary incontinence.*
Infection
    documentation of, 2, 3(t)

Infection (*Continued*)
congenital maldevelopment and, 166, 167(t)
etiologic agents in, 3(t)
immunosuppression and, 1250
mycobacterial, in non-domestic animals, 604–606
of burn wound, 192
treatment of, 194
of respiratory system, control of, 213
urinary tract, 1158–1161. See also *Urinary tract, infections of.*
Infectious diseases, 1247–1317
ocular signs of, 594–595(t)
of neonate, 80
of non-domestic carnivores, 713–715, 713(t)
of reptiles, 625–633
diagnosis and treatment of, 631–632
taxonomic distribution of, 626–631
of tropical fish, 611–615
Infectious myocarditis, 318
Infertility
canine, 1226–1231
female, 1229–1231
male, 1227–1229
feline, 1231–1237
Infiltrative myocardial disease, 317
Inflammation
anemia and, 414
cytology of, 19–21, 19(t), *20*
effects of glucocorticoids on, 988
inhibition of, in glomerulo-nephropathy, 1060
Inflammatory effusions, 258, 258(t)
Inflammatory muscle disease, canine, 779–782
infectious causes of, 782
Influenza, 738
avian, 675
Inguinal hernia, 94(t)
Inhalation, water, 182–186
Inhalation anesthesia, for rabbits and rodents, 708–709
Inhalation injury, 186–191
classification of, 188(t)
initial treatment of, 189(t)
physical examination in, 187(t)
sequelae of, 190, *190*
Inhalation pneumonia, 242
Inhalation therapy, in feline respiratory disease, 1282
Inorganic phosphates, in calcium oxalate urolithiasis, 1182
Insecticides, poisoning with, 147–148. See also under individual agents.
teratogenic, 169, 169(t)
Insemination, artificial, of cats, [VI:1252]
of dogs, [VI:1245]
Insulin
dosage of, 1013, 1014(t)
preparations of, 1012(t)
requirement of, exercise and, 1015
therapy, 1012, 1013, *1013*, 1014(t), 1018
Intermittent positive-pressure ventilation, of caged birds, 655

Intervertebral disk disease, canine, [VI:841]
Intestinal biopsy, 966
in malassimilation syndrome, 932
Intestinal immunity, active, 910–912
Intestinal impactions, in aquatic turtles, 644
Intestinal lymphangiectasia, 934
Intestinal malabsorption, 934
Intestinal motility, in diarrhea, 914–916
modifiers of, 916–918, 916(t), 917(t)
Intestine(s)
peristalsis in, 914
rhythmic segmentation of, 914, *915*
small, obstruction of, [VI:952]
Intracranial injury, 815–820, *819*
Intraocular tumors, 585–586
Intravenous fluids, contents of, 51(t)
Intubation, endotracheal, of rabbit, 709–710
intragastric, of laboratory animals, 762
Iridocyclitis, 571–574
causes of, 572(t)
Iris
atrophy of, 574, 575
colobomas of, 571
congenital abnormalities of, 570
cysts of, 575
hypoplasia of, genetic etiology of, 590
Irish terriers, sex-linked myopathy in, 790
Ischemic myocardial disease, 317
Islet cell tumors, functional pancreatic, 1020–1023
Ixodes holocyclus, 777

Jaundice, 877
diagnosis of, use of bilirubin in, 877(t)
Johne's disease, 606
Joint(s)
canine, degenerative diseases of, 796
elbow, osteochondrosis in, 809–813, *810–812*
genetic disorders of, 85–86(t)
knee, osteochondritis dissecans of, 813, *813*
lesions of, in oil-soaked birds, 691
luxations of, in birds, 667–669, *667, 668*
shoulder, osteochondritis dissecans of, 808–809
stifle, osteochondritis dissecans of, 813, *813*
synovial fluid in, normal values of, 1329(t)

Kaolin, for diarrhea, 918
Kennel
breeding, control of brucellosis in, 1304
diseases in, 72–75

Kennel (*Continued*)
reproductive considerations in, 75–76
preventive medicine in, 67–76
Kennel cough, 229, 1276–1278
in non-domestic carnivores, 714
vaccine for, 1251, 1255
Keratitis, 561–564
chronic, *534,* 563
ulcerative, 561
Keratoconjunctivitis, herpetic, 552
Keratoconjunctivitis sicca, 554–556, 563
Ketamine, use of, in renal failure, 1120
Ketoacidosis, diabetic, 1016–1019, [V:822]
Kidneys, 1042–1121. See also *Renal* entries.
decreased size of, 1130
diseased, response to diuretics, 1092
disorders of, in burns, 193
hollow fiber artificial, 1112
neonatal, anatomy and physiology of, 1085
neoplasms of, 1203–1208, 1204–1206(t)
role of, in congestive heart failure, 347
in drug elimination, 1114, 1115(t)
susceptibility of, to toxins, 1048
traumatic injury of, 1045
tubular-interstitial disease of, chronic, 1076–1079
Kitten mortality complex, 81, 1313–1316
Knee, osteochondritis dissecans of, 813, *813*
Knott technique, modified, 329

Laboratory animals
blood collection in, 746–749(t), 749–750
care and treatment of, 741–767
communicable diseases in, 767
drug dosages for, 764–766(t), 767
ectoparasites in, 751
fecal analysis in, 751
intragastric intubation and artificial alimentation of, 762
physical examination of, 741–743
routes of medication in, 762
sexing of, 743, *744–745,* 745(t)
surgery and anesthesia in, 767
urine collection and analysis in, 750
virus diagnostic testing in, 750, 751(t)
Labrador retrievers, myopathy with myotonia and muscle fiber deficiency in, 790
Lacrimal apparatus, diseases of, 553–558
Lacrimal drainage system, 556–558
cannulization of, 508
Lactation, blood parameters in, canine, 1323(t)
feline, 1324(t)
inappropriate, 1225

Lactulose, in hepatic encephalopathy, 828
Lagomorphs, manual restraint of, 744
Lagophthalmus, 548
Laparoscopy, diagnostic, in birds, 659–661, *660, 661*
    in small animal medicine, 969–973, *970, 972*
Laparotomy, in adrenocortical tumor, 979, 983
Laryngeal collapse, canine, 223
Laryngeal malformations, 94(t)
Laryngeal paralysis, canine, 222
    in young Bouviers, 290–291
Laryngeal spasm, in cats, 227
Laryngeal trauma, 217
Laryngeal tumors, 251
Laryngoscopy, 206
Lavage, gastric, 106
LE cell test, 394
Lead poisoning, 125(t), 126, 136–141
    in caged birds, 143
    in cats, 140, 143
    in dogs, 141
    in parrots, 141
    in New Zealand, 141–144
Leeches, of aquatic turtles, 645
Lens
    classification of, 566(t)
    coloration of, 566
    diseases of, 565–570
    growth of, 565
    opacities of, transient, 569
    subluxations and luxations of, 566
Leptospirosis, canine, vaccine for, 1255
    chronic interstitial nephritis and, 1076
Leukemia, feline. See *Feline leukemia virus.*
    lymphatic, clinical staging of, 421(t)
Leukocyte(s), normal values for, 1321(t)
Leukocyte antigens, dog, histocompatibility test for, 401
Levamisole, 263, 264, 267
    for canine heartworm disease, 331
Libido, loss of, in cats, 1232–1233
Lidocaine, 358
Light reflex, 511–517, *511, 512*
Limbic system, effect of progestins on, 846
Lincomycin, properties of, 7(t)
Linguatula serrata, 266
Lipid metabolism, effect of glucocorticoids on, 989
    in liver disease, 882, 882(t)
Liver
    biopsy of, 883
        in feline liver disease, 894
    cirrhosis of, 884
    clinical pathology of, 875–885
    disease of, anemia of, 414
        biochemistries in, 876(t)
        blood coagulation defects and, 879, 879(t)
        feline, 891–895
        hypoglycemia and, 1025
        laboratory findings in, 883–885, 883(t), 884(t)
        lipid metabolism in, 882, 882(t)
        neoplastic, laboratory findings in, 883, 883(t), 884(t)

Liver (*Continued*)
    disorders of, in burns, 193
    fatty, 884
    functional mass of, reduced, 879–882
    tests of synthesizing and detoxifying ability of, 882–883
Lizards, infectious agents in, 628
    venomous, 176
Loop diuretics, 1090
Lovebirds, psittacosis in, treatment of, 683
Lungs, adverse effects of drugs on, 213
    normal fluid movement in, 244, *245*
    tumors of, 252–253
Lupus erythematosus
    discoid, 439
        cutaneous manifestations of, 433(t), 435
    systemic, 393, 439
        cutaneous manifestations of, 433(t), 435
    systemic canine, [VI:463]
        polyarthritis in, 798–800
Lupus erythematosus cell test, 394
Luteinizing hormone, immunization with, for canine contraception, 1033
Luxations, lens, 566
    of bird joints, 667–669, *667, 668*
Lymph node aspirates, cytologic evaluation of, 24–27, *25–27*
Lymphadenitis, granulomatous, cytology of, 26, *26*
    subacute, cytology of, 26, *26*
Lymphangiectasia, intestinal, 934
Lymphatic leukemia, clinical staging of, 421(t)
Lymphatic system, genetic disorders of, 87(t)
Lymphatics, peripheral, diseases of, 337–340
Lymphedema, 337–340
    primary, 339
    secondary, 338
Lymphocyte blastogenesis (transformation) technique, 398
Lymphocyte rosette assays for T cells, 399
Lymphocytic choriomeningitis, 738
    human infection with, 1267
Lymphoid neoplasms, feline, treatment of, 408, 409(t)
Lymphoma, canine cutaneous, 493–495
    malignant, cytology of, 26, *26*
    of kidneys, 1205, 1206(t)
Lymphoproliferative disorders, feline, 407
    treatment of, 408, 409(t)
Lymphosarcoma
    canine, 419–422, 421(t)
        clinical staging of, 421(t)
        drug combinations for, 421(t)
    cutaneous, 494
    feline, induction-remission chemotherapy of, 409, 409(t)
    ocular involvement due to, 586

Macchiavello staining method, for psittacosis, 679

Macrolides, properties of, 7(t)
Macrophages, 908
Magnesium oxide, in calcium oxalate urolithiasis, 1183
Malabsorption, 930, 934–935
Malassimilation syndrome, 930–935
Maldigestion, 930, 932–934
Malignant disease, immunotherapy of, 426–430
Malignant neoplasia, cytology of, 21, 21(t), *22, 23*
Malnutrition, in oil-soaked birds, 691
Mammary glands, hypertrophy of, 1226
    non-neoplastic disorders of, 1224–1226
Mange, demodectic, 437
    notoedric, 470
    otodectic, 470
    sarcoptic, human infection with, 1267
Mannitol, in shock, 42
Marburg disease, 737
Marcus Gunn sign, 514
Masticatory muscle myositis, canine, 779–781, *781*
Mastitis, 1224
    in kennels, 75
Mastocytoma, cryotherapy of, 496
Mating, in kennels, 76
Matrix-nucleation theory, of calculogenesis, 1177
Measles virus, in non-human primates, 739
    vaccine for, 1252, 1253(t)
Mediastinoscopy, 207
Medication, routes of, in laboratory animals, 762
Medroxyprogesterone acetate, 846
Megaesophagus, generalized, 957
Megaureter, 1129
Megestrol acetate, 846
    as canine contraceptive, 1032
    for prevention of estrus, 1238
Melanoma, of anterior uvea, 585
Melena, 932
Membrane immunoglobulin assay, for B cells, 400
Mercurial diuretics, 357
Metabolism
    disorders of, 974–1039
        episodic weakness and, 792(t), 794–795
        genetic, 89(t)
        hepatic encephalopathy and, 823, 824(t)
        inherited, [VI:868]
        ocular signs of, 596(t)
    in shock state, 34
    in teratogenesis, 168
Metaldehyde poisoning, 125(t), 126, 135–136
Metastrongyles, in lungs, 262–264, 267
Metestrus, 1031
Methemoglobinemia, 419
Methenamine, 1165
Methoxyflurane, nephrotoxicity of, 1050
Methylene blue, as urinary antiseptic, 1166
    in calcium oxalate urolithiasis, 1182
Methylphenidate, in cataplexy, 840

Metritis, acute, 1214–1215
  feline, 1234
  in kennels, 75
Mibolerone, as canine contraceptive, 1033
  for estrus prevention, 1238, 1239(t)
Mice, diseases of, 758–760(t)
  physiologic data on, 742(t)
  sexing of, 745, 745(t)
Microbronchitis, 283
Microfilariae, detection and identification of, in blood, 329
Microphthalmia, genetic etiology of, 588
Micturition, anatomy and physiology of, 1122, 1123
  encouraging of, 1167–1168
  inappropriate, 1136
Midbrain, effect of progestins on, 846
Migration inhibition factor (MIF), 399
Mineral poisoning, 123
Mineral requirements, in renal failure, 1099
Miotics, 519
  topical, for canine glaucoma therapy, 520(t)
Mismating injections, 1240
Mites, nasal, 266
  respiratory system, in psittacine birds, 703
Mitral valve, chronic fibrosis of, 298–301
  congenital insufficiency of, 305
Mixed leukocyte reaction (MLR), 401
Molluscum contagiosum, 738
Monitoring, in shock, techniques of, 44–48
  of fluid therapy, 52
Monkey(s), restraint and physical examination of, [VI:721]
  viral diseases in, 734–737
    transmitted from humans, 739
Monkey B-virus encephalitis, 1266
Monkeypox, 736
  benign epidermal, 736
Mott cells, 25, 25
Mouth. See Oral cavity.
Mouth rot, in aquatic turtles, 643
Mucin deficiency sicca, 556
Mural endocarditis, 305–307
Muscle disease, inflammatory canine, 779–782
  infectious causes of, 782
Muscle relaxants, use of, in renal failure, 1120
Musculoskeletal disorders, 768–853
Mutagenesis, 161–171
  potential causes of, 164–171, 167(t), 169(t)
Myasthenia gravis, 792, 792(t), 793
  anticholinesterase therapy in, 793(t)
Mycetoma, 481
Mycobacterial infections, in non-domestic animals, 604–606
Mycoplasma, canine respiratory disease and, 1277
Mycoplasma-associated conjunctivitis, 552
Mycosis, opportunistic, 477–481
  subcutaneous, 477–481
  systemic, 481–485
Mycosis fungoides, 494

Mycotic disease, of cats, 472
Mycotic infection, nasal, canine, 219
Mycotic pneumonia, 239
Mycotoxicosis, 123
Mycotoxins, teratogenic, 169(t)
Mydriasis, 507
Mydriatic agents, 518
Myelopathy, fibrocartilaginous embolic ischemic, [VI:908]
Myeloproliferative disorders, 416
  feline, 408
    treatment of, 410
Myiasis, of aquatic turtles, 645
Myocardial contractility, improvement of, 373
Myocardial disease, 316–321
  acquired secondary, 317–319
    treatment of, 319–321
  congenital, 316–317
    treatment of, 319
  infiltrative, 317
  ischemic, 317
Myocardial function, in shock, 34
Myocardial toxicity, hyperkalemic, treatment of, 986
Myocardiopathy, non-infectious, 319
Myocarditis, infectious, 318
  non-infectious, 319
Myofascitis, 874
Myoglobinuria, in racing greyhound, 783–787
Myopathy, with Cushing's disease, 790, 791
  sex-linked, in Irish terriers, 790
  with myotonia and muscle fiber deficiency, in Labrador retrievers, 790
Myositis, idiopathic, canine, 779–782
  masticatory muscle, 779–781, 781
Myositis complex, 584
Myotonia, canine, 787–791, 788, 789

Narcolepsy, diagnosis and treatment of, 837–841
Narcotic analgesics, in diarrhea, 916, 916(t)
  in renal failure, 1119
Nasal arthropods, 266
Nasal aspergillosis, 479
  serology of, 208
Nasal disease, chronic, in dogs, 219–223
Nasal flushing, in dog, 215
Nasal fold irritation, genetic etiology of, 589
Nasal foreign bodies, 218
Nasal hypopigmentation, 488
Nasal mites, 266
Nasal pentastomids, 266
Nasal sinus tumors, 249
Nasal solar dermatitis, canine, 438, 440–443
Nasal trauma, 216, 217
Nasolacrimal system, genetic disorders of, 589
Nasopharyngeal tumors, 251
Near-drowning, 182–186
Nematode(s)
  filarioid, 326, 326(t)
  in lungs, 262–264, 266

Nematode(s) (Continued)
  in tracheobronchial tree, 229
  in urinary tract infection, 1141–1143
  of aquatic turtles, 645
  of fish, 614
  prevalence of, in pound vs. owned dogs, 936(t)
Neonatal deaths, 79–82
  causes and treatment of, [VI:44]
  congenital anomalies and, 73
Neonate, clinical nephrology of, 1085–1087
  hypoglycemia of, 1024
  in kennels, diseases of, 72
Neoplasia. See also Carcinoma; Tumors; and specific tumor types.
  anemia and, 414
  benign, cytology of, 23, 24(t)
  discrete cell, cytology of, 23, 23
  in caged birds, [V:585]
  intranasal, feline, 228
  intraocular, 585–586
    primary and secondary, 573
  lymph node, cytology of, 26, 27
  lymphoid, feline, treatment of, 408, 409(t)
  malignant, cytology of, 21, 21(t), 22, 23
  nasal, canine, 220
  nonendocrine, ectopic hormone production by, [VI:1061]
  ocular signs of, 597(t)
  of eyelids, 549
  of kidney, 1203–1208, 1204–1206(t)
  of liver, laboratory findings in, 883, 883(t), 884(t)
  of reproductive tract, [VI:1263]
  of respiratory tract, 249–253
    chemotherapeutic agents used in, 251(t)
    of psittacine birds, 703
    remote effects of, 253
  of ureter, 1208, 1208(t)
  of urethra, 1211–1212, 1211(t)
  of urinary bladder, 1208–1211, 1209(t)
  of urinary tract, 1203–1212
  orbital, 584, 586–587
  urothelial, vs. polypoid cystitis, 1138(t)
Neoplastic effusions, 259(t), 261
Nephritis, chronic interstitial, 1076–1079
Nephroblastoma, 1204, 1204–1205(t), 1206
  chemotherapy of, 1207
Nephrology, clinical neonatal, 1085–1087
Nephroma, embryonal, 1204, 1204–1205(t), 1206
  chemotherapy of, 1207
Nephropathy, hypercalcemic, 1051, 1067–1072
  toxic, 1047–1052
Nephrotic syndrome, 1053, 1055–1056, 1055, 1096
Nephrotoxicity, mechanisms of, 1048
Nervous system, metabolic disorders of, inherited, [VI:868]
Neurodermatitis, feline, 491

Neuroleptics, for birds, 655(t)
Neurologic disorders, 768–853
    of aquatic turtles, 645
Neuromuscular disorders, effect on
    micturition, 1124(t), 1126
    episodic weakness and, 792–794,
        792(t)
    genetic, 92–93(t)
Neuro-opthalmology, 510–517
Neurotoxins, in Australian elapid
    venom, 179
Neutropenia, 414
    cyclic, in gray collie dogs, 415
"New tank syndrome," 608
Newcastle disease, 674, 702
    vaccine for, 1275(t)
Nictitating membrane
    eversion of, 553
        double, 508
        genetic etiology of, 590
    protrusion of, 538, 552
Night howling, canine, 851
Nitrification, of aquarium water, 608,
    609
Nitrate, in aquarium water, 608, 610,
    611(t)
Nitrite, toxicity of, to tropical fish,
    609, 610, 611(t)
Nitrite test, for urine culture, 1156,
    1156(t)
Nitroblue tetrazolium test, 397
Nitrogen, in parenteral
    hyperalimentation solutions, 927
Nocardiosis, 486
Nose, collie, 438
Notoedric mange, 470
Nuclear sclerosis, 566
Nutrition
    canine, 77
    deficiencies of, ocular signs of,
        597(t)
    during uremic crisis, 1104–1106
    feline, 77, 78(t)
    in kennels, 69
    in management of gastrointestinal
        problems, 919–929
    of non-domestic carnivores,
        718–719, 719(t)
Nutrition-related disorders, in
    congenital maldevelopment, 167
Nutritional hypercalcitoninism,
    [VI:1048]
Nutritional problems, in captive
    reptiles, [VI:778]
Nystagmus, genetic etiology of, 588
Nystatin, properties of, 7(t)

Obesity, 1034–1039
    alterations in cardiorespiratory
        system due to, 341
Obstruction, airway, cardiopulmonary
    resuscitation for, 295, 295(t), 296
    of small intestine, [VI:952]
    urethral, 1191–1193
Obstructive effusions, 258(t), 260
Ocular color changes, 505
Ocular dermoids, genetic etiology of,
    588
Ocular discharge, 505
    thick, 530
    watery, 529

Ocular disorders, feline, [VI:656]
    immunologically mediated,
        [VI:638]
    in aquatic turtles, 643
Ocular emergencies, 542–546
Ocular examination, 506–510
Ocular pain, 505
Ocular staining, 508
Ocular therapeutics, 517–527
Oil-soaked birds, management of,
    687–692
Oil toxicity, in birds, 691
Oligospermia, canine, 1228
    feline, 1236
Oncology, 389–430
Onychectomy, 728
O'nyong-nyong fever, 740, 740(t)
o,p'-DDD chemotherapy, in
    hyperadrenocorticism, 982
Ophthalmic disorders, of genetic
    etiology, 587–593
Ophthalmic drugs, 517–527
Ophthalmic examination, 505–510
Ophthalmologic diseases, 504–598
Ophthalmologic problems, 528,
    529–541
Ophthalmoscopy, 509
Optic nerve hypoplasia, genetic
    etiology of, 592
Oral cavity, 855–875
    developmental problems in,
        858–859
    microbiology of, 859, 859(t)
    prehensile dysfunction of, 873–875
Oral hygiene, 869
Orbit
    diagnostic techniques for, 583
    diseases of, 583–584
    inflammation of, 583
    tumors of, 584, 586–587
Orbital bleeding technique, in
    laboratory animals, 750
Orchitis, canine, [VI:1255]
Organophosphate poisoning, 125(t),
    126, 147–148
Ornithosis, 676
    of pigeons, treatment of, 683, 683(t)
Orteca, 736
Osmotic diuresis, mechanics of, 1093
Osmotic diuretics, 1089, 1091
    in intracranial injury, 818
Osteoarthritis, [V:707]
Osteoarthropathy, cranial mandibular,
    875
Osteochondritis dissecans
    of hock, 813–814, 814
    of knee, 813, 813
    of medial condyle of humerus,
        811–813, 812
    of shoulder joint, 808–809
    of stifle, 813, 813
Osteochondroma, of trachea, 252
Osteochondrosis, canine, 807–815,
    808
    of elbow joint, 809–813, 810–812
Osteolysis, with tumor metastases,
    1068(t), 1070
Osteomyelitis, septic, 1068(t), 1070
Otitis externa, 461–466, [VI:848]
Otitis media, [VI:848]
Otodectic mange, 470
Otoscope technique, for sexing birds,
    656, 657, 658

Ovarian hormones, 1030–1031
Ovaries, 1030
Ovariohysterectomy, 1239, 1240
Overgrooming, feline, 851
Overhydration, with renal failure,
    1044
Oxygen, fish requirement of, 611,
    611(t)
    humidified, in smoke inhalation
        pneumonia, 242
Oxygen therapy, for respiratory
    emergencies, 277
    in hypertrophic cardiomyopathy,
        313
    in shock, 43
Oxygen toxicity, 278

Pacheco's parrot disease, 704–705
Pad culture test, for urine, 1156,
    1156(t)
Pain, in poisoning, 114
    ocular, 505
Palpation, in shock, 45
    of thorax, 205
Pancreatic islet cell adenocarcinoma,
    functional, canine, 1020–1023
Pancreatitis, acute, [VI:973]
    diabetic ketoacidosis and, 1018
Pancytopenia, 415
Panleukopenia, feline, 1286–1288
    control of, in catteries, 1270
    vaccines for, 1256, 1257(t), 1259
Panniculitis, nodular, 433(t), 435
Pannus, 563
Papanicolaou stains, of cytologic
    slide, 18
Papilloma, cryotherapy of, 496
    of urinary bladder, 1208, 1209(t)
Paracentesis, abdominal, cytologic
    specimen from, 18
Paragonimus kellicotti, 265
Parainfluenza virus, canine, infectious
    tracheobronchitis and, 1276
    vaccine for, 1253(t), 1254
Parakeet, physical examination,
    laboratory and medication
    techniques and hospitalization
    procedures for, [V:533]
Paralysis
    coonhound, 773–776
    radial-brachial, [V:658]
    tick, 178, 773–776
    in Australia, 777–779
Paramyxovirus, in non-human
    primates, 739
Paranasal sinus tumors, 249
Paraphimosis, in kennels, 75
Parasites
    copepod, 614
    helminth, preventive and control
        measures for, 947–948
    in kennels, 71
    of aquatic turtles, 644
    of caged birds, [VI:682]
        control of, 1273
        imported, 676
    of canine urinary tract, 1141–1143
    of cats, 469–471
    of non-domestic carnivores, 719
        treatment of, 726–729(t)
    of respiratory tract, 262–268
        in psittacine birds, 703

Parasites (*Continued*)
  protozoan, preventive and control measures for, 947–948
  sporozoan, of fish, 613
Parasiticides, for tropical fish, 615
Parasitism, gastrointestinal, 935–948
Parathyroid glands, [VI:1038]
Parenchymal disease, pulmonary, radiographic diagnosis of, 284–289, 286–289(t)
Paredrine test, 516
Parrots, herpesvirus infection of, 704–705
  lead poisoning in, 141
  psittacosis in, treatment of, 681–683
Parvovirus, canine, 1294
  vaccine for, 1253(t), 1254, 1295
Patent ductus arteriosus, [VI:400]
Pectin, for diarrhea, 918
Pediatrics, 77–82
  of non-domestic carnivores, 715–717
Pediculosis, in cats, 470
Pemphigoid, bullous, 433(t), 434
Pemphigus erythematosus, 432, 433(t), 439
Pemphigus foliaceus, 432, 433(t), 439
Pemphigus vegetans, 432, 433(t)
Pemphigus vulgaris, 432, 433(t)
Penicillamine, in cystinuria, 1176
  in lead poisoning, 139
  nephrotoxicity of, 1051
Penicillins, 14
  properties of, 6(t)
  nephrotoxicity of, 1050
Penicillium disease, serology of, 208
Pentastomids, nasal, 266
Peptic ulcers, gastric, 959
Percussion, of thorax, 205
Periapical disease, 869–871
Perianal fistulas, 952–954
Pericardial disease, 321–325
Pericardiocentesis, 323
Pericarditis, 319, 321, 322
Periodontal disease, 863–869, *864*, *865*
Periodontium, normal, *856*, 861–862, *861*
Peristalsis, intestinal, 914
Peritoneal dialysis, current status of, 1106–1111
  in hypothermia, 199, 200
Peritonitis, feline infectious, 229, 713, 1288–1292
  control of, in catteries, 1271
Pesticides, 124, 125(t). See also under individual agents.
  teratogenic, 168
Pets, exotic. See *Exotic pets.*
Pet-associated zoonoses, 1265–1268
Phaeohyphomycosis, 480
Phagocytic index, 396
Phagocytosis, in bronchopulmonary clearance, 209
Pharyngostomy, in feline respiratory disease, 1280
Pharynx, trauma of, 217
Phenobarbital, in epilepsy, 836, 837
Phenolic chemicals, poisoning from, [VI:145]
Phenothiazines, 501(t)
  use of, in renal failure, 1119

Phenytoin, 358
  in epilepsy, 836, 837
Phosphate(s), cellulose and inorganic, in calcium oxalate urolithiasis, 1182
Phosphate binders, intestinal, 1104
Phosphorus, abnormalities of, in renal failure, 1045
Phycomycosis, 480
Physical disorders, 104–201
Physical fitness for dogs, 53–64
Physiological data, normal, 1319(t)
Pigeons, herpesvirus infection of, 705
  ornithosis in, treatment of, 683, 683(t)
Pigment, hereditary abnormalities of, 487–490
Pilocarpine, for estrus prevention, 1239
Pilocarpine test, 515
Pinna, alopecia of, 489
Piperazine, 501(t)
Pitressin Tannate, for ADH deficiency, 1008, *1009*, *1010*
Pituitary, evaluation of function of, in hyperadrenocorticism, 976–977
PKW method, 330
Plague, fowl variant, 675
  in humans, 1266
Plants, poisonous, sources of, 150(t)
Plant toxins, 123
Plaque, 863
Plasma, chemical constituents of, 1325–1327(t)
  in shock, 41
Plasma proteins, in Basenji, 1327(t)
  in cats, 1327(t)
Pleural effusions, 253–261
  classification and etiologies of, 258–259(t)
  fluid evaluation in, 256
  patterns of, 257–261
Pleural friction rub, 236(t), 237
Pneumonia, 235–243
  allergic, 240, 287
  aspiration, 241
  bacterial, 237–239
  following smoke inhalation, 242
  foreign body, 213
  inhalation, 242
  mycotic, 239
  radiographic classification of, 235
Pneumonitis, feline, 229, 1299–1302, *1300, 1301*
  control of, in catteries, 1270
  human infection with, 1267
  vaccine for, 1257(t), 1258, 1260, 1302
Pneumonyssus caninum, 266
Pneumoperitoneum, introduction of, in laparoscopy, 971
Pneumothorax, 270–272, *271*
  tension, 272
Pododermatitis, canine, 467–469
Poison(s)
  absorbed, antidotes against, 107, 109–112(t)
  elimination of, 112
  classification of, 123–124
  man-made sources of, 123
  natural, 123
  unabsorbed, antidotes against, 107, 108–109(t)

Poison control centers and diagnostic laboratories, 114
Poisoning(s), 105–114. See also *Toxicoses.*
  anticoagulant, 125(t), 131–134, 132(t)
  antifreeze, 125(t), 126, 144–146
  ANTU, 125, 125(t), [VI:117]
  arsenic, 125(t), [VI:134]
  carbamate, 126, 147–148
  chlorinated hydrocarbon, 125(t), [VI:141]
  compound 1080, 125, 125(t), [VI:119]
  emergency intervention in, 105–112
  from phenolic chemicals, [VI:145]
  fungicide, [VI:143]
  herbicide, 126, [VI:143]
  in small animals, common, 122–128
    emergency kit for treatment of, 201
    frequency of, 124–128, 125(t)
    potential sources of, 149, 150–153(t)
  insecticide, 147–148
  instructions to clients in, 105
  laboratory diagnosis of, 115–121, 117–118(t)
  lead, 125(t), 126, 136–144
  metaldehyde, 125(t), 126, 135–136
  sodium fluoroacetate, 125, 125(t), [VI:119]
  strychnine, 125(t), 126, 129–131
  supportive measures in, 112–114
  thallium, 125, 125(t), [VI:124]
  toad, [VI:173]
  warfarin, 125(t), 131–134, 132(t)
  zinc phosphide, 125(t), 126
Poisonous plants, sources of, 150(t)
Poliomyelitis, in non-human primates, 739
Polyarthritis, canine, 795–802
  differential diagnosis of, 796(t)
  inflammatory infectious, 797–798
  inflammatory non-infectious, 798–802
  non-inflammatory, 796–797
Polydipsia, with chronic interstitial nephritis, 1077
Polymyopathy, episodic weakness and, 792(t), 793
Polymyositis, canine, 781
Polymyxins, properties of, 7(t)
Polyneuritis, canine, [VI:825]
Polyps, colonic, 960
Polyradiculoneuritis, acute, 773–776
Polyuria
  differentiation of, 1080–1085, *1081*
    by vasopressin concentration test, 1080, 1083
    by water deprivation test, 1080, 1082, *1082*
    partial, 1084
  verification of, 1080
  with chronic interstitial nephritis, 1077
Portal vein anomaly, congenital, hepatic encephalopathy and, 825
Portography, jejunal catheterization for, 826, *826*
Portosystemic disease, laboratory findings in, 884, 884(t)
Positive pressure breathing, 277

Posterior caval syndrome, 328
Potassium, abnormalities of, in renal
    failure, 1044
    sinus bradycardia and, 377, 379,
        380
Pox, avian, 702
Prausnitz-Küstner test, in canine
    atopic disease, 453
Precipitation-crystallization theory, of
    calculogenesis, 1177
Pregnancy
    blood parameters in, canine, 1323(t)
        feline, 1324(t)
    diagnosis of, 76
    prevention of, 1239–1240
    termination of, 1240–1241
Primates, restraint and physical
    examination of, [VI:721]
    virus diseases of, 733–741, 734(t),
        735(t)
Primidone, in epilepsy, 836, 837
Probe freezing, in cryosurgery, 66
Procainamide, 358
Proestrus, 1031
Progestins, effect on limbic system
    and midbrain, 846
    for behavior control, 845, 847–853,
        848–849(t)
Progestogens, for estrus prevention,
    1237
Prolapse, uterine, 1223–1224
    uveal, 544
Propranolol, 313, 314, 358
Prostaglandins, for pregnancy
    termination, 1241
Prostatic disease, medical
    management of, 1146–1150
    signs of, 1147(t)
Prostatitis, bacterial, in urinary tract
    infection, 1160
Protein
    dietary restriction of, in hepatic
        encephalopathy, 827, 828
    metabolism of, effect of
        glucocorticoids on, 989
    requirements of, in renal failure,
        1099, 1100
    serum levels of, in malassimilation
        syndrome, 932
    total, in cerebrospinal fluid, 771
        reduction of, in chronic active
            hepatitis, 886
Prothrombin time, as liver test, 882
Prototheosis, 480
Protozoa, of aquatic turtles, 644
    of fish, external, 613
        internal, 614
Protozoan infections, 944–946
Protozoan parasites, preventive and
    control measures for, 947–948
Pruritus, food-induced, in cats, 471
Pseudocyesis, in kennels, 75
Pseudohermaphroditism, 1241–1243
    feline, male, 1231
    urinary incontinence and, 1133
Pseudohyperparathyroidism, 1004,
    1068(t), 1069
Pseudorabies, 1296–1298
    canine, 1297
    feline, 1297
Psittacine birds, import regulations
    for, 684–686
    psittacosis in, treatment of, 681–683
    respiratory disease in, 697–704

Psittacine herpesvirus infection, 675
Psittacosis, 677–686, 1265
    control of, in aviaries, 1275
    in humans, 686, 1265
Puerperal tetany, 1027–1029,
    1027–1029, 1045
Pulmonary contusion, 272, 272
Pulmonary edema, 243–249
    alveolar, 286
    cardiogenic, 246
    causes of, 244, 244(t)
    non-cardiogenic, 246, 246
    therapy of, 247–249, 247(t)
Pulmonary embolism, due to adverse
    drug reaction, 213
Pulmonary function, in shock, 35–37
Pulmonary infiltrates with
    eosinophils, 240, 287
Pulmonary insufficiency, progressive,
    35, 36(t)
Pulmonary parenchymal disease,
    radiographic diagnosis of, 284–289,
    286–289(t)
Pulmonary radiographs, interpretation
    of, 279–289
Pulmonic stenosis, 302–303, [VI:403]
Pulp, disease of, 859–860
Pulse, in shock, monitoring of, 45
Pupillary changes, 505
Pupillary membranes, persistent, 571
    genetic etiology of, 591
Pupillary reactions, 510–517
Puppy
    diseases of, in kennels, 73
    hypoglycemia of, 1024–1025
    in adoption shelter, control of
        infectious diseases in, 1269
    normal physiologic values for, 79(t)
    whelping of, 76
"Puppy-dog dermatitis," human
    infection with, 1267
Puppy viremia, in kennels, 73
Pustular dermatitis, of neonate, in
    kennels, 73
Pyelonephritis, 1076
Pyodermas, in neonate, 80
Pyogranulomatous effusions, 259(t),
    261
Pyometra, canine, 1216–1219
    feline, 1235
Pyridoxine, in calcium oxalate
    urolithiasis, 1183
Pyruvate, in calcium oxalate
    urolithiasis, 1183

Q fever, in humans, 1266
Quinidine, 357

Rabbits
    anesthesia for, 706–710, 707–709(t)
    diseases of, 752–753(t)
    endotracheal intubation of, 709–710
    manual restraint of, 744, 749
    physiologic data on, 742(t)
    sexing of, 744, 745(t)
Rabies
    monkey, 738
    pathogenesis of, 1261
    treatment of, 1264
    vaccine for, 1261–1265
        canine, 1252, 1253(t)
        feline, 1257(t), 1258, 1260

Racing dog, cardiovascular system of,
    347–351
Radial-brachial paralysis, [V:658]
Radial immunodiffusion, 396, 397,
    400
Radiation, congenital
    maldevelopment and, 165
Radiation toxicity, [VI:184]
Radioallergosorbent test, 400
    in canine atopic disease, 453
Radiodensities, pulmonary, 285–289
Radiographs
    abdominal, in canine pyometra,
        1217
    avian, in respiratory disease, 698
        technique and interpretation of,
            649–653, 651, 652(t)
    diagnostic, for rodents, 751, 762(t)
    in canine heartworm disease, 328
    in feline liver disease, 892–893
    in heart failure, acute, 361
    in lower airway disease, 283–284
    in pleural effusion, 254
    in pneumonia, 235
    in prostatic disease, 1147
    of exotic pets, [VI:756]
    pulmonary, interpretation of,
        279–289
    thoracic, 206, 281
        in pulmonary edema, 245, 246
Radioimmunoassay, of plasma T$_4$
    concentration, 996, 996, 997
Radioimmunosorbent test, 400
Radiology, exotic animal, [VI:756]
Rales, 236
Raptors, herpesvirus infections in,
    705–706
RAST, 400
    in canine atopic disease, 453
Rats, diseases of, 758–760(t)
    physiologic data on, 742(t)
    sexing of, 745, 745(t)
Reactive hyperplasia, cytology of, 23,
    24(t), 25
Record keeping, in kennels, 70
Rectum, biopsy of, 967
Regurgitation, 956
Rehabilitation centers, veterinary
    involvement in, 601–604
Renal amyloidosis, 1063–1066
Renal calculi, 1169
Renal cyst, capsulogenic, 1073
Renal disease, anemia of, 414
    primary, hypercalcemia in, 1071
Renal disorders, drug therapy in,
    1114–1117, 1115(t), 1116(t)
Renal failure, 1042–1043
    acute, 1071
        with incomplete recovery, 1076
    anesthesia in, 1117–1121
    body fluid abnormalities in,
        1043–1045
    chronic, 1071, 1103–1104
    drug therapy in, 1116, 1116(t)
    oliguric and anuric, 1087–1090
    polyuric, anabolic steroid therapy
        of, 1102
        characteristics of, 1091
        diet therapy in, 1097–1101,
            1100(t)
        diuresis in, 1091–1093
            osmotic, 1092–1093
        salt and sodium bicarbonate
            therapy of, 1094–1096

Renal failure (*Continued*)
  postrenal, 1042
  prerenal, 1042
  primary, 1042
  secondary hyperparathyroidism and, 1004
Renal function, anesthetic drug effects on, 1118
  normal parameters in, 1328(t)
  in shock, 37–38
Renal function tests, normal parameters in, 1328(t)
Renal insufficiency, disorders in drug disposition in, 1115
  in chronic active hepatitis, 889
  stable polyuric, 1095
Renal lesions, of hypercalcemia, 1069
Renal trauma, 1045
Renal tumors, 1203–1208, 1204–1206(t)
Reo-like virus, canine, vaccine for, 1255
Reovirus, 738
  canine respiratory disease and, 1277
Reproduction, in kennels, 75–76
Reproductive tract, neoplasms of, [VI:1263]
Reptiles
  anesthesia of, 618–620
  antibiotic therapy in, 647–649
  captive, amputations in, 624–625
    bacterial diseases of, [VI:787]
    celiotomy of, 623–624
    cryosurgery of, 625
    fracture repair in, 624
    fungal diseases of, [VI:787]
    hematology of, [VI:792]
    management problems in, [VI:778]
    nutritional problems in, [VI:778]
    surgery in, 620–625
  infectious diseases of, 625–633
    diagnosis and treatment of, 631–632
    taxonomic distribution of, 626–631
  respiratory disease in, 633–637
    diagnosis of, 635–636, 635(t)
    signs of, 634, 635(t)
  respiratory system of, 634, *634*
  salmonellosis in, [VI:799]
Respiration, in shock, monitoring of, 45
  stimulation of, 212
Respiratory disease, 202–291
  canine, 214–223. See also *Canine upper respiratory disease.*
  diagnostic approach to, 203–208
    special procedures for, 206–208
  feline, 224–228, 714. See also *Feline upper respiratory disease.*
  in psittacine birds, 697–704
  of puppy, in kennels, 74
  of reptiles, 633–637
    diagnosis of, 635–636, 635(t)
    signs of, 634, 635(t)
  of upper tract, in brachycephalic dogs, 221
  physical examination in, 204–205
Respiratory disease complex, canine, 1276–1278
  vaccines for, 1253(t), 1254
  feline, 1279–284

Respiratory disorders, in burns, 193
Respiratory emergencies, therapy for, 277–279
Respiratory infections, in aquatic turtles, 641
  upper, control of, in catteries, 1270
Respiratory sounds, auscultation of, 205
Respiratory support measures, in poisoning, 113
Respiratory syncytial virus, human, 738
Respiratory tract
  clinical pharmacology of, 208–213
  neoplasms of, 249–253
    chemotherapeutic agents used in, 251(t)
    in psittacine birds, 703
    remote effects of, 253
  parasitic diseases of, 262–268
Resuscitation, human cardiopulmonary, 293–296, 293(t), 294, 295(t), 296
Retinal atrophy, central progressive, 582
  progressive, 581
Retinal degeneration, feline central, 582
  genetic etiology of, 591
  peripheral cystoid, 580
Retinal disease, 579–582
Retinal dysplasia, genetic etiology of, 591
Retinal separation (detachment), 580
Retinitis, 580
Retinopathy, taurine deficient, 582
Retro-orbital abscess, 583
Rewarming, techniques, for hypothermia, 198, 198(t), 200
Rhabdomyolysis, exertional, in racing greyhound, 783–787
Rheumatoid arthritis, 392, *392*
  canine, 800–802
Rheumatoid factor (RF) test, 392, *392*
Rhinitis
  C. neoformans, 227
  chronic, canine, 219
  feline, 227
  traumatic, feline, 226
Rhinoscopy, 206
Rhinosporidiosis, 479
Rhinotracheitis, feline viral, 224, 225(t), 229, 872, 1279–1284
  control of, in catteries, 1270
  vaccines for, 1257, 1257(t), 1259, 1283
Rhinovirus, 738
Rhonchi, 236(t), 237
Rib fractures, 274, *275*
Ringworm, 437
  control of, in catteries, 1271
  in non-domestic carnivores, 715
RIST, 400
Rodent(s), anesthesia for, 706–710, 707–709(t)
  diagnostic radiography for, 751, 762(t)
  manual restraint of, 744
Rodent botfly, 266
Rodenticides, 125, 125(t)
  chemical structures of, *132*
Romanowsky stains, of cytologic slide, 18
Rose bengal dye test, 508, 527

Rose-Waaler test, 392, *392*
Rota-like virus, canine, vaccine for, 1255

Salicylates, teratogenicity of, 170
Salmonellosis
  feline, 1305–1307
  in non-domestic carnivores, 715
  in reptiles, [VI:799]
  in aquatic turtles, 646
Sarcoma, cytology of, 22, *22*
Sarcoptic mange, human infection with, 1267
Scaling, of calculus, 866, *866*, *867*
Schirmer tear test, 507, 527
Sclera, lacerations of, 544
Sclerosis, nuclear, 566
Scorpion stings, 178
Screening tests, dexamethasone, 977(t), 978
  for significant bacteriuria, 1154–1157, 1156(t)
Seborrheic dermatitis, 438
Seizures, 830–837
  differential diagnosis of, 831, 832(t)
  epileptic, 830, 831–833, [VI:853]
    treatment of, 835–837
  motor, 833
  psychomotor, 833
  recognizing of, 830
  treatment of, 835–837
Semen
  canine, constituents of, 1329(t)
  collection of, in cats, [VI:1252]
    in dogs, [VI:1245]
  evaluation of, in infertility, 1227
Septal defect, atrial, 316, [VI:394]
  ventricular, 316, [VI:395]
Septicemia, of neonate, in kennels, 72
Septicemic conditions, in aquatic turtles, 643
Serum, chemical constituents of, 1325–1327(t)
  chemistry abnormalities of, with glucocorticoids, 990
  examination of, for microfilariae, 329
Serum protein electrophoresis, in liver disease, 881, 881(t)
Sexing, of birds, by laparoscopy, 659
  otoscope technique for, 656, *657*, *658*
  of laboratory animals, 743, *744–745*, 745(t)
Sheather's sugar centrifugal flotation technique, 946
Shell rot, in aquatic turtles, 644
Shelters, animals. See *Adoption shelters.*
Shipping, of small animals, regulations for, 1316–1317, 1317(t)
Shock
  causes of, 32(t)
  clinical signs of, 38, 38(t)
  dynamics of, 33, *33*
  in burns, 192
    treatment of, 194
  initial evaluation of, 38
  metabolism in, 34
  monitoring techniques in, 44–48
  pathophysiology and management of, 32–48

Shock (*Continued*)
    pulmonary function in, 35–37
    regional blood flow in, 34–35
    renal function in, 37–38
    treatment of, 38–44
        general precautions in, 44
Shock syndrome, definition of, 32
Shoulder joint, osteochondritis
    dissecans of, 808–809
Sick sinus syndrome, 377, 379
Silica urolithiasis, canine, 1184–1186,
    1185
Simian vacuolating virus, 740
Sinoventricular rhythm, 377, 379, 380
Sinus, nasal, tumors of, 249
    paranasal, tumors of, 249
    urachal, 1145
Sinus arrest, 377, *378*, *380*
Sinus bradycardia, 377, *378*
Sinus tachycardia, 382, *382*
Sinusitis, traumatic, feline, 226
Skin, diseases of, in aquatic turtles,
    646
        autoimmune, 432–436, 433(t)
        genetic disorders of, 94(t)
Skin grafts, in burn treatment, 194
Skin tests
    delayed hypersensitivity (type IV),
        401
    for inhalant allergens, in respiratory
        disease, 207
    in canine atopic disease, 451, 451(t)
    types I and III, 401
Smallpox, in non-human primates,
    739
Smoke inhalation, resulting in
    pneumonia, 242
Snake(s), infectious agents in,
    629–631
    poisonous, 174–176
Snake venoms, 174, 181(t)
Snakebite, 174–176
    clinical signs and diagnosis of, 175,
        180
    in Australia and New Guinea,
        179–182
    severity of, factors contributing to,
        174
    signs of, comparative frequency of,
        180, 180(t)
    treatment of, 175, 180–182
Sneezing, 210
    paroxysmal, 226
Sodium, retention of, reduction of,
    374
    serum, alterations of, effect on
        heart, 345
        in renal failure, 1044
Sodium bicarbonate therapy, in urate
    urolithiasis, 1174
    of polyuric renal failure, 1094–1096
Sodium chloride therapy, in urate
    urolithiasis, 1173
    of polyuric renal failure, 1094–1096
Sodium fluoroacetate poisoning, 125,
    125(t) [VI:119]
Soft palate malformation, 94(t)
Solar dermatitis, canine nasal, 438,
    440–443
Somogyi effect, *1013*, 1015
Spastic colon syndrome, 952
Spastic pupil syndrome, 517
Spaying, 731
Sphingolipidoses, 821(t)
Spider bites, 177–178

Spinal cord, progressive cervical
    compression of, [V:674]
    trauma to, evaluation and therapy
        of, [VI:837]
Spirocerca lupi, 267
Splanchnic circulation, in shock, 35,
    36
Sporotrichosis, 477
Sporozoan parasites, of fish, 613
Spray freezing, in cryosurgery, 66
Sputum, collection of, 207
Squamata, infectious agents in,
    628–631
Status epilepticus, 834
Stenosis, aortic, 303–305, [VI:392]
    pulmonic, 302–303, [VI:403]
Sterilization, 731
Steroids. See also *Corticosteroids*.
    anabolic, in polyuric renal failure,
        1102
    effect of, on central nervous
        system, 846–847
    selection of, in ocular therapy, 520
Steroid therapy, alternate-day,
    992–994
Stifle, osteochondritis dissecans of,
    813, *813*
Stings, of venomous animals, 174–178
Stomach
    biopsy of, 965
        endoscopic, 959
    decompression of, 898
    dilation of, 896–901
    foreign bodies in, 958
    mucosal aspect of, endoscopic
        examination of, 957–960
Stomatitis, 871–872
    feline, 871
    necrotic or ulcerative, in aquatic
        turtles, 643
    Vincent's, 871
    vs. respiratory disease, in reptiles,
        636
Storage diseases, 821–822, 821(t)
Strabismus, genetic etiology of, 588
Streptothricosis, 436
Stress, heat, 195–197
Stroke, heat, 195–197
Strongyloides stercoralis, 266
Struvite urolithiasis, 1168–1172
Strychnine poisoning, 125(t), 126,
    129–131
Subconjunctival hemorrhage, 542, 551
Subcorneal pustular dermatosis, 438,
    443–445
Sugar cataracts, 568
Sulfonamide, 15
    in ocular therapy, 521
    nephrotoxicity of, 1049
    properties of, 8(t)
Sulfonamide potentiators, 15
    properties of, 8(t)
Sunscreens, topical, 442
Supraventricular tachyarrhythmia,
    382–385
Surgery
    avian, [VI:711]
    elective, in diabetes mellitus, 1015
    in aquatic turtles, 646
    in captive reptiles, 620–625
    in feline urologic syndrome,
        1201–1203
    in laboratory animals, 767
    in non-domestic carnivores,
        728–733

Susceptibility, to disease, genetic,
    95(t)
SV$_5$ parainfluenza virus, infectious
    tracheobronchitis and, 1276
    vaccine for, 1254
SV40, 740
Swimming puppy syndrome, [VI:905]
Synechiae, 574
Synovial fluid, in canine arthritis,
    801(t)
    normal values in, 1329(t)
Systemic disease
    eye and, 593, 594–598(t)
    fungal, 239
        processing clinical specimens for,
            478
        serology of, 208

T cells, 908
    lymphocyte rosette assays for, 399
T-cell system, deficiencies of,
    397–400
Tachyarrhythmia, 381–388
    supraventricular, 382–385
    ventricular, 385–387
    with heart failure, control of, 375
Tachycardia, atrial, 383, *384*
    sinus, 382, *382*
    ventricular, 386, *387*
Tail chasing, 851
Tanapox, 736
Tannic acid, for diarrhea, 918
Tapetum, absence or
    underdevelopment of, 579
Tapeworms, 942–944
Tattooing, in canine nasal solar
    dermatitis, 442
Taurine deficiency, and retinopathy,
    582
Tear film, abnormalities of, 554–556
Tear substitutes, 525, 525(t)
Technicon SMA, 1325(t), 1326(t)
Teeth
    cavities in, 860–861, *861*
    chemical composition of, 855(t)
    deciduous, development and
        retention of, 855–858
    loose, 862–863
    permanent, eruption of, 856(t)
        relation of, *857*
    polishing of, 868
    scaling technique for, 866, *866*, *867*
Telogen effluvium, alopecia and, 492
Temperature, body, control of, in
    poisoning, 113
    in shock, monitoring of, 45
Tendon injuries, in birds, 672, *672*
Tension pneumothorax, 272
Tentorial herniation, 816, 817(t), *818*,
    818(t)
Teratogenesis, 161–171
    potential causes of, 164–171, 167(t),
        169(t)
Terriers, Irish, sex-linked myopathy
    in, 790
Testes, tumors of, [VI:1054]
Testicles, cryptorchid, 1244–1245
Testosterone, implants of, for canine
    contraception, 1033
    in treatment of pyometra, 1218
Tetany, puerperal, 1027–1029,
    1027–1029, 1045

Tetracyclines, 15
  nephrotoxicity of, 1049
  properties of, 6–7(t)
Tetralogy of Fallot, [VI:397]
Thalidomide, teratogenicity of, 170
Thallium intoxication, 125, 125(t), [VI:124]
Theophylline, 211
  pharmacodynamics of, 355–356
Thermal injury, 191–194
  inhalation, 186. See also *Inhalation injury.*
Thermal solubility test, for Bence Jones protein, 396
Thiabendazole, in *Filaroides osleri* infection, 263
Thiacetarsamide sodium, for canine heartworm disease, 331, 332
  in *Filaroides osleri* infection, 263
  nephrotoxicity of, 1051
Thiazide diuretics. See *Diuretics, thiazide.*
Thoracic cage, open wounds of, 274
Thoracic radiographs, 206, 281
  in pulmonary edema, 245, 246
Thoracic tube drainage, in pneumothorax, 271, 272
Thoracic wall, traumatic injuries to, 274
Thoracocentesis, 255, 259
  cytologic specimen from, 18
  in acute heart failure, 365
  in hemothorax, 275
  in pneumothorax, 271
Thoracoscopy, 207
Thorax, palpation of, 205
  percussion of, 205
  traumatic injury to, 268–276
Thrombocytopenia, 415
Thrombocytopenic purpura, [VI:445]
  immunologic, 393
Thromboembolism, aortic, feline, acquired heart disease and, [V:305]
Thrush, 871
Thyroid glands, enlargement of, in budgerigars, 704
  tumors of, [VI:1020]
Thyroiditis, autoimmune (lymphocytic), 394
Thyroxine, in treatment of hypothyroidism, 997
  radioimmunoassay of plasma concentration of, 996, 996, 997
Tick(s), of aquatic turtles, 645
Tick paralysis, 178, 773–776
  in Australia, 777–779
Timidity, canine, 850
Tissues, chemical analysis of, in poisoning, 115–121, 117–118(t)
Toad poisoning, [VI:173]
Tonography, 509
Tonometry, 509
Tonsils, 872–873
Topical anesthetic agents, ophthalmic, 519
Tortoise, infectious agents in, 626–628
  respiratory system of, 634, 634
Total hemolytic complement assay, 397
Total solids, in shock, monitoring of, 46
Toxascaris leonina, 937
Toxemia, of neonate, in kennels, 72
Toxic milk syndrome, 81

Toxicants. See also *Poison(s).*
  specimens for diagnosis of, 116, 117–118(t)
Toxicity, drug, ocular signs of, 597(t)
  radiation, [VI:184]
Toxicology services, 118–121
Toxicosis. See also *Poisoning(s).*
  laboratory diagnosis of, 115–121, 117–118(t)
Toxins, cerebral, hepatic encephalopathy and, 823, 824(t)
  natural, 123
Toxocara canis, 266, 937, 941
Toxocara cati, 266, 937
Toxoplasma gondii, 267
  life cycle of, 1308, 1308
Toxoplasmosis, 1307–1311
  control of, in catteries, 1271
  in non-domestic carnivores, 715
Tracheal collapse, 94(t), 233–235, 233(t), 282, 283
  cervical vs. thoracic, 234
Tracheal hypoplasia, 94(t)
Tracheal tears, 218
Tracheal trauma, 217, 269, 269, 270
Tracheal tumors, 251
Tracheitis, 229–232
Tracheobronchial tree, canine and feline diseases of, 229–235
Tracheobronchitis, 229, 283, 284
  infectious canine, 229, 1276–1278
Training for dogs, 53–64
  basic principles of, 53–55
  clinical syndromes associated with, 60–62
  diet and performance in, 62–64
  management of, 57–60
  types of, 55–57, 55(t)
Training response, 53
  rates of, 53
  specificity of, 54
Transtracheal aspiration, 207
Transudates, pure, 257, 258(t)
Trematodes, of aquatic turtles, 645
  of fish, 613, 614
Trichiasis, 547
Trichrome stains, of cytologic slide, 18
Tricuspid valve, insufficiency of, 301–302
Tropical fish, infectious diseases of, 611–615
  medical care of, 606–615
Tuberculosis, in aviaries, 1274
  in non-domestic animals, 604–606
Tumors. See also *Neoplasia.*
  adrenocortical, hyperadrenocorticism due to, 976
    therapy of, 983
  conjunctival, 553
  corneal, 564
  intraocular, 585–586
  laryngeal, 251
  lung, 252–253
  nasopharyngeal, 251
  of nasal sinus, 249
  of paranasal sinus, 249
  of testes, [VI:1054]
  orbital, 584, 586–587
  pancreatic islet cell, 1020–1023
  renal, 1203–1208, 1204–1206(t)
  thyroid, [VI:1020]
  tracheal, 251
Tumor specific antigens (TSA), 426

Turtles
  aquatic, diseases of, 641–646
    medical care of, 637–647
    surgery of, 646
  infectious agents in, 626–628

Ulcer(s), corneal, 533, 543, 561
  eosinophilic, in cats, cryotherapy of, 496
  peptic, 959
Ulcerative colitis, 949–952
Ulcerative keratitis, 561
Ulcerative shell disease, in aquatic turtles, 644
Ulna, fragmentation of coronoid process of, 811–813, 811, 812
Umbilical hernia, 94(t)
Urachal cyst, 1144, 1145
Urachal sinus, 1145
Urachus
  congenital diseases of, 1143–1145, 1144
  patent, 1133
  persistent, 1143, 1144
Urate urolithiasis, 1172–1174
Urease, antibodies to, for hepatic encephalopathy, 828, 829
Uremia, anesthetic drug effects on, 1118
Uremic bone disease, 1078
Uremic crisis, decompensated, 1095
  nutrition during, 1104–1106
Uremic syndrome, 1079–1080, 1080(t)
Ureter, ectopic, 1128–1133, 1132
  neoplasms of, 1208, 1208(t)
  traumatic rupture of, 1046
Ureteroectasia, 1129
Urethra
  abnormalities of, and incontinence, 1130
  calculi in, 1169
  massage of, 1191
  neoplasms of, 1211–1212, 1211(t)
  obstruction of, relief of, 1191–1193
  retrograde irrigation of, 1191
  traumatic rupture of, 1047
Urethrorectal fistulas, 1133
Urethrostomy, 1202
Uric acid, pathway of synthesis of, 1172, 1173
Urinalysis, in laboratory animals, 750
  semiquantitative values in, 1328(t)
Urinary incontinence
  estrogen-responsive, 1133–1135
  iatrogenic, 1136
  neurogenic, 1122–1127, 1123, 1125
  non-neurogenic, 1128–1136
  obstructive (paradoxical), 1135
  urge, 1135–1136
Urinary system, avian, diseases of, [VI:703]
  emergency treatment of, 1042–1047
Urinary tract, 1122–1212
  canine, parasites of, 1141–1143
  infections of, 1158–1161
    ancillary treatment of, 1164–1168
    antimicrobial treatment of, 1162–1163, 1163(t)
    bacterial, struvite urolithiasis and, 1168
    neonatal, 1086
    vs. inflammation, 1154
  neoplasms of, 1203–1212
Urination, inappropriate, feline, 851

Urine
  alkaline, struvite urolithiasis and, 1169
  alkalinization of, in cystinuria, 1176
  bacteria in screening tests for, 1154–1157, 1156(t)
  collection of, by cystocentesis, 1150–1153, 1152, 1153, 1192
    in laboratory animals, 750
  constituents of, 1328(t)
  crystalloid in, increasing solubility of, 1198
    reduction of, 1197
  culture of, 1159
    quantitative, laboratory methods for, 1155
      screening methods for, 1155, 1156(t)
      vs. qualitative, 1155
  output of, in shock, monitoring of, 47
  parameters of, in liver disease, 876(t)
    normal, 1328(t)
  pH of, and calcium oxalate urolithiasis, 1182
  production and concentration of, 1007, 1083
  spraying of, in cats, 852, [VI:1259]
  stasis of, 1167
  struvite supersaturation of, alteration of, 1197–1199
  volume of, altering of, 1167
    augmentation of, 1199
Urogenital system, genetic disorders of, 96(t)
Urolithiasis
  calcium oxalate, 1177–1184, 1179–1181(t)
  cystine, 1175–1176
  silica, canine, 1184–1186, 1185
  struvite, 1168–1172
  urate, 1172–1174
Urologic syndrome, feline. See Feline urologic syndrome.
Urothelial neoplasms, vs. polypoid cystitis, 1138(t)
Uterus, prolapse of, 1223–1224
Uvea, anterior, diseases of, 570–575
  melanomas of, 585
  prolapse of, lacerations with, 544
Uveal tract, diseases of, [VI:638]
Uveitis, 536–537, [VI:638]
  anterior, 571–574
    feline, 573, 573(t)

Vaccination. See Immunization.
Vaccines
  avian, 1275(t)
  canine, 1252–1255, 1253(t)
  feline, 1256–1261, 1257(t), 1260(t)
  future trends in, 1251
  nature of, immune response and, 1249
  route of administration of, immune response and, 1249
Vagal dysrhythmia, 377, 378
Vagina, bacterial flora of, 1220, 1221(t)
  hyperplasia of, 1222–1223
  swabbing of, sampling technique for, 1220, 1220
Vaginitis, canine, 1219–1222

Valley Fever, 482
Valvular endocarditis, 305–307
Valvular heart disease, 297–307
Varicella virus, in non-human primates, 739
Variola, in non-human primates, 739
Vasodilators, for acute heart failure, 364(t), 366
  in dilated cardiomyopathy, 314
  in shock, 42, 43(t)
Vasopressin concentration test, 1080, 1083
Vasopressors, in shock, 42, 43(t)
Venipuncture, in laboratory animals, 749
Venoms
  Australian elapid, pathogenesis of, 179–182
  Hymenoptera, 177
  snake, 174, 181(t)
  spider, 177
Ventilation, artificial, in pulmonary edema, 248
  for respiratory emergencies, 277–279
Ventricular bigeminy, 385, 386
Ventricular premature beats, 385, 386
Ventricular septal defects, 316, [VI:395]
Ventricular tachyarrhythmia, 385–387
Ventricular tachycardia, 386, 387
Vervet monkey disease, 737
Vesicular breath sounds, 236, 236(t)
Vesicourachal diverticulum, 1144, 1144
Viral diseases, neutropenia and, 414
  of imported birds, 674–675
  of primates, 733–741, 734(t), 735(t)
Viral enteritis, canine, 1292–1295
Viral infection, control of, in aviaries, 1275
  of neonate, 81
  of respiratory tract, in psittacine birds, 702
Viremia, puppy, in kennels, 73
Virus. See also names of specific viruses.
  and infectious feline upper respiratory disease, 224, 226
  and tracheobronchial diseases, 229
  congenital maldevelopment and, 166, 167(t)
  diagnostic testing for, in laboratory animals, 750, 751(t)
  feline leukemia, disease complex of, 404–410
Virus neutralizing antibody test, 407
Vision, decreased, 505
  loss of, 540–541
Vitamin(s)
  A, deficiency of, in psittacine birds, 700
    in reptiles, 636, 636(t)
  B6, in calcium oxalate urolithiasis, 1183
  D, intoxication with, 1068(t), 1070
  D2, in hypoparathyroidism, 1001
  in parenteral hyperalimentation, 929
  K therapy, in warfarin poisoning, 134
  requirements for, in renal failure, 1099, 1101
  therapy, in feline respiratory disease, 1281

Vitiligo, 488
Vitreal disease, 579
Vitreous floaters, 579
Volume replacement. See Fluid therapy.
Volvulus, 896–901
von Gierke's disease, 1024

Warfarin poisoning, 125(t), 131–134, 132(t)
Warts, feline infectious, 714
Washings, bronchial, 207
Wasp stings, 177
Water, contamination of, 124
  quality problems of, in aquarium, 608–611
  retention of, reduction of, 374
Water balance, effect of glucocorticoids on, 989
Water composition, of parenteral hyperalimentation, 928
Water deprivation test, 1007, 1080, 1082, 1082
  partial, 1084
Water imbalance, in renal failure, 1043
Water inhalation, 182–186
Water loss, in diabetic ketoacidosis, 1017
Weakness, episodic, 791–795, 792(t)
Weight, conversion of, to body-surface area, 1320(t)
  reduction of, 1036–1039, 1037(t), 1038(t), 1038
Wet blood smear, for microfilariae, 329
Wheeze, 236(t), 237
Whelping, 76
Whipworms, 942
Wild animals, restraint mortality in, [VI:723]
Wings, disorders of, 665, 666
Worms. See also Nematodes.
  esophageal, of dogs, 267
Wound, burns, 191–192
  treatment of, 193–194
  aquatic turtles, 644

Xanthochromia, of cerebrospinal fluid, 769
Xylazine, use of, in renal failure, 1120
D-Xylose absorption, in malassimilation syndrome, 932

Yaba virus, 736
Yaba-like disease, 736
Yellow fever, 739, 740(t)

Zinc phosphide poisoning, 125(t), 126
Zinc-responsive dermatitis, 439
Zinc-responsive dermatoses, 472–476
Zoo animals, hematology of, [VI:765]
Zoonoses, pet-associated, 1265–1268
Zoonotic dirofilariasis, 334
Zootoxins, 123, 150(t)
Zygomatic gland mucoceles, 584
Zygomycosis, 480